THE AMERICAN PSYCHIATRIC PUBLISHING

Textbook of Child and Adolescent Psychiatry

Third Edition

THE AMERICAN PSYCHIATRIC PUBLISHING

Textbook of Child and Adolescent Psychiatry

Third Edition

Edited by

Jerry M. Wiener, M.D.
Mina K. Dulcan, M.D.

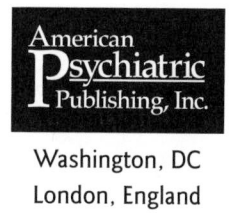

Washington, DC
London, England

Manufactured in the United States of America on acid-free paper
07 06 05 04 03   5   4   3   2   1
Third Edition

Typeset in Adobe's New Baskerville and Goudy Sans Medium

American Psychiatric Publishing, Inc.
1000 Wilson Boulevard
Arlington, VA 22209-3901
www.appi.org

Library of Congress Cataloging-in-Publication Data
Textbook of child and adolescent psychiatry / edited by Jerry M. Wiener, Mina K.
  Dulcan.– 3rd ed.
      p. ; cm.
  Includes bibliographical references and index.
  ISBN 1-58562-057-2 (alk. paper)
   1. Child psychiatry. 2. Adolescent psychiatry. I. Wiener, Jerry M., 1933- II. Dulcan,
Mina K.
  [DNLM: 1. Mental Disorders–Adolescent. 2. Mental Disorders–Child. 3. Mental
Disorders–Infant. WS 350 T355 2004]
  RJ499.T47 2004
  618.92′ 89–dc21
                                                              2003056098

British Library Cataloguing in Publication Data
A CIP record is available from the British Library.

Contents

I

The Field of Child and Adolescent Psychiatry

An Overview

II

Assessment and Diagnosis

III

Developmental Disorders

IV

Schizophrenia, Other Psychotic Disorders, and Mood Disorders

V

Attention-Deficit and Disruptive Behavior Disorders

VI

Anxiety Disorders

VII

Eating Disorders

VIII

Disorders Affecting
Somatic Function

IX

Other Disorders and Special Issues

X

Treatment

Contributors

Lisa Amaya-Jackson, M.D., M.P.H.
Director, Trauma Treatment Service, Department of Psychiatry, Duke University Medical Center, Durham, North Carolina

Thomas F. Anders, M.D.
Professor of Psychiatry, M.I.N.D. Institute, University of California, Davis, Sacramento, Callifornia

Sandra L. Barrueco, Ph.D.
Postdoctoral Fellow, Kennedy Krieger Institute, Johns Hopkins University, Baltimore, Maryland

Myron L. Belfer, M.D., M.P.A.
Professor of Psychiatry, Department of Social Medicine, Harvard Medical School, Boston, Massachusetts

Jules Bemporad, M.D.
Professor of Clinical Psychiatry, New York Medical College, Valhalla, New York

Eugene V. Beresin, M.D.
Director, Child and Adolescent Psychiatry Residency Training Program, Massachusetts General Hospital/McLean Hospital; Associate Professor of Psychiatry, Harvard Medical School, Boston, Massachusetts

Irving N. Berlin, M.D.
Emeritus Professor and Director, Division of Child and Adolescent Psychiatry, University of New Mexico School of Medicine, Albuquerque, New Mexico

Gail A. Bernstein, M.D.
Endowed Professor in Child and Adolescent Anxiety Disorders; Head, Program in Child and Adolescent Anxiety and Mood Disorders, Division of Child and Adolescent Psychiatry, University of Minnesota Medical School, Minneapolis, Minnesota

Joseph Biederman, M.D.
Chief, Joint Program in Pediatric Psychopharmacology, Massachusetts General Hospital, McLean Hospital; Professor of Psychiatry, Harvard Medical School, Boston, Massachusetts

Héctor R. Bird, M.D.
Professor of Clinical Psychiatry, Columbia University College of Physicians and Surgeons; Deputy Director, Department of Child Psychiatry, New York State Psychiatric Institute, New York, New York

Bruce Black, M.D.
Director, Comprehensive Psychiatric Associates, Wellesley, Massachusetts; Assistant Professor of Psychiatry, Tufts University School of Medicine, New England Medical Center, Boston, Massachusetts

Susan J. Bradley, M.D.
Consultant Psychiatrist, Child and Adolescent Gender Identity Clinic, Child Psychiatry Program, Centre for Addiction and Mental Health; Professor, Department of Psychiatry, University of Toronto, Toronto, Ontario, Canada

Larry K. Brown, M.D.
Associate Professor of Psychiatry, Brown University School of Medicine; Director, Outpatient Services, Child and Family Psychiatry, Rhode Island Hospital, Providence, Rhode Island

Kristin Bruning, M.D.
Clinical Assistant Professor, Psychiatry and Human Behavior, Brown University School of Medicine; Staff Psychiatrist, Child and Family Psychiatry, Rhode Island Hospital, Providence, Rhode Island

Donna J. Champine, M.D.
Clinical Assistant Professor of Psychiatry, Department of Psychiatry, University of Michigan Medical School, Ann Arbor, Michigan

Valerie E. Charat, Ed.M.
Harvard Graduate School of Education, Cambridge, Massachusetts

Irene Chatoor, M.D.
Professor of Psychiatry and Pediatrics, George Washington University School of Medicine; Vice Chair of Psychiatry and Director, Infant and Toddler Mental Health Center, Children's National Medical Center, Washington, D.C.

Brent Collett, Ph.D.
Postdoctoral Fellow in Pediatric Psychology, University of Washington School of Medicine, Department of Child Psychiatry and Behavioral Medicine, Children's Hospital and Regional Medical Center, Seattle, Washington

Martha E. Crotts, M.D.
Private practice, Rockford, Illinois

Arman K. Danielyan, M.D.
Children's Hospital of Cincinnati, Cincinnati, Ohio

Peter T. Daniolos, M.D.
Residency Training Director and Medical Director, Center for Autism Spectrum Disorders, Department of Psychiatry and Behavioral Sciences, Children's National Medical Center; Assistant Professor of Psychiatry, Behavioral Sciences, and Pediatrics, George Washington University School of Medicine, Washington, D.C.

Craig L. Donnelly, M.D., M.A.
Director, Pediatric Psychopharmacology, Associate Professor of Psychiatry and Pediatrics, Section of Child and Adolescent Psychiatry, Department of Psychiatry, Dartmouth Medical School, Lebanon, New Hampshire

Mina K. Dulcan, M.D.
Margaret C. Osterman Professor of Child Psychiatry; Head, Department of Child and Adolescent Psychiatry, Children's Memorial Hospital; Director, Warren Wright Adolescent Program, Northwestern Memorial Hospital; Professor of Psychiatry and Behavioral Sciences and Pediatrics; Chief, Child and Adolescent Psychiatry, Northwestern University, Feinberg School of Medicine, Chicago, Illinois

Lisa A. Efron, Ph.D.
Assistant Professor of Psychology and Behavioral Sciences, Children's National Medical Center, Washington, D.C.

Carl Feinstein, M.D.
Professor of Child Psychiatry, Stanford University Department of Psychiatry, Division of Child and Adolescent Psychiatry, Stanford, California

Jennifer B. Freeman, Ph.D.
Assistant Professor (Research) of Psychiatry and Human Behavior, Brown University School of Medicine; Staff Psychologist, Division of Child and Family Psychiatry, Rhode Island Hospital, Providence, Rhode Island

Gregory K. Fritz, M.D.
Professor and Director of Child and Adolescent Psychiatry, Brown University School of Medicine; Director, Child and Family Psychiatry, Rhode Island Hospital, Providence, Rhode Island

Christina M. Fucci, B.A.
Clinical Research Assistant, Division of Child and Family Psychiatry, Rhode Island Hospital, Providence, Rhode Island

Abbe M. Garcia, Ph.D.
Postdoctoral Research Fellow, Department of Psychiatry and Human Behavior, Brown University School of Medicine, Providence, Rhode Island

Laurence L. Greenhill, M.D.
Professor of Psychiatry, Division of Child Psychiatry, New York State Psychiatric Institute, Columbia University College of Physicians and Surgeons, New York, New York

Stanley I. Greenspan, M.D.
Clinical Professor of Psychiatry, Behavioral Sciences, and Pediatrics, George Washington University School of Medicine; Chairman, Interdisciplinary Council on Developmental and Learning Disorders; Supervising Child Psychoanalyst, Washington Psychoanalytic Institute, Washington, D.C.

Jeffrey M. Halperin, Ph.D.
Professor of Psychiatry, Queens College, City University of New York, New York

XiaoYan He, M.D.
Assistant Professor of Clinical Psychiatry, University of California, Davis; Child and Adolescent Psychiatrist, Kaiser Permanente—South Sacramento, Sacramento, California

Robert L. Hendren, D.O.
Professor of Psychiatry; Executive Director, M.I.N.D. Institute; Chief, Child and Adolescent Psychiatry, University of California, Davis, Sacramento, California

David B. Herzog, M.D.
Director, Eating Disorders Unit, Massachusetts General Hospital; President, Harvard Medical School Eating Disorders Center; Professor of Psychiatry (Pediatrics), Harvard Medical School, Boston, Massachusetts

Steven L. Jaffe, M.D.
Professor of Child and Adolescent Psychiatry, Emory University School of Medicine; Clinical Professor, Morehouse School of Medicine; Director, Child and Adolescent Programs, Peachford Hospital, Atlanta, Georgia

Paramjit T. Joshi, M.D.
Chair, Department of Psychiatry and Behavioral Sciences, Children's National Medical Center; Professor of Psychiatry, Behavioral Sciences, and Pediatrics, George Washington University School of Medicine, Washington, D.C.

Lawrence C. Kaplan, M.D.
Director, Division of Genetics and Child Development, Children's Hospital at Dartmouth, Lebanon, New Hampshire; Associate Professor of Pediatrics, Dartmouth Medical School, Hanover, New Hampshire

Mai Karitani, A.B.
Clinical Research Assistant, Division of Child and Family Psychiatry, Rhode Island Hospital, Providence, Rhode Island

Alan E. Kazdin, Ph.D.
Professor and Director, Child Study Center, and John M. Musser Professor of Psychology, Yale University School of Medicine, New Haven, Connecticut

Paulina F. Kernberg, M.D.
Director, Child and Adolescent Psychiatry Training, The New York Presbyterian Hospital–Cornell Medical Center, Westchester Division; Professor of Psychiatry, Weill Medical College of Cornell University, White Plains, New York

Clarice J. Kestenbaum, M.D.
Professor of Clinical Psychiatry and Director of Training, Division of Child and Adolescent Psychiatry, Columbia University College of Physicians and Surgeons, New York, New York

Robert A. King, M.D.
Professor of Child Psychiatry and Medical Director, Tourette's/OCD Clinic, Yale Child Study Center, Yale University, New Haven, Connecticut

Anlee D. Kuo, J.D., M.D.
Forensic Fellow, Psychiatry and the Law Program, Department of Psychiatry, University of California, San Francisco, California

Ann E. Layne, Ph.D.
Postdoctoral Fellow, Division of Child and Adolescent Psychiatry, University of Minnesota Medical School, Minneapolis, Minnesota

James F. Leckman, M.D.
Neison Harris Professor of Child Psychiatry and Pediatrics, Yale Child Study Center, New Haven, Connecticut

Henrietta L. Leonard, M.D.
Professor of Psychiatry and Human Behavior, Brown University School of Medicine; Director of Training, Child and Adolescent Psychiatry, Rhode Island Hospital, Providence, Rhode Island

Bennett L. Leventhal, M.D.
Professor of Psychiatry and Pediatrics; Director of Child and Adolescent Psychiatry; and Chairman, Department of Psychiatry, University of Chicago, Chicago, Illinois

Dorothy Otnow Lewis, M.D.
Professor of Psychiatry, New York University School of Medicine, New York, New York; Clinical Professor of Psychiatry, Yale Child Study Center, Yale University, New Haven, Connecticut

Melvin Lewis, M.B., B.S., F.R.C.Psych., D.C.H.
Professor of Child Psychiatry and Pediatrics, Yale Child Study Center, Yale University, New Haven, Connecticut

John S. March, M.D., M.P.H.
Chief, Division of Childhood and Adolescent Psychiatry, Departments of Psychiatry and Psychology: Social and Health Sciences, Duke University Medical Center, Durham, North Carolina

Jon McClellan, M.D.
Associate Professor, University of Washington, Child Study and Treatment Center, Lakewood, Washington

Edgardo Menvielle, M.D.
Assistant Professor of Psychiatry and Behavioral Sciences, George Washington University School of Health Sciences, Washington, D.C.

David A. Mrazek, M.D., F.R.C.Psych.
Chair, Departent of Psychiatry and Psychology, Mayo Clinic; Professor of Psychiatry and Pediatrics, Mayo Medical School, Rochester, Minnesota

David J. Mullen, M.D.
Associate Professor of Psychiatry, University of New Mexico; Executive Medical Director, UNM Children's Psychiatric Hosital, Albuquerque, New Mexico

Kerim Munir, M.D., M.P.H., D.Sc.
Director, Mental Health and Developmental Disabilities (MH/DD) Program, Division of General Pediatrics, and Associate in Psychiatry, Department of Psychiatry, Children's Hospital, Boston, Massachusetts

Kathleen Myers, M.D., M.P.H.
Associate Professor, University of Washington School of Medicine; Director, Consultation-Liaison Psychiatry, Department of Child Psychiatry and Behavioral Medicine, Children's Hospital and Regional Medical Center, Seattle, Washington

Theodore A. Petti, M.D., M.P.H.
Professor of Psychiatry and Director, Division of Child and Adolescent Psychiatry, Robert Wood Johnson Medical School, University of Medicine and Dentistry of New Jersey, Piscataway, New Jersey

Cynthia R. Pfeffer, M.D.
Professor of Psychiatry and Director, Childhood Bereavement Program, Weill Medical College of Cornell University, White Plains, New York

Jennifer M. Phillips, Ph.D.
Staff Psychologist, Stanford University Department of Psychiatry, Division of Child and Adolescent Psychiatry, Stanford, California

David Pruitt, M.D.
Professor, Psychiatry and Pediatrics, and Division Director, Child and Adolescent Psychiatry, University of Maryland College of Medicine, Baltimore, Maryland

Judith L. Rapoport, M.D.
Chief, Child Psychiatry Branch, National Institute of Mental Health, National Institutes of Health, Bethesda, Maryland

Gloria Reeves, M.D.
Assistant Professor, Division Child and Adolescent Psychiatry, University of Maryland College of Medicine, Baltimore, Maryland

Adelaide S. Robb, M.D.
Associate Professor of Psychiatry and Behavioral Sciences, Children's National Medical Center, Washington, D.C.

Jay A. Salpekar, M.D.
Director of Outpatient Services, Department of Psychiatry and Behavioral Sciences, Children's National Medical Center; Assistant Professor of Psychiatry, Behavioral Sciences, and Pediatrics, George Washington University School of Medicine, Washington, D.C.

John E. Schowalter, M.D.
Albert J. Solnit Professor of Child Psychiatry and Pediatrics; Chief, Child Psychiatry, Yale Child Study Center, Yale University, New Haven, Connecticut

Robert K. Schreter, M.D.
Associate Professor of Psychiatry, University of Maryland School of Medicine, Baltimore, Maryland

David Shaffer, M.B., B.S., F.R.C.P.
Irving Philips Professor of Child and Adolescent Psychiatry, Columbia University College of Physicians and Surgeons, New York State Psychiatric Institute, New York, New York

Theodore Shapiro, M.D.
Professor Emeritus of Psychiatry, Weill Cornell Medical College, Division of Child-Adolescent Psychiatry, Payne Whitney Clinic, New York Presbyterian Hospital, New York, New York

G. Pirooz Sholevar, M.D.
Clinical Professor of Psychiatry, Jefferson Medical College, Thomas Jefferson University, Philadelphia, Pennsylvania

John B. Sikorski, M.D.
Clinical Professor, Department of Psychiatry, University of California, San Francisco, California

Ramon Solhkhah, M.D.
Director, Division of Child and Adolescent Psychiatry, St. Luke's-Roosevelt Hospital Center; Assistant Professor of Clinical Psychiatry, Columbia University, New York, New York

Thomas Spencer, M.D.
Assistant Director, Pediatric Psychopharmacology, Massachusetts General Hospital; Professor of Psychiatry, Harvard Medical School, Boston, Massachusetts

Mark A. Stein, Ph.D.
Professor of Psychiatry, University of Chicago, Chicago, Illinois

Susan E. Swedo, M.D.
Chief, Pediatrics and Developmental Neuropsychiatry Branch, National Institute of Mental Health, National Institutes of Health, Bethesda, Maryland

David Szydlo, M.D., Ph.D.
Associate Research Scientist, Yale Child Study Center, Yale University School of Medicine; Director of Education and Curriculum Development, National Center for Children Exposed to Violence, Yale University School of Medicine, New Haven, Connecticut

Ludwik S. Szymanski, M.D.
Director of Psychiatry, Emeritus, Institute for Community Inclusion, Children's Hospital; Associate Professor of Psychiatry, Harvard Medical School, Boston, Massachusetts

Luke Y. Tsai, M.D.
Professor of Psychiatry and Pediatrics, University of Michigan Medical School; Director, Developmental Disorders Clinic, University of Michigan Medical Center, Ann Arbor, Michigan

Thomas Walsh, M.D.
Clinical Associate Professor of Psychiatry and Behavioral Sciences, George Washington University School of Health Sciences, Washington, D.C.

Bruce Waslick, M.D.
Associate Clinical Professor of Psychiatry, Division of Child Psychiatry, New York State Psychiatric Institute, Columbia University College of Physicians and Surgeons, New York, New York

Elizabeth B. Weller, M.D.
Professor of Psychiatry and Pediatrics, Department of Psychiatry, University of Pennsylvania; Department of Child and Adolescent Psychiatry, The Children's Hospital of Philadlephia, Philadelphia, Pennsylvania

Ronald A. Weller, M.D.
Senior Lecturer, Department of Psychiatry, University of Pennsylvania, Philadelphia, Pennsylvania

Jerry M. Wiener, M.D.
Leon Yochelson Professor of Psychiatry and Behavioral Sciences, and Professor of Pediatrics, Department of Psychiatry, George Washington University School of Medicine, Washington, D.C. (deceased)

Timothy Wilens, M.D.
Director of Pediatric Substance Abuse Unit, Pediatric Psychopharmacology, Massachusetts General Hospital; Associate Professor of Psychiatry, Harvard Medical School, Boston, Massachusetts

Daniel T. Williams, M.D.
Clinical Professor of Psychiatry, Columbia College of Physicians and Surgeons; Consultant, Pediatric Neuropsychiatry Service, Columbia-Presbyterian Medical Center, New York, New York

Joseph L. Woolston, M.D.
Professor, Child Psychiatry and Pediatrics, Yale Child Study Center, Yale University School of Medicine, New Haven, Connecticut

Maurizio Zambenedetti, M.D.
Assistant Professor of Psychiatry, New York University School of Medicine, New York, New York

Kenneth J. Zucker, Ph.D.
Head, Child and Adolescent Gender Identity Clinic, Child Psychiatry Program; Psychologist-in-Chief, Centre for Addiction and Mental Health; Professor, Departments of Psychiatry and Psychology, University of Toronto, Toronto, Ontario, Canada

Preface

The American Psychiatric Publishing Textbook of Child and Adolescent Psychiatry aims to be both scholarly and practical. It is comprehensive, but not so lengthy or detailed that the child and adolescent psychiatrist in training or the practitioner looking for an update is daunted or exhausted. The Textbook can serve as a core text for a child psychiatrist or a reference for pediatricians, family physicians, general psychiatrists, advanced-practice child psychiatric nurses, and psychiatric social workers. Each chapter presents a summary of a core topic and blends clinical wisdom with evidence-based practices in assessment and treatment.

This third edition has been updated and revised throughout, in recognition of the accelerating progress in research on developmental psychopathology. DSM-IV has been replaced by DSM-IV-TR (Text Revision), fortunately not as monumental a change as from DSM-III-R to DSM-IV. Many of our most experienced chapter authors remain, with refreshed chapters. Senior authors have been encouraged to add junior faculty as coauthors, as part of the mentoring and faculty development process. Chapters new to this edition include "Role of Culture, Race, and Ethnicity" (Héctor Bird, M.D.), "Economic Issues" (Robert Schreter, M.D.), "Diagnostic Interviews" (Jack McClellan, M.D.), "Clinical Genomic Testing" (David Mrazek, M.D.), and "Milieu Treatment: Inpatient, Partial, Residential" (Ted Petti, M.D.). New principal authors of completely rewritten chapters include Kathleen Myers, M.D. ("Rating Scales"), Mark Stein, Ph.D. ("Psychological and Neuropsychological Testing"), Craig Donnelly, M.D. ("Pediatric Posttraumatic Stress Disorder"), David Szydlo, M.D. ("Bulimia Nervosa"), David Pruitt, M.D. ("Adjustment and Reactive Disorders"),

Steve Jaffe, M.D. ("Substance Abuse Disorders"), Paramjit Joshi, M.D. ("Physical Abuse of Children" and "Sexual Abuse of Children"), and Adelaide Robb, M.D. ("Group Psychotherapy"). Returning contributors Bob Hendren, D.O. ("Laboratory and Diagnostic Testing"), Luke Tsai, M.D. ("Schizophrenia and Other Psychotic Disorders"), and Elizabeth Weller, M.D. ("Mood Disorders in Adolescents"), have also written additional chapters for this edition. A study guide with questions and answers based on this text is being published as a companion volume.

Jerry Wiener, M.D., was a giant in child psychiatry. Although his own education and training were classical, he was always alert to the latest empirical findings that might benefit children and families. He sought to integrate clinical wisdom and scientific research to promote both improved patient care and advocacy for children and families. Although trained as a psychoanalyst, he wrote the first textbook on pediatric psychopharmacology, because "it needed to be done." He personally taught many child and adolescent psychiatrists who became prominent academicians and community clinicians. His example, mentoring, and publications have benefited all child psychiatrists. Jerry held key administrative roles, including over 20 years as the chair of the Department of Psychiatry and Behavioral Sciences at George Washington University School of Medicine, president of both the American Academy of Child and Adolescent Psychiatry and the American Psychiatric Association, and chairman of the editorial board of the American Psychiatric Press. His expertise and authority were widely recognized. When we learned that Jerry had been called to consult regarding Elián González, we knew that decisions would be informed by expert advice in the best interests of Elián. Jerry left us without warning, and much too soon. We all miss him and feel the loss of his ever-fresh wisdom and guidance.

The third edition of the *Textbook of Child and Adolescent Psychiatry* caps and commemorates the contributions of Jerry Wiener to the entire field of child and adolescent psychiatry. Before his illness, Jerry shaped this new edition, commissioned the chapters, and edited many of them. When Jerry called to ask me to "help a little" with this edition, it was a great honor. Jerry's requests were always difficult to resist, so I speedily accepted his invitation, with the plan to be involved with this edition in a small way and then take primary responsibility for the fourth edition. Even while undergoing treatment, Jerry continued to encourage authors and edit chapters. In the wake of his untimely death, many people rallied to ensure that the book would be completed as Jerry had planned. Louise Wiener gathered up all of the completed and in-process chapters from Jerry's offices at home and at George Washington University. Her generosity enabled the staff at American Psychiatric Publishing, Inc. (APPI), to determine the status of each chapter and pick up where Jerry left off. Tina Coltri-Marshall, Editorial Assistant, masterfully organized the project, communicated with chapter authors, and put every-thing into shape. Bob Hales, M.D., Editor-in-Chief of APPI Books, not only made major contributions to editing the remaining chapters, but provided almost daily support and encouragement to me, APPI staff, and authors. Some chapters had already been received at APPI, some were lost in process and had to be recovered (thank goodness for computers with data storage devices!), and some remained to be completed. Several were reassigned, and I am especially grateful to those new authors who rose to the occasion on short notice. APPI staff members John McDuffie, Editorial Director; Pam Harley, Managing Editor, Books Department; Roxanne Rhodes, Senior Editor; Robin Simpson, Acquisitions Coordinator; Bob Pursell, Director of Sales and Marketing; and Katie Duffy, Marketing Associate, make the best team for which an editor could wish.

My husband, Richard Wendel, graciously supported my efforts in this unexpected "opportunity," and my intrepid assistant, Jean Stiman, rose to every occasion, as always.

Onward and upward!

Mina K. Dulcan, M.D.
Children's Memorial Hospital
Northwestern University
Feinberg School of Medicine
Chicago, Illinois

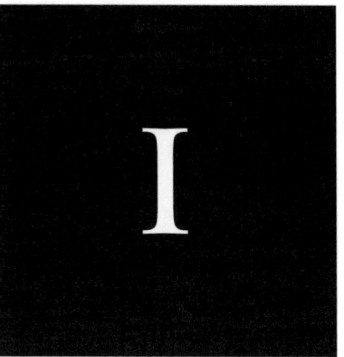

The Field of Child and Adolescent Psychiatry

An Overview

Development of the Subspecialty of Child and Adolescent Psychiatry in the United States

Irving N. Berlin, M.D.

This chapter ties together some of the historical influences that ultimately led to the establishment of the subspecialty of child and adolescent psychiatry and the proximate events and people responsible for the subspecialty boards in child psychiatry. Many of the pioneers in child and adolescent psychiatry were personally known to me. I mention their significant contributions. I bring into historical perspective the development of psychotherapy and some of the other therapeutic methods utilized in our field, as well as aspects of early research significant to the growth of this subspecialty. The current trends toward managed care and cost containment in health and mental health care require new activities for the subspecialty and its practitioners.

Role of the Academy of Child Psychiatry

Child psychiatry as a subspecialty began with the formation of the Academy of Child Psychiatry. Its founders were all members of the American Orthopsychiatric Association (often called Ortho). Ortho was founded by psychiatrists in 1924 as a place to discuss clinical issues, especially those having to do with children and adolescents. Karl Menninger, David Levy, and Sheldon Glueck were among the founders. A decade later, Ortho became an interdisciplinary organization (Crutcher 1943; Lowrey 1955; Witmer 1940). In 1951, George Gardner was president of

Ortho, and James Cunningham was president of the American Association of Psychiatric Clinics for Children (Lowrey 1955). This latter organization had become the standard-setting body for child psychiatric practice and training in clinics in the United States. On May 7, 1951, when Ortho was meeting in Cincinnati, Ohio, George Gardner and Mabel Ross convened a meeting of the leading child psychiatrists who were present. These distinguished child psychiatrists were either directors of child guidance clinics or faculty of the several medical schools with affiliated child psychiatry clinics. Gardner, for example, was director of the Judge Baker Child Guidance Center in Boston and a member of the Harvard Medical School faculty in the Department of Psychiatry (American Academy of Child Psychiatry 1962; Lowrey 1944).

The child psychiatrists who met together were Drs. Spafford Ackerly, Frederick Allen, Lauretta Bender, Jules Coleman, James Cunningham, Frank Curran, George Gardner, Margaret Gerard, Reynold Jenson, Leo Kanner, Othilda Krug, William Langford, Hyman Lippman, Edward Liss, John Rose, Mabel Ross, and Stanislaus Szurek. This group agreed to meet in Atlantic City, New Jersey, on February 24, 1952, and to issue a call to all child psychiatrists in the United States to plan the formation of the Academy of Child Psychiatry. At this second meeting, 96 child and adolescent psychiatrists, some of them psychoanalysts, met to discuss the purpose and function of an academy of child psychiatry. They elected 17 members under the temporary chairmanship of George Gardner, with Frank

Curran as acting secretary, to meet and draw up a constitution, goals of the organization, and criteria for membership.

At a third meeting, on May 12, 1952, in Atlantic City, the constitution was discussed and modified, as were the purpose of the organization and criteria for membership. Six members of the organizing committee became the first council. George Gardner was the first president; Frederick Allen, the president-elect; Frank Curran, the secretary; and Mabel Ross, the treasurer. The first meeting of the Academy of Child Psychiatry was held in February 1953 in Cleveland, Ohio (American Academy of Child Psychiatry 1962).

Characteristics of the Academy of Child Psychiatry

The Academy of Child Psychiatry was clearly a medical organization whose purpose was to delineate the scope of child psychiatry and its practice. It also emphasized the need to have such specialty practice recognized by medicine and psychiatry. It set standards of training and practice; there was a desire to stimulate physicians to enter the field of child psychiatry. The academy also endorsed the promotion and advancement of prevention, treatment, research, and teaching in child psychiatry.

The constitution and bylaws established two classes of membership: fellows and associate members. Membership was by invitation only. To become a fellow, one had to be a physician who was trained in psychiatry, a member of the American Psychiatric Association, and certified or eligible for certification by the American Board of Psychiatry and Neurology. Individuals who began their training in child psychiatry after 1946 had to be diplomates of the board and had to have 2 years' training in child psychiatry in addition to their general psychiatry training. The setting for training in child psychiatry had to be deemed adequate by the organization. Invitations to membership required 5 years of practice in the field; one had to have made a significant contribution to child psychiatry and also demonstrated competence in the field as a practitioner, teacher, trainer, researcher in child psychiatry, or administrator of a clinic or a governmental child psychiatry office. The associate members were distinguished physicians who had made significant contributions to the field but could not meet the specifications of train-

ing and certification (American Academy of Child Psychiatry 1962).

In 1969, the academy of scholars concept, which had excluded a growing number of child psychiatrists from the Academy of Child Psychiatry, altered when the group became a general membership organization by approval of the new membership criteria. Applications were encouraged from those who, after completing general psychiatry training, completed their child psychiatry training in an accredited program. Each applicant had to demonstrate that his or her current professional interests and work were in child psychiatry. This change made the academy more representative of child psychiatry in the nation and made it a more influential organization on behalf of children (Berman 1970; Slaff 1989).

Role of the American Psychiatric Association

There was simultaneous activity in the American Psychiatric Association, which also contributed to the establishment of a subspecialty in child psychiatry. In 1943, the American Psychiatric Association established the Committee on Psychopathology of Childhood. In 1949, it became the Committee on Child Psychiatry. The members of that committee included many of the founders and charter members of the Academy of Child Psychiatry. In 1952, this committee, chaired by Dr. George Gardner, petitioned the council of the American Psychiatric Association for endorsement of subspecialty certification in child psychiatry. That petition was turned down. In 1957, the Committee on Child Psychiatry, together with a committee from the American Academy of Child Psychiatry, gained the endorsement of the American Psychiatric Association to request that the American Board of Psychiatry and Neurology form a subspecialty board in child psychiatry (American Psychiatric Association 1964).

Creation of the Committee on Certification in Child Psychiatry

In 1958, the American Board of Psychiatry and Neurology requested that the six members of the council of the Academy of Child Psychiatry meet with the board to work out the mechanism for a subspecialty committee on certification in child psychiatry. The Committee on Certification in Child Psychiatry was created in 1959. Frederick Allen was chairman, William Langford was vice chairman, and Franklin Robinson was secretary. Frank Curran, Othilda Krug, and Hyman Lippman were the other board members, with James Hugh as the representative from the American Board of Pediatrics (American Psychiatric Association 1964).

In 1960, the Subcommittee on Child Psychiatry of the Residency Review Committee in Psychiatry was established. The group developed training and accreditation criteria and began to accredit child psychiatry training programs (Wiener 1988).

Other Factors in the Development of Child Psychiatry as a Subspecialty

Child guidance clinics were formed after World War I because of the large number of psychiatric casualties. The Commonwealth Fund and the Rockefeller Foundation began to sponsor the development of child guidance clinics to prevent mental illness in the late 1920s and early 1930s. In the mid-1930s, the rise of Hitler in Germany and his invasion of Austria resulted in an exodus of psychoanalysts from Germany and Austria to the United States. This also was the time of the Great Depression. The only positions open to these psychoanalysts were in the child guidance clinics and the universities. Thus began a melding of psychoanalytical ideas about psychotherapy of children with ideas developed in the many child guidance clinics, especially ideas from the earlier work of Healy (Healy and Bronner 1936; Levy 1968).

The pattern of service delivery in Frederick Allen's Philadelphia Child Guidance Clinic was typical. In the early 1930s and 1940s, a psychiatrist treated the child, a social worker consulted with the mother or parents, and a psychologist did the testing. Family involvement in the child guidance clinics evolved, in part, from Adolf Meyer's convictions that one could study and understand the whole child only by also working with the family, as well as from Healy and Bronner's work with delinquents (Berlin 1964; Crutcher 1943; Healy and Bronner 1936). In 1930, Adolf Meyer asked Leo Kan-

ner to form the first "pediatric psychiatry clinic." The child psychiatry section of the Harriet Lane Pediatric Clinic at Johns Hopkins was the precursor of later university divisions of child psychiatry (Kanner 1960b).

In 1935, Kanner published the first textbook on child psychiatry. It was the first official use of the term *child psychiatry*. In 1942, Allen's first book, *Psychotherapy With Children,* was published. In the late 1930s and early 1940s, Adelaide Johnson and Stanislaus Szurek at the Institute for Juvenile Research in Chicago began to test the effectiveness of collaborative therapy for both the neurotic child and his or her parents (Szurek et al. 1942). In 1948, under Frederick Allen's leadership, 54 child guidance clinics banded together to form the American Association of Children's Psychiatric Clinics to develop standards for clinic operations, services, and training. Once the Committee on Certification was formed, this organization no longer had influence on child psychiatrists' training and eventually gave up its standard-setting and clinic evaluation functions.

An important stimulus to child psychiatry as a subspecialty occurred in 1949 with the creation of the National Institute of Mental Health (NIMH), directed by Dr. Robert Felix. From the NIMH training branch came the stipends for training in psychiatry, child psychiatry, psychology, and social work (American Psychiatric Association 1964).

In 1963, a conference on training in child psychiatry was called, sponsored by the American Psychiatric Association and the Association of American Medical Colleges. In its deliberations, the conference sought to lay out the essentials of a curriculum and to specify areas that were necessary to child psychiatry training, as well as areas that might be elective. At the time of this conference, there were about 200 board-certified child psychiatrists, most of them members of the Academy of Child Psychiatry, and perhaps another 200 individuals in training.

As a participant in that conference, I can recall the comments and presentations from pioneers in the field such as Frank Curran, George Gardner, Irene Josselyn, Leo Kanner, Othilda Krug, and Eveoleen Rexford. I was struck by the dedication of this group of eminent child psychiatrists and by the sense of intimacy, good humor, and respect that permeated their relationships. It should be noted that of this group, more than half were in charge of university child psychiatric inpatient and outpatient facilities (American Psychiatric Association 1964).

Evolution of Various Therapies and Research: Influence on the Development of the Subspecialty

■ Psychotherapy

For many years, psychoanalysis formed the theoretical base of child psychiatry. Influenced by Anna Freud (1928, 1946) and Melanie Klein (1932), play therapy began as an effort to discover the unconscious conflicts revealed in a child's play. In contrast, Allen (1942) and others emphasized the therapeutic effect of the formation of a new and healthier relationship between an adult and the child. In 1947, Virginia Axline, a student of Carl Rogers, published her book *Play Therapy.* She emphasized the priority of helping children work through conflicts, without much interpretation, by empathic understanding of the child's problems and by communicating that awareness. In 1950, Erik Erikson published *Childhood and Society,* which brought ego psychology (introduced by Anna Freud in 1946) into the forefront as an important factor in understanding development and psychopathology in children and adolescents. Solomon (1948) introduced structured play techniques, Levy (1939, 1959) described release therapy and reported on his demonstration clinic to treat disturbed mothers and young children, and Lippman (1961) synthesized many of these ideas.

■ Family and Group Therapy

Beginning with Ackerman's work in 1958, family therapy began to have its effect on psychiatry and child psychiatry. In the late 1950s and 1960s, Bateson, Bowen, Jackson, Laing, Lidz, Wynne, and others began to develop family therapy theory. The books of Ackerman (1958) and Satir (1963) on clinical applications of family therapy were major influences on its growth (Whiteside 1979).

Group therapy had its start with the work of Slavson (1934). He described group activity therapy with latency-aged children. In 1936, Bender and Waltman described their work with psychotic children in group therapy. In 1954, Gisela Konopka, a professor of social work, wrote her book on group therapy with adolescent girls. Throughout the 1950s, 1960s, and 1970s, many child psychiatrists helped develop the theory and practice of group therapy with children and adolescents (Kraft 1979).

■ Behavior Therapy

Behavior therapy has been described as starting with the work of Pavlov on conditioned reflexes in animals. The noted psychologist Watson applied learning principles to alter children's behavior patterns. Thorndike's learning theory described the "law of effect," which emphasized the influence of reinforcing consequences on behavior. Skinner used these ideas to develop the behavioral psychology of operant conditioning. Wolpe (1952) helped develop the methodology. The development of social learning theory by Ferster along with Zigler and others provided new explanations of development and psychopathology. The behavior therapy methods described by Luria and Lazarus include cognitive learning theory and practice (McGee and Saidel 1979). Imitative learning through modeling, as described by Bandera and Walters (1963) and others, provided a cognitive awareness of how behavior can be altered through emulation. The disaffection with psychoanalysis because it was not demonstrably effective is believed to have been responsible for the development of behavior therapy, primarily by academic psychologists (Krasner 1971; McGee and Saidel 1979).

■ Mental Health Consultation and Crisis Intervention

Child psychiatrists and child and adult analysts have developed both the theory and applications of the models for mental health consultation and crisis intervention. Lindemann (1944), one of the pioneers, worked primarily in the area of crisis intervention with families and individuals who experienced overwhelming stress. Lindemann devised methods of helping victims of tragic experiences, such as the Boston Coconut Grove fire in 1947. Although the original methodology was akin to consultation methods (i.e., helping individuals to fully share their feelings of terror and their fear of death), more recently, the treatment of children and families who experience catastrophic events has been dealt with as a field of its own, with different therapeutic strategies utilizing psychodynamic, behavioral, and pharmacological techniques (Eth and Pynoos 1985; Lindemann 1944; Terr 1985).

Many of the pioneers who developed mental health consultation methodology were child psychiatrists: Jules Coleman (1947) at Yale, Viola Bernard (1954) at Columbia, Gerald Caplan (1955) at the Harvard School of Public Health, and Irving Berlin (1956) at the University of California. The method of consultation consisted of identifying the particular problem a consultee or teacher had with a "client" or student and helping the consultee to become more effective in dealing with the student's problem, which impinged on the consultee's psychopathology and resulted in the impasse in his or her work with the student. The consultee was helped to become effective in dealing with the student's problems by involving the consultee in problem-solving interventions. Simultaneously, consultees would unconsciously deal with their own pathology. Thus, consultation is therapeutic, that is, a helpful intervention, but not therapy.

These efforts led to the teaching and training of child psychiatry residents to conduct school and agency mental health consultation.

■ Delinquency Research and Treatment Strategies

Since the 1800s, delinquency has been one of the most serious, poorly understood, and poorly treated phenomena in childhood and especially adolescence.

William Healy (1915), a neurologist, was encouraged by those working with the courts in Chicago, Illinois, and by philanthropists influenced by Adolf Meyer and William James, to study and try to treat delinquency. In 1909, Healy founded the Juvenile Psychopathic Institute in Chicago, later named the Institute for Juvenile Research. This was the first child guidance clinic in America. In 1915, he published his first findings in *The Individual Delinquent* (Healy 1915). In 1917, Healy and his collaborator, Augusta Bronner, dissatisfied with the role of the juvenile court in Chicago, were encouraged to move to Boston. There they founded the Judge Baker Foundation, later named the Judge Baker Guidance Center. In his first book, Healy described the role of social and developmental factors in the etiology of delinquency. He emphasized the team concept of having a psychiatrist, psychologist, and social worker collaborate both in gathering data and in working with the delinquent child and his or her family. *New Light on Delinquency and Its Treatment,* by Healy and Bronner, was published in 1936. In this volume, they documented the role of dysfunctional families and adverse social conditions, such as poverty and ghetto living, as being significant to the origins of delinquency (Gardner 1972).

The understanding and treatment of delinquents were also of major concern to child psychiatrists and analysts. Szurek (1942) and Johnson (1949) described "superego lacunae" in adolescents resulting from unconscious parental permission for delinquent acts. This thesis was amplified in Johnson and Szurek's (1952) work on the genesis of antisocial behavior. Rexford and Van Amerongen (1957) and Josselyn (1958) reported their clinical work with impulsive acting-out in children. The talented educator and psychoanalyst Fritz Redl, together with Wineman, studied delinquent adolescent boys and wrote *Children Who Hate* in 1951 (Redl and Wineman 1951) and *Controls From Within* in 1952 (Redl and Wineman 1952). In 1959, Redl wrote *The Life Space Interview* (Redl 1959b). Redl pioneered the use of group therapy with delinquents, first in his famous Michigan summer camp and later at Pioneer House in Detroit. He also described many of the principles of residential treatment (Redl 1959a). The studies of juvenile delinquency by Glueck (1959) and Glueck and Glueck (1970) implicated poverty as one of its causes. Noshpitz (1962), who had worked with Redl, described his studies of hyperaggressive children. Always a great concern of American society, delinquent antisocial behavior has been studied since the early 1800s and is still an important area of research. It was only with the pioneering work of Kempe et al. (1962) that the role of physical abuse as an etiological factor in some delinquent behavior became clear.

■ The Psychotic Child

In 1942, Bender described her experiences beginning in 1935 at Bellevue Hospital in New York City as the director of one of the first child psychiatric wards for the treatment of childhood schizophrenia. Her extremely astute observations pointed to a combination of genetic and environmental etiological factors. Kanner (1943) described early infantile autism and the "refrigerator-like" characteristics of these children's parents, which he later noted to be an inaccurate conclusion. In 1952, Margaret Mahler described autistic and symbiotic infantile psychoses. Previously, Potter (1933) and Bradley (1941) had described the characteristics of schizophrenia in children whom they treated in hospital settings (Bender 1942; Kanner 1943, 1960b; Mahler 1952). Fish et al. (1968) also described the various characteristics and classification of childhood schizophrenia.

Bettelheim and Sylvester (1949) of the orthogenic school in Chicago coined the term *milieu* to describe their setting. Jones (1953) described the therapeutic community. Bettelheim (1950) was one of the major proponents of a psychotherapeutic approach to childhood psychoses. In California, Ekstein and Wallerstein (1956) and Szurek (1956) described their inpatient psychotherapeutic treatment efforts with psychotic children (i.e., intensive psychotherapy with the child). For Szurek, and others, treatment involved both the child and the parents. The biological genetic determinants of childhood psychoses have become most manifest in the last two decades. Bender (1942), Fish and Alper (1962), and Goldfarb (1956) are among the researchers who described some of these early biological manifestations. Kallmann (1938) studied adult identical twins with schizophrenia and their family backgrounds and discovered and confirmed a genetic link in adult schizophrenia. Chapman (1957) described infantile autism in twins.

■ Research Important to Child Psychiatry as a Subspecialty

Piaget's (1926) important research in cognitive development laid a foundation for later research. In 1941, at the Yale Child Study Center, Gesell and Amatruda developed the first scales for measuring developmental stages of physical, cognitive, and psychological development (Kanner 1960a). Infant psychiatry, as it is known today, began with the early illuminating research of René Spitz. In his first book, he described the results of early deprivation of mothering in infancy (Spitz 1945). Later, he clearly delineated the devastating effects of prolonged separation from the mother in the second half of the first year (Spitz 1946). Bergman and Escalona (1949) described the effects of separation and stress on young children. Levy (1937) described primary affect hunger in young children. Bowlby's (1951) seminal work for the World Health Organization and his later volumes on attachment (Bowlby 1969, 1973) further emphasized the critical nature of the mother-child relationship in infancy. The words *attachment* and *bonding* became important descriptions of a close relationship between an infant, child, adolescent, and adult that supported normal development (Bowlby 1969, 1973). Brazelton et al. (1966) were able to observe and capture on film the early competence of the infant and how the infant's interaction with the mother influenced maternal behavior. Spock's (1946) book on baby and child care introduced psychodynamic

principles of development to the general public and became a best-seller.

A number of longitudinal studies produced important data. Prospective studies by Chess et al. (1963) and Thomas et al. (1968) on temperamental differences in children and the resulting impact on the environment and on the child throughout life are some of these pioneering efforts. These researchers coined the term *mother-child fit* (Chess et al. 1963; Thomas et al. 1968). Werner et al. (1971) did a prospective study on a cohort of infants born on the island of Kauai and studied them for 30 years. These researchers were able to document the effects of neurological dysfunction in infancy on the subsequent development of these children. They learned, as did others, that unlike some of the children in the cohort—whose developmental, learning, and social problems led to psychopathology—a few children in the same cohort, with early neurological signs and raised in very poor social and home environments, did very well; these individuals were called invulnerable children.

Psychopharmacological research, beginning with the discoveries of chlorpromazine and lithium, was important to the development of the field of child psychiatry. Subsequent research on the use of various pharmacotherapeutic agents in "minimal brain dysfunction" (now called attention deficit disorder or attention-deficit/hyperactivity disorder), childhood psychoses, childhood and adolescent depressions, Tourette's syndrome, anorexia and bulimia nervosa, and obsessive-compulsive disorder has made pharmacotherapy very important in child and adolescent psychiatry (Campbell 1979).

Impact of Sociopolitical Forces on the Recent History of Child Psychiatry

Child psychiatrists always have regarded child psychiatry as a medical subspecialty, particularly of general psychiatry.

Psychiatry has developed primarily as a result of the growing concern with mental illness in the adult population. The child and adolescent populations have benefited incidentally. Historians of the development of child psychiatry—such as Crutcher (1943), Lowrey (1944), and Levy (1968)—described the concerns raised by the large number of psychiatric casualties among United States soldiers during World War I. Philanthropic foundations such as the Commonwealth Fund and the Rockefeller Foundation began to fund the development of child guidance clinics throughout the United States as a preventive effort. The hope was that treating seriously disturbed young children would result in a healthier adult population. In general, however, throughout the history of the United States, mental health concerns about children have been rare, and the mental health needs of children have been largely ignored.

The assassination of President John F. Kennedy by Lee Harvey Oswald (who was described as having been severely mentally ill in childhood but never treated) resulted in the creation in 1965 of the congressional Joint Commission on the Mental Health of Children to study the origins and causes of mental illness in children and adolescents. The joint commission's report (Joint Commission on the Mental Health of Children 1970) detailed the findings of the various task forces and special committees, which spent 5 years studying various aspects of mental illness in children. The leadership of the commission, two renowned researchers in child development—Dr. Reginald Lourie, president, and Dr. Julius Richmond, vice president—encouraged a focus on the first 3 years of life as being critical to prevention of and early intervention in mental illness of children.

Each task force emphasized that without such a focus the mental health of many young children and adolescents would be seriously impaired. The report presented data to substantiate task force findings and a design to accomplish the required prevention or early intervention (Joint Commission on the Mental Health of Children 1970). Berlin (1975) elaborated on these early interventions and prevention methods in the Joint Commission's report.

By the mid-1970s, the political forces that endorsed and funded the Joint Commission were no longer influential, and these very important recommendations were largely ignored. Head Start and Early Periodic Screening, Diagnosis and Treatment were proven to be effective programs but were not fully funded. There was a growing movement to reduce the costs of treating the mentally ill and mentally retarded. The rationale for the widespread deinstitutionalization of these populations was that there would be community services—including treatment facilities, housing, and support services—available to serve the individuals turned out of the large institutions of care. These promises, like many others to enhance the care of the mentally

ill and retarded who flooded communities after the large institutions were closed, were never fulfilled. Society spawned a large mentally ill homeless population. Many of the homeless families included young children.

The political climate nationally and in most states reflected the fact that the health and mental health of children and adolescents had very low priority. Community mental health centers with their child treatment components, once considered major resources for the mental health of poor and minority communities (Langsley et al. 1981), were being closed throughout the nation.

We are now in the age of managed care. Child and adolescent mental health and child, adolescent, and adult health care are being examined in terms of nonexistent standards of cost-effectiveness. Poorly designed and conducted outcome studies are used to determine cost-effectiveness. It is clear that any concern for adequate health and mental health care for children, adolescents, and adults is being replaced by a primary concern for cost containment.

Child psychiatry is currently involved in an effort to carefully examine the criteria for each of the modalities used in the treatment of the various child and adolescent disorders currently described under the diagnostic criteria in DSM-IV-TR (American Psychiatric Association 2000).

On the national level, there is a major effort to contain the costs of health care without regard for need. This effort confronts child psychiatry with severe reductions in funds for the treatment of mentally ill children, adolescents, and families (Schetky 1995). There appear to be corporate directives that only the "least costly treatments" that require the least amount of treatment time (e.g., pharmacotherapy) be used. The various psychotherapeutic methods, whether delivered through individual or milieu therapy, are rapidly being made unavailable to children and their families because of cost concerns (I.N. Berlin, unpublished data, January 1992–January 1995; Schetky 1995).

Physicians, psychiatrists, and child psychiatrists are besieged with demands to express their concerns about many federal and state legislative efforts to ignore pain and individual and family dysfunction in the face of costs of treatment. Child psychiatrists, perhaps for the first time, are involved in meeting with insurance companies, managed care organizations, and health maintenance organizations to clarify and assert the need for and value of mental health treatment in children, adolescents, and families. Thus, child psychiatry is engaged in advocating for the patients it serves (AACAP Advocates for Patients 1995). In her 2000 presidential address to the American Academy of Child and Adolescent Psychiatry, Kestenbaum (2000) expressed her concern for the health care and mental health care of children in the twenty-first century.

Conclusion

The subspecialty of child psychiatry has a long history, beginning with the child guidance movement in the late 1920s and 1930s. After World War II, the large number of draftees rejected for psychiatric reasons and the great frequency of mental illness in the armed services led to a resurgence of interest in the mental health of children and adolescents. Child psychiatry in the 1950s and 1960s to a large extent moved from the child guidance clinics to the university medical schools. The purely psychotherapeutic treatment model was altered as basic research in the epidemiology of mental illnesses and in the biological and biochemical aspects of mental illnesses, especially genetic research, began to shed light on important variables in the etiology of mental illness. Psychopharmacological treatment became common for certain mental illnesses of childhood and adolescence. Child and adolescent psychiatry as a subspecialty has now come a long way. The NIMH has taken a leading role in promoting research on the diagnosis and treatment of mental illness in children (Shaffer et al. 2000). At the same time, managed care and cost containment of health care and mental health care, especially Medicare and Medicaid, seriously threaten the health and mental health of large segments of the population. New concerns and activities are now required of child psychiatrists.

References

AACAP advocates for patients. News of The American Academy of Child and Adolescent Psychiatry, Vol 26, No 6, November–December 1995, pp 2–4

Ackerman NW: The Psychodynamics of Family Life. New York, Basic Books, 1958

Allen F: Psychotherapy With Children. New York, WW Norton, 1942

American Academy of Child Psychiatry: The History of the American Academy of Child Psychiatry. J Am Acad Child Psychiatry 1:196–202, 1962

American Psychiatric Association: Career Training in Child Psychiatry. Washington, DC, American Psychiatric Association, 1964

American Psychiatric Association: Diagnostic and Statistical Manual of Mental Disorders, 4th Edition, Text Revision. Washington, DC, American Psychiatric Association, 2000

Axline VM: Play Therapy. New York, Ballantine Books, 1947

Bandera A, Walters R: Social Learning and Personality Development. New York, Holt Rinehart, 1963

Bender L: Childhood schizophrenia. Nervous Child 1:138–140, 1942

Bender L, Waltman AS: The use of puppet shows as a psychotherapeutic method for behavior problems in children. Journal of the American Orthopsychiatric Association 6:341–348, 1936

Bergman P, Escalona SK: Unusual sensitivities in very young children, in The Psychoanalytic Study of the Child, Vol III/IV. Edited by Freud A, Glover E, Greenacre P, et al. New York, International Universities Press, 1949, pp 333–352

Berlin IN: Some learning experiences as a psychiatric consultant in the schools. Ment Hyg 40:215–236, 1956

Berlin IN: A history of challenges in child psychiatry training. Ment Hyg 48:558–565, 1964

Berlin IN: Advocacy for Child Mental Health. New York, Brunner/Mazel, 1975

Berman S: Epilogue and a new beginning. J Am Acad Child Psychiatry 9:193–201, 1970

Bernard V: Psychiatric consultation in the social agency. Child Welfare 33:3–8, 1954

Bettelheim B: Love Is Not Enough: The Treatment of Emotionally Disturbed Children. Glencoe, IL, Free Press, 1950

Bettelheim B, Sylvester E: Milieu therapy: indications and illustrations. Psychoanal Rev 36:54–67, 1949

Bowlby J: Maternal Care and Mental Health, Monograph No 2. Geneva, World Health Organization, 1951

Bowlby J: Attachment and Loss, Vol 1: Attachment. New York, Basic Books, 1969

Bowlby J: Attachment and Loss, Vol 2: Separation, Anxiety, and Anger. London, Hogarth Press, 1973

Bradley C: Schizophrenia in Childhood. New York, Macmillan, 1941

Brazelton TB, School ML, Robey JF: Visual responses in the newborn. Pediatrics 37:284–290, 1966

Campbell M: Psychopharmacology, in Basic Handbook of Child Psychiatry, Vol 3. Edited by Noshpitz JD. New York, Basic Books, 1979, pp 376–408

Caplan G: The role of the social worker in preventive psychiatry. Medical Social Work 4:144–159, 1955

Chapman AH: Early infantile autism in identical twins: report of a case. Archives of Neurology and Psychiatry 78:621–623, 1957

Chess S, Thomas A, Rutter M, et al: Interaction of temperament and environment in the production of behavioral disturbances. Am J Psychiatry 120:142–147, 1963

Coleman JV: Psychiatric case consultation in case work agencies. Am J Orthopsychiatry 17:533–539, 1947

Crutcher R: Child psychiatry: a history of its development. Psychiatry 6:191–201, 1943

Ekstein R, Wallerstein J: Observations on the psychology of borderline and psychotic children. Psychoanal Study Child 11:166–235, 1956

Erikson EH: Childhood and Society. New York, WW Norton, 1950

Eth S, Pynoos RS (eds): Post-Traumatic Stress Disorder in Children. Washington, DC, American Psychiatric Press, 1985

Fish B, Alper M: Abnormal states of consciousness and muscle tone in infants born to schizophrenic mothers. Am J Psychiatry 119:439–445, 1962

Fish B, Shapiro T, Campbell M, et al: A classification of schizophrenic children under five years. Am J Psychiatry 124:1415–1423, 1968

Freud A: Introduction to the Technique of Child Analysis. New York, Nervous and Mental Disease Publishing, 1928

Freud A: The Ego and the Mechanisms of Defense. New York, International Universities Press, 1946

Gardner GE: William Healy 1869–1963. J Am Acad Child Psychiatry 11:1–29, 1972

Glueck S: The Problem of Delinquency. Boston, MA, Houghton, Mifflin, 1959

Glueck S, Glueck E: Toward a Typology of Juvenile Offenders. New York, Grune & Stratton, 1970

Goldfarb W: Receptor preference in schizophrenic children. Archives of Neurology and Psychiatry 76:643–652, 1956

Healy W: The Individual Delinquent. Boston, MA, Little, Brown, 1915

Healy W, Bronner AF: New Light on Delinquency and Its Treatment. New Haven, CT, Yale University Press, 1936

Johnson A: Sanctions for superego lacunae of adolescents, in Searchlight on Delinquency. Edited by Eissler KR. New York, International Universities Press, 1949, pp 225–245

Johnson A, Szurek SA: The genesis of antisocial acting out in children and adults. Psychoanal Q 21:323–343, 1952

Joint Commission on the Mental Health of Children: Crisis in Child Mental Health. New York, Harper & Row, 1970

Jones M: The Therapeutic Community: A New Treatment Method in Psychiatry. New York, Basic Books, 1953

Josselyn IM: A type of predelinquent behavior. Am J Orthopsychiatry 28:606–612, 1958

Kallmann FJ: The Genetics of Schizophrenia. New York, Augustin, 1938

Kanner L: Child Psychiatry. Springfield, IL, Charles C Thomas, 1935

Kanner L: Autistic disturbances of affective contact. Nervous Child 2:217–250, 1943

Kanner L: Arnold Gesell's place in the history of developmental psychology and psychiatry, in Child Development and Child Psychiatry. Edited by Shagass C, Pasamanick B. Washington, DC, American Psychiatric Association, 1960a, pp 1–9

Kanner L: Child psychiatry: retrospect and prospect. Am J Psychiatry 117:15–22, 1960b

Kempe CH, Silverman FN, Steele BF, et al: The battered child syndrome. JAMA 181:17–24, 1962

Kestenbaum C: How shall we treat children in the 21st century? J Am Acad Child Adolesc Psychiatry 39:1–10, 2000

Klein M: The Psychoanalysis of Children. New York, WW Norton, 1932

Konopka G: Group Work in the Institution: A Modern Challenge. New York, Whiteside & Wimorrow, 1954

Kraft I: Group therapy, in Basic Handbook of Child Psychiatry, Vol 3. Edited by Nosphitz JD. New York, Basic Books, 1979, pp 159–180

Krasner L: Behavior therapy. Annu Rev Psychol 222:483–531, 1971

Langsley DG, Berlin IN, Yarvis RM: Handbook of Community Mental Health. New York, Medical Examination Publishing, 1981

Levy DM: Primary affect hunger. Am J Psychiatry 94:643–652, 1937

Levy DM: Release therapy. Am J Orthopsychiatry 9:713–736, 1939

Levy DM: The Demonstration Clinic for the Psychological Study and Treatment of Mother and Child in Medical Practice. Springfield, IL, Charles C Thomas, 1959

Levy DM: Beginnings of the child guidance movement. Am J Orthopsychiatry 38:799–804, 1968

Lindemann E: Symptomatology and management of acute grief. Am J Psychiatry 101:141–148, 1944

Lippman HS: Treatment of the Child in Emotional Conflict. New York, Blakiston, 1961

Lowrey LG: Psychiatry for children: a brief history of developments. Am J Psychiatry 101:375–388, 1944

Lowrey LG: The contribution of orthopsychiatry to psychiatry: brief historical note. Am J Orthopsychiatry 25:475–478, 1955

Mahler MS: On child psychosis and schizophrenia: autistic and symbiotic infantile psychoses, in The Psychoanalytic Study of the Child, Vol 7. Edited by Eissler RS, Freud A, Glover E. New York, International Universities Press, 1952, pp 286–305

McGee JP, Saidel DH: Individual behavior therapy, in Basic Handbook of Child Psychiatry. Edited by Noshpitz JD. New York, Basic Books, 1979, pp 72–107

Noshpitz JD: Notes on the theory of residential treatment. J Am Acad Child Psychiatry 1:284–296, 1962

Piaget J: The Language and Thought of the Child. New York, Harcourt Brace, 1926

Potter H: Schizophrenia in children. Am J Psychiatry 8:1253–1270, 1933

Redl F: The concept of a therapeutic milieu. Am J Orthopsychiatry 29:721–736, 1959a

Redl F: A strategy and technique of the life space interview. Am J Orthopsychiatry 29:1–18, 1959b

Redl F, Wineman D: Children Who Hate. Glencoe, IL, Free Press, 1951

Redl F, Wineman D: Controls From Within: Techniques for the Treatment of the Aggressive Child. Glencoe, IL, Free Press, 1952

Rexford EN, Van Amerongen ST: The influence of unsolved maternal oral conflicts upon impulsive acting out in young children. Am J Orthopsychiatry 27:75–87, 1957

Satir V: Conjoint Family Therapy: A Guide. Palo Alto, CA, Science and Behavior Books, 1963

Schetky DH: The inequities of managed care. News of the American Academy of Child and Adolescent Psychiatry, Vol 26, No 5, September–October, 1995, p 20

Shaffer D, Fisher P, Lucas CP, et al: NIMH Diagnostic Interview for Children Version IV (NIMH DISC-IV): description, differences from previous versions, and reliability of some common diagnoses. J Am Acad Child Adolesc Psychiatry 39:28–38, 2000

Slaff B: History of child and adolescent psychiatry ideas and organizations in the United States: a twentieth century review. Adolesc Psychiatry 16:31–52, 1989

Slavson SR: An Introduction to Group Therapy. New York, Commonwealth Fund, 1934

Solomon JC: Play techniques. Am J Orthopsychiatry 18:402–413, 1948

Spitz R: Hospitalism: an inquiry into the genesis of psychiatric conditions in early childhood. Psychoanal Study Child 1:53–74, 1945

Spitz R: Anaclitic depression. Psychoanal Study Child 2:313–342, 1946

Spock B: Baby and Child Care. New York, Pocket Books, 1946

Szurek SA: Notes on the genesis of psychopathic personality trends. Psychiatry 5:1–6, 1942

Szurek SA: Childhood schizophrenia: psychotic episodes and psychotic maldevelopment. Am J Orthopsychiatry 26:519–543, 1956

Szurek SA, Johnson A, Falstein E: Collaborative psychiatric therapy of parent-child problems. Am J Orthopsychiatry 12:511–516, 1942

Terr LC: Psychic trauma in children and adolescents. Psychiatr Clin North Am 8:815–835, 1985

Thomas A, Chess S, Birch HG: Temperament and Behavior Disorders in Children. New York, New York University Press, 1968

Werner EE, Bierman JM, French FE: The Children of Kauai. Honolulu, HI, University of Hawaii Press, 1971

Whiteside MF: Family therapy, in Basic Handbook of Child Psychiatry. Edited by Noshpitz JD. New York, Basic Books, 1979, pp 117–158

Wiener JM: The future of child and adolescent psychiatry: if not now, when? J Am Acad Child Adolesc Psychiatry 27:8–10, 1988

Witmer HC: Psychiatric Clinics for Children. New York, Commonwealth Fund, 1940

Wolpe J: Experimental neurosis as learned behavior. Br J Psychol 43:243–268, 1952

Overview of Development From Infancy Through Adolescence

Melvin Lewis, M.B., B.S., F.R.C.Psych., D.C.H.

Human development starts with genetic potential and blossoms through the interaction between the individual and the caring others in the individual's environment. Certain species characteristics may strongly influence the emergence and form of particular patterns of functioning. For example, the prolonged relative biological helplessness of the human infant is associated with characteristic patterns of attachment behavior, which presumably have great survival value. Furthermore, functions that are closely tied to central nervous system maturation (e.g., motor development) appear to be more robust and resistant to environmental influences than, for example, the capacity to develop relationships, which is exquisitely sensitive to environmental influences, particularly the competence of the mothering person.

Some central nervous system maturational events, such as electroencephalographic changes and associated behaviors (e.g., the shift from a perceptual mode to a symbolic-linguistic mode around age 17 months), appear to be relatively discontinuous. Other characteristics, such as the temperament of the individual ("easy," "slow to warm up," and "difficult" temperaments), appear to be relatively stable characteristics that are present from birth onward.

For convenience, we tend to focus on discrete elements within disciplines such as the neurosciences, developmental psychology, and psychoanalysis (see Figure 2–1). However, development is a complex phenomenon, and ultimately all the discrete elements must be integrated into a theory of the whole person. As yet, no single theory is completely satisfactory.

At the same time, several general concepts are helpful in attempts to organize understanding of the development of the child. *Maturation* is the sequential emergence and linear growth of specific capacities; *development* is the totality of full blossoming and the multiple, interlocking uses of these functions and skills brought about by interaction between the individual and the environment. Viewed in this way, development is the result of the mutually interacting influences of endowment, maturation, environment, memory, and experiential factors.

The concept of *stages* is particularly useful because it enables one to analyze behavior, just as classification in biology serves as a basis for subsequent analysis and understanding (Figure 2–2).

Piaget (1958) suggested that eight principles underlie the development of stages:

1. A stage, or structure, is characterized as a whole and not just as the juxtaposition of parts. The concept of definable stages signifies behavioral characteristics that have some degree of stability and autonomy.
2. There is an invariant sequence of succession from one stage to another.
3. Although multiple and interrelated lines of stage development are present, each line may also have its own trajectory (from preparatory level to a level of more or less completion) and rate of develop-

Sections of this chapter are modified from Lewis M, Volkmar F: *Clinical Aspects of Child and Adolescent Development,* 3rd Edition. Baltimore, MD, Lea & Febiger, 1990.

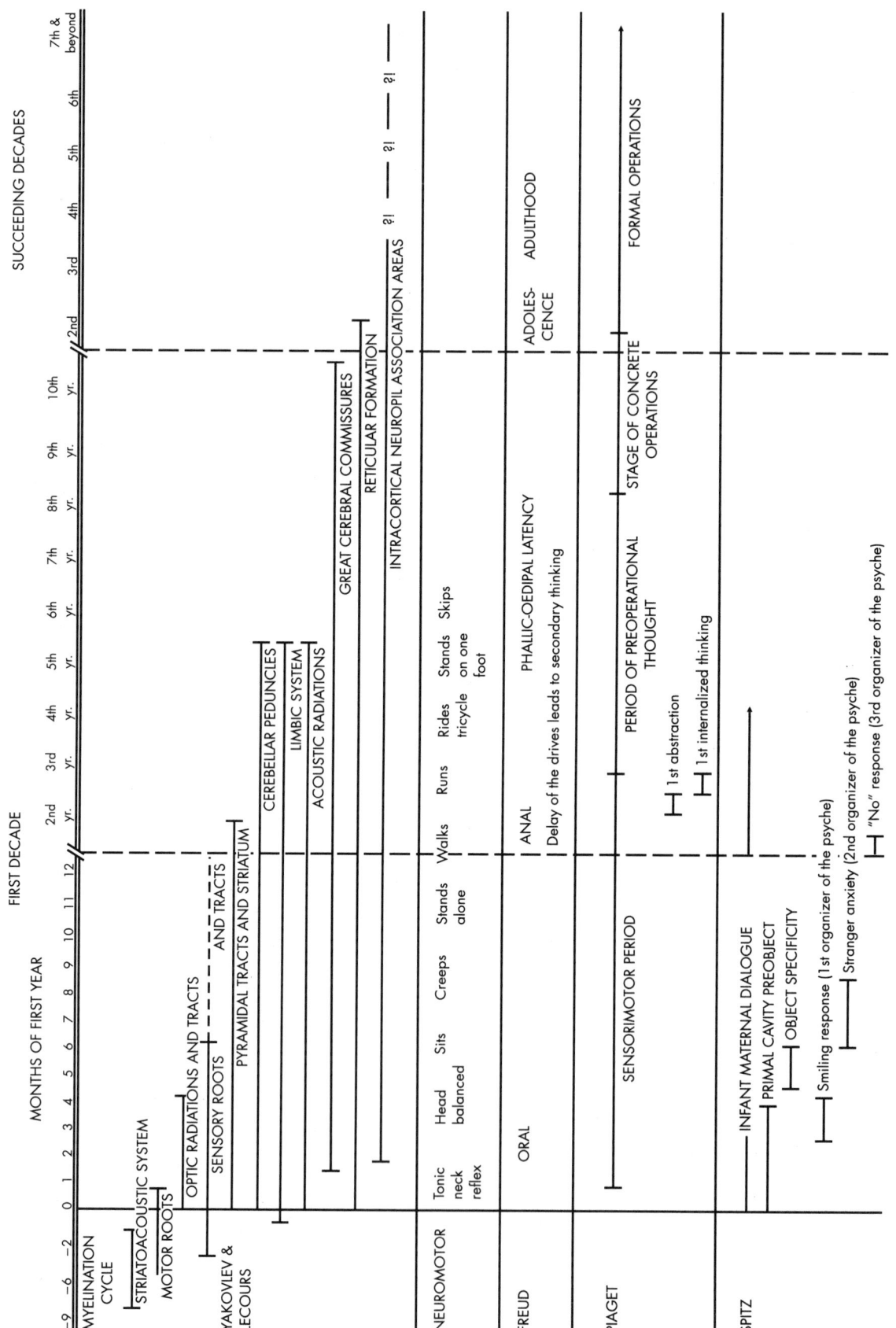

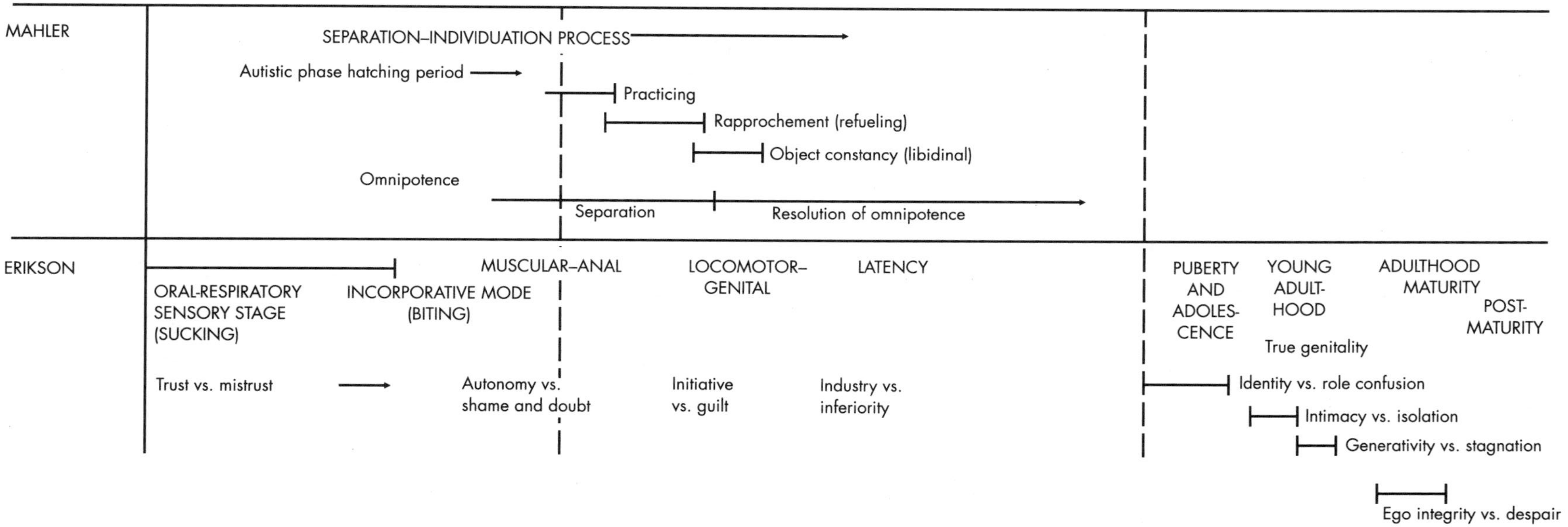

Figure 2–1. Temporal correspondence of several neurological and psychological developmental sequences.

Source. Reprinted from Meyersburg HA, Post RM: "An Holistic Developmental View of Neural and Psychological Processes: A Neurobiologic-Psychoanalytic Integration." *British Journal of Psychiatry* 135:139–155, 1979. Used with permission from the *British Journal of Psychiatry*.

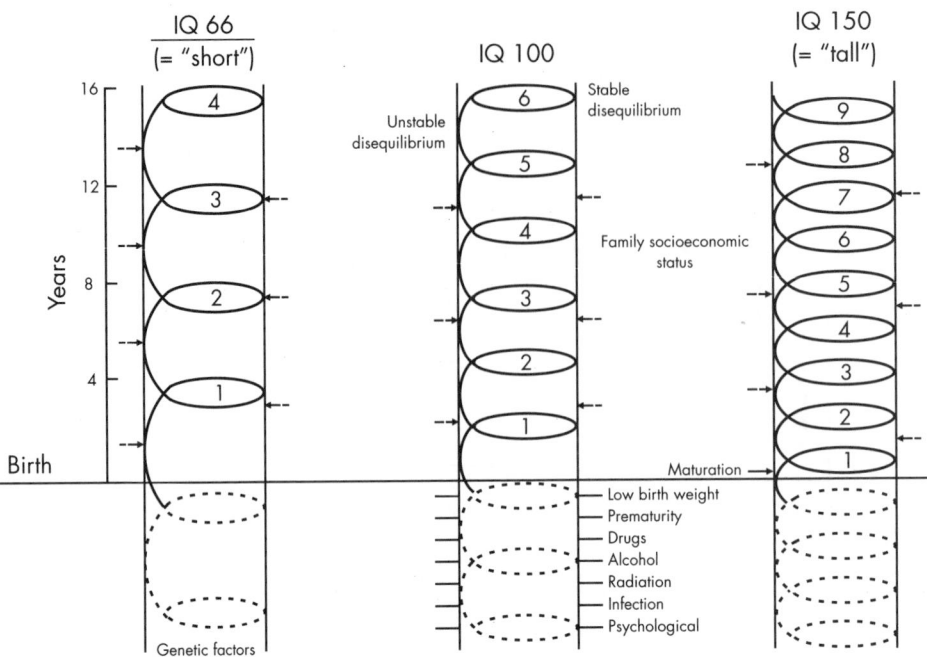

Figure 2–2. A stage model for cognitive development.

The horizontal arrows represent environmental events impinging on the individual, who is represented as a pair of vertical lines. The individual's cognitive development appears as an internal ascending spiral, in which the numbered loops represent successive stages of cognitive growth.

Source. Reprinted from Zigler E, Cascione R: "Overview of Cognitive, Behavioral, and Communicative Disorders, in *The Physician and the Mental Health of the Child, II: The Psychological Concomitants of Illness.* Edited by Grossman HJ, Stubblefield RL. Monroe, WI, American Medical Association, 1980.

ment, giving rise at any given moment to a multi-leveled organism.

4. Each successive stage in normal development represents an advance from the previous stage (i.e., the change is qualitative, not just quantitative).

5. Each later stage supersedes all earlier stages, in that structures constructed earlier become an integral part of structures that follow.

6. Each stage proceeds in the direction of increasing complexity of organization, from a state of relative globality to a state of increasing differentiation and integration.

7. Biogenetic, environmental, experiential, and psychological factors contribute to and facilitate development, which includes coping and adaptive functions.

8. There are presumed critical or sensitive periods during which conditions are ideal for the emergence and development of important functions, such as attachment, gender identity, and language. However, during such sensitive periods, the emerging function is also more vulnerable.

Theories of developmental stages imply the development of a mental structure. Thus, psychoanalysis (Freud), psychosocial development (Erikson), and cognitive development (Piaget)—which together can be called the structural theories—postulate a genetically determined capacity for the development of patterns or systems of behavior in which the child acts on the environment from the very beginning. The overall behavior patterns that then emerge are qualitatively different from one another but also exhibit continuity. The clinical implication of such structural theories is that some kind of reorganization within the child is required (e.g., resolution of intrapsychic conflict, alteration of the family homeostasis, and acquisition of new schema).

On the other hand, some theories of function and behavior do not appear to have a strong developmental point of view and rely instead on certain principles of reaction. Such reactive theories postulate that the child reacts in particular ways to environmental stimuli. Major examples of this type of theory are stimulus-response theory, learning theories, classical conditioning theory, and operant conditioning theory. The clinical implication of such reactive theories is that because it is regarded as learned behavior, the symptom is removed (i.e., the symptom is the disorder) and the disorder is cured through relearning or environmental change.

Although development is a complex process involving biological, psychological, cultural, and social factors, for convenience the study of development is usually approached along the lines of some of its major functional components (see Figure 2–1).

The maturational and developmental lines discussed below include motor sequence, the senses, emotions, language development, cognitive development, memory, moral thinking, attachment, psychosexual phases, relationships, and temperament. A summary of developmental tasks and an account of developmental concepts concerning body image and psychological aspects of illness and death are also provided.

Motor Sequence

Gesell and Amatruda (1941/1964) observed that most children creep, can be pulled to their feet, and have a crude prehensile release by the time they are 10 months old. Within the next 2 months, they can walk with help and can grasp a small pellet. By age 2 years, they are running with ease, although not with great skill.

A steady increase in motor skills can be observed in most children. By age 3 years, a child can stand on one foot, dance, and jump, and he or she is also more dexterous than before and can build a tower of 10 cubes. Ambidexterity gives way to lateralization some time during the third year, although handedness may not be firmly established for several years. Leg, eye, and ear dominance also may not become firmly established until the seventh, eighth, or ninth year, respectively, or even later.[1]

Children become increasingly agile as they grow and develop during the period of early childhood (e.g., learning to skip on alternate feet). Perceptual-motor skills also improve at this time: a child at age 2 years can copy a circle; by age 3 years, a cross; by age 5 years, a square; and by age 7 years, a diamond. Memory also improves with brain maturation: by age 6 years, the child can count five digits forward and three digits backward. Between ages 6 and 11 years, the child not only learns new motor skills, such as balancing on a bicycle, but at some point, perhaps around age 9 years, does so with ease—the skill becomes an automatic, established unselfconscious act requiring no effort of concentration.

The Senses

Within a few hours after birth, the infant pays most attention to high-contrast visual stimuli (Kessen 1967). By age 1 week, infants prefer to look at strongly patterned shapes, for example, a face, especially one in motion (e.g., nodding) (Fantz et al. 1975). With a "visual cliff" procedure, depth perception can be demonstrated by age 2 months (Campos et al. 1970). Color perception can also be demonstrated at this time (Bornstein 1975). The newborn can discriminate the particular smell of the mother virtually at birth (Engen et al. 1963) and can also discriminate the four basic tastes—sweet, acidic, salty, and bitter (Kobre and Lipsett 1972). The newborn clearly experiences pain (e.g., on circumcision) (Porter et al. 1988). Infants hear at birth and respond preferentially to the mother's voice by age 1 week (Mills and Melhuish 1974). The newborn indeed seems to be especially tuned in to human speech (Ferald 1984).

Early maturation and development of each of the inborn capacities described above presumably had great survival value for the human infant. Such functions facilitate attachment and enhance full communication. Impairment of sight and hearing are particularly difficult handicaps for the developing child and family.

---

[1]*Laterality* is a measurable, specialized, central function of a paired faculty such as eyes, ears, hands, and feet. *Preference* is the subjective, self-reported experience of an individual and need not be the same as objectively measured laterality. The preference of an individual may be related more to the acuity of the peripheral organ (e.g., the ear) than to anything else. *Dominance* is the term used for the concept of cerebral hemisphere specialization (e.g., information processing, language, and speech lateralization). Hemispheric lateralization appears to proceed sequentially from gross and fine motor skills to sensorimotor skills to speech and language (Leong 1976). Handedness is commonly consolidated around age 5 years; footedness, around age 7 years; eye preference, around age 7 or 8 years; and ear preference, around age 9 years (Touwen 1980).

Emotions

Emotions are complex phenomena having subjective, perceptual, and cognitive—as well as neurophysiological, expressive, and motoric—components interacting with one another and with the environment. Similar patterns of facial expression for emotions—such as apparent bliss, surprise, fear, distress, anger, sadness, and disgust—have been observed in infants in many cultures (Darwin 1872/1975; Izard 1977). The development of emotions appears to proceed through a progressive differentiation from more or less global affective states (e.g., generalized excitement) to more specific emotions such as anger or delight, depending in part on the infant's experience of social interaction and increasing maturation. Attempts to control emotions are seen in children in nursery school (age 3 years).

The expression of pleasure occurs early. A reflex half-smile (without involvement of the eye muscles) can be seen in the newborn. However, these reflex smiles, although correlated perhaps with internal states, do not necessarily reflect pleasure (Korner 1969). Whole-face smiles in response to positive social interaction occur at about age 4–6 weeks (Sroufe and Waters 1976) and increasingly become involved in the attachment behaviors of infants that promote social reciprocity. Smiling also is seen when the infant seems to have mastered some task (e.g., performing a secondary or tertiary circular reaction—see under "Cognitive Development" below). Laughter is the next expression of pleasure to appear, usually around age 4 months, and is often seen in response to peek-a-boo games.

Anxiety occurs in infants in response to sudden stimulus changes. Fear and anxiety in response to the experience of cognitive discrepancy at the sight of a stranger (Kagan 1971, 1984) occur at age 8 months, followed by separation anxiety when the security provided by the presence and proximity of an attachment figure is threatened. Repeated separations and threats of abandonment may give rise to anger, sadness, and the so-called affectionless character (Bowlby 1951). Anger is often seen in response to frustration and restraint, perhaps peaking in the second year when autonomy is threatened. However, it may also be seen in school-age children and adolescents when the same conflict occurs. Guilt, which involves awareness of a transgression and a feeling of remorse, may be observed in 2-year-olds as part of a developmental sequence that includes a change in the child's explanations in relation to the development of his or her moral thinking (see the section "Moral Development" below).

Preschool children fear animals, frightening dreams, and natural phenomena such as thunder and lightning. School-age children fear harm to the body, and adolescents may exhibit social anxiety. Most of these fears tend to diminish with age.

Presumably, all affects can serve adaptive and protective functions. However, excessive affects can be disorganizing, and affective deprivation may give rise to an emotionally blunted personality.

Language Development

The sequence for the emergence of actual sounds is broadly the same in all children everywhere (Lenneberg 1967; Lewis 1963). Children vocalize and respond to sounds from birth, possibly even prenatally. The infant can be soothed specifically by the voice of his or her mother (primary caregiver) as early as the first few weeks. The early phonetic characteristics of discomfort—cries of the infant—appear to be the vocal manifestations of the infant's total reaction to discomfort, determined in part by the physiological contraction of the facial muscles. By age 6 weeks, the infant begins to utter repetitive strings of sound called *babbling*. In doing so, the infant finds satisfaction in producing at will sounds that at first occurred involuntarily. Skill is acquired in making sounds, and the sounds of others are imitated as nearly as possible.

Up to about 5 months the infant tends to use "filler syllables," which are usually nasals and which gradually decrease as multiple syllable utterances occur (Aoyama 2001). Thus the number of filler syllables increases up through 20 months, after which, at 21.1 months, it drops dramatically.

The nearer the approximation of the infant's sounds to those of the parents, the more marked will be the parents' approval and the greater will be the infant's incentive to repeat such sounds. In this way, the phonetic pattern of the child's mother tongue is acquired. What is important in these earliest weeks is that the frequency and variety of sounds may already be restricted through inadequate stimulation by the caring adult.

The capacity to discriminate among different sounds is present in the newborn (Friedlander 1970). Almost from the beginning, the infant seems to be programmed to move in rhythm to the human voice (Condon and Sander 1974) and will orient with eyes, head, and body to animate sound stimuli (Mills 1974). Subsequent language development correlates most closely with motor development, although the two functions are not necessarily causally related in any specific way. Crying, which is present during fetal life, soon becomes differentiated during the first few months into recognized cries related to hunger, discomfort, pain, pleasure, and other stimuli (Wolff 1969). As crying decreases, cooing increases, and vowel sounds (e.g., "ooh") begin to dominate. Consonants begin to appear at about age 5 months and words at about age 1 year, with a range of 8–18 months (Morley 1965). At the same time, by age 1 year, the infant discriminates between and responds to differences in language, depending on who is speaking and how that person is speaking (e.g., the intonation and the amount of repetition used). Vocabulary gradually increases to approximately 200 words by age 2 years. Nouns appear first, then verbs, adjectives, and adverbs. Pronouns appear by the time the child is age 2 years and conjunctions, after age 2½ years. By this time, too, the child's understanding of language has increased immensely. Play at this stage in effect represents the child's "inner language." Between ages 2 and 4 years, the child has acquired, or learned, most of the fundamental (as opposed to the academic) rules of grammar, although how this is done is not known.

Linguistic shifts occur continuously. For example, at age 6 or 7 years, children shift from making syntagmatic responses to making paradigmatic responses (Francis 1972). Syntagmatic associations are response items that are in a grammatical class different from that of the stimulus, that is, the words just "go together" (e.g., hot-bath or apple-eat). Paradigmatic associations are response items that belong to the same grammatical class as the stimulus (e.g., hot-cold or apple-pear). Also, before age 6 or 7 years, children link temporal succession to succession of enunciation; for example, a young child will interpret the sentence "The girl goes upstairs when the boy has parked the car" to mean that the girl goes upstairs first and the boy parks the car afterward (Ferreiro 1971). After age 6 or 7 years, the child is no longer tied to this concrete perception of sequence. Furthermore, sometime between ages 5 and 10 years, children become more conscious of the struc-

ture of the language they use (Nelson 1977).

Finally, the child is able to speak and understand language independently of the context in which it occurs. Around age 12 years, when the child is in the stage of logical operations, language becomes a means of knowing.

The theory of language development is in a state of flux. The child apparently has a built-in capacity to abstract various universal relationships and regularities in the particular language heard, and he or she uses this capacity to construct an operation by which principles can be applied to formulate an infinite number of sentences. Such an operation for language is obviously far more economical and powerful than anything the child might accrue or learn from simple imitation. Moreover, the capacity for this operational work seems not only to be related to the child's general cognitive capacities but also to be an integral part of the child's uniquely human condition.

As the child develops and moves from stage to stage, he or she develops the capacity to react to increasingly complex stimuli, starting with intonation and moving through articulation of specific sounds to special syntactic and semantic stimuli. In this way, the child learns a linguistic code. All children appear to follow the same sequence in the development of phonology, syntax, and semantics. Chomsky's (1957) theory of generative transformational grammar suggests that in some way, perhaps through "innate intellectual structures," the child develops a basic grammar that can generate an infinite number of sentences and an optional transformational grammar that transforms the basis of a sentence into its various forms (e.g., passive and interrogative).

Alternatively, these inner structures may derive from the sensorimotor schemes (Piaget 1954). Indeed, the formation of such schemas during the long sensorimotor stage may be essential for the subsequent emergence of language and linguistic competence. Language in this view is one expression of what Piaget called the *semiotic function* (Inhelder 1971). Early schemas of experience precede symbolic language, and language comprehension precedes language production (children understand words and sentences long before they can say them) (Lovell and Dixon 1967).

There is no satisfactory psychoanalytic theory for language acquisition (Wolff 1967). The child begins to use language as a symbolic instrument, initially—and necessarily—through the help of the mothering person, who is referred to throughout this chapter as the mother. For example, the mother uses a word (e.g., "Dada" or "Mama," then "Daddy" or "Mommy") as a symbol, and in so doing she helps in the organization of the symbolizing process that is taking place within the infant. She does not create that process within the infant; she facilitates its development. Initially, of course, considerable overextension occurs; a child may call all men Daddy (or all four-legged animals doggie) until further accommodation of the concepts, or schemas, of Daddy (or doggie) occurs.

It is very likely that the mother's spoken words are initially experienced by the infant as tones and rhythms rather than as words with meanings, and as such they are part of the unprecedented kinesthetic, tactile, visual, auditory, olfactory, and gustatory bombardment that the infant tries to assimilate and organize into schemas. Eventually, the child's percept of mother, for example, already linked to the word *mother,* becomes better defined. In this sense, mothers are sensitive language teachers of their children (Moerk 1974). The sensitive timing, repetition, and associated pleasurable affects with which the mother uses words for labeling, shaping, and so on serve to stimulate the development of language. (Curiously, mothers seem to talk more to their baby girls than to their baby boys [Halverson and Waldrop 1970].)

Reinforcement may be more important for phonetic and semantic development than for syntactic development (R. Brown and Hanlon 1970). The best stimulus for syntactic development appears to be a rich conversational interchange without any attempt to modify the child's utterances (Cazden 1966).

Children continue to learn phonology, syntax, and semantics throughout the school years. The utterances of young children appear to depend on the support of the nonlinguistic environment. For example, if one asks a child a question out of context, the child often "draws a blank" (Bloom 1975). Young children tend to respond more readily when they are asked to talk about events that are in a more immediately perceived context (R. Brown and Bellugi 1964).

Cognitive Development

The beginning of thinking is in the body. The infant reacts to a sensory stimulus with a motor reaction: when a finger is placed in the infant's hand, the infant will grasp; when a nipple is placed in the infant's mouth, he or she will begin sucking; when a pattern is placed in front of the infant's eyes, he or she will respond by looking. This sensorimotor pattern is the earliest kind of thinking, and it starts with innate patterns of behavior such as grasping, sucking, looking, and gross body activity.

The basic element in Piaget's theory of the child's cognitive development is the *schema,* which consists of a pattern of behavior in response to a particular stimulus from the environment. However, the schema is more than just a response, because the child also acts on the environment. For example, the infant sucks in response to a nipple. The schema of sucking then becomes increasingly complex as the child reacts to and acts on a wider range of environmental stimuli. Thus, when the thumb is put into the mouth, the schema of sucking evoked by a nipple is gradually broadened to include this new and similar but not identical stimulus, the thumb. The new object (the thumb) is said to be *assimilated* into the original schema. At the same time, sucking behavior has to be slightly modified because the thumb is different in shape, taste, and other characteristics from the nipple. This act of modification, which Piaget called *accommodation,* results in a new equilibrium. These two processes, assimilation and accommodation, proceed in ever-increasing complexities.

Four major stages of development are described in Piaget's theory:

1. Sensorimotor stage (from birth to 2 years)
2. Preoperational stage (from 2 years to 7 years)
3. Concrete operational stage (from 7 years to adolescence)
4. Formal operational stage (adolescence)

In the sensorimotor stage (birth to 2 years), six substages are discernible:

1. In the first month, the infant exercises a function, such as looking or grasping, simply because the function exists.
2. During the next 3–4 months (from age 1 to 4½ months), new schemas are acquired that usually center on the infant's own body (e.g., his or her thumb) (*primary circular reactions*).
3. Sometime between ages 4½ and 8 or 9 months, the infant tries to produce an effect on the object he or she sees or grasps. That is, he or she now includes events or objects in the external environment (e.g., a rattle) (*secondary circular reactions*).

4. By ages 8 to 11½ months, the infant begins to be aware of the existence of unperceived objects hidden, for example, behind a pillow or in peek-a-boo games. This is also the time of so-called stranger anxiety. The mental image of the object has now achieved some degree of permanence in the infant's mind (*object permanence*), a phenomenon probably related to increased metabolic rate in the prefrontal cortex at that time (Chugani et al. 1987).

5. In the first half of the second year (age 11 or 12–18 months), the child explores an object and its spatial relationship more thoroughly, for example, by putting smaller objects into and taking them out of larger ones.

   a. The child initiates changes that produce variations in the event itself, for example, dropping bread and then toys from different heights or different positions (*secondary circular reactions*).

   b. The child actively searches for novel events, constituting *tertiary circular reactions*.

6. By the end of the second year (age 18–24 months), the child shows some evidence of reasoning; mental trial and error replaces trial and error in action. For example, the child uses one toy as an instrument to get another.

The use of toys and play for a child is essentially a form of thinking. External objects (play items) are organized in such a way as to represent the child's internal symbolization of events and fantasies. Piaget called this evocation of past events and fantasies in the present play *deferred imitation,* a characteristic of symbolic thought.

The preoperational stage, occurring approximately between ages 2 and 7 years, clearly reflects progress over the preceding stage of sensorimotor intelligence. Two substages are described: 1) *symbolic activity* and make-believe play and 2) *decentration.*

The substage of symbolic activity and make-believe play occurs between ages 2 and 4 years. In this substage, symbolic thought and representation develop. Language becomes increasingly important as the child learns to distinguish between actual objects and the labels used to represent them. As a result, the child gradually becomes able to reason symbolically rather than motorically, as was the case in the preceding sensorimotor period, when the infant was limited to the pursuit of concrete goals through action.

However, despite these significant advances, there are striking cognitive limitations to preoperational thinking that distinguish it from the logical thought processes emerging in the subsequent concrete and, ultimately, formal operational stages. Principally, the child's judgments in the early preoperational stage are dominated by the child's perceptions of events, objects, and experiences. Furthermore, the child can attend to only one perceptual dimension or attribute at a time. The concept of time is also not available to a child at this preoperational stage. Sequences and daily routines can be recognized (e.g., mealtime, playtime, sleep time, day and night, and Daddy's or Mommy's going and coming), but the child has no concept of an hour, a minute, a week, or a month.

The preoperational child is also extremely egocentric. By that, Piaget did not mean that the child is selfish per se. Rather, Piaget used the term *egocentric* to refer to a certain cognitive limitation during the preoperational stage, namely, that the young child is conceptually unable to view events and experiences from any point of view but his or her own. The child is clearly the center of his or her own representational world. Similarly, the child is unable to differentiate clearly between the self and the world, between the subjective realm of thoughts and feelings and the objective realm of external reality.

In addition, at the preoperational stage, the child's reasoning is neither inductive nor deductive but what Piaget termed *transductive.* That is, the young child tends to relate the particular to the particular in an alogical manner. Events may be viewed as related not because of any inherent cause-and-effect relationship but simply on the basis of spatial or temporal contiguity or juxtaposition. Furthermore, the child at this stage is unaware of and therefore unconcerned about possible logical contradictions.

The substage of decentration occurs between ages 4 and 7 years. In this substage, an increased accommodation to reality gradually takes over, and the child's own interests, perception, and points of view progressively decenter. The decentering comes about partly because of the child's increased social involvement (e.g., at school). Social interaction virtually demands that the child use language, and the child discovers that what he or she thinks is not necessarily the same as what the child's peers think. The child begins to recognize other points of view.

The concrete operational stage usually occurs between ages 7 and 11 years. The child at this stage is no longer bound by the configuration perceived at a given moment. Two variables (e.g., height and width) can now be taken into account at once. Piaget (1952) performed what is now a classic experiment. One form of Piaget's experiment follows. The child is first asked to make sure that the amounts of water in two identical beakers are the same. The water from one of the beakers is then transferred into a tall, narrow cylinder. The child is asked whether the remaining beaker contains the same amount of water as the cylinder. A child who is in the preoperational stage may say "no" and, if asked why, may say either that the cylinder contains more water "because it's higher" or that the beaker contains more water "because it's wider." A child who is at the concrete operational stage will be able to say, "Yes, the amount of water is the same" and, if asked why, will be able to say, "because it's narrower in the cylinder and wider in the beaker" and (perhaps) "because it's the same water that had been in the other beaker."

The child has mastered what Piaget called the concept of *conservation*. The child learns to apply the concept of conservation not only to volume but also to number, class, length, weight, and area.

These types of conservation occur at different ages. The conservation of objects occurs quite early, usually by the end of the sensorimotor period. Quantity is conserved at ages 6–8 years and weight at ages 9–12 years. Probably the variation in age at which different conservations are achieved is related to how easily the property can be dissociated from the child's own action. According to Piaget (1958), "It is more difficult to…equalize…objects whose properties are less easy to dissociate from one's own action, such as weight, than to apply the same operation to properties which can be objectified more readily, such as length" (p. 249).

Age 6 or 7 years marks a key turning point in the child's thinking. After age 6 or 7 years, the child is no longer bound by his or her perception and can apply reasoning. It is the age at which the child starts first grade. It also corresponds in psychoanalytic theory to the time when the oedipal struggle is thought to be resolved and the superego consolidated. Feelings can be distanced, thought about, and put into context. Also, the child can more readily distinguish between fantasy and reality.

In short, the major advance in the concrete operational stage is that the child can apply basic logical principles to the realm of concrete experiences and events without being bound by his or her perceptions. Gradually, logical thought processes become orga-

nized into an increasingly complex and integrated network through which the surrounding world is confronted and responded to systematically.

Piaget (1969) observed that in the formal operational stage, "the great novelty that characterizes adolescent thought and that starts around the age of 11 to 12, but probably does not reach its point of equilibrium until the age of 14 or 15,…consists in the possibility of manipulating ideas in themselves and no longer in merely manipulating objects" (p. 23). The young adolescent can now use hypotheses, experiment, make deductions, and reason from the particular to the general. The adolescent is no longer tied to the environment. He or she in essence can now make theoretical statements independent of specific content and can apply this way of thinking to many kinds of data.

The result is a further release from the concrete world: "The most distinctive property of formal thought is this reversal of direction between reality and possibility; instead of deriving a rudimentary type of theory from the empirical data, as is done in concrete inferences, formal thought begins with a theoretical synthesis implying that certain relations are necessary and this proceeds in the opposite direction" (Piaget 1958, p. 251).

Pragmatically, Piaget provided a set of cognitive developmental norms that are useful to the clinician. For example, preschool children are often preoccupied with superpowerful and giant figures such as dinosaurs and doll-figure heroes and heroines that represent the perceived powerful and idealized human figures in the child's life. This symbolic representation is evident in the symbolic play of young children. The clinician can then use this information as a means of understanding the concerns, conflicts, wishes, and anxieties of a child and may choose, at a particular moment in psychotherapy, to interpret to the child the meaning of the play as gathered from the child's associations (e.g., verbalizations, activities) within the symbolic play. At the same time, Piaget's system offers an explanation of the preoperational child's difficulties in resolving emotional as well as intellectual problems. For such a child, fantasy and reality may be poorly differentiated and affects more difficult to conceptualize (conserve).

The school-age child in the concrete operational stage is trying to construct an orderly and lawful world and is becoming socialized. These processes can be seen, for example, in the child's use of rules in games, such as checkers and Monopoly, and in the child's acceptance of symbols such as paper money and the hierarchical implications in games like checkers (e.g., "king").

Piaget's system is particularly helpful in school consultation for the child in the concrete operational stage.

Memory

Memory is increasingly viewed as a highly complex process consisting of numerous interacting systems that function at different levels. Such systems include attention (Mirsky et al. 1991) and motivation systems, as well as the actions of neurotransmitters and hormones. Throughout the course of development, changes within each system give rise to qualitative and quantitative changes to—and therefore shifts in—the interrelationships among the many systems that contribute to the functioning of memory.

■ Neurobiology of Memory

During fetal development an astonishing, orderly, massive migration of cells occurs, starting in a proliferative zone near the cerebral ventricle and ending in various locations of the cerebral cortex. This migration was found to continue throughout the middle third of gestation, at which time neurogenesis appeared to be complete; that is, no further neurogenesis was found to occur (Rakic 1996; Rakic et al. 1994). One theory put forth to account for this one-time maximum number of new cells is that this phenomenon, if true, might be an essential prerequisite for the preservation of cognitive experiences (e.g., memory) (Rakic 1985).

Although a profusion of synapses may form among these neurons laid down during the fetal period, and although some cells may die at different times, in this classic view no new cells are formed. However, Gould and colleagues asserted that the neocortex in primates continues to acquire a large number of new neurons and in fact does so on a daily basis throughout the life cycle.

At present a majority of scientists in the field continue to support the classical view that neurogenesis is completed during the fetal period. For example, Nowakowski and Hayes (2000) published a comment on the 1999 finding by Gould et al. of the formation of new neurons. They concluded that although Gould and colleagues had made an intriguing case for continuing neurogenesis, the burden of proof had not been met. In the same publication, Gould and Gross responded that the description of their work was inaccurate and that the criticism of their inferences was unjustified by data, logic, or literature. Gould and Gross also asserted that their study results did support their view that new neurons continued to be added to the adult neocortex and that this took place throughout the life cycle of the individual. The significance of this dispute in relation to human memory is unclear at present, and the matter requires further research.

At the molecular level, memory formation involves synaptic calcium ion and neurotransmitter exchanges that occur in the lollipop-shaped spines found on dendrites in many parts of the brain, including the prefrontal- and frontal-lobe cortices and the hippocampus (trisynaptic circuit). Of the 30 or more neurotransmitters in the central nervous system (Coyle 1985), at least 6—including norepinephrine, dopamine, serotonin, acetylcholine, γ-aminobutyric acid (GABA), and possibly an opiate peptide system—may influence memory function either directly or secondarily through induced hormonal activity. For example, release of norepinephrine in the neural projection that proceeds from the locus ceruleus to the forebrain may increase vigilance and attention at the moment of learning and remembering. Although the locus ceruleus is but one comparatively small structure in the human adult brain, containing fewer than 9,000–15,000 cells, it connects with the amygdala, hippocampus, hypothalamus, and thalamus, all of which are critically involved in some aspect of memory.

Regarding hormonal effects on memory, adults with posttraumatic stress disorder may experience short-term memory deficits as a result of damage to the hippocampus caused by stress-induced increases in circulating glucocorticoids (Bremner et al. 1993). In infants, the hippocampus may be particularly susceptible to stress-induced glucocorticoid damage because the hippocampus is in a vulnerable stage of neurogenesis for the first 9–12 months of postnatal life. Similarly, in one study, a trend toward higher 24-hour urinary free cortisol excretion was found among stressed sexually abused girls compared with control subjects (De Bellis et al. 1993).

Research has yielded an increasingly complex and intricate picture of the loci of memory functions. For long-term memory, the hippocampus appears to be particularly important. Positron emission tomographic scans administered after a word-recall test show increased blood flow in the right posterior medial temporal lobe (perhaps more than in the left posterior medial temporal lobe) in the area occupied by the hippocampus and the parahippocampal gyrus (Squire et al. 1992). Lesions of the hippocampus (in field CA1) lead to anterograde amnesia (e.g., as tested by story or diagram recall) but little, if any, retrograde amnesia (Zola-Morgan et al. 1986). It appears that declarative memory-knowledge of facts and ideas alone is impaired in this kind of amnesia; procedural memory-knowledge of skills remains intact.

Memory for pattern recognition appears to require an intact parietal lobe, temporal lobe, hippocampus, thalamus, and midbrain (Petersen et al. 1985; Posner et al. 1988). Visual word forms are processed in the occipital lobe (Posner et al. 1988). Mental imagery and the arrangement of shapes take place in the left hemisphere more than in the right hemisphere (Kosslyn 1988). Semantic language tasks are processed in the anterior left frontal lobe. Words presented in auditory form are processed in the left temporoparietal cortex (Geschwind 1965). Auditory memory and attention (e.g., digit span memory as tested in the mental status examination) appear to involve the left supramarginal and angular gyri.

Specific memory functions may be confined to specific domains. According to Squire (1987):

> Each specialized system has its own specific, short-term, working-memory capacity and also the capacity to retain in long-term memory specific features or dimensions of information. Each specialized system thereby stores the product of its own processing. Long-term memory of even a single event depends on synaptic change in a distributed ensemble of neurons, which themselves belong to many different processing systems, and the ensemble acting together constitutes memory for the whole event. (p. 241)

■ Information Processing and Memory

Information processing theories have in common the concept of cognition as a data processing system analogous to a computer (Newell et al. 1958). In short, the mental processes are defined in terms of a sequence of problem-solving steps that transform sensory or perceptual input into cognitive or behavioral output.

One model (Miller 1989) proposes that relatively large amounts of information are contained in a small number of units (seven) by items being grouped together into composite units. This process, called "chunking," is regarded as a central strategy for managing (processing) information. Chunks are aggregates of related facts, concepts, or precepts that enlarge with experience. These chunks become hierarchically integrated, one within another, something like Russian dolls (Yates 1991) or perhaps more like the chess master who "chunks" sets and relations among the moves of chess pieces and consequently remembers whole games of chess. In essence, chunking is the process by which representations, procedures, and memories that occur together are automatically accessed simultaneously.

Chunking occurs in what is now called *short-term memory*. For example, a child perceives an auditory sensation, which is instantaneously scanned for pattern recognition (e.g., it may immediately be recognized as speech). Information processing theory suggests that this speech pattern is then transferred into short-term memory, where it may last for about a minute or two and then evaporate, or it may undergo some other process and last longer. Other processes might include a rehearsal strategy such as repetition (e.g., as one repeats a telephone number aloud to enable remembering it). One of three things may then happen to the item:

1. It may be emitted or discharged in a behavioral-affective response (e.g., one makes the telephone call).
2. It may be stored (i.e., remembered) in long-term memory.
3. It may remain temporarily in short-term memory for further processing of the kind mentioned above. Within the context of short-term memory, new information may also interact with relevant information retrieved from long-term memory.

Working memory is the term used when all of the active processes described above (chunking, rehearsal, discharge, and storage) are taking place.

Long-term memory appears to involve two types of knowledge:

1. *Declarative knowledge* (a "knowing that" kind of memory), which is knowledge of facts, concepts, and ideas that are nodal, with links between nodes representing associations between ideas. This kind of knowledge is accessible to consciousness and can be

declared. Amnesia due to brain damage usually results in a loss of this kind of declarative knowledge.

2. *Procedural knowledge* (or "how-to" implicit knowledge), which is knowledge of how to perform certain skills—such as riding a bicycle, reading (Anderson 1983), certain conditioned responses, and perhaps subliminal sound or image retention—all of which soon become automatized. This kind of knowledge is usually unconscious and is usually not lost in the amnesia commonly found in brain damage. However, because procedural memory is mediated by the basal ganglia, lesions of the basal ganglia will consequently disrupt procedural memory and will cause impairment of motor memory and deficits in learning new motor skills, as in Huntington's disease and parkinsonism.

Retrieval of ideas or images from long-term memory presumably involves a *spreading activation* through the declarative network. The firing off of a node presumably influences the direction of the activation. Firing off may occur with repeated conversations, which then may lead to reactivation of memory.

Another model is called *neuroconnectionism* (Johnson-Laird 1988), in which the long-term memory for an experience is distributed over many processing units, perhaps spread widely in different parts of the brain, including the prefrontal cortex (Goldman-Rakic 1987). One additional model (Sternberg 1984) involves interaction among performance components (e.g., encoding) and knowledge acquisition components (e.g., selective encoding, as in distinguishing between relevant and irrelevant information), and a metacomponent that coordinates these two sets of components (e.g., Is more knowledge required? Is the problem recognized?).

In essence, information theory proposes a number of networks that are called forth for various tasks—a model that is in contrast to, for example, the Piagetian developmental structural concept of a hierarchical organization of mental operations (e.g., concrete operations and formal operations). Unfortunately, to date, information theory lacks a truly developmental perspective. Whereas information theory can explain differences between, for example, a novice and an experienced adult, this theory does not yet account for all the steps from infancy through childhood and adolescence to adulthood.

■ Memory and Maturation

Memory seems to develop in spurts. For example, there seems to be a developmental shift and enhancement of memory between ages 8 and 12 months, perhaps in relation to central nervous system maturation (Kagan 1971, 1984). Clinically, this also corresponds to the time when one commonly sees children become anxious when around strangers.

Very soon after birth, an infant recognizes and remembers the mother's voice, smell, taste, and touch; as mentioned earlier, the infant can remember the mother's smell virtually at birth. From an evolutionary perspective, these capacities can be understood in terms of their value for attachment and survival. However, initially, memory is short. A 1-month-old infant can remember a mobile for about 24 hours (Weizmann et al. 1971). By age 5 or 6 months, an infant can remember for several weeks an object seen only for a few minutes (L.J. Cohen and Gelber 1975). Memory subsequently increases in duration as memories accumulate and as memory becomes less context dependent. Evidence of early memory is seen in phenomena such as object permanence, object constancy, stranger reaction, attachment behaviors, and separation anxiety. Memories of the past gradually lead to predictions of the future (e.g., the infant anticipates that the mother is about to leave by observing her preparatory actions).

During the school-age years, children quickly acquire a wider repertoire of metacognitive strategies to improve memory, and today, good teachers help each child identify his or her best metacognitive strategy.

Children's short-term memory for things that they understand may be as good as, if not better than, adults' short-term memory (Johnson and Foley 1984; Loftus and Davies 1984); however, such memories are vulnerable because of children's susceptibility to suggestions. Some researchers (R.L. Cohen and Harnick 1980; Dale et al. 1978; S. Murray, "The Effect of Post-Event Information on Children's Memories for an Illustrated Story," unpublished manuscript, 1983) found in the laboratory that asking leading questions increased the likelihood that subjects of all ages would incorporate the memory of specific information contained in those questions into answers given 2 weeks later (R.L. Cohen and Harnick 1980; S. Murray, unpublished manuscript, 1983). In an attempt to observe children in a more realistic setting, Goodman et al. (1987) studied children receiving inoculations in their doctors' offices. The researchers found the children to be highly accurate in their recall of events, but they also found that 3- and 4-year-olds were more suggestible than 5- and 6-year-olds. The latter showed some suggestibility, but mostly to detail about the room rather than to information about persons or actions. Children seem to notice items that adults might consider irrelevant, but they also make more errors of omission than do adults (Neisser 1984). Sometimes children try to fill gaps in their memories by confabulating, although in some instances the apparent confabulation may be the result—neurobiologically speaking—of faulty or inaccurate recall. And perhaps because children lack previous knowledge, they may have difficulty relating events and organizing disparate elements into a cohesive whole (Johnson and Foley 1984). However, as noted by Kobasigawa (1974), if given external prompts or cues, children can perform quite well on recall, a fact that a clever attorney might use when he or she asks leading questions of a child witness.

Recall in children may be confounded by a number of factors related to cognitive and emotional development. For example, children younger than age 6 years may, in some situations, confuse fact with fantasy. Johnson and Foley (1984) found that young children had some difficulty in discriminating between what they had done and what they had thought of doing. However, the researchers concluded that children at this age were able to differentiate their own thoughts from another person's actions. Young children are also often concrete in their thinking.

Young children may quite correctly describe events in relation to holidays, seasons, birthdays, meals, or television programs (Hudson 1990). Older children have been shown in some studies to be quite accurate with regard to frequency of occurrence or temporal sequence of events (A.L. Brown 1975; Hasher and Zacks 1979). Recent studies have reported that some children as young as 16 months can remember sequentially (i.e., temporally). In general, however, young children, ages 4–6 years, are able to locate events spatially but have difficulty dating events in real time compared with children age 10 years and older, who generally have acquired the concept of time units and sequences and therefore can more easily order events temporally (Goldstone and Goldfarb 1966).

Children may also interpret certain events according to their stage of psychosexual development. Thus, the very young child may perceive a sexual act as an aggressive attack. The degree of awareness of social mores will also affect how the child perceives abuse and how much guilt is later experienced.

■ Childhood Psychiatric Stress Disorders and Memory

Findings concerning memory in infants and children are especially important clinically in posttraumatic stress disorder (Terr 1988) and in children's accounts of alleged sexual abuse (Schetky and Green 1988). However, it has been suggested that even vivid and seemingly accurate recall of sexual abuse, including incest, may have little or no relation to any external event and that such memories may instead be almost entirely the product of fantasy. This was the so-called second position Freud took after his disavowal of his earlier "seduction theory," notwithstanding 1) the abundant evidence of the then-prevailing high rate of sexual assault of children; 2) the phenomenon of delayed recall; and 3) the knowledge that many adults find it painful to face the reality that so many children are brutally abused, leading them to label the recall as fantasy. Clinically, of course, any simple all-or-none dichotomy is plainly wrong and can lead to disastrous treatment. The significance, meaning, and interpretation of memory in the context of treatment are far more complicated than simply determining what is "real" versus what is "fantasy" (which in any event is itself usually far from simple).

It is very likely that what we call a memory is not just the simple recall of a thing or an event but the representation of multiple processes—including perceptions, fantasy formation, and affects—that are aroused by, or that come to be associated with, an "event" (or even a nonevent). From the point of view of psychopathology and treatment, still other processes are involved, including defenses that are subsequently mobilized against the anxiety that arises when a memory and its associated affects emerge during treatment.

■ Infantile Amnesia and Memory

To adopt a comprehensive approach toward understanding memory, several different perspectives—psychoanalytic, neurobiological, information processing, cognitive development, developmental shift, and evolutionary—need to be taken into consideration.

Psychoanalytic Theory

Notwithstanding the strong evidence of robust memory during infancy, few people remember much, if anything, from their first few years of life. To account for this apparent phenomenon, psychoanalysts proposed the concept of infantile amnesia due to repression of the beginnings of sexual life, with the expectation that repressed memories from that period will be recovered in some form during analysis. Freud (1899/1962, 1905/1953, 1917/1963, 1933/1964) somewhat poetically referred to this phenomenon as "the veil of amnesia," which he variously placed as covering what he called "youth," meaning a period lasting from birth to age 5, 6, 8, or even 10 years.

Neurobiological Research

Neurobiological findings, on the other hand, suggest that forgetting in the context of so-called infantile amnesia may in some instances, of a weakening of neural connections through lack of reinforcement (a kind of disuse atrophy). Alternatively, the forgetting may be a result of some actual loss of the neural connections that contained parts of the initial memory, perhaps through a process similar to the loss that occurs during development through synapse elimination, axonal competition, and cell death (Squire 1987). New learning may also alter prior memory, perhaps in conjunction with or as a result of morphological and synaptic neurotransmitter changes. Reinforcement of the axonal network might lead to reactivation and could thus contribute to, or even be a component of, the apparent "lifting of repression" and the subsequent "recovery" of at least portions of the absent memory in infantile amnesia.

Information Processing Contributions

Information theory meanwhile suggests that so-called infantile amnesia may be in part a reflection of developmental factors. Thus, the memory system that enables long-lasting declarative memory (as opposed to nonconscious, procedural memory) is not yet established in the infant—at least not during the first year of life (Nadel and Zola-Morgan 1984; Schacter and Moscovitch 1984). Ontogenetically, declarative memory develops later than procedural memory and perhaps after the very period when there is so-called infantile amnesia.

Developmental Shift Hypothesis

Memory is not simply one neurological system. Moreover, developmental shifts in memory often occur during childhood. More particularly, different memory processes may operate at different stages of development. These multilevel processes are known to occur in other developmental-behavioral phenomena such as attachment behaviors. For example, expanding on Hofer's (1987) view of two components of attachment—one that does not develop and one that does develop—Pipp and Harmon (1987) commented that some other mental structures such as primary process and sensorimotor thought are maintained as they are throughout development, whereas others such as secondary process and operational thought change with development. In the same way, it is possible that the earliest memory processes are physiological (so-called tissue memories) and are maintained virtually unchanged throughout development. They would be manifested by preverbal, affective, sensory, and motoric memory patterns, whereas later memory functions would change extensively with development, allowing memory to be expressed through more complex processes, including language.

Infantile amnesia may also be a reflection of a developmental shift from one memory system to another—from an early memory system encoded mostly in action and affect to a memory system encoded mostly in words and verbal categories. The earlier system may remain active and influence perception but might not be available in the form of language.

Lastly, what is said about a so-called event may become incorporated into the memory for that event.

Evolution and Memory

From an evolutionary point of view, MacLean's (1990) conceptualization of the triune brain in his study of the human brain may also contribute to the understanding of memory. In the triune brain model, the three basic evolutionary formations or layers—reptilian, paleomammalian, and neomammalian—retain some ancestral relationship to the brain functions found in reptiles, early mammals, and recent mammals, respectively. Most important, each of the three neural formations has unique structure and chemistry, and each has its own kind of memory (MacLean 1990).

Accordingly, an early form of procedural memory may be the oldest form of memory with roots in the preserved components of the paleomammalian (limbic system) middle layer of the triune brain that overlays part of the basal nuclei found in the evolutionarily oldest reptilian layer.

The paleomammalian middle level is presumably also the level from which functions such as nursing, mothering, and early play patterns emerge (including perhaps sensorimotor activity). This middle level is layered or covered by the third, most recent layer, the neomammalian complex (consisting of the neocortex and thalamic nuclei). This third layer has in part given rise to the more complex functions of memory, association, and language.

Moral Development

Moral behavior derives in part from the basic cultural rules governing social action that the child assimilates and internalizes, and moral development is the increase in the degree to which the internalization and accommodation of these basic cultural rules have occurred.

Fear of punishment is prominent in young children. The next attribute to develop is an urge to confess. By age 12 or 13 years, most children seem to react directly with guilt and internal self-criticism when faced with the fact of their transgression, although this reaction often occurs at a much younger age.

Piaget's (1965) view on the moral development of the child can be conceptualized in the context of the major stages of cognitive development, as outlined below:

- *Preoperational stage:* The morality is one of constraints—rules of behavior are viewed as natural laws handed down by the child's parents. Violation brings retribution or unquestioned punishment, and no account is taken of motives.
- *Concrete operational stage:* The morality is one of acceptance—rules of behavior become a matter of mutual acceptance, with complete equality of treatment, but no account is taken of special circumstances.
- *Formal operational stage:* The morality is one of cooperation—rules can be constructed as required by the needs of the group as long as they can be agreed on. Motives are now taken into account, and circumstances may temper the administration of justice.

As the child advances through these stages, progressive decentering occurs. Building on Piaget's views, Kohlberg (1964) suggested three major levels of development of moral judgment: premorality, morality of conventional role-conformity, and morality of self-accepted moral principles (Table 2–1).

Table 2–1. Kohlberg's three major levels of development of moral judgment

Level I: Premorality (or preconventional morality)
Type 1. Punishment and obedience orientation (i.e., obedience to parents' superior force)
Type 2. Naïve instrumental hedonism (i.e., agreement to obey only in return for some reward)

Level II: Morality of conventional role-conformity
Type 3. Good-boy morality of maintaining good relations, approval of others (i.e., conformity to rules in order to please and gain approval)
Type 4. Authority-maintaining morality (i.e., adherence to rules for the sake of upholding social order)

Level III: Morality of self-accepted moral principles
Type 5. Morality of social contract, of individual rights, and of, for example, democratically accepted law (with a reliance on a legalistic "social contract")
Type 6. Morality of individual principles of conscience (there is voluntary compliance based on ethical principles; this level is probably not reached until early adolescence, and it may not be reached at all)

Interestingly, Jurkovic (1980) noted that delinquent children differ in their level of moral development just as they do in their personality and behavioral style: "Not only do they vary from one another in stages of moral development, but they also fluctuate in their own reasoning level on different moral problems" (p. 724).

Numerous criticisms of Kohlberg's (1964) work have been made. Some of the stages, especially the later stages, have not been reliably substantiated, and many believe that descriptions of some stages are too politicized in favor of a liberal viewpoint. Others think that the stages described are, in any event, bound by culture, the historic moment, middle-class status, and male gender of the subjects. As a result of these criticisms, Kohlberg attempted some revisions. For example, Kohlberg (1978) and Colby (1978) subsequently identified two types of reasoning at each stage: type A emphasizes literal interpretation of the rules and roles of society, whereas type B is a more consolidated form and refers to the intent of normative standards. However, in general, Kohlberg (1978) essentially held to the same hierarchical sequence and idealized end point.

More recently, Gilligan (1982) offered a different view of moral development in which an expanding connection with and concern for others was thought to represent an alternative developmental pathway and goal. This alternative and equally valid pathway has been demonstrated more often in girls than in boys; that is, in general, girls seem to have "a greater sense of connection and concern with relationships more than with rules" (p. 202).

Attachment Behavior

Attachment is an affectional tie that one person forms with another person, binding them together in space and enduring over time. Attachment is discriminating and specific. One may be attached to more than one person, but there is usually a gradient in the strength of such multiple attachments (Schaffer and Emerson 1964). Attachment implies affect, predominantly affection or love.

Bonding implies a selective attachment (L.J. Cohen 1974) that is maintained even when there is no contact with the person with whom the bond exists.

Attachment behavior is behavior that promotes proximity to or contact with the specific figure or figures to whom the person is attached. Attachment behavior includes signals (crying, smiling, vocalizing), locomotion (looking, following, and approaching), and contacts (clambering up, embracing, and clinging). Sucking, clinging, following, crying, and smiling are used by the time a child is age 8 or 9 months. Attachment behavior is strongest in toddlers; bonding is most secure in older children (Rutter 1976b).

Bowlby (1969) proposed that the biological function of attachment behavior is to protect the infant from danger, especially the danger of attack by predators. The system may be activated by hormonal state, by environmental stimulus, and by central nervous system excitation. The system is terminated in response to a specific terminating signal (e.g., attachment achieved) or by habituation. The attachment behavior system is in equilibrium with other important behavior systems (e.g., exploratory behavior, which is elicited by stimuli that have novelty and complexity or change and may draw the infant away from the mother).

At least 15 kinds of attachment behavior have been described (Ainsworth 1963), including differential crying, smiling, and vocalization; greeting responses, such as lifting of arms and hand clapping; crying when the mother leaves; scrambling over the mother; following the mother; clinging and kissing; and exploration away from the mother when the mother is a secure base, with rapid return to the mother as a haven of safety.

These attachment behaviors may vary in intensity, and in certain pathological states, such as infantile autism, they may all be absent.

■ Summary of Phases in the Development of Attachment

First Phase (Undiscriminating Social Responsiveness, 0–3 Months)

From the beginning, the infant has some capacity to respond differentially to different stimuli and thus to discriminate them:

- *Primitive behaviors:* Sucking, grasping
- *Orienting behaviors:* Visual fixation, visual tracking, listening
- *Signaling behaviors:* Smiling, crying, vocalizing, rooting, postural adjustment

Second Phase (Discriminating Social Responsiveness, 3–7 Months)

The infant discriminates between familiar figures (mother and one or two others) and those who are relatively unfamiliar.

In the first subphase, discrimination between and differential responses to figures close at hand occur (e.g., differential smiling, vocalization, and crying). In the second subphase, discrimination between figures at a distance appears (e.g., as evidenced by differential greeting and crying when a particular figure leaves the room).

Third Phase (Active Initiative in Seeking Proximity and Contact, 7 Months–3 Years)

When the infant is about age 7 months, a striking increase occurs in the infant's initiative in promoting proximity and contact. Voluntary movements of the infant's hands and arms are now conspicuous in attachment behavior. Following, approaching, clinging, and similar behaviors become more prominent. The infant is now attached.

The range of stimuli to which the infant is most responsive includes the range commonly emanating from human adults, including visual stimuli, auditory stimuli, and stimuli associated with feeding. Yet the infant does not initially discriminate among the persons presenting these stimuli.

When the infant does begin to discriminate among persons, this is done more readily through some modalities than others (e.g., tactile-kinesthetic discrimination first, then auditory discrimination, and then visual discrimination at approximately 8 weeks).

In psychoanalytic theory, the infant at this stage is said to have an *anaclitic* (leaning on) type of object relation. In cognitive-developmental theory, the infant at this stage is said to be at the fourth subphase of sensorimotor development and to have acquired object permanence.

It is interesting that Spitz (1965) talked of three "organizers" as a concept to account for the factors that govern the process of transition from one level of development to the next:

1. The first organizer is the smiling response, which is the visible manifestation of a certain degree of organization in the psychic apparatus.
2. The second organizer is the 8-month anxiety, which marks a new stage in development.
3. The third organizer is the achievement of the sign of negation and of the word *no*. In Spitz's view, it is the first abstraction, or symbol, formed by the child, usually at the beginning of the second year (around 15 months), when the infant turns his or her head away to refuse food (a response that has its origins in the rooting reflex).

Fourth Phase (Goal-Directed Partnership, 3 Years)

The infant in the fourth phase infers something about the mother's *set goals* and attempts to alter those goals to fit better with his or her own goals in regard to contact, proximity, and interaction, provided the mother does not dissemble her set goals (e.g., to leave the infant at nursery school).

■ Necessary Conditions for the Development of Attachment

The following conditions are prerequisites for the development of attachment: 1) sufficient interaction

with the mother, 2) the ability of the infant to discriminate his or her mother or other attachment figure from other persons, and 3) the ability of the infant to have at least begun to conceive of a person as having a permanent and independent existence even when that person is not present to the infant's perception.

An infant's goal-corrected behavior probably becomes increasingly smooth and effective in parallel with the later stages of development of the concept of object, which, according to Piaget, is completed around age 18 months. Piaget (1958) suggested that the concept of persons as permanent objects evolves in homologous stages but in advance of the development of the concept of things as permanent objects, presumably because an infant finds people the most interesting of objects.

■ Factors That Influence the Development of Attachment

Four factors influence the development of attachment. The first factor concerns sensitive phases in the development of infant-mother attachment. The sensitive phase during which attachments are most readily formed spans a period of months in the middle of the first year. It probably starts in the neonatal period. Provence and Lipton (1962) showed that infants kept in an institution until they are ages 8–24 months find it difficult to become attached to a foster mother later and that 24 months seems to be the upper limit of the sensitive phase for becoming attached for the first time. The second factor concerns infant-care practices such as feeding practices. The third factor concerns maternal care, infant behavior, and mother-infant interaction. The mother's contribution to attachment is affected by factors such as her hormonal state, her parity and experience, and her personality. The infant's contribution is affected by factors such as wakefulness and activity level, crying, temperament, genetic makeup, and organic makeup. The final factor influencing the development of attachment concerns maternal deprivation.

Strong attachments occur under the following five conditions:

1. When the interaction has a certain degree of intensity, as when a sensitive, responsive parent gives a great deal of attention to the child, talks with the child, and, especially, plays with the child (Stayton and Ainsworth 1973).

2. When the parent responds regularly and readily to the child's needs as signaled, for example, by crying. The child is likely to become strongly attached to a parent who can recognize and respond to the child's signals.
3. When the number of caregivers is limited. The fewer the caregivers, the greater the attachment.
4. When the child's own contribution is strong; that is, when the child's needs and signals are strong.
5. When the child is in the early sensitive phase (of imprinting), during his or her first 2 years.

Finally, several clinical types of attachment have been described, including *secure, insecure-avoidant, insecure-resistant,* and *insecure-disorganized/disoriented* (Main and Solomon 1986).

Clinically, attachment theory is useful as a basis for providing appropriate care of premature infants and very young children in the hospital, deciding on adoption practices and child placement, and understanding certain aspects of child abuse and delinquency.

Although a full discussion is beyond the scope of this chapter, it is important to note an increasingly large body of molecular neurobiological research involving the roles of oxytocin and vasopressin in relation to social memory and social attachment. The genes involved appear to have been robustly conserved throughout evolution—from fish, reptiles, birds, and mammals—in complex neural pathways that extend from olfactory bulbs through to the amygdala and cortex (Insel 1997; Leckman and Herman 2002).

Psychosexual Development

By age 2 years, children know their own sex (i.e., boy or girl) and recognize clearly whether others are boys or girls. By age 5 years, the child knows that one's sex is (more or less) permanent. Sex role behaviors are shaped and influenced through stereotyping by others, beginning at birth. Self-stereotyping and further socialization increase with peer relationships and are manifested in play and toy preferences. However, same-sex play in children is not necessarily predictive of adult sexual identity. Green (1987) reported that boys who play more like girls excessively, who cross-dress, and who prefer or wish to be a girl *may* be more likely to become homosexual but are not definitely so.

Some boys also may have a genetic predisposition to homosexuality (Bailey and Pillard 1991).

■ Psychoanalytic Views

In psychoanalytic theory, the sexual aim of a young infant is said to be to obtain pleasure and relief from discomfort by the most immediate means possible. The infant draws pleasure from a wide variety of visual, tactile, kinesthetic, and auditory stimuli.

Oral Phase

By far the most sensitive region in the infant—and apparently the greatest source of pleasure—is the mouth. The object of the sexual instinct is thought to be the body of the infant, seen in *autoerotic* (self-stimulating) activities such as mouthing and sucking. Questions have been raised about some of the psychoanalytic viewpoints subsumed under the heading of "orality" (Sandler and Dare 1970). Moreover, Freud noted that "the phylogenetic foundation has so much the upper hand over personal accidental experience that it makes no difference whether a child has really sucked at the breast or has been brought up on the bottle and never enjoyed the tenderness of a mother's care. In both cases the child's development takes the same path" (Freud 1940/1969, pp. 188–189).

It is important to note that certain genetic factors and biological orienting patterns are in operation before any psychological mechanisms. For example, the suck reflex is coordinated to the cyclical flow of breast milk (Dubignon and Campbell 1969), and by age 6 days the infant can selectively orient to smell, preferring mother's milk (Macfarlane 1975).

Anal Phase

As the infant develops and as speech and the capacity for symbol formation emerge, the child begins to experience feelings about separateness and worth. A sense of autonomy develops that has to be reconciled with ambivalent feelings, all at about the same time that new skills are acquired, only one of which is sphincter control. During this process, according to psychoanalytic theory, the anal mucosa is said to become "erotogenized" and may serve in part the aims of the ambivalent feelings just mentioned. Indeed, the young child may express his or her ambivalence in the (pleasurable) holding in and letting go of feces during bowel movements. However, this ambivalence may also be expressed in the controlling and clinging behaviors seen in some 2- and 3-year-old children. This suggests that the alleged central role of the anal mucosa at this stage has probably been exaggerated, reflecting perhaps the practices that prevailed at the time Freud made his observations.

Phallic-Oedipal Phase

When the child is between ages 3 and 6 years, behavior that is more clearly recognizable as sexual appears. The child at this stage is very much aware of the anatomical differences between the sexes and is curious about pregnancy, childbirth, and death. Sometimes this interest is represented in the play of the child. For example, play with toys that involves filling and emptying, opening and shutting, fitting in and throwing away, and building up and knocking down blocks has been interpreted as representing a curiosity about the body and sexual functions.

Opportunities for the sequential development of play in childhood thus become as important for the sexual development of the child as they are for other purposes (e.g., problem solving, mastery of body skills, functional pleasure in play, coping with anxiety, facilitating relationships, and communication purposes). The child at this stage is said to experience intense sexual and aggressive urges toward both parents, but the aim is less well defined. Boys and girls may become absorbed by fairy-tale or television characters that serve to represent the children's own fantasies. Such fantasies also emerge in the dreams of children. Children at this age may also play at being mothers and fathers or doctors and nurses—working toward a partial fulfillment of their sexual aims, which at this time may be partially fused with their aggressive fantasies. Boys and girls may inflict pain on each other in keeping with their understanding of the sexual act as an act of violence. They also may be quite exhibitionistic and possessive, especially of the parent of the opposite sex. Hostility toward the same-sex parent seems to be influenced by certain characteristic family patterns of relationships present in a particular society (Honigmann 1954).

Latency Phase

Between ages 6 and 12 years, during the elementary-school years, concepts of inevitability regarding birth, death, and sex differences become clarified, and the sense of time and the ability to differentiate between fantasy and reality become established. Defense mechanisms, which in general bar from consciousness certain unacceptable impulses and fantasies and at the same time provide some substitute gratification, are strengthened. The child consolidates earlier reactions, such as shame against exhibitionistic urges, disgust against messiness, and a sense of guilt that serves to contain sexual and aggressive wishes. The child's play at this time is usually characterized by organization, whether in a board game or a team game. Sex play, far from being dormant, continues actively, especially with voyeuristic tendencies and the urge to touch. The sex play often may be more discreet at this age (i.e., adults may see it less often); however, it also may be quite overt, with much interest and curiosity (Reese 1966). The object of the sexual instinct may be a peer, but the actual playmate may be of either sex.

■ Puberty and Adolescence

Pubertal Maturation

Pubertal maturation sequences are shown in Figure 2–3 and Table 2–2.

Early-maturing females and late-maturing males are more likely to receive negative peer and adult evaluations than on-time females and early-maturing males (Tobin-Richards et al. 1983). Physically attractive adolescents are stereotyped more extensively than unattractive adolescents (Langlois and Stephen 1981), and unattractive adolescents seem to have more adjustment and behavioral problems than their attractive counterparts (Lerner and Lerner 1977). Adolescents are likely to be agents in their own development.

Cultural Perspectives on Adolescence

Adolescence as a phase of development existed in some form long before it was recognized and conceptualized in the United States by G. Stanley Hall in 1904. For example, at the time of the Sumerian culture of 4000 to 3000 B.C., the first case of juvenile delinquency was recorded on clay tablets (Kramer 1959). The *Oxford English Dictionary* traces the word itself to the fifteenth century. In *Emile* (1762), Rousseau noted, "We are born, so to speak, twice over; born into existence, and born into life; born a human being and born a man."

In all cultures and in all times the period has been marked by rites of passage. In simple cultures where

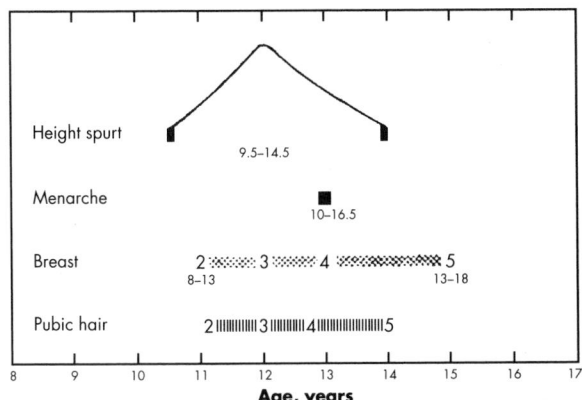

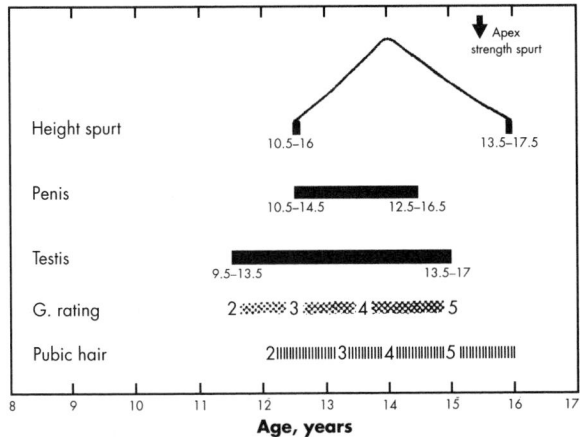

Figure 2–3. Diagram of sequence of events at adolescence in girls (top) and boys (bottom).

The average boy and girl are represented. The range of ages within which each charted event may begin and end is given by the figures placed directly below its start and finish. G. rating=genital rating.

Source. Reprinted from Marshall WA, Tanner JM: "Variations in the Pattern of Pubertal Changes in Boys." *Archives of Disease in Childhood* 45:13–23, 1970 (originally redrawn from Tanner JM: *Growth at Adolescence*, 2nd Edition. Oxford, Blackwell, 1962). Copyright 1970, British Medical Association. Used with permission.

young men and women are needed to do adult work, the period of initiation is short. The initiation rites vary from culture to culture, but they often involve periods of fasting or other ordeals.

During puberty, the young adolescent struggles to achieve body mastery, to control sexual and aggressive urges, to separate from the family, to find new and appealing sexual relationships, and to achieve a sense of identity. In the course of this struggle, the sexual behavior of the adolescent may range from an indiscrim-

inate regression (toward expressions of earlier forms of the sexual drive, manifested in impulsive behavior, messiness, and alternating labile affects) to petting and mutual masturbation (which may be heterosexual or homosexual) and, eventually, intercourse. Sometimes, earlier aims and objects are temporarily gratified and used (e.g., in isolated acts of fellatio or in exhibitionistic behavior).

Ultimately, a mature primacy of the genital zone is established, with an appropriate object choice and an appropriate achievement of new sexual aims such as a love relationship, sexual intercourse, orgasm, discharge, and childbirth.

Rutter (1971, 1976a) reviewed the scientific literature on normal psychosexual development. He concluded that Freud's description of the oral and anal stages is too narrow and somewhat misleading, that the oedipal situation is not universal, that Freud's description of the latency period is wrong in most respects, and that Freud's concept of an innate sex drive that has a quantifiable energy component is only a half-truth. Rutter noted that current evidence is insufficient to decide among the various psychological theories of sexual development.

Although it is true that the level of scientific reliability and validity in psychoanalytic research is generally low, clinical experience still has a very compelling, supportive quality. In any event, Freud himself was very acutely aware that in the future, findings from "organic biology and chemistry" might well supplant the psychoanalytic hypotheses of his time (Freud 1920/1955, p. 60). Examples of Freud's prescient thinking in this regard are shown by the following quotations:

Even when investigation shows that the primary exciting cause of a phenomenon is psychical, deeper research will one day trace the path further and discover an organic basis for the mental event. (Freud 1900/1953, pp. 41–42)

All our provisional ideas in psychology will... someday be based on an organic substructure. This makes it probable that it is special substances and chemical processes which perform the operations of sexuality. (Freud 1914/1957, p. 78)

Biology is truly a land of unlimited possibilities. We may expect it to give us the most surprising information and we cannot guess what answers it will return....They may be of a kind which will blow away the whole of our artificial structure of hypotheses. (Freud 1920/1955, pp. 3–64)

Table 2–2. Genital maturity stages in boys and sexual maturity stages in girls

Classification of genitalia maturity stages in boys

Stage	Pubic hair	Penis	Testes
1	None	Preadolescent	
2	Slight, long, slightly pigmented	Slight enlargement	Enlarged scrotum, pink, texture altered
3	Darker, starts to curl, small amount	Penis longer	Larger
4	Resembles adult type, but less in quantity, coarse, curly	Larger, glans and breadth increase in size	Larger, scrotum dark
5	Adult distribution spread to medial surface of thighs	Adult	Adult

Classification of sexual maturity stages in girls

Stage	Pubic hair	Breasts
1	Preadolescent	Preadolescent
2	Sparse, lightly pigmented, straight, medial border of labia	Breast and papilla elevated as small mound; areolar diameter increased
3	Darker, beginning to curl, increased amount	Breast and areola enlarged, no contour separation
4	Coarse, curly, abundant but amount less than in adult	Areola and papilla form secondary mound
5	Adult feminine triangle, spread to medial surface of thighs	Mature; nipple projects, areola part of general breast contour

Source. Reprinted from Daniel WA Jr.: *Adolescents in Health and Disease.* St. Louis, MO, Mosby, 1977; originally adapted from Tanner JM: *Growth at Adolescence,* 2nd Edition. Oxford, England, Blackwell Scientific Publications, 1962. Used with permission.

In view of the intimate connection between the things that we distinguish as physical and mental, we may look forward to a day when paths of knowledge and, let us hope, of influence will be opened up, leading from organic biology and chemistry to the field of neurotic phenomena. (Freud 1926/1959, p. 231)

The future may teach us to exercise a direct influence, by means of particular chemical substances, on the amounts of energy and their distribution in the mental apparatus. It may be that there are other still undreamt-of possibilities of therapy. (Freud 1940, p. 182)

The phylogenetic foundation has so much the upper hand over personal accidental experience that it makes no difference whether a child has really sucked at the breast or has been brought up on the bottle and never enjoyed the tenderness of a mother's care. In both cases the child's development takes the same path. (Freud 1940, pp. 188–189)

Relationships

In psychoanalytic theory, relationships are said to start with the virtual biological unity of the mother-infant couple. This period has been subdivided by some psychoanalysts (Mahler 1967) into so-called autistic, symbiotic, and separation-individuation phases.

A prototypical early stage is said to be a part-object or need-fulfilling, anaclitic type of relationship based on the child's needs. This type of relationship generally ends when object constancy is achieved. Ambivalent relationships then develop, characterized by clinging behavior and attempts to dominate the love object.

A phallic-oedipal phase is said to follow, characterized by possessiveness of the parent of the opposite sex and jealousy of and rivalry with the parent of the same sex. In the postoedipal period, a lessening of drive urgency is said to occur, and the apparent object of the transference changes from parents to other adults (e.g., teachers). Sublimation is seen, and a disillusionment with the parents can be observed.

In preadolescence, a temporary, partial return to earlier attitudes and behaviors occurs, especially toward earlier part-object, need-fulfilling, and ambivalent relationships.

Finally, in adolescence a true interest is invested in persons outside the family.

Temperament

In the course of their clinical observations and research for their New York Longitudinal Study, Thomas and Chess (1977) became fascinated with what they perceived as the individual styles that characterized each child—or rather, the peculiar shaping and reshaping of these styles as the child and his or her family develop. This phenomenon came to be known as the *temperament* of the child.

Chess and Thomas (1986) identified nine categories of behavior that constitute the individual's temperament: 1) activity level, 2) rhythmicity (hunger, elimination, sleep–wake), 3) approach or withdrawal response, 4) adaptability to a change in the environment, 5) threshold of responsiveness, 6) intensity of any given reaction, 7) mood (quality, quantity), 8) degree of distractibility, and 9) persistence in the face of obstacles.

About 1 child in 10 was found to have a so-called difficult temperament, and about 1 in 6 was in a slow-to-warm-up group. About two-fifths of the children studied were found to have a so-called easy temperament.

The New York Longitudinal Study showed, among other things, that the consistency of the interactional process between temperament and environment constituted a kind of continuity. This continuity also allowed some plasticity in development. Although this plasticity in turn might make some kinds of predictions uncertain, it also suggested that early parental errors and even specific emotional trauma to the child do not necessarily have fixed, inevitable consequences and that therapeutic intervention could help at any stage of development. It also suggested that subsequent improved and positive experiences following a therapeutic intervention might in themselves have a further therapeutic effect.

These ideas challenged some previously held views on the causes of various developmental and clinical phenomena. In particular, Thomas et al. (1968) added the important idea that the child, far from being a passive recipient or simply a responder to various stimuli, is an active initiator and contributor to his or her own experience and development. They also found that this activity on the part of the child was determined to an extent by the child's temperament and that the child's particular developmental characteristics contributed in important ways to some of the behavior disorders seen in children.

Also new was the notion of variations in style originating in the genotype of an individual and brought out and modified by the individual child's active interaction with the environment. In other words, just as there are breeds in some other species, one could see various strains of genotypical styles among human beings (such as fearful, shy, timid, bold, outgoing, and aggressive), with each strain modified and capable of being shaped by experience, teaching, and learning.

A practical and central concept Thomas and Chess (1977) devised to study and understand the child's struggle for mastery was the "goodness of fit" in the complex interactions over time between the child's temperament and the environment.

In this clinical perspective, temperament is not seen as a theory of development; rather, it is regarded as but one attribute of an individual—albeit an important one. Clinically, these concepts and findings of temperament studies are useful in understanding and relieving certain parent–child problems.

For an account of other research contributions on the topic of temperament, see Kagan 2002.

Developmental Tasks

Finally, development can be thought about in terms of its meaning for the individual from infancy through adolescence (Figure 2–4).

The developmental task of the very young infant is to achieve adaptation to the outside world. Sometime between ages 1½ and 3 years it becomes clear that a child is tackling several other developmental tasks. First, a fundamental task is to achieve greater physical independence. The maturation of the child's neuromuscular system is central to feelings of self-worth. The child also makes a shift from a passive to an active position. Furthermore, the child now can think instead of act by using language with symbols and concepts. Whereas the young child at first uses few words, mostly in the service of direct discharge of feelings (primary process), the child later uses language more independently of immediate need. Along with this development, definite attitudes toward people are formed, especially toward those who set limits. It is toward such persons that the child may behave in a "negativistic" manner. For example, the child may say, "I don't want to" and "No!" when a parent makes a request or sets a limit. It is as though the child is defining autonomy through oppositional behavior. However, in some instances, the behavior may be a manifestation of anxiety as the child struggles against a regressive

	1.	2.	3.	4.	5.	6.	7.	8.
I. INFANCY	Trust vs. mistrust							
II. EARLY CHILDHOOD		Autonomy vs. shame, doubt			Unipolarity vs. premature self-differentiation			
III. PLAY AGE			Initiative vs. guilt		Bipolarity vs. autism			
IV. SCHOOL AGE				Industry vs. inferiority	Play identification vs. (oedipal) fantasy identities			
V. ADOLESCENCE	Time perspective vs. time diffusion	Self-certainty vs. identity consciousness	Role experimentation vs. negative identity	Anticipation of achievement vs. work paralysis	Work identification vs. identity foreclosure — Identity vs. identity diffusion	Sexual Identity vs. bisexual diffusion	Leadership polarization vs. authority diffusion	Ideological polarization vs. diffusion of ideals
VI. YOUNG ADULT					Solidarity vs. social isolation	Intimacy vs. isolation		
VII. ADULTHOOD							Generativity vs. self-absorption	
VIII. MATURE AGE								Integrity vs. disgust, despair

Figure 2–4. Erikson's life-cycle chart.

Source. Reprinted from Erikson E: *Identity and the Life Cycle.* New York, W.W. Norton, 1979. Copyright 1980 by W.W. Norton & Company, Inc. Copyright 1959 by International Universities Press, Inc. Used by permission of W.W. Norton & Company, Inc.

pull. In other instances, the behavior may be a direct discharge of aggression against the parent, especially if the parent–child relationship is an ambivalent one.

Perhaps the crux of the school-age period of development is the child's move toward greater separation, independence, and autonomy at a time when he or she is still capable of being demanding, intrusive, and negativistic. The extent to which the child successfully emerges from this stage depends on many factors, including the degree to which the parents facilitate or hinder the child's progress.

When adolescence arrives, at least four major groups of developmental tasks can be defined: 1) defining oneself (identity), 2) achieving separation and coming to terms with specific feelings about one's family, 3) developing love relationships, and 4) achieving mastery over one's impulses, body functions, and capacities.

Developing Concepts of Body, Illness, and Death

■ Concept of Body

Judging from the infant's facial expressions and vocal sounds, in the beginning, the infant seems to be aware of and react to pleasurable body states and feelings and states of discomfort arising from hunger, thirst, wetness, pain, temperature extremes, fatigue, and illness. The infant soon learns that his or her body has a separate existence but does not initially appear to recognize any well-defined boundary.

The infant clearly sees and touches his or her body, at first randomly and then intentionally. For example, as early as age 3 weeks, the infant can reliably put his or her thumb in the mouth and appears to develop a schema of thumb. Such schemata increase in complexity, especially during the sensorimotor stage of cognitive development. The infant also experiences a wide range of sensory stimuli, including those accompanying being fed, burped, bathed, diapered, cuddled, tickled, whirled in the air, spoken and sung to, and confronted almost nose to nose by strange, seemingly contorted faces.

By age 3–6 months, the infant can smile appreciatively when shown a moving mask consisting of forehead, eyes, and nose, indicating the infant's capacity for pattern recognition—in this case, the elements of a face. The infant also begins to discriminate between sensations that come from within and those that come from the outside (what is me and what is not me). Gradually, the infant perceives, constructs, and recognizes the mothering person's face, and the mothering person's face becomes associated with all the actions of the mother that satisfy the infant. Meanwhile, the infant is further exploring and differentiating among the parts of his or her own body. The infant takes pleasure in peek-a-boo games, which help the child begin to acquire object permanence—the sense of what is here, what is hidden but continues to exist, and what is absent. The infant begins to change from watching his or her image in a mirror as though it were some other child to recognizing his or her own image. The infant remembers this image and, usually by 8 or 9 months, has at least a rudimentary sense of self. All these developments—leading up to a firm sense of self and body and to the child's attachment to the important figures in his or her life—flourish in the context of reliable, predictable, loving, responsive, and stimulating parenting and the advent of language.

By the time a child is age 2 or 3 years, the child's image of his or her body is more defined. The typical 3-year-old can name body parts such as eyes, nose, and mouth, and a 4-year-old usually can draw a simple representation of the body—usually a single circle with dots for eyes and nose, a curved line for the mouth, hair (by which the child usually identifies the sex), lines representing limbs that spring from the circle, and an indeterminate number of digits at the end of each limb. The child also often seems to have the idea that the body is a kind of sac filled with fluid that sometimes oozes out. If the child grazes his or her knee and some blood oozes out, the 3-year-old may become upset at the loss of fluid. The child at this age is often readily reassured by the application of a bandage strip, which seems to seal the leak and hides the wound from view.

Later, the child will acquire some concept of internal organs, usually from the conversations of older persons. However, the internal organs are usually stereotyped (e.g., hearts that look like the representations on valentine cards). At this stage, the child's drawings depict bodies with floating organs, and the child has no clear idea of their function or physiology. By age 5 or 6 years, the child represents the body more accurately in his or her drawings, with distinct head and torso; more body parts, such as eyebrows and ears; and more detail, such as clothing.

Sometimes the child's inner mental image of his or her body is represented in play, especially play that involves toys that can be filled and emptied, open and shut, fitted together and pulled apart, messed and cleaned, and hoarded or discarded. As the child's cognitive development, learning, and experience increase, the child's knowledge of his or her body gradually becomes increasingly accurate, although gaps in knowledge and misconceptions may persist through adolescence and even adulthood.

■ Concepts of Illness

Although neonates have no concept of illness, they feel and react to painful attacks on the body (e.g., circumcision of a newborn requires that the infant be anesthetized). Perhaps the earliest idea of illness in the child at age 2 or 3 years is as a form of punishment (*immanent justice*) that has been visited on the child for misdeeds, committed or imagined, which also may be a source of guilt. Next the child develops a primitive concept of contagion: illness is caused by a bug or germ, which you might catch. As the child imagines it, the germ is caught by touching something dirty or by eating something that is bad for you. How the germ brings about the symptoms of the illness remains a mystery to the child, who may nonetheless invent a theory. By age 5 or 6 years, the child can and will ask questions and should receive simple, straightforward, truthful answers.

■ Psychological Reactions to Acute Illness

Every child has a psychological reaction to his or her own illness and to illness in siblings and parents. The intensity of the reaction may vary with the child's developmental level and premorbid psychological state, the seriousness of the illness, and the reactions of the family. Factors that increase the child's likelihood of having an intense psychological reaction to illness can be divided into those that are specific to the child and those that are specific to the family and the child's relationship with his or her parents.

Factors specific to the child include 1) age, especially when it is less than 4 years; 2) premorbid psychopathology; 3) severe illness; 4) chronic illness and multiple hospitalizations; 5) difficult, painful treatment; and 6) poor preparation for hospitalization or treatment.

Factors specific to the child's relationship with his or her parent or parents include 1) relationships char-

acterized by parental neglect, abuse, ambivalence, hostility, rejection, unpredictability, or inconsistency; 2) psychiatric disturbance in either parent; and 3) maladaptive parental reactions to illness, such as unrealistic expectations or feelings of helplessness and pessimism.

Additional risk factors that may intensify the child's psychological reactions to illness include exposure to illness factors (e.g., disfigurement, loss of autonomy, and immobilization) and parents' reactions of loss, grief, guilt, depression, anxiety, exhaustion, isolation, marital strain, financial drain, and secrecy about the illness (often found in families with acquired immunodeficiency syndrome [AIDS]).

Manifestations of the child's normal psychological reactions to illnesses may include the folowing:

- *Biopsychological symptoms,* such as malaise, reduced threshold for pain, irritability, loss of appetite, and sleep disturbance.
- *Increased attachment behaviors,* such as clinging and demanding behavior and intensified separation anxiety.
- *Regression,* expressed as thumb sucking, returning to baby speech, and wetting or soiling.
- *Passivity,* with marked feelings of helplessness and powerlessness.
- *Frightening fantasies* about the illness and treatment, fear of mutilation and bodily harm, and overwhelming guilt.
- *Excessive anxiety,* with intense mobilization of psychological defense mechanisms, such as denial, or symptoms of phobic reactions or conversion disorder.
- *Reactivation* of premorbid psychiatric symptoms.

These reactions may intensify when children are exposed to serious illness in a parent or sibling.

■ Psychological Reactions to Chronic Illness

Most chronically ill children seem to cope adequately and do not develop mental health, social, or school adjustment problems. Certain risk factors associated with chronic illness of any kind may nevertheless adversely affect the child's and the family's coping capacities, and these factors may also affect the child who is exposed to stresses brought on by chronic illnesses in a family member.

Factors that must be considered in any assessment of psychological risk for the child include the strengths or weaknesses of the adaptive capacities of the child, including the child's temperament and cognitive-developmental stage; the adaptive capacities of the parents; how well the child and his or her parents fit together; the positive or negative aspects of the sociocultural context of the hospitalization; and the depth and duration of discomfort and pain experienced or observed. Other general psychosocial factors that may affect, but not necessarily cause, an adverse psychological outcome are lower socioeconomic status, poor diet, unhygienic living conditions, and violent environment.

Chronic illness in a child sometimes entails recurrent or long-term hospitalization. When this occurs, new stresses arise, including loss of autonomy and a sense of decreased competence, relative immobilization, impaired functioning, body intrusion, invasion of privacy, and disfigurement. Parents of a chronically ill child are likely to experience fatigue, guilt, depression, and anxiety, as well as marital stress and economic loss. The whole family may become isolated. Children who are younger than 5 years may experience difficulty in attachments as a result of recurrent hospitalization. Sometimes, staff members who are caring for a chronically ill child—particularly one who is inexorably deteriorating—may become discouraged, frustrated, and angry and may displace these feelings onto the child, with undesirable effects on the child and his or her family.

■ The Child's Cognitive Understanding of Death

Very young children may see, experience, and understand the death of someone they know and love as an abandonment, which, the child may reason, has come about because of his or her own misbehavior. This cognitive idea is similar to the child's initial immanent justice concept of illness. This experience and reasoning may evoke feelings of guilt, anger, sadness, and loss. These thoughts and feelings are important to the young child, who needs help in understanding that the death of the loved person is not the child's fault.

School-age children who have acquired or are acquiring the concepts of universal inevitability, finality, irreversibility, and the causality of death can mourn more successfully and can use their increased cognitive and emotional maturity to deal more effectively with the feelings of sadness, anger, and guilt that are aroused by the experience of a death in the family. At the same time, the death of a loved person may exacerbate the school-age child's concerns about harm to his or her body. These concerns may continue until the normative developmental tasks of adolescence are resolved.

Many other risk factors may adversely influence the psychological outcome for a child when a death occurs (Osterweis et al. 1984):

- Loss to a child before age 5 years or during early adolescence
- Loss of a mother for a girl before age 11 years or loss of a father for an adolescent boy
- Premorbid psychological difficulties in the child or lack of prior knowledge about death
- A conflictual relationship with the deceased or a poor subsequent relationship between the child and the stepparent
- A surviving parent who is psychologically vulnerable and excessively dependent on the child, or an environment that is unstable and inconsistent
- Lack of adequate family or community support, or a surviving parent who lacks access to available supports
- A death that was not expected or prepared for (e.g., the result of suicide or homicide)

■ Mourning

Children and adolescents have a wide range of reactions to the illness and death—from whatever cause—of a parent or sibling. It is important to recognize this individuality, especially during the mourning process (Furman 1974; Krementz 1981).

Young children may believe that the family member did not really die (especially if the death was sudden and in a remote hospital) and will one day come back from some faraway place, or the child may have a fantasy of being seen by or reunited with the absent parent, who the child may believe is now in heaven. Young children tend to mourn on a piecemeal basis, extended over time; thus, a child will most feel the loss when a fun time previously shared with the parent (e.g., a birthday celebration or a vacation) does not happen. This event becomes a time for more mourning. Later, a child may pretend the dead parent is just "away" and will daydream or recall memories of past times with the parent. It is not unusual for a child to want to keep something that belonged to the now-dead parent—an article of clothing, a piece of jewelry, a pen or pencil, a book or pocketknife—as a way of holding onto the memory of the parent or a token of identification with the lost parent.

Children usually hesitate to share fantasies or memories of the dead parent with other children for fear of being teased. A child may feel embarrassed, ashamed, or uncomfortably unique, gripped by the sense that he or she alone has a dead parent. These feelings—along with emotions such as anger, anxiety, sadness, and loneliness—may also be kept secret. If a child becomes caught in the web of a family's secret, he or she will avoid expressing feelings and opinions for fear of upsetting the living parent.

Children work to overcome grief in part by expressing to themselves or to others—sometimes during play—their feelings of sadness. A child may also exhibit various mechanisms of defense, including denial. Children who lack sufficient opportunity to share feelings, or whose opportunity is actively blocked, may resort unconsciously—or even consciously—to behavioral manifestations of their anxiety, frustration, and anger, engaging in disruptive behaviors such as marked oppositionality, temper tantrums, antisocial conduct, and high-risk behavior.

The child or adolescent also must deal with the grief reactions of the surviving parent, including withdrawal, avoidance, denial, and anger. Roles in the family may change. The child may become the substitute for the lost parent and may take on some parental or even marital roles—perhaps caring for siblings or comforting the surviving parent. The child may feel a sense of urgency and desperation as well as guilt in striving to perform the parental role while still being in need of parenting himself or herself.

Children and adolescents must also deal with the many changes that may occur in the family, including new partners for the surviving parent, sometimes through remarriage. The surviving parent may have to change jobs or locations, and the family's standard of living may decline.

The child or adolescent may become fearful that the surviving parent may die. A child who fears being left alone may react by becoming oversolicitous of the surviving parent, by being angry, or by acting out anxieties and guilt about the safety of the surviving parent by courting precarious or dangerous situations. Such displacement of fears, anxieties, and guilt at the same time gives the child a transient feeling of being in control instead of suffering passively the anxiety of an anticipated and dreaded abandonment.

In short, children and adolescents react to the death of a parent in a variety of ways: some cry a lot, some deny the death, some try to avoid thinking about it in the hope of continuing with their lives, and some clamor for attention through their behavior. These and other reactions may be determined in part by the previous relationship with the now-dead parent, the relationship with surviving family members, and the inner life and temperament of the child. In any event, the young person's unique way of reacting to the death of a parent should be respected and understood by those trying to help the child or adolescent deal with his or her feelings.

References

Ainsworth MDS: The development of infant-mother interaction among the Ganda, in Determinants of Infant Behavior, Vol 2. Edited by Foss BM. London, Methuen, 1963, pp 67–112

Anderson JR: The Architecture of Cognition. Cambridge, MA, Harvard University Press, 1983

Aoyama K: Filler syllables in early language development. Paper presented at the Yale Child Study Center, November 21, 2001

Bailey JM, Pillard RC: A genetic study of male sexual orientation. Arch Gen Psychiatry 48:1089–1096, 1991

Bloom L: Language development review, in Review of Child Development Research, Vol 4. Edited by Horowitz FR. Chicago, IL, University of Chicago Press, 1975, pp 245–303

Bornstein MH: Qualities of color vision in infancy. J Exp Child Psychol 19:401–419, 1975

Bowlby J: Maternal Care and Mental Health. Geneva, World Health Organization, 1951

Bowlby J: Attachment (Attachment and Loss, Vol 1). New York, Basic Books, 1969

Bremner JD, Scott TM, Delaney RC, et al: Deficits in short-term memory in posttraumatic stress disorder. Am J Psychiatry 150:1015–1019, 1993

Brown AL: The development of memory: knowing about and knowing how to know. Adv Child Dev Behav 10:104–152, 1975

Brown R, Bellugi N: Three processes in the child's acquisition of syntax. Harv Educ Rev 34:133–151, 1964

Brown R, Hanlon C: Derivational complexity and order of acquisition in child speech, in Cognition and the Development of Language. Edited by Hayes JR. New York, Wiley, 1970, pp 11–53

Campos JJ, Langer A, Krowitz A: Cardiac responses on the visual cliff in prelocomotor human infants. Science 170:196–197, 1970

Cazden C: Subcultural differences in child language: an interdisciplinary review. Merrill Palmer Q 12:185–219, 1966

Chess S, Thomas A: Temperament in Clinical Practice. New York, Guilford, 1986

Chomsky N: Syntactic Structures. The Hague, Mouton, 1957

Chugani HT, Phelps ME, Mazziotta JL: Positron emission tomography study of human brain functional development. Ann Neurol 22:487–497, 1987

Cohen LJ: The operational definition of human attachment. Psychol Bull 81:107–217, 1974

Cohen LJ, Gelber E: Infant's visual memory, in Infant Perception: From Sensation to Cognition, Vol 1: Basic Visual Processes. Edited by Cohen L, Salapatek P. New York, Academic Press, 1975, pp 347–403

Cohen RL, Harnick AH: The susceptibility of child witnesses to suggestion. Law Hum Behav 4:201–210, 1980

Colby A: Evolution of a moral-developmental theory, in New Directions for Child Development: Moral Development. Edited by Damon W. San Francisco, CA, Jossey-Bass, 1978, pp 89–104

Condon WS, Sander LW: Neonate movement is synchronized with adult speech: interactional participation and language acquisition. Science 183:99–101, 1974

Coyle JL: Introduction to the phenomenology of the synapse, in Psychiatry Update: American Psychiatric Association Annual Review, Vol 4. Edited by Hales RE, Frances AJ. Washington, DC, American Psychiatric Press, 1985, pp 6–16

Dale PS, Loftus E, Rathburn R: The influence of the form of the question of eyewitness testimony on preschool children. J Psycholinguist Res 7:269–277, 1978

Darwin C: The Expression of Emotions in Man and Animals (1872). Chicago, IL, University of Chicago Press, 1975

De Bellis MD, Chrousos GP, Dorn L, et al: Blunted plasma ACTH responses to the ovine corticotropin-releasing hormone stimulation test in sexually abused girls. Biol Psychiatry 33:103A, 1993

Dubignon J, Campbell D: Sucking in the newborn during a feed. J Exp Child Psychol 7:282–298, 1969

Engen T, Lipsitt LP, Kaye H: Olfactory responses and adaptation in the human neonate. J Comp Physiol Psychol 56:73–77, 1963

Fantz RL, Fagan JF, Miranda SB: Early visual selectivity, in Infant Perception: From Sensation to Cognition, Vol 1: Basic Visual Processes. Edited by Cohen L, Salapatek P. New York, Academic Press, 1975, pp 249–345

Ferald A: The perceptual and affective salience of mothers' speech to infants, in The Origin and Growth of Communication. Edited by Feagaus LC, Garvey R, Golinkoff MT, et al. Norwood, NJ, Ablex, 1984

Ferreiro E: Les Relations Temporelles Dans la Langue de L'enfant [Temporal Relations in the Language of the Infant]. Geneva, Droz, 1971

Francis H: Toward an explanation of paradigmatic-syntagmatic shift. Child Dev 43:949–959, 1972

Freud S: Screen memories (1899), in The Standard Edition of the Complete Psychological Works of Sigmund Freud, Vol 3. Translated and edited by Strachey J. London, Hogarth Press, 1962, pp 303–322

Freud S: The interpretation of dreams (first part) (1900), in The Standard Edition of the Complete Psychological Works of Sigmund Freud, Vol 4. Translated and edited by Strachey J. London, Hogarth Press, 1953, pp 1–610

Freud S: Three essays on the theory of sexuality (1905), in The Standard Edition of the Complete Psychological Works of Sigmund Freud, Vol 7. Translated and edited by Strachey J. London, Hogarth Press, 1953, pp 125–143

Freud S: On narcissism: an introduction (1914), in The Standard Edition of the Complete Psychological Works of Sigmund Freud, Vol 14. Translated and edited by Strachey J. London: Hogarth Press, 1957, pp 67–102

Freud S: Introductory lectures on psychoanalysis, part III (1917), in The Standard Edition of the Complete Psychological Works of Sigmund Freud, Vol 16. Translated and edited by Strachey J. London, Hogarth Press, 1963, pp 243–448

Freud S: Beyond the pleasure principle (1920), in the Standard Edition of the Complete Psychological Works of Sigmund Freud, Vol 18. Translated and edited by Strachey J. London, Hogarth Press, 1955, pp 7–64

Freud S: The question of lay analysis (1926), in The Standard Edition of the Complete Psychological Works of Sigmund Freud, Vol 20. Translated and edited by Strachey J. London, Hogarth Press, 1959, pp 179–258

Freud S: New lectures on psychoanalysis (1933), in The Standard Edition of the Complete Psychological Works of Sigmund Freud, Vol 22. Translated and edited by Strachey J. London, Hogarth Press, 1964, pp 1–182

Freud S: An outline of psychoanalysis (1940), in The Standard Edition of the Complete Psychological Works of Sigmund Freud, Vol 23. Translated and edited by Strachey J. London, Hogarth Press, 1969, pp 144–207

Friedlander BZ: Receptive language development in infancy: issues and problems. Merrill Palmer Q 16:7–51, 1970

Furman E: A Child's Parent Dies: Studies in Childhood Bereavement. New Haven, CT, Yale University Press, 1974

Geschwind N: Disconnexion syndromes in animals and man. Brain 88:237–294, 1965

Gesell AO, Amatruda CS: Stages and sequences of development (1941), in Developmental Diagnosis, 11th Edition. New York, Harper & Row, 1964, pp 8–14

Gilligan C: In a Different Voice: Psychological Theory and Women's Development. Cambridge, MA, Harvard University Press, 1982

Goldman-Rakic P: Circuitry of the prefrontal cortex: short-term memory and the regulation of behavior by representational knowledge, in Handbook of Physiology: Higher Functions of the Nervous System. Edited by Blum F. Bethesda, MD, American Physiological Society, 1987

Goldstone S, Goldfarb JL: The perception of time by children, in Perceptual Development in Children. Edited by Kidd AH, Rivoire JL. New York, International Universities Press, 1966, pp 445–486

Goodman GS, Aman C, Hirschman J: Child sexual and physical abuse: children's testimony, in Children's Eyewitness Memory. Edited by Ceci S, Toglia MP, Ross D. New York, Springer-Verlag, 1987

Gould E, Gross CG: Response to Goodman et al, in Perceptual Development in Children. Edited by Kidd AH, Rivoire JL. New York, International Universities Press, 1966

Gould E, Reeves AJ, Graziano MS, et al: Neurogenesis in the neocortex of adult primates. Science 286:548–552, 1999

Green A: The "Sissy" Boy Syndrome and the Development of Homosexuality. New Haven, CT, Yale University Press, 1987

Hall GS: Adolescence: Its Psychology, and Its Relation to Physiology, Anthropology, Sociology, Sex, Crime, Religion and Education. New York, Appleton, 1904

Halverson CF, Waldrop MF: Maternal behavior towards own and other preschool children: the problems of "ownness." Child Dev 41:839–845, 1970

Hasher L, Zacks RT: Automatic and effortful process in memory. J Exp Psychol Gen 108:356–388, 1979

Hofer MA: Early social relationships: a psychologist's view. Child Dev 58:633–647, 1987

Honigmann JJ: Culture as Personality. New York, Harper, 1954

Hudson JA: The emergence of autobiographical memory in mother-child conversation, in Knowing and Remembering in Young Children. Edited by Fivush R, Hudson JA. New York, Cambridge University Press, 1990

Inhelder B: The sensory-motor origins of knowledge, in Early Childhood: The Development of Self-Regulatory Mechanisms. Edited by Walcher DN, Peters DL. New York, Academic Press, 1971, pp 141–155

Insel TR: A neurobiological basis of social attachment. Am J Psychiatry 154:726–735, 1997

Izard C: Human Emotions. New York, Plenum, 1977

Johnson MK, Foley MA: Differentiating fact from fantasy: the reliability of children's memory. J Soc Issues 40:33–50, 1984

Johnson-Laird PN: The Computer and the Mind: An Introduction to Cognitive Science. Cambridge, MA, Harvard University Press, 1988

Jurkovic GJ: The juvenile delinquent as a moral philosopher: a structural-developmental perspective. Psychol Bull 88:709–727, 1980

Kagan J: Change and Continuity in Infancy. New York, Wiley, 1971

Kagan J: The Nature of the Child. New York, Basic Books, 1984

Kagan J: The contribution of temperament to developmental profiles, in Child and Adolescent Psychiatry: A Comprehensive Textbook, 3rd Edition. Edited by Lewis M. Philadelphia, PA, Lippincott Williams & Wilkins, 2002, pp 211–220

Kessen W: Sucking and looking: two organized congenital patterns of behavior in the newborn, in Early Behavior: Comparative and Developmental Approaches. Edited by Stevenson HW, Hess EH, Rheingold HL. New York, Wiley, 1967

Kobasigawa A: Utilization of retrieval cues by children to recall. Child Dev 45:127–134, 1974

Kobre KR, Lipsett LP: A negative contrast effect in newborns. J Exp Child Psychol 14:81–91, 1972

Kohlberg L: Development of moral character. Review of Child Development Research 1:400–404, 1964

Kohlberg L: Revisions in the theory and practice of moral development, in New Directions in Child Development: Moral Development. Edited by Damon W. San Francisco, CA, Jossey-Bass, 1978, pp 83–88

Korner AF: Neonatal startles, smiles, erections, and reflex sucks as related to state, sex, and individuality. Child Dev 40:1039–1053, 1969

Kosslyn SM: Aspects of a cognitive neuroscience of mental imagery. Science 240:1621–1626, 1988

Kramer SN: History Begins at Sumer. Garden City, New York, Doubleday, 1959

Krementz J: How It Feels When a Parent Dies. New York, Knopf, 1981

Langlois JH, Stephan CW: Beauty and the beast: the role of physical attraction in peer relationships and social behavior, in Developmental Social Psychology: Theory and Research. Edited by Brehm SS, Kassin SM, Gibbons SX. New York, Oxford University Press, 1981, pp 152–168

Leckman JF, Herman AE: Maternal behavior and developmental psychopathology. Biol Psychiatry 51:27–43, 2002

Lenneberg EH: Biological Foundation of Language. New York, Wiley, 1967, pp 128–130

Leong C: Lateralization in severely disabled readers in relation to functional cerebral development and synthesis of information, in The Neuropsychology of Learning Disorders. Edited by Knights RM, Baker DJ. Baltimore, MD, University Park Press, 1976, pp 221–231

Lerner RM, Lerner JV: Effects of age, sex, and physical attractiveness on child–peer relations, academic performance, and elementary school adjustment. Dev Psychol 13:585–590, 1977

Lewis M: Language, Thought and Personality in Infancy and Childhood. New York, Basic Books, 1963

Loftus EF, Davies GM: Distortion in memory of children. J Soc Issues 40:51–67, 1984

Lovell K, Dixon EM: The growth of the control of grammar in imitation, comprehension, and production. J Child Psychol Psychiatry 8:31–39, 1967

Macfarlane A: Olfaction in the development of social preference in the human neonate. CIBA Found Symp (33):103–117, 1975

MacLean PD: The Triune Brain in Evolution: Role in Paleocerebral Functions. New York, Plenum, 1990

Mahler MS: On human symbiosis and the vicissitudes of individuation. J Am Psychoanal Assoc 15:740–763, 1967

Main M, Solomon J: Discovery of an insecure, disorganized/disoriented attachment pattern: procedures, findings and implications for the classification of behavior, in Affective Development in Infancy. Edited by Yogman M, Brazelton TB. Norwood, NJ, Ablex, 1986, pp 95–124

Miller PH: Theories of Developmental Psychology, 2nd Edition. New York, WH Freeman, 1989

Mills M, Melhuish E: Recognition of mother's voice in early infancy. Nature 252:123–124, 1974

Mirsky AF, Anthony BJ, Duncan CC, et al: Analysis of the elements of attention: a neuropsychological approach. Neuropathol Rev 2:109–145, 1991

Moerk E: Changes in verbal child-mother interactions with increasing language skills of the child. J Psycholinguist Res 3:101–116, 1974

Morley ME: The Development and Disorders of Speech in Childhood, 2nd Edition. Edinburgh, Livingston, 1965

Nadel L, Zola-Morgan S: Infant amnesia: a neurobiological perspective, in Infant Memory. Edited by Moscovitch M, Saroka E. New York, Plenum, 1984, pp 145–172

Neisser Y: The control of information pickup in selective looking, in Perception and Its Development. Edited by Pick AD. Hillsdale, NJ, Erlbaum, 1984, pp 201–219

Nelson KE: Aspects of language acquisition and use from 2 to age 20. J Am Acad Child Psychiatry 16:584–607, 1977

Newell A, Shaw J, Simon HA: Elements of a theory of human problem solving. Psychol Rev 65:151–166, 1958

Nowakowski RS, Hayes NL: New neurons: extraordinary evidence or extraordinary conclusion? (comment). Science 288:771, 2000

Osterweis M, Solomon F, Green M (eds): Bereavement: Reactions, Consequences and Care. Washington, DC, National Academy Press, 1984

Petersen SE, Robinson DL, Keys W: Pulvinar nuclei of the behaving rhesus monkey: visual responses and their modulation. J Neurophysiol 54:867–886, 1985

Piaget J: The Child's Conception of Number. Translated by Gattegno C, Hodgson FM. London, Routledge & Kegan Paul, 1952

Piaget J: Language and thought from a genetic point of view. Acta Psychol 10:88–98, 1954

Piaget J: The Growth of Logical Thinking. New York, Basic Books, 1958

Piaget J: The Moral Development of the Child. New York, Free Press, 1965

Piaget J: The intellectual development of the adolescent, in Adolescence: Psychosocial Perspectives. Edited by Caplan G, Lebovici S. New York, Basic Books, 1969, pp 22–26

Pipp S, Harmon RJ: Attachment as regulation: a commentary. Child Dev 58:648–652, 1987

Porter FL, Porges SQ, Marshall RE: Newborn pain cries and vagal tones: parallel changes in response to circumcision. Child Dev 59:495–505, 1988

Posner MI, Petersen SE, Fox PT, et al: Localization of cognitive operations in the human brain. Science 240:1627–1637, 1988

Provence S, Lipton RC: Infants and Institutions. New York, International Universities Press, 1962

Rakic P: Limits of neurogenesis in primates. Science 227:154–156, 1985

Rakic P: Development of the cerebral cortex in human and nonhuman primates, in Child and Adolescent Psychiatry: A Comprehensive Textbook. Edited by Lewis M. Baltimore, MD, Williams & Wilkins, 1996, pp 9–30

Rakic P, Cameron RS, Komura H: Recognition, adhesion, transmembrane signaling and cell motility in guided neuronal migration. Curr Opin Neurobiol 4:63–69, 1994

Reese HW: Attitudes toward the opposite sex in late childhood. Merrill Palmer Quarterly 12:157–163, 1966

Rutter M: Normal psychosexual development. J Child Psychol Psychiatry 11:259–283, 1971

Rutter M: Other family influences, in Child Psychiatry. Edited by Rutter M, Hersov L. Oxford, Blackwell, 1976a, pp 74–108

Rutter M: Separation, loss and family relationships, in Child Psychiatry. Edited by Rutter M, Hersov L. Oxford, Blackwell, 1976b, pp 47–73

Sandler J, Dare C: The psychoanalytic concept of orality. J Psychosom Res 14:211–222, 1970

Schacter DL, Moscovitch M: Infants, amnesias, and dissociable memory systems, in Infant Memory. Edited by Moscovitch M, Saroka E. New York, Plenum, 1984, pp 173–216

Schaffer HR, Emerson PE: Patterns of response to physical contact in early human development. J Child Psychol Psychiatry 5:1–13, 1964

Schetky D, Green A: Child Sexual Abuse: A Handbook for Health Care Professionals. New York, Brunner/Mazel, 1988

Spitz R: The First Year of Life. New York, International Universities Press, 1965

Squire LR: Memory and Brain. New York, Oxford University Press, 1987

Squire LR, Ojamann JG, Miezin FM, et al: Activation of the hippocampus in normal humans: a functional anatomical study of memory. Proc Natl Acad Sci U S A 89:1837–1842, 1992

Sroufe LA, Waters E: The ontogenesis of smiling and laughter: a perspective on the organization of development in infancy. Psychol Rev 83:173–189, 1976

Stayton DJ, Ainsworth MD: Individual differences in infant responses to brief everyday separations as related to other infant and maternal behaviors. Dev Psychol 9:226–235, 1973

Sternberg RJ: Mechanisms of cognitive development: a componential approach, in Mechanisms of Cognitive Development. Edited by Sternberg RJ. New York, WH Freeman, 1984, pp 163–186

Terr L: What happens to early memories of trauma? A study of twenty children under age five at the time of documented traumatic events. J Am Acad Child Adolesc Psychiatry 27:96–104, 1988

Thomas A, Chess S: Temperament and Development. New York, Brunner/Mazel, 1977

Thomas A, Chess S, Birch HG: Temperament and Behavior Disorders in Children. New York, New York University Press, 1968

Tobin-Richards MH, Boxer AM, Peterson AC: The psychological significance of pubertal change: sex differences in perception of self during early adolescence, in Girls at Puberty. Edited by Brooks-Gunn J, Peterson AC. New York, Plenum, 1983, pp 127–154

Touwen BCL: Laterality, in Scientific Foundations of Developmental Psychiatry. Edited by Rutter M. London, Heinemann, 1980, pp 154–164

Weizmann F, Cohen L, Pratt J: Novelty, familiarity and the development of infant attention. Dev Psychol 4:149–154, 1971

Wolff P: Cognitive consideration for a psychoanalytic theory of language acquisition, in Motives and Thought: Psychoanalytic Essays in Honor of David Rappaport. Edited by Holt R. New York, International Universities Press, 1967, pp 300–343

Wolff P: The natural history of crying and other vocalizations of early infancy, in Determinants of Infant Behavior. Edited by Foss BM. London, Methuen, 1969

Yates T: Theories of cognitive development, in Child and Adolescent Psychiatry: A Comprehensive Textbook. Edited by Lewis M. Baltimore, MD, Williams & Wilkins, 1991, pp 109–129

Zola-Morgan S, Squire LR, Amaral DG: Human amnesia and the medial temporal region: enduring memory impairment following a bilateral lesion limited to field CA 1 of the hippocampus. J Neurosci 6:2950–2957, 1986

Role of Culture, Race, and Ethnicity in Child and Adolescent Psychiatry

Héctor R. Bird, M.D.

Clinicians and investigators alike agree on the need to consider culture and ethnicity in both assessment and treatment (Giordano 1973; Papajohn and Spiegel 1975). It is important to differentiate three characteristics of individuals and groups that, although distinct, are in many ways related, may overlap, and are often used interchangeably: culture, ethnicity, and race. *Culture* refers to learned and widely shared ideas, attitudes, values, and beliefs that influence behavior. Lewis-Fernandez and Kleinman (1995) define culture as a dynamic process, highly influenced by differences in gender, race, class, ethnicity, and age. Culture therefore involves a system of standards for behavior, a cluster of meanings that are shared by members of a group that serve to interpret experience and guide action. Culture is transmitted through verbal and nonverbal learning and has a historical element because values, knowledge, and beliefs are handed down from one generation to the next. The transmission often comes with some changes and transformations, but these are changes that occur within the context of the culture itself. In this sense the concept of culture is dynamic and longitudinal and evolves over time.

Ethnicity is one aspect of culture. It is related to culture but refers primarily to nationality and national identification. Like culture, it comprises group-shared patterns of social interaction and shared values, behaviors, perceptions, and use of language. However, ethnicity has a greater degree of specificity than culture, which is a broader concept. The concept of *race*, unlike that of ethnicity, is biologically defined, and differentiation by race has been generally based on skin color

and other observable physical or anatomical features. Racial identification is complicated by the large numbers of individuals of mixed race.

Although the concept of race is frequently used interchangeably with that of ethnicity (Wilkinson and King 1987), and ethnicity with that of culture, there is some merit in keeping the basic notions of each concept separate and distinct. A great deal of confusion exists in the use of the three concepts. For example, there are individuals who are culturally and ethnically Hispanic but racially of black or mixed race; others are racially Asian but culturally North American. The term *African American* refers specifically to someone of black race who is born in the United States; immigrants from the West Indies who are black identify themselves as West Indians rather than as African Americans. Likewise, individuals of Hispanic ethnicity can be at differing levels of cultural assimilation or adaptation dependent on their use of language or the changes that may have taken place in their customs and cultural attitudes.

In somewhat oversimplified terms, race can be seen as being defined in the context of biology and genetics. The geographic origin of the individual or his or her immediate ancestors determines ethnicity. Culture is defined by the standards of behavior and meanings shared by members of a given group (usually an ethnic group, but it can be broader and encompass several ethnic groups). All three concepts are deeply intertwined and in many ways overlapping. However, it is important to keep in mind that self-perception and identity are greatly influenced by the attitudes of the predominant or dominant society toward a particular racial, ethnic, or cultural group. This fact alone consigns large numbers of individuals to minority status, and minority status usually—although not always—places those individuals at a societal disadvantage. When such a situation exists, there can be a profound impact on self-esteem and identity and a conscious or unconscious thrust toward modifying racial features (to the extent that these can be modified) or modifying ethnic identification and cultural values to conform with those of the dominant society.

The Cultural Controversies

Cross-cultural psychiatry has been of concern to clinicians who treat patients with psychopathology and to clinical researchers who investigate cultural phenomena from a clinical perspective. Cross-cultural psychiatry is also of interest to anthropologists and sociologists, whose foci include the broader implications of culture and concern over the societal and personal impact of labeling people as being "disordered." Each of these perspectives has long-standing traditions of research behind it. Nonetheless, the approach to cultural issues has generally been dichotomized along those lines. Those who are clinicians or clinical researchers tend to be more empirically oriented and quantitative, to have a greater need for categorization and therefore a more concrete conceptualization of culture, and to be somewhat dismissive of cultural issues. The anthropological and sociological viewpoint, on the other hand, tends to be more ethnographic and descriptive and therefore tends to dwell more on symbols and semantic differences. Both perspectives have led to the development of numerous formulations regarding the cultural relativism of human behavior and the meanings of behavior that for many years have been at the forefront of thinking in cross-cultural psychiatry. These formulations reflect widely divergent views that range from nihilism and the belief that diagnoses do not really exist to the assignment of psychiatric diagnoses through literal applications of criteria in widely different settings without due consideration of the culture of the subjects being studied, evaluated, or treated.

Clinicians tend to position themselves at different points on this spectrum; fortunately there are few who would adhere to either extreme—that is, either the view that due to cultural considerations there is no such thing as universally applicable psychiatric disorders or psychiatric diagnoses or the view that cultural issues should be altogether disregarded in the assessment of psychiatric conditions. One viewpoint that is frequently expressed is that different cultural groups experience specific "culturally valid" conditions that constitute the diagnostic entities that should be considered for each group. Although in fact a number of conditions appear to exist in certain cultural settings and are considered to be culture-specific syndromes (e.g., *susto* among Mexicans and Central Americans, *ataque de nervios* among Caribbean Hispanics, *taijin-kyofusho* among Japanese adolescents, or *irijua* among Peruvian children), these generally seem to be culturally tainted variants of different known disorders (such as panic attacks, social phobia, or depression) that are more universal. The important notion to bear in mind is that the more common conditions that clinicians confront may have different characteristics in different cultural and ethnic groups and that even when there are certain symptoms in common across groups, the same condition may exhibit specific characteristics that are unique to a particular cultural group and that are not universally applicable. Nevertheless, there seem to be sets of core symptoms of different psychiatric disorders that are universally applicable across cultures.

In a simple example, one might argue that a condition in culture A would be characterized by symptoms *a, b, c, d, e, f,* and *g,* whereas in culture B the same condition is characterized by symptoms *a, b, c,* and *d,* but according to those familiar with this culture, individuals manifesting that condition in culture B seldom exhibit symptoms *e, f,* or *g.* Instead, an additional set of symptoms *h, i,* and *j* is commonly observed as part of the diagnosis in culture B but seldom occurs in culture A. Some argue that the condition in each culture should be defined and named differently. The proponents of this view would depart from standard definitions of disorder and either leave out, substitute, or add symptomatic criteria to the necessary conditions for the diagnosis in each cultural group.

The underlying and foremost consideration in all of this is the issue of misclassification, which might in turn lead to inadequate therapy. Moreover, the issue must be approached in a somewhat different manner in research than it is in clinical work. Wakefield (1996), arguing about this issue from within a single culture, questioned whether diagnostic criteria as presented in the DSM validly distinguish real disorders from the vast array of problematic human conditions that, although not disorders, can be considered problems in living. He argues that in many of the DSM categories, a strict application of the criteria produces a great possibility that individuals with no disorders may be mistakenly diagnosed as having disorders and therefore results in the likelihood of producing many false-positive diagnoses. The issue is compounded in cross-cultural work, in which the application of different diagnostic criteria needs to include consideration of issues relevant to the person being assessed as well as to the clinician carrying out the assessment. In clinical work, culturally sensitive clinicians can minimize these biases by exercising their judgment; by taking context into account; and by using their knowledge of the culture, their sensitivity, and their intuition to adjust or interpret the diagnostic criteria. They can thereby tailor their assessments and interventions to the specific individual who comes to clinical attention.

Overdiagnosis and misdiagnosis become even more problematic in other circumstances, especially in research. Participants for a clinical research protocol are selected with strictly defined and highly operationalized inclusion criteria that rarely take cultural nuances into consideration. In epidemiological survey research, for example, large samples of the population are surveyed with structured instruments that do not have the potential to fine-tune the criteria or to take context into account. In these instances, truly heterogeneous groups of individuals who may not really share an underlying pathology are ultimately classified as homogeneous. Study results concerning etiology, biological correlates or treatment response, and other outcomes may become muddled and equivocal if the instruments used for classification are overinclusive or have a tendency to misclassify subjects. In epidemiological research, the field survey data may provide policymakers with inflated or inaccurate estimates of the real prevalence of a disorder. Misclassification and overinclusiveness may also confuse and muddle the assessment of risk factors and other correlates of psychopathology.

For purposes of cross-cultural research, it is critical to apply criteria uniformly in different settings. It behooves investigators to subsequently take cultural nuances and cultural variations into account in explaining their results. This perspective, albeit oversimplified, allows a common point of departure. A compelling rationale for the need for a common language in psychiatric research was provided by Wing (1985):

The central methodologic issue in psychiatric research ... is how, in the absence of simple physiological or biochemical indices, to construct techniques that will ensure a useful degree of comparability between studies. This is not just a matter of achieving "reliability" between a few close collaborators, but the much more difficult task of ensuring that teams working independently, perhaps in different countries and using different languages, can replicate each other's studies, thus adding to the stock of knowledge available to investigators all over the world.

From both a clinical and an epidemiological perspective, the use of a common language and consensus categories of disorder are essential and critical for the proper study of cultural and contextual differences in the distributions of disorders and for proper diagnosis and treatment to occur. This principle must be safeguarded for the purpose of achieving comparability across studies carried out in different cultural settings. Robins (1994) commented that one of the five foci that Sartorius considered critical to the World Health Organization (WHO) mental health program was the development of such a common language as a basic element of cross-cultural research. The WHO took a major step in this direction in 1969 when it undertook the International Pilot Study for Schizophrenia (World Health Organization 1973), which compared the disorder in nine countries, using identical criteria and identical instruments to elicit the symptoms of the disorder.

The term *common language* includes an agreement on concepts by investigators and clinicians alike. As a consequence, the recent nosological systems have undergone extensive field trials to test the diagnostic criteria in many countries, both developed and underdeveloped, in both the East and the West. The task forces for the *International Statistical Classification of Diseases and Related Health Problems,* 10th Revision (ICD-10; World Health Organization 1993), primarily in Europe, and DSM-IV (American Psychiatric Association 1994), in the United States, cooperated to try to bring the two diagnostic systems together to reduce the competition and the conceptual conflicts that had divided ICD-9 (World Health Organization 1977) from DSM-III and DSM-III-R (American Psychiatric Association 1980, 1987).

Robins (1994) also observed that one result of the WHO effort was that for the first time there is something very close to a common language for the assessment of many psychiatric disorders. There are shared concepts, and their expression has been formulated in clear language that is easy to understand. Assessment instruments developed to ascertain diagnoses based on DSM-III-R, DSM-IV, and ICD-10 criteria have been translated into many languages, and concerted efforts have been made to convey the original meanings in content, degree, and connotations. As a result of such efforts, it is less important whether a syndrome is conceived, diagnosed, and labeled as conduct disorder or depression rather than being thought of as defensive misbehavior or socially caused human misery. Only when an explicitly operationalized syndrome of symptomatology is defined can one begin to ask the more substantive and important question of whether there are other variables that account for differences in rates in different cultural settings and circumstances or among individuals from different cultures and to ensure that such variables are assessed or measured. Factors such as social adversity or cultural influences may well be the risk factors or the etiological factors associated with the syndrome. Cultural differences in risk factors can be determined only if the presence or absence of the syndrome is defined by using similar parameters in the cultures that are being compared.

Various examples provide some evidence about the subtlety of cultural differences regarding the presence of symptomatic criteria in different cultural settings. Studies carried out by Achenbach and other investigators throughout the world have employed the Children's Behavior Checklist for one purpose or another in a wide variety of cultural settings. The places where it has been used include Australia, Belgium, Canada, Chile, China, France, Germany, Greece, India, Israel, Jamaica, Kenya, the Netherlands, Puerto Rico, Sweden, and Thailand. The specific studies are reviewed in detail in other publications (see Bird 1996; de Groot et al. 1994; Verhulst and Achenbach 1995). The relevance of these studies to this topic is that cross-cultural comparisons across different settings have yielded relatively small differences in problem rates and syndrome structures among children in all of these widely disparate settings. Moreover, the studies have shown considerable similarity in the associations between problem behaviors and gender and socioeconomic status, as well as similar correlations between reports by different types of informants (Achenbach et al. 1987). The studies in different cultural settings that had sufficiently large samples of children in the clinical range yielded factor structures that are very close to those initially described by Achenbach and Edelbrock (1981), so this finding provides additional confirmatory evidence for the contention that psychopathology does not differ dramatically from culture to culture. In clinical work these issues are not as pressing. Clinicians have greater latitude on the issue of categorization, and clinical decisions are not necessarily based purely on the determination of the presence or absence of symptoms. However, many of the issues relevant to research are also relevant to clinical practice.

Issues in Assessment and Treatment of Children and Adolescents

From the foregoing it can be seen that there may be divergence in the ways that disorders and psychiatric symptoms are labeled in different cultures (Murphy 1976). However, when broadly defined, the major psychiatric syndromes and symptom clusters in Axis I of DSM-IV-TR (American Psychiatric Association 2000), as well as the personality types delineated in Axis II, appear to exist in all societies (Konner 1995). Nonetheless, race, culture, and ethnicity undoubtedly influence the expressions of psychopathology. They shape patterns of child rearing, styles of family and social interaction, social class assumptions, peer relations, societal standards, and individual personal cognitive styles and personality structures. Particularly important is the fact that cultural attitudes influence the threshold of tolerance for certain behaviors or feelings and the way that emotional states are seen as being either normal or deviant. Environmental factors and material conditions also affect human behavior and psychopathology, but their influence is always contextualized by cultural meaning.

Several questions are relevant to an examination of the divergent meanings and interpretations attributable to race, ethnicity, or culture (Wilkinson and King 1987). As social concepts, race and ethnicity cannot be interpreted apart from the environmental context in which they are placed. When are we speaking exclusively of cultural patterns? When is ethnicity an indicator or a strongly correlated covariant of socioeconomic status? What are the socially relevant differences between race and ethnicity?

As a result of revolutionary changes in the means of transportation and communication and because of the migration resulting from European colonial expansion, the nineteenth and twentieth centuries witnessed spiraling increases in social mobility and in mobility of large numbers of people across national and international geographic boundaries. Until relatively recently in history, most individuals lived and died in the same location or immediate region where they were born and raised. Although the influences of culture, ethnicity, and race on psychopathology were topics of controversy and discussion throughout the twentieth century, it is only in the past one or two decades that certain notions about their importance have been systematically integrated into the fields of psychiatry and child psychiatry. For the first time in the development of the psychiatric nosology, DSM-IV incorporated a significantly greater systematic attempt than had previously been made to consider culture in the formulation of diagnosis. It addressed some of the difficulties that may be encountered in applying diagnostic criteria across different cultures. In their diagnostic formulations, clinicians are encouraged to systematically describe the individual's cultural and social reference group and to stipulate the ways in which the cultural context is relevant to the diagnostic formulation and may be relevant to subsequent clinical care. Although the inclusion of this guideline is a concrete step in the right direction, the extent to which it is followed may leave much to be desired.

Presented in Appendix I of DSM-IV-TR are several cultural parameters that may be relevant to the diagnostic formulation. It is equally important to consider these parameters during the course of treatment. The first is the cultural identification of the individual. The ethnic or cultural reference group of an individual must be determined by asking patients and subjects what ethnicity they consider themselves to be. This becomes more critical when operating within a multicultural environment where there are sizable numbers of immigrants or ethnic minorities, as often happens in clinical settings in large urban communities. It is also more complicated in child and adolescent psychiatry when each of a child's parents may have a different cultural background. It is imperative to determine children's cultural and ethnic self-identification and their involvement both with their parents' cultures of origin and with their host culture, their abilities to use their parents' native language, and the language or languages in which they are most proficient. This may be a source of inner conflict in immigrant children who are pressured to become proficient in the use of English and at the same time are expected to retain an-

other language or languages to communicate with their parents and other relatives.

Another important area of inquiry is the possibility of cultural explanations for the individual's presenting symptoms. This determination requires that the clinician have some degree of awareness of the predominant idioms of distress in a particular cultural group or of the ways in which symptoms are used to express the need for emotional or social support (e.g., "nerves," somatic complaints, possession by spirits, the "evil eye"). It behooves clinicians to familiarize themselves with the cultural idioms of the groups that seek their clinical attention. Furthermore, each cultural group seems to have a normative, assumed level of severity of symptoms beyond which an individual is considered to be deviant from the norm. It is important to know the meaning and the perceived severity of the individual's symptoms vis-à-vis the reference group and the perceived causes or explanatory models that are used in the particular culture.

Another area that requires some elaboration in assessment and treatment is the existence of cultural factors in the psychosocial environment. Available social supports, religious affiliation and participation, kinship networks, and group solidarity among members of disadvantaged minorities are known to provide emotional buffers to stress and to the development of psychopathology (Kessler et al. 1985). It is also critical to assess the influence of cultural elements that are likely to affect the relationship between the patient and the clinician. It is important to be aware of the problems that differences in culture and social status may create during the diagnostic and treatment processes.

From a clinical perspective, it is known that belonging to an ethnic minority group can be a source of stress. Individuals in minority groups are very often subject to prejudice and discrimination, which they have to contend with from very early in life. Prejudice and discrimination often lead to marginalization and to the need for minorities to cluster in ghettos, where the impact of prejudice and discrimination is reduced but where environmental circumstances and quality of life are poor. Minority and immigrant children often find themselves in an extremely ambivalent situation with regard to acculturation. Their taking on values of the dominant society generates intrafamilial conflict so that a shift of allegiances takes place. As a result, the child is much more strongly influenced by peer pressures. Acculturation involves a loss that threatens personal identity. Research has shown that the healthiest outcomes are obtained by those who learn to negotiate between the cultures that influence them and whose adaptation is bicultural.

Minority children also face other sources of stress in their environment, such as generally lower socio-economic status and varying degrees of socioeconomic deprivation and other social ills; inaccessibility to proper health care and mental health care; living in high-risk environments where they are exposed to violence, criminality, and drugs; school situations that may not be sensitive to their particular needs; and problems with the use of multiple languages (often they fail to master either language satisfactorily).

Another issue is the cultural biases inherent in the assessment of cognitive functioning and learning abilities in children who speak different languages. The lack of adequate norms and the lack of tests that are truly culturally unbiased make the results of these assessments suspect. Clinicians should be hesitant, for example, to make major clinical decisions about special-class placements purely on the basis of these tests, as this happens more frequently than it should.

The developmental assessment should be based on consideration of what is universal for the human race and what may be culturally unique; furthermore (and this is more difficult), it should evaluate how the universals are modified by cultural factors. Konner (1995) outlined five cross-cultural universal factors in human development that have been noted in the literature and that have been related to varying stages of physiological maturation and development. The first is the emergence of socialization, which is manifested by social smiling and which occurs during the first 4 months of life as the basal ganglia and cortical motor circuits mature. The second is the onset of attachments, manifested by fears of separation and of strangers. This tends to occur in the second half of the first year of life (6–12 months) and co-occurs with the maturation of the major fiber tracts of the limbic system. The third is the emergence of language, which starts during the second year and increases in complexity after that. The emergence of language coincides and seems to be associated with the maturation of the thalamic projection to the auditory cortex—among other circuits that become established and that permit the perception, integration, and repetition of the spoken word—and subsequently the mental representation of words and concepts. The fourth is the observable sex difference in physical aggressiveness that is observed during early and middle childhood, with male children on average manifesting greater physical aggressiveness than the average female child. This is thought to be due in part to prenatal androgenization of the hypothalamus. Finally, there is the emergence of adult sexual motivation and functioning in adolescence, which goes in parallel with the maturation of the hypothalamic-pituitary-gonadal axis in puberty and which in turn is also associated with the prenatal androgenization of the hypothalamus related to aggressivity.

Konner (1995) also notes that other probable cross-cultural universals in development have been proposed, but they are not as well established; more importantly, they have not been related to any of the underlying neurophysiological changes that come with maturation. These include a scheme of phases of moral development in childhood that appears to have cross-cultural universality. The universals serve a very important purpose in that they provide a baseline for understanding how subsequent variations in social experience act on the individual to produce potentially lasting changes. This is where culture and context become paramount in importance. For example, at around the same time in their development, all children who have comparable cognitive and social functioning will acquire languages. However, there will be cultural and ethnic differences in the semantic content of the language they acquire. Konner (1995) also sees the development of the social smile as a function of myelination, but he elaborates further on the related sociocultural component, which can lead to cultural differences. For example, infants whose smiles are favorably responded to will smile more than others. There are therefore cultures of lesser or greater expressivity, and this level of expressivity becomes a cultural trait that is transmitted across generations through learning and imitation. Clinicians are familiar with the frequent labeling of individuals from Mediterranean cultures as being *hysterical* or those from Asian cultures as having *constricted or flat affect* based purely on their level of emotional expressivity.

The Issue of Acculturation

Children from cultural backgrounds different from those of a dominant majority need to contend with two processes: enculturation and acculturation (Berry et al. 1986; Canino and Spurlock 2000). Enculturation involves acquiring the norms and values of one's own cultural group. Acculturation involves one of two processes: assimilation, which is the desire and the attempt by the minority group member to give up his or her own identity and culture and replace it with that of the dominant majority; and biculturalism, whereby the individual retains important cultural values from his or her cultural background while taking on characteristics of the host culture, resulting in a combination of cultural identifications (Oetting and Beauvais 1990; Rogler et al. 1991). A major limitation in attempting to relate acculturation to psychopathology has been the use of a unidimensional notion of acculturation that equates acculturation with assimilation and that fails to tap biculturalism or its related concepts. For example, in a study that relates acculturation in Puerto Rican youths to antisocial behavior (Sommers et al. 1993), high acculturation (in the form of assimilation) was associated with participation in interpersonal violence and theft, but lower acculturation was associated with participation in illicit drug use. These results, which are difficult to interpret, are probably attributable to the measurement of acculturation as a unitary dimension. The distinction between assimilation and biculturalism as alternative forms of acculturation is critical.

High acculturation (in the form of assimilation) has been correlated with greater risk for psychopathology and delinquent behavior among Hispanic adolescents (Friedrich and Flannery 1995; Rogler et al. 1991; Vega et al. 1993). More-assimilated second- and third-generation youths are at greater risk for delinquency than those who have remained unacculturated. A hypothetical pathway by which acculturation might influence the risk for antisocial behavior would be that when acculturated youths exhibit more assertiveness and independence, they have more conflicts (intergenerational acculturative stress) with and greater distancing from their parents (Oetting and Beauvais 1990, 1990–1991; Szapocznik et al. 1989). Conflict and distancing may lead to a weakening of attachment to parents and decreased responsivity to parental monitoring, which in turn render the youths more susceptible to the influence of deviant peers.

Characteristic Differences Among Ethnic Groups

It is important for clinical practitioners to be aware of some of the cultural patterns observed among different ethnic minorities in the United States. However, it must be emphasized that any delineation of the characteristic elements of any culture is a generalization that is subject to a great degree of individual variability. Even within an ethnic group there may be many subgroup differences that need to be taken into account. Therefore, in this context, reference is made here to the prevailing patterns without implying that there is homogeneity within each group or a clear-cut dichotomy between the cultural assumptions existing in any cultural setting. Rotheram and Phinney (1986) suggested four important dimensions along which one can assess the social interaction patterns within different cultural and ethnic groups. These are 1) the degree of interpersonal affiliation in terms of dependence versus interdependence, 2) activity versus passivity, 3) authoritarianism versus egalitarianism, and 4) level of emotional expressiveness in the style of communication (i.e., expressive/overt/personal versus restrained/formal/impersonal).

■ African Americans

African Americans constitute the largest minority group in the United States. Culturally, African Americans are said to exhibit a high degree of loyalty to their kin (Norton 1983). They are generally highly religious and giving. Although many of the traditional family assumptions and ties suffered in the migrations from the South to large urban centers in the North, extended kinship networks seem to provide a high degree of emotional support for the traditional African American family. Several centuries of oppression and discrimination may have led to passive or passive-aggressive interpersonal styles of relating that are often observed. A collective sense of outrage about injustices and the burden of prejudice that has accumulated over generations (Burkey 1978) leads to repressed rage and frequent expressions of anger that are not fully grasped by the dominant majority. However, Spurlock (1982) warned against stereotyping African Americans in ways that lead to dismissing their psychiatric symptoms.

Community surveys have consistently shown that on the average, African Americans experience higher levels of social, emotional, and financial distress than whites. However, when socioeconomic status is statistically controlled, these differences disappear (Canino and Spurlock 2000). Canino and Spurlock (2000) suggest that being from the African American ethnic minority and having certain life experiences associated with it are not themselves causal in generating mental health problems. It may well be that although there are factors that create greater risk, there may also be ethnic factors that help protect against the adverse mental health effects of those stresses. For example, the stress-buffering effect of group solidarity among members of this ethnic group has long been emphasized. This buffering could hypothetically occur in at least two ways: 1) The group can provide and reinforce cognitions that place the responsibility for adversity on structural conditions, such as the experience of prejudice and discrimination, and thereby minimize or reduce self-blame for the lack of (for example) financial achievement. 2) The group allegiance also provides a source of emotional support that can buffer the effects of life stresses in a variety of ways. There is insufficient research in this area, and efforts need to be directed at elucidating the risk factors and the factors that promote resilience.

■ Hispanics

Hispanics do not constitute a homogeneous ethnic group. Any comparison between Hispanics in the United States and the mainline Anglo culture must consider the subtle and sometimes not-so-subtle differences that exist among different Hispanic subgroups. Many of these differences relate to the ethnic background of different individuals across several generations (Canino and Spurlock 2000). For example, Argentineans of Italian background may be more like Italian Americans than they are like Peruvians of Inca background.

In general terms, the typical Hispanic culture is said to be one in which families are closely knit, interpersonally organized along an authoritarian hierarchy in which acquiescence is encouraged and at the level of the individual characterized by high levels of emotional expressiveness. Close family attachments and responsibilities are fostered. Typically, the needs and objectives of the family as a group take precedence over individual goals and objectives (Hofstede 1990; Triandis et al. 1982), and a high degree of loyalty and solidarity among family members is expected (Marin and Marin 1991). One generally finds strict family monitoring and close supervision of young persons occurring within the context of a pervasive authoritarian orientation that fosters acquiescence to parents, teachers, close relatives, or significant societal institutions. Much greater control is exerted over girls than boys.

Such a pattern may influence the manifestations of certain types of psychopathology. For example, it is generally believed that cultures in which religious and family values are emphasized and in which children are closely supervised have low rates of conduct disorder (Robins and McEvoy 1990). One finds in the Hispanic culture two strong elements that are traditionally associated with decreased risk for antisocial behavior: social control (Hirschi 1969) based on strong family attachments (Hagan 1989) and direct parental control based on strict discipline and coercion (Patterson 1982). The prevailing social and cultural context is different in mainline American culture, where there tends to exist a highly individualistic orientation, greater latitude in child-rearing norms, more flexible disciplinary practices, and an emphasis on the development of autonomy and self-sufficiency rather than acquiescence. The individualistic orientation in traditional Anglo culture, in which people's social behavior is primarily motivated by personal objectives, contrasts sharply with the collectivistic and familial orientation of Hispanic cultures. For a Hispanic, resettling on the United States mainland involves a change in social context that creates cultural conflict and exerts a push toward assimilation, including a shift from a collectivistic to an individualistic orientation and a loosening of family networks and bonds (Rogler 1994).

■ Asian Americans

Asian Americans have a number of racial physiognomic characteristics in common, but like Hispanics they originate from widely different ethnic groups (e.g., Chinese, Japanese, Korean, Vietnamese), which may differ among themselves almost to the same extent that each of them differs from the dominant culture in the United States. Even within a supposedly single ethnic group, such as the Chinese, there is broad variability depending on the regional and language backgrounds (e.g., Cantonese, Toishanese, Mandarin, Shanghainese, Taiwanese, Fookienese, and others) (Gaw 1982) or the literary and religious traditions that prevail (e.g., Confucianism, Taoism, or Buddhism among the Chinese [Gaw 1993] or Shintoism in Japan, to which external influences of Confucianism, Buddhism, and Christianity have been added over the centuries [Fujii et al. 1993]).

The stereotype of individuals descended from Asian cultures is that they are strongly hierarchical, exhibiting great deference and respect for the more highly educated and for those who achieve. Kinship bonds extend to distant relatives and in some cultures to religiously defined relationships (Araneta 1982). As a group, Asian Americans tend to be highly respectful of their elders. Disobedience to one's parents and resistance to authority are considered highly undesirable. Individually, there is an expectation to display a low level of affective expression, at least in public, and the overt expression of emotion, especially negative emotions, is frowned on.

■ Native Americans

Native Americans are another case in point. From the moment that European colonizers stepped on American soil, the observable differences between different Native American tribes were patent. There are approximately 550 federally recognized tribes and Alaska native villages, and a recognition of specific tribal or village origin is a key aspect of identity (Norton 1999). In general terms, Native Americans tend to rely on nonverbal communication (Canino and Spurlock 2000). Negative feelings are not openly expressed (Katz 1981). The culture emphasizes self-control, independence, and social responsibility (LaFromboise and Bigfoot 1988). Competition is discouraged and collaboration is valued. Allegiance to the family and the community at large at the expense of the self is fostered (Yates 1987). Parents tend to encourage their children's independence and to make them responsible for themselves from relatively early in life. Noninterfering parents may resist participation in their child's treatment and may come across to a clinician as uninvolved (Canino and Spurlock 2000; Yates 1987). Simultaneously, however, a high degree of social responsibility is expected, and personal gain is subservient to the improvement of the family or clan (Berlin 1986). Distress may be communicated by abnormal interpersonal relations rather than by a report of a feeling state, such as anxiety or depression (Norton 1999). Not caring about others has been noted to be a more serious indicator of depression than dysphoric mood (O'Nell 1996).

Conclusion

This chapter emphasizes the importance of drawing distinctions between the notions of culture, ethnicity, and race as characteristics of individuals and groups that are in many ways related, may overlap, and are often used interchangeably. An individual's self-perception, identity, and self-esteem are greatly influenced by the attitudes of the predominant or dominant society toward a particular racial, ethnic, or cultural group. Based on race, culture, and ethnicity, large numbers of individuals in the United States are relegated to minority status, and minority status usually—although not always—places these individuals at a societal disadvantage, with significant impact on self-esteem and identity.

Cultural formulations of psychopathology reflect widely divergent views, ranging from nihilism and a negation of the very existence of psychiatric diagnoses to the assignment of psychiatric diagnoses through literal applications of criteria in widely different settings without due consideration of the cultural nuances that have a bearing on psychopathology in the subjects being studied, evaluated, or treated. The major concern is the issue of misclassification, which might in turn lead to inappropriate labeling and inadequate therapy. Although there may be divergence in the ways that different cultures label disorders and psychiatric symptoms, when broadly defined, the major psychiatric syndromes and symptom clusters in Axis I of DSM-IV-TR, as well as the personality types delineated in Axis II, appear to exist in all ethnic, racial, and cultural groups. However, race, culture, and ethnicity undoubtedly influence the manifestations of psychopathology. They shape patterns of child rearing, styles of family and social interaction, social class assumptions, peer relations, societal standards, and individual personal cognitive styles and personality structures.

Recent diagnostic systems include systematic attempts to consider culture in the formulation of diagnosis. Before making diagnostic assessments and interventions, clinicians must consider the individual's cultural identification, possible cultural explanations of his or her presenting symptoms, and cultural factors present in the psychosocial environment; they must also assess the influence of cultural elements that are likely to affect the relationship between the patient and the clinician.

It is critical for clinical practitioners to be aware of some of the cultural patterns observed among different ethnic minorities in the United States and to become thoroughly familiar with the cultural assumptions of the patients they treat. This effort must not rely on stereotypical assumptions but must be done through a systematic inquiry carried out with each individual patient treated. Any delineation of the characteristic elements of a culture is a generalization that is subject to a great degree of individual variability; furthermore, there are within-group as well as between-group differences that need to be considered.

References

Achenbach T, Edelbrock C: Behavioral problems and competencies reported by parents of normal and disturbed children aged 4 through 16. Monogr Soc Res Child Dev 46(188):1–82, 1981

Achenbach TM, McConaughy SH, Howell CT: Child-adolescent behavioral and emotional problems: implications of cross-informant correlations for situational specificity. Psychol Bull 101:213–232, 1987

American Psychiatric Association: Diagnostic and Statistical Manual of Mental Disorders, 3rd Edition. Washington, DC, American Psychiatric Association, 1980

American Psychiatric Association: Diagnostic and Statistical Manual of Mental Disorders, 3rd Edition, Revised. Washington, DC, American Psychiatric Association, 1987

American Psychiatric Association: Diagnostic and Statistical Manual of Mental Disorders, 4th Edition. Washington, DC, American Psychiatric Association, 1994

American Psychiatric Association: Diagnostic and Statistical Manual of Mental Disorders, 4th Edition, Text Revision. Washington, DC, American Psychiatric Association, 2000

Araneta EG: Filipino Americans, in Cross-Cultural Psychiatry. Edited by Gaw AC. Littleton, MA, Wright-PSG, 1982, pp 55–68

Berlin IN: Psychopathology and its antecedents among American Indian adolescents, in Advances in Clinical Child Psychology. Edited by Lahey BB. New York, Plenum, 1986, pp 125–152

Berry JW, Trimble JB, Olmedo EL: Assessment of acculturation in field methods, in Field Methods in Cross-Cultural Research (Cross-Cultural Research and Methodology Series Vol 8). Edited by Lonner WJ, Berry JW. Beverly Hills, CA, Sage, 1986, pp 291–324

Bird H: Epidemiology of childhood disorders in a cross-cultural context. J Child Psychol Psychiatry 37:35–49, 1996

Burkey RM: Ethnic and Racial Groups: The Dynamics of Dominance. Menlo Park, CA, Cummings, 1978

Canino I, Spurlock J: Culturally Diverse Children and Adolescents: Assessment, Diagnosis and Treatment, 2nd Edition. New York, Guilford, 2000

de Groot A, Koot H, Verhulst FC: The cross-cultural generalizability of the CBCL cross-informant syndromes. Psychol Assess 6:225–230, 1994

Friedrich AH, Flannery DJ: The effects of ethnicity and acculturation on early adolescent delinquency. Journal of Child and Family Studies 4:69–87, 1995

Fujii JS, Fukushima SN, Yamamoto J: Psychiatric care of Japanese Americans, in Culture, Ethnicity, and Mental Illness. Edited by Gaw AC. Washington, DC, American Psychiatric Press, 1993, pp 305–345

Gaw AC: Chinese Americans, in Cross-Cultural Psychiatry. Edited by Gaw AC. Littleton, MA, Wright-PSG, 1982, pp 1–30

Gaw AC: Psychiatric care of Chinese Americans, in Culture, Ethnicity, and Mental Illness. Edited by Gaw AC. Washington, DC: American Psychiatric Press, 1993, pp 245–280

Giordano J: Ethnicity and Mental Health. New York, Institute of Pluralism and Group Identity, 1973

Hagan J: Structural Criminology. New Brunswick, NJ, Rutgers University Press, 1989

Hirschi T: Causes of Delinquency. Berkeley, University of California Press, 1969

Hofstede G: Culture's Consequences. Beverly Hills, CA, Sage, 1990

Katz P: Psychotherapy with native adolescents. Can J Psychiatry 26:455–459, 1981

Kessler RC, Price RH, Wortman CB: Social factors in psychopathology: stress, social support and coping processes. Annu Rev Psychol 36:531–572, 1985

Konner M: Contributions of the sociocultural sciences, 4.1, anthropology and psychiatry, in Comprehensive Textbook of Psychiatry, 6th Edition. Edited by Kaplan HI, Sadock BJ. Baltimore, MD, Williams & Wilkins, 1995, 337–354

LaFromboise TD, Bigfoot DS: Cultural and cognitive considerations in the prevention of American Indian adolescent suicide. J Adolesc 11:139–153, 1988

Lewis-Fernandez R, Kleinman A: Cultural psychiatry: theoretical, clinical, and research issues. Psychiatr Clin North Am 18:433–448, 1995

Marin G, Marin BV: Research With Hispanic Populations (Applied Social Research Methods Series, Vol 23). Newbury Park, CA, Sage, 1991

Murphy JM: Psychiatric labeling in cross-cultural perspective. Science 191:1019–1023, 1976

Norton DG: Black family life patterns: the development of self and cognitive development of black children, in The Psychosocial Development of Minority Group Children. Edited by Powell GJ. New York, Brunner/Mazel, 1983, pp 187–193

Norton IM: American Indians and mental health: issues in psychiatric assessment and diagnosis, in Cross Cultural Psychiatry. Edited by Herrera JM, Lawson WB, Sramek JJ. New York, Wiley, 1999, pp 77–85

Oetting ER, Beauvais F: Adolescent drug use: findings of national and local surveys. J Consult Clin Psychol 58:385–394, 1990

Oetting ER, Beauvais F: Orthogonal cultural identification theory: the cultural identification of minority adolescents. Int J Addict 25:655–685, 1990–1991

O'Nell TD: Disciplined Hearts: History, Identity and Depression in an American Indian Community. Berkeley, CA, University of California Press, 1996

Papajohn J, Spiegel J: Transition in Families. San Francisco, CA, Jossey-Bass, 1975

Patterson GR: Coercive Family Process. Eugene, OR, Castalia, 1982

Robins LN: Cross-cultural issues in diagnosis, in Search for a Common Language in Psychiatric Assessment. Edited by Hoppe SK, Holtzman WH. Austin, TX, WHO Collaborating Center, Hogg Foundation for Mental Health, 1994, pp 21–35

Robins L, McEvoy L: Conduct problems as predictors of substance abuse, in Straight and Devious Pathways from Childhood to Adulthood. Edited by Robins L, Rutter M. New York, Cambridge University Press, 1990

Rogler LH: International migrations: a framework for directing research Am Psychol 49:701–708, 1994

Rogler LH, Cortes DE, Malgady RG: Acculturation and mental health status among Hispanics. Am Psychol 46:585–597, 1991

Rotheram MJ, Phinney JS: Introduction: definitions and perspectives in the study of children's ethnic socialization, in Children's Ethnic Socialization: Pluralism and Development. Edited by Phinney JS, Rothram MJ. Newbury Park, CA, Sage, 1986

Sommers I, Fagan J, Baskin D: Sociocultural influences on the explanation of delinquency for P.R. youths. Hisp J Behav Sci 15:36–62, 1993

Spurlock J: Black Americans, in Cross-Cultural Psychiatry. Edited by Gaw AC. Littleton, MA, Wright-PSG, 1982, pp 163–178

Szapocznick J, Santiesteban D, Rio A, et al: Family effectiveness training: an intervention to prevent problem behaviors in Hispanic adolescents. Hisp J Behav Sci 11:4–27, 1989

Triandis HC, Marin G, Betancourt H, et al: Dimensions of familism among Hispanic and mainstream Navy recruits (Technical Report No 14). Champaign, University of Illinois Department of Psychology, 1982

Vega WA, Gil AG, Warheit GJ, et al: Acculturation and delinquent behavior among Cuban American adolescents: toward an empirical model. Am J Community Psychol 21:113–125, 1993

Verhulst FC, Achenbach TM: Empirically based assessment and taxonomy of psychopathology: cross-cultural applications. Eur Child Adolesc Psychiatry 4:61–76, 1995

Wakefield JC: DSM-IV: are we making diagnostic progress? Contemporary Psychology 11:646–652, 1996

Wilkinson D, King G: Conceptual and methodological issues in the use of race as a variable: policy implications. Milbank Q 65 (suppl 1):56–71, 1987

Wing JK: Case identification and risk prediction in psychiatric epidemiology: methodological issues, in Prevalence of Mental Disorders: Proceedings of the International Symposium on Psychiatric Epidemiology. Edited by Yeh EK, Rin H, Yeh CC, et al. Taipei, Republic of China Department of Health, 1985, pp 31–55

World Health Organization: The International Pilot Study of Schizophrenia, Vol 1. Geneva, World Health Organization, 1973

World Health Organization: International Classification of Diseases, 9th Revision. Geneva, World Health Organization, 1977

World Health Organization: ICD-10, The ICD-10 Classification of Mental and Behavioural Disorders: Diagnostic Criteria for Research. Geneva, World Health Organization, 1993

Yates A: Current status and future directions of research on the American Indian child. Am J Psychiatry 144:1135–1142, 1987

Economic Issues in Child and Adolescent Psychiatry

Robert K. Schreter, M.D.

In the mid-1980s, spiraling health care costs in the United States reached $750 billion annually, consuming 14% of the gross domestic product. Payers for this care (employers, government, and consumers) began to demand cost containment and accountability (Schreter et al. 1994). This provided an opportunity to for-profit managed care enterprises. These organizations entered the marketplace using cost-cutting strategies to limit covered conditions and treatments, reduce the units of service, decrease the fees paid for these services, and ration care under the pressure of risk-sharing arrangements.

During much of the 1990s, health care expenditures stabilized. But by the year 2000, health care costs resumed their 10% escalation, reaching an annual cost of $1 trillion. All the constituents in the health care marketplace (consumers, employers, government, insurers, physicians, and the uninsured) voiced their discontent with the cost and quality of health care and demanded change. To anticipate the transformations that will take place in child mental health care in response to these demands, it is useful to examine the payers who finance most of the care.

Government-Funded Programs

The public sector pays for health care through Medicare, Medicaid, the Indian Health Service, and the Department of Veterans Affairs at the federal level; through Medicaid, public hospitals, and grants at the state level; and through local allotments (Sharfstein et al. 1993). Approximately 28% of health care costs are borne by the federal government, 28% are borne by state and local governments, and 44% are borne by private payers and insurers (Pruitt and Kiser 1998).

Legislation passed in 1965—including Medicare, Medicaid, and the Community Mental Health Centers Act (1963)—positioned the federal government as the major source of funding for mental health care. Medicare is a form of universal health coverage for all people age 65 and over who are eligible for Social Security and for those under 65 who have been receiving Social Security disability payments for at least 2 years (Stolene and Sharfstein 1996). States can design their own programs under broad federal guidelines and are required to match federal contributions. All eligible people are enrolled in Part A (hospital insurance) and may voluntarily enroll in Part B (supplemental medical insurance) by paying a premium deducted from their Social Security payment (Sharfstein et al. 1995). Medicaid, enacted with the Medicare program in 1965, is a joint federal and state program to cover the costs of care for indigent patients. Although there are mandatory services (mandates) under Medicaid, each state is permitted to determine eligibility requirements (as a percentage of the federally recognized poverty level) and to expand the menu of services beyond the federal mandates. The Community Mental Health Centers Act provided seed money to support the development of a broad range of community-based services to be made available to eligible individuals within a catchment area (a circumscribed geographic area). Importantly, the following five services were expected to be part of each proposal: inpatient services, outpatient services, day treatment, emergency services, and consultation and education services. Thus, the Community Mental Health Centers Act set in motion the development of the continuum of care that has been further expanded in the era of managed care. The Child and Adolescent Service Systems Program was created at the national level to help each state develop and operationalize its own comprehensive continuum of care with public dollars.

Government also funds mental health services for children and adolescents as the insurer/protector of last resort through its support of state mental health programs and public hospitals. These facilities operate as the "safety net" that can catch the uninsured and underinsured, including children with severe emotional disturbance and their parents with serious mental illness.

Employer-Sponsored Insurance

The purpose of casualty insurance is to protect against catastrophic losses. Insurers offer coverage to large populations of patients for a fixed premium. The size of the premium is based on the anticipated risk or amount the insurer predicts it will have to pay out for the care of the lives covered under the program. When the covered population is large, the insurer is able to spread the anticipated risk over many individuals (including those who will not collect on their benefit), thereby spreading the risk and reducing the cost to individual enrollees and families. When the covered population is small or contains an unusual number of high utilizers of expensive mental health services, the few costly cases can consume all of the available dollars. It is possible to protect against this with risk adjustments, rates that take into account the health and previous experience of the covered population. Adverse selection is said to occur when a large number of individuals who consume services collect in a single plan, raising costs so high that the plan becomes unaffordable.

Private employer–sponsored health insurance was born in 1929 in Baylor, Texas, when 1,500 schoolteachers started an enterprise that grew into Blue Cross, which paid for hospital costs. Later, Blue Shield was created to pay for professional fees. Especially after World War II, health insurance became inextricably associated with employment when employees surrendered wage increases in exchange for health care coverage during labor negotiations. After 1954, when the federal government permitted this fringe benefit to escape taxation, union and management negotiators were encouraged to continue to include health care benefits as an employer obligation.

Powerful economic forces have converged to make the cost of health insurance greater than most employers and employees are willing to pay. When health insurance was designed to protect against catastrophic events (high cost, long term), mental health services were not included as covered benefits. Over time, employees demanded first-dollar, full-dollar coverage that decreased their out-of-pocket costs and removed any disincentive to utilize health services. The deinstitutionalization movement, which moved patients with chronic mental illnesses out of state-supported custodial-care hospitals further increased health care costs. Blue Cross/Blue Shield as well as other insurers responded to this movement of patients into the community by including mental health coverage for inpatient and outpatient services in its benefit packages. As Barton (1966) observed, "service follows the dollars," and general hospitals began to open their own inpatient psychiatric units to capture this newly available revenue stream. Because these new benefit packages reimbursed for inpatient care at a much higher level than for outpatient services, they unintentionally favored the use of this much more expensive treatment option. With no one involved in the system responsible for containing costs, an inflationary spiral ensued.

One of the first efforts by the insurance industry to contain costs was to introduce "inside limits" into the behavioral health benefit. This was achieved by reducing coverage for mental health services compared with medical or surgical care. For example, by covering fewer conditions, requiring consumers of behavioral health care to pay more of the initial cost of the care (higher deductible) and a greater percentage of the cost of the care (higher co-payment), dollars could be saved. Additional inside limits included capping the numbers of outpatient visits and inpatient days per episode and lifetime, and implementing other annual and lifetime maximum benefits. The result is that, by tradition, mental health services have been viewed as different from overall health care and are reimbursed at a lower rate.

During the 1980s, the cost of health insurance escalated 10% per year. A disproportionate amount of this escalation was for mental health and substance services, which rose 32.4% between 1986 and 1988, compared with a 20.1% increase for all health care (Frank et al. 1991). Importantly, child and adolescent services accounted for 72% of this increase, placing the psychiatric benefit and child and adolescent services in jeopardy. When inside limits proved inadequate to contain costs, payers turned to managed care and carve-out managed behavioral health organizations.

Managed Care

The health maintenance organization (HMO) is the prototype managed care organization (MCO). HMOs provide for the total health and mental health care of large populations of individuals, of whom only some will become patients, for a predetermined amount of money paid prospectively in monthly installments over a calendar year. This fixed payment, or capitation, is paid on a per-member per-month basis or as a lump-sum payment on referral to cover the cost of an episode of care (case rate). These two elements—the population-based perspective and prospective payment—are two hallmarks of managed care. Because the MCO must operate under a global budget, it must shepherd limited resources to cover all illness arising in the covered population without running out of money by the end of the year.

MCOs and managed behavioral health organizations (MBHOs) employ a range of approaches to contain costs. One strategy is to reduce access and utilization of services. Access to care can be restricted by placing gatekeepers between patients and specialty services to limit referrals. Plans can limit utilization by requiring precertification or concurrent review of care and can deny care for not meeting the plan's criteria for medical necessity.

A second approach to cost containment is to decrease the costs of care. Patients can be channeled to the least expensive providers (social workers and psychologists instead of child psychiatrists). Medical and counseling functions can be split into independent services, with the more expensive child psychiatrist permitted only 15-minute medication management checks. Patients can be referred only to the least expensive level of care (partial hospital or intensive outpatient programs instead of acute inpatient facilities). MCOs aggressively negotiate discounted fees with facilities and practitioners. Practitioners and facilities must routinely agree to 30%–50% discounts in many localities to receive managed care referrals. Practitioners and facilities that agree to accept discounted

rates are organized into preferred provider panels and networks. Patients pay limited co-payments when they utilize these preferred providers but pay higher out-of-pocket costs when they exercise the right to choose out-of-network providers. Recently, MCOs have been unable to sustain this downward pressure on pricing and have become more reliant on provider profiling, the auditing of provider performance (utilization of services tracked in inpatient days, outpatient services, and the cost of an episode of care by age and diagnosis).

A third approach by MCOs to contain costs relies on reversing the financial incentives by placing physicians and institutions at financial risk for the cost of the services they provide. This is achieved by replacing retrospective fee-for-service reimbursement with various forms of prospective payment. A report by the Hay Group (1999) revealed that psychiatry has been more profoundly affected by this and other managed care strategies than any other branch of medicine. This study showed that between 1988 and 1998, the amount of money spent on mental health services had decreased by 54% compared with a decrease of 7% for all other medical specialties.

Social Services

Title XX of the Social Securities Act channels federal dollars to the states to provide for children in need of protection who would be denied services as a consequence of poverty. In *Making Sense of Federal Dollars*, De-Woody (1994) reports that Title XX dollars are used for the following purposes:

- To achieve or maintain economic support to prevent, reduce, or eliminate dependency
- To prevent or remedy neglect, abuse, or exploitation of children and adults who are unable to protect their own interests or to preserve, rehabilitate, or reunite families
- To prevent or reduce inappropriate institutional care by providing for community-based care, home-based care, or other forms of less-intensive services
- To secure referral or admission for institutional care when other forms of care are not appropriate, or to provide services to individuals in institutions

Although Title XX dollars serve a large number of children with a mental health diagnosis, the funds do not routinely support the actual cost of their care in the mental health system. When they are used to support mental health care, these funds are often used to pay for staff members working with abused or neglected youths or adults; to support room, board, and foster care services for children and adolescents; or to treat parents and families in the service of reunification.

Juvenile Justice

Departments of juvenile justice are given funds earmarked for the mental health needs of children in detention in penal facilities or other court-ordered placements. Most of these dollars are spent outside of the correctional system to contract for beds and placement in residential treatment centers under subcontract arrangements. An examination of the roles of the department of juvenile justice, the departments of social services, and the department of mental health in each state reveal that all three often provide for the care of the same children, who move back and forth among all three systems. Interestingly, a child in a residential treatment center can have some days covered by one agency and some days and services covered by another. The department of juvenile justice provides for children only during the period of their detention.

Education

Federal legislation mandates that each school system address the academic and emotional needs of its students. Federal dollars flow to the states and then to each board of education to fund mainstream and special education. Each jurisdiction combines these dollars with funds from other sources to support their initiatives—hire tutors or build a freestanding facility for children with severe emotional disturbance. Special-education dollars address the needs not only of children with severe emotional disturbance but also of those with developmental disabilities, learning disabilities, and physical impairments. Federal legislation mandates minimal standards that each school system must follow. However, how each school interprets these standards is crucial, and the range of services differs from jurisdiction to jurisdiction.

An interesting new trend is the movement of behavioral health care out of the child psychiatrist's office and into the school. In addition to counseling offered by school counselors, innovative programs in prevention, dealing with violence, screening for treatable conditions, and teacher education are being developed. Health suites are being expanded to provide onsite psychiatric evaluation, crisis intervention, psychotropic medication, and family treatment. Educational offerings for students now include programs in substance abuse awareness and family planning.

Social Security Disability

Supplemental Security Income (SSI) goes to families of children who are developmentally impaired or disabled, including children with severe emotional disturbance, mental retardation, autism, pervasive developmental disorder, and, more recently, attention-deficit/hyperactivity disorder. To receive support, children and adolescents must qualify according to age-specific criteria that define the nature of the disability. Typically, a physician performs an examination, on the basis of which a Social Security administrator determines the percentage of the child's disability. This disability is translated into monthly payments made to the child's family—roughly between $350 and $500 per month in many localities. Before age 18, SSI payments go to parents. Theoretically, these payments are intended to compensate parents for the time away from work and the additional costs associated with addressing their child's special needs.

Are Our Systems Broken?

Six constituents dominate the health care marketplace: consumers, employers, government, insurers, physicians, and the uninsured. Each participant brings different expectations and dissatisfactions, but all agree that the current system is in need of reform.

■ Consumers

Consumers want unencumbered access to high-quality service, freedom to choose their providers, a minimum of administrative hassle, and little out-of-pocket expense. Too often these expectations go unmet. Patients who seek services in the private sector through their employer-sponsored plans find access to care blocked by managed care cost-containment strategies. Patients seeking care financed under public support experience an additional set of problems in gaining access to care. When states turned to Managed Medicaid to contain costs, they began to dismantle their community mental health and state hospital systems, which had previously functioned as the safety net. When patients do not qualify for private health care benefits or exhaust their benefits and convert to state-funded support, they too often discover that the safety net no longer exists.

For both private and public systems of care, underfunding is a huge problem. In the private sector before the emergence of managed care, mental health services accounted for an estimated 6% of total health care expenditures. Currently, the proportion of the health care dollar devoted to mental health services has decreased to approximately 3% (Hay Group 1999). Similarly, states and municipalities are no longer willing and able to maintain government spending at levels adequate to meet current needs. Because of this, programs have been discontinued and hospitals and systems have been closed.

As a consequence of this underfunding, neither private nor public systems have been able to adequately address some of the unique needs of children that distinguish them from adult patients. Child cases are more likely to be complex because of the confounding issues arising from their dependence, family disorganization, and educational status. Children routinely require longer inpatient stays and more often need foster and residential placements at the time of discharge. Because there is rarely risk adjustment in the insurance premiums, the special needs of these children go unmet because there are no additional funds available for their care. To obtain this necessary care, families sometimes turn their children with the most serious conditions over to the state (i.e., declare them one-person households) so they can qualify for inpatient or residential care through departments of mental health or other government-sponsored programs.

Finally, the absence of parity raises the same barriers to children who need behavioral health services as it does to adults. Parity refers to the situation in which benefits, services, and reimbursement for mental health and substance abuse are identical to those in all other areas of health care. The existence of inside limits and the "carve-out" nature of behavioral health care have led to greater restrictions on services and a greater percentage of the cost of care being shifted to patients and their families.

■ Employers

Employers are looking to alter or shed their role as the middleman in employee health care. Under the current system, employers hire consulting firms, which design health benefit packages. Insurers and health plans are invited to bid against each other for the right to serve the employee population. This arrangement initially reversed the inflationary rise in health care costs; in one year it actually produced savings that dropped directly to the corporate bottom line. But managed care is no longer generating savings. This undermines the willingness of employers to deal with the negative consequences of providing health care as an employee benefit. One negative consequence of employer-provided health care plans is that companies have to defend themselves against their employees' complaints of inadequate access, denial of care, and administrative lapses such as failure to be timely or accurate in patient reimbursement or provider payments.

Another negative consequence that employers are eager to avoid is increased risk of involvement in the medicolegal confrontations that are working their way through the courts. Presently, MCOs are protected by the so-called ERISA [Employee Retirement Income Security Act] preemption, which prevents them from being held liable for untoward medical consequences. Employers are very much aware of the changing mood of state legislators and the decisions by the courts to weaken this protection. These employers fear that they will be forced to share responsibility with their MCO partners, who may claim that they are only doing what the employers hired them to do. Employers are also apprehensive about being caught in the net thrown by plaintiffs' attorneys, who are modeling HMO class action suits on their successful assault on the tobacco industry.

■ Government

Government participates in health care in two important ways, as purchaser and as regulator/policymaker. In an effort to make their diminishing funds go as far as possible, governments have turned to MCOs to manage Medicare and Medicaid dollars. Like private-sector payers, government purchasers are beset by consumer complaints about lack of access and less-than-adequate quality.

Furthermore, having dismantled the safety net, governments find themselves in a vulnerable position. They would be unable to gear back up quickly enough to address patient needs should managed care abandon public-sector child and adolescent mental health the way it has left Managed Medicare. The result is that government has nowhere else to turn but to managed care despite its concerns about the quality of its product and fear of a managed care pullout.

Governments would appear to have more leverage than private purchasers in their dealings with MCOs and MBHOs because of their ability to set policy and enact legislative mandates about what services are covered. However, experience has proved that mandates are not always effective. HMOs have protection from some mandates, self-insured companies are not bound by them, and the uninsured have no coverage at all.

■ Insurers

In health care, the term *insurer* can be used to describe traditional indemnity carriers (e.g., Aetna and Cigna), MCOs when they accept risk (e.g., United Health Care and Kaiser), and health plans (e.g., Blue Cross/Blue Shield). Commercial insurers are in the business of calculating risks, predicting costs, and designing and selling products that provide them with profit. As a consequence of the merger and acquisition frenzy of the 1990s, the boundaries between insurer and provider have become blurred, and many insurers find themselves providing mental health services through a variety of contractual arrangements. When these various forms of insurer/MCO/MBHO relationships were profitable and public outcry was muted, insurers and their partners were content. However, the financial reversals and public protest against managed care are forcing these conservative corporate giants to reconsider the strategy of straying so far from their core business.

Most important, insurers are losing money in these health care ventures. In addition, their reputations and signature insurance products are being tainted by the bad public relations generated by their own health care ventures and those of their partner MCOs and MBHOs. Finally, as cost, competition, and other pressures increase, insurers sometimes suspect that their best interests are being sacrificed to the self-interest of their health care partners.

■ Physicians

The new health care marketplace has been difficult for physicians, encouraging them to abandon both the private and public managed care sectors. Increasing numbers of psychiatrists are refusing to participate in private managed networks, which require them to discount their fees by as much as 30%–50%. Child and adolescent psychiatrists, because of their short supply relative to demand, are able to prosper by taking only full-fee, carriage-trade patients. Physician opt-out is particularly damaging to MCOs because their inadequate networks place them in violation of their contractual obligation to the payer.

The withdrawal from private managed care mirrors child psychiatry's earlier withdrawal from the public sector, where fee discounts can approach 50%–60% in some localities. And salaries in public mental health systems are often far below those in other sectors of the marketplace, discouraging child and adolescent psychiatrists from participating as salaried employees.

Child and adolescent psychiatrists are often placed at a disadvantage because neither public nor private systems recognize or reimburse for the additional costs of treating children. These costs are associated with the need to consult with parents, pediatricians, teachers, and other systems of care. Consultation and liaison are especially important for children and adolescents because these patients often require multimodal services.

■ The Uninsured

There are an estimated 42–45 million uninsured Americans, of whom 60% are employed full-time or part-time in occupations or with companies that do not include health care as a benefit. Forty percent of these uninsured are children. Pressure is building in many sectors of the marketplace and in many constituencies to examine the question of whether health care is a right or a privilege and to address this inequality in access to adequate health care for every citizen of the United States.

Proposed Solutions:
If It's Broken, Fix It

With so many players in the health care marketplace calling for reform, it is reasonable to anticipate fundamental change. The solutions that have been proposed fall into three main categories: reform of health care financing, redesign of clinical care and clinical services, and changes in structures and systems.

■ Health Care Financing Reform

Single Payer

Single-payer health care financing is essentially an expansion of Medicare. In this model, a single government entity would be responsible for paying for all health care services: hospital/facility and professional services. Intermediaries may continue to exist to handle administrative aspects of the system as in the current Medicare plan. Single-payer financing offers the opportunity to spread risk over a large population, to expand coverage to include many of the uninsured, and to reduce administrative overhead. It would permit a greater percentage of the premium dollar to be devoted to clinical care because of administrative savings and the elimination of corporate profit as a cost. Administrative overhead can now consume up to 15% or more of each dollar spent on health care. Under single-payer financing, payment for health care would shift from premium dollars to tax dollars.

Most proposals for single-payer financing involve replacing business-sponsored private health plans as well as public-sector insurance. The benefit package would be modeled on typical employer packages and care would be managed. A recent study conducted for the State of Vermont concluded, "the Single Payer model would cover all Vermont residents, including the estimated 51,390 uninsured persons in the state, while actually reducing total health spending in Vermont by $118.1 million in 2001 (i.e., 5%)" (Sheils and Haught 2001).

Defined-Contribution Health Plan

In the defined-contribution health plan (DCHP) arrangement, the employer defines or caps the contribution it is willing to make toward the cost of an employee's health benefit. The employee is responsible for selecting a mix of health insurance options and other employee benefits to meet his or her needs. The employer may either assemble various health care plan options from which the employee may choose or contract with an outside vendor who assembles these options and assists the employee directly. The employer contribution is made at the beginning of each year on

a "use it or lose it" basis and is not carried over into the next year. Under DCHP, the employer ceases to be the payer and shifts the risks and responsibilities to the employee.

Medical Savings Account

Medical savings accounts offer contributors the opportunity to put money aside in a tax-sheltered account to be drawn on in time of need. Because these accounts will be small, especially in the beginning, contributors are expected to purchase catastrophic coverage with a high deductible. Unlike the DCHP, money in medical savings accounts carries over from year to year, is portable, and can increase in value depending on investment options. Spending is entirely discretionary and can be directed into or out of the benefit plan. One risk associated with medical savings accounts is that the young and healthy are the least likely to participate, which would create distortions in the risk pool.

Subcapitation for Selected Populations

Patients with special needs are often the least well served in the existing health care system. Some of these patients are identified by the nature or severity of their illness—for example, severe emotional disturbance or mental retardation. Others are grouped by characteristics such as age or circumstance, for example, preschool children of depressed or psychotic mothers or adolescents residing in a center city. Creative thinkers have proposed arrangements in which providers such as behavioral group practices, hospital systems, or academic medical centers carve out these defined populations and care for them on a capitated basis. Recognizing the dangers involved in these kinds of financial arrangements, providers must be certain that they have adequate actuarial and contractual protections.

■ Clinical Care and Clinical Services Redesign

The Continuum of Care

Until the 1980s, insurers reimbursed only for inpatient care and outpatient services, creating a perverse incentive to utilize only these two levels of care. The earliest efforts at cost containment by managed care targeted hospital services because of their great cost relative to outpatient care.

Clinicians have responded by developing a continuum of care with a range of services midway between acute inpatient and traditional outpatient services (Schreter et al. 1997). Hospitals and entrepreneurial physicians have created 3-day admission units, subacute facilities, group homes and specialized foster placements, full- and half-day treatment settings, therapeutic schools, community-based ambulatory teams, delivery of services in schools, and visiting nurse programs. Insurers have been willing to pay for these treatment alternatives because they are less expensive. These programs make it possible to discharge patients "quicker and sicker" and divert patients from hospitals into lower levels of care.

Treatment Guidelines

Payers for care recognize that relying on independent clinical decision making results in care that is random in the selection of treatment options, subject to wide regional variations in cost and practice pattern, and unreliable for predicting outcome. Payers, especially those large enough to be responsible for people scattered over wide geographic areas, now insist on the same standardization from health care providers that they expect from all other vendors from whom they purchase a product. This standardization is possible only through the application of guidelines. Ideally these guidelines should be based on best practice shown to reduce hospitalization, prevent relapse, and promote wellness—all of which translate into decreased cost. Existing treatment guidelines represent the consensus of experts from the field. Treatment guidelines of the future will be informed by actual data that compare the efficacy of treatment alternatives.

Disease Management

The Disease Management Association of America defines its product as "a system of coordinated health care interventions and communications for populations with conditions in which self care efforts are significant." The programs are designed to promote wellness by managing risk in patients and in the population to improve outcome in quality and cost of health care. These goals are achieved through the following means:

- Early detection of vulnerable or affected individuals
- Reliance on evidence-based practice guidelines

- Close collaboration with physicians and support services
- Patient education to empower self-management
- Process and outcomes measurement, evaluation, and management
- Use of a routine reporting/feedback loop (may include communication with patient, physician, health plan, school, other service providers, and support agencies)

Case Management

Future Health Corporation of Baltimore, Maryland, defines case management as "a holistic collaborative process which assesses, plans, implements, coordinates, monitors, and evaluates the options and services required to meet an individual's needs." The case manager relies on communication and the organization of appropriate resources to empower the patient to achieve positive outcomes in health, quality of care, and cost. Future Health identifies six activities that are essential for quality case management:

1. Assess data about the patient's physical, psychological, sociocultural, cognitive, developmental, and functional abilities to identify individual needs.
2. Create an individualized treatment plan including specific objectives, goals, and actions designed to meet the patient's needs.
3. Implement specific case-management activities and/or interventions that will lead to accomplishing the goals set forth in the care plan.
4. Coordinate the resources necessary to accomplish these goals set forth in a case-management plan.
5. Monitor activities and services from all involved sources to enable the case manager to determine the plan's effectiveness.
6. Evaluate the plan's effectiveness in reaching the stated outcomes and goals and modify the plan as appropriate.

At its best, case management coordinates care over the entire clinical and service continuum, including the home, workplace, hospital, ambulatory facility, and community. Case managers routinely interact with all relevant components of the child's or adolescent's health care system such as third-party payers, family members, employers, insurers, teachers, health care providers, and others in the patient's support system. Clinicians and health care planners have long been aware that 20% of patients consume 80% of health care dollars (Patterson 1994). Forward-thinking systems have focused their case-management services on these high-risk, high-cost patients.

Disease Prevention and Wellness

Until recently, cost-containment measures focused exclusively on treating illness. This approach can contribute only so much to overall public health and cost containment in health care. Clinicians and budget designers may derive a greater long-term benefit from a focus on wellness and prevention (Schreter 1998). One set of wellness programs focuses on empowering patients to eliminate behaviors that jeopardize their health, such as smoking, abuse of alcohol and other substances, and physical and sexual abuse of children. Each of these behaviors contributes significantly to the prevalence of psychiatric disorder and care costs in America. Another set of programs can be designed to help individuals, who are currently in good health, to make lifestyle choices that prolong their well-being. Such wellness interventions might include healthy diets, stress management workshops, violence prevention programs, and Head Start programs for young children. For-profit managed care companies are reluctant to invest in these programs because it can take 5 years to reap rewards and their contracts often expire in 2 or 3 years.

■ Structural and Systems Changes

Integration of Services and Fusing of Funds

The recent managed care experiment has proved that it is possible to focus on a limited area of health care costs, make them the object of intense cost-cutting efforts, and reduce expenditures in the target area. The carve-out approach has unintended costs and consequences that result from its reliance on fragmentation. Employers are discovering that their employees adapt to decreased reimbursement for medical services by shifting costs to workers' compensation and disability insurance. Decreased spending on the medical side is contributing to greater absenteeism and reduced performance of workers who attend their job but perform below optimal levels. Importantly, this increased absenteeism and decreased performance can result from illness affecting family members as well as the employee, such as in the cases of parents of inadequately treat-

ed asthmatic or academically underachieving children. Employers are beginning to recognize the cost benefit to them of highly integrated programs that coordinate rather than fragment the variety of services they provide as employee benefits. These services include medical benefits, workers' compensation, short- and long-term disability, employee-assistance programs, wellness initiatives, coverage for pharmaceuticals, and risk management, which currently exist in independent silos.

A similar opportunity exists with child and adolescent services in the public sector (Kiser et al. 2001). The lack of integration among the different funding sources, services, and systems contributes to gaps, duplications, and restricted access when money is available but is in the wrong pot. The failure to integrate dollars and services also leads to cost shifting. For example, large numbers of psychiatrically ill and substance-abusing children and adolescents have been shifted, along with the cost of their care, from the mental health sector to the courts, jails, and juvenile justice system.

Highly Focused Medical Enterprises

Evidence is mounting in support of the claim that higher-quality care at lower cost with fewer complications can be delivered in highly focused, intense medical enterprises. Superiority in cost and outcome that results from intensity has been documented with treatment delivered by specialists compared with generalists (Alsever 1995), with integrated teams of clinicians instead of independent providers (Levetan et al. 1995), with units dedicated to the treatment of single conditions rather than scattered hospital beds (Advisory Board 1997a), and even within the hospitals devoted to a single service (Heskett 1992).

Shouldice Hospital in Toronto, Canada, offers an example of the relationship between intensity and outcome in surgical care (Advisory Board 1997b). This hospital provides only hernia repairs at rates of 7,000/year and 600/surgeon, compared with the U.S. hospital rate of 150/year and typically 30/surgeon. Shouldice can boast infection rates that are only 17% and recurrence rates that are only 8% of those in the typical hospital program at a comparative cost of approximately 50% of its competitors. The organization of inpatient and outpatient delivery systems into "focused factories" also offers advantages in administrative efficiency and the opportunity to benefit from economies of scale. In her book *Market Driven Health Care: Who*

Wins, Who Loses in the Transformation of America's Largest Service Industry, Harvard Business School professor Regina Herzlinger predicts that health care will go the way of other business sectors, in which highly sophisticated companies (e.g., Staples, Toys "R" Us, Home Depot) gained market dominance through mastery of a single niche, concentration on a specific product, and an unrelenting emphasis on consistency, reliability, low cost, and customer satisfaction (Herzlinger 1997).

Rather than generalists, focused health care factories will likely turn to intensivists who will practice as individuals and in teams in inpatient and outpatient settings. This will permit them to benefit from repetition and from an infrastructure that supports best practices.

Outcomes Data Research

As the cost of health care increases, payers are demanding accountability for clinical outcomes and costs. Currently, MCOs assess hospital care by tracking lengths of stay by diagnosis, readmission rates in the first 30 days after discharge, and suicide rates per thousand covered lives. Organizing clinical care around treatment guidelines makes it possible to actually compare the clinical outcomes of different treatment approaches—which treatments prove more effective for which patients in the hands of which providers in both the short term and the long term. Tracking outcome by monitoring meaningful measures of clinical performance will take us a step closer to actual evidence-based health care.

Continuous Quality Improvement

Continuous quality improvement (CQI) programs attempt to support quality by identifying specific indicators, which are monitored over time. The results are then fed back into the system to promote ongoing quality enhancement. A recent report by the Institute of Medicine (2000) that between 44,000 and 98,000 Americans die unnecessarily in hospitals each year because of medical errors offers an interesting lesson in CQI. At present, physicians and hospitals remain quite secretive about possible errors and systems failures, fearing damage to their reputations and malpractice suits. Applying a CQI approach to this situation would have physicians reporting these errors and deaths to an organization resembling the Federal Aeronautics Administration, which would promise them immunity from prosecution in exchange for access to the information about untoward occurrences. These data could then be studied to isolate causes and trends. A corrective action would be created and implemented. Finally, the situation would be reevaluated to determine whether the corrective action and systems reengineering led to a genuine quality improvement.

Creation of an Equitable System for Allocating Resources

The robust epidemiology of mental health disorders guarantees that there will be more illness than resources made available to treat all affected individuals without regard to cost. The Epidemiologic Catchment Area study revealed that 20% of Americans, including children and adolescents, had a diagnosable psychiatric disorder that required treatment in any given year (Regier et al. 1993). It was estimated that only 20% of these individuals received care. This high demand exists over the entire spectrum of health care. The needs and expectations of an aging population; the occurrence of severe disorders earlier in childhood and adolescence; and the availability of ever newer and more expensive technologies, services, and medicines ensure that it will not be possible to avoid the challenge of selecting from among competing social claims and claimants. The name for this process may change to avoid the baggage associated with "managed care" and "rationed care," but the need to prioritize and allocate will persist. In fact, two prominent health care economists, Reinhardt and Enthoven, have recommended the establishment of a politically independent commission modeled on the Federal Reserve Board that would evaluate medical treatments and decide which costs outweigh the benefits (Weinsline 2001).

Conclusion

Delivering health care, allocating health care resources, and designing the funding mechanisms to support this care should be viewed as an evolutionary process. No one can say with confidence where health care is heading. Some of the approaches reviewed in this chapter will likely shape the next generation of health care. In this next phase, success will most likely come to systems that manage care, not dollars, with interventions supported by evidence of superior outcome and quality.

References

The Advisory Board: Cost Re-engineering Report. Washington, DC, The Advisory Board, 1997a

The Advisory Board: Culture of Intensity: Emergence of a Focused Medical Enterprise. Washington, DC, The Advisory Board, 1997b, p 29

Alsever R: Specialists versus primary care: not an easy question. Physician Executive 21:39–41, 995

Barton WE: Trends in community mental health programs. Hosp Community Psychiatry 17:253–258, 1966

Community Mental Health Centers Construction Act of 1963 (Publ Law 88-164)

DeWoody M: Making sense of federal dollars: a funding guide for social service providers. Washington, DC, Child Welfare League of America, 1994

Frank RG, Salkever DS, Sharfstein SS: A new look at rising mental health insurance costs. Health Aff (Millwood) 10:116–123, 1991

Hay Group: Health care plan design and cost trends: 1988 through 1998. Report prepared for the National Association of Health Systems and the Association of Behavioral Group Practices. Arlington, VA, Hay Group, 1999

Herzlinger RE: Market-Driven Health Care: Who Wins, Who Loses in the Transformation of America's Largest Service Industry. Reading, MA, Addison-Wesley, 1997

Heskett J: Shouldice Hospital Limited, in Creating New Health Care Ventures: The Role of Management. Edited by Herzlinger RE. Gaithersburg, MD, Aspen, 1992, p 392

Institute of Medicine Committee on Quality of Health Care in America: To Err Is Human: Building a Safer Health System. Edited by Kohn LT, Corrigan JM, Donaldson MS. Washington, DC, National Academy Press, 2000

Kiser LJ, Lefkowitz PM, Kennedy LL: The Integrated Behavioral Continuum: Theory and Practice. Washington, DC, American Psychiatric Press, 2001

Levetan CS, Salas JR, Wilets IF, et al: Impact of endocrine and diabetes team consultation on hospital length of stay for patients with diabetes. Am J Med 99:22–28, 1995

Patterson DY: Outpatient services, in Allies and Adversaries: The Impact of Managed Care on Mental Health Services. Edited by Schreter RK, Sharfstein SS, Schreter LA. Washington, DC, American Psychiatric Press, 1994, pp 51–60

Pruitt DB, Kiser LJ: Health insurance and child/adolescent psychiatry, in Handbook of Child and Adolescent Psychiatry. Edited by Noshpitz JD, Adams P, Bleiberg E. New York, Wiley, 1998, pp 485–491

Regier DA, Narroe WE, Rae DS, et al: The defacto US mental and addictive disorders service system. Epidemiologic Catchment Area prospective 1-year prevalence rates of disorders and services. Arch Gen Psychiatry 50:85–94, 1993

Schreter RK: Uncertain market opens doors for new strategies in promoting wellness. Psychiatric Practice and Managed Care Newsletter 4, 1998

Schreter RK, Sharfstein SS, Schreter CA: Allies and Adversaries: The Impact of Managed Care on Mental Health Services. Washington, DC, American Psychiatric Press, 1994

Schreter RK, Sharfstein SS, Schreter CA: Managing Care, Not Dollars: The Continuum of Mental Health Services. Washington, DC, American Psychiatric Press, 1997

Sharfstein SS, Stoline AM, Goldman HH: Psychiatric care and health insurance reform. Am J Psychiatry 150:7–18, 1993

Sharfstein SS, Webb WL, Stoline AM: Economics of psychiatry, in Comprehensive Textbook of Psychiatry/VI. Edited by Kaplan HI, Sadock BJ. Baltimore, MD, Williams & Wilkins, 1995, pp 2677–2689

Sheils JF, Haught RA: Analysis of the cost and impact of universal health care coverage under a single payer model for the state of Vermont. Report prepared for the Vermont HRSA State Planning Grant, Office of Vermont Health Access. August 28, 2001. Vermont Government Web site, http://www.dsw.state.vt.us/districts/ovha/AnalysisoftheCosts.pdf. Accessed June 16, 2003

Stoline AM, Sharfstein SS: Funding the continuum of care: a rational social policy for the care and support of persons with schizophrenia, in Handbook of Mental Health Economics and Health Policy, Vol 1: Schizophrenia. Edited by Moscarelli M, Rupp A, Sartorius N. New York, Wiley, 1996, pp 485–492

Weinsline M: Curbing the high cost of health. New York Times, July 29, 2001, p 5

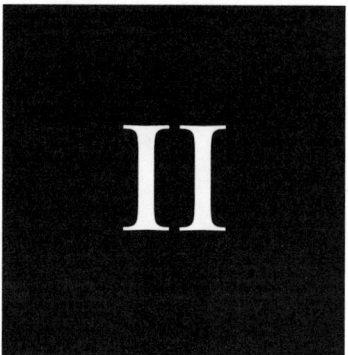

Assessment and Diagnosis

Classification of Child and Adolescent Psychiatric Disorders

Jerry M. Wiener, M.D.
Mina K. Dulcan, M.D.

Diagnostic classification of childhood psychiatric disorders had its formal beginning with the publication by Leo Kanner (1935) of the first English-language textbook of child psychiatry. Kanner placed all disorders in categories of "personality difficulties." In the third (and final) edition of his textbook, Kanner (1957) addressed the limitations of then available diagnostic classification, particularly the insufficiency of descriptive categories. In Kanner's discussion of phenomenology, personality problems were categorized as related to physical illness, psychosomatic problems, and behavior problems. The latter grouping was the largest, including categories such as eating behavior (e.g., anorexia nervosa, rumination), sleeping behavior (e.g., nightmares, sleepwalking, narcolepsy), speech and language habits, scholastic performance, sexual behavior, anger, jealousy, fear, anxiety attacks, hypochondriasis, obsession and compulsion, hysteria, delinquency (a large chapter), hospitalism, schizophrenia (including a chapter on Kanner's concept of early infantile autism), and suicide. By that edition, the influence of psychoanalytic theory was considerably in evidence, as was a wealth of astute observation, clinical wisdom, and sound advice. The classification system was largely phenomenological, with little conceptual framework.

The first edition of the DSM (American Psychiatric Association 1952) was published in 1952 by the American Psychiatric Association (APA). Of the 28 members of the APA committee that was responsible for developing DSM-I, none were identified primarily with child and adolescent psychiatry. There were only four categories in the nomenclature for which childhood or adolescence was a specific condition: 1) chronic brain syndrome associated with birth trauma; 2) schizophrenic reaction, childhood type; 3) special symptom reactions such as learning disturbance, enuresis, and somnambulism; and 4) the adjustment reactions (habit disturbance, conduct disturbance, neurotic traits) of infancy, childhood, and adolescence. It is not surprising that DSM-I had little if any impact on the practice of psychiatry in general or on child and adolescent psychiatry in particular, because it was neither strongly phenomenological nor conceptual in organization.

The Group for the Advancement of Psychiatry (GAP) Committee on Child Psychiatry published its classification in 1966 (Group for the Advancement of Psychiatry 1966). It is interesting to note that the appendix of that classification identified 24 previous systems containing various degrees of detail and differences in approach. The GAP classification provided a broad, inclusive biopsychosocial and developmental framework within which to include interactive, etiological, and phenomenological considerations. Innovations in the GAP classification were new categories of healthy response and developmental deviations in maturational rate or sequence, use of a symptom list, and modifying of diagnoses as acute or chronic and mild, moderate, or severe.

DSM-II

DSM-II (American Psychiatric Association 1968) was intended to coincide with the *International Classification of Diseases,* 8th Revision (ICD-8; World Health

Organization 1969). DSM-II tried to avoid terms that carry with them implications regarding either the nature of a disorder or its causes and to be "explicit about causal assumptions when they are integral to a diagnostic concept" (p. viii). DSM-II reflected the growing importance of biological theories and research findings in understanding mental disorders and the growing challenge to psychoanalytic theory as either sufficiently or even predominantly explanatory. Descriptive phenomenology assumed a larger role than it had previously.

DSM-II did represent progress in the classification of child and adolescent disorders. Mental retardation was placed as the first category. Schizophrenia, childhood type, remained, as did an expanded section of "special symptoms" and transient situational disturbances. The major change was the addition of "behavior disorders of childhood and adolescence," including the following:

- Hyperkinetic reaction of childhood
  (or adolescence)
- Withdrawing reaction of childhood
  (or adolescence)
- Overanxious reaction of childhood
  (or adolescence)
- Runaway reaction of childhood
  (or adolescence)
- Unsocialized aggressive reaction of childhood
  (or adolescence)
- Group delinquent reaction of childhood
  (or adolescence)
- Other reaction of childhood
  (or adolescence)

The addition of this category was an important recognition of a broader and more specific range of psychopathologies in children and adolescents.

DSM-III

American Psychiatric Association 1980) represented and became the hallmark of the dramatic changes that had occurred in psychiatry during the previous 20 years. Except when etiology was clearly known, as in organic mental disorders, no assumptions as to etiology were included. DSM-III was comprehensively categorical, provided specific diagnostic criteria for each disorder, and introduced a five-part multiaxial system

that allowed for the coding of physical disorders, psychosocial stressors, and the highest level of adaptive functioning in the past year (in addition, of course, to the coding of disorders on Axis I and Axis II).

For the field of child and adolescent psychiatry, DSM-III introduced as its first Axis I category "Disorders Usually First Evident in Infancy, Childhood, or Adolescence," which included the following:

- Mental retardation
- Attention-deficit disorder (with and without hyperactivity)
- Conduct disorder (with five subtypes)
- Anxiety disorders (separation anxiety, avoidant, and overanxious disorders)
- Other disorders of infancy, childhood, or adolescence (reactive attachment, schizoid, oppositional, and identity disorders, and elective mutism)
- Eating disorders
- Stereotyped movement disorders (tic disorders and Tourette's disorder)
- Other disorders with physical manifestations (stuttering, enuresis, encopresis, and sleepwalking and sleep terror disorders)
- Pervasive developmental disorders (including infantile autism)

"Specific developmental disorders" (e.g., developmental reading or arithmetic disorder) were to be coded on Axis II. Diagnoses such as schizophrenia, affective disorders, organic disorders, and anxiety disorders now were to be made in children and adolescents by applying the same criteria required for the diagnosis in adults.

The major principles guiding DSM-III-R (American Psychiatric Association 1987) were the same as for DSM-III. Some important changes occurred in the sections covering disorders usually first evident in infancy, childhood, or adolescence. First, because developmental disorders usually begin in childhood and persist into adulthood, a new category was created on Axis II. These disorders included 1) mental retardation, 2) pervasive developmental disorders (autistic disorder), and 3) specific developmental disorders (including academic, language, and motor skills disorders).

DSM-IV

As in the two previous editions (DSM-III and DSM-III-R, American Psychiatric Association 1980, 1987), relevant disorders in DSM-IV (American Psychiatric Association 1994) and its Text Revision (DSM-IV-TR; American Psychiatric Association 2000) are listed in two ways: some under disorders "usually first diagnosed in infancy, childhood, or adolescence" and others in subsequent sections that are applicable to all age groups and use the same diagnostic criteria as for adults (e.g., affective, schizophrenic, and anxiety disorders). As DSM-IV makes clear, "The provision of a separate section for disorders that are usually first diagnosed in infancy, childhood, or adolescence is for convenience only and is not meant to suggest that there is any clear distinction between 'childhood' and 'adult' disorders.... For most (but not all) DSM-IV disorders, a single criteria set is provided that applies to children, adolescents, and adults" (p. 37).

The disorders in the section titled "Disorders Usually First Diagnosed in Infancy, Childhood, or Adolescence" include

- Mental retardation
- Learning disorders (LDs)
- Motor skills disorder
- Communication disorders
- Pervasive developmental disorders (PDDs)
- Attention-deficit and disruptive behavior disorders (DBDs)
- Feeding and eating disorders of infancy or early childhood
- Tic disorders
- Elimination disorders
- Other disorders of infancy, childhood, or adolescence

A number of changes in DSM-IV apply to childhood. The overarching category of developmental disorders coded on Axis II is dropped. PDDs and LDs (formerly academic skills disorders), motor skills disorder, and communication disorders (formerly language and speech disorders) have been moved to Axis I from Axis II. PDD in DSM-IV has a great deal of subclassification to improve differential diagnosis and provide greater specificity and now includes

- Autistic disorder
- Rett's disorder—a syndrome with onset after a period of normal development associated with severe mental retardation and progressive loss of function
- Childhood disintegrative disorder—a syndrome of marked aggression and loss of function following at

least 2 years of apparently normal functioning, also termed *Heller's syndrome* and *infantile dementia*
- Asperger's disorder—a syndrome very similar to high-functioning autism but differing in the absence of any clinically significant delay in development of language, communication, cognitive skills, or age-appropriate self-help and adaptive skills
- PDD not otherwise specified

The diagnostic criteria for LDs remain essentially the same as in DSM-III-R, but the terminology is simplified and the exclusion criteria have been modified to allow for the presence of a neurological condition. LD now includes

- Reading disorder (formerly developmental reading disorder)
- Mathematics disorder (formerly developmental arithmetic disorder)
- Disorders of written expression (formerly developmental expressive writing disorder)
- LD not otherwise specified

The communication disorders category now includes the previous two DSM-III-R categories of language and speech disorders and speech disorders not elsewhere classified and is subdivided into

- Expressive language disorder (formerly developmental expressive language disorder)
- Mixed receptive-expressive language disorder (formerly developmental receptive language disorder)
- Phonological disorder (formerly developmental articulation disorder)
- Stuttering, including a much expanded criteria set and discussion (the term *cluttering* in DSM-III-R has been eliminated from DSM-IV)
- Communication disorder not otherwise specified

The category attention-deficit and disruptive behavior disorders replaces the previously simplified category of DBDs. This category now is subdivided into

- Attention-deficit/hyperactivity disorder (ADHD), which now includes the undifferentiated type previously listed in DSM-III-R (see below) and subclassifies ADHD into
  1. Combined type
  2. Predominantly inattentive type
  3. Predominantly hyperactive-impulsive type

- ADHD not otherwise specified
- Conduct disorder—DSM-III-R categories of group, solitary, and undifferentiated are dropped in favor of childhood-onset or adolescent-onset (after age 10 years) type with mild, moderate, and severe specifiers; the criteria are reorganized into thematically related groups, and "stays out at night" and "intimidates others" have been added
- Oppositional defiant disorder
- DBD not otherwise specified; an addition

The category of anxiety disorders of childhood or adolescence is eliminated, being subsumed under the disorders of infancy, childhood, or adolescence (see below) and anxiety disorders (see Table 5–1).

The category of feeding and eating disorders of infancy or early childhood is a new category, reflecting the displacement of anorexia nervosa and bulimia nervosa to a separate eating disorders section and allowing for a broader inclusion of early-onset eating problems. This new category now includes

- Pica
- Rumination disorder
- Feeding disorder of infancy or early childhood— the persistent failure to eat adequately, with weight loss or failure to gain weight and a number of associated features

The category of gender identity disorders (GIDs) has been removed from the section of disorders usually first diagnosed in infancy, childhood, or adolescence and reclassified under the section "Sexual and Gender Identity Disorders," with the categories "in children," "in adolescents or adults," and not otherwise specified. The category of transsexualism has been dropped from DSM-IV and is subsumed under GID with specifiers.

The tic disorders category is left essentially unchanged in DSM-IV, with only a drop in the upper limit of age at onset from 21 to 18 years, and includes

- Tourette's disorder
- Chronic motor or vocal tic disorder
- Transient tic disorder
- Tic disorder not otherwise specified

The elimination disorders category has some relatively minor changes in duration specifiers and terminology, including

Table 5–1. Relevant DSM-III-R disorders that were deleted for DSM-IV or subsumed into other DSM-IV categories

Cluttering
Overanxious disorder of childhood
Avoidant disorder of childhood
Undifferentiated attention-deficit disorder
Identity disorder
Transsexualism

- Encopresis (previously "functional encopresis")
  1. With constipation and overflow incontinence
  2. Without constipation and overflow incontinence
- Enuresis (previously "functional enuresis")
  1. Nocturnal only
  2. Diurnal only
  3. Nocturnal and diurnal

Other disorders of infancy, childhood, or adolescence in DSM-III-R included elective mutism, identity disorder, reaction attachment disorder, and stereotypy/habit disorder. This category has been reorganized in DSM-IV and now includes

- Separation anxiety disorder
- Selective mutism, which includes a number of new provisions to reduce false-positive diagnoses
- Reactive attachment disorder of infancy or early childhood, for which two subtypes have been added—the inhibited type and the disinhibited type (indiscriminate and diffuse attachments)—to allow for compatibility with ICD-10 (*International Classification of Diseases and Related Health Problems*, 10th Revision; World Health Organization 1992)
- Stereotypic movement disorder, previously stereotypy/habit disorder; the specifier "with self-injurious behavior" is added if the behavior results in self-damage requiring treatment
- Disorders of infancy, childhood, or adolescence not otherwise specified

Eating disorders now constitute a separate category in DSM-IV incorporating anorexia nervosa and bulimia nervosa, which were in the DSM-III-R section "Disorders Usually First Evident in Infancy, Childhood, or Adolescence." The category of anorexia nervosa is now subdivided into restricting and binge-eating/purging types. Bulimia nervosa is not given as a diagnosis if the bingeing behavior occurs during episodes of anorexia nervosa. Subtypes of bulimia nervosa include purging and nonpurging types.

In the DSM-IV section on anxiety disorders, social phobia subsumes the DSM-III-R category of avoidant disorder of childhood or adolescence. DSM-IV includes criteria and discussion for a childhood onset. Generalized anxiety disorder in DSM-IV now subsumes DSM-III-R overanxious disorder of childhood and requires "excessive" anxiety and worry rather than "unrealistic" worries. The DSM-IV discussion of diagnostic features, age features, and criteria includes considerations specific or relevant to childhood onset.

Finally, there is a significant change in the use of Axis IV, which in DSM-III-R was termed "severity of psychosocial stressors" and included severity ratings, coding, and types of stressors to be considered. DSM-IV conceptualizes Axis IV as "psychosocial and environmental problems," grouped together as indicated in Table 5–2. Coding and severity rating scales are dropped from DSM-IV. It is recognized that these psychosocial and environmental factors affect the diagnosis, treatment, and prognosis of Axis I and Axis II disorders and furthermore play a role in the onset or exacerbation of a psychiatric disorder. These factors, ranging from a death in the family to homelessness to illiteracy to legal problems, obviously must be considered in any management plan and are of particular importance in childhood- and adolescent-onset disorders.

Table 5–2. DSM-IV Axis IV psychosocial and environment problems

Problems with primary support group
Problems related to the social environment
Educational problems
Occupational problems
Housing problems
Economic problems
Problems with access to health care services
Problems related to interaction with the legal system/crime
Other psychosocial and environmental problems

DSM-IV-TR

DSM-IV-TR (Text Revision) was published by the American Psychiatric Association in 2000 to reflect new research since the publication of DSM-IV. With very few exceptions, changes were made only in the text of the manual, not in the criteria themselves. The goal was to correct errors and ambiguities and to use empirical data to update and clarify sections of the manual describing symptoms, associated features, etiology, comorbidity, course, and prognosis. An exception to the rule of not changing criteria was made in the "Tic Disorders" section (including Tourette's disorder): The requirement for "clinically significant distress or impairment" that was added to the majority of disorders in DSM-IV has been removed.

Other Diagnostic Criteria Sets

Two other diagnostic systems have been developed for special populations of patients or professionals who have not been well served by the DSM or ICD models. A collaboration between the American Academy of Pediatrics and the American Psychiatric Association (including representatives of the American Academy of Child and Adolescent Psychiatry) developed the *Diagnostic and Statistical Manual for Primary Care* (DSM-PC), Child and Adolescent Version (American Academy of Pediatrics 1996). This is designed to be used by pediatricians and family physicians to classify emotional and behavioral problems seen in office practice. It includes a system for coding "Situation" that might be producing a child's symptoms and three clusters of "Child Manifestations": Developmental Variations, Problems Requiring Intervention, and Disorders (for those children who meet DSM-IV criteria for a disorder).

The DSM system has very limited utility for infants and toddlers. The Zero to Three/National Center for Clinical Infant Programs (1994) published a diagnostic classification system specifically tailored for very young children.

Toward DSM-V

Because each new version of the DSM disrupts clinicians' work, clinical administrative systems, and research, a decision has been made that DSM-V will be published no sooner than 2010. The American Psychiatric Association has convened work groups to develop white papers setting out the issues to be considered for various age groups and diagnoses and to specify what new research is required to clarify and improve our diagnostic system.

References

American Academy of Pediatrics: The Classification of Child and Adolescent Mental Diagnoses in Primary Care: Diagnostic and Statistical Manual for Primary Care (DSM-PC) Child. Chicago, IL, American Academy of Pediatrics, 1996

American Psychiatric Association: Diagnostic and Statistical Manual: Mental Disorders. Washington, DC, American Psychiatric Association, 1952

American Psychiatric Association: Diagnostic and Statistical Manual of Mental Disorders, 2nd Edition. Washington, DC, American Psychiatric Association, 1968

American Psychiatric Association: Diagnostic and Statistical Manual of Mental Disorders, 3rd Edition. Washington, DC, American Psychiatric Association, 1980

American Psychiatric Association: Diagnostic and Statistical Manual of Mental Disorders, 3rd Edition, Revised. Washington, DC, American Psychiatric Association, 1987

American Psychiatric Association: Diagnostic and Statistical Manual of Mental Disorders, 4th Edition. Washington, DC, American Psychiatric Association, 1994

American Psychiatric Association: Diagnostic and Statistical Manual of Mental Disorders, 4th Edition, Text Revision. Washington, DC, American Psychiatric Association, 2000

Group for the Advancement of Psychiatry: Psychopathological Disorders in Childhood: Theoretical Considerations and a Proposed Classification, Vol 6. New York, Group for the Advancement of Psychiatry, 1966

Kanner L: Child Psychiatry. Baltimore, MD, Charles C Thomas, 1935

Kanner L: Child Psychiatry, 3rd Edition. Baltimore, MD, Charles C Thomas, 1957

World Health Organization: International Classification of Diseases, 8th Revision. Geneva, World Health Organization, 1969

World Health Organization: International Statistical Classification of Diseases and Related Health Problems, 10th Revision. Geneva, World Health Organization, 1992

Zero to Three/National Center for Clinical Infant Programs Diagnostic Classification Task Force: Diagnostic Classification of Mental Health and Developmental Disorders of Infancy and Early Childhood. Arlington, VA, The Zero to Three/National Center for Clinical Infant Programs, 1994

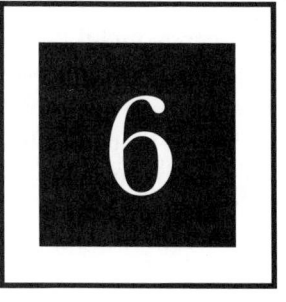

Concepts of Diagnostic Classification

David Shaffer, M.B., B.S., F.R.C.P.

History

It is likely that the need to order objects and concepts is as old as humankind itself. Early classifications of medical and psychological phenomena figure prominently in the 2,500-year-old writings of Hippocrates and Aristotle. It is interesting that these two scientists, working in the same general time period, should have chosen two distinct approaches to the problem of ordering that have persisted until modern times. Hippocrates created simple lists of diseases and symptoms that he had observed or that had been described to him. Aristotle sought to order all manner of phenomena according to theoretical beliefs of how they came about (Shaffer 2001). Grouping according to theory has undoubted heuristic value and is part of the process of discovery, but when used in practice and not as a hypothesis to be tested, it has the potential for serious error. It could be argued that the pervasive use of theory-based systems that characterized the Dark Ages held back progress in physiology and medicine for countless centuries. The influence of unproven theories almost certainly pushed psychological medicine into a newer dark age, and the advent of the atheoretical DSM-III, DSM-III-R, and DSM-IV of the American Psychiatric Association (1980, 1987, 1994) was a liberating milestone for a new era of evidence-based psychiatry.

The later versions of DSM and *International Classification of Diseases and Related Health Problems* (ICD) owe much to the advances in psychiatric phenomenology made around the end of the nineteenth century and the start of the twentieth by Kraepelin (1883), Bleuler (1911), and Jaspers (1913). Their astute observations had significant impact on the principal value of diagnostic classification, which is to advance communication within the limits of the period. Psychiatric training took place in large hospitals and asylums, and each had its own scheme for naming and ordering disorders for statistical purposes. Institutional nomenclatures were taught to trainees who, in due course, took them with them when they moved out to new practices or hospitals. This process resulted in frequent changes and adaptations, and inconsistencies developed, even among related systems (Raines 1952). The *Bellevue Hospital Nomenclature* (Bellevue 1911) emerged as the most influential of the North American systems, ultimately becoming the basis of the *Nomenclature of Diseases and Conditions* developed by the U.S. Public Health Service (1916) and shortly afterward by the American Medico-Psychological Association (1917), the precursor to the American Psychiatric Association.

However, the problem of multiple systems persisted, and in 1928, the New York Academy of Medicine convened a conference to develop a single standard nomenclature. The chairperson, Haven Emerson, summarized the problem: "Hospitals, health organizations, and insurance companies have been obliged to devise their own nomenclatures or, having borrowed an existing one, have promptly proceeded to modify it beyond recognition. A confusing multiplicity of effort has been due to the absence of any central guiding influence…the

This work was made possible by National Institute of Mental Health (NIMH) Research Training Grant MH16434 and NIMH Center Grant MH43878–01A1 to the Center to Study Youth Depression, Anxiety, and Suicide.

terminology employed has represented the personal choice of the author and has, therefore, been open to individual criticism and continuous alteration" (Emerson 1933). Reflecting the influence of hospitals and asylums, contemporary nomenclatures placed most emphasis on psychotic and organic conditions. The sole diagnosis for children was "problem state in children," listed under maladjustment (Logie 1933).

In 1950, the American Psychiatric Association and the recently formed National Institute of Mental Health joined forces to develop the first Diagnostic and Statistical Manual (DSM; American Psychiatric Association 1952). The system was based on then-current concepts of etiology and assumed psychogenicity for all disorders "without clearly defined physical cause." Conditions such as learning difficulties and enuresis were grouped as "adjustment reactions."

In 1968, DSM-II (American Psychiatric Association 1968) was released and was the last of the American Psychiatric Association classification systems to base itself on presumed etiology. The dominant theoretical influence was Adolf Meyer's (1957) view that mental disorders represented reactions of the personality to psychological, social, and biological factors (Spitzer 1980), and almost all of the listed conditions were labeled "reactions."

The field of child psychiatry was largely neglected in both DSM-I (American Psychiatric Association 1952) and DSM-II (American Psychiatric Association 1968). The latter provided for three groups of childhood disorders: behavior disorders, hyperkinetic reaction, and withdrawing and overanxious reactions. The behavior disorders were further divided into runaway, unsocialized aggressive, and group-delinquent reactions. This brief list was profuse in comparison with ICD-8 (World Health Organization 1969), which appeared at the same time as DSM-II and included only one childhood disorder category, "psychiatric disorder of childhood."

The years that followed saw momentous changes in psychiatric classification. Spitzer et al. (1978) developed the Research Diagnostic Criteria for the Collaborative Depression Study, which required uniform inclusion and exclusion criteria across all of its multiple sites. These criteria were descriptive and written in easily replicated operational terms to maximize reliability. The use of criteria would become one of the most distinctive features of DSM-III, edited by Spitzer (American Psychiatric Association 1980). In the field of child psychiatry, Rutter et al. (1969) drew up a considerably expanded list of psychiatric disorders of childhood that was eventually incorporated into ICD-9 (World Health Organization 1977). These disorders became the basis for the disorders listed in DSM-III and included neurodevelopmental, as well as emotional and behavioral, disorders. When DSM-III (American Psychiatric Association 1980) appeared, the number of diagnostic categories applicable to children had increased from 4 in DSM-I to 48 (American Psychiatric Association 1980). With the exception of adjustment and organic disorders, DSM-III avoided reference to any model of causation or to any symptom that required a clinician's inference. Opponents of the system argued that strict adherence to behavioral-descriptive principles would reduce the clinician's appreciation of the complexity of the patient's environmental and developmental history (see Rutter and Shaffer 1980). However, it was almost certainly this atheoretical aspect of the new generation of DSMs that allowed for their broad and universal acceptance among clinicians trained in very different ways in very different parts of the globe.

The Value of a Classification System

■ Communication

The major task of a classification system is to facilitate communication among interested clinicians, investigators, and those involved in public health planning, surveillance, and quality control. To do this, it must be reliable. Different users evaluating similar patients should come to the same diagnostic conclusions. Reliability will be greater if the classification is based on clearly defined observable or reportable phenomena (e.g., signs and symptoms) rather than on features that require interpretation or inference (e.g., subconscious or unrevealed cognitive or affective states). Criteria that are phrased in specific, unambiguous language and that precisely state frequency, duration, and indicators of impairment are more likely to be used reliably than those that employ general or ambiguous terms such as *often*, *lengthy*, or *severe*. Reliability is also influenced by the structure of the system. Shorter lists of categories or criteria are easier to navigate and to use consistently than are long lists. Users tend to select from only a part of a long and complicated listing rather than to choose consistently from the whole array of possibilities.

The value of communicating the contents of the classification system is enhanced if it does more than describe the patient's current mental and behavioral state. Knowledge of the diagnosis should allow the professional to make inferences about 1) likely etiology, 2) probable natural history, 3) expected response to specified types of treatment, and 4) the nature of other clinical conditions that are commonly associated with the condition.

This function (communication) requires that the system not attempt to classify every aspect of a disorder that might be encountered by the clinician, as in a conventional formulation. A classification system that encompassed all aspects of the individual would be as limitless, complex, and ultimately meaningless as a classification system for human beings that took account of all possible variations and combinations of hair color, nose length, blood pressure, and clothing preference. Rather, it should emphasize the salient features that the individual holds in common with others.

A large body of research from clinical, epidemiological, and natural history studies indicates that the symptom-based approach is valid and useful and does not just capture surface phenomena or a description of current mental state. Thus, the two groups into which most child psychiatric patients fall—children with antisocial symptoms (the disruptive, behavior, or conduct disorders) and children who experience distress from depressive and/or anxious feeling states (the internalizing or emotional disorders)—differ with respect not only to symptoms but also to demographics, past experiences, prognosis, and response to treatment. The disruptive disorders include attention-deficit/hyperactivity disorder, which on its own may be associated with any environmental disadvantage. However, it is very frequently comorbid with oppositional defiant disorder (Lahey and Applegate 2001) for which the following generalizations apply. Children with a disruptive or conduct disorder are predominantly boys, have often been reared in a disturbed home where they received little supervision and harsh punishment, and frequently have parents who are unhappily married, delinquent, and/or alcoholic. Many of these children will resist known treatments and have a poor long-term prognosis, being especially likely to develop adult sociopathy. By contrast, children with emotional (anxiety and affective) symptoms are as likely to be girls as boys, their family circumstances and

rearing experiences are not grossly different from those of control subjects, and most will respond well to intervention and, with or without treatment, tend to do well in the long term. If they go on to develop a psychiatric disorder as adults, it is likely to be an anxiety or mood disorder rather than sociopathy.

■ Heuristic

A diagnostic system expressed in operational and reproducible terms, such as those in DSM-IV and its Text Revision, DSM-IV-TR (2000), promotes the discovery of new knowledge. A category, even if it was first arrived at by consensus among experts rather than through empirical research, can be tested and, if faulty, can be changed. As an example, the DSM-III (American Psychiatric Association 1980) diagnosis of attention deficit without hyperactivity was designed for what was predicted would be a very small group of non-hyperactive inattentive children who would not be appropriately described by the designation attention-deficit/hyperactivity disorder (ADHD). When the diagnosis was first defined, little or nothing was known about children with that diagnosis, but its presence in the system stimulated research that validated its existence and led to elaborated clinical descriptions (Cantwell and Baker 1989; Lahey and Applegate 2001; Lahey et al. 1987), and it was retained in DSM-III-R and in DSM-IV. By contrast, the "identity disorder" placed into DSM-III and DSM-III-R was found to overlap almost completely with existing mood and anxiety disorder categories and was ultimately deleted.

■ Public Health and Treatment

As information accrues about the course of a disorder and about its treatability, it becomes possible to develop diagnosis-based quality-control criteria such as expected form and duration of treatment. These become useful for planning and for quality control and can be a spur to forms of professional education that stress evidence-based treatment for specific disorders.

Problems in Diagnostic Systems

■ Misdiagnosis and Labeling

The diagnostic process, although conducted to help the clinician determine the best treatment and predict outcome, is prone to error that might harm the patient. Given the trend to develop more diagnosis-specific treatments, it follows that a wrong diagnosis might lead to an inappropriate treatment. No matter how careful and sensitive the clinician is in relaying the implications of a diagnosis, qualifications and uncertainties may not be heard or heeded, and this might lead to lower expectations or inappropriate restriction of educational or social opportunity by others. The fact that the diagnostic process is subject to error and misunderstanding calls for the professional to be as careful as possible in arriving at a diagnosis and in conveying information to a child and family; it is important to make sure that the communication has indeed been understood and to lay out specifically how the diagnosis should alter, if at all, any expectations for learning and behavior.

The authors of DSM-IV attempted to reduce unwanted effects related to diagnosis. For example, the diagnosis of conduct disorder carries with it implications of therapeutic futility, poor prognosis, and criminality. It was decided that this diagnosis should be given sparingly and only in very severe cases of behavior disturbance. The threshold for meeting the criteria was increased between DSM-III-R (American Psychiatric Association 1987) and DSM-IV (American Psychiatric Association 1994, 1998), whereas the criteria for the related, but less stigmatizing, category of oppositional defiant disorder (ODD) were broadened. The result was a reduction in the prevalence of conduct disorder and an increase in the prevalence of ODD (Angold and Costello 2001).

■ Comorbidity

Comorbidity between different diagnoses is poorly understood (Angold et al. 1999). Comorbidity can arise

- For purely structural reasons such as the presence of similar criteria in different disorders. This has been a problem in DSM-IV-TR and in earlier versions. In DSM-IV-TR, irritability is a sufficient criterion in hypomania, yet it is present in no fewer than five other diagnoses, and agitation, distractibility, and reduced need for sleep are present in no fewer than four (Carlson 1999).
- Because the presence of one disorder has led to another as a complication, such as when depression occurs in a youth with a conduct disorder who repeatedly experiences losses and unpleasant, puni-

tive sanctions (Shaffer et al. 1996; Zoccolillo 1992) or when children with social phobia are predisposed to depression by the lack of support their phobia generates (Regier et al. 1998; Schatzberg et al. 1998).

- Because there is an etiological relationship between the two disorders. Some have held this to be the explanation for why the high rates of comorbidity between ADHD and ODD arise—because ADHD predisposes to ODD (Klein and Mannuzza 1991; Loeber et al. 1992, 1995; Mannuzza et al. 1989, 1998.)
- Because of common environmental or biological antecedents.
- Because (of greatest concern for nosologists) comorbidity reflects errors of diagnostic definition—that is, that the lines around different disorders have been drawn at the wrong places and that what appear to be two commonly co-occurring disorders are, in reality, manifestations of a single disorder.

■ Revisions

It is a tribute to the powerful heuristic value of criterion-based classification systems that they appear to generate both debate and data and, as a result, are subject to frequent revision. With each revision, new findings emerge that have direct implications for the existing classification scheme. The process of revision is inconvenient, and each new version requires an expensive educational effort for mental health professionals. A revision can render diagnostic instruments obsolete and make studies adhering to one set of criteria difficult to compare with those adhering to a different set. Seemingly small changes in the criteria can result in large and unpredictable shifts in the prevalence of a disorder. For example, a number of children whose impairment previously had met DSM-III criteria for conduct disorder did not meet criteria for DSM-III-R conduct disorder (Piacentini et al. 1989). Conversely, a number of children whose symptoms previously had not met criteria for infantile autism in DSM-III did meet criteria for autistic disorder in DSM-III-R (Volkmar et al. 1988). As a result of these effects, the revisions to DSM-III that appeared in DSM-III-R and the short interval between DSM-III-R and DSM-IV were broadly criticized as cutting the ground beneath established investigators and clinicians (Gift 1988; Zimmerman 1988). It was agreed that the delay before DSM-V was introduced would be longer than the two previous intervals.

Different Approaches to Classification

■ Categorical Systems

DSM-IV-TR and ICD-10 are examples of categorical systems. An individual will either meet criteria and carry the diagnosis or will not and will be declared free of the disorder. The advantage of a categorical system is that it represents the way that both clinicians and patients think of a disorder. The present/absent categorization is clear and seems precise and, as such, should increase reliability.

However, categorical diagnoses also carry distinct disadvantages:

- Disorders do not always present themselves in as complete a form as are represented by the diagnostic definitions. They might start with a single symptom and only meet full diagnostic criteria after some time. The categorical diagnoses in DSM and ICD have not found any good way of dealing with early features of a disorder.
- Diagnostic criteria differ in their potential for causing impairment. Thus, a child who meets fewer criteria than are required to make a diagnosis may nonetheless be disabled because of the criteria that he or she does meet.
- The number and type of symptoms will commonly vary with the age and sex of the patient. For example, an inability to wait one's turn in line or not speak out of turn (ADHD in DSM-IV-TR) might be clinically significant in middle childhood but is much less likely to be so in very young children. Many of the features of separation anxiety disorders are normal and expected in young children. The perpetration of rape and of theft with confrontation are rare in girls.

DSM has dealt with this problem by increasing the number of criteria to cover both genders and a wider age range. This, in turn, sometimes increases the number of criteria to a figure that cannot easily be remembered. Thus, in DSM-IV-TR, there are 16 criteria for ADHD, 14 for autistic disorder, and 8 for separation anxiety disorder. Diagnostic criteria are governed by specific rules or algorithms. The criteria themselves are built around specific parameters (e.g., duration, length). This process is rarely informed by any empirical information, and the rules and parameters are usually arrived at by consensus among experienced clinicians. However, it is not uncommon for a clearly impaired patient to have fewer, less-frequent, or briefer symptoms than are specified by the criteria. In other instances—and this is especially so with the anxiety disorders—a patient might meet the criteria for the disorder but be seemingly unimpaired. It is clear that symptoms alone might not determine the degree of suffering or impairment that is experienced. Those factors are as yet undiscovered, however.

■ Dimensional Classification Systems

An alternative approach to classifying psychiatric disorder has been widely used in child psychiatry and is exemplified by the work of Achenbach (2001) and of Boyle et al. (1996). The dimensional approach starts with the collection of a large inventory of symptoms from both clinical and community samples. A statistical procedure, such as factor analysis, is applied to the data, and factors, or dimensions of naturally occurring symptoms, are then identified. The symptom groups will usually vary somewhat between boys and girls and with age. The distribution of factor scores is compared in both clinical and nonclinical samples, and normative and clinically significant scores are produced for different ages and genders. The scores on all the factors can be profiled.

Regardless of the child-adolescent population or the source of the symptom information, two principal groupings usually emerge from this procedure: a group of intercorrelated disruptive (externalizing) behaviors and a group of emotional and affective (internalizing) symptoms.

The dimensional approach has been especially popular among researchers of child psychopathology, who have a long tradition of using comprehensive symptom inventories that lend themselves to dimensional analysis. Further, very few disturbed children present with pathognomonic or unusual symptoms that are never encountered among nondisturbed children. Child psychiatric symptoms are, in most cases, similar to normal behaviors, differing only in number, duration, or the stage of development at which they occur. The dimensional approach is conceptually sympathetic to this notion of continuum.

The advantage of the dimensional/empirical approach is that it reflects what happens in nature and does not rely on the clinical lore or anecdotal information that is typically used when formulating categorical diagnoses. Furthermore, although the dimensional system uses cutoff points or thresholds to designate a "case," these points are based on comparison with the normal population rather than on an arbitrary number of criteria selected by experts, as is usually the case in the categorical systems.

The disadvantages of the dimensional/empirical approach include the following:

- Being a "case" becomes a function of deviation from normal scores rather than impairment or interference with functioning, the criterion used in everyday practice by clinicians.
- The items in the inventories are usually written simply, with few if any qualifiers, such as "Have you been feeling depressed?" rather than "Have you been feeling depressed for at least 2 weeks, most of the day, nearly every day?" It therefore becomes difficult to relate responses on symptom inventories to DSM or ICD criteria.
- Factor structure differs across different age and sex groups. This makes it difficult to compare or even group different sex and age groups because each will have a different symptom profile.
- The information is usually collected on a single instrument. One consequence of this is that scores on the individual factors or dimensions are usually highly correlated. For example, the correlation between internalizing and externalizing dimensions in the latest standardization of the Achenbach Youth Self Report is considerable. The odds ratio for simultaneously exceeding both cutoffs is 7 (Roussos et al. 2001). This makes it difficult to differentiate within a group of children with a disorder. Most youth with a high score on the internalizing dimension will also have a high score on the externalizing dimension.
- Finally, despite their allegedly greater accuracy in reflecting nature, there is little evidence that dimensional profiles are equal to or superior to the categorical diagnostic systems in predicting outcome or identifying antecedents.

■ Nonbehavioral Classification: Multiaxial Systems

Clinically relevant information, such as IQ, personality, degree of impairment, and associated physical illnesses, can also be organized systematically following definitional rules. Rutter et al. (1975) originally proposed

that multiple relevant domains be represented on a separate axis (multiaxial) and that clinicians be encouraged to make a rating on each (Janca et al. 1996; Mezzich and Mezzich 1985; Williams 1985a). Attempts also have been made to develop classification systems for other psychological constructs such as Anna Freud's Hampstead Index of defensive styles (Freud 1970; Group for the Advancement of Psychiatry 1974; Perry et al. 1998). The Hampstead Index is long and complex and was designed to be applied to extensive analytic case records; thus, it cannot readily be applied in a new case or in the same case after an initial evaluation.

Advantages

The principal advantages of a multiaxial approach are that it results in clinicians recording more relevant information that is more easily retrieved and that it encourages clinicians to review systematically the areas covered by the different axes. When child psychiatrists were asked to rate the diagnoses of a mentally retarded child with psychiatric symptoms, they were much more likely to code both the psychiatric disorder and the intellectual deficit when offered a multiaxial framework than when simply given instructions to code all abnormalities present. Other studies subsequently replicated this (Mezzich and Mezzich 1985; Williams 1985b), and multiaxial classification has now become the rule in many clinical settings in many nations (Mezzich 2002). It appears particularly useful in the psychiatric assessment of individuals with associated physical illness (Fava et al. 2001).

DSM-IV-TR provides five axes. *Axis I* includes clinical syndromes. *Axis II* is for reporting personality disorders and mental retardation. *Axis III* contains general medical conditions. *Axis IV* is used to report psychosocial and environmental problems that have been present in the year before the evaluation. *Axis V* is for reporting the degree of impairment that results from the psychiatric disorder. Although most child psychiatrists and other professionals routinely use Axis I, only a few regularly make ratings on Axes IV and V (Setterberg et al. 1991). Both Axis I and Axis II are used to report clinical psychiatric disorders, but Axis II is reserved for personality disorders and mental retardation. The rationale offered in DSM-IV-TR (p. 26) is to ensure that consideration will be given to these diagnoses. DSM-IV-TR makes it clear that no difference in pathogenesis or treatment approaches is to be inferred from the placement of personality disorders on Axis II.

Psychosocial Factors

A number of different approaches have been used to code psychosocial circumstances and stressors on Axis IV. The approach taken by DSM-III and DSM-III-R was to list codes for the severity of psychosocial stressors considered to be relevant to the psychiatric disorder on Axis IV. The word *relevant* did not distinguish between stressors that had a causal influence on the disorder and those that arose as a result of the disorder; in practice, that distinction is difficult to make. DSM-IV-TR tries to simplify by doing away with codes and simply listing nine groupings (eight plus "other") of "psychosocial and environmental problems that may affect the diagnosis, treatment, and prognosis of mental disorders (Axes I and II)." Although this is appealing to most clinicians, the relationship between psychosocial problems and etiology is not always clear. Regardless, additional psychosocial problems invariably influence clinical management. It may be difficult to recall the order of stressors and behavior or emotional problems accurately because 1) most childhood disorders and many stressors are chronic, 2) distortions occur as part of a search for meaning, and 3) the influence of subclinical premorbid states on an individual's functioning (which may lead to stress) is difficult to reconstruct. However, differentiating between stressors with and without causal significance is important because a disorder that clearly follows a stressor, such as a bereavement response, may have a better prognosis than one that arises spontaneously.

A second approach creates categories for different types of psychosocial stressors (Shaffer et al. 1991; van Goor Lambo et al. 1990). Two problems arise with this approach. First, if the stressors are described at a very general level, then the same stressor will be designated in a wide variety of cases, and the coding has no discriminating value. Second, if stressors are described in more specific terms, then reliability falls to unacceptably low levels (Shaffer et al. 1991).

A third approach is to use a continuous "psychosocial adversity index" (Rey et al. 1987; Shaffer et al. 1975) that groups psychosocial stressors together in a single weighted index of severity.

A fourth approach rates the adequacy of the child's psychosocial support from the family, school, and broader society (Shaffer et al. 1989). Although the expectation is that this will predict treatment compliance and natural history, the reliability and validity of this method have yet to be determined.

Conclusion

The way psychopathology is classified exerts a profound influence on how clinical problems are evaluated and managed. Classification sets the direction of and the parameters for a good deal of academic and scholarly activity. It determines the adequacy of communication among parties involved in the diagnosis and treatment of children. The systems in use are imperfect in many ways. Some categories have been formulated as informed guesses. Some are a compromise between established custom and new and not yet fully digested information. Others have stood the test of time. Although the introduction of frequent revisions may be disturbing and a nuisance, it is also a sign of the vitality of current classification systems and how actively they intersect with new knowledge and experience.

References

Achenbach TM: Challenges and benefits of assessment, diagnosis, and taxonomy for clinical practice and research. Aust N Z J Psychiatry 35(3):263–271, 2001

American Medico-Psychological Association: Proceedings of the American Medico-Psychological Association at Seventy-Third Annual Meeting. American Journal of Insanity 74:254–271, 1917

American Psychiatric Association: Diagnostic and Statistical Manual: Mental Disorders. Washington, DC, American Psychiatric Association, 1952

American Psychiatric Association: Diagnostic and Statistical Manual of Mental Disorders, 2nd Edition. Washington, DC, American Psychiatric Association, 1968

American Psychiatric Association: Diagnostic and Statistical Manual of Mental Disorders, 3rd Edition. Washington, DC, American Psychiatric Association, 1980

American Psychiatric Association: Diagnostic and Statistical Manual of Mental Disorders, 3rd Edition, Revised. Washington, DC, American Psychiatric Association, 1987

American Psychiatric Association: Diagnostic and Statistical Manual of Mental Disorders, 4th Edition. Washington, DC, American Psychiatric Association, 1994

American Psychiatric Association: DSM-IV Sourcebook, Vol 4. Washington, DC, American Psychiatric Association, 1998

American Psychiatric Association: Diagnostic and Statistical Manual of Mental Disorders, 4th Edition, Text Revision. Washington, DC, American Psychiatric Association, 2000

Angold A, Costello EJ: The epidemiology of disorders of conduct: nosological issues and comorbidity, in Conduct Disorders in Childhood and Adolescence. Edited by Hill J, Maughan B. Cambridge, UK, Cambridge University Press, 2001, pp 126–168

Angold A, Costello EJ, Erkanli A: Comorbidity. J Child Psychol Psychiatry 40:57–87, 1999

Bellevue: Bellevue Hospital Nomenclature. New York, Bellevue Board of Trustees, 1911

Bleuler PE: Dementia Praecox oder Gruppen der Schizophrenia. Handbuch der Psychiatrie, Vol 1, Sect 4. Edited by Aschaffenburg G. Leipzig and Vienna, Franz Deuticke, 1911

Boyle MH, Offord DR, Racine Y, et al: Identifying thresholds for classifying childhood psychiatric disorder: issues and prospects. J Am Acad Child Adolesc Psychiatry 35: 1440–1448, 1996

Cantwell DP, Baker L: Stability and natural history of DSM-III childhood diagnosis. J Am Acad Child Adolesc Psychiatry 28:691–700, 1989

Carlson GA: Juvenile mania versus ADHD. J Am Acad Child Adolesc Psychiatry 38:353–354, 1999

Emerson H: Preface, in National Conference on Nomenclature of Disease: A Standard Classified Nomenclature of Disease. Edited by Logie HB. New York, Commonwealth Fund, 1933, pp xi–xvii

Fava GA, Mangelli L, Ruini C: Assessment of psychological distress in the setting of medical disease. Psychother Psychosom 70(4):171–175, 2001

Freud A: The symptomatology of childhood: a preliminary attempt at classification. Psychoanal Study Child 26:19–41, 1970

Gift TE: Changing diagnostic criteria. Am J Psychiatry 145: 1414–1415, 1988

Group for the Advancement of Psychiatry: Psychopathological Disorders in Childhood: Theoretical Considerations and a Proposed Classification (Report No 62). New York, Group for the Advancement of Psychiatry, 1974

Janca A, Kastrup MC, Katschnig H, et al: The ICD-10 multiaxial system for use in adult psychiatry: structure and applications. J Nerv Ment Dis 184(3):191–192, 1996

Jaspers K: Allgemeine Psychopathologie: Ein Leitfaden für Studierende, Ärzte, und Psychologen. Berlin, Verlag von Julius Springer, 1913

Klein RG, Mannuzza S: Long-term outcome of hyperactive children: a review. J Am Acad Child Adolesc Psychiatry 30:383–387, 1991

Kraepelin E: Compendium der Psychiatrie. Leipzig, Verlag von Ambr. Abel, 1883

Lahey BB, Applegate B: Validity of DSM-IV ADHD. J Am Acad Child Adolesc Psychiatry 40:502–504, 2001

Lahey BB, Schaughency EA, Hynd GW, et al: Attention deficit disorder with and without hyperactivity: comparison of behavioral characteristics of clinic-referred children. J Am Acad Child Adolesc Psychiatry 26:718–723, 1987

Loeber R, Green SM, Lahey BB, et al: Developmental sequences in the age of onset of disruptive child behaviors. Journal of Child and Family Studies 1:21–41, 1992

Loeber R, Green SM, Keenan K, et al: Which boys will fare worse? Early predictors of the onset of conduct disorder in a six-year longitudinal study. J Am Acad Child Adolesc Psychiatry 34:499–509, 1995

Logie HB (ed): National Conference on Nomenclature of Disease: A Standard Classified Nomenclature of Disease. New York, Commonwealth Fund, 1933

Mannuzza S, Klein RG, Konig PH, et al: Hyperactive boys almost grown up. IV. Criminality and its relationship to psychiatric status. Arch Gen Psychiatry 46:1073–1079, 1989

Mannuzza S, Klein RG, Bessler A, et al: Adult psychiatric status of hyperactive boys grown up. Am J Psychiatry 155:493–498, 1998

Meyer A: Psychobiology: A Science of Man. Springfield, IL, Charles C Thomas, 1957

Mezzich JE: International surveys on the use of ICD-10 and related diagnostic systems. Psychopathology 35(2–3):72–75, 2002

Mezzich AC, Mezzich JE: Perceived suitability and usefulness of DSM-III vs DSM-II in child psychopathology. J Am Acad Child Adolesc Psychiatry 24:281–285, 1985

Perry JC, Hoglend P, Shear K, et al: Field trial of a diagnostic axis for defense mechanisms for DSM-IV. J Personal Disord 12(1):56–68, 1998.

Piacentini JC, Abikoff HA, Klein RG, et al: Teacher ratings of DSM-III-R disruptive behavior disorders: symptom and syndrome prevalence in a normative population. Paper presented at the annual meeting of the American Academy of Child and Adolescent Psychiatry, New York, October 1989

Raines GN: Foreword, in Diagnostic and Statistical Manual of Mental Disorders. Washington, DC, American Psychiatric Association, 1952, pp v–xi

Regier DA, Rae DS, Narrow WE, et al: Prevalence of anxiety disorders and their comorbidity with mood and addictive disorders. Br J Psychiatry 34(suppl):24–28, 1998

Rey JM, Plapp JM, Stewart G, et al: Reliability of the psychosocial axes of DSM-III in an adolescent population. Br J Psychiatry 150:228–234, 1987

Roussos A, Francis K, Zoubou V, et al: The standardization of Achenbach's Youth Self-Report in Greece in a national sample of high-school students. Eur Child Adolesc Psychiatry 10(1):47–53, 2001

Rutter M, Shaffer D: DSM-III: A step forward or back in terms of the classification of child psychiatric disorders? J Am Acad Child Adolesc Psychiatry 19:371–394, 1980

Rutter M, Lebovici S, Eisenberg L, et al: A triaxial classification of mental disorders in childhood. J Child Psychol Psychiatry 10:41–61, 1969

Rutter ML, Shaffer D, Shepard M: A Multiaxial Classification of Child Psychiatric Disorders. Geneva, World Health Organization, 1975

Schatzberg AF, Samson JA, Rothschild AJ, et al: McLean Hospital depression research facility: early onset phobic disorders and adult-onset major depression. Br J Psychiatry 34(suppl):29–34, 1998

Setterberg S, Ernst M, Rao U, et al: Child psychiatrists' views of DSM-III-R: a survey of usage and opinions. J Am Acad Child Adolesc Psychiatry 30:652–658, 1991

Shaffer D: Classification and categorization revisited, in Research and Innovation on the Road to Modern Child Psychiatry, Vol 1, Festschrift for Professor Sir Michael Rutter. Edited by Green J, Yule W. London, Gaskell and Association of Child Psychology and Psychiatry, 2001, pp 104–114

Shaffer D, Chadwick O, Rutter M: Psychiatric outcome of localized head injury in children, in Outcome of Severe Damage to the Central Nervous System (CIBA Foundation Symposium Series, No 34). Edited by Porter R, Fitzsimons DW. Amsterdam, Elsevier, 1975, pp 191–213

Shaffer D, Campbell M, Cantwell D, et al: Child and adolescent psychiatric disorders in DSM-IV: issues facing the work group. J Am Acad Child Adolesc Psychiatry 28:830–835, 1989

Shaffer D, Gould M, Rutter R, et al: Reliability and validity of a psychosocial axis in patients with a child psychiatric disorder. J Am Acad Child Adolesc Psychiatry 30:109–115, 1991

Shaffer D, Fisher P, Dulcan MK, et al: The NIMH Diagnostic Interview Schedule for Children, version 2.3 (DISC-2.3): description, acceptability, prevalence rates, and performance in the MECA study. J Am Acad Child Adolesc Psychiatry 35:865–877, 1996

Spitzer R: Introduction to DSM-III, in Diagnostic and Statistical Manual of Mental Disorders, 3rd Edition. Washington, DC, American Psychiatric Association, 1980, pp 1–12

Spitzer R, Endicott J, Robins E: Research Diagnostic Criteria (RDC) for a Selected Group of Functional Disorders. New York, Biometrics Research, 1978

United States Public Health Service: Nomenclature of Diseases and Conditions. Washington, DC, U.S. Public Health Service, Government Printing Office, 1916

van Goor Lambo G, Orley J, Poustka F, et al: Classification of abnormal psychosocial situations: a preliminary report of a revision of a WHO scheme. J Child Psychol Psychiatry 31:229–241, 1990

Volkmar FR, Bregman J, Cohan DJ, et al: DSM-III and DSM-III-R diagnoses of autism. Am J Psychiatry 145:1404–1408, 1988

Williams JB: The multiaxial system of DSM-III: where did it come from and where should it go? I: its origins and critiques. Arch Gen Psychiatry 42(2):175–180, 1985a

Williams JB: The multiaxial system of DSM-III: where did it come from and where should it go? II: empirical studies, innovations, and recommendations. Arch Gen Psychiatry 42:181–186, 1985b

World Health Organization: International Classification of Diseases, 8th Revision. Geneva, World Health Organization, 1969

World Health Organization: International Classification of Diseases, 9th Revision. Geneva, World Health Organization, 1977

Zimmerman M: Why are we rushing to publish DSM-IV? Arch Gen Psychiatry 45:1135–1138, 1988

Zoccolillo M: Co-occurrence of conduct disorder and its adult outcomes with depressive and anxiety disorders: a review. J Am Acad Child Adolesc Psychiatry 31:547–556, 1992

Clinical Assessment in Infancy and Early Childhood

Stanley I. Greenspan, M.D.

Recent understanding of both normal and disturbed emotional functioning in infants and young children makes it possible to explore new comprehensive approaches to understanding early development and implementing patterns of assessment, treatment, and prevention (Greenspan 1992; Greenspan and Wieder 1998; Interdisciplinary Council on Developmental and Learning Disorders Clinical Practice Guidelines Workgroup 2000). Descriptions of adaptive and maladaptive emotional milestones can be added to the well-known sensorimotor and cognitive milestones (Greenspan 1979, 1981, 1987, 1989 1992, 1997b; Greenspan and Wieder 1998; Greenspan et al. 2001; Interdisciplinary Council on Developmental and Learning Disorders Clinical Practice Guidelines Workgroup 2000). The importance of early assessment is indicated by studies of cumulative risk, which suggest that family and interactive patterns during infancy correlate with later cognitive and behavioral performance at age 4 years. For example, children with four or more infancy risk factors have a 24-fold increase in the probability of marginal IQ scores in comparison with children who have only one or two risk factors (Sameroff et al. 1986).

The following approach to emotional assessment includes a guide that can be used for screening or as an outline for a comprehensive evaluation. Basic concepts relevant to assessment in infancy include 1) the importance of considering multiple lines of development (compared with only physical or cognitive), 2) the components of a comprehensive approach, and 3) the sequence of normal and disturbed emotional development.

Multiple Lines of Development

The view of the infant as developing along multiple rather than single lines (i.e., physical, cognitive, socioemotional, and familial) is perhaps self-evident; however, the implications of this approach are not always obvious. For example, babies who have been nutritionally compromised improve physically and gain weight more efficaciously when nutrition is provided together with adequate social interaction. An approach that focuses only on cognitive stimulation to enliven a withdrawn baby may lead to further withdrawal if the infant has an undiagnosed sensory hypersensitivity. In contrast, use of a gradual, soothing, individually tailored approach may be more effective.

Components of a Comprehensive Clinical Approach

A comprehensive clinical approach views infants in a context that includes not only multiple lines of development but also the parents, other family members, and relevant variations in social structures, including poverty. A comprehensive approach would include, for example, the parents' predominant attitudes and feelings, family relationships, and other crucial contextual factors, such as the system of health and mental health services and relevant community structures. More isolated intervention strategies, although working to stimulate an infant's cognitive capacities, may limit involvement by parents to helping only with issues such as food and housing or cognitive stimulation.

A comprehensive clinical approach must begin with the assessment of a number of conceptually related categories, discussed below, that take into account multiple lines of development that reflect the full complexity of clinical phenomena.

■ Prenatal and Perinatal Variables

Prenatal and perinatal variables, especially insults such as rubella, maternal drug and alcohol use, and poor maternal nutrition, all have some effect on the infant's constitutional status and development tendencies. Prenatal variables include familial genetic patterns; the mother's status during pregnancy, including nutrition, physical health and illness, personality functioning, mental health, and degree of stress; characteristics of familial and social support systems; characteristics of the pregnancy; and the delivery process, including complications, time in various stages, and the infant's status after birth. Perinatal variables include the mother's perceptions of her infant, the mother's reports of the emerging daily routine, and observations of the infant and mother–infant interaction.

■ Parental, Familial, and Environmental Variables

Evaluations of parents, other family members, and individuals who relate closely to the family are made along a number of dimensions, including each member's personality organization and developmental needs, child-rearing capacity, and family interaction patterns. Evaluations of the support system (extended family, friends, and community agencies) used or available to the family and of the total home environment (both animate and inanimate components) also are included. Of special importance is the capacity of the parents and family to calm and regulate the infant, reach out and foster attachment, perceive basic status of pleasure and discomfort, respond with balanced empathy (i.e., without either overidentification or isolation of feeling), perceive and respond flexibly and differently to the infant's cues, foster organized and complex interactions, and support representational elaboration and differentiation.

■ Primary Caregiver and Caregiver–Infant/ Child Relationship Variables

The interaction between the infant and his or her important nurturing figures is evaluated. Included are the status of the caregiver (e.g., teenage mother, single-parent family); the quality of shared attention, comfort, and regulation; the capacity for joint pleasure and intimacy; and the flexibility in tolerating tension and being able to return to a state of intimacy. Later, it is important to evaluate the capacity for reciprocal interaction to form complex emotional and behavioral patterns and to construct and differentiate mental representations.

■ Infant Variables: Physical, Neurological, Physiological, and Cognitive

Infant variables include the infant's genetic background and status immediately after birth, including the infant's general physical integrity (size, weight, general health), neurological integrity, physiological tendencies, rhythmic patterns, and levels of alertness and activity. Special attention should be paid to the infant's individual differences, including sensory hypo- or hyperreactivity, motor tone, motor planning, sensory processing (DeGangi et al. 1993; Porges and Greenspan 1990), and cognitive level and style. Attention also should be paid to how these factors could foster or hinder the child's capacities to experience stimulation and regulate and organize experience; develop human relationships; interact in cause-and-effect reciprocal patterns; form complex behavioral, emotional, and cognitive patterns; and construct representations to guide behavior, feelings, and thinking.

■ Infant Variables: Formation and Elaboration of Emotional Patterns and Human Relationships

The relationships between the infant and caregivers are additional infant variables. These help the infant develop the capacity for a range of emotions (from dependency to assertiveness) and relationship patterns, in the context of a sequence of organizational stages. The organizational stages include the capacity for shared attention and engagement, purposeful interactions, complex and organized social and emotional patterns, construction of representations, and differentiation of internal representations along self versus nonself time and space dimensions (Greenspan 1981, 1989).

Sequence of Adaptive and Maladaptive Emotional Development

The examination of multiple aspects of development of the infant and family has made it possible to formulate developmental stages that focus on the infant's social and emotional functioning. Although there are no large-scale studies of disturbed affective patterns of infants and young children at different ages, there is extensive literature on the emotional development of presumed normal infants. Interestingly, since the 1980s, there has been considerably greater documentation of normal emotional development in infants than probably in any other age group.

It now is well documented that the infant is capable, either at birth or shortly thereafter, of organizing experience in an adaptive fashion. He or she can respond to pleasure and displeasure (Lipsitt 1966); change behavior as a function of its consequences (Gewirtz 1965, 1969); form intimate bonds and make visual discriminations (Klaus and Kennell 1976; Meltzoff and Moore 1977); organize cycles and rhythms, such as the sleep–wake cycle and alertness states (Sander 1962); evidence a variety of affects or affect proclivities (Ekman 1972; Izard 1978; Tomkins 1963a, 1963b); and demonstrate organized social responses in conjunction with increasing neurophysiological organization (Emde et al. 1976). From the early months, the infant demonstrates a unique capacity to enter into complex social and affective interactions (Brazelton et al. 1974; Stern 1974a, 1974b, 1977). That the organization of experience broadens during the early months of life to reflect increases in the capacity to experience and tolerate a range of stimuli, including stable responses to social interactions and personal configurations, is also consistent with empirical data (Brazelton et al. 1974; Emde et al. 1976; Escalona 1968; Murphy and Moriarty 1976; Sander 1962; Sroufe 1979; Stern 1974a, 1974b).

Increasingly complex patterns continue to emerge as the infant develops further, as indicated by complex emotional responses such as surprise (Charlesworth 1969) and affiliation; wariness and fear (Ainsworth et al. 1974; Bowlby 1969; Sroufe and Waters 1977); exploration and refueling patterns (Mahler et al. 1975); behavior suggesting functional understanding of objects (Werner and Kaplan 1963); and the eventual emergence of symbolic capacities (Bell 1970; Gouin-Decarie 1965; Piaget 1962).

In addition to the studies on normal infant emotional development, important observations on disturbed development fill out the emerging picture of early emotional development. Constitutional and maturational patterns that influence the formation of early relationship patterns were already noted in the early 1900s, with descriptions of "babies of nervous inheritance who exhaust their mothers" and infants with "excessive nerve activity and a functionally immature" nervous system (Cameron 1919).

Winnicott (1931), as a pediatrician, began describing the environment's role in early relationship problems. His work was followed in the 1940s by the now well known studies describing the severe developmental disturbances of infants brought up in institutions or in other situations of emotional deprivation (Bakwin 1942; Bowlby 1951; Hunt 1941; Lowery 1940; Spitz 1945). Spitz's (1945) films resulted in laws in the United States prohibiting permanent placement of infants in institutions.

Both the role of individual differences based on constitutional maturational and early interactional patterns and the "nervous" infants described by Rachford (1905) and Cameron (1919) again became a focus of inquiry, as evidenced by the observations of Burlingham and Freud (1942); by Bergman and Escalona's (1949) descriptions of infants with "unusual sensitivities"; by Murphy and Moriarty's (1976) description of patterns of vulnerability; by Thomas and Chess's (1977) temperament studies; by Cravioto and DeLicardie's (1973) descriptions of the role of infant-individual differences in malnutrition; and by the impressive emerging empirical literature on infants (Brazelton et al. 1974; Emde et al. 1976; Gewirtz 1961; Lipsitt 1966; Rheingold 1966, 1969; Sander 1962; Stern 1974a, 1974b). More integrated approaches to understanding disturbances in infancy have been emphasized in descriptions of selected disorders and clinical case studies (Fraiberg 1979; Greenspan 1987; Provence 1983).

To further understanding of both adaptive and disturbed infant functioning, an in-depth study of normal and disturbed developmental patterns in infancy was undertaken to develop a systematic comprehensive classification of infant and family patterns. Table 7–1 summarizes observations of these patterns (Greenspan 1979, 1981, 1989).

Table 7–1. Developmental basis for psychopathology and adaptation in infancy and early childhood

Stage-specific tasks and capacities	Capacities		Environment (caregiver)	
	Adaptive	Maladaptive (pathological)	Adaptive	Maladaptive
Homeostasis (0–3 months) (self-regulation and interest in the world)	Internal regulation (harmony) and balanced interest in world	Unregulated (e.g., hyperexcitable); withdrawn (apathetic)	Invested, dedicated, protective, comforting; predictable; engaging and interesting	Unavailable, chaotic, dangerous, abusive; hypostimulating or hyperstimulating; dull
Attachment (2–7 months)	Rich, deep, multisensory emotional investment in animate world (especially with primary caregivers)	Total lack of or nonaffective, shallow, impersonal involvement (e.g., autistic patterns) with animate world	In love and woos infant to "fall in love"; affective multimodality, pleasurable involvement	Emotionally distant, aloof, and/or impersonal (highly ambivalent)
Somatopsychological differentiation (3–10 months) (purposeful, cause-and-effect signaling or communication)	Flexible, wide-ranging, affective multi-system-contingent (reciprocal) interactions (especially with primary caregivers)	Random and/or chaotic or narrow, rigid, and stereotyped behavior and affects	Reads and responds contingently to infant's communications across multiple sensory and affective systems	Ignores infant's communications (e.g., overly intrusive, preoccupied, or depressed) or misreads infant's communications (e.g., projection)
Behavioral organization, initiative, and internalization (9–24 months)	Complex, organized, assertive, innovative, integrated behavioral and emotional patterns	Fragmented, stereotyped, and polarized behavior and emotions (e.g., withdrawn, compliant, hyperaggressive, or disorganized toddler)	Admiring of toddler's initiative and autonomy yet available, tolerant, and firm; follows toddler's lead and helps toddler organize diverse behavioral and affective elements	Overly intrusive, controlling; fragmented, fearful (especially of toddler's autonomy); abruptly and prematurely "separates"

Table 7–1. Developmental basis for psychopathology and adaptation in infancy and early childhood *(continued)*

Stage-specific tasks and capacities	Capacities		Environment (caregiver)	
	Adaptive	Maladaptive (pathological)	Adaptive	Maladaptive
Representational capacity, differentiation, and consolidation (1½–4 years) (the use of ideas to guide language, pretend play, and behavior and eventually thinking and planning)	Formation and elaboration of internal representations (imagery); organization and differentiation of imagery pertaining to self and nonself; emergence of cognitive insight; stabilization of mood and gradual emergence of basic personality functions	No representational (symbolic) elaboration; concrete, shallow, and polarized behavior and affect; sense of self and others fragmented and undifferentiated or narrow and rigid; reality testing, impulse regulation, mood stabilization compromised or vulnerable (e.g., borderline psychotic and severe character problems)	Emotionally available to phase-appropriate regressions and dependency needs; reads, responds to, and encourages symbolic elaboration across emotional behavioral domains (e.g., love, pleasure, assertion) while fostering gradual reality orientation and internalization of limits	Fearful of or denies phase-appropriate needs; engages child only in concrete (nonsymbolic) models generally or in certain realms (e.g., around pleasure) and/or misreads or responds noncontingently or nonrealistically to emerging communications (e.g., undermines reality orientation; overly permissive or punitive)
Capacity for limited and multiple extended representational systems (middle childhood through adolescence)	Enhanced and eventually optimal flexibility to conserve and transform complex and organized representations of experience in the context of expanded relationship patterns and phase-expected developmental tasks	Derivative representational capacities limited or defective, as are latency and adolescent relationships and coping capacities	Supports complex, phase- and age-appropriate experiential and interpersonal development (i.e., into triangular and post-triangular patterns)	Conflicted over child's age-appropriate propensities (e.g., competitiveness, pleasure orientation, growing competence, assertiveness, and self-sufficiency); becomes aloof or maintains symbiotic tie; withdraws from or overengages in competitive or pleasurable strivings

Source. Adapted from Greenspan 1981.

Monitoring developmental progress with explicit guidelines facilitates the early identification of those infants, young children, and families who are progressing in a less-than-optimal way. For example, it is now possible to evaluate infants who continue to have difficulty regulating their state and developing the capacity for focused interest in their immediate environments or who fail to develop a positive emotional interest in their caregivers. It also is possible to assess an infant's difficulty in learning cause-and-effect interactions and complex emotional and social patterns or the infant's inability, by age 2 or 3 years, to create representations or symbols and, by age 3 or 4 years, to differentiate these to guide emotions and behavior.

In exploring the factors that may be contributing to less-than-optimal patterns of development, the focus on multiple aspects of development offers many advantages. Some infants, for example, may evidence a motor delay because of familial patterns in which explorativeness and the practice of the motor system are discouraged. In other infants, there may be a maturational variation that, together with family patterns, is contributing to a motor lag. In still other cases, genetic and/or maturational factors may explain the delay. Even with a symptom as common as a motor lag, unless all aspects of all contributing factors are explored, important contributing factors may go unrecognized. The focus on multiple aspects of development, in the context of clearly delineated developmental and emotional landmarks, opens the door to comprehensive assessment, diagnosis, and preventive intervention strategies. Such a comprehensive approach offers a developmental perspective on many of the severe disorders of early childhood, including autism and pervasive developmental disorder; mild-to-moderate disorders, such as conduct, anxiety, and attentional disorders; and different forms of global lags in cognition (e.g., mental retardation), as well as any specific lags in receptive or expressive language, motor regulation, or sensory reactivity and processing (Greenspan 1989, 1992, 1997a, 1997b; Greenspan and Wieder 1998).

The Developmental, Individual-Difference, Relationship-Based Model

The different variables that must be dealt with in clinical assessments in infancy and early childhood are best conceptualized in terms of what has been described as the developmental, individual-difference, relationship-based (DIR) model. The DIR model attempts to facilitate understanding of children and their families by identifying, systematizing, and integrating the essential functional developmental capacities. These include 1) the child's functional-emotional developmental level; 2) the child's individual differences in sensory reactivity, processing, and motor planning; and 3) the child's relationships and interactions with caregivers, family members, and others.

■ Functional Developmental Capacities

Functional Emotional Developmental Level

The child's functional emotional developmental level examines how children integrate all their capacities (motor, cognitive, language, spatial, sensory) to carry out emotionally meaningful goals. The support for these functional emotional developmental levels is reviewed elsewhere (Greenspan 1979, 1989, 1992, 1997b). These capacities include the ability to

- Attend to multisensory affective experience and, at the same time, organize a calm, regulated state (e.g., looking at, listening to, and following movement of a caregiver)
- Engage with and show affective preference and pleasure for a caregiver or caregivers (e.g., joyful smiles and affection with a stable caregiver)
- Initiate and respond to two-way presymbolic gestural communication (e.g., back-and-forth use of smiles and sounds)
- Organize chains of two-way social problem-solving communications (opening and closing many circles of communication in a row), maintain communication across space, integrate affective polarities, and synthesize an emerging prerepresentational organization of self and other (e.g., taking Dad by the hand to get a toy on the shelf)
- Create and functionally use ideas as a basis for creative or imaginative thinking, giving meaning to symbols (e.g., pretend play, using words to meet needs: "Juice!")
- Build bridges between ideas as a basis for logic, reality testing, thinking, and judgment (e.g., engage in debates, opinion-oriented conversations, and/or elaborate, planned pretend dramas)

Individual Differences in Sensory Modulation, Sensory Processing, and Motor Planning

These biologically based individual differences are the result of genetic, prenatal, perinatal, and maturational variations and/or deficits and can be characterized in at least four ways:

1. Sensory modulation, including hypo- and hyper-reactivity in each sensory modality, including touch, sound, smell, vision, and movement in space
2. Sensory processing in each sensory modality, including auditory processing and language and visuospaatial processing; includes the capacity to register, decode, and comprehend sequences and abstract patterns
3. Sensory-affective processing in each modality (e.g., the ability to process and react to affect, including the capacity to connect "intent" or affect to motor planning and sequencing, language, and symbols); this capacity may be especially relevant for autism spectrum disorders (Greenspan and Wieder 1998)
4. Motor planning and sequencing, including the capacity to sequence actions, behaviors, and symbols (including symbols in the form of thoughts, words, visual images, and spatial concepts)

Relationships and Interactions

Relationship and affective interaction patterns include developmentally appropriate, or inappropriate, interactive relationships with caregiver, parent, and family patterns. Interaction patterns between the child and caregivers and family members bring the child's biology into the larger developmental progression and can contribute to the negotiation of the child's functional developmental capacities. Developmentally appropriate interactions mobilize the child's intentions and affects and enable the child to broaden his or her range of experience at each level of development and move from one functional developmental level to the next. In contrast, interactions that do not deal with the child's functional developmental level or individual differences can undermine progress. For example, a caregiver who is aloof may not be able to engage an infant who is underreactive and self-absorbed.

The DIR model examines the developmental capacities of children in the context of their unique biologically based processing profile and their family relationships and interactive patterns. As a functional approach, it uses the complex interactions between biology and experience to explain behavior. Implementation of an appropriate assessment of all the relevant functional areas requires a number of sessions with the child and family. These sessions must begin with discussions and observations.

The assessment process, which is described in detail elsewhere (Greenspan 1992; Greenspan and Wieder 1998), includes 1) two or more clinical observations, of 45 minutes each, of child–caregiver and/or clinician–child interactions; 2) developmental history and review of current functioning; 3) review of family and caregiver functioning; 4) review of current programs and patterns of interaction; 5) consultation with speech pathologists, occupational and physical therapists, educators, and mental health colleagues, including the use of structured tests on an as-needed, rather than routine, basis; and 6) biomedical evaluation.

■ The Functional Developmental Profile

The assessment leads to an individualized functional profile that captures each child's unique developmental features and serves as a basis for creating individually tailored intervention programs (i.e., tailoring the program to the child rather than fitting the child to a general program). The profile describes the child's functional developmental capacities and contributing biological processing differences and environmental interactive patterns, including the different interaction patterns available to the child at home, at school, with peers, and in other settings. The profile should include all areas of challenge, not simply the ones that are more obviously associated with symptoms of one or another syndrome or disease. For example, the preschooler's lack of ability to symbolize a broad range of emotional interests and themes in either pretend play or talk is just as important, if not more important, than that same preschooler's tendency to be perseverative or self-stimulatory. In fact, clinically it is often the case that as the child's range of symbolic expression broadens, perseverative and self-stimulatory tendencies decrease.

The functional approach to creating a profile enables the clinician to consider each functional challenge separately, explore different explanations for it, and resist the temptation to assume difficulties are

Table 7–2. Outline for the evaluation of the emotional development of infants and young children

I. General parenting patterns (by history and/or direct observation)

1. *Tends to engage his or her infant pleasurably* in a relationship (e.g., by looking, vocalizing, gentle touching) rather than tending to ignore the infant (e.g., by being depressed, aloof, preoccupied, withdrawn, indifferent) — Yes/No/Unsure

2. *Tends to comfort his or her infant*, especially when the infant is upset (e.g., by relaxed, gentle, firm holding and rhythmic vocal or visual contact), rather than tending to make the infant more tense (by being overly worried, tense, or anxious or mechanical or anxiously over- or understimulating) — Yes/No/Unsure

3. *Tends to find appropriate levels of stimulation to interest his or her infant in the world* (e.g., by being interesting, alert, and responsive, including offering appropriate levels of sounds, sights, and touch—including the caregiver's face—and appropriate games and toys) rather than being hyperstimulating and intrusive (e.g., picking at and poking or shaking infant excessively to gain his or her attention) — Yes/No/Unsure

4. *Tends to read and respond to his or her infant's emotional signals and needs in most emotional areas* (e.g., responds to the infant's desire for closeness as well as need to be assertive, explorative, and independent) rather than either misreading signals or responding to only one emotional need (e.g., can hug when baby reaches out but hovers over baby and cannot encourage assertive exploration, or vice versa) — Yes/No/Unsure

5. *Tends to encourage his or her infant to move forward in development* rather than overprotecting, "holding on," or infantilizing. For example: — Yes/No/Unsure
   a. Helps baby crawl, vocalize, and gesture by actively responding to infant's initiative and encouragement rather than overanticipating infant's needs and doing everything for infant
   b. Helps toddler make shift from proximal, physical dependency (e.g., being held) to feeling secure while being independent (e.g., keeps in verbal and visual contact with toddler as he or she builds a tower across the room)
   c. Helps 2- to 3-year-old child shift from motor discharge and gestural ways of relating to the use of "ideas" through encouraging pretend play (imagination) and language around emotional themes (e.g., gets down on floor and plays out dolls hugging each other or separating from each other or soldiers fighting with each other)
   d. Helps 3- to 4-year-old child take responsibility for behavior and deal with reality rather than "giving in" all the time

II. General infant tendencies (all ages)

1. Is able to be calm and/or calm down and is not excessively irritable, clinging, active, or panicked — Yes/No/Unsure
2. Is able to take an interest in sights, sounds, and people and is not excessively withdrawn, apathetic, or unresponsive — Yes/No/Unsure
3. Is able to focus his or her attention and is not excessively distractible — Yes/No/Unsure
4. Enjoys a range of sounds, including high and low pitch, loud and soft, and different rhythms, and is not upset or confused by sounds — Yes/No/Unsure
5. Enjoys various sights, including reasonably bright lights, visual designs, facial gestures, and moving objects, and is not upset or confused by various sights — Yes/No/Unsure
6. Enjoys being touched (on face, arms, legs, stomach, trunk, and back) and bathed and clothed and is not bothered by things touching his or her skin — Yes/No/Unsure
7. Enjoys movements in space (e.g., being held and moved up and down, side to side), does not get upset with movement, and does not crave excessive movement — Yes/No/Unsure
8. Enjoys a range of age-appropriate foods and is not bothered (e.g., with abdominal pains, skin rashes, or other symptoms) by any age-appropriate, healthy food as part of a balanced diet — Yes/No/Unsure
9. Is comfortable and asymptomatic around household odors and materials and not bothered by any routine levels of household odors such as cleaning materials, paint, oil or gas fumes, pesticides, plastics, composite woods (e.g., plywood), and synthetic fabrics (e.g., polyester) — Yes/No/Unsure

Table 7–2. Outline for the evaluation of the emotional development of infants and young children *(continued)*

III. By age 4 months
Calms down and takes an interest in the world, and falls in love (as illustrated by a special interest and joy in the caregiver)

A. Primary-emotional

1. Responds to environment by brightening to *sights* (by becoming alert, calm, and focused on objects rather than ignoring or becoming overexcited by bright lights or interesting objects) — Yes/No/Unsure
2. Responds to environment by brightening to *sounds* (same as above) — Yes/No/Unsure
3. Looks at person with great interest — Yes/No/Unsure
4. Responds to social overtures with some vocalization, smile, or arm or leg movements — Yes/No/Unsure

B. Emotional

1. Looks at a person with a special joyful smile — Yes/No/Unsure
2. Smiles joyfully when spoken to — Yes/No/Unsure
3. Smiles joyfully in response to interesting facial expressions — Yes/No/Unsure
4. Vocalizes back when spoken to — Yes/No/Unsure
5. Maintains focused interest on caregiver (e.g., looking, listening, and showing some pleasure) for 1 minute or more — Yes/No/Unsure
6. Calms down when comforted — Yes/No/Unsure
7. Sleeps for intervals of 4 hours or more at night — Yes/No/Unsure
8. Enjoys being touched (e.g., being stroked on arms, legs, stomach) — Yes/No/Unsure
9. Enjoys being cuddled and held firmly — Yes/No/Unsure

C. Cognitive, sensory, or motor

1. Cognitive
   a. Shows selective attention to (special interest in) some sights or sounds — Yes/No/Unsure
   b. Coos with two or more different sounds — Yes/No/Unsure
   c. Enjoys moderate movement in space (up and down, side to side) and neither gets upset with gentle movement nor craves excessive movement — Yes/No/Unsure
   d. Follows moving object or person easily — Yes/No/Unsure
   e. Turns head in the direction of a pleasant sound (rattle or voice) — Yes/No/Unsure

2. Sensory
   a. Holds and waves a small rattle — Yes/No/Unsure
   b. Keeps hands mostly open when quiet and alert — Yes/No/Unsure

3. Motor
   a. Lifts head by leaning on elbows while on stomach — Yes/No/Unsure
   b. Holds head steady when sitting supported on caregiver's lap — Yes/No/Unsure

IV. By age 8 months
Communicates intentionally (cause and effect) and begins to learn how people act and things work

A. Primary-emotional

1. Initiates simple interaction (e.g., expectantly looks for the caregiver to respond to facial expressions) — Yes/No/Unsure
2. Responds to gestures with gestures (e.g., when the caregiver goes to pick the child up, the child responds by raising arms and leaning forward) — Yes/No/Unsure

B. Emotional

1. Initiates joy and pleasure (woos caregiver spontaneously) — Yes/No/Unsure
2. Initiates comforting (e.g., reaches up to be held) — Yes/No/Unsure
3. Responds to simple social games, such as peek-a-boo or pat-a-cake, with pleasure and smiles or laughs when the caregiver does something silly like duck his or her head or pretend to sneeze — Yes/No/Unsure
4. Shows assertiveness by reaching out for or going after an interesting toy that was taken away or put out of reach — Yes/No/Unsure
5. Shows special interest in and cautiousness toward new people or unusual objects (e.g., usually examines from a distance before approaching) — Yes/No/Unsure

Table 7–2. Outline for the evaluation of the emotional development of infants and young children *(continued)*

C. Cognitive, sensory, motor, or language	
1. Cognitive	Yes/No/Unsure
a. Focuses on toy, object, or person for 2 minutes or more	Yes/No/Unsure
b. Explores a new toy (e.g., turns it to look at its different parts; mouths, shakes, and bangs toy on a surface)	Yes/No/Unsure
c. Likes to make things happen (bangs spoon on a pot, bangs two toys together, knocks down a stand-up toy)	Yes/No/Unsure
d. Follows an object as it goes out of sight (e.g., mother's face, food, or a toy that falls to the floor) and searches for it when out of sight (e.g., looking under a chair for a favorite ball)	Yes/No/Unsure
2. Sensory	
a. Reaches out and grasps an object or toy on a table while on the caregiver's lap	Yes/No/Unsure
b. Picks up small objects, such as cereal O's or raisins	Yes/No/Unsure
c. Drinks from a cup or glass held by an adult	Yes/No/Unsure
3. Motor	
a. Rolls back to stomach	Yes/No/Unsure
b. Sits unsupported and plays from that position	Yes/No/Unsure
c. Creeps or crawls	Yes/No/Unsure
d. Pulls to stand in the crib or while holding on to furniture	Yes/No/Unsure
4. Language	
a. Imitates sounds (e.g., tongue click, fake cough, raspberry)	Yes/No/Unsure
b. Makes sounds from the front of mouth (*da, ba, ma*) and begins repeating them	Yes/No/Unsure

V. By age 12 months

Begins to develop a complex sense of self by organizing behavior and emotion

A. Primary-emotional	
1. Initiates complex interactions (e.g., hands caregiver a toy to get him or her to make it go, rolls a ball back and forth, uses gestures or vocalization to communicate the need for a desired object or food)	Yes/No/Unsure
B. Emotional	
1. Uses complex behavior to establish closeness (e.g., pulls the caregiver's leg *and* reaches up to be picked up)	Yes/No/Unsure
2. Asserts self through organized behavior, such as pointing and vocalizing at desired toy or exploring for desired objects or people	Yes/No/Unsure
3. Responds to limits set by the caregiver's voice or gesture	Yes/No/Unsure
4. Recovers from distress after 10–15 minutes	Yes/No/Unsure
5. Seems to know how to get the caregiver to react (which actions make the caregiver laugh, which actions make him or her mad)	Yes/No/Unsure
C. Cognitive, sensory, motor, or language	
1. Cognitive	
a. Plays on own in a focused, organized manner for 10 minutes or more	Yes/No/Unsure
b. Copies simple gestures (waving bye-bye, shaking head no)	Yes/No/Unsure
c. Uses hands and eyes more than mouth to examine a new object or toy	Yes/No/Unsure
d. Looks at simple pictures in a book with the caregiver's help	Yes/No/Unsure
2. Sensory	
a. Drops objects, such as blocks or toys, into a container	Yes/No/Unsure
b. Feeds self small finger foods	Yes/No/Unsure
c. Chews small food, such as pieces of dry cereal, without choking	Yes/No/Unsure
3. Motor	
a. Throws a ball forward	Yes/No/Unsure
b. Walks while holding on to furniture	Yes/No/Unsure
4. Language	
a. Understands simple words, such as *shoe*, or commands, such as "give me a kiss"	Yes/No/Unsure
b. Uses sounds for specific objects, such as *ba-ba* for *bath* or *dup* for *cup*.	Yes/No/Unsure
c. Jabbers	Yes/No/Unsure

Table 7–2. Outline for the evaluation of the emotional development of infants and young children *(continued)*

VI. By age 18 months
Continues to develop a complex sense of self by intentional planning and exploration

A. Primary-emotional
1. Shows intentional planning and exploration in interactions and play (e.g., chooses a toy, finds   Yes/No/Unsure
caregiver, and indicates with word or gesture that caregiver is the play partner)
2. Communicates needs and feelings across the room as well as close up, in gestures or words, with   Yes/No/Unsure
touch or holding (e.g., can look at caregiver's admiring glance or hear reassuring word, smile
happily, and return to organized play), or indicates interest in having caregiver join in play

B. Emotional
1. Uses gestures and vocalizations to get caregiver's interest and a sense of closeness from across the   Yes/No/Unsure
room
2. Asks easily for help from adults with play activities, to get food, and so on   Yes/No/Unsure
3. Balances a desire for independence and closeness (e.g., explores across the room and then   Yes/No/Unsure
comes back for a touch or cuddle)
4. Shows assertiveness by organizing complex behavior to meet own needs (e.g., going to   Yes/No/Unsure
refrigerator, opening door, and pointing to food) or by refusing to comply with an adult or
another child by saying no and doing something else
5. Protests or is angry, using voice and gestures without having to cry, hit, or bite   Yes/No/Unsure
6. Recovers from anger or upset within 15 minutes   Yes/No/Unsure
7. Uses role-playing as part of complex play (e.g., cooking with pots or washing dishes in play sink,   Yes/No/Unsure
driving toy fire engine with firefighter's hat on)

C. Cognitive, sensory, motor, or language
1. Cognitive
a. Searches for a desired object, such as a toy, in more than one place   Yes/No/Unsure
b. Plays on own in a focused, organized manner for 15 minutes or more   Yes/No/Unsure
c. Shows intentional planning and exploration by choosing a toy and then going to get it for   Yes/No/Unsure
play and exploration
d. Uses objects such as stuffed animals and toy telephones in play (e.g., putting animal to sleep,   Yes/No/Unsure
pretending to talk on the telephone)
e. Is able to imitate something seen a few minutes earlier   Yes/No/Unsure
2. Sensory
a. Recognizes many simple pictures in a favorite book   Yes/No/Unsure
b. Recognizes pictures of familiar objects (e.g., a dog, a baby, a ball)   Yes/No/Unsure
c. Chews a variety of foods   Yes/No/Unsure
d. Is interested in puzzles and blocks and tries to order them   Yes/No/Unsure
3. Motor
a. Walks with a sense of security   Yes/No/Unsure
b. Tries to catch a ball rolled in his or her direction   Yes/No/Unsure
c. Navigates well around furniture   Yes/No/Unsure
d. Scribbles with a pencil or crayon   Yes/No/Unsure
4. Language
a. Understands simple commands   Yes/No/Unsure
b. Uses a variety of words to convey intentions and to label things   Yes/No/Unsure

VII. By age 2–2½ years
Creates new feelings and ideas

A. Primary
1. Engages in pretend play (e.g., feeds doll and puts doll to sleep, has cars or trucks race)   Yes/No/Unsure
2. Uses words and/or gestures to express what is wanted   Yes/No/Unsure

Table 7–2. Outline for the evaluation of the emotional development of infants and young children *(continued)*

   B. Emotional

      1. Uses words or gestures to get caregiver to participate in play (e.g., "Come here," "Hold dolly")   Yes/No/Unsure

      2. Uses words to communicate desire for closeness (e.g., "hug")   Yes/No/Unsure

      3. Uses simple repetitive play sequences to indicate interest in closeness (e.g., dolls being cuddled)   Yes/No/Unsure

      4. Uses words for expressions of assertiveness ("Me want," "Give me")   Yes/No/Unsure

      5. Uses simple repetitive play sequences to indicate interest in assertiveness (e.g., a truck race)   Yes/No/Unsure

      6. Communicates anger with gestures, words, or wordlike sounds with insistence that caregiver comply   Yes/No/Unsure

      7. Recovers from anger or temper tantrum after 10 minutes   Yes/No/Unsure

   C. Cognitive, sensory, motor, or language

      1. Cognitive

         a. Plays in a focused, organized manner for 20 minutes or more   Yes/No/Unsure

         b. Searches for favorite toy where it was the day before   Yes/No/Unsure

         c. Engages in pretend play alone   Yes/No/Unsure

      2. Sensory

         a. Does simple shape puzzles with a few pieces   Yes/No/Unsure

         b. Plays with blocks with some order or design (builds a tower or lines up blocks in a train)   Yes/No/Unsure

         c. Copies a circle   Yes/No/Unsure

      3. Motor

         a. Catches a large ball from a couple of feet away using arms and hands   Yes/No/Unsure

         b. Balances momentarily on one foot   Yes/No/Unsure

         c. Jumps with both feet off the ground   Yes/No/Unsure

         d. Walks up steps putting two feet on each step before going to the next   Yes/No/Unsure

         e. Runs   Yes/No/Unsure

      4. Language

         a. Uses simple two-word sentences ("Go bye-bye," "More milk")   Yes/No/Unsure

         b. Understands simple questions ("Is Mommy home?")   Yes/No/Unsure

VIII. By age 3–3½ years

Uses emotional thinking

   A. Primary

      1. Enjoys pretend play that conveys human dramas, which become more complex so that one pretend sequence leads to another (e.g., instead of repetition where the doll goes to bed, gets up, and goes to bed, the doll goes to bed, gets up, and then gets dressed; or the cars race, crash, and then go to get fixed)   Yes/No/Unsure

      2. Knows what is real and what is not real (e.g., knows that cartoons are "pretend")   Yes/No/Unsure

   B. Emotional

      1. Uses another person's help and some toys to play out complex pretend drama dealing with closeness, nurturing, or caregiving (taking care of a stuffed animal or doll that has fallen down and hurt itself)   Yes/No/Unsure

      2. Uses another person's help and some toys to play out pretend drama dealing with assertiveness, exploration, or aggression (e.g., a truck race, monsters and soldiers fighting, a trip to Grandma's house)   Yes/No/Unsure

      3. Follows rules   Yes/No/Unsure

      4. Remains calm and focused for 30 minutes or more   Yes/No/Unsure

      5. Feels optimistic and confident   Yes/No/Unsure

      6. Realizes how behavior, thoughts, and feelings can be related to consequences (if behaves nicely, makes caregiver pleased; if misbehaves, must face consequences; if tries hard, learns to do something)   Yes/No/Unsure

      7. Uses relationship between feelings, behavior, and consequences to be assertive (e.g., bargains, "Eat broccoli later!")   Yes/No/Unsure

      8. Interacts in socially appropriate way with adults   Yes/No/Unsure

      9. Interacts in socially appropriate way with peers   Yes/No/Unsure

Table 7–2. Outline for the evaluation of the emotional development of infants and young children *(continued)*

C. Cognitive, sensory, motor, or language	
1. Cognitive	
a. Plays in a focused, organized manner without another person for 20 minutes or more	Yes/No/Unsure
b. Enjoys pretend play elements that are logically connected (e.g., "Dolly gets a time-out because she messed up")	Yes/No/Unsure
2. Sensory	
a. Puts pop beads together	Yes/No/Unsure
b. Uses spatial designs that become more complex and have interrelated parts (e.g., a block house has rooms or maybe furniture, or cars have different places to go, such as the store and the house or garage)	Yes/No/Unsure
c. Draws a person by putting indications of facial features or limbs on a circular shape	Yes/No/Unsure
3. Motor	
a. Walks up stairs alternating feet	Yes/No/Unsure
b. Catches a large ball using both hands	Yes/No/Unsure
c. Kicks a ball	Yes/No/Unsure
4. Language	
a. Uses sentences that become complex, with logical connecting words between phrases (e.g., *because* or *but* is used: "No like fish because icky")	Yes/No/Unsure
b. Asks "Why?" although not necessarily interested in the answer and may repeat	Yes/No/Unsure

necessarily tied together as part of a syndrome (unless all alternative explanations have been ruled out). For example, hand-flapping is often related to motor problems and is seen when children with a variety of motor problems become excited or overloaded. Many conditions, including cerebral palsy, autism, hypotonia, and dyspraxia, involve motor problems and, at times, hand-flapping. Yet this symptom is often assumed to be uniquely a part of the autistic spectrum. Similarly, sensory over- or under-reactivity is present in many disorders and developmental variations, yet it often also is assumed to be a unique part of autism. The functional approach does not detract from understanding existing syndromes. In fact, over time it may clarify what symptoms are unique to particular syndromes, lead to new classifications, and further tease out biological and functional patterns.

Constructing the child's profile of functional capacities through appropriate clinical assessments enables the clinician to tailor the intervention program to the child's and family's unique features, rather than have the child fit the program, based on some broad but nonspecific diagnostic criteria.

To facilitate screening and comprehensive evaluations, Table 7–2 provides a guide to emotional development in the context of sensorimotor, cognitive, and language development. (See Greenspan 1992 for a fuller discussion of this table and the principles it is based on.)

Conclusion

The framework presented here, both theoretical and practical, may also prove useful for guiding the comprehensive clinical evaluations that are indicated when an infant's emotional progress is lagging or shifting into a disordered configuration. The clinician may use careful history taking, clinical interviews, observations of infant–caregiver and family interaction, and formal testing of sensorimotor and cognitive abilities to determine 1) whether the infant and family have reached a certain emotional milestone (e.g., attachment, purposeful communication, representational capacities) and 2) whether there are constrictions in the emotional domains engaged at that level. For either a deficit or a constriction, the clinician can determine the relative contributions of family, parent, infant–parent interaction, and infant constitutional–maturational factors.

In addition, determining overall developmental level and behavioral and emotional range at that level helps the clinician pinpoint the nature of the psychopathology (Greenspan 1981). Symptoms such as sleep problems, eating difficulties, or impulsive behavior may be part of an overall developmental lag or deficit or a constriction in the range of emotional domains engaged in by the infant and family. In this way, the clinician can assess and treat emotional problems in infancy as part of a normative preventive developmental framework for emotional stages.

References

Ainsworth M, Bell SM, Stayton D: Infant-mother attachment and social development: socialization as a product of reciprocal responsiveness to signals, in The Integration of the Child into a Social World. Edited by Richards M. Cambridge, UK, Cambridge University Press, 1974, pp 99–135

Bakwin H: Loneliness in infants. Am J Dis Child 63:30–42, 1942

Bell SM: The development of the concept of the object as related to infant-mother attachment. Child Dev 41:219–311, 1970

Bergman P, Escalona S: Unusual sensitivities in very young children. Psychoanal Study Child 3–4:333–352, 1949

Bowlby J: Maternal care and mental health. WHO Monograph No. 51. Geneva, World Health Organization, 1951

Bowlby J: Attachment and Loss, Vol 1. London, Hogarth Press, 1969

Brazelton TB, Koslowski B, Main M: The origins of reciprocity; the early mother-infant interaction, in The Effect of the Infant on Its Caregiver. Edited by Lewis M, Rosenblum L. New York, Wiley, 1974, pp 49–76

Burlingham D, Freud A: Young Children in Wartime: A Year's Work in a Residential War Nursery. London, Allen & Unwin, 1942

Cameron HS: The Nervous Child. London, Oxford Medical Publications, 1919

Charlesworth WR: The role of surprise in cognitive development, in Studies in Cognitive Development: Essays. Edited by Elkind D, Flavell JH. London, Oxford University Press, 1969, pp 257–314

Cravioto J, DeLicardie E: Environmental correlates of severe clinical malnutrition and language development survivors from kwashiorkor or marasmus. PAHO Scientific Publication No. 251. Washington, DC, Pan American Health Organization, 1973

DeGangi GA, Porges SW, Sickel RZ, et al: Four-year follow-up of a sample of regulatory disordered infants. Infant Mental Health Journal 14:330–343, 1993

Ekman P: Universals and Cultural Differences in Facial Expressions of Emotion. Lincoln, NE, University of Nebraska Press, 1972

Emde RN, Gaensbauer TJ, Harmon RJ: Emotional expression in infancy: a biobehavioral study. Psychol Issues 37 (monograph), 1976

Escalona S: The Roots of Individuality. Chicago, IL, Aldine, 1968

Fraiberg S: Treatment modalities in an infant mental health program. Paper presented at the annual meeting of the National Center for Clinical Infant Programs, Washington, DC, December 5–7, 1979

Gewirtz JL: A learning analysis of the effects of normal stimulation, privation and deprivation on the acquisition of social motivation and attachment, in Determinants of Infant Behavior, Vol 1. Edited by Foss BM. London, Methuen, 1961, pp 28–35

Gewirtz JL: Levels of conceptual analysis in environment-infant interaction research. Merrill-Palmer Q 15:9–47, 1969

Gouin-Decarie T: Intelligence and Affectivity in Early Childhood: An Experimental Study of Jean Piaget's Object Concept and Object Relations. New York, International Universities Press, 1965

Greenspan SI: Intelligence and adaptation: an integration of psychoanalytic and Piagetian developmental psychology. Psychol Issues 13 (monograph), 1979

Greenspan SI: Psychopathology and adaptation in infancy and early childhood: principles of clinical diagnosis and preventive intervention. Clinical Infant Reports 1 (monograph), 1981

Greenspan S[I]: A model for comprehensive preventive intervention services for infants, young children and their families, in Infants in Multirisk Families. Edited by Wieder S, Lieberman A, Nover R, et al. New York, International Universities Press, 1987, pp 377–390

Greenspan SI: The Development of the Ego: Implications for Personality Theory, Psychopathology, and the Psychotherapeutic Process. New York, International Universities Press, 1989

Greenspan SI: Infancy and Early Childhood: The Practice of Clinical Assessment and Intervention with Emotional and Developmental Challenges. Madison, CT, International Universities Press, 1992

Greenspan SI: Developmentally Based Psychotherapy. Madison, CT, International Universities Press, 1997a

Greenspan SI: The Growth of the Mind and the Endangered Origins of Intelligence. Reading, MA, Addison Wesley Longman, 1997b

Greenspan SI, Wieder S: The Child with Special Needs: Encouraging Intellectual and Emotional Growth. Reading, MA, Perseus Books, 1998

Greenspan SI, DeGangi GA, Wieder S: The Functional Emotional Assessment Scale (FEAS) for Infancy and Early Childhood: Clinical and Research Applications. Bethesda, MD, Interdisciplinary Council on Developmental and Learning Disorders, 2001

Hunt JM: Infants in an orphanage. Journal of Abnormal Psychology and Social Psychology 36, 1941

Interdisciplinary Council on Developmental and Learning Disorders Clinical Practice Guidelines Workgroup: Interdisciplinary Council on Developmental and Learning Disorders' Clinical Practice Guidelines: Redefining the Standards of Care for Infants, Children, and Families with Special Needs. Bethesda, MD, Interdisciplinary Council on Developmental and Learning Disorders, 2000

Izard CE: On the development of emotions and emotion-cognition relationships in infancy, in The Development of Affect. Edited by Lewis M, Rosenblum L. New York, Plenum, 1978

Klaus M, Kennell J: Maternal-Infant Bonding: The Impact of Early Separation or Loss on Family Development. St. Louis, MO, CV Mosby, 1976

Lipsitt L: Learning processes of newborns. Merrill-Palmer Q 12:45–71, 1966

Lowery LG: Personality disorders and early institutional care. Am J Orthopsychiatry 10:546–555, 1940

Mahler MS, Pine F, Bergman A: The Psychological Birth of the Human Infant: Symbiosis and Individuation. New York, Basic Books, 1975

Meltzoff A, Moore K: Imitation of facial and manual gestures by human neonates. Science 198:75–78, 1977

Murphy LB, Moriarty A: Vulnerability, Coping, and Growth. New Haven, CT, Yale University Press, 1976

Piaget J: The stages of intellectual development of the child, in Childhood Psychopathology. Edited by Harrison S, McDermott J. New York, International Universities Press, 1962, pp 157–166

Porges SW, Greenspan SI: Regulatory-disordered infants: a common theme. Presented at the National Institute on Drug Abuse RAUS Review Meeting on Methodological Issues in Controlled Studies on Effects of Prenatal Exposure to Drugs of Abuse, Richmond, VA, June 8–9, 1990

Provence S (ed): Infants and Parents: Clinical Case Reports (Clinical Infant Reports No 2). New York, International Universities Press, 1983

Rachford BK: Neurotic Disorders of Childhood. New York, E. B. Treat and Company, 1905

Rheingold H: The development of social behavior in the human infant. Monogr Soc Res Child Dev 31(1):1–17, 1966

Rheingold H: Infancy, in Encyclopedia of the Social Sciences. Edited by Sills D. New York, Macmillan, 1969

Sameroff A, Seifer R, Barocas R, et al: IQ scores of 4-year-old children: social-environmental risk factors. Pediatrics 29:343–350, 1986

Sander L: Issues in early mother-child interaction. J Am Acad Child Adolesc Psychiatry 1:141–166, 1962

Spitz RA: Hospitalism: an inquiry into the genesis of psychiatric conditions in early childhood. Psychoanal Study Child 1:53–74, 1945

Sroufe LA: Socioemotional development, in Handbook of Infant Development. Edited by Osofsky J. New York, Wiley, 1979

Sroufe LA, Waters E: Attachment as an organizational construct. Child Dev 48:1184–1199, 1977

Stern D: The goal and structure of mother-infant play. J Am Acad Child Psychiatry 13:402–421, 1974a

Stern D: Mother and infant at play: the dyadic interaction involving facial, vocal, and gaze behaviors, in The Effect of the Infant on Its Caregiver. Edited by Lewis M, Rosenblum L. New York, Wiley, 1974b

Stern D: The First Relationship: Mother and Infant. Cambridge, MA, Harvard University Press, 1977

Thomas A, Chess S: Temperament and development. New York, Brunner/Mazel, 1977

Tomkins S: Affect, Imagery, Consciousness, Vol 1. New York, Springer, 1963a

Tomkins S: Affect, Imagery, Consciousness, Vol 2. New York, Springer, 1963b

Werner H, Kaplan B: Symbol Formation. New York, Wiley, 1963

Winnicott DW: Clinical Notes on the Disorders of Childhood. London, Heineman, 1931

The Clinical Interview of the Child

Clarice J. Kestenbaum, M.D.

The clinical interview always has been the sine qua non of the psychiatric evaluation. As MacKinnon and Michels (1971) observed in *The Psychiatric Interview in Clinical Practice*, a "clear understanding of the psychopathology and psychodynamics is the foundation of the psychiatric interview" (p. 1). The foremost goal of the clinical interview is to establish a diagnosis. The interviewer may begin an intake session with a particular hypothesis about the nature of the patient's problem, but with each new piece of evidence the patient presents, the hypothesis formulation may change in midinterview. For example, the therapist may view an overactive child as possibly having attention-deficit/hyperactivity disorder but soon discover that nightmares and phobias point to an anxiety disorder.

Despite advances in molecular genetics, breakthroughs in cellular pathology, and new knowledge about mind–brain synergy, our understanding of the etiology of disorders has not changed very much. "Clinical syndromes continue to be defined by patterns of symptoms and course of illness, using the methods of Hippocrates, Sydenham, and other great physicians," according to McClellan and Werry (2000, p. 19). They stated, furthermore, that "the lack of understanding regarding the exact nature and etiology of psychiatric disorders requires that diagnoses be made based solely on recognized patterns or clusters of symptoms. Although helpful, this has all the diagnostic precision of 'fever.'...Although the clinical interview remains the accepted standard of psychiatric assessment, research suggests that clinicians' diagnoses are fraught with numerous biases" (p. 20).

Thus, a variety of structured interviews have been developed so that evidence-based research designs can be both reliable and valid (see Chapter 13, "Rating Scales," in this volume). For an in-depth understanding of the complex factors that constitute an integra-tion of psychopathology and psychodynamics inherent in any given individual, however, the clinical interview remains the best instrument we have.

In the assessment of an adult, the chief informant is the patient. Additional information may, of course, be requested from other physicians, hospital records, or psychological tests, but usually the skilled interviewer can obtain a psychiatric history and perform a mental status examination in one or two sessions if the adult is reasonably cooperative. The task facing the child psychiatric interviewer, however, is far more complex. The interviewer first must take into account the child's age, cognitive level of development, and willingness to discuss problems. The examination of the child alone rarely, if ever, can serve as the only source of information sufficient for making a diagnosis, but the examiner can certainly form a valuable diagnostic impression.

Children between ages 3 and 6 years can usually provide correct information when questions are asked in a way commensurate with their developmental level (Bjorklund and Muir 1988; Ornstein et al. 1991). The interviewer must be careful about making assumptions about the validity of a child's report in highly charged situations, such as custody cases or cases involving child abuse allegations. Younger children are suggestible and may repeat information fed to them by a hostile parent involved in an angry divorce, despite their own observations to the contrary (Ceci et al. 1987). However, additional information is also needed that the child cannot supply: a developmental history (including genetic background), a broad understanding of the home environment, and some knowledge of the significant people in the child's life. A thorough assessment from the school and other aspects of the child's world often is needed for a comprehensive evaluation, including current or past events (e.g., the death of a parent, effects of divorce, or a traumatic event such as a fire or automobile accident) that may have a lasting impact on future development.

School reports as well as pediatric records (including a neurological examination when indicated) may be sent to the diagnostician before the first visit. A psychological evaluation may already have been obtained or may be requested by the evaluator. Evaluation of family functioning is important. A family interview at some point in the evaluation process helps to determine the quality of the parent–child "fit"; for example, depression in the mother, alcoholism in the father, and a disruptive home environment may become more apparent.

A more detailed discussion concerning history taking and the family interview is available elsewhere (see Chapters 10, "The Parent Interview," and 11, "Initial and Diagnostic Family Interviews," in this volume).

The clinical interview with the child should be considered as one piece of a puzzle that is ready to be assembled when all other data are gathered. In presenting a detailed method of approaching a child and the child's family, from the initial telephone call to the final presentation of the findings, Gardner (1985) observed that "the initial interview and intensive evaluation should provide an in-depth understanding of the child's problems and also establish a good relationship or at least communication with the child and family members…without which the likelihood of a successful psychotherapy is minimal" (p. 371).

The evaluation process can take many weeks. A clinician who has the time and has no concerns about third-party payers may see the child optimally four or five times before completing the evaluation. The interview technique depends on the orientation of the interviewer and is highly personal. I recall one senior psychiatrist's response to the question "What is the best way to learn interview technique?" He answered, "Twenty-five years of clinical experience." Child psychoanalysts such as Anna Freud (1946) and D. W. Winnicott (1971) have made valuable contributions to the understanding of the process of child psychodynamic assessment. Good reviews of such techniques include *The Child Mental Status Examination* (Goodman and Sours 1967), *Psychiatric Examination of Children* (Simmons 1981), *The Clinical Interview of the Child* (Greenspan and Greenspan 1991), *Psychodynamic Psychotherapy of Children: An Introduction to the Art and the Techniques* (Coppollilo 1987), and "Taking a History" (Canino 1985).

In many cases, the clinical interview is performed under less than optimal circumstances. A court-referred adolescent or a child hospitalized on a pediatric ward may need an emergency consultation when other informants and data are not available. Sometimes a single interview is all the clinician is allowed, even though a diagnostic impression must be formulated. In terms of diagnostic reliability, Bird et al. (1992) found that clinicians were less likely to assign certain comorbid diagnoses than were computer algorithms using DSM-IV (American Psychiatric Association 1994) diagnostic criteria. To make a valid diagnosis, one needs a thorough familiarity with child development, psychopathology, and the current DSM-IV-TR (American Psychiatric Association 2000) diagnostic criteria. Structured interviews such as the Child Assessment Schedule (Hodges et al. 1982) and the Diagnostic Interview Schedule for Children (Costello et al. 1984) and semistructured interviews such as the Children's Version of the Schedule for Affective Disorders and Schizophrenia (Chambers et al. 1985) have been successfully designed for research purposes. Other instruments are typically used in epidemiological surveys, where trained lay interviewers, not clinicians, administer the instrument. These include the National Institute of Mental Health Diagnostic Interview Schedule for Children (Shaffer et al. 2000), the Children's Interview for Psychiatric Syndromes (Weller et al. 2000), and the Diagnostic Interview for Children and Adolescents (Reich 2000). However, they do not allow for gathering data on the full range of feelings, personality organization, and coping mechanisms, as does the free-range clinical interview. For these reasons, a semistructured clinical interview—the Mental Health Assessment Form (MHAF; Kestenbaum and Bird 1978)—was developed to provide a bridge between the structured questionnaire and the open-ended clinical interview. The MHAF may be used with children between ages 6 and 12 years. (There is a supplement for adolescents.) It can be performed in a relatively brief period, 45 minutes, or extended for several sessions, depending on the clinical situation.

Cards or questionnaires are not used. The "structure" is in the mind of the examiner. The examiner must be familiar with child developmental principles and psychopathology because the MHAF was designed to be used by clinicians with a certain level of training and experience.

The interview itself involves an inquiry into all areas of a child's life and functioning, including specific questions about 1) the child in his or her family (a description of home and family life problems in family relationships), 2) the child in school (including sports, hobbies, homework, and relationships with teachers and peers), 3) the child's fantasy life (quality and content of fantasies and dreams, as well as problem-solving ability), and 4) the child's personality organization (self-concept, overall mood, perceptions, coping mechanisms).

The MHAF consists of 189 items divided into two major sections (Table 8–1). Part I is scored according to observable data and is primarily a mental status examination. It is subdivided into five major areas: 1) physical appearance, 2) motoric behavior and speech, 3) relatedness during the interview, 4) affect, and 5) language and thinking. Part II scores information derived from the content of the interview. Both historical and developmental data elicited from the child during the interview are included. Part II also deals with the child's self-concepts and perceptions in his or her world. It is divided into six major areas: 1) feeling states, 2) interpersonal relations, 3) symbolic representation (fantasies and dreams), 4) self-concept, 5) conscience/moral judgment, and 6) general level of adaptation.

General level of adaptation includes positive attributes: personality characteristics such as skills or talents, interests (e.g., hobbies), perseverance (stick-to-itiveness), frustration tolerance, creativity, imagination, sense of humor, empathy, ability to cope with stress (e.g., actual events by history such as separations, hospitalizations, illnesses), and problem-solving ability (when given an imaginary situation).

The rater must use both clinical experience and theoretical knowledge to determine whether the particular item is to be scored within the expectable range or to determine the degree of deviance from age-group norms. There is a section at the end of the form for descriptive information as well as a global assessment score for the current level of function (Shaffer et al. 1983).

The questions designed specifically for the MHAF interview can be geared toward younger or older children and take into account degrees of cooperation and resistance. Suggested questions are presented in an open-ended manner (Table 8–2). The examiner is advised to follow the child's lead and not stay rigidly within a given framework. He or she may return at any time to topics that were brushed aside or ignored the first time around (Bird and Kestenbaum 1988).

Table 8–1. Outline of the Mental Health Assessment Form

Part I—Mental status

I. *Physical appearance*
    A. General attractiveness
    B. Physical characteristics
    C. Physical maturation
    D. Observable deviations in physical characteristics
    E. Grooming and dress
    F. Gender differentiation

II. *Motoric behavior and speech*
    A. Motor activity
    B. Motor coordination
    C. Presence of unusual motoric patterns, habit patterns, and mannerisms
    D. Speech

III. *Relatedness during interview*
    A. Quality of relatedness as judged by nonverbal behavior
    B. Quality of relatedness as judged by verbal behavior
    C. Social interaction

IV. *Affect*
    A. Inappropriate affect
    B. Constriction of affect
    C. Elated affect
    D. Depressed affect
    E. Labile affect
    F. Overanxious affect
    G. Angry affect
    H. Histrionic affect

V. *Language and thinking*
    A. Overall intelligence
    B. Cognitive functions
    C. External reality testing
    D. Use of language
    E. Thought process
    F. Attention span

Part II—Content of the interview

VI. *Feeling states*
    A. Depression
    B. Elation
    C. Mood disturbance (other)
    D. Anger
    E. Anxiety
    F. Irritability
    G. Impulsivity

VII. *Interpersonal relations*
    A. The child's relationship with his or her family
    B. The child's relationship with other adult authority figures
    C. The child's relationship with peers
    D. The child's relationship with pets

Table 8–1. Outline of the Mental Health Assessment Form *(continued)*

    E. Modes of interaction with others
    F. Aggressive behavior
    G. Sexual behavior

VIII.*Symbolic representation*
    A. Fantasies
    B. Dreams

IX. *Self-concept*
    A. Dissatisfaction with self
    B. Comparison of self with peers
    C. Comparison of self with ideal self

X. *Conscience/moral judgment*
    A. Deficit in development of conscience
    B. Antisocial behavior

XI. *General level of adaptation*
    A. Personality characteristics
    B. Defense mechanisms
    C. Maladaptive solutions in dealing with anxiety

Interviewing the Younger Child (Age 5–9 Years)

There is no "best way" to interview children. Various techniques are derived from practicing a variety of established approaches with a number of children and adding new approaches that have proved helpful in establishing rapport with young children in a relatively brief period (no checklists). What follows is a distillate of my clinical experience.

In most circumstances, the clinician interviews one or both parents, before meeting with the child, to ascertain the nature of the presenting problem, to obtain pertinent information, and to suggest ways of informing the child about the nature of the psychiatric examination. In those instances when the child refuses to leave the parent (usually a manifestation of separation anxiety), the parent is invited into the consultation room. Otherwise, the child is interviewed alone.

Most children spend a few minutes examining the strange surroundings, such as children's books, drawing materials, a dollhouse with simple furniture and little dolls, several hand puppets in full view, and a few standard games. An explanation may be given about the nature of the interview, with some reassurance if necessary.

Table 8–2. Questions suggested for the semistructured interview

School

What grade are you in?
What is your best subject? Which is the worst? Are you better in subjects in which you have to figure things out or ones that require memory?
Have you ever been held back in school?

Interpersonal relations: family

Who lives at home with you?
Do you have brothers and sisters?
How do you all get along?
Who else is in your family?
When you have a problem, whom do you tell about it?
Does he or she help you with your problem?
Who is the closest person to you in your family?
Who gives you the most problems? Tell me about that.
How do you get along with your mother/father?
Who is your favorite?

Dependence/independence with family members

Do your parents tell you what to do, or can you make some of your decisions?
What are the rules at home about going out alone or getting home, bringing friends home, etc.?
Have you ever been away from home at sleep-away camp or at a friend's home? How did you feel about being away?
What happens at home when you do something wrong or break the rules?

Interpersonal relations: other adults

What kind of relationship do you have with other adults (grown-ups) outside the family (e.g., teachers, coach, minister, counselor)?
Is there someone you especially admire?
Which adults do you respect the least?

Interpersonal relations: peers

Do you have friends?
Are most of your friends about your age?
Do you have friends who are older? Younger?
Do you have a best friend?
How long has he or she been your best friend?
What sort of things do you do together?
Why did you pick him or her as your best friend?
How do you feel when something good/bad happens to one of your friends?
Do you do what most kids want to do, or do they do what you want?
What happens when you can't get your own way?

Table 8–2. Questions suggested for the semistructured interview *(continued)*

Future plans

What would you like to be when you grow up?

Why do you think you would enjoy that?

Do you know anyone who is a (occupation)?

How good are your chances of becoming a (occupation)?

What would you do if you couldn't be a (occupation)?

Have you ever had an after-school or summer job?

What did/do you do with the money you made/make?

Gender concepts and behavior

What are the advantages of being a boy/girl?

What are the disadvantages?

Do you like being a boy/girl?

Suppose you could start all over again. Would you rather be a boy/girl?

Self-concept

If I asked your parents what they think about you, what would they say? Suppose I asked your friends?

If you could change anything about yourself, what would you change?

How do you compare yourself with your friends (in sports, looks, intelligence, personality)?

Do you like the way you are? Do people like you?

Conscience

What was your best deed?

What is the worst thing you've ever done?

Did it get you into trouble?

How did you feel?

Did you ever take something that didn't belong to you? What?

What happened? How did you feel?

How do you feel when you do something you know is wrong?

Do you ever do it again?

Feeling states: general

How do you feel most of the time (happy/sad)?

How do you feel now compared with the way you usually feel?

What sort of things make you happy? Sad?

What things do you enjoy doing most of all?

What was the happiest time in your life?

Feeling states: anxiety

What things make you nervous?

What is the scariest thing that's ever happened to you?

What happens when you get scared like that?

When you are scared, does it bother you in other ways, such as you can't sleep or you get headaches?

Do you ever feel scared like that for no reason at all?

What does that feel like?

Table 8–2. Questions suggested for the semistructured interview *(continued)*

Feeling states: depression

What is the saddest thing that ever happened to you?

Do you ever feel sad even if there's no good reason? Tell me about that.

Do you ever think of dying? Have you ever thought of killing yourself? Have you ever tried to kill yourself?

When you feel sad like that, does it ever last many days in a row? How many days?

When you feel sad like that, does it bother you in other ways, such as you can't sleep or you have no appetite? Does that last many days in a row? How many days?

Did you ever feel the opposite, like you're on top of the world, for no reason at all? Tell me about it (duration, severity, other descriptive symptoms).

Feeling states: anger

What do you do when you really want something and you don't get your way?

Do you have a "short fuse" (lose your temper easily)?

What sort of things make you angry?

What do you do when you get very angry?

Do you ever get into fights? With whom?

(If yes) Do you fight alone or in a group?

Reality testing

Do you think there are people who can predict the future?

Do you believe in extrasensory perception (ESP)? Have you had experiences like that? Some people, when they get very nervous, have funny experiences. Did you ever hear voices inside/outside your head? Were you fully awake? What did they say (frequency, severity)? What do you think that was?

Some kids have told me that they think their minds are controlled by something or someone else. Others believe someone is looking at them or talking about them when it really isn't so. Did something like that ever happen to you?

Fantasy

Do you have an active imagination?

When you're bored in school and looking out the window, what do you think about?

Make believe we just heard a loud noise outside the window. Can you make up a story about what happened?

Do you dream a lot?

How often do you dream?

Are most of your dreams good dreams or bad dreams?

Tell me about a dream that you remember.

Did you ever or do you have a make-believe friend? Tell me about him or her.

Do you keep a diary of your secret thoughts?

Table 8–2. Questions suggested for the semistructured interview *(continued)*

Other

What do you think the future will be like?

What do you think happens to people after they die?

Do you play sports? Are you good in sports?

Do you have any hobbies?

Do you have any special talents (e.g., drawing, music)?

The interview can begin with a question about why the child has been brought to see the psychiatrist. For example, this is how the interview with Marjorie, age 7 years, began:

Marjorie: I don't know.

Dr. K: Did your mother explain that I am the kind of doctor who helps children with their feelings and troubles?

Marjorie: No.

Dr. K: Well, I am. Some children have the kind of troubles everyone can see. For instance, if there's a child in school who bullies other children, or yells or throws things in class, or gets into fights…

Marjorie: Billy's like that. He's always in the principal's office.

Dr. K: Yes, exactly. I might see someone like Billy to help him with his problem controlling himself. But I also see children who have problems no one can see—worries about their parents going away, bad dreams, sad feelings.

Marjorie said nothing, but her solemn nod let me know my words made an impression.

After such an introduction, I shift gears and ask neutral questions about the child's home, family members, and pets. I might ask the child to draw a floor plan of his or her house or apartment—his or her room, the distance from the parents' room, the approximate distance to the school—and perhaps a rough sketch of his or her family. In 5 minutes, I will have already observed the child enough to score (mentally) the first part of the MHAF: general attractiveness, motor activity and coordination, presence or absence of tics, quality of speech, and relatedness to me (usually determined by eye contact, shyness, withdrawal, and general affect). I can estimate the child's overall level of intelligence by his or her vocabulary and comprehension, ability to follow directions, and graphomotor skill in drawing. Of course, if there seems to be a problem in cognitive functioning, I will order a psychologi-

cal examination if one has not already been obtained. I usually turn the conversation to the subject of favorite activities, friends, playmates, and sleepovers.

In Marjorie's case, her parents were concerned about school avoidance and somatic complaints, and the child was not forthcoming about her worries and particularly avoided questions about school:

Dr. K: Marjorie, do you see that boy puppet over there? Reach in that bag and take out some of those people.

Marjorie: Those are finger puppets. (She took two puppets that represented children.)

Dr. K: I'll take these two (adult figures). Hi. I'm Ms. Smith, your teacher. What are your names?

Marjorie (with a little prodding): Mary and Susie.

Dr. K (whispering to her): Which one knows all the right answers and which one has trouble? (Marjorie responds by pointing to each puppet.) All right, children. Today we'll have math. How much is 2 + 2? How do you spell *cat?*

Marjorie (answering for puppet figures): Four, but only Mary can spell *cat.* Susie can't read.

(After several minutes of simple questions, I introduced a third puppet: the good wizard.)

Dr. K: I am the wizard who can grant all your wishes. What would you want more than anything in the world, Susie?

Marjorie: To be smart.

In my experience, for a child with school problems, nothing so readily establishes the distinction between a learning disability and attention-deficit or conduct disorder as this kind of fantasy play. Further testing in Marjorie's case and appropriate academic intervention coupled with brief psychotherapy for herself and her family proved extremely helpful.

Another technique that can be used with younger children is asking projective make-believe questions. For example, the same question brought forth very different responses from a dysthymic 8-year-old and a psychotic child of the same age:

Dr. K: Billy, make believe you are looking out the window and you hear an enormous crash. What do you see?

Billy: Two cars crash into each other.

Dr. K: And then what happens?

Billy: The ambulance comes.

Dr. K: And then what?

Billy: Nothing. Everyone is dead.

Most nondepressed children, unlike Billy, manage to get the passengers to a hospital where everyone is eventually saved. In response to the same question, Mark, a psychotic child, gave a very bizarre answer:

> *Mark:* A monster from outer space throws a bomb and the whole world is killed and all the people in it and you and me too and then he eats all the pieces up and the ocean is all bloody and he drinks it and it's delicious.

Another projective technique is a variant of Winnicott's (1971) "squiggles" game—that is, drawing a scribbled design and asking the child to use his or her imagination, to complete the drawing by turning it into anything he or she thinks of, and to tell a story about the completed picture.

Asking for a description of a favorite television program is another useful tactic. Does the child relate the story in a logical, sequential fashion, or are cognitive deficits evident?

Overall mood can be elicited by the appearance of the "mood machine." Facing the child, I extend one arm, bent 90 degrees at the elbow:

> *Dr. K:* John, pretend my arm is a pendulum. On one side we have "happiness," on the other side "sadness," and straight up is "neutral." [I swing my arm slowly.] Now, when my arm reaches the place that describes how you feel most of the time, yell, "Stop!"

I then ask the child to describe the happiest and saddest events in his or her life. I often inquire about dreams and, when possible, ask the child to draw a picture of the dream. This drawing can lead to inquiry about perceptual distortions, such as familiar objects taking on frightening aspects, illusions at night, hypnagogic phenomena, or hallucinations.

Eliciting feelings about family members should be done after rapport has been established. The parent with whom the child feels closest or safest can then be determined, as can the examiner's own impression of the "fairness" of discipline, any overly strict or punitive parenting, and any actual child abuse. (Rarely will an abused child actually accuse the parent of physical or sexual abuse in the first session.)

Interviewing the Older Child (Age 10–12 Years)

There is no explicit age cutoff at which the interviewer knows with certainty whether to begin with the version

of the MHAF designed for younger children or to shape questions according to the presumed cognitive level of the preadolescent or adolescent youngster. Some 10-year-olds do far better when interviewed with the use of techniques usually reserved for younger children; others conduct themselves like teenagers. A sensitive interviewer will know when to shift gears. In general, I begin with the chief complaint. Frequently, the older child also will deny having any problems:

> *James (age 10):* My parents said I had to come or I could not watch TV.
> *Dr. K:* Boy, they must really think there's a problem. What do you think about it?
> *James:* Nothing. Ask them!
> *Dr. K:* I did already, but you know, I'm not so interested in their opinion as I am yours. The fact that they think there's a problem and even insist on your coming when you think there's no problem at all…well, even that's a problem! Besides, whatever you tell me is a one-way street. I want to hear all sides, but I don't repeat back to them what you say. I like to form my own opinion.

Usually this type of opening is sufficient to establish some degree of rapport.

After inquiries about interests and school activities, children are asked to describe their friends (or enemies). Then I might inquire about peer relationships; for example, "If I asked your best friend about you, what would he (she) say?"

For preadolescents, self-esteem is very much connected to body image. When asked "If there is anything you could change about yourself, what would it be?" most very young adolescents discuss their pimples, hair color, braces, or unsightly blemishes. If the answer is "everything," depression is a major diagnostic consideration.

It is important to obtain some idea about the development of empathy. Exploring feelings about animals is usually a useful approach. The clinician should inquire about family pets—their names, personality characteristics, and children's identifications with their pets. Other questions probing for empathic feelings bring forth a variety of responses:

> *Dr. K:* What would you do if a new girl appeared in class one day in the middle of the term?
> *Jill (age 11):* Well, I'd go over to her and tell her my name and introduce her to my friends and show her where the bathroom is and all.
> *Dr. K:* Why would you do that?

Jill: Well, I went to a new school once, and I felt all scared and alone, and so I'd know how she feels.

George (age 10, responding to the same question, except that the newcomer is a boy): Well, I wouldn't hit him or anything...not on the first day.

Questions about superego or conscience formation usually bring myriad responses:

Dr. K: Let's suppose that a man is walking down the street in front of you and a ten-dollar bill slips from his pocket and lands on the sidewalk. What would you do?

Arthur (age 11): I'd pick it up and call, "Hey, mister, you dropped your money!" Maybe I'd get a reward.

Jim (age 10): I'd keep it. Finders keepers!

Martha (age 11): I'd run over and give it back.

Dr. K: What if he crossed the street and cars were coming?

Martha: I'd wait for the light to change and try to find him.

Dr. K: What if you couldn't?

Martha: Well, I'd take it to the police and ask if anyone lost ten dollars.

Most children find the type of interview I have described reassuring and nonpressured. I usually try to end the session on an upbeat note with a statement such as "I think we can put our heads together and figure out what we want to do." If psychotherapy is indicated and the evaluating psychiatrist is not available for treatment, the child should be told that as the consultant, you will find the right person to help with the problem. The consultant should always explain what the next step will be, whether it is further testing, a second interview, a family interview, or a visit with the parents alone.

Summing-Up Session

When all information has been gathered and a diagnostic impression is made, a treatment plan is formulated. Next, an appointment is set up with the parents to discuss options.

Often several treatment modalities may be indicated: psychotherapy with parental counseling, psychoanalysis, pharmacological intervention combined with therapy, family therapy, tutoring, or language and learning therapy. The recommendation could be a change of school, residential placement, or hospital-

ization. It is important that parents are helped to feel comfortable discussing their finances and the range of possibilities so that the best arrangement can be instituted, taking individual circumstances into account. When acting as a consultant, one must be available for helping with the disposition and facilitation of treatment, particularly in the event that the child or family is not satisfied with the referral. Setting the fee, establishing rules, discussing vacations, and the like take place during the summing-up session. Once a treatment plan has been selected, the child is invited to participate in the subsequent planning (for instance, the session time should not compete with a regular after-school activity) and to discuss the reasons for the type of treatment offered.

In an excellent chapter on general issues in clinical assessment, Diamond (1988) discussed parental reluctance to accept treatment recommendations, a reluctance that is usually reflected in whining, silent, or uncooperative children.

Conclusion

The semistructured interview I describe in this chapter is only one aspect of the total evaluation. It provides a reliable and comprehensive assessment of the signs and symptoms of psychiatric disorder, as well as positive attributes and strengths of the patient. Moreover, such an interview is therapeutic in that a relationship is established from the outset, an important factor if further psychotherapy is the recommended intervention. Used together with the information based on physical examination, history, and cognitive functioning, in addition to the problems reported by patients and their parents, it provides a valid psychiatric diagnosis that can result in an optimal psychotherapeutic intervention.

References

American Psychiatric Association: Diagnostic and Statistical Manual of Mental Disorders, 4th Edition. Washington, DC, American Psychiatric Association, 1994

American Psychiatric Association: Diagnostic and Statistical Manual of Mental Disorders, 4th Edition, Text Revision. Washington, DC, American Psychiatric Association, 2000

Bird H, Kestenbaum CJ: A semi-structured approach to clinical assessment, in Handbook of Clinical Assessment of Children and Adolescents, Vol 1. Edited by Kestenbaum CJ, Williams DT. New York, New York University Press, 1988, pp 19–30

Bird HP, Gould MS, Staghezza BM: Patterns of diagnostic comorbidity in a community sample of children. Paper presented at the annual meeting of Research in Child and Adolescent Psychopathology, Sarasota, FL, 1992

Bjorklund DF, Muir JE: Children's development of free recall memory: remembering on their own. Annals of Child Development 5:79–123, 1988

Canino IA: Taking a history, in The Clinical Guide to Child Psychiatry. Edited by Shaffer D, Ehrhardt AA, Greenhill LL. New York, Free Press, 1985, pp 393–408

Ceci SS, Ross DF, Tuglia MP: Suggestibility of children's memory: psychological implications. J Exp Psychol Gen 116:338–349, 1987

Chambers WJ, Puig-Antich J, Hirsch M, et al: The assessment of affective disorders in children and adolescents by semi-structured interview: test-retest reliability of the K-SADS-P. Arch Gen Psychiatry 42:696–702, 1985

Coppollilo H: Psychodynamic Psychotherapy of Children: An Introduction to the Art and the Techniques. Madison, CT, International Universities Press, 1987

Costello AJ, Edelbrock CS, Dulcan M: Report on the NIMH Diagnostic Interview Schedule for Children (DISC). Washington, DC, National Institute of Mental Health, 1984

Diamond CB: General issues in the clinical assessment of children and adolescents, in Handbook of Clinical Assessment of Children and Adolescents, Vol 1. Edited by Kestenbaum CJ, Williams DT. New York, New York University Press, 1988, pp 43–55

Freud A: The Psychoanalytic Treatment of Children. London, Imago, 1946

Gardner RA: The initial clinical evaluation of the child, in The Clinical Guide to Child Psychiatry. Edited by Shaffer D, Ehrhardt AA, Greenhill LL. New York, Free Press, 1985, pp 371–392

Goodman JD, Sours JA: The Child Mental Status Examination. New York, Basic Books, 1967

Greenspan SI, Greenspan NT: The Clinical Interview of the Child, 2nd Edition. Washington, DC, American Psychiatric Press, 1991

Hodges K, McKnew D, Cytryn L, et al: The Child Assessment Schedule (CAS) Diagnostic Interview: a report on reliability and validity. J Am Acad Child Psychiatry 21:468–473, 1982

Kestenbaum CJ, Bird HR: A reliability study of the Mental Health Assessment Form for school-age children. J Am Acad Child Psychiatry 17:338–347, 1978

MacKinnon R, Michels R: The Psychiatric Interview in Clinical Practice. Philadelphia, PA, WB Saunders, 1971

McClellan JM, Werry SM: Introduction: research psychiatric diagnostic interviews for children and adolescents. J Am Acad Child Adolesc Psychiatry 39:19–27, 2000

Ornstein PA, Larus DM, Clubb PA: Understanding children's testimony: implications of research on the development of memory. Annals of Child Development 8:145–176, 1991

Reich W: Diagnostic Interview for Children and Adolescents (DICA). J Am Acad Child Adolesc Psychiatry 39:59–66, 2000

Shaffer D, Gould MS, Brasic J, et al: A Children's Global Assessment Scale (C-GAS). Arch Gen Psychiatry 40:1228–1231, 1983

Shaffer D, Fisher P, Lucas CP, et al: NIMH Diagnostic Interview Schedule for Children Version IV (NIMH DISC-IV): description, differences from previous versions, and reliability of some common diagnoses. J Am Acad Child Adolesc Psychiatry 39:28–38, 2000

Simmons JK: Psychiatric Examination of Children, 3rd Edition. Philadelphia, PA, Lea & Febiger, 1981

Weller EB, Weller RA, Fristad MA, et al: Children's Interview for Psychiatric Syndromes (ChIPS). J Am Acad Child Adolesc Psychiatry 39:76–84, 2000

Winnicott DW: Therapeutic Consultations in Child Psychiatry. New York, Basic Books, 1971

The Clinical Interview of the Adolescent

Robert A. King, M.D.
John E. Schowalter, M.D.

The psychiatric evaluation of an adolescent is intended to obtain as full a picture as possible of the current difficulties in the overall context of the strengths and weaknesses of the adolescent and his or her family (King et al. 2000). Although formal psychological testing, structured instruments, laboratory data, and information gathered from school may be useful adjuncts, the heart of this clinical endeavor is the diagnostic interview with the adolescent and family.

The Prologue

It is important early on to clarify who is the moving force in seeking consultation and what is the adolescent's attitude toward the process. By seeking out a therapist, an adult patient acknowledges, at least implicitly, a problem and a desire for assistance. In contrast, the primary school–age child most often is simply brought by the parents. The adolescent's situation lies somewhere in between. Many adolescents take a cautious and ambiguous stance as to whether there is any problem for which help is wanted or instead there is mere passive compliance with a parental initiative.

Several considerations must guide the clinician in deciding whether the first interview should be with the adolescent, the parents, or all together. Seeing the adolescent first underlines his or her active participation in the process and serves to allay anxiety that the therapist and parents will collude against or gang up on the youngster. However, some adolescents will protest that this casts them in the role of being the problem or

the patient, when in their view the difficulty lies instead with their parents or between family members. The clinician must make clear that he or she is not out to assign blame but rather to help understand the difficulties the adolescent and the family have been confronting and to hear the views of all concerned. This usually requires both individual and family interviews. In most cases, the adolescent should be seen before the parents, but the parents may have to be seen first if they have difficulty getting their child to come for the first appointment.

The parents also should be seen alone to hear their concerns, to assess their explicit and implicit reasons for seeking assistance at this time, and to obtain a developmental and family history. (Details of the family interview are discussed elsewhere [see Chapter 11, "Initial and Diagnostic Family Interviews," in this volume].) The interview with the parents also yields valuable data concerning their view of the role played by the adolescent and the symptomatology in the psychic economy of the parents as individuals, as a couple, and in the family as a whole.

It often is useful at some point in the evaluation to interview the adolescent and parents together. The clinician frames the meeting's purpose as a forum in which family members can talk together; active structuring of this meeting may be needed to prevent the session from deteriorating into a "you hold him while I hit him" session in which the parents tell the therapist what is wrong with their child. Without the interviewer's active intervention, the adolescent may become very guarded or adversarial when seen with the parents. A family interview provides a useful opportunity to see how family members interact and to scrutinize overt and covert alliances and conflicts, shared family assumptions, coping patterns, and convergent and divergent areas of concern, as well as the family's ability to work together therapeutically and to make constructive use of the clinician's skills.

Confidentiality

Adolescents generally are very sensitive to the extremity of some of their thoughts and actions. Many fear that this information might be divulged by the clinician to their parents or to other authority figures. It is important from the outset for the parents and the adolescent to know that therapist–patient interactions are confidential. The exception is when the therapist believes that the patient or someone else is in danger. This rule should be spelled out at the beginning not only for general clarity but also to emphasize that it is a generic and not a specific response to a particular patient or disclosure. Patients sometimes want the clinician to tell something to parents or others "because you can say it much better than I can." Such a spokesperson role occasionally may be indicated, but its use should be preceded by a careful discussion and should occur in the adolescent's presence.

Developmental Issues and Interview Behavior

The clinician's approach to the interview with the adolescent is informed by an understanding of the developmental tasks and dynamics of adolescence and by the characteristic patterns used by adolescents to relate to adults and to manage their conflicts and anxiety (King 2002; Meeks and Bernet 2001; Mishne 1986). In the process of reworking and loosening dependent and libidinal ties to parents, adolescents turn, at times with a vengeance, to peers as objects of support and longing. Although some nonparental adults may be admired and turned to for guidance or identification, the adolescent's relationship with most adults is colored by a strong push toward autonomy and a great wariness of feeling vulnerable, dependent, or controlled. Even many adolescents who consciously want help approach a clinical evaluation with anxiety about revealing problems that they may regard as shameful weaknesses and with concerns about being criticized, controlled, or overwhelmed or becoming regressively dependent. These apprehensions may take the form of bland denials of any difficulties or insistence that either "everything is okay" or "I can handle it by myself."

Narcissistic vulnerability and difficulty tolerating ambivalence, internal conflicts, or painful feelings lead many adolescents to portray their problems as arising from outside rather than from within themselves. Adolescents often externalize one side or another of their conflicted feelings. A youngster may focus on bitter complaints of parental overprotectiveness while ignoring inner insecurities or wishes to be taken care of. Many adolescents deal with anxiety, guilt, shame, and other painful affects by means of counterphobic maneuvers or reversal of affect. For example, frightened teenagers may pick fights rather than take flight, and it is not unusual for sad adolescents to feel primarily angry during an interview. The clinician must learn to look beyond the adolescent's surface behavior and develop a capacity to notice when the youngster "doth protest too much."

An unrealistic faith in the "omnipotence of thought" is also characteristic of many adolescents who want to believe that even long-standing maladaptive patterns can be overcome simply by resolving to do things differently. Exploration of a problem area may thus be resisted with the sincere protestation, "Oh, I don't do that anymore" (i.e., not since yesterday). Adolescents' moods are labile, and their time perspective is short. Today's insoluble crisis, eternal passion, or irreversible decision may be forgotten by next week. Therefore, it is useful to evaluate an adolescent over time to assess which issues are transient and which are enduring. Of course, a propensity to frequent, albeit transient, upsets is in itself an important vulnerability to note.

Personal Issues for the Interviewer

Work with adolescents makes special demands on the clinician and is not to everyone's taste. Recall of and comfort with one's own adolescence are an enormous advantage. Enjoying teenagers is a prime prerequisite, followed by tact, flexibility, and a sense of humor. Schopenhauer once described friendship as "the art of distances." The same might be said of interviewing adolescents. Conveying a genuine and benign interest in the adolescent is essential. Condescension, aloofness, or excessive passivity in the interviewer is likely to be fatal. On the other hand, most adolescents will be frightened by overfamiliarity, seductiveness, or failure of the clinician to maintain an adult role.

Adolescents' narcissism is exquisitely tender, and one must learn how to talk frankly yet tactfully about vulnerable areas in such a way that adolescents do not feel they are being criticized. In the face of some adolescents' insistence that "you are either for me or against me," the clinician's task is to convey a genuine empathic interest in the adolescent's own view of the situation without collusively implying uncritical acceptance of that view.

Clinicians who work with adolescents need a good knowledge of their own adolescence and what they have made of that experience. Clinicians also must be aware of their feelings and biases about parenting. For example, at moments, the clinician may feel tempted to identify strongly with the patients' struggles against authority or feel a twinge of envy at their seeming freedom of sexual or aggressive expression; on the other hand, the clinician may find that certain adolescents or situations stir censorious or confrontational impulses or an identification with beleaguered or embattled parents. In short, the interviewer may feel either pressured to regress to an adolescent's viewpoint or propelled into a defensive parental stance.

The Interview

In the interview, the clinician is interested in several aspects of the presenting problem (King et al. 2000). What is the nature of the difficulty the adolescent is experiencing, and what areas of adaptive functioning are affected and to what degree? How does the adolescent think about the problem—as one lying entirely within, as a problem between himself or herself and others, or as a difficulty coming solely from without? Is the difficulty acute or long-standing? Which elements of the problem seem reactive, and which appear related to intrapsychic conflict or character? Do the symptoms provide important secondary gains for the patient or family? If chronic medical illness or constitutionally based developmental difficulties (such as dyslexia) are present, what has the adolescent made of them?

Beyond the manifest problem, the clinician also must assess the adolescent's personality structure and level of psychosexual development. Of particular importance are ego functions such as the capacity to tolerate frustration or anxiety, the degree of psychological-mindedness, the quality of mood regulation, and vulnerability to regression or impulsivity. This broader assessment of the adolescent's strengths and weaknesses is best accomplished in the course of reviewing how the adolescent is coping with the major adaptive tasks in the various realms of his or her life: school, family, and friends. It is important to inquire matter-of-factly about sadness, suicidality, eating habits, drug and alcohol use, and the presence of possible legal difficulties.

The degree to which one performs a formal, as opposed to an informal, mental status examination depends on variables such as the severity of the disorder, the reason for the evaluation, the time available, and the experience of the interviewer. A more formal approach is likely to be used when a disorder is severe, when precise documentation is required, or when there are concerns about the possibility of psychosis, dementia, or an organic brain syndrome. Basic areas to be covered in both formal and informal mental status examinations include the adolescent's general appearance, behavior, ability to relate, mood perceptions, thought content and coherence, memory, general information, intelligence, judgment, and insight.

To obtain a full picture, it is important not to limit the interview to areas of difficulty (King et al. 2000). The adolescent should know that the interviewer is interested in learning about him or her as a whole person, including areas of strength, enjoyment, and accomplishment. Adolescents may become defensive or blandly deny difficulties in the face of a too-exclusive focus on pathology. The experienced and empathic diagnostician conveys a genuine interest in learning about the nature, quality, and depth of the young person's interests, hobbies, and recreations. Rather than demonstrating or feigning one's familiarity with the latest rock group, sports cars, or athletic team, it is preferable to let the adolescent teach one about his or her particular interests. In so doing, the adolescent can enjoy a sense of mastery and control and some sense of parity with the adult examiner. At the same time, the clinician can learn what blend of interests, identifications, sublimations, and direct instinctual and narcissistic gratifications animates the adolescent. The temptation to make early interpretations is best resisted. Even, perhaps especially, if accurate, they are more likely to scare the patient away than to impress him or her with the interviewer's sagacity.

A closely related area is that of values, ideals, and aspirations (Kernberg 1978). What are the adolescent's values, and who are the adolescent's models for emulation or disidentification? Are these values congruent or in conflict with those of the patient's family, subculture, or larger society? What is the adolescent's sense of the future, and what aspirations, realistic or not, does the adolescent have for it?

The world of friends and peers is another related area for exploration. With whom does the patient "hang out"? What do they do for fun? How do they get along? Friends may be chosen on many grounds, including shared interests, admired virtues, or repudiated aspects of the adolescent's self. Friends may function as sources of support or admiration, as partners for sexual or aggressive exploitation, as collusive companions in regression or delinquency, as targets for projection, and so on. Asking the adolescent to tell one what a close friend is like provides an opportunity to learn how the adolescent thinks about people and relationships and to assess his or her capacity for empathy. Adolescents' own concerns are often more readily revealed in displacement: "I have a friend who is always…" It is sometimes helpful to ask whether a friend is bothered by or involved with something the adolescent has denied but is likely involved in himself or herself.

The topic of peer friendships leads naturally to the topic of dating and sexual relationships. This area requires tact and a good measure of rapport with the patient. Even so, one may not always receive a fully candid response during the diagnostic phase. Beyond the usual issues of privacy, this area of adolescents' lives is usually filled with concern and uncertainty, no matter how enlightened they may consider themselves to be. Does the teenager date, and is there anyone of either sex with whom he or she is close? What is the other person like, and what attracted each to the other? How has the relationship gone? Are there patterns in regard to the type of person found attractive and to the course of past relationships? When the patient has romantic daydreams (as we all do), what are they like? What is the script? Have any of the patient's relationships developed into sexual ones? Has the adolescent had other sexual experiences? Here one wants to be open to hearing about possible episodes of sexual abuse and concerns about sexual orientation. The goal goes beyond assessing the patient's popularity, experience, and ease with intimacy. Rather, the clinician is interested in the patient's "preconditions for loving" and the influences guiding object choice, as well as the extent to which recurrent anxiety, envy, ambivalence, sadomasochism, or issues of exploitation or narcissistic gratification interfere with the capacity for intimacy.

The Epilogue

Because of the adolescent's natural concern, it is important that the clinician summarize the findings at the end of the initial interviews. This summary should occur after the patient has been invited to add anything about which the interviewer has not asked and to say what he or she believes to be the best approach to be taken. Although this response may be quite different from what the clinician plans to propose, it is better to know areas of disagreement and resistance earlier than later.

Almost always, it is better first to share the recommendations and the reasons for them with the adolescent alone. An exception is when hospitalization is mandatory and parental support and quick action are required. Otherwise, it is useful to get the adolescent's reactions, to discuss any potential confidentiality questions, and to make any adjustments that seem indicated for the initial plan. The subsequent summarization for the parent or parents should be in the adolescent's presence.

References

Kernberg O: The diagnosis of borderline conditions in the adolescent. Adolesc Psychiatry 6:298–319, 1978

King RA: Adolescence, in Child and Adolescent Psychiatry: A Comprehensive Textbook, 3rd Edition. Edited by Lewis M. Baltimore, MD, Lippincott Williams & Wilkins, 2002

King RA, Schwab-Stone M, Peterson B, et al: Psychiatric assessment of the infant, child, and adolescent, in Kaplan and Sadock's Comprehensive Textbook of Psychiatry, 7th Edition,Vol 2. Edited by Kaplan HI, Kaplan VA. Baltimore, MD, Lippincott Williams & Wilkins, 2000, pp 2558–2586

Meeks JE, Bernet W: The Fragile Alliance: An Orientation to Psychotherapy of the Adolescent, 5th Edition. Malabar, FL, Krieger Publishing, 2001

Mishne JM: Clinical Work With Adolescents. New York, Free Press, 1986

The Parent Interview

Bennett L. Leventhal, M.D.
Martha E. Crotts, M.D.

The most commonly performed procedure in all of medicine is the clinical interview. The capacity to perform this critical clinical procedure is inherent to good practice, and in no other specialty is it more significant than in child and adolescent psychiatry. The clinical interview must be adapted to accommodate the effective examination of both individuals who present with vastly different developmental capacities and third parties who are unique sources of information about the identified patient. The parents of the child or adolescent patient are usually the most important of these third parties. By providing information about the child and family, the parents enable the clinician to understand not only the child's behavior but also the functioning of the family, the individuals, the environment, and the whole system in which the child exists (Group for the Advancement of Psychiatry 1957).

Although clinicians generally agree that it is vitally important to interview parents as part of the clinical process, there is some controversy, both theoretically and methodologically. On the one hand, there is Freud (1909/1955), who learned quite a bit about his famous patient, Little Hans, primarily from Hans's father. On the other hand, some family therapists view assessment and intervention with the child and parents as a simultaneous event and, consequently, may not even rely on the individual parent interview as part of their clinical process (Walsh 1983).

Rutter and Cox (1985) emphasized the importance of children's experiences in their family lives. They clearly identified not only the role of parents in modifying children's behaviors but also the role of children in shaping parental behaviors. Additionally, they pointed out that there are different types of parenting that interact in a unique way with a particu-

lar child's development, behaviors, and other characteristics, thus implying the necessity for interviewing parents in any evaluation or treatment process.

Whatever one's point of view, the parent interview is an essential part of an evaluation or other clinical process involving children and adolescents. In some recently developed circumstances surrounding health care, in particular managed behavioral health, the opportunity for careful data collection may be limited. This may in turn limit other aspects of the clinical process. With these extrinsic factors in mind, carefully considering the role and function of work with parents is all the more critical in contemporary practice.

Clinicians must be concerned about the utility of the information acquired from the parent interview when working with children and adolescents. Does the parent interview provide a valid account of the information necessary to formulate a diagnosis, establish a treatment plan, and monitor the treatment of a given child? When one thinks broadly about ways to interview parents—that is, the use of structured interviews, unstructured interviews, and parent report scales—one recognizes that there is enormous variability in the quantity and quality, and therefore in the reliability and validity, of the information obtained. Indeed, studies have shown that parental reports often are temporally distorted and that parents may deny a particular problem or may be unable to recall pertinent past behavior (Chess et al. 1966). Mednick and Shaffer (1963) arrived at similar conclusions as a result of their studies of mothers' retrospective reports collected in a pediatric setting. Maternal interviews were compared with pediatric records, and the mothers' reports were found to be discrepant 21%–62% of the time for facts about discrete experiences, such as breast-feeding, childhood illnesses, and the age at completion of toilet training.

Kashani et al. (1985) also found low agreement between parents and children on all DSM-III-R (American Psychiatric Association 1987) Axis I disorders. Interestingly, the patterns of disagreement were generally consistent in that children reported more anxiety and depressive symptoms, whereas parents stressed more externalizing symptoms, such as oppositional behavior and short attention span. The authors concluded that multiple sources of information might help the clinician arrive at a clearer clinical picture. Weissman et al. (1987) reviewed numerous studies and identified discrepancies between parent and child reports on the nature, extent, and severity of children's symptoms. Irrespective of the interview setting, the diagnostic criteria, the method of interview, or the symptom scales, the authors found that children reported far more information about all their disorders. Indeed, Weissman et al. recommended that at least in certain types of studies, one should consider interviewing only the child, if a choice has to be made. In contrast, Orvaschel et al. (1981) found that parents were more accurate in providing factual time-related information. Using an early version of the Diagnostic Interview Schedule for Children (DISC) and the Diagnostic Interview Schedule for Children—Parent (DISC-P, the parent interview), Edelbrock et al. (1985) studied age differences in the reliability of interviews of children. Not surprisingly, these investigators found that the reliability of a child's report increased with the child's age and with the presence of overt behaviors such as aggression and hyperactivity. The importance of parental collaboration was most evident in the results of structured parent interviews for younger children. In general, parents were believed to be more reliable than their children until the children reached age 10 years, after which there was little or no difference in the reliability of parent and child reports.

Despite reported discrepancies, parents can and do provide essential information about a child's birth, development, medical history, and current functioning and symptoms, as well as marital and family history. Diagnostic and clinical work with children are invariably "more than the classification of a child in a nosologic system based on the clinical observation and the description of the presenting signs and symptoms of deviant behavior" (Group for the Advancement of Psychiatry 1957, p. 399). Although so-called factual information about children and their functioning is impor-

tant, other information that is not so concrete and not so obvious may be inconsistently collected, evaluated, and incorporated in the evaluation process. It is critical to remember that parental involvement and parental interviews do not just provide factual information; they are essential in forming the relationship among the clinician, the patient, and the family. An alliance with the parents is very important in reaching a consensus about the nature of parenting and family problems and in developing and implementing a treatment plan (Simmons 1987).

Simmons (1987) warned the clinician to identify clearly who is the patient. The child may be presented as the identified patient. However, careful discussion with the parents and child and examination of each parent, the marital couple, the family, the child's school, and the family's community are necessary to assess the child and to develop an intervention plan. Therefore, most clinicians agree that the parent interview is but one component of an evaluation that must be placed into the clinical context. Data gathered from the parents, and from other parties, may be affected greatly by the attitude parents hold toward a referral for therapy, toward the child, and toward other matters in the child's life. Furthermore, it appears essential, in most clinical settings, to evaluate features such as parental temperament, personality organization, and psychopathology to place the data that the parents provide into a clinical context that also includes the child's role in the parents' struggles, unconscious and conscious wishes for the child, and other dynamic issues (Greenspan and Greenspan 2003).

What, then, is the function of the parent interview? Certainly the gathering of information about the child's history and the child's present functioning is crucial. Equally important, however, is the opportunity for the clinician to develop an alliance. This alliance may be the key to sustaining the evaluation and treatment process and to fostering the child's relationship with the clinician. Developing an alliance with parents during the interview process is not simply a matter of collecting information; it is also important to give them information. The clinician can and should identify strengths and weaknesses in the child and help the parents clarify what they already know. The clinician also can give parents information about normal child development and the clinical process. In this way, the parent interview becomes a collaborative effort.

Parent interviews are conducted in a variety of settings; therefore, it is important for the clinician to identify the purpose of the interview beforehand. Some interviews are part of a diagnostic process, whereas others are a component of individual, family, or parent-oriented treatment. Furthermore, some interviews take place under scheduled circumstances, whereas others are in an acute setting, such as an emergency room, or are part of the inpatient, pediatric, or psychiatric consultation. Each of these interviews has a different tone and a separate set of goals.

Depending on the purpose of the interview, a variety of formal, partially or fully structured instruments could be used as a part of the interviewing process. Although formal interviewing instruments can never replace the parent interview conducted by an experienced clinician, these instruments can provide supplemental information. Instruments are generally divided into two types: 1) those that are administered by the clinician or trained staff and 2) those that are self-administered. Instruments administered by the clinician may be of either a semistructured or a structured variety. In general, these instruments can provide clinicians and researchers a systematized means of gathering information, which may be helpful in assessing a child or guiding treatment. Examples of semistructured instruments include the Schedule for Affective Disorders and Schizophrenia for School-Aged Children (Kiddie-SADS or K-SADS; Ambrosini 2000) and the Interview Schedule for Children and Adolescents (ISCA; Sherrill and Kovacs 2000). Both of these instruments include an interview of the parents, beginning with an unstructured portion during which presenting complaints and their duration are discussed. The semistructured portion is then administered, consisting of clusters of questions organized around specific diagnostic categories. Examples of structured instruments include the Diagnostic Interview for Children and Adolescents—Parent (DICA-P; Reich 2000) and the DISC-P (Shaffer et al. 2000). The DICA-P allows somewhat more latitude for the interviewer than the DISC-P. Both may be used in either epidemiological or clinical settings. These instruments consist of a set framework of interview questions that are organized in diagnostic modules. For more information on semistructured and structured child psychiatric diagnostic instruments, see Chapter 12 ("Diagnostic Interviews").

Self-administered instruments or rating scales can be completed by the parent before or after the in-person interview. An example of this type would be the Child Behavior Checklist (CBCL) (http://www.aseba.org/index.html), developed by Achenbach and Edelbrock in the early 1980s as a screening device for psychiatric illness in children, and extensively revised since then, with nationally representative norms. Some rating scales, such as the CBCL, assess a wide range of symptoms. Others are used to evaluate specific symptom clusters or diagnoses. Rating scales are discussed in detail in Chapter 13 ("Rating Scales").

An additional option is to use family measurement instruments for data collection from parents. These instruments are numerous and varied with regard to their emphases. Each one has its own set of characteristics that can be used by the clinician to meet the needs of a specific clinical problem or interview situation. Areas in which they can be of assistance include exploration of parental roles and parent–child interactions, among other aspects of family functioning. Family assessment measures are covered in more detail in Chapter 11 ("Initial and Diagnostic Family Interviews") and in the American Psychiatric Association's *Handbook of Psychiatric Measures*, specifically the chapter entitled "Family and Relational Issues Measures" (Messer and Reiss 2000).

Whether self-administered or administered by staff or the clinician, formal instruments can be completed and their results available for use at the time of the interview. When used in this manner, they may serve as efficient tools in the current health care environment, in which time is of the essence.

Components of an Interview

All good parent interviews incorporate some degree of structure, which is ultimately the responsibility of the interviewer; therefore, all parent interviews require careful thought and planning. Each interview has five components: 1) preliminaries, 2) prologue, 3) interview proper, 4) closing, and 5) epilogue.

The clinician must establish the goals for each particular interview and set a tentative agenda in advance. Although it may seem a bit prosaic, one must remember that each interview begins with a beginning and that that beginning sets the tone for the balance of the process.

■ Preliminaries

The preliminary phase is the planning for the interview process. The first tasks of this phase are to identify the patient and the purpose of the interview, in order to determine the interview type and goals. For example, if the interview is to be diagnostic, then the collection of information may be the most critical component of the interview; if the interview is to be therapeutic, then the means of intervention and the goals of the treatment must be clearly understood before the intervention is to begin. The content of the interview differs significantly according to the age and diagnostic category of the identified patient. Once these preliminary tasks have been completed, the clinician must ascertain that the amount of time available and other conditions are suitable to meet the interview objectives.

■ Prologue

The prologue is the introductory phase of the parent interview. It begins with introductions, which must be respectful of the parental role and competence, and details the circumstances of the interview. Similarly, introductions must clearly identify the clinician and his or her role while also setting the ground rules regarding matters such as confidentiality. During this portion of the interview, it is useful to assess both the parents' and the clinician's expectations for the interview and to get some indications about, for example, parental defensiveness, shame, guilt, and embarrassment:

> It is never easy to think of a child as having these sorts of problems. You may even be embarrassed or scared. Despite this, you have been able to come for help. Now I would like to help you understand what is happening so we can make a plan to solve the problems facing both you and your child.

■ Interview Proper

The interview proper is the opportunity to establish an empathic relationship with the parents while collecting data and making the appropriate intervention. Even in a parent interview, it is important to attend to the more traditional elements of the psychiatric evaluation. Transference, countertransference, resistance, defenses, strengths, weaknesses, and similar matters that specifically relate to the parents require careful assessment. The clinician simultaneously must assess family matters, including traditions, locus of control, discipline, family dynamics, communication, and other matters that more commonly are associated with parent and family functioning. At the same time, the interviewer must help parents to manage their anxiety and to maintain an appropriate sense of responsibility for the child.

■ Closing

The closing portion of the parent interview is the clinician's opportunity to reassure the parents and reinforce their control and competence. It is also a time for answering questions that the parents may have and articulating the next step in the clinical process:

> At this point, there are several possibilities to explain the current situation. These are 1)..., 2)..., 3)..., and 4).... I would like to suggest that we do the following to answer the remaining questions and establish a treatment plan. I realize that this may seem a bit overwhelming or confusing, so please be sure that I have satisfactorily answered your questions before we proceed.

■ Epilogue

Finally, each clinician must allow some time to review the interview. By carefully reconsidering the data that have been acquired and the response to interventions, the clinician can review the validity of the plans and the next step. Similarly, planning for future clinical activity can be assessed before the report of the interview is generated. Although the epilogue may be the end of the parent interview, it also may be the beginning of further clinical activity with the parents and the child.

■ Source of Referral

It is always useful during the course of an interview to assess parental attitudes about the referral and the source of referral and why parents have accepted the referral for an evaluation at a particular time. This information not only may guide the clinical process but also may help identify problems that are of particular interest to the patient and the family. For example, a family forced into an evaluation by an outside agency or the legal system may perceive the evaluation very differently from a family in which there is an extensive history of psychiatric illness that is being manifested by the child, who is the identified patient. Whatever the case, understanding the basis for referral and the relationship that exists between the family and the referral source is important. It is equally important to consider the relationship between the clinician and the referral source as the clinical process unfolds.

■ Impression of Parents

In addition to collecting information about the whys and wherefores of the referral, it is important to derive at least a general impression of the parents, if not a detailed understanding of their past, personality organization, and established family patterns. This allows the clinician to develop a preliminary conceptual framework in which to place the child's and the parents' functioning in a family context. It is also important to gain some appreciation not only of the parents' role in shaping the lives of their children but also of the children's capacity to shape the parental role (Rutter and Cox 1985).

Types of Interviews and Settings

■ Diagnostic Interview

In the diagnostic or history-taking interview, the information to be collected from parents is both factual and impressionistic. Because of the discrepancies between parental reports and actual occurrences (as documented in, for example, medical and school records and records from previous evaluations or testing), it is important, whenever possible, to review additional sources of information. Several authors have offered detailed outlines of historical information to guide the interviewer (Canino 1985; French 1979). These and many other structured and unstructured interview schedules outline extensive variables, such as pregnancies, labor and delivery, birth, infancy, medical history, and family history, that provide more information:

> I want to be of help to *you* in determining why your child is having these problems. We will have to work together as we search for answers to your good questions and concerns.

■ Medical Consultation Setting

In medical consultation settings, the parents are important informants about the child's premorbid functioning and the impact of the child's illness on the child and the family. Even in this setting, it is important to identify who is the patient. This is particularly problematic because sometimes the consulting professional may not know who should be the focus of the consultation or may have an agenda that is completely different from that of the patient or the parents. Often, consultation requests are quite focused, and the

parent interview must be targeted. For example, an adolescent patient may be identified as noncompliant with the treatment when, in fact, the source of conflict originates in ambivalent relationships between the primary treating physician and the parents, who are highly involved and may try to control the medical treatment process. Therefore, the focus during the parent interview, although manifestly directed toward the child's medical care, may be more directly related to the parents' sense of control, frustration, and incompetence in the clinical situation. For example, a pediatric colleague who has evaluated a 10-year-old with vague stomach pains, contacted the child psychiatry consultation-liaison team, and reviewed the case with the consultants might tell the parents:

> There is nothing physically wrong with your son, so I am asking the psychiatrist to see you. . . . It is very hard for you and your doctors to see your child in pain and not understand the cause. There are often multiple causes. The psychiatrist can help us solve this problem for your child.

■ Emergency Setting

In emergency settings, where the clinician must make relatively rapid decisions about assessment and treatment and particularly is concerned about protecting a child from danger, entirely different forms of parent interviews are necessary. Whether the risk of self-injury or injury to others is the question, or whether the child is a possible victim of physical or sexual abuse, the scope and direction of the parent interview change. Clearly, in the emergency setting, the focus of the interview must be on assessing the risk of danger and establishing a safe and protective environment for the child. In some circumstances, extraordinary levels of parental defensiveness, anxiety, guilt, and avoidance of conflict may be present. In addition, because legal culpability for the events may be in question, careful attention must be given to details such as evasiveness of the parents. Although building an alliance with parents and assessing overall parent functioning are important, these can be dealt with in a cursory fashion until fundamental safety issues and other crucial matters are addressed:

> I realize that this has been a very difficult day for you and your daughter. Even though she is 15 years old and capable of using good judgment, she is now in a great deal of distress. As much as you might now wish to take her home and care for her there, we must determine what will ensure her immediate safety.

■ Forensic Interviews (Including Custody Evaluations)

Custody evaluations and other forensic interviews have a particular tone set for the interview a priori. In the forensic setting, parents and clinicians are often faced with profoundly adversarial relationships, which may focus not only on a marital struggle but also on the different opinions (e.g., the parents', the lawyers', the court's) regarding parenting. Indeed, forensic interviews also may contribute to a great deal of hostility and criticism about a particular parent's parenting and multiple accusations about the veracity of the history. Furthermore, there is often defensiveness, if not outright fabrication, in reporting parental activities in the life of the child. As such, a parent interview in the forensic setting may leave the clinician feeling responsible to ascertain "absolute truth." This is virtually impossible. Instead, the clinician must stand outside the legal wrangling and focus on consistent patterns of behavior that have existed over time. Forensic interviews most often are repeated, and multiple sources of information are essential to get a reasonably clear, if not accurate, picture of the patterns of the parents' and child's behavior. In most forensic settings, there is an adversarial system that leads to labeling "winners" and "losers." Despite their best efforts, clinicians are often cast in this light as well. One must try not to place oneself in this position or take this attribution to heart. Finally, the court's or the family's acceptance or rejection of the clinician's recommendations cannot be seen as a measure of the clinician's success or failure in the case. Success can be measured only by the subsequent outcome for the child, not just for the parents:

> I have been appointed by the court to conduct an evaluation to determine what will be in the best interest of your child. This is a struggle between adults, and the sooner the adults resolve it, the easier it will be for your child. As one of two parents, you are one of the two most important people in your child's life and in this evaluation process. Therefore, I need your assistance and cooperation. I would very much like to hear anything that you have to offer about your child. I will take whatever time is required to collect the necessary information to make recommendations to you and the court. Please feel free to tell me or give me whatever you feel is important.

■ Other Settings

There are other settings in which child psychiatrists are asked to interview parents as part of the diagnostic or treatment process. Commonly, clinicians are asked to consult with pediatricians, family practitioners, or other mental health professionals concerning psychopharmacological interventions. Before the consultation, a great deal of information may be provided by other professionals, and often the parents arrive in these settings with strong feelings that they are being criticized or that the situation is rapidly becoming desperate. Still others approach the medication consultation with the notion that a medication to definitively treat their child may be available. The medication consultation with parents necessitates not only careful gathering of a child history and family history but also careful assessment of parental expectations. These expectations must be dealt with directly, along with provision of detailed information about the treatment process. The parents must be carefully and accurately informed about the types of medications to be used, the potential side effects and serious consequences related to these medications, and the real therapeutic potential. Because medication consultations are often stressful and the information itself is critical, the parent interview in this case often takes on an instructive format, which must be carefully tested before the patient and family are sent on their way.

Conclusion

Fundamentally, the parent interview is a pedagogic process. It is an opportunity for the parents to teach the clinician about themselves, their roles as parents, the child, and the family. The parent interview also is an opportunity for the clinician to teach parents about the clinical process and perhaps about the parents themselves and their child. For all of this teaching to take place, each party must be open to the process. It is the interviewer's responsibility not only to ensure that his or her mind is open but also to establish the same receptivity in the parents. Without this receptivity, the parent interview offers little reliable information and contributes little to the clinical enterprise.

Clarence Darrow once said, "The first half of our lives is ruined by our parents and the second half is ruined by our children." The same can be said for the clinical process with parents and children. However, if we avoid ruining our work with the parents, then our work with the children will more likely be successful.

References

Ambrosini PJ: Historical development and present status of the Schedule for Affective Disorders and Schizophrenia for School-Age Children (K-SADS). J Am Acad Child Adolesc Psychiatry 39:49–58, 2000

American Psychiatric Association: Diagnostic and Statistical Manual of Mental Disorders, 3rd Edition, Revised. Washington, DC, American Psychiatric Association, 1987

Canino IA: Taking a history, in The Clinical Guide to Child Psychiatry. Edited by Shaffer D, Ehrhardt AA, Greenhill LL. New York, Free Press, 1985, pp 393–408

Chess S, Thomas A, Birch HG: Distortions in developmental reporting made by parents of behaviorally disturbed children. J Am Acad Child Psychiatry 5:226–234, 1966

Edelbrock C, Costello AJ, Dulcan NM, et al: Age differences in the reliability of the psychiatric interview of the child. Child Dev 56:265–275, 1985

French AP: Disturbed Children and Their Families: Innovations in Evaluation and Treatment. New York, Human Sciences Press, 1979

Freud S: Analysis of a phobia in a five-year-old boy (1909), in The Standard Edition of the Complete Psychological Works of Sigmund Freud, Vol 10. Translated and edited by Strachey J. London, Hogarth Press, 1955, pp 1–149

Greenspan SI, Greenspan NT: The Clinical Interview of the Child, 2nd Edition. Washington, DC, American Psychiatric Publishing, 2003

Group for the Advancement of Psychiatry: The Diagnostic Process in Child Psychiatry (Rep No 38). New York, Group for the Advancement of Psychiatry, 1957

Kashani JH, Orvaschel H, Burk JP, et al: Informant variance: the issue of parent-child disagreement. J Am Acad Child Psychiatry 24:437–441, 1985

Mednick SA, Shaffer JBP: Mothers' retrospective reports in child-rearing research. Am J Orthopsychiatry 33:457–461, 1963

Messer SC, Reiss D: Family and relational issues measures, in Handbook of Psychiatric Measures. Washington, DC, American Psychiatric Association, 2000, pp 239–260

Orvaschel H, Weissman MM, Padian N, et al: Assessing psychopathology in children of psychiatrically disturbed parents: a pilot study. J Am Acad Child Psychiatry 20:112–122, 1981

Reich W: Diagnostic Interview for Children and Adolescents (DICA). J Am Acad Child Adolesc Psychiatry 39:59–66, 2000

Rutter M, Cox A: Other family influences, in Child and Adolescent Psychiatry: Modern Approaches. Edited by Rutter M, Hersov L. London, Blackwell, 1985, pp 58–81

Shaffer D, Fisher P, Lucas CP, et al: NIMH Diagnostic Interview Schedule for Children Version IV (NIMH DISC-IV): description, difference from previous versions, and reliability of some common diagnoses. J Am Acad Child Adolesc Psychiatry 39:28–38, 2000

Sherrill JT, Kovacs M: Interview Schedule for Children and Adolescents (ISCA). J Am Acad Child Adolesc Psychiatry 39:67–75, 2000

Simmons JE: Psychiatric Examination of Children. Philadelphia, PA, Lea & Febiger, 1987

Walsh F: Family therapy: a systemic orientation to treatment, in Handbook of Clinical Social Work. Edited by Rosenblatt A, Waldfogel D. San Francisco, CA, Jossey-Bass, 1983, pp 466–489

Weissman MM, Wickramaratne P, Warner V, et al: Assessing psychiatric disorders in children: discrepancies between mothers' and children's reports. Arch Gen Psychiatry 44:747–753, 1987

Initial and Diagnostic Family Interviews

G. Pirooz Sholevar, M.D.

The diagnostic family interview is an invaluable tool for the psychiatrist in the development of diagnostic and therapeutic goals. The multiple goals of the family interview may vary depending on the clinician's theoretical orientation or the nature of the problem and can shape the structure, form, and content of the session. The diagnostic interview can take place as the initial contact with the family, regardless of the nature of the presenting "problem"; it can be part of the comprehensive assessment of a symptomatic child or adult; or it can occur when therapeutic efforts of any type are partially or totally ineffective. The interview can occur in an outpatient or inpatient setting.

The assessment of the total family is important because a person is part of a larger emotional unit—the family—rather than an autonomous psychological entity. In treating a patient, a psychiatrist may fail to recognize how the problematic relationship between child and parents, or between parents and grandparents, contributes to the disorder and may therefore prescribe a prolonged and relatively ineffective course of individual or conjoint family therapy. A broader evaluation of the problems addressing multiple sets of variables can result in more successful treatment choices.

The diagnostic family interview is guided by the theoretical orientation of the clinician. A psychodynamic family therapist would pay special attention to traumatic events, developmental failures, and intrafamilial transference reactions, which may shape the contemporary interactions and identity of the family members in a decisive manner. The behavioral family therapist would focus on the antecedents and consequences of the problematic behavior and collect extensive data in this area. A communications orienta-

tion would lead to an interest in the homeostatic mechanisms and rules that maintain the family transactions. A multigenerational family therapist would be most interested in the level of differentiation and the pathological loyalty and indebtedness between the parents and their families of origin.

The goals of clinicians vary and may include 1) learning of family and individual variables that may play the decisive role in shaping the behavior of a problematic family member; 2) assessing the adequacy of family functioning, structure, and development according to the family life cycle; and 3) conducting an initial family treatment session when the necessity of such a course has been recognized by the family or by the referral source.

These multiple goals can influence the clinician's strategy. For the first goal, the clinician pays equal attention to the interpersonal, individual, and intrapsychic data. For the second goal, the systematic exploration of the family structure is complemented by interventions aimed at testing the flexibility of the family system and rules to determine whether the most leverage and the least defensiveness can be gained in individual or in family treatment. For the third goal, raising the positive expectancies of the family as a group may assume the first priority.

Stages of the Initial Family Interview

The diagnostic family interview is commonly divided into three segments: 1) social stage, 2) multidimensional inquiry into the presenting problem, and 3) exploration of the structure and developmental phase of the family (Haley 1977; Minuchin 1974).

In the *social stage* of the interview, the clinician acts as a host to the family according to the prevailing customs. The clinician puts the family at ease by engaging in mutual introductions, asking the family to introduce themselves by name, matching the names with family members, and inviting them to make themselves comfortable in the office. The family should be provided with adequate seating, preferably in a conversational living-room arrangement, and with play material, table, and chairs for young children. Zilbach (1986) recommended that the clinician crouch down to establish eye-to-eye contact with young children when they enter the office and remember that some young children may be afraid of handshakes or physical touching. A few minutes may be spent in small talk, inquiring, for example, if the family had any difficulty with transportation or finding the office.

In the *multidimensional inquiry stage*, the clinician asks the family to describe the problem that has prompted the clinical contact. The clinician can share prior information about the family with them, which may exhibit the clinician's interest and open style. Such information can include what the psychiatrist has learned in the initial telephone call about the presenting problem and recent events involving the family. The family members generally feel very comfortable with the initial part of this stage of evaluation because their statements are largely prerehearsed and allow them to present their "official" image to the clinician. The initial inquiry may be directed to the father, in recognition of the often tenuous motivation of many fathers to be in the therapeutic setting, or to the mother, as the person who may be most knowledgeable about the family life and problems. After hearing the views of one parent, the clinician should ask the other parent to describe the problem. The therapist should then inquire about the views of different family members on problematic areas in the family. It is preferable to elicit the views of the siblings of the identified patient about the problem areas in the family before moving to the identified patient, because an early solicitation of the patient's views may increase defensiveness and further polarize the family.

The clinician should be prepared to encounter resistance from the family members against broadening the focus of the explorations and establishing a true multidirectional partiality (Boszormenyi-Nagy 1972).

Such resistances will become apparent when one or both parents demand a solution to the presenting problem from the therapist or instruct the therapist on what to do (e.g., prescribe medication for a child's hyperactivity). Understanding such attempts as signs of a high level of family tension, the clinician should avoid confrontation with the parents and gently underline the importance of understanding everyone's viewpoint on family life as a necessary step for establishing a corrective course of action for the problems.

The family's manner of negotiating boundaries with the clinician as a member of the outside world may be exhibited by a readiness to include the therapist immediately in their conflicts, projections, and blaming. The emergence of an intense, negative transference to the therapist can give rise to countertransferential feelings, which should be used as a clue to the level of family health and pathology.

While listening to the family's presentation of the problem, the therapist should observe carefully the family's relatively unconstrained nonverbal behavior. The observation of any restless behavior in the children following a look at one of the parents and interruption, qualification, or negation of messages by one or multiple family members are the signals used to regulate family transactions and should provide the interviewer with useful clues about family structure to be tested in the next stage of the family interview. By the end of the second stage, each family member should have experienced a sense of participation in the interview and the opportunity for input in the evaluation. However, an excessive accommodation to some family members, particularly the autocratic and tyrannical ones, may undermine the potential trust of the scapegoated and peacemaking members because the family members may assume an alliance between the therapist and the victimizers against the scapegoated victims.

The *stage of exploration of family structure* through observation of family interactions provides the clinician with valuable clues, including the level of differentiation, boundary formation, and boundary flexibility of different family subsystems and family members. The clinician is particularly interested in the functional adequacy of different family subsystems. The common family subsystems include the marital or parental, parent–child, and sibling subsystems. Grandparental involvement, very common in certain ethnic and socioeconomic groups, would add grandparent–parent and grandparent–grandchild subsystems.

Assessment and Diagnosis

In the advanced phase of the family interview, the clinician devises active interventions or interpretations to test the flexibility and adequacy of different family subsystems, such as the marital or parental subsystem. Some family therapists may ask some family members to discuss in the session a potentially conflictual subject, which will reveal their hidden disagreements and their flexibility in family negotiation and compromise formation. Generally, most clinically referred families show observable deficiencies in at least one of the family subsystems, such as the parent–child subsystem, while proving adequate and resourceful in other subsystems, such as the marital or parental and sibling subsystems.

The strategy of broadening the focus of exploration extends the reach of the clinician beyond the problems of the identified patient to other functional and dysfunctional aspects of the family life. Depending on the level of tension in the family and the skill of the family therapist, the session may oscillate between two competing forces: the family pushing to focus on the identified patient when the tension mounts and the therapist attempting to discuss other family issues involving different family subsystems.

While attempting to broaden the focus on a problem, the psychiatrist may uncover hidden or apparent marital problems. Generally, an early focus on marital difficulties is correlated with a high rate of dropout from treatment and with negative therapeutic outcome due to heightened family tension. Additionally, the family may present the marital problems in an attempt to diffuse the therapeutic efforts directed at the identified child, without genuine motivation to deal with marital issues (Montalvo and Haley 1973).

Maintaining the family's motivation to return for treatment is an important therapeutic goal. Therefore, at the time of heightened tension during the sessions, the therapist may choose to retreat from uncomfortable family topics until the tension is reduced.

With a family with a rigid structure, siding with and confronting family members in the first session may result in the interruption of the family evaluation. The clinician should always be aware of the unity of the family system as a natural group with strong ties of loyalty, common history, and rigid homeostatic rules dictating the behavior of each family member. A close and intricately functioning family can close ranks readily and extrude the therapist if the family's tolerance is exceeded through the therapist's incorrect assessment of the family's power or the therapist's status.

Specific Procedural Considerations

The benefits of the diagnostic family interview include the recognition of subtle parental pathology, different aspects of individual and family dysfunction, and, most important, powerful dysfunctional interlocking relationships and loyalties. Such dysfunctional relationships can play a decisive role in reducing the adaptation of the family and producing symptoms in one or multiple family members.

For the initial family session, all members of the household and significant others should be invited, including young children, toddlers, and infants, who are an important source of diagnostic data about the family. The invitation should be extended in a matter-of-fact manner, emphasizing the importance of all family members' views for a full understanding of the problem. Simple statements such as "I'd like to meet you all, including the little ones" can readily communicate the clinician's goal. The success of the invitation depends on the conviction of the clinician about the importance of family interactional data. The clinician should avoid any lengthy telephone discussion to justify the participation of all family members because a prolonged explanation based on general assumptions may make the therapist seem lacking in confidence. Once the family members recognize the importance of the family interview to the diagnostic process, they usually comply. The common parental fear about the "contamination" of younger children and "well" siblings by their exposure to the problems of the identified patient readily yields to the clinician's reassurance. Other sources of fear in the family include the parents' fear of blame for the child's problems and the fear that the entire family may be pronounced "sick." The clinician can reduce the family's fears by emphasizing the consultative nature of the diagnostic family interview, which does not imply any commitment to treatment on the family's part. The refusal of an adolescent to attend a diagnostic family interview usually indicates parental apprehension about the session or weakness of parental authority.

The family assessment can occur during one or multiple family sessions. The diagnostic interview preferably should be scheduled for 1½ hours to allow a systematic, unhurried evaluation of the family. One should be prepared for a high rate of cancellation for the initial family interview, with little hope of receiving remuneration for the canceled session.

Assessment of family structure should include determining the characteristic constellations of family conflicts, patterns of control, clarity of parental authority and generational boundaries, expression of feelings, and family rigidity, including the brittleness of family defenses. Structural flexibility of the family includes the accessibility of alternative action patterns.

Assessment of family functioning should include exploring the family's instrumental-adaptive function, which is geared toward enhanced adaptation and problem resolution, and the family's expressive-integrative function, which is geared toward expressing affect and providing comfort. The lack of balance between these two functions can result in an imbalanced family system with reduced adaptability. The elucidation of multigenerational dynamic and relational patterns may be an important factor, particularly with chronically and severely dysfunctional families.

The diagnostic family interview can be extended into interviews with family subgroups, such as parents, children, or one child, for exploration of other important information that may not be readily shared in a conjoint session. The intimate aspects of the parental relationship, such as the parents' sexual functioning, can be explored in such an interview. When the children are seen alone, they may reveal phobias, eating disorders, or elimination problems that may be too embarrassing to reveal in a diagnostic family session.

In the advanced stage of the initial interview, the impact of the clinician on the family may move family members beyond a rigid or stalemated position into a more flexible mode of family functioning characteristic of earlier stages of their family life. The early and ready occurrence of this phenomenon indicates flexibility in the family system and a favorable therapeutic outcome.

Additional guidelines for family assessment (Weber et al. 1985) include the following:

- Establish structure in the interview to counter the common tendencies of dysfunctional families toward chaos, a high level of blame, and "silencing" of their members. Reframing, the restatement of a problem in a positive rather than a negative way, and diffusing attacks by demonstrating a dyadic or triadic view of the problems are effective techniques to establish an empathic atmosphere.
- Maintain objectivity, avoid taking sides or closing topics prematurely, and elicit the views of all family members.
- Address the transactional patterns that are clearly burdensome to many family members and therefore more amenable to change (Gordon and Davidson 1981).
- Understand the roles of different family members within the family unit. The roles of "scapegoat," "tyrant," "martyr," and "baby" are common in families with symptomatic children and adolescents.
- Uncover the explicit and implicit rules that govern family interaction.
- Determine the family's problem-solving behavior.
- Understand the nature of boundaries, splits, alliances, and coalition formations in the family.
- Assess the level of concordance between the developmental and chronological stages of the family.
- Assess the concordance between the value system of the family and the surrounding community.
- Help the family to transcend the repetitive, immediate, and trivial problems and to recognize the underlying patterns and major issues.

Goals of the Diagnostic Interview

A significant goal of the diagnostic family interview is to help the family recognize and acknowledge its strengths as a family and the assets of family members, particularly the index patient. The commonly observed emphasis of the family on negative attributes of the index patient is a manifestation of the family's negative view of itself as a family that is projected onto the index patient. Recognizing the assets of the index patient, which is usually resisted by the family as a whole, is generally followed by recognizing the many assets and resources of the family and enhancing the family's problem-solving capacity as a result of a heightened optimism and confidence.

■ Role of Closure

Closing the diagnostic family interview is an important component of the assessment. When the diagnostic family interview is part of a comprehensive evaluation, it is best to delay the therapeutic recommendation until the closing conference. In circumstances other than a comprehensive evaluation, the diagnostic family interview should be closed by highlighting the points of convergence among the problems of the index patient, the information gathered from different family members, the transactional patterns in the family system, and the referral information. The clinician should attempt to integrate and summarize data while highlighting the family's assets, positive attributes, and affectionate feelings for one another, which would enhance their optimism and confidence for undertaking a therapeutic endeavor. An experienced family therapist highlights the family's assets, knowing well that the family is aware of its conflictual interactions and relationships but barely is cognizant of those assets that are the key to therapeutic success. An inexperienced family therapist tends to focus on family problems to demonstrate his or her observational acumen; this focus may inadvertently make the family feel severely disturbed and discouraged.

Family History and Its Role in the Diagnostic Process

Significant experiences in the past, such as the early death or suicide of a grandparent when a parent was very young, significant financial losses, or other events traumatic for the family, may influence family orientation and mythology and directly or indirectly relate to the family's problems. For example, an overly solicitous father of a young man revealed that the year before his son's bar mitzvah, the son was involved in a serious accident requiring prolonged hospitalization and cancellation of the bar mitzvah plans. The oversolicitousness, related to the accident's impact, irritated the new stepmother, who had not known about the collision.

The gradual unfolding of historical information in the family session is an important aspect of the family interview and generally reveals the affectively charged and dynamically significant past experiences of the family. This phenomenon of "living family history" (Ackerman 1958) exceeds the validity of the historical data obtained in a formal chronological, developmental history. The living family history may reveal past deprivations, successes, failures, hidden strengths, and weaknesses of the family that may be related to the current crisis (Sholevar 1985).

Most family therapists gather historical material as it arises in the family interview and occasionally probe specific issues in the past that appear to be related to current problems. The information can be gathered along chronological or analogical lines. Multigenerational family therapists gather such information within a multigenerational context. Family data may reveal that some of the current dysfunctions are a prolonged attempt at solving past problems, at times spanning many generations.

Collecting diagnostic information about disruptive childhood disorders within a developmental framework is essential for the psychiatrist who works with children and adolescents. In cases of oppositional defiant disorder and conduct disorder, important areas of inquiry are history of criminality or mental illness in the parents, prenatal maternal smoking and substance abuse, the level of parent–infant bonding, attention to and reinforcements of prosocial behavior, presence of coercive family processes, and the adequacy of parental monitoring practices (see Chapter 53, "Family Therapy," in this volume). Assessment of the level of cooperation and alliance between the family and other social systems such as school and peers has received increasing attention lately (see Chapter 53) (Henggeler et al. 1999; Sholevar 2001). Inquiry into exposure of family members to domestic violence or violence in the community can help the psychiatrist assess the level of stress or potential for violence in the family (McAdams and Foster 2002). In cases of attention-deficit/hyperactivity disorder (ADHD), the parental level of positive attentiveness, enhancement of attentiveness and focusing capacity in the child, reinforcement of prosocial and adaptive behavior, and protection of the child's self-esteem are some of the important areas for evaluation. The predominance of a negative interaction between parents and child should alert the psychiatrist to inadequate familial management of ADHD (see Chapter 53). Parents' poor management of their own ADHD—whether limited to their childhood or still present in adulthood—may make them especially vulnerable to transmitting some maladaptive and counterproductive parenting practices.

Family Life Cycle and Developmental Issues

The concept of the *family life cycle*, analogous to the life cycle of individuals, means that family issues are different at various stages in a family's life. This model describes a series of stages and their corresponding family tasks (Sholevar 1994). The most commonly accepted models, those by Carter and McGoldrick (1980) and Zilbach (1988), describe the stages of coupling, becoming three with the arrival of the first child, and growing into a family with young children. These stages are followed by a partial or more complete separation of the adolescent family members from the rest of the family, succeeded by the death of one partner, and continuing until the death of the other partner. At each stage of the life cycle, the family structure is rearranged to facilitate the adaptation and mastery of family members. The concept of the *family life spiral* and its intergenerational dimension is that issues overlap in different generations. The family assumes a centripetal shape around birth and during the early life of the children and a centrifugal shape as the children move into adolescence (Combrinck-Graham 1985). The family life cycle models, used differentially by family theorists, describe the emotional problems characteristic of periods of the life cycle that manifest when the family becomes stagnant. The family crisis when older adolescents leave home is a common clinical problem (Table 11–1) (Duvall 1962; Haley 1973; Terkelson 1980; Zilbach 1988).

Establishment of a Therapeutic System and Joining Operations

Minuchin (1974) termed the therapist's methods of creating a therapeutic system and positioning himself or herself as its leader as *joining operations*. Joining operations, or maneuvers, are a prerequisite for subsequent family change and are necessary because the clinician encounters an organized family system. The accommodation by the therapist to the family system is necessary to "join" them. Joining maneuvers include

- *Contact* with each family member so that each feels heard, understood, and respected.
- *Attention* to the needs of younger, less articulate, or disruptive family members. The therapist's accommodation to the children and to their style of communication is an important but neglected area for many family therapists, who tend to be more responsive to the adult family members. Attention to children's communication, play, and art can enhance the children's alliance with the clinician.

Working with different family subgroups can be an important restructuring tool (Scharff and Scharff 1987; Zilbach 1986).

- *Mimesis*, which is the accommodation of the therapist to the family's style, affective range, and tempo of communication. The therapist should accept the family's organization and experience the strength of its transactional pattern, the pain and pleasure of different family members, and the family's resistance to the interventions.
- *Maintenance*, which refers to the accommodation techniques that provide planned support for the family structure. For example, the therapist may exhibit respect for a strong relationship between a mother and her children by making his or her contact with the children through the mother or by praising the complementarity between husband and wife where the husband defers to the wife's leadership. The maintenance operation may involve the active confirmation and support of the subsystems, such as the executive parental position.
- *Tracking*, which is an accommodation technique by which the therapist follows the contents of the family's communication and encourages family members to continue their expressions, asks clarifying questions, makes approving comments, and requests amplification of certain points. Tracking can apply to the actions or verbal communication of the family.

The therapeutic challenge to the family should not endanger its return for the next session. Therefore, the initial joining maneuvers may be away from the therapeutic goal and in the service of the temporary alliance with the family members and rules. Joining is more related to the initial phase of the treatment and establishing a family diagnosis, in contrast to the *restructuring* methods that belong to the therapeutic phase proper.

Psychodynamic Family Data

In addition to attending to observable and conscious communications, the psychodynamically oriented family therapist is equally attentive to the manifestations of the unconscious life of the family. The unconscious system is considered the repository of repressed object relations derived from past and present family experiences rooted in the basic need for attachment to others. The psychodynamic family therapist pays

Table 11–1. Family development: stages of the family life cycle

Stage	Developmental task
Early stages: forming and nesting	
Stage I Coupling	
Family stage marker	The family begins at the establishment of a common household by two people, which may or may not include marriage.
Family task	Individual independence to couple/dyadic interdependence
Stage II Becoming three	
Family stage marker	The second phase in family life is initiated by the arrival and subsequent inclusion/incorporation of the first child/dependent member.
Family task	Interdependence to incorporation of dependence
Substage A: first year of life	
Family tasks	Development of "parental identity"
	Enhancement of bonding between the child and each parent
Substage B: the family and toddler	
Family tasks	Enhancement of autonomy
	Enhancement of gender role and identity
Substage C: the oedipal constellation	
Family tasks	Differential interaction with parents of each sex
	Enhancement of identification with parent of same sex
Middle stages: family expansion/separation process	
Stage III Entrances	
Family stage marker	The third phase is signaled by the exit of the first child/dependent member from the intrafamilial world to the larger world. This occurs at the point of entrance into school or other extrafamilial environment.
Family task	Dependence to facilitation of beginning separations, partial independence/expansion
Stage IV Expansion	
Family stage marker	This phase is marked by the entrance of the last child/dependent member of the family into the community.
Family task	Support and facilitation of continuing separations/expansion
Stage V Exits	
Family stage marker	This phase starts with the first complete exit of a dependent member from the family. This is achieved by the establishment of an independent household, which may include marriage or another form of independent household entity.
Family task	Partial separations to first complete independence
Late stages: finishing	
Stage VI Becoming smaller/extended	
Family stage marker	Ultimately, the moment comes for the exit of the last child/dependent member from the family.
Family task	Continuing expansion of independence
Stage VII Endings	
Family stage markers	The final years start with the death of one spouse/partner and continue up to the death of the other partner.
Family task	Facilitation of family mourning and working through final separations

Source. Adapted from Zilbach 1988.

special attention to creating a "holding environment" in the treatment—a mode of functioning that contains the emerging family anxiety and therefore minimizes the need for projection and suppression. Two other important aspects of psychodynamic family therapy are transference phenomena among family members and the clinician's own countertransference feelings. The emergence of a strong transference reaction toward the therapist in the diagnostic sessions is generally indicative of more severe psychopathology and possibly requires early transference interpretation. The therapeutic use of countertransference feeling as a tool requires constant scrutiny and self-examination by the therapist to understand the nature of the family's communication (Scharff and Scharff 1987).

Psychodynamic family therapists are particularly allied with psychodynamically oriented psychiatrists because of their mutual emphasis on the concordance between the developmental level of behavior in the patient and transactions in the family. Two special levels of arrest in relational development are excessive infantile dependency among family members and excessive oppositional and defiant behavior and power play. The goal of the treatment is to enhance cooperation, reciprocity, and tenderness characteristic of a more mature (genital) level of interaction and development among family members.

Family Interactional Diagnosis

The family diagnosis is a working hypothesis that encapsulates the clinician's observations of the family interactions, structure, and presenting problems. Dysfunctions in family interactions and structure may be correlated with diagnosable disorders in a child or "primary relationship disorders" in the family, with no symptomatology in individual family members. The clinician's assessment specifically emphasizes the family as a whole and the course of the family in the future; this view contrasts with other approaches that focus on the past and problems, especially in an individual.

Minuchin (1974) emphasized the following six major areas in family assessment:

1. The family structure, its preferred transactional pattern, and the available alternatives
2. The role of the symptoms in the maintenance of the family's preferred transactional pattern

3. The family system's flexibility and capacity for autonomous restructuring by reshuffling the system's alliances and coalitions to deal with stress
4. The family system's resonance and sensitivity to individual members' actions and feelings and their threshold for the activation of corrective or repressive measures
5. The family life context, including sources of support and stress in the family network
6. The family's developmental stage and its concordance with the family members' chronological stage

The interactional diagnosis is formed by gathering different classes of verbal and nonverbal information. The diagnosis must be made after the therapist has entered and joined the family, because the diagnosis cannot be made from outside. The therapeutic joining with the family introduces alternative transactional patterns that are an important indicator of prognosis and therapeutic outcome.

Therapeutic Contract

The contracting phase is an important step before the therapist initiates formal family therapy. The contract between the therapist and the family refers to agreed-on issues and goals for treatment. In addition to accepting the family's wish for help with the presenting problem, the therapist recommends the broader goal of alteration in family interactions underlying the problem, such as disciplining methods used with the children. Later on, the goals can expand to include, for example, resolving disagreements between the parents about their views on child rearing or other issues.

Many treatment failures are due to inadequate contracting between the family and the therapist. The problems of contracting include covert disagreement between the therapist and the family, within the family, or between the family and referral sources (e.g., the department of human services or the court system).

Family Evaluation Scales

Family evaluation scales may augment the clinical interview by providing standardized self-report data that can highlight the areas of family dysfunction. A comparison of family evaluation scales is available elsewhere (see Chapter 13, "Rating Scales"). Several scales are commonly used:

- The Beavers-Timberlawn Family Evaluation Scale (Lewis et al. 1976) is an observer-rated scale that addresses the structural dimensions of power hierarchy, parental coalition, family mythology, goal-directed negotiations, permeability, conflict, self-disclosure, and invasiveness. The controls and sanctions that are measured are overt power and responsibility.
- The Family Adaptability Cohesion Evaluation Scale (FACES III; Olson 1986, 1991; Olson et al. 1982) is a self-report instrument that addresses the structural dimensions of systems feedback, negotiation, family roles, boundaries, coalitions, space, decision making, and time. The controls and sanctions include assertiveness, control, discipline, rules, and independence.
- The Family Assessment Device (Epstein and Bishop 1981) is based on McMaster's problem-centered model of family therapy (Miller et al. 1994). This self-report instrument assesses the structural dimensions of problem solving, communication, roles, and general functioning.
- The Family Environment Scale (Moos and Moos 1980) measures social climates of all types of families, with subscales in areas such as family cohesion, expressiveness, conflict, independence, and achievement. It has been used widely in many research projects.
- The Card Sorting Procedure (Reiss 1981) is an observer-rated instrument that addresses the structural dimensions of configuration, coordination, and closure.

Case Example

The following initial family interview describes the basic family evaluation process but also demonstrates two additional factors: 1) the impact of ethnic characteristics of the family and 2) the interface between family evaluation and hospitalization.

> Present in the sessions were Ricardo, a 15-year-old; his 9-year-old sister, Lisa; the mother, Ms. F; and the mother's boyfriend, Mr. J. Ricardo had been hospi-

talized for the third time in the past 3 years at the same hospital for conduct problems and dangerous behavior. His father moved back to the Dominican Republic when Ricardo was a few months old and subsequently died when Ricardo was 7 years old. Ricardo had visited his father for several months at a time at 1- to 2-year intervals before age 7. The consulting family therapist, Dr. S, was told that Mr. J has moved out of the house and probably was no longer involved with the family. Therefore, Dr. S was not sure that Mr. J would attend the session.

Opening Phase of the Interview

The mother was a slender, attractive woman; Ricardo was a large, overweight boy; Lisa was a well-dressed, attractive girl who carried herself like a princess; and Mr. J was a tall, muscular, handsome, and exceptionally articulate African American man who was casually dressed but carried a briefcase.

Dr. S was introduced to all the family members by Ricardo's psychiatrist and social worker and shook hands with everyone as they entered the room. Mr. J inquired immediately about where Dr. S was going to sit and was encouraged to choose his own seat. The family seated themselves, with Mr. J on the outside, the mother next to him, and Ricardo next to the mother. Lisa immediately moved away from the family to write on the blackboard; she continued to draw circles, write the names of her friends in the circles, erase them, and rewrite them. She interrupted this activity only to answer direct questions in a pleasant, cooperative, and eager fashion. Mr. J started the session by asking about where the offices of Ricardo's psychiatrist and the social worker were located now and sent his regards to another hospital staff member. He then directly asked Dr. S, "What are we going to talk about?" He wanted to know if we were going to talk about the "child's issues, adult–child issues, adult issues, the circumstances around hospitalization, etc." Dr. S responded by smiling and saying, "All of the above."

As soon as a comment was made about Lisa, Dr. S used the occasion to ask Lisa about how she was doing, what grade she was in, her activities, and her friends. Lisa clearly was pleased and proud that she was doing well in school, had many friends, and was free of any problems. Mr. J then proceeded, in a very long, articulate speech, to state that Ricardo was doing well and learning well in the hospital classroom and to describe the hospitalization as a way of getting Ricardo out of the neighborhood to prevent his hanging around with the wrong crowd. He was not interrupted by Ms. F or anyone in the family, although after 10 minutes Ricardo started to show signs of restlessness. At that point, Dr. S inquired if the reason for hospitalization was to get Ricardo out of a bad neighborhood or if there were some behavioral problems requiring hospitalization. Mr. J became somewhat quiet at that point, which allowed Dr. S to inquire about Ms. F's point of view. Ms. F spoke in relatively broken English, despite having been raised in the United States, and appeared very passive. Mr. J attempted to interrupt Ms. F on several occasions, but Dr. S encouraged her to go on and asked Mr. J gently to allow Ms. F to finish her statements. In response to direct inquiries, Ms. F eventually revealed that Ricardo was hospitalized because of dangerous behavior such as throwing large bags of garbage from a roof to where young children were walking by and reckless use of a BB gun around his young cousins, which frightened the family.

Commentary: It was quite clear that the mother is a very passive and ghostlike figure in the family and that Mr. J is a very central and dominant force. Dr. S was puzzled by the contradiction between the preliminary information, which indicated that Mr. J had moved outside of the family and was uninvolved with them, and the observation about his central position in the family.

Second Phase of the Interview

Dr. S inquired if Mr. J lived with the family. Mr. J became momentarily anxious but explained that he had moved away from the family because he was disappointed that Ms. F had not become more of a person, obtained a job, furthered her education, and "blossomed." Mr. J and Ms. F continued dating while living apart, but, according to Mr. J, Ms. F still had not yet blossomed. Mr. J's underlying assumption was that Ricardo's nonaccomplishments, poor school performance, noncompliance, and maladjustment were related to the mother's unproductivity, lack of goals, and insufficient self-definition.

Commentary: The second phase revealed a major point of stress in the family. Mr. J, who had been the central and dominant figure in the family for 3 years, moved out of the house around the time of Ricardo's hospitalization. Furthermore, it revealed an underlying conflict between the adults that had brought about Mr. J's departure. At the same time, Mr. J's behavior in the session and his continued involvement with the family and Ricardo exhibited his strong commitment to both the children and Ms. F.

The plan for the next stage was to include Ricardo in the process and solicit his point of view, further explore the differences between Mr. J and Ms. F, and assess the two adults' ability to negotiate their differences.

Third Phase of the Interview

Dr. S noticed Ricardo's mild restlessness but praised him for his patience and invited him to join the group and share his ideas. Before Dr. S addressed the teenager's problematic behavior, Ricardo proudly described his adjustment to the hospital setting, effective use of the hospital classroom, and his positive response to medication (Mellaril). The problematic behavior was then discussed, and Ricardo subtly acknowledged that before his hospital admission his behavior had been dangerous. Next, in the "living family history," the family described the circumstances leading to Ricardo's hospitalization and Mr. J's departure from the family's house; they revealed that both events occurred approximately at the same time.

The family then became confused and could not accurately identify the dates of Ricardo's hospitalization and Mr. J's departure. Mr. J then stated strongly, "Ricardo was hospitalized before I left the house," revealing his strong guilt feelings about the possibility that his moving out could have precipitated Ricardo's decompensation and hospitalization. Once the sequence of events was clarified, Dr. S explored the feelings of different family members about Mr. J's departure. Ricardo described "feeling depressed" about Mr. J's moving out. He explained that his depression was extremely deep but volunteered that he was not suicidal. Having established the connection between Ricardo's strong depressive reaction and Mr. J's departure, Dr. S asked Lisa about her reaction. Lisa became openly attentive to the content of the session at this point and stated that she was very depressed and referred to having had a "dream." Dr. S quickly inquired about the dream, which occurred within 6 months of the departure of Mr. J. In the dream, Lisa returns home from school and, to her great delight, finds that Mr. J is back home, although she expects him to be absent.

Lisa described and enacted in the session her ritualized greeting for Mr. J. She would shake her head, swing her braided hair from side to side, and tap her feet. In her dream, Lisa acts the same way when she returns home and finds Mr. J is back, and she reenacted this scene. The family united in a joyful moment of laughter, which was understood to be reminiscent of better days when they were all happily united at home.

Ricardo clearly connected the regression in his behavior, the maladaptive and dangerous behavior, to his deep feeling of depression in anticipation of Mr. J's departure. Lisa shared Ricardo's feeling of depression about Mr. J's leaving. Dr. S inquired about Ms. F's reaction to Mr. J's departure. She gave a faint, affectless smile saying that she did not have any feeling, implying that the event did not have much effect on her. Mr. J was listening quietly and attentively. Ms. F's comments came through as a clear put-down and lack of appreciation for Mr. J's enormous contributions to the family and the child rearing.

Commentary: The mother appeared to be in denial of her feelings of loss and grief, which enhanced Ricardo's acting-out and Lisa's excessive psychological departure from the family into her peer group and school. Dr. S suspected that Mr. J felt that his contributions were not valued by Ms. F and possibly the family.

Fourth Phase of the Interview

Mr. J expressed his deep devotion to the children and his wish to help them along, describing himself as exceptionally caring and involved with many children. He acted as a father figure to many children in his large family and neighborhood. His interest in children dated to the departure of his father when Mr. J was very young. His mother became solely responsible for the total care of the children while being the breadwinner for the family, and Mr. J assisted his mother with the children.

Dr. S emphasized Mr. J's importance to the children and to the family as a whole, as well as his competence and interest in caring for and connecting with the children, and touched on Mr. J's frustration about Ms. F's lack of progress in becoming a more competent person, woman, and mother, as well as partner for him. However, Dr. S wondered why all of Mr. J's expectations for the family could not be achieved, considering his skills with and enormous attachment, dedication, and contributions to the family. Following up on Mr. J's deep interest in being a father figure to Ricardo and the other children, Dr. S praised Mr. J's commitment to self-improvement and success, excellent physical health, and muscular build before Mr. J revealed that he was carrying his gym shoes in his briefcase. Dr. S then asked Mr. J if he took Ricardo to the gym so that they could work out together.

At the conclusion of the session, Lisa psychologically rejoined the family, Ricardo's behavior was placed in the context of the tensions and conflicts in the family, and Ms. F became somewhat animated and recognized the potential for gain if she moved forward according to Mr. J's expectations. The accomplishment of Mr. J's goals for the mother would have helped her become a competent leader in the family. Mr. J was very proud and pleased that his enormous contributions to the family were recognized, that he was not viewed as someone who had deserted the children, and that he had not been instrumental in bringing about Ricardo's decompensation. As the family prepared to leave the room, Mr. J asked for Dr. S's business card and inquired where he was teaching.

■ Discussion

The family was using the defensive maneuver of isolating the context of the events leading to the presenting problem from the problem itself. They denied intrafamilial conflicts and externalized the origin of the problem into the bad neighborhood and negative peer pressure. Connecting the two events—Ricardo's hospitalization and Mr. J's leaving—made it clear that the tensions eventually leading to Mr. J's departure had been building for several months and therefore predated the deterioration in Ricardo's behavior. In this way, the presenting problems were placed into their true context, which was the inability of Ms. F and Mr. J to negotiate their differences. Mr. J was further humiliated by his own family and by his peers for acting as a "sucker," raising the children of someone who did not do her own share.

During the session, it was revealed that Ricardo's father moved back to "the islands" because he was depressed. His death, in the Dominican Republic, occurred while he was in his 30s and seemed to be related to multiple depressive episodes, with the possibility of suicide.

The interconnection between genetic predisposition to depression—with possible seasonal features—and conduct disorders and depression in Ricardo was emphasized as an issue requiring exploration and resolution in family and individual treatment. The strong reaction of Ricardo to Mr. J's departure possibly also was related to his unresolved grief over the loss of his father, further complicated by Ms. F's inability to deal with loss.

An important contributing factor to Mr. J's conflict with Ms. F was the cultural context of the family. Being an African American man, Mr. J was deeply committed to "upward mobility," self-enhancement, and improvement in one's circumstances. Ms. F, in contrast, reflected the more relaxed cultural expectation of a woman in a Dominican family. Furthermore, her poor acculturation and limited assimilation to U.S. culture left her isolated, vulnerable, and lacking in skills. She was clearly inhibited and ambivalent about enhancing her skills and pursuing success rigorously, despite having been enrolled in school to become a beautician.

Mr. J's high expectations of Ms. F were partly rooted in his comparison of Ms. F with his mother, who was a hard-driving, competent woman functioning as a mother and father to the children. Compared to Mr. J's mother, Ms. F appeared as highly lacking, which made Mr. J conflicted about being attracted to her.

The interface between psychiatric hospitalization and family functioning was apparent in multiple ways. Ricardo, as well as the family, considered the hospital as a second line of support when the family was no longer able to contain Ricardo's problems. The family clearly viewed the hospital as a Hispanic family would view the grandmother (*comadre*) for the care of the children when the family is no longer able to deal with the problems. Ricardo felt very comfortable returning to the hospital when the home situation proved depressive and a void was created by the departure of Mr. J. The task of inpatient family therapy was to enhance the familial resources to reabsorb Ricardo rather than allowing the hospital or institution to care for him or declaring the family hopeless.

Conclusion

The initial family interview is a highly valuable tool for determining the interpersonal and interactional characteristics of the family and its contributions to psychopathology in a child or an adult family member. Furthermore, the family interview allows the child psychiatrist to demonstrate the hidden resources of the family, enhancing the family's positive expectancies and countering the feelings of despair and antagonism in the family.

References

Ackerman NV: The Psychodynamics of Family Life: Diagnosis and Treatment of Family Relationships. New York, Basic Books, 1958

Boszormenyi-Nagy I: Loyalty implications of the transference model in psychotherapy. Arch Gen Psychiatry 27:374–380, 1972

Carter EA, McGoldrick M: The family life cycle and family therapy, in The Family Life Cycle. Edited by Carter EA, McGoldrick M. New York, Gardner Press, 1980, pp 3–20

Combrinck-Graham L: A model of family development. Fam Process 24:139–150, 1985

Duvall EM: Family Development. Chicago, IL, JB Lippincott, 1962

Epstein NB, Bishop DS: Problem-centered systems therapy of the family, in Handbook of Family Therapy. Edited by Gurman AS, Kniskern DP. New York, Brunner/Mazel, 1981, pp 444–482

Gordon SB, Davidson N: Behavioral parent training, in Handbook of Family Therapy. Edited by Gurman AS, Kniskern DP. New York, Brunner/Mazel, 1981, pp 517–555

Haley J: Uncommon Therapy. Toronto, ON, WW Norton, 1973

Haley J: Conducting the first interview, in Problem-Solving Therapy. San Francisco, CA, Jossey-Bass, 1977, pp 9–47

Henggeler SW, Rowland MD, Randall J et al: Home-based multisystemic therapy as an alternative to the hospitalization of youth in psychiatric crisis. J Am Acad Child Adolesc Psychiatry 38:1331–1339, 1999

Lewis JM, Beavers WR, Grossett JT, et al: No Single Thread. New York, Brunner/Mazel, 1976, pp 83–98

McAdams CR, Foster VA: The safety session. Journal of Family Counseling and Therapy 10:49–56, 2002

Miller I, Kabacoff R, Epstein N, et al: Development of a clinical rating scale for the McMaster Model of Family Functioning. Fam Process 33:53–69, 1994

Minuchin S: Families and Family Therapy. Cambridge, MA, Harvard University Press, 1974

Montalvo B, Haley J: In defense of child therapy. Fam Process 12:227–244, 1973

Moos R, Moos B: Family Environment Scale Manual. Palo Alto, CA, Consulting Psychologists Press, 1980

Olson D: Circumplex Model VII: validation studies and FACES III. Fam Process 25:337–351, 1986

Olson D: Commentary: three-dimensional circumplex model and revised scoring of Faces III. Fam Process 30:74–79, 1991

Olson DH, McCubbin HI, Barnes H, et al: FACES III: Family Adaptability and Cohesion Evaluation Scales. St. Paul, MN, University of Minnesota, Family Social Science, 1982

Reiss D: The Family's Construction of Reality. Cambridge, MA, Harvard University Press, 1981

Scharff D, Scharff J: Object Relations Family Therapy. Northvale, NJ, Jason Aronson, 1987

Sholevar GP: Marital assessment, in Contemporary Marriage. Edited by Goldberg DC. Homewood, IL, Dorsey, 1985, pp 290–311

Sholevar GP: Family development and life cycle, in Psychiatry, Vol 2. Edited by Michaels R. Philadelphia, PA, JB Lippincott, 1994, pp 1–9

Sholevar GP: Family therapy for conduct disorders. Child Adolesc Psychiatr Clin N Am 10:501–517, 2001

Terkelson KG: Toward a theory of the family life cycle, in The Family Life Cycle. Edited by Carter EA, McGoldrick M. New York, Gardner Press, 1980, pp 21–52

Weber T, McKeever J, McDaniel SH: The beginner's guide to the problem-oriented first family interview. Fam Process 24:357–364, 1985

Zilbach JJ: Young Children in Family Therapy. New York, Brunner/Mazel, 1986

Zilbach JJ: The family life cycle: a framework for understanding children in family therapy, in Children in Families: Ecological and Treatment Perspectives. Edited by Combrinck-Graham L. New York, Guilford, 1988, pp 46–66

Diagnostic Interviews

Jon McClellan, M.D.

The practice of psychiatry, perhaps more than any other medical specialty, is dictated by the scope and limitations of its diagnostic system. The field has not shared the enormous scientific and technological advances affecting other medical specialties, primarily because the complex mechanisms underlying brain function and mental illness remain elusive. Mid-nineteenth-century breakthroughs in cellular pathology and bacteriology did little to advance the field (with the exception of syphilis, pellagra, and a few other diseases). Similarly, molecular genetics has only yet defined a few mental disorders, such as Alzheimer's-type dementia, fragile X syndrome, and Rett's disorder. Psychiatric practice remains embedded in clinically defined syndromes based primarily on subjective symptom reports and course of illness.

The evolution of medical science is dependent on a valid diagnostic nosology. The success of research examining biological properties underlying pathophysiological states is dependent on the ability to distinguish distinct clinical entities on the basis of presenting history, pattern of illness, and symptomatology. Efforts to unravel the human genome in part require the recognition of valid phenotypes, especially for more complex illnesses with polygenic inheritance. This likely includes all major psychiatric illnesses.

Thus, a mainstay of psychiatric research continues to focus on the refining of diagnostic categories, tools, and techniques. The DSM and ICD (*International Classification of Diseases and Related Health Problems*) systems commenced the epoch of psychiatric diagnostic classification. Prior to these classification schemas, although syndromes such as schizophrenia, depression, manic depression (now called bipolar disorder), and autism were well described, the application of diagnoses was often variable and unreliable. A major advantage was the atheoretical basis of the DSM and ICD systems that emphasized clinically defined syndromes, with criteria based on symptomatology and pattern of illness. This moved the field away from diagnostic formulations based on unproven theoretical doctrines and ill-defined constructs such as defense mechanisms and ego formation.

Through several iterations and revisions, the DSM and ICD systems remain the foundation of psychiatric diagnosis and treatment. Criteria-based diagnoses confer great advantages by improving reliability and ensuring that similar definitions are used by different clinicians and across sites, enhancing communication for clinical, administrative, and research purposes. However, despite their utility, the validity of many of the diagnostic categories remains unknown, especially for those specific to child psychiatry. The lack of understanding regarding the exact nature and etiology of psychiatric disorders requires that diagnoses be made solely on the basis of recognized patterns or clusters of symptoms. Although helpful, this approach has all the diagnostic precision of the term *fever*.

History of the Psychiatric Interview

The clinical interview, the primary diagnostic tool for psychiatry, has evolved over time. Early physicians such as Kraeplin and Bleuler promoted an indirect approach, with the clinician allowing the patient to set the course and content of the interview (Costello 1996). Freud, and the theories underlying classical psychoanalysis, emphasized an even more passive style, with the intent to eliminate interviewer biases. Clinicians were taught to observe unfettered discourse and play (in children) without direct questioning, which was felt to be a potential contaminant (Costello 1996).

Since the advent of the DSM and ICD diagnostic systems, the focus on interviewing has shifted to a more disease-oriented approach. As noted above, this change was prompted in part by the recognized lack of clinician reliability in diagnosing recognized illnesses (e.g., schizophrenia, autism) and in part by the recognized lack of an etiological model on which to base a diagnostic system (Costello 1996). Psychiatric diagnoses are defined by using a medical model, wherein each illness is assumed to be a distinct psychopathological entity, with definable symptom criteria. This allows clinicians, researchers, and administrative bodies (e.g., third-party payers, medical records departments) to communicate broadly about diagnostic entities with some expectation that the disorders are the same, or at least similar, across settings.

The subjective and variable nature of the symptom reports used to generate psychiatric diagnoses remains a limitation. Information derived from patients, their families, and other observers (e.g., teachers) is subtle, complex, and often conflicting (Achenbach et al. 1987). Clinicians' diagnoses are potentially fraught with numerous biases (Angold and Fisher 1999), including

- Making diagnoses before all relevant information is collected
- Collecting information selectively when confirming and/or ruling out a diagnosis
- Neglecting to be systematic in collecting and organizing information
- Allowing the clinician's particular expertise (e.g., a physician in a mood disorders clinic diagnosing most patients' disorders as depression, regardless of each patient's clinical presentation) to influence diagnosis assignment
- Assuming correlations between symptoms and illnesses that in reality are spurious or nonexistent (e.g., equating all irritability with mania)

The creation of diagnostic criteria helped structure the diagnostic process. However, even when the same diagnostic criteria are used, disagreement may occur for any of the following reasons (Costello 1996):

- Differences in wording of the questions used to identify symptoms
- Differences in how clinicians interpret the responses

- Differences in responses the patient may make to different interviewers or to the same interviewer at different times

Structured Diagnostic Interviews

To address these limitations, various diagnostic tools have been developed to enhance the reliability of the information gathered and the diagnosis assignment. The two types of diagnostic tools commonly used by clinicians and researchers are diagnostic interviews and questionnaires. Questionnaires are usually completed by patients, parents, or other significant individuals (e.g., teachers) and generally focus on broader domains of psychopathology but may focus more narrowly on specific illness states or symptoms. For a thorough discussion of questionnaires and checklists pertinent to child and adolescent psychopathology, see Chapter 13 ("Rating Scales").

Structured diagnostic interviews are designed to elicit information from children and/or their parents about various aspects of functioning and mental health, including specific inquiries about symptom criteria for different psychiatric disorders. They are primarily used for psychiatric research, both in epidemiological surveys and in clinical studies. The instruments vary as to whether they are administered by clinicians or trained interviewers, although some researchers have research assistants administer measures originally designed for use by clinicians. Structured interviews were first developed to examine mental health problems in adults; interviews for use with children and adolescents and their families were subsequently developed. Many of the available measures have evolved over several versions, dating back to DSM-III (American Psychiatric Association 1980).

■ Interview Characteristics and Relevant Concepts

There are several characteristics and concepts relevant to the development, choice, use, and interpretation of structured diagnostic interviews.

Validity

Validity reflects the degree to which a measure or classification system accurately characterizes the entity it is examining. Descriptors of various types of validity (Volkmar 1996) include

- Face validity, or how well a category as defined appears to describe a recognized illness
- Predictive validity, or how well the category predicts a pertinent aspect of care, such as treatment needs or prognosis
- Construct validity, or whether the category has meaning in terms of what it is designed to describe (see below)

Childhood psychiatric disorders generally have face validity but not necessarily construct or predictive validity (Spitzer and Cantwell 1980). Some categories are better than others, with only a few disorders having been adequately studied (e.g., attention-deficit/hyperactivity disorder). Diagnostic validity is difficult to assess in psychiatry. Given the lack of biological markers, diagnoses made using a structured interview are often compared with those made by experienced clinicians. This is problematic because clinicians are notoriously unreliable at diagnostic assessments and may not represent the gold standard (Robins 1985). Furthermore, because the same diagnostic criteria define both methods, the validity of a diagnostic tool is not independent from the diagnostic criteria it assesses.

Some authors assess the construct validity of their diagnostic instruments as a method of inferring validity. Comparison is often made with a series of other measures that assess predictive and/or concurrent features of the disorder, using a strategy referred to as a nomological network (Cronbach and Meehl 1955). For example, the results of a diagnostic interview are compared with several pertinent theoretically related attributes, such as patterns and stability of diagnoses, independent ratings of psychopathology, service utilization, and family psychiatric history. Thus, by a process akin to triangulation, researchers examine the validity of a measure by determining its proximity to that of other theoretically related measures or attributes. The inferred validity of each measure supports the validity of the entire construct.

This method avoids the problems associated with defining a diagnostic gold standard. However, the diagnostic construct is only as valid as the measures or attributes used to define it. Validity of diagnostic concepts and constructs is often examined by comparing the results of diagnostic interviews with related questionnaires (e.g., determining the association between a diagnosis of major depressive disorder on a structured interview and the score on a depression rating scale). Because the same symptoms are assessed by both measures, the instruments are not truly independent. This type of validity test is commonly used, but it represents a circular logic that simply reifies the diagnostic criteria rather than establishing the validity of the disorder or the measure.

Another challenge is distinguishing between syndrome specificity and severity. Many measures used to predict validity assess functional impact (e.g., academic or social impairment). Although a diagnosis may be a good indicator of impairment, this is not unexpected, because impairment is usually one of the diagnostic criteria. Furthermore, although functional impairment is an important health issue, it does not imply specificity. The actual validity of the disorder itself—or the diagnostic criteria that define it—remains illusory.

Reliability

Reliability reflects agreement, including how often different interviewers assign the same diagnosis (interrater reliability), how consistently respondents report the same symptoms or diagnoses over time (test-retest reliability), and how internally consistent the measure is (i.e., the degree to which different sections of the measure give similar information; Verhulst and Koot 1992).

Differences in diagnostic reliability may be due to 1) differences in the information collected, 2) theoretical biases held by diagnosticians, and/or 3) variations in symptoms that individuals with disorders will experience over time (Volkmar 1996). Diagnostic tools must be reliable to be useful, but reliability does not ensure validity (Volkmar 1996). The two concepts are often confused. A diagnostic category may be reliably defined but not valid. Conversely, a disorder may be valid, but the diagnostic criteria, or the instruments used to assess for its presence, may not be reliable.

For categorical variables, reliability is generally measured using either percent agreement or the kappa statistic (κ) for categorical variables (Verhulst and Koot 1992). The kappa statistic controls for the fact that high rates of agreement may be misleading when a disorder is rare, because most of the agreement will be for noncases. For continuous variables, either the product-moment correlation coefficient (r) or the intraclass correlation coefficient (ICC) is used to measure rater agreement. Cronbach's coefficient alpha is used to assess the internal consistency of a scale, which reflects how well different items measure similar information (Verhulst and Koot 1992).

The methods used by investigators to establish reliability on a diagnostic interview raise some interesting questions. For example, establishing reliability at one site often means establishing agreement with the senior investigator. Many studies simply have other examiners watch and score the same interviews. It is not difficult to reach agreement regardless of whether one agrees with the conclusions. There is no guarantee that the same results would be obtained at another program. This is especially true for diagnoses that are considered controversial (e.g., juvenile bipolarity). Although the interviews were designed to improve reliability, the rules used to interpret symptoms and assign a diagnosis remain in part dependent on the views of the person using the measure, with some instruments more prone to this influence than others (see below). Research is needed to establish the reliability of measures across different centers, including nonacademic community programs.

Interview Type

The available diagnostic interviews are often described in terms of their degree of structure—that is, how closely interviewers must follow an outlined script (Costello 1996). In a highly structured interview, the interviewer asks set questions using specified wording, and the subject's responses are recorded as given. Semistructured interviews allow interviewers to use their own probe questions and/or incorporate other sources of information to assess symptoms and interpret the subject's responses. Angold and Fisher (1999) questioned this distinction, suggesting that it is the degree of decision-making process allowed by the interviewer that is structured, rather than the questions themselves. Using this model, interviews can be characterized as 1) respondent-based, in which the interviewer follows a set script without interpreting the subject's response, and/or 2) interviewer-based, in which the interview serves as a tool to guide the interviewer's questioning, including definitions of symptoms and patterns of disorders that the interviewer uses to decide whether a symptom is present. These two methods are not necessarily mutually exclusive, and many interviews have elements of both.

■ Defining Cases

The goal of the psychiatric interview is to identify whether an individual has an illness. Theoretically, using the current categorical model, psychiatric disorders are either present or absent. However, in practice, how cases are defined will depend on the nature and application of diagnostic criteria. Therefore, in any sample, individuals will be either disordered or nondisordered (reflecting the true population prevalence rates) and will be classified as either cases or noncases (depending on the diagnostic criteria). Although it is hoped that these two concepts are related, being a case is not necessarily the same as being truly disordered (Zarin and Earls 1993). This model assumes that the disorder actually does exist in nature, an assumption that may not hold true for any given illness as the neuroscience underlying psychopathology evolves.

In assessing a diagnostic instrument's utility at assigning cases, the following concepts are important:

- *Sensitivity:* The percentage of individuals in a sample who have the disorder who are accurately identified by the interview
- *Specificity:* The percentage of individuals in a sample who do not have the disorder who are accurately identified by the interview as being nondisordered
- *Predictive value positive:* The percentage of individuals in the defined sample positively identified by the interview who actually have the disorder
- *Predictive value negative:* The percentage of individuals in the defined sample identified by the interview as not having the disorder who are in fact nondisordered

The predictive value, both positive and negative, is important because it represents the conditional probability of having or not having a disorder, on the basis of the assessment procedure results. These values are influenced by the overall prevalence of the condition being investigated, whereas sensitivity and specificity are theoretically independent of prevalence rates (although clinicians' awareness of prevalence rates, and therefore assumptions about the frequency with which a disorder is diagnosed, may influence sensitivity and specificity ratings) (Robins 1985). Therefore, the probability of correctly diagnosing a rare condition using a given diagnostic tool may be low, even if the tool has acceptable sensitivity and specificity ratings.

Figure 12–1 demonstrates these concepts, using a hypothetical sample. (This example was previously published by McClellan and Werry [2000] and is adapted from one developed by Zarin and Earls [1993].) Diagnostic criteria met are plotted against the number of individuals with and without the "true" disorder. There is no single cutoff (i.e., number of criteria met) that accurately categorizes each individual. Setting different diagnostic criteria changes how cases are defined (Table 12–1). When five criteria is the diagnostic cutoff, there are 20 false negatives and 50 false positives. When four criteria is the cutoff, there are only 5 false negatives but 100 false positives. The trade-off between false positives and false negatives is unavoidable and important to recognize. Diagnostic decision making must prioritize whether it is better to recognize all cases and accept the risk of overdiagnosis or to establish more conservative criteria and risk false negatives.

As demonstrated in Table 12–2, prevalence rates greatly affect positive and negative predictive values. In a hypothetical example, the accuracy of a diagnostic instrument is examined for a disorder with two different prevalence rates, 20% and 5%. The sensitivity and specificity rates are arbitrarily set to approximately 95%. These are far better rates than for any of the available diagnostic interviews, leading to the assumption that a high rate of accuracy would be expected. However, when the prevalence rate is 5%, the predictive value positive is only 51% (i.e., of those individuals identified as "cases," only one-half actually had the disorder). This is a problem for disorders that have relatively low base rates within the population. Note that in this example, the "low" prevalence rate of 5% in reality reflects the rate of common illnesses (e.g., attention-

deficit/hyperactivity disorder) in the general population. Although high sensitivity and specificity ratings increase the likelihood that those with and without the disorder are correctly identified, a high rate of false positives is still found for rare or uncommon disorders. This fact also holds true for predicting other types of rare events, such as predicting suicides or acts of isolated violence in adolescents.

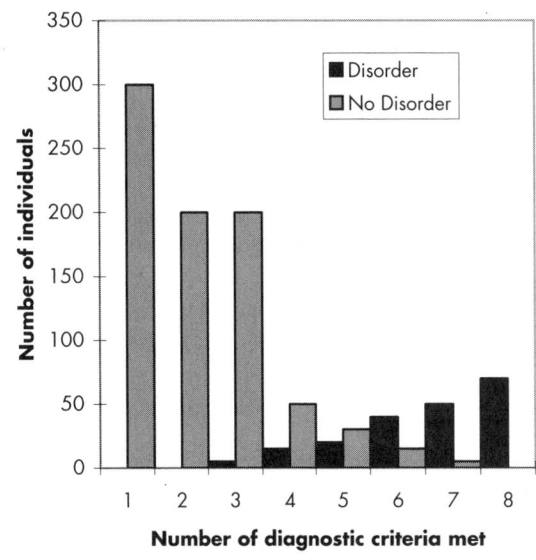

Figure 12–1. Hypothetical sample: number of individuals with or without the "true disorder," by number of diagnostic criteria met.

Illustration of the difference between "caseness," as defined by criteria, and true rates of disorder. There is no "true" diagnostic criteria cutoff that accurately categorizes all individuals.

Source. Previously published by McClellan and Werry 2000 in a version adapted from Zarin and Earls 1993.

Table 12–1. Impact of diagnostic criteria on defining "caseness" in a hypothetical sample

Cutoff	Disorder	No disorder	Total	Sensitivity	Specificity	Predictive value positive	Predictive value negative
Meets 5 criteria							
Cases	180	50	230	90	94	78	97
Noncases	20	750	770				
Total	200	800	1,000				
Meets 4 criteria							
Cases	195	100	295	98	88	66	99
Noncases	5	700	705				
Total	200	800	1,000				

Note. This table represents the hypothetical sample presented in Figure 12–1.

Table 12–2. Impact of prevalence rates on instrument ratings

Cutoff	Disorder	No disorder	Total	Sensitivity	Specificity	Predictive value positive	Predictive value negative
Prevalence rate=20%							
Cases	190	40	230	95	95	83	99
Noncases	10	760	770				
Total	200	800	1,000				
Prevalence rate=5%							
Cases	48	47	95	96	95	51	100
Noncases	2	903	905				
Total	50	950	1,000				

Note. These examples highlight the effect of prevalence rates on predictive value, positive and negative. The predictive value positive is the percentage of individuals identified as being a "case" that truly have the disorder. The predictive value negative is the percentage of individuals identified as being a "noncase" that truly do not have the disorder. False positives are more likely with disorders that have low prevalence rates in the population.

■ Interview Instruments

Table 12–3 outlines characteristics of the structured diagnostic interviews most often used with children and adolescents. The choice of interview generally depends on the purpose (e.g., epidemiological versus treatment study), type of interviewer (clinician versus lay interviewer), training requirements, past familiarity or use of the instrument, and costs.

Respondent-based interviews capture the patient's response without interpretation by the interviewer. This limits variability in how information is obtained. They are typically used in epidemiological surveys, where trained lay interviewers, not clinicians, administer the measure. The National Institute of Mental Health (NIMH) Diagnostic Interview Schedule for Children (DISC) (Shaffer et al. 2000) is the most widely tested measure, having undergone several multicenter field trials to establish its use for the NIMH epidemiological study. It is generally administered by trained lay interviewers, which lowers the cost, making it useful for large epidemiological studies examining for prevalence rates of disorder within a population.

In interviewer-based interviews (Angold and Fisher 1999), the concepts to be explored are defined with a range of possible answers, but interviewers are allowed to phrase questions in their own words and/or develop their own probes to elicit further information. Depending on the methods being used, the interviewer may also incorporate information obtained from other sources (e.g., other informants, medical records) prior to making a decision about a particular symptom or di-

agnosis. Some of the interviews have screening questions so that entire topics can be skipped if the initial inquiry is negative. Interviewer-based interviews require some clinical decision making on the part of the interviewer, are often used in studies of clinical populations, and are presumably more tolerable to clinicians.

Among the interviewer-based instruments, the Child and Adolescent Psychiatric Assessment (CAPA; Angold and Costello 2000), the Schedule for Affective Disorders and Schizophrenia for School-Aged Children (K-SADS; Ambrosini 2000), and the Diagnostic Interview for Children and Adolescents (DICA; Reich 2000) have been most studied. The CAPA has an extensive glossary to aid decision making and provides separate ratings of symptomatology and psychosocial impairment. The K-SADS has been used extensively in child psychiatry research, especially in the area of mood disorders, and includes individual ratings of symptom impairment. The DICA can be used either by clinicians as an interviewer-based instrument or by lay interviewers as a respondent-based measure.

The Interview Schedule for Children and Adolescents (ISCA; Sherrill and Kovacs 2000); the Children's Interview for Psychiatric Syndromes (ChIPS; Weller et al. 2000); and the Structured Clinical Interview for DSM-IV, Childhood Diagnoses (KID-SCID; Matzner et al. 1997) have less research supporting their reliability and validity and are not used as widely. All, however, are promising tools. The ISCA has been used to study mood and anxiety disorders in youth. There is a version for young adults, which is potentially useful for longitudinal follow-up studies. Because the ISCA is

Table 12–3. Structured diagnostic interviews most often used with children and adolescents

Instrument	Disorders covered	Informant	Age range (years)	Type	Time (minutes)	Interviewer qualifications	Special issues
Child and Adolescent Psychiatric Assessment (CAPA; Angold and Costello 2000)	ANX, BEH, EAT, ELIM, MOOD, SCH, SOM, SUB, TIC	Child, parent	9–17	Interviewer	60–150	Bachelor's degree plus training program	Glossary used to define symptoms and severity ratings; Spanish version available
Related Instruments							
YAPA (Young Adult Psychiatric Assessment)		Patient	18+				
PAPA (Pre-school Age Psychiatric Assessment)		Parent	3–6				
NIMH Diagnostic Interview Schedule for Children Version IV (NIMH DISC-IV; Shaffer et al. 2000)	ANX, BEH, EAT, ELIM, MOOD, SCH, SUB, TIC	Child, parent	6–17	Respondent	70–120	Trained lay interviewer	Computerized voice and Spanish versions available
Versions							
DISC-Y (Youth)			9–17				
DISC-P (Parent)			6–17				
Schedule for Affective Disorders and Schizophrenia for School-Aged Children (K-SADS; Ambrosini 2000)	ANX, BEH, EAT, MOOD, SCH, SUB	Child, parent	6–18	Interviewer	75–90	Trained clinician	Although designed for clinicians, many researchers use trained interviewers
Versions							
K-SADS-E (epidemiological)	Also assesses ELIM and TIC						
K-SADS-P/L (Present and Lifetime)							
K-SADS-P (present state) Washington University K-SADS	Expands definitions of *mania*						
Diagnostic Interview for Children and Adolescents (DICA; Reich 2000)	ANX, BEH, EAT, ELIM, MOOD, PSYCH, SOM, SUB, TIC	Child, parent	6–17	Respondent/ interviewer	60–120	Trained lay interviewer	Used as both structured and semistructured interview
Structured Clinical Interview for DSM-IV, Childhood Diagnoses (KID-SCID) (Matzner et al. 1997)	ANX, BEH, MOOD, SCH, SOM, SUB	Child, parent	?–17	Interviewer	60–120	Clinician	Only preliminary data available

Table 12–3. Structured diagnostic interviews most often used with children and adolescents *(continued)*

Instrument	Disorders covered	Informant	Age range (years)	Type	Time (minutes)	Interviewer qualifications	Special issues
Interview Schedule for Children and Adolescents (ISCA; Sherrill and Kovacs 2000)	ANX, BEH, EAT, ELIM, MOOD, PSYCH, SOM, SUB, TIC	Child, parent	8–17	Interviewer	120 (parent), 60 (child)	Clinician	Organized around symptom reports
Follow-Up Interview Schedule for Adults (FISA)		Young adults	18+		60–120		Designed for longitudinal research
Children's Interview for Psychiatric Syndromes (ChIPS; Weller et al. 2000)	ANX, BEH, EAT, ELIM, MOOD, SCH, SUB	Child, parent	6–18	Respondent	40	Trained lay interviewer	Primarily a screening tool
Dominic-R (Valla et al. 2000)	ANX, BEH, DEP	Child	6–11	Pictorial	15–25	Trained lay interviewer	Pictorial depiction of DSM-III-R symptoms; versions for African American and French-speaking children available
Pictorial Instrument for Child and Adolescent Psychiatry (PICA-III-R; Ernst et al. 2000)	ANX, BEH, MOOD, PSYCH	Child	4–7	Pictorial	40–60	Clinician	Not available yet for DSM-IV-TR

Note. ANX=anxiety disorders (often includes posttraumatic stress disorder); BEH=disruptive behavior disorders; DEP=depressive disorders; EAT=eating disorders; ELIM=encopresis and enuresis; MOOD=mood disorders (depressive and bipolar); NIMH=National Institute of Mental Health; PSYCH=nondiagnostic screen for psychotic symptoms; SCH=schizophrenia and psychotic disorders; SOM=somatoform disorders; SUB=substance abuse/dependence; TIC=tic disorders. Type of interview: respondent=answers coded on the basis of responses (also described as structured); interviewer=interviewer allowed to make clinical judgments regarding respondent's answers (also called semistructured). Interview times are approximate and may vary depending on the case and interviewer.

structured around symptom reports rather than diagnostic categories, it can be used to explore alternative ways of defining disorders. The ChIPS is respondent-based and can be administered in a relatively short period of time. Therefore, it may be useful as a screening tool in, for example, a clinic setting. The KID-SCID is an adaptation of the adult SCID (First et al. 1996), which is widely used for studies of mood and psychotic disorders.

Two measures, the Dominic-R (Valla et al. 2000, 2002) and the Pictorial Instrument for Child and Adolescent Psychiatry (PICA-III-R; Ernst et al. 2000), use pictures as cues to inquire about symptoms. Each picture has an accompanying question the interviewer uses to prompt the child for a response. These measures were developed because younger children may not provide reliable responses with standard question-and-answer interviews. However, the pictorial methods entail difficulties in assessing certain concepts important to diagnosis, such as duration and severity. The Dominic-R is computerized and highly structured but does not include inquiries about frequency, duration, or age of onset of symptoms. The PICA-III-R is designed for use by clinicians and allows other inquiries and/or clinical judgment to characterize symptoms. To date, there is not a DSM-IV-TR (American Psychiatric Association 2000) version of the PICA-III-R. Neither of these measures has been extensively studied, but both may offer a potentially useful and innovative method for obtaining reliable diagnostic information from younger children.

Discussion

Structured diagnostic interviews are useful tools that have improved the reliability of diagnostic assignment. Although most often used by researchers, these instruments would likely enhance practice if adopted by clinicians in community settings. When using these instruments, it is important to recognize the limitations.

Perhaps most important is that the validity of a diagnostic interview is no greater than the validity of the diagnoses themselves. Although children and adolescents with psychiatric disorders can be reliably differentiated from control subjects without disorders, the distinction between disorders is less clear (Reeves et al. 1987). The lack of a definitive gold standard for identifying disorders remains a significant impediment. If structured diagnostic interviews are the gold standard (which researchers often assume), how can their validity be examined? Diagnostic criteria were originally created in an attempt to describe recognized disorders, yet unwittingly, they have become the disorders. The same criteria used to define a disorder are used to validate its existence. The challenge is distinguishing between the validity of a disorder and the criteria or measure that defines it. Ultimately, making that distinction will require the identification of external markers for disorders, separate from phenomenological criteria.

There are several methodological limitations associated with the use of structured diagnostic interviews. All diagnostic tools have error, and use of even those with excellent ratings of sensitivity and specificity will result in misdiagnosis. Slight variations in wording, or in diagnostic criteria, may produce significant changes in prevalence estimates (Regier et al. 1998). For example, in a large-scale epidemiological study, estimates of the prevalence rates for children having any psychiatric disorder ranged from 5.4% to 50.4%, depending on degree to which functional impairment was required (Shaffer et al. 1996).

In addition, the presence of a diagnosis may not adequately characterize clinical significance, as defined by either treatment needs or level of impairment (Frances 1998; Regier et al. 1998). One difficulty is in the ability to discriminate between individuals with actual disorders and individuals with typical yet problematic responses to some type of event or stimulus. Human beings have a fairly consistent repertoire of responses to stress, regardless of the source (a final common pathway). Symptoms may represent transient adaptive changes in mood, behavior, and/or physiological measures rather than evidence for a distinct pathological state (Regier et al. 1998). Many symptoms are not necessarily specific to any single disorder (e.g., irritability, sleep problems, aggression).

Another difficulty is that children may overreport rare or unusual phenomena, such as obsessive-compulsive, psychotic, or manic symptoms, using structured diagnostic interviews (Breslau 1987; Weller et al. 1996). This is likely due to the child's either misinterpreting the question or not being aware of the concept being described. In general, younger children lack the prerequisite attention span, abstract awareness (including timelines for duration criteria), and verbal skills necessary to understand the concepts involved (Valla et al. 2000). Clinical judgment generally is touted to be the mechanism for differentiating non-specific experiences or problems from qualitatively specific psychiatric symptoms. Yet the lack of reliability across clinicians challenges this notion. Glossary-based interviews (e.g., the CAPA, K-SADS) address this by developing clear definitions and training the interviewers to recognize the distinctions.

Disagreement between diagnostic instruments is an area of concern that has not been well studied. Different interviews, or different versions of the same instrument, may vary significantly in estimates of prevalence rates or in defining whether a specific individual is a "case" (Regier et al. 1998; Rutter 1997). Boyle et al. (1997) compared a parent-completed questionnaire to a nonclinician-administered structured interview in a sample of public school children. Although the overall reliability between the two measures was acceptable, substantial disagreement occurred for specific diagnoses. There is a paucity of research comparing one structured diagnostic interview with another or examining which instruments are superior for certain diagnoses or clinical issues.

The noted low rates of agreement between different informants (e.g., parent–child, parent–teacher) represent another challenge (Achenbach et al. 1987; Rutter 1997). It is generally taught that youth are thought to be better at describing their own internalizing states, whereas adults are better at describing acting-out behaviors in children. Research is needed to clarify when and if this is the case. Poor agreement does not necessarily imply error. Some differences are expected, because children's behavior depends to some extent on the setting and situation (Achenbach et al. 1987).

Given these methodological difficulties, it is generally recommended that research studies use multiple diagnostic tools, with repeated measures over time, to minimize error (Rutter 1997). Some studies use best-estimate procedures, with experienced clinicians determining diagnostic status after reviewing all available information (Leckman et al. 1982). This method reflects that of clinical decision making and the integration of multiple sources of information into diagnostic formulations. However, this procedure can be time-consuming and costly. Furthermore, consensus agreement at one center does not guarantee that the same diagnosis would be made at a different center.

There are no universally accepted algorithms dictating how to combine different types of information. For example, are both child and parent reports of symptoms necessary for diagnosis? If not, which informant's information takes precedence? How do the responses of other informants, such as teachers, influence the findings? These are complex processes normally characterized as clinical judgment. Psychiatric decision making is dependent on the integration of information from diverse sources and perspectives, including the patient and family interviews, the mental status examination, collateral informants (e.g., teachers), and other treatment providers. These decision-making processes must be quantified in a manner that translates to different settings and situations.

The utility of diagnostic interviews in clinical settings outside of academic centers must be examined. By compelling clinicians to follow standard diagnostic and interviewing methods, structured interviews promote more consistent diagnostic practices and help justify therapeutic interventions and outcomes. These are important issues as the field moves toward evidence-based practices. Computerized instruments and medical records allow the integration of clinical care and information management systems, thus promoting the inclusion of standardized assessments and treatment protocols into routine care.

Conclusion

There are a number of structured diagnostic interviews available to assess psychiatric illnesses in youth. The choice of instrument depends in part on the purpose (e.g., epidemiological vs. clinical intervention study), diagnoses to be addressed, training requirements, interviewer characteristics (lay interviewer vs. clinician), and time needed to administer. Structured diagnostic interviews have helped advance the field by enhancing reliability and improving consistency of diagnostic practices across sites. Though primarily used for research, they also have potential utility for clinical settings.

Although structured diagnostic interviews represent a significant improvement over unstructured nonstandardized approaches, the results remain dependent on, and interwoven with, the skills and fidelity of the person administering the interview and the validity of the diagnosis being assessed. Thus, further work is needed to improve the efficiency and accuracy of these instruments, but their ultimate utility is dependent on advances in the understanding of mechanisms underlying childhood psychopathology.

References

Achenbach TM, McConaughy SH, Howell CT: Child/adolescent behavioral and emotional problems: implications of cross-informant correlations for situational specificity. Psychol Bull 101:213–232, 1987

Ambrosini PJ: Historical development and present status of the Schedule for Affective Disorders and Schizophrenia for School-Age Children (K-SADS). J Am Acad Child Adolesc Psychiatry 39:49–58, 2000

American Psychiatric Association: Diagnostic and Statistical Manual of Mental Disorders, 3rd Edition. Washington, DC, American Psychiatric Association, 1980

American Psychiatric Association: Diagnostic and Statistical Manual of Mental Disorders, 4th Edition, Text Revision. Washington, DC, American Psychiatric Association, 2000

Angold A, Costello E: The Child and Adolescent Psychiatric Assessment (CAPA). J Am Acad Child Adolesc Psychiatry 39:39–48, 2000

Angold A, Fisher PW: Interviewer-based interviews, in Diagnostic Assessment in Child and Adolescent Psychopathology. Edited by Shaffer D, Lucas CP, Richters JE. New York, Guilford, 1999, pp 34–64

Boyle MH, Offord DR, Racine YA, et al: Adequacy of interviews vs checklists for classifying childhood psychiatric disorder based on parent reports. Arch Gen Psychiatry 54:793–799, 1997

Breslau N: Inquiring about the bizarre: false positives in Diagnostic Interview Schedule for Children (DISC), ascertainment of obsessions, compulsions and psychotic symptoms. J Am Acad Child Adolesc Psychiatry 26:639–655, 1987

Costello AJ: Structured interviewing, in Child and Adolescent Psychiatry, A Comprehensive Textbook, 2nd Edition. Edited by Lewis M. Baltimore, MD, Williams & Wilkins, 1996, pp 457–464

Cronbach L, Meehl P: Construct validity in psychological tests. Psychol Bull 52:281–302, 1955

Ernst M, Cookus BA, Moravec BC: Pictorial Instrument for Children and Adolescents (PICA-III-R). J Am Acad Child Adolesc Psychiatry 39:94–99, 2000

First MB, Gibbon M, Spitzer RL, et al: User's Guide for the Structured Clinical Interview for DSM-IV Axis I Disorders—Research Version. New York, Biometrics Research Department, New York State Psychiatric Institute, 1996

Frances A: Problems in defining clinical significance in epidemiological studies. Arch Gen Psychiatry 55:116, 1998

Leckman JF, Sholomskas D, Thompson WD, et al: Best estimate of lifetime psychiatric diagnosis: a methodological study. Arch Gen Psychiatry 29:879–883, 1982

zMatzner F, Silva R, Silvan M, et al: Preliminary test-retest reliability of the KID-SCID. Scientific proceedings, American Psychiatric Association meeting, 1997. Available at: http://cpmcnet.columbia.edu/dept/scid/kid-scid.htm. Accessed April 16, 2003

McClellan JM, Werry JS: Introduction: research psychiatric diagnostic interviews for children and adolescents. J Am Acad Child Adolesc Psychiatry 39:19–27, 2000

Reeves JC, Werry JS, Elkind GS, et al: Attention-deficit conduct, oppositional, and anxiety disorders in children, II: clinical characteristics. J Am Acad Child Adolesc Psychiatry 26:144–55, 1987

Regier DA, Kaelber CT, Rae DS, et al: Limitations of diagnostic criteria and assessment instruments for mental disorders: implications for research and policy. Arch Gen Psychiatry 55:109–115, 1998

Reich W: Diagnostic Interview for Children and Adolescents (DICA). J Am Acad Child Adolesc Psychiatry 39:59–66, 2000

Robins LN: Epidemiology: reflections on testing the validity of psychiatric interviews. Arch Gen Psychiatry 42:918–924, 1985

Rutter M: Child psychiatric disorder: measures, causal mechanisms and interventions. Arch Gen Psychiatry 54:785–789, 1997

Shaffer D, Fisher P, Dulcan MK, et al: The NIMH Diagnostic Interview Schedule for Children Version 2.3 (DISC-2.3): description, acceptability, prevalence rates, and performance in the MECA Study. J Am Acad Child Adolesc Psychiatry 35:865–877, 1996

Shaffer D, Fisher P, Lucus CP, et al: NIMH Diagnostic Interview Schedule for Children Version IV (NIMH DISC-IV): description, differences from previous versions and reliability of some common diagnoses. J Am Acad Child Adolesc Psychiatry 39:28–38, 2000

Sherrill JT, Kovacs M: Interview Schedule for Children and Adolescents (ISCA). J Am Acad Child Adolesc Psychiatry 39:67–75, 2000

Spitzer RL, Cantwell DP: The DSM-III classification of the psychiatric disorders of infancy, childhood and adolescence. J Am Acad Child Adolesc Psychiatry 19:356–370, 1980

Valla JP, Bergeron L, Berube H: The Dominic-R, a pictorial interview for 6- to 11-year-old children. J Am Acad Child Adolesc Psychiatry, 39:85–93, 2000

Valla JP, Kovess V, Chan Chee C, et al: A French study of the Dominic Interactive. Soc Psychiatry Psychiatr Epidemiol 37:441–448, 2002

Verhulst FC, Koot HM: Child Psychiatric Epidemiology: Concepts, Methods and Findings. Newbury Park, CA, Sage Publications, 1992

Volkmar FR: Classification in child and adolescent psychiatry: principals and issues, in Child and Adolescent Psychiatry, A Comprehensive Textbook, 2nd Edition. Edited by Lewis M. Baltimore, MD, Williams & Wilkins, 1996, pp 417–422

Weller EB, Weller RA, Svadjian H: Mood Disorders, in Child and Adolescent Psychiatry, A Comprehensive Textbook, 2nd Edition. Edited by Lewis M. Baltimore, MD, Williams & Wilkins, 1996, pp 650–665

Weller EB, Weller RA, Fristad M, et al: Children's Interview for Psychiatric Syndromes (ChIPS). J Am Acad Child Adolesc Psychiatry 39:76–84, 2000

Zarin DA, Earls F: Diagnostic decision making in psychiatry. Am J Psychiatry 150:197–206, 1993

Rating Scales

Kathleen Myers, M.D., M.P.H.
Brent Collett, Ph.D.

This chapter discusses the use of rating scales in psychiatric assessment. The term *rating scale* refers to any instrument that provides rapid assessment of a behavior or psychological dimension, yielding a numerical score that is easily interpreted to complement clinical care. The emphasis here is in on scales that assess the externalizing and internalizing problems routinely encountered in clinical practice. The text discusses general issues regarding the functioning and applications of rating scales, whereas the tables provide information regarding the availability of technical data supporting the functioning of these scales. All scales presented here have adequate functioning documented for their intended purposes.

Advantages and Disadvantages of Rating Scales

The value of rating scales is indicated by their inclusion in the Practice Parameters of the American Academy of Child and Adolescent Psychiatry. These scales have multiple uses, such as community screening, monitoring at-risk youths, selecting homogeneous groups for treatment, and evaluating outcome. They provide systematic coverage and quantification of behaviors for comparison of youths with self and peers over time, setting, and context. They may allow youths to more easily reveal sensitive symptoms, such as compulsions, or secretive behaviors, such as arson. Rating scales provide cost-efficient documentation for evidence-based treatment.

Perhaps the greatest difficulty with rating scales is the user's unrealistic expectations (Myers and Winters 2002a; Piacentini 1993). Clinicians often inaccurately assume that an elevated score equates to diagnosis.

Many scales were developed as modified adult measures and may not provide a suitable response format or tap youths' experience, as the ability to report one's experience varies with development. Finally, many popular scales do not have established technical adequacy. It may then be difficult to determine how well that scale differentiates clinical groups, how reliable scores are, and how suitable the scale may be for a specific youth.

Individual and situational factors can also affect a scale's performance. Youths who seek social acceptance may underreport ("denial" or "lying"), whereas those who feel overwhelmed may overreport ("faking") symptoms. Adult respondents may convey their own distress with the youth or may portray their child as having few problems. Validity scales may be included to assess this issue. Poor agreement is noted among adults who rate a youth in different settings, such as teachers and parents, and only moderate agreement is achieved among adults in the same environment, such as mothers and fathers in the home. These disparities reflect both differences in reporters' perceptions and variations in youths' behavior as a function of context. Not surprisingly, there is also great disparity between youths' self-reports and adults' reports. This highlights the need for collecting information from multiple informants and the importance of viewing scales as a means of communication when interpreting scores.

Psychometric Properties of Rating Scales

Rating scales do not yield "the truth"; rather, they measure a construct, and all measurement is subject to error. Psychometric properties estimate this error and help to determine whether a scale is appropriate for an application (Piacentini 1993).

Reliability refers to the consistency with which a scale's items measure the same construct and the consistency with which the scale measures that construct in the same way every time. Lack of reliability is termed *random error*. Coefficients exceeding 0.80 support reliability but also mean that a considerable portion of the scale's score is due to random error. *Internal reliability*, or *internal consistency*, represents the degree to which individual items are consistent with each other. Items that are not internally consistent detract from the scale. *Test-retest reliability*, or *stability*, assesses whether a scale is stable over time. If the construct measured has not changed, then repeated measurements should be similar. This might be difficult to determine for a state construct that waxes and wanes, such as suicidality or aggression. If stability has not been established, then it is difficult to determine whether measured change is real or represents random error in the scale. *Interrater reliability* represents the agreement, or *concordance*, between different informants.

Validity pertains to whether the scale accurately assesses what it was designed to assess. Lack of validity is referred to as *systematic error*. Validity must be assessed against multiple criteria over time. *Content validity* assesses whether the scale's items represent the construct being measured. *Face validity* is a type of content validity that is determined by subjectively judging whether items measure the content area. *Criterion validity* is assessed in relation to other scales with established validity in measuring the same construct. There are two subtypes: *Predictive validity* asks whether the scale correlates with an event that will occur in the future; *concurrent validity* refers to a scale's correlation with an event assessed at the same time the scale is administered. There are two types of concurrent validity: *Discriminant validity* compares scores for groups that do have a problem with scores for those who do not have a problem; *convergent validity* is the extent of correlation with some other relevant variable. In contrast, *divergent validity* measures the extent to which a measured construct diverges from another unrelated variable, such as whether a scale measuring depression correlates poorly with a scale measuring conduct disorder. *Construct validity* examines whether the scale taps a theoretical construct and is usually determined through statistical procedures, such as factor analysis.

Even when a scale has excellent technical proper-

ties, more than one scale should be used, as different scales tap different aspects of the problem and better approximate "the truth." These scales should demonstrate at least fair (>0.6) convergent validity, but not so high (>0.95) that they measure the same aspects of the problem. Psychometric properties should be "matched" to the scale's intended application. For example, screening requires high sensitivity. Monitoring requires good stability, sensitivity, and a response format that detects response variation. Finally, cutoff scores vary according to development, culture, and clinical status. Thus, caution is needed in using scales that were developed with groups that differ from the target subjects.

Broad-Band Rating Scales

Broad-band scales (Table 13–1) assess a variety of problems across broad dimensions of youths' behavior and subjective experience. They have excellent utility for initial evaluation, as they can be quickly completed by multiple informants in different settings and help to focus further evaluation. Broad coverage is important in initial evaluation, as youths referred for specific concerns generally have other problems needing attention. Despite their utility, broad-band scales have some limitations. Their length often precludes repeated administrations. Because some subscales overlap with diagnostic constructs, clinicians may misconstrue high scores as diagnosis. Finally, owing to their breadth and a need to minimize respondent burden, these scales contain few items per subscale—that is, they lack depth. Thus, they are best used to identify problems needing further evaluation with interviews, observations, or narrow-band scales.

The Child Behavior Checklist (CBCL; Achenbach and Rescorla 2000, 2001) is the most popular broad-band scale used in research and clinical work and has been the gold standard among behavior rating scales since its development in the 1960s. In addition to the parent report form, the CBCL scales include the Teacher Report Form (TRF), the Youth Self-Report (YSR), and the Child Behavior Checklist 1½–5 (CBCL 1½–5) and Caregiver–Teacher Report Form (C-TRF) for preschoolers. These scales have recently been updated with new normative data and several modifications to item content and subscale structure. The age ranges for the CBCL and TRF have shifted slightly, as

Table 13–1. Psychometric properties of broad-band rating scales

Scale (ages for use)	Type of scale, number of items and subscales	Availability of normative data and reliability data	Availability of validity data	Other
Child Behavior Checklist (CBCL) / Teacher Report Form (TRF) (6–18 years): copyright held by Achenbach System of Empirically Based Assessment (ASEBA) (Achenbach and Rescorla 2001)	Parent–teacher report: 120 items; 8 problem subscales, 6 DSM-IV-TR subscales, 3 composite scales	Normative data available IC: yes (parent and teacher) TR: yes (parent and teacher) IR: yes (parent–parent; teacher–teacher; parent–teacher)	CONV: yes (parent and teacher with nonclinical samples) DIVG: NR DISC: yes (parent and teacher for clinical vs. nonclinical samples)	Administration time: 15–20 minutes Computer scoring Extensive data available >60 translations
Child Behavior Checklist 1½–5 (CBCL 1½–5) / Caregiver–Teacher Report Form (C-TRF) (1½–5 years): copyright held by ASEBA (Achenbach and Rescorla 2000)	Parent, teacher, caregiver report: 102 problem items; 8 language items, 310 vocabulary words, 7 problem subscales, 5 DSM-IV-TR subscales, 2 language subscales, 3 composite scales	Normative data available IC: yes (parent and teacher) TR: yes (parent and teacher) IR: yes (parent–parent, teacher–teacher, parent–teacher)	CONV: yes (parent and teacher with various clinical and nonclinical samples) DIVG: NR DISC: yes (parent and teacher for clinical vs. nonclinical samples and for language—delayed vs. nondelayed samples)	Administration time: 15–20 minutes Computer scoring
Youth Self-Report (YSR) (11–18 years): copyright held by ASEBA (Achenbach and Rescorla 2000)	Self-report: 105 problem items; 8 problem subscales, 6 DSM-IV-TR subscales, 3 composite scales	Normative data available IC: yes TR: yes IR: yes (youth–parent and youth–teacher)	CONV: NR DIVG: NR DISC: yes (clinical vs. nonclinical)	Administration time: 15–20 minutes Computer scoring Multiple translations

Note. CONV = convergent validity; DISC = discriminant validity; DIVG = divergent validity; IC = internal consistency reliability; IR = interrater reliability; TR = test-retest reliability; NR = not reported.

has the age range for the downward extension for toddlers and preschoolers. A new innovation for the CBCL 1½–5 is a language scale, intended to provide brief screening of this dimension given the frequent overlap between language delays and behavior problems among young children. Additionally, all of the scales can now be scored in accordance with DSM-IV-TR (American Psychiatric Association 2000) diagnoses.

The CBCL, TRF, and YSR include subscales that measure a range of internalizing and externalizing behaviors, consistent with earlier versions of these scales. Subscale scores are derived for several specific problem areas. The revised versions also offer scores for selected DSM-IV-TR diagnoses. Composite scores for Internalizing, Externalizing, and Total Problems are also provided. As with earlier versions, a series of items assesses youths' adaptive functioning in home, community, and school settings.

Subscales for the CBCL 1½–5 and C-TRF cover internalizing and externalizing problems typical of this developmental stage. As with the scales for older youths, subscale scores are derived for a variety of specific behavior problems and selected DSM-IV-TR diagnoses. As noted above, there is also a language development scale. Composite scores for Internalizing, Externalizing, and Total Problems are also calculated.

A few issues with clinical interpretation of the CBCL scales warrant mention. Several problem-behavior items in the CBCL system include blanks for respondents to provide specific manifestations of a youth's problem. When interpreting children's scores, it is important to review these responses to ensure that the respondent has accurately understood the items. It should be noted that the labels for the CBCL subscales may be misleading. For example, the Aggressive Behavior subscale describes oppositional and defiant behaviors, with few items describing actual aggression. Scores on the Thought Problems subscale can be affected by a variety of cognitive problems, and this should not be considered equivalent to an index of thought disorder. These problems underscore the need to review a scale's items to ascertain what they really measure. Finally, the controversy regarding the use of DSM-IV-TR with young children suggests caution in using these subscales for the CBCL 1½–5 and C-TRF.

Overall, the CBCL has immense utility because of its rapid coverage of a wide range of problems in various settings, for youths of different ethnicities, along with an emphasis on youths' adaptive skills. Its computer scoring further increases its utility by integrating the various reporter forms and obviating cumbersome hand scoring.

Rating Scales Assessing Externalizing Behaviors

Externalizing behaviors are publicly observable, and youths displaying these behaviors are referred *because* of problems they pose to parents and teachers in multiple situations. Youths tend to underestimate their misbehaviors, so adults are considered the optimal informants on narrow-band scales that focus on one specific externalizing construct, or behavior (Table 13–2). Ratings are generally obtained from multiple adults to describe youths' behaviors across perspectives and settings and perhaps to understand the ecological aspects of youths' behaviors. These scales are more likely than scales that assess internalizing symptoms to demonstrate developmental relevance, or suitability, as they were developed for elementary-school children on the basis of their behaviors at home and school. Suitability of these scales for younger and older ages is less clear. Further, research in this area has focused almost exclusively on externalizing behavior in boys, and less is known about the suitability of current assessment and conceptualization approaches for girls.

■ Attention-Deficit/Hyperactivity Rating Scales

Ongoing interest in honing the measurement of attention-deficit/hyperactivity disorder (ADHD), particularly during interventions, has led to several scales being updated to DSM-IV-TR criteria (Collett et al., 2003). These scales are very similar to one another. Their basis in diagnostic criteria ensures construct validity. Furthermore, factor analyses showed subscales of inattention and hyperactivity/impulsivity consistent with the DSM construct of ADHD. They all have parent and teacher report forms. They vary in the number of items used to assess ADHD symptoms and as to whether the scale also measures comorbid disorders. Choosing among them then hinges on the intended application, other scales included in the assessment, the best reporter available, and the need for adolescent self-report. Beyond these factors, an application should be matched with a scale's characteristics, such

Table 13–2. Psychometric properties of scales assessing externalizing behaviors

Scale (ages for use)	Type of scale, number of items and factors	Availability of normative data and reliability data	Availability of validity data	Other
Conners' Rating Scales—Revised (CRS-R) (3–17 years): copyright held by Multi-Health Systems, Inc. (Conners 1997)	Parent, teacher, and adolescent reports: 80 items (parent), 59 items (teacher), 87 items (adolescent); 7 factors (parent), 6 factors (teacher), 6 factors (adolescent) Global index ADHD index DSM-IV-TR symptom subscales	Normative data available IC: yes (parent, teacher, and adolescent for clinical and nonclinical samples) TR: yes (parent, teacher, and adolescent for clinical and nonclinical samples) IR: yes (parent–teacher, parent–adolescent, teacher–adolescent, all for clinical and nonclinical samples)	CONV: NR DIVG: NR DISC: yes (ADHD vs. nonclinical samples) SENS and SPEC: yes (for parent, teacher, and adolescent versions)	Administration time: 20–30 minutes Quick-score forms; computer, fax, mail-in scoring French translation
Swanson, Nolan, and Pelham-IV questionnaire (SNAP-IV) (5–11 years): copyright held by KC Publishing; available online at http://www.adhd.net (Swanson 1992)	Parent–teacher report: 90 items, full version; 31 items, ADHD+ODD version; 2 factors	Limited normative data available IC: yes (teacher for clinical and nonclinical samples) TR: NR IR: yes (parent–teacher for clinical and nonclinical samples)	No validity data available	Administration time: 20–30 minutes, full version; 5–10 minutes, ADHD+ODD version No self-report
ADHD Rating Scale-IV (ADHD RS-IV) (5–18 years): copyright held by Guilford Press (DuPaul et al. 1998)	Home (parent) and school (teacher) report: 18 items; 2 factors	Normative data available IC: yes (home and school for nonclinical samples) TR: yes (home and school for nonclinical samples) IR: yes (parent–teacher for nonclinical samples)	CONV: yes (nonclinical sample) DIVG: NR DISC: yes (ADHD vs. nonclinical sample; ADHD vs. clinical control; ADHD-I vs. ADHD-C) SENS and SPEC: yes (home and school versions)	Administration time: 5–10 minutes Spanish translation
Home Situations Questionnaires (HSQ) (4–11 years): copyright held by Guilford Press (Barkley 1997)	Parent report: 16 items; 2 factors	Normative data available IC: yes (parent for nonclinical samples) TR: yes (parent for nonclinical sample) IR: yes (mother–father for nonclinical sample)	CONV: yes (nonclinical samples) DIVG: NR DISC: yes (ADHD vs. nonclinical samples)	Administration time: 5–10 minutes Adolescent version available Rates for problems and their severity

Table 13–2. Psychometric properties of scales assessing externalizing behaviors *(continued)*

Scale (ages for use)	Type of scale, number of items and factors	Availability of normative data and reliability data	Availability of validity data	Other
School Situations Questionnaires (SSQ) (4–11 years): copyright held by Guilford Press (Barkley 1997)	Teacher report scale: 12 items; 2 factors	Normative data available IC: yes (teacher for nonclinical samples) TR: yes (teacher for clinical and nonclinical samples) IR: NR	CONV: yes (clinical and nonclinical samples) DIVG: NR DISC: yes (ADHD vs. nonclinical samples)	Administration time: 5–10 minutes Adolescent and other modified versions available Rates for problems and their severity

Note. ADHD = attention-deficit/hyperactivity disorder; ADHD-I=ADHD, inattentive type; ADHD-C=ADHD, combined type; CONV=convergent validity; DISC=discriminant validity; DIVG=divergent validity; HSQ=Home Situations Questionnaire; IC=internal consistency reliability; IR=interrater reliability; ODD=oppositional defiant disorder; SENS=sensitivity; SPEC=specificity; TR=test-retest reliability; NR=not reported.

as adequacy of the normative data and psychometric strengths and weaknesses.

The Conners' Rating Scale—Revised (CRS-R; Conners 1997) is an updated version of the popular Conners' Rating Scale (CRS). It addresses prior deficits in the factor structure, normative base, and empirical support of the CRS. Consistent with past versions, the CRS-R covers core ADHD subscales as well as a variety of comorbid problems, such as oppositional defiant disorder (ODD) and conduct disorder (CD). The multiple indices assessing these constructs, along with the normative base, strong psychometrics, and multiple uses, make the CRS-R excellent for comprehensive assessment. Its discriminant validity (Conners et al. 1998a, 1998b) and good sensitivity also make it effective in group assignment and screening, although the lower sensitivity for the teacher version may produce false negatives in school screening. Stability and availability of the abbreviated version facilitate efficient treatment monitoring (Rugino and Copley 2001). Disadvantages relate to poorer functioning for the comorbidity indices relative to the ADHD indices. Overall, the CRS-R is the standard measure of ADHD.

The Swanson, Nolan, and Pelham-IV Questionnaire (SNAP-IV; Swanson 1992) was among the first DSM-based rating scales and has been updated with each DSM revision. The short version includes core ADHD subscales along with summary questions in each domain. An extended version adds symptom criteria for common comorbid DSM-IV-TR disorders. Rather than using the full SNAP-IV, clinicians often extract selected indices or subscales for specific applications. The SNAP-IV and scoring information are posted on a Web site (http://www.adhd.net), making this scale a popular and cost-efficient option for clinical work. This is reinforced by the SNAP-IV's sensitivity to treatment effects (MTA Cooperative Group 1999). A disadvantage relates to the limited normative and psychometric data. However, because the SNAP-IV's ADHD and ODD subscales resemble other ADHD scales that are based on DSM-IV-TR, their psychometric support may also support the SNAP-IV (Swanson et al. 2001; J.M. Swanson, personal communication, November 2002).

The ADHD Rating Scale-IV (ADHD RS-IV; DuPaul et al. 1998) is an updated version of the ADHD Rating Scale (ADHD RS). It impressively differentiates children with ADHD from clinical controls and also differentiates the hyperactive/impulsive and the inattentive subtypes. Thus, the ADHD RS-IV is a good choice for establishing severity and designating group membership, especially in evaluating the subtypes. Additionally, its brevity and sensitivity to treatment make it an excellent choice for repeated administrations during treatment (Michelson et al. 2002). This scale is particularly useful for research applications.

■ General Disruptive Behavior Scales

In contrast to the plethora of ADHD scales based on DSM-IV-TR, there are few diagnosis-based scales assessing other disruptive disorders, such as ODD and CD. However, several scales assess general externalizing behaviors without direct connection to DSM-IV-TR (Collett et al., in press). Some of these scales, such as the Eyberg Child Behavior Inventory and the Sutter-Eyberg Student Behavior Inventory—Revised (Eyberg and Pincus 1999) have a long history of research and clinical use, particularly in evaluation of youths' behaviors across home and school settings. Others, such as the New York Teacher Rating Scale (Miller et al. 1995) and Antisocial Process Screening Device (Frick and Hare 2001) are newer scales with great potential for clinical practice, as they assess specific aspects of behaviors. New scales measuring aggression, such as the Children's Aggression Scale—Parent and Teacher Versions (Halperin et al. 2002), should also soon be integrated into clinical practice. However, because these scales are not yet routinely used in practice, they are not fully reviewed here.

The Home Situations Questionnaire (HSQ) and School Situations Questionnaire (SSQ) (Barkley 1997) are unique observer-rated scales for younger children that do have established applicability for clinical practice. They focus on the environmental context in which deviant behaviors occur, rather than emphasizing the frequency of behavior problems. The scales include common household or classroom situations and ask respondents to indicate whether the behavior is problematic in that setting. For situations rated as problematic, respondents then rate their severity. These scales' utility lies in assessing effects of youths' behaviors on daily life, not in assessing any disorder. Thus, they are best used as adjuncts to diagnosis-based or construct-driven scales. The data they yield are used to prioritize targets for intervention, evaluate situational precipitants, and assess times of the day that may relate to interventions. These scales are sensitive to treatment gains achieved through medication and behavioral interventions (Barkley et al. 1988). However, caution is warranted when interpreting an individual's scores with respect to the normative data that are outmoded. Modifications of the HSQ and SSQ specific to ADHD-related symptoms (DuPaul and Barkley 1992) and relevant to adolescents (Adams et al. 1995) have been made.

Rating Scales Assessing Internalizing Symptoms

Internalizing symptoms are not readily observable by others. They represent youths' subjective distress and are best assessed by youths' self-report. Most of the narrow-band scales for rating internalizing symptoms now have parallel parent report and/or teacher report forms that broaden the perspective of youths' difficulties, including revealing adults' failure to appreciate youths' distress (Table 13–3). A few scales are clinician rated and integrate youths' and adults' responses. They are increasingly used in treatment studies because of their greater accuracy and the inadequate sensitivity of self-report scales to treatment (Emslie et al. 1997; Keller et al. 2001).

Several aspects intrinsic to internalizing symptoms affect the functioning of these scales. Youths' feelings of depression, anxiety, or suicidality wax and wane. Thus, to accurately detect these changes during treatment, a scale with good stability is needed. Another difficulty relates to the overlap of internalizing symptomatology. Most depression rating scales detect anxiety and suicidality, and vice versa. Therefore, a scale with good discriminative and divergent validity is especially valuable in measuring internalizing symptoms.

■ Rating Scales Assessing Mood and Related Symptoms

Most depression rating scales were developed in the 1980s when depressive disorders in youth were elucidated (Myers and Winters 2002b). Few of these scales continue to be widely used. Their shortcomings relate to laxity in the construct they tap, so that these scales may better measure distress than depression. Also, diagnosing depression in youths can be difficult, as depressive symptoms are common in both clinical and community samples, and these scales detect other internalizing constructs. Sorting out the interaction of internalizing symptoms can be difficult because there

is a dearth of scales measuring suicidality for youth (Winters et al. 2002). Many juvenile studies have used suicide scales developed with adults, but they do not function well with youths (Spirito et al. 1996). Recently developed scales for youth, such as the Child-Adolescent Suicidal Potential Scale (Pfeffer et al. 2000) and the Reasons for Living Inventory for Adolescents (Osman et al. 1998), have not yet amassed a critical literature elucidating their utility. By contrast, a large literature is devoted to scales assessing hopelessness. Hopelessness is correlated with depression and powerfully predicts suicidality. Thus, hopelessness scales may help to tease out the relationships among depression-related constructs.

The Beck Depression Inventory (BDI; Beck 1993) is the most popular depression rating scale for adolescents, with high utility in multiple diverse applications across ethnicity. It assesses the same aspects of depression with adolescents that it assesses with adults: cognitive, behavioral, affective, and somatic. The BDI functions well, although less predictably, with clinical than with community samples. Most impressively, the BDI may discriminate outpatient depressed teens from those with anxiety and conduct disorders, making it a preferred scale for complementing diagnostic assessment (Bennett et al. 1997). Decreasing scores as youths recover from depression also make the BDI useful for monitoring treatment. However, cutoff scores vary with gender, clinical status, and ethnicity. Disadvantages relate to the lack of adult report forms to provide broader contextual perspectives of youths' behavior.

The Children's Depression Inventory (CDI; Kovacs 1992) is a downward extension of the BDI to preadolescents, although it is often used with teens. It is the most studied and popular scale of juvenile depression and has great utility. Five subscales are most often found: Dysphoric Mood, Acting Out, Loss of Personal and Social Interest, Self-Deprecation, Vegetative Symptoms (Craighead et al. 1998). The Acting Out subscale demonstrates how children's misbehaviors are related to their depressive cognitions. For adolescents these two issues appear independent. The role of the factors is unclear, and total scores are usually used. The CDI functions well, has predictive validity, and detects treatment effects (Emslie et al. 1997). However, sensitivity, specificity, and discriminant validity are poor, and the CDI may really measure distress. Nevertheless, its ongoing diverse applications and use in exploring the conceptual and cultural aspects of depres-

Table 13–3. Psychometric properties of scales assessing internalizing symptoms

Scale (ages for use)	Type of scale, number of items and factors	Availability of normative data and reliability data	Availability of validity data	Other
Beck Depression Inventory (BDI) (adolescents): copyright held by Psychological Corporation (Beck 1993)	Self-report scale: 21 items; 1 factor	No normative data IC: yes (clinical and nonclinical samples) TR: yes (various clinical and nonclinical samples) IR: NR	CONV: yes (clinical and nonclinical) DIVG: NR DISC: yes (clinical and nonclinical) SENS and SPEC: yes (clinical sample)	Administration time: <10 minutes to complete and score Brief version available No parent report form
Children's Depression Inventory (CDI) (7–18 years): copyright held by Multi-Health Systems, Inc. (Kovacs 1992)	Self-report scale: 27 items; 5 factors	Normative data available IC: yes (multiple samples) TR: yes (clinical and nonclinical samples) IR: yes (clinical samples)	CONV: yes (multiple samples) DIVG: NR DISC: yes (multiple samples) SENS and SPEC: yes (multiple samples)	Administration time: <20 minutes to complete and score Parent, teacher, and brief versions available
Children's Depression Rating Scale (CDRS) (6–12 years): copyright held by Western Psychological Services (Poznanski and Mokros 1999)	Clinician-administered scale: 17 items; 1 factor	No normative data IC: yes (clinical samples) TR: yes (various clinical samples) IR: yes (various clinical samples)	CONV: yes (various clinical samples) DIVG: NR DISC: NR	Administration time: 45–70 minutes to complete and score Integrates youth and parent scores Brief version available
Beck Hopelessness Scale (BHS) (adults and adolescents): copyright held by Psychological Corporation (Beck 2003)	Self-report scale: 20 items; 3 factors	No normative data IC: yes (clinical samples) TR: NR IR: NR	CONV: yes (clinical samples) DIVG: NR DISC: yes (clinical samples)	Administration time: <15 minutes to complete and score No parent report
Hopelessness Scale for Children (HSC) (children and adolescents): available from Alan Kazdin, Ph.D., at alan.kazdin@yale.edu (Kazdin 2003)	Self-report scale: 17 items; 1 factor	No normative data IC: yes (clinical samples) TR: yes (clinical samples) IR: NR	CONV: yes (clinical samples) DIVG: NR DISC: yes (clinical samples)	Administration time: <15 minutes to complete and score
Mania Rating Scale (MRS) (adults, but now being used with children and adolescents): available from Young et al. (1978)	Clinician-administered scale: 11 items; 1 factor	No normative data IC: yes (clinical samples) TR: NR IR: NR	CONV: yes (various clinical samples) DIVG: yes (various clinical samples) DISC: yes (various clinical samples)	Administration time: 15 minutes to complete and score, but considerable time to gather data

Table 13–3. Psychometric properties of scales assessing internalizing symptoms (continued)

Scale (ages for use)	Type of scale, number of items and factors	Availability of normative data and reliability data	Availability of validity data	Other
Multidimensional Anxiety Scale for Children (MASC) (children and adolescents): copyright held by Multi-Health Systems, Inc. (March 1997)	Self-report scale: 39 items; 4 factors	No normative data IC: yes (clinical samples) TR: yes (clinical samples) IR: yes (clinical samples)	CONV: yes (clinical and nonclinical samples) DIVG: yes (clinical and nonclinical samples) DISC: yes (clinical samples)	Administration time: <25 minutes to complete and score Parent and brief versions available
Screen for Child Anxiety Related Emotional Disorders (SCARED) (9–19 years): available from Boris Birmaher, M.D. (Birmaher 2003)	Self-report scale: 41 items; 5 factors	No normative data IC: yes (clinical samples) TR: yes (clinical samples) IR: yes (clinical samples)	CONV: yes (clinical samples) DIVG: NR DISC: yes (clinical samples) SENS and SPEC: yes (clinical samples)	Administration time: <15 minutes to complete and score Parent and brief versions available
Pediatric Anxiety Rating Scale (PARS) (5–15 years): available from Mark Riddle, M.D. (Riddle 2003)	Clinician-administered scale: 50 checklist items, 7 severity items	No normative data IC: yes (clinical samples) TR: yes (clinical samples) IR: yes (clinical samples)	CONV: yes (clinical samples for clinician, parent, and child ratings) DIVG: yes (clinical samples for clinician and parent ratings) DISC: NR	Administration time: 30 minutes for first administration, then 15 minutes for subsequent administrations Integrates youth and parent scores
Social Phobia Anxiety Inventory for Children (SPAI-C) (9–14 years): copyright held by Multi-Health Systems, Inc. (Beidel et al. 1988)	Self-report scale: 26 items; 3 factors	Normative data available IC: yes (clinical and nonclinical samples) TR: yes (clinical and nonclinical samples) IR: NR	CONV: yes (clinical and nonclinical samples) DIVG: yes (clinical and nonclinical samples) DISC: NR SENS and SPEC: yes (clinical and nonclinical samples)	Administration time: 30 minutes to complete and score
Fear Survey Schedule for Children—Revised (FSSC-R) (children and adolescents): copyright held by Thomas Ollendick, Ph.D. (Ollendick 2003)	Self-report scale: 80 items; 5 factors	Normative data available IC: yes (nonclinical samples) TR: yes (nonclinical samples) IR: NR	CONV: yes (nonclinical samples) DIVG: yes (nonclinical samples, girls) DISC: yes (nonclinical samples)	Administration time: 30 minutes to complete and score Parent and brief versions available Use total score or subscale scores
Child Posttraumatic Stress Disorder—Reaction Index (CPTS-RI) (8–18 years): available from Robert Pynoos, M.D. (Pynoos 2003)	Clinician-administered scale or self-report scale: 20 items; 3 factors	No normative data IC: yes (clinical sample of traumatized children) TR: yes (clinical sample of traumatized teens) IR: yes (clinical sample of traumatized teens)	CONV: yes (clinical samples of traumatized children) DIVG: NR DISC: NR SENS: yes (clinical sample of traumatized children)	Administration time: 20–45 minutes to complete and score Training required

Note. CONV = convergent validity; DISC = discriminant validity; DIVG = divergent validity; IC=internal consistency; IR = interrater reliability; SENS = sensitivity; SPEC = specificity; TR=test-retest reliability; NR = not reported.

sion attest to the CDI's ability to keep "reinventing itself" (Barreto and McManus 1997).

The Children's Depression Rating Scale—Revised (CDRS-R; Poznanski and Mokros 1999) is a clinician-rated scale patterned on the Hamilton Depression Rating Scale but developed specifically for children and widely used with teens. It has three unique features: It integrates information from both the child and parent to produce three scores, includes behaviors observed during the interview, and contains several items that are not specific to depression. Thus, the CDRS-R's construct differs somewhat from depression as defined by DSM-IV-TR. There is some evidence that the CDRS-R discriminates depressed from other youths, a distinct advantage. Its impressive interrater reliability supports the alleged superiority of clinician-rated scales over lay scales. The short form facilitates screening and longitudinal assessments (Overholser et al. 1995). Use of the CDRS-R in combination with self-reports and global ratings offers comprehensive yet efficient assessment that is sensitive to treatment (Emslie et al. 1997; Weisz et al. 1987).

The Beck Hopelessness Scale (BHS; Beck 2003; Beck and Steer 1989) was developed for adults but has been widely used with teens. The three subscales identified with adults are inconsistently noted with adolescents: Feelings about the Future, Loss of Motivation, and Future Expectations (Aish and Wasserman 2001). The BHS strongly discriminates suicidal from nonsuicidal adolescents and predicts suicide attempts independent of depression, a major strength (Morano et al. 1993). It has good utility for group assignment, longitudinal assessment, and screening. However, its utility for monitoring treatment is unclear because of the lack of stability data and its 2-point scoring format.

The Hopelessness Scale for Children (HSC; Kazdin 2003; Kazdin et al. 1986) is a downward modification of the BHS. Although widely used with adolescents, the HSC functions better with children than teens (Thurber et al. 1996). The HSC has discriminated suicidal from nonsuicidal children, but such discrimination may be confounded by depression in children. Nevertheless, it should function well in screening and phenomenological applications. The HSC has demonstrated some sensitivity to interventions despite a 2-point response format (Grizenko 1997). Overall, the HSC enjoys an extensive literature supporting its use with suicidal as well as nonsuicidal youths.

The Mania Rating Scale (MRS; Young et al. 1978) is a clinician-administered scale with minimal evidence of its functioning with youths found to have bipolar disorder (Fristad et al. 1995; Youngstrom et al. 2002). The MRS is completed by the clinician after interviewing youths, their parents, and possibly staff. Thus, considerable time is expended gathering information needed to create a rating with this brief scale. It has shown some ability to discriminate bipolar disorder from ADHD, and some divergent validity in relation to ADHD and depression (Gracious et al. 2002). The MRS has also shown some sensitivity to treatment with mood stabilizers (Soutullo et al. 1998). However, the MRS has not yet been adequately examined to establish its suitability with children or adolescents or its utility for clinical applications. Nonetheless, it is increasingly used with youths found to have bipolar disorder. Caveat emptor.

■ Rating Scales Assessing Anxiety Symptoms

Anxiety was among the first juvenile symptoms evaluated with rating scales (Myers and Winters 2002b). Older scales had questionable suitability and focused on trait versus state anxiety, a construct with questionable clinical relevance. Several newer scales have overcome these difficulties. In particular, they have good stability, as well as discriminant and divergent validity to help in differentiating anxiety from other internalizing symptoms.

The Multidimensional Anxiety Scale for Children (MASC; March 1997; March et al. 1997) was developed with heterogeneous clinical and community samples. It assesses a spectrum of anxiety symptoms with four major subscales, three of which can be subdivided: Physical Symptoms (Tense/Restless and Somatic/Autonomic), Social Anxiety (Humiliation/Rejection and Public Performance Fears), Harm Avoidance (Perfectionism and Anxious Coping), and Separation Anxiety. Two factors match the DSM-IV-TR diagnoses of social phobia (SocPh) and separation anxiety disorder (SAD), whereas the total score matches generalized anxiety disorder (GAD). This is the first scale to validate the hypothesized division of anxiety into physical symptoms and approach/avoidance behaviors. Its strengths include an Inconsistency Index that identifies invalid profiles, an Anxiety Disorders Index that discriminates anxious youths with 88% accuracy (March et al. 1999), and evidence that the MASC's construct diverges from depression and from other anxiety disorders. Its 4-point scoring is sensitive to treatment. Overall, the MASC has become the preferred child anxiety rating scale.

The Screen for Child Anxiety Related Emotional Disorders (SCARED; Birmaher 2003; Birmaher et al. 1997, 1999) was developed with youths presenting to a mood and anxiety disorders clinic. Its five factors conform to DSM-IV-TR disorders: GAD, SAD, SocPh, somatic/panic, and school phobia. This scale shows some divergence from both disruptive behaviors and depression, as well as sensitivity to treatment (Research Unit on Pediatric Psychopharmacology Anxiety Study Group 2002). It has functioned well with community and clinical samples. The SCARED could challenge the MASC because of its broader diagnostic coverage, but further work is needed to establish its niche, particularly with nonclinical samples.

The Pediatric Anxiety Rating Scale (PARS; Research Unit on Pediatric Psychopharmacology Anxiety Study Group 2002; Riddle 2003) is a new scale that already has a niche because of its clinician-administered format. Most of its items were derived from DSM-IV-TR to measure GAD, SAD, and SocPh. The PARS rates frequency, severity, and impairment with a complicated scoring system, reducing overall utility, although the valuable data it yields would be difficult to otherwise ascertain. Scores on the PARS do not vary with age or gender, unusual for a scale measuring internalizing symptoms. Although developed for pharmacological trials, it is not yet clear whether the PARS detects generic treatment response or specific anxiolytic effects. Despite these uncertainties, combination of the PARS with youth self-report scales should provide comprehensive but efficient assessment of anxiety in many venues.

The Social Phobia and Anxiety Inventory for Children (SPAI-C; Beidel et al. 1988, 2000) differs from the aforementioned scales in that it measures a specific anxiety construct: social anxiety. It has three subscales: Assertiveness, Traditional Social Encounters, and Public Performance. Its moderate validities support the assertion that the SPAI-C measures a construct that differs from other anxiety disorders. This is one of few scales to discriminate among anxiety disorders. The SPAI-C correctly classifies 67% of youths with SocPh and 74% with other anxiety disorders. However, its sensitivity to treatment needs clarification, as it has detected benefits of medication (Compton et al. 2001) but not psychotherapy (Masia et al. 2001). The special focus of this rigorously examined scale has found many uses with school and clinical samples.

The Fear Survey Schedule for Children—Revised (FSSC-R; Ollendick 2003; Ollendick et al. 1989) represents an update of the well-established and popular Fear Survey Schedule for Children (FSSC). It assesses both the number and intensity of fears in five subscales: Fear of Failure and Criticism, Fear of the Unknown, Fear of Injury and Small Animals, Fear of Danger and Death, Medical Fears. The FSSC-R—especially the Fear of Failure and Criticism subscale—appears able to discriminate phobic from nonphobic children, as well as to discriminate among phobias. Generally, the FSSC-R performs similarly across ethnicity, nationality, culture, and religion. Its youth and parent report forms have many diverse applications, and the scale has little competition.

The Child Posttraumatic Stress Disorder—Reaction Index (CPTSD-RI; Pynoos 2003) is the most widely used measure of posttraumatic stress disorder (PTSD) symptoms in youth. It is a clinician-administered scale that can also be used as a self-report. Its three subscales are based on the DSM-III-R definition of PTSD: reexperiencing/numbing, fear/anxiety, and concentration/sleep. The scale functions well across culture in relation to various types of trauma, from abuse to medical procedures to war. Higher scores correlate with greater traumatization, and the CPTSD-RI has shown sensitivity to psychotherapy (Salloum et al. 2001). This flexible scale offers considerable utility in clinical and large-scale applications, although other scales are providing some competition (Ohan et al. 2002).

Conclusion

The scales presented here do not substitute for diagnostic assessment and good clinical judgment. They augment diagnostic assessment and individualize assessment for specific applications. They offer the clinician a better understanding of youths' difficulties, quantify those difficulties in a manner that can be readily understood, and follow the response of those difficulties to treatment. Rating scales help to establish evidenced-based treatments that better ensure accountability in clinical practice and appropriate treatments for our young patients.

References

Achenbach TM, Rescorla LA: Manual for the ASEBA school-age forms & profiles. Burlington, VT, University of Vermont, Research Center for Children, Youth, and Families, 2000. Available from the Achenbach System of Empirically Based Assessment (ASEBA), 1 South Prospect Street, room 6436, Burlington, VT 05401-3456; phone: (802) 656-8313 or (802) 656-2608; http://www.aseba.org. Accessed May 1, 2003.

Achenbach TM, Rescorla LA: Manual for the ASEBA preschool forms & profiles. Burlington, VT, University of Vermont, Research Center for Children, Youth, and Families, 2001. Available from the Achenbach System of Empirically Based Assessment (ASEBA), 1 South Prospect Street, room 6436, Burlington, VT 05401-3456; phone: (802) 656-8313 or (802) 656-2608; http://www.aseba.org. Accessed May 1, 2003.

Adams CD, McCarthy M, Kelly ML: Adolescent versions of the Home and School Situations Questionnaires: initial psychometric properties. J Clin Child Psychol 24:377–385, 1995

Aish AM, Wasserman D: Does Beck's Hopelessness Scale really measure several components? Psychol Med 31:367–372, 2001

American Psychiatric Association: Diagnostic and Statistical Manual of Mental Disorders, 4th Edition, Text Revision. Washington, DC, American Psychiatric Association, 2000

Barkley RA: Defiant Children: A Clinician's Manual for Assessment and Parent Training, 2nd Edition. New York, Guilford, 1997

Barkley RA, Fischer M, Newby RF, et al: Development of a multimethod clinical protocol for assessing stimulant drug response in children with attention deficit disorder. J Clin Child Psychol 17:14–24, 1988

Barreto S, McManus M: Casting the net for "depression" among ethnic minority children from the high-risk urban communities. Clin Psychol Rev 17:823–845, 1997

Beck AT: Beck Depression Inventory (BDI) Manual, 2nd Edition. San Antonio, TX, Psychological Corporation, 1993. Available from Psychological Corporation, 19500 Bulverde Road, San Antonio, Texas 78259; phone: (800) 872-1726; http://www.psychcorp.com. Accessed May 1, 2003.

Beck AT: The Beck Hopelessness Scale (BHS), 2003. Available from the Beck Institute at beckinst@gim.net

Beck AT, Steer RA: Clinical predictors of eventual suicide: a 5- to 10-year prospective study of suicide attempters. J Affect Disord 17:203–209, 1989

Beidel DC, Turner SM, Morris TL: Social Phobia and Anxiety Inventory for Children (SPAI-C). North Tonawanda, NY, Multi-Health Systems, 1988. Available from Multi-Health Systems, Inc., 908 Niagara Falls Boulevard, North Tonawanda, NY 14120-2060; phone: (800) 456-3003; http://www.mhs.com. Accessed April 30, 2003

Beidel DC, Turner SM, Hamlin K, et al: The Social Phobia and Anxiety Inventory for Children (SPAI-C): external and discriminative validity. Behav Ther 31:75–87, 2000

Bennett DS, Ambrosini PJ, Bianchi M, et al: Relationship of Beck Depression Inventory factors to depression among adolescents. J Affect Disord 45:127–134, 1997

Birmaher B: Screen for Child Anxiety Related Emotional Disorders (SCARED), 2003. Available from the Division of Child Psychiatry, Western Psychiatric Institute and Clinic, 3811 O'Hara Street, Pittsburgh, PA 15213; e-mail: birmaherb@msx.upmc.edu.

Birmaher B, Khetarpal S, Brent D, et al.: The Screen for Child Anxiety Related Emotional Disorders (SCARED): scale construction and psychometric characteristics. J Am Acad Child Adolesc Psychiatry 36:545–553, 1997

Birmaher B, Brent DA, Chiappetta L, et al: Psychometric properties of the Screen for Child Anxiety Related Emotional Disorders (SCARED): a replication study. J Am Acad Child Adolesc Psychiatry 38:1230–1236, 1999

Collett BR, Ohan JL, Myers KM: Ten-year review of rating scales, V: scales assessing attention-deficit/hyperactivity disorder. J Am Acad Child Adolesc Psychiatry 42:1015–1037, 2003

Collett BR, Ohan JL, Myers KM: Ten-year review of rating scales, VI: scales assessing disruptive behavior disorders and externalizing behaviors. J Am Acad Child Adolesc Psychiatry (in press)

Compton SN, Grant PJ, Chrisman AK, et al: Sertraline in children and adolescents with social anxiety disorder: an open trial. J Am Acad Child Adolesc Psychiatry 40:564–571, 2001

Conners CK: Conners' Rating Scales—Revised, Technical Manual. North Tonawanda, NY, Multi-Health Systems, 1997. Available from Multi-Health Systems, Inc., 908 Niagara Falls Boulevard, North Tonawanda, NY 14120-2060; (800) 456-3003; http://www.mhs.com. Accessed April 30, 2003

Conners C, Sitarenios G, Parker JD, et al: The revised Conners' Parent Rating Scale (CPRS-R): factor structure, reliability, and criterion validity. J Abnorm Child Psychol 26:257–268, 1998a

Conners C, Sitarenios G, Parker JD, et al: Revision and restandardization of the Conners' Teacher Rating Scale (CTRS-R): factor structure, reliability, and criterion validity. J Abnorm Child Psychol 26:279–291, 1998b

Craighead W, Smucker MR, Craighead LW, et al: Factor analysis of the Children's Depression Inventory in a community sample. Psychol Assess 10:156–165, 1998

DuPaul GJ, Barkley RA: Situational variability of attention problems: psychometric properties of the Revised Home and School Situations Questionnaires. J Clin Child Psychol 21:178–188, 1992

DuPaul GJ, Power TJ, Anastopoulos AD, et al: ADHD Rating Scale-IV: Checklist, Norms, and Clinical Interpretation. New York, Guilford, 1998

Emslie GJ, Rush J, Weinberg WA, et al: A double-blind, randomized, placebo-controlled trial of fluoxetine in children and adolescents with depression. Arch Gen Psychiatry 54:1031–1037, 1997

Eyberg SM, Pincus D: Eyberg Child Behavior Inventory and Sutter-Eyberg Student Behavior Inventory—Revised, Professional Manual. Odessa, FL, Psychological Assessment Resources, Inc., 1999. Available from Psychological Assessment Resources, Inc., 16204 N. Florida Avenue, Lutz, FL 33549; phone: (813) 968-3003; http://www.parinc.com. Accessed May 1, 2003.

Frick PJ, Hare RD: Antisocial Process Screening Device (APSD), north Tonawanda, NY, Multi-Health Systems, Inc., 2001. Available from Multi-Health Systems, Inc., 908 Niagara Falls Boulevard, North Tonawanda, NY 14120-2060; phone: (800) 456-3003; http://www.mhs.com. Accessed April 30, 2003.

Fristad MA, Weller RA, Weller EB: The Mania Rating Scale (MRS): further reliability and validity studies with children. Ann Clin Psychiatry 7:127–132, 1995

Gracious BL, Youngstrom EA, Findling RL, et al: Discriminative validity of a parent version of the Young Mania Rating Scale. J Am Acad Child Adolesc Psychiatry 41:1350–1359, 2002

Grizenko N: Outcome of multimodal day treatment for children with severe behavior problems: a five-year follow-up. J Am Acad Child Adolesc Psychiatry 36:989–997, 1997

Halperin JM, McKay KE, Newcorn JH: Development, reliability, and validity of the children's aggression scale—parent version. J Am Acad Child Adolesc Psychiatry 41: 245–252, 2002

Kazdin AE: The Hopelessness Scale for Children (HSC), 2003. Available from Alan E. Kazdin, Ph.D., Yale University; phone: (203) 432-9993; alan.kazdin@yale.edu.

Kazdin AE, Rodgers A, Colbus D: The Hopelessness Scale for Children: psychometric characteristics and concurrent validity. J Consult Clin Psychol 54:241–245, 1986

Keller MB, Ryan ND, Strober M, et al: Efficacy of paroxetine in the treatment of adolescent major depression: a randomized, controlled trial. J Am Acad Child Adolesc Psychiatry 40:762–772, 2001

Kovacs M: Children's Depression Inventory Manual. North Tonawanda, NY, Multi-Health Systems, 1992. Available from Multi-Health Systems, Inc., 908 Niagara Falls Boulevard, North Tonawanda, NY 14120-2060; phone: (800) 456-3003; http://www.mhs.com. Accessed April 30, 2003

March JS: Manual for the Multidimensional Anxiety Scale for Children (MASC). North Tonawanda, NY, Multi-Health Systems, 1997. Available from Multi-Health Systems, Inc., 908 Niagara Falls Boulevard, North Tonawanda, NY 14120-2060; phone: (800) 456-3003; http://www.mhs.com. Accessed April 30, 2003

March JS, Parker JD, Sullivan K, et al: The Multidimensional Anxiety Scale for Children (MASC): factor structure, reliability, and validity. J Am Acad Child Adolesc Psychiatry 36:554–565, 1997

March JS, Sullivan K, Parker J: Test-retest reliability of the Multidimensional Anxiety Scale for Children. J Anxiety Disord 13:349–358, 1999

Masia CL, Klein RG, Storch EA, et al: School-based behavioral treatment for social anxiety disorder in adolescents: results of a pilot study. J Am Acad Child Adolesc Psychiatry 40:780–786, 2001

Michelson D, Albert AJ, Busner J, et al: Once-daily atomoxetine treatment for children and adolescents with attention deficit hyperactivity disorder: a randomized, placebo-controlled study. Am J Psychiatry 159:1896–1901, 2002

Miller LS, Klein RG, Piacentini J, et al: The New York Teacher Rating Scale for disruptive and antisocial behavior. J Am Acad Child Adolesc Psychiatry 34:359–370, 1995

Morano CD, Cisler RA, Lemerond J: Risk factors for adolescent suicidal behavior: loss, insufficient familial support, and hopelessness. Adolescence 28:851–865, 1993

MTA Cooperative Group: A 14-month randomized clinical trial of treatment strategies for attention-deficit/hyperactivity disorder: the MTA Cooperative Group. Multimodal Treatment Study of Children with ADHD. Arch Gen Psychiatry 56:1073–1086, 1999

Myers K, Winters NC: Ten-year review of rating scales, I: overview of scale functioning, psychometric properties, and selection. J Am Acad Child Adolesc Psychiatry 41:114–122, 2002a

Myers K, Winters NC: Ten-year review of rating scales, II: scales for internalizing disorders. J Am Acad Child Adolesc Psychiatry 41:634–659, 2002b

Ohan JL, Myers K, Collett BR: Ten-year review of rating scales, IV: scales assessing trauma and its effects. J Am Acad Child Adolesc Psychiatry 41:1401–1422, 2002

Ollendick TH: The Fear Survey Schedule for Children—Revised, 2003. Available from Thomas H Ollendick, Ph.D., Department of Psychology, Child Study Center, 460 Turner Street, Suite 207, Virginia Polytechnic Institute and State University, Blacksburg, VA 24061-0355; fax: (540) 231-4250; phone: (540) 231-6451; tho@vt.edu

Ollendick TH, King NJ, Frary RB: Fears in children and adolescents: reliability and generalizability across gender, age and nationality. Behav Res Ther 27:19–26, 1989

Osman A, Downs WR, Kopper BA, et al: The Reasons for Living Inventory for Adolescents (RFL-A): development and psychometric properties. J Clin Psychol 54:1063–1078, 1998

Overholser JC, Brinkman DC, Lehnert KL, et al: Children's Depression Rating Scale—Revised: development of a short form. J Clin Child Psychol 24:443–452, 1995

Piacentini J: Checklists and ratings scales, in Handbook of Child and Adolescent Assessment, Vol 167. Edited by Ollendick TH. Boston, MA, Allyn & Bacon, 1993, pp 82–97

Pfeffer CR, Jiang H, Kakuma T: Child-Adolescent Suicidal Potential Index (CASPI): a screen for risk for early onset suicidal behavior. Psychol Assess 12:304–318, 2000

Poznanski EO, Mokros HB: Children's Depression Rating Scale—Revised (CDRS-R). Los Angeles, CA, Western Psychological Services, 1999. Available from Western Psychological Services, 12031 Wilshire Boulevard 90025-1251; phone: (800) 648-8857; http://www.wpspublish.com. Accessed May 2, 2003

Pynoos RS: The Child Posttraumatic Stress Disorder—Reaction Index (CPTSD-RI), 2003. Available from Robert Pynoos, M.D., Trauma Psychiatry Service, University of California, Los Angeles, 300 UCLA Medical Plaza, Los Angeles, CA 90024-6968; rpynoos@npih.medsch.ucla.edu

Research Unit on Pediatric Psychopharmacology Anxiety Study Group: The Pediatric Anxiety Scale (PARS): development and psychometric properties. J Am Acad Child Adolesc Psychiatry 41:1061–1069, 2002

Riddle M: The Pediatric Anxiety Rating Scale (PARS), 2003. Available from Mark A. Riddle, M.D., Division of Child and Adolescent Psychiatry, Johns Hopkins Medical Institutions, Children's Center, Suite 346, 600 North Wolfe Street, Baltimore, MD 21287-3325; mriddle@jhmi.edu

Rugino TA, Copley TC: Effects of modafinil in children with attention-deficit/hyperactivity disorder: an open-label study. J Am Acad Child Adolesc Psychiatry 40:230–235, 2001

Salloum A, Avery L, McClain RP: Group psychotherapy for adolescent survivors of homicide victims: a pilot study. J Am Acad Child Adolesc Psychiatry 40:1261–1267, 2001

Soutullo CA, Casuto LS, Keck PE: Gabapentin in the treatment of adolescent mania: a case report. J Child Adolesc Psychopharmacol 8:81–85, 1998

Spirito A, Sterling CM, Donaldson DL, Arrigan ME: Factor analysis of the suicide intent scale with adolescent suicide attempters. J Pers Assess 67:90–101, 1996

Swanson J: School-Based Assessments and Interventions for ADD Students. Irvine, CA, KC Publishing, 1992

Swanson JM, Kraemer HC, Hinshaw SP, et al: Clinical relevance of the primary findings of the MTA: success rates based on severity of ADHD and ODD symptoms at the end of treatment. J Am Acad Child Adolesc Psychiatry 40:168–179, 2001

Thurber S, Hollingsworth DK, Miller LA: The Hopelessness Scale for Children: psychometric properties with hospitalized adolescents. J Clin Psychol 52:543–545, 1996

Weisz JR, Weiss B, Wasserman AA, et al: Control-related beliefs and depression among clinic-referred children and adolescents. J Abnorm Psychol 96:58–63, 1987

Winters NC, Myers K, Proud L: Ten-year review of rating scales. III: Scales for suicidality, cognitive style, and self-esteem. J Am Acad Child Adolesc Psychiatry 41:1050–1181, 2002

Young R, Biggs J, Ziegler V, et al: A rating scale for mania: reliability, validity and sensitivity. Br J Psychiatry 133:429–435, 1978

Youngstrom EA, Danielson CK, Findling RL, et al: Factor structure of the Young Mania Rating Scale for use with youths ages 5 to 17 years. J Clin Child Adolesc Psychol 31:567–572, 2002

Psychological and Neuropsychological Testing

Mark A. Stein, Ph.D.

Sandra L. Barrueco, Ph.D.

Jeffrey M. Halperin, Ph.D.

Psychological evaluation is a process that results in quantifiable measurement of behavior within and across a range of psychological and neuropsychological domains, such as cognitive, academic, attention, and socioemotional functioning. Such quantifiable measurement is coupled with information on relative standings with normative, clinical, and other criterion groups and supplemented with observations and interpretations to serve important functions in child and adolescent psychiatry. For example, psychological and neuropsychological evaluations aid in the formulation of a diagnosis, determination of comorbid diagnoses, measurement of a child's degree of impairment or level of adaptive development, and quantification of a child's strengths and weaknesses. Such information is imperative to the development of specific targeted interventions, as well as to the development of recommendations to enhance areas of strength and compensate areas of weakness. In addition, establishment of an initial baseline evaluation allows for later retesting to monitor a child's development over time and for evaluation of the effectiveness of an intervention.

According to Meyer et al. (2001), "Psychological testing is a relatively straightforward process wherein a particular scale is administered to obtain a specific score.... In contrast, psychological assessment is concerned with the clinician who takes a variety of test scores, generally obtained from multiple test methods, and considers the data in the context of history, referral information, and observed behavior to understand the person being evaluated, to answer the referral

questions, and then to communicate findings" (p. 143). Hunsley (2002) pointed out that despite the common use of psychological and neuropsychological assessment, there is relatively little research on the validity of the assessment *process* per se relative to the voluminous support for the validity of individual tests (Matarazzo 1990). For example, a recent meta-analysis of 125 studies of test validity concluded that many psychological tests demonstrated validity similar to medical tests, such as pulse oximetry, cardiac stress tests, and magnetic resonance imaging studies (Meyer et al. 2001, 2002). Yet research is needed on the incremental validity of measures (i.e., what a specific test adds to the evaluation when used with other measures) and on the treatment utility of measures and the assessment process (i.e., the degree to which the addition of psychological test results will lead to improved treatment planning or outcome) (Garb et al. 2002). It is logical to assume that if more measures are used, a greater understanding about a child's development will be acquired. It is also logical to assume that if a specific learning disability or mood disorder is identified through the process of psychological testing, this will lead to improved outcomes through treatment. As yet, there is little systematic research to test these important assumptions.

Although relatively less research has been conducted on the assessment process than on individual tests themselves, the process of assessment is a critical component of psychological and neuropsychological evaluations. Accordingly, this chapter reviews the assessment process and commonly used psychology and neuropsychology measures appropriate for children or adolescents.

Evaluation Process and Techniques

Psychological evaluation involves much more than merely obtaining test scores. An evaluation has multiple essential and interrelated components: the development of testing questions; the selection of testing materials; test administration; test results interpretation; case formulation and recommendations; and the provision of results and recommendations. These steps are reviewed succinctly here; see Kamphaus and Frick (1996) and Sattler (2002) for more thorough discussions of the evaluation process.

■ Development of the Testing Questions

An essential first step in a psychological or neuropsychological evaluation is the development of a refined list of hypotheses or questions to be answered by the psychological evaluation. Increasing the specificity of the questions increases the efficiency and clinical utility of the testing process. For example, the testing plan that is developed for the question "Does this child have a reading disability and/or attentional difficulties?" or "What is this adolescent's language comprehension development?" would be more focused and efficient than the testing plan developed for questions such as "Can psychopathology be ruled out?" or perfunctory remarks such as "We need a psychological evaluation."

■ Selection of Testing Materials

Test selection is based on numerous factors, including the referral question, the age or developmental level of the child, and characteristics of the test itself, including the scientific rigor with which a test has been developed and empirically validated. The training and orientation of the psychologist also influence measure selection. Thus, the measures used for one evaluation can differ substantially from the measures selected for another evaluation, although most comprehensive psychological evaluations of children and adolescents include measures of intelligence, achievement, and emotional or personality functioning. In most clinical

situations, several tests or a comprehensive testing battery will be used to attempt to answer the referral questions. In addition, constructs of traits of interest (e.g., impulsivity, working memory, reading) are often assessed with several different measures to increase confidence in the findings.

One of the most important features of selecting a measure is consideration of the *standardization* sample and validation procedures for the test, because tests vary considerably in their construction, degree of structure, scoring, and degree of standardization. Such procedures involve the administration of the test during development to large samples of children and/ or adolescents to obtain information about its normative values at each age and grade level. Because the nature, rate, and degree of change are so rapid in children and adolescents, it is critical to evaluate the performance of individual children in relation to other children of similar age and/or grade levels. In addition, because there have been rapid and dramatic social and educational changes, tests are now more frequently revised to provide a more accurate normative comparison. Consequently, it is important that the most recent revision of a test is administered.

Testing procedures are also evaluated for their *validity* (i.e., the test is measuring what it is intended to measure) and *reliability* (i.e., the stability of the test under different conditions and different times). The provision of valid and reliable measurements of the domain or domains under examination is an essential criterion in test selection. Because published tests vary considerably in their psychometric characteristics (i.e., reliability, validity), it is important to review and evaluate such evidence before administering the test. Typically, this information is contained in the test manual. Specific standards for reviewing and evaluating the psychometric properties of psychological tests have been developed by the American Educational Research Association et al. (1999) and are taught to neuropsychologists, clinical psychologists, and school and educational psychologists during their training. It should be noted, however, that there is considerable variability in the degree to which psychological assessment of children and adolescents is emphasized in graduate training programs, internships, and postdoctoral fellowships. A detailed discussion of test construction, criteria for determining reliability and validity, and normative applicability is available elsewhere (e.g., Anastasi 1988; Cureton et al. 1995; Kelley et al. 1996). For the purposes of this chapter, it is imperative to know that psychologists must consider the psychometric properties (i.e., the extent to which each measure they use has been developed, evaluated, and standardized) prior to administration and interpretation.

Another critical component considered when selecting measures for an evaluation is the degree of correspondence between the child's characteristics and the characteristics of the *standardization sample*, which is the sample used to standardize the test. Therefore, the psychological examiner must be aware of the subject's age or developmental stage, language and cultural background, or any sensory or motor impairments that would invalidate or require alteration of the testing process. The match between the cultural and language milieus of the patients and the standardization sample should be considered during test selection and interpretation. The process of a simple translation or simple adaptation for people of another culture can alter or negate the validity and reliability of a standardized measure.

■ Test Administration

The issues of reliability and validity extend beyond the test standardization process and test selection into the entire testing process. To maximize the likelihood that the child's performance is a true reflection of his or her functioning, the examiner must work on establishing a positive atmosphere while also optimizing the child's performance through the creation of a structured environment. Importantly, a careful balance must be achieved between individualizing the testing sessions to obtain adequate performance, by taking account of the developmental and emotional functioning of each child, and maintaining the administration practices that were used in the standardization of the measure.

During the testing process, the examiner should note and describe the child's or adolescent's attitude toward testing, his or her affect and mood, relatedness, presence of any unusual behaviors or verbalizations, and any difficulties in attentional, impulsive, visual, auditory, linguistic, and/or motor functioning. It is also important to note factors outside the testing situation that may influence the testing performance, such as medication status, sleep, and nutritional status (e.g., whether the child ate breakfast or was complaining of hunger). Such observations not only provide insight into the contributing factors of children's and adolescents' performances but also are essential in obtaining a comprehensive understanding of their

strengths and weaknesses in the context of the clinical situation.

Occasionally, children's weaknesses can impair their functioning during portions of the testing to such a degree that it may invalidate some or all of the results. For example, children with attention-deficit/ hyperactivity disorder (ADHD) may have particular difficulty attending to sign functions on mathematical written subtests of academic achievement batteries and, as a result, obtain poor scores on this particular measure of aptitude. Severe difficulties with attention and impulsivity may also adversely affect children's performance on tests that require adequate reaction time, auditory memory, or attention to detail. Having observed a particular child's impulsive responding on a mathematical measure, for example, often leads examiners to further investigate whether the child's performance reflects his or her impulsivity, whether it reflects a separate mathematical weakness, or whether both weaknesses may be present. This is often conducted by asking the child to review his or her work for errors, by presenting the problems aloud to the child, and/or by comparing the child's performance on the subtest with performance on other mathematical tests that make fewer demands on the attentional system.

■ Interpretation, Case Formulation, and Recommendations

Observations and, at times, further examination (e.g., testing the limits) are critical to the interpretation of results as valid indicators of children's ability in each of the domains tested. In some instances, the goal of testing is to determine ability or potential, and the best possible performance is desired. However, in other situations the goal is to assess current functioning or more typical performance. Importantly, although a particular test score or the full evaluation may be rightfully identified as an underestimate of a child's underlying ability, the results still provide critical information for psychologists and psychiatrists on the child's current level of functioning in the school and/or home environment. In turn, this information on the degree of functioning and impairment can be utilized to formulate and develop a treatment plan. (See Chapter 17, "Diagnosis and Diagnostic Formulation," for more on the process of diagnostic formulation.)

In addition to the information conveyed by a total, standard, or summary score, psychologists also attend to the variability or pattern within and among individual scales to gain additional information and generate hypotheses. According to Matarazzo (1990), the challenge in psychological assessment is to assess human potential, not deficit, and the assessment of intelligence "is never conducted in isolation, but is always conducted as an assessment of the whole personality" (p. 22). For example, in intelligence testing, the pattern and variability of subtest scores and intrasubtest performance can be more clinically relevant than the total IQ score, especially when the overall IQ is within the average range. Test variability, particularly patterns of strengths and weaknesses, can potentially inform both the diagnostic formulation and the treatment plan in clinical populations. However, this information should be viewed cautiously. On average, the reliability and validity of each of the subtests are lower than the reliability and validity of the composite score. Because of this reduction, some strongly contend that the variability among subtests should not be interpreted at all (e.g., Macmann and Barnett 1994; McDermott et al. 1992). Others have developed systematic, hierarchical approaches to the interpretation of total scores and subtests that balance the extraction of meaning from subtest variability with the extra caution that must be taken when doing so (e.g., Kaufman 1994).

Regardless of whether psychologists decide to interpret the subtest scores, one aspect of test interpretation that must be stressed is the consideration and integration of all sources of available information. This includes the performance of children on, across, and within each measure, as well as the information obtained through parent history taking, supplementary teacher interviews, records review, and observation. When scores are not consistent among measures of similar developmental domains, psychologists use their clinical judgment to determine the reasons for differences and to describe the implications and relevance of such variability to the referral question.

Referral questions may be answerable in degrees, depending on the test battery and experience of the tester (A. Bloom, personal communication, May 2002). For example, when the question is whether a learning disorder is present, traditional batteries of IQ and achievement tests typically allow for rather general and robust statements (e.g., "IQ–achievement discrepancies"). On occasion, such traditional batteries permit a bit of specificity as to the nature of the learning disorder (e.g., language-based vs. perceptual). As indicated previously, traditional tests such as the Wechsler Intelligence Scale for Children—Third Edition

(WISC-III) and Wechsler Individual Achievement Test—Second Edition (WIAT-II) should be approached very cautiously when it comes to subtest pattern analyses. Depending on the skills of the examiner, other specific measures (e.g., phonological awareness) may be used to further refine diagnostic specificity.

Once the results of the evaluation are interpreted, specific recommendations are often made to target the areas of weakness and to support and build on areas of strength and coping processes. For example, recommendations may call for the participation (or continued participation) in specialized academic programs or tutoring; in individual, family, and/or group therapy; in a behavioral modification program; or in a psychotropic medication trial. For children or adolescents who are exhibiting self-injurious behavior or who are experiencing extreme difficulty functioning in their environments, recommendations are also made regarding the level of care (e.g., inpatient unit, day treatment, structured daily evening programs, or less intensive outpatient programs) that they should receive. Optimally, all treatment recommendations are made with regard to both evidence-based best practices for the specific problem(s) in question and the individual characteristics of the child and family.

Data and observations from psychological testing may also lead to recommendations for further evaluation. For example, observations of staring spells may lead to a neurological referral, observations of fine motor difficulties may lead to an occupational therapy referral, observations of difficulties discriminating sounds or visual objects may lead to an audiology or ophthalmology referral, and verbal or speech deficits may lead to a speech and language referral.

Psychologists often also recommend a specified time interval for follow-up assessment—abbreviated assessments to track the development of the child, to screen for other problems the child may be at risk for at a later age (e.g., reading disability, depression), and to provide updated recommendations. Such follow-up assessments should be scheduled at an appropriate time interval to minimize practice effects on the tests, as well as the inconvenience and cost of "overtesting."

■ Provision of Results and Recommendations

The final step in testing is the provision of the results and recommendations, usually in two formats. First, psychologists engage in a discussion with parents and/ or children and adolescents, if appropriate, about the findings and the recommendations. This feedback session should not consist of a one-way presentation of information and suggestions from the psychologists to the caregivers; rather, it is an opportunity for mutual discussion about the test results, implications regarding prognosis, and the course of action that should be undertaken. (See Stein and Pearl [1998] for a thorough discussion and a model for providing feedback, and Chapter 17, "Diagnosis and Diagnostic Formulation," for a discussion of the presentation of findings and recommendations.)

The second medium through which psychologists provide results and recommendations is a written report, which often becomes part of the child's medical or school record. A testing report provides a summary of the evaluation and is often used for communicating findings to the referring psychiatrist, parents, school systems, pediatricians, and/or other mental health professionals. Psychological reports should be brief and sharply focused and should answer the referral question in a succinct manner that is free of jargon. Just as with tests, evaluation reports should be composed of numerous components. The format of the report will vary with the setting but should be guided by the purpose and intended audience of the report. However, most testing reports will contain the elements displayed in Table 14–1.

Psychological and Neuropsychological Measures for Children and Adolescents

An important step in the process of psychological and neuropsychological testing is selecting which tests to use from the large number that have been developed and evaluated. Some of the most commonly used measures that have demonstrated adequate levels of reliability and validity for use with children and/or adolescents are described below. (For more detailed descriptions of these tests and other measures, see Sattler 2002.)

■ Tests of Cognitive Development and Functioning

One of the most well researched and common tests used in clinical applications with children and adoles-

Table 14–1. Checklist for information that should be present in testing reports

✔ Reason for referral: presenting problems and specific evaluation questions
✔ Identifying information
✔ Developmental and familial history
✔ Behavioral observations and statement regarding reliability of the findings
✔ Tests administered
✔ Test results
✔ Interpretation
✔ Recommendations
✔ Signature of psychologist who wrote the report

cents is the IQ test. Intelligence tests (e.g, IQ tests) aim to provide information about the individual's repertoire of cognitive knowledge and abilities at a particular point in time. This information is often represented in numerical form, called the *intelligence quotient* (IQ). William Stern (1914) developed the original IQ score, consisting of the ratio of mental age to chronological age. Current tests use the concept of the deviation IQ, in which the individual's position relative to the normal distribution for his or her age group is calculated. Most IQ tests will take 45 to 90 minutes to administer and require a high degree of examiner skill. Specialized training is often required to test very young children.

In most cases, the scores from intelligence tests are quite stable for children after age 5 (Zigler et al. 1984). Importantly, IQ scores are only modest predictors of overall adjustment (Zigler and Farber 1985) but are strongly associated with academic achievement (McCall 1977). An adequate assessment of overall intellectual function, using any of several standard intelligence tests, serves as marker for comparison purposes for other, more specific tests. For example, one would interpret an average score on a test of language function differently for a child with a low-average IQ as compared with one with a superior IQ. Furthermore, although generally lacking specificity, most intelligence tests are composed of a wide array of subtests that provide a broad evaluation of diverse cognitive domains. As such, the initial administration of a standard intelligence test, when integrated with the referral question and clinical observations, allows for the generation of more specific hypotheses regarding the nature of the cognitive difficulties. These hypotheses can then be tested through the use of more specific neuropsychological tests.

In addition, examining children's performance on tests of intellectual functioning is necessary for the assessment of clinical problems, particularly in the diagnosis of mental retardation, giftedness, and specific learning disabilities. In addition to assisting in the identification of disorders or areas of weakness, the performance of children on intelligence tests can also indicate the degree to which their intellectual functioning may serve as a protective factor or prognostic indicator.

There are also several brief measures of intelligence appropriate for screening or research purposes, such as the Wechsler Abbreviated Intelligence Scale (Wechsler 1999) or Kaufman Brief Intelligence Scale (Kaufman and Kaufman 1990). These tests have the advantage of being relatively quick to administer and are strongly associated with the longer measures of intellectual functioning. However, they have limited clinical utility because of the small number of domains that are sampled.

Table 14–2 summarizes several of the tests of cognitive functioning that are available.

■ Tests of Academic Achievement

Tests of academic achievement (Table 14–3) are frequently included in assessments of children and adolescents to identify learning and other disorders and to aid in educational placement and planning. It is important to note that the achievement test *score* provides only a piece of the story. In addition to the level of functioning, a key component of the information gathering is to determine the underlying processes that result in errors. Thus, it is imperative to insist that the child continue to attempt items well after he or she is making errors, if possible. By analyzing the errors, one can begin to determine the degree to which deficiencies are due to phonological difficulties, visual or auditory processing errors, lack of familiarity with words or the rules of the language, or perhaps even memory.

Objectively assessing a child's level of academic achievement through individualized testing is more reliable than group-administered achievement tests or grades frequently given by schools (Anastasi 1976). Group-administered tests are subject to influence by multiple extraneous factors and are therefore less valid than individually administered achievement tests.

In selecting an achievement test, the examiner must choose between screening measures that assess several academic functions, such as the Wide Range Achievement Test (WRAT) (Wilkinsen 1993), and more comprehensive and detailed measures of learning processes.

■ Tests of Adaptive Functioning

Learning the degree to which children are functioning in their environments not only provides psychologists a more comprehensive clinical picture but also is critical for determining the appropriateness of a diagnosis of mental retardation. According to definitions in DSM-IV-TR (American Psychiatric Association 2000), individuals are identified as being mentally retarded if their standardized IQ score is below 70 *and* if they demonstrate significant deficits in adaptive functioning. Children's adaptive functioning is also relevant to many psychiatric disorders, such as for children with ADHD and/or pervasive developmental disorders. For example, individuals with ADHD display marked deficits in adaptive functioning relative to their intelligence (Stein et al. 1995). Importantly, identifying adaptive weaknesses can lead to targeted psychosocial treatments. In some individuals, adaptive functioning may serve as a strength or protective factor, especially if encouraged.

One of the most common measures of adaptive functioning is the Vineland Adaptive Behavior Scales (VABS; Sparrow et al. 1984). The VABS assesses four domains: communication, daily living skills, socialization, and motor skills. The Parent Interview version is most frequently used; however, a classroom version is also available.

Projective Tests of Socioemotional Functioning

Projective tests are based on the projective hypothesis (Frank 1939; Murray 1938), which posits that one's needs, interests, coping style, and personality organization will determine the pattern of responses to relatively ambiguous perceptual stimuli. The tests described in Table 14–4 are among the most widely used measures of socioemotional functioning and, for adolescents, personality functioning. Importantly, many of these measures have not yet demonstrated ade-

Table 14–2. Selected measures of intellectual and cognitive functioning for children and adolescents

Measure	Ages	Brief description
Bayley Scales of Infant Development—Second Edition (BSID-II; Bayley 1969, 1993)	1–42 months	The BSID-II is a standardized developmental test battery for infants and toddlers. The three domains measured are cognitive development, motor development, and behavior.
Differential Abilities Scale (DAS; Elliot 1994)	2.5–17 years	The DAS is a multifaceted yet flexible cognitive battery, yielding a General Conceptual Ability (GCA) score; cluster scores in verbal and nonverbal ability at preschool level; and verbal reasoning, nonverbal reasoning, and spatial ability at school-age level.
Kaufman Assessment Battery for Children (K-ABC; Kaufman and Kaufman 1983)	2.6–12.5 years	The K-ABC makes a clear distinction between fluid nonverbal intelligence (mental processing scales) and crystallized knowledge (achievement scales). Because the mental processing composite does not include tests of verbal ability, it is weakened in estimating overall intellectual capacity, but its use may be advantageous for the assessment of ethnic subgroups and cultural minorities, who may perform more poorly on language-based measures.
Leiter International Performance Scale—Revised	2 years–adult	The International Performance Scale—Revised is a standardized, nonverbal test of intelligence often used to evaluate language-handicapped and non–English-speaking children.
McCarthy Scales of Children's Abilities (McCarthy 1972)	2.5–8.5 years	The McCarthy Scales comprise a verbal scale, perceptual-performance scale, quantitative scale, memory scale, motor scale, and an overall general cognitive scale, which yields a general cognitive index, equivalent to an IQ standard score.
Stanford-Binet Intelligence Scale, Fourth Edition (SBFE; Thorndike et al. 1986)	2–17 years	The SBFE is also a widely used battery of verbal and nonverbal cognitive ability that is particularly useful with younger or developmentally impaired children.
Wechsler Intelligence Scale for Children—Third Edition (WISC-II; Wechsler 1991)	6–16 years	The WISC-III, the most widely used IQ test for children, assesses four factors: verbal comprehension, perceptual organization, freedom from distractibility, and processing speed.
Wechsler Preschool and Primary Scale of Intelligence—Third Edition (WPPSI-III; Wechsler 2002)	3–7 years	The WPPSI-III, a widely used test of verbal and nonverbal cognitive ability for preschoolers, is very similar to the other Wechsler scales in format.
Woodcock-Johnson Tests of Cognitive Ability—Third Edition (WJ-III; Woodcock et al. 2002)	2 years–adult	The WJ-III, a comprehensive battery of subtests tapping multiple cognitive domains, is often utilized by school systems.

quate levels of reliability and validity to be used for diagnostic purposes (Gittelman-Klein 1986). However, some proponents say that in the hands of skilled clinicians, these techniques can be helpful in generating clinical hypotheses and recommendations. Therefore, these measures are used frequently in clinical settings. At present, empirically derived checklists or dimensional measures of psychopathology and structured diagnostic interviews are the most often utilized tools for assessment of socioemotional functioning.

Neuropsychological Testing

The primary goals of a comprehensive neuropsychological assessment are to evaluate a wide array of cognitive and behavioral functions and to interpret the data within the context of a thorough understanding of brain–behavior relationships. The field of clinical neuropsychology has primarily evolved from studies of neurologically intact adults who subsequently sustained brain damage. The study of such patients has

Table 14–3. Selected measures of academic achievement for children and adolescents

Measure	Ages	Brief description
Gray Oral Reading Test—Third Edition (Wiederholt and Bryant 1992)	7–17 years	The Gray Oral Reading Test is a test of reading ability and behavior. Children are asked to read passages of increasing difficulty so that their fluency, accuracy, and comprehension of passages can be assessed.
Wechsler Individual Achievement Test—Second Edition (WIAT-II; Wechsler 2001)	5–19 years	The WIAT-II, a comprehensive measure of reading, math, and written language skills, was co-normed with the WISC-III.
Wide Range Achievement Test—Third Edition (WRAT-3; Wilkinson 1993)	5 years–adult	The WRAT-3 is a quick screening measure that evaluates spelling, math, and reading decoding skills.
Woodcock-Johnson Tests of Achievement—Third Edition (WJ-III; Woodcock et al. 2002)	4 years–adult	The WJ-III is a comprehensive measure of reading, math, written language, and knowledge base; it was standardized on a large national population.

tremendously furthered our understanding of the behavioral sequelae of neurological dysfunction in humans. Furthermore, the knowledge gained and procedures developed from work with brain-damaged adults have had a substantial influence on the assessment of neuropsychological disorders in children. This transfer, however, is most relevant to and appropriate for children and adolescents with acquired neurological disorders. Yet much of pediatric neuropsychology, and particularly those aspects most relevant to clinical assessments in child and adolescent psychiatric settings, involves children with developmental disorders. Unlike most neurology patients, frank brain damage or a localized lesion is rarely observed in these children. More importantly, in the vast majority of these children, one is assessing not an initially "normal" brain that has been damaged but rather the impact of deviant developmental processes on brain function. Thus, the clinical psychologist or neuropsychologist is rarely looking for the "site of lesion" or the clinical manifestations of a localized neurological insult. Rather, the examination covers an array of cognitive processes with the goal of providing a refined picture of these children's cognitive and behavioral functioning.

Because diverse cognitive, behavioral, and neurological functions interact throughout development, one rarely finds, when evaluating children with developmental disorders, a single, highly specific deficit that accounts for their difficulties. Therefore, it is essential that the neuropsychologist or psychologist take a broad perspective and consider a wide array of domains and processes. Although specific tests in every domain may not be necessary, the thoughtful evalua-

tion should consider each area and allow for a comprehensive picture of the child's absolute (as compared to norms) and relative (as compared to him- or herself) strengths and weaknesses. Although neuropsychological data alone are rarely adequate for establishing a psychiatric diagnosis, they can be extremely helpful for understanding key aspects of an individual's difficulties and play a central role in treatment planning. Domains typically considered during a neuropsychological evaluation of children and adolescents are 1) overall cognitive function, 2) motor function, 3) perception, 4) visuomotor integration, 5) language, 6) learning and memory, 7) academic abilities, and 8) executive functions. Each of these domains is reviewed in more detail below.

First, however, it should be pointed out that neuropsychologists and psychologists vary somewhat in their approach to the assessment of these diverse cognitive and behavioral functions. Many use well-standardized, comprehensive neuropsychological test batteries such as those described in Table 14–5. The use of a standardized comprehensive test battery has the advantages of 1) increasing the probability of adequate coverage across a wide array of domains, 2) being familiar to most practitioners, and 3) having been standardized across a single normative sample. This latter point reduces the likelihood that strengths and weaknesses that emerge from the assessment are due to unique characteristics of diverse normative samples rather than true subject differences.

Nevertheless, some experts contend that the fixed format of comprehensive neuropsychological test batteries is too rigid and that testing should be tailored to

Table 14–4. Selected measures of socioemotional functioning for children and adolescents

Measure	Ages	Brief description
Children's Apperception Test (CAT; Bellak and Bellak 1974)	3–10 years	The CAT consists of 10 cards depicting animals in ordinary human situations, because young children are apt to identify easily with animals. The CAT—Human Figures (CAT-H) (Bellak and Bellak 1965) consists of human figures and situations that parallel those of the original CAT. Children are asked to develop stories based on the ambiguous pictures; these stories are reviewed for their content and themes.
Human Figure Drawing (Koppitz 1968)	2 years and above	The Human Figure Drawing test aims to assess psychological factors such as self-concept and self-esteem through children's drawings of humans.
Roberts Apperception Test for Children (Roberts and McArthur 1982)	6–15 years	The Roberts Apperception Test for Children has advantages over older apperception tests in that its stimuli are more modern in appearance, it offers a wider range of everyday interpersonal familial events, and it has an objective scoring system.
Rorschach Inkblot Test (Rorschach 1921)	8 years and above	The Rorschach Inkblot Test consists of 10 symmetrical inkblots presented to the subject. The most commonly used scoring system was designed by Exner and Weiner (1995). This scoring system yields information on individuals' characteristics in the domains of perception, cognition, and emotion. The method and content of responses are also analyzed for socioemotional meaning.
Sentence-completion tests	3 years and above	Sentence-completion tests are semistructured, open-ended measures designed to elicit information about children's feelings, conflicts, and concerns about themselves and others. They can reveal both conscious and unconscious sentiments and thoughts. The most popular sentence-completion test is the Rotter Incomplete Sentences Blank (Lau 1989; Rotter et al. 1954), followed by the Rohde Sentence Completion Method (Rohde 1957).
Thematic Apperception Test (TAT; Murray 1943)	7 years and above	The TAT requires children to construct a story based on each of a series of ambiguous pictures, which provides data about their socioemotional, interpersonal, and personality functioning.

the individual patient (e.g., Baron et al. 1995; Hammeke et al. 1978). Fixed test batteries may require excessive testing in some domains (which may not be necessary for certain patients) and may not provide enough in-depth testing in other areas that are appropriate for other patients. Therefore, many clinical neuropsychologists and psychologists prefer to choose from a wide array of tests those to use with a particular patient. This more tailored approach may have several advantages for the skilled examiner, but it must be used cautiously because many smaller neuropsychological tests may not have adequate norms from representative samples, and the reliability and validity of many tests may not have been adequately assessed. Further, there is always the risk of missing a key domain for assessment.

Whether one uses a standardized or a specially selected battery of tests, a comprehensive neuropsychological assessment should evaluate a wide array of domains, including overall intellectual and academic

Table 14–5. Selected measures of general neuropsychological functioning for children and adolescents

Measure	Ages	Brief description
Halstead-Reitan Neuropsychological Test Battery for Children (Reitan 1979)	9–14 years	The Halstead-Reitan comprises numerous cognitive and perceptual-motor subtests. It is often used for evaluating children suspected to have brain damage. Information on the test's reliability and validity is scarce, and norms are limited.
Luria-Nebraska Neuropsychological Battery for Children (LNNB-C; Golden 1981)	8–12 years	The LNNB-C is designed to assess cognitive deficits and to aid in planning rehabilitation programs.
NEPSY Developmental Neuropsychological Assessment (NEPSY; Korkman et al. 1998)	3–12 years	The NEPSY is extensively normed to assess five basic neuropsychological domains. Several subtests cover each of the following functional domains: attention and executive functions, language, sensorimotor, visuospatial, and memory.

functioning, as reviewed above. The following domains are also important components of many neuropsychological assessments.

■ Tests of Motor Function

The assessment of motor function generally begins from the moment that the child is first seen. During the clinician's walk with the child from the waiting room to the test office, the child's gait, posture, and overall stance are carefully observed. Important clues regarding motor problems, ranging from subtle awkwardness and clumsiness to overactivity to more severe disturbances of gait (e.g., toe walking), or coordination may be apparent. The careful observer also looks for tics and other forms of movement problems. In addition to clinical observations, particular instruments, most of which involve timed measurements, are well suited for detecting more subtle problems in fine and gross motor coordination, speed, and dexter-

ity. Careful use of these measures not only allows for the evaluation of motoric difficulties that can lead to anything from poor handwriting to an inability to ride a bicycle but also allows for a systematic comparison of the two sides of the body, which may reflect lateralized cerebral deficits. Table 14–6 describes selected measures of motor function commonly used with children.

■ Tests of Perception

Although most neuropsychological evaluations focus primarily on visual perception, it is important to also consider auditory and tactile/somatosensory modalities. Basic sensory and perceptual deficits can lead to a wide array of difficulties in children, including problems of language (auditory), reading (visual or auditory), kinesthesis, or social behaviors. Table 14–7 describes measures often used to assess various perceptual domains in children.

Table 14–6. Selected measures of motor function for children and adolescents

Measure	Ages	Brief description
Dynamometer Grip Strength and Tapping Tests (Finlayson and Reitan 1976; Reitan and Wolfson 1985)	6 years–adult	These tests from the Halstead-Reitan Battery assess strength and motor speed of the index finger for each hand.
Grooved Pegboard (Klove 1963)	5 years–adult	The Grooved Pegboard is a brief test of unimanual visuomotor planning, motor speed, and dexterity.
Purdue Pegboard (Costa et al. 1963; Gardner and Broman 1979; Tiffin 1968; Wilson et al. 1982)	2 years–adult	The Purdue Pegboard is a brief test of unimanual and bimanual fine motor speed and dexterity. Subjects are timed as they place small pegs in holes on dominant, nondominant, and bimanual trials.

Table 14–7. Selected measures of perceptual function for children and adolescents

Measure	Ages	Brief description
Gestalt Closure Test (Kaufman and Kaufman 1983)	5–12.5 years	The Gestalt Closure subtest of the Kaufman Assessment Battery for Children is an untimed measure of visual perception that requires the child to identify degraded pictures of common objects.
Judgment of Line Orientation (JLO; Benton et al. 1977)	7 years–adult	The JLO is a motor-free untimed measure of spatial perception and orientation requiring judgment as to the spatial directionality and size of angles.
Reitan-Klove Sensory-Perceptual Examination (Reitan and Davison 1974)	5 years–adult	The Reitan-Klove Sensory-Perceptual Examination measures perception of tactile, auditory, and visual stimuli.
Tactile Perception Test (TPT; Reitan and Wolfson 1985; Spreen and Gaddes 1969)	5–13 years	The TPT assesses tactile form recognition and memory for shapes and spatial location.

Table 14–8. Selected measures of visuomotor integration for children and adolescents

Measure	Ages	Brief description
Developmental Test of Visual-Motor Integration (VMI; Beery 1989)	3–18 years	The VMI is a developmentally normed drawing test assessing visual planning, organization, graphomotor control, and visuomotor integration. It requires the child to copy increasingly complex line drawings.
Rey-Osterrieth Complex Figure Test and Recognition Trial (RCFT; Meyers and Meyers 1995; Waber and Holmes 1985)	6 years–adult	The RCFT requires the individual to copy and then redraw from memory a complex geometric figure. It assesses visuospatial construction ability, visual memory, and visual organization.
Visual-Motor Gestalt Test (Bender 1938; Canter 1976)	5 years–adult	The Visual-Motor Gestalt Test requires the individual to copy a series of line drawings.

■ Tests of Visuomotor Integration

Visuomotor integration difficulties, which are impairments in the ability to use visual information to accurately guide motor responses, are highly prevalent among clinically referred children. Although deficiencies in the integration process can arise from problems of either visual/perceptual processing or motoric output, visuomotor integration difficulties often represent a disconnection or poor processing between the input and output. Thus, visuomotor integration can be manifested in numerous behaviors ranging from being able to copy a simple figure to hitting a baseball. Visuomotor integration is generally evaluated through a variety of tasks assessing graphomotor skills (copying figures) and construction skills (e.g., with blocks). In younger children, addi-tional measures requiring eye–hand coordination, such as throwing a ball into a basket, are sometimes used. Table 14–8 describes measures often used to assess visuomotor integration.

■ Tests of Learning and Memory

Learning and memory involve a heterogeneous set of brain regions that are differentially associated with distinct processes, so a neuropsychological assessment may be recommended for children experiencing learning difficulties. In general, memory is divided into short-term versus long-term, verbal versus visual, and storage versus retrieval. An overlapping and related function, working memory, is considered below under "Tests of Executive Functions." Although there is no clear demarcation between short-

and long-term memory, in general, short-term memory involves processes that are maintained via rehearsal, prior to the time of storage, whereas long-term memory refers to material that is accessed at some point after storage has taken place and rehearsal has terminated. Learning and memory tests explore the capacity to integrate novel information and facility in retrieving acquired data (Rieger and Baron 1997a, 1997b). Most memory tests require the individual to recall previously presented material, but it is difficult to determine whether a lack of recall reflects the fact that the information was not adequately encoded and stored or whether it is instead a problem with accessing previously learned and stored information. Standardized cueing and recognition paradigms help to differentiate these processes. Table 14–9 describes selected tests of learning and memory for children and adolescents.

■ Tests of Executive Functions

Executive functions represent a heterogeneous set of cognitive abilities that are mediated by neural circuits involving prefrontal cortical regions and are critical to allowing the individual to adapt to an ever-changing environment. Under the umbrella of executive functions are multiple overlapping subdomains, including regulation of attention/attentional control, inhibitory control, working memory, planning, cognitive flexibility/shifting sets, response preparation/organization of motor output, organizational skills, resistance to in-

terference, and regulation of affect. Deficits within these subdomains have been associated with a wide array of childhood psychiatric disorders, including ADHD, Tourette's disorder, and autism. However, it is important to recognize that most measures of executive functions involve synthesis or organization of many of the more specific processes described above. As such, it is difficult to confidently diagnose executive function deficits in the context of more basic cognitive deficits. Table 14–10 describes selected measures of executive functions for children and adolescents.

Recently, a molar measure of executive functions based on parent or teacher report has been developed, the Behavior Rating Inventory of Executive Functioning (BRIEF; Gioia et al. 2000). The BRIEF is completed by parents or teachers and provides indices of behavioral regulation and metacognition, each of which is subdivided into more discrete subscales.

Children's attention/concentration functioning is an important domain to assess. Continuous performance tests, such as the Test of Variables of Attention (TOVA), Conners, or Gordon, are popular with clinicians because they provide an objective measure of distractibility and impulsivity, which is sensitive to stimulant medication effects. Caution is warranted in using these measures for diagnostic purposes in isolation, however, because of their limited diagnostic specificity (Reinecke et al. 1999). Examples of executive functioning tests that aid in assessment of aspects of attentional capacity include WISC-III subtests (arithmetic, coding, digit span), as well as the tests described in Table 14–11.

Table 14–9. Selected measures of learning and memory function for children and adolescents

Measure	Ages	Brief description
Benton Visual Retention Test—Fifth Edition (Sivan 1991)	8 years–adult	The Benton Visual Retention Test assesses visual memory by requiring the subject to reproduce line drawings of geometric figures after a brief delay.
California Verbal Learning Test—Children's Version (CVLT-C; Delis et al. 1994)	5–17 years	The CVLT-C assesses varied aspects of list learning and memory, including the ability to learn through repeated trials, learning strategies, and the effect of interference. Long-term storage and retrieval are assessed after a time delay.
Rey-Osterrieth Complex Figure Test and Recognition Trial (RCFT; Meyers and Meyers 1995; Waber and Holmes 1986)	6 years–adult	The RCFT requires the individual to copy and then redraw from memory a complex geometric figure. It assesses the use of cues for assisting with retrieval.
Wide Range Assessment of Memory and Learning (WRAML; Sheslow and Adams 1990)	5–17 years	The WRAML assesses verbal and visual memory, with multiple measures in each domain to assess immediate and delayed recall as well as delayed recognition memory.

Table 14–10. Selected measures of executive functions for children and adolescents

Measure	Ages	Brief description
Continuous performance tests (Conners 1995; Gordon 1983; Gordon et al 1986; Greenberg and Crosby 1992)	4 years–adult	Numerous versions of continuous performance tests are available that vary somewhat with regard to task demands and stimulus parameters. All require the subject to monitor rapidly presented stimuli and to respond (or not respond) to a predetermined target stimulus.
Digit span test (Wechsler 1991)	6 years–adult	The digit span test assesses the ability to hold and manipulate verbal information. Whereas the digits-forwards segment primarily assesses attention and memory span, the digits-backwards segment is a sensitive measure of working memory.
Rey-Osterrieth Complex Figure Test and Recognition Trial (RCFT; Meyers and Meyers 1995; Osterrieth and Rey 1944; Waber and Holmes 1985, 1986)	6 years–adult	The RCFT requires the individual to copy and then redraw from memory a complex geometric figure. In addition to assessing visuospatial construction ability and visual memory, it is particularly sensitive to aspects of visual organization.
Stroop Color and Word Test (Golden 1978; Stroop 1935)	7 years–adult	The Stroop test measures the ability to shift perceptual set and to inhibit an automatic response in favor of a more effortful one.
Tower of London (TOL; Culbertson and Zillmer 1998)	7–12 years	The TOL evaluates the child's ability to plan a series of moves according to a set of rules to replicate patterns produced by the examiner.
Trail Making Test (Reitan 1979; Reitan and Davison 1974)	5 years–adult	The Trail Making Test of the Halstead-Reitan Neuropsychological Test Battery is a brief, two-part pencil-and-paper test assessing visual scanning, graphomotor speed, cognitive flexibility, temporal sequencing, and planning.
Wisconsin Card Sorting Test—Revised and Expanded (WCST; Heaton et al. 1993)	6 years–adult	The WCST requires the subject to discover a rule and then shift cognitive set when the rule changes. The test assesses preservation, abstract reasoning, and failure to maintain set.

Table 14–11. Selected measures of attention and impulsivity

Measure	Ages	Brief description
California Verbal Learning Test—Child Version (CVLT-C; Delis et al. 1994)	5–16 years	The CVLT-C assesses many aspects of verbal list learning and memory, including the ability to learn through repeated trials, learning strategies, organizational ability, working memory, and sensitivity to proactive and retroactive interference. Long-term storage and retrieval of verbal information are assessed after a timed delay.
Children's Memory Scales (CMS; Cohen 1997)	5–16 years	The CMS assesses verbal and visual memory and learning skills.
Gordon Diagnostic System (Gordon et al. 1986)	4–16 years	The Gordon Diagnostic System tests the ability to sustain attention and exert self-control.
Test of Variables of Attention (TOVA) (computerized) (Greenberg et al. 1997)	5 years–adult	The computerized TOVA is a 20-minute test of sustained visual attention, vigilance, impulsivity, and distractibility.
Wide Range Assessment of Memory and Learning (WRAML; Sheslow and Adams 1990)	5–17 years	The WRAML assesses verbal and visual memory skills, with multiple measures in each subdomain to assess immediate and delayed recall as well as delayed recognition memory.

■ Tests for Language Disorders

Disorders of language are common in children and adolescents encountered through psychiatric referrals and may be manifested in a variety of ways. Language difficulties may initially present as academic/ learning problems or as social/communication difficulties. On the basis of lesion data from adults, neuropsychologists oftentimes divide language disorders into receptive and expressive subtypes. This practice stems from the fact that, in adults, posterior left cortical lesions typically result in disorders of language reception and comprehension, whereas more anterior lesions often result in expressive language difficulties (Luria 1973). However, this dichotomy does not work particularly well for characterizing developmental language disorders. In children, receptive difficulties rarely exist without expressive disorders. Although there may be advantages to dichotomizing expressive and receptive abilities, it is often beneficial to differentially examine linguistic processes such as phonology, syntax, semantics, pragmatics, and perhaps naming. More often than not, one will find that a deficit in most of these latter domains will be present in both language reception and expression. Thus, a child who experiences difficulties with syntax will likely experience these difficulties in both comprehension and expression. Table 14–12 describes several examples of neuropsychological tests of various language functions.

Table 14–12. Selected measures of language function for children and adolescents

Measure	Ages	Brief description
Boston Naming Test (Halperin et al. 1989; Kaplan et al. 1983)	6 years–adult	The Boston Naming Test assesses the ability to name pictured objects.
Clinical Evaluation of Language Fundamentals 3 (CELF-3; Semel et al. 1995)	3–7 years; 6–21 years	The CELF-3 measures both receptive and expressive language and identifies language skills in the areas of form and content that characterize mature language use.
Controlled Oral Word Association Test (Halperin et al. 1989; Spreen and Benton 1977)	6 years–adult	The Controlled Oral Word Association Test requires the subject to rapidly produce as many words as possible that begin with a particular letter or belong to a given semantic category (e.g., animals).
Detroit Tests of Learning Aptitude—Oral Directions (Hammill 1998)	6–17 years	Detroit Tests of Learning Aptitude—Oral Directions is a worksheet task requiring pencil-and-paper execution of detailed directions presented orally.
Expressive One-Word Picture Vocabulary Test—Revised (Gardner 1990)	2–12 years; 12–16 years	The Expressive One-Word Picture Vocabulary Test—Revised is a test of one-word picture naming, requiring subjects to verbally label drawings of objects.
Multilingual Aphasia Examination—Third Edition (MAE 3; Benton et al. 1994)	6 years–adult	The MAE 3 measures the presence, severity, and qualitative aspects of aphasic disorder.
Oral Vocabulary (subtest of the Woodcock-Johnson Tests of Cognitive Ability—Revised [WJ-R])	4 years–adult	The Oral Vocabulary subtest of the WJ-R is a test of synonym and antonym production, requiring single-word oral responses.
Peabody Picture Vocabulary Test-III (Dunn and Dunn 1997)	2 years–adult	The Peabody Picture Vocabulary Test-III assesses one-word receptive vocabulary, requiring the subject to select one of four pictures that best depicts a spoken word. Assesses one-word receptive vocabulary.
Picture Vocabulary (WJ-R)	4 years–adult	The Picture Vocabulary subtest of the WJ-R is a test of one-word picture naming, requiring subjects to verbally label drawings of objects.

Table 14–12. Selected measures of language function for children and adolescents *(continued)*

Measure	Ages	Brief description
Preschool Language Scale—Third Edition (PLS-3; Zimmerman et al. 1992)	Birth–6.11 years	The PLS-3 is a test designed to measure receptive and expressive language of children and to identify and describe maturational lags.
Rapid Automatized Naming (RAN; Denckla 1989)	5–13 years	The RAN is a timed measure of rapid color, number, object, and letter naming in response to a page of pictured stimuli.
Token Test for Children (DiSimoni 1978)	6–13 years	In the Token Test for Children, using colored tokens of varying shapes, the child must follow verbal commands of increasing complexity.
Verbal Analogies (Woodcock-Johnson Tests of Cognitive Ability—Third Edition [WJ-III]) (Woodcock et al. 2002)	4 years–adult	The Verbal Analogies subtest of the WJ-III is a test requiring oral completion of analogies.

Table 14–13. Selected measures of phonological awareness and auditory processing for children and adolescents in English

Measure	Ages	Brief description
Incomplete Words (subtest of the Woodcock-Johnson Tests of Cognitive Ability—Revised [WJ-R])	4 years and above	The Incomplete Words subtest of the WJ-R measures auditory closure. Subjects hear standardized audiotaped words with missing phonemes and must identify the words.
NEPSY Phonological Processing	3–12 years	Phonological Processing is an oral measure of the ability to analyze common words into sound components through deletion of specific phonemes or substitution of phonemes.
Lindamood Auditory Conceptualization Test—Revised (Lindamood and Lindamood 1979)	4 years–adult	The Lindamood Auditory Conceptualization Test—Revised measures speech sound discrimination and perception of number, order, and sameness or difference of speech sounds in sequences.
Phoneme Segmentation Test	6–12 years	The Phoneme Segmentation Test is an oral measure of the ability to analyze sound components of real words through deletion of initial or end sounds and through comparison of initial versus medial versus end phonemes in words.
Phonological Awareness Test (Robertson and Salter 1995)	5–9 years	The Phonological Awareness Test assesses phonological constructs such as rhyming, segmentation, and decoding.
Sound Blending (WJ-R)	4 years and above	The Sound Blending subtest of the WJ-R measures the ability to integrate and say whole words after hearing parts of the words via audiotape.

■ Tests of Phonological Awareness and Auditory Processing

Phonological awareness and auditory processing ability are components of language development and have been implicated as a critical skill in reading develop-ment. Thus, measures assessing these components are often used in evaluations of children with possible reading disorder, as well as of children who are experiencing speech and language difficulties (Table 14–13). For more on phonological awareness, reading disorders, and learning disorders, see Pennington (1991).

Conclusion

Psychological assessment is composed of careful attention to and examination of multiple components: formulating the question, test selection, test administration, observation, and interpretation of test findings. A vast number of psychological and neuropsychological tests are now available for a variety of age groups, diagnostic and cultural subgroups, and clinical purposes. Reliability, validity, and clinical utility vary considerably from test to test and are dependent on a host of factors related to the test, the child, the examiner, the clinical situation, and the purpose of testing or clinical question. Care should be given to selecting a psychologist or neuropsychologist with appropriate training and experience who can administer, interpret, and communicate findings relevant to your clinical or research needs. When used appropriately, psychological and neuropsychological testing are valuable tools in clinical, academic, and research settings. Whether data obtained from psychological and neuropsychological assessment confirm a clinical hypothesis related to diagnosis or comorbidity; help educate others about how best to assist, "reach," or communicate with a child; or document the efficacy of a specific treatment, it is hoped that greater specification and precision in measuring behavior and cognition will lead to increased understanding of the child and ultimately improve clinical care.

References

American Educational Research Association, American Psychological Association, and National Council on Measurement in Education: Standards for Educational and Psychological Testing. Washington, DC, American Educational Research Association, 1999

American Psychiatric Association: Diagnostic and Statistical Manual of Mental Disorders, 4th Edition, Text Revision. Washington, DC, American Psychiatric Association, 2000

Anastasi A: Psychological Testing, 4th Edition. New York, Macmillan, 1976

Anastasi A: Psychological Testing, 6th Edition. New York, Macmillan, 1988

Baron IS, Fennel EB, Voeller KS: Pediatric Neuropsychology in the Medical Setting. New York, Oxford University Press, 1995

Bayley N: Bayley Scales of Infant Development (BSID). San Antonio, TX, Psychological Corporation, 1969

Bayley N: Bayley Scales of Infant Development—revised (BSID-II). San Antonio, TX, Psychological Corporation, 1993

Beery KE: Revised administration, scoring and teaching manual for the Developmental Test of Visual-Motor Integration. Cleveland, OH, Modern Curriculum Press, 1989

Bellak L, Bellak S: Children's Apperception Test—Human Figures. Larchmont, NY, CPS, 1965

Bellak L, Bellak S: Children's Apperception Test, Revised Edition. Larchmont, NY, CPS, 1974

Bender L: A visual-motor gestalt test and its clinical use (monograph no. 3). New York, American Orthopsychiatric Association, 1938

Benton AL, Varney NR, Hamsher K. de S: Manual of Judgment of Line Orientation. Iowa City, IA, University of Iowa, 1977

Benton AL, Hamsher KS, Sivan A: Multilingual Aphasia Examination. Iowa City, IA, AJA Associates, 1994

Canter A: The Canter Background Interference Procedure for the Bender-Gestalt Test: Manual for Administration, Scoring and Interpretation. Nashville, TN, Counselor Recordings and Tests, 1976

Cohen M: Children's Memory Scale. San Antonio, TX, Psychological Corporation, 1997

Conners CK: The Conners Continuous Performance Test. North Tonawanda, NY, Multi-Health Systems, 1995

Costa LD, Vaughan HG, Levita E et al: The Purdue Pegboard as a predictor of the presence and laterality of cerebral lesions. J Consult Psychol 27:133–137, 1963

Culbertson WC, Zillmer EA: The Tower of London: a standardized approach to assessing executive functioning in children. Arch Clin Neuropsychol 13:285–301, 1998

Cureton EE, Cronbach LJ, Meehl PE, et al: Validity, in Educational Measurement: Origins, Theories, and Explications, Vol 1: Basic Concepts and Theories. Edited by Ward AW, Stoker HW, Murray-Ward M. Lanham, MD, University Press of America, 1995, pp 125–243

Delis DC, Kramer JH, Kaplan E, et al: The California Verbal Learning Test—Children's Version (CVLT-C). New York, Psychological Corporation, 1994

Denckla MB: Executive function: the overlap zone between attention deficit hyperactivity disorder and learning disabilities. International Pediatrics 4:155–160, 1989

DiSimoni F: The Token Test for Children. Boston, MA, Teaching Resources Corporation, 1978

Dunn LM, Dunn LM: Peabody Picture Vocabulary Test, Third Edition. Examiner's Manual and Norms Booklet. Circle Pines, MN, AGS Publishing, 1997

Elliot C: Differential Abilities Scale. San Antonio, TX, Psychological Corporation, 1994

Exner JE Jr, Weiner I: The Rorschach: A Comprehensive System, Vol 3, 2nd Edition: Assessment of Children and Adolescents. New York, Wiley, 1995

Finlayson MA, Reitan RM: Handedness in relation to measures of motor and tactile–perceptual function in normal children. Percept Mot Skills 43:475–481, 1976

Frank LK: Projective methods for the study of personality. J Psychol 8:389–413, 1939

Garb HN: Studying the Clinician: Judgment Research and Psychological Assessment. Washington, DC, American Psychological Association, 1998

Gardner MF: Expressive One-Word Picture Vocabulary Test—Revised. Novato, CA, Academic Therapy Publications, 1990

Gardner RA, Broman M: The Purdue Pegboard: normative data on 1334 school children. J Clin Child Psychol 8:156–162, 1979

Gioia GA, Isquith PK, Guy SC, et al: Behavior Rating Inventory of Executive Function (BRIEF)—Parent Form. Odessa, FL, Psychological Assessment Resources, 2000

Gittelman-Klein R: Questioning the clinical usefulness of projective psychological tests for children. J Dev Behav Pediatr 7:378–382, 1986

Golden CJ: Manual for the Stroop Color and Word Test. Chicago, IL, Stoetling, 1978

Golden CJ: A standardized version of Luria's neuropsychological tests: a quantitative and qualitative approach to neuropsychological evaluation, in Handbook of Clinical Neuropsychology. Edited by Filskov SB, Boll TJ. New York, Wiley-Interscience, 1981, pp 608–642

Gordon M, McClure FD, Post EM: Interpretive Guide to the Gordon Diagnostic System. DeWitt, NY, Gordon Systems, Inc, 1986

Greenberg LM, Crosby RD: A summary of developmental normative data on the Test of Variables of Attention (TOVA). Minneapolis, MN, University of Minnesota, 1992

Greenberg L, Leark RA, Dupuy TR, et al: Tests of Variables of Attention. Version 7.03. Los Alamitos, CA, Universal Attention Disorders, 1997

Halperin JM, Healy JM, Zeitschick E et al: Developmental aspects of linguistic and mnestic abilities in normal children. J Clin Exp Neuropsychol 11:518–528, 1989

Hammeke TA, Golden CJ, Purisch AD: A standardized, short, and comprehensive neuropsychological test battery based on the Luria neuropsychological evaluation. Int J Neurosci 8:134–141, 1978

Hammill DD: Detroit Tests of Learning Aptitude (DTLA-4). Austin, TX, PRO-ED, 1998

Heaton RK, Chelune GJ, Talley JL, et al: Wisconsin Card Sorting Test Revised and Expanded. Odessa, FL, Psychological Assessment Resources, 1993

Hunsley H: Psychological testing and psychological assessment: a closer examination. Am Psychol 57(2):139–140, 2002

Kamphaus RW, Frick PJ: Clinical assessment of child and adolescent personality and behavior. Needham Heights, MA, Allyn & Bacon, 1996

Kaplan EF, Goodglass H, Weintraub S: The Boston Naming Test, 2nd edition. Philadelphia, PA, Lea & Febiger, 1983

Kaufman AS: Intelligent Testing with the WISC-III. New York, Wiley, 1994

Kaufman AS, Kaufman NL: Interpretive Manual for the Kaufman Assessment Battery for Children. Circle Pines, MN, AGS Publishing, 1983

Kaufman AS, Kaufman NL: Kaufman Brief Intelligence Test (K-BIT). Circle Pines, MN, AGS Publishing, 1990

Kelley TL, Cronbach LJ, Rajaratnam N, et al: Reliability, in Educational Measurement: Origins, Theories, and Explications, Vol. 1: Basic Concepts and Theories. Edited by Ward AW, Stoker HW, Murray-Ward M. Lanham, MD, University Press of America, 1996, pp 245–286

Klove H: Clinical neuropsychology, in The Medical Clinics of North America. Edited by Forster FM. New York, WB Saunders, 1963, pp 1647–1658

Koppitz EM: Psychological Evaluation of Children's Human Figure Drawings. Orlando, FL, Grune & Stratton, 1968

Korkman M, Kirk U, Kemp S: A Developmental Neuropsychological Assessment (NEPSY). New York, Psychological Corporation, 1998

Lau MI: New validity, normative and scoring data for the Rotter Incomplete Sentences Blank. J Pers Assess 53:607–620, 1989

Lindamood C, Lindamood P: Lindamood Auditory Conceptualization Test. Circle Pines, MN, AGS Publishing, 1979

Luria AR: The Working Brain: An Introduction to Neuropsychology. New York, Basic Books, 1973

Macmann GM, Barnett DW: Structural analyses of correlated factors: lessons from the verbal-performance dichotomy of the Wechsler scales. School Psychology Quarterly 9:161–197, 1994

Matarazzo JD: Wechsler's Measurement and Appraisal of Adult Intelligence. New York, Oxford University Press, 1972

Matarazzo JD: Psychological assessment versus psychological testing: validation from Binet to the school, clinic, and courtroom. Am Psychol 45:999–1017, 1990

McCall RB: Childhood IQ's as predictors of adult educational and occupational status. Science 197:482–483, 1977

McCarthy D: Manual for the McCarthy Scales of Children's Abilities. San Antonio, TX, Psychological Corporation, 1972

McDermott PA, Fantuzzo JW, Glutting JJ, et al: Illusions of meaning in the ipsative assessment of children's ability. Journal of Special Education 25:504–526, 1992

Meyer GI, Finn SE, Eyde LD, et al: Psychological testing and psychological assessment: a review of evidence and issues. Am Psychol 56:128–165, 2001

Meyer GI, Finn SE, Eyde LD, et al: Amplifying issues related to psychological testing and assessment. Am Psychol 57:140–141, 2002

Meyers JE, Meyers KR: Rey Complex Figure Test and Recognition Trial (RCFT). Odessa, FL, Psychological Assessment Resources, 1995

Murray HA: Explorations in Personality. New York, Oxford University Press, 1938

Murray HA: Thematic Apperception Test Manual. Cambridge, MA, Harvard University Press, 1943

Osterrieth P, Rey A: Le test de copie d'une figure complexe. Archives de Psychologie 30:206–356, 1944

Pennington BF: Diagnosing Learning Disorders: A Neuropsychological Framework. New York, Guilford, 1991

Reinecke MA, Beebe D, Stein MA: The WISC-III Freedom from Distractibility Factor: it's (probably) not freedom from distractibility. J Am Acad Child Adolesc Psychiatry 38:322–328, 1999

Reitan RM: Halstead-Reitan Neuropsychological Test Battery. Tucson, AZ, Reitan Neuropsychology Laboratory, 1979

Reitan RM, Davison LA: Clinical Neuropsychology: Current Status and Applications. Washington, DC, Winston, 1974

Reitan RM, Wolfson D: The Halstead–Reitan Neuropsychological Test Battery: Theory and Interpretation. Tucson, AZ, Neuropsychology Press, 1985

Rieger RE, Baron IS: Psychological and neuropsychological testing, in Handbook of Child and Adolescent Psychiatry, Vol 5. Edited by Noshpitz JD, Greenspan S, Wieder S, et al. New York, Wiley, 1997a

Rieger RE, Baron IS: Psychological and neuropsychological testing, in Textbook of Child and Adolescent Psychiatry, 2nd Edition. Edited by Wiener JM. Washington, DC, American Psychiatric Press, 1997b, pp 133–152

Roberts GE, McArthur DS: Roberts Apperception Test for Children. Los Angeles, CA, Western Psychological Services, 1982

Robertson G, Salter W: Phonological Awareness Test. East Moline, IL, LinguiSystems, 1995

Rohde AR: The Sentence Completion Method: Its Diagnostic and Clinical Application to Mental Disorders. New York, Ronald, 1957

Rorschach H: Psychodiagnostik. Translated by HH Verlag. Bern, Switzerland, Bircher, 1921

Rotter JB, Rafferty JE, Lotsoff AB: The validity of the Rotter Incomplete Sentences Blank, High School Form. J Consult Psychol 18:105–111, 1954

Sattler JM: Assessment of Children: Behavioral and Clinical Applications. San Diego, CA, JM Sattler, 2002

Semel E, Wiig EH, Secord WA: Clinical Evaluation of Language Fundamentals 3 (CELF-3). San Antonio, TX, Psychological Corporation, 1995

Sheslow D, Adams W: Wide Range Assessment of Memory and Learning: Administration Manual. New York, Jastak Assessment Systems, 1990

Sivan AB: Benton Visual Retention Test—Fifth Edition. Odessa, FL, Psychological Assessment Resources, 1991

Sparrow SS, Balla DA, Cicchetti D: Vineland Adaptive Behavior Scales—Interview Edition: Expanded and Survey Forms. Circle Pines, MN, American Guidance Service, 1984

Spreen O, Benton AL: Neurosensory Center Comprehensive Examination for Aphasia—Revised Edition (NCCEA). Victoria, BC, Canada, University of Victoria, 1977

Spreen O, Gaddes WH: Developmental norms for 15 neuropsychological tests age 6 to 15. Cortex 5:171–191, 1969

Stein MA, Pearl PL: How to conduct a feedback. ADHD Report 9:10–13, 1998

Stein MA, Szumowski E, Blondis T, et al: Adaptive skills dysfunction in ADD and ADHD Children. J Child Psychol Psychiatry 36:663–670, 1995

Stern W: The Psychological Methods of Testing Intelligence. Translated by Whipple WP. Baltimore, MD, Warwick & York, 1914

Stroop JR: Studies of interference in serial verbal reaction. J Exp Psychol 18:643–662, 1935

Tiffin J: Purdue Pegboard: Examiner Manual. Chicago, IL, Science Research Associates, 1968

Thorndike R, Hagen E, Sattler J: Technical Manual for Stanford-Binet Intelligence Scale, 4th Edition. Chicago, IL, Riverside, 1986

Waber DP, Holmes JM: Assessing children's copy product of the Rey-Osterrieth Complex Figure. J Clin Exp Neuropsychol 7:264–280, 1985

Waber DP, Holmes JM: Assessing children's memory productions of the Rey-Osterrieth Complex Figure. J Clin Exp Neuropsychol 8:565–580, 1986

Wechsler D: Wechsler Intelligence Scale for Children—3rd Edition. San Antonio, TX, Psychological Corporation, 1991

Wechsler D: Wechsler Abbreviated Scale of Intelligence (WASI). San Antonio, TX, Psychological Corporation, 1999

Wechsler D: Wechsler Individual Achievement Test—Second Edition (WIAT-II). San Antonio, TX, Psychological Corporation, 2001

Wechsler D: Wechsler Preschool and Primary Scale of Intelligence—Third Edition. San Antonio, TX, Psychological Corporation, 2002

Wiederholt JL, Bryant BR: Gray Oral Reading Test—Diagnostic. Austin, TX, PRO-ED, 1992

Wilkinsen GS: Wide Range Achievement Test (WRAT)—3rd Edition. Wilmington, DE, Wide Range, 1993

Wilson BC, Iacovello JM, Wilson JJ, et al: Purdue Pegboard performance of normal preschool children. J Clin Neuropsychol 4:19–26, 1982

Woodcock RW, McGrew K, Mather N: Woodcock-Johnson Psycho-Educational Battery—Third Edition. Itasca, IL, Riverside Publishing, 2002

Zigler E, Farber EA: Commonalities between the intellectual extremes: giftedness and mental retardation, in The Gifted and Talented: Developmental Perspectives. Edited by Horowitz FD, O'Brien M. Washington, DC, American Psychological Association, 1985, pp 387–408

Zigler E, Balla D, Hodapp R: On the definition and classification of mental retardation. American Journal of Mental Deficiency 89:215–230, 1984

Zimmerman IL, Steiner VG, Pond RE: Preschool Language Scale—3rd Edition. San Antonio, TX, Psychological Corporation, 1992

Laboratory and Diagnostic Testing

Robert L. Hendren, D.O.

XiaoYan He, M.D.

Systematic assessment and objective measurement are essential in psychiatric evaluation. A thorough review of the history and a clinical interview are cornerstones in the evaluation and management of behavioral and emotional disturbances in children. In addition, careful medical evaluation and laboratory testing are important for three reasons: 1) to identify an unrecognized medical condition that may be causing the psychiatric symptoms, 2) to determine baseline values of physiological parameters that may be affected by psychotropic medications, and 3) to identify any medical condition that may be complicated by medication treatment. With a rapidly growing number of tests and technical instruments available to physicians treating psychiatric disorders in both the hospital setting and outpatient practice, learning about and effectively using laboratory and diagnostic tests is challenging yet crucial. Decisions about testing must be made for individual circumstances because clear guidelines are rarely available. This chapter focuses on the utility of the more commonly considered laboratory tests and neuroimaging studies in both initial assessment and clinical management.

Laboratory Testing in Initial Assessment

■ Baseline Laboratory Tests

The potential value of a laboratory test depends on its sensitivity in detecting a specific disorder and the prevalence of the disorder in the relevant population. In the child or adolescent with negative medical history and physical examination findings for whom the expected risk for a specific medical disorder is low, the likelihood that a laboratory test will identify a true positive finding is minimal. However, when there is a positive medical history or physical findings suggesting a medical illness, specific laboratory tests should be used as clinically necessary. Some experts recommend the following laboratory tests as part of a comprehensive examination and/or premedication workup: 1) complete blood count (CBC), differential, and hematocrit; 2) urinalysis; 3) blood urea nitrogen (BUN) level; 4) serum electrolytes for sodium, potassium, chloride, calcium, phosphate, and carbon dioxide content; 5) liver function tests for aspartate aminotransferase (AST), alanine aminotransferase (ALT), alkaline phosphatase, and bilirubin; and 6) lead level in children younger than age 7 years when risk factors are present and in older children when indicated (Green 2001). However, the utility of routine laboratory tests is not clear. Sheline and Kehr (1990) studied 252 psychiatric inpatients to evaluate how often screening test findings revealed important clinical information. Although 49% of the patients had a coexisting medical illness, in only 6% did laboratory test findings lead to changes in clinical management. Anfinson and Kathol (1992) noted that whereas screening tests frequently generate abnormal results, in only 0.8%–4.0% are findings clinically significant. In their review, no specific laboratory tests were recommended on a routine basis.

Given this background, certain laboratory tests can provide valuable information to confirm or validate diagnoses. Careful consideration should be given to obtaining the following tests for individuals at increased risk for particular medical problems.

Hematological Measures

It is suggested that a CBC should always be a part of a routine screen (Green 2001). The CBC is sensitive to a wide range of medical problems that can cause, complicate, or mimic psychiatric conditions. Selective screening should be considered for individuals at increased risk for anemia, such as cow's milk–fed infants, toddlers, adolescent girls, pregnant teens, and recent immigrants from developing countries. Iron deficiency and iron deficiency anemia are still relatively common in toddlers, adolescent girls, and women of childbearing age (Ania et al. 1994). Anemia can be associated with a wide range of mental status changes, including asthenia, depression, and psychosis. Obtaining follow-up hematocrit and hemoglobin values is recommended if the screening red blood cell (RBC) count is abnormal. The white blood cell (WBC) count should be considered in the baseline screening before initiating certain psychotropic medications, such as clozapine, lithium, and carbamazepine, as well as in treatment monitoring. A WBC differential is recommended if clinical manifestations of infectious diseases or leukemia are present. Additional discussion of hematological measures can be found in Rosse et al. (1989) and Speicher (1998).

Biochemical Measures

Serum electrolytes. Neuropsychiatric complications may be the cause or result of serum electrolyte abnormalities. For instance, hyponatremia may be the result of the syndrome of inappropriate secretion of antidiuretic hormone (SIADH), psychogenic polydipsia, or carbamazepine use. Clinicians should consider the resulting hyponatremia as a possible cause of anorexia, depression, irritability, lethargy, or confusion. Another example is hypokalemia, which can be associated with significant weakness and electrocardiographic changes. When an adolescent girl presents with binge-purge behavior, self-induced vomiting, or laxative abuse, testing potassium level and treating hypokalemia can be lifesaving.

Renal Function Tests

Abnormal BUN levels may be associated with various mental status changes. For patients who are taking lithium, tests for BUN levels, creatinine clearance, and 24-hour urine protein levels are frequently used in pretreatment and follow-up evaluation. Urinalysis is important in the evaluation of certain organic mental disorders secondary to disorders such as diabetes, SIADH, and hepatobiliary disease.

Liver Function Tests

Abnormal liver enzyme values may be associated with certain psychiatric conditions. In patients with bulimia, testing for serum amylase levels has been proposed as a method to help monitor binge-purge activities. Baseline serum amylase levels for patients who engage in severe bingeing are reportedly higher than for control subjects without eating disorders or those with nonbulimic anorexia (Green 2001).

Baseline liver function should be assessed prior to initiating anticonvulsant treatment, especially valproate and carbamazepine therapy. Liver function should be monitored more often during the first several weeks of therapy and every 6–12 months afterward (Janicak et al. 2001).

Neuroendocrine Tests

Thyroid hormone is responsible for normal growth and development. Abnormalities in the concentration of thyroid hormones can result in psychiatric symptoms, including anxiety, depression, panic, restlessness, mental retardation, and psychosis. Laboratory tests to detect thyroid dysfunction include serum thyroxine (T_4), triiodothyronine (T_3), resin uptake, thyroid-stimulating hormone (TSH), and serum T_3 levels. Significant differences in basal thyroid hormone and T_4 elevations are reported in adolescents with depression and those with mania compared with control subjects (Sokolov et al. 1994). However, most studies report normal thyroid function (TSH) in depression in both adolescents (Khan 1987; Kutcher et al. 1991) and prepubertal children (Garcia et al. 1991).

Kutcher (1997) suggested that there is no evidence to support the use of basal neuroendocrine laboratory testing for either screening or diagnostic purposes in child and adolescent psychiatric patients. He further suggested that special stimulation tests, such as the dexamethasone suppression test (DST), the thyrotropin-releasing hormone (TRH) test, and the corticotropin-releasing hormone (CRH) test, have not demonstrated diagnostic validity for any child and adolescent psychiatric disorder. However, if family and clinical history or physical examination findings indicate a possible thyroid disorder, a screening test for T_4 and T_3 resin uptake are recommended (Leo et al. 1997).

Abnormal thyroid function can result in behavior that may resemble attention-deficit/hyperactivity disorder (ADHD; Weiss and Stein 1999). Three thyroid disorders have been reported to be associated with ADHD-like symptoms: hyperthyroidism, hypothyroidism, and the syndrome of resistance to thyroid hormone (Pear et al. 2001). Several studies have concluded that routine TSH screening in children with nonfamilial ADHD is not indicated (Elia et al. 1994; Toren et al. 1997; Valentine et al. 1997). However, it is indicated for children with a family history of thyroid disorder or physical signs of goiter, low birth weight, growth retardation, and speech and hearing impairment (Zametkin et al. 1998).

Other neuroendocrine tests, including those for plasma cortisol and catecholamines, amylase and lipase, antidiuretic hormone (ADH), growth hormone, prolactin, and testosterone and estrogen, are used for evaluation of a variety of endocrine disorders that may manifest as psychiatric symptoms.

Baseline Drug Screening

Serum toxicology and urine toxicology are commonly used to determine whether a patient is using one or more psychoactive substances. Drug screening is limited by the time needed to obtain results and the risk of false-positive and false-negative results. Positive results may not prove substance abuse or dependence but do indicate substance use. Negative results are not sufficient to rule out substance use. A positive result on an immunoassay screen test should be followed by confirmation by a more sensitive method (Bukstein 1997). A drug screen should be requested for adolescents who present with new-onset psychosis, behavioral changes, or severe anxiety, and when substance abuse is suspected.

Baseline Electrocardiogram

Various medical conditions and psychotropic medications predispose patients to cardiac risks. Baseline electrocardiography (ECG) should be considered when elements of risk are present. For instance, a pretreatment electrocardiogram should be obtained for patients with known cardiac disease or at high cardiac risk (e.g., family history of sudden death or cardiac arrhythmia, hypertension, or cardiac diseases) when psychotropic medication with cardiac effects is being considered. Some antipsychotics, especially thioridazine,

are known to cause QTc interval prolongation. Ziprasidone is a newer atypical antipsychotic medication that prolongs QT interval more than do haloperidol, olanzapine, quetiapine, and risperidone but less than do mesoridazine and thioridazine (FDA 2000). Data on the effect of ziprasidone on ECG indicate an approximately 20-ms increase in the QT interval but no cases of mortality from overdose, torsade de pointes, or excess in sudden death and unexpected deaths (Goodnick 2001). However, it is important to ask apparently healthy patients if they have had syncope, a family history of sudden death, or long QT syndrome. If any of these are present, a pretreatment electrocardiogram should be obtained (Glassman and Bigger 2001). Tricyclic antidepressants (TCAs) can cause cardiac arrhythmia, so ECG should be considered to monitor possible adverse effects on cardiac function with these medications.

There is some controversy about cardiac monitoring with α-adrenergic agents such as clonidine. The American Academy of Child and Adolescent Psychiatry practice parameters for ADHD (Dulcan 1997) suggest baseline and monitoring ECG, whereas the American Heart Association says this is not necessary (Gutgesell et al. 1999).

■ Special Populations

Suicide Attempters

Clinicians should order blood toxicology workups for patients who have overdosed on prescribed or abused drugs. The severity of specific organ involvement can be assessed by the appropriate tests. An electrocardiogram should be obtained for patients who have overdosed with a TCA. Liver function tests are important for assessing patients who have overdosed with acetaminophen, and serum electrolyte values are needed to assess anion gap in cases of aspirin overdose. Radiological assessment may help evaluate damage caused by a self-inflicted injury.

Children With Unexplained Weight Loss

Children and adolescents with a history of starvation, bingeing, and/or purging who are being evaluated for symptoms of weight loss, depression, or anxiety need a medical and laboratory assessment to determine the degree of weight loss and to identify a potential medical emergency, especially for those with a history of anorexia nervosa and/or bulimia nervosa.

Hypercarotenemia is a common finding in patients with anorexia nervosa, especially in those in the restrictor subtype. Measuring serum beta-carotene value in patients with restricting or purging anorexia provides supporting evidence for the diagnosis, especially in atypical presentations (Boland et al. 2001). However, the significance of elevated beta-carotene levels for prognosis and treatment of anorexia nervosa is unproven. Recent research implicates an association of disturbed neuropeptide Y release and pathological behavior in patients with bulimia nervosa. Significantly higher levels of plasma leptin and neuropeptide Y in patients with bulimia and significantly lower levels in patients with anorexia than in control subjects have also been reported (Baranowska et al. 2001). Nevertheless, measurement of neuropeptide Y in children and adolescents with eating disorders is not recommended for diagnosis or treatment. Increased serum cholesterol and decreased free T_4 levels are found in patients with bulimia nervosa; however, the mechanism and consequences of the abnormality are uncertain (Pauporte and Walsh 2001).

Patients with anorexia nervosa often have functional cardiac abnormalities secondary to their nutritional depletion, including decreased left ventricular mass and varying degrees of left ventricular systolic dysfunction. A study measuring myocardial performance index (MPI) for global ventricular function in patients with anorexia nervosa (Eidem et al. 2001) found a significantly elevated left ventricular MPI, which indicated a subclinical degree of ventricular impairment. The study suggested the potential clinical utility of MPI in the early identification of subclinical left ventricular dysfunction in patients with anorexia nervosa.

Serum and urine electrolyte tests should be used routinely in assessment of children and adolescents with weight loss. Laboratory screening for serum hypokalemia and hypochloremia should be considered for individuals with bulimia nervosa (Wolfe et al. 2001). The ratio of urine sodium to chloride has been reported to predict bulimic behavior (Crow et al. 2001) better than do traditional screening tests such as that for serum hypokalemia.

For patients with eating disorders, a CBC with differential count should be obtained to monitor anemia and leukopenia, as should findings for serum electrolyte (especially potassium and BUN) and amylase levels and urinalysis (Rosse et al. 1989). Additional tests, including ECG and TSH and those for other pituitary hormones, may be useful to assess effects of starvation, laxative abuse, dehydration, and abnormal electrolyte levels.

An enlarged parotid gland associated with an elevated amylase level is commonly observed in patients who binge and vomit. The serum amylase level is an excellent way to monitor vomiting in patients with bulimia who deny purging (Halmi 1999).

Profound osteopenia is a serious complication of anorexia nervosa. Patients with anorexia nervosa are at high risk for fracture (Espallargues et al. 2001) and osteoporosis (Zipfel et al. 2001). The clinician who treats adolescents with eating disorders should educate them regarding the danger of bone fragility and the risk of fracture and should consider X-ray examination to determine the reduction of bone density and size if the patient's history and condition indicate.

Children With Neurodevelopmental Disorders

The benefits of genetic diagnosis in children with neurodevelopmental disorders include 1) recognition of recurrent risk, which is useful in genetic counseling; 2) prediction of prognosis; 3) elimination of unnecessary laboratory tests; 4) establishment of guidelines for disorder management; and 5) family support (i.e., cooperation with family's request to identify etiologic factors) (Carey and McMahon 1999).

In fragile X syndrome, a fragile site on the X chromosome is usually detected by cytogenetic testing in individuals with mental retardation but not in the individuals with only emotional or learning problems. With the discovery of the *FMR1* gene, DNA testing can identify not only individuals affected by fragile X syndrome but also all carriers. Screening schoolchildren with learning disabilities for fragile X syndrome has been suggested (Slaney et al. 1995), and a saliva DNA test as an alternative to the blood DNA test for such a screening program has been evaluated (Hagerman et al. 1994).

Examination of karyotype (morphology and number of chromosomes) is important in the evaluation of possible sex chromosomal abnormality. Girls with an abnormal number of X chromosomes have psychosocial, educational, and behavioral problems. In Turner syndrome (45, XO), deficits in nonverbal abilities, visuospatial processing, visual memory, and visual construction are clear and consistent findings. These individuals have lower self-esteem, poor peer relationships and social skills, and short attention span. Boys with Klinefelter syndrome (47, XXY) have cognitive deficits in verbal ability and language processing.

Prader-Willi syndrome is caused by absence of the normally active paternal inherited gene at chromosome 15 (q11–13) region, or by deletion. Prader-Willi syndrome can be diagnosed most efficiently by a molecular diagnostic test using southern hybridization and methylation-sensitive probes, fluorescent in situ hybridization, and polymerase chain reaction technique (Dykins and Cassidy 1999). Establishing the diagnosis of Williams syndrome is another example of the clinical benefit of molecular genetics in child and adolescent psychiatry (Morris and Mervis 1999).

Wilson's disease is an autosomal-recessive inherited disorder of abnormal copper metabolism, which results in decreased intellectual functioning, inappropriate behavior, anxiety, depression, psychosis, and movement disorder. However, it is not diagnosed by genetic tests. Serum ceruloplasmin, serum, and urine copper tests are usually used to evaluate patients for Wilson's disease. It is critical for clinicians to consider Wilson's disease in the differential diagnosis of psychotic young adults with a movement disorder, because the disease is treatable.

Neuroimaging and Electroencephalographic Evaluation

Neuroimaging technology, including structural magnetic resonance imaging (MRI), magnetic resonance spectroscopy (MRS), functional MRI, positron emission tomography (PET), and single-photon emission computed tomography (SPECT), have great promise for neurodevelopmental diagnosis and treatment, but they are not yet valid diagnostic instruments in child and adolescent psychiatry (Hendren et al. 2000). Although each of these modalities has particular advantages in biomedical research, magnetic resonance technology is the most suited to assessment and research in child and adolescent psychiatry (Pine 2001). In clinical practice, use of MRI should be seriously considered in all cases in which there is a rapid onset of severe psychopathology, in which there are significant abnormal findings on neurological examination, in which there are seizures, or in which certain genetic syndromes are present (Hoon and Melhem 2000).

Neuroimaging may become useful in early identification of psychiatric disorders, determining the diagnosis, treatment matching, and prognosis prediction and thus improving outcomes (Nemeroff 2001). Difficulties with neuroimaging research that limit its routine application currently include inadequate normative data; imprecise definitions of structures measured; nonstandardized and slow, tedious measurements; vague hypotheses; and lack of control for age, sex, and diagnostic imprecision.

Structural MRI creates images of brain structures that can be measured to determine volumes in a region of interest (Frank and Pavlakis 2001). Structural changes occur over months and years in psychiatric disorders. MRS is a measure of metabolism and reflects changes that occur over weeks and months (Stoll et al. 2000). Functional MRI measures oxygen consumption in brain regions of interest and reflects changes that occur over minutes or hours on the basis of a task–response paradigm (O'Tuama et al. 1999).

PET has limited use in children because of the expense and risk associated with the isotopes necessary for the procedure and the paucity of children without a disorder who have been studied as normal control subjects (O'Tuama et al. 1999). SPECT uses less radioactive isotope and is therefore less expensive and has less perceived risk in children, but it does not have the spatial resolution of PET. Although some authors promote the use of SPECT in diagnosis and treatment matching (Amen 2001), there are no analyses in the scientific peer-reviewed literature of the validity of SPECT for this purpose.

Electroencephalography (EEG) is indicated when a seizure disorder is a possibility and may identify relationships to decreased cognitive function (Ballaban-Gil and Tuchman 2000). Minor, nonspecific abnormalities occur in up to 30% of children and do not require treatment. Quantitative EEG may play a role in the evaluation of youngsters with learning disorders and ADHD (Chabot et al. 2001), but it is not in common use. Magnetoencephalography uses magnetic resonance technology that allows electroencephalographic evaluation of deeper limbic structures than is possible with conventional EEG (Otsubo and Snead 2001). However, the technique has not yet fully found its place in child psychiatry research.

Laboratory Tests in Treatment Management

One of the goals of initial laboratory testing is to obtain baseline information for patients who are likely to receive psychotropic medications. Following are guidelines for monitoring several commonly used psychotropic medications.

■ Tricyclic Antidepressants

TCAs are commonly associated with adverse effects on blood pressure and heart rate (Walsh et al. 1999). Pretreatment baseline measurement and regular monitoring of blood pressure, pulse, and ECG are therefore essential. Biederman et al. (1995) reported desipramine-associated sudden death in children between ages 4 and 14 years, which has led to a careful examination of the potential cardiac effects of tricyclics in children. Several subsequent reports of sudden death associated with imipramine and desipramine (Varley and McClellan 1997) have further increased interest in investigation of TCAs' cardiac effects in children and adolescents.

Johnson et al. (1996) found no consistent pattern of electrocardiographic interval changes related to dosage, age, treatment duration, or plasma levels of desipramine and imipramine in children. Although some argue that ECG should not be routinely used until the dose is above 2.5–3.5 mg/kg, it is recommended currently that routine ECG be done before initiating TCA treatment and that follow-up ECG be done when clinically indicated (Zametkin et al. 1998).

The American Psychiatric Association Task Force on the Use of Laboratory Tests in Psychiatry (1985) concluded that blood-level measurements of TCAs are unequivocally useful. TCA blood level might be ordered for 1) patients who have questionable compliance, 2) patients who have a poor response to a "typical" dose, 3) patients who experience side effects at a very low dose, 4) patients who are potentially very sensitive to side effects, and 5) patients for whom treatment is urgent and who require a potentially therapeutic medication level in as short a time as possible. Therapeutic blood levels of TCA are described by the task force as follows: Total imipramine and its metabolite, desmethylimipramine, should exceed 150 ng/mL; for nortriptyline, a therapeutic range is between 50 and 150 ng/mL; for desipramine, the therapeutic level should be above 125 ng/mL. TCA blood levels are generally obtained 9–12 hours after the last dose, and blood for determining them should be drawn when TCA dosage is at a steady state (at least 5 days after initiation or change in medication dosage).

■ Selective Serotonin Reuptake Inhibitors, Monoamine Oxidase Inhibitors, Neuroleptics, and Stimulants

Currently, no baseline laboratory tests are indicated before the initiation of selective serotonin reuptake inhibitors or monoamine oxidase inhibitors if findings from the review of systems are negative for medical disorders. A urine pregnancy test should be ordered for a sexually active female adolescent. For patients who are about to take neuroleptics, especially pimozide and clozapine, a CBC, liver function test, and electrocardiogram are necessary for monitoring their adverse effects. No laboratory tests are indicated for routine use of stimulants. However, with evidence linking pemoline to liver failure (Marotta and Roberts 1998; Safer et al. 2001), a baseline liver function test should be obtained and liver function should be closely monitored; parents and patients should be educated about the risks and the signs and symptoms of liver toxicity (Adcock et al. 1998).

■ Lithium

Lithium can have significant adverse effects on the thyroid, kidney, heart, and developing fetus and may cause a benign elevation of the CBC. It is recommended that pretreatment evaluation include a CBC, serum electrolytes test, BUN test, serum creatinine test, thyroid function tests, urinalysis, and an electrocardiogram (Morihisa et al. 1999). For sexually active female patients, a urine pregnancy test should be ordered.

For acute mania, a therapeutic lithium level is suggested for adults, from a lower range of 0.8–1.0 mEq/L to an upper range of 1.4–1.5 mEq/L (Carroll et al. 1987), but no therapeutic range is established for children and adolescents. A steady-state lithium level is generally obtained 4 or 5 days after the last dosage change. The lithium blood level should be checked every 5 days until an adequate therapeutic concentration is achieved or adverse effects preclude further increases (Janicak et al. 2001). For maintenance therapy, lower lithium levels of 0.6–1.0 mEq/L are recommended (Gelenberg et al. 1989).

The optimal frequency of follow-up laboratory tests has not been established. However, laboratory work is warranted if adverse effects increase or the patient's health status changes.

■ Anticonvulsants

Carbamazepine has been implicated in aplastic anemia, leukopenia, thrombocytopenia, and anemia as well as slow atrioventricular conduction. Pretreatment laboratory work should include liver function tests, an electrocardiogram, and hematological measures, including CBC and platelet count, serum iron assay, and reticulocyte count. Hematological measures should be repeated weekly for the first 3 months of treatment because of the risk of carbamazepine-related aplastic anemia, agranulocytosis, leukopenia, and thrombocytopenia (Zametkin et al. 1998). A urine pregnancy test should be obtained for sexually active teenagers. A CBC should be immediately obtained if there are any signs or symptoms of bone marrow suppression such as fever, malaise, sore throat, and petechiae. A therapeutic carbamazepine level for psychiatric disorders has not been established, but a laboratory level of 8–12 ng/mL is used when treating partial complex seizures. Carbamazepine level monitoring, especially in the first several weeks of therapy, is crucial because of the phenomenon of autometabolism and potential drug interactions.

For patients taking valproic acid, baseline liver function tests are recommended because of potential hepatotoxicity. An elevated incidence of birth defects in children whose mothers took valproic acid prior to or during their pregnancy suggests that a urine pregnancy test should always be obtained before initiation of treatment. A therapeutic level of 50–125 µg/mL for the treatment of mania has been suggested (Bowden et al. 1996). Measuring the serum level of valproic acid is important for predicting adverse effects and monitoring compliance.

References

Adcock KG, MacElroy DE, Wolford ET, et al: Pemoline therapy resulting in liver transplantation. Ann Pharmacother 32:422–425, 1998

Amen DG: Why don't psychiatrists look at the brain? NeuroPsychiatry Reviews 2:1,19–21, 2001

American Psychiatric Association Task Force on the Use of Laboratory Tests in Psychiatry: Tricyclic antidepressants blood level measurements and clinical outcome: an APA Task Force report. Am J Psychiatry 142:155–162, 1985

Anfinson TJ, Kathol RG: Screening laboratory evaluation in psychiatric patients: a review. Gen Hosp Psychiatry 14:248–257, 1992

Ania BJ, Suman VJ, Fairbanks VF, et al: Prevalence of anemia in medical practice: community versus referral patients. Mayo Clin Proc 69:730–733, 1994

Ballaban-Gil K, Tuchman R: Epilepsy and epileptiform EEG: association with autism and language disorders. Ment Retard Dev Disabil Res Rev 6:300–308, 2000

Baranowska B, Wolinska-Witort E, Wasilewska-Dziubinska E, et al: Plasma leptin, neuropeptide Y (NPY) and galanin concentrations in bulimia nervosa and in anorexia nervosa. Neuroendocrinol Lett 22:365–358, 2001

Biederman J, Thisted RA, Greenhill LL, et al: Estimation of the association between desipramine and the risk for sudden death in 5- to 14-year-old children. J Clin Psychiatry 56:87–93, 1995

Boland BB, Beguin C, Zech F, et al: Serum beta-carotene in anorexia nervosa patients: a case-control study. Int J Eat Disord 30: 299–305, 2001

Bowden CL, Janicak PG, Orsulak P, et al: Relationship of serum valproate concentration to response in mania. Am J Psychiatry 153:765–770, 1996

Bukstein O: Practice parameters for the assessment and treatment of children and adolescents with substance use disorders. J Am Acad Child Adolesc Psychiatry 36(10 suppl):140S–156S, 1997

Carey JC, McMahon WM: Neurobehavioral disorders and medical genetics, in Handbook of Neurodevelopmental and Genetic Disorders in Children. Edited by Goldstein S, Reynolds CR. New York, Guilford, 1999, pp 38–60

Carroll JA, Jefferson JW, Greist JH: Psychiatric uses of lithium for children and adolescents. Hosp Community Psychiatry 38:927–928, 1987

Chabot RJ, diMichele F, Prichep L, et al: The clinical role of computerized EEG in the evaluation and treatment of learning and attention disorders in children and adolescents. J Neuropsychiatry Clin Neurosci 13:171–186, 2001

Crow SJ, Rosenberg ME, Mitchell JE, et al: Urine electrolytes as markers of bulimia nervosa. Int J Eat Disord 30:279–287, 2001

Dulcan M: Practice parameters for the assessment and treatment of children, adolescents, and adults with attention-deficit/hyperactivity disorder. J Am Acad Child Adolesc Psychiatry 36(10 suppl):85S–121S, 1997

Dykins EM, Cassidy SB: Prader-Willi syndrome, in Handbook of Neurodevelopmental and Genetic Disorders in Children. Edited by Goldstein S, Reynolds CR. New York, Guilford, 1999, pp 525–554

Eidem BW, Cetta F, Webb JL, et al: Early detection of cardiac dysfunction: use of the myocardial performance index in patients with anorexia nervosa. J Adolesc Health 29:267–270, 2001

Elia J, Gulotta C, Rose SR, et al: Thyroid function and attention-deficit/hyperactivity disorder. J Am Acad Child Adolesc Psychiatry 33:169–172, 1994

Espallargues M, Sampietro-Colom L, Estrada MD, et al: Identify bone mass–related risk factors for fracture to guide bone densitometry measurements: a systematic review of the literature. Osteoporos Int 2:811–822, 2001

FDA Briefing Document for Zeldox Capsules (Ziprasidone). New York, Pfizer Inc, July 18, 2000, p 116

Frank Y, Pavlakis SG: Brain imaging in neurobehavioral disorders. Pediatr Neurol 25:278–287, 2001

Garcia MR, Ryan ND, Rabinovitch H, et al: Thyroid stimulating hormone response to thyrotropin in prepubertal depression. J Am Acad Child Adolesc Psychiatry 30:398–406, 1991

Gelenberg AJ, Kane JM, Keller MB, et al: Comparison of standard and low levels of lithium for maintenance treatment of bipolar disorder. N Engl J Med 321:1489–1493, 1989

Glassman AH, Bigger TJ Jr: Antipsychotic drugs: prolonged QTc interval, torsade de pointes, and sudden death. Am J Psychiatry 158:1774–1782, 2001

Goodnick PJ:. Ziprasidone: profile on safety. Expert Opin Pharmacother 2:1655–1662, 2001

Green WH: Child and Adolescent Clinical Psychopharmacology, 3rd Edition. Philadelphia, PA, Lippincott Williams & Wilkins, 2001, pp 22–26

Gutgesell H, Atkins D, Barst R, et al: AHA Scientific Statement: cardiovascular monitoring of children and adolescents receiving psychotropic drugs. J Am Acad Child Adolesc Psychiatry 38:1047–1050, 1999

Hagerman RJ, Wilson P, Staney LW, et al: Evaluation of school children at high risk for fragile X syndrome utilizing buccal cell FMR-1 testing. Am J Med Genet 51:474–481, 1994

Halmi KA: Eating disorders: anorexia nervosa, bulimia nervosa, and obesity, in Textbook of Psychiatry, 3rd Edition. Edited by Hales RE, Yudofsky SC, Talbott JA. Washington, DC, American Psychiatric Press, 1999, pp 983–1002

Hendren RL, DeBacker I, Pandina G: Review of neuroimaging studies of child and adolescent psychiatric disorders from the past ten years. J Am Acad Child Adolesc Psychiatry 39:815–828, 2000

Hoon AH, Melhem ER: Neuroimaging: applications in disorders of early brain development. J Dev Behav Pediatr 21:291–302, 2000

Janicak PG, Davis JM, Preskorn SH, et al: Principles and Practice of Psychopharmacotherapy, 3rd Edition. Philadelphia, PA, Lippincott Williams & Wilkins, 2001

Johnson A, Guiffre RM, O'Malley K: ECG changes in pediatric patients on tricyclic antidepressants, desipramine, and imipramine. Can J Psychiatry 41:102–106, 1996

Khan AU: Biochemical profile of depressed adolescents. J Am Acad Child Adolesc Psychiatry 26:873–878, 1987

Kutcher SP: Child and Adolescent Psychopharmacology. Philadelphia, PA, WB Saunders, 1997

Kutcher S, Malkin D. Silverberg J, et al: Nocturnal cortisol, thyroid stimulating hormone, and growth hormone secretory profiles in depressed adolescents. J Am Acad Child Adolesc Psychiatry 30:407–414, 1991

Leo RJ, Batterman-Faunce JM, Pickhardt D, et al: Utility of thyroid screening in adolescent psychiatric inpatients. J Am Acad Child Psychiatry 36:103–111, 1997

Marotta PJ, Roberts EA: Pemoline hepatotoxicity in children. J Pediatr 132:894–897, 1998

Morihisa JM, Rosse RB, Cross CD, et al: Laboratory and other diagnostic tests in psychiatry, in Textbook of Psychiatry, 3rd Edition. Edited by Hales RE, Yudofsky SC, Talbott JA. Washington DC, American Psychiatric Press, 1999, pp 281–316

Morris CA, Mervis CB: Williams syndrome, in Handbook of Neurodevelopmental and Genetic Disorders in Children. Edited by Goldstein S, Reynolds CR. New York, Guilford, 1999, pp 555–590

Nemeroff CB: The development of new technologies in medicine: what will the impact be in psychiatry? CNS Spectrums 6:21, 2001

Otsubo H, Snead OC: Magnetoencephalography and magnetic source imaging in children. J Child Neurol 16:227–235, 2001

O'Tuama LA, Dickstein DP, Neeper R, et al: Functional brain imaging in neuropsychiatric disorders of childhood. Child Neurol 14:207–221, 1999

Pauporte J, Walsh BT: Serum cholesterol in bulimia nervosa. Int J Eat Disord 30:294–298, 2001

Pear PL, Weiss RE, Stein MA: Medical mimics: medical and neurological conditions simulating ADHD. Ann N Y Acad Sci 931:97–112, 2001

Pine DS: Functional magnetic resonance imaging in children and adolescents, in Advances in Brain Imaging. Edited by Morihisa JM. (Review of Psychiatry Series, Vol 20, No 4; Oldham JM, Riba MB, series editors.) Washington, DC, American Psychiatric Publishing, 2001, pp 53–82

Rosse RB, Giese AA, Deutsch SI, et al: A Concise Guide to Laboratory and Diagnostic Testing in Psychiatry. Washington, DC, American Psychiatric Association, 1989

Safer DJ, Zito JM, Gardner JE: Pemoline hepatotoxicity and postmarketing surveillance. J Am Acad Child Adolesc Psychiatry 40:622–629, 2001

Sheline Y, Kehr C: Cost and utility of routine admission laboratory testing for psychiatric inpatients. Gen Hosp Psychiatry 12:329–334, 1990

Slaney SF, Wilkie AOM, Hirst MC, et al: DNA testing for fragile X syndrome in schools for learning difficulties. Arch Dis Child 72:33–37, 1995

Sokolov S, Kutcher S, Joffe R: Basal thyroid indices in adolescent depression and bipolar disorder. J Am Acad Child Adolesc Psychiatry 33:469–475, 1994

Speicher CE: The Right Test: A Physician's Guide to Laboratory Medicine, 3rd Edition. Philadelphia, PA, WB Saunders, 1998

Stoll AL, Renshaw PF, Yurgelunn-Todd DA, et al: Neuroimaging in bipolar disorder: what have we learned? Biol Psychiatry 48:505–517, 2000

Toren P, Karasik A, Eldar S, et al: Thyroid function in attention deficit hyperactivity disorder. J Psychiatr Res 31:359–363, 1997

Valentine J, Rossi E, O'Leary P, et al: Thyroid function in a population of children with attention deficit hyperactivity disorder. J Paediatr Child Health 33:117–120, 1997

Varley CK, McClellan J: Case study: two additional sudden deaths with tricyclic antidepressants. J Am Acad Child Adolesc Psychiatry 36:390–394, 1997

Walsh BT, Greenhill LL, Giardina EG, et al: Effects of desipramine on autonomic input of the heart. J Am Acad Child Adolesc Psychiatry 38:1186–1192, 1999

Weiss RE, Stein MA: Thyroid function and attention deficit hyperactivity disorder, in Attention Deficit Disorders and Hyperactivity in Children and Adults. Edited by Accardo PJ, Blondis TA, Whitman BY, et al. New York, Marcel Dekker, 1999, pp 419–430

Wolfe BE, Metger ED, Levine JM, et al: Laboratory screening for electrolyte abnormalities and anemia in bulimia nervosa: a controlled study. Int J Eat Disord 30:288–293, 2001

Zametkin AJ, Ernst M, Silver R: Laboratory and diagnostic testing in child and adolescent psychiatry. J Am Acad Child Adolesc Psychiatry 37:464–472, 1998

Zipfel S, Seibel MJ, Lowe B, et al: Osteoporosis in eating disorders: a follow-up study of patients with anorexia and bulimia nervosa. J Clin Endocrinol Metab 86:5227–5233, 2001

Clinical Genomic Testing

16

David A. Mrazek, M.D., F.R.C.Psych.

The use of genotyping to improve psychopharmacological treatment has reached a new level of feasibility and usefulness. Considerable progress has also been made in linking atypical polymorphisms to traditional psychotic diagnoses. In the early 1990s, genetic testing could clarify the diagnosis of phenylketonuria and fragile X syndrome, but testing provided little insight into the treatment of most child psychiatric patients. With the development of low-cost, high-throughput genotyping, pharmacogenomics has increasingly become a practical adjunct to medication management and is now available at a number of major academic medical centers. With the continued development of microarray technologies, it will soon be practical to routinely genotype multiple genes that code for neurotransporters, neurotransmitter receptors, and the enzymes that metabolize psychotropic medications. These results will make it possible to individualize the selection of appropriate psychotropic medications.

Overwhelming evidence has established the heritability of the majority of child and adolescent disorders. However, psychiatric illnesses are complex in nature; very few psychiatric syndromes are the result of a single gene mutation. This chapter considers polymorphisms of known susceptibility genes that have been shown to affect psychopharmacotherapy:

- Cytochrome P450 genes, which affect the treatment of children requiring psychotropic medications
- The dopamine transporter and dopamine receptor, which affect the treatment response of children with attention-deficit/hyperactivity disorder (ADHD)
- The serotonin transporter gene
- The serotonin receptor gene
- The tryptophan hydroxylase (*TPH*) gene and catecholamine-*O*-methyltransferase (*COMT*) genes, which are associated with an increased risk of suicide

This chapter also discusses the ethical issues that have been raised as a consequence of our current ability to identify children at increased risk for differential medication response. Testing in adolescence for the gene responsible for Huntington's disease is considered as a model for ethical decision making.

It is well established that virtually all common psychiatric illnesses are, to some degree, heritable. However, environmental factors play a significant role in the expression of all of these disorders. The classic literature supporting this position has been well reviewed (Rutter et al. 1999a, 1999b). The research designs that have been used to establish heritability have predominantly been twin studies. However, adoption studies have also been helpful because this design provides a unique opportunity to examine gene–environment interactions. Finally, informative family studies continue to be useful in the clarification of differential patterns of transmission.

No common child psychiatric disease is the result of a single atypical gene. However, many forms of mental retardation are the result of chromosomal abnormalities. Classic examples are Down syndrome and fragile X syndrome. Huntington's disease remains the best example of a single autosomal gene polymorphism that affects mental status.

Polymorphisms Associated With Complex Psychiatric Illnesses

Traditional psychiatric illnesses, such as ADHD, depression, autism, and bipolar disorder, are genetically complex illnesses. These diseases occur as a result of the interaction of many atypical gene products that are derived from multiple genes. Although this conceptual framework has been evolving since the 1990s, the insight that psychiatric illnesses are the result of the interactions of a discrete set of definable atypical gene products represents a distinctly new frame of reference.

ADHD provides a good model to illustrate these principles. This disorder has been traditionally defined as requiring six of nine symptoms of inattention or six of nine symptoms of hyperactivity and impulsiveness. By definition, two children could carry this diagnosis and have only three symptoms in common. Furthermore, many of these symptoms, such as "talks excessively," are nonspecific and often occur as isolated difficulties in children with no psychiatric disorder. Thus, from a genetic perspective, the phenotype of ADHD is extremely variable. As a consequence of our current diagnostic practice, children with many different biological characteristics are grouped together as having an ADHD diagnosis.

Until quite recently, the molecular genetic research methodologies used to study the genetic basis of psychiatric diseases were those that had been effectively employed to find genes that were associated with a discrete phenotype such as cystic fibrosis. It has gradually been understood that these designs are not appropriate for the study of diseases that are the result of multiple gene interactions. The application of these single-gene analytic strategies to study complex illnesses has led to the reporting of inconsistent results that have varied across geographic populations and ethnic groups. More recently, the simultaneous measurement of many genes has been advocated by an increasing number of investigators (Comings et al. 2000a, 2000b, 2001). Although there continue to be major problems in the interpretation of the data derived from the genotyping of multiple susceptibility genes, this strategy is conceptually innovative and, for the first time, allows for the discovery of gene–gene interactions.

The distinction between a candidate gene and susceptibility gene has not been consistently articulated in the literature. However, a susceptibility gene for a complex disorder represents only a component of the cause of the illness. In contrast, the term *candidate gene* has often been used to refer to a single gene that is believed to be linked to a specific illness. Traditionally investigators have searched for *the* gene that is responsible for depression or autism. Given that multiple genes are almost certainly responsible for these illnesses, the search for a single candidate gene has not been very successful.

Diagnostic genomic testing is justified on the basis of clinical utility. The results of the testing must provide a clinical course of action based on a more precise understanding of the genomic characterization for an individual patient. In the case of pharmacogenomics, there is now a consensus that such testing is indicated to achieve specific clinical goals (Lerer 2002).

■ Cytochrome P450 Genes

The *2D6* gene, a P450 gene that codes for the 2D6 enzyme, is located on the long arm of the twenty-second chromosome (22g13.1). The 2D6 enzyme is primarily responsible for the metabolism of fluoxetine, paroxetine, clomipramine, desipramine, amitriptyline, nortriptyline, and risperidone and plays an important role in the metabolism of many other psychotropic medications. Given the frequency with which these medications are prescribed in the treatment of children with mood or anxiety disorders, atypical metabolism of these medications can have significant clinical implications.

The *2D6* gene is one of the most highly variable genes that is commonly genotyped. More than 70 variants have been reported, and there is great variation in the frequency of these atypical alleles in different ethnic groups. In Caucasian samples, the range of patients who have one of the atypical *2D6* polymorphisms associated with poor metabolism is between 5% and 10%, depending on the precise ethnic background of the individual patient. In contrast, relatively few Asians have *2D6* polymorphisms that result in poor metabolism, but many have alleles that modestly decrease the rate of metabolism. Even beyond these pharmacogenomic implications of *2D6* genomic variation, independent links have been demonstrated with clinical symptoms, such as dyskinesias associated with treatment with antipsychotics (Ellingrod et al. 2000).

A classic indication for pharmacogenomic testing is to prevent toxic drug reactions. Given the relatively high percentage of the population that has atypical 2D6 enzyme activity and that these individuals will have atypical serum levels of many psychotropic medications, identifying poor 2D6 metabolizers to avoid negative medication reactions is a clear indication for genomic testing. The 2D6 enzyme produced by the *2D6* gene metabolizes more than a dozen psychotropic medications. The 2D6 enzyme also metabolizes codeine, which is frequently used to control moderate pain, and dextromethorphan, which is a popular cough suppressant (Lin et al. 2001). Some advocates of pharmacogenomic testing have suggested that the time has come for all individuals to know the status of their *2D6* genes, given the large number of drugs that are metabolized by the 2D6 enzyme.

The psychiatric treatment strategies available to manage treatment of those with poor metabolism must be different than for those with normal alleles (Coutts and Urichuk 1999; Kirchheiner et al. 2001). The dangers of using drugs metabolized by the 2D6 enzymes in young children are greater than in adults because young children are less able to identify side effects or to independently discontinue medications when they begin to develop toxic symptoms. This clinical concern is illustrated by the case example below, in which the reported death from fluoxetine toxicity of a 9-year-old child highlights the potential risks of using medications in patients with atypical metabolism (Sallee et al. 2000).

> Clinical signs of toxicity were misinterpreted as being the expression of a seizure-related syndrome. Unfortunately, before the origin of the seizures was determined, the child went into status epilepticus followed by cardiac arrest. At autopsy, serum levels of fluoxetine and its princip[al] active metabolite, norfluoxetine, were sevenfold greater than expected. Genotypic analysis of tissue obtained at autopsy revealed that the child was homozygous for a *2D6* polymorphism that was functionally inactive and consequently the child was unable to produce any active enzyme to metabolize the fluoxetine.

Other cytochrome P450 genes that have clinical psychiatric relevance include *1A2*, *2B6*, *2C19*, *2C9*, and *3A4*. The specific influences of the allelic variations of each of these genes are beyond the scope of this chapter. However, the ability to genotype the entire family of P450 genes is an important step in being able to select the most appropriate psychotropic medication for each individual patient. The clinical significance of this new technology is reflected in the suggestion that individuals obtain a P450 "passport" that could be determined in childhood and would subsequently be made available to the patient's physicians in the same way that information regarding blood type is certified (Brockmoller et al. 2000).

■ The Dopamine Transporter and Dopamine Receptor Genes

Dopamine Transporter Gene

The dopamine transporter (*DAT1*) gene is located on the short arm of the fifth chromosome at 5p15.3. A specific polymorphism of the *DAT1* gene has been found to occur more frequently in children with ADHD (Cook et al. 1995). Specifically, a form of the gene that was created as a result of the insertion of 10 repetitions of the same three nucleotides was found to be associated with ADHD symptoms. This finding has been confirmed by a number of other teams of investigators (Gill et al. 1997; Waldman et al. 1998). More recently, this "ten-repeat" polymorphism and two other versions of the dopamine transporter gene have been associated with ADHD symptoms (Barr et al. 2001). As with other susceptibility genes, links between these polymorphisms and other psychiatric diagnoses have been reported. These associations include Tourette's disorder and alcohol dependence (Vandenbergh et al. 2000).

Studies have also begun appearing that indicate that variation in medication response can be predicted on the basis of *DAT1* gene polymorphisms. Specifically, children who are homozygous for the ten-repeat allele have been reported to be less responsive to stimulant medication (Winsberg and Comings 1999).

Dopamine Receptor 2

The dopamine 2 receptor (*DRD2*) gene is located on the long arm of the eleventh chromosome at 11q23. Despite early reports of a polymorphism associated with alcoholism, no consistent associations with psychiatric illnesses have yet been established.

Dopamine Receptor 3

The dopamine 3 receptor (*DRD3*) gene is located on the long arm of the third chromosome at the 3q13.3 location. Although it has not been associated with ADHD, a link to schizophrenia has been demonstrated. Two polymorphisms have been identified on the basis of a mutation in the first exon, or coding region, of the gene. The normal form is referred to as the "serine polymorphism," or "allele 1," and the atypical form is referred to as the "glycine polymorphism," or "allele 2." The link to schizophrenia was originally reported in individuals homozygous for the glycine polymorphism (Crocq et al. 1992). This association is most clearly seen in selected families with a well-documented family history of schizophrenia (Nimgaonkar et al. 1993). A more recent meta-analysis has confirmed this link and has led to the recommendation of using genomic testing for the identification of individuals at risk for schizophrenia who might benefit from preventive intervention (Williams et al. 1998).

There have also been some studies of the association between the glycine polymorphism and an increased risk for tardive dyskinesia in schizophrenic patients (Steen et al. 1997). This finding was extended to include subjects who were either homozygous or heterozygous for the glycine allele (Segman et al. 1999).

Dopamine Receptor 4

The dopamine receptor 4 (*DRD4*) gene is located on the short arm of the eleventh chromosome at 11p15.5. *DRD4* is a highly variable gene. Many of these alleles are created by the insertion of a specific sequence of 48 nucleotide base pairs that is repeated multiple times. The identified versions of this gene range from an allele with just 2 repetitions of this sequence to a polymorphism that has 11 repetitions. Because these "repeats" occur in an exon of the gene, each form of the gene produces a protein of a different size. The length of these proteins varies from 32 amino acids for the "two-repeat," or the 2R, form of the gene to 176 amino acids for the "eleven-repeat," or 11R, version. The most common allele iin the U.S. population is the "four-repeat," or 4R, polymorphism. The 4R version of the gene has an allelic frequency of 65%. Therefore, the most common genotype in the population is 4R homozygous, which is often considered to be the "normal" allele. The next most common form of this gene is the "seven-repeat," or 7R, polymorphism. The 7R polymorphism has a frequency of 19% reported in U.S. samples. The 2R allele accounts for about 9% of the allele frequency. Other less common forms of the gene, such as the 3R, 5R, and 6R, code for altered proteins. Most studies of the 7R polymorphism have focused on the relationship between this form of the gene and the diagnosis of ADHD.

Individuals who carry the 7R allele of the DRD4 gene appear to be less sensitive to endogenous dopamine as a consequence of their D_4 receptors being less effective in the recognition of dopamine molecules. This hypothesized blunting of the dopamine response is consistent with the therapeutic effect of methylphenidate, which is believed to raise synaptic dopamine levels.

Several studies have reported that children with the diagnosis of ADHD are more likely to be carrying a copy of the 7R allele of the *DRD4* gene. However, not all children who meet the ADHD diagnostic criteria carry this allele. Faraone et al. (1999) reported finding an association between having the 7R allele of *DRD4* and being found to have ADHD. The probability of a subject who had ADHD but did not possess the 7R allele was 0.58. If an individual had one copy of the 7R allele, the probability rose to 0.73. All of the individuals with two copies of the 7R alleles were found to have ADHD. An association between the 7R allele of *DRD4* and having ADHD has also been reported in a nonclinical sample (Curran et al. 2001), although this relationship was not demonstrated in a large birth cohort (Mill et al. 2002).

Polymorphisms of the Serotonin Transporter and Serotonin Receptor Genes

■ The Serotonin Transporter Gene

The serotonin transporter (*5HTT*) gene is located on the long arm of the seventeenth chromosome at 17q12. The *5HTT* gene plays a central role in serotonergic transmission and is one of the sites of action of the serotonin reuptake inhibitors. Two common polymorphisms have been described as the long ("*l*") and short ("*s*") forms of the gene (Lesch et al. 1996). The short form is the result of a deletion in the promotor region of the gene that results in a 25%–59% reduction in the gene expression of the *5HTT* gene. In the original reports describing these alleles, the frequency of the long form was 57% and the frequency of the short form was 43%. Therefore, it can be calculated that approximately half of the population is heterozygous for these alleles. Other, rarer forms of this gene, such as an even longer promoter region polymorphism ("*lj*"), have been reported in isolated populations (Michaelovsky et al. 1999).

The *5HTT* gene has been linked to a number of different psychiatric illnesses that are mediated by serotonin (Murphy et al. 2001). The homozygous long form of the gene was found to be associated with obsessive-compulsive disorder (Bengel et al. 1999; McDougle et al. 1998). However, replication of this finding has been inconsistent, and more recent studies have found the association with the homozygous long form of the gene to be limited to patients with obsessive-compulsive disorder with counting rituals who also had comorbid tics (Cavallini et al. 2002).

Another important series of association studies have linked the *5HTT* gene to suicide in depressed patients. The long allele was originally reported to be so linked (Du et al. 1999). However, subsequent studies have demonstrated a link between subjects with the homozygous short form of the gene and more violent suicidal behavior (Bellivier et al. 2000; Bondy et al. 2000). An association between the short allele and repetitive suicidal behavior was also found in a U.S. alcoholic cohort (Gorwood et al. 2000). The short allele was also found to occur more commonly in a Western European cohort that had made violent suicide attempts (Courtet et al. 2001).

The association between the alleles of *5HTT* and autism has been less consistent. Original reports suggested an association with the short allele in a U.S. sample (Cook et al. 1997) and with the long allele in a German sample (Klauck et al. 1997). Subsequently, it was hypothesized that variation in severity of autistic features might be differentially linked to the long or short form of the gene (Tordjman et al. 2001). If the long form of the gene ultimately proves to be linked to autism, it would suggest that the molecular mechanism by which the *5HTT* gene contributes to the clinical presentation of autism is through enhanced uptake of serotonin (Yirmiya et al. 2001).

Even more recently, a link between the presence of an association of the short form of the *5HTT* gene and greater amygdala neuronal activity has been demonstrated using a functional magnetic resonance imaging paradigm that includes the use of a fearful stimulus (Hariri et al. 2002). Given that the short form of the gene has been associated with the occurrence of fear- and anxiety-related symptoms, this new study links both the genotype and the clinical symptoms to neuronal activity in the amygdala. A recent primate study of early rearing behavior found that the mothers who were heterozygous for the *5HTT* gene and had one copy of the long form and one copy of the short form demonstrated increased "affective responding" when compared with mothers with two copies of the long form (Champoux et al. 2002).

The *5HTT* gene has been demonstrated to predict therapeutic response to serotonin reuptake inhibitors. The presence of a copy of the long form of the gene was initially shown to predict a positive response to fluvoxamine (Smeraldi et al. 1998) and a positive response to paroxetine (Zanardi et al. 2000). A subsequent study of the relationship between these genotypes and paroxetine response confirmed the better response of subjects who were homozygous for the long form of the gene (Pollock et al. 2000).

■ The Serotonin Receptor Genes

Although many serotonin receptor genes have been studied, there are fewer linkages between polymorphisms of these genes and either clinical syndromes or therapeutic responses. Recently, the serotonin 5-HT$_{2A}$ receptor gene, which is located on the long arm of chromosome 13 at 13qX, appears to hold some promise for clinical assessment. However, there are multiple polymorphisms of this gene, which makes translation of research findings to clinical practice more challenging. For example, a polymorphism of a T at position 102 was shown to be linked to mood disorder (Zhang et al. 1997). However, this same T allele at position 102 has also been linked to schizophrenia (Williams et al. 1997). Furthermore, a promoter polymorphism of this same gene has been linked both to obsessive-compulsive disorder (Enoch et al. 2001; Walitza et al. 2002) and specific eating disorders (Enoch et al. 1998; Nishiguchi et al. 2001; Sorbi et al. 1998).

An association between a different polymorphism of serotonin 5-HT$_{2A}$ receptor gene at 452 and medication response has also been reported (Masellis et al. 1998). Subjects with an allele that codes for tyrosine at 452 are less likely to respond to clozapine than are subjects who code for histamine at 452. Although this association is promising, it is not sufficiently well established to be considered in clinical management.

The Tryptophan Hydroxylase Gene

The *TPH* gene is an important central nervous system gene that has long been known to produce the rate-limiting enzyme in the synthesis of serotonin. Two alleles, the "*U*" or "*A*" form (*TPH*1779A*) and the "*L*" or "*C*" form (*TPH*1779C*), have been described. Mann et al. (1997) reported an association between the *U* allele and greater frequency of suicide. Several confirmations followed. However, Nielsen et al. (1998) reported an association between the *L* allele and suicidality in impulsive offenders. This *L* allele was also linked to alcohol abuse. Paoloni-Giacobino et al. (2000) reported that another intron 7 polymorphism was associated with suicidality. Two more recent studies have focused on different aspects of the relationship between suicide and these polymorphisms. Turecki et al. (2001) demonstrated three polymorphisms linked to suicidal behavior and again specifically demonstrated that the strongest association was with suicide by violent means. Abbar et al. (2001) reported variations in intron 7, 8, and 9 that were all linked to suicide by violent means. These associations were enhanced if subjects had a history of depression. Finally, homozygosity for the *L* allele of the *TPH* gene was found less commonly in depressed patients with a history of a suicide attempt, supporting the findings in the original reports (Souery et al. 2001).

As with other susceptibility genes, polymorphisms of the *TPH* gene have been associated with other psychiatric illnesses. Specifically, Bellivier et al. (1998) reported association between specific *TPH* genotypes and manic depressive illness. Within this population, there was not an association with suicidality. Subsequently, Kirov et al. (1999) commented that there was a significantly increased frequency of the *U* (*TPH*1779A*) allele in patients with bipolar disorder (52%) when compared with control subjects (36%). This finding has not been consistently replicated in other bipolar samples. Of particular interest has been association between the intron-7 allele and poor impulse control. In this regard, the *U* allele has been suggested to be linked to early smoking initiation (Lerman et al. 2001). Sullivan et al. (2001) also found an association between *TPH* gene polymorphisms and initiation of smoking but not between such polymorphisms and nicotine dependence.

The possibility of finding polymorphisms that would predict medication response continues to be one of the key rationales for genomic screening. In that regard, *TPH* alleles have been linked to response to lithium. Specifically, subjects with *TPH* genes homozygous for the *U* allele did worse when treated with lithium than heterozygous *U/L* individuals or subjects who were homozygous for *L*.

The Catecholamine-*O*-Methyltransferase Gene

The *COMT* gene is located on the long arm of the twenty-second chromosome at 22q11.2. Since the mid-1970s, it has been known that individuals vary in their ability to metabolize catecholamines, and there has been presumptive evidence of three phenotypes: high activity, intermediate activity, and low activity (Weinshilboum et al. 1999). Subsequently, this has been shown to be the result of a single-point mutation that produces an enzyme with a single differentiating amino acid. The high-activity genotype consists of individuals who have two copies of the high-activity gene. This gene has the amino acid valine at the critical coding site and produces a thermostable enzyme. The low-activity genotype consists of individuals with two copies of the low-activity gene. This gene has the amino acid serine at the key coding site and is thermolabile. The intermediate phenotype results from having one high-activity allele and one low-activity allele. Some studies have found that heterozygous subjects resemble high-activity subjects, which suggests that a single copy of the high-activity gene can largely compensate for the low-activity allele. This enzyme is responsible for the metabolism of dopamine in the prefrontal cerebrum as well as metabolism of serotonin and norepinephrine in other sites in the central nervous system.

The *COMT* gene has long been considered a susceptibility gene because of the metabolic function of the COMT enzyme. Individuals with high-activity enzymatic capability are conceptualized as having less accessible dopamine, whereas those with low activity would have greater central dopamine concentration. This variability in dopamine concentration provides an explanation for why different genotypes result in variable behavior (Lachman et al. 1996). There is an ethnic variation in the distribution of these two alleles. In European samples, there is often a nearly equal distribution of the high-activity and the low-activity alleles. However, in Asian and African samples, the gene frequency of the low-activity allele is much lower (Palmatier et al. 1999).

A number of studies have linked the low-activity allele to psychotic symptoms. This has been quite elegantly demonstrated in patients with velocardiofacial disorder. All of these patients lack one entire copy of the gene (Lachman et al. 1996). Therefore, as a group, they would produce less enzyme. However, those individuals with this disorder who also have a low-activity allele for their only copy of this gene have been shown to be more likely to have psychotic features (Graf et al. 2001). This association was reported for a large sample of schizophrenic subjects (Egan et al. 2001). Another polymorphism affecting the activity of the enzyme produced by this gene further supports a link between low activity and schizophrenia (Shifman et al. 2002).

Links between *COMT* gene polymorphisms and other illnesses have been less conclusive but are still conceptually interesting. For example, subjects who are homozygous for the low-activity allele have been reported to be more at risk for alcoholism, which is explained as the result of their experiencing the euphoric effects of alcohol more intensely. A number of studies have looked for an association between the activity level of the *COMT* gene and symptoms of obsessive-compulsive disorder, although no conclusive result has been established (Alsobrook et al. 2002; Karayiorgou et al. 1997, 1999; Schindler et al. 2000). Most studies have reported that subjects who are homozygous for the low-activity alleles are at greater risk, but this has not always proved to be true for both men and women in individual studies. The pathophysiological mechanism for these symptoms would be an increased dopamine level in these individuals.

A link between psychotic ideation and high-activity homozygosity has recently received support. Additionally, a link to a possible mechanism for symptom expression has been shown by demonstrating a decrease in prefrontal activation on functional magnetic resonance imaging (Weinberger et al. 2001). The presence of even one high-activity allele was shown to be associated with poorer neurocognitive function as measured by standard testing (Malhotra et al. 2002).

Ethical Issues Related to Genomic Testing

Much concern has been expressed about the ethics of genomic testing (Farmer et al. 2000). Identifying atypical polymorphisms does provide both new clinical information about an individual's health status and data that predict prognosis. Therefore, there has been appropriate discussion regarding implications for privacy. However, these privacy concerns are very similar for all medical information linked to an individual patient. When these concerns are analyzed, the ethics issues that pertain to the use of genomic information are very similar to those that guide the use of data derived from laboratory or radiological procedures. A positive test result that has medical implications will in all likelihood have personal and interpersonal consequences.

Four principles that have been put forward as critical elements for medical testing apply equally to genomic testing:

1. There should be adequate informed consent, with information provided for the patient regarding both benefits and risks.
2. The decision to have a test must be voluntary.
3. Test results must be accurate.
4. Knowledge derived from the test must provide some potential medical or psychological benefit.

There is reasonable consensus on all but the fourth principle.

The issue of testing for the Huntington's disease gene has become a classic example. The test is highly accurate. It is uniformly agreed within the medical community that there should be no coercion regarding the decision to be tested. Informed consent is relatively straightforward. There is some documented physical risk in having the test, given that some patients have become depressed and even suicidal on learning that they have the gene that will ultimately result in developing the illness. However, the discussions that have been of most interest have focused on the other risks and benefits of testing. On the positive side of the argument, proponents provide poignant examples of individuals who have needed to know whether they had the gene in order to make life choices and prepare for a shorter anticipated life span. On the negative side, there is no currently available intervention to delay the onset of the illness, nor is there any effective early treatment. A reasonable current practice is to allow the individual who is at risk to make the decision about whether to be tested. At least one in four relatives of patients with Huntington's disease choose to know what their fate will be. To deny them this information is currently viewed as inappropriately paternalistic. However, these results should be provided in a supportive environment to allow response to the patients' concerns.

Although this gene responsible for Huntington's disease does not produce the protein responsible for central nervous system dysfunction until adulthood, the developmental implications of living with the risk of carrying the gene for this debilitating illness is relevant to treating child psychiatric patients.

One critical issue for child psychiatrists is whether children have the right to know their genotype. Currently, the recommendation of the American Academy of Pediatrics is that children should not be tested if there is no available treatment for the condition. One aspect of the argument is that if parents decide to have their child tested, this action will foreclose the possibility of the child's later choosing not to know. Of course, this same argument could be applied to any pediatric laboratory or radiological evaluation that did not have a clear and immediate treatment indication. The ethical issue becomes more difficult if the child expresses an interest in having genomic information in order to make a life decision. In the case of Huntington's disease, a 15-year-old girl would be cognitively able to fully understand the implications of having an affected genotype. Her decision to develop a sexual relationship and bear a child may well be affected by whether she will develop this illness. Her own capacity to care for the child will be influenced by the development of Huntington's disease, and the chance that her child will develop the illness would be either zero or 50%, depending on the results of her own genotypic assessment. From a societal perspective, providing her the opportunity of having this information would be highly desirable, whereas coercing her to know her status would be contrary to our currently accepted ethical guidelines.

The ethical issues related to screening for common psychiatric conditions have been addressed in the Nuffield Council on Bioethics Report. The council concluded in 1998 that the time had not arrived to embark on genomic testing of mental disorders. Since then, there has been an explosion of new studies that have identified informative polymorphisms of many susceptibility genes. However, a major limitation in the area of screening for common psychiatric illnesses is that no one gene is likely to be responsible for more than a fraction of the risk for the actual onset of the illness. Just as identifying an elevated cholesterol level does not imply that the patient will develop coronary artery disease, finding a patient homozygous for the seven-repeat *DRD4* allele does not mean that he or she will invariably develop ADHD. However, being homozygous for the seven-repeat *DRD4* allele does imply that the patient has an increased risk for the condition and that appropriate surveillance is indicated.

A final consideration is that caution must be used in assessing bioethical risks associated with psychiatric illnesses. It has been effectively argued that to treat psychiatric disorders differently from other medical disorders would be a form of "discrimination against those who suffer from mental illness" (Farmer et al. 2000). In fact, genetic research findings related to psychiatric illness have clearly reduced, rather than increased, the stigma that has been associated with schizophrenia and bipolar disorder, which are now more appropriately understood as illnesses of the brain rather than failures of character.

References

Abbar M, Courtet P, Bellivier F, et al: Suicide attempts and the tryptophan hydroxylase gene. Mol Psychiatry 6:268–273, 2001

Alsobrook JP 2nd, Zohar AH, Leboyer M, et al: Association between the COMT locus and obsessive-compulsive disorder in females but not males. Am J Med Genet 114:116–120, 2002

Barr CL, Xu C, Kroft J, et al: Haplotype study of three polymorphisms at the dopamine transporter locus confirm linkage to attention-deficit/hyperactivity disorder. Biol Psychiatry 49:333–339, 2001

Bellivier F, Leboyer M, Courtet P, et al: Association between the tryptophan hydroxylase gene and manic-depressive illness. Arch Gen Psychiatry 55:33–37, 1998

Bellivier F, Szoke A, Henry C, et al: Possible association between serotonin transporter gene polymorphism and violent suicidal behavior in mood disorders. Biol Psychiatry 48:319–322, 2000

Bengel D, Greenberg BD, Cora-Locatelli G, et al: Association of the serotonin transporter promoter regulatory region polymorphism and obsessive-compulsive disorder. Mol Psychiatry 4:463–466, 1999

Bondy B, Erfurth A, de Jonge S, et al: Possible association of the short allele of the serotonin transporter promoter gene polymorphism (*5-HTTLPR*) with violent suicide. Mol Psychiatry 5:193–195, 2000

Brockmoller J, Kirchheiner J, Meisel C, et al: Pharmacogenetic diagnostics of cytochrome P450 polymorphisms in clinical drug development and in drug treatment. Pharmacogenomics 1:125–251, 2000

Cavallini MC, Di Bella D, Silliprandi F, et al: Exploratory factor analysis of obsessive-compulsive patients and association with *5-HTTLPR* polymorphism. Am J Med Genet 114:347–353, 2002

Champoux M, Bennett A, Shannon C, et al: Serotonin transporter gene polymorphism, differential early rearing, and behavior in rhesus monkey neonates. Mol Psychiatry 7:1058–1063, 2002

Comings DE, Gade-Andavolu R, Gonzalez N, et al: Comparison of the role of dopamine, serotonin, and noradrenaline genes in ADHD, ODD and conduct disorder: multivariate regression analysis of 20 genes. Clin Genet 57:178–196, 2000a

Comings DE, Gade-Andavolu R, Gonzalez N, et al: Multivariate analysis of associations of 42 genes in ADHD, ODD and conduct disorder. Clin Genet 58:31–40, 2000b

Comings DE, Gade-Andavolu R, Gonzalez N, et al: The additive effect of neurotransmitter genes in pathological gambling. Clin Genet 60:107–116, 2001

Cook EH Jr, Stein MA, Krasowski MD, et al: Association of attention-deficit disorder and the dopamine transporter gene. Am J Hum Genet 56:993–998, 1995

Cook EH Jr, Courchesne R, Lord C, et al: Evidence of linkage between the serotonin transporter and autistic disorder. Mol Psychiatry 2:247–250, 1997

Courtet P, Baud P, Abbar M, et al: Association between violent suicidal behavior and the low activity allele of the serotonin transporter gene. Mol Psychiatry 6:338–341, 2001

Coutts RT, Urichuk LJ: Polymorphic cytochromes p450 and drugs used in psychiatry. Cell Mol Neurobiol 19:325–354, 1999

Crocq MA, Mant R, Asherson P, et al.: Association between schizophrenia and homozygosity at the dopamine D_3 receptor gene. J Med Genet 29:858–860, 1992

Curran S, Mill J, Sham P: QTL association analysis of the *DRD4* exon 3 *VNTR* polymorphism in a population sample of children screened with a parent rating scale for ADHD symptoms. Am J Med Genet 105:387–393, 2001

Du L, Faludi G, Palkovits M, et al: Frequency of long allele in serotonin transporter gene is increased in depressed suicide victims. Biol Psychiatry 46:196–201, 1999

Egan MF, Goldberg TE, Kolachana BS, et al: Effect of *COMT Val108/158 Met* genotype on frontal lobe function and risk for schizophrenia. Proc Natl Acad Sci U S A 98:6917–6922, 2001

Ellingrod VL, Schultz SK, Arndt S: Association between cytochrome P4502D6 (*CYP2D6*) genotype, antipsychotic exposure, and abnormal involuntary movement scale (AIMS) score. Psychiatr Genet 10:9–11, 2000

Enoch MA, Kaye WH, Rotondo A, et al: 5-HT$_{2A}$ promoter polymorphism: *1438G/A*, anorexia nervosa, and obsessive-compulsive disorder. Lancet 351:1785–1786, 1998

Enoch MA, Greenberg BD, Murphy DL, et al: Sexually dimorphic relationship of a 5-HT$_{2A}$ promoter polymorphism with obsessive-compulsive disorder. Biol Psychiatry 49:385–388, 2001

Faraone SV, Biederman J, Mennin D, et al: Bipolar and antisocial disorders among relatives of ADHD children: parsing familial subtypes of illness. Am J Med Genet 81:108–116, 1998

Faraone SV, Biederman J, Weiffenbach B, et al: Dopamine D_4 gene 7-repeat allele and attention deficit hyperactivity disorder. Am J Psychiatry 156:768–770, 1999

Farmer AE, Owen MJ, McGuffin P: Bioethics and genetic research in psychiatry. Br J Psychiatry 176:105–108, 2000

Gill M, Daly G, Heron S, et al: Confirmation of association between attention deficit hyperactivity disorder and a dopamine transporter polymorphism. Mol Psychiatry 2:311–313, 1997

Gorwood P, Batel P, Ades J, et al: Serotonin transporter gene polymorphisms, alcoholism, and suicidal behavior. Biol Psychiatry 48:259–264, 2000

Graf WD, Unis AS, Yates CM, et al: Catecholamines in patients with 22q11.2 deletion syndrome and the low-activity *COMT* polymorphism. Neurology 57:410–416, 2001

Hariri AR, Mattay VS, Tessitore A, et al: Serotonin transporter genetic variation and the response of the human amygdala. Science 297:400–403, 2002

Karayiorgou M, Altemus M, Galke BL, et al: Genotype determining low catechol-*O*-methyltransferase activity as a risk factor for obsessive-compulsive disorder. Proc Natl Acad Sci U S A 94:4572–4575, 1997

Karayiorgou M, Sobin C, Blundell ML, et al: Family-based association studies support a sexually dimorphic effect of COMT and MAOA on genetic susceptibility to obsessive-compulsive disorder. Biol Psychiatry 45:1178–1189, 1999

Kirchheiner J, Brosen K, Dahl ML, et al: *CYP2D6* and *CYP2C19* genotype-based dose recommendations for antidepressants: a first step towards subpopulation-specific dosage. Acta Psychiatr Scand 104:173–192, 2001

Kirov G, Owen MJ, Jones I, et al: Tryptophan hydroxylase gene and manic-depressive illness. Arch Gen Psychiatry 56:98–99, 1999

Klauck SM, Poustka F, Benner A, et al: Serotonin transporter (*5-HTT*) gene variants associated with autism? Hum Mol Genet 6:2233–2238, 1997

Lachman HM, Papolos DF, Saito T, et al: Human catechol-*O*-methyltransferase pharmacogenetics: description of a functional polymorphism and its potential application to neuropsychiatric disorders. Pharmacogenetics 6:243–250, 1996

Lerman C, Caporaso NE, Bush A, et al: Tryptophan hydroxylase gene variant and smoking behavior. Am J Med Genet 105:518–520, 2001

Lesch KP, Bengel D, Heils A, et al: Association of anxiety-related traits with a polymorphism in the serotonin transporter gene regulatory region. Science 274:1527–1531, 1996

Lin KM, Smith MW, Ortiz V: Culture and psychopharmacology. Psychiatr Clin North Am 24:523–538, 2001

Malhotra AK, Kestler LJ, Mazzanti C, et al: A functional polymorphism in the *COMT* gene and performance on a test of prefrontal cognition. Am J Psychiatry 159:652–654, 2002

Mann JJ, Malone KM, Nielsen DA, et al: Possible association of a polymorphism of the tryptophan hydroxylase gene with suicidal behavior in depressed patients. Am J Psychiatry 154:1451–1453, 1997

Masellis M, Basile V, Meltzer HY, et al: Serotonin subtype 2 receptor genes and clinical response to clozapine in schizophrenia patients. Neuropsychopharmacology 19:123–132, 1998

McDougle CJ, Epperson CN, Price LH, et al: Evidence for linkage disequilibrium between serotonin transporter protein gene (*SLC6A4*) and obsessive compulsive disorder. Mol Psychiatry 3:270–273, 1998

Michaelovsky E, Frisch A, Rockah R, et al: A novel allele in the promoter region of the human serotonin transporter gene. Mol Psychiatry 4:97–99, 1999

Mill JS, Caspi A, McClay J, et al: The dopamine D_4 receptor and the hyperactivity phenotype: a developmental-epidemiological study. Mol Psychiatry 7:383–391, 2002

Murphy DL, Li Q, Engel S, et al: Genetic perspectives on the serotonin transporter. Brain Res Bull 56:487–494, 2001

Nielsen DA, Virkkunen M, Lappalainen J, et al: A tryptophan hydroxylase gene marker for suicidality and alcoholism. Arch Gen Psychiatry 55:593–602, 1998

Nimgaonkar VL, Zhang XR, Caldwell JG, et al: Association study of schizophrenia with dopamine D_3 receptor gene polymorphisms: probable effects of family history of schizophrenia? Am J Med Genet 48:214–217, 1993

Nishiguchi N, Matsushita S, Suzuki K, et al: Association between 5HT$_{2A}$ receptor gene promoter region polymorphism and eating disorders in Japanese patients. Biol Psychiatry 50:123–128, 2001

Nuffield Council on Bioethics: Mental Disorders and Genetics: The Ethical Context. London, Nuffield Council on Bioethics, 1998

Ozdemir V, Kashuba ADM, Basile VS, et al: Pharmacogenetics of psychotropic drug metabolism, in Pharmacogenetics of Psychotropic Drugs. Edited by Lerer B. Cambridge, UK, Cambridge University Press, 2002, pp 157–180

Palmatier MA, Kang AM, Kidd KK: Global variation in the frequencies of functionally different catechol-O-methyltransferase alleles. Biol Psychiatry 46:557–567, 1999

Paoloni-Giacobino A, Mouthon D, Lambercy C, et al: Identification and analysis of new sequence variants in the human tryptophan hydroxylase (TpH) gene. Mol Psychiatry 5:49–55, 2000

Pollock BG, Ferrell RE, Mulsant BH, et al: Allelic variation in the serotonin transporter promoter affects onset of paroxetine treatment response in late-life depression. Neuropsychopharmacology 23:587–590, 2000

Rutter M, Silberg J, O'Connor T, et al: Genetics and child psychiatry, I: advances in quantitative and molecular genetics. J Child Psychol Psychiatry 40:3–18, 1999a

Rutter M, Silberg J, O'Connor T, et al: Genetics and child psychiatry, II: empirical research findings. J Child Psychol Psychiatry 40:19–55, 1999b

Sallee FR, DeVane CL, Ferrell RE: Fluoxetine-related death in a child with cytochrome P-450 2D6 genetic deficiency. J Child Adolesc Psychopharmacol 10:27–34, 2000

Schindler KM, Richter MA, Kennedy JL, et al: Association between homozygosity at the COMT gene locus and obsessive compulsive disorder. Am J Med Genet 96:721–724, 2000

Segman R, Neeman T, Heresco-Levy U, et al: Genotypic association between the dopamine D_3 receptor and tardive dyskinesia in chronic schizophrenia. Mol Psychiatry 4:247–253, 1999

Shifman S, Bronstein M, Sternfeld M, et al: A highly significant association between a COMT haplotype and schizophrenia. Am J Hum Genet 71:1296–1302, 2002

Smeraldi E, Zanardi R, Benedetti F, et al: Polymorphism within the promoter of the serotonin transporter gene and antidepressant efficacy of fluvoxamine. Mol Psychiatry 3:508–511, 1998

Sorbi S, Nacmias B, Tedde A, et al: 5-HT$_{2A}$ promoter polymorphism in anorexia nervosa (letter). Lancet 351:1785, 1998

Souery D, Van Gestel S, Massat I, et al: Tryptophan hydroxylase polymorphism and suicidality in unipolar and bipolar affective disorders: a multicenter association study. Biol Psychiatry 49:405–409, 2001

Steen VM, Lovlie R, MacEwan T, et al: Dopamine D_3-receptor gene variant and susceptibility to tardive dyskinesia in schizophrenic patients. Mol Psychiatry 2:139–145, 1997

Sullivan PF, Jiang Y, Neale MC, et al: Association of the tryptophan hydroxylase gene with smoking initiation but not progression to nicotine dependence. Am J Med Genet 105:479–484, 2001

Tordjman S, Gutknecht L, Carlier M, et al: Role of the serotonin transporter gene in the behavioral expression of autism. Mol Psychiatry 6:434–439, 2001

Turecki G, Zhu Z, Tzenova J, et al: TPH and suicidal behavior: a study in suicide completers. Mol Psychiatry 6:98–102, 2001

Vandenbergh DJ, Thompson MD, Cook EH, et al: Human dopamine transporter gene: coding region conservation among normal, Tourette's disorder, alcohol dependence and attention-deficit hyperactivity disorder populations. Mol Psychiatry 5:283–292, 2000

Waldman ID, Rowe DC, Abramowitz A, et al: Association and linkage of the dopamine transporter gene and attention-deficit hyperactivity disorder in children: heterogeneity owing to diagnostic subtype and severity. Am J Hum Genet 63:1767–1776, 1998

Walitza S, Wewetzer C, Warnke A, et al: 5-HT$_{2A}$ promoter polymorphism—1438G/A in children and adolescents with obsessive-compulsive disorders. Mol Psychiatry 7:1054–1057, 2002

Weinberger DR, Egan MF, Bertolino A, et al: Prefrontal neurons and the genetics of schizophrenia. Biol Psychiatry 50:825–844, 2001

Weinshilboum RM, Otterness DM, Szumlanski CL: Methylation pharmacogenetics: catechol-O-methyltransferase, thiopurine methyltransferase, and histamine N-methyltransferase. Annu Rev Pharmacol Toxicol 39:19–52, 1999

Williams J, McGuffin P, Nothen M, et al: Meta-analysis of association between the 5-HT$_{2a}$ receptor T102C polymorphism and schizophrenia. EMASS Collaborative Group. European Multicentre Association Study of Schizophrenia (letter). Lancet 349:1221, 1997

Williams J, Spurlock G, Holmans P, et al: A meta-analysis and transmission disequilibrium study of association between the dopamine D$_3$ receptor gene and schizophrenia. Mol Psychiatry 3:141–149, 1998

Winsberg BG, Comings DE: Association of the dopamine transporter gene (DAT1) with poor methylphenidate response. J Am Acad Child Adolesc Psychiatry 38:1474–1477, 1999

Yirmiya N, Pilowsky T, Nemanov L, et al: Evidence for an association with the serotonin transporter promoter region polymorphism and autism. Am J Med Genet 105:381–386, 2001

Zanardi R, Benedetti F, Di Bella D, et al: Efficacy of paroxetine in depression is influenced by a functional polymorphism within the promoter of the serotonin transporter gene. J Clin Psychopharmacol 20:105–107, 2000

Zhang HY, Ishigaki T, Tani K, et al: Serotonin2A receptor gene polymorphism in mood disorders. Biol Psychiatry 41:768–773, 1997

Diagnosis and Diagnostic Formulation

Theodore Shapiro, M.D.

When a family consults with a child and adolescent psychiatrist for help and diagnosis for their child, the parties enter the consultation with at least two different sets of presuppositions. In accord with his or her professional group, the psychiatrist has decided to apply the specialized categorization used to convey knowledge among peers. The diagnosis is also informed by recent research and current therapeutic interventions. This taxonomy—or, in the best case, nosology—corresponds to the most recent knowledge and practice within the medical profession. However, the therapeutic goals of parents and children who seek professional help may be quite different from those of the psychiatrist. In general, parents come to a child and adolescent psychiatrist because they perceive that something is awry in their child, and they cannot understand, control, or deal with the behaviors and suffering that are adversely affecting development. They also believe that the child psychiatrist has a means of examining and discovering "what is wrong," hoping that an intervention exists to remedy the discomfort or to change maladaptive behavior. Insofar as these two aims coincide, the psychiatrist constructs a formulation that includes a diagnosis and a treatment plan and encourages the family's collaboration in treatment.

History and Examination

The child psychiatrist must make a diagnosis in accord with the currently accepted scheme—DSM-IV-TR (American Psychiatric Association 2000)—and must also construct a dynamic formulation of the case that includes a guide for further action (Shapiro 1989); that is, data accumulated from the history, from other multiple sources of information, and from examination of the child must be tied together in a dynamic matrix. Thus, the case formulation to be implemented must be responsive both to professional and social contingencies and to the family's specific needs at a particular point in time. The child psychiatrist also must simultaneously consider biological, social, developmental, and psychological factors for a comprehensive and contextual history and examination of the child. This task of formulation is especially demanding in child and adolescent psychiatry because many sources of information about the child or adolescent must be consolidated. The child and adolescent psychiatrist must consider the following:

- The role of the child as an organism and a person with the disorder or possibly as a designated patient or a symptom bearer in a family or community
- The biological and psychosocial immaturity of the child in the family and the fact that the youngster is brought by family members or surrogates whose auxiliary function to the ego of that child changes with each stage of development
- The organismic contribution, which is evident not only in genetic disposition but also in perinatal insults that lead to developmental disability
- The child's embeddedness in a family network and a protected developmental path, which differ for children and adults and also differ across cultures and socioeconomic conditions

Taken together, these four domains constitute the ecology of the consultation as it pertains to the developing human child, in whom genes and social surroundings meet and are individually expressed and synthesized.

In view of these general issues, the clinician will ultimately be asked at which level his or her efforts should be dispatched to effect a plan for intervention. Is a useful therapy available at the organismic level, or is a family or social intervention possible, that can address the issues that prompted consultation? If one does intervene after diagnostic assessment, an additional dynamic formulation must be added to help guide expectations and plans in the context of what is possible for a particular child and family (Group for the Advancement of Psychiatry 1974; Shapiro 1989). Clinicians dare not move from diagnosis to treatment that cannot be delivered. Moreover, they must bring their acumen to the level of the community, which includes mastering the most recent developments from biological, social, and intrapsychic research. Parents expect that because they are physicians, psychiatrists will bring the best and most recent biological information to bear on their formulations.

Role of DSM in Diagnostic Assessment

Since the publication of DSM-III (American Psychiatric Association 1980)—and continuing through the releases of DSM-III-R (American Psychiatric Association 1987), DSM-IV (American Psychiatric Association 1994), and DSM-IV-TR (American Psychiatric Association 2000)—the American Psychiatric Association and the American Academy of Child and Adolescent Psychiatry have followed a diagnostic approach that is essentially based on cross-sectional categories describing specific syndromes on Axis I (see Cantwell 1988). This approach was adopted because empirical description is relatively easier to use than elaborate theoretical structures that subsume other nomenclatures. However, this diagnostic scheme offers little guidance to the clinician in organizing his or her ideas about etiological or nosological distinctions (see McClellan and Werry 2000; Wakefield 1992). Dimensional issues, which are so vital to a developmental point of view of childhood, are also excluded, diminishing similarities among children in the service of discriminant validity (Achenbach 1988; Nurcombe et al. 1989). The widely used Child Behavior Checklist (CBCL) (Achenbach

and Edelbrock 1983) provides not diagnoses but factors (e.g., externalizing and internalizing) that can be further distinguished into other factors. Nonetheless, discrete syndromes have been described in children, with adequate correspondence to observations (validity), that compare well with adult diagnoses.

Well-researched instruments are available in structured and semistructured interviews of the child and the parent that permit diagnosis as well (McClellan and Werry 2000). However, in both children and adults there are high rates of comorbidity. Whenever a child receives a particular psychiatric diagnosis, the developmental status of the child must be noted so that the effects of immaturity in coping mechanisms on the diagnosis and on the rapidity of behavioral regression and recovery can be accounted for. Recently there has been an increased tendency to diagnose bipolar disorder before puberty or to cluster attentional, oppositional, and conduct problems under a larger rubric of disruptive disorders with more uncertain outcome. Clinicians also use a multiaxial scheme and a dynamic formulation to approximate a complete description of a child. Axis II and Axis III (providing a modifier for the Axis I diagnosis) allow the developmental, biological, and medical disturbances to be brought into focus. Axis IV permits a similar consideration for social dimensions of stress. Axis V gives a rough categorization of chronicity based on the highest level of functioning recorded during the previous year.

These formulations are based on a medical model that, in its most mature stage, presumes that diagnostics leads to therapeutics or that diagnosis and prognosis are tightly interwoven. These presumptions are only partially achieved in child psychiatry (and, for that matter, in general psychiatry). Child psychiatrists not only are struggling with issues concerning the discriminant validity of diagnoses but also are attempting to determine whether the taxonomy has continuing significance over the life span of the child (e.g., predictive validity and comorbidity). Furthermore, both pharmacological and behavioral treatments have targeted symptoms rather than disorders.

In gathering data during the early stages of history and observation, clinicians must arrive at a differential diagnosis and determine whether the criteria for a specific disorder are fulfilled and whether the exclusion criteria are present to establish an Axis I or Axis II diagnosis. This process permits clinicians to incorporate information derived from epidemiological and biological research, as well as follow-up research, to achieve professional concordance in the clinical setting. Recent advances in the understanding of etiology have taken the field further into medical modeling. Pediatric autoimmune neuropsychiatric disorder associated with streptococcal infections (Swedo et al. 1997, 1998) is now recognized as a poststreptococcal autoimmune disease with symptoms of obsessive-compulsive disorder or Tourette's syndrome (Swedo et al. 1997), and posttraumatic stress disorder represents a clearly defined etiologic determinant of irritability and anxiety in some children.

A confounding factor in diagnosis, a high rate of comorbidity as noted above, suggests to the psychiatrist that surface descriptions of symptom constellations may not correspond to organismic segmentation at a biological level. Even syndromes as discrete as attention-deficit/hyperactivity disorder (ADHD) have high comorbidity with conduct disorder, learning disabilities, and some anxiety disorders, and now there is ample evidence that bipolar disorder may be comorbid with ADHD (Geller et al. 2001; Wozniak et al. 1995). Moreover, clinicians are better at judging functional competence by the use of global schemes such as the Children's Global Assessment Scale (Green et al. 1994) than they are at judging the severity of symptoms. Therefore, patients with diagnoses may not have severe expression of symptoms but may have functional failures in other areas of ego expression and adaptation that elicit attention.

Another confounding factor is the determination of what constitutes a mental disorder in a child. The difficulty in applying the mental disorder rule to a developing organism, as described in all DSMs, is reflected in the reluctance to make a personality disorder diagnosis during adolescence. Richters and Cicchetti (1993) examined the "conduct disorder rubric" using Huckleberry Finn as a metaphor to explore how clinicians attribute intrinsic and extrinsic weight to diagnostic judgments. These investigators claim good success in unraveling the underlying matrix of such judgments, but they suggest that Wakefield's (1992) idea of harmful dysfunction would be a useful frame of reference for the newly popular evolutionary biology:

> A condition is a disorder if and only if (a) the condition causes some harm or deprivation of benefit to the person as judged by the standards of the person's culture…, and (b) the condition results from the inability of some internal mechanism to perform its natural function, wherein a natural function is an effect that is part of the evolutionary explanation of the existence and structure of the mechanism. (Wakefield 1992, p. 384)

These are but two recent developments that clinicians must confront when thinking about labeling and working toward a helpful solution to individual clinical problems. Indeed, if the evolutionary biology stance and theory take hold as a better means of examining children in a modern context, existing taxonomies such as DSM-III, DSM-III-R, and DSM-IV may need to be reexamined. In their review of diagnostic instruments, McClellan and Werry (2000) note that in the collaborative Multisite Multimodal Treatment Study symptoms identified by research instruments alone do not determine caseness. Instead clinicians need to make an additional judgment regarding severity (or, in other words, degree of maladaptation). In their proposal of new considerations for future nomenclature, Jensen et al. (1997) used ADHD as an example of the expression of evolutionary variation in a spectrum of attentional types.

These developments strongly indicate that much remains to be said about the clinical case outside of the framework of DSM. The additional power of a formulation based on other paradigms is necessary to establish whether the most central locus of problems is within the child, within the family, within society, or bound to the biological substrate that prompts the behaviors of the child. The completeness of both—a best-bet diagnosis based on a clear differential diagnosis and a dynamic construction for treatment based on a psychosocial structural theory—should provide a comprehensive diagnostic formulation that addresses the individual needs of the patient and his or her family, who are in need and in pain and who wish to obtain some type of relief or help from the psychiatrist. Similar surface descriptors, as used in DSM-IV-TR, should not deceive psychiatrists into concluding that all patients with similar symptoms ought to receive the same diagnosis and treatment. The sensitivity and specificity dimension of diagnosis requires that psychiatrists learn how to recognize false positives.

Therefore, arriving at an Axis I diagnosis and its complementary dynamic formulation permits the physician to act within the scope of a professional role and to use all the knowledge available to the field and to provide a framework for action. Within such a framework, interventions can then be directed at relieving the patient's suffering and reducing the maladaptive impact that a childhood disturbance or disorder has on the patient, the family, and the school.

Differential Diagnosis

As noted above, there are many approaches to diagnosis. DSM-IV-TR includes many categories that essentially coalesce around four varieties of disorders (conduct, emotion, development, and adjustment) and a subset of highly specific focal problems (Table 17–1). To these must be added various disorders with more specialized symptom pictures: tic disorders; disorders of eating, of gender identity, of elimination, and of speech; and other disorders.

Clinicians begin a diagnostic formulation in a practical way by making a simple determination: Are the behaviors that are most prominent externalizing or internalizing? The differential diagnosis in the line of externally directed behaviors (alloplastic disorders) essentially includes conduct disorders with symptoms of aggression, lying, stealing, and antisocial behavior—conduct that may lead to confrontations with the law in later life, such as in delinquency or minor disturbances of behavior within and outside the family. These behaviors constitute oppositional disorders and what have become known as status offenses: behaviors such as running away, which would be an offense under the law only if the individual is a minor (Group for the Advancement of Psychiatry 1989). As noted, the disruptive disorder cluster during middle childhood may await further parceling out as the child matures.

Disorders of emotion (autoplastic disorders) are primarily anxiety disorders and depressive disorders. Most prominent among the childhood anxiety disorders is a separation disturbance that is sometimes called a shyness disorder and that was previously classified under school reluctance or school phobia (Shapiro and Jegede 1973). Generalized anxiety disorder is another consideration for diffusely anxious and phobic children; then, if the child fits categorically within the panic disorder group in late adolescence, this diagnosis could be established. In so doing, the child psychiatrist should keep in mind the possibility of "contagion" (Last et al. 1987) or temperamental diathesis (Kagan et al. 1990). The higher rate of disorders of emotion in girls requires further study, as does the higher rate of externalizing disorders in boys.

Depression (Birmaher et al. 1996) is a relatively new diagnosis for prepubertal children. It is certainly increasing, according to epidemiological studies (Kas-

Table 17–1. Differential diagnosis

Disorders of
Conduct
Emotion
Development
Adjustment
Eating
Gender identity
Tics
Elimination
Speech
Other

Acute
Social upheaval/yes-no

Chronic
Reality disorganizing/preserving

hani et al. 1987). We encounter children who fit criteria for major depressive disorder, once thought to be a third-decade illness. Psychiatrists also know much more about the tendency for recurrence of major depression and dysthymia in children (Kovacs 1996; Lewinsohn et al. 2000). Other disturbances, such as anorexia nervosa and bulimia nervosa, may show associated depressive symptoms, and some suggest that depression is the disorder to be treated pharmacologically as an adjunctive approach. Although clinicians are reluctant to make personality disorder diagnoses in young children, clinical judgments about temperament are made, and the "difficult child" may be seen as a resultant of one line of clinical investigation (Chess and Thomas 1987). In fact, a study of inhibited children (Kagan et al. 1990) suggested a temperamental precursor to anxiety disorders and even inferences of genetic predisposition. Moreover, the presence of panic disorder and major depression in parents has significant effects on offspring (Biederman et al. 2001).

The developmental disorders category includes pervasive developmental disorders and autism, learning disabilities, and ADHD, all located on Axis I. All have specific features that earmark them as developmentally significant because they are characterized by the persistence of certain immaturities of younger children even though chronological age is advanced. These disorders also show deviance, insofar as the developmental profile of the disorders taken together creates an uneven pattern among developmental lines. Mental retardation, by contrast, involves uniform delays across the adaptive functions and is coded on Axis II. As noted above, oppositional disorder, conduct disorders, and learning disabilities commonly co-occur with ADHD (Beitchman et al. 1986; Cantwell and Baker 1989). The clinician should keep in mind that comorbidity is prominent in childhood, and two Axis I or II diagnoses should not be eschewed in the name of the tradition of medical parsimoniousness.

Disorders of adjustment represent a large group of Axis I diagnoses related to Axis IV severity. They should be short-lived (less than 6 months) and must have clear precipitants. However, DSM-IV-TR allows for longer periods of disorder. One can view posttraumatic stress disorder as an adjustment disorder that takes a larger toll on the individual's adaptive capacity with respect to immature status and the prolongation of symptoms beyond the adjustment period. Clinicians must also look for formes frustes of these disorders, and the special characteristics of these disorders in children may not include flashbacks, visualizations, and so on. The children may also demonstrate habitual replaying of games and fantasies to master the original traumas (Pynoos and Nader 1989; Terr 1983). Laor et al. (2001) showed the significant effect of parenting on children's symptoms 5 years after exposure to war trauma.

In addition to these determinations in the differential diagnosis on Axis I, clinicians determine whether a disorder is acute or chronic and whether it is disorganizing or preserving of reality. The latter feature provides another dimension that permits psychiatrists to consider psychosis when it can be diagnosed with the adult diagnostic schema as well as the childhood diagnostic schema.

After a differential diagnosis has been determined, options for prescription are available, but not all is told about the child by way of arriving at a diagnosis (Cantwell 1980, 1988). An additional diagnostic formulation is necessary to pull together the data that have been gathered. A caution is warranted in this age of structured and semistructured interviews and diagnostic checklists, because each of these instruments was designed for research purposes to accomplish specific tasks. Some structured interviews, such as the CBCL, do not correlate with DSM-IV-TR diagnoses. Others, such as the Diagnostic Interview for Children and Adolescents (Herjanic and Campbell 1977), are designed for specific age groups and provide diagnoses but do not offer clear routes to other vital information to round out the diagnostic formulation. Clin-

ical interviews have been measured against structured interviews (Rutter et al. 1981) and have been found to enable patients to elaborate their subject states, whereas structured interviews are highly inclusive and do not omit information that may slip by in the open-ended approach. Nonetheless, Rutter's Parent Questionnaire was modified (Goodman 1994) to include exploration of children's strengths as an acknowledgment of such deficiency. McClellan and Werry (2000, p. 26) note that the DSM diagnostic formulation has clear utility and is easy to conceptualize, but that "does not mean it exists in nature."

Formulation and Summary

Because children are developmentally immature and are unable to fend for themselves biologically and psychosocially, the family or its surrogates are routinely consulted so that they may provide information for the working formulation to guide action and convince patients to participate fully in a plan. This formulation for treatment must be organized in a useful way for the clinician and must be communicated to the parents, who decide if and how recommendations are to be carried out. To make such a formulation, the physician is advised to subdivide the available data on the patient into psychosocial and developmental features found during the examination (Table 17–2).

Table 17–2. Formulation and summary of features found during examination

Biological
  Family
  Perinatal
  Injury

Social
  Family
  Peer
  Community

Psychological
  Conflict (intrapsychic)
  Identification
  Self-esteem regulation

Developmental
  Phase/stage-related behavior
  Reinforcing factors

While cataloging the relevant biological features of the life of the child or adolescent, the clinician considers familial factors—including diseases and disorders in first-degree relatives, genetic history, and important facts about developmental delays within the family—that correlate with specific disorders. For example, Rutter and Folstein (1977) suggested that in autism the heritable features may be language delay and deviance, which combine with accidental perinatal stress factors. A family history of language delay should therefore be highlighted in the biological background of the diagnostic formulation. It is well known, for example, that hypoxia during the first trimester (as evidenced by bleeding or other symptoms) is significant postnatally and that chromosomal anomalies are relevant to developmental deviance. In fact, during the perinatal period itself, fetal distress and meconium staining are notable, as are disturbances in the immediate postnatal period. Hyperbilirubinemia or intracranial bleeding and low birth weight warrant attention for their impact on development. Anything that intrudes on brain integrity throughout the early life span—which could include toxic-metabolic states or infections such as meningitis, viral encephalitis, diabetic coma, or malnutrition—should alert clinicians. As noted above (see "Role of DSM in Diagnostic Assessment"), the recent discovery that the autoimmune response to streptococcal infection may be a precursor to obsessive-compulsive disorder and Tourette's syndrome indicates that swift action is required to interrupt the prolonged effect of such insults. These biological factors are significant for etiological inferences concerning biological insult and should be summarized for review in the diagnostic formulation. They also should be used to suggest contributions to the origins of current conditions.

Social disturbances are pertinent to the widening cone of human contacts as the infant develops. Initially, the immediate caregiving, nurturing environment is important, but this environment gradually expands as the child develops and begins to appreciate more people as being relevant in the surroundings. This expanding surround includes parents and surrogate caregivers; ultimately, when the child begins school, it also includes teachers and a widening array of peers with whom the child interacts. Finally, the community at large becomes the proximally relevant world of the adolescent. Disturbances in each of these areas—communities; objects of identification in early childhood, in early adolescence, and in school circumstances;

crushes; heroes; drugs; and intrusions by the family such as incest, abuse, and overly rigorous or lax child rearing—may take their toll on the child.

The social role of the child also becomes important in determining whether illness will ensue or whether the disorder is in the child or in the family (McDermott and Char 1974). The community may also become a figurative toxigenic agent in poverty-stricken areas, where schooling may be inferior or where delinquency and sociopathy reign. The likelihood of psychiatric diagnosis later in life is correlated with social disadvantage in youth. In addition, the potentially toxic effect of wealth or charismatic parents on some children should not be overlooked.

The psychological and intrapsychic vantage point may be addressed from data obtained in the interview of the child and from one's observations of family dynamics. It must be established whether symptoms appear to be meaningful to the child, represent symbolic transformations that are related to identifications, or are signs of maladaptive self-esteem regulation (Shapiro and Esman 1985). These three areas are easily tapped through the direct interview and through modification of the interview process by the use of special techniques such as figure drawings, symbolic play, kinetic family drawings, squiggle games, and dreams. These are all essential variant procedures that can be adapted to specific goals in clinical practice.

The notion of acting out is a central dynamic proposition based on the idea that fantasies (either unknown or known to the child) determine overt behavior. These symbolic actions can be seen as externalizing behaviors of conduct disorder in children so disposed or as phobic anxiety behaviors, which also may partially result from identification with parents, siblings, or peers. As noted above (see "Differential Diagnosis"), it is not clear whether the high rate of anxiety and panic disorders observed in mothers of anxious children is related to inheritance or contagion (Last et al. 1987). The clinician's examination determines what kinds of conflict have been resolved and represented in what kinds of behavior or symptoms. The standard diagnostic assessments that focus on simple differential diagnosis do not permit the elaboration of such formulations. Thus, the nature of the net cast determines what will be caught: Examiners who do not look will not find these features.

Although these externalizing behaviors are meaningful, clinicians also must consider whether they are components of development that signify way stations in the progress of childhood. Because certain appropriate behaviors are expected in each stage and phase of life, symptoms may be expected to occur as transient phenomena of the developmental course and as expressions of disorders as well. Thus, the degree of maladaptation and severity should be weighed.

For example, a child's secure attachment to the parent is healthy, but separation anxiety also must be expected at age 10–18 months. However, separation anxiety that occurs during school years as a symptom needing intervention is maladaptive and inappropriate. The reinforcing factors that permit certain behaviors to arise or prevail at each developmental stage must be examined. For example, some parents really do not take *any* direct disciplinary action toward their children for fear that such action is overly aggressive and punitive. Frequently, these parents have had difficult and harsh rearing themselves. The notion that the developmental path will be traversed without parental guidance or discipline is another fact to be taken into account in symptom formation in early childhood. It is well known that abusing parents have themselves frequently been abused.

Pulling together the biological, social, psychological, and developmental features of the history, contact with teachers and others, and examination of the child, the psychiatrist can present to the caregiver a coherent picture in the follow-up visit or informing consultation. The diagnostic formulation may still lack coherence and be incomplete, however, despite the newfound orderliness. The dynamic formulation has traditionally been a feature of the psychoanalytical dynamic vantage of psychiatry. If this latter dimension is added to the consultative effort, psychiatrists must apply several principles that would make the enterprise clinically reasonable.

Dynamic Formulation

Clinically oriented dynamic formulations are conceptually related to models derived from freudian psychoanalysis and the derivative dynamic and cognitive therapies (Shapiro 1989, 1995). Four fundamental notions are essential to this vantage point (Shapiro and Esman 1985):

1. The existence of unconscious mental function is assumed.

2. Observable symptoms and signs may be driven by internalized conflicts that may be out of awareness or by habitual patterns designed to cope with the deficit.
3. Symptoms have meaning and significance to the child and are decipherable in terms of his or her life and experience. They also may be secondary elaborations of deficiency or physical defect.
4. A central need exists to displace internalized conflicts and maladaptive interpersonal relationships onto the therapist as transferential behaviors.

The dynamic formulation includes a summary paragraph describing the complaints of the patient, diagnosis, and precipitating events (Table 17–3). Biological factors include genetics, social deprivation, traumatic facts, and other external sources of data that would contribute to coherence of the current symptoms.

Table 17–3. Dynamic formulation

Summary paragraph
Nondynamic factors
Dynamic formulation
Predictive responses

The dynamic formulation itself should help the clinician interpret the patient's presenting symptoms and his or her behavior. These integrative inferences are based either on models of ego-psychological factors, developmental lines (Freud 1963), and separation-individuation (Mahler et al. 1975) or on any of the coherent dynamic schemes that help to account for the meaning of behavior. The dynamic formulation also includes predictive responses concerning future therapeutic interactions.

The following three vignettes of children at three stages of life are drawn from an article on dynamic formulation (Shapiro 1989).

Sammy, a 3.5-year-old boy, speaks at an age-appropriate level and in relevant sentences. He has no stereotypies but seems withdrawn and unrelated. His play is restricted, and his graphomotor skills are poor. He meets criteria for pervasive developmental disorder not otherwise specified, having been markedly isolated in his earlier years and echolalic because he began to speak late at age 2.5 years. Recently, he has shown increasing representational play but has become hypervigilant, not permitting his mother to leave, clinging to her, and screaming as she tries to separate.

Sammy's developmental disorder involves his object constancy and attachment to his mother. He has begun to differentiate and is attempting to maintain a stable representation of his mother. He is not yet able to do so. As his other developmental areas improve, and his linguistic and cognitive skills emerge, his crisis in emotional removal becomes a central problem.

Therapeutically, the clinician must anticipate modifications in treatment to include the mother and permit her to stay longer at his special school until Sammy can be taught techniques to remain secure in his mother's absence. She and his father must be engaged in a continuing encounter with a therapist or group to accept Sammy's developmental problems, help him to advance, and plan for special schooling. Their own despair and hope must be dealt with as they are helped to negotiate the real world for Sammy.

The interplay of faulty cognition, attachment behavior, and object relations in a developmental disorder creates numerous problems. The clinician must continue to be alert to this interaction to help a child adapt to his or her surroundings and to permit parents to hope while realistically guiding the disabled child in a complex, specialized world. Even if one were to add new behavioral reinforcements, the meaning of the behaviors to parents adds new dimensions to the parents' worry, guilt, and even conflict. The best treatment involves approaching these issues.

> Jerry, a 7-year-old boy, was hitting his peers and had become a petty thief. These maladaptive behaviors were associated with talking back to his parents after he had been in a new school for 3 months. Academically, he could not yet read, but his mathematics skills were at a grade-appropriate level. The diagnoses of conduct disorder (Axis I) and learning disability (Axis I) were made. No symptoms of anxiety, sadness, or other mental disturbances were present.
>
> Jerry's family had moved to a new school district a year ago after the father was terminated from his former job. The father found a new position in a neighboring town, but family discord and difficulty developed before the move. The mother was overwhelmed by Jerry's withdrawal and disciplinary problems. She also was burdened by having to care for Jerry's 4-year-old sister, who was born when he was almost 3 years old. He continually complained about diminished contact with his mother, who was busy with his sister, and responded sullenly to his father's eruptive and punitive interventions. The father had, in turn, been increasingly angry and demanding of the mother (Axis IV).

Developmentally, Jerry had been a normal full-term spontaneous delivery, with a paternal family history of learning difficulties. His mother was educated and sensitive but was easily overwhelmed. Developmental landmarks were on time, and although Jerry's response to his sister's birth had seemed casual, he changed from being an assertive and overactive boy to a withdrawn, eruptive, naughty child.

Jerry's current behavior is seen as an identification with the aggressor in a setting of experienced withdrawal of love by his mother, the object of his oedipal desires and his most steady internalized support. He has a strong regressive pull toward imitating his sister's infantile behavior, whereas he also tries to compensate and reassert his masculine role maladaptively based on imitation of his father's violent assertive displays. The recurrent jeopardy of losing his mother's affection since his sister's birth was reexperienced when they moved, causing him to overidentify with father's aggressiveness as he symbolically steals to undo his passive helplessness in not being able to learn and in trying to make friends.

Therapeutically, one would expect initial bravado and assertiveness with an insistent need to win. Jerry's move toward the therapist or tutor will be controlling and assertive until the underlying emotions can be elicited and confronted with permission for expression and until his more regressive wishes are interpreted. Jerry needs continuing support for his deficits in learning by resource room or tutoring. Counseling for the parents should be entertained. They could be directed toward better toleration of his assertive behavior through seeing it as mock masculinity, and his regressive demands may be better tolerated as a plea for love at his sister's level and considered nonpunitively.

This case of a child with learning disabilities and conduct disorder, if approached only from the standpoint of symptom clusters, might lead the clinician to some understanding of the social impact of the child's circumstance only if Axis IV were considered. The stressors of the move, the father's eruptiveness, and the mother's irritability might turn attention to the environment. However, in considering treatment, the parents' anger at the child, their inability to see his needs, and their focal attention to their own egocentric needs require family therapy to interrupt their pattern of neglect and even mistreatment of Jerry. He could not be expected to show them the way, given his developing maladaptive internalized patterns, which only accentuate his "bad boy" image. On the other hand, the patterns are not so firmly internalized that one would treat the child first.

Ron, an 8-year-old with impulsivity, excessive activity, and restlessness, was diagnosed as having ADHD. He seems to be insatiable in his wish to have things, constantly pleading with his mother to buy toys and wishing to take home toys of others. However, even when he does get some of the things requested, he tends to break them and to spoil events that he has longed for. He shows bravado with other children and assertiveness, which makes him unpopular, but sometimes he acts the clown in the classroom, seeking the attention of other children.

Ron has a high IQ despite his attentional problems and seems to have been able to compensate by learning quickly. He scores either at or above an age-appropriate level on his achievement tests. Treatment with methylphenidate was begun this year, but he still has altercations with his mother and father that end in screaming matches during which they tell him how he "spoils everything." After each tearful encounter, he can be comforted and is remorseful.

Ron's developmental history is marked by his mother's first-trimester bleeding and a bilirubin level of 15 mg/dL postnatally.

This child has achieved landmarks, with background difficulties in mastering his impulsiveness and distractibility. He too readily falls into a pattern with his parents in which his neediness for them and the things that they provide degenerates into accusations about his inability to enjoy things. The accusations are externally projected guilt representing a harsh superego serving inhibitions of forbidden wishes. He easily entered latency, permitting learning, but is constantly tormented by the need to act out his guilt feelings by spoiling his good times to elicit the final comforting. The miscarried struggles between him and his parents, however satisfying at some level, signify a maladaptive pattern stimulated from within and participated in by the parents.

In treatment, one would see a continuation of the oral hunger in settings of disappointment and frustration of need. Ron will also try to get the therapist to turn on him, fight with him, reprimand him, and hold him down in a continuing sadistic struggle that mimics his internal struggle with his superego. Although he compensates well for his impulsivity and is helped by his medication, his problems with control continue because they are symbolically driven by conflict. Parental counseling could help also. A psychoeducational approach might lead to more capacity to sympathize.

Children with ADHD are more than drug-responsive, attentionally deficient patients. They also regress, arrest, and progress in a human environment. Moreover, the drug's dynamic interaction with Ron's body and his tendency toward symptom formation are relevant to management. As noted in the literature, these children need more than medicine—they require multimodal treatment.

Conclusion

After reading these cases, one can see that differential diagnosis and traditional clinical diagnostic formulation alone do not complete the descriptions of children and their interactions with their bodies, worlds, and inner lives. To proceed therapeutically and to answer questions about what made the family seek help, what they want from therapists, and what therapists can provide, dynamic formulation is necessary. Only through this approach can the diagnostic formulation as a whole be used to inform parents, with the prospect of intervening appropriately and helpfully. The dynamic formulation does not represent a commitment to a specific treatment, but it should serve as a guide to a well-formulated intervention plan.

History has shown a progression of diagnostic approaches to children and adolescents. Whichever approach is adopted, specialized knowledge of the role of development is needed to manage and treat patients and their families.

References

Achenbach TM: Integrating assessment and taxonomy, in Assessment and Diagnosis in Child Psychopathology. Edited by Rutter M, Tuma AH, Lann IS. New York, Guilford, 1988, pp 300–346

Achenbach TM, Edelbrock CS: Manual for the Child Behavior Checklist and Revised Child Behavior Profile. Burlington, VT, University of Vermont, Department of Psychiatry, 1983

American Psychiatric Association: Diagnostic and Statistical Manual of Mental Disorders, 3rd Edition. Washington, DC, American Psychiatric Association, 1980

American Psychiatric Association: Diagnostic and Statistical Manual of Mental Disorders, 3rd Edition, Revised. Washington, DC, American Psychiatric Association, 1987

American Psychiatric Association: Diagnostic and Statistical Manual of Mental Disorders, 4th Edition. Washington, DC, American Psychiatric Association, 1994

American Psychiatric Association: Diagnostic and Statistical Manual of Mental Disorders, 4th Edition, Text Revision. Washington, DC, American Psychiatric Association, 2000

Beitchman J, Nair R, Clegg M, et al: Prevalence of psychiatric disorders in children with speech and language disorders. J Am Acad Child Psychiatry 25:528–535, 1986

Biederman J, Faraone SV, Hirshfeld-Becker DR, et al: Patterns of psychopathology and dysfunction in high-risk children of parents with panic disorder and major depression. Am J Psychiatry 158:49–57, 2001

Birmaher B, Ryan ND, Williamson DE, et al: Child and adolescent depression: a review of the past 10 years. Part II. J Am Acad Child Adolesc Psychiatry 35:1575–1583, 1996

Cantwell DP: The diagnostic process and diagnostic classification in child psychiatry: DSM-III. J Am Acad Child Psychiatry 19:345–355, 1980

Cantwell DP: DSM-III studies, in Assessment and Diagnosis in Child Psychopathology. Edited by Rutter M, Tuma AH, Lann IS. New York, Guilford, 1988, pp 3–36

Cantwell DP, Baker L: Stability and natural history of DSM-III childhood diagnoses. J Am Acad Child Adolesc Psychiatry 28:691–700, 1989

Chess S, Thomas A: Know Your Child. New York, Basic Books, 1987

Freud A: The concept of development lines, in The Psychoanalytic Study of the Child, Vol 18. New York, International Universities Press, 1963, pp 245–266

Geller B, Zimerman B, Williams M, et al: Bipolar disorder at prospective follow-up of adults who had prepubertal major depressive disorder. Am J Psychiatry 158:125–127, 2001

Goodman R: A modified version of the Rutter Parent Questionnaire including extra items on children's strengths: a research note. J Child Psychol Psychiatry 35:1483–1494, 1994

Green B, Shirk S, Hanze D, et al: The Children's Global Assessment Scale in clinical practice: an empirical evaluation. J Am Acad Child Adolesc Psychiatry 33:1158–1164, 1994

Group for the Advancement of Psychiatry: From Diagnosis to Treatment in Child Psychiatry. Northvale, NJ, Jason Aronson, 1974

Group for the Advancement of Psychiatry: How Old Is Old Enough? Washington, DC, American Psychiatric Press, 1989

Herjanic B, Campbell W: Differentiating psychiatrically disturbed children on the basis of a structured interview. J Abnorm Child Psychol 5:127–134, 1977

Jensen PS, Mrazek D, Knapp PK, et al: Evolution and revolution in child psychiatry: ADHD as a disorder of adaptation. J Am Acad Child Adolesc Psychiatry 36:1672–1679, 1997

Kagan J, Reznick JS, Snidman N, et al: Origins of panic disorder, in Neurobiology of Panic Disorder. Edited by Ballenger J. New York, Wiley, 1990, pp 71–87

Kashani JH, Carlson GA, Beck NC, et al: Depression, depressive symptoms, and depressed mood among a community sample of adolescents. Am J Psychiatry 144:931–934, 1987

Kovacs M: Presentation and course of major depressive disorder during childhood and later years of the life span. J Am Acad Child Adolesc Psychiatry 35:705–715, 1996

Laor N, Wolmer L, Cohen DJ: Mother's functioning and children's symptoms 5 years after a SCUD missile attack. Am J Psychiatry 158:1020–1026, 2001

Last CG, Hersen M, Kasdin AE, et al: Psychiatric illness in mothers of anxious children. Am J Psychiatry 144:1580–1583, 1987

Lewinsohn PM, Rohde P, Seeley JR, et al: Natural course of adolescent major depressive disorder in a community sample: predictors of recurrence in young adults. Am J Psychiatry 157:1584–1591, 2000

Mahler MS, Pine F, Bergman A: The Psychological Birth of the Human Infant. New York, Basic Books, 1975

McClellan JM, Werry JS: Introduction: research psychiatry diagnostic interviews for children and adolescents. J Am Acad Child Adolesc Psychiatry 39:19–27, 2000

McDermott J, Char WF: The undeclared war between child psychiatry and family therapy. J Am Acad Child Psychiatry 13:422–436, 1974

Nurcombe B, Seifer R, Scioli A: Is major depressive disorder in adolescence a distinct diagnostic entity? J Am Acad Child Adolesc Psychiatry 28:333–342, 1989

Pynoos R, Nader K: Children's memory and proximity to violence. J Am Acad Child Adolesc Psychiatry 28:236–241, 1989

Richters J, Cicchetti D: Mark Twain meets DSM-III-R: conduct disorder, development, and the concept of harmful dysfunction. Devel Psychopathol 5:5–29, 1993

Rutter M, Folstein S: Genetic influences and infantile autism. Nature 265:726–728, 1977

Rutter M, Cox A, Egert S, et al: Psychiatric interviewing techniques, V: experimental study: eliciting information. Br J Psychiatry 139:29–37, 1981

Shapiro T: The psychodynamic formulation in child and adolescent psychiatry. J Am Acad Child Adolesc Psychiatry 28:675–680, 1989

Shapiro T: Developmental issues in psychotherapy research. J Abnorm Child Psychol 23:31–43, 1995

Shapiro T, Esman A: Psychotherapy with children and adolescents: still relevant in the 1980s? Psychiatr Clin North Am 8:909–921, 1985

Shapiro T, Jegede RO: School phobia: a Babel of tongues. J Autism Child Schizophr 3:168–186, 1973

Swedo SE, Leonard HL, Mittleman BB, et al: Identification of children with pediatric autoimmune neuropsychiatric disorders associated with streptococcal infections by a marker associated with rheumatic fever. Am J Psychiatry 154:110–112, 1997

Swedo SE, Leonard HL, Garvey M, et al: Pediatric autoimmune neuropsychiatric disorders associated with streptococcal infections: a clinical description of the first fifty cases. Am J Psychiatry 155:264–271, 1998

Terr L: Chowchilla revisited: the effects of psychic trauma four years after a school bus kidnapping. Am J Psychiatry 140:1543–1550, 1983

Wakefield JC: The concept of mental disorder: on the boundary between biological fact and social values. Am Psychol 47:373–388, 1992

Wozniak J, Biederman J, Kiely K, et al: Mania-like symptoms suggestive of childhood-onset bipolar disorder in clinically referred children. J Am Acad Child Adolesc Psychiatry 34:867–876, 1995

Presentation of Findings and Recommendations

Héctor R. Bird, M.D.

The postassessment (or "informing") interview is a crucial aspect of the diagnostic process in child and adolescent psychiatry (Group for the Advancement of Psychiatry 1957). Its main purposes are to share the clinician's observations with the child's parents, to elaborate further on parental feelings and perceptions, and to discuss the clinician's recommendations so as to arrive collaboratively at a plan that will be helpful to both the child and his or her family. It is generally the parents who have brought the child to treatment, and it is they who will need to implement the clinician's recommendations. If treatment is indicated, the parents must work out the practical arrangements to enable their child to see the clinician and to subsidize the cost of treatment.

Parents generally approach this interview with a great deal of anxiety. Guilt is the underlying emotion generating their anxiety, and parents bring this guilt with them into the office. Quite often, guilt is externalized as anger toward their child and often toward the clinician. Parents view their child as their product (not entirely inaccurately), but this leads them to see their child's failings and difficulties as their own failure and to view their child's pathology as an affront to the adequacy of their parenting abilities. For many parents, the postassessment interview is the day of reckoning on which the "guilty" verdict will be passed by the all-knowing professional—the moment when all their parental flaws and all their mistakes and faulty child-rearing practices will be exposed. The parents generally arrive at the office on the defensive, anticipating an accusatory finger pointed at them, with a view of the clinician as their adversary. Thus, the clinician's first task is to provide these anxious parents with reassurance and support (Cox 1994).

One important way to provide support and reassurance to the parents is by conveying that regardless of the developmental, behavioral, or emotional difficulties, their child is basically a good person. Although the parents may believe that they have "failed" in bringing up their child (and in some respects, this may indeed be true), it is important to make them feel that there are equally many things that they have done "right." This first step in the information-sharing process must heavily emphasize the child's observed assets: "Johnny is a very nice kid. He's engaging... sensitive...good at relating to others...witty... affectionate...has a great sense of humor.... There's a lot about him to be proud of." At this stage, one must be cautious to maintain a balance between the positive and the negative. To deny any kind of parental influence on the child's difficulties and to attribute everything to genetics or to temperament can be as detrimental as pointing the accusatory finger at the parents and placing the blame entirely on the way they have brought up their child. The parents must be brought to the realization that they have as much to do with what are perceived as their child's positive characteristics as they may have to do with what are seen as their child's liabilities. If this balance of positive and negative is achieved, the parents will be more receptive to the information shared with them.

The informing interview should not be a lecture in which the clinician does all the talking. The next step is to move into the problem areas and to summarize what has happened since the onset of the consultation process: "When you first came to see me three weeks ago, your major concerns seemed to be that Johnny's work in school had gone downhill and that his teachers complained that he does not pay attention in class. …I wonder what your thoughts about this have been since we last met." In this interview it is important to share what has happened since the parents were last seen during the diagnostic process. How has their child reacted to the diagnostic interviews? What has his or her behavior been like? Has he or she given the parents any feedback about the meetings with the clinician? Have there been any observable changes in the child's behavior or emotional state?

It is also important that the parents understand that what is "wrong" with their child is not simply the maladaptive behavior that is manifested but that these behaviors are closely linked to the child's emotions and cognitions. This understanding is often facilitated by an elaboration of those insights about their child, about themselves, and about family interactions that may have been gained during the diagnostic process. It is thus crucial to de-emphasize how the child behaves and to emphasize how the child feels and sees the world. Many parents require more than one session to explore their motivations, to relieve their guilt about having failed or their anger at their child, and, when treatment is indicated, to overcome their resistance to treatment.

Another important factor that serves to reassure the parents and to gain their confidence and alliance is for the clinician to be perceived as a reliable and competent professional whose observations and recommendations can be trusted. From their brief contact during the diagnostic process, the parents may have developed fantasies about the clinician, some of which may already be transference reactions. When a recommendation for treatment is being made, it is pertinent to explain to parents, "I have a feeling that I can be helpful to your child, but I have known your child for only a few days, and you have known your child all his or her life. From what you have observed about me, do you think I am the kind of person whom he or she will find helpful?" Although this is in many ways a leading question, given that most parents would find it difficult to reply "No, you are not," this line of questioning opens up a dialogue and communicates to parents that the clinician is not an all-powerful, all-knowing expert who will rescue their child. Rather, it conveys that the clinician sees possible limitations to his or her capacities, as well as the need to have a good fit between patient and therapist.

To enhance communication with the parents, the clinician should avoid technical jargon and should provide observations and comments in lay terms. Even with highly educated parents, technical terms may not necessarily have the same meaning as they have for a trained professional. Greenspan (1981) recommended that information about the child be addressed in a developmental context. It is easier for parents to accept a statement such as "Your child relates to others more like a two-year-old would" than "There is a disturbance in the way your child relates to other children," or "Your child is extremely immature in the way that he or she relates to others."

The clinician should limit the content of the interview with the parents to those areas that will help the patient and should limit the extent to which either parent may discuss individual problems to the exclusion of the identified patient.

The postdiagnostic interview with parents whose child's prognosis is poor, such as an autistic child or a child with mental retardation, is particularly sensitive. Regardless of the diagnosis or prognosis that can be anticipated, it is obviously impossible for any clinician to predict the future unequivocally for an individual patient. It behooves the clinician to be well versed in the literature and in recent findings about the disorder at hand so that a realistic appraisal of what or what not to expect can be communicated. The clinician should not feed into the parents' denial mechanisms by minimizing the severity of the psychopathology, but by the same token, the parents should not be allowed to leave the clinician's office in hopelessness and despair. Follow-up sessions are indicated with such parents to help them shape their expectations. Prognosis is poor only when the real outcome is much worse than the anticipated outcome. Outcome must be dissected into its component parts. If the child is intellectually dull and the family expects him or her to have a brilliant career, then prognosis is extremely poor. If the parents can tone down their level of expectation and can see their child as a productive member of society in a more modest role, then the prognostic statement can be more favorable.

Confidentiality

Clearly, a child's family, particularly the parents, constitutes the child's most important source of social support. Often the clinician is hesitant to use this source of support to its fullest because of restricted conceptions of confidentiality that preclude discussion of the child's problems with the parents. This barrier often impairs the clinician's ability to find the most effective approach to helping the patient (Barth 1986).

The child clinician's task is complicated because the therapeutic alliance is twofold: the therapeutic contract must be negotiated with the child and with both parents. Particularly for a child whom one expects to have in treatment, a goal of the informing interview is to ensure that there is an alliance with the parents as well as the child. The alliance with the parents will serve to maintain the child in treatment when resistance surfaces. In an intact family, the clinician must share the results of the evaluation with both parents and must accommodate both parents in setting up appointments. When there is a marital separation, the quality of the relationship between the parents dictates whether separate appointments are needed. Even under those circumstances, it is desirable that both parents share the session with the clinician. An observation of their interaction can provide the clinician with a firsthand view of circumstances that the child faces on a daily basis.

From the very first contact with the patient, the clinician should inform the patient of the process that will be followed. Both the child and the family should know that the child will be interviewed individually, that there may be a family interview, and that after a number of sessions the clinician will meet with the parents to convey results of the evaluation and recommendations. The child should be made aware that the purpose of this informing interview is to share information so that his or her parents can be more helpful and that the interview is not a forum to manipulate the parents or to chide them on the patient's behalf.

The clinician can promise confidentiality within certain limits, and the child must know these limits from the outset. As a general rule, the clinician can promise confidentiality to a child with the proviso that information which, in the clinician's judgment, is potentially self-destructive or destructive to others will be shared with those who can protect the child. In those instances, the clinician specifically breaches confidentiality to protect the child and those around him or her. The rubrics "self-destructive" and "destructive to others" include issues such as suicidality, antisocial behaviors, sexual promiscuity, and use of drugs or alcohol. To most children and adolescents, these limitations to confidentiality are reassuring and promote a sense of safety as well as confidence rather than mistrust in the clinician. Before meeting with the parents, the clinician should ask the patient about information

that the patient wants to keep confidential, and this information should be kept confidential as long as the aforementioned proviso is upheld. The clinician also should inquire whether the patient would like the clinician to emphasize a particular topic while meeting with the parents. This inquiry often promotes, from an early stage, a view of the clinician as a helping agent (Adams 1982; Simmons 1969).

Confidentiality is qualitatively different for younger children than for adolescents. Younger children find it difficult to conceive of events or circumstances that their parents either do not know or should not know. It usually is not necessary to include younger children in the postdiagnostic interview, and most children accept that the clinician must meet with parents privately.

Adolescence, however, is the second stage of separation-individuation, and regardless of whether it is acknowledged by the adolescent, the issues of privacy and confidentiality are of paramount importance, possibly of greater importance than they are for adult patients (Bird 1995). Any real or imagined breach of the adolescent's confidence may irreversibly block the patient's capacity to ever trust a particular clinician. As a general rule, the adolescent should be given the option to be present at meetings with the parents for the purpose of presenting findings and making recommendations. Some adolescents choose to be present; others presumably do not care. However, the choice should be theirs, and parents should be advised at the outset that their children are allowed to make this decision. Regardless of an adolescent's choice, before the informing interview, the clinician should specifically discuss with the adolescent what the parents will be told at the meeting. The adolescent then can provide the clinician with specific feedback and can discuss details that will be shared with the parents. This discussion with the adolescent also has therapeutic purpose in that it conveys to the adolescent the clinician's impressions and recommendations, as well as the clinician's opinion that the adolescent is the central person in the entire process. This approach places the clinician and the patient on the same team.

Therapeutic Alliance

The therapeutic alliance that the clinician hopes to establish with the patient must be preceded by a therapeutic alliance with the patient's parents. Either parent, as a senior member of the family and one who controls the family resources, is in a position to sabotage the clinician's efforts and to act out any resistance to treatment. For this reason, parents' collaboration is essential. Several factors are relevant to a family's remaining in therapy, including the therapist's activity and directiveness, the congruence between family expectations and the therapist's response, and the family's ability to influence the consultation. Parents, and patients in general, seem to prefer active and directive clinicians. This is particularly true of families who attend low-cost clinics, but this preference probably applies to families at all socioeconomic and educational levels. Studies of adults have shown that when therapists provided feedback that the patients' communications had been perceived, these patients were more likely to continue in therapy after the initial consultation (Roter 1989). The experience in child psychiatry is similar to what is generally experienced in medicine: Patient compliance and satisfaction are strongly related to the physician's providing adequate feedback and information. It appears that sharing information in this way enhances patients' sense of empowerment and their conviction that they will be active participants in the therapeutic process.

The way that findings and recommendations are discussed with the family can have therapeutic and prognostic implications. The informing interview is a critical aspect of the diagnostic process. If this interview is handled poorly, it can lead to premature closure of a process that is potentially beneficial and therapeutic to the child and family. When done thoughtfully and sensitively, the informing interview can relieve parental anxiety and guilt, provide alternative ways for parents to view and deal with their children's difficulties, and establish an alliance between the clinician and family (Duehn and Proctor 1977; Stevenson 1971).

References

Adams PL: A Primer of Child Psychotherapy, 2nd Edition. Boston, MA, Little, Brown, 1982

Barth RP: Social and Cognitive Treatment of Children and Adolescents. San Francisco, CA, Jossey-Bass, 1986

Bird H: Psychiatric treatment of adolescents, in Kaplan and Sadock's Comprehensive Textbook of Psychiatry, 6th Edition. Edited by Kaplan HI, Sadock BJ. Baltimore, MD, Williams & Wilkins, 1995, pp 2439–2446

Cox AD: Interviews with parents, in Child and Adolescent Psychiatry: Modern Approaches. Edited by Rutter M, Taylor E, Hersov L. Oxford, UK, Blackwell Scientific, 1994, pp 34–50

Duehn WD, Proctor EK: Initial clinical interaction and premature discontinuance in treatment. Am J Orthopsychiatry 47:284–290, 1977

Greenspan SI: The Clinical Interview of the Child. New York, McGraw-Hill, 1981

Group for the Advancement of Psychiatry (GAP): The Diagnostic Process in Child Psychiatry (Report No 38). New York, Group for the Advancement of Psychiatry, 1957

Roter D: Which facets of communication have strong effects on outcome: a meta-analysis, in Communicating With Medical Patients. Edited by Stewart M, Roter D. London, Sage, 1989, pp 183–196

Simmons JE: Psychiatric Examination of Children. Philadelphia, PA, Lea & Febiger, 1969

Stevenson I: The Diagnostic Interview, 2nd Edition. New York, Harper & Row, 1971

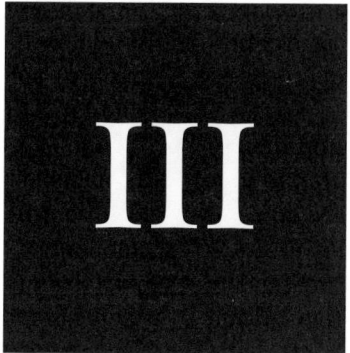

Developmental Disorders

Mental Retardation

Ludwik S. Szymanski, M.D.

Lawrence C. Kaplan, M.D.

Mental retardation, even though it is listed as a mental disorder in DSM-IV-TR (American Psychiatric Association 2000), is different from other mental disorders. First, it is not a "usual" illness, in that it does not have a single etiology or course or pathognomonic features. It is a term that refers to a person whose level of functioning (cognitively and adaptively) is below a certain cutoff point.

In this chapter, we discuss mental retardation both as a psychosocial phenomenon and as a biomedical phenomenon. We then address the psychiatry of mental retardation—that is, diagnosis and treatment of mental disorders that might be comorbid with it. The focus is primarily on children and adolescents, although the material presented here often applies to adults with mental retardation as well.

Mental Retardation as a Psychosocial Phenomenon

■ Evolution of the Concept and Definition of Mental Retardation

An early definition of mental retardation was suggested by Sir Anthony Fitzherbert, who wrote in 1534: "And he who shall be said to be a sot and idiot from his birth is such a person who cannot account or remember 20 pence, nor can he tell who was his father or mother, nor how old he is, etc.,…" (Scheerenberger 1983, p. 36). The modern precursor of psychological testing was first developed in France by Alfred Binet and his student, Theodore Simon, in 1905. Its purpose was not to measure intelligence and to classify people on this basis but to detect children who would have difficulty learning in regular classes in Paris (Scheerenberger 1983, p. 142). However, soon after these tests were introduced to the United States by Goddard in 1908, their use became widespread as a primary means to diagnose mental retardation by low test scores. In 1916 Lewis Terman, head of department of psychology in Stanford University, introduced to the United States the concept of an intelligence quotient (IQ), which has been used to classify people on the basis of its scores, with 90–110 for normal or average intelligence. However, measuring cognitive abilities is a complex issue, with many factors, such as cultural and linguistic background, being involved. This topic is dealt with in detail in Chapter 14 ("Psychological and Neuropsychological Testing") in this volume.

Since 1921, the American Association on Mental Retardation (AAMR)—and its forerunners—has periodically published manuals on classification and terminology. The traditional cutoff for the diagnosis of mental retardation was an IQ 2 standard deviations (SD) below the mean for the test being used. The fifth edition of the manual, published in 1959, contained sections on measuring both intelligence and a second dimension—deficits in adaptive behavior. The latter is now included in all the current standard definitions of mental retardation, although some researchers have called for the return to a unidimensional definition based on only the IQ (Zigler et al. 1984). In the 1959 edition, the IQ cutoff was changed to 1 SD below the mean (equal to an IQ of about 85), thus making about 15% of the population eligible for the diagnosis. Because of the concern about such a broad definition, it was changed again in 1973 to 2 SD below the mean, thus eliminating the category of "borderline retardation." The "developmental period" for the age at onset was set at age 18 years or younger.

The 1983 edition of the American Association on Mental Deficiency's *Classification in Mental Retardation* (Grossman 1983) was edited to be consistent with the *International Classification of Diseases*, 9th Revision (ICD-9; World Health Organization 1977), and DSM-III (American Psychiatric Association 1980). The basic definition of mental retardation was unchanged, but it was clarified that in making the diagnosis, one should consider the ±5 points of error inherent in the psychometric tests.

The nature of mental retardation is still controversial. According to one view (Ellis and Cavalier 1982), people with mental retardation are deficient in at least one of the cognitive processes required for intelligent behavior. Instead of focusing on discrete deficiencies, Detterman (1987) viewed mental retardation as characterized by deficits in those abilities that are important in the functioning of the complex system of characteristics that together define human intelligence. A developmental approach (Zigler 1969; Zigler and Balla 1982) views the central problem in mental retardation as being the slower development and the lower ultimate level that the individual achieves rather than a deficiency in basic cognitive processes. Whitman (1990) perceived mental retardation as a "self-regulatory disorder," in that people with this condition are unable to generalize their knowledge to situations outside those of training. Szymanski et al. (1989) conceptualized mental retardation as a final common pathway of a central nervous system (CNS) dysfunction that may have varied causation.

The 2002 Definition of the American Association on Mental Retardation

In 2002, the AAMR published its current manual, *Mental Retardation: Definition, Classification, and Systems of Supports*, 10th Edition, with the following definition:

> Mental retardation is a disability characterized by significant limitations both in intellectual functioning and in adaptive behavior as expressed in conceptual, social, and practical adaptive skills. This disability originates before age 18. (p. 8)

"Significant limitations" in intellectual functioning are defined as an IQ standard score at least 2 SD below the mean of an individually administered assessment instrument. The standard error of measurement for the instrument, usually between 3 and 5 points, has to be taken into account. In contrast to the previous definition (American Association on Mental Retardation 1992) and that from DSM-IV (American Psychiatric Association 1994), 3 general types of adaptive behavior are listed instead of 10 specific adaptive skills. For the diagnosis of mental retardation to apply, the performance on a standardized instrument should be at least 2 SD below the mean in one of these types or in an overall score. The importance of clinical judgment is highlighted, not as a substitute for the use of an appropriate measurement but for assessment of the results, drawing conclusions, and planning for treatment and needed supports. Significant limitations both in intellectual functioning and in adaptive behavior have to be documented. Thus, a person can be diagnosed as having mental retardation of higher or lower severity than that which the IQ score alone would indicate, depending on the level of adaptive skills. A person with an IQ of 68 might not be diagnosed as having mental retardation if he or she has basic academic skills, lives almost independently, and holds a regular job. The reverse may be true for a person who has an IQ of 75 but poor adaptive skills.

This definition refers to the current level of functioning, regardless of etiology; therefore, mental retardation is not necessarily viewed as a lifelong condition. It is required that the limitations be seen in the context of person's environment, culture, language diversity, and coexisting limitations, such as physical, sensory, and behavioral. The AAMR definition (American Association on Mental Retardation 2002, p. 9) uses a "multidimensional" (essentially biopsychosocial) approach to mental retardation that includes five dimensions:

1. Intellectual abilities
2. Adaptive behavior
3. Participation, interactions, and social roles
4. Health (physical and mental)
5. Context (including environment and culture)

Thus, this definition stresses the importance of comorbidity of mental disorders with mental retardation in determining the person's functioning.

The focus of the AAMR recent definitions is not solely on the deficiencies and abnormalities related to the diagnosis. Instead, it sees the functioning of the individual with mental retardation as resulting from interaction of the individual's capabilities, the environment, and available supports. Thus, even if there is a defined etiology, such as Down syndrome due to trisomy 21, the actual level of associated mental retardation will be influenced by factors such as presence of associated disabilities (e.g., sensory impairments), educational and other opportunities, attitudes of caregivers, and level of stimulation.

The DSM-IV-TR Definition

The DSM-IV-TR definition of mental retardation (Table 19–1) is similar to the 1992 AAMR definition. It uses an IQ cutoff of 70, retains the subdivision into four levels of severity (mild, moderate, severe, and profound) based on the IQ score (Table 19–2), and lists 10 types of adaptive behaviors. No general diagnosis or coding of mental retardation is available. Separate codes are used for each of the severity levels. Mental retardation is coded on Axis II.

Related Terms

Developmental disability. *Developmental disability* is a term defined by the Developmental Disabilities Assistance and Bill of Rights Amendments of 1996. Its definition is not identical to that for the term *mental retardation*. It often appears in statutes concerning educational and other entitlements. Its main points are these:

- The disability is due to mental and/or physical impairment.
- It is manifested before age 22 years.
- It is likely to continue indefinitely.
- It results in substantial functional limitations in three or more major life activities.
- It reflects the individual's need for lifelong or extended special services or supports that are individualized and coordinated.

If this term is applied to children younger than 5 years, it means presence of substantial developmental delay or specific congenital or acquired conditions, with a high probability that developmental disabilities will result if services are not provided (University of Minnesota 2000).

Dual diagnosis. The term *dual diagnosis* has been used by some professionals in the field of mental retardation to denote people with diagnosed mental retardation and a comorbid mental disorder. Use of this term might be confusing because most mental health professionals employ it to denote comorbidity of mental illness and substance abuse disorder.

■ Diagnostic Criteria and Clinical Findings

Various initial clinical presentations can raise the question of mental retardation and initiate the diagnostic process. For example, certain disorders associated with retardation might be diagnosed in routine neonatal screening, and then early treatment might effectively prevent retardation (e.g., phenylketonuria, congenital hypothyroidism). If the retardation is part of a syndrome with an obvious physical phenotype, the expressed features might be the first clue to a diagnosis such as Down syndrome, which is usually made in the neonatal period or, increasingly, prenatally. Sometimes the diagnostic process might be initiated because of a comorbid disorder (e.g., seizures), in the course of which a CNS pathology might be discovered. Such associated physical findings are usually more common if the retardation is more severe. Generally, the milder the retardation, the later the diagnosis is made. The first concern might arise when the infant or toddler fails to reach developmental milestones as expected, usually in motor and language development. In some cases, another developmental disorder comorbid with the retardation, such as autism, might be the focus, and the retardation might not be noticed initially. Some children's retardation will not be diagnosed until early school years, when academic failure becomes obvious. Even then, the initial concern might be about other manifestations, such as disruptive behavior, until detailed psychological assessment discloses the intellectual impairment. It is important to remember that, by definition, mental retardation is not necessarily a lifelong disorder. Some individuals may meet the criteria for mild mental retardation during school years because of failure in academic learning, but with proper services and training, they can acquire adaptive and independence skills to the level that these criteria are no longer met.

■ Differential Diagnosis

In *learning disorders* and *communication disorders*, the impairments are usually more circumscribed and limited to a specific domain, unlike the generalized impairment in intellectual and adaptive skills that characterizes mental retardation. These disorders can coexist with mental retardation if the specific impairments are in excess of those usually seen at this level of mental

Table 19–1. DSM-IV-TR diagnostic criteria for mental retardation

A. Significantly subaverage intellectual functioning: an IQ of approximately 70 or below on an individually administered IQ test (for infants, a clinical judgment of significantly subaverage intellectual functioning).

B. Concurrent deficits or impairments in present adaptive functioning (i.e., the person's effectiveness in meeting the standards expected for his or her age by his or her cultural group) in at least two of the following areas: communication, self-care, home living, social/interpersonal skills, use of community resources, self-direction, functional academic skills, work, leisure, health, and safety.

C. The onset is before age 18 years.

Code based on degree of severity reflecting level of intellectual impairment:

317	**Mild Mental Retardation:**	IQ level 50–55 to approximately 70
318.0	**Moderate Mental Retardation:**	IQ level 35–40 to 50–55
318.1	**Severe Mental Retardation:**	IQ level 20–25 to 35–40
318.2	**Profound Mental Retardation:**	IQ level below 20 or 25
319	**Mental Retardation, Severity Unspecified:**	when there is strong presumption of mental retardation but the person's intelligence is untestable by standard tests

Source. Reprinted from the *Diagnostic and Statistical Manual of Mental Disorders*, 4th Edition, Text Revision. Washington, DC, American Psychiatric Association, 2000. Copyright 2000, American Psychiatric Association. Used with permission.

Table 19–2. Mental retardation: degrees of severity

Severity	Approximate IQ range
Mild	50–55 to 70
Moderate	35–40 to 50–55
Severe	20–25 to 35–40
Profound	Below 20–25

retardation. *Pervasive developmental disorders* are characterized by qualitative impairments in social interaction and communication, whereas children with otherwise uncomplicated mental retardation do relate to others, even if in a manner immature for their age. *Dementia* is diagnosed if specific multiple cognitive impairments, including memory impairment, are present and represent decline from the previous level of functioning. Dementia may be diagnosed at any age, whereas criteria for mental retardation require an age at onset before 18 years. Theoretically, both dementia and mental retardation might be diagnosed if the insult to the brain was postnatal, but because of difficulty in establishing premorbid level of functioning, such double diagnosis is not recommended before age 4–6 years, or in cases in which the condition is sufficiently described by the diagnosis of mental retardation alone.

■ Epidemiology

Historically, the estimates of the prevalence of mental retardation have varied, depending on the definition and the methodology used. One approach was to calculate the prevalence of individuals with an IQ score below the cutoff expected according to the normal distribution. With the early definitions based on an IQ of 1 SD or below, the prevalence was thought to be about 15% of the population. This was lowered to 3% when the criterion of 2 SD was used and the IQ score was the sole diagnostic criterion. The modern approach is to use the IQ and adaptive-behavior–based definition and to conduct a study of unselected populations. With this approach, the prevalence was estimated to be about 1% of the general population. A review of epidemiological studies found the estimated prevalence of mild mental retardation to be 0.37%–0.59%, and of moderate, severe, and profound mental retardation combined, 0.3%–0.4% (McLaren and Bryson 1987). As might be expected, the prevalence is highest among school-age children because they are faced with academic learning tasks that require cognitive abilities. The prevalence declines in the adult age group, when good adaptive skills, particularly for work, assume more importance. Mental retardation is also more prevalent in males than in females (1.6:1).

The data from the National Health Interview Survey for 1994–1995 indicate that the combined prevalence of mental retardation and developmental disabilities in the United States is 1.58% of the population (excluding people living in residential settings of four or more people). This number is useful in reflecting the number of people in need of support services. The prevalence of mental retardation alone was estimated to be 0.78% (University of Minnesota 2000).

People with mental retardation often have associated medical, neurological, and sensory disorders. Seizure disorders are estimated to occur in 15%–30%, motor handicaps (including cerebral palsy) in 20%–30%, and sensory impairments in 10%–20% of this population (McLaren and Bryson 1987). The prevalence of these associated disorders is higher when the retardation is more severe.

Mental Retardation as a Biomedical Phenomenon

■ Pathoetiology

It is helpful to consider mental retardation as a developmental and behavioral manifestation of variations in the form, function, and adaptation of the CNS (Leroy 1992). The health professional also must consider the contribution of other organ systems, as well as the important effect of the environment on human beings, each of whom has unique responses to the various stresses and challenges of life.

With rapid advances in the prenatal and early postnatal detection of certain conditions, and with improvements in medical and educational supports, a number of clinical conditions traditionally associated with particular patterns of mental retardation appear to be quite different from their earlier descriptions (Curry et al. 1997; Mayes et al. 1985). This underscores the importance of seeing mental retardation as a reflection of embryonic, perinatal, and postnatal influences, with the balance among these characterizing the individual's actual clinical status (Kaplan 1985).

Three basic etiological categories can assist the clinician in formulating diagnoses (Table 19–3):

Table 19–3. Etiological categories of mental retardation

Errors in morphogenesis of the central nervous system
Malformation and malformation syndromes
In utero neurological disease altering form and posture (deformations)
Disruption (injury) to developing central nervous system

Alterations in the intrinsic biological environment
Inborn errors in metabolism
Non-inborn changes in metabolism

Extraordinary extrinsic influences or events
Hypoxia
Trauma
Poisoning

---

1. Prenatal errors in morphogenesis of the CNS and/or other systems severe enough to alter normal development
2. Alterations in the intrinsic biological environment of an individual such that the function of the CNS is also altered (such alterations may be established prenatally but can evolve postnatally)
3. Extraordinary extrinsic influences, resulting in a drastic change in mental function

Errors in Morphogenesis

In this group of conditions, embryonic development and fetal development are altered (Table 19–4) (Jones 1997; Jones and Rubinson 1983). Approximately 4% of live-born infants are found, in the first year of life, to have major errors in morphogenesis. In a study by Holmes (1980), 2.4% of newborns had a major anomaly, and nearly 60% of these were associated with genetic or in utero causes.

Errors in morphogenesis may be due to malformations (failure of tissue to form normally from the time of conception), deformations (alteration of normally forming tissues by abnormal mechanical forces), and disruptions (in utero injury or toxicity to tissues) (Hudgins and Cassidy 1999). These events have common processes but differ in terms of the mechanisms by which form and function of the CNS are affected.

Malformations are usually sporadic or multifactorial (Cohen 1982; Wuu et al. 1991). Examples of multiple malformation syndromes include Brachmann-de Lange syndrome, Prader-Willi syndrome (Butler et al. 1986; Hawley et al. 1985; Kaplan et al. 1987), Pena-Shokeir syndrome (an autosomal-recessive disorder involving severe mental retardation and upper motor neuron disease), and Down syndrome (Hall 1986; Pueschel and Pueschel 1992). Implied in all of these examples is the concept that some signal or operator, such as an identified gene or chromosome or an unidentified stimulus that produces a recognizable pattern of abnormal morphogenesis, has directed a cascade of abnormal CNS growth and development. Myelodysplasia (spina bifida), which may be associated with mental retardation, represents a particularly striking example of a multiple malformation syndrome (Kaplan 1998). Despite the involvement of multiple organ systems, the primary error in morphogenesis resides in the formation or differentiation of the early neural tube, and the general effect is abnormal innervation of multiple organs.

Table 19–4. Abnormalities of central nervous system morphogenesis

Etiology	Example	Pathology	Diagnostic considerations	Degree of mental retardation (MR)	Management considerations
Malformations					
Single gene recessive	Pena-Shokeir syndrome	Heterogeneous, muscle atrophy; abnormal spinal cord, cerebral dysgenesis	Neurogenic arthrogryposis; pulmonary hypoplasia; hypertelorbitism; phenotype overlaps with trisomy 18; autosomal recessive; decreased fetal movement	Severe to profound	Pulmonary insufficiency; seizures; swallowing difficulties; over half of instances are autosomal recessive
	Seckel's syndrome	Microcephaly; cerebral dysgenesis	Severely short stature; prominent nose; hyperactivity common; severe microcephaly	Severe to profound	Generally healthy; performance is variable
	Smith-Lemli-Opitz syndrome	Cerebral dysmorphogenesis; hypoplasia of frontal lobes, brainstem, cerebellum; irregular gyral patterns, heterotopia	Ptosis; anteverted nostrils; syndactyly of second and third toes; hypospadias; cryptorchidism in males	Severe	Feeding difficulties—20% of newborn survivors die in first year; irritability; significant multisystem management challenges
Single gene dominant	Tuberous sclerosis	Glioma, angioma in cortex and white matter basal ganglia, periventricular mineralization, phakomata, fibrous angiomatous skin lesions, cystlike lesions in phalanges	Hamartomatous skin nodules, seizures, phakomata, bone lesions on x-ray	Frequent; greater with severe seizures	Seizures in early childhood, difficult to manage, occasional hypsarrhythmia, widely variable expression
X-linked recessive	Menkes' syndrome	Cortical degeneration, gliosis, atrophy; intracranial vascular dysplasia; tortuosity; sparse, stubby, "kinky" hair; defect in intestinal copper absorption	Progressive cerebral deterioration with seizures; twisted and fractured hair	Progresses to severe	Death usually by age 3 years; hair normal at birth but loss of pigmentation by 6 weeks
	Fragile X syndrome	Fragile site represents a mutation of the *FMR1* gene; maternal carrier state important; previously thought to affect only males, but females can also be affected	Developmental delay often mistaken for autism; mild connective tissue dysplasia; macroorchidism; large-appearing ears that measure normal size; gaze aversion common	Mild to moderate in 80% of affected males	Expressive language delay frequent in those younger than age 3 years; emotional lability; can have hyperactivity

Table 19–4. Abnormalities of central nervous system morphogenesis (*continued*)

Etiology	Example	Pathology	Diagnostic considerations	Degree of mental retardation (MR)	Management considerations
Multifactorial	Neural tube defects, including spina bifida	Includes hydrocephalus; Arnold-Chiari II malformation; spina bifida, abnormalities in neural tube closure by 18–28 days' gestation	Wide spectrum of clinical features; unshunted hydrocephalus typically progresses, increasing chances for MR; hydrocephalus does not always correlate with definite MR	Variable, with mild hydrocephalus; cognitive function can be normal; coincident CNS pathology affects developmental outcome	Multidisciplinary attention needed, including orthopedics, pediatrics, child development, urology, neurosurgery, nursing, social work; habilitative potential frequently excellent with coordinated care
Sporadic/unknown	Cornelia de Lange's syndrome	Unknown cerebral dysgenesis; microcephaly	Synophrys; thin, down-turned upper lip; hirsutism; micromelia; cardiac, renal, genitourinary abnormalities	Variable; severe MR correlates with complexity of other organ systems	Growth retardation is very common; seizures in 20%; coloboma and blindness may occur; possible "mild" form with significant behavioral disabilities
	Williams syndrome	Deletion of an elastin gene allele located on chromosome 7	Prominent lips; stellate iris pattern; hoarse voice; supravalvular aortic stenosis; calcium metabolism problems	Average IQ 56 (41–80); expressive language delay	Often but not always loquacious, personable; may develop spasticity later in life; typically hypotonic in infancy and may fail to thrive
	Molecular and chromosomal defects	Prader-Willi syndrome (Labhart syndrome)	>70% of clinical diagnosis associated with deletion of long arm of chromosome 15 at q11q13 detected by high-resolution chromosome analysis or fluorescent studies (FISH)	Hypotonia; obesity; small hands and feet; hyperphagia common; narrow forehead; downward-slanted palpebral fissures	IQ range 20–80; often but not always have behavioral problems; typically presents with failure to thrive in infancy and hypotonia; hypotonia persists; eventually becomes hyperphagic and can develop obesity early in life

Table 19–4. Abnormalities of central nervous system morphogenesis *(continued)*

Etiology	Example	Pathology	Diagnostic considerations	Degree of mental retardation (MR)	Management considerations
	Down syndrome	Trisomy 21; D/G chromosomal translocation	Microcephaly; brachycephaly; Brushfield spots; hypotonia; medial epicanthal folds; small ears; endocardial cushion defect common	IQ range 25–50, occasionally higher	Intensive positive experience with early infant stimulation; Alzheimer's disease symptomatology encountered frequently; Down syndrome growth charts are available
	Trisomy 18 syndrome	Trisomic chromosome 18	Microcephaly; micrognathia; ventricular septal defect; hypotonia; short sternum; highly lethal condition	Profound	Mosaicism for extra chromosome 18 often associated with better outcome; 10% survival past first year of life
	Cri du chat syndrome	5p- (partial deletion of chromosome 5)	Catlike cry; microcephaly; downward-slanted palpebral fissures	Severe to profound	Diagnosis difficult to make in older individuals
	Angelman's syndrome	60%–80% of affected individuals have interstitial deletion of chromosome 15q11q13 (molecular/FISH)	Ataxic movements; paroxysmal laughter; cerebral palsy common	Severe to profound	Seizures common; evidence for progressive loss of function after first decade; possible parkinsonian-like dementia in adulthood
Deformations	Arthrogryposis secondary to CNS malformation	CNS abnormality results in diminished fetal movement, leading to contractures at birth	Neuropathy and myopathy must be ruled out	Often none, but related to degree of CNS pathology	Contractures often improve after birth, especially with physical therapy
Disruptions	Porencephaly	Vascular disruption of brain in utero	Vascular disruption of brain in utero	Mild to severe	Motor impairment common

Note. CNS=central nervous system; FISH= fluorescence in situ hybridization.

Deformations are changes in the form or growth of tissues and organ systems that have been influenced by unusual mechanical forces (Dunn 1976). These deformations may be due to an abnormally shaped uterus compressing the developing calvarial bones and resulting in simple cosmetic changes in the shape of the head (plagiocephaly) or to abnormal fetal movement that may result in fixed contractures at birth, hip dislocation, or clubfoot (Clarren et al. 1979; Graham 1988). Rarely do deformations, per se, cause mental retardation, but identifying them is helpful because they may point to underlying congenital neurological conditions that are associated with mental retardation.

Disruptions involve catastrophic gestational damage to the embryo or fetus or possibly the steady "undoing" of formed and forming tissues and organ systems. This category of errors in morphogenesis includes effects of the large and growing group of teratogens, chemicals, and toxins that can disrupt normal morphogenesis. These include well-known substances such as alcohol, the largest cause of preventable mental retardation in the United States today; the anticoagulant sodium warfarin (Coumadin); and cocaine and crack, substances with largely unknown effects but that appear to be involved in significant long-term effects even in the absence of distinct physical findings at birth (Kaplan 1985; Weiner et al. 1988; Zuckerman et al. 1989). Also included in the group of disruptions are certain viruses, particularly toxoplasmosis, rubella, and cytomegalovirus, and, less commonly, the effects of maternal hyperthermia and intrauterine vascular accidents involving either placenta or fetal cerebral blood vessels (Hoyme et al. 1981).

For all of the mechanisms of abnormal morphogenesis outlined, the effect on the developing CNS may follow an identifiable pattern or may be variable and depend on the extent, duration, and intensity of the abnormal genetic, environmental, and/or physical influences. These general categories require careful consideration of family history and of drug and toxin use during the pregnancy. It is in these categories also that the clinician is likely to see patterns among children based on their physical appearance and possibly on their developmental outcome. An example of this concept can be seen in males with fragile X syndrome in whom the sex-linked mode of inheritance often can be identified when taking a family history but also in whom specific phenotypic features can be identified. In this example of a malformation syndrome, mutations of the *FMR1* gene on the X chromosome in these affected individuals supports the idea of inheritance of a gene for mental retardation through the maternal X chromosome (Laird 1987). A similar gene–chromosome behavioral–developmental association may also be true for Angelman's syndrome, involving abnormalities in the molecular structure of chromosome 15 (Kaplan et al. 1987; Kishino et al. 1997).

The identification of these general groups also permits the clinician to understand which conditions involving mental retardation may be preventable. Examples include fetal alcohol syndrome, in which abstinence from alcohol is the prevention, and fetal rubella syndrome, in which maternal immunity against the rubella virus is preventive (Hanshaw 1970; Katz et al. 1998).

Alterations in the Intrinsic Biological Environment

As summarized in Table 19–5, there are several circumstances under which changes in the brain's biochemical environment lead to mental retardation. These include genetically determined enzyme deficiencies (Leroy 1992), such as phenylalanine hydroxylase deficiency, resulting in the mental retardation of phenylketonuria, or homocystinuria, which is associated with mental retardation as well as ophthalmological and growth changes (Levy 1973; Scriver and Clow 1980). Precise diagnosis is important in these conditions because of the possibility of prevention or arrest of the mental retardation (Nichols 1988).

Another cause of mental retardation in an otherwise normal CNS is the cerebral edema encountered in Reye's syndrome, a hepatic encephalopathy (Baethmann et al. 1988). Another is the potential injury to cortical tissue encountered in profound hypoglycemia.

Although the mechanisms of certain conditions are not understood, the natural history of children with certain clinical diagnoses still aids the choice of a strategy to evaluate them. For example, Rett's disorder presents the challenge of the female with loss of milestones within the first 2 years of life progressing to dementia and with autismlike behavior, for which no biochemical marker has yet been identified (Holm 1985; Lindberg 1991). Nonetheless, the abnormal movements seen in these children and their slow clinical deterioration suggest that the nature of this condition is neurodegenerative rather than, for example, related to a congenital, structural CNS abnormality.

Table 19–5. Alterations in the intrinsic biological environment

Etiology	Example	Pathology	Diagnostic considerations	Degree of mental retardation (MR)	Management considerations
Inborn errors of metabolism					
Autosomal recessive	Galactosemia	Disorder of carbohydrate metabolism; galatose-1-phosphate uridyl transferase	Normal at birth; failure to thrive, vomiting by first week; jaundice, hepatosplenomegaly; cataracts	Moderate MR; may be severe if untreated	Dietary restriction may reduce degree of disability; prenatal diagnosis is possible
	Phenylketonuria	Disorder of amino acid metabolism; phenylalanine hydroxylase deficiency	Usually normal at birth, then onset of vomiting, irritability in first 2 months; developmental delay, seizures, microcephaly, spasticity if not treated with phenylalanine-free diet	Severe to profound if untreated	Diagnosed as part of routine newborn metabolic screening; phenylalanine-restricted diet prevents MR; prenatal diagnosis is possible; possible learning difficulties if diet lapses
	Homocystinuria	Methionine metabolism defect	Normal at birth; onset of symptoms at 6–10 months; developmental delay, seizures, glaucoma, lens dislocation, thromboembolic disease, cerebrovascular accidents	Moderate to severe	Dietary management reduces morbidity; cofactor therapy possible, may reduce degree of disability
	Niemann-Pick disease	Sphingomyelinase lipid metabolism defect	Different forms are known; hepatosplenomegaly; cherry-red maculae; motor and cognitive deterioration after normal milestones	Profound MR possible	Some forms associated with no MR; others are lethal

Effects of Extraordinary Extrinsic Influences

As illustrated in Table 19–6, a number of accidental and environmental factors may contribute to the pathogenesis of mental retardation. Obvious examples include perinatal asphyxia, neonatal airway obstruction with profound hypoxemia, anesthesia complications, near drownings, poisonings, and trauma. In each case, the specific circumstances, lost response, and environmental response interact to determine the final outcome (Kuban 1994; Seshia et al. 1983; Truwit et al. 1992). Although few data precisely correlate specific clinical and historical factors with the degree of CNS and behavioral impairment, developmental prognosis can be built in part on the sense one has of both the duration of injury and the effectiveness of interventions.

Frequently, a child or an adult with mental retardation secondary to a catastrophic event presents with obvious upper motor neuron disease, especially secondary to profound hypoxia. One must not conclude, however, that mental retardation will always occur together with the obvious motor impairment. Numerous individuals with cerebral palsy are delayed in certain developmental domains but do not have mental retardation.

Finally, although insults to an otherwise normal brain are usually static in nature and occur in the context of a single accident, the so-called plasticity of the human CNS contributes to the wide variability seen in the outcome of specific types of injury and should be taken into consideration in the evaluation process. This might explain, for example, why the child commencing a course of rehabilitation after head trauma may later recover some skills.

■ Medical Evaluation of the Child With the Question of Mental Retardation

The algorithm in Figure 19–1 emphasizes the importance of a systematic approach in the identification and evaluation of mental retardation (Kaplan 1989).

Family and Gestational Histories

Maternal obstetrical history should include attention to miscarriages or infertility, drug and chemical exposure, and fetal movement in particular. Additional history of fetal distress or premature labor can also be helpful. Parents usually can accurately report diminished fetal activity or problems in the size of the fetus, and this should alert the clinician to review or request further prenatal obstetrical data. A family history of mental retardation may provide very helpful information, especially in males (fragile X syndrome). In obtaining a drug or alcohol history, it is useful to ask about both the amount and the frequency of exposure.

General Physical Examination

The finding of three or more minor anomalies (phenotypic features that are obvious but not medically consequential) should alert the examiner to the possibility of a syndrome of abnormal morphogenesis. A finding of microcephaly in the newborn tells the examiner that brain growth and development were prenatally abnormal, raising the possibility of a malformation syndrome or of gestational disruption to the CNS. This finding should lead the clinician to obtain head ultrasound and cranial computed tomography (CT) scan or a magnetic resonance imaging (MRI) scan if these are available. Abnormal scalp hair patterns are also often helpful in predicting cerebral dysgenesis because these patterns reflect the growth of the brain and resultant stretching of the scalp (Jones 1997; Smith and Gong 1973). Their abnormal appearance often implies problems of brain growth as early as the eighteenth week of gestation.

Midface asymmetry, especially undergrowth and abnormalities of the facial midline, may point to an underlying CNS malformation resulting in mental retardation. Close-set eyes (for measurement of which standard tables are available) often are encountered when a problem of the midline axis of the brain is present (Feingold and Bassert 1974). However, none of these findings is pathognomonic for the diagnosis of mental retardation. Rather, these are clues that mental retardation may occur, and its likelihood is greater when the dysgenesis is severe.

The neurological examination or neurodevelopmental evaluation should include careful attention to the symmetry of movements, the pitch of the infant's or child's cry, and response to stimuli (e.g., a bell or hand clapping). Often a high-pitched cry suggests long-standing prenatal insults. The child with irregular movements, extreme irritability, or hyperactive startle response may also be at risk for developmental disabilities. It should be pointed out, however, that although failure to respond to sounds or visual stimuli may signal that the child is deaf or blind, neither diagnosis implies mental retardation.

Table 19–6. Extraordinary extrinsic influences affecting the central nervous system

Etiology	Example	Pathology	Diagnostic considerations	Degree of mental retardation (MR)	Management considerations
Hypoxia	Near drowning	Hypoxemia; cerebral edema; hypothermia	Long recovery common; prognosis dependent on status at scene of accident and time until onset of CPR	Wide variability dependent on water temperature, length of immersion, resuscitation	Rehabilitation may require counseling and support; parental guilt a major concern; uncertain deficits in some patients
	Neonatal asphyxia	Cerebral ischemia; hypoglycemia; acute renal failure	Obstetrical history helpful; CT scan may show infarction or edema; seizures and persistence of hypotonia are poor prognostic signs	Wide variability	Motor disability common
	Obstruction of the airway	Acute complete blockage of airway resulting in hypoxia	Inability to ventilate	Wide variability; may cause severe to profound MR	Motor disability common
Trauma	Blunt head trauma, fractures	Hematoma; edema; "tearing" of brain tissue	History requires careful attention; examination often uncovers evidence of intentional abuse; consider other causes of developmental delay in suspected abuse cases	Variable	Requires formal neurorehabilitation; long-term sequelae may be evident years after injury
Poisoning	Lead	Insidious effects in children, typically due to pica (lead, solder, brass alloys)	Early effects include weight loss, vomiting, abdominal pain, headache; late effects include seizures, MR, coma, increased intracranial pressure	Can be severe, but variable	Variable, including learning disabilities

Note. CPR=cardiopulmonary resuscitation; CT=computed tomography.

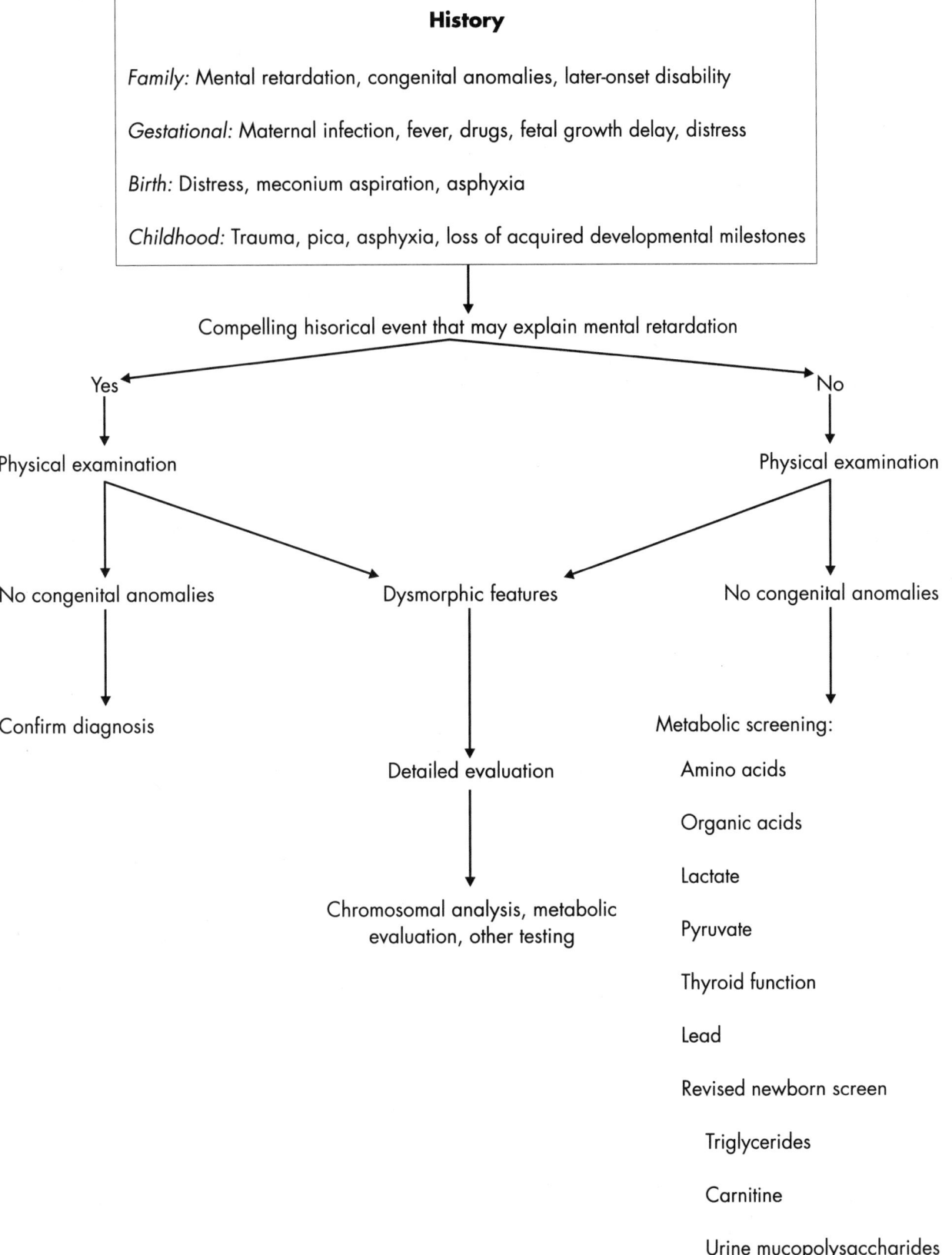

Figure 19–1. Diagnostic approach to mental retardation for all ages.

Laboratory Investigations

A number of screening studies are available. The urine amino acid screen plays an important role in the identification of conditions that may be treated through diet (e.g., phenylketonuria) (Wilcken et al. 1980).

Another study is chromosome analysis including, when indicated, the fragile X study. Providing pertinent history and physical findings will help the laboratory to determine which specific culture and staining methods to use (Hagerman and Silverman 1996).

Serum levels of lactate, pyruvate, bicarbonate, and venous pH recently have become recognized as being helpful in identifying any inborn errors of metabolism, especially if the individual has been acidotic.

When pica or significant lead exposure is suspected in the child with mental retardation, determining the blood level of lead can be critical. Anemia also may be significant (Needleman et al. 1990).

MRI is particularly helpful in assessing gray and white matter differentiation, posterior fossa structures, and myelination. The CT scan has become the standard for the evaluation of ventricular enlargement and, when interpreted by an experienced specialist, defines much of what MRI can provide.

A number of mental retardation conditions for which laboratory studies can be helpful are indicated in specific clinical presentations. Examples of these include the hyperammonemia of urea-cycle disorders and biotinidase deficiency associated with seizures and developmental delay.

■ Relation of Specific Mental Retardation Conditions to Molecular Genetic Analysis

Since the 1990s, advances in molecular genetics and refinements in cytogenetic technology have increased the accuracy of diagnosis for a number of syndromes associated with mental retardation (Delach et al. 1995). These techniques include fluorescence in situ hybridization (FISH), other specific DNA marker methods, and the application of quantitatively calibrated DNA probes to differentiate among clinical entities that share abnormal microscopic features on standard karyotype analysis.

Unlike high-resolution banding, these newer molecular techniques define abnormal regions of the human genome—DNA molecules that correlate with certain clinical features. Furthermore, these molecular variations allow geneticists to search for similar patterns in parents and other relatives, thereby enhancing their ability to provide genetic counseling regarding the possibility of recurrence.

Prader-Willi syndrome represents an example of a condition in the diagnosis of which specific DNA markers has replaced extended prophase (high-resolution) banding techniques. This syndrome is characterized by hypotonia, obesity, developmental and behavioral problems (including mental retardation), hyperphagia (typically after the first year of life), hypogonadism in males, and dysmorphic features (including a narrow-appearing forehead, downslanting palpebral fissures, small-appearing hands and feet, and downturning of the corners of the mouth). Children often present in the neonatal period with low muscle tone and failure to thrive, a feature seen in a number of conditions (Kaplan et al. 1987). Before DNA probes were available for the q11–q12 region of chromosome 15, banding procedures identified microdeletions in this region in approximately 50% of children with clinical features of Prader-Willi syndrome. DNA analysis now enables molecular confirmation of the diagnosis in most cases (Tantravahi et al. 1989).

Angelman's syndrome also frequently presents with hypotonia and failure to thrive in infancy but evolves gradually to include ataxia, spasticity and other movement disorders, and mental retardation (Knoll et al. 1990). Phenotypically, children with Angelman's syndrome have prognathism and a tendency in some of these children toward excitability and uncontrolled laughter, prompting use of the unfortunate term *happy puppet syndrome.*

Before a chromosome 15 deletion similar to that found in children with Prader-Willi syndrome was identified, Angelman's syndrome was diagnosed in children on the basis of clinical features. FISH studies now accurately identify subtle molecular differences in the q11–q12 region of chromosome 15 between these two entities (Delach et al. 1995). The molecular analysis has shown that in Prader-Willi syndrome, the deletion is of the chromosome of paternal origin, and in Angelman's syndrome, the deletion is of the chromosome of maternal origin.

The fragile X syndrome of X-linked mental retardation was initially identified by a constriction at the end of the long arm of the X chromosome (site Xq27.3), resulting in the appearance of a fragment being broken off, or fragile. This cytogenetic finding is thought to occur in 1 of 250 males and in 1 of 2,500 females (Harris 1995). Fragile X syndrome is the most common inherited form of mental retardation. In the past few years, analysis with DNA probes has identified the *FMR1* gene, with an unstable DNA sequence of CGG. In individuals without fragile X syndrome, this sequence has up to 54 repeats; in carriers, 52–230 (premutation); and in affected individuals, more than 230 (full mutation). The premutation inherited by a daughter from her mother tends to increase in length (expansion) and may result in full mutation in the next generation. The expansion does not occur in father-to-daughter transmission. The clinical features in affected prepubertal males include mental retardation, language impairment, gaze aversion, self-stimulatory behaviors, and a presentation similar to that of attention-deficit/hyperactivity disorder (ADHD). Initially, this clinical presentation suggested that many of these individuals had autistic disorder, but review of later studies did not support this association (J.C. Harris 1995). In carrier females, learning disabilities and/or mild mental retardation are seen. Physical phenotype, most obvious in postpubertal males, includes large testes, midfacial underdevelopment (resulting in long, narrow face), and large ears. Currently, the DNA studies are used for definite diagnosis, and they are extremely useful in determining carrier state in maternal relatives as well as in females with developmental difficulties and a family history of mental retardation. Some of the clinical features of fragile X syndrome seen in adults may not be noted in young children, particularly macroorchidism. Thus, a family history of mental retardation and speech and language disorder/autism further justifies obtaining the DNA study. It is important, however, to remember that routine karyotype analysis still has utility, because a number of aneuploidy and polyploidy chromosome anomalies are not diagnosable by molecular studies. Examples of these include XXY syndrome and XYY syndrome.

The support and treatment of children and adults with conditions such as Prader-Willi syndrome, Angelman's syndrome, and fragile X syndrome are most effective as a multidisciplinary effort. The input from geneticists, nutritionists, developmental psychologists, and physical, occupational, and speech therapists is as essential as the contribution of the developmental pediatrician and child psychiatrist. Nutritional management requires collaboration between these and other professionals. This collaboration is particularly important in helping parents understand the sensitive relationship between potential compulsive eating patterns and the child's self-image and response to educational strategies.

Other conditions that are diagnosed by molecular studies include Williams syndrome and a variety of conditions involving deletions (e.g., cri du chat syndrome) for which DNA probes now exist. Rett's disorder, although not associated with any known molecular abnormality, may represent another example of a unique clinical entity, similar in presentation among unrelated individuals, for which a molecular marker eventually will be found. Like the conditions described, it is characterized by discrete clinical features (loss of developmental milestones, which accelerates in the second decade of life; atypical hand movements; progressive dementia) with similar natural history in affected individuals. No biochemical marker has yet been identified; however, the fact that this condition occurs only in females suggests that the X chromosome is involved (Kerr 1991).

■ Treatment

Some physicians perceive the treatment of people with mental retardation as unrewarding because this condition usually cannot be cured. However, the ultimate objective of a physician is not only to cure illness but also to help the patient to achieve the best feasible quality of life (QOL) and function as an individual and as a member of society. This is true for most illnesses, including mental retardation.

The treatment of mental retardation has three aspects. First, the treatment is directed at the underlying cause, such as early diet in phenylketonuria or thyroid replacement in congenital hypothyroidism. Second, the treatment also focuses on associated physical and mental disorders to improve the person's functioning. Third, the treatment includes proper education and habilitation. We briefly discussed the first two aspects in the previous section; we discuss the third one in the section that follows.

■ Education and Habilitation: Society's Attitudes, Past and Present

Children with mental retardation were identified already in ancient times, primarily because of physical disabilities, deformations, and disorders associated with severe mental retardation. In Sparta and in Rome, infanticide of obviously deformed newborns was common. On the other hand, ancient texts, especially the Bible, called for kindness to people with disabilities such as blindness and deafness (Scheerenberger 1983). One can presume that the recognition of mental retardation was based on observable deficits in adaptive behaviors and depended on societal expectations of an individual at a given age and in a given culture. A child who had little or no communication skills and no self-help skills (whose condition we would now diagnose as severe or profound mental retardation) would be recognized in all cultures as exceptional. On the other hand, children with milder impairments would not be as noticeable in less-developed, preindustrial societies or settings, where it would be easier to absorb them into simple but productive jobs. In fact, for centuries, some children with mental retardation who survived to adulthood secured valued and protected positions as court fools (Scheerenberger 1983). In the Middle Ages, on one hand, some religious views linked mental retardation (or rather deformities) with sin, witchcraft, and work of the devil (Scheerenberger 1983, p. 32). On the other hand, many people with mental retardation found refuge (together with the poor and those with mental illness) in hostels run by religious institutions.

The reform in the care of people with mental illness instituted by Pinel at the end of the eighteenth century reflected also on the care of those with mental retardation (which was not readily differentiated then from mental illness). Itard, who was a student of Pinel and physician at the institute for deaf-mutes, acquired his fame through his work with Victor, the "Wild Boy of Aveyron," a feral child. Victor appears to have had at least functional mental retardation. Itard created for him what would be called today an early program of individualized special education that included enrichment; cognitive, emotional, and sensory stimulation; and positive reinforcement (although with limited results). Edouard Seguin, who was also Pinel's student, developed a "physiological method" specifically for the education of children with mental retardation that included systematic development of physical, cognitive, sensory, and social skills.

In colonial America and during the early years of the United States, the fate of people with mental retardation was not much different from that in Europe. Dorothea Dix, in her report to the Massachusetts Legislature in 1843, described people with mental retardation kept in inhumane conditions in jails and poorhouses (Scheerenberger 1983, p. 100). In 1839 Dr. Samuel Gridley Howe, who directed a state school for the blind in Massachusetts, accepted a student who had also mental retardation. Owing largely to his efforts, Massachusetts funded the first U.S. public residential school for children with mental retardation. Another one was a private school started in 1847, in Barre, Massachusetts, by Dr. Wilbur. A year later, Seguin immigrated to the United States and became very influential in the development of education of children with mental retardation. He envisioned the role of residential facilities as solely educational, with the goal of eventually returning the student to the community. Yet soon this role changed. With progress in neurology, mental retardation came to be seen as incurable, and, with mass psychological testing of largely poor and uneducated people, as a cause of criminality and social ills. The institutions came to be seen as a place to protect children with mental retardation from society, and later as a place to protect society from them (Donaldson and Menolascino 1977). With discharges limited, the population of institutions aged, although children continued to be admitted, partly due to lack of services in the community and partly due to physicians' recommendations to place mentally retarded children in institutions as soon as possible, before the parents could develop attachment to them. However, at no time did more than 10% of people with mental retardation live in institutions.

In the past, it was customary to speak about the care of individuals with mental retardation. That reflected the view that they had to be cared for indefinitely because they were unable to care for themselves. This was the custodial approach, as opposed to the present active treatment approach, which seeks to help the individual achieve the highest feasible level of development and independent functioning in mainstream society rather than in segregated, protected settings. Instead of discussing care, we refer now to the services or supports needed for the individual to achieve the highest possible QOL, which is becoming the dominant concept in this field (Schalock and Begab 1990). The current approaches were influenced by several developments. The first was a bill of rights adopted in 1968 by the International League of Societies for the Mentally Handicapped. The second was the concept of the developmental model, which holds that all individuals with mental retardation, regardless of the degree and nature of their impairment, can learn, even if they do it in a unique manner and at their own speed (Wolfensberger 1972). The third development was of the "normalization principle," which referred to providing people with mental retardation "patterns and conditions of everyday life which are as close as possible to the norms and patterns of the mainstream of society" (Nirje 1969, p. 181), although this principle did not specifically include integration into society (Wolfensberger 1995). Adoption of the normalization principle was followed by a trend toward deinstitutionalization. At the peak of institutionalization in 1967, 194,650 people lived in large, state-operated institutions. This number declined to 52,801 in 1998. The largest decrease was in the child and adolescent populations. In many states now, children are not admitted at all to these facilities. By 1999, eight states had closed all institutions. In contrast, the number of people living in community-based settings for fewer than six people increased dramatically (Braddock et al. 2000).

These changes were enabled by an increase in services in the community for people with mental retardation. Previously, special education for children with mental retardation was limited, usually in separate schools, which were often unavailable to those with severe disabilities. Public Law 94–142 of 1975 made appropriate public education available to all who needed it (Table 19–7). At first the concept of *mainstreaming* was popular: placing the child in some "regular" classes, usually for nonacademic subjects. The current standard is *inclusion*. It refers to placing a child in an age-appropriate regular classroom and providing in that classroom all services necessary because of the child's limitations. There should be collaboration between special-education and regular teachers, synchronization of the topics being taught (e.g., the child with mental retardation learns the concept of counting during the algebra class), employment of nondisabled peers as teaching buddies, provision of an individual teaching aide, provision of appropriate special therapies (such as speech therapy), and all teaching aids and other measures required to enable the child to participate in all class activities. For adults, in the workplace, inclusion refers to a job in a "normal" environment (rather than in a segregated special workshop), with provision of necessary supports and supervision, preferably "natural," by local, properly trained co-workers.

Table 19–7. Case and statute laws related to rights of disabled people

Case or statute	Year	Coverage
Wyatt v. Stickney	1971	People with mental disabilities in institutions have the right to habilitation; case set its minimum standards; required least restrictive alternative
Donaldson v. O'Connor	1974	Civilly committed people have the right to treatment
O'Connor v. Donaldson	1975	Nondangerous people with mental disorder who can live in the community should not be civilly committed
Individuals with Disabilities Education Act (IDEA; originally Public Law 94–142)	1975	All disabled children (including mentally ill and retarded) from birth to age 21 years have the right to appropriate public education and related services, maximal possible mainstreaming, family support
Halderman v. Pennhurst (and follow-up cases)	1975	Closure of institutions: could not provide minimally adequate habilitation in least restrictive environment; moved residents to appropriate community settings
Civil Rights of Institutionalized Persons Act (CRIPA)	1980	U.S. Department of Justice can sue states if rights of residents in state institutions are violated
Youngberg v. Romeo (and follow-up cases)	1984	Institutionalized people have the right to safety, training, and freedom from unnecessary restraints
Americans with Disabilities Act (ADA)	1990	Discrimination against disabled people who are otherwise qualified is forbidden; requires reasonable accommodations
IDEA amendments (IDEA 1997)	1997	Extension of early intervention programs; mental retardation is specifically mentioned as one of the impairments
Developmental Disabilities Assistance and Bill of Rights (Public Law 106–402)	2000	Ensures for individuals with disabilities and their families a role in design of programs, access to community services, supports, self-determination

As a result of these attitudinal changes, children and adolescents with mental retardation and other disabilities are now expected to attend public schools, live at home, and participate in age-appropriate community activities, and adults are expected to live as independently as possible in the community, in supported apartments, or in group homes and to gain employment in normal settings (Kiernan and Stark 1986).

Table 19–7 summarizes some of the landmark court decisions and legislation on the basis of which these changes have been brought about. However, the legal field is constantly changing because of new court decisions reinterpreting existing legislation and new state-level statutes. Therefore, clinicians should be aware of the current laws and regulations in their jurisdictions, in order to inform the families of children with disabilities whom they see about their right to services and to advocate for them.

A recent development has been resistance, by self-advocates who have disabilities, their families, and some professionals, to the use of the term *mental retardation*, which acquired a pejorative meaning. In the United Kingdom and many other English-speaking countries, the term *intellectual disability* has replaced *mental retardation*. In 2001 in the United States, a consortium of organizations led by the AAMR recognized that fact and also the reality that any new term will become pejorative unless accompanied by changes in society's attitudes. A campaign to change these attitudes is being planned, and child and adolescent psychiatrists and other mental health clinicians could play a major role in it.

Psychiatry of Mental Retardation

Both mental retardation and mental illness are manifested by behaviors that deviate from norms for the particular sociocultural group and age. These behaviors often are not understood, may be unpredictable, and evoke emotional reactions in others, including fear. Society's emotional responses to people with mental illness and mental retardation alike led to measures such as isolating the afflicted individuals and shaped policies regarding their care. These measures, in turn, influenced the roles of professionals, including psychiatrists and other physicians. Table 19–8 summarizes the evolution of the roles of psychiatry in the field of mental retardation in modern times; detailed reviews are available elsewhere (Donaldson and Menolascino 1977; Menolascino 1983).

■ Personality Development and Developmental Crises

A common misconception about people with mental retardation is that they are a homogeneous group with similar characteristics, behaviors, and personality patterns. However, people with mild mental retardation are more similar to people without this condition than they are to people who have severe or profound impairments. Philips (1966) listed several of these misconceptions about mental retardation and behavior:

> That the maladaptive behavior of the retarded child is a function of his retardation, rather than of his interpersonal relationships;…that emotional disorder in the retarded is different in kind from that in a normal child;…that certain symptoms and specific maladaptive behavior patterns in a retarded child are the result of organic brain damage. (p. 112)

Some of the stereotypes about people with mental retardation include lack of inhibitions and moral sense, rigidity, and attention seeking (Reiss 1994). Systematic studies confirmed Philips's suspicion about the role of environmental factors, especially negative experiences and failures, in shaping the personality traits of children who have mental retardation (Zigler and Burack 1989). A personality feature frequently found in children with mental retardation (but not unique to them) is negative self-concept, probably related to failures in life or to messages of rejection and failure received from significant people and society (Reiss 1994; Szymanski and Crocker 1985, 1989). These children often expect failure, especially when faced with new tasks.

Recent research in molecular genetics has also led to increased interest in genetic determinants of behavior in mental retardation–associated syndromes. This is discussed in detail below, in the section "Genetics and Behavior: Behavioral Phenotypes."

Infancy and Preschool Period

Much of the behavior and functioning of children with mental retardation at this stage will depend on whether an etiology is recognized (e.g., Down syndrome) or an associated disability is present (e.g., congenital heart defect, sensory defect). Infants and young chil-

Table 19–8. Evolution of attitudes toward mental retardation

Period	Society's attitudes	Psychiatrists' roles
Mid- to late nineteenth century	Optimism, belief in education, "moral training" in special schools to return the person to society	Psychiatrists in forefront of progress as leaders, educators, and diagnosticians; precursor of the American Association on Mental Retardation founded in 1876 by psychiatrists
End of nineteenth century to beginning of twentieth century	Focus on neuropathology; retardation seen as incurable defect; therapeutic nihilism; protecting people with mental retardation from society	Roles change to those of diagnostician, neuropathologist, and administrator
Early to mid-twentieth century	Introduction of intelligence tests, which discover mildly retarded "morons"; assumption of link with antisocial behavior; protecting society: custodial institutionalization, sterilization; "Tragic Interlude"	Psychiatrists become administrators; people with mental retardation seen as unable to benefit from psychiatric treatment (i.e., psychoanalytical therapy); early pioneers (e.g., Howard Potter) study, describe, and treat mental disorders in people with mental retardation
Early second half of twentieth century	Recognition of rights of people with mental retardation to public education, treatment, and life in community; concept of normalization	Studies on mental illness in people with mental retardation; psychiatrists become interested in this field, chiefly as psychopharmacologists but also as therapists and diagnosticians
Current	Implementation of right of all handicapped children to education; deinstitutionalization and community living and working for adults	Psychiatrists increasingly treat people with mental retardation using all treatment modalities and are accepted as team members

Source. Partly based on Donaldson and Menolascino (1977) and Kanner (1964).

dren who have uncomplicated mental retardation may respond less readily to their parents, show fewer or delayed attachment behaviors, and appear to be less active (Buckhalt et al. 1978; Cicchetti and Sroufe 1978; Stone and Chesney 1978). In comparison with normally developing, healthy infants of the same mental or chronological age, those with mental retardation tend to be more compliant and less vocally interactive (Hanzlik and Stevenson 1986). Other reasons for psychiatric referral in this age group include eating and sleeping problems and irritability. Not infrequently, when mental retardation has been diagnosed or suspected, the family may still hope for a diagnosis of a mental disorder instead, as it might be seen as treatable, perhaps more acceptable, and leading to better services.

Early social interaction with peers also may be difficult for these children. They may have considerable communication difficulties, may lack age-expected self-care skills, and may be overtly rejected. Various mental disorders may be diagnosed in this age group. At the Developmental Evaluation Center of the Chil-

dren's Hospital in Boston, Massachusetts, of 100 children younger than 6 years who were referred because of developmental and/or behavioral concerns, the following diagnoses were made: pervasive developmental disorders in 45%, ADHD in 12%, and posttraumatic stress disorder (after abuse) in 8% (Szymanski 1989).

School-Age Period

During the school-age period, the expected mastery of various academic, social, and independence skills will be difficult for youngsters with mental retardation. Some children with mild mental retardation that has not yet been diagnosed are subjected to age-appropriate expectations that they cannot meet. As a result of this pressure, they may develop behavioral problems, which may bring them to the attention of a psychiatrist. These may include impulsivity, inattention, overactivity, and aggressive behavior. Inclusionary placement in regular classes is rapidly becoming a standard. However, such placement without proper support and preparation might lead to anxiety, depression, and behavioral problems if the child tries to engage in the same activities as peers or becomes disruptive to gain attention and avoid difficult tasks.

Adolescence

The most difficult developmental challenge in adolescence is the need for the child and for the family to accept that the cognitive impairment is permanent and will not be modified substantially by yet another educational program (Szymanski and Crocker 1989). Paradoxically, less disabled children may be more disadvantaged because they are more aware of their deficiencies and employ maladaptive defenses. The usual gap between physical puberty and emotional readiness for adult roles is even more accentuated because most of these youngsters have normal physical development. Realistic planning for the future is impeded by the uncertainty about their own abilities, low self-image, unwillingness to plan for a less-than-"normal" future, and lack of habilitation services. Developing mature peer and peer-group relationships is even more difficult. A latency-age child may be accommodated by nondisabled peers in concrete play and interaction in peripheral and protected roles. However, it is much more difficult to participate in an adolescent group interaction that requires communication skills, pragmatic language in particular, as well as cognitive, and abstraction skills.

The sexual revolution has not yet reached the mental retardation field, and old misconceptions and myths abound. These include notions such as that people with mental retardation are uninhibited and are unable to learn social mores or are not interested in sexuality.

The defenses used during adolescence, as in earlier stages, may include passivity (withdrawal, task avoidance, regression) or acting out (aggressive behavior, delinquency, noncompliance). Depression is frequent and may underlie disruptive behaviors. Unfortunately, these youngsters, in their quest for social acceptance, may become victims of sexual and other exploitation by their peers who do not have mental retardation. In one notorious case, a young woman with mild mental retardation was sexually exploited by a group of high school students. Yet in court, she stated that they were her friends and that she agreed to those activities.

The best intervention here is prevention through early sexuality education, starting with helping the adolescent to develop a positive self-image and progress-ing to teaching social interaction skills and, finally, to teaching about sexuality, which should include principles of appropriate relevant social behaviors. In the past, many states' statutes permitted sterilization of people with mental retardation, either involuntarily or by legal guardian's permission, and many abuses occurred, such as when parents had their children sterilized even though mental retardation was only suspected, not confirmed. At present, the general approach is that no sterilization of minors or legally incompetent adults is permitted, except for rare cases when court permission is obtained. Usually, proof is required that a significant danger of sexual activity or abuse resulting in pregnancy exists that cannot be prevented by noninvasive means. People who have mental retardation but are competent to make such decisions might themselves consent to having sterilization or an abortion.

■ Parental Reactions and Adaptation

Initial Reactions

Children whose retardation is diagnosed at birth or in early infancy usually have severe retardation and an associated physical syndrome or impairment. The child's health problems may be overwhelming, and often the diagnosis is unexpected. In most of these cases, the parents are told about the diagnosis by a physician, and the manner in which they are informed is crucial (Lynch and Staloch 1988). In particular, the physician should take adequate time for this informing conference, listen to the parents' concerns, express empathy and compassion but not pity or personal value judgments, and provide detailed and helpful information about available services and what the parents can do to promote the child's development. Above all, parents should never be told that nothing can be done for the child; such statements are untrue and destructive.

In the past, parents were expected to have a pathological depressive reaction to the birth of a child with mental retardation. Early researchers saw such a child as a loss of the ideal object: the expected normal child (Solnit and Stark 1961). Others recognized that parental sadness was not necessarily a pathological depression but an adaptive reaction, a "chronic sorrow" (Olshansky 1962). Some studies have shown that there is no significant difference in the occurrence of psychopathology in parents of infants with mental retardation and in parents of those without it (Harris and

McHale 1989). Similarities have been drawn to the stage model of mourning, in which the parents are expected to go through stages of adaptation such as shock, denial, anger, sadness, reorganization, and adaptation, but more recent research suggests that such orderly schemas may not always apply. Some parents may have various intermixed reactions, whereas others may have generally negative initial reactions, followed by denial, and ending with adjustment (Mary 1990).

Later Adaptation

Mild retardation unassociated with physical abnormalities is usually diagnosed later in life, often only when the child begins school. The parents usually are already aware of the child's developmental problems. Some parents who believe the child's developmental delay is caused by emotional problems may have sought psychiatric consultation. By the time the child is of school age, the parents usually have developed an attachment to the child and also are aware of the child's strengths, which may attenuate their reaction to the diagnosis. Some families, however, may persist in denial and subject the child to continuous "shopping" for a new, more acceptable diagnosis and tests and unsuccessful therapies to cure the retardation. A relatively recent development has been an increase in the diagnosis of pervasive developmental disorder not otherwise specified (PDDNOS), often not justified by clinical presentation, leaving comorbid significant mental retardation undiagnosed and the parents hopeful that child's presumed high intelligence will become apparent when autistic symptoms recede.

Parental adjustment to a child's retardation is a multidimensional process that depends on many factors (Frey et al. 1989). Parents need adequate explanations for the child's condition and concrete help in finding the needed services. Their uncertainty about the child's future care is often the most stressful issue. Environmental factors, which are most important, include availability of medical, educational, and other services; access to understanding and helpful professionals; and availability of a support network, such as The Arc (formerly the Association for Retarded Citizens). The earlier view was that a high rate of marital problems existed in these families, but current clinical experience seems to be more positive (perhaps because of better available services for these children and families). Many families, in fact, derive considerable

and healthy gratification from their child who has mental retardation.

Family adaptation will, of course, be influenced by the balance between the innate strengths of the family, the available supports and services, and child-related factors such as severity of the handicap, communication skills, the need for medical care, and behavioral and emotional problems. The family's adaptation is an ongoing process because new challenges appear at each developmental stage.

The role of brothers and sisters (especially older ones) is most important, as role models and often as protectors. Many, as adults, report that the experience of having a handicapped sibling made them more empathetic and better people. Many also choose careers in helping professions, such as speech therapy or social work. However, their adjustment may be compromised if they are subjected to undue pressure from the parents to assume responsibility for the care of the disabled sibling.

■ Mental Disorders and Mental Retardation

Epidemiology

There is a general agreement that children and adolescents with mental retardation are at higher risk for developing psychopathology than their peers without mental retardation. However, there are no reliable and reproducible prevalence data on the subject; available reports on studies note quite diverse results because of methodological problems. A common problem has been the selection of study cohort. Earlier studies were done on selected groups with a built-in bias, such as patients in institutions or those referred to mental health clinics. As could be expected, these studies reflected a high prevalence of mental disorders. Other methodological problems included use of different definitions of mental retardation, use of different diagnostic criteria for various mental disorders, and diagnostic techniques that varied from retrospective reviews of charts to detailed psychiatric interviews with patients and multiple informants. Other studies relied on psychopathology diagnostic instruments, although these could be designed for purposes other than yielding a specific psychiatric diagnosis (review: Dykens 2000). In the early and classic study on an unselected population—the Isle of Wight study by Rutter et al. (1970)—the prevalence of psychopathology in children ages 9–11 years with mental retardation was 30%–42%, compared with 6%–7% in subjects without mental retardation. Gillberg et al. (1986) studied a representative sample of subjects ages 13–17 years through direct and parental interviews. In 57% of those with mild and 64% with severe mental retardation, symptoms met DSM-III (American Psychiatric Association 1980) criteria for affective, anxiety, attention-deficit, conduct, schizophrenia, somatoform, and pervasive developmental disorders. Stromme and Diseth (2000) in Norway screened a cohort of children born within 5 years of each other. Of these chidren, 178 were found to have mental retardation, assessed through psychiatric interview with the child, semistructured interview with the parent, and chart review. Psychiatric diagnosis according to ICD-10 (*International Classification of Diseases and Related Health Problems*, 10th Revision; World Health Organization 1992) was made in 37% (in 42% of those with severe retardation and in 33% with mild retardation). The most common diagnoses were hyperkinesis and pervasive development disorder (PDD). Significantly, in one-third of children in whom a diagnosis was made, the disorder had been unrecognized, even though the children had been previously examined by a child psychiatrist. In another population-based study, Linna et al. (1999), in a sample of 8-year-old children in Finland, found that 1.5% were attending special-education programs (remarkably close to National Health Interview Survey data on prevalence of combined mental retardation and developmental disorder in the United States). Prevalence of psychiatric symptoms was studied by three screening instruments. Depending on the instrument used, between 32.2% and 34.2% of the children were identified as possibly having a psychiatric disturbance, and 11% as having depression. In summary, it now is generally agreed that virtually all types of mental disorders may occur among people with mental retardation and that the prevalence of such disorders is three to four times higher in those with mental retardation than in the general population.

A number of factors have been considered in efforts to explain why people with mental retardation are at high risk for developing mental disorders (Dykens 2000). The lowered cognitive skills might make them less able to solve problems and deal with the stresses inherent in everyday life, resulting in anxiety, aberrant behavior, and/or withdrawal. Poor language skills may lead to using behavior, especially disruptive, as means of communication. They have repeated experiences of failure, and most are aware that their peers are more capable, leading to poor self-image and learned helplessness, which might be associated with depression (Dagnan and Sandhu 1999). Zigler and Burack (1989) described "outerdirectedness": a tendency to look first to others for solution and approval. Poor pragmatic skills and social skills will put them at risk for social rejection, abuse, and exploitation. Other risk factors might include the neuropathology underlying the mental retardation and associated disabilities, which might also contribute to certain aberrant behaviors.

Genetics and Behavior: Behavioral Phenotypes

Historically, there had been a tendency to see certain behavioral patterns as typical for people with mental retardation. Usually these were inappropriate behaviors, sometimes even contradictory, such as passive and aggressive, asexual and sexually disinhibited. People with Down syndrome were described as charmers, attention-seeking, "Prince Charming." At their extreme, these views led to the belief that maladaptive behaviors of people with mental retardation were genetically determined and contributed to the eugenic movement in the early part of the twentieth century, with its resulting involuntary sterilization of people with mental retardation. In the later backlash, these views were seen as stereotyping, and behaviors of these people as due only to the attitudes of other people in their environment. At the present, it seems that there has been a partial return to the earlier views. No one denies that environment exerts a powerful influence in shaping a person's behavior, but as there have been developments in molecular genetics, increasing attention has been paid to genetic factors. The concept of behavioral phenotypes has become increasingly popular. It has been defined by Dykens (1995) as "the heightened probability or likelihood that people with a given syndrome will exhibit certain behavioral and developmental sequelae relative to those without the syndrome" (p. 523). Most of these behaviors are not unique to the particular syndrome (such as hyperactivity), but some might be, such as extreme overeating in people with Prader-Willi syndrome or extreme self-biting of hands and mouth in Lesch-Nyhan syndrome (Dykens 2000). Some of these behaviors (or at least their frequency and intensity) may be associated with the type of the genetic abnormality. For example, maladaptive behaviors are more frequent or intense in people with Prader-Willi syndrome due to paternal deletion on chromosome 15 than in those with maternal uniparental disomy (Dykens 2000). Thus, these patients offer a unique opportunity to study genetic underpinning of behavior.

Diagnosis of Comorbid Mental Disorders: Use of Diagnostic Criteria and Clinical Findings

The multiaxial approach first introduced by DSM-III has enabled a systematic approach to description of the patient in addition to the traditional "code diagnosis," consisting only of the standardized term and coding for the mental disorder. Although this is a step in the right direction, this approach may not be enough for individuals who have mental retardation. They often have multiple disabilities, associated disorders, and multiple factors that cause, trigger, or maintain the maladaptive behaviors. Thus, to adequately describe such individuals, diagnostic understanding rather than code diagnosis is needed. A brief but comprehensive statement covering the formal diagnosis as well as the environmental, psychological, and biomedical issues and the person's needs for support is necessary. This could follow the five dimensions outlined in the AAMR diagnostic manual (American Association on Mental Retardation 2002).

Because the same mental disorders found in the general population are seen in people who have mental retardation, the standard diagnostic criteria—DSM-IV-TR (American Psychiatric Association 2000)—should be used. In most people with mild mental retardation, there are sufficient communicative skills to permit making the diagnosis and using the criteria in the same manner as in people who do not have mental retardation. If the person's communicative language is significantly impaired, it might be difficult to satisfy the diagnostic criteria that are based on communication with the patient, so the diagnosis must be based primarily on history from caregivers and observations of overt behaviors (as noted below in discussions of specific diagnostic categories).

■ Psychiatric Clinical Assessment

Comprehensive Context

The diagnostic evaluation of children and adolescents who have mental retardation is similar to the evaluation of those without it, in that it is based on a developmental approach and follows principles of sound psy-

chiatric practice. (See also Part II of this volume, "Assessment and Diagnosis"). Considering the multiplicity of cognitive and other deficiencies most of these individuals have, the assessment should be done within a framework of comprehensive understanding of the patient's biomedical and psychosocial problems. Past psychological, medical, neurological, linguistic, and other evaluations should be reviewed and new ones requested, if needed. The diagnostician should be careful not to focus only on the questions of the caregivers that led to the referral (both verbalized and "hidden" agendas) but should review the whole spectrum of the patient's functioning and problems (Szymanski 1977, 1980b).

Referral

Children and adolescents with mental retardation are referred for psychiatric evaluation for a variety of reasons, just like those without mental retardation (AACAP 1999). These may include disruptive and aggressive behaviors, noncompliance at school, poor attention span, and overactivity. The parents are often concerned about their child's delay in development and learning and feel that these are due to a treatable psychiatric problem, whether the diagnosis of mental retardation had been made in the past or not. Not infrequently, and depending on school policies in the particular locality, the parents prefer to have a diagnosis of a mental disorder (especially a PDD) rather than of mental retardation because the former may result in the child receiving better educational supports. Some children are referred because of symptoms of emotional distress (such as depressed mood or anxiety) or a lack of age-appropriate social skills. Not infrequently the referral is initiated by several people, for different and sometimes contradictory reasons. For example, a teacher might expect a diagnosis of mental disorder and a prescription for medication "for aggression," whereas a parent might want a recommendation for a transfer to a better school.

Patient's History

A detailed and comprehensive patient history is essential. It should be obtained from all involved (e.g., parents, sitters, teachers, therapists, classroom aides), as they usually have different and complementary information. This should include the following (AACAP 1999):

1. *Presenting symptoms:* detailed behavioral description with specific examples; variability in time, place, and with different people; change in symptom nature over time; correlation with environmental events, antecedents, and consequences (how the problems are handled by caregivers).

2. *Past history and personality patterns:* premorbid and current; strengths and weaknesses in adaptive skills, academic learning, attention span, activity level, self-care, social interactions, leisure/recreation, self-direction, self-preservation, language, including verbal and nonverbal. Unusual behavioral patterns, such as stereotypies, rituals, and self-injury, should be explored. Not infrequently, individuals without verbal language use behaviors, often disruptive, to communicate their needs, and these might be the reason for referral.

3. *Psychiatric history:* past evaluations, diagnoses, treatments; medication history (including dosages, results, and adverse effects); use of nonestablished treatments; review of past reports if available.

4. *Education/work history:* description of programs attended; mainstreaming/inclusion (description and child's response), supports from teachers/supervisors, peers' attitudes; review of the individualized education program (IEP) is desirable.

5. *Health and developmental history:* family history of developmental and mental disorders, pregnancy, developmental history, illnesses and treatments, etiological workup to date (review results).

6. *Past assessments:* review cognitive and other psychological tests, profile of strengths and weaknesses (rather than global IQ); request new testing if needed.

7. *Family and environmental history:* knowledge of and reaction to child's disabilities, management of them (promoting independence vs. dependence), effects of child's disabilities on family's life, siblings' reaction and roles, long-term expectations and plans for child's care, role of cultural background.

Interviewing Techniques

These techniques have been described elsewhere in detail (AACAP 1999; Reiss 1994; Szymanski 1977, 1980b). The three crucial factors are

1. The interviewer's attitude (understanding of mental retardation, empathy but not pity, support without paternalism)

2. The interviewer's ability to adapt the communication style to the patient's communication skills

3. The interviewer's ability to set structure and limits as well as support and be directive while promoting spontaneous expression

Verbal interviewing techniques can be used with most patients, perhaps with the caregivers "translating" to help the interviewer understand the patient, if there are articulation problems. The questions must be as neutral as possible, because people with mental retardation commonly fear that they will make a mistake and tend to agree with clues in leading questions or, if given a choice of answers, select the last possibility they hear. It is essential to establish, rather than assume, that the patient understands the questions. For example, "Did you hear voices of someone who was not there?" might be answered "Sure, I did," but "What do you mean?" might elicit "My mother was in another room and called me." Nonverbal techniques such as play, drawing, and various activities are helpful, but as much as possible they should be appropriate to the child's chronological age. People with mental retardation are sensitive to being treated as eternal children or as "stupid" and might be insulted if an age-inappropriate activity is suggested or very simple questions are asked of them. For this reason it might be better, with more verbal people, to avoid standard questions of a "formal" mental status and disguise them instead within a casual conversation. The patient's knowledge, understanding, and feelings about the disability should be explored; the best time to do so is after first asking about strengths and abilities. General behavior—social communication, attention, activity level, any unusual behaviors, and mood—must be observed. A visit to the patient's natural environment and unobtrusive behavioral observations may be helpful in difficult cases. Even in the office, an unobtrusive initial observation in the waiting room will provide valuable information.

Psychometric Instruments

Psychometric instruments have been developed to assess psychopathology and maladaptive behaviors in people of various ages who have mental retardation of varying severity (O'Brien et al. 2001). Some instruments not specifically designed for people with mental retardation are nevertheless useful with them. The Reiss Screen for Maladaptive Behavior (Reiss 1988) and its child and adolescent version, the Reiss Scales

(Reiss and Valenti-Hein 1990), are based on interviews with informants and produce an overall score reflecting severity and subscores for types of psychopathology. The Child Behavior Checklist (Achenbach 1991), designed to measure a wide range of behavior problems, has been used also to assess psychopathology in children with mental retardation and uses caregivers as informants. The Aberrant Behavior Checklist (Aman et al. 1985), also based on history provided by informants, is intended for evaluation of medication effects rather than for measurement of psychopathology. There are also a number of instruments for assessment of specific mental disorders. In general, the various scales might be useful for research purposes, screening (e.g., for referral to a psychiatrist), and follow-up assessment (e.g., to measure treatment effectiveness) rather than as primary diagnostic instruments.

Assessment of Clinical Data

The data obtained during diagnostic evaluation must be viewed in the context of the child's total clinical presentation (behavioral, psychological, and physical), developmental and communication level, associated disabilities (especially sensory and neurological), environmental and cultural factors and events, education, and experience. For example, a boy who is withdrawn and talks to himself may be hallucinating, may be rejected by his peers and feel depressed and lonely, may be trying to attract his teacher's attention, or may be talking to an imaginary friend, who might be appropriate to his developmental but not chronological age. An "expanded diagnosis" should be produced, integrating these data and including, in addition to a formal diagnostic label, a review of the patient's strengths, liabilities, and needs for support in all applicable domains; factors initiating and maintaining the problem; and a comprehensive treatment plan (American Association on Mental Retardation 1992; Szymanski and Crocker 1989). The possibility of an underlying general medical disorder must always be considered. Individuals with mental retardation might not be able to report on their signs and symptoms; some disorders with psychiatric manifestations are more common in certain conditions (e.g., thyroid disorders in Down syndrome); a physical discomfort in a nonverbal person might be communicated via overt behaviors; and, as a group, these individuals frequently receive medications that have behavioral and emotional side effects.

The Use of DSM-IV-TR Terminology

Formal DSM-IV-TR diagnosis should be possible with most people who have mild mental retardation. With those having more severe disability, especially if they have no communication skills, a nonspecific diagnosis within the appropriate category might be used (e.g., not otherwise specified) if no sufficient information is available from the history and/or the patient.

Professionals in the mental retardation field generally agree that DSM-IV-TR is not particularly well suited for use with people with significant limitations, especially in verbal communication. It is not well adapted for use with people on various developmental levels, including children (see also Chapter 7, "Clinical Assessment in Infancy and Early Childhood").

The Concept of Behavior Disorder

The concept of behavior disorder is neither well defined nor recognized by DSM-IV-TR. It is listed in ICD-10. Commonly it is used administratively to denote people whose undesirable behaviors are to be managed by nonmedical means, whereas those with "official" psychiatric diagnosis are to be treated with medications. Obviously such a simplistic approach is neither scientific nor useful. Another common practice holds that the diagnosis of behavior disorder should be used for people in whom a formal psychiatric diagnosis cannot be made and whose behavior appears to be a response to environmental antecedents. However, because of difficulties in making a diagnosis in people with severe mental retardation, it becomes all too easy to just label them in this manner. Furthermore, even in well-defined disorders there is an element of learned behavior. Presumably this term might be used to describe behavioral problems that occur solely in certain situations (e.g., aggression only at school in an overcrowded classroom) and disappear when the conditions there are corrected.

■ Diagnosis of Specific Mental Disorders: Review of the Issues

Diagnosis of mental disorders in people with mild cognitive difficulties and reasonable communication skills is similar to the diagnosis of comparable disorders in the general population. The higher the severity of the retardation and the greater the degree of communication impairments, the more difficult it is to make the diagnosis. Although it might still be possible to diagnose the general category of the mental disorder, it may be difficult to specify an exact subcategory. Reiss (1994) listed several factors that might be responsible for this difficulty: 1) the unreliability of self-report by the patient (or unavailability if the patient is nonverbal); 2) the patient's wish to deny the retardation and difficulties (the "cloak of competence" mechanism, described by Edgerton 1967); 3) "psychosocial masking" (in which symptom expression is modified by life experiences and concreteness); 4) baseline exaggeration (in which the onset of a mental disorder might lead to a relapse of preexisting maladaptive behavior) (Sovner 1986); 5) "diagnostic overshadowing" (a tendency of psychologists to underdiagnose mental disorders if they know that the patient has mental retardation [Reiss et al. 1982]).

In this section, we focus on the modifications of usual diagnostic approaches that are necessary in specific categories of mental disorders because of comorbid mental retardation. The most common reason for such modifications is not mental retardation per se but rather the associated impairment in communication skills.

Disorders Usually First Diagnosed in Infancy, Childhood, or Adolescence

Pervasive developmental disorders. A common differential diagnostic question is whether the patient has mental retardation or autism. However, the diagnoses of retardation and autism are not mutually exclusive; in fact, they frequently coexist, with 75%–80% of children with autism also having mental retardation and usually being initially referred to developmental disabilities clinics because the first concern is developmental delay. Both disorders may be associated with the same pathology (e.g., congenital rubella or tuberous sclerosis). Diagnosis of a PDD may be very difficult in people with profound mental retardation, although with prolonged observation one might discern in them some nonverbal social communication with familiar caregivers (see also Chapter 20, "Autistic Disorder," and Chapter 21, "Other Pervasive Developmental Disorders"). The PDD category now comprises five disorders: 1) autistic disorder, 2) Asperger's disorder, 3) Rett's disorder, 4) childhood disintegrative disorder, and 5) PDDNOS (including atypical autism). Mental retardation is commonly present in all except (by definition) Asperger's disorder.

Diagnostic confusion commonly arises if the child has self-stimulatory behaviors and significant delay in language development. This constellation is frequently seen in children with mental retardation who do not have autistic disorder. They usually do not show the core symptoms of autistic disorder: qualitative impairments in reciprocal social relationships and social communication. They usually relate well, especially to familiar people, albeit more appropriately to their developmental rather than chronological age. Some patients, especially those with poor language skills, may avoid contact with people whom they do not understand. Such avoidance is sometimes mistaken for social withdrawal, but careful observation of the child on several occasions in nondemanding situations and detailed developmental history will usually lead to the correct diagnosis.

Attention-deficit/hyperactivity disorder and disruptive disorders. Overactivity and poor attention had been considered typical for children and adolescents with mental retardation, and they remain one of the most frequent reasons for referral for psychiatric consultation. However, it is thought that the prevalence of ADHD is similar among people with mental retardation and those without it and ranges from 4% to 11% (Feinstein and Reiss 1996). Most of the DSM-IV-TR criteria for ADHD are based on observable behaviors, and therefore generally it can be diagnosed as in people without mental retardation (see Chapters 26, "Attention-Deficit/Hyperactivity Disorder"; 27, "Conduct Disorder and Oppositional Defiant Disorder"; and 28, "Conduct and Antisocial Disorders in Adolescence," in this volume). The symptoms should be evaluated in the context of the person's developmental level, as required by these criteria (although no developmental norms are available). For example, short attention span in an adolescent with profound mental retardation may actually be developmentally appropriate. Care should be exercised to recognize inattentiveness due to unwillingness to pay attention to a task, disobedience, and disruptive behaviors that are situation specific (i.e., occur only in one setting). These behaviors are usually a reaction to environmental factors such as lack of structure or a boring or difficult activity and may be a normal reaction to an abnormal situation. In such cases, the treatment is milieu change rather than medication. ADHD-like symptoms may be also a part of some behavioral phenotypes, such as fragile X, or a side effect of medications, such as barbiturates (still sometimes used for seizures), and may be confused with akathisia due to neuroleptics.

Children with mental retardation and ADHD, similarly to those without mental retardation, often have associated behavioral and emotional symptoms, such as depression, anxiety, noncompliance, and poor social skills (Pearson et al. 2000). The few long-term studies that are available indicate that variety of problems may continue through adolescence, even if the child was treated with medications, and many require psychiatric hospitalization (Handen et al. 1997).

Conduct disorders occur frequently. Disobedience and noncompliance are common reasons for referral. As with ADHD, the diagnostic assessment should consider developmental level, child's understanding of the rules that he or she is breaking, and appropriateness of the expectations of the caregivers and of the educational program (if the problems happen primarily in the school).

Feeding and eating disorders. Pica and rumination disorder, not uncommon in people with severe and profound mental retardation, are separate diagnostic categories in DSM-IV-TR. In the presence of mental retardation, they are diagnosed if the problem is severe enough to be the focus of clinical attention. Care should be exercised to assess for the presence of underlying physiological disorder, such as gastroesophageal reflux and peptic ulcers caused by *Helicobacter pylori* (the latter disorder having been reported quite frequently in institutional populations). Some cases of pica were reported in which a zinc or iron deficiency was present, and the symptoms abated with dietary supplementation (Lofts et al. 1990). Anorexia has been described in people with mental retardation, including Down syndrome.

Mental Disorders Due to a General Medical Condition

This category replaced the various categories of "organic" mental disorders, which had been used indiscriminately on the premise that brain disorder responsible for the mental retardation is the cause of all associated behavioral disorders. However, all recent editions of DSM clearly require that to use the "organic" diagnosis, the neuropathology must be present and its causative relation to the behavioral manifestations must be proven. The fact that the child has mental retardation and perhaps an associated neurological disorder (e.g., seizures) does not justify an automatic diagnosis of an "organic" disorder. Diagnosis of this type

might be inferred from the nature of the clinical symptoms (e.g., if they are typical for a temporal lobe pathology, which has been demonstrated) and whether a chronological correlation between the onset of behavioral and neurological manifestations is found.

The specific diagnosis of this category is listed on Axis I, and the underlying medical condition, on Axis III. Disorders in this category are found in several places in DSM-IV-TR. Within the general categories such as mood disorder, the diagnosis of *mood disorder due to a general medical condition* can be made if the criteria for "due to a general medical condition" are met.

Schizophrenia and Other Psychotic Disorders

Schizophrenia and mental retardation were often confused in the past, and people with severe mental retardation were sometimes thought to have psychosis because of their bizarre, self-stimulatory behaviors.

The diagnosis of schizophrenia and other psychotic disorders in people who have mild mental retardation and are verbal usually can be made in the same manner as in people without mental retardation, and the diagnosis of subtypes of schizophrenia is possible. However, documenting delusions and hallucinations is difficult if not impossible in people with severe mental retardation, especially if they are nonverbal, and the diagnosis may not be possible (Reid 1993). In some people without sufficient language to report delusions or hallucinations, the presence of grossly disorganized behavior coexisting with negative symptoms might be sufficient evidence for the diagnosis of schizophrenia (although not of its specific subtype) or of psychotic disorder not otherwise specified.

Results of most studies of epidemiology of psychotic disorders in children with mental retardation are difficult to evaluate because the studies used diverse methodologies and diagnostic criteria. Earlier studies were mostly of selected groups, such as clinic patients. In a referred group of 60 children and adolescents, Reid (1980) diagnosed childhood psychosis in 8%. In the neurodevelopmental psychiatry clinic at the Children's Hospital in Boston, psychotic disorder was diagnosed (by DSM-III criteria) in 3 of 413 (0.7%) patients younger than 18 years. In an unselected sample of 144 children ages 13–17 years, Gillberg et al. (1986) diagnosed schizophrenia in 1% of those with mild and in 1.5% of those with severe mental retardation. Currently the estimates of prevalence of schizophrenia in people with mental retardation range from about 1%, as accepted for the general population (Reiss 1994), to about 2%–3% (Bregman 1991; Fraser and Nolan 1994). In a follow-up study of an unselected cohort of 18-year-old Swedish conscripts, low IQ was found to be a risk factor for development of schizophrenia later in life (David et al. 1997).

Children with a psychotic disorder may be first referred to the psychiatrist owing to a suspicion of mental retardation because psychosis may be associated with cognitive deficiencies (Russell and Tanguay 1981). A syndrome considered to be an early stage of childhood schizophrenia, and in which cognitive functioning may be compromised, has been described (Cantor 1988). Infants or toddlers with this syndrome manifest sleep disturbance, hypotonia in the second year of life, social withdrawal, unusual behaviors such as rocking, and fears. Some of them may have standard intelligence test scores within the mild mental retardation range. However, because thought disorder may not yet be recognizable, the diagnosis of PDD is typically used in addition to mental retardation (Kestenbaum et al. 1989). When these children reach late latency, symptoms of thought disorder are usually clear enough to permit a formal diagnosis of schizophrenia.

With recent interest in behavioral phenotypes, it was found that there is an increased risk for psychotic disorders in certain mental retardation syndromes, especially velocardiofacial syndrome and Prader-Willi syndrome (Dykens 2000).

Depressive Disorders

For many years, there were doubts whether depression could occur in people with mental retardation. One view held that they could not become depressed because they had no ability to realize their shortcomings and to develop low self-esteem. An opposite view was that they were very much at risk for depression because they had been, most likely, rejected by their mothers (Gardner 1967). In earlier studies of prevalence of mental disorders in children and adolescents with mental retardation, depression was not mentioned. Sovner and Hurley (1983) showed, in a literature review, that depression does occur in this population. In the neurodevelopmental psychiatry clinic at the Children's Hospital in Boston, in a referred sample of 277 children and adolescents with mild and moderate mental retardation, a mental disorder with significant components of depression was diagnosed in 14% (Szymanski 1988). In an unselected sample of 144 chil-

dren ages 13–17 years, Gillberg et al. (1986) diagnosed major affective disorder in 4% of those with mild and in 1.5% of those with severe mental retardation. This could have been an underestimate, because people with less prominent dysphoric symptoms were included in another category. The current general view is that mood disorders among people with mental retardation are about as frequent as or more frequent than in the general population (Reiss 1994). However, in many instances, mood disorders remain undiagnosed (Feinstein and Reiss 1996). Caregivers may overlook depression in these individuals because their behavior may not be disturbing to others and because, in fact, they may be easier to manage. However, children with mental retardation might show depressive symptoms more often than those with average intelligence (Schloss et al. 1988), possibly linked to their learned helplessness, poor self-image, and lack of peer supports (Dagnan and Sandhu 1999) (as discussed above under *Epidemiology*, in the section "Mental Disorders and Mental Retardation"). Suicide can also occur among children, adolescents, and adults with mental retardation (Patja et al. 2001; Walters et al. 1995).

Another obstacle to diagnosis is the lack of language skills sufficient to reflect the traditional symptoms of depression (e.g., poor self-image and hopelessness). However, of the nine symptoms listed in the first group of DSM-IV-TR criteria for a major depressive episode (five or more are required for a diagnosis), seven can be satisfied on the basis of observation and history, even if the patient is not verbal: depressed or irritable mood, diminished interest in activities, significant weight loss or gain, insomnia or hypersomnia, psychomotor agitation or retardation, fatigue, and diminished ability to concentrate. The mood changes may be reported by the patient or by others. Children and adolescents with mild mental retardation and good language skills usually can describe the same symptoms as those without mental retardation. They may, however, use simple and concrete description; for example, they may say that they feel sick and weak, rather than depressed, or complain that no one likes them, rather than say that they feel worthless (AACAP 1999). Depression in this population has also been found to be strongly associated with aggressive behavior (Reiss and Rojahn 1993). Such behaviors could be a method of affective expression in people with limited language or even a form of self-defense against caregivers' expectations and pressure to perform and comply. Depression has been also reported in people with Down syndrome (Szymanski and Biederman 1984) and as being related to menstrual cycles in women with mental retardation. As in people without mental retardation, depression may occur in conjunction with psychotic features, making diagnosis more difficult.

The differential diagnosis of depression versus dementia often emerges in people with mental retardation—especially in people with Down syndrome, because of its association with Alzheimer's disease. However, this is not an issue with children and adolescents. Clinical dementia in individuals with Down syndrome does not occur before the fourth or even fifth decade of life and is associated with loss of skills and memory. This contrasts with depression, in which there is diminished interest and productivity but no actual loss of skills. Another important differential diagnosis is with thyroid disorders, to which people with Down syndrome are prone. Depressive symptoms may be also a side effect of some β-blockers, such as propranolol, sometimes used in treatment of aggressive behavior in people with mental retardation.

Bipolar Disorder

Manic symptoms may be noticed more readily than depression because they are usually disturbing to caregivers. Otherwise, problems with the diagnosis are similar to those listed for depressive disorders. The symptoms have to be evaluated in the context of premorbid abilities and behavior. For example, a nonverbal adolescent with significant mental retardation would not exhibit grandiosity, pressured speech, flight of ideas, and buying sprees, but there may be noticeable insomnia, hyperactivity, screaming, increased masturbation, distractibility, and irritability leading to aggression. Inappropriately elevated mood may be expressed through yelling, laughter, and dancing. People familiar with the individual will notice a mood change. Teachers usually notice behavior problems, noncompliance, inattentiveness, and noncompletion of assignments. Bipolar disorder is probably underdiagnosed in the many individuals who are referred primarily because of periodic disruptive behaviors. In some, these behaviors may represent a bipolar disorder; in others, they may be a reaction to usual life stresses that occur periodically, such as staff and school changes. In facilities where behavioral data are collected, usually these are on occurrence of disruptive behaviors, rather than on actual mood changes, which would be a better indicator of mood disorder. In some children and adoles-

cents with severe mental retardation, the mood changes are rapid-cycling, as often as every few days (Jan et al. 1994).

Anxiety Disorders

These disorders have been reported in people with mental retardation, although the prevalence reports are conflicting. In children, adolescents, and young adults with mild mental retardation, generalized anxiety disorder has manifestations generally similar to those in comparable populations without mental retardation, and it can be diagnosed through patient self-report and interview with the caregivers (Masi et al. 2000). Phobias and panic disorders occur as well in this population (Feinstein and Reiss 1996). As with other disorders, higher-functioning, verbal people can provide reports that make the diagnosis more reliable, whereas in those with significant mental retardation, it has to be inferred from behavioral observations and caregiver reports. It is quite possible that anxiety disorders are often undiagnosed in the many patients referred because of behavior problems such as noncompliance, hyperactivity, and short attention. Anxiety and social avoidance are part of certain behavioral phenotypes, most notably fragile X syndrome.

Obsessive-Compulsive Disorder

The diagnosis of obsessive-compulsive disorder requires that the compulsions be a response to the obsessions and thus that the anxiety and distress underlying the obsessions be identified. This can usually be done for people with mild mental retardation and sufficient language skills. In those with significant mental retardation and poor or no language, the diagnosis is often inferred from the person's repetitive, ritualistic behaviors. However, such behaviors are often seen in people with significant mental retardation as well as with autistic disorder, and it is not clear whether they represent an obsessive-compulsive disorder.

Posttraumatic Stress Disorder

This diagnosis is an important one to consider in this population and probably is often unnoticed. It is usually related to sexual abuse. Ryan (1994) described 51 persons with developmental disabilities who also met DSM-III-R criteria (American Psychiatric Association 1987) for posttraumatic stress disorder. The diagnosis usually requires the patient's verbal reports but it might be suspected in nonverbal individuals if symptoms such as excessive masturbation, loss of toilet training, sleep disorder, avoidance of places or people possibly associated with the abuse, heightened arousal, and vigilance appear. The history of the traumatic experience is needed, but people with poor verbal skills may have problems in describing it. One should keep in mind that people with mental retardation may subjectively perceive the traumatic event as threatening, even if it would not be perceived as such by a person of similar age without mental retardation. Children and adolescents with mental retardation are at a particular risk for sexual abuse. They are considered "safe" victims because they may have problems in reporting the abuse. Perpetrators' usual defense is that the victim is too mentally retarded to be able to testify. Retarded victims may actually cooperate with the perpetrator, because of their tendency to trust others and to relate indiscriminately and the belief that by cooperating they will make a friend.

Self-Injurious Behaviors and Stereotypic Behaviors

A variety of repetitive and seemingly nonfunctional behaviors may occur as part of other mental disorders or independently; in either case, they are a frequent reason for psychiatric referral and the focus of treatment. Healthy young children may engage in such behaviors (Werry et al. 1983), but in people with mental retardation and/or autism, these behaviors may be of high intensity and persist into adulthood. These may include body rocking, head banging, and hand shaking. Because this is a very heterogeneous group, there is no single treatment approach, and accurate differential diagnosis is essential (Gualtieri 1989). If association with another mental disorder can be ruled out and the behavior is the focus of treatment, the DSM-IV-TR category of stereotypic movement disorder can be used. If there is tissue damage that requires medical treatment, the specifier "with self-injurious behavior" is added. The self-injurious behaviors (SIBs) may lead to serious damage (e.g., retinal detachment and blindness due to head banging, or self-biting that may lead to virtual limb amputation), may severely compromise the patient's functioning, and may be even life-threatening. Severe stereotypic motor disorder, both with and without self-injury, occurs with higher prevalence among people with severe or profound mental retardation who live in institutions. In some cases the individual appears to want to prevent the SIB, such as through self-restraining (holding hands inside the clothing) or even asking to be restrained. In assessing the SIB it is important to rule out physical discomfort due to a medical problem; for example, head banging might be due to migraine headache or earache from otitis. They also are associated with disorders such as autism, blindness, and certain behavioral phenotypes, such as Lesch-Nyhan and fragile X syndromes. Detailed discussion of the etiology and mechanism of SIBs is beyond the scope of this chapter. An excellent review is provided by Harris (1995).

Aggression

Aggressive behavior is one of the most common reasons for psychiatric referral of people of all ages who have mental retardation; *aggressive behavior* is also one of the most misused terms, including behaviors as diverse as swearing (verbal aggression) and life-threatening violence. There is no discrete disorder called aggression. Rather, aggression can be seen as a final common pathway related to various causes and mechanisms. It can be associated with psychopathology, such as psychosis, ADHD, paranoid traits, personality and conduct disorders, and affective disorders (Connor and Steingard 1996; Reiss 1994). It can be a learned behavior, such as behavior related to exposure to aggressive role models, to certain antecedents, or to consequences such as reactions of the caregivers that will reinforce the aggressive behavior. It can be related to neuropathology, such as head injury, and to certain seizure disorders (although then it is usually not goal directed). Frequently aggression becomes a means of communication for nonverbal people. In most cases, there are concomitant factors. For example, a depressed individual might refuse to go to a day program but is forced to. He resists physically, resulting in caregiver-directed aggression. He is treated with an antidepressant and the depression lifts, but he also becomes manic, so the aggression gets worse. The medication is adjusted and the manic episodes subside. However, in the meantime, he has learned that aggressive behavior helps him to avoid tasks in the day program and be permitted to sit in the office all day. This reinforces the aggression and maintains it. Thus, comprehensive diagnostic assessment, biomedical, psychiatric, and psychosocial, is a precondition to treatment (Connor and Steingard 1996; Harris 1995, p. 478). An important part of assessment is defining operationally and behaviorally the aggressive behavior that is of concern, then collecting reliable data on its occurrence in various settings.

■ Treatment of Mental Disorders in People With Mental Retardation

The principles of psychiatric treatment are the same whether the patient has mental retardation or not. As is the rule in child psychiatry (which is by its nature a developmental psychiatry), the specific techniques and approaches should be individualized according to the individual's unique personal needs and developmental level. These are addressed below.

Designing a Treatment Program

Several special issues must be kept in mind in the treatment of children and adolescents with mental retardation. These individuals usually have deficiencies in a number of interrelated areas that must be treated in concert. They are involved with many caregivers and professionals who may have different views of them, different expectations, and different complaints but whose cooperation in and understanding of the treatment plan are essential. Unfortunately, many mental health professionals often limit themselves to symptomatic pharmacological treatment of individual disruptive behaviors, a tactic that is even supported by health insurers as a cheapest solution (even if short-term). Thus, the following guidelines are important to the success of the treatment:

- Comprehensive diagnostic psychiatric assessment is a precondition. A psychiatric diagnosis should be made whenever appropriate. As described previously, this should include comprehensive understanding of the person's environment and of strengths, disabilities, and needs in all domains (as discussed above under "Psychiatric Clinical Assessment"). The caregivers' concerns must be understood and their cooperation ensured.
- Biomedical, psychological, and environmental factors that could have initiated and/or maintained the problem—such as inappropriate school or residential placement, lack of appropriate supports, or inconsistent management by caregivers—should be explored. Up-to-date assessment, including etiology, of the mental retardation and associated disabilities is needed. The current medications should be

assessed for effectiveness, side effects, and interactions.
- Clear goals of treatment should be established, regularly reviewed, and updated as necessary (see "General Treatment Goals" below).
- Comprehensiveness of the treatment program is essential; all the patient's needs, not only the disruptive behaviors, should be addressed. These may include psychiatric and medical problems, self-care skills, communication skills, interpersonal relating, education and/or work, and recreation. Collaboration of the psychiatrist with all members of the treatment team responsible for each of those aspects is essential.
- Choice of psychiatric interventions should be guided by the best risk–benefit ratio. They should be integrated with the patient's total treatment program, including medical, educational, behavioral, and habilitative interventions. The least intrusive approaches should be chosen first.
- Behaviors and skills that will be an index of progress should be identified, and means of monitoring them should be established. All involved professionals and caregivers should agree on the treatment goals and approaches. They should form a de facto interdisciplinary team with the mental health clinician, even if their communication is mainly by phone or e-mail.
- Adverse treatment effects should be monitored regularly, because the patient may not be able to report them.
- Human rights and legal requirements (such as obtaining legal informed consent for use of medications) should be respected.

General Treatment Goals

The older approach was to see suppression of undesirable behaviors as the goal of psychiatric treatment of people with mental retardation, thus rendering them quiet and cooperative with caregivers. In recent years the concept of QOL has become popular (Schalock and Begab 1990). At first it was thought that objective measures such as the state of the person's health and health care and the quality of housing and services were the best measure of QOL. At the present, the importance of the subjective satisfaction of the individual—in other words, the individual's happiness—is recognized as essential to the QOL and an important goal of treatment (Szymanski 2000). Assessing it may not be easy with people who do not have sufficient language skills. For them, a variety of indicators, such as objective ones and subjective impressions of caregiving team members, will reflect the QOL, including the individual's sense of satisfaction with his or her own life. The goal of achieving this sense has to be reconciled with the realities of life and with goals of the parents of the disabled child or adolescent. Many measures should be taken to enable people with mental retardation to develop an optimal QOL and sense of self-satisfaction. A most important goal of these measures is the facilitation of a sense of self-worth, leading to a positive self-image that may prevent development of learned helplessness, passivity, or maladaptive defenses. Learning self-care and independence-related skills is essential. Thus, even young children should be taught chores that they can do and that help them feel that they are useful family members. Adolescents need prevocational, vocational, money-management, and independent-travel training. Appropriate and early sexuality education, combined with an honest discussion of limitations, social skills training, and an opportunity to interact with appropriate peers, may prevent sexual acting out and sexual victimization. All of these measures will eventually be helpful in preventing future psychosocial dysfunction (Szymanski 1987).

Psychotherapies

Psychotherapy with people with mental retardation has been around for many years. Already in the 1950s, an anthology of papers on this topic was published (Stacey and DeMartino 1957). Most of the available research to date has been based on case studies; although it has been positive about the results of psychotherapy, most authors agree on the need for more controlled outcome research (Hurley 1989; Reiss 1994).

The available literature agrees on the following guidelines as essential to the success of both individual and group therapy:

- The therapist should be willing, trained, flexible, supportive, eclectic, and able to serve as a "real person," a role model, and a teacher for the patient.
- The patient should have basic skills of verbal or nonverbal communication, and the therapist should communicate in a manner commensurate with the patient's communication skills and developmental level but treat the patient respectfully according to chronological age. A great deal of repetition is necessary.
- The therapy often must be directive, concrete, and structured but permitting spontaneous expression, and focused on issues of importance to the patient. Nonverbal communication through means such as play may be very helpful, but choice of activity materials should be commensurate with patient's age and self-image, as people with mental retardation are very sensitive to being treated as younger than they are. Play activities may be useful in modeling real-life situations and learning ways of handling them.
- An eclectic approach is needed, using reality-oriented cognitive techniques, behavior modification, role modeling, family supports, and, to a lesser degree, psychodynamic exploration.
- The therapy should be a part of a comprehensive treatment program, with all involved working as a team and the therapist providing information to and receiving input from other caregivers.
- A hierarchy of specific and realistic goals should be set up. In particular, the patient should acquire a constructive understanding of his or her disabilities, balanced by an appreciation of his or her strengths, leading to development of a positive self-image.

Details of the various therapeutic techniques helpful with people who have mental retardation may be found elsewhere (Hollins 2001; Reiss 1994; Sigman 1985; Stavrakaki and Klein 1985; Szymanski 1980a).

The term *counseling* is often used to describe a supportive approach by any caregiver, focused on day-to-day events.

Group psychotherapy and multiple-family group psychotherapy may be most useful with adolescents and young adults (Szymanski and Rosefsky 1980; Szymanski and Kiernan 1983). In the latter mode of therapy, both the patients and their families participate. Both approaches, especially the latter, provide a microcosm of society and an opportunity to learn to relate to one's peers and to use them as a source of support.

Behavior Modification

In behavior modification, essentially the same techniques are used as for people without mental retardation (see Chapter 52, "Cognitive-Behavior Modification," in this volume). As with other treatments, allowances have to be made to accommodate patients' developmental level and communication skills. For example, nonverbal, severely handicapped individuals may need a reward immediately after the desired behavior occurs, in order to recognize the connection between reward and behavior, rather than have the reward be significantly delayed. Various forms of behavioral approaches are effective with this population in teaching skills and appropriate behaviors as well as in eliminating the inappropriate ones (Reiss 1994). The focus should be not only on eliminating objectionable behaviors but also on teaching appropriate replacement behaviors. Ignoring inappropriate behaviors works only if sufficient social and other rewards are given for appropriate ones. A consistent and structured treatment plan, hierarchy of goals to be achieved, and means to monitor progress are necessary, especially in more complex situations. The treatment should be generalized to other settings and caregivers, such as through training parents to apply the same techniques at home that are used at school.

Aversive techniques (punishment) at present are generally used only in exceptional circumstances. These are limited to dangerous SIBs and aggression that did not respond to thorough application of other treatments; they are used only for a short period of time.

Family-Directed Interventions

The families of people with mental retardation are no longer considered a priori patients in need of psychotherapy. Of course, some may need it, if they have psychopathology that requires it, just as for families of children without mental retardation (see Chapter 53, "Family Therapy"). However, all families of people with mental retardation will benefit from appropriate supports. They should be seen as members of the treatment team. Most families ask for information from the professional, or at least a referral to one who can provide it, about such things as the nature of child's problems, genetics, appropriate expectations, behavioral management techniques, entitlements for education and other services, and resources and support groups. On the other hand, in the era of the Internet and family empowerment, many parents have a great deal of knowledge about the child's disability, meaning that the professional may learn from them as well.

Many families may need support in alleviating guilt feelings, if these are present, or modifying overprotec-

tive or overdemanding attitudes toward the child. Optimally the families should be able to integrate the child into family life and expect him/her to do chores, even if minimal and with hands-on help, to let the child feel like a valued family member. Psychiatrists may be particularly effective in helping the parents recognize the child's strengths and learn to derive gratification regardless of the level of disability. Having an opportunity to watch the psychiatrist interact and play with the child is often very helpful. Parents of older adolescents need help in recognizing their child's need for independence and reconciling it with the need for protection.

Pharmacotherapy

In this section, only certain aspects of pharmacotherapy relevant to people with mental retardation are reviewed. For additional information, see Chapter 50 ("Psychopharmacology"). For many years, psychotropic drugs, particularly antipsychotics, were used unnecessarily in institutionalized patients to make the patients more docile and easier to handle, even though their disruptive behaviors could actually represent a good adaptation to an understaffed facility and to the lack of constructive programs and care. In some institutions, more than 50% and up to 86% of residents were given psychotropic drugs, mostly antipsychotics. In the past several decades, a great deal of progress has occurred as a result of improved general care and services as well as new statutes and court decisions that regulated the use of psychotropics in this population. The use of psychotropics in children in the community is considered to be high also. Common mistakes include treating single nonspecific symptoms, without prior diagnostic understanding; continuing the treatment without evidence of effectiveness; using medications alone, without other interventions; and using medications as a substitute for education and training.

Research on the use of these agents in children and adolescents with mental retardation has been limited. Many studies were not controlled and were done on heterogeneous groups with various etiologies of the mental retardation. However, there is no evidence that just the presence of low IQ changes the mechanism of drug action and its effectiveness, although this might vary in different syndromes associated with mental retardation. The frequency of side effects in this population might not be the same as for populations without mental retardation (AACAP 1999). People with Down syndrome might be very sensitive to anticholinergic drugs, which may lead to cognitive impairment and delirium. Lithium might also lead to cognitive dulling; because of irregular fluid intake, there is higher risk of toxicity. Sedative-hypnotic drugs may have the paradoxical effect of behavioral disinhibition.

The attitude of mental retardation professionals and of the general public is often antimedication. Statutes and regulations have often equated use of drugs with aversive and intrusive measures, to be avoided by all means. In fact, some treatment programs pride themselves on being "drug free." This has been changing, however. The recent guidelines of Centers for Medicare and Medicaid Services (formerly the Health Care Financing Administration) state that psychotropics might be useful and that denying them to people with mental retardation, if they would be indicated, is inappropriate. These individuals are at high risk for mental disorders, and they have the right to the best available treatments, including drugs, that may improve their QOL. The main points of these guidelines are

- Comprehensive diagnostic evaluation *prior* to drug initiation (and not afterward, to justify drug use)
- Baseline behavioral data
- Prior trial of less intrusive treatments if applicable; medication to be used only as part of a comprehensive treatment/habilitation program; use of the lowest effective dose
- Avoidance of reducing patient's functioning as a result of the medication
- Careful monitoring of side effects
- Continuation of the drug only if it is clearly proven effective and safe

Thus, the use of the drugs should be guided by the same principles as for any medical treatment for the population at large in general and for psychotropic drugs in particular. Drugs are justified if they help to achieve the best possible QOL for the patient (not necessarily the total elimination of all symptoms) and if the benefits clearly outweigh the adverse effects.

For an excellent review of current knowledge of psychopharmacology in the field of mental retardation, see Reiss and Aman (1998).

Antipsychotics. In people with mental retardation, antipsychotic drugs have a long history of use for virtually any behavioral symptoms rather than for their principal indications: psychosis (schizophrenia in particular), Tourette's disorder, and dangerously aggressive behavior or SIB. Even if they control the behavioral symptoms, there is always concern about long-term side effects, especially tardive dyskinesia. It also should be kept in mind that people with mental retardation might be more at risk for tardive akathisia and dyskinesia; when antipsychotics are abruptly discontinued, behavioral symptoms, such as irritability, insomnia, and weight loss, may emerge (Gualtieri et al. 1986). At present, atypical antipsychotics, because of their effectiveness and more favorable side effect profile, are the drugs of choice. There are case reports of the effectiveness of risperidone in children and adolescents with psychosis, SIB, and aggression (Dosen 2001).

Antidepressants. In children, tricyclic antidepressants had also been used for the treatment of ADHD and symptomatic relief of nocturnal enuresis, but at present, owing to their cardiotoxic side effects, their use is not recommended. Newer antidepressants, chiefly selective serotonin reuptake inhibitors (SSRIs), are used now as first-line agents for the treatment of depression and obsessive-compulsive symptoms and, recently, ADHD and anxiety disorders. Case reports on their effectiveness in children and adolescents with mental retardation are appearing (Dosen 2001; Sovner et al. 2001). They have been found in preliminary studies to be helpful, at least temporarily, for SIBs in some individuals. The choice of the particular SSRI will largely depend on the side effect profile.

Lithium. Lithium was the first drug effective for the treatment of mania. At the present, because of side effects, it has been largely replaced by anticonvulsants as the first-line treatment. In people with mental retardation, it has been found to be useful occasionally in the treatment of aggressive behaviors (Langee 1990; McCracken and Diamond 1988). As with other drugs, side effects must be closely monitored because the patient may not be able to report them. In people with mental retardation, side effects may be more troublesome, and obtaining cooperation in appropriate fluid intake may be a problem.

Anticonvulsants. Other than their most common use in treatment of seizure disorders, anticonvulsants have been increasingly used in the general population, as well as in people with mental retardation, as mood stabilizers, and they have been reported as useful in controlling aggressive behavior (Glue 1989; Langee 1989; Sovner 1991). An important point is that because seizures are often comorbid with mental retardation, if there is an associated behavioral problem, one of these drugs might be helpful for both conditions. Hyponatremia and water intoxication are important side effects of carbamazepine that are sometimes overlooked. It also appears that phenobarbital, although helpful in controlling seizures, might result in hyperactivity and behavior problems, especially in people with brain damage, epilepsy, and mental retardation (Alvarez 1998).

Anxiolytics.   Although the primary indication is short-term treatment of anxiety, anxiolytics have been used periodically in people with mental retardation for long-term treatment of aggressive behavior. However, there is no clear evidence of their effectiveness in such situations. People with mental retardation who receive benzodiazepines are described as at risk for cognitive and memory impairments. Paradoxical reactions, such as behavioral disinhibition and increase in stereotypic behaviors and SIBs, might occur. Some studies reported that buspirone was effective, with few side effects. SSRIs are also tried sometimes as anxiolytics (review; AACAP 1999).

Stimulants.   Controversy exists in the literature about the effectiveness of stimulants, primarily methylphenidate, in the presence of mental retardation. Lack of effectiveness in some studies may have been related to incorrect diagnosis, when a developmentally age-appropriate or situationally related inattentiveness was mistaken for ADHD. Also, one can expect, at best, improvement in attention and hyperactivity but not acquisition of appropriate behaviors, which requires behavioral intervention. There is concern about side effects, particularly tics, especially in people who already exhibit stereotypic behaviors. Clonidine has been used for the treatment of ADHD in this population, and it may be effective in reducing overactivity. It is available in patch form, which may be important with people unwilling to take oral medication. However, monitoring blood pressure and pulse rate requires some cooperation.

Beta-blockers.   Since the appearance of reports on the effectiveness of propranolol in the treatment of rage episodes after brain damage (Williams et al. 1982), β-blockers have been used quite extensively for the treatment of "generic" aggression in people with mental retardation. This approach has had mixed results, probably related to the heterogeneity of the behavioral problems being treated. Because depression might be a side effect, the person's disruptive behavior, together with global functioning, might decrease, but so does general level of functioning.

Other agents.   Naltrexone, an opiate receptor antagonist, has been studied in the treatment of SIBs in adults with severe mental retardation, on the basis of the hypothesis that the endogenous opioid system has a role in its pathogenesis. The results have been mixed, and it appears that naltrexone might be effective in no more than half of all who receive it, and in some it may exacerbate the SIB.

Nonestablished treatments.   Some families have tried treating their children's mental retardation with various diets and regimens of vitamins, minerals, and other nutritional supplement combinations, such as megavitamin treatment; vitamin B_6 with magnesium; and gluten-free, yeast-free, and casein-free diets. However, there are no empirical studies supporting these treatments' effectiveness, and results of initial reports have not been subsequently reproduced. With some supplements, there is a danger of side effects, such as with very high doses of fat-soluble vitamins. It is important that clinicians specifically ask families about use of such agents.

■ Roles of Psychiatrists in the Mental Retardation Field

The Position Statement on Psychiatry and Mental Retardation issued by the American Academy of Child and Adolescent Psychiatry (AACAP 1988) lists four roles for psychiatrists in this field:

1. Provision of clinical services to people with mental retardation
2. Prevention of mental disorders through early diagnosis and provision of emotional supports to the child and the family
3. Research
4. Learning skills that are also useful in the practice of psychiatry in general

The common theme of these roles is participation in an interdisciplinary developmental team (Cushna et al. 1980). The role of the modern psychiatrist on such a team is one of an equal member, not necessarily a leader or an uninvolved consultant. Because of their roots in the biomedical and psychosocial aspects of medicine, psychiatrists can function in the unique role of a synthesizer, helping the team to integrate the contributions of various disciplines (West 1973). In particular, psychiatrists should not limit themselves to the role of medication specialists, even if other disciplines attempt to cast them in such a role. A psychiatric physician should do not a "medication review" (one of the common reasons for referring a patient with mental retardation) but a "patient review," which focuses on all aspects of diagnosis and treatment. In summary, the field of mental retardation can be seen as an archetype for modern psychiatry anchored in the integration of biological and psychological medicine.

References

Achenbach TM: Manual for the Child Behavior Checklist and 1991 Profile. Burlington, VT: University of Vermont, 1991

Alvarez N: Barbiturates in the treatment of epilepsy in people with intellectual disability. J Intellect Disabil Res 42 (suppl 1):16–23, 1998

Aman MG, Singh NN, Stewart AW, et al: The Aberrant Behavior Checklist: a behavior rating scale for the assessment of treatment effects. Am J Ment Defic 89:485–491, 1985

American Association on Mental Retardation: Mental Retardation: Definition, Classification, and Systems of Supports, 9th Edition. Washington, DC, American Association on Mental Retardation, 1992

American Association on Mental Retardation: Mental Retardation: Definition, Classification, and Systems of Supports, 10th Edition. Washington, DC, American Association on Mental Retardation, 2002

American Academy of Child and Adolescent Psychiatry [AACAP]: Practice parameters for the assessment and treatment of children, adolescents, and adults with mental retardation and comorbid mental disorders. J Am Acad Child Adolesc Psychiatry 38(12, suppl):5S–31S, 1999

American Academy of Child and Adolescent Psychiatry [AACAP], Committee on Mental Retardation and Developmental Disabilities: The roles and responsibilities of child and adolescent psychiatry in the field of developmental disabilities. American Academy of Child and Adolescent Psychiatry Newsletter, winter 1988, p 7

American Psychiatric Association: Diagnostic and Statistical Manual of Mental Disorders, 3rd Edition. Washington, DC, American Psychiatric Association, 1980

American Psychiatric Association: Diagnostic and Statistical Manual of Mental Disorders, 3rd Edition, Revised. Washington, DC, American Psychiatric Association, 1987

American Psychiatric Association: Diagnostic and Statistical Manual of Mental Disorders, 4th Edition. Washington, DC, American Psychiatric Association, 1994

American Psychiatric Association: Diagnostic and Statistical Manual of Mental Disorders, 4th Edition, Text Revision. Washington, DC, American Psychiatric Association, 2000

Baethmann A, Maier-Hauff K, Kempski O, et al: Mediators of brain edema and secondary brain damage. Crit Care Med 16:972–976, 1988

Braddock D, Hemp R, Parish S, et al: The state of the states in developmental disabilities: 2000 study summary. Chicago, IL, University of Illinois at Chicago, Department of Disability and Human Development, 2000

Bregman J: Current developments in the understanding of mental retardation, part II: psychopathology. J Am Acad Child Adolesc Psychiatry 30:861–872, 1991

Buckhalt J, Rutherford B, Goldberg K: Verbal and nonverbal interaction of mothers with their Down's syndrome and nonretarded infants. Am J Ment Defic 82:337–343, 1978

Butler MG, Meany FJ, Palmer CG: Clinical and cytogenetic survey of 39 individuals with Prader-Labhart-Willi syndrome. Am J Med Genet 23:793–809, 1986

Cantor S: Childhood Schizophrenia. New York, Guilford, 1988

Cicchetti D, Sroufe A: An organizational view of affect: illustration from the study of Down's syndrome infants, in The Development of Affect. Edited by Lewis M, Rosenblum LA. New York, Plenum, 1978, pp 309–350

Clarren SK, Smith DW, Hansen JW: Helmet treatment for plagiocephaly and congenital muscular torticollis. J Pediatr 94:43–46, 1979

Cohen MM Jr: The Child With Multiple Birth Defects. New York, Raven, 1982

Connor DF, Steingard, RJ: A clinical approach to the pharmacotherapy of aggression in children and adolescents. Ann N Y Acad Sci 794:290–307, 1996

Corbett JA, Harris E, Robinson R: Epilepsy, in Mental Retardation and Developmental Disabilities, Vol 7. Edited by Wortis J. New York, Brunner/Mazel, 1975, pp 79–111

Curry C, Stevenson R, Aughton D: Evaluation of mental retardation: recommendations of a consensus conference. Am J Med Genet 72:468–477, 1997

Cushna B, Szymanski LS, Tanguay PE: Professional roles and unmet manpower needs, in Emotional Disorders of Mentally Retarded Persons. Edited by Szymanski LS, Tanguay PE. Baltimore, MD, University Park Press, 1980, pp 3–17

Dagnan D, Sandhu S: Social comparison, self-esteem and depression in people with intellectual disability. J Intellect Disabil Res 43:372–379, 1999

David AS, Malmberg A, Brandt L, et al: IQ and risk for schizophrenia: a population-based cohort study. Psychol Med 27:1311–1323, 1997

Delach J, Rosengren S, Kaplan L, et al: Comparison of high resolution chromosome banding and fluorescence in situ hybridization (FISH) for the diagnosis of Prader-Willi syndrome and Angelman syndrome. Genetics 52:85–91, 1995

Detterman DK: Theoretical notions of intelligence and mental retardation. Am J Ment Defic 92:2–11, 1987

Donaldson JY, Menolascino FJ: Past, current, and future roles of child psychiatry in mental retardation. J Am Acad Child Psychiatry 3:352–374, 1977

Dosen A: Pharmacotherapy in mentally retarded children, in Treating Mental Illness and Behavior Disorders in Children and Adults With Mental Retardation. Edited by Dosen A, Day K. Washington, DC: American Psychiatric Publishing, 2001, pp 429–450

Dunn PM: Congenital postural deformities. Br Med Bull 93:71–76, 1976

Dykens EM: Measuring behavioral phenotypes: provocations from the "new genetics." Am J Ment Retard 99:522–532, 1995

Dykens EM: Annotation: psychopathology in children with intellectual disability. J Child Psychol Psychiatry 41:407–417, 2000

Edgerton RB: The Cloak of Competence: Stigma in the Lives of Mentally Retarded. Berkeley, CA, University of California Press, 1967

Ellis NR, Cavalier AR: Research perspectives in mental retardation, in Mental Retardation: The Developmental-Difference Controversy. Edited by Zigler E, Balla D. Hillsdale, NJ, Lawrence Erlbaum, 1982, pp 121–152

Feingold M, Bassert WH: Normal values. Birth Defects 10:1–5, 1974

Feinstein C, Reiss AL: Psychiatric disorder in mentally retarded children and adolescents: the challenges of meaningful diagnosis. Child Adolesc Psychiatr Clin N Am 5:827–852, 1996

Fraser W, Nolan M: Psychiatric disorders in mental retardation, in Mental Health in Mental Retardation. Edited by Bouras N. Cambridge, MA, Cambridge University Press, 1994, pp 83–84

Frey KS, Greenberg MT, Fewell RR: Stress and coping among parents of handicapped children: a multidimensional approach. Am J Ment Retard 94:240–249, 1989

Gardner WI: Occurrence of severe depressive reactions in the mentally retarded. Am J Psychiatry 124:142–144, 1967

Gillberg C, Persson E, Grufman M, et al: Psychiatric disorders in mildly and severely mentally retarded urban children and adolescents: epidemiological aspects. Br J Psychiatry 149:68–74, 1986

Glue P: Rapid cycling affective disorder in the mentally retarded. Biol Psychiatry 26:250–256, 1989

Graham JM Jr: Smith's Recognizable Patterns of Human Deformation. Philadelphia, PA, WB Saunders, 1988

Grossman HJ (ed): Classification in Mental Retardation. Washington, DC, American Association on Mental Deficiency, 1983

Gualtieri CT: The differential diagnosis of self-injurious behavior in mentally retarded people. Psychopharmacol Bull 25:358–363, 1989

Gualtieri CT, Schroeder SR, Hicks RE, et al: Tardive dyskinesia in young mentally retarded individuals. Arch Gen Psychiatry 43:335–340, 1986

Hagerman RJ, Silverman AC (eds): Fragile-X Syndrome: Diagnosis, Treatment, and Research. Baltimore, MD, Johns Hopkins University Press, 1996

Hall JG: Invited editorial comment: analysis of Pena-Shokeir phenotype. Am J Med Genet 25:99, 1986

Handen BJ, Janosky J, McAuliffe S: Long-term follow-up of children with mental retardation/borderline intellectual functioning and ADHD. J Abnorm Child Psychol 25:287–295, 1997

Hanshaw GB: Developmental abnormalities associated with congenital CMV infection. Advances in Teratology 4:64–93, 1970

Hanzlik JR, Stevenson MB: Interaction of mothers with their infants who are mentally retarded, retarded with cerebral palsy, or nonretarded. Am J Ment Defic 90:513–520, 1986

Harris JC: Developmental Neuropsychiatry. Oxford, UK, Oxford University Press, 1995

Harris VS, McHale SM: Family life problems, daily caregiving activities, and the psychological well-being of mothers of mentally retarded children. Am J Ment Retard 94:231–239, 1989

Hawley PD, Jackson LG, Kurnit DM: Sixty-four patients with Brachmann-de Lange syndrome: a survey. Am J Med Genet 20:453–459, 1985

Hollins S: Psychotherapeutic methods, in Treating Mental Illness and Behavior Disorders in Children and Adults With Mental Retardation. Edited by Dosen A, Day K. Washington, DC, American Psychiatric Publishing, 2001, pp 27–44

Holm VA: Rett's syndrome: a progressive developmental disability in girls. J Dev Behav Pediatr 6:32–36, 1985

Holmes LB: Congenital malformations, in Manual of Neonatal Care. Edited by Doherty JP, Stark AR. Boston, MA, Little, Brown, 1980, pp 91–96

Hoyme EH, Higginbottom MC, Jones KL: Vascular etiology of disruptive structural defects in monozygotic twins. Pediatrics 67:288–291, 1981

Hudgins L, Cassidy S: Congenital anomalies, in Developmental Behavioral Pediatrics, 3rd Edition. Edited by Levine MD, Carey WB, Crocker AC. Philadelphia, PA, WB Saunders, 1999, pp 249–262

Hurley AD: Individual psychotherapy with mentally retarded individuals: a review and a call for research. Res Dev Disabil 10:261–275, 1989

Jan JE, Abroms IF, Freeman RD, et al: Rapid cycling in severely multidisabled children: a form of bipolar affective disorder? Pediatr Neurol 10:34–39, 1994

Jones KL: Smith's Recognizable Patterns of Human Malformation, 5th Edition. Philadelphia, PA, WB Saunders, 1997

Jones KL, Rubinson LK: An approach to the child with structural defects. J Pediatr Orthop 4:238–244, 1983

Kanner L: History of the Care and Study of the Mentally Retarded. Springfield, IL, Charles C Thomas, 1964

Kaplan LC: Congenital Dandy Walker malformation associated with first trimester warfarin: a case report and literature review. Teratology 32:333–336, 1985

Kaplan LC: Assessment and management of infants and children with multiple congenital anomalies, in Developmental Disabilities: Delivery of Medical Care for Children and Adults. Edited by Rubin IL, Crocker AC. Philadelphia, PA, Lea & Febiger, 1989, pp 97–116

Kaplan LC: Neural tube defects, in Manual of Neonatal Care. Edited by Cloherty JP, Start AR. Boston, MA, Little, Brown, 1998

Kaplan LC, Wharton R, Elias E, et al: Clinical heterogeneity associated with deletions in the long arm of chromosome 15: report of three new cases and their possible genetic significance. Am J Med Genet 28:45–53, 1987

Katz SL, Gershon AA, Hotez PJ, et al (eds): Krugman's Infectious Diseases of Children, 10th Edition. St. Louis, MO, Mosby, 1998

Kerr AM: Rett syndrome: British longitudinal study, in Mental Retardation and Medical Care. Edited by Roosendaal JJ. Proceedings of the European Congress on Mental Retardation and Medical Care, Zeist, Uitgeverij Kerokebosch, April 21–24, 1991

Kestenbaum CJ, Canino IA, Pleak RR: Schizophrenic disorders of childhood and adolescence, in American Psychiatric Press Review of Psychiatry, Vol 8. Edited by Tasman A, Hales RE, Frances AJ. Washington, DC, American Psychiatric Press, 1989, pp 242–261

Kiernan WE, Stark JA (eds): Pathways to Employment for Adults With Developmental Disabilities. Baltimore, MD, Paul H Brookes, 1986

Kishino T, Lalande M, Watstaff J: UBE3A/E6-AP mutations cause Angelman syndrome. Nat Genet 15:70, 1997

Knoll JH, Nichols RD, Magenis RE, et al: Angelman syndrome: three molecular classes identified with chromosome 15q11q13 specific DNA markers. Am J Hum Genet 47:149–155, 1990

Kuban KCK, Leviton A: Cerebral palsy. N Engl J Med 330:188–195, 1994

Laird CD: Proposed mechanism of inheritance and expression of the human fragile-X syndrome of mental retardation. Genetics 117:587–590, 1987

Langee HR: A retrospective study of mentally retarded patients with behavioral disorders who were treated with carbamazepine. Am J Ment Retard 93:640–643, 1989

Langee HR: Retrospective study of lithium use for institutionalized mentally retarded individuals with behavior disorders. Am J Ment Retard 94:448–452, 1990

Leroy JG: Heredity, development and behavior, in Developmental-Behavioral Pediatrics, 2nd Edition. Edited by Levine MD, Carey WB, Crocker AC. Philadelphia, PA, WB Saunders, 1992, pp 193–212

Levy HL: Genetic screening. Adv Hum Genet 4:1–3, 1973

Lindberg B: Understanding Rett Syndrome. Toronto, Ontario, Canada, Hogrefe & Huber, 1991

Linna SL, Moilanen I, Ebeling H, et al: Psychiatric symptoms in children with intellectual disability. Eur Child Adolesc Psychiatry 8(suppl 4):77–82, 1999

Lofts RH, Schroeder SR, Maier RH: Effects of serum zinc supplementation on pica behavior of persons with mental retardation. Am J Ment Retard 95:103–109, 1990

Lynch EC, Staloch NH: Parental perceptions of physicians' communication in the informing process. Ment Retard 26:77–81, 1988

Mary NL: Reactions of black, Hispanic, and white mothers to having a child with handicaps. Ment Retard 28:1–5, 1990

Masi G, Favilla L, Mucci M: Generalized anxiety disorder in adolescents and young adults with mild mental retardation. Psychiatry 63:54–64, 2000

Mayes LC, Kirk V, Haywood N, et al: Changing cognitive outcome in preterm infants with hyaline membrane disease. Am J Dis Child 139:20–24, 1985

McCracken JT, Diamond RP: Bipolar disorder in mildly retarded adolescents. J Am Acad Child Adolesc Psychiatry 27:494–499, 1988

McLaren J, Bryson SE: Review of recent epidemiological studies of mental retardation: prevalence, associated disorders, and etiology. Am J Ment Retard 92:243–254, 1987

Menolascino FJ: Bridging the gap between mental retardation and mental illness, in Mental Retardation and Mental Health: Bridging the Gap. Edited by Menolascino FJ, McCann BM. Baltimore, MD, University Park Press, 1983, pp 3–64

Needleman HL, Schell A, Bellinger D, et al: The long-term effects of exposure to low doses of lead in childhood. An 11-year follow-up report. N Engl J Med 322:83–88, 1990

Nichols EK: Human Gene Therapy. Cambridge, MA, Harvard University Press, 1988

Nirje B: The normalization principle and its human management applications, in Changing Patterns in Residential Services for the Mentally Retarded. Edited by Kugel R, Wolfensberger W. Washington, DC, President's Committee on Mental Retardation, 1969, p 181

Nyhan WL: Behavioral phenotypes in organic genetic disease. Presidential address to the Society for Pediatric Research 6:1–9, 1972

O'Brien G, Pearson J, Berney T, et al: Measuring behavior in developmental disability: a review of existing schedules. Dev Med Child Neurol 87(suppl):1–72, 2001

Olshansky L: Chronic sorrow: a response to having a mentally defective child. Social Casework 43:190–193, 1962

Patja K, Iivanainen M, Raitasuo S, et al: Suicide mortality in mental retardation: a 35-year follow-up study. Acta Psychiatr Scand 103:307–311, 2001

Pearson DA, Lachar D, Loveland KA, et al: Patterns of behavioral adjustment and maladjustment in metal retardation: comparison of children with and without ADHD. Am J Ment Retard 105:236–251, 2000

Philips I: Children, mental retardation and emotional disorder, in Prevention and Treatment of Mental Retardation. Edited by Philips I. New York, Basic Books, 1966, pp 111–122

Pueschel SM, Pueschel JK (eds): Biomedical Concerns in Persons With Down Syndrome. Baltimore, MD, Paul H Brookes, 1992

Reid AH: Psychiatric disorders in mentally handicapped children: a clinical and follow-up study. J Ment Defic Res 24:287–298, 1980

Reid AH: Schizophrenic and paranoid syndromes in persons with mental retardation: assessment and diagnosis, in Mental Health Aspects of Mental Retardation. Edited by Fletcher RJ, Dosen A. New York, Lexington Books, 1993, pp 98–110

Reiss S: The Reiss Screen for Maladaptive Behavior Test Manual. Worthington, OH, IDS Publishing, 1988

Reiss S: Handbook of Challenging Behavior: Mental Health Aspects of Mental Retardation. Worthington, OH, IDS Publishing, 1994

Reiss S, Aman M: Psychotropic Medication & Developmental Disabilities: The International Consensus Handbook. Columbus, OH, Ohio State University, 1998

Reiss S, Rojahn J: Joint occurrence of depression and aggression in children and adults with mental retardation. J Intellect Disabil Res 37:287–294, 1993

Reiss S, Valenti-Hein D: Reiss Scales for Children's Dual Diagnosis: Test Manual. Worthington, OH, IDS Publishing, 1990

Reiss S, Levitan GW, Szyszko J: Emotional disturbance and mental retardation: diagnostic overshadowing. Am J Ment Def 86:567–574, 1982

Russell AT, Tanguay PE: Mental illness and mental retardation: cause or coincidence? Am J Ment Defic 85:570–574, 1981

Rutter M, Graham P, Yule W: A neuropsychiatric study in childhood, in Clinics in Developmental Medicine, Vols 35–36. London, Heinemann Medical Books, 1970

Ryan R: Posttraumatic stress disorder in persons with developmental disabilities. Community Ment Health J 30:45–54, 1994

Schalock RL, Begab MJ (eds): Quality of Life: Perspectives and Issues. Washington, DC, American Association on Mental Retardation, 1990

Scheerenberger RC: A History of Mental Retardation. Baltimore, MD, Paul H Brookes, 1983

Schloss PJ, Epstein MH, Cullinan D: Depression characteristics among mildly handicapped students. Journal of the Multihandicapped Person 1:293–302, 1988

Scriver CL, Clow CL: Phenylketonuria: epitome of human biochemical genetics (2 parts). N Engl J Med 303:1336–1394, 1980

Seshia SS, Johnston R, Kasian G: Non-traumatic coma in childhood: clinical variables in prediction of outcome. Dev Med Child Neurol 25:493–501, 1983

Sigman M: Individual and group psychotherapy with mentally retarded adolescents, in Children With Emotional Disorders and Developmental Disabilities. Edited by Sigman M. Orlando, FL, Grune & Stratton, 1985, pp 259–276

Singh NN, Ellis CR, Mulick JA, et al: Vitamin, mineral and dietary treatments, in Psychotropic Medication and Developmental Disabilities: The International Consensus Handbook. Edited by Reiss S, Aman M. Columbus, OH, Ohio State University, 1998, pp 311–320

Smith DW, Gong BT: Scalp hair patterning as a clue to early fetal brain development. J Pediatr 83:374–378, 1973

Solnit A, Stark M: Mourning and a birth of a defective child. Psychoanal Study Child 16:523–537, 1961

Sovner R: Limiting factors in the use of DSM-III criteria with mentally ill/mentally retarded persons. Psychopharmacol Bull 22:1055–1059, 1986

Sovner R: Use of anticonvulsant agents for treatment of neuropsychiatric disorders in the developmentally disabled, in Mental Retardation: Developing Pharmacotherapies. Edited by Ratey JJ. Washington, DC, American Psychiatric Publishing, 1991, pp. 83–106

Sovner R, Hurley AD: Do the mentally retarded suffer from affective illness? Arch Gen Psychiatry 40:61–67, 1983

Sovner R, Pary R, Dosen A, et al: Antidepressant drugs, in Treating Mental Illness and Behavior Disorders in Children and Adults with Mental Retardation. Edited by Dosen A, Day K. Washington, DC, American Psychiatric Publishing, 2001, pp 179–200

Stacey CL, DeMartino MF: Counseling and Psychotherapy with the Mentally Retarded. Glencoe, IL, Free Press, 1957

Stavrakaki C, Klein C: Psychotherapies with the mentally retarded. Psychiatr Clin North Am 9:733–743, 1985

Stone NW, Chesney BH: Attachment behaviors in handicapped infants. Ment Retard 16:8–12, 1978

Stromme P, Diseth TH: Prevalence of psychiatric diagnoses in children with mental retardation: data from a population-based study. Dev Med Child Neurol 42:266–270, 2000

Szymanski LS: Psychiatric diagnostic evaluation of mentally retarded individuals. J Am Acad Child Psychiatry 16:67–87, 1977

Szymanski LS: Individual psychotherapy with retarded persons, in Emotional Disorders of Mentally Retarded Persons. Edited by Szymanski LS, Tanguay PE. Baltimore, MD, University Park Press, 1980a, pp 131–148

Szymanski LS: Psychiatric diagnosis of retarded persons, in Emotional Disorders of Mentally Retarded Persons. Edited by Szymanski LS, Tanguay PE. Baltimore, MD, University Park Press, 1980b, pp 61–81

Szymanski LS: Prevention of psychosocial dysfunction in persons with mental retardation. Ment Retard 25:215–218, 1987

Szymanski LS: Integrative approach to diagnosis of mental disorders in retarded persons, in Mental Retardation and Mental Health. Edited by Stark JA, Menolascino FJ, Albarelli MH, et al. New York, Springer-Verlag, 1988, pp 124–139

Szymanski LS: Psychiatric diagnoses in developmentally delayed young children, in Scientific Proceedings of the Annual Meeting of the American Academy of Child and Adolescent Psychiatry, Vol 5. Washington, DC, American Academy of Child and Adolescent Psychiatry, 1989, pp 41–42

Szymanski LS: Happiness as a goal of treatment. Journal of the American Association on Mental Retardation 105:352–362, 2000

Szymanski LS, Biederman J: Depression and anorexia nervosa of persons with Down syndrome. Am J Ment Defic 89:246–251, 1984

Szymanski LS, Crocker AC: Mental retardation, in Comprehensive Textbook of Psychiatry, 4th Edition. Edited by Kaplan HI, Sadock BJ. Baltimore, MD, Williams & Wilkins, 1985, pp 1635–1671

Szymanski LS, Crocker AC: Mental retardation, in Comprehensive Textbook of Psychiatry, 5th Edition. Edited by Kaplan HI, Sadock BJ. Baltimore, MD, Williams & Wilkins, 1989, pp 1728–1771

Szymanski LS, Kiernan WE: Multiple family group therapy with developmentally disabled adolescents and young adults. Int J Group Psychother 33:521–534, 1983

Szymanski LS, Rosefsky QB: Group psychotherapy with retarded persons, in Emotional Disorders of Mentally Retarded Persons. Edited by Szymanski LS, Tanguay PE. Baltimore, MD, University Park Press, 1980, pp 173–194

Szymanski LS, Rubin IL, Tarjan G: Mental retardation, in American Psychiatric Press Review of Psychiatry, Vol 8. Edited by Tasman A, Hales RE, Frances AJ. Washington, DC, American Psychiatric Press, 1989, pp 217–241

Tantravahi U, Nicholls RD, Stroh H, et al: Quantitative calibration and use of DNA probes for investigating chromosome abnormalities in the Prader-Willi syndrome. Am J Med Genet 33:78–87, 1989

Truwit CL, Barkovitch AJ, Kock TK, et al: Cerebral palsy: MR findings in 40 patients. Am J Neuroradiol 13:67–78, 1992

University of Minnesota, the College of Education and Human Development: MR/DD Data Brief, Vol 2, No. 1, p 5, 2000. Available at: http://rtc.umn.edu/nhis/databrief2/index.html. Accessed July 2003

Walters AS, Barrett RP, Knapp LG, et al: Suicidal behavior in children and adolescents with mental retardation. Res Dev Disabil 16:85–96, 1995

Weiner L, Morse BA, Garrido T: FAS-FAE: focusing prevention on women at risk. Int J Addict 24:385–395, 1988

Werry JS, Carlielle J, Fitzpatrick J: Rhythmic motor activities (stereotypies) in children under five: etiology and prevalence. J Am Acad Child Psychiatry 22:329–336, 1983

West LJ: The future of psychiatric education. Am J Psychiatry 130:521–528, 1973

Whitman TL: Self-regulation and mental retardation. Am J Ment Retard 94:347–362, 1990

Wilcken B, Smith A, Brown DA: Urine screening for aminoacidopathies: is it beneficial? Results of a long-term follow-up of cases detected by screening one million babies. J Pediatr 97:492–496, 1980

Williams DT, Mehl R, Yudofsky S, et al: The effects of propranolol on uncontrolled rage outbursts in children and adolescents with organic brain dysfunction. J Am Acad Child Psychiatry 21:129–135, 1982

Wolfensberger W: The Principle of Normalization in Human Services. Toronto, Ontario, Canada, National Institute on Mental Retardation, 1972

Wolfensberger W: Of "normalization," lifestyles, the Special Olympics, deinstitutionalization, mainstreaming, integration, and cabbages and kings. Ment Retard 33:128–131, 1995

World Health Organization: International Classification of Diseases, 9th Revision. Geneva, World Health Organization, 1977

World Health Organization: International Classification of Diseases and Related Health Problems, 10th Revision. Geneva, World Health Organization, 1992

Wuu KD, Chiu PC, Li Sy, et al: Chromosomal and biochemical screening on mentally retarded school children in Taiwan. Jpn J Human Genet 36:267–274, 1991

Zigler E: Developmental vs difference theories of mental retardation and the problem of motivation. Am J Ment Defic 73:536–556, 1969

Zigler E, Balla D: Introduction: the developmental approach to mental retardation, in Mental Retardation: The Developmental-Difference Controversy. Edited by Zigler E, Balla D. Hillsdale, NJ, Lawrence Erlbaum, 1982, pp 3–26

Zigler E, Burack J: Personality development and the dually diagnosed person. Res Dev Disabil 10:225–240, 1989

Zigler E, Balla D, Hodapp R: On the definition and classification of mental retardation. Am J Ment Defic 89:215–230, 1984

Zuckerman B, Frank DA, Hingson R, et al: Effects of maternal marijuana and cocaine use on fetal growth. N Engl J Med 23:762–768, 1989

Autistic Disorder

Luke Y. Tsai, M.D.

Definition and Diagnostic Criteria

■ Historical Background

In 1943, Kanner described a group of 11 children with a previously unrecognized disorder. He noted a number of characteristic features in these children, such as an inability to develop relationships with people, extreme aloofness, a delay in speech development, and noncommunicative use of speech. Other features included repeated simple patterns of play activities and islets of ability. He described these children as having "come into the world with innate inability to form the usual, biologically provided affective contact with people" (Kanner 1943, p. 250). Despite the variety of individual differences that appeared in the case descriptions, Kanner believed that only two features were of diagnostic significance: autistic aloneness and obsessive insistence on sameness. He adopted the term *early infantile autism* to describe this disorder and called attention to the fact that its symptoms were already evident in infancy.

During the next decade, clinicians in the United States and in Europe reported patients with similar features (Asperger 1944/1991; Despert 1951; van Krevelen 1952). However, controversy continued over the definition of the disorder because the name *autism* was ill chosen. It led to confusion with Bleuler's (1911/1950) use of the same term to describe schizophrenia in adults. This confusion led many clinicians to use terms such as *childhood schizophrenia, borderline psychosis, symbiotic psychosis,* and *infantile psychosis* as interchangeable diagnoses. Each label had its definition and roots in a particular view of the nature and causation of autism.

In an attempt to clarify the confusion, Eisenberg and Kanner (1956) reduced the essential symptoms to two: extreme self-isolation and preoccupation with the pres-

ervation of sameness. The peculiar abnormality of language was considered to be secondary to the disturbance of human relatedness and, hence, not essential. They also expanded the age at onset to the first 2 years of life. Their efforts, however, were sometimes taken as a license to ignore age at onset as a necessary diagnostic criterion or to change the criteria altogether (Rutter 1978). For example, Schain and Yannet (1960) omitted preservation of sameness from their criteria; Creak et al. (1961) used nine diagnostic points to encompass all forms of childhood psychoses, including Kanner's (1943) infantile autism, within a single diagnosis (schizophrenic syndrome of childhood); and Ornitz and Ritvo (1968) emphasized disturbances in perception as a primary symptom that was not included by Kanner.

Rutter (1968) critically analyzed the existing empirical evidence and proposed four essential characteristics of infantile autism: 1) a lack of social interest and responsiveness; 2) impaired language, ranging from absence of speech to peculiar speech patterns; 3) bizarre motor behavior, ranging from rigid and limited play patterns to more complex ritualistic and compulsive behavior; and 4) early onset, before age 30 months. These features were present in nearly all children with autism. There were many other specific features, but they were unevenly distributed. In 1978, the Professional Advisory Board of the National Society for Children and Adults with Autism further formulated a definition of the syndrome of autism as a behavioral syndrome that manifested itself before age 30 months and had the following essential features: 1) disturbances of developmental rates and sequences; 2) disturbances of responses to any sensory stimuli; 3) disturbances of speech, language, cognition, and nonverbal communication; and 4) disturbances of the capacity to relate appropriately to people, events, and objects (Ritvo and Freeman 1978). This definition and the definitions of Kanner (1943) and Rutter (1968) paved the way for two sets of criteria that were widely used by clinicians all over the world: ICD-9-CM (*International Classification of Diseases and Related Health Problems*, 9th Revision, Clinical Modification) (U.S. Department of Health and Human Services 1980) and DSM-III (American Psychiatric Association 1980).

■ Diagnostic Concepts

Although ICD-9-CM and DSM-III had similar definitions and diagnostic criteria for infantile autism, differences in the concept of autism were apparent. In ICD-9-CM, infantile autism was classified as a subtype of "psychoses with origin specific to childhood," whereas in DSM-III and DSM-III-R (American Psychiatric Association 1987), infantile autism was viewed as a type of pervasive developmental disorder (PDD, defined as a group of severe, early developmental disorders characterized by delays and distortions in the development of social skills, cognition, and communication). In DSM-III, PDDs included infantile autism (i.e., the onset of the disorder was before age 30 months), childhood-onset PDD (i.e., the onset of the disorder was after age 30 months), atypical PDD (i.e., autism-like condition that could not be classified as infantile autism or childhood-onset PDD), and residual infantile autism (i.e., a condition that no longer met the full criteria for infantile autism but that was once diagnosed as such). However, empirical data published after 1980 showed no significant differences (except age at onset) between individuals with infantile autism and those with childhood-onset PDD.

In DSM-III-R, the category childhood-onset PDD was eliminated. In addition, it was found to be difficult to differentiate between atypical PDD and residual infantile autism. The DSM-III-R Pervasive Developmental Disorders Work Group therefore decided to take a combining approach and to include only two subcategories under PDDs: autistic disorder (roughly corresponding to infantile autism) and PDD not otherwise specified (PDDNOS).

In 1994, the American Psychiatric Association published DSM-IV (with its Text Revision, DSM-IV-TR, published in 2000), which continues to adopt the diagnostic term *pervasive developmental disorders*. In DSM-IV and DSM-IV-TR, these disorders included 1) autistic disorder, 2) Rett's disorder, 3) childhood disintegrative disorder, 4) Asperger's disorder, and 5) PDDNOS (including atypical autism). These texts also offer operational diagnostic criteria for all of the subtypes of PDDs except PDDNOS. It is obvious that the concept of PDDs in DSM-IV and DSM-IV-TR is a "splitters" approach. This approach supports the taxonomic validity of each subtype and aims to facilitate research in the subclassification of these disorders. Although the DSM-IV and DSM-IV-TR diagnostic criteria for PDDs are based on a field study (Volkmar et al. 1994), it is expected that these criteria will not satisfy everyone and will be revised when improved understanding and further knowledge are gained. Nonetheless, it is hoped that refinement of the criteria would not only ensure more reliable diagnosis but also provide further support for the taxonomic validity of the various subtypes of PDDs. This chapter focuses on autistic disorder. The other subtypes of PDDs are discussed in Chapter 21 ("Other Pervasive Developmental Disorders") in this volume.

■ DSM-IV Diagnostic Criteria

Although the concept of PDDs was retained in DSM-III-R, the diagnostic criteria for autistic disorder were revised considerably. The DSM-III criteria were descriptive, whereas the menu-like scheme of DSM-III-R criteria required the presence of a minimum number of criteria in each of the three cardinal areas of deficits. The revised criteria were much more concrete, observable, and operational than those in DSM-III. The revised criteria did not require raters to determine subjectively whether a "pervasive impairment" or a "gross deficit" was present; hence, clinicians no longer hesitated to use the diagnosis of autistic disorder in older and higher-functioning autistic individuals. DSM-III-R broadened the diagnostic concept of autism from that in DSM-III, allowing for the gradation of behavior seen in autistic individuals. The DSM-IV and DSM-IV-TR diagnostic criteria for autistic disorder resemble those of DSM-III-R, but the total number of diagnostic criteria has been reduced from 16 to 12, and the required minimum number for a diagnosis of autistic disorder also has been reduced from 8 to 6 (Table 20–1). These changes were made to facilitate the use of the criteria by clinicians while the diagnostic validity and reliability are maintained at a high level.

Diagnostic Rating Scales

Several commonly used diagnostic rating scales have been developed for clinicians and investigators to

Table 20–1. DSM-IV-TR diagnostic criteria for autistic disorder

A. A total of six (or more) items from (1), (2), and (3), with at least two from (1), and one each from (2) and (3):

  (1) qualitative impairment in social interaction, as manifested by at least two of the following:

    (a) marked impairment in the use of multiple nonverbal behaviors such as eye-to-eye gaze, facial expression, body postures, and gestures to regulate social interaction

    (b) failure to develop peer relationships appropriate to developmental level

    (c) a lack of spontaneous seeking to share enjoyment, interests, or achievements with other people (e.g., by a lack of showing, bringing, or pointing out objects of interest)

    (d) lack of social or emotional reciprocity

  (2) qualitative impairments in communication as manifested by at least one of the following:

    (a) delay in, or total lack of, the development of spoken language (not accompanied by an attempt to compensate through alternative modes of communication such as gesture or mime)

    (b) in individuals with adequate speech, marked impairment in the ability to initiate or sustain a conversation with others

    (c) stereotyped and repetitive use of language or idiosyncratic language

    (d) lack of varied, spontaneous make-believe play or social imitative play appropriate to developmental level

  (3) restricted repetitive and stereotyped patterns of behavior, interests, and activities, as manifested by at least one of the following:

    (a) encompassing preoccupation with one or more stereotyped and restricted patterns of interest that is abnormal either in intensity or focus

    (b) apparently inflexible adherence to specific, nonfunctional routines or rituals

    (c) stereotyped and repetitive motor mannerisms (e.g., hand or finger flapping or twisting, or complex whole-body movements)

    (d) persistent preoccupation with parts of objects

B. Delays or abnormal functioning in at least one of the following areas, with onset prior to age 3 years: (1) social interaction, (2) language as used in social communication, or (3) symbolic or imaginative play.

C. The disturbance is not better accounted for by Rett's disorder or childhood disintegrative disorder.

Source. Reprinted from the *Diagnostic and Statistical Manual of Mental Disorders*, 4th Edition, Text Revision. Washington, DC, American Psychiatric Association, 2000. Copyright 2000, American Psychiatric Association. Used with permission.

screen individuals for suspected autistic disorder and to diagnose the disorder: the Autism Behavior Checklist (ABC), Autism Diagnostic Interview-Revised (ADI-R), Autism Diagnostic Observation Schedule (ADOS), Pre-Linguistic Autism Diagnostic Observation Schedule (PL-ADOS), Autism Screening Questionnaire (ASQ), Autism Spectrum Disorder Screening Questionnaire (ASDSQ), Checklist for Autism in Toddlers (CHAT), and Childhood Autism Rating Scales (CARS). All these scales have been tested for their validity and reliability.

Clinical Features

■ Age at Onset

Several studies have demonstrated that children younger than 3 years can be reliably identified as potentially having PDDs (Baird et al. 2000; Lord 1995; Stone et al. 1999).

Kanner (1943) described autism as beginning shortly after birth. In a study of parental recognition of developmental abnormalities in a sample of 82 consecutive referrals, De Giacomo and Fombonne (1998) found that the mean age of children was 19.1 months when the parents first became concerned and that the first professional advice was sought when children were 24.1 months old.

Other investigators, however, have observed that in perhaps one-third of the autistic children, parents reported a clinical picture indistinguishable from that of Kanner's original autism, which arose after a period of seemingly normal development (up to age 2 years). Whether early development in these children had been truly normal in all aspects is difficult to determine. Subtle signs occurring during the first 2 years of life may have been forgotten, overlooked, or denied by the parents because of difficulty in recall, anxiety, or lack of knowledge of normal child development. Nonetheless, a few investigators had reported the onset of typically autistic behavior in the third to fifth year of life. In Rutter and Lockyer's (1967) series of 63 autistic children, 4 had an onset between ages 3 and 5.5 years. Lotter (1966) found a similar history among the autistic children identified in his survey: a "setback in development" occurred in 3 of 32 children between ages 3 and 4.5 years. Such a pattern is classified as PDDNOS in DSM-IV and DSM-IV-TR, whereas it is described as atypical autism in the ICD-10 classification (World Health Organization 1992).

Davidovitch et al. (2000) interviewed 39 mothers of autistic children and found that 19 (47.5%) of the autistic children regressed in verbal and nonverbal communication and social abilities but not in motor abilities. Mean age of regression was 24 months, with 11 children who regressed before that age and 8 who regressed after that age. There was little difference between those children who regressed and those who did not in maternal perceptions and reports of development, family, and medical history. Kobayashi and Murata (1998) studied setback phenomenon (regression) in 179 children for whom precise records about infancy were available. They found a significantly higher rate of epilepsy and a significantly lower level of language development on entering elementary school among the setback group compared with the non-setback group.

■ Deficits in Social Behavior

Social deficits were considered by Kanner (1943) to be central to the pathogenesis of autism. Autistic infants tend to avoid eye contact and to show little conventional interest in the human voice. They do not assume an anticipatory posture or put up their arms to be picked up in the way that children do who are not autistic. They are indifferent to affection and seldom show facial responsiveness. As a result, parents often suspect that the child is deaf. In more intelligent autistic individuals, lack of social responsiveness may not be obvious until well into the second year of life.

In early childhood, autistic children continue to show deviation in eye contact, but they may enjoy a tickle or may passively accept physical contact, such as lap sitting. They do not develop a bonding relationship with their parents. They generally do not follow their parents around the house. They tend to lack social referencing and to not look toward an adult in the presence of an ambiguous and unfamiliar stimulus. Most autistic children do not show normal separation

or stranger anxiety. Adults usually are treated as interchangeable, so that these children may approach a stranger almost as readily as they do their parents. They generally are not interested in being with or playing with other children, or they may even actively avoid other children.

In middle childhood, greater awareness of the attachment to parents and other familiar adults may develop. However, serious social difficulties continue. These children show a lack of interest in playing group games, and they are unable to form peer relationships. Some of the least handicapped may become passively involved in other children's games or physical play. However, this apparent sociability is usually superficial.

As autistic children grow older, they may become affectionate and friendly with their parents and siblings. However, they seldom initiate social contacts and they show an apparent lack of positive interest in people. Some of the less severely impaired autistic individuals may desire friends. However, a lack of response to other people's interests and emotions as well as a lack of appreciation of humor often result in the autistic youngster's saying or doing socially inappropriate things that usually prevent the development of friendships.

■ Problems in Communication

Impairment in Nonverbal Communication

Autistic infants show their needs through crying and screaming. In early childhood, they may develop the concrete gesture of pulling adults by the hand to the object that is desired or wanted. This is often done without a socially appropriate facial expression. Nodding and shaking of the head are seldom seen either as a substitute for or as an accompaniment of speech. They generally do not participate in imitative games. These children are less likely than other children to copy or follow their parents' activities.

In middle and late childhood, they use gestures infrequently, even when they understand other people's gestures fairly well. A small number of autistic children do develop imitative play skills, but these tend to be stereotyped repetitive actions based on their own experience.

Generally speaking, autistic children are able to show their emotions of joy, fear, or anger, but they tend to show only the extreme of emotions. Facial expressions that ordinarily reinforce meaning are usually absent. Some autistic people appear wooden and expressionless much of the time.

Impairment in Understanding of Speech

Comprehension of speech is impaired to various degrees. Severely retarded autistic people may never develop any awareness of the meaning of speech. Children who are less severely impaired may follow simple instructions given in an immediate present context or with the aid of gestures. When impairment is mild, only the comprehension of subtle or abstract meanings may be affected. Humor and idiomatic expressions can be confusing for even the brightest autistic person.

Impairment in Speech Development

Many autistic people have an impaired amount or pattern of babble in their first year. Nearly half of Kanner's subjects were still mute by age 5 years (Eisenberg and Kanner 1956). About one-half of autistic patients remain mute for their entire lives (Ricks and Wing 1976). When speech has developed, it usually reveals many abnormalities. Meaningless immediate or delayed echolalia may be the only kind of speech acquired in some autistic individuals. However, although the echolalic speech may be produced quite accurately, the child often has little or no comprehension of its meaning. When echolalia is extreme, distorted syntax and fragmented speech patterns result. Other autistic people may develop appropriate use of phrases copied from others. This is often accompanied by pronoun reversal in the early stages of language development.

Often the mechanical production of speech is impaired. The speech may be like that of a robot, characterized by a monotonous, flat delivery with little lability, change of emphasis, or emotional expression. Some children may use speech primarily for self-stimulatory purposes. Such speech tends to be repetitive in nature, with words, phrases, or sounds being produced over and over without any apparent relation to the environment or ongoing activity. Problems of pronunciation are common in young autistic children, but these tend to diminish with increasing age. There may be a marked contrast between clearly enunciated echolalic speech and poorly pronounced spontaneous speech. There may be chanting or singsong speech, with odd prolongation of sounds, syllables, and words. A question-like intonation may be used for propositional statements. Odd respiratory rhythms may produce staccato speech in some autistic individuals.

Immature and abnormal grammatical constructions are often present in the spontaneous speech of autistic people. Words and phrases may be used idiosyncratically, or phrases may be telegraphic and distorted. Words of similar sound or related meaning may be muddled. Autistic people may label objects by their use or else coin words of their own. Prepositions, conjunctions, and pronouns often are dropped from phrases or are used incorrectly.

When functional speech develops, it tends not to be used in the usual way for social communication. Usually autistic people rely on stereotyped phrases and repetition when they talk. Their speech almost always fails to convey imagination, abstraction, or subtle emotion. Their language skills are generally poor in talking about anything outside the immediate context. They tend to talk about their special interests, and the same information tends to recur whenever the same subject is raised. The most advanced autistic people may be able to exchange concrete pieces of information that interest them, but once the conversation departs from this level, they become lost and may withdraw from social contact. In general, the ordinary to-and-fro chatter of a reciprocal interaction is lacking. Thus, they give the impression of talking *to* someone rather than *with* someone.

■ Unusual Patterns of Behavior

Autistic children's unusual responses to their environment may take several forms. All of the items of behavior mentioned here are common in autistic children, but a single child seldom shows all the features at one time.

Resistance to Change

Autistic children are disturbed by changes in the familiar environment, and tantrums may follow even a minor change in everyday routine. Many autistic children line up toys or objects and become very distressed if these are disturbed. The behavior is twice as common in retarded autistic children as in autistic youngsters with normal intelligence (Bartak and Rutter 1976). Almost all autistic children resist learning or practicing a new activity.

Ritualistic or Compulsive Behaviors

Ritualistic or compulsive behaviors usually involve rigid routines (e.g., insistence on eating particular foods) or stereotyped, repetitive motor acts, such as hand clapping or finger mannerisms (e.g., twisting, flicking movements carried out near the face). Some children develop preoccupations, such as spending a great deal of time memorizing weather information, state capitals, or birth dates of family members. In adolescence, some of these behaviors may develop into obsessional symptoms (e.g., repeatedly asking the same question, which must be answered in a specific manner) and compulsive behaviors (e.g., compulsive touching of certain objects). Ritualistic or compulsive behaviors are more often displayed by nonretarded people with autism than by retarded people with autism (Bartak and Rutter 1976).

Abnormal Attachments

Many autistic children develop intense attachments to odd objects (e.g., pipe cleaners, small plastic toys). The child may carry the object at all times and protest or throw tantrums if it is removed; if the object is not eventually returned to the child, he or she frequently chooses a new object.

Unusual Responses to Sensory Experiences

Children with autism may have a fascination with lights, patterns, sounds, spinning objects, and tactile sensations. Objects often are manipulated without regard for their usual functions. Young autistic children may perseveringly line up, stack, or twirl objects. They may repetitively flush toilets or turn on and off light switches. They may have a continuing preoccupation with certain features of objects, such as their texture, taste, smell, color, or shape. These children are often either underresponsive or overresponsive to sensory stimuli. Thus, they may be suspected of being deaf, nearsighted, or blind. Rosenhall and colleagues (1999) noted mild to moderate hearing loss in 7.9% and unilateral hearing loss in 1.6% of 199 autistic children and adolescents who could be tested appropriately. Pronounced to profound bilateral hearing loss or deafness was diagnosed in 3.5% of the subjects. Hyperacusis was common, affecting 18%. Autistic children may actively avoid gentle physical contact but react with intense pleasure to rough games. Some autistic children may follow extreme food fads.

■ Disturbance of Motility

The typical motor milestones may be delayed, but they are often within normal range. Young autistic children usually have difficulties with motor imitation, especially when they have to learn by watching and when the movements have to be reversed in direction. Many young autistic children are markedly overactive, but they may become underactive in adolescence. The autistic child often displays grimacing, hand flapping or twisting, toe walking, lunging, jumping, darting or pacing, body rocking and swaying, and head rolling or banging. Some of these movements appear to be involuntary. In some cases, they may appear intermittently, whereas in other cases, they are continuously present. They are usually interrupted by episodes of immobility and odd posturing, with head bowed and arms flexed at the elbow. Many children with autism exhibit body-tensing movements when they are excited about or absorbed in some sensory experience, such as watching a spinning toy. Using a standardized test, the Test of Motor Impairment—Henderson Revision, Manjiviona and Prior (1995) noted that about 67% of nine autistic children showed a clinically significant level of motor impairment. Motor coordination deficits in autistic subjects had also been observed by other investigators (Ghaziuddin and Butler 1998).

■ Intelligence and Cognitive Deficits

Most autistic children are mentally retarded (Rutter 1978). About 40%–60% of autistic children have an IQ below 50; only 20%–30% have an IQ of 70 or more. Because a significant number of autistic children either do not have functional speech or are untestable, the validity of testing their intelligence is questionable. Several observations argue against the notion that autism masks the intellectual potential of these children. First, Hingtgen and Churchill (1971) showed that low IQ scores are not a function of poor motivation, because even when motivation was greatly increased through operant techniques, intellectual performance remained well below normal. Second, both short-term (Alpern and Kimberlin 1970) and long-term (Lockyer and Rutter 1969) studies have shown that autistic children who fail to score on IQ tests do so because they are severely retarded, not because they are unwilling to attempt the tasks. Third, a number of autistic children had major improvements in autism during the follow-up period but no changes in IQ (Lockyer and

Rutter 1969). Fourth, follow-up studies have shown that retardation present at the time of initial diagnosis tends to persist (Freeman et al. 1985).

A Wechsler Adult Intelligence Scale (WAIS) profile characterized by a verbal IQ lower than performance IQ (VIQ<PIQ) with the lowest subtest score on comprehension and highest on block design had been associated with autistic disorder. However, a study of 81 high-functioning subjects with autistic order by Siegel et al. (1996) found that autistic individuals could demonstrate a wide range of ability levels and patterns on the Wechsler scales, without a single characteristic prototype.

Although autistic children with low IQ and those with high IQ are similar in terms of the main symptoms associated with autism, those with a low IQ show a more severely impaired social development and are more likely to display deviant social responses, such as touching or smelling people, stereotypies, and self-injury (Bartak and Rutter 1976). One-third of mentally retarded autistic youngsters develop seizure disorders; this condition is less prevalent in those who are not retarded (Rutter 1978). The prognosis is both worse and different for autistic people with low IQ (Rutter 1970). Because the difference in outcome according to IQ is so marked, it is essential to obtain an accurate assessment of intelligence during the initial evaluation of every autistic child.

Earlier studies (Creak et al. 1961) suggested that the retardation accompanying autism is differentiated from general retardation by islets of normal or near-normal intellectual function, revealed particularly on performance tests or in special abilities of the idiot savant type. Kanner (1943) noted the excellent rote memories of autistic children. The most common areas of special skills tend to be musical, mechanical, and mathematical abilities. Rutter and Lockyer (1967) noted that in contrast to a clinic control group matched for IQ, autistic children generally had a superior performance on the subtests requiring manipulative or visuospatial skills or immediate memory, whereas they did poorly on tasks demanding symbolic or abstract thought and sequential logic. Other studies have shown that cognition in autistic children is impaired, particularly in capacity for imitation, comprehension of spoken words and gestures, flexibility, inventiveness, rule formation and application, and information use. The impairment is both more severe and more extensive than in nonautistic children of comparable IQ (for review, see Werry 1979).

Mentally retarded autistic children tend to have a wider cognitive deficit that involves general difficulties in sequencing and feature extraction, whereas in normally intelligent autistic children, the deficits mainly affect verbal and coding skills (Rutter 1977).

■ Associated Features

The affective expression of autistic people may be flattened, excessive, or inappropriate to the situation. Their mood often is labile. Sobbing, crying, or screaming may be unexplained or inconsolable. Inappropriate laughing and giggling may occur for no obvious reason. Real dangers, such as moving vehicles or heights, may not be appreciated by a young autistic child, but the same child may be terrified of harmless objects or situations, such as a stuffed animal or visiting a relative's house. Peculiar habits, such as hair pulling or biting parts of the body, are sometimes present, particularly in mentally retarded autistic children. Lack of dizziness after spinning has often been observed, and some autistic children love to spin themselves for long periods. Excessive water drinking behavior (polydipsia) has also been observed (Terai et al. 1999).

Epilepsy has been noted in 4%–42% of autistic people (Giovanardi et al. 2000). Several reports have suggested that many autistic individuals first develop seizures in adolescence (Deykin and MacMahon 1979; Rutter 1984). Volkmar and Nelson (1990) reported that the risk that autistic people will develop seizures is highest during early childhood. A prospective study of epilepsy in children with autistic spectrum disorder found that about 5% of those with an autistic condition had epilepsy. Most had onset of seizures before age 1 year (Wong 1993). In a retrospective study of 60 patients (mean age 17 years 2 months), the prevalence of electroencephalographic paroxysmal abnormalities without epilepsy was 6.7% (4 patients); seizure onset was after age 12 years in 40 patients (66.7%). The most common type of epilepsy was partial in 45% (Rossi et al. 1995) to 65.2% (Giovanardi et al. 2000) of subjects. Rossi et al. (1995) noted that electroencephalographic paroxysmal abnormalities were mostly focal and multifocal. Females with autism seemed to be more frequently affected by seizures than were males (Elia et al. 1995).

At some stage during childhood, particularly before 8 years of age, the majority of autistic children studied have been reported to have sleep problems, including one or more of the following: extreme sleep latencies (difficulty falling asleep), lengthy periods of night waking, shortened night sleep, and early waking (Elia et al. 2000b; Patzold et al. 1998; Richdale and Prior 1995; Taira et al. 1998; Takase et al. 1998). Other investigators, however, raised the question of parental oversensitivity to sleep disturbance of their autistic children (Hering et al. 1999; Schreck and Mulick 2000; Tsai 1997).

Comorbid Psychiatric Disorders

Many investigators have found that in addition to the core autistic symptomatologies (i.e., impairment in social interaction; impairment in communication; and restricted repetitive and stereotyped patterns of behavior, interests, and activities), many autistic individuals develop other behavioral and/or psychiatric symptoms that may be considered clinical manifestations of comorbid psychiatric disorders. In summary, 64% had poor attention and concentration; 36%–48% were hyperactive; 43%–88% had morbid or unusual preoccupation; 37% had obsessive phenomena; 16%–86% engaged in compulsions or rituals; 50%–89% had stereotyped utterance; 68%–74% had stereotyped mannerism; 17%–74% had anxiety or fears; 9%–44% showed depressive mood, irritability, agitation, and inappropriate affect; 11% had sleep problems; 24%–43% had a history of self-injury; and 8% presented with tics (Ando and Yoshimura 1979; Chung et al. 1990; Fombonne 1992; Le Couteur et al. 1989; Rumsey et al. 1985b; Rutter and Lockyer 1967). These investigators, however, did not specifically examine the incidence of diagnosable psychiatric disorders in their samples.

On the basis of the observations as described above, the DSM-III, DSM-III-R, and DSM-IV/DSM-IV-TR diagnostic classification systems consider some of these behavioral and/or psychiatric symptoms (e.g., abnormalities of posture and motor behavior, odd responses to sensory input or fascination with some sensations, self-injurious behavior, excessive fearfulness in response to harmless objects or events, generalized anxiety and tension, abnormalities of mood, abnormalities in sleeping) to be "associated features" of autistic disorder. On the other hand, the DSM classifications considered the symptoms of motor stereotypies (e.g., hand clapping; peculiar hand movements; and

rocking, dipping, and swaying movements of the whole body) and verbal stereotypies (e.g., repetition of words or phrases) to be diagnostic criteria for autistic disorder (under the categories of markedly restricted repertoire of activities and interests and of qualitative impairments in communication, respectively). However, these motor and verbal stereotypies are frequently noted in individuals with Tourette's disorder and have been considered as diagnostic features of Tourette's disorder.

Research on the specific relationship between these associated features and autistic symptoms is sparse or nonexistent. It is not clear whether these emergent behavioral and psychiatric symptoms are developmentally related symptoms and behaviors of autistic disorder or whether they should really be considered symptoms of comorbid psychiatric disorders.

Because of difficulties in communicating with other people, as well as in showing appropriate affect, autistic individuals do not appear to resist their compulsions, to complain about the compulsive acts, or to manifest distress. This increases the possibility that clinicians may hesitate to diagnose additional psychiatric disorders in people with autistic disorder. Nevertheless, some case reports have described other specific types of psychiatric disorders occurring in autistic individuals. These include reports of unipolar and bipolar affective disorders (Ghaziuddin and Tsai 1991; Ghaziuddin et al. 1995; Gillberg 1985; Kerbeshian and Burd 1996; Komoto et al. 1984; Lainhart and Folstein 1994; Steingard and Biederman 1987), anxiety disorder (Muris et al. 1998), anorexia nervosa (Fisman et al. 1996), obsessive-compulsive disorder (McDougle et al. 1990; Simons 1974; Tsai 1992a), schizophrenia (Clarke et al. 1989; Petty et al. 1984; Volkmar and Cohen 1991), and Tourette's disorder (Barabas and Matthews 1983; Baron-Cohen et al. 1999b; Burd et al. 1987; Comings and Comings 1991; Realmuto and Main 1982; Sverd 1991; Sverd et al. 1993). Given the relatively high frequencies of the associated features and the increasing number of case reports of autism associated with other major psychiatric disorders, a significant number of individuals with autistic disorder may also have coexisting major psychiatric disorders (Tsai 1996).

To allow effective treatment of people with autistic disorder who may also have one or more comorbid psychiatric disorders, the current diagnostic criteria of certain psychiatric disorders and assessment techniques must be modified and refined. For example, the diagnosis of obsessive-compulsive disorder may be considered in lower-functioning autistic individuals even in the absence of clear ego dystonicity, or the diagnosis of major depression may be considered in non-verbal and/or lower-functioning autistic people even in the absence of subjectively reported depressed mood, worry, guilty feeling, and suicidal ideation.

Yet some of the additional behavioral and/or psychiatric symptoms in autistic people as described above have been viewed as results of these individuals' inability to cope with environmental demands and physical discomfort. Thus, these symptoms have been viewed as "maladaptive behaviors" of autistic disorder and have been treated mainly with behavioral modification techniques. However, if these associated behavioral and/or psychiatric symptoms are considered as symptoms of various comorbid psychiatric disorders, pharmacotherapy can be a safe and efficacious treatment for these symptoms in autistic people (Tsai 2001).

Other Comorbid Medical Disorders

Some medical disorders have been observed to have an increased rate of co-occurrence with autistic disorder:

- Among patients with tuberous sclerosis (TSC), 20%–25% also meet criteria for autistic disorder (Baker et al. 1998; Gutierrez et al. 1998; Smalley 1998).
- In a sample of 25 Swedish patients with Mobius syndrome, a condition characterized by involvement of the sixth and seventh cranial nerves, six patients also met criteria for autism (Miller et al. 1998).
- About 7% of individuals with Down syndrome also had autistic disorder (Kent et al. 1999). Many parents of these children had faced considerable difficulties in obtaining the additional diagnosis of autistic disorder (Howlin et al. 1995).
- In a study of 17 congenitally blind children, four had a definite or likely autism, based on the Autism Behavior Checklist completed by the parents and teachers (Goodman and Minne 1995). Other investigators had also reported autism in congenitally blind children (Ek et al. 1998; Hobson et al. 1999). Ek et al. (1998) reported that in 15 of the 27 children with blindness, the cause was retinopathy of

prematurity and suggested that the association between the retinopathy and autism was most probably mediated by brain damage and was largely independent of the blindness per se.
- A population-based study found the prevalence of Angelman's syndrome to be 4 in 49,000 Swedish children. All 4 children in the study with Angelman's syndrome also met full criteria for the diagnosis of autistic disorder (Steffenburg et al. 1996).

Differential Diagnosis

Autism should be distinguished from the following conditions, some of which are described in detail in other chapters in this volume.

■ Asperger's Disorder

Asperger's disorder (see also Chapter 21, "Other Pervasive Developmental Disorders," in this volume) is a syndrome described by Asperger (1944/1991) as an abnormal personality trait that is not evident until the third year of life. The main features are a lack of social intuition, leading to naive and tactless behavior and difficulty with social relationships; normal intelligence but with poor coordination and visuospatial perception; and obsessive preoccupation or circumscribed interest patterns. Wing (1981) reported that the picture described by Asperger could be seen in some adults who clearly had classic autism as children but who had made progress in language and other skills. This finding suggested that Asperger's disorder be considered as a mild form of autism. DSM-IV and DSM-IV-TR, however, classify Asperger's disorder as distinct from autism. If additional features described by Asperger (1944/1991) and other clinicians (e.g., extremely argumentative with a condescending attitude, verbally abusing other children, hitting other children, and lashing out and knocking objects over, interested in violence) (Gillberg 2000) but not included in DSM-IV-TR would also be considered as diagnostic features of Asperger's disorder, autistic disorder could be much more easily differentiated from Asperger's disorder.

■ Rett's Disorder

Children with Rett's disorder (see also Chapter 21, "Other Pervasive Developmental Disorders," in this volume) develop "autistic features" during the rapid developmental regression stage (usually appears at age 1–2 years). The features include no sustained interest in people or objects; stereotypic responses to environmental stimuli; absent or very limited interpersonal contact; manifestation of great anxiety and apparent fear when confronted with an unfamiliar situation, or even without evident stimulation; loss of already acquired elements of language; stereotypic hand movements, such as hand-washing movements in front of the mouth or chest and rubbing motions of the hands; and repetitive blows on the teeth, grabbing of the tongue, and other movements (Hagberg et al. 1983). However, the clinical course is quite different from that of autism, with Rett's disorder progressing from relatively normal development up to about age 6 months to various forms of progressive neurological impairment, a progression not seen in autism. Further, a methyl-CpG-binding protein 2 mutation can be found in almost every patient with classical Rett's disorder but not in patients with autistic disorder.

■ Childhood Disintegrative Disorder

Childhood disintegrative disorder (see also Chapter 21, "Other Pervasive Developmental Disorders," in this volume) is a childhood disorder that is similar to Heller's (1930/1954) account of dementia infantilis: a progressive intellectual deterioration with, ultimately, the appearance of neurological signs. In this condition, development usually appears normal or near normal up to age 3 or 4 years, at which time profound regression and behavioral disintegration take place. Children with childhood disintegrative disorder have loss of speech and language, loss of social skills, and loss of interest in objects. These children have impaired interpersonal relationships and develop stereotypies and mannerisms. Sometimes these disorders develop after some clear-cut organic brain disease. More often, no clinical signs of neurological damage are apparent, but the subsequent course and postmortem studies often reveal some kind of organic cortical degeneration (Rutter 1977). The patterns of symptomatology differ in crucial aspects from those of autism.

■ General Mental Retardation

People with general mental retardation (see also Chapter 19, "Mental Retardation," in this volume) often have behavioral abnormalities similar to those

seen in people with autism. Wing (1975) found that about one-fourth of the severely retarded children in one area of London had a lack of affect, resistance to change, stereotypies, and bizarre responses to sensory input, but few could be called classically autistic. Furthermore, in general mental retardation, generalized delays in development occur across many areas. Some children, especially those with Down syndrome, are quite sociable and can communicate in gesture and mime. Moreover, in some studies, autistic children were found to be different from matched groups of children with mental retardation. In a study of face recognition, Klin et al. (1999) found that children with mental retardation performed significantly better than children with autistic disorder. The autistic children made less use of meaning in their memory processes, were impaired in their use of concepts, and were limited in their abilities of coding and categorizing (Hermelin and O'Connor 1970).

■ Developmental Language Disorder

Children with a developmental language disorder (see also Chapter 22, "Developmental Disorders of Learning, Motor Skills, and Communication," in this volume) may show some autistic behavior, especially before age 5 years (Wing 1969). They may develop disturbances in relating and social responses, but they do not manifest the perceptual disturbances (e.g., sensory hyperreactivity or hyporeactivity) that are characteristic of autistic children (Ornitz and Ritvo 1976). However, children with language disorder are much more likely to be able to relate to others by nonverbal gestures and expressions. When they do acquire speech, they also demonstrate communicative intent and emotion, characteristics that are not present in verbal autistic children. Furthermore, children with a language disorder have some imaginative play, which is markedly deficient in autistic children (Bartak et al. 1975). Cantwell et al. (1989) reported an interim follow-up study of a group of "higher-functioning" boys with autism and a control group of boys with severe receptive developmental language disorder. They noted that in middle childhood very few of the autistic boys had good language skills at follow-up evaluation, whereas nearly one-half of the group with language disorder was communicating well, a striking difference in view of the initial general similarity.

Courchesne et al. (1989) studied event-related brain potential in nonretarded autistic children, in children with a receptive developmental language disorder, and in nonimpaired children. Their findings suggest that higher-functioning autism may be differentiated from receptive developmental language disorder by using quantitative neurophysiological measures.

■ Obsessive-Compulsive Disorder

Bartak and Rutter (1976) noted that about 68% of the 14 nonretarded autistic children in their study had shown rituals. About 80% of these children also had "quasi-obsessive" behaviors. Difficult adaptation to new situations was found in about 74% of these children. Although Mesibov and Shea (1980) described ritualistic and compulsive behaviors as most intense during middle childhood and tending to decrease during adolescence and adulthood, Rumsey et al. (1985b) reported that stereotyped, repetitive movements were highly prevalent (78%) and were directly observable among the nine higher-functioning autistic men they studied. The movement most frequently observed involved the hands or arms with individual finger movement, rotating movements or whole-body rocking, and pacing.

Some of these obsessive and/or compulsive symptoms have obvious similarities to those seen in obsessive-compulsive disorder (see also Chapter 30, "Obsessive-Compulsive Disorder," in this volume). However, in a case-controlled study, McDougle et al. (1995) found that the autistic subjects, as compared with the obsessive-compulsive subjects, were significantly less likely to experience thoughts with aggressive, contamination, sexual, religious, symmetric, and somatic content and were less likely to engage in cleaning, checking, and counting behaviors. Repetitive behaviors in the form of ordering, hoarding, telling or asking, touching, tapping, and rubbing occurred significantly more frequently in the autistic patients compared with the patients with obsessive-compulsive disorder.

■ Tourette's Disorder

Compulsive and ritualistic behaviors (e.g., keeping objects neatly arranged and routines unchanged; compulsive touching of people and things nearby; compulsive shouting and swearing; echoing of words, sounds, and actions) that can occur in the Gilles de la Tourette syndrome (or the syndrome of chronic multiple tics)

resemble some phenomena that occur in autism (see also Chapter 37, "Tic Disorders," in this volume). Sometimes separating symptoms of Tourette's disorder from the symptoms of autism can be difficult. However, the examination of the total behavior pattern and developmental history should make the diagnosis clear. Individuals with Tourette's disorder are aware of their disorder. They are frightened and distressed because they do not feel that they can control it. They usually do not have significantly delayed and deviant language and speech development, and their tics often have a waxing and waning pattern.

■ Schizophrenia

One well-established finding is that autistic children almost never develop a thought disorder with delusions and hallucinations (see also Chapter 23, "Schizophrenia and Other Psychotic Disorders," in this volume). Children with childhood-onset schizophrenia can be differentiated from children with autistic disorder on the basis of age at onset, developmental history, family history, and clinical features. For almost all autistic children and adolescents, the age of disorder onset is before 5 years, whereas the onset of schizophrenia in childhood is most often during preadolescence or adolescence. Eggers (1978) reported that the early development in slightly half of the schizophrenic children was unremarkable. There is no evidence that children with a DSM-IV-TR diagnosis of childhood-onset schizophrenia have severe developmental deficits, whereas all autistic children and adolescents, including those with higher functioning, have a clear history of PDD. A study by Asarnow et al. (1987) of patterns involving intellectual functioning (Wechsler Intelligence Scale for Children, revised factor scores [Wechsler 1974]) found that schizophrenic and autistic children did not differ significantly on the verbal and perceptual organization factors but that the schizophrenic children had significantly lower scores on the freedom-from-distraction factor (including attention, short-term memory, visuomotor coordination, speed of responding, and mental arithmetic) than the nonretarded (higher-functioning) autistic children. The comprehension subtest was the only one on which the autistic children scored significantly lower than did the schizophrenic children. The incidence of schizophrenia is increased in the families of children with schizophrenia but not in those with autism (Kolvin et al. 1971).

■ Selective Mutism

In selective mutism (see also Chapter 31, "Specific Phobia, Panic Disorder, Social Phobia, and Selective Mutism," in this volume), the child refuses to speak in almost all social situations, despite the ability to comprehend spoken language and to speak. The child may communicate by gestures, nodding or shaking the head, or, in some cases, by monosyllabic or short, monotone utterances. The same child may talk normally at home with family members. Autistic children retain their characteristic language abnormalities in all situations. In any case, the whole pattern of behavior is markedly different in the two conditions.

■ Congenital Peripheral Blindness or Partial Sightedness

Children with congenital peripheral blindness or partial sightedness may show self-stimulation and stereotyped movements like those seen in autism. Blind children, however, usually develop an interest in their environment and do not have disturbances in relating to other people. As described earlier, in the section "Other Comorbid Medical Disorders," although some individuals with blindness had been diagnosed as having comorbid autistic disorder, the majority of the blind population under study did not have such a comorbid condition.

■ Landau-Kleffner Syndrome

Landau-Kleffner syndrome (LKS) is a neurological syndrome in which children's development is normal until, usually, age 3–5 years, and then, without evident cause, the children have an abrupt or gradual loss of language ability. The regression of language development involves a profound impairment in both language comprehension and expression and may first manifest as deafness or inattentiveness to sound, sometimes called auditory agnosia. In many children with LKS, the regression of language development is closely preceded, accompanied, or followed by the onset of seizure disorders and/or electroencephalographic abnormalities (Hirsch et al. 1990; Landau and Kleffner 1957; Stefanatos et al. 1995). The syndrome is also called *acquired aphasia with convulsive disorder in children, acquired epileptiform aphasia of childhood,* and *acquired epileptica aphasia.*

In about 25% of autistic individuals, difficulties are not apparent until after the second birthday (Short and Schopler 1988). Some of these children may have actual regression in language development and have electroencephalographic abnormalities or a seizure disorder. Although some investigators argue that for such patients the disorder diagnosis should be LKS instead of autistic disorder or PDDNOS (Stefanatos et al. 1995), other researchers disagree with this point of view (Volkmar et al. 1996).

No systematic investigation has specifically examined the diagnostic differences between LKS and autistic disorder or PDDNOS. However, available published data indicate that nonverbal skills and social interaction skills tend to be preserved in LKS. The behavioral problems with restricted repetitive and stereotyped patterns of behavior, interests, and activities are not as prominent in LKS as in autistic disorder. Neurophysiological studies using single-photon emission computed tomography (SPECT) show that LKS is associated with disseminated physiological disturbances most often affecting perisylvian language areas in the left hemisphere, whereas brain metabolic studies of autistic children have failed to reveal a diagnostically significant pattern of disturbance (Stefanatos et al. 1995). In many subjects with LKS, characteristic multifocal spikes and spike-and-wave discharges with marked activation of these discharges occur during sleep (Hirsch et al. 1990; Stefanatos et al. 1995), an electroencephalographic pattern rarely presented in autistic disorder.

The age at onset of LKS is usually much later than that of autistic disorder. Children with autistic disorder usually have delayed language development, whereas children with LKS have normal language development before the onset of LKS. The available data indicate that subjects with LKS most likely would not qualify for a diagnosis of autistic disorder. However, some subjects with LKS may qualify for a diagnosis of PDDNOS as defined by DSM-IV-TR.

■ Tuberous Sclerosis

TSC is an autosomal-dominant disorder with a variable penetrance characterized by benign tumors (hamartomas) and malformations (hamartias) of one or more organs, most notably, the brain, retina, heart, and kidneys (Gomez 1991). The predominant neurological manifestations are mental retardation, seizures, and psychiatric and behavioral problems, including autism, attention-deficit/hyperactivity disorder, aggressiveness, and anxiety disorders (Smalley et al. 1992).

As described earlier, estimated frequencies of autism among patients with TSC range from 20% to 25% (Baker et al. 1998; Gutierrez et al. 1998; Smalley 1998), whereas the frequency of TSC among patients with autism is about 0.4%–3.0% (in autistic subjects with seizures, it is 8%–14%) (Gillberg et al. 1994; Smalley et al. 1992). It is apparent that there is a significant association between autism and TSC.

The diagnosis of TSC is not difficult in patients who have the classic manifestations of seizures, mental retardation, facial angiofibromas, multiple ungual fibromas, and calcified subependymal nodules. In individuals who have subtle findings or mild forms of TSC, the diagnostic criteria established by the National Tuberous Sclerosis Association are helpful (Roach et al. 1992). Thus, the diagnostic question is not actually who has TSC, but who among the patients with TSC also has autistic disorder or PDDNOS/atypical autism.

■ Fragile X Syndrome

Fragile X syndrome has been recognized as a cause of nonspecific mental retardation. This syndrome is inherited in an X-linked recessive manner. Some studies reported that individuals with fragile X syndrome were described as autistic or having autistic features that were most apparent in childhood. Hagerman (1992) reported that 15% of individuals with fragile X syndrome also had autistic disorder. Bailey et al. (1998) reported that 14 of 57 boys (approximately 25%) with fragile X syndrome scored above the cutoff for autism on the Childhood Autism Rating Scale.

However, the prevalence of the fragile X anomaly among autistic people has been reported to be between 0% and 20% (Piven et al. 1991b), with a general consensus that the actual prevalence is 2%–5% (Hallmayer et al. 1994). A question had been raised regarding the differential diagnosis between fragile X syndrome and autistic disorder. A carefully designed study of 58 mentally retarded men with fragile X syndrome matched for age, cognitive level, living conditions, and length of institutionalization with 58 mentally retarded men without fragile X syndrome (Maes et al. 1993) reported that the core features of autism, namely social indifference and severely disturbed social relations, generally were not found in the fragile X group. The adults with fragile X syndrome had average interpersonal and communicative skills. They were more sensitive to social contact and attention from others

and approached not only new physical environments but also other people with great openness and interest (Maes et al. 1993). It appears that individuals with a nonautistic fragile X syndrome have clinical features that are clearly distinguishable from those of autistic disorder. In subjects with fragile X syndrome and autistic features, the possibility of fragile X syndrome with a comorbid condition of autistic disorder or PDDNOS should be considered.

■ Psychosocial Deprivation

Although psychosocial deprivation is commonly mentioned as a possible cause of autism, no data from systematic studies have yet been presented to support such a view. However, some studies reported children who had been in a deprived environment over several years, resulting in severe retardation in all aspects of development, who then made rapid strides in development when they were rescued from that environment and placed in a caring and stimulating environment. They showed no evidence of autism (Wing 1976). Thus, a careful history and observation of a rapid response to environmental stimulation should differentiate this condition from autism.

Epidemiology

■ Prevalence

DSM-IV-TR suggests the prevalence of autistic disorder to be 2–5 per 10,000 children in the United States (American Psychiatric Association 2000). Epidemiological studies in North America, Europe, Japan, and Israel have estimated the prevalence of autism to be between 0.15 and 34 per 10,000 children (Chakrabarti and Fombonne 2001; Davidovitch et al. 2001; Fombonne and du Mazaubrun 1992; Fombonne et al. 1997b; Hillman et al. 2000; Honda et al. 1996; Kielinen et al. 2000; Lotter 1966; Matsuishi et al. 1999; Powell et al. 2000; Ritvo et al. 1989a; Sponheim and Skjeldal 1998; Steffenburg and Gillberg 1986; Sugiyama and Abe 1989; Treffert 1970; Wing and Gould 1979). The trend is for more recent studies to report a higher frequency. Honda et al. (1996) reported that on the basis of ICD-10 criteria, the cumulative incidence and prevalence were 16.2 per 10,000 children and 21.1 per 10,000 children, respectively, in the northern part of Yokohama, Japan. Matsuishi et al.

(1999) reported an incidence of 34 per 10,000 children, based on DSM-III-R criteria, in another Japanese sample. Chakrabarti and Fombonne (2001) reported a prevalence of 16.8 per 10,000 children between ages 2.5 and 6.5 years who lived in Staffordshire, England. In a sample in northern Finland, Kielinen and colleagues (2000) reported the cumulative incidence to be 6.1 per 10,000 in children between ages 15 and 18 years and 20.7 per 10,000 in children between ages 5 and 7 years.

Gillberg and Wing (1999) reviewed all English-language articles on the prevalence of autism published between 1966 and 1997. The earlier studies reported prevalence of fewer than 5 per 10,000 children, whereas the later ones showed a mean rate of about 10 per 10,000 children. Those studies that included some children born before 1970 tended to have low rates and those that included only children born in 1970 and after tended to have high rates. It is speculated that the earlier low rates were obtained by applying stricter diagnostic criteria.

In an extensive review of the prevalence of autism, Fombonne (1999) noted a median prevalence of 5.2 per 10,000 children worldwide. The prevalence significantly increased with publication year. The median rate was 7.2 per 10,000 children for 11 surveys carried out worldwide since 1989, suggesting changes in case definition and improved recognition as the reasons for higher rates.

It is not clear whether prevalence rates of autism in cities differ from those in rural districts. Treffert (1970) reported that no statistically significant difference was found between the rural and urban prevalence rates. However, some studies have found higher rates in urban areas (Hoshino et al. 1982; Steffenburg and Gillberg 1986).

The prevalence of autistic disorder in children with mental retardation is reported to be 8.9%–11.7% (Nordin and Gillberg 1996).

■ Sex Ratio

All studies of autism have shown a predominance of boys over girls. Ratios of 3 or 4 boys to 1 girl have consistently been reported (Tsai 1986). In addition, several studies have found that autistic girls tend to have a greater degree of morbidity—that is, more often, a greater proportion of autistic females than autistic males are severely impaired (Tsai 1986). Females with autism seemed to be more frequently affected by sei-

zures than were males (Elia et al. 1995). Boutin et al. (1997) noted that females with autism and patients with low IQ and autism had more first-degree relatives with cognitive disability. Volkmar et al. (1993) reported that the sex differences were primarily confined to IQ, and the other matrices of severity of autism were not prominent. However, in a study of 21 males and 21 females with autism who were higher functioning, McLennan et al. (1993) found that the autistic males were rated to be more severely autistic than the females on several measures of early social development but not in any other areas.

These findings indicate that there may be significant sex differences in the occurrence and the severity of autism, and they warrant further study.

■ Socioeconomic Class

Kanner (1943) originally observed that families of his patients were predominantly of an upper socioeconomic status. However, later population studies (Schopler et al. 1979; Tsai et al. 1982; Wing 1980) did not support Kanner's idea. As pointed out by Tsai et al. (1982), most of the studies showing high socioeconomic class bias were conducted before 1970, and those showing no bias were carried out after that date. When the possible effects of parental educational and occupational achievements and patterns of referral were controlled, autistic people were found in all socioeconomic classes.

Etiology

■ Known Medical Conditions

There is general agreement that autistic disorder has an organic basis, but there is less agreement on the frequency with which it is associated with known medical conditions. After a review of the literature, Rutter et al. (1994) concluded that the rate of known medical conditions in autism is probably about 10%, and that the rate is higher in autistic disorder associated with profound mental retardation and in atypical autism. In a French epidemiological survey, Fombonne and colleagues (1997b) concluded that known medical disorders (excluding epilepsy and sensory impairments) were associated with less than 10% of the cases of autism. Gillberg and Coleman (1996) reported a higher rate of 24.4% having known comorbid medical conditions but found a similar trend for higher rates of medical disorders among autistic individuals with severe mental retardation. Barton and Volkmar (1998) retrospectively reviewed medical records of 211 subjects with autism and found that the prevalence of medical conditions suspected to have an association with autism varied between 10% and 15% and, with a less strict definition of *medical condition*, between 25% and 37%. Nonetheless, these medical conditions or disorders were not considered to be causes of autistic disorder.

■ Congenital Factors

Results of numerous studies show that many autistic children have organic brain disorders. A wide variety of neurological disorders have been reported: cerebral palsy, congenital rubella, toxoplasmosis, TSC, cytomegalovirus infection, lead encephalopathy, meningitis, encephalitis, severe brain hemorrhage, many types of epilepsy, and others. Many of these neurological or congenital disorders derive from prenatal, perinatal, and neonatal complications. Several investigators have reported that such complications (reduced optimality) appear with increased frequency in the histories of autistic patients. These factors include increased maternal age, firstborn children and those born fourth or later, bleeding after the first trimester, maternal use of medication, and meconium in amniotic fluid (Tsai 1987). Juul-Dam et al. (2001) also reported an association of unfavorable events in pregnancy, delivery, and the neonatal phase and autism. Burd and colleagues (1999) identified five variables (decreased birth weight, low maternal education, later start of prenatal care, having a previous termination of pregnancy, and increasing father's age) associated with increased risk of autism.

On the other hand, Lord et al. (1991) proposed that pre- and perinatal factors play less of a role in autism in higher-functioning individuals. Piven et al. (1993) found that the reported association between optimality and autism in autistic probands and their siblings might be the result of failure to control for birth order. Bolton et al. (1997) noted that the optimality score was significantly elevated in both autistic probands and those with Down syndrome and concluded that obstetric adversities associated with autism either represented an epiphenomenona of the condition or derived from some shared risk factor(s). Other investigators reported no significant obstetric adversity

in mothers of autistic subjects (Cryan et al. 1996; Deb et al. 1997).

Because of the lack of uniformity in applying diagnostic criteria to autism as well as to the selection of obstetric complications, the findings on the association between optimality and autism should be accepted cautiously. Also, the data reviewed here do not indicate a unifying pathological process in autism.

■ Genetic Factors

Research since the 1980s has convincingly indicated that autism is a genetic disorder. This conclusion is based mainly on data from family studies, twin studies, and chromosome studies. Autism has been reported to be associated with various chromosomal abnormalities: a duplication of the short arm of chromosome X (Rao et al. 1994); deletion of the short arm of chromosome X (Thomas et al. 1999); supernumerary XYY (Nicolson et al. 1998) and XXY (Konstantareas and Homatidis 1999); partial duplication of the short arm of chromosome Y (Blackman et al. 1991); translocation with both chromosomes X and 8 (Ishikawa-Brush et al. 1997); deletion of the distal portion of the long arm of chromosome 2 (2q37) (Ghaziuddin and Burmeister 1999); chromosome 4 duplication (4)p12-p13 (Sabaratnam et al. 2000); balanced translocation between chromosomes 4 and 12 (Nasr and Roy 2000); translocation of chromosome 7 (Vincent et al. 2000); ring chromosome 7 (Schroer et al. 1998); partial duplication of the short arm of chromosome 11 (Herault et al. 1994); pericentric inversion of chromosome 12 (Schroer et al. 1998); trisomy 13 (Konstantareas and Homatidis 1999); balanced 13;16 translocation (Schroer et al. 1998); partial trisomy of chromosome 15 (Gillberg et al. 1991); partial tetrasomy of chromosome 15 (Hotopf and Bolton 1995), chromosome 15q11–13 (Baker et al. 1994), and chromosome 18q (Seshadri et al. 1992); inversion-duplication of chromosome 15 (Borgatti et al. 2001; Flejter et al. 1996; Konstantareas and Homatidis 1999; Schroer et al. 1998); mosaic trisomy of chromosome 17 (Shaffer et al. 1996); mosaicism for a duplication of the long arm and a deletion of the short arm of chromosome 18 (Ghaziuddin et al. 1993); interstitial deletion of chromosome 20 (20p11.22-p11.23) (Michaelis et al. 1997; Schroer et al. 1998); chromosomes 20 and 22 translocation (Carratala et al. 1998); Ring chromosome 22 (Assumpcao 1998; MacLean et al. 2000) and 22q13.3 deletion (Goizet et al. 2000); and complex chromosome rearrangement of chromosomes 1, 7, and 21 (Lopreiato and Wulfsberg 1992). The significance of these associations is not clear because these findings are all from case reports. Nonetheless, these case reports may support the idea that autism is genetically heterogeneous, with variability of clinical features.

Some genetic syndromes are associated with autism, including phenylketonuria (Knoblock and Pasamanick 1975), fragile X syndrome, and TSC. Some investigators have found a high prevalence of fragile X syndrome in people with autism (Bloomquist et al. 1985), but others have been unable to replicate this finding (Payton et al. 1989). As described earlier, about 20%–25% of patients with TSC also meet criteria for autistic disorder (Baker et al. 1998; Smalley 1998). The mechanism underlying the association of autism and TSC is unclear. It is speculated that the presence of autism may arise if TSC gene mutations occur at critical stages of neural development in the brain (Smalley 1998).

As mentioned earlier, one study found 4 of 49,000 Swedish children to have Angelman's syndrome. All 4 children also met full criteria for the diagnosis of autistic disorder (Steffenburg et al. 1996). Maternal truncation mutation in the *UBE3A/E6-AP* gene in chromosome 15q11–13 has been known to cause Angelman's syndrome. This finding suggests that the possible gene for autism may be identified in the 15q11–13 region (Herzing et al. 2001).

Several studies have shown that between 2% and 7% of the siblings of children with autism have the same condition (Bolton et al. 1994; Chudley et al. 1998; Ritvo et al. 1989b; Smalley 1991; Tsai et al. 1981). When this estimated incidence is compared with the risk for autism in general population, the rate of autism in siblings is 50 times higher.

Ritvo et al. (1985) reported a study involving 281 families enrolled in the University of California, Los Angeles Registry for Genetic Studies in Autism. They included (by parental report) 22 sets of monozygotic twins concordant for autism; 18 sets of dizygotic twins, of whom 2 sets were concordant for autism; and 46 sets of nontwin siblings concordant for autism. On the basis of these preliminary findings, it was suggested that a subgroup of autistic people might develop this syndrome by way of a recessive gene transmission. The data on which the suggestion was based, however, were from a highly selected group of subjects. Twenty-one pairs (11 monozygotic and 10 dizygotic) of twins and 1 set of identical triplets were identified in the Nordic countries (Denmark, Finland, Iceland, Norway, and Sweden) (Steffenburg et al. 1989). The concordance for autism by pair was 91% in the monozygotic and 0% in the dizygotic pairs. In most of the pairs discordant for autism, the autistic twin had been under more perinatal stress. It was concluded that the results supported the hypothesis that autism had a hereditary component and that perinatal complication was a contributory factor in some cases.

Folstein and Rutter (1977) studied 21 same-sex autistic twin pairs and found that 4 of 11 monozygotic twin pairs (36%) were concordant for autism, as compared with 0 of 10 (0%) dizygotic twins. Discordance was usually associated with definite or suggestive evidence of organic brain dysfunction in the affected twin. This first British twin sample was reexamined along with a second total-population British sample of autistic twins and triplets. In the combined sample of 44 sets of twins and triplets, 60% of monozygotic pairs were concordant for autism, compared with no dizygotic pairs. When a broader spectrum of related cognitive or social abnormalities was applied to the sample, 92% of the monozygotic pairs were concordant for the spectrum, compared with 10% of the dizygotic pairs. The findings indicate that autism is under a high degree of genetic control and suggest that multiple genetic loci are involved (Bailey et al. 1995). The findings also suggest that autism might develop because of a combination of genetic predisposition and biological impairment.

On the basis of the findings from their twin study, Folstein and Rutter (1977) suggested that autism is one manifestation of an underlying genetic liability to cognitive dysfunction; that is, a cognitive disorder may present in its mildest form as learning disabilities and in its most severe form as autism. To date, family studies of autism seem to provide some support for such a hypothesis. The sibling data show that between 6% and 24% of the siblings of autistic probands have cognitive disorders (including autism, mental retardation, and learning disability) and/or speech-language disorders (August et al. 1981; Bolton et al. 1994; Freeman et al. 1986; Piven et al. 1990).

Szatmari et al. (1995) reported that rates of cognitive impairments and psychiatric symptoms were not found more frequently in parents or relatives of probands with PDD compared with relatives of control subjects. Other investigators have reported that parents of autistic children had increased rates of anxiety disorder (Piven et al. 1991a), major depressive disorder (Bolton et al. 1998; DeLong and Nohria 1994; Piven and Palmer 1999; Smalley et al. 1995), social phobia (Piven and Palmer 1999; Smalley et al. 1995), motor tics and obsessive-compulsive disorder (Bolton et al. 1998), and higher rates of particular characteristics (rigidity, aloofness, hypersensitivity to criticism, and anxiousness), speech and pragmatic language deficits, and limited friendships (Piven et al. 1997b). Murphy et al. (2000) noted significantly increased expression of anxiety, impulsiveness, aloofness, shyness, oversensitivity, irritability, and eccentricity among relatives of subjects with autism. Gillberg et al. (1992) reported that mothers of autistic subjects tended to have schizoaffective disorder and that Asperger's disorder was more common among first-degree relatives of children with autism compared with control subjects. Plumet et al. (1995) reported that the brothers of a group of autistic females had a lower verbal performance. Folstein et al. (1999) found that parents of autistic children scored slightly but significantly lower on the WAIS-R Full Scale and Performance IQ and on the Word Attack Test from the Woodcock-Johnson battery compared with parents of control subjects. There was no difference, however, between siblings of those in the group with autism and siblings of control subjects with Down syndrome. However, Fombonne et al. (1997a), reported that the parents and siblings of autistic probands had slightly superior verbal performance to the parents and siblings of control subjects with Down syndrome. These findings suggest some association between autism and other major psychiatric disorders and verbal performance, but more study is needed to define the genetic implications.

With the recent advancement of molecular genetic techniques, a number of whole-genome screenings for linkage have been carried out in several samples of autistic subjects. Strong evidence for linkage to autism has been identified for chromosomes 1p, 2q, 3, 4p, 4q, 5p, 6q, 7q, 8, 10q, 11, 12, 15q11-q13, 16p, 17q, 18q, 19p, 19q, 22q, and Xp (Auranen et al. 2000; International Molecular Genetic Study of Autism Consortium 2001a; Liu et al. 2001; Philippe et al. 1999). Several studies seemed to exclude the gene effect causing autism on the X chromosome (Hallmayer et al. 1996), particularly at Xq27.3 region (Klauck et al. 1997a). Rogers et al. (1999) reported that it was unlikely that loci in the HLA (human leukocyte antigen) region on chromosome 6p would contribute genetically to the cause of autistic disorder to any significant extent.

However, two chromosomes have received the most attention: 7q and 15q. Several studies focused on chromosome 7q in autistic subjects have been carried out; these identified chromosome band 7q31–33 as the likely susceptibility locus (Ashley-Koch et al. 1999; Barrett et al. 1999; International Molecular Genetic Study of Autism Consortium 2001b; Warburton et al. 2000; Wassink et al. 2001). Several other studies have found evidence in support of linkage to the 15q11–13 region (Bass et al. 2000; Cook et al. 1998; Craddock and Lendon 1999; Maddox et al. 1999; Martin et al. 2000; Repetto et al. 1998; Rineer et al. 1998; Wolpert et al. 2000) and 15q22–23 region (M. Smith et al. 2000). Furthermore, the duplication of 15q11–13 was found to be maternally inherited (Cook et al. 1997b; Martinsson et al. 1996; Schroer et al. 1998). Salmon et al. (1999), however, believed that the role of 15q11–13 is minor, at best, in the majority of individuals with autism. Lauritsen et al. (1999) proposed some candidate regions on chromosomes 7q21 and 10q21.2.

Several genes have been proposed as candidates for association with autism. Cook et al. (1997a) provided evidence of linkage and association between the serotonin transporter gene (*HTT*) in the 15q11–13 region and autism. Yirmiya et al. (2001) also showed evidence for an association between the polymorphism of the serotonin transporter region and autism. Other investigators, however, were not able to replicate this finding (Klauck et al. 1997b; Maestrini et al. 1999; Persico et al. 2000b; Zhong et al. 1999). Tordjman et al. (2001) noted that transmission of *HTT* promoter alleles did not differ between probands with autism and their unaffected siblings. However, allelic transmission in probands depended on severity of impairment in the social and communication domains. It was concluded that *HTT* promoter alleles by themselves do not convey risk for autism but rather modify the severity of autism in the social and communication domains. Other candidate genes or genetic markers that have been proposed include *ATP10C* in the 15q11–13 region (Herzing et al. 2001), c-Harvey-*ras* (H-*ras*) markers (Herault et al. 1995), adenosine deaminase 2 (*ADA2*) alleles (Persico et al. 2000a), an allele of the *ADA* Asp8Asn polymorphism (Bottini et al. 2001), *HOXA1* (Ingram et al. 2000), longer triplet repeats in the 5′ untranslated regions (5′UTRs) of the reelin (*RELN*) gene (Persico et al. 2001), GXAlu marker of the neurofibromatosis type 1 (*NF1*) gene (Mbarek et al. 1999; not supported by Plank et al. 2001), and the third hypervariable region (HVR-3) of

HLADRB1 alleles (Warren et al. 1996). Careful replication studies are necessary before it can be determined that all the proposed markers and candidate genes have a role in the development of autism.

The data available to date show reasonable evidence that genetic factors play a major contributory role in a subgroup of autistic individuals. However, several genomewide screens for susceptibility genes have been performed with limited concordance of linked loci. These data seem to indicate that there are numerous genes of weak effect involved in the development of autistic disorder and/or that autistic disorder is genetically heterogeneous. Nonetheless, presently the most interesting chromosome regions being studied for possible links to autistic disorder are chromosomes 7q31–35, 15q11–13, and 16p13.3 (Lauritsen and Ewald 2001).

■ Immunological Factors

Several studies have suggested the possibility of an immune defect in autistic disorder. Chess (1977) reported an increased frequency of autism in individuals with congenital rubella. Deykin and MacMahon (1979) found that autism was associated with prenatal rubella or influenza infection in about 5% of patients.

Young et al. (1977) studied the cerebrospinal fluid (CSF) immunoglobulin levels in 15 autistic children and found no abnormalities of glucose, protein cells, or folate. They concluded that the hypothesis that a slow virus plays a role in autism is not supportable.

Stubbs (1976) gave rubella vaccine challenge to 15 autistic children and 8 age-matched control subjects. The vaccine challenge did not differentiate autistic children from the control subjects. However, 5 of the 13 autistic children who had previously been given the vaccine had undetectable hemagglutination-inhibition antibody titers, whereas all 6 control subjects who had previously been given the vaccine had detectable titers. Stubbs (1976) speculated that these autistic children had an altered immune response or an immune defect.

Warren et al. (1986) reported several immune system abnormalities in 31 autistic patients. In a further study of the activity of the natural killer cell (a large granular lymphocyte and a likely part of basic defense mechanism against virus-infected cells and malignancy), 12 (39%) of the autistic subjects were found to have significantly reduced natural killer cell activity (Warren et al. 1987). Warren et al. (1994) also investigated the complement C4B protein concentration in the plasma of 42 autistic subjects. The plasma concentration of C4B protein was significantly decreased in these subjects. In an additional study of autoimmune processes in autism, Warren et al. (1995) found that 14 of 26 autistic subjects (54%) had DR+ T cells, an indicator of activated T cells, the presence of which was inversely correlated to a decreased plasma level of the C4B protein. These findings were interpreted as suggesting that decreased protein concentration of C4B may be associated with autism.

Gupta et al. (1998) examined Th1-like and Th2-like cytokines in CD4+ and CD8+ T cells in children with autism and found an imbalance of cytokines. They speculated that such an imbalance is a cause of autism.

Denney et al. (1996) reported that children with autism had a lower percentage of helper-inducer cells and a lower helper:suppressor ratio, with both measures inversely related to the severity of autistic symptoms.

Scifo et al. (1996) found that naltrexone improved autistic children's behaviors and caused alterations in the distribution of the major lymphocyte subsets, with a significant increase of the T-helper-inducers (CD4+CD8–) and a significant reduction of the T-cytotoxic-suppressor (CD4+CD8+), resulting in a normalization of the CD4:CD8 ratio. The findings were interpreted as meaning that the mechanisms underlying opioid–immune interactions are altered and may play a role in the development of autism.

On the basis of the observation that reactivity to human myelin had been implicated in a number of central nervous system disorders such as multiple sclerosis, Guillain-Barré syndrome, and acute disseminated encephalomyelitis, Weizman et al. (1982) investigated the cell-mediated immune response to human myelin basic protein (a component of myelin) by using the macrophage migration inhibition factor test in 17 autistic patients and 11 control subjects with other mental disorders. Of the 17 autistic subjects, 13 (76%) had inhibition of macrophage migration, whereas none of the control subjects was found to have such a response. The results were thus interpreted to suggest that a cell-mediated autoimmune response to brain antigen exists in some autistic individuals. This hypothesis was supported by a report that described 19 of 33 autistic subjects (58%) as testing positive for antibodies to myelin basic protein—a rate more than six times higher than in nondisabled and retarded control subjects (Singh et al. 1993). In a further study, Singh et al. (1997) found a significant increase in incidence of autoantibodies to neuron-axon filament protein and autoantibodies to glial fibrillary acidic protein in autistic subjects. It was speculated that these autoantibodies might be related to autoimmune pathology of autism. Singh et al. (1998) further reported an association between virus serology and brain autoantibody in autistic subjects and proposed a hypothesis that virus-induced autoimmune response might play a causal role in autism. Connolly et al. (1999) found immunoglobulin G (IgG) antibrain autoantibodies in 27% of sera and immunoglobulin M (IgM) autoantibodies in 36% of sera from children with autistic spectrum disorder. The findings were speculated to mean that autoimmunity might play a role in the pathogenesis of language and social development abnormalities in a subset of children with autism.

Monoclonal antibody D8/17–positive cells were found in 14 of 18 patients (78%) with autism. As severity of repetitive behaviors significantly correlated with D8/17 expression, Hollander et al. (1999) suggested that D8/17 expression could serve as a marker for compulsion severity within autism.

Westall and Root-Bernstein (1983), however, called for attention to be paid to the serotonin-binding sites. This suggestion seemed to be supported by Todd and Ciaranello (1985), who reported that about one-third of the autistic children in their study had an unusual antibody circulating in their blood and spinal fluid. This antibody appeared to attack the receptor for serotonin (5-hydroxytryptamine [5-HT]). In a further study, Todd et al. (1988, p. 647) concluded that "if an antibody-mediated autoantigen recognition is important in, or related to, established infantile autism, only a few antigens are involved."

All these findings seem to suggest that depressed immune function, autoimmune mechanism, or faulty immune regulation (deficiency in some components of immune system and excesses in others) may be associated with the etiology of autism. However, the interpretation of the reported data is hampered by conceptual and methodological differences between studies. Both the clinical significance of the immune changes and the causal connection between immune changes and autistic symptoms remain to be elucidated by more extensive studies.

■ Neurological Factors

Neurological abnormalities have been reported in 30%–50% of several series of autistic patients (DeMyer et al. 1973; Tsai et al. 1981), including hypotonia or hypertonia, disturbance of body schema, clumsiness, choreiform movements, pathological reflexes, myoclonic jerking, drooling, abnormal posture and gait, dystonic posturing of hands and fingers, tremor, ankle clonus, emotional facial paralysis, and strabismus. These are all signs of dysfunction in the basal ganglia, particularly the neostriatum, and closely related structures of the medial aspects of the frontal lobe or limbic system.

Several investigators have reported that some individuals with autism (between 12% and 46%) had macrocephaly (head circumference in the 97th percentile or higher) (Davidovitch et al. 1996; Fidler et al. 2000; Lainhart et al. 1997; Piven et al. 1995; Woodhouse et al. 1996). Fidler et al. (2000) also noted that the first-degree relatives of these patients also had a higher rate of macrocephaly when compared against a published normative sample. However, Courchesne et al. (1999) reported that the brain weight was normal in most postmortem studies of autistic subjects. Rare cases of microcephaly have also been observed. Other investigators questioned the specificity of macrocephaly to autism (Ghaziuddin et al. 1999).

On the basis of the analogy to signs and conditions seen in adults with certain forms of brain damage, Damasio and Maurer (1978) proposed that autism results from dysfunction in a system of bilateral central nervous system structures that include the ring of mesolimbic cortex located in the medial frontal and temporal lobes, the neostriatum, and the anterior and medial nuclear groups of the thalamus. They suggested that such dysfunction might involve macroscopic or microscopic cerebral changes consequent to a variety of causes, such as perinatal viral infection, insult to the periventricular watershed area, or genetically determined neurochemical abnormalities. Although this hypothesis is plausible, it must be verified.

■ Neuroanatomical Factors

Neuropathology Studies

Very few neuropathology studies have been done in autistic people. Postmortem brain studies of seven patients revealed negative findings (Darby 1976; Williams et al. 1980). However, a few positive findings also have been reported (Bailey et al. 1998; Bauman 1991; Ritvo et al. 1986; Rodier et al. 1996), including increased cell-packing density and reduced nerve cell size bilaterally in the limbic system; variable loss of Purkinje cells, sometimes accompanied by gliosis; loss of granule cells in the neocerebellum; developmental abnormalities of the brainstem (near-complete absence of the facial nucleus and superior olive, along with shortening of the brainstem between the trapezoid body and the inferior olives); and megalencephalic brains. The cerebral cortex seems to be involved in autism. Because these studies examined only limited brain structures of a few autistic subjects without use of control subjects, the cause-and-effect meaning and the specificity of these findings are unclear. Nevertheless, the findings provide some direction (i.e., posterior cerebral fossa) for in vivo neuroanatomical imaging studies of autism and provide information on when the autism-causing injury to the brain most likely occurs.

Computed Tomography Scan Studies

Computed tomography (CT) studies have identified gross abnormalities (e.g., porencephalic cyst) in a minority of autistic patients (Damasio et al. 1980; Gillberg and Svendsen 1983). However, study findings are contradictory and inconsistent. Some studies that showed abnormalities such as reversed hemispheric asymmetry (Hier et al. 1979) and ventricular enlargement (Rosenbloom et al. 1984) have been challenged by other studies that have not reported such abnormalities (Creasey et al. 1986; Prior et al. 1984; Rumsey et al. 1988).

Magnetic Resonance Imaging Studies

Magnetic resonance imaging (MRI) is rapidly replacing CT as the method of choice for obtaining detailed anatomical information about the brain. MRI studies have reported cerebellar hypoplasia and/or a small brainstem, including the midbrain, pons, and medulla oblongata, in autistic patients (Ciesielski et al. 1997; Courchesne et al. 1988, 1994a, 1994c; Gaffney et al. 1987a, 1987b, 1988; Hashimoto et al. 1992a, 1992b, 1993a, 1993b, 1995; Levitt et al. 1999; Murakami et al. 1989; Piven et al. 1992; Saitoh and Courchesne 1998; Saitoh et al. 1995) smaller amygdala (Aylward et al. 1999); reduced size of corpus callosum (Egaas et al. 1995; Hardan et al. 2000; Piven et al. 1997a; Saitoh et al. 1995); smaller area dentate within the limbic system (Saitoh et al. 2001); reduced volume of hippocampus (Aylward et al. 1999); smaller right anterior cingulated

gyrus (Haznedar et al. 1997); significantly increased total brain, total tissue, and total lateral ventricle volumes (Piven et al. 1995, 1996a); increased volume of the caudate nuclei (Sears et al. 1999); and increased total volume of cerebellum and cerebellar hemispheres (Hardan et al. 2001). Other studies, however, have not found any abnormalities in the posterior fossa structures of the brain, particularly the cerebellum (Garber and Ritvo 1992; Garber et al. 1989; Hardan et al. 2001; Holttum et al. 1992; Hsu et al. 1991; Kleiman et al. 1992; Minshew et al. 1986; Piven et al. 1997c), or in the hippocampus (Piven et al. 1998).

Harris et al. (1999) studied the neuroanatomical contributions to slowed orienting of attention in autistic children. Degree of slowed attention orienting to visual cues was significantly correlated with degree of cerebellar hypoplasia. Pierce and Courchesne (2001) reported that measures of decreased exploration were significantly correlated with the magnitude of cerebellar hypoplasia of lobules VI–VII and that measures of rates of stereotyped behavior were significantly negatively correlated with area measures of cerebellar lobules VI–VII and positively correlated with frontal lobe volume in autistic subjects.

In a study of 22 boys with low-functioning autism, Elia et al. (2000a) reported a significant negative correlation between the midsagittal area of the cerebrum and age and a positive correlation between the midsagittal area of the midbrain and some subscales of the Psychoeducational Profile—Revised.

Howard et al. (2000) found that people with high-functioning autism had neuropsychological profiles characteristic of effects of amygdala damage, and that the same individuals also had abnormalities of medial temporal lobe brain structure, notably bilateral enlarged amygdala volumes.

On the other hand, Ciesielski and Knight (1994) found that the abnormal MRI cerebellar morphology was similar for both the high-functioning autistic subjects and those who had had childhood leukemia and had been treated with radiotherapy and intrathecal chemotherapy. The abnormal MRI macromorphology of the vermis may be nonspecific to autism. Nonetheless, the finding of cerebellar abnormalities is consistent with microscopic postmortem findings described above. Although the link between the cerebellar abnormalities and autism has yet to be determined, MRI technology has provided an exciting new avenue for future in vivo studies of the brain.

Differences in MRI study results may have been

due to subjects' ages, subjects' cognitive functioning level, the number of subjects, and the area measurement method used.

Functional Magnetic Resonance Imaging Studies

Using functional magnetic resonance imaging (fMRI), Baron-Cohen et al. (1999a) found that attempting to judge from the expression of another person's eyes what that other person might be thinking or feeling activated the frontotemporal regions but not the amygdala of autistic subjects. These results seemed to provide support for the social brain theory of normal function and the amygdala theory of autism (Baron-Cohen et al. 2000).

Ring et al. (1999) employed the Embedded Figures Task and fMRI in a study of autistic patients' brain activation patterns. Although the normally developed control subjects showed activated prefrontal areas, the autistic subjects showed greater activation of ventral occipitotemporal regions. The findings suggest that normal people invoke a greater contribution from the working memory system while the autistic subjects depend to an abnormally large extent on visual systems for object feature analysis.

Critchley et al. (2000) found that autistic subjects differed significantly from control subjects in the activity of cerebellar, mesolimbic, and temporal lobe cortical regions of the brain when processing facial expression. Autistic subjects did not activate a cortical "face area" when explicitly appraising expressions or the left amygdalar region and left cerebellum when implicitly processing emotional facial expression.

Using fMRI as subjects performed visually paced finger movement, Muller et al. (2001) found that in general, the autistic group had less pronounced activation compared with control subjects. The control subjects showed greater activation in perirolandic and supplementary motor areas, whereas the autistic subjects had greater activation in posterior and prefrontal cortices.

Magnetic Resonance Spectroscopy Studies

Magnetic resonance spectroscopy (MRS) is a fairly new research technology that has potential to provide insights into the molecular metabolic pathology of neuropsychiatric disorders. Minshew et al. (1993) used MRS to study 11 high-functioning autistic individuals. The pilot study found that the autistic group had de-

creased levels of phosphocreatine and esterified ends. As neuropsychological and language test performance of these subjects declined, levels of the most labile energy phosphate compound and of membrane building blocks decreased and levels of membrane breakdown products increased. These results indicate alterations in brain energy and phospholipid metabolism in autism that correlate with neuropsychological and language deficits. These findings also seem to be consistent with neuropathological and neurophysiological findings in autism. Otsuka et al. (1999) used MRS to examine the right hippocampus–amygdala region and left cerebellar hemisphere of 27 autistic patients between ages 2 and 18 years. The N-acetylaspartate (NAA) concentration was significantly decreased. It was speculated that the decreased NAA concentration might be due to neuronal hypofunction or immature neurons. Chugani et al. (1999) reported that autistic children had lower levels of NAA in the cerebellum. The significance of these findings is unclear, but this research approach merits further exploration.

Positron Emission Tomography Studies

Rumsey et al. (1985a), using positron emission tomography (PET), reported substantially elevated use of glucose throughout many parts of the brain in 10 autistic men compared with control subjects. Heh et al. (1989) reported no significant differences in mean cerebellar glucose metabolism between 7 adult patients with autism and 8 age-matched control subjects, although all mean glucose rates for the autistic patients were either equal to or greater than those of the control subjects. Zilbovicius et al. (2000) reported that autistic patients tended to have a highly significant hypoperfusion in both temporal lobes centered in the associative auditory and adjacent multimodal cortex. Haznedar et al. (2000) noted significant glucose metabolic reductions in both the anterior and posterior cingulate gyri.

Using PET to study five high-functioning autistic adults, Muller et al. (1998) found that the activation in the right dentate nucleus and in the left frontal area 46 was reduced during verbal, auditory, and expressive language and enhanced during motor speech. This finding may indicate impairment of the dentatothalamocortical pathway. Muller et al. (1999) also reported a reversed hemispheric dominance during verbal auditory stimulation; a trend toward reduced activation of the auditory cortex during acoustic stimulation; and reduced cerebellar activation during use of nonverbal auditory perception and possibly expressive language. These findings were considered as compatible with previous findings of cerebellar anomalies.

Siegel et al. (1992) used [^{18}F]fluoro-2-deoxyglucose PET to assess regional cerebral glucose metabolic rate (GMR) in 16 high-functioning autistic adults and 26 nonautistic control subjects. Autistic subjects had an abnormal anterior rectal gyrus asymmetry, in which the left side was larger than the right, which is the reverse of the normal asymmetry in that region. The autistic group also showed a low GMR in the left posterior putamen and a high GMR in the right posterior calcarine cortex. Brain regions with GMRs greater than 3 standard deviations from the normal mean were more prevalent in the autistic group than in the control group. Siegel et al. (1995) later observed negative correlations of medial frontal GMR with attentional performance on continuous performance test in autistic subjects, suggesting that neuronal inefficiency in that region might contribute to poor continuous performance test execution.

In a study of serotonin synthesis in the dentatothalamocortical pathway in seven boys and one girl with autism, Chugani et al. (1997) found asymmetries of serotonin synthesis in the frontal cortex, thalamus, and dentate nucleus of the cerebellum in all seven boys but not in the one girl. Decreased serotonin synthesis was found in the frontal cortex and thalamus in five of the seven boys (71%) and in the right frontal cortex and thalamus in the two remaining boys (29%). In all seven boys, elevated serotonin synthesis in the contralateral dentate nucleus was observed. These serotonergic abnormalities in a brain pathway were considered as one mechanism underlying the pathophysiology of autism.

Schifter et al. (1994) used [^{18}F]fluoro-2-deoxyglucose PET, MRI, and CT to study 13 autistic children. Of the 13 patients, 7 (54%) had normal findings on both PET and MRI or CT, 4 (31%) had abnormal findings on both PET and MRI, and 2 (15%) had anatomical anomalies that were noted only after PET findings had been obtained. Although the meaning of these findings remains to be determined, it appears that PET should become increasingly important for researchers studying autism.

Zilbovicius et al. (1992) measured regional cerebral blood flow with SPECT in 21 autistic children; no cortical regional abnormalities were found. In another study of five autistic children, Zilbovicius et al. (1995) used SPECT twice during the children's development: at age 3–4 years and 3 years later. A transient frontal hypoperfusion was found in the autistic children at age 3–4 years. However, by age 6–7 years, these children's frontal perfusion had attained normal values. These results indicate a delayed frontal maturation in childhood autism.

George et al. (1992) used SPECT to study four autistic young adults and four nonautistic age-matched control subjects. Total brain perfusion was significantly decreased in the autistic subjects. The autistic subjects had significantly decreased blood flow in the right lateral temporal and right, left, and midfrontal lobes compared with control subjects.

Chiron et al. (1995) used [^{133}Xe]SPECT to study 18 autistic children between the ages of 4 and 17 years. The regional cerebral blood flow (rCBF) in autistic subjects was decreased in the left hemisphere, particularly in the region of the sensorimotor and language-related cortex.

Mountz et al. (1995) used [^{99m}Tc]HMPAO SPECT to investigate the rCBF in 6 young, severely impaired autistic children. Abnormally low rCBF values were found in the temporal and parietal lobes, with the left cerebral hemisphere showing greater rCBF abnormalities than the right.

Starkstein et al. (2000) measured rCBF using [^{99m}Tc]HMPAO SPECT in 30 autistic patients and noted significantly low perfusion in the following brain regions: right temporal lobe (basal and inferior areas), occipital lobes, thalami, and left basal ganglia.

Hashimoto et al. (2000) performed SPECT in 22 autistic patients and reported that the rCBF in both laterotemporal and dorsomediolateral areas decreased significantly in autistic patients. The rCBf was significantly higher in the right temporal and right parietal lobes than that in the left ones. Inversely, the rCBF in the frontal and occipital lobes was significantly higher on the left side than on the right side. A positive correlation between rCBF and IQ was observed in the left laterotemporal and both dorsomediolateral frontal areas, and a negative one was noted in the cerebellar vermis area.

Ohnishi et al. (2000) assessed the relationship between rCBF and symptom profiles in 23 autistic children and found decreased rCBF in the bilateral insula, superior temporal gyri, and left prefrontal cortices. Impairments in communication and social interaction were thought to be related to the altered perfusion in the medial prefrontal cortex and anterior cingulate gyrus, and the obsessive desires for sameness were associated to altered perfusion in the right mediotemporal lobe.

■ Neurophysiological Factors

There are two rather disparate neurophysiological hypotheses of autism. The first, which considers a primary cortical dysfunction in autism, emphasizes the autistic symptoms of language and communication and assumes an underlying specific cognitive disorder that is presumably of cortical origin. More specifically, this hypothesis suggests that autism results from a disorder of hemispheric lateralization—that is, that the neural substrates in the left hemisphere necessary for sequential forms of information processing fail to develop (Prior 1979).

The cortical dysfunction hypothesis of autism has received some support from the fact that a significant proportion of autistic people have electroencephalographic abnormalities (Dawson et al. 1995; Elia et al. 1995; Ritvo et al. 1970; Rossi et al. 1995; Tsai and Tsai 1984; Waldo et al. 1978). Dawson et al. (1995) noted that compared with normally developing children, the autistic children had reduced electroencephalographic power in the frontal and temporal regions, and the differences were more prominent in the left than the right hemisphere. However, in general, these abnormalities tend to involve bilateral brain hemispheres and are characterized by focal or diffused spike, slow wave, or slow dysrhythmic patterns. The type of abnormality does not appear to be specific.

The cortical dysfunction hypothesis is also supported by the event-related brain potential study, which reported an abnormally small amplitude of the P3b, a component of the event-related brain potential (Kemner et al. 1995; Lincoln et al. 1993), and markedly smaller amplitude of N1c wave at bitemporal sites and pronounced peak latency delay (around 20 ms), particularly on the left side of the superotemporal gyrus (Bruneau et al. 1999).

Sleep electroencephalographic studies in autistic children (Tanguay et al. 1976) have found that the eye movements of autistic children were more like those of nonautistic infants than those of age-matched control subjects. Computerized quantitative electroencephalographic studies indicate an abnormal pattern of cerebral lateralization in autistic individuals (Cantor et al. 1986). Maturational deviation has also been indicated in several auditory evoked-response studies of autistic children (Fein et al. 1981; Lelord et al. 1973; Tanguay et al. 1982). These findings may indicate a defective integration between the visual and auditory pathways in autistic children.

The second hypothesis proposes a primary brainstem dysfunction in autism. This hypothesis has been developed through observation of the impaired ability of autistic children in modulating their own responses to sensory input and consequently their own motor output (Ornitz 1983). The hypothesis suggests a rostrally directed sequence of pathophysiological influences originating in the brain, substantia nigra, and nonspecific nuclei of the thalamus (Ornitz 1985).

The hypothesis of brainstem dysfunction in autism is somewhat supported by autonomic response studies (Hutt et al. 1975); vestibular nystagmus studies (for review, see Ornitz 1985) except in high-functioning autism, which seems to have normal postrotary nystagmus as reported by Goldberg et al. (2000); and brainstem auditory evoked-potential studies (e.g., prolongation of the early auditory evoked-response interpeak latencies) (Martineau et al. 1992b; Maziade et al. 2000; McClelland et al. 1992; Novick et al. 1980; Rumsey et al. 1984; Tanguay et al. 1982; Wong and Wong 1991).

■ Biochemical Factors

The results obtained from neuropathology and brain imaging studies strongly suggest that the cerebral defect in autism is microscopic or functional, without major gross neuroanatomical pathology. Thus, the neurochemical correlates in autism must be examined.

Serotonin Studies

Serotonergic activity in the brain has been linked to body temperature, pain, sensory perception, sleep, sexual behavior, motor function, neuroendocrine regulation, appetite, learning, memory, and immune response (Young et al. 1982). Many studies consistently have reported that about one-third of autistic individuals have hyperserotonemia (Anderson et al. 1987). There are three possible explanations for this condition: 1) enhanced platelet uptake, storage, or volume; 2) increased synthesis; and 3) decreased catabolism.

Geller et al. (1988) reported no significant difference in platelet volumes between autistic subjects and control subjects. The platelet volumes and blood 5-HT concentration also did not correlate. Marazziti et al.

(2000) investigated the 5-HT transporter by means of the specific binding of [^{3}H]paroxetine in 20 autistic children and adolescents. The results showed a significantly higher density of [^{3}H]paroxetine binding sites in autistic subjects than in healthy control subjects, suggesting the presence of serotonergic dysfunction in autism.

Although some previous studies found that the platelets' handling of 5-HT appeared to be normal in autism (Anderson et al. 1985; Boullin et al. 1982), other studies indicated that the role of the platelets might need to be reexamined (Katsui et al. 1986; Rotman et al. 1980). Furthermore, the autistic probands and their first-degree relatives had strong familial resemblance. There was positive correlation of both platelet-rich plasma 5-HT and platelet-poor (free) plasma 5-HT between autistic probands and their first-degree relatives (Cook et al. 1988; Kuperman et al. 1985; Leboyer et al. 1999; Wright et al. 1989). The platelet-rich plasma 5-HT levels of autistic subjects with affected siblings (i.e., with either autistic disorder or PDDNOS) were significantly higher than those of the autistic subjects without affected siblings, and autistic subjects without affected siblings had 5-HT levels significantly higher than those of control subjects. The results suggest that 5-HT levels in autistic subjects may be associated with genetic liability to autism (Piven et al. 1991c).

McBride et al. (1998) found that autistic children had significantly higher 5-HT plasma concentrations than control subjects did and that white children had significantly lower 5-HT levels than black or Latino youngsters. Postpubertal subjects had lower 5-HT concentrations than prepubertal subjects. These findings suggest that future studies must pay attention to the importance of controlling and matching for race and pubertal status.

The studies of 5-HT synthesis in autism have been conflicting. Several studies have not found any difference between autistic and nonautistic subjects (Minderaa et al. 1987). However, Croonenberghs et al. (2000) recently found that the plasma concentrations of tryptophan, the precursor of 5-HT, were significantly lower in 13 postpubertal autistic subjects than in healthy control subjects. Nevertheless, there was no significant difference between the groups in the serum concentration of 5-HT. The ratio of serum tryptophan to large neutral amino acids is considered a reliable marker of tryptophan availability for brain serotonin synthesis. D'Eufemia et al. (1995) found a significantly lower serum ratio in the autistic subjects compared with the nonautistic control subjects.

The occurrence of hyperserotonemia in autistic people does not appear to be the result of decreased catabolism of 5-HT. Although there was a preliminary finding of negative correlation between whole-blood 5-HT levels and verbal-expressive/symbolic abilities in 18 autistic patients and their first-degree relatives (Cuccaro et al. 1993), no consistent correlations have been found between blood levels of 5-HT and any autistic behaviors or symptoms. Moreover, hyperserotonemia has also been found in some children with severe retardation. The mechanism and importance of hyperserotonemia in autism are unclear. Furthermore, the CSF concentration of the 5-HT metabolite 5-hydroxyindoleacetic acid (5-HIAA) in autistic children was not significantly different from that seen in the control group of children without neurological impairment (Narayan et al. 1993).

Dopamine Studies

The brain dopaminergic system is considered to affect several functions and behaviors, including cognition, motor function, eating and drinking behaviors, sexual behavior, neuroendocrine regulation, and selective attention. Campbell (1977) reported that neuroleptics, which are dopamine receptor–blocking agents, modulated several symptoms involving the motor system (e.g., hyperactivity, stereotypies, aggression, and self-injury) and made autistic children more compliant and receptive to special-education procedures. On the other hand, dopamine agonists, such as stimulants, worsen preexisting stereotypies, aggression, and hyperactivity in autistic children (Young et al. 1982).

Studies of dopamine in autism have focused on the measurement of homovanillic acid (HVA), the main metabolite of dopamine. Cohen et al. (1974) and Narayan et al. (1993) found that the autistic children did not differ from other diagnostic groups in CSF level of HVA. However, the levels were found to be higher in the more severely impaired children, especially those with greater locomotor activity and more severe stereotypies. Leckman et al. (1980) also did not find a difference in CSF HVA between "child psychosis (largely autism)" and "perceptual cognitive disorder" diagnostic groups. Gillberg and Svennerholm (1987) found elevated CSF HVA levels in autistic subjects. Two studies found no difference in plasma HVA levels between the autistic children and control subjects

(Launay et al. 1987; Minderaa et al. 1989). However, HVA concentrations have not been shown to correlate with any autistic behaviors or symptoms.

Epinephrine and Norepinephrine Studies

Epinephrine and norepinephrine are often discussed concurrently because of their similar effects on behavior. They are associated with cardiovascular function, respiratory function, appetite, activity level, arousal, attention, anxiety, response to stress, movement, sleep, memory, and learning (Young et al. 1982).

Plasma norepinephrine level has been reported to be elevated in autistic subjects (Lake et al. 1977), but in platelets, both epinephrine and norepinephrine levels were significantly lower in the autistic group compared with the control group (Launay et al. 1987).

No difference in CSF levels, plasma levels, and urinary excretion of MHPG (3-methoxy-4-hydroxyphenylglycol), as well as urinary excretion rates of epinephrine, norepinephrine, and vanillylmandelic acid, has been found between autistic subjects and control subjects (Minderaa et al. 1994; Young et al. 1982).

Other Monoamine Studies

Martineau et al. (1992a) reported that the urinary levels of dopamine and its derivatives HVA, 3,4-dihydroxyphenylacetic acid (DOPAC), 3-methoxytyramine (3MT), epinephrine, norepinephrine, and 5-HT and its metabolite 5-HIAA in autistic children between ages 2 and 12.5 years decreased significantly with age. The results suggest a maturation defect of the monoaminergic system in autism.

In summary, because it is believed that the catecholamine and indoleamine systems may be in dynamic balance and that disturbances in one or both systems may be involved in adult schizophrenia, it is important to pursue the studies of catecholamine in autism.

Dopamine β-Hydroxylase

Conflicting results have been reported from the study of dopamine β-hydroxylase, the enzyme that controls the conversion of dopamine to norepinephrine. M. Goldstein et al. (1976) and Lake et al. (1977) found decreased dopamine β-hydroxylase activity in autistic subjects compared with control subjects, whereas Young et al. (1980) found no difference. The real meaning of blood dopamine β-hydroxylase activity is unclear because most nonautistic people also exhibit a wide range of this activity without evident effect.

Catechol-O-Methyltransferase and Monoamine Oxidase

Two metabolic enzymes, catechol-O-methyltransferase and monoamine oxidase, may change norepinephrine activity. Giller et al. (1980) found no difference between autistic children and control subjects in catechol-O-methyltransferase activity in cultured fibroblasts and in red blood cells. Monoamine oxidase activity also appeared to be normal in autistic subjects (Young et al. 1982).

Peptides

Trygstad et al. (1980) described several different urinary peptides' profile patterns, each said to be characteristic of a different behavioral abnormality. The characteristic profile for autism was initially shown in 20 patients, with a variation of ±30% for each peak. However, in an attempt to replicate such a finding from 69 urine samples obtained from three groups of young adult men (autistic, mentally handicapped, and not impaired), no consistent patterns of urinary chromatographic profile were identified (Couteur et al. 1988).

Nevertheless, the findings are intriguing, and further study may develop patterns with high specificity that may be used as diagnostic markers. Isolation and identification of any factors present in the chromatographic fractions may also contribute to the understanding of the pathogenesis of autism.

Brain Opioids

An endorphin hypothesis was proposed based on the analogy between opiate addiction and autism (Kalat 1978) and the similarity between opiate-induced psychosocial distortion in animals and clinical manifestations of autism (Panksepp 1979). Ross et al. (1987) reported higher levels of CSF β-endorphin in baseline measures of autistic children compared with control samples; Gillberg et al. (1990) found low levels of CSF β-endorphin in autistic subjects; Nagamitsu et al. (1997) reported that CSF levels of β-endorphin in autistic subjects did not differ from those of age-matched controls.

Sandman et al. (1991) reported low levels of plasma β-endorphin in autistic individuals; Brambilla et al.

(1997), Tordjman et al. (1997), and Cazzullo et al. (1999) reported increased plasma β-endorphin levels in autistic subjects. Leboyer et al. (1999) found familial aggregation of elevated plasma β-endorphin levels. Willemsen-Swinkels et al. (1996b) found that the β-endorphin levels of the autistic subjects with severe self-injurious behavior were significantly lower than those of autistic subjects without self-injurious behavior. These findings suggest that severe self-injurious behavior plays a more significant role than autism in plasma β-endorphin levels.

■ Other Biomedical Factors

A number of other abnormal biomedical measures in autistic people have been reported. Sankar (1971) reported significantly lower blood adenosine triphosphatase activity in assays of red blood cells from autistic children. Katz and Liebman (1970) found that CSF creatine phosphokinase activity was elevated in some autistic children, as well as in children with meningitis; this finding suggests that autistic children with increased CSF creatine phosphokinase may represent a subgroup of children whose autism is due to brain insult from infection. Rolf et al. (1993) reported significantly decreased levels of the amino acids aspartic acid, glutamine, glutamic acid, and γ-aminobutyric acid in 18 drug-free autistic patients. Moreno-Fuenmayor et al. (1996) reported that the mean plasma glutamic, aspartic acid, and taurine values were elevated in autistic children. The CSF glial fibrillary acidic protein in autism and autism-like conditions was significantly increased (Ahlsen et al. 1993). Concentrations of CSF gangliosides were significantly increased in autistic subjects (Lekman et al. 1995; Nordin et al. 1998). The mean thyroid-stimulating hormone basal and peak levels were significantly lower in 41 autistic subjects than in control subjects (Hashimoto et al. 1991). Page and Coleman (2000) suggested that about 20% of autistic people are hyperuricosuric individuals and that their purine synthesis is increased. Plasma levels of testosterone and adrenal androgen were found to be normal in postpubertal autistic subjects (Tordjman et al. 1995). On the whole, the significance of these findings is far from clear, but these studies merit further exploration.

■ Vaccination Factor

The hypothesis that measles, mumps, and rubella (MMR) vaccines cause autism was first raised by reports of cases in which developmental regression occurred soon after MMR vaccination. However, several major epidemiological studies failed to find any evidence to support a causal association between MMR vaccine and autism (Farrington et al. 2001; Kaye et al. 2001; Taylor et al. 1999). Concern has also been raised about possible association between MMR vaccine–induced mercury (thimerosal) exposure and autism (Bernard et al. 2001). The available evidence, however, does not support such a hypothesis (Halsey et al. 2001).

■ Other Biological Factors

Gastrointestinal Abnormalities

Horvath et al. (1999) reported high rates of reflux esophagitis, chronic gastritis, and chronic duodenitis in 36 children with autism. Unrecognized gastrointestinal disorders were considered to be a contributing factor to the behavioral problems of nonverbal autistic subjects.

Abnormal Intestinal Permeability

An altered intestinal permeability was found in 9 of 21 autistic subjects (43%). It was speculated that an altered intestinal permeability could represent a possible mechanism for the increased passage through the gut mucosa of peptides derived from food, with subsequent behavioral abnormalities in these patients (D'Eufemia et al. 1996).

Food Allergy

Lucarelli et al. (1995) found high levels of immunoglobulin A (IgA) antigen-specific antibodies for casein, lactalbumin, and β-lactoglobulin and IgG and IgM for casein in 36 autistic subjects. They speculated that food allergy might cause autism.

Xenobiotic Influences

Edelson and Cantor (1998) studied 20 children with autism and found that 100% of them had liver detoxification profiles outside of normal, and that 16 of 18 subjects (89%) with blood analysis available showed evidence of levels of toxic chemicals exceeding the adult maximum tolerance. They proposed that the interaction of xenobiotic toxins with immune dysfunction and continuous and/or progressive endogenous toxicity in these children caused the development of their autism.

Summary of Other Biological Factors

These hypotheses are intriguing but were based on findings from studies with very small sample sizes, so more studies are needed.

■ Neuropsychological Factors

Several studies suggest that autistic people may have a diminished or altered capacity for selectively channeling information for further internal attention and processing, as well as differential hemispheric involvement in attentional deficits (Courchesne 1987; Dawson et al. 1988). Courchesne et al. (1994b) reviewed autopsy, MRI, and neurophysiological findings and proposed that in autism, cerebellar maldevelopment may contribute to an inability to execute rapid attention shifts, which undermines social and cognitive development. Deficit in shifting attention has also been reported by other investigators (Swettenham et al. 1998; Townsend et al. 1996; Wainwright and Bryson 1996). However, Pascualvaca et al. (1998) reported that all of the 23 children with autism demonstrated ability to shift their attention.

Investigators have found that autistic individuals had deficits of face recognition (Boucher et al. 1998; Celani et al. 1999; Klin et al. 1999), voice recognition (Boucher et al. 1998), and emotion recognition (Bormann-Kischkel et al. 1995; Celani et al. 1999). Based on results of tasks used in studies of amygdala dysfunction in autism, Adolphs et al. (2001) suggested that such dysfunction might contribute to an impaired ability to link visual perception of socially relevant stimuli with retrieval of social knowledge and with elicitation of social behavior. However, Loveland et al. (1997) reported that people with autism could use affective information from multiple sources to recognize emotions in much the same ways as people of comparable developmental level without autism.

A deficit in theory of mind ability (i.e., the ability to make inferences about others' mental states) has been described as the core deficit in autism (Baron-Cohen et al. 1997; Jolliffe and Baron-Cohen 1999; Ozonoff et al. 1991; Ziatas et al. 1998). However, other investigators reported that autism did not involve a specific impairment in theory of mind ability (Yirmiya and Shulman 1996) and that theory of mind deficits are not

unique to autism (Buitelaar et al. 1999; Dahlgren and Trillingsgaard 1996; Yirmiya et al. 1998). Further, Rieffe et al. (2000) studied the understanding of atypical emotions in 23 high-functioning children with autism spectrum disorders (mean age, 9 years 3 months) and concluded that the theory of mind ability of such children might be intact.

There is growing interest in the studying of the precursors to the ability of conceiving other people's minds. Investigators have found that autistic individuals have deficits in two candidate precursors, imitation and joint attention (Charman et al. 1997; Roeyers et al. 1998).

Many studies have shown that autistic individuals perform at a much lower level than control subjects on tests of executive functioning, defined as tasks requiring subjects to hold information in mind while suppressing a prepotent response (Bennetto et al. 1996; Ozonoff et al. 1991). A significant proportion of parents and siblings of autistic children have been observed to also have impaired executive functioning (Hughes et al. 1997, 1999). However, other investigators reported that executive functioning in autistic children was not impaired (Griffith et al. 1999; Russell et al. 1999) or impairment was not universally presented (Liss et al. 2001).

■ Birth Season Factor

Some investigators had proposed that birth in particular months may be a risk for autism. Barak et al. (1995) suggested that being born in March or August may be a risk factor for development of autistic disorder in Israel. Stevens et al. (2000) noted a significant elevation of persons with autism born in March within a Boston sample. However, other investigators failed to replicate such a finding (E.C. Landau et al. 1999; Yeates-Frederikx et al. 2000).

■ Psychogenic Factors

Kanner's (1943) original description of autism, as well as a number of subsequent reports by other investigators, had suggested that parents of autistic children were highly intelligent, were preoccupied with abstractions, had limited interest in people, and were emotionally cold. Some studies reported findings of disturbances in family dynamics (Reiser 1963a, 1963b), unconscious parental hostility and rejection (Bettelheim 1967), parental perplexity, and lack of parent–

child communicative clarity (Goldfarb et al. 1972). These investigators suggested that autism might be a response to these parental personality characteristics, to deviant parent–child interactions, or to severe early stress of various kinds. However, findings that support these psychogenic hypotheses are from samples in which autism and schizophrenia in childhood were not differentiated, from projective tests, and from selected family observations. Similar techniques and other well-controlled studies have produced largely negative findings (Ornitz and Ritvo 1976). The conclusion that no psychological or social factors cause autistic disorder seems warranted.

■ Summary of Etiology

As yet, no specific causes of autistic disorder have been identified. Neurobiological investigations in autism have found various abnormalities. However, no single measure of the abnormalities has been found consistently, and the etiological implications of the findings are far from clear, possibly because autistic disorder is a behavior-defined syndrome that includes several distinct conditions. It is anticipated that if this is the case, future studies will determine a range of biological etiologies for the subgroups constituting autistic disorder.

Treatment

So far, no cure for autism has been developed, because its etiology is still unknown. However, comprehensive intervention, including parental counseling, behavior modification, special education in a highly structured environment, sensory integration training, speech therapy, social skills training, and medications, has demonstrated significant treatment effects in many autistic individuals (American Academy of Child and Adolescent Psychiatry 1999; Tsai 2001).

■ Special-Education Intervention

Emphasis is now placed on treatments to promote the autistic child's more normal social and linguistic developments and on minimization of the child's maladaptive behaviors (e.g., hyperactivity, stereotypies, self-injury, aggressiveness), which interfere with or are incompatible with the child's functioning and learn-

ing. There has been an increasing focus on early identification and treatment of preschool autistic children through special-education programs in highly structured environments (preschools or day-care centers) and on working closely with the family members of autistic children to help them cope better with the problems faced at home and to increase positive interaction (Jocelyn et al. 1998; Kobayashi et al. 2001; Koegel et al. 1996; Ozonoff and Cathcart 1998; Zanolli et al. 1996).

There has been an increasing focus on providing education services/interventions through "regular education programs" (i.e., inclusion education) with strong special-education support (Mesibov and Shea 1996). Some general student peers have demonstrated their usefulness and effectiveness in helping their autistic classmates to increase reading fluency, make correct responses to reading comprehension questions and social interactions, and decrease inappropriate behaviors (H. Goldstein et al. 1992; Kamps et al. 1992, 1994; Laushey and Heflin 2000; Pierce and Schreibman 1997; Roeyers 1996; Schleien et al. 1995; Zanolli et al. 1996).

Educational treatment should be intensive and sustained and should emphasize acquisition of self-care, social, and job skills. It is critical that each student's educational intervention plan be truly individualized and take into consideration both the student's weaknesses/deficits and strengths/talents. The educational curriculum has to be individualized and unconventional because it has become clear that when autistic students are taught using an appropriate individualized educational plan, they are happier and learn faster. When their downtime decreases, their performance gets better and their productivity increases. Ultimately, their self-esteem also increases.

■ Computer-Based Treatment

A computer-based intervention with a motivating multimedia program has been demonstrated to increase reading and communication skills in children with autism (Heimann et al. 1995) and to increase their ability to construct correct sentences and to use more appropriate vocal responses (Yamamoto and Miya 1999). Some investigators have attempted to use virtual reality technologies to teach autistic children new coping skills that may then be generalized in their everyday lives (Max and Burke 1997; Strickland 1997).

■ Behavior Therapy

Extensive research in behavior therapy since the 1960s has shown that many autistic children can be taught special skills in the areas of social adaptation and cognitive and motor skills. Their maladaptive behavior can also be ameliorated significantly. Lovaas et al. (1976) reviewed the principles involved in behavior therapy with autistic children. A few points are emphasized here: First, behavior therapy programs should be designed for individual children because autistic children vary greatly in their handicaps and family circumstances. Some treatment approaches that work for certain patients may not work for others. Second, autistic children have an impaired ability to generalize from one situation to another, so the skills they have learned in a hospital or school tend not to transfer to the home or other settings. It is crucial in treatment to plan the approach specifically to ensure that the changes in the child's clinical state are being carefully monitored, that the problems in each setting are dealt with, and that steps are taken to encourage generalization of behavior changes. Third, because one of the treatment goals is to promote the child's social development, long-term residential treatment is a definite drawback.

Intensive behavior therapy in early childhood is critical, and some preliminary data seemed to show long-lasting positive effects (McEachin et al. 1993; Sheinkopf and Siegel 1998; T. Smith et al. 1997, 2000a, 2000b). A home-based approach, which trains parents, siblings, and local special education teachers to carry out behavior therapies, has been instrumental in achieving maximum results (Hemsley et al. 1978; Knott et al. 1995). It is critical that parents and siblings of autistic patients have the appropriate mental conditions to carry out such therapies. Some studies reported that parents and siblings of autistic individuals had significant personality adjustment difficulties, with a high degree of anxiety (Weiss 1991), and they tended to have higher scores on depression and stress ratings than did control subjects (Gold 1993; Koegel et al. 1992). Several factors have been identified as significantly influencing adjustment of families with an autistic child: the severity of the child's disorder, mother's social support, mother's perceived locus of control, and family service agency affiliation (Henderson and Vandenberg 1992).

■ Speech and Language Therapies

Licensed speech and language therapists have developed many different treatments, most of which are aimed at stimulating the individual's natural ability for and interest in learning language. The treatments customarily take place in one-to-one sessions held 2 or 3 hours per week. However, no scientific studies have evaluated whether any form of speech and language therapy helps individuals with autism. Speech and language therapy sessions should also include peers, siblings, and parents so that the therapist can assess the learning effect on the autistic children (i.e., whether the child applies the newly learned skills in other settings with other people).

■ Social Skills Training

Both individual and group social skills training may be helpful to older and higher-functioning individuals with autism. Some autistic individuals seem to enjoy meeting with other people who have similar difficulties. The therapist working with these individuals should facilitate such social contacts within the context of an activity- or special interest–oriented group. However, the therapist should also create or facilitate opportunities for these individuals to meet with nonautistic friends or peers so that they have opportunities to learn or to practice appropriate social skills. Autistic individuals tend not to learn social skills naturally. They have to be taught to recognize social cues and how to react to them. They need to be told how to monitor and modify their own inappropriate social behaviors. These skills can be taught through role modeling, role playing, social stories, cartooning, and video recordings, using rules, visual cues, and positive behavioral reinforcement. To ensure success, the first step is to identify specific measurable target behaviors that must be learned. It is important to teach one skill at a time and then build a repertoire. Each new skill to be learned should be broken into smaller components or steps. The new skill should be taught using multiple methods and building in ways that would ensure generalizing such a skill in many different situations or settings.

Group social skills training sessions must be structured with very specific rules. At the outset, carefully scripted rules that specify appropriate responses should be taught and discussed. The students would then be taught to know when they are being unintentionally insulting, tactless, or inappropriate. Alternative and appropriate skills should be taught and practiced with positive reinforcement strategies (i.e., rewards) to increase use of the newly learned social skills. Autistic individuals usually do not possess a sense of humor, tell jokes, or use metaphors. They tend to interpret words and phrases literally. It is important to teach how to appreciate humor, jokes, metaphors, and irony, as well as to practice discerning when to appropriately use them.

■ Sociodramatic Play Therapy

Teaching sociodramatic play, using a variation of Pivotal Response Training, to autistic children has produced positive changes in play, language, and social skills (Thorp et al. 1995).

■ Cognitive Therapy

Individual cognitive psychotherapy may be helpful to higher-functioning autistic individuals. The focus of therapy is to help them understand the social behavior of other people and to see how their own behavior can be viewed as unusual. Additional therapeutic group experiences can provide these individuals with more insight into their disabilities, helping them to accept their limitations in some areas and to discover their strengths and potentials in others. Thus, cognitive therapy can also prevent depression in these individuals.

■ Sensorimotor Therapies

One of the oldest and most popular notions about children with development delays, including those with autism, is that they have difficulty processing sensory input from the environment and/or translating such input into effective action. In this view, children may be over- or underaroused by normal levels of sensory input. Consequently, according to theorists, such children have difficulty perceiving and responding to environmental events. Moreover, they try to moderate their arousal levels by engaging in ritualistic behaviors such as rocking their bodies back and forth. Nevertheless, no one knows whether these behaviors are in fact due to suboptimal arousal and, if so, what physiological problems cause the suboptimal arousal. Because of this fundamental gap in sensorimotor theories, investigators have had no systematic way to develop treatments that might improve arousal levels, relying instead on speculation.

Sensory Integration Therapy

In sensory integration therapy (SIT), a therapist stimulates an individual's skin and vestibular systems. This stimulation consists of activities such as swinging in a hammock suspended from the ceiling, spinning in circles on specially constructed chairs, brushing parts of the individual's body, and engaging in physical activities that require balance. A number of informal case reports and poorly designed studies have indicated that SIT may be helpful for autistic individuals. It may increase the ability to integrate sensory information efficiently. Improvements in motor coordination, language development, emotional adjustment, and self-confidence, plus reduction of hyper- or hyporesponsiveness to sensory stimuli, are possible benefits. However, scientifically sound research has not confirmed the reported findings. Hence, there is no information on the treatment length that is required to yield significantly positive results, if any. Nonetheless, because SIT resembles play and most children with autism enjoy it, SIT can be used as a reward or positive reinforcer to enhance speech/communication and social skills training. Furthermore, SIT may offer enjoyable and healthy physical activity, which is as important for autistic patients as for typically developing children.

Deep pressure was applied to six autistic children who received two 20-minute sessions a week for 6 weeks. There was a significant reduction in tension and marginally significant reduction in anxiety for autistic children compared with control subjects (Edelson et al. 1999). Case-Smith and Bryan (1999) reported positive behavioral changes in five preschool children with autism who underwent 10 weeks of SIT.

Auditory Integration Training

Auditory integration training (AIT) begins with obtaining an audiogram to determine the frequencies at which a child's hearing appears to be too sensitive. Various compact discs are selected containing music determined to be the best for the person receiving the therapy. The music is then played on a standard compact disc player and fed through an electronic device. In turn, that device has been set in accordance with the person's audiogram to amplify and/or filter each frequency of the sound spectrum. The person listens to the music through standard headphones. The treatment consists of 20 half-hour sessions at a rate of 2 per day over a period of 10 days.

However, the measure of hypersensitive hearing based on the audiogram has been criticized by audiologists as an unreliable and invalid measure. Furthermore, among practitioners of AIT, the application of the "filtering" component has been inconsistent. As with other alternative treatments for autism, some patients' parents reported positive effects after AIT. However, parental reports should be viewed cautiously. Bettison (1996) found that helping people with autism learn to listen to various kinds of music via a music player (e.g., a compact disc player) and a headphone set for the same amount of time daily as in AIT can produce much the same effects as those produced by expensive AIT. Mudford et al. (2000) failed to demonstrate any behavior benefits in 16 autistic children who received AIT. In 1998, the American Academy of Pediatrics stated that there was not enough information to support the claims that AIT improved communication skills in autistic children.

■ Music Therapy

The implementation of music therapy involves interactions of the therapist, client, and music that initiate and sustain musical and nonmusical change processes. As the musical elements of rhythm, melody, and harmony are elaborated across time, the therapist and client can develop a relationship that optimizes the quality of life. Music therapy may include many activities, among them singing, movement to music, and playing instruments.

Proponents of music therapy believe that it can help individuals with developmental disabilities, including autism, because it requires no verbal interaction, although it may eventually facilitate it; because music is structured, and it can facilitate structure in the environment in which it is experienced; because sound stimulus can aid in sensory integration because it involves all the senses; because the vestibular system is also stimulated when rhythmic movement is included in the therapy; because music naturally facilitates play and therefore enhances learning through play; and because music therapy can aid in socialization and influence behavior.

In general, music therapists hope to improve various aspects of an individual's physical and mental health and to foster desired changes in behavior. A qualified music therapist makes a careful assessment of the individual's present capabilities and, on that basis, defines program goals, both short- and long-term. Music therapy can be carried out in a private setting, but it can also be incorporated into school. An interested parent could also learn techniques for using music as a teaching tool at home. Music therapy has been used for many years to treat autistic individuals. It has not "cured" any individual with autism, but it does seem to improve the quality of life of some autistic people.

■ Pharmacotherapy

Psychotropic and anticonvulsant medication and vitamin treatment have frequently been given to autistic patients. Aman et al. (1995) surveyed the prevalence and pattern of medication therapy among autistic individuals in North Carolina. In all, 33.8% of the survey sample (taken from the caseloads of 838 care providers) was taking some psychotropic drug or vitamin for autism or associated behavior/psychiatric problems. More than 50% of the sample was taking some psychotropic, antiepileptic, vitamin, or "medical" agent. Recently, Martin et al. (1999b) reviewed the rates and pattern of psychotropic drug use in 109 high-functioning children, adolescents, and adults with PDD enrolled in the Yale Child Study Center's Project on Social Learning Disabilities. In all, 55% were taking psychotropics, with 29.3% taking two or more medications simultaneously. Antidepressants were the most commonly used drugs (32.1%), followed by stimulants (20.2%) and neuroleptics (16.5%).

Pharmacotherapy does not alter the natural history or course of autistic disorder. It can be helpful, however, in controlling specific symptoms such as hyperactivity, withdrawal, stereotypies, self-injury, aggressiveness, and sleep disorders. This subject has been reviewed by Tsai (2001).

Neuroleptics

Low-potency typical neuroleptics, such as chlorpromazine, have little or no therapeutic effect because they cause excessive sedation, even at low doses. On the other hand, haloperidol, a high-potency neuroleptic, has demonstrated both short- and long-term efficacy in 40 young autistic children (ages 2.6–7.2 years) (Campbell et al. 1983). Haloperidol was significantly superior to placebo in reducing symptoms of withdrawal and stereotypies in these children. The combination of haloperidol and contingent reinforcement was found to be most effective in facilitating the acquisition of imitative speech. A long-term study of haloperidol by Campbell et al. (1983) reported that the effect lasts for 6 months to 2.5 years. At optimal doses, no adverse effects were noted. When above-optimal or regulated doses were given, excessive sedation was most common, followed by acute dystonic reaction. However, since the introduction of newer atypical neuroleptics, the role of haloperidol in autistic disorder has decreased and has been limited mostly to the treatment of tic disorders. When it is used, patients must be very carefully monitored for any side effects.

Agonists, Antagonists, and Blockers

Fenfluramine, an antiserotonergic anorectic, was initially reported as showing positive effects, but subsequent data from a multicenter study (Campbell et al. 1988b) and an independent study failed to show any positive effect (Leventhal et al. 1993).

Naltrexone, an opiate antagonist, has been reported to have positive effects on hyperactivity, social relatedness, and self-injury (Campbell et al. 1989, 1993; Herman et al. 1987; Kolmen et al. 1995, 1997). However, other investigators did not find such effects (Gillberg 1995; Willemsen-Swinkels et al. 1995, 1996a; Zingarelli et al. 1992). Naltrexone treatment did not lead to improvement in communication skills (Feldman et al. 1999). Willemsen-Swinkels et al. (1995) reported increased incidence of stereotyped behavior with naltrexone treatment.

Clomipramine, a 5-HT reuptake blocker with unique antiobsessional properties, has been shown to be effective in reducing compulsive and ritualistic behaviors, stereotypies, and aggressive and impulsive behaviors and in improving social relatedness (Gordon et al. 1993; McDougle et al. 1992). However, Sanchez et al. (1996) reported that clomipramine was not therapeutic and was associated with serious side effects.

Fluoxetine, another 5-HT reuptake blocker, also has been reported to reduce overall autistic symptoms (Buchsbaum et al. 2001; Cook et al. 1992; DeLong et al. 1998; Fatemi et al. 1998) but also to induce significant side effects, including restlessness, hyperactivity, agitation, vivid dreams, decreased appetite, and insomnia (Cook et al. 1992; Fatemi et al. 1998).

Fluvoxamine, another 5-HT reuptake blocker, was reported as more effective than placebo in a short-term treatment of symptoms of autism (i.e., social relatedness, repetitive thoughts and behavior, maladaptive behavior, and aggression) in 15 adults (McDougle et al. 1996).

Sertraline, another 5-HT reuptake blocker, was reported as effective in reducing self-injury and aggression in mentally retarded autistic patients (Hellings et al. 1996) and in transition-associated anxiety and agitation in autistic children (Steingard et al. 1997).

A low dosage of venlafaxine, a potent inhibitor of neuronal serotonin and norepinephrine reuptake, was reported as effective in six subjects with autism. Improvement was noted in repetitive behaviors and restricted interests, social deficits, communication and language function, inattention, and hyperactivity (Hollander et al. 2000).

Clonidine, an α_2-adrenergic receptor agonist, showed effectiveness in reducing several hyperarousal behaviors and in improving social relationships in some autistic patients. However, clonidine also caused significant drowsiness and decreased activity levels (Fankhauser et al. 1992; Jaselskis et al. 1992).

Risperidone, a potent 5-HT_{2A}-dopamine D_2 antagonist with additional dopamine antagonistic properties, seemed to reduce repetitive behavior, aggression, anxiety or nervousness, depression, irritability, self-injury, and overall behavioral symptoms (Findling et al. 1997b; Fisman and Steele 1996; Horrigan and Barnhill 1997; McDougle et al. 1998; Perry et al. 1997; Posey et al. 1999; Purdon et al. 1994; Zuddas et al. 2000). However, weight gain seems to be common (Findling et al. 1997b; Horrigan and Barnhill 1997; Zuddas et al. 2000). The rate of increase lessened over a period of time, and after drug withdrawal, considerable weight loss was observed in the patients who had previously shown the most significant weight increase (Zuddas et al. 2000).

Quetiapine fumarate is an antagonist at multiple neurotransmitter receptors in the brain: serotonin 5-HT_{1A}, 5-HT_2, dopamine D_1 and D_2, histamine H_1, and α_1-adrenergic and α_2-adrenergic receptors. In an open-label quentiapine treatment in six autistic children, Martin et al. (1999a) reported that there was no significant improvement as rated on the Clinical Global Impression Scale and that quetiapine was poorly tolerated and associated with serious side effects.

Olanzapine is a selective monoaminergic antagonist to the following receptors: serotonin $5\text{-HT}_{2A/2C}$, dopamine D_1 through dopamine D_4, muscarinic M_1

through muscarinic M_5, histamine H_1, and adrenergic. Five of six children treated with olanzapine showed improved scores on the Clinical Global Impression Scale (Malone et al. 2001). Weight gain is common with olanzapine treatment.

Stimulants

The use of stimulants in autism has not received extensive evaluation. Quintana et al. (1995) reported modest but statistically significant improvement with the use of methylphenidate in 10 autistic children. Handen et al. (2000) reported that 8 of 13 autistic children (62%) showed a positive response to methylphenidate, based on a minimum 50% decrease on the Conners Hyperactivity Index. Stimulants are frequently reported to exacerbate irritability, insomnia, and aggression in clinical populations (Posey and Mc-Dougle 2000).

Anticonvulsants

Anticonvulsants have been used to treat autistic symptoms. Hollander et al. (2001) reported that 10 of 14 autistic patients (71%) taking divalproex sodium were rated as having sustained response to treatment. It appeared that the responders were those who had associated features of affective instability, impulsivity, and aggression as well as those with a history of electroencephalographic abnormalities or seizures.

Natural and Synthetic Hormones

Secretin is a peptide hormone that stimulates pancreatic secretion. After the initial report of positive effect of secretin treatment of three autistic subjects (Horvath et al. 1998), many children with autism have received secretin treatment. However, several large-sample controlled studies have failed to demonstrate any significant positive treatment effect for autism (Chez et al. 2000; Coniglio et al. 2001; Dunn-Geier et al. 2000; Roberts et al. 2001; Sandler et al. 1999), and a worsening in autistic symptoms during secretin treatment was noted by Robinson (2001).

The effects of neuropeptide ORG 2766, a synthetic analogue of adrenocorticotropic hormone, were studied in 34 autistic children. ORG 2766 was reported to increase the amount and quality of social interaction (Buitelaar et al. 1992a, 1992b). However, in a later study of 50 children with autism between ages 7 and 15 years and with a Performance IQ above 60, ORG 2766 failed to improve social and communicative behavior at the group level. Future studies should examine whether ORG 2766 differentially affects various subtypes of autism (Buitelaar et al. 1996).

Other Medications and Supplements

Niaprazine is a histamine H_1-receptor antagonist with marked sedative properties. Niaprazine was administered at 1 mg/kg/day for 60 days in 25 subjects with autism. A positive effect was noted in 13 patients (52%), particularly for hyperkinesias, unstable attention, resistance to change and frustration, mild anxiety, aggression, and sleep problems (Rossi et al. 1999).

R-THBP (6R-L-erythro-5,6,7,8-tetrahydrobiopterin), a cofactor for tyrosine hydroxylase in the biosynthetic pathway of catecholamines and serotonin, was reported as effective in improving autistic children's social functioning—mainly eye contact and desire to interact and in the number of words or sounds that the children used (Fernell et al. 1997; Komori et al. 1995).

The efficacy of pyridoxine (vitamin B_6) plus magnesium has been controversial. Some short-term (2-week to 30-day) studies reported positive results (Pfeiffer et al. 1995; Tsai 1992b). However, interpretation of these findings must be tempered because of methodological problems inherent in many of the studies (Pfeiffer et al. 1995). Other investigators could not confirm such findings (Findling et al. 1997a; Tolbert et al. 1993).

N,N-dimethylglycine (DMG), a dietary supplement, has been reported, in nonmedical literature, to be beneficial in children with autism. Two recently published studies failed to find any significant difference between groups given DMG and those given placebos (Bolman and Richmond 1999; Kern et al. 2001).

Summary

Larger samples and long-term studies are needed before final conclusions about the efficacy of all these drugs can be drawn.

■ Pharmacotherapy for Clinical Conditions

The following clinical conditions in autistic disorder and associated psychiatric disorders are potentially drug responsive. For some conditions, the administration of certain drugs has been based on well-documented research, but for others, further research is required. I base these suggestions on my limited clinical and empirical experiences and those of a few other investigators because little research has been done in this field.

In unusual behaviors such as resistance to change, stereotypies, ritualistic and compulsive behaviors, and abnormal attachments, haloperidol, clomipramine, or selective serotonin reuptake inhibitors may be considered (Anderson et al. 1984; Gordon et al. 1993; Mehlinger et al. 1990; Tsai 2001).

In patients with severe hyperactivity, attention-deficit/hyperactivity disorder and impulsivity, clonidine (Ghaziuddin et al. 1992; Jaselskis et al. 1992), guanfacine, or imipramine may be considered in low- or midlevel-functioning autistic individuals with or without other neurological disorders, such as seizure disorders and Tourette's disorder. Haloperidol may be considered for patients who do not respond to clonidine, guanfacine, or imipramine. In high-functioning individuals without other neurological disorders, stimulants may be tried first. Guanfacine, clonidine, and imipramine may be considered in patients who do not respond to stimulants or in those who have other neurological disorders (Tsai 2001).

In autistic patients with tic-like symptoms, haloperidol and pimozide should be tried first because they are more potent than clonidine. Risperidone and fluoxetine have been reported to be effective in the treatment of tic disorders. In some cases, the combination of haloperidol or pimozide with fluoxetine may be needed (Tsai 2001).

For treatment of social withdrawal in people with autistic disorder, naltrexone and fluoxetine may be considered (Campbell et al. 1989; Tsai 2001).

In depressed individuals with autism and a strong family history of unipolar affective illness, tricyclic antidepressants, such as desipramine, or other 5-HT reuptake blockers may be considered (Ghaziuddin and Tsai 1991). Close monitoring of the drug response is critical in these patients because my associate and I and other clinicians have noted that the depressive episode became a hypomanic episode in some patients. Lithium may be the drug of choice in maniclike patients with a family history of bipolar affective illness.

Some autistic individuals may become aggressive and physically attack other people. Some of the aggressive behaviors may be related to frustrations. Most of the aggressive behaviors, however, do not seem to have any clear cause. They are of great concern because of their devastating effect. For individuals who demonstrate frequent aggressive behaviors and who do not respond to behavioral interventions, risperidone or olanzapine may be the drug of choice. Trazodone, carbamazepine, lithium, and propranolol may be considered in patients who do not respond to risperidone or olanzapine treatment (Tsai 2001).

Self-injurious behavior such as head banging, finger, hand, or wrist biting, and scratching of face or extremities may occur in lower-functioning autistic individuals. A selective serotonin reuptake inhibitor or naltrexone may be the drug of first choice (Campbell et al. 1988a; Herman et al. 1987; Tsai 2001). Haloperidol or trazodone may be considered for individuals who do not respond to naltrexone treatment.

Unusual sleeping patterns are common in autistic children. Some children develop complete reversed sleep pattern; that is, they sleep during the day and wake during the night. The key to solve such a problem is to reverse the sleep cycle through a well-planned regimen. Some autistic children seem to need a much longer time to settle down for sleep (i.e., have initial insomnia) and/or need less sleep than most nonautistic children. Children with these sleep disturbances tend to keep the entire family awake every night. Melatonin may be the drug of first choice (Jan et al. 1994; Tsai 2001). Some autistic children may respond to antihistamines, such as diphenhydramine and hydroxyzine, or to clonidine. In other, more severe cases, tricyclic antidepressants, such as imipramine or trazodone (Gualtieri 1991; Tsai 2001), may be considered.

In autistic individuals who develop clear delusions, hallucinations, and bizarre behaviors, including catatonia, an atypical neuroleptic (e.g., risperidone, olanzapine, quetiapine) may be the drug of first choice (Tsai 2001). Other antipsychotic medications, such as haloperidol, thiothixene, and loxapine, are the second-line drugs of choice.

Because the above information was developed mainly from experience with small samples of autistic children treated with psychotropic medications, a great deal of work remains to be done to verify these medications' efficacy in adolescents and adults with autistic disorder.

■ Summary of Treatment

As yet, no single treatment modality can alter the course of autism. Achieving significant treatment goals for autistic children requires comprehensive treatment programs, which include behavior modification and special education in a highly structured environment. Pharmacotherapy may be useful to control behaviors that are not responsive to behavior modification or special-education techniques.

Clinical Course and Prognosis

The general picture of autism is of a disorder with a chronic course. Although social, conceptual, linguistic, and obsessive difficulties frequently persist, they do so in forms that are rather different from those shown in early years. In a 12-year prospective study of 53 autistic children, 68% achieved scores within their original IQ group, 23% moved into higher IQ groups, and 9% moved down to lower IQ groups. The Vineland Adaptive Behavior Scores (VABS) were consistently lower than cognitive scores, and maladaptive behaviors were found to occur with equal frequency in the high-, medium-, and low-IQ groups (Freeman et al. 1991). In a further study, Freeman et al. (1999) observed that autistic subjects improved with age in all domains of VABS. The rate of growth in communication and daily living skills was related to initial IQ, whereas rate of growth in social skills was not. In a group of preschool autistic children reevaluated at a mean age of 10–13 years, Sigman et al. (1999) found little change in the diagnosis of autism but sizable improvements in intellectual and language abilities. Harris and Handleman (2000) reexamined the educational placement of 27 preschool autistic children 4 to 6 years later. It was found that having a higher IQ at intake and being of younger age were both predictive of being in a regular education class after discharge from an intensive treatment program, whereas having a lower IQ and being older at intake were closely related to placement in a special-education classroom.

A small group of autistic children—11% in Rutter and Lockyer's (1967) study and 22% in Gillberg's (1991) study—showed a progressive deterioration during adolescence, characterized by a general intellectual decline. Between 7% and 28% of autistic children who had shown no clinical evidence of neurological disorder in early childhood first developed seizures in adolescence or early adulthood. The seizures were usually major but tended to occur infrequently (Rutter 1977). During adolescence, hyperactivity is often replaced by marked underactivity and lack of initiative and drive. Some autistic people may have increased anxiety and tension. They may have sexual curiosity (Konstantareas and Lunsky 1997) that may lead to socially embarrassing behavior, such as masturbation in public or self-exposure (Van Bourgondien et al. 1997). A Japanese follow-up study of 201 young adults reported that about 31.5% had some marked deterioration during adolescence but that 43.2% had shown marked improvement during that period (Kobayashi et al. 1992). On the basis of data from the California developmental disabilities registry, Shavelle and Strauss (1998) reported that people with autism have an increased mortality risk that increases with age. The mortality ratio for females was strikingly higher than for males.

In an extensive review of follow-up studies of children with psychosis, Lotter (1978) found that between 5% and 17% of autistic children had a good outcome, as assessed from a judgment of overall social adjustment; that is, they had a normal or near-normal social life and satisfactory functioning at school or work. In a Swedish sample, Gillberg (1991) also found that a minority of people with autism had a productive, self-supporting adult life. However, even those with good adjustment generally continued to have difficulties in relationships and some oddities of behavior. In Lotter's study, between one-sixth and one-fourth of autistic people had an intermediate outcome; that is, they had some degree of independence and only minor problems in behavior, but they still needed supervision and could not retain a job. Between 61% and 74% had a generally poor outcome, remaining severely handicapped and unable to lead any kind of independent life. Gillberg (1991) also reported that about two-thirds of the individuals with autism remained dependent on others throughout life. Ballaban-Gil et al. (1996), in a study of 54 adolescents and 45 adults, reported that behavior difficulties continued to be a problem in 69% of the subjects; 90% of both adolescents and adults had persisting social deficits; only 35% achieved normal or near-normal fluency; and only 29% had achieved normal or near-normal comprehension of oral language. Piven et al. (1996b) reported significant change over time in autistic behaviors, generally in the direction of improvement, particularly in communication and social behaviors. Mawhood et al. (2000) found that at about age 23 or 24 years, autistic subjects showed significant improvement in verbal IQ and receptive language scores. However, about 74% had severe social difficulties (Howlin et al. 2000).

Earlier studies showed that between 39% and 74% of autistic people were placed in institutions. These studies, however, monitored autistic people to only about age 30 years. Obviously, placement depends on age and on local patterns of available services. The effect of age on institutional placement is evident in the Rutter and Lockyer (1967) study; at the first follow-up, 44% were so placed; 6 years later, the proportion had risen to 54%. Nonetheless, the University of North Carolina program Treatment and Education of Autistic and Related Communication Handicapped Children (Division TEACCH) has found that when community services are available and provide adequate educational and vocational training, only a minority (i.e., 8%) of autistic individuals are placed in institutions (Schopler et al. 1982). Ballaban-Gil et al. (1996) noted that 53% of 45 autistic adults lived in residential placement; only 11% of adults were employed on the open market, all in menial jobs, an additional 16% were employed in sheltered workshops. Howlin et al. (2000) reported that by age 23 or 24 years, many autistic adults still lived with their parents, few had close friends or permanent jobs, and ratings of social interaction indicated abnormalities in a number of different areas.

Three factors were consistently related to outcome: 1) IQ, 2) the presence or absence of speech, and 3) the severity of the disorder. IQ alone best predicts only those with poor outcome. A high nonverbal score with no subsequent language development is of no predictive value, whereas if language subsequently develops, the nonverbal score is a useful guide to later general IQ scores (Rutter 1970). One additional factor, work/school status, was found to be the best predictor of work or academic performance at follow-up (DeMyer et al. 1973). Other variables have been reported to be significantly associated with outcome (although the correlations are less strong than for the previous three variables): 1) amount of time spent in school, 2) rating of social maturity, 3) rating of social behavior, 4) developmental milestones, and 5) comorbid neuropsychiatric disorders.

Conflicting findings have been reported for several variables in relation to outcome: sex, brain dysfunc-

tion or damage, and the category "untestable child." Factors that were unrelated to outcome included birth weight, perinatal complications, age at onset, history of a period of normal development before onset, late development of seizures, socioeconomic class, broken home, family history of mental illness, and type of treatment.

Research Issues

A range of neurobiological abnormalities associated with autistic disorder has been found, although the replicability of specific findings has not been high. The inconsistent findings may be the result of a number of factors, including the use of different diagnostic criteria for patient selection; failure to control for developmental factors (i.e., many studies included both children and adults); lack of suitable control groups (i.e., most studies used nonretarded rather than mentally retarded control subjects and hence failed to control for concomitant mental retardation found in most of the autistic subjects); failure to control for concomitant medical disorders (particularly central nervous system pathologies); and use of medications that may significantly affect a subject's neurochemical or neurophysiological responses. Nevertheless, the lack of consistent and specific findings can also be viewed as supporting evidence for the existence of many different subgroups within autistic disorder.

Future neurobiological research should do the following: 1) focus on the question of specificity and selectivity within each of the subgroups; 2) avoid combining high-functioning autistic subjects with those who have Asperger's disorder, as many studies did in the past; 3) integrate many levels of inquiry for neurobiological information associated with autism; 4) put more emphasis on developing agreeable, reliable, and valid diagnostic instruments to identify comorbid psychiatric disorders in autistic individuals; and 5) involve collaboration between multiple research centers from various countries to study various races and ethnic groups.

The amount of research into pharmacotherapy for autistic disorder has steadily increased since the 1980s. However, studies have been complicated by various factors, including a tremendous range of syndrome expression, uncommunicative subjects, treatment with multiple medications combined with nonpharmacological interventions, failure to include behavioral measures, and absence of long-term outcome measures.

Future psychopharmacological research should emphasize the use of a randomized, double-blind, placebo-controlled, crossover design; the involvement of multicenters with extensive cross-site training; and the use of uniform diagnostic criteria to study medication treatment in autistic children and adolescents. Communication problems may be solvable by several strategies, including careful questioning of care providers; specially adapted and sensitive rating scales with good clinician reliability; laboratory tests; and physical examinations. The broad heterogeneity of subjects will require that outcome measures be sensitive to individual change over a wide spectrum of treatment response and side effects.

Future psychopharmacological investigations should focus on the efficacy of combined treatments such as pharmacotherapy with behavior therapy or group therapy, because it is highly unlikely that curative medications for autism will be developed in the near future.

References

Adolphs R, Sears L, Piven J: Abnormal processing of social information from faces in autism. J Cogn Neurosci 13:232–240, 2001

Ahlsen G, Rosengren L, Belfrage M, et al: Glial fibrillary acidic protein in the cerebrospinal fluid of children with autism and other neuropsychiatric disorders. Biol Psychiatry 33:734–743, 1993

Alpern GD, Kimberlin CC: Short intelligence test ranging from infancy levels through childhood levels for use with the retarded. Am J Ment Defic 75:65–71, 1970

Aman MG, Van Bourgondien ME, Wolford PL, et al: Psychotropic and anticonvulsant drugs in subjects with autism: prevalence and patterns of use. J Am Acad Child Adolesc Psychiatry 34:1672–1681, 1995

American Academy of Child and Adolescent Psychiatry: Practice parameters for the assessment and treatment of children, adolescents, and adults with autism and other pervasive developmental disorders. J Am Acad Child Adolesc Psychiatry 38(12, suppl):32S–54S, 1999

American Psychiatric Association: Diagnostic and Statistical Manual of Mental Disorders, 3rd Edition. Washington, DC, American Psychiatric Association, 1980

American Psychiatric Association: Diagnostic and Statistical Manual of Mental Disorders, 3rd Edition, Revised. Washington, DC, American Psychiatric Association, 1987

American Psychiatric Association: Diagnostic and Statistical Manual of Mental Disorders, 4th Edition. Washington, DC, American Psychiatric Association, 1994

American Psychiatric Association: Diagnostic and Statistical Manual of Mental Disorders, 4th Edition, Text Revision. Washington, DC, American Psychiatric Association, 2000

Anderson GM, Schlicht KR, Cohen DJ: Two-dimensional high-performance liquid chromatographic determination of 5-hydroxyindoleacetic acid and homovanillic acid in urine. Anal Biochem 144:27–31, 1985

Anderson GM, Freedman DX, Cohen DJ, et al: Whole blood serotonin in autistic and normal subjects. J Child Psychol Psychiatry 28:885–900, 1987

Anderson LT, Campbell M, Grega DM, et al: Haloperidol in the treatment of infantile autism: effects on learning and behavior symptoms. Am J Psychiatry 141:1195–1202, 1984

Ando H, Yoshimura I: Effects of age on communication skill levels and prevalence of maladaptive behaviors in autistic and mentally retarded children. J Autism Dev Disord 9:83–93, 1979

Asarnow RF, Tanguay PE, Bott L, et al: Patterns of intellectual functioning in non-retarded autistic and schizophrenic children. J Child Psychol Psychiatry 28:273–280, 1987

Ashley-Koch A, Wolpert CM, Menold MM, et al: Genetic studies of autistic disorder and chromosome 7. Genomics 61:227–236, 1999

Asperger H: Die autistischen psychopathen im kindesalter (1944), in Autism and Asperger Syndrome. Translated by Frith U. Cambridge, UK, Cambridge University Press, 1991, pp 37–92

Assumpcao FB Jr: Brief report: a case of chromosome 22 alteration associated with autistic syndrome. J Autism Dev Disord 28:253–256, 1998

August GJ, Stewart MA, Tsai L: The incidence of cognitive disabilities in the siblings of autistic children. Br J Psychiatry 138:416–422, 1981

Auranen M, Nieminen T, Majuri S, et al: Analysis of autism susceptibility gene loci on chromosomes 1p, 4p, 6q, 7q, 13q, 15q, 16p, 17q, 19q, and 22q in Finnish mutiplex families. Mol Psychiatry 5:320–322, 2000

Aylward EH, Minshew NJ, Goldstein G, et al: MRI volumes of amygdala and hippocampus in non–mentally retarded autistic adolescents and adults. Neurol 53:2145–2150, 1999

Bailey A, Le Couteur A, Gottesman I, et al: Autism as a strong genetic disorder: evidence from a British twin study. Psychol Med 25:63–77, 1995

Bailey A, Luthert P, Dean A, et al: A clinicopathological study of autism. Brain 121(Pt 5):889–905, 1998

Bailey DB Jr, Mesibov GB, Hatton DD, et al: Autistic behavior in young boys with fragile X syndrome. J Autism Dev Disord 28:499–508, 1998

Baird G, Charman T, Baron-Cohen S, et al: A screening instrument for autism at 18 months of age: a 6-year follow-up study. J Am Acad Child Adolesc Psychiatry 39:694–702, 2000

Baker P, Piven J, Schwartz S, et al: Brief report: duplication of chromosome 15q11–13 in two individuals with autistic disorder. J Autism Dev Disord 24:529–535, 1994

Baker P, Piven J, Sato Y: Autism and tuberous sclerosis complex: prevalence and clinical features. J Autism Dev Disord 28:279–285, 1998

Ballaban-Gil K, Rapin I, Tuchman R, et al: Longitudinal examination of the behavioral, language, and social changes in a population of adolescents and young adults with autistic disorder. Pediatr Neurol 15:217–223, 1996

Barabas G, Matthews WS: Coincident infantile autism and Tourette syndrome: a case report. J Dev Behav Pediatr 4:280–281, 1983

Barak Y, Ring A, Sulkes J, et al: Season of birth and autistic disorder in Israel. Am J Psychiatry 152:798–800, 1995

Baron-Cohen S, Jolliffe T, Mortimore C, et al: Another advanced test of theory of mind: evidence from very high functioning adults with autism or Asperger syndrome. J Child Psychol Psychiatry 38:813–822, 1997

Baron-Cohen S, Ring HA, Wheelwright, et al: Social intelligence in the normal and autistic brain: an fMRI study. Eur J Neurosci 11:1891–1898, 1999a

Baron-Cohen S, Scahill VL, Izaguirre J, et al: The prevalence of Gilles de la Tourette syndrome in children and adolescents with autism: a large scale study. Psychol Med 29:1151–1159, 1999b

Baron-Cohen S, Ring HA, Bullmore ET, et al: The amygdala theory of autism. Neurosci Biobehav Rev 24:355–364, 2000

Barrett S, Beck JC, Bernier R, et al: Autosomal genomic screen for autism: collaborative linkage study of autism. Am J Med Genet 88:609–615, 1999

Bartak L, Rutter M: Differences between mentally retarded and normally intelligent autistic children. J Autism Child Schizophr 6:109–120, 1976

Bartak L, Rutter M, Cox A: A comparative study of infantile autism and specific developmental receptive language disorder. I. the children. Br J Psychiatry 126:127–145, 1975

Barton M, Volkmar F: How commonly are known medical conditions associated with autism? J Autism Dev Disord 28:273–278, 1998

Bass MP, Menold MM, Wolpert, et al: Genetic studies in autistic disorder and chromosome 15. Neurogenetics 2:219–226, 2000

Bauman M: Microscopic neuroanatomic abnormalities in autism. Pediatr 31:791–796, 1991

Bennetto L, Pennington BF, Rogers SJ: Intact and impaired memory functions in autism. Child Dev 67:1816–1835, 1996

Bernard S, Enayati A, Redwood L, et al: Autism: a novel form of mercury poisoning. Med Hypotheses 56:462–471, 2001

Bettelheim B: The Empty Fortress: Infantile Autism and the Birth of the Self. New York, Free Press, 1967

Bettison S: The long-term effects of auditory training on children with autism. J Autism Dev Disord 26:361–374, 1996

Blackman JA, Selzer SC, Patil S, et al: Autistic disorder associated with an iso-dicentric Y chromosome. Dev Med Child Neurol 33:162–166, 1991

Bleuler E: Dementia Praecox oder Gruppe der Schizophrenien (1911). Translated by Zinkin J. New York, International Universities Press, 1950

Bloomquist HK, Bohman M, Edvinsson SO, et al: Frequency of fragile X syndrome in infantile autism: a Swedish multicenter study. Clin Genet 27:113–117, 1985

Bolman WM, Richmond JA: A double-blind, placebo-controlled, crossover pilot trial of low dose dimethylglycine in patients with autistic disorder. J Autism Dev Disord 29:191–194, 1999

Bolton P, Macdonald H, Pickles A, et al: A case-control family history study of autism. J Child Psychol Psychiatry 35:877–900, 1994

Bolton PF, Murphy M, Macdonald H, et al: Obstetric complication in autism: consequences or causes of the condition? J Am Acad Child Adolesc Psychiatry 36:272–281, 1997

Bolton PF, Pickles A, Murphy M, et al: Autism, affective and other psychiatric disorders: patterns of familial aggregation. Psychol Med 28:385–395, 1998

Borgatti R, Piccinelli P, Passoni D, et al: Relationship between clinical and genetic features in "inverted duplication chromosome 15" patients. Pediatr Neurol 24:111–116, 2001

Bormann-Kischkel C, Vilsmeier M, Baude B: The development of emotional concepts in autism. J Child Psychol Psychiatry 36:1243–1259, 1995

Bottini N, De Luca D, Saccucci P, et al: Autism: evidence of association with adenosine deaminase genetic polymorphism. Neurogenetics 3:111–113, 2001

Boucher J, Lewis V, Collis G: Familiar face and voice matching and recognition in children with autism. J Child Psychol Psychiatry 39:171–181, 1998

Boullin D, Freeman BJ, Geller E, et al: Toward the resolution of conflicting findings. J Autism Dev Disord 12:97–98, 1982

Boutin P, Maziade M, Merette C, et al: Family history of cognitive disabilities in first-degree relatives of autistic and mentally retarded children. J Autism Dev Disord 27:165–176, 1997

Brambilla F, Guareschi-Cazzullo A, Tacchini C, et al: Beta-endorphin and cholecystokinin 8 concentration in peripheral blood mononuclear cells of autistic children. Neuropsychobiology 35:1–4, 1997

Bruneau N, Roux S, Adrien JL, et al: Auditory associative cortex dysfunction in children with autism: evidence from late auditory evoked potentials (N1 wave–T complex). Clin Neurophysiol 110:1927–1934, 1999

Buchsbaum MS, Hollander E, Hazenedar MM, et al: Effect of fluoxetine on regional cerebral metabolism in autistic spectrum disorder: a pilot study. Int J Neuropsychopharmacol 4:119–125, 2001

Buitelaar JK, Van Engeland H, de Kogel KH, et al: The adrenocorticotrophic hormone (4–9) analog ORG 2766 benefits autistic children: report on a second controlled clinical trial. J Am Acad Child Adolesc Psychiatry 31:1149–1156, 1992a

Buitelaar JK, Van Engeland H, de Kogel KH, et al: The use of adrenocorticotrophic hormone (4–9) analog ORG 2766 in autistic children: effects on the organization of behavior. Biol Psychiatry 31:1119–1129, 1992b

Buitelaar JK, Dekker ME, van Ree JM, et al: A controlled trial with ORG 2766, an ACTH-(4–9) analog, in 50 relatively able children with autism. Euro Neuropsychopharmacol 6:13–19, 1996

Buitelaar JK, van der Wees M, Swaab-Barneveld H, et al: Theory of mind and emotion-recognition functioning in autistic spectrum disorders and in psychiatric control and normal children. Dev Psychopathol 11:39–58, 1999

Burd L, Fisher WW, Kerbeshian J, et al: Is development of Tourette disorder a marker for improvement in patients with autism and other pervasive developmental disorders? J Am Acad Child Adolesc Psychiatry 26:162–165, 1987

Burd L, Severud R, Kerbeshian J, et al: Prenatal and perinatal risk factors for autism. J Perinat Med 27:441–450, 1999

Campbell M: Treatment of childhood and adolescent schizophrenia, in Psychopharmacology in Childhood and Adolescence. Edited by Wiener JM. New York, Basic Books, 1977, pp 101–118

Campbell M, Perry R, Bennett WG, et al: Long-term therapeutic efficacy and drug-related abnormal movements: a prospective study of haloperidol in autistic children. Psychopharmacol Bull 19:80–83, 1983

Campbell M, Adams P, Perry R, et al: Naltrexone in infantile autism. Psychopharmacol Bull 24:135–139, 1988a

Campbell M, Adams P, Small AM, et al: Efficacy and safety of fenfluramine in autistic children. J Am Acad Child Adolesc Psychiatry 4:434–439, 1988b

Campbell M, Overall JE, Small AM, et al: Naltrexone in autistic children: an open dose range tolerance trial. J Am Acad Child Adolesc Psychiatry 28:200–206, 1989

Campbell M, Anderson LT, Small AM, et al: Naltrexone in autistic children: behavioral symptoms and attentional learning. J Am Acad Child Adolesc Psychiatry 32:1283–1291, 1993

Cantor DS, Thatcher RW, Hrybyk M, et al: Computerized EEG analyses of autistic children. J Autism Dev Disord 16:169–187, 1986

Cantwell DP, Baker L, Rutter M, et al: Infantile autism and developmental dysphasia: a comparative follow-up into middle childhood. J Autism Dev Disord 19:19–31, 1989

Carratala F, Galan F, Moya M, et al: A patient with autistic disorder and a 20/22 chromosomal translocation. Dev Med Child Neurol 40:492–495, 1998

Case-Smith J, Bryan T: The effect of occupational therapy with sensory integration emphasis on preschool-age children with autism. Am J Occup Ther 53:489–497, 1999

Cazzullo AG, Musetti MC, Musetti L, et al: Beta-endorphin levels in peripheral blood mononuclear cells and long-term naltrexone treatment in autistic children. Eur Neuropsychopharmacol 9:361–366, 1999

Celani G, Battacchi MW, Arcidacono L: The understanding of the emotional meaning of facial expressions in people with autism. J Autism Dev Disord 29:57–66, 1999

Chakrabarti S, Fombonne E: Pervasive developmental disorders in preschool children. JAMA 285:3093–3099, 2001

Charman T, Sweettenham J, Baron-Cohen S, et al: Infants with autism: an investigation of empathy, pretend play, joint attention, and imitation. Dev Psychol 33:781–789, 1997

Chess S: Follow-up report on autism in congenital rubella. J Autism Dev Disord 7:69–81, 1977

Chez MG, Buchanan CP, Bagan BT, et al: Secretin and autism: a two-part clinical investigation. J Autism Dev Disord 30:87–94, 2000

Chiron C, Leboyer M, Leon F, et al: SPECT of the brain in childhood autism: evidence for a lack of normal hemispheric asymmetry. Dev Med Child Neurol 37:849–860, 1995

Chudley AE, Gutierrez E, Joycelyn LJ, et al: Outcomes of genetic evaluation in children with pervasive developmental disorder. J Dev Behav Pediatr 19:321–325, 1998

Chugani DC, Muzik O, Rothermel R, et al: Altered serotonin synthesis in the dentatothalamocortical pathway in autistic boys. Ann Neurol 42:666–669, 1997

Chugani DC, Sundram BS, Behen M, et al: Evidence of altered energy metabolism in autistic children. Prog Neuropsychopharmacol Biol Psychiatry 23:635–641, 1999

Chung SY, Luk SL, Lee P, et al: A follow-up study of infantile autism in Hong Kong. J Autism Dev Disord 20:221–232, 1990

Ciesielski KT, Knight JE: Cerebellar abnormality in autism: a nonspecific effect of early brain damage? Acta Neurobiol Exp (Warsz) 54:151–154, 1994

Ciesielski KT, Harris RJ, Hart BL, et al: Cerebellar hypoplasia and frontal lobe cognitive deficits in disorders of early childhood. Neuropsychologia 35:643–655, 1997

Clarke DJ, Littlejohns CS, Corbett JA, et al: Pervasive developmental disorders and psychosis in adult life. Br J Psychiatry 155:692–699, 1989

Cohen DJ, Shaywitz BA, Johnson WK, et al: Biogenic amines in autistic and atypical children: cerebrospinal fluid measure of homovanillic acid and 5-hydroxyindole acetic acid. Arch Gen Psychiatry 31:845–853, 1974

Comings DE, Comings BG: Clinical and genetic relationship between autism–pervasive developmental disorder and Tourette syndrome: a study of 19 cases. Am J Med Genet 39:180–191, 1991

Coniglio SJ, Lewis JD, Lang C, et al: A randomized, double-blind, placebo-controlled trial of single-dose intravenous secretin as treatment for children with autism. J Pediatr 138:649–655, 2001

Connolly AM, Chez MG, Pestronk A, et al: Serum autoantibodies to brain in Landau-Kleffner variant, autism, and other neurologic disorders. J Pediatr 134:607–613, 1999

Cook EH Jr, Leventhal BL, Freedman DX: Free serotonin in plasma: autistic children and their first-degree relatives. Biol Psychiatry 24:488–491, 1988

Cook EH Jr, Rowlett R, Jaselskis C, et al: Fluoxetine treatment of children and adults with autistic disorder and mental retardation. J Am Acad Child Adolesc Psychiatry 31:739–745, 1992

Cook EH Jr, Courchesne RY, Lord C, et al: Evidence of linkage between the serotonin transporter and autistic disorder. Mol Psychiatr 2:247–250, 1997a

Cook EH Jr, Lindgren V, Leventhal BL, et al: Autism or atypical autism in maternally but not paternally derived proximal 15q duplication. Am J Hum Genet 60:928–934, 1997b

Cook EH Jr, Courchesne RY, Cox NJ, et al: Linkage-disequilibrium mapping of autistic disorder. Am J Hum Genet 62:1077–1083, 1998

Courchesne E: A neurophysiological view of autism, in Neurobiological Issues in Autism. Edited by Schopler E, Mesibov GB. New York, Plenum, 1987, pp 285–324

Courchesne E, Yeung-Courchesne R, Press GA, et al: Hypoplasia of cerebellar vermal lobules VI and VII in autism. N Engl J Med 318:1349–1354, 1988

Courchesne E, Lincoln AJ, Yeung-Courchesne R, et al: Pathophysiologic findings in nonretarded autism and receptive developmental language disorder. J Autism Dev Disord 19:1–17, 1989

Courchesne E, Saitoh O, Yeung-Courchesne R, et al: Abnormality of cerebellar vermian lobules VI and VII in patients with infantile autism: identification of hypoplastic and hyperplastic subgroups with MR imaging. AJR Am J Roentgenol 162:123–130, 1994a

Courchesne E, Townsend J, Akshoomoff NA, et al: Impairment in shifting attention in autistic and cerebellar patients. Behav Neurosci 108:848–865, 1994b

Courchesne E, Townsend J, Saitoh O: The brain in infantile autism: posterior fossa structures are abnormal. Neurology 44:214–223, 1994c

Courchesne E, Muller RA, Saitoh O: Brain weight in autism: normal in the majority of cases, megalencephalic in rare cases. Neurology 52:1057–1059, 1999

Couteur AL, Trygstad O, Evered C, et al: Infantile autism and urinary excretion of peptides and protein-associated peptide complexes. J Autism Dev Disord 18:181–190, 1988

Craddock N, Lendon C: Chromosome Workshop: chromosomes 11, 14, and 15. Am J Med Genet 88:244–254, 1999

Creak M, Cameron K, Cowie V, et al: Schizophrenic syndrome in childhood. BMJ 2:889–890, 1961

Creasey H, Rumsey J, Schwartz M, et al: Brain morphometry in autistic men as measured by volumetric computed tomography. Arch Neurol 43:669–672, 1986

Critchley HD, Daly EM, Bullmore ET, et al: The functional neuroanatomy of social behaviour: changes in cerebral blood flow when people with autistic disorder process facial expressions. Brain 123(pt 11):2203–2212, 2000

Croonenberghs J, Delmeire L, Verkerk R, et al: Peripheral markers of serotonergic and noradrenergic function in post-pubertal, Caucasian males with autistic disorder. Neuropsychopharmacology 22:275–283, 2000

Cryan E, Byrne M, O'Donovan A, et al: A case-control study of obstetric complications and later autistic disorder. J Autism Dev Disord 26:453–460, 1996

Cuccaro ML, Wright HH, Abramson RK, et al: Whole-blood serotonin and cognitive functioning in autistic individuals and their first-degree relatives. J Neuropsychiatry Clin Neurosci 5:94–101, 1993

Dahlgren SO, Trillingsgaard A: Theory of mind in non-retarded children with autism and Asperger's syndrome: a research note. J Child Psychol Psychiatry 37:759–763, 1996

Damasio AR, Maurer RG: A neurological model for childhood autism. Arch Neurol 35:777–786, 1978

Damasio H, Maurer RG, Damasio AR, et al: Computerized tomographic scan findings in patients with autistic behavior. Arch Neurol 37:504–510, 1980

Darby JC: Neuropathologic aspects of psychosis in children. J Autism Child Schizophr 6:339–352, 1976

Davidovitch M, Patterson B, Gartside P: Head circumference measurements in children with autism. J Child Neurol 11:389–393, 1996

Davidovitch M, Glick L, Holtzman G, et al: Developmental regression in autism: maternal perception. J Autism Dev Disord 30:113–119, 2000

Davidovitch M, Holtzman G, Tirosh E: Autism in the Haifa area: an epidemiological perspective. Isr Med Assoc J 3:188–189, 2001

Dawson G, Finley C, Phillips S, et al: Reduced P3 amplitude of the event-related brain potential: relationship to language ability in autism. J Autism Dev Disord 18:493–504, 1988

Dawson G, Klinger LG, Panagiotides H, et al: Subgroup of autistic children based on social behavior display distinct patterns of brain activity. J Abnorm Child Psychol 23:569–583, 1995

Deb S, Prasad KB, Seth H, et al: A comparison of obstetric and neonatal complications between children with autistic disorder and their siblings. J Intellect Disabil Res 41 (pt 1):81–86, 1997

De Giacomo A, Fombonne E: Parental recognition of developmental abnormalities in autism. Eur Child Adolesc Psychiatry 7:131–136, 1998

DeLong R, Nohria C: Psychiatric family history and neurological disease in autistic spectrum disorders. Dev Med Child Neurol 36:441–448, 1994

DeLong GR, Teague LA, McSwain Kamran M: Effects of fluoxetine treatment in young children with idiopathic autism. Dev Med Child Neurol 40:551–562, 1998

DeMyer M, Barton S, DeMyer W, et al: Prognosis in autism: a follow-up study. J Autism Child Schizophr 3:199–246, 1973

Denney DR, Frei BW, Gaffney G: Lymphocyte subsets and interleukin-2 receptors in autistic children. J Autism Dev Disord 26:87–97, 1996

Despert JL: Some considerations relating to the genesis of autistic behavior in children. Am J Orthopsychiatry 21:335–350, 1951

D'Eufemia P, Finocchiaro R, Celli M, et al: Low serum tryptophan to large neutral amino acids ratio in idiopathic infantile autism. Biomed Pharmacother 49:288–292, 1995

D'Eufemia P, Celli M, Finocchiaro R, et al: Abnormal intestinal permeability in children with autism. Acta Paediatr 85:1076–1079, 1996

Deykin E, MacMahon B: The incidence of seizures among children with autistic symptoms. Am J Psychiatry 126:1310–1312, 1979

Dunn-Geier J, Ho HH, Auersperg E, et al: Effect of secretin on children with autism: a randomized controlled trial. Dev Med Child Neurol 42:796–802, 2000

Edelson SB, Cantor DS: Autism: xenobiotic influences. Toxicol Ind Health 14:553–563, 1998

Edelson SM, Edelson MG, Kerr DC, et al: Behavioral and physiological effects of deep pressure on children with autism: a pilot study evaluating the efficacy of Grandin's Hug Machine. Am J Occup Ther 53:145–152, 1999

Egaas B, Courchesne E, Saitoh O: Reduced size of corpus callosum in autism. Arch Neurol 52:794–801, 1995

Eggers C: Course and prognosis of childhood schizophrenia. J Autism Child Schizophr 8:21–36, 1978

Eisenberg L, Kanner L: Early infantile autism 1943–55. Am J Orthopsychiatry 26:556–566, 1956

Ek U, Fernell E, Jacobson L, et al: Relation between blindness due to retinopathy of prematurity and autistic spectrum disorders: a population-based study. Dev Med Child Neurol 40:297–301, 1998

Elia M, Musumeci SA, Ferri R, et al: Clinical and neurophysiological aspects of epilepsy in subjects with autism and mental retardation. Am J Ment Retard 100:6–16, 1995

Elia M, Ferri R, Musumeci SA, et al: Clinical correlates of brain morphometric features of subjects with low-functioning autistic disorder. J Child Neurol 15:504–508, 2000a

Elia M, Ferri R, Musumeci SA, et al: Sleep in subjects with autistic disorder: a neurophysiological and psychological study. Brain Dev 22:88–92, 2000b

Fankhauser MP, Karumanchi VC, German ML, et al: A double-blind, placebo-controlled study of the efficacy of transdermal clonidine in autism. J Clin Psychiatry 53:77–82, 1992

Farrington CP, Miller E, Taylor B: MMR and autism: further evidence against a causal association. Vaccine 19:3632–3635, 2001

Fatemi SH, Realmuto GM, Khan L, et al: Fluoxetine in treatment of adolescent patients with autism: a longitudinal open trial. J Autism Dev Disord 28:303–307, 1998

Fein D, Skoff B, Mirsky AF: Clinical correlates of brainstem dysfunction in autistic children. J Autism Dev Disord 11:303–315, 1981

Feldman HM, Kolmen BK, Gonzaga AM: Naltrexone and communication skills in young children with autism. J Am Acad Child Adolesc Psychiatry 38:587–593, 1999

Fernell E, Watanabe Y, Adolfsson Y, et al: Possible effects of tetrahydrobiopterin treatment in six children with autism: clinical and position emission tomography data—a pilot study. Dev Med Child Neurol 39:313–318, 1997

Fidler DJ, Bailey JN, Smalley SL: Macrocephaly in autism and other pervasive developmental disorders. Dev Med Child Neurol 42:737–740, 2000

Findling RL, Maxwell K, Scotese-Wojtila L, et al: High-dose pyridoxine and magnesium administration in children with autistic disorder: an absence of salutary effects in a double-blind, placebo-controlled study. J Autism Dev Disord 27:467–478, 1997a

Findling RL, Maxwell K, Wiznitzer M: An open clinical trial of risperidone monotherapy in young children with autistic disorder. Psychopharmacol Bull 33:155–159, 1997b

Fisman S, Steele M: Use of risperidone in pervasive developmental disorders: a case series. J Child Adolesc Psychopharmacol 6:177–190, 1996

Fisman S, Steele M, Short J, et al: Case study: anorexia nervosa and autistic disorder in an adolescent girl. J Am Acad Child Adolesc Psychiatry 35:937–940, 1996

Flejter WL, Bennett-Baker PE, Ghaziuddin M, et al: Cytogenetic and molecular analysis of inv dup(15) chromosomes observed in two patients with autistic disorder and mental retardation. Am J Med Genet 61:182–187, 1996

Folstein S, Rutter M: Infantile autism: a genetic study of 21 twin pairs. J Child Psychol Psychiatry 18:297–321, 1977

Folstein S, Santangelo SL, Gilman SE, et al: Predictors of cognitive test patterns in autism families. J Child Psychol Psychiatry 40:1117–1128, 1999

Fombonne E: Diagnostic assessment in a sample of autistic and developmentally impaired adolescents. J Autism Dev Disord 22:563–581, 1992

Fombonne E: The epidemiology of autism: a review. Psychol Med 29:769–786, 1999

Fombonne E, du Mazaubrun C: Prevalence of infantile autism in four French regions. Soc Psychiatry Psychiatr Epidemiol 27:203–210, 1992

Fombonne E, Bolton P, Prior J, et al: A family study of autism: cognitive patterns and levels in parents and siblings. J Child Psychol Psychiatry 38:667–683, 1997a

Fombonne E, du Mazaubrun C, Cans C, et al: Autism and associated medical disorders in a French epidemiological survey. J Am Acad Child Adolesc Psychiatry 36:1561–1569, 1997b

Freeman BJ, Ritvo ER, Needleman R, et al: The stability of cognitive and linguistic parameters in autism: a five-year prospective study. J Am Acad Child Psychiatry 24:459–464, 1985

Freeman BJ, Ritvo ER, Yokota A, et al: Autism, forme fruste: psychometric assessments of first-degree relatives, in Biological Psychiatry. Edited by Shagass E, Perris C, Struwe G, et al. New York, Elsevier Science, 1986, pp 1487–1488

Freeman BJ, Rahbar B, Ritvo ER, et al: The stability of cognitive and behavioral parameters in autism: a twelve-year prospective study. J Am Acad Child Adolesc Psychiatry 30:479–482, 1991

Freeman BJ, Del'Homme M, Guthrie D, et al: Vineland Adaptive Behavior Scale scores as a function of age and IQ in 210 autistic children. J Autism Dev Disord 29:379–384, 1999

Gaffney G, Kuperman S, Tsai L, et al: Midsagittal magnetic resonance of autism. Br J Psychiatry 151:831–833, 1987a

Gaffney G, Tsai L, Kuperman S, et al: Cerebellar structure in autism. Am J Dis Child 141:1330–1332, 1987b

Gaffney GR, Kuperman S, Tsai LY, et al: Morphological evidence of brainstem involvement in infantile autism. Biol Psychiatry 24:578–586, 1988

Garber HJ, Ritvo ER: Magnetic resonance imaging of the posterior fossa in autistic adults. Am J Psychiatry 149:245–247, 1992

Garber HJ, Ritvo ER, Chiu LC, et al: A magnetic resonance imaging study of autism: normal fourth ventricle size and absence of pathology. Am J Psychiatry 146:532–534, 1989

Geller E, Yuwiler A, Freeman BJ, et al: Platelet size, number, and serotonin content in blood of autistic, childhood schizophrenic, and normal children. J Autism Dev Disord 18:119–126, 1988

George MS, Costa DC, Kouris K, et al: Cerebral blood flow abnormalities in adults with infantile autism. J Nerv Ment Dis 180:413–417, 1992

Ghaziuddin M, Burmeister M: Deletion of chromosome 2q37 and autism: a distinct subtype? J Autism Dev Disord 29:259–263, 1999

Ghaziuddin M, Butler E: Clumsiness in autism and Asperger syndrome: a further report. J Intellect Disabil Res 42(Pt 1):43–48, 1998

Ghaziuddin M, Tsai L: Depression in autistic disorder. Br J Psychiatry 159:721–723, 1991

Ghaziuddin M, Tsai L, Ghaziuddin N: Clonidine for autism. J Child Adolesc Psychopharmacol 2:1–2, 1992

Ghaziuddin M, Sheldon S, Tsai L, et al: Abnormalities of chromosome 18 in a girl with mental retardation and autistic disorder. J Intellect Disabil Res 37:313–317, 1993

Ghaziuddin M, Alessi N, Greden JF: Life events and depression in children with pervasive developmental disorders. J Autism Dev Disord 25:495–502, 1995

Ghaziuddin M, Zaccagnini J, Tsai L, et al: Is megalencephaly specific to autism? J Intellect Disabil Res 43(pt 4):279–282, 1999

Gillberg C: Asperger's syndrome and recurrent psychosis: a case study. J Autism Dev Disord 15:389–397, 1985

Gillberg C: Outcome in autism and autistic-like conditions. J Am Acad Child Adolesc Psychiatry 30:375–382, 1991

Gillberg C: Endogenous opioid and opiate antagonists in autism: brief review of empirical findings and implications for clinicians. Dev Med Child Neurol 37:239–245, 1995

Gillberg C: Autism and Asperger Syndrome. Cambridge, UK, Cambridge University Press, 2000

Gillberg C, Coleman M: Autism and medical disorders: a review of the literature. Dev Med Child Neurol 38:191–202, 1996

Gillberg C, Svendsen P: Childhood psychosis and computed tomographic brain scan findings. J Autism Dev Disord 13:19–32, 1983

Gillberg C, Svennerholm L: CSF monoamines in autistic syndromes and other pervasive developmental disorders of early childhood. Br J Psychiatry 151:89–94, 1987

Gillberg C, Wing L: Autism: not an extremely rare disorder. Acta Psychiatr Scand 99:399–406, 1999

Gillberg C, Terenius L, Hagberg B, et al: CSF beta-endorphins in childhood neuropsychiatric disorders. Brain Dev 12:88–92, 1990

Gillberg C, Steffenburg S, Wahlstrom J, et al: Autism associated with marker chromosome. J Am Acad Child Adolesc Psychiatry 30:489–494, 1991

Gillberg C, Gillberg IC, Steffenburg S: Siblings and parents of children with autism: a controlled population-based study. Dev Med Child Neurol 34:389–398, 1992

Gillberg IC, Gillberg C, Ahlsen G: Autistic behavior and attention deficits in tuberous sclerosis: a population based study. Dev Med Child Neurol 36:50–56, 1994

Giller EL Jr, Young JG, Breakfield XO, et al: Monoamine oxidase and catechol-O-methyltransferase activities in cultured fibroblasts and blood cells from children with autism and the Gilles de la Tourette syndrome. Psychiatry Res 2:187–197, 1980

Giovanardi Rossi P, Posar A, Parmeggiani A: Epilepsy in adolescents and young adults with autistic disorder. Brain Dev 22:102–106, 2000

Goizet C, Excoffer E, Taine L, et al: Case with autistic syndrome and chromosome 22q13.3 deletion detected by FISH. Am J Med Genet 96:839–844, 2000

Gold N: Depression and social adjustment in siblings of boys with autism. J Autism Dev Disord 23:147–163, 1993

Goldberg MC, Landa R, Lasker A, et al: Evidence of normal cerebellar control of the vestibulo-ocular reflex (VOR) in children with high-functioning autism. J Autism Dev Disord 30:519–524, 2000

Goldfarb W, Levy DM, Meyers DI: The mother speaks to her schizophrenic child: language in childhood schizophrenia. Psychiatry 35:217–226, 1972

Goldstein H, Kaczmarek L, Pennington R, et al: Peer-mediated intervention: attending to, commenting on, and acknowledging the behavior of preschoolers with autism. J Appl Behav Anal 25:289–305, 1992

Goldstein M, Mahanand P, Lee J, et al: Dopamine-beta-hydroxylase and endogenous total 5-hydroxyindole levels in autistic patients and controls, in The Autistic Syndrome. Edited by Coleman M. Amsterdam, The Netherlands, Elsevier/North-Holland, 1976, pp 57–63

Gomez MR: Phenotype of the tuberous sclerosis complex with a revision of diagnostic criteria, in Tuberous Sclerosis and Allied Disorders: Clinical, Cellular, and Molecular Studies. Edited by Johnson WG, Gomez MR. New York, New York Academy of Sciences, 1991, pp 1–7

Goodman R, Minne C: Questionnaire screening for comorbid pervasive developmental disorders in congenitally blind children: a pilot study. J Autism Dev Disord 25:195–203, 1995

Gordon CT, State RC, Nelson JE, et al: A double-blind comparison of clomipramine, desipramine, and placebo in the treatment of autistic disorder. Arch Gen Psychiatry 50:441–447, 1993

Griffith EM, Pennington BF, Wehner EA, et al: Executive functions in young children with autism. Child Dev 70:817–832, 1999

Gualtieri CT: Neuropsychiatry and Behavioral Pharmacology. New York, Springer-Verlag, 1991

Gupta S, Aggarwal S, Rashanravan B, et al: Th1- and Th-2-like cytokines in CD4+ and CD8+ T cells in autism. J Neuroimmunol 85:106–109, 1998

Gutierrez GC, Smalley SL, Tanguay PE: Autism in tuberous sclerosis complex. J Autism Dev Disord 28:97–103, 1998

Hagberg BA, Aicardi J, Dias K, et al: A progressive syndrome of autism, dementia, ataxia, and loss of purposeful hand use in girls: Rett's syndrome—report of 35 cases. Ann Neurol 14:471–479, 1983

Hagerman R: Medical aspects of the fragile X syndrome, in The Fragile X Child. Edited by Schopmeyer BB, Lowe F. San Diego, CA, Singular Publishing Group, 1992, pp 19–29

Hallmayer J, Pintado E, Lotspeich L, et al: Molecular analysis and test of linkage between the FMR-1 gene and infantile autism in multiplex families. Am J Hum Genet 55:951–959, 1994

Hallmayer J, Hebert JM, Spiker D, et al: Autism and the X chromosome. Multipoint sib-pair analysis. Arch Gen Psychiatry 53:985–989, 1996

Halsey NA, Hyman SL, Conference Writing Panel: Measles-mumps-rubella vaccine and autistic spectrum disorder: report from the New Challenges in Childhood Immunizations Conference convened in Oak Brook, IL, June 12–13, 2000. Pediatrics 107:E84, 2001

Handen BL, Johnson CR, Lubetsky M: Efficacy of methylphenidate among children with autism and symptoms of attention-deficit hyperactivity disorder. J Autism Dev Disord 30:245–255, 2000

Hardan AY, Minshew NJ, Keshavan MS: Corpus callosum size in autism. Neurology 55:1033–1036, 2000

Hardan AY, Minshew NJ, Harenski K, et al: Posterior fossa magnetic resonance imaging in autism. J Am Acad Child Adolesc Psychiatry 40:666–672, 2001

Harris NS, Courchesne E, Townsend J, et al: Neuroanatomic contributions to slowed orienting of attention in children with autism. Brain Res Cogn Brain Res 8:61–71, 1999

Harris SL, Handleman JS: Age and IQ at intake as predictors of placement for young children with autism: a four- to six-year follow-up. J Autism Dev Disord 30:137–142, 2000

Hashimoto T, Aihara R, Tayama M, et al: Reduced thyroid-stimulating hormone response to thyrotropin-releasing hormone in autistic boys. Dev Med Child Neurol 33:313–319, 1991

Hashimoto T, Murakawa K, Miyazaki M, et al: Magnetic resonance imaging of the brain structures in the posterior fossa in retarded autistic children. Acta Paediatr Scand 81:1030–1034, 1992a

Hashimoto T, Tayama M, Miyazaki M, et al: Reduced brain-stem size in children with autism. Brain Dev 14:94–97, 1992b

Hashimoto T, Tayama M, Miyazaki M, et al: Brainstem and cerebellar vermis involvement in autistic children. J Child Neurol 8:149–153, 1993a

Hashimoto T, Tayama M, Miyazaki M, et al: Brainstem involvement in high functioning autistic children. Acta Neurol Scand 88:123–128, 1993b

Hashimoto T, Tayama M, Murakawa K, et al: Development of the brainstem and cerebellum in autistic patients. J Autism Dev Disord 25:1–18, 1995

Hashimoto T, Sasaki M, Fukumizu M, et al: Single-photon emission computed tomography of the brain in autism: effect of the developmental level. Pediatr Neurol 23:416–420, 2000

Haznedar MM, Buchsbaum MS, Metzger M, et al: Anterior cingulated gyrus volume and glucose metabolism in autistic disorder. Am J Psychiatry 154:1047–1050, 1997

Haznedar MM, Buchsbaum MS, Wei TC, et al: Limbic circuitry in patients with autism spectrum disorder studied with positron emission tomography and magnetic resonance imaging. Am J Psychiatry 157:1994–2001, 2000

Heh CWC, Smith R, Wu J, et al: Positron emission tomography of the cerebellum in autism. Am J Psychiatry 146:242–245, 1989

Heimann M, Nelson KE, Tjus T, et al: Increasing reading and communication skills in children with autism through an interactive multimedia computer program. J Autism Dev Disord 25:459–480, 1995

Heller T: Dementia infantilis (1930). Translated by Hulse WC. J Nerv Ment Dis 119:471–477, 1954

Hellings JA, Kelley LA, Gabrielli WF, et al: Sertraline response in adults with mental retardation and autistic disorder. J Clin Psychiatry 57:333–336, 1996

Hemsley R, Howlin P, Berger M, et al: Treating autistic children in a family context, in Autism: A Reappraisal of Concepts and Treatment. Edited by Rutter M, Schopler E. New York, Plenum, 1978, pp 371–421

Henderson D, Vandenberg B: Factors influencing adjustment in the families of autistic children. Psychol Rep 71:167–171, 1992

Herault J, Martineau J, Petit E, et al: Genetic marker in autism: association study on short arm of chromosome 11. J Autism Dev Disord 24:233–236, 1994

Herault J, Petit E, Martineau J, et al: Autism and genetics: clinical approach and association study with two markers of HRAS gene. Am J Med Genet 60:276–281, 1995

Hering E, Epstein R, Elroy S, et al: Sleep patterns in autistic children. J Autism Dev Disord 29:143–147, 1999

Herman BH, Hammock MK, Arthur-Smith A, et al: Naltrexone decreases self-injurious behavior. Ann Neurol 22:550–552, 1987

Hermelin B, O'Connor N: Psychological Experiments with Autistic Children. Oxford, UK, Pergamon, 1970

Herzing LB, Kim SJ, Cook EH Jr, et al: The human aminophospholipid-transporting ATPase gene *ATP10C* maps adjacent to *UBE3A* and exhibits similar imprinted expression. Am J Hum Genet 68:1501–1505, 2001

Hier DE, LeMay M, Rosenberger PB: Autism and unfavorable left-right asymmetries of the brain. J Autism Dev Disord 9:153–159, 1979

Hillman RE, Kanafani N, Takahashi TN, et al: Prevalence of autism in Missouri: changing trends and the effect of comprehensive state autism project. Mo Med 97:159–163, 2000

Hingtgen JN, Churchill DW: Differential effects of behavior modification in four mute autistic boys, in Infantile Autism. Edited by Churchill DW, Alpern CD, DeMyer M. Springfield, IL, Charles C Thomas, 1971, pp 185–199

Hirsch E, Marescaux C, Maquet P, et al: Landau-Kleffner syndrome: a clinical and EEG study of five cases. Epilepsia 31:756–767, 1990

Hobson RP, Lee A, Brown R: Autism and congenital blindness. J Autism Dev Disord 29:45–56, 1999

Hollander E, DelGiudice-Asch G, Simon L, et al: B lymphocyte antigen D8/17 and repetitive behaviors in autism. Am J Psychiatry 156:317–320, 1999

Hollander E, Kaplan A, Cartwright C, et al: Venlafaxine in children, adolescents, and young adults with autism spectrum disorders: an open retrospective clinical report. J Child Neurol 15:132–135, 2000

Hollander E, Dolgoff-Kaspar R, Cartwright C, et al: An open trial of divalproex sodium in autism spectrum disorders. J Clin Psychiatry 62:530–534, 2001

Holttum JR, Minshew NJ, Sanders RS, et al: Magnetic resonance imaging of the posterior fossa in autism. Biol Psychiatry 32:1091–1101, 1992

Honda H, Shimizu Y, Misumi K, et al: Cumulative incidence and prevalence of childhood autism in children in Japan. Br J Psychiatry 169:228–235, 1996

Horrigan JP, Barnhill LJ: Ridperidone and explosive aggressive autism. J Autism Dev Disord 27:313–323, 1997

Horvath K, Stefanatos G, Sokolski KN, et al: Improved social and language skills after secretin administration in patients with autistic spectrum disorders. J Assoc Acad Minor Phys 9:9–15, 1998

Horvath K, Papadimitriou JC, Rabsztyn A, et al: Gastrointestinal abnormalities in children with autistic disorder. J Pediatr 135:533–535, 1999

Hoshino Y, Kumashiro H, Yshima Y, et al: The epidemiological study of autism in Fukushima-ken. Folia Psychiatr Neurol Jpn 36:115–124, 1982

Hotopf M, Bolton P: A case of autism associated with partial tetrasomy. J Autism Dev Disord 25:41–49, 1995

Howard MA, Cowell MA, Boucher J, et al: Convergent neuroanatomical and behavioural evidence of an amygdala hypothesis of autism. Neuroreport 11:2931–2935, 2000

Howlin P, Wing L, Gould J: The recognition of autism in children with Down syndrome: implications for intervention and some speculation about pathology. Dev Med Child Neurol 37:406–414, 1995

Howlin P, Mawhood L, Rutter M: Autism and developmental receptive language disorder—a follow-up comparison in early adult life, II: social, behavioural, and psychiatric outcomes. J Child Psychol Psychiatry 41:561–578, 2000

Hsu M, Yeung-Courchesene R, Courchesne E, et al: Absence of magnetic resonance imaging evidence of pontine abnormality in infantile autism. Arch Neurol 48:1160–1163, 1991

Hughes C, Leboyer M, Bouvard M: Executive function in parents of children with autism. Psychol Med 27:209–220, 1997

Hughes C, Plumet MH, Leboyer M: Towards a cognitive phenotype for autism: increased prevalence of executive dysfunction and superior spatial span amongst siblings of children with autism. J Child Psychol Psychiatry 40:705–718, 1999

Hutt C, Forrest SJ, Richer J: Cardiac arrhythmia and behavior in autistic children. Acta Psychiatr Scand 51:361–372, 1975

Ingram JL, Stodgell CJ, Hyman SL, et al: Discovery of allelic variants of HOXA1 and HOXB1: genetic susceptibility to autism spectrum disorders. Tetratology 62:393–405, 2000

International Molecular Genetics Study of Autism Consortium (IMGSAC): A genomewide screen for autism: strong evidence for linkage to chromosomes 2q, 7q, and 16p. Am J Hum Genet 69:570–581, 2001a

International Molecular Genetics Study of Autism Consortium (IMGSAC): Further characterization of autism susceptibility locus AUTS1 on chromosome 7q. Hum Mol Genet 10:973–982, 2001b

Ishikawa-Brush Y, Powell JE, Bolton P, et al: Autism and multiple exostoses associated with an X;8 translocation occurring within the GRPR gene and 3 to the SDC2 gene. Hum Mol Genet 6:1241–1250, 1997

Jan JE, Espezel H, Appleton RE: The treatment of sleep disorders with melatonin. Dev Med Child Neurol 36:97–107, 1994

Jaselskis CA, Cook EH, Fletcher KE, et al: Clonidine treatment of hyperactive and impulsive children with autistic disorder. J Clin Psychopharmacol 12:322–327, 1992

Jocelyn LJ, Casiro OG, Beattie D, et al: Treatment of children with autism: a randomized controlled trial to evaluate a caregiver-based intervention program in community daycare centers. J Dev Behav Pediatr 19:326–334, 1998

Jolliffe T, Baron-Cohen S: The Strange Stories Test: a replication with high-functioning adults with autism or Asperger syndrome. J Autism Dev Disord 29:395–406, 1999

Juul-Dam N, Townsend J, Courchesne E: Prenatal, perinatal, and neonatal factors in autism, pervasive developmental disorder–not otherwise specified, and the general population. Pediatrics 107:E63, 2001

Kalat JW: Speculations on similarities between autism and opiate addiction. J Autism Child Schizophr 8:477–479, 1978

Kamps DM, Leonard BR, Vernon S, et al: Teaching social skills to students with autism to increase peer interactions in an integrated first-grade classroom. J Appl Behav Anal 25:281–288, 1992

Kamps DM, Barbetta PM, Leonard BR, et al: Classwide peer tutoring: an integration strategy to improve reading skills and promote peer interactions among students with autism and general education peers. J Appl Behav Anal 27:49–61, 1994

Kanner L: Autistic disturbances of affective contact. Nervous Child 2:217–250, 1943

Katsui T, Okuda M, Usuda S, et al: Kinetics of H-serotonin uptake by platelets in infantile autism and developmental language disorder (including five pairs of twins). J Autism Dev Disord 16:69–76, 1986

Katz RM, Liebman W: Creatine phosphokinase activity in central nervous system disorders and infections. Am J Dis Child 120:543–546, 1970

Kaye JA, del Mar Melero-Montes M, et al: Mumps, measles, and rubella vaccine and the incidence of autism recorded by general practitioners: a time trend analysis. BMJ 322:460–463, 2001

Kemner C, Verbaten MN, Cuperus JM, et al: Auditory event-related brain potentials in autistic children and three different control groups. Biol Psychiatry 38:150–165, 1995

Kent L, Evans J, Paul M, et al: Comorbidity of autistic spectrum disorders in children with Down syndrome. Dev Med Child Neurol 41:153–158, 1999

Kerbeshian J, Burd L: Case study: comorbidity among Tourette's syndrome, autistic disorder, and bipolar disorder. J Am Acad Child Adolesc Psychiatry 35:681–685, 1996

Kern JK, Miller VS, Cauller PL, et al: Effectiveness of N,N-dimethylglycine in autism and pervasive developmental disorder. J Child Neurol 16:169–173, 2001

Kielinen M, Linna SL, Moilanen I: Autism in northern Finland. Eur Child Adolesc Psychiatry 9:162–167, 2000

Klauck SM, Munstermann E, Bieber-Martig B, et al: Molecular analysis of the FMR-1 gene in a large collection of autistic patients. Hum Genet 100:224–229, 1997a

Klauck SM, Pouska F, Benner A, et al: Serotonin transporter (5-HTT) gene variants associated with autism? Hum Mol Genet 6:2233–2238, 1997b

Kleiman MD, Neff S, Rosman NP: The brain in infantile autism: are posterior fossa structures abnormal? Neurology 42:753–760, 1992

Klin A, Sparrow SS, de Bildt A, et al: A normal study of face recognition in autism and related disorders. J Autism Dev Disord 29:499–508, 1999

Knoblock H, Pasamanick B: Some etiologic and prognostic factors in early infantile autism and psychosis. Pediatrics 55:182–191, 1975

Knott F, Lewis C, Williams T: Sibling interaction of children with learning disabilities: a comparison of autism and Down's syndrome. J Child Psychol Psychiatry 36:965–976, 1995

Kobayashi R, Murata T: Setback phenomenon in autism and long-term prognosis. Acta Psychiatr Scand 98:296–303, 1998

Kobayashi R, Murata T, Yoshinaga K: A follow-up study of 201 children with autism in Kyushu and Yamaguchi areas, Japan. J Autism Dev Disord 22:395–411, 1992

Kobayashi R, Takenoshita Y, Kobayashi H, et al: Early intervention for infants with autistic spectrum disorder in Japan. Pediatr Int 43:202–208, 2001

Koegel RL, Schreibman L, Loos LM, et al: Consistent stress profiles in mothers of children with autism. J Autism Dev Disord 22:205–216, 1992

Koegel RL, Bimbela A, Schreibman L: Collateral effects of parent training on family interactions. J Autism Dev Disord 26:347–359, 1996

Kolmen BK, Feldman HM, Handen BL, et al: Naltrexone in young autistic children: a double-blind, placebo-controlled crossover study. J Am Acad Child Adolesc Psychiatry 34:223–231, 1995

Kolmen BK, Feldman HM, Handen BL, et al: Naltrexone in young autistic children: replication study and learning measures. J Am Acad Child Adolesc Psychiatry 36:800–802, 1997

Kolvin I, Ounsted C, Humphrey M, et al: Six studies in the childhood psychoses. Br J Psychiatry 118:381–419, 1971

Komori H, Matsuishi T, Yamada S, et al: Cerebrospinal fluid biopterin and biogenic amine metabolites during oral R-THBP therapy for infantile autism. J Autism Dev Disord 25:183–193, 1995

Komoto J, Usui S, Hirata J: Infantile autism and affective disorder. J Autism Dev Disord 14:81–84, 1984

Konstantareas MM, Homatidis S: Chromosomal abnormalities in a series of children with autistic disorder. J Autism Dev Disord 29:275–285, 1999

Konstantareas MM, Lunsky YJ: Sociosexual knowledge, experience, attitude, and interests of individuals with autistic disorder and developmental delay. J Autism Dev Disord 27:397–413, 1997

Kuperman S, Beeghly JH, Burns TL, et al: Serotonin relationships of autistic probands and their first-degree relatives. J Am Acad Child Psychiatry 24:189–190, 1985

Lainhart JE, Folstein SE: Affective disorders in people with autism: a review of published cases. J Autism Dev Disord 24:587–601, 1994

Lainhart JE, Piven J, Wzorek M, et al: Macrocephaly in children and adults with autism. J Am Acad Child Adolesc Psychiatry 36:282–290, 1997

Lake CR, Ziegler MG, Murphy DL: Increased norepinephrine levels and decreased dopamine-beta-hydroxylase activity in primary autism. Arch Gen Psychiatry 34:553–556, 1977

Landau EC, Cicchetti DV, Klin A, et al: Season of birth in autism: a fiction revision. J Autism Dev Disord 29:385–393, 1999

Landau WM, Kleffner FR: Syndrome of acquired aphasia with convulsive disorder in children. Neurology 7:523–530, 1957

Launay JM, Bursztejn C, Ferrari P, et al: Catecholamine metabolism in infantile autism: a controlled study of 22 autistic children. J Autism Dev Disord 17:333–347, 1987

Lauritsen M, Ewald H: The genetics of autism. Acta Psychiatr Scand 103:411–427, 2001

Lauritsen M, Mors O, Mortensen PB, et al: Infantile autism and associated autosomal chromosome abnormalities: a register-based study and a literature survey. J Child Psychol Psychiatry 40:335–345, 1999

Laushey KM, Heflin LJ: Enhancing social skills of kindergarten children with autism through the training of multiple peers as tutors. J Autism Dev Disord 30:183–193, 2000

Leboyer M, Philipppe A, Bouvard M, et al: Whole blood and plasma beta-endorphin in autistic probands and their first-degree relatives. Biol Psychiatry 45:158–163, 1999

Leckman JF, Cohen DJ, Shaywitz BA, et al: CSF monoamine metabolites in child and adult psychiatric patients. Arch Gen Psychiatry 37:677–681, 1980

Le Couteur A, Rutter M, Lord C, et al: Autism Diagnostic Interview: a standardized investigator-based instrument. J Autism Dev Disord 19:363–387, 1989

Lekman A, Skjeldal O, Sponheim E, et al: Gangliosides in children with autism. Acta Paediatr 84:787–790, 1995

Lelord G, Laffont F, Jusseaume P, et al: Comparative study of conditioning of averaged evoked responses by coupling sound and light in normal and autistic children. Psychophysiology 10:415–425, 1973

Leventhal BL, Cook EH, Morford M, et al: Clinical and neurochemical effects of fenfluramine in children with autism. J Neuropsychiatry Clin Neurosci 5:307–315, 1993

Levitt JG, Blanton R, Capetillo-Cunliffe L, et al: Cerebellar vermis lobules VIII–X in autism. Prog Neuropsychopharmacol Biol Psychiatry 23:625–633, 1999

Lincoln AJ, Courchesne E, Harms L, et al: Contextual probability evaluation in autistic, receptive developmental language disorder, and control children: event-related brain potential evidence. J Autism Dev Disord 23:37–58, 1993

Liss M, Fein D, Allen D, et al: Executive functioning in high-functioning children with autism. J Child Psychol Psychiatry 42:261–270, 2001

Liu J, Nyholt DR, Magnussen P, et al: A genomewide screen for autism susceptibility loci. Am J Hum Genet 69:327–340, 2001

Lockyer L, Rutter M: A five- to fifteen-year follow-up study of infantile psychosis, III: psychological aspects. Br J Psychiatry 115:865–882, 1969

Lopreiato JO, Wulfsberg EA: A complex chromosome rearrangement in a boy with autism. J Dev Behav Pediatr 13:281–283, 1992

Lord C: Follow-up of two-year-olds referred for possible autism. J Child Psychol Psychiatry 36:1365–1382, 1995

Lord C, Mulloy C, Wendelboe M, et al: Pre- and perinatal factors in high-functioning females and males with autism. J Autism Dev Disord 21:197–209, 1991

Lotter V: Epidemiology of autistic conditions in young children. I. Prevalence. Soc Psychiatry 1:124–137, 1966

Lotter V: Follow-up studies, in Autism: A Reappraisal of Concepts and Treatment. Edited by Rutter M, Schopler E. New York, Plenum, 1978, pp 475–495

Lovaas OI, Schreibman L, Koegel RL: A behavior modification approach to the treatment of autistic children, in Psychopathology and Child Development. Edited by Schopler E, Reichler RJ. New York, Plenum, 1976, pp 291–310

Loveland KA, Tunali-Kotoski B, Chen YR, et al: Emotion cognition in autism: verbal and nonverbal information. Dev Psychopathol 9:579–593, 1997

Lucarelli S, Frediani T, Zingoni AM, et al: Food allergy and infantile autism. Paminerva Med 37:137–141, 1995

MacLean JE, Teshima IE, Szatmari P, et al: Ring chromosome 22 and autism: report and review. Am J Med Genet 90:382–385, 2000

Maddox LO, Menold MM, Bass MP, et al: Autistic disorder and chromosomes 15q11-q13: construction and analysis of a BAC/PAC contig. Genomics 62:325–331, 1999

Maes B, Fryns JP, Van Walleghem M, et al: Fragile-X syndrome and autism: a prevalent association or a misinterpreted connection? Genet Couns 4:245–263, 1993

Maestrini E, Lai C, Marlow A, et al: Serotonin transporter (5-HTT) and gamma-aminobutyric acid receptor subunit beta3 (GABR3) gene polymorphisms are not associated with autism in the IMGSA families. The International Molecular Genetic Study of Autism Concertium. Am J Med Genet 88:492–496, 1999

Malone RP, Cater J, Sheikh RM, et al: Olanzapine versus haloperidol in children with autistic disorder: an open pilot study. J Am Acad Child Adolesc Psychiatry 40:887–894, 2001

Manjiviona J, Prior M: Comparison of Asperger syndrome and high-functioning autistic children on a test of motor impairment. J Autism Dev Disord 25: 23–39, 1995

Marazziti D, Muratori F, Cesari A, et al: Increased density of the platelet serotonin transporter in autism. Pharmacopsychiatry 33:165–168, 2000

Martin A, Koenig K, Scahill L, et al: Open-label quetiapine in the treatment of children and adolescents with autistic disorder. J Child Adolesc Psychopharmacol 9:99–107, 1999a

Martin A, Scahill, Klin A, et al: Higher-functioning pervasive developmental disorders: rates and pattern of psychotropic drug use. J Am Acad Child Adolesc Psychiatry 38:923–931, 1999b

Martin ER, Menold MM, Wolpert CM, et al: Analysis of linkage disequilibrium in gamma-aminobutyric acid receptor subunit genes in autistic disorder. Am J Med Genet 96:43–48, 2000

Martineau J, Barthelemy C, Jouve J, et al: Monoamines (serotonin and catecholamines) and their derivatives in infantile autism: age-related changes and drug effects. Dev Med Child Neurol 34:593–603, 1992a

Martineau J, Roux S, Garreau B, et al: Unimodal and cross-modal reactivity in autism: presence of auditory evoked responses and effects of the repetition of auditory stimuli. Biol Psychiatry 31:1190–1203, 1992b

Martinsson T, Johannesson T, Vujic M, et al: Maternal origin of the dup (15) chromosome in infantile autism. Eur Child Adolesc Psychiatry 5:185–192, 1996

Matsuishi T, Yamashita Y, Ohtani Y, et al: Brief report: incidence of and risk factors for autistic disorder in neonatal intensive care unit. J Autism Dev Disord 29:161–166, 1999

Mawhood L, Howlin P, Rutter M: Autism and developmental receptive language disorder: a comparative follow-up in early adult life, I: cognitive and language outcomes. J Child Psychol Psychiatry 41:547–559, 2000

Max ML, Burke JC: Virtual reality for autism communication and education, with lessons for medical training simulators. Stud Health Technol Inform 39:46–53, 1997

Maziade M, Merette C, Cayer M, et al: Prolongation of brainstem auditory-evoked responses in autistic probands and their unaffected relatives. Arch Gen Psychiatry 57:1077–1083, 2000

Mbarek O, Marouillat S, Martineau J, et al: Association study of the NF1 gene and autistic disorder. Am J Med Genet 88:729–732, 1999

McBride PA, Anderson GM, Hertzig ME, et al: Effects of diagnosis, race, and puberty on platelet serotonin levels in autism and mental retardation. J Am Acad Child Adolesc Psychiatry 37:767–776, 1998

McClelland RJ, Eyre DG, Watson D, et al: Central conduction time in childhood autism. Br J Psychiatry 160:659–663, 1992

McDougle CJ, Price LH, Goodman WK: Fluvoxamine treatment of coincident autistic disorder and obsessive-compulsive disorder: a case report. J Autism Dev Disord 20:537–543, 1990

McDougle CJ, Price LH, Volkmar FR, et al: Clomipramine in autism: preliminary evidence of efficacy. J Am Acad Child Adolesc Psychiatry 31:746–750, 1992

McDougle CJ, Kresch LE, Goodman WK, et al: A case-controlled study of repetitive thoughts and behavior in adults with autistic disorder and obsessive-compulsive disorder. Am J Psychiatry 152:772–777, 1995

McDougle CJ, Naylor ST, Cohen DJ, et al: A double-blind, placebo-controlled study of fluvoxamine in adults with autistic disorder. Arch Gen Psychiatry 53:1001–1008, 1996

McDougle CJ, Holmes JP, Carlson DC, et al: A double-blind, placebo-controlled study of risperidone in adults with autistic disorder and other pervasive developmental disorders. Arch Gen Psychiatry 55:633–641, 1998

McEachin JJ, Smith T, Lovaas OI: Long-term outcome for children with autism who received early intensive behavioral treatment. Am J Ment Retard 97:359–372, 1993

McLennan JD, Lord C, Schopler E: Sex differences in higher functioning people with autism. J Autism Dev Disord 23:217–227, 1993

Mehlinger R, Scheftner WA, Poznanski E: Fluoxetine and autism (letter). J Am Acad Child Adolesc Psychiatry 29:985, 1990

Mesibov GB, Shea V: Social and interpersonal problems of autistic adolescents and adults. Paper presented at the annual meeting of the Southeastern Psychological Association, Washington, DC, March 1980

Mesibov GB, Shea V: Full inclusion and students with autism. J Autism Dev Disord 26:337–346, 1996

Michaelis RC, Skinner SA, Deason R, et al: Interstitial deletion of 20p: new candidate region for Hirschsprung disease and autism? Am J Med Genet 71:298–304, 1997

Miller MT, Stromland K, Gillberg C, et al: The puzzle of autism: an ophthalmologic contribution. Trans Am Ophthalmol Soc 96:369–385, 1998

Minderaa RB, Anderson GM, Volkmar FR, et al: Urinary 5-hydroxyindoleacetic acid and whole blood serotonin and tryptophan in autistic and normal subjects. Biol Psychiatry 22:933–940, 1987

Minderaa RB, Anderson GM, Volkmar FR, et al: Neurochemical study of dopamine functioning in autistic and normal subjects. J Am Acad Child Adolesc Psychiatry 28:190–194, 1989

Minderaa RB, Anderson GM, Volkmar FR, et al: Noradrenergic and adrenergic functioning in autism. Biol Psychiatry 36:237–241, 1994

Minshew NJ, Payton JB, Wolf GL, et al: NMR imaging of autistics: implication for neurobiology (abstract). Ann Neurol 20:417, 1986

Minshew NJ, Goldstein G, Dombrowski SM, et al: A preliminary MRS study of autism: evidence for undersynthesis and increased degradation of brain membranes. Biol Psychiatry 33:762–773, 1993

Moreno-Fuenmayor H, Borjas L, Arrieta A, et al: Plasma excitatory amino acids in autism. Invest Clin 37:113–128, 1996

Mountz JM, Tolbert LC, Lill DW, et al: Functional deficits in autistic disorder: characterization by technetium-99m-HMPAO and SPECT. J Nucl Med 36:1156–1162, 1995

Mudford OC, Cross BA, Breen S, et al: Auditory integration training for children with autism: no behavioral benefits detected. Am J Ment Retard 105:118–129, 2000

Muller RA, Chugani DC, Behen ME, et al: Impairment of dentate-thalamo-cortical pathway in autistic men: language activation data from positron emission tomography. Neurosci Lett 245:1–4, 1998

Muller RA, Behen ME, Rothermel RD, et al: Brain mapping of language and auditory perception in high-functioning autistic adults: a PET study. J Autism Dev Disord 29:19–31, 1999

Muller RA, Pierce K, Ambrose JB, et al: Atypical patterns of cerebral motor activation in autism: a functional magnetic resonance study. Biol Psychiatry 49:665–676, 2001

Murakami JW, Courchesne E, Press GA, et al: Reduced cerebellar hemisphere size and its relationship to vermal hypoplasia in autism. Arch Neurol 46:689–694, 1989

Muris P, Steerneman P, Merckelbach H, et al: Comorbid anxiety symptoms in children with pervasive developmental disorders. J Anxiety Disord 12:387–393, 1998

Murphy M, Bolton PF, Pickles A, et al: Personality traits of the relatives of autistic probands. Psychol Med 30:1411–1424, 2000

Nagamitsu S, Matsuishi T, Kisa, et al: CSF beta-endorphin levels in patients with infantile autism. J Autism Dev Disord 27:155–163, 1997

Narayan M, Srinath S, Anderson GM, et al: Cerebrospinal fluid levels of homovanillic acid and 5-hydroxyindoleacetic acid in autism. Biol Psychiatry 33:630–635, 1993

Nasr A, Roy M: Association of balanced chromosomal translation (4;12)(q21.3; q15), affective disorder and autism. J Intellect Disabil Res 44 (Pt 2):170–174, 2000

Nicolson R, Bhalerao S, Sloman L: 47,XYY karyotypes and pervasive developmental disorders. Can J Psychiatry 43:619–622, 1998

Nordin V, Gillberg C: Autism spectrum disorder in children with physical or mental disability or both, I: clinical and epidemiological aspects. Dev Med Child Neurol 38:297–313, 1996

Nordin V, Lekman A, Johansson M, et al: Gangliosides in cerebrospinal fluid in children with autism spectrum disorders. Dev Med Child Neurol 40:587–594, 1998

Novick B, Vaughn HG Jr, Kurtzberg D, et al: An electrophysiologic indication of auditory processing defects in autism. Psychiatry Res 3:107–114, 1980

Ohnishi T, Matsuda H, Hashimoto T, et al: Abnormal regional cerebral blood flow in childhood autism. Brain 123(Pt 9): 1838–1844, 2000

Ornitz EM: The functional neuroanatomy of infantile autism. Int J Neurosci 19:85–124, 1983

Ornitz EM: Neurophysiology of infantile autism. J Am Acad Child Psychiatry 24:251–262, 1985

Ornitz EM, Ritvo ER: Perceptual inconstancy in early infantile autism. Arch Gen Psychiatry 18:76–98, 1968

Ornitz EM, Ritvo ER: The syndrome of autism: a critical review. Am J Psychiatry 133:609–621, 1976

Otsuka H, Harada M, Mori K, et al: Brain metabolites in the hippocampus-amygdala region and cerebellum in autism: an 1H-MR spectroscopy study. Neuroradiol 41:517–519, 1999

Ozonoff S, Cathcart K: Effectiveness of home program intervention for young children with autism. J Autism Dev Disord 28:25–32, 1998

Ozonoff S, Pennington BF, Rogers SJ: Executive function deficits in higher-functioning autistic individuals: relationship to theory of mind. J Child Psychol Psychiatry 32:1081–1105, 1991

Page T, Coleman M: Purine metabolism abnormalities in hyperuricosuric subclass of autism. Biochim Biophys Acta 1500:291–296, 2000

Panksepp J: A neurochemical theory of autism. Trends Neurosci 2:174–177, 1979

Pascualvaca DM, Fantie BD, Papageorgiou M, et al: Attentional capacities in children with autism: is there a general deficit in shifting focus? J Autism Dev Disord 28:467–478, 1998

Patzold LM, Richdale AL, Tonge BJ: An investigation into sleep characteristics of children with autism and Asperger's disorder. J Paediatr Child Health 34:528–533, 1998

Payton JB, Steele MW, Wenger SL, et al: The fragile X marker and autism in perspective. J Am Acad Child Adolesc Psychiatry 28:417–421, 1989

Perry R, Pataki C, Munoz-Silva DM, et al: Risperidone in children and adolescents with pervasive developmental disorder: pilot trial and follow-up. J Child Adolesc Psychopharmacol 7:167–179, 1997

Persico AM, Militerni R, Bravaccio C, et al: Adenosine deaminase alleles and autistic disorder: case-control and family-based association studies. Am J Med Genet 96:784–790, 2000a

Persico AM, Militerni R, Bravaccio C, et al: Lack of association between serotonin transporter gene promotor variants and autistic disorder in two ethnically distinct samples. Am J Med Genet 96:123–127, 2000b

Persico AM, D'Agruma L, Maiorano N, et al: Reelin gene alleles and halotypes as a factor predisposing to autistic disorder. Mol Psychiatry 6:150–159, 2001

Petty LK, Ornitz EM, Michelman JD, et al: Autistic children who become schizophrenic. Arch Gen Psychiatry 41:129–135, 1984

Pfeiffer SI, Norton J, Nelson L, et al: Efficacy of vitamin B_6 and magnesium in the treatment of autism: a methodology review and summary of outcomes. J Autism Dev Disord 25:481–493, 1995

Philippe A, Martinez M, Guilloud-Bataille M, et al: Genome-wide scan for autism susceptibility genes. Paris Autism Research International Sibpair Study. Hum Mol Genet 8:805–812, 1999

Pierce K, Courchesne E: Evidence for a cerebellar role in reduced exploration and stereotyped behavior in autism. Biol Psychiatry 49:655–664, 2001

Pierce K, Schreibman L: Multiple peer use of pivotal response training to increase social behaviors of classmates with autism: results from trained and untrained peers. J Appl Behav Anal 30:157–160, 1997

Piven J, Palmer P: Psychiatric disorder and the broad autism phenotype: evidence from a family study of multiple-incidence autism families. Am J Psychiatry 156:557–563, 1999

Piven J, Gayle J, Chase G, et al: A family history of neuropsychiatric disorders in adult siblings of autistic individuals. J Am Acad Child Adolesc Psychiatry 29:177–183, 1990

Piven J, Chase GA, Landa R, et al: Psychiatric disorders in the parents of autistic individuals. J Am Acad Child Adolesc Psychiatry 30:471–478, 1991a

Piven J, Gayle J, Landa R, et al: The prevalence of fragile X in a sample of autistic individuals diagnosed using a standardized interview. J Am Acad Child Adolesc Psychiatry 30:825–830, 1991b

Piven J, Tsai GC, Nehme E, et al: Platelet serotonin, a possible marker for familial autism. J Autism Dev Disord 21:51–59, 1991c

Piven J, Nehme E, Simon J, et al: Magnetic resonance imaging in autism: measurement of the cerebellum, pons, and fourth ventricle. Biol Psychiatry 31:491–504, 1992

Piven J, Simon J, Chase GA, et al: The etiology of autism: pre-, peri- and neonatal factors. J Am Acad Child Adolesc Psychiatry 32:1256–1263, 1993

Piven J, Arndt S, Bailey J, et al: An MRI study of brain size in autism. Am J Psychiatry 152:1145–1149, 1995

Piven J, Arndt S, Bailey J, et al: Regional brain enlargement in autism: a magnetic resonance imaging study. J Am Acad Child Adolesc Psychiatry 35:530–536, 1996a

Piven J, Harper J, Palmer P, et al: Course of behavioral change in autism: a retrospective study of high-IQ adolescents and adults. J Am Acad Child Adolesc Psychiatry 35:523–529, 1996b

Piven J, Bailey J, Ranson BJ, et al: An MRI study of the corpus callosum in autism. Am J Psychiatry 154:1051–1056, 1997a

Piven J, Palmer P, Landa R, et al: Personality and language characteristics in parents from multiple-incidence autism families. Am J Med Gene 74:398–411, 1997b

Piven J, Saliba K, Bailey J, et al: An MRI study of autism: the cerebellum revisited. Neurol 49:546–551, 1997c

Piven J, Bailey J, Ranson BJ, et al: No difference in hippocampus volume detected on magnetic resonance imaging in autistic individuals. J Autism Dev Disord 28:105–110, 1998

Plank SM, Copeland-Yates SA, Sossey-Alaoui K, et al: Lack of association of the (AAAT) 6 allele of the GX Alu tetranucleotide repeat in intron 27b of *NF1* gene with autism. Am J Med Genet 105:404–405, 2001

Plumet MH, Goldblum MC, Leboyer M: Verbal skill in relatives of autistic females. Cortex 31:723–733, 1995

Posey DJ, McDougle CJ: The pharmacotherapy of target symptoms associated with autistic disorder and other pervasive developmental disorders. Harv Rev Psychiatry 8:45–63, 2000

Posey DJ, Walsh KH, Wilson GA, et al: Risperidone in the treatment of two very young children with autism. J Child Adolesc Psychopharmacol 9:273–276, 1999

Powell JE, Edwards A, Edwards M, et al: Changes in the incidence of childhood autism and other autistic spectrum disorders in preschool children from two areas of the West Midlands, UK. Dev Med Child Neurol 42:624–628, 2000

Prior MR: Cognitive abilities and disabilities in infantile autism: a review. J Abnorm Child Psychol 7:357–380, 1979

Prior MR, Tress B, Hoffman WL, et al: Computed tomographic study of children with classic autism. Arch Neurol 41:482–484, 1984

Purdon SE, Lit W, Labelle A, et al: Risperidone in the treatment of pervasive developmental disorder. Can J Psychiatry 39:400–405, 1994

Quintana H, Brimaher B, Stedge D, et al: Use of methylphenidate in the treatment of children with autistic disorder. J Autism Dev Disord 25:283–294, 1995

Rao PN, Klinepeter K, Stewart W, et al: Molecular cytogenetic analysis of a duplication in Xp in a male: further delineation of a possible sex influencing region on the X chromosome. Hum Genet 94:149–153, 1994

Realmuto GM, Main B: Coincidence of Tourette's disorder and infantile autism. J Autism Dev Disord 12:367–372, 1982

Reiser DE: Psychosis of infancy and early childhood, as manifested by children with atypical development, I. N Engl J Med 269:790–798, 1963a

Reiser DE: Psychosis of infancy and early childhood, as manifested by children with atypical development, II. N Engl J Med 269:844–850, 1963b

Repetto GM, White LM, Bader PJ, et al: Interstitial duplications of chromosome region 15q11q13: clinical and molecular characterization. Am J Med Genet 79:82–89, 1998

Richdale AL, Prior MR: The sleep/wake rhythm in children with autism. Eur Child Adolesc Psychiatry 4:175–186, 1995

Ricks DM, Wing L: Language, communication and the use of symbols, in Early Childhood Autism. Edited by Wing L. Oxford, UK, Pergamon, 1976, pp 93–134

Rieffe C, Meerum Terwogt M, Stockmann L: Understanding atypical emotions among children with autism. J Autism Dev Disord 30:195–203, 2000

Rineer S, Finucane B, Simon EW: Symptoms among children and young adults with isodicentric chromosome 15. Am J Med Genet 81:428–433, 1998

Ring HA, Baron-Cohen S, Wheelwright S, et al: Cerebral correlates of preserved cognitive skills in autism: a functional study of embedded figures task performance. Brain 122:1305–1315, 1999

Ritvo ER, Freeman BJ: Current research in the syndrome of autism: introduction—the National Society of Autistic Children's definition of the syndrome of autism. J Am Acad Child Psychiatry 17:565–575, 1978

Ritvo ER, Ornitz EM, Walter RD, et al: Correlation of psychiatric diagnoses and EEG findings: a double-blind study of 184 hospitalized children. Am J Psychiatry 126:988–996, 1970

Ritvo ER, Freeman BJ, Mason-Brothers A, et al: Concordance for the syndrome of autism in 40 pairs of afflicted twins. Am J Psychiatry 142:74–77, 1985

Ritvo ER, Freeman BJ, Scheibel AB, et al: Lower Purkinje cell counts in the cerebella of four autistic subjects: initial findings of the UCLA-NSAC autopsy research report. Am J Psychiatry 143:862–866, 1986

Ritvo ER, Freeman BJ, Pingree C, et al: The UCLA–University of Utah epidemiologic survey of autism: prevalence. Am J Psychiatry 146:194–196, 1989a

Ritvo ER, Jorde LB, Mason-Brothers A, et al: The UCLA–University of Utah epidemiologic survey of autism: recurrence risk estimate and genetic counseling. Am J Psychiatry 146:1032–1036, 1989b

Roach ES, Smith M, Huttenlocher P, et al: Report of the diagnostic criteria committee of the National Tuberous Sclerosis Association. J Child Neurol 7:221–224, 1992

Roberts W, Weaver L, Brian J, et al: Repeated doses of porcine secretin in the treatment of autism: a randomized, placebo-controlled trial. Pediatrics 107:E71, 2001

Robinson TW: Homeopathic secretin in autism: a clinical pilot study. Br Homeopath J 90:86–91, 2001

Rodier PM, Ingram JL, Tisdale B, et al: Embryological origin for autism: developmental anomalies of the cranial nerve motor nuclei. J Comparat Neurol 370:247–261, 1996

Roeyers H: The influence of nonhandicapped peers on the social interaction of children with pervasive developmental disorder. J Autism Dev Disord 26:303–320, 1996

Roeyers H, Van Oost P, Bothuyne S: Immediate imitation and joint attention in young children with autism. Dev Psychopathol 10:441–450, 1998

Rogers T, Kalaydjieva L, Hallmayer J, et al: Exclusion of linkage to the HLA region in ninety mutiplex sibships with autism. J Autism Dev Disord 29:195–201, 1999

Rolf LH, Haarmann FY, Grotemyer KH, et al: Serotonin and amino acid content in platelets of autistic children. Acta Psychiatr Scand 87:312–316, 1993

Rosenbloom S, Campbell M, George AE, et al: High resolution CT scanning in infantile autism: a quantitative approach. J Am Acad Child Psychiatry 1:72–77, 1984

Rosenhall U, Nordin V, Sandstrom M, et al: Autism and hearing loss. J Autism Dev Disord 29:349–357, 1999

Ross DL, Klykylo WM, Hitzemann R: Reduction of elevated CSF beta-endorphin by fenfluramine in infantile autism. Pediatr Neurol 3:83–86, 1987

Rossi PG, Parmeggiani A, Bach V, et al: EEG features and epilepsy in patients with autism. Brain Dev 17:169–174, 1995

Rossi PG, Posar A, Parmeggiani A, et al: Niaprazine in the treatment of autistic disorder. J Child Neurol 14:547–550, 1999

Rotman A, Caplan R, Szekeley GA: Platelet uptake of serotonin in psychotic children. Psychopharmacology 67:245–248, 1980

Rumsey JM, Grimes AM, Pikus AM, et al: Auditory brainstem responses in pervasive developmental disorders. Biol Psychiatry 19:1403–1418, 1984

Rumsey JM, Duara R, Grady C, et al: Brain metabolism in autism: resting cerebral glucose utilization rates measured with positron emission tomography. Arch Gen Psychiatry 42:448–455, 1985a

Rumsey JM, Rapoport JL, Sceery WR: Autistic children as adults: psychiatric, social and behavioral outcomes. J Am Acad Child Psychiatry 24:465–473, 1985b

Rumsey JM, Creasy ES, Stepanek IS, et al: Hemispheric asymmetries, fourth ventricular size, and cerebellar morphology in autism. J Autism Dev Disord 18:127–137, 1988

Russell J, Jarrold C, Hood B: Two intact executive capacities in children with autism: implications for the core executive dysfunction in the disorder. J Autism Dev Disord 29:103–112, 1999

Rutter M: Concepts of autism: a review of research. J Child Psychol Psychiatry 9:1–25, 1968

Rutter M: Autistic children: infancy to adulthood. Semin Psychiatry 2:435–450, 1970

Rutter M: Infantile autism and other child psychoses, in Child Psychiatry: Modern Approaches. Edited by Rutter M, Hersov L. Oxford, UK, Blackwell Scientific, 1977, pp 717–747

Rutter M: Diagnosis and definition, in Autism: A Reappraisal of Concepts and Treatment. Edited by Rutter M, Schopler E. New York, Plenum, 1978, pp 1–25

Rutter M: Autistic children growing up. Dev Med Child Neurol 26:122–129, 1984

Rutter M, Lockyer L: A five to fifteen year follow-up study of infantile psychosis, I: description of sample. Br J Psychiatry 113:1169–1182, 1967

Rutter M, Bailey A, Bolton P, et al: Autism and known medical conditions: myth and substance. J Child Psychol Psychiatry 35:311–322, 1994

Sabaratnam M, Turk J, Vroegop P: Case report: autistic disorder and chromosomal abnormality 46, XX duplication (4)p12-p13. Eur Child Adolesc Psychiatry 9:307–311, 2000

Saitoh O, Courchesne E: Magnetic resonance imaging study of the brain in autism. Psychiatry Clin Neurosci 52(suppl):S219–S222, 1998

Saitoh O, Courchesne E, Egaas B, et al: Cross-sectional area of posterior hippocampus in autistic patients with cerebellar and corpus callosum abnormalities. Neurol 45:317–324, 1995

Saitoh O, Karns CM, Courchesne E: Development of hippocampal formation from 2 to 42 years: MRI evidence of smaller areas dentate in autism. Brain 124(pt 7):1317–1324, 2001

Salmon B, Hallmayer J, Rogers T, et al: Absence of linkage and linkage disequilibrium to 15q11-q13 markers in 139 multiplex families with autism. Am J Med Genet 88:551–556, 1999

Sanchez LE, Campbell M, Small AM, et al: A pilot study of clomipramine in young autistic children. J Am Acad Child Adolesc Psychiatry 35:537–544, 1996

Sandler AD, Sutton KA, DeWeese J, et al: Lack of benefit of a single dose of synthetic human secretin in the treatment of autism and pervasive developmental disorder. N Engl J Med 341:1801–1806, 1999

Sandman CA, Barron JL, Chicz-DeMet A, et al: Plasma beta-endorphin and cortisol levels in autistic patients. J Autism Dev Disord 21:83–88, 1991

Sankar DV: Studies on blood platelets, blood enzymes, and leukocyte chromosome breakage in childhood schizophrenia. Behav Neuropsychiatry 2:2–10, 1971

Schain RJ, Yannet H: Infantile autism: an analysis of 50 cases and a consideration of certain relevant neurophysiologic concepts. J Pediatr 57:560–567, 1960

Schifter T, Hoffman JM, Hatten HP, et al: Neuroimaging in infantile autism. J Child Neurol 9:155–161, 1994

Schleien SJ, Mustonen T, Rynders JE: Participation of children with autism and nondisabled peers in a cooperatively structured community art program. J Autism Dev Disord 25:397–413, 1995

Schopler E, Andrews CE, Strupp K: Do autistic children come from upper-middle-class parents? J Autism Dev Disord 9:139–152, 1979

Schopler E, Mesibov GB, Baker A: Evaluation of treatment for autistic children and their parents. J Am Acad Adolesc Child Psychiatry 21:262–267, 1982

Schreck KA, Mulick JA: Parental report of sleep problems in children with autism. J Autism Dev Disord 30:127–135, 2000

Schroer RJ, Phelan MC, Michaelis RC, et al: Autism and maternally derived aberrations of chromosome 15q. Am J Med Genet 76:327–336, 1998

Scifo R, Cioni M, Nicolosi A, et al: Opioid–immune interaction in autism: behavioural and immunological assessment during a double-blind treatment with naltrexone. Ann Ist Super Sanita 32:351–359, 1996

Sears LL, Vest C, Mohamed S, et al: An MRI study of the basal ganglia in autism. Prog Neuropsychopharmacol Biol Psychiatry 23:613–624, 1999

Seshadri K, Wallerstein R, Burack G: 18q-chromosomal abnormality in a phenotypically normal 2½-year-old male with autism. Dev Med Child Neurol 34:1005–1009, 1992

Shaffer LG, McCaskill C, Hersh JH, et al: A clinical and molecular study of mosaicism for trisomy 17. Hum Genet 87:69–72, 1996

Shavelle RM, Strauss D: Comparative mortality of person with autism in California, 1980–1996. J Insur Med 30:220–225, 1998

Sheinkopf SJ, Siegel B: Home-based behavioral treatment of young children with autism. J Autism Dev Disord 28:15–23, 1998

Short AB, Schopler E: Factors relating to age of onset. J Autism Dev Disord 18:207–216, 1988

Siegel BV Jr, Asarnow R, Tanguay P, et al: Regional cerebral glucose metabolism and attention in adults with a history of childhood autism. J Neuropsychiatry Clin Neurosci 4:406–414, 1992

Siegel BV Jr, Nuechterlein KH, Abel L, et al: Glucose metabolic correlates of Continuous Performance Test performance in adults with a history of infantile autism, schizophrenia, and controls. Schizophrenia Res 17:85–94, 1995

Siegel DJ, Minshew NJ, Goldstein G: Wechsler IQ profiles in diagnosis of high-functioning autism. J Autism Dev Disord 26:389–406, 1996

Sigman M, Ruskin E, Arbeile S, et al: Continuity and change in the social competence of children with autism, Down syndrome, and developmental delays. Monogr Soc Res Child Dev 64:1–114, 1999

Simons JM: Observations on compulsive behavior in autism. J Autism Child Schizophr 4:1–10, 1974

Singh VK, Warren RP, Odell JD, et al: Antibodies to myelin basic protein in children with autistic behavior. Brain Behav Immun 7:97–103, 1993

Singh VK, Warren R, Averett R, et al: Circulating autoantibodies to neuronal and glial filament proteins in autism. Pediatr Neurol 17:88–90, 1997

Singh VK, Lin SX, Yang VC: Serological association of measles virus and human herpesvirus-6 with brain autoantibodies in autism. Clin Immunol Immunopathol 89:105–108, 1998

Smalley SL: Genetic influences in autism. Psychiatr Clin North Am 14:125–139, 1991

Smalley SL: Autism and tuberous sclerosis. J Autism Dev Disord 28:407–414, 1998

Smalley SL, Tanguay PE, Smith M, et al: Autism and tuberous sclerosis. J Autism Dev Disord 22:339–355, 1992

Smalley SL, McCracken J, Tanguay P: Autism, affective disorder, and social phobia. Am J Med Genet 60:19–26, 1995

Smith M, Filipek PA, Wu C, et al: Analysis of a 1-megabase deletion in 15q22-q23 in an autistic patient: identification of candidate gene for autism and of homologous DNA segments in 15q22-q23 and 15q11-q13. Am J Med Genet 96:765–770, 2000

Smith T, Eikeseth S, Klevstrand M, et al: Intensive behavioral treatment for preschoolers with severe mental retardation and pervasive developmental disorder. Am J Ment Retard 102:238–249, 1997

Smith T, Buch GA, Gamby TE: Parent-directed, intensive early intervention for children with pervasive developmental disorder. Res Dev Disabil 21:297–309, 2000a

Smith T, Groen AD, Wynn JW: Randomized trial of intensive early intervention for children with pervasive developmental disorder. Am J Ment Retard 105:269–285, 2000b

Sponheim E, Skjeldal O: Autism and related disorders: epidemiological findings in a Norwegian study using ICD-10 diagnostic criteria. J Autism Dev Disord 28:217–227, 1998

Starkstein SE, Vazquez S, Vrancic D, et al: SPECT findings in mentally retarded autistic individuals. J Neuropsychiatr Clin Neurosci 12:370–375, 2000

Stefanatos GA, Grover W, Geller E: Case study: corticosteroid treatment of language regression in pervasive developmental disorder. J Am Acad Child Adolesc Psychiatry 34:1107–1111, 1995

Steffenburg S, Gillberg C: Autism and autistic-like conditions in Swedish rural and urban areas: a population study. Br J Psychiatry 149:81–87, 1986

Steffenburg S, Gillberg C, Hellgren L, et al: A twin study of autism in Denmark, Finland, Iceland, Norway and Sweden. J Child Psychol Psychiatry 30:405–416, 1989

Steffenburg S, Gillberg C, Steffenburg U, et al: Autism in Angelman syndrome: a population-based study. Pediatr Neurol 14:131–136, 1996

Steingard R, Biederman J: Lithium responsive manic-like symptoms in two individuals with autism and mental retardation. J Am Acad Child Adolesc Psychiatry 26:932–935, 1987

Steingard R, Zimnitzky B, DeMaso DR, et al: Sertraline treatment of transition-associated anxiety and agitation in children with autistic disorder. J Child Adolesc Psychopharmacol 7:9–15, 1997

Stevens MC, Fei DH, Waternouse LH: Season of birth effects in autism. J Clin Exp Neuropsychol 22:399–407, 2000

Stone WL, Lee EB, Ashford L, et al: Can autism be diagnosed accurately under 3 years? J Child Psychol Psychiatry 40:219–226, 1999

Strickland D: Virtual reality for the treatment of autism. Stud Health Technol Inform 44:81–86, 1997

Stubbs EG: Autistic children exhibit undetectable hemagglutination-inhibition antibody titers despite previous rubella vaccination. J Autism Child Schizophr 6:269–274, 1976

Sugiyama T, Abe T: The prevalence of autism in Nagoya, Japan: a total population study. J Autism Dev Disord 19:87–96, 1989

Sverd J: Tourette syndrome and autistic disorder: a significant relationship. Am J Med Genet 39:173–179, 1991

Sverd J, Montero G, Gurevich N: Cases for an association between Tourette syndrome, autistic disorder, and schizophrenia-like disorder. J Autism Dev Disord 23:407–413, 1993

Swettenham J, Baron-Cohen S, Charman T, et al: The frequency and distribution of spontaneous attention shifts between social and nonsocial stimuli in autistic, typically developing, and nonautistic developmental delayed infants. J Child Psychol Psychiatry 39:747–753, 1998

Szatmari P, Jones MB, Fisman S, et al: Parents and collateral relatives of children with pervasive developmental disorders: a family history study. Am J Med Genet 60:282–289, 1995

Taira M, Takase M, Sasaki H: Sleep disorder in children with autism. Psychiatr Clin Neurosci 52:182–183, 1998

Takase M, Taira M, Sasaki H: Sleep–wake rhythm of autistic children. Psychiatr Clin Neurosci 52:181–182, 1998

Tanguay PE, Ornitz EM, Forsythe AB, et al: Rapid eye movement (REM) activity in normal and autistic children during REM sleep. J Autism Child Schizophr 6:275–288, 1976

Tanguay PE, Edwards RM, Buchwald J, et al: Auditory brainstem evoked responses in autistic children. Arch Gen Psychiatry 39:174–180, 1982

Taylor B, Miller E, Farrington CP, et al: Autism and measles, mumps, and rubella vaccine: no epidemiological evidence for a causal association. Lancet 353:2026–2029, 1999

Terai K, Munesue T, Hiratani M: Excessive water drinking behavior in autism. Brain Dev 21:103–106, 1999

Thomas NS, Sharp AJ, Browne CE, et al: Xp deletion associated with autism in three females. Hum Genet 194:43–48, 1999

Thorp DM, Stahmer AC, Schreibman L: Effects of sociodramatic play training on children with autism. J Autism Dev Disord 25:265–282, 1995

Todd RD, Ciaranello RD: Demonstration of inter- and intraspecies differences in serotonin binding sites by antibodies from an autistic child. Proc Natl Acad Sci U S A 82:612–616, 1985

Todd RD, Hickok IM, Anderson GM, et al: Antibrain antibodies in infantile autism. Biol Psychiatry 23:644–647, 1988

Tolbert L, Haigler T, Waits MM, et al: Brief report: lack of response in an autistic population to a low dose clinical trial of pyridoxine plus magnesium. J Autism Dev Disord 23:193–199, 1993

Tordjman S, Anderson GM, McBride PA, et al: Plasma androgens in autism. J Autism Dev Disord 25:295–304, 1995

Tordjman S, Anderson GM, McBride PA, et al: Plasma beta-endorphin, adrenocorticotropin hormone, and cortisol in autism. J Child Psychol Psychiatry 38:705–715, 1997

Tordjman S, Gutknecht L, Carlier M, et al: Role of the serotonin transporter gene in behavioral expression of autism. Mol Psychiatry 6:434–439, 2001

Townsend J, Harris NS, Courchesne E: Visual attention abnormalities in autism: delayed orienting to location. J Int Neuropsychol Soc 2:541–550, 1996

Treffert DA: Epidemiology of infantile autism. Arch Gen Psychiatry 22:431–438, 1970

Trygstad OE, Reichelt KL, Foss I, et al: Patterns of peptides and protein-associated peptide complexes in psychiatric disorders. Br J Psychiatry 136:59–72, 1980

Tsai LY: Infantile autism and schizophrenia in childhood, in The Medical Basis of Psychiatry. Edited by Winokur G, Clayton P. Philadelphia, PA, WB Saunders, 1986, pp 331–351

Tsai LY: Pre-, peri-, and neonatal factors in autism, in Neurobiological Issues in Autism. Edited by Schopler E, Mesibov GB. New York, Plenum, 1987, pp 179–189

Tsai LY: Diagnostic issues in high-functioning autism, in High-Functioning Individuals With Autism. Edited by Schopler E, Mesibov GB. New York, Plenum, 1992a, pp 11–40

Tsai LY: Medical treatment in autism, in Autism: Identification, Education, and Treatment. Edited by Berkell DE. Hillsdale, NJ, Lawrence Erlbaum, 1992b, pp 151–184

Tsai LY: Brief report: comorbid psychiatric disorders of autistic disorder. J Autism Dev Disord 26:159–163, 1996

Tsai LY: Sleep problems and effective treatment in children with autism. Proceedings of the Autism Society of America National Conference, pp 183–184, 1997

Tsai LY: Taking the Mystery Out of Medication in Autism/Asperger Syndromes. Arlington, TX, Future Horizons Inc., 2001

Tsai LY, Tsai MC: Using EEG diagnosis to subtype autistic syndrome. Paper presented at the International Conference on the National Society for Children and Adults with Autism, San Antonio, TX, July 1984

Tsai LY, Stewart MA, August G: Implication of sex differences in the familial transmission of infantile autism. J Autism Dev Disord 11:165–173, 1981

Tsai Ly, Stewart MA, Faust M, et al: Social class distribution of fathers and children enrolled in the Iowa autism program. J Autism Dev Disord 12:211–222, 1982

U.S. Department of Health and Human Services: International Classification of Diseases, 9th Revision, Clinical Modification. Washington, DC, U.S. Department of Health and Human Services, 1980

Van Bourgondien ME, Reichle NC, Palmer A: Sexual behavior in adults with autism. J Autism Dev Disord 27:113–125, 1997

van Krevelen DA: Early infantile autism. Acta Paedopsychiatr 91:81–97, 1952

Vincent JB, Herbrick, JA, Gurling HM, et al: Identification of a novel gene on chromosome 7q31 that is interrupted by a translocation breakpoint in an autistic individual. Am J Hum Genet 67:278–281, 2000

Volkmar FR, Cohen DJ: Comorbid association of autism and schizophrenia. Am J Psychiatry 148:1705–1707, 1991

Volkmar FR, Nelson DS: Seizure disorders in autism. J Am Acad Child Adolesc Psychiatry 29:127–129, 1990

Volkmar FR, Szatmari P, Sparrow SS: Sex difference in pervasive developmental disorders. J Autism Dev Disord 23:579–591, 1993

Volkmar FR, Kline A, Siegel B, et al: Field trial for autistic disorder in DSM-IV. Am J Psychiatry 151:1361–1367, 1994

Volkmar FR, Cook EH Jr, Lord C, et al: Autism and related conditions (letter). J Am Acad Child Adolesc Psychiatry 35:401–402, 1996

Wainwright JA, Bryson SE: Visual-spatial orienting in autism. J Autism Dev Disord 26:423–438, 1996

Waldo MC, Cohen DJ, Caparulo BK, et al: EEG profiles of neuropsychiatrically disturbed children. J Am Acad Child Psychiatry 17:656–670, 1978

Warburton P, Baird G, Chen W, et al: Support for linkage of autism and specific language impairment to 7q3 from two chromosome rearrangement involving 7q31. Am J Med Genet 96:228–234, 2000

Warren RP, Margaretten NC, Pace NC, et al: Immune abnormalities in patients with autism. J Autism Dev Disord 16:189–197, 1986

Warren RP, Foster A, Margaretten NC: Reduced natural killer cell activity in autism. J Am Acad Child Adolesc Psychiatry 26:333–335, 1987

Warren RP, Burger RA, Odell D, et al: Decreased plasma concentrations of the C4B complement protein in autism. Arch Pediatr Adolesc Med 148:180–183, 1994

Warren RP, Yonk J, Burger RW, et al: DR-positive T cell in autism: association with decreased plasma levels of the complement C4B protein. Neuropsychobiology 31:53–57, 1995

Warren RP, Odell JD, Warren WL, et al: Strong association of the third hypervariable region of HLA-DR beta 1 with autism. J Neuroimmunol 67:97–102, 1996

Wassink TH, Piven J, Vieland VJ, et al: Evidence supporting WNT2 as an autism susceptibility gene. Am J Med Genet 105:406–413, 2001

Wechsler D: Wechsler Intelligence Scale for Children—Revised. New York, Psychological Corporation, 1974

Weiss SJ: Personality adjustment and social support of parents who care for children with pervasive developmental disorders. Arch Psychiatr Nurs 5:25–30, 1991

Weizman A, Weizman R, Szekely GA, et al: Abnormal immune response to brain tissue antigen in the syndrome of autism. Am J Psychiatry 139:1462–1465, 1982

Werry JS: The childhood psychoses, in Psychopathological Disorders of Childhood, 2nd Edition. Edited by Quay HC, Werry JS. New York, Wiley, 1979, pp 43–89

Westall FC, Root-Bernstein RS: Suggested connection between autism, serotonin, and myelin basic protein. Am J Psychiatry 140:1260–1261, 1983

Williams RS, Hauser SL, Purpura DP, et al: Autism and mental retardation. Arch Neurol 37:749–753, 1980

Willemsen-Swinkels SH, Buitelaar JK, Nijhof GJ, et al: Failure of naltrexone hydrochloride to reduce self-injurious and autistic behavior in mentally retarded adults: double-blind placebo-controlled studies. Arch Gen Psychiatry 52:766–773, 1995

Willemsen-Swinkels SH, Buitelaar JK, van Engeland H: The effect of chronic naltrexone treatment in young autistic children: a double-blind placebo-controlled crossover study. Biol Psychiatry 39:1023–1031, 1996a

Willemsen-Swinkels SH, Buitelaar JK, Weijnen FG, et al: Plasma beta-endorphin concentrations in people with learning disability and self-injurious and/or autistic behavior. Br J Psychiatry 168:105–109, 1996b

Wing L: The handicaps of autistic children: a comparative study. J Child Psychol Psychiatry 10:1–40, 1969

Wing L: A study of language impairments in severely retarded children, in Language, Cognitive Deficits and Retardation. Edited by O'Conner N. London, Butterworths, 1975, pp 87–112

Wing L: Diagnosis, clinical description and prognosis, in Early Childhood Autism. Edited by Wing L. Oxford, UK, Pergamon, 1976, pp 15–64

Wing L: Childhood autism and social class: a question of selection. Br J Psychiatry 137:410–417, 1980

Wing L: Asperger's syndrome: a clinical account. Psychol Med 11:115–129, 1981

Wing L, Gould J: Severe impairments of social interaction and associated abnormalities in children: epidemiology and classification. J Autism Dev Disord 9:11–29, 1979

Wolpert CM, Menold MM, Bass MP, et al: Three probands with autistic disorder and isodicentric chromosome 15. Am J Med Genet 96:365–372, 2000

Wong V: Epilepsy in children with autistic spectrum disorder. J Child Neurol 8:316–322, 1993

Wong V, Wong SN: Brainstem auditory evoked potential study in children with autistic disorder. J Autism Dev Disord 21:329–340, 1991

Woodhouse W, Bailey A, Rutter M, et al: Head circumference in autism and other pervasive developmental disorders. J Child Psychol Psychiatry 37:665–671, 1996

World Health Organization: The International Statistical Classification of Diseases and Related Health Problems, 10th Revision. Geneva, World Health Organization, 1992

Wright HH, Carpenter R, Brennan W, et al: Elevated blood serotonin in autistic probands and their first degree relatives. J Autism Dev Disord 19:397–407, 1989

Yamamoto J, Miya T: Acquisition and transfer of sentence construction in autistic students: analysis by computer-based teaching. Res Dev Disabil 20:355–377, 1999

Yeates-Frederikx MH, Nijman H, Logher E, et al: Birth parents in mentally retarded autistic patients. J Autism Dev Disord 30:257–262, 2000

Yirmiya N, Shulman C: Seriation, conservation, and theory of mind abilities in individuals with autism, individuals with mental retardation, and normally developing children. Child Dev 67:2045–2059, 1996

Yirmiya N, Erel O, Shaked M, et al: Meta-analyses comparing theory of mind abilities of individuals with autism, individuals with mental retardation, and normally developing individuals. Psychol Bull 124:283–307, 1998

Yirmiya N, Pilowsky T, Nemanov L, et al: Evidence for an association with serotonin transporter region polymorphism and autism. Am J Med Genet 105:381–386, 2001

Young JG, Caparulo BK, Shaywitz BA, et al: Childhood autism: cerebrospinal fluid examination and immunoglobulin levels. J Child Psychiatry 16:174–179, 1977

Young JG, Kyprie RM, Ross NT, et al: Serum dopamine-beta-hydroxylase activity: clinical applications in child psychiatry. J Autism Dev Disord 10:1–14, 1980

Young JG, Kavanagh ME, Anderson GM, et al: Clinical neurochemistry of autism and associated disorders. J Autism Dev Disord 12:147–165, 1982

Zanolli K, Daggett J, Adams T: Teaching preschool age autistic children to make spontaneous initiations to peers using priming. J Autism Dev Disord 26:407–422, 1996

Zhong N, Ye L, Ju W, et al: 5-HTTLPR variants not associated with autistic spectrum disorders. Neurogenetics 2:129–131, 1999

Ziatas K, Durkin K, Pratt C: Belief term development in children with autism, Asperger syndrome, specific language impairment, and normal development: links to theory of mind development. J Child Psychol Psychiatry 39:755–763, 1998

Zilbovicius M, Garreau B, Tzourio N, et al: Regional cerebral blood flow in childhood autism: a SPECT study. Am J Psychiatry 149:924–930, 1992

Zilbovicius M, Garreau B, Samson Y, et al: Delayed maturation of the frontal cortex in childhood autism. Am J Psychiatry 152:248–252, 1995

Zilbovicius M, Boddaert N, Belin P, et al: Temporal lobe dysfunction in childhood autism: a PET study. Am J Psychiatry 157:1988–1993, 2000

Zingarelli G, Ellman G, Hom A, et al: Clinical effects of naltrexone on autistic behavior. Am J Ment Retard 97:57–63, 1992

Zuddas A, Di Martino A, Muglia P, et al: Long-term risperidone for pervasive developmental disorder: efficacy, tolerability, and discontinuation. J Child Adolesc Psychopharmacol 10:79–90, 2000

Other Pervasive Developmental Disorders

Luke Y. Tsai, M.D.

As described in Chapter 20 ("Autistic Disorder"), DSM-III (American Psychiatric Association 1980) classification of pervasive developmental disorders (PDDs) had four subtypes: infantile autism, residual autism, childhood-onset PDD and atypical PDD. After the publication of DSM-III, reports suggested that other developmental disorders such as Asperger's disorder (Wing 1981), Rett's disorder (Gillberg 1987), and disintegrative psychosis (Rutter 1985) should also be considered as separate subgroups of PDDs. However, the DSM-III-R (American Psychiatric Association 1987) Work Group on Pervasive Developmental Disorders did not believe there was sufficient evidence for the taxonomic validity of the additional subgroups of PDDs to justify the establishment of separate diagnostic categories, preferring instead pervasive developmental disorder not otherwise specified (PDD-NOS).

This decision generated a number of significant controversies, particularly the concern that further research into the taxonomic validity of the subtypes of PDDs other than autistic disorder would become virtually impossible because all these different disorders are being grouped together in a way such that they all will lose crucial diagnostic distinctions (Tsai 1992). DSM-IV and its Text Revision, DSM-IV-TR (American Psychiatric Association 1994, 2000), now have included the additional diagnostic categories (i.e., Asperger's disorder, Rett's disorder, childhood disintegrative disorder) as subtypes of PDDs. PDD-NOS is retained as another subtype of PDDs, with an emphasis that PDDNOS also includes atypical autism.

Asperger's Disorder

■ Definition and Diagnostic Criteria

Asperger's disorder was first described in 1944 by Hans Asperger, a Viennese pediatrician. Asperger regarded the syndrome he described as a personality disorder, and he used the term *autistic psychopathy*. According to Asperger's observation, individuals with Asperger's disorder usually began to speak at approximately the same time as children without this disorder. A full command of grammar was acquired sooner or later. The child might have difficulty in using pronouns correctly. The content of speech was usually abnormal and pedantic and consisted of lengthy disquisitions on favorite subjects. Often a word or phrase was repeated over and over again in a stereotyped fashion. Other features he described were impaired two-way social interaction, totally ignoring demands of the environment, repetitive and stereotyped play, and isolated areas of interests. Asperger observed these children talking back to or sassing teachers, verbally abusing other children, hitting other children, and lashing out and knocking objects over. These children seemed to act out to gain pleasure from their actions, with no regard for the feelings of others or the consequences of their actions. Asperger believed that the condition was never recognized in infancy and early childhood and that those with the syndrome had excellent, logical abstract thinking and were capable of originality and creativity in chosen fields.

Asperger's disorder was unknown in the English literature until Wing (1981) published an influential review and series of case reports. Whereas speech was less commonly delayed in the patients reported on by Asperger (1944/1991), Wing (1981) observed that half of her sample of 34 patients with Asperger's disorder had been slow to begin talking. Wing also found that careful questioning often elicited a history of a lack of communication behaviors in infancy and that the apparent originality and special abilities were best explained by reliance on rote memory skills. Wing suggested that Asperger's disorder be considered as a part of the "autistic continuum." She believed that Asperger's disorder could be a mild variant of autism in relatively bright children. Both DSM-III and DSM-III-R adopted Wing's (1981) view of Asperger's disorder and did not offer any specific definition and diagnostic criteria for it. Tantam (1988) proposed that the term *Asperger's syndrome* be used to refer to individuals without cognitive and language delays but who have severely impaired social understanding and reciprocity, pragmatic difficulties, and unusual circumscribed interests. The proposal has been adopted by the *International Statistical Classification of Diseases and Related Health Problems*, 10th Revision (ICD-10; World Health Organization 1992), DSM-IV, and DSM-IV-TR diagnostic schemes, although the term *Asperger's disorder* is being used as the diagnostic category (Table 21–1).

The validity of Asperger's disorder as a distinct subtype of PDD continues to be the topic of considerable debate. Some researchers continue to believe that Asperger's disorder is better regarded as the highest-functioning end of the PDD continuum, rather than as a valid subtype of PDD (Kurita 1997; Mayes et al. 2001; Miller and Ozonoff 1997; Myhr 1998; Prior et al. 1998), although others believe that subtypes of PDD, including Asperger's disorder, can be identified on the basis of variables relatively independent of the defining characteristics (Ehlers et al. 1997; Ghaziuddin et al. 1995a; Klin et al. 1995; Ramberg et al. 1996; Szatmari et al. 1995; Ziatas et al. 1998).

The following information on Asperger's disorder must be viewed cautiously because it is derived from studies using diagnostic criteria that cannot ensure complete separation of Asperger's disorder and higher-functioning autistic disorder or atypical autism. In fact, Gillberg (1989, p. 529) admitted that "despite the diagnostic criteria used, it could be merely my own clinical notion that Asperger's syndrome seemed to be a more appropriate label in some cases and infantile autism in others." Many studies quoted in this chapter combined individuals with autistic disorder and those

Table 21–1. DSM-IV-TR diagnostic criteria for Asperger's disorder

A. Qualitative impairment in social interaction, as manifested by at least two of the following:
  (1) marked impairment in the use of multiple nonverbal behaviors such as eye-to-eye gaze, facial expression, body postures, and gestures to regulate social interaction
  (2) failure to develop peer relationships appropriate to developmental level
  (3) a lack of spontaneous seeking to share enjoyment, interests, or achievements with other people (e.g., by a lack of showing, bringing, or pointing out objects of interest to other people)
  (4) lack of social or emotional reciprocity
B. Restricted repetitive and stereotyped patterns of behavior, interests, and activities, as manifested by at least one of the following:
  (1) encompassing preoccupation with one or more stereotyped and restricted patterns of interest that is abnormal either in intensity or focus
  (2) apparently inflexible adherence to specific, nonfunctional routines or rituals
  (3) stereotyped and repetitive motor mannerisms (e.g., hand or finger flapping or twisting, or complex whole-body movements)
  (4) persistent preoccupation with parts of objects
C. The disturbance causes clinically significant impairment in social, occupational, or other important areas of functioning.
D. There is no clinically significant general delay in language (e.g., single words used by age 2 years, communicative phrases used by age 3 years).
E. There is no clinically significant delay in cognitive development or in the development of age-appropriate self-help skills, adaptive behavior (other than in social interaction), and curiosity about the environment in childhood.
F. Criteria are not met for another specific pervasive developmental disorder or schizophrenia.

Source. Reprinted from the *Diagnostic and Statistical Manual of Mental Disorders*, 4th Edition, Text Revision. Washington, DC, American Psychiatric Association, 2000. Copyright 2000, American Psychiatric Association. Used with permission.

with Asperger's disorder into one group to be compared with other control groups.

■ Clinical Findings

Some young children with Asperger's disorder precociously learn numbers, letters, and decoding words.

They are interested in human relationships and like to be with people but are unable to carry through social interactions with sufficient success to make relationships easy. They have been described as approaching others only to have their needs met, having a very clumsy social approach, engaging in one-sided social interactions, and having difficulty sensing or being detached from the feelings of others (Szatmari et al. 1989). Using standardized interviewer-rated assessment of social functioning, Green et al. (2000) noted severe impairment in practical social functioning despite good cognitive ability and no significant early language delay in 20 male adolescents with Asperger's disorder.

Children with Asperger's disorder like to talk. However, their speech may be marked by poor prosody, frequent abnormalities in inflection (either flat and monotonous or exaggerated), and conversation often described as stilted, gauche, thought disordered, or centered on preoccupying idiosyncratic interests. Ghaziuddin and Gerstein (1996) reported that pedantic speech is quite common in adolescents with Asperger's disorder. Szatmari et al. (1989) noted that children with Asperger's disorder have markedly impaired nonverbal expression and limited use of gestures to communicate.

On standardized neurocognitive measures, children with Asperger's disorder showed significant impairments on subtests for both verbal IQ (about 86) and performance IQ (about 88) (Szatmari et al. 1990). They performed quite well on tests requiring good rote memory, but their scores showed deficits on tests that depended on abstract concepts or sequencing in time (Wing 1981). On the basis of results of the Rorschach inkblot test, subjects with Asperger's disorder seemed to have greater levels of disorganized thinking, appeared to have more complex inner lives involving elaborate fantasies, and tended to be more focused on their internal experience than subjects with higher-functioning autistic disorder (Ghaziuddin et al. 1995a).

Some investigators emphasize delayed motor milestones and motor clumsiness and argue for including these features as diagnostic criteria. Other investigators, however, question the diagnostic validity and reliability of these clinical features as they had been defined in the literature (Ghaziuddin and Butler 1998; Ghaziuddin et al. 1994). Manjiviona and Prior (1995) compared the motor impairment levels of children with Asperger's disorder and children with high-func-tioning autistic disorder using a standardized test, the Test of Motor Impairment—Henderson Revision. The two groups did not differ on either total or subscale impairment scores. About 50% of children with Asperger's disorder and 67% of children with autistic disorder showed a clinically significant level of motor impairment.

Patients with Asperger's disorder may have an increased risk for being underweight and having disturbed eating behavior (Hebebrand et al. 1997; Sobanski et al. 1999).

■ Comorbid Psychiatric Disorders

Other psychiatric disorders such as Tourette's disorder (Berthier et al. 1993; Kadesjo and Gillberg 2000; Marriage et al. 1993; Ringman and Jankovic 2000; Searcy et al. 2000), attention-deficit/hyperactivity disorder (Ghaziuddin et al. 1998), affective illness or depression (Ghaziuddin et al. 1998; Tantam 1988, 1991; Wing 1981), anxiety disorder (Tantam 1991), obsessive-compulsive disorder (Tantam 1991), and schizophrenia (Tantam 1991) have been associated with Asperger's disorder.

The etiological meaning of these associations is not yet clear. Comorbid conditions may be markers for underlying neurobiological disorders, so there is a great need for in-depth study into this area.

■ Differential Diagnosis

Autistic Disorder

The differential diagnosis between high-functioning autistic disorder (see also Chapter 20, "Autistic Disorder," in this volume) or atypical autism and Asperger's disorder may or may not be made easily, depending on how the conditions are defined. On the one hand, if one adheres to the current DSM-IV-TR definition of Asperger's disorder that emphasizes a lack of a general delay in language development, individuals with Asperger's disorder should be easily differentiated from those with autistic disorder or atypical autism, because by definition these latter individuals all should have a history of delayed speech development. On the other hand, Wing's (1981) and Gillberg and Gillberg's (1989) definitions of Asperger's disorder do not consider language delay as a critical exclusion criterion, nor do some other investigators (Mayes et al. 2001; Tsai 2000).

The DSM-IV-TR definition of Asperger's disorder specifies intact cognitive function. By this criterion, the differential diagnosis between Asperger's disorder and autistic disorder with an IQ below 70 should not be difficult to make. However, some individuals with clinical features of Asperger's disorder and mild mental retardation have been noted (Asperger 1944/1991; Gillberg and Gillberg 1989; Tsai 2000), clouding the differential diagnosis.

The following findings from clinical studies may be helpful in differentiating Asperger's disorder and autistic disorder:

- Individuals with Asperger's disorder and people with high-functioning autistic disorder or atypical autism differ in their ability to decode nonverbal social information and in their use of vocal intonation to communicate effectively (Szatmari et al. 1989).
- Neuropsychological profiles also can be used to differentiate between Asperger's disorder and high-functioning autistic disorder (e.g., Asperger's disorder may be associated with higher verbal IQ than found in high-functioning autism) (Klin et al. 1995; Ramberg et al. 1996).
- On the Wechsler Intelligence Scale for Children—Revised, the Asperger's disorder group had good verbal ability and troughs on Object Assembly and Coding, whereas the autistic disorder group had a peak on Block Design (Ehlers et al. 1997).
- On the Rorschach inkblot test, adolescents with Asperger's disorder were observed as having higher levels of disorganized thinking than adolescents with high-functioning autistic disorder. The Asperger group also tended to have more individuals classified as "introversive" with more complex inner lives involving elaborate fantasies (Ghaziuddin et al. 1995a).
- On false belief, belief term comprehension, and belief term expression tasks, the Asperger's disorder group performed better than the autistic group (Ziatas et al. 1998).
- As described above, individuals with Asperger's disorder tend to be argumentative and aggressive and have a condescending attitude, features very rarely seen in individuals with autistic disorder.

Oppositional Defiant Disorder

Individuals with oppositional defiant disorder (see also Chapter 27, "Conduct Disorder and Oppositional Defiant Disorder," in this volume) have a pattern of recurrent negative, defiant, disobedient, and hostile behavior toward authority figures or peers. They tend to have many of the following behaviors: anger, argumentativeness, defiance toward and noncompliance with the requests or rules of adults, deliberately doing things that will annoy other people, often blaming others, being irritable and spiteful or vindictive (American Psychiatric Association 1994). Many of these behaviors also are present in Asperger's disorder, making it sometimes difficult to differentiate between the two disorders. However, people with Asperger's disorder also tend to have pedantic, tangential, and circumstantial speech; unusual interests in certain topics or activities; and unusual neuropsychological profiles, as described above. Future research should identify neurobiological markers that can reliably differentiate between these two disorders.

Affective Disorders

When prepubertal children develop Asperger's disorder, not infrequently the main features are mood-related symptoms or behaviors (see also Chapter 24, "Mood Disorders in Prepubertal Children," and Chapter 25, "Mood Disorders in Adolescents," in this volume). They tend to have quick and frequent mood swings when things are not under their control. They can become angry and aggressive. These symptoms tend to be interpreted as the irritability of a depressive disorder. On the other hand, their condescending attitude easily can be seen as grandiosity, and their pedantic talks about their special interests can be viewed as pressured speech. Clinically, it is not unusual that prepubertal children receive a diagnosis of "mood disorder" before they receive the diagnosis of Asperger's disorder. Many of these children have failed to respond to several medications for mood disorder. It is unclear whether these "mood features" should be considered as a part of Asperger's disorder or instead as features of comorbid affective disorder. The frequency and interval of the mood swings are quite variable and can be daily for many years. The pedantic speech and condescending attitude also present daily for many years. Affective disorders tend to be episodic. Nonetheless, there are individuals with Asperger's disorder who also develop clear-cut affective disorders.

Schizophrenia

Individuals with schizophrenia in childhood (see also Chapter 23, "Schizophrenia and Psychotic Disorders," in this volume) usually have a rather clear deterioration of daily functioning. Other features such as thought disorder, delusions, and hallucinations also are present in schizophrenia. Asperger's disorder usually has an early onset, but those children who have it make steady developmental progress. Although some case reports indicate that individuals with Asperger's disorder may be at greater risk for developing a thought disorder (Volkmar et al. 1988), no delusions or hallucinations, as seen in schizophrenia, are present. The incidence of schizophrenia or other psychoses is not increased in family members of subjects with Asperger's disorder. Nonetheless, some individuals with Asperger's disorder may develop schizophrenia as a comorbid disorder (Tantam 1991).

Schizoid Personality or Schizotypal Personality

It may be very difficult to differentiate individuals with Asperger's disorder from children who later develop schizoid personality disorder or schizotypal personality disorder, or from adults with schizoid personality disorder or schizotypal personality disorder whose childhood history is unclear or unavailable. Nonetheless, individuals with Asperger's disorder have more severe impairment in social interaction, emotional reciprocity, and communication skills and have more stereotyped behaviors and unusual interests. Individuals with Asperger's disorder also tend to be argumentative and aggressive.

Obsessive-Compulsive Disorder

Asperger's disorder and obsessive-compulsive disorder (see also Chapter 30, "Obsessive-Compulsive Disorder," in this volume) share repetitive and stereotyped patterns of behavior. In contrast to obsessive-compulsive disorder, Asperger's disorder is characterized by a more severely impaired social interaction and a more restricted pattern of interests and activities. Although most individuals with Asperger's disorder have normal language development, they tend to have pedantic, tangential, and circumstantial speech. They also have significant difficulties in the pragmatics of communication.

■ Epidemiology

Prevalence

Information on the prevalence of Asperger's disorder is somewhat limited. In the epidemiological study carried out by Wing and Gould (1979) in the United Kingdom, the prevalence was 0.6 per 10,000 for children with a combination of Asperger's disorder and mild mental retardation. An additional 1.1 per 10,000 children had been described as autistic in early life but later showed features of Asperger's disorder.

In a Swedish epidemiological study (Gillberg and Gillberg 1989) among children with normal intelligence, prevalence rates of 10–26 per 10,000 were considered minimum figures. Another 0.4 per 10,000 Swedish teenagers had the combination of Asperger's disorder and mild mental retardation. Ehlers and Gillberg (1993) conducted a total population study of Asperger's disorder by using a two-stage procedure. With Gillberg's criteria, the study showed a minimum prevalence of 36 per 10,000 Swedish children (age 7–16 years) and a male-to-female ratio of 4:1. When children with suspected and possible Asperger's disorder were included, the prevalence rose to 71 per 10,000 children and the male-to-female ratio dropped to 2.3:1. These rates might have been lower if DSM-IV-TR criteria for Asperger's disorder were applied to the total population sample, because the DSM-IV-TR diagnostic criteria for Asperger's disorder are more stringent than those used by Ehlers and Gillberg (1993).

Sex Ratio

Boys outnumber girls in all the studies of Asperger's disorder. The current ratio has ranged from 3.8 to 10.5 boys to every girl (Szatmari et al. 1990; Wing 1981).

Social Class

There seems to be a trend toward greater prevalence in higher social classes. Wing (1981), however, also pointed out that the parents from higher social classes tend to have a special interest in Asperger's disorder and, hence, would make an effort to seek further information or service from special clinics.

■ Etiology

Birth Factors

Nearly half of the patients seen by Wing (1981) had a history of pre-, peri-, or postnatal complications such as anoxia at birth. However, other investigators reported that the rate of complications during pregnancy or the neonatal period in the patients with Asperger's disorder was about the same as that in the control group (Ghaziuddin et al. 1995b; Szatmari et al. 1989).

Genetic Factors

Asperger (1944/1991) considered the syndrome to have a genetic etiology. He reported that its characteristics tended to occur in families, especially in fathers, of those with the syndrome. Wing (1981) noted that 5 of 16 fathers and 2 of 24 mothers of children with Asperger's disorder had behavior resembling that found in Asperger's disorder. Gillberg (1989) reported that fathers often had very similar clinical features to those of their sons with Asperger's disorder. The 28 patients with Asperger's disorder in the study by Szatmari et al. (1989) came from 26 families. These patients included a pair of identical twins and another pair who were brothers. A fifth child with Asperger's disorder had a retarded autistic brother; another subject had a sister with schizophrenia. At this time the evidence for genetic factors is only suggestive.

Neurological Factors

No consistent or particular neurological factors have been identified, except that motor clumsiness seemed to be a fairly common feature (Manjiviona and Prior 1995).

Neurophysiological Factors

In the series of 23 Swedish children with Asperger's disorder (Gillberg 1989), 5 of the 20 boys examined with auditory brainstem response had a prolonged brainstem transmission time (I–V interval). Six of the 21 children examined with electroencephalography (EEG) had abnormal waking-state electroencephalographic findings.

Godbout et al. (2000) investigated sleep patterns in eight patients with Asperger's disorder and noted decreased sleep time in the first two-thirds of the night, increased number of shifts into rapid eye movement (REM) sleep from a waking epoch, signs of REM sleep disruption, and decreased electroencephalographic sleep spindles. It is speculated that defective sleep control systems may be associated with the clinical picture of Asperger disorder.

Neuroanatomical Factors

Eighteen children with Asperger's disorder in Gillberg's (1989) study were examined with computed tomography (CT) scans. Three of the 18 children had slight or moderate atrophy of the brain (internal, frontal-general, and occipital). Jones and Kerwin (1990) reported left temporal lobe damage seen in a CT scan of an adult with Asperger's disorder. Berthier et al. (1990) reported a CT study in two patients with Asperger's disorder. One patient had left frontal macrogyria; the other had bilateral opercular polymicrogyria. Ozbayrak et al. (1991) reported a cerebral blood flow study with left occipital hypoperfusion shown in single-photon emission computed tomography (SPECT) of a patient with Asperger's disorder. In a magnetic resonance imaging (MRI) study of seven males with concurrent Asperger's disorder and Tourette's disorder and nine age-matched males with Tourette's disorder, five males in the former group and one male from the latter group had abnormal findings on MRI scans suggesting cortical and subcortical abnormalities (Berthier et al. 1993).

Using functional magnetic resonance imaging (fMRI) to study the superior temporal gyrus and amygdala function in patients with Asperger's disorder, Baron-Cohen et al. (1999) reported findings suggesting deficits in amygdala function in Asperger's disorder. When fMRI was used to investigate the activation pattern during a task involving social judgment, 4 of 9 children with Asperger's disorder did not show signal intensity change, whereas all 8 control subjects did (Oktem et al. 2001). Critchley et al. (2000) reported that subjects with autistic spectrum disorder (i.e., autism and Asperger's syndrome) differed significantly from controls in the fMRI activity of cerebellar, mesolimbic, and temporal lobe cortical regions of the brain when consciously and unconsciously processing facial emotions. Schultz et al. (2000) noted abnormal ventral temporal cortical fMRI activity during face discrimination among individuals with autism or Asperger's disorder.

A positron emission tomography (PET) study of five patients with Asperger's disorder noted findings that suggest that a highly circumscribed region of left medial prefrontal cortex may be involved in Asperger's disorder (Happe et al. 1996)

Neuropsychological Factors

Theory of mind (the ability to attribute mental states to others) tests have been used to investigate possible causes of Asperger disorder. Individuals with Asperger's disorder were noted to have subtle mind-reading deficits (Baron-Cohen et al. 1997); to have impaired local coherence (Jolliffe and Baron-Cohen 1999a); to perform less well on Happe's Strange Stories Test, which assesses the ability to interpret a nonliteral statement (Jolliffe and Baron-Cohen 1999b); to have impaired spatial working memory (Morris et al. 1999); to have impaired creativity and imagination (Craig and Baron-Cohen 1999, 2000); to have a tendency to deteriorate over time with respect to logical reasoning abilities (Nyden et al. 2001); and to have marked deficits in social cognition (Klin 2000).

Episodic memory in a group of adults with Asperger's disorder was noted to be moderately impaired even when overall recognition performance was not (Bowler et al. 2000).

Children and adolescents with Asperger's disorder were able to recognize simple emotions, but they performed poorly at recognizing emotions when faces were paired with mismatching words, suggesting that children with Asperger's disorder may be using compensatory strategies, such as verbal mediation, to process facial expressions of emotion (Grossman et al. 2000).

Summary

Too few studies of Asperger's disorder have been done to determine specific etiological associations. Nonetheless, some evidence suggests neurobiological involvement.

■ Treatment

As in autistic disorder, the treatment of individuals with Asperger's disorder requires intervention at multiple levels. However, there is very little published information on treatment.

Psychological

Family counseling should be provided to parents and should include a careful explanation of the disorder, realistic expectations of the child, and resources for obtaining support. Individual cognitive psychotherapy and group social skills training may be helpful to older children, adolescents, and adults. Some individuals with Asperger's disorder seem to enjoy meeting with other people with similar difficulties. The therapist working with these individuals should facilitate such social contact within the context of groups oriented toward an activity or a special interest (Tsai 1996).

Educational

Therapists should work with staff members at the child's school, particularly to help them recognize the need for special education services. Tests measuring comprehension and abstract problem-solving skills are needed to elucidate fully the type of learning disability seen in these children. Both the learning disability and social skills deficits often can be treated by using cognitive-behavioral techniques. Early application of special motor or visuomotor skills training may be helpful for some clumsy individuals and may prevent further development of motor deficiency. Early application of occupational therapy may provide some skills that can be used in vocational training. Vocational training should begin as early as possible and should be based on a thorough neuropsychological assessment, so that individuals with Asperger's disorder receive training for and placement in jobs in which they perform at their maximum potential and in which they enjoy the working environment (Tsai 1996).

In children with Asperger's disorder who experience mild to severe distress in the presence of some sounds, both auditory integration training and listening to selected unmodified music may be beneficial (Bettison 1996).

Pharmacological

Although little information is available about pharmacological treatment of individuals with Asperger's disorder, medication can be useful for symptoms of attention deficit, hyperactivity, tics, anxiety, depression, delusions and/or hallucinations, or obsessive-compulsive behaviors. I have successfully treated these conditions in some individuals with Asperger's disorder with stimulants (e.g., methylphenidate), antidepressants (e.g., fluoxetine), and medications for obsessive-compulsive disorder (e.g., clomipramine, serotonin reuptake inhibitors). However, I have seen some older adolescents and adults with Asperger's disorder with comorbid mental conditions who refused to accept diagnostic conclusions and would not cooperate with any interventions, including medications.

■ Clinical Course and Prognosis

Asperger's disorder tends to be recognized somewhat later if no obvious motor delays or motor clumsiness is present. In a survey study of 156 children with Asperger's disorder in England, the parents' report showed that although the parents' concerns emerged when their children were about 30 months old, the average age of their children when the diagnosis was confirmed was about 11 years (Howlin and Asgharian 1999). Gillberg et al. (1996) reviewed a number of screening and diagnostic tools and concluded that Asperger's disorder is not usually suspected, screened for, or diagnosed until children are of school age. Difficulties in social interaction become more apparent then, and idiosyncratic or circumscribed interests (e.g., a fascination with bridges or maps) begin to occupy much of these children's time.

In a 2-year follow-up study of nonverbal IQ in children, some with Asperger's disorder and others with autism, Szatmari and Streiner (1996) noted a significant drop in nonverbal IQ in the Asperger's disorder group. This drop appeared to be a function of high initial nonverbal IQ scores that fell over time because of increasing complexity of problem-solving tests. However, children with Asperger's disorder had better social skills and fewer autistic symptoms than did children with autism (Szatmari et al. 2000a).

Asperger (1944/1991) reported that only 1 of more than 200 patients with Asperger's disorder (less than 0.5%) developed symptoms of schizophrenia. In Wing's (1981) series of 18 patients with Asperger's disorder, 3 subjects developed schizophrenic or psychotic symptoms. Tantam (1991) noted that 10 of 85 adults with Asperger's disorder developed psychosis or schizophrenia. Gillberg (1991) stated that a wide variety of "bizarre" and "borderline" behaviors occurred in late adolescence and adult life in patients with Asperger's disorder but that classic schizophrenia was rare. Tantam (1991) noted that 30 of the 85 adults with Asperger's disorder (about 35%) developed psychiatric disorders.

Some reports have implied that patients with Asperger's disorder may be predisposed to violent behavior (Ghaziuddin et al. 1991). Scragg and Shah (1994) reported that about 1.5% of patients in a secure (forensic) hospital met diagnostic criteria for Asperger's disorder. A case of aggression and sexual offense in an adolescent with Asperger's disorder has been reported (Kohn et al. 1998). My clinical impression is that there is a fairly high frequency of aggressive behaviors in patients referred for evaluation and treatment. An extensive review of the literature does not support the speculation that violence is common in Asperger's disorder, however (Ghaziuddin et al. 1991). A possible reason for the low prevalence in the literature is that Asperger's disorder is a relatively new diagnostic category, so that the true prevalence of aggressive and violent behaviors have not been studied adequately. Community-based studies, using clear operationalized diagnostic criteria for both Asperger's disorder and violence, are needed to determine the prevalence of violence in patients with this syndrome.

A 30-year follow-up study of patients with Asperger's disorder and with autism showed that in adulthood, the Asperger's disorder group had a better outcome than did the autism group regarding education, employment, autonomy, marriage, reproduction, and the need for continuing medical and institutional care (Larsen and Mouridsen 1997).

Szatmari et al. (1989) reported that individuals with Asperger's disorder seemed to improve with maturity, even into adulthood. Asperger (1944/1991) and Gillberg (1991) also described the outcome for children with the syndrome as good. However, Wing (1981) described the outcome as rather poor. The abnormalities associated with the disorder often persist into adolescence and adulthood (American Psychiatric Association 1994), and they appear to represent individual characteristics that are not greatly affected by environmental influences. Tantam (1991) reported that in 93 adults with Asperger's disorder, 11% had obtained higher education; 22% were employed; 16% were in residential care; 7% lived independently; 71% lived with parents; and 1% was married.

■ Research Issues

It is clear that the syndrome Asperger originally described is not captured by contemporary diagnostic criteria (i.e., DSM-IV-TR and ICD-10 criteria) (Miller and Ozonoff 1997). In turn, the diagnostic validity of Asperger's disorder as defined by DSM-IV-TR/ICD-10 criteria continues to be a topic of debate. Much more research is needed to substantiate the diagnostic validity and reliability of the criteria for Asperger's disorder. A well-designed and carefully controlled total-population study based on DSM-IV-TR criteria for Asperger's disorder, autistic disorder, and PDDNOS is necessary to include all possible cases to more clearly determine continuities or distinguishing features of these disorders. Comprehensive assessment procedures, including behavioral evaluation, social and adaptive functioning assessment, neuropsychological testing, speech evaluation, motor coordination assessment, neurophysiological evaluation, neuroimaging studies (fMRI and PET), patterns of comorbidity, and associated psychopathology in family members, should be carried out. Only after the diagnostic validity and reliability of the criteria for Asperger's disorder are established can patterns of comorbidity, possible causes, and effective psychological and educational interventional strategies be investigated and established.

Rett's Disorder

■ Definition and Diagnostic Criteria

Rett's disorder is a condition characterized by a specific developmental course, characteristic neurological features, and a variety of unusual behaviors and developmental findings. The disorder was originally described by Rett (1966/1977), who reported—in German—his findings in 22 patients. However, the disorder did not gain wide recognition until 1983, when a series of 35 cases from a pool of French-Portuguese-Swedish patients was reported in English (Haas 1988).

Diagnostic criteria for Rett's disorder have been developed by a group representing the Centers for Disease Control and Prevention (CDC), the Association of University Centers on Disabilities (formerly the American Association of University Affiliated Programs), and the International Rett Syndrome Association (IRSA) (Trevathan and Moser 1988). These criteria are based on the "Vienna criteria" for the diagnosis of Rett's disorder (Hagberg et al. 1985) and were adopted by a panel of international experts at the 1984 Rett Syndrome Conference. The criteria contain three categories: 1) necessary criteria, 2) supportive criteria, and 3) exclusive criteria.

The *necessary criteria* include apparently normal prenatal and perinatal development; apparently normal psychomotor development through the first 5 months (in some cases, development may appear to be normal up to 18 months); normal head circumference at birth; deceleration of head growth between ages 5 and 48 months; loss of acquired purposeful hand skills between ages 5 and 30 months; development of stereotypic hand movements such as handwringing/squeezing, clapping/tapping, mouthing, and washing/rubbing automatisms after purposeful hand skills are lost; development of severely impaired expressive and receptive language; presence of appar-

ently severe psychomotor retardation; appearance of gait apraxia and truncal apraxia/ataxia between ages 1 and 4 years; temporal social withdrawal; and diagnosis tentative until age 2–5 years (Hagberg et al. 1985; Trevathan and Moser 1988).

The *supportive criteria* include breathing dysfunction, such as periodic apnea during wakefulness, intermittent hyperventilation, breath-holding spells, and forced expulsion of air or saliva; electroencephalographic abnormalities; seizures; spasticity, often with associated development of muscle wasting; dystonia; peripheral vasomotor disturbances; scoliosis; growth retardation; and hypotrophic small feet. Although most patients with Rett's disorder display many of the supportive criteria, diagnosis is possible in the absence of all the supportive criteria, especially in young patients.

The *exclusive criteria* include evidence of intrauterine growth retardation, organomegaly or other signs of storage disease, retinopathy at birth, evidence of perinatally acquired brain damage, existence of identifiable metabolic or other progressive neurological disorder, and acquired neurological disorders resulting from severe infections or head trauma. The presence of one or more of these excludes the diagnosis of Rett's disorder, regardless of whether all of the necessary criteria are present.

In DSM-IV-TR, Rett's disorder is classified as a separate subcategory of PDDs, and the DSM-IV-TR diagnostic criteria are primarily based on the necessary criteria of the IRSA-CDC criteria (Table 21–2).

The IRSA-CDC diagnostic criteria for Rett's disorder are restricted to include only typical patients to ensure a homogeneous patient population for future clinical and epidemiological research. Although female sex was considered by Hagberg and associates (1985) as one of the inclusion criteria of Rett's disorder, the IRSA-CDC criteria do not include it. This decision was made in consideration of males in whom the condition may be undiagnosed (Trevathan and Moser 1988). However, some studies reported patients who had several features suggestive of Rett's disorder but did not satisfy all the official criteria; either they lacked a history of normal development for several months followed by a period of definite deterioration or they had congenital or acquired encephalopathy of a known etiology (Goutieres and Aicardi 1986, 1987; Zappella et al. 1998). Many clinicians have used the controversial term *forme fruste Rett syndrome* to describe what they consider atypical and abortive vari-

Table 21–2. DSM-IV-TR diagnostic criteria for Rett's disorder

A. All of the following:
   (1) apparently normal prenatal and perinatal development
   (2) apparently normal psychomotor development through the first 5 months after birth
   (3) normal head circumference at birth
B. Onset of all of the following after the period of normal development:
   (1) deceleration of head growth between ages 5 and 48 months
   (2) loss of previously acquired purposeful hand skills between ages 5 and 30 months with the subsequent development of stereotyped hand movements (e.g., hand-wringing or hand washing)
   (3) loss of social engagement early in the course (although often social interaction develops later)
   (4) appearance of poorly coordinated gait or trunk movements
   (5) severely impaired expressive and receptive language development with severe psychomotor retardation

Source. Reprinted from the *Diagnostic and Statistical Manual of Mental Disorders*, 4th Edition, Text Revision. Washington, DC, American Psychiatric Association, 2000. Copyright 2000, American Psychiatric Association. Used with permission.

ants of Rett's disorder. Zappella et al. (1998) proposed to use *Rett complex* to include cases ranging from severe with classical presentation to considerably milder variants.

The diagnosis of Rett's disorder is clinically difficult before 3 years of age, especially in atypical cases, but molecular analysis of the mutations in the gene encoding X-linked methyl-CpG-binding protein 2 (MECP2) (described later in this chapter) will assist diagnosis in some patients. Mutations in *MECP2* seem to be the main cause for Rett's disorder. It can be expected that approximately 80% of patients who fulfill the criteria for Rett's disorder have *MECP2* mutations. Therefore, analysis of *MECP2* should be performed to support the clinical diagnosis if Rett's disorder is suspected. It has been suggested that a two-tiered strategy be applied to identify *MECP2* mutations. Denaturing high-performance liquid chromatography is used for initial screening of nucleotide variants and is followed by confirmatory sequencing analysis. If a definite mutation is not identified, then the entire *MECP2* coding region is sequenced to reduce the risk of a false negative (Buyse et al. 2000).

■ Associated Clinical Features

Abnormalities of the sleep-wake cycle have been observed in patients with Rett's disorder, and the abnormalities appear to continue into late childhood and adolescence. Compared with age-matched peers, these patients had significantly more total sleep, significantly less nighttime sleep, more disrupted sleep, and significantly more daytime sleep (Piazza et al. 1990). The abnormalities involved both the phasic and tonic components of sleep and the observation of the components of REM stage in non-REM (NREM) stage. These abnormalities aggravated with age, disturbances in percentage of sleep stage, nocturnal variation of tonic and phasic components of sleep, and REM–NREM cycles (Segawa and Nomura 1992).

Compared with a group of healthy controls of similar age range, girls with Rett's disorder had significantly lower heart variability (marker of autonomic disarray) (Guideri et al. 1999) and had prolonged QT intervals (Ellaway et al. 1999a; Guideri et al. 1999; Sekul et al. 1994), a serious and potentially lethal cardiac disorder.

Cooke et al. (1995) reported that patients with Rett's disorder had significantly lower serum total thyroxine (T_4) concentrations, which was associated with decreased concentration of thyroid-stimulating hormone (TSH). They also observed a delay in peak glucose and insulin concentrations.

In a study of 36 patients, with an average age of 8 years 7 months, with Rett's disorder, 64% had orthopedic problems: 45% had spinal deformities and 36% had joint contractures (Loder et al. 1989). The occurrence of scoliosis in Rett's disorder appears to be age dependent, with a reported incidence of 36%–100%. The onset of scoliosis is usually before age 8 years (Huang et al. 1994). However, Lidstrom et al. (1994) argued that the development of scoliosis was dependent more on stage of disease (i.e., stage IV) than on age. Holm and King (1990) reported that the scoliosis curves ranged from 10 to 86 degrees at a mean age of 14.9 years.

Haas et al. (1997) studied bone density in 20 subjects with Rett's disorder and found that bone mineral density, bone mineral content, and spine mineral density were significantly reduced in these girls and concluded that subjects with Rett's disorder were at risk for osteoporosis.

Julu et al. (2001) analyzed breathing rhythms in 47 cases with Rett's disorder. Respiratory rhythm was found to be normal during sleep and abnormal in the waking state. Forced and apneustic breathing were prominent among 5- to 10-year-olds, and Valsalva breathing was prominent in those older than age 18 years, who were also most likely to breathe normally. Inadequate and exaggerated breathing was noted to be associated with vacant spells.

In a study of oral manifestations in 17 subjects with Rett's disorder with a mean age of 7.3 years, Ribeiro et al. (1997) found that the most frequent oral habits were digit/hand sucking and/or biting (100%), bruxism (82%), mouth breathing (41%), drooling (29%) and tongue thrusting (29%).

Feeding problems are common in Rett's disorder because of characteristic oropharyngeal abnormalities. In a study of 20 individuals with Rett's disorder between ages 1.5 and 33 years, Morton et al. (1997) noted that all of the subjects had reduced movement of the mid- and posterior tongue, with premature spillover of food and liquid from the mouth into the pharynx. They also showed delayed pharyngeal swallow. Those individuals with the most general neurological impairment tended to have the worst feeding problems and were smaller and malnourished. Motil et al. (1999) reported that oropharyngeal dysfunction and gastroesophageal dysmotility were present in 100% and 69%, respectively, of 13 subjects with Rett's disorder between ages 3.7 and 25.7 years. Abnormalities of oropharyngeal function included poor tongue mobility, reduced oropharyngeal clearance, and laryngeal penetration of liquids and solid food during swallowing. Esophageal dysmotility included absent primary or secondary waves, delayed emptying, atony, spasm, and gastroesophageal reflux. Gastric dysmotility included diminished peristalsis or atony.

Although stereotyped hand movements in Rett's disorder tend to be symmetrical and midline, Elian and de M Rudolf (1996) reported that the hand movements were asymmetrical and nonmidline in 44% of 25 girls with Rett's disorder. The hand movements in these girls appeared to change with changing emotional or mental states.

Guerrini et al. (1998) observed myoclonus in 9 of 10 females between ages 3 and 20 years with Rett's disorder. Multifocal, arrhythmic, and asynchronous jerks mainly involved distal limbs. The severity of myoclonus did not correlate with that of other symptoms or with age.

■ Differential Diagnosis

Autistic Disorder

In the past, children with Rett's disorder were frequently regarded as autistic (Olsson and Rett 1985, 1990; Percy et al. 1988). For example, Witt-Engerström and Gillberg (1987) reported that 78% of children with Rett's disorder previously had received diagnoses of infantile autism (see also Chapter 20, "Autistic Disorder," in this volume). Several independent studies of behavioral observations reported qualitative and quantitative differences between patients with Rett's disorder and those with autism.

Gillberg (1987) used a comprehensive questionnaire containing a number of semistructured questions and 130 items concerned with early characteristics of perceptual, motor, and emotional development in children. Eight mothers of eight young girls (ages 3–9 years) with Rett's disorder were interviewed using the questionnaire. Although considerable overlap was found between early symptoms in Rett's disorder and infantile autism, there were indications that certain features might differentiate the two disorders. For example, three items were typical of autism but were rare in Rett's disorder: 1) "played only with hard objects," 2) "did not like to be disturbed 'in her world,'" and 3) "was very pleased when left completely to herself."

Olsson and Rett (1985) compared the behavior of girls with Rett's disorder with those with infantile autism. Visual, acoustic, tactile, and gustatory stimuli and social contact were used for the comparison. The following behaviors were observed only in patients with Rett's disorder, not in patients with autism: slow movements plus hypoactivity, uniform stereotypic movements of hands with a broad-base stance, stereotypic "washing movements" of hands, stereotypic wetting of hands with saliva, stereotypic bringing together of hands, consistent isolated stretching and flexing of the middle finger joints, episodic hyperventilation via mouth, no chewing. Among behavior that is characteristic of autism, the following five traits were not seen in the patients with Rett's disorder: 1) predominant rejection of caressing and tenderness, 2) conspicuous physical hyperactivity in terms of continuous grabbing and concomitant locomobility, 3) excessive attachment to certain objects, 4) rotation of small objects, and 5) stereotypic playing habits. Thus, the authors demonstrated that Rett's disorder and autism could be differentiated based on behavioral observations.

Percy et al. (1988) analyzed motor and behavioral characteristics of 15 patients with Rett's disorder. The authors found that children with Rett's disorder differed from children with autism in having ataxia, breath-holding, hyperventilation, bruxism, simplicity of stereotypies, and hand apposition. On the other hand, children with autism differed from those with Rett's disorder in terms of overactivity, complex repetitive movements, and inappropriate vocalization. It is apparent that the course is different with Rett's disorder, progressing to various forms of neurological impairment that are not seen in autism.

MECP2 mutation or polymorphisms (described later in this chapter) are most likely absent in autistic disorder (Vourc'h et al. 2001).

Levels of cerebrospinal fluid (CSF) nerve-growth factor (NGF) were normal in autism but low to negligible in Rett's disorder. CSF NGF could be used as a biochemical marker for differentiation of patients with autism from those with Rett's disorder (Riikonen and Vanhala 1999).

Disintegrative Disorder

Although patients with Rett's disorder and most individuals with childhood disintegrative disorder both have a phase of developmental deterioration or disintegration and no subsequent dementia, only patients with Rett's disorder develop severe lower-motor neuron and basal ganglia dysfunction, which forces the patients into a wheelchair-bound life. These motor signs completely distinguish Rett's disorder from childhood disintegrative disorder.

Infantile Neuronal Ceroid Lipofuscinosis

In the first stage (at age 1–2 years) of infantile neuronal ceroid lipofuscinosis (INCL), rapid regression occurs with loss of acquired fine motor skill, learned words, and communication. It can be difficult to distinguish from Rett's disorder. However, careful observers will note transient drop spells, loss of head control, and irregular myoclonias in INCL. MRI scans usually show early atrophy and hyperdensity in the thalami in INCL but not in Rett's disorder (Vanhanen et al. 1994). For accurate diagnosis of INCL, a biopsy with characteristic electromagnetic findings of "snowball" aggregate is necessary. After age 3 years, a clinical differentiation becomes possible because of the presence of visual failure, rapid deterioration of head control, hyperexcitability, and trunk-limb extension tonus in INCL (Hagberg and Witt-Engerström 1990).

■ Epidemiology

Prevalence

Using both the Vienna criteria and the IRSA-CDC criteria and on the basis of findings from Swedish (Hagberg and Witt-Engerström 1987), Scottish (Kerr and Stephenson 1985), Portuguese (Hagberg and Witt-Engerström 1987), U.S. (Kozinetz et al. 1993), Italian (Pini et al. 1996), Australian (Leonard et al. 1997), and Norwegian (Skjeldal et al. 1997) studies, the estimated prevalence of Rett's disorder ranges from 0.44 to 2.1 per 10,000 females. In the Australian study, of those older than 5 years, 68% had classical Rett's disorder and 32% had atypical Rett's disorder.

Today, Rett's disorder is known to exist in all races and probably all countries (Hagberg 1989). More than 2,000 cases of Rett's disorder have been recognized worldwide. The many pathognomonic examples of its clinical expression have convinced clinicians of the existence of this unique syndrome (Tsai 1994).

Sex Ratio

Initially, Rett's disorder was considered a disorder only of females. However, there have been a few case reports of males with Rett's disorder (Christen and Hanefeld 1995; Clayton-Smith et al. 2000; Coleman 1990; Hagberg and Witt-Engerström 1987; Jan et al. 1999; Philippart 1990; Schanen et al. 1998). Males with Rett's disorder appear to represent a heterogeneous phenotype. Their clinical features may meet many but not all of the necessary diagnostic criteria of classic Rett's disorder. For evaluating males with idiopathic developmental regression, autistic features, and loss of hand function, less restrictive criteria are required so as to include variants (Jan et al. 1999).

Social Class

Rett's disorder is known to exist in all classes of families. There is no evidence suggestive of prevalence in any particular social class.

■ Etiology

Genetic Factors

Although twin studies demonstrate a high concordance rate of Rett's disorder in monozygotic twins

(Hagberg 1989; Percy 1992), the fact that probably fewer than 1% of Rett's disorder cases are familial speaks in favor of a spontaneous mutation as the most common cause of Rett's disorder (Buhler et al. 1990).

Amir et al. (1999) first identified mutations in the gene encoding X-linked MECP2 at Xq28 in about 50% of patients with Rett's disorder. Since then *MECP2* mutations have been found in 35%–100% of patients with typical Rett's disorder (Auranen et al. 2001; Bienvenu et al. 2000; De Bona et al. 2000; Huppke et al. 2000; Inui et al. 2001; Laccone et al. 2001; Vacca et al. 2001; Van den Veyver and Zoghbi 2000; Xiang et al. 2000) as well as in 20%–40% of patients with atypical Rett's disorder (Bourdon et al. 2001; Buyse et al. 2000; Cheadle et al. 2000; Hoffbuhr et al. 2001). Furthermore, more than 30 different types of *MECP2* mutations have been identified in different samples of Rett's disorder (Amano et al. 2000; Amir et al. 2000; Bienvenu et al. 2000; Cheadle et al. 2000; Hoffbuhr et al. 2001; Huppke et al. 2000; Laccone et al. 2001; Nielsen et al. 2001). It is conceivable that Rett's disorder may be further classified into many subtypes.

However, *MECP2* mutations also have been identified in boys who do not present a Rett's disorder phenotype (Hoffbuhr et al. 2001; Meloni et al. 2000; Villard et al. 2000; Wan et al. 1999). The pathobiology of *MECP2* could be a prototype for other disorders of neurodevelopment (Orrico et al. 2000; Percy 2000; Wan et al. 1999).

Although Nielsen et al. (2001) reported that there was no consistent correlation between the type of mutation and the clinical presentation of the patient or the X-inactivation pattern in peripheral blood, other investigators suggested that the mutation type strongly affected disease severity (Amir et al. 2000; Amir and Zoghbi 2000; Cheadle et al. 2000; Hoffbuhr et al. 2001; Shahbazian and Zoghbi 2001).

It appears that 99.5% of all instances of Rett's disorder are due to sporadic de novo mutations in the *MECP2* gene, mostly from the fathers, and that the familial cases of Rett's disorder are due to X-chromosomal inheritance from a carrier mother (Trappe et al. 2001). Hence, the recurrence risk is higher in maternal-origin cases and lower in paternal-origin cases (Girard et al. 2001; Trappe et al. 2001).

In summary, abnormal gene expression may underlie the Rett's disorder, so discovering which genes are misregulated in the absence of functional MECP2 is crucial for understanding the pathogenesis of Rett's disorder.

Neuropathological Factors

Neuropathological studies have found diffuse cortical atrophy; mild loss of pyramidal neurons in frontal and temporal areas and in the visual cortex; increased cell-packing density in cerebral cortex with decreased size of neurons; reduced cortical dendrities in the temporal lobe and in the visual cortex; severe cortical cell hypochromia in the entorhinal cortex, hippocampus, and fascia dentate; underpigmentation in certain nigral structures; decreased immunoreaction for prolactin and growth hormone in the pituitary gland, increased β-endorphins in the thalamus and cerebellum; severe cerebellar degeneration affecting the Purkinje cells and their axons; and degeneration in the descending corticospinal tracts, gliosis, decreased anterior horn cells, and decreased neurons in the dorsal root ganglion (Armstrong 1992; Armstrong et al. 1995, 1998; Bauman et al. 1995; Belichenko et al. 1997; Hagberg 1989; Jellinger et al. 1988; Johnston et al. 1995; Kerr et al. 1997; Kitt and Wilcox 1995; Leontovich et al. 1999; Oldfors et al. 1988, 1990; Percy 1993)

At present, investigators disagree about the locus of the lesions. However, there appears to be a consensus that the main lesion of Rett's disorder is in the particular subcortical area that occurs early in the development of the central nervous system (Segawa 1992).

Neuroanatomical Factors

CT studies have shown findings ranging from normal (Trevathan and Naidu 1988) to various brain structural abnormalities, including slight changes (Nielsen et al. 1990) and atrophy of cortex, thalamus, and brainstem (Nihei and Naitoh 1990; Nomura et al. 1984; Yoshikawa et al. 1990).

MRI studies also showed inconsistent findings (Nihei and Naitoh 1990), including craniofacial disproportion, bilateral atrophy of the frontotemporal lobes, and cerebellar atrophy (Murakami et al. 1992; Reiss et al. 1993; Subramaniam et al. 1997; Yano et al. 1991).

A cerebral magnetic resonance spectroscopy study found an increased cerebral regional concentration of total choline, indicating gliosis, and decreased levels of *N*-acetyl aspartate, reflecting reduced neuronal and dendritic tree size (Horska et al. 2000).

SPECT studies have found reduced blood flow to the prefrontal and temporoparietal association regions, reflecting the widespread functional disturbances in the brains of patients with Rett's disorder (Bjure et al. 1997; Lappalainen et al. 1997; Nielsen et al. 1990). SPECT studies also found low dopamine D_2 receptor levels (Naidu et al. 1992) and high binding potential for [^{123}I]iodolisuride (a specific D_2 ligand) and D_2 receptors, suggesting reduced dopaminergic neurotransmission as a possible cause of Rett's disorder (Chiron et al. 1993).

PET studies found impaired oxidative metabolism in the temporal, posteroparietal, and occipital regions (Naidu et al. 1992; Yoshikawa et al. 1990). A SPECT study revealed a considerable global reduction in cerebral perfusion (Burroni et al. 1997).

In summary, neuroradiological studies generally appear to be able to provide in vitro evidence to support the neuropathological findings described above, though there is no neuroradiological marker for the cause of Rett's disorder.

Neurophysiological Factors

Electroencephalographic findings seem to be normal in the premonitory stage (birth to age 1.5 years). In the acute exacerbation stage (age 1.5–5 years), occipital dominant alpha wave–like activity persists for a few years. When the patient is about 4 years old, the electroencephalographic background activity in the waking stage shows irregularity. Frequent seizure activity is noted on sleep electroencephalograms. In the chronic stage (after age 6 years), a monotonous theta rhythm dominates the waking tracing. After age 20 years, the monotonous theta rhythm tends to be more localized to the centroparietal area. The rhythm is not influenced by either opening or closing of the eyes but is attenuated by a loud noise, suggesting a dysfunction of the ascending reticular activating system in the brainstem (Ishizaki 1992; Ishizaki et al. 1989; Lappalainen et al. 1997; Trevathan and Naidu 1988). Niedermeyer et al. (1997) observed unusual and prominent rhythmical activity present in waking and/or sleep, suggesting a dysfunction of the motor cortex in Rett's disorder.

Studies of auditory and visual evoked responses have shown conflicting results (Bader et al. 1989; Kalmanchey 1990; Stach et al. 1994).

A study of brainstem frequency-following response (a short-latency evoked response providing unique information concerning the early processing of auditory inputs) found considerable intersubject latency variability and poor intrasubject repeat reliability, suggesting developmental arrest rather than a neurodegenerative process in Rett's disorder (Galbraith et al. 1996).

Somatosensory evoked response studies have obtained findings suggesting involvement of the spinal cord and the spinothalamic system (Guerrini et al. 1998; Kimura et al. 1992).

Nomura et al. (1997) noted that some patients showed absence of sympathetic skin response and that some showed asymmetrical involvement of parameters of the sympathetic skin response, indicating autonomic nervous system involvement at various levels, from the central to the peripheral nervous system.

Neurochemical Factors

It has been suggested that changes in specific neurotransmitter systems, particularly cholinergic neurons, in the thalamus, cerebellum, and basal ganglia may underlie the progressive deterioration in motor and cognitive function in Rett's disorder (Wenk et al. 1993).

When two studies found low CSF levels of β-phenylethylamine (Satoi et al. 2000) and a decreased number and activity of dopamine terminals in the basal ganglia (Wenk 1995), this seemed to indicate dopamine system impairment. However, a further study by Wenk (1996) found relatively normal dopaminergic neuronal function in Rett's disorder.

Gamma-aminobutyric acid receptor density was significantly increased in the caudate of young patients with Rett's disorder. The results showed regional, receptor-subtype, and age-specific alteration in amino acid neurotransmitter receptors in the basal ganglia; the observed changes may correlate with age-related clinical stages of Rett's disorder (Blue et al. 1999).

Wenk and Hauss-Wegrzyniak (1999) reported that the number of choline acetyltransferase–positive neurons was significantly decreased, resulting in decreased production of choline acetyltransferase protein, which is necessary for the production of the neurotransmitter acetylcholine.

Other studies reported elevated CSF β-endorphin (Brase et al. 1989; Myer et al. 1992; Nagamitsu et al. 1997) and CSF glutamate levels (Hamberger et al. 1992; Lappalainen and Riikonen 1996); low levels of CSF NGF (Lappalainen et al. 1996; Lipani et al. 2000; Vanhala et al. 1998); and abnormalities of purine and pyridine metabolism (Rocchigiani et al. 1995).

Chatterjee et al. (1990) reported two double-blind studies showing the presence of an unusual glycosphingolipid in 70% of the patients with Rett's disorder and in approximately 10% of the patients with other disorders. However, this glycosphingolipid was absent from the plasma of control subjects. New information suggests a disturbance in the ganglioside pattern that leads to a reduction in GD1a and GT1b gangliosides in the cerebrum and cerebellum (Leckman et al. 1991, 1999). The corresponding reduction in these gangliosides in the CSF, if shown to be specific for Rett's disorder, could be used as a diagnostic marker (Percy 1992).

Immunological Factors

Fiumara et al. (1999) investigated humoral and cell-mediated immunity and found a reduced percentage of CD8+ suppressor-cytotoxic cells, resulting in an increased CD4+/CD8+ ratio; low levels of natural killer cells; and an absence of antineuronal and antimyelin ganglioside antibodies, antinuclear antibodies, anti-striated muscle antibodies, and anti–smooth muscle antibodies. The etiological meaning of these findings is unclear.

Substance P (a tachykinin peptide) immunoreactivity expression was significantly decreased in many of the brain regions involved in the control of autonomic nervous system, suggesting that substance P may contribute to the autonomic dysfunction in Rett's disorder (Deguchi et al. 2000; Matsuishi et al. 1997).

Messahel et al. (2000) investigated urinary neopterin and biopterin levels and found that the neopterin levels were raised in a proportion of young girls but not in older women. They also found that the biopterin levels were not different from those in control subjects but remained low, whereas control subjects' biopterin levels increased with age. These results suggest an inherited fault in tetrahydrobiopterin metabolism, increasing the risk both of developing Rett's disorder and of developing an immune activation during the regression phase of Rett's disorder.

Summary

To date, the only consistent finding in investigations into the cause of Rett's disorder is *MECP2* mutations. There is no consistent characteristic alteration in biochemical, immunological, neurophysiological, neurotransmitter, or morphological markers.

■ Treatment

Treatment of patients with Rett's disorder requires that the primary care clinician collaborate with members of allied disciplines and community agencies that serve children with special needs and their families. Treatment encompasses a comprehensive medical, therapeutic, educational, and psychosocial approach.

Psychological

In a study of parental stress, the parents of 29 girls with Rett's disorder reported more stress, lower marital satisfaction, and certain adaptations in family functioning compared with norms (Perry et al. 1992). Family counseling should be provided to parents and should include a careful explanation of the disorder and its prognosis, realistic expectations of the child, and resources for obtaining support. Family members who are not the primary caretakers must learn to recognize the signs of burnout and know how to step in and provide relief (Weisz 1990). If the parents can no longer keep the child at home, the child psychiatrist should also help the parents select an alternative arrangement, such as foster care or a group home.

Educational

Special education (including prevocational and vocational training) and related services (e.g., physical therapy, special transportation to school) are needed, as are medical and/or psychiatric consultations with the classroom teacher and other teaching staff involved in the child's education or care.

Teachers and other caregivers should be trained to recognize communicative behaviors (e.g., facial expression, eye gaze, vocalization, gestures, walking toward a desired item or activity) displayed by children with Rett's disorder. These children should be taught to use pictures, photographs, communication boards, and specially designed computers to communicate with other people. Speech and language therapy should be included in the child's individual education plan. Music therapy has been shown to promote these children's desire to interact with other people (Zappella 1986). Special education in a regular education or inclusive setting can provide the context for many typical social interactions and facilitate social relationships between students with Rett's disorder and regular peers.

Communicational

In a study of six girls with Rett's disorder, mothers were trained to read familiar and unfamiliar storybooks in their homes. Group and individual data collected from the six girls indicated that they became more active and successful participants in the interactions during storybook reading (Koppenhaver et al. 2001).

Behavioral

Operant conditioning procedures have been shown to reestablish functional self-feeding skills (Piazza et al. 1993); reinforcing incompatible behaviors seems to decrease stereotyped hand movements (Hanks 1986); and preventing reinforcement delivery may reduce the motivation to engage in aberrant behavior (Roane et al. 2001).

Medical

Haas et al. (1986) reported improved weight gain in conjunction with diminished stereotyped hand movements and better seizure control (even in seizures refractory to medications) when a high-calorie, high-fat ketogenic diet was implemented. Many patients with Rett's disorder do not consume adequate fluids and fiber, which may result in constipation (Hunter 1987). The medical treatment team should include a nutritionist to provide consultations to parents and caregivers of individuals with Rett's disorder.

Pharmacological

Appropriate anticonvulsants should be given to children who develop epilepsy, which is common during the rapid developmental regression stage (between ages 1 and 2 years). Several investigators have reported that carbamazepine seems to be the most effective anticonvulsant, especially in patients with a predominance of complex partial seizures (Trevathan and Naidu 1988).

In an open pilot study of lamotrigine in girls with the classical form of Rett's disorder or the milder forme fruste variants, two of three girls with epilepsy responded relatively well to treatment, and for one of them, even bad tantrums disappeared. Lamotrigine made another four girls happier, more alert, more able to concentrate, and more at ease in interpersonal contact (Stenbom et al. 1998). Kumandas et al. (2001) also reported that lamotrigine successfully controlled seizures in two girls, and their stereotyped hand movements and autistic behaviors also markedly decreased.

A study of treatment with bromocriptine (a dopamine agonist) showed improvements in communication, sleep pattern, facial expression, and motor abilities and reduction of stereotypic hand activities, bouts

of hyperpnea, and grinding of the teeth. However, these improvements failed to recur after the "washout" phase of the study (Zappella et al. 1990).

Levodopa and levodopa/carbidopa have been found to have some benefits in a few patients in the later stages of the disorder, when increasing rigidity appeared (Percy and Hagberg 1993).

Magnesium orotate or citrate has been reported to decrease hyperventilation, hand stereotypies, and episodes of agitation (Egger et al. 1992).

Naltrexone was given to 25 patients with Rett's disorder, and there were positive effects on certain respiratory characteristics, including decreased disorganized breathing during wakefulness. However, deleterious effects, including declines in motor function and more rapid progression of the clinical stages, were also noted (Percy et al. 1994).

In a randomized controlled trial of L-carnitine in 35 subjects with Rett's disorder, both parents/caregivers and clinicians conducting medical follow-up detected improvements in subjects' well-being and showed an improvement on the Hand Apraxia Scale (Ellaway et al. 1999b).

Melatonin has produced positive effect in the treatment of sleep disorders in patients with Rett's disorder (McArthur and Budden 1998; Miyamoto et al. 1999).

Most patients become wheelchair-bound during the late motor deterioration stage. General treatment should be directed toward correction of malnutrition, anemia, and electrolyte disturbances that may be caused by the patient's immobilized status. Exercise and physical therapy should be done to prevent muscle weakness and wasting. Daily walking with assistance, weight-bearing and weight-shifting exercises, and gait training should be encouraged. Hydrotherapy has helped to improve range of motion and reduce discomfort (Hanks 1986; Lieb-Lundell 1988). The skin over the coccyx and ischial tuberosities must be inspected daily. Elbow orthotics and hand splints may be used to decrease stereotypic hand movements and to increase hand-to-toy contact (Aron 1990; Sharpe 1992). Surgical treatment has successfully reduced thoracolumbar curvature (scoliosis), preventing curve progression and improving spinal balance for sitting and walking (Harrison and Webb 1990).

■ Clinical Course and Prognosis

Rett's disorder must be viewed primarily as a progressive neurological disorder with variable clinical presentations that depend on the patient's age and the stage of the disease. Hagberg and Witt-Engerström (1986) proposed a four-stage model:

1. The *early-onset stagnation stage* occurs between age 6 months and 1.5 years, with a median age of 10–11 months (Engerström 1992).
2. The *rapid developmental regression stage* usually occurs at age 1–2 years and lasts for 13–19 months (Engerström 1992).
3. The *pseudostationary stage* usually occurs at age 3–4 years, but it can be delayed and persists many years or even decades.
4. The *late motor deterioration stage* often occurs during school age or early adolescence.

During the stagnation stage, head growth decelerates, hypotonia develops, and loss of interest in play activity occurs. Linear growth declines, with both height and weight below the 2.5th percentile for those of healthy young children (Thommessen et al. 1992). Hagberg et al. (2000) reported that in classic types, the mean head circumference fell to 2 standard deviations (SDs) below the norm at age 4 years and that after age 8 years, it stabilized at close to 3 SDs. In forme fruste variants, the mean head circumference was within normal limits. Body height in those with the classic types deviated by up to 2 SDs at age of 6 years and was highly correlated to decline in head growth. The head growth was also correlated to the severity of motor disability; that is, a marked deceleration in head growth was related to maximum gross and fine motor disability, whereas normal head growth was related to well-preserved gross motor function and some preserved fine motor function (Hagberg et al. 2000; Stenbom et al. 1995).

Many investigators report that "autistic features" develop during the rapid developmental regression stage. In addition, 80% of patients develop seizures, including complex partial, atypical absence, generalized tonic or tonic-clonic, atonic, and/or myoclonic seizures. After age 2 years, the electroencephalographic findings are typically abnormal, usually with a slow, poorly organized waking background. Some patients engage in self-abusive behavior, such as chewing their fingers and slapping their face (Trevathan and Moser 1988). Steffenburg et al. (2001) reported that in a series of 53 females with Rett's disorder, ages 5–55 years, a history of seizure was present in 50 (94%), 45 of whom had 5-year active epilepsy. The median age at seizure onset was 4 years. Partial complex seizures were the most common seizure type, occurring in 27 (54%). It was noted that after adolescence, the severity of seizure tended to decrease (i.e., lower seizure frequency and relatively more partial seizures). Of those who had had epilepsy for 10 years, 8% were seizure-free for 1 year; of those who had had it for 27 years, 40% were seizure-free for 1 year.

Cooper et al. (1998) reported that the proportion of abnormal electroencephalographic records increased from 6 of 18 (33%) during the first 6 months of the regression period to 44 of 59 (75%) in the later period to 6 years, the increase in abnormality following rather than preceding the onset of regression. Epileptogenic activity was commonly present without clinical seizure. Eleven vacant spells were monitored and were not epileptic but related to the breathing abnormality.

Glaze et al. (1998) conducted video/polygraphic/electroencephalographic monitoring sessions in 82 females, ages 2–30 years, with Rett's disorder. The parents of 23 (42%) of the 55 patients with a history of seizures identified events during monitoring that were not associated with seizure discharges but that they felt were representative of the child's typical "seizures." These "nonseizure" events included episodes of motor activity, such as twitching, jerking, head turning, falling forward, and trembling, as well as episodes of staring, laughing, pupil dilatation, breath holding, and hyperventilation. It was concluded that the occurrence of epileptic seizures tended to be overestimated.

During the pseudostationary stage, most patients develop respiratory dysfunction, bruxism, truncal ataxia or apraxia with an unusual jerky quality, and early scoliosis. Many patients also have episodes of apnea during wakefulness. However, respiratory patterns are usually regular during sleep (Marcus et al. 1994). On the other hand, during the pseudostationary stage, patients with Rett's disorder begin to show a return of interest in interacting with other people (Engerström 1992).

Most patients in the late motor deterioration stage experience tetraparetic weakness, muscle wasting, limb distortion, and severe scoliosis. The combination of lower-motor neuron and basal ganglia dysfunction forces the patient into a wheelchair-dependent life. A Swedish series of 30 adult patients, ages 22–44 years (median age, 27 years), with Rett's disorder revealed that 24 (80%) had severe invalidism and were more or less completely immobilized (Witt-Engerström and

Hagberg 1990). However, by adulthood, epilepsy in many patients with Rett's disorder spontaneously attenuates.

In a survey of 107 families of children with Rett's disorder, the children had a high prevalence of behavioral and emotional problems, including episodes of anxiety (76%), low mood (70%), and self-injurious behavior (49%). Epilepsy occurred in more than one-half of the children, but it was not clearly associated with behavioral and emotional problems. These problems tended to diminish with increasing age (Sansom et al. 1993).

In most of the patients monitored until at least age 15 years, autistic traits became less prominent than evidenced during the initial phase of the disorder (Hagberg 1989; Hagberg et al. 1983). ICD-10 also states that in Rett's disorder, social interest tends to be maintained and social interactions often develop later. Gillberg (1987) reported that eye contact improved and sometimes became very intense. The girls with Rett's disorder did not object to human interaction and usually did not protest if their world was "disturbed." The automatisms also tended to become slower and more simplified in adulthood. Woodyatt and Ozanne (1993) reported improved eye contact, social interaction, and communication intentionality during adolescence. The IRSA-CDC criteria define the communication dysfunction and social withdrawal as "temporal" features. It is not clear, however, whether "temporal" means that all the patients with Rett's disorder eventually regain communicative and social skills that match their mental age. In a study of six subjects, ages 2–13 years, with Rett's disorder, the level of communication was found to be at a preintentional level, which was consistent with the subjects' profound intellectual disability (Woodyatt and Ozanne 1992). Furthermore, most girls with Rett's disorder did not show intentional communication to communicative partners (von Tetzchner 1997; Woodyatt and Ozanne 1997).

Most patients with Rett's disorder survive at least into their 40s. However, sudden, unexplained death of patients with Rett's disorder is not uncommon, possibly as a result of brainstem dysfunction, with respiratory arrest (Hagberg 1989) or cardiac abnormalities, including longer QT intervals and more T-wave abnormalities (Guideri et al. 1999; Sekul et al. 1994). Kerr et al. (1997) reported that the mortality rate in Rett's disorder was 1.2% per annum, and that among the deaths, 48% occurred in debilitated people, 13% were from natural causes, 13% occurred among people with prior severe seizures, and 26% were sudden and unexpected.

Because Rett's disorder is a relatively newly recognized disorder, many questions remain about its course, necessitating further follow-up studies.

■ Research Issues

Because many different types of *MECP2* mutations have been identified, future research should focus on linking each type of mutation with clinical presentations. Such an approach will enable further subclassifications of Rett's disorder.

Future neuroimaging studies should employ serial longitudinal scans of very young children manifesting early signs of the clinical syndrome. Such studies will help to elucidate the neuropathological pathways to the debilitating clinical manifestation of Rett's disorder.

Future research should also investigate at what stage of Rett's disorder the clinical features begin to resemble severe or profound mental retardation more than PDDs. In other words, it is necessary to determine whether Rett's disorder should be considered as a subtype of PDDs only during certain stages of the disorder.

Future research should also focus on developing effective comprehensive treatment, including medication and nonmedication interventions.

Childhood Disintegrative Disorder

■ Definition and Diagnostic Criteria

Heller (1930/1979) reported 28 cases of dementia in young children whose development had been entirely normal until age 3 or 4 years. The term *dementia infantilis* was used to describe the disorder, which is recognized as a syndrome (Heller's syndrome) in textbooks of pediatric neurology and child psychiatry. Rutter et al. (1969) used the term *disintegrative psychosis of childhood* to describe children with Heller's syndrome. The authors argued that most children with Heller's syndrome, after the initial process of disintegration, remained static. Some children even made small advances in social behavior by means of educational treatment. In only a few cases was there progressive loss of intellectual capacity as seen in the various types of degenerative neurological disorders.

Fewer than 100 cases of Heller's syndrome or disintegrative psychosis have been reported (Volkmar

1994). The diagnostic category of disintegrative psychosis of childhood was included in ICD-9 (World Health Organization 1977), and it roughly follows Heller's account of dementia infantilis. Disintegrative psychosis, however, was not included in either DSM-III or DSM-III-R classifications of PDDs. It has been viewed as a relatively rare disorder that apparently is a nonspecific organic brain syndrome consisting of a dementia plus other behavioral abnormalities, such as rapid loss of language and social skills. Rutter (1985) has criticized this view as "an unjustified inference" because "there are well-reported cases of children with a clear-cut clinical picture of disintegrative psychosis but without any unambiguous evidence of brain disease or damage" (p. 56).

Several lines of data support the validity of disintegrative psychosis (Kurita 1988; Mouridsen et al. 1998; Volkmar 1992; Volkmar and Rutter 1995). Both ICD-10 and DSM-IV/DSM-IV-TR include childhood disintegrative disorder (a new term for disintegrative psychosis) as a subcategory of PDDs. It is defined as a disorder with a marked regression in multiple areas of functioning following at least 2 years of apparently normal development and the onset of characteristic abnormalities in social, communicative, and behavioral functioning (Table 21–3). It is likely that this diagnostic category is heterogeneous and may include patients with disintegrative psychosis, Heller's syndrome (or dementia infantilis), and symbiotic psychosis. For the present, it seems highly desirable to retain childhood disintegrative disorder as a separate category so that the conditions can be identified for further study of the relationship between these conditions and other PDDs.

■ Clinical Findings

Individuals with childhood disintegrative disorder have remarkably consistent clinical features. Their general development usually is normal or near normal up to, in most cases, age 3 or 4 years (American Psychiatric Association 2000). In most instances, without any obvious antecedent illness, these children become anxious, irritable, negativistic, and disobedient; have frequent outbursts of temper without provocation; and throw their toys. In some cases, the disorder develops after measles, encephalitis, or another clear-cut brain disease (e.g., metachromatic leukodystrophy, Schilder's disease) that damages the central nervous system (American Psychiatric Association 2000;

Table 21–3. DSM-IV-TR diagnostic criteria for childhood disintegrative disorder

A. Apparently normal development for at least the first 2 years after birth as manifested by the presence of age-appropriate verbal and nonverbal communication, social relationships, play, and adaptive behavior

B. Clinically significant loss of previously acquired skills (before age 10 years) in at least two of the following areas:
(1) expressive or receptive language
(2) social skills or adaptive behavior
(3) bowel or bladder control
(4) play
(5) motor skills

C. Abnormalities of functioning in at least two of the following areas:
(1) qualitative impairment in social interaction (e.g., impairment in nonverbal behaviors, failure to develop peer relationships, lack of social or emotional reciprocity)
(2) qualitative impairments in communication (e.g., delay or lack of spoken language, inability to initiate or sustain a conversation, stereotyped and repetitive use of language, lack of varied make-believe play)
(3) restricted, repetitive, and stereotyped patterns of behavior, interests, and activities, including motor stereotypies and mannerisms

D. The disturbance is not better accounted for by another specific pervasive developmental disorder or by schizophrenia.

Source. Reprinted from the *Diagnostic and Statistical Manual of Mental Disorders*, 4th Edition, Text Revision. Washington, DC, American Psychiatric Association, 2000. Copyright 2000, American Psychiatric Association. Used with permission.

Rutter 1985). Two distinctive patterns of onset have been reported in the literature: abrupt onset (over days to weeks) and gradual onset (over weeks to months) (Volkmar 1994). Over the course of a few months, these children have a complete loss of speech and language (Kurita 1996). Language comprehension and cognitive function are impaired. Social skills are lost and interpersonal relationships impaired. These children become disinterested in the environment and develop motor restlessness and stereotyped repetitive movements and mannerisms, with grimacing and tics. During this regressive period, the children become incontinent and need to be fed. Functionally, all these children are severely mentally retarded, but some children retain "islands" of relatively good abilities in some areas. General physical and neurological examinations usually reveal no abnormal physical signs. After the regression phase, the children are stable for many years. However, they are overactive, with poor attention span, isolation, and obsessive behavior. Their comprehension of language is rather limited, as is their expressive language. Volkmar (1992) reported that as many as 40% of patients may regain the ability to speak in single words, with 20% regaining the capacity to speak in sentences. These patients generally have relatively good motor abilities.

In a follow-up study of 13 patients with disintegrative disorder, Mouridsen et al. (1999a) noted that 77% of the patients had epilepsy and that in 50% the epilepsy was of the psychomotor variant. IQ scores did not seem to relate to the presence or absence of epilepsy.

■ Differential Diagnosis

Childhood disintegrative disorder must be differentiated from other PDDs. Millichap (1987) suggested that Rett's disorder be regarded as a type of Heller's dementia (i.e., disintegrative disorder), but only patients with Rett's disorder have *MECP2* mutations and have developed severe lower-motor neuron and basal ganglia dysfunction.

Sometimes it may be difficult to differentiate between autistic disorder with speech loss (see also Chapter 20, "Autistic Disorder," in this volume) and disintegrative disorder. Mouridsen et al. (2000) found very little in the neurobiological background of either group to support a clear distinction between disintegrative disorder and autistic disorder. Nonetheless, the patients with disintegrative disorder have clearer regression after more satisfactory development than do the patients with autistic disorder with speech loss. Three to 4 years after regression, patients with disintegrative disorder are significantly more severely retarded than those with autistic disorder (Kurita et al. 1992).

In Asperger's disorder, in general there is no delay in language development, no significant cognitive impairment, and no marked loss of developmental skills.

Infancy- and childhood-onset dementia occurs as a consequence of the direct physiological effects of a general medical condition (e.g., head trauma), whereas childhood disintegrative disorder typically occurs in the absence of an associated general medical condition (American Psychiatric Association 2000).

■ Epidemiology

Prevalence

No detailed, large-scale epidemiological studies have yet been carried out, so the exact prevalence of childhood disintegrative disorder is unknown. It is apparently rare. The 10 cases identified in Volkmar and Cohen's (1989) study represent 6% of the larger sample of autistic individuals; that is, childhood disintegrative disorder may be about one-tenth as common as autistic disorder. Burd et al. (1989) reported a prevalence of 0.11 in 10,000.

Sex Ratio

There were eight boys and two girls in the study by Evans-Jones and Rosenbloom (1978). All 10 patients with disintegrative disorder in Volkmar and Cohen's (1989) study were boys. Volkmar (1994) described a male-to-female ratio of 8:1 based on cases reported since 1977. It is clear that males predominate in disintegrative disorder.

Social Class

Earlier case reports tended to relate childhood disintegrative disorder to middle to upper social classes because of referral bias. More recent data do not indicate that this disorder occurs more frequently in any particular socioeconomic group (Evans-Jones and Rosenbloom 1978; Volkmar 1994).

■ Etiology

Stress Factors

Evans-Jones and Rosenbloom (1978) reported that the deterioration often seemed to follow some life events. However, Rutter (1985) noted that these events were no more than the usual stresses that all children are subjected to at one time or another.

Birth Factors

Evans-Jones and Rosenbloom (1978) reported no significant perinatal history in their series of cases.

Genetic Factors

Autism and disintegrative disorder cosegregating within a sibship was reported by Zwaigenbaum et al. (2000). Evans-Jones and Rosenbloom (1978) did not find any significant family history in their study. As noted above, no particular socioeconomic group was preponderant in their series of patients. Chromosome studies have not identified any abnormality (Volkmar and Cohen 1989).

Neuropathological Factors

Malamud (1959) reported a postmortem study that showed clear-cut evidence of cerebral degenerative disease suggestive of late infantile forms of cerebral lipidosis. Creak (1963) also noted lipidosis in 2 patients with disintegrative psychosis. Findings on CT scans that were performed in 5 of the 10 patients in the Volkmar and Cohen (1989) study were all normal.

Neurophysiological Factors

Evans-Jones and Rosenbloom (1978) studied 10 children with disintegrative psychosis. The electroencephalographic findings were abnormal in 5 patients; however, no constant pattern emerged. The electroencephalographic findings of the 9 patients in Hill and Rosenbloom's (1986) series were all normal. In the study by Volkmar and Cohen (1989), electroencephalographic findings were normal in 6, borderline in 2, and clearly abnormal in 2 of the 10 patients.

Summary

The clinical features and course of childhood disintegrative disorder and electroencephalographic abnormalities with seizure disorders in most of the patients with childhood disintegrative disorder suggest that an underlying basic neurobiological dysfunction is present, but the cause is currently unknown in most cases.

■ Treatment

Psychological

Once the diagnosis is established, family counseling should be provided and aimed at relieving parents' guilt and minimizing the ambivalent feelings of the family members.

Educational

Special educational and behavioral treatments are essential for controlling and minimizing aberrant behaviors as well as maximizing the child's potential.

Medical

Children with disintegrative disorder need more general health care, including frequent clinic visits, proper diet and nutrition, prevention of infections, dental care, and physical fitness, than children who do not have disintegrative disorder. Medications such as haloperidol, benzodiazepines, and anticonvulsants have been used to modify behavior but generally have not been effective.

■ Clinical Course and Prognosis

There is a strikingly uniform 6- to 9-month duration of progressive loss of abilities. This is followed by a plateau and then a limited improvement. Hill and Rosenbloom (1986) reported a follow-up study of nine individuals with disintegrative psychosis followed up for 11–16 years. Eight continued to fulfill the criteria for a diagnosis of disintegrative psychosis. Two of the nine children developed grand mal seizures. However, none of the patients had shown continuing regression when reviewed 11–16 years later. Burd et al. (1998) reported a prospective 14-year outcome for two individuals with disintegrative disorder and noted that both patients continued to have a severe PDD, mental retardation, and seizure disorder and were nonverbal. Both required residential care.

An increased frequency of electroencephalographic abnormalities and seizure disorder appears common in this disorder (American Psychiatric Association 2000).

The prognosis of disintegrative disorder is usually very poor. In the patients with neurolipidoses and leukodystrophies, progressive deterioration leads to death. In the other instances, the children's lack of speech persists, and they are moderately or severely mentally retarded. They continue to be wholly dependent individuals, and their social and behavioral difficulties remain relatively constant throughout life. However, after the initial diagnosis of disintegrative disorder is made, they seem to be given more heterogeneous diagnoses during the follow-up period (Mouridsen et al. 1999b).

■ Research Issues

Future research should examine the prevalence of childhood disintegrative disorder and compare its clinical course with that of autistic disorder with loss of speech. This research would require that research centers work together. Any data that indicate significant differences between the two conditions will provide strong support for the diagnostic validity of childhood disintegrative disorder. Data from larger samples will facilitate the search for neurobiological factors that cause childhood disintegrative disorder, as well as ensure more effective treatment or prevention of childhood disintegrative disorder.

Pervasive Developmental Disorder Not Otherwise Specified (Including Atypical Autism)

■ Definition and Diagnostic Criteria

DSM-IV-TR states that PDDNOS should be used when there is a severe and pervasive impairment in the development of reciprocal social interaction or verbal and nonverbal communication skills, or when stereotyped behavior, interests, and activities are present, but the criteria are not met for a specific PDD, schizophrenia, schizotypal personality disorder, or avoidant personality disorder (American Psychiatric Association 2000, p. 84).

However, DSM-IV-TR does not offer specific diagnostic criteria for PDDNOS. There are at least five subgroups of individuals within PDDNOS:

1. *Atypical autism:* young children who have not yet developed full-blown autistic disorder; individuals who "almost but not quite" meet the full criteria for autistic disorder (i.e., broader autism phenotype or lesser variant autism) (Piven et al. 1997; Szatmari et al. 2000b); patients who have a late onset (i.e., after age 3 years) of autistic disorder
2. *Residual autism:* individuals who had a history of having autistic disorder but presently do not meet the criteria for autistic disorder (i.e., still having some autistic features subsequent to effective interventions and/or natural development)
3. *Atypical Asperger's disorder:* young children who have not yet developed full-blown Asperger's disorder and individuals who "almost but not quite" meet the full criteria for Asperger's disorder
4. Mixed features of atypical autism and atypical Asperger's disorder
5. *Comorbid autism:* children with a medical or neurological disorder (e.g., tuberous sclerosis) associated with some "autistic features"

Thus, PDDNOS is actually a heterogeneous group of conditions that share autistic-like clinical features. Mahoney et al. (1998) and Allen et al. (2001) find very little difference between children with PDDNOS and those with autistic disorder and question the specificity of these diagnostic subtypes of PDD.

■ Clinical Findings

As a single diagnostic entity, as defined by DSM, very little is known about PDDNOS except that it is "more common than Autistic Disorder in the general population" (American Psychiatric Association 1987, p. 34). Epidemiological studies find that atypical autism appears to occur most often in individuals with profound retardation and in individuals with a severe specific developmental disorder of receptive language, some of whom show social, emotional, and/or behavioral symptoms that overlap with childhood autism (World Health Organization 1992). Clinical studies seem to identify a higher-functioning group of individuals with atypical autism.

No systematic study specifically based on DSM-III-R, DSM-IV, or DSM-IV-TR definitions and diagnostic criteria for PDDNOS has been done. The information on PDDNOS presented here is derived mainly from the limited studies that used DSM-III diagnostic criteria for childhood-onset PDD and atypical PDD.

Dahl et al. (1986) studied 390 children younger than 72 months; 24 were considered to have childhood-onset PDD. They had impaired human relationships, bizarre motor behavior, and confused and bizarre thinking. On the measures of cognitive functioning, these children showed a wide spread between the various sector means. There were no islets of intelligence. In general, the childhood-onset PDD group was noted to be more heterogeneous; many of these children showed clinical characteristics similar to those seen in children with infantile autism. Sparrow et al. (1986) reported similar findings in a follow-up study of 11 children with atypical PDD and 14 children without PDD. The atypical and control groups had similar cognitive measures; that is, both groups fell into the average to high-average range. However, poorer motor development and relatively impaired socialization and communication behaviors were much more characteristic of children with atypical PDD than of their age-matched peers without PDD. The children with atypical PDD had a tenuous, brittle, and shallow manner of relating to others; major difficulties interacting with similar-aged peers; high levels of anxiety; perseveration; and fascination with odd or idiosyncratic substances or objects.

Serra et al. (1999) studied children with PDDNOS and age-, sex- and intelligence-matched control subjects without PDDNOS by giving three structured emotional role-taking tasks and by asking them to give two spontaneous descriptions of peers. The results showed that the two groups did not differ with respect to their ability to infer other people's emotions in the structured role-taking tasks. However, significant differences were found for the unstructured description task: the children with PDDNOS used fewer inner, psychological characteristics to describe peers.

In various reports, children with PDD were somewhat heterogeneous, were similar to children with autistic disorder, and were significantly impaired in relationship, communication, cognition, and behavior (Dahl et al. 1986). Similar findings were reported by Sparrow et al. (1986). A number of additional studies of early-onset and/or atypical PDD have reported various combination of low IQ, impaired speech/language development such as echolalia, perseveration, withholding, idiosyncrasies, disordered relationships with parents and peers, rituals and mannerisms, unusual and/or intense fears, inappropriate affect, oppositional behavior, and motor coordination delays and/or deficits (Ghaziuddin and Butler 1998; Levine and Demb 1987; Rescorla 1988).

■ Differential Diagnosis

Because PDDNOS has a vague definition, diverse subtypes, and unclear diagnostic boundaries, making the differential diagnosis between PDDNOS and other mental disorders can be a very challenging task for even experienced practitioners, and in terms of treatment and prognosis it is unclear what clinical relevance this differential represents.

The differential diagnosis between autistic disorder (see also Chapter 20, "Autistic Disorder," in this volume) and atypical autism is mainly by the quantitative measure of the diagnostic criteria. Nonetheless, some clinical studies seem to find some significant differences between the two disorders in some clinical variables. For example, Njardvik et al. (1999) noted that the group with PDDNOS/atypical autism demonstrated better positive nonverbal social skills than the group with autism; Stella et al. (1999) reported that factor-based scales created from the Childhood

Autism Rating Scale (CARS) were able to distinguish subjects with PDDNOS from subjects with autistic disorder.

In Asperger's disorder, there should not be a delay in cognitive and language development. In atypical autism, there is delayed as well as deviant development in language. In lower-functioning atypical autism, there is severe or profound impairment of cognition. Kurita (1997) compared patients with Asperger's disorder and high-functioning atypical autism on 64 clinical variables, including obstetric risk factors, early developmental landmarks, IQ, autistic symptoms on the CARS-TV (CARS—Tokyo Version), epileptic electroencephalographic abnormalities, and epilepsy. The Asperger's disorder group did not differ significantly from high-functioning atypical autism group on the CARS-TV in any but total score and four item scores (imitation, visual responsiveness, auditory responsiveness, and nonverbal communication), in which the Asperger's disorder group scored significantly lower than the high-functioning atypical autism group.

Many individuals with severe or profound mental retardation (see also Chapter 19, "Mental Retardation," in this volume) are mute and have stereotypies. The distinction of atypical autism from severe or profound mental retardation can be difficult. However, individuals with severe or profound mental retardation tend to maintain their interest in other people and welcome social interactions.

The observation of "thought disorders" in children with atypical PDD could support the view that this disorder is a variant of schizophrenia in childhood (see also Chapter 23, "Schizophrenia and Other Psychotic Disorders," in this volume). However, several points argue against such a notion. First, no deterioration from a previous level of functioning occurs in these children. Second, no clear evidence of delusions or hallucinations is present in any of the children. Third, no evidence of family history of schizophrenia or other types of psychoses is found in these children.

It may be very difficult to differentiate children who later develop schizoid personality disorder or schizotypal personality disorder, and adults with schizoid or schizotypal personality disorder whose childhood history is unclear or unavailable, from people with PDDNOS. Nonetheless, individuals with PDDNOS have more severely impaired social awareness, emotional reciprocity, and communication skills, as well as more stereotyped behaviors and unusual interests.

For the differential diagnosis from expressive and mixed receptive-expressive language disorders, obsessive-compulsive disorder, Tourette's disorder, selective mutism, and congenital peripheral blindness or partial sightedness, see the discussion in Chapter 20, "Autistic Disorder," in this volume. As described in Chapter 20, some medical or neurological disorders (e.g., fragile X syndrome, Landau-Kleffner syndrome, tuberous sclerosis) may be comorbid with PDDNOS.

■ Epidemiology

Prevalence

Lotter (1966) surveyed the entire population of 8- to 10-year-old children in Middlesex, United Kingdom, and found the rate of atypical autism to be about 5 per 10,000. Various studies of atypical autism/atypical PDD in various countries and locales have yielded prevalence rates ranging from a high of 16 per 10,000 to a low of 1.99 per 10,000 children (Burd et al. 1987; Levine and Demb 1987; Steffenburg and Gillberg 1986; Wing and Gould 1979). These diverse prevalence rates of atypical autism readily illustrate the problem caused by the use of an imprecise definition, lack of reliable explicit diagnostic criteria for atypical autism, and reliance on inexperienced clinicians' judgment and recall for case identification.

Sex Ratio

PDDNOS appears to be considerably more common in boys than in girls, with ratios ranging from 5:1 to 2:1 (Dahl et al. 1986; Sparrow et al. 1986; Volkmar et al. 1988). However, in the survey study by Steffenburg and Gillberg (1986), there was a higher proportion of girls. It is apparent that different definitions and diagnostic criteria used in these studies yielded somewhat different sex ratios.

Social Class

The families of children with childhood-onset PDD were somewhat better educated and of higher socioeconomic status (i.e., 50% from the top two categories of socioeconomic status) than the families of children in the other diagnostic groups. Levine and Demb (1987) also noted that the educational level of the atypical PDD group tended to be higher than that of other clinic patients. The significance of the finding is not clear; it requires further study with a large-scale sample.

■ Etiology

Atypical autism has been associated with the genetic disorder tuberous sclerosis (Bolton and Griffiths 1997). Steffenburg and Gillberg (1986) reported that 12% of the atypical autism group had specific neurological disorders (e.g., tuberous sclerosis). There were case reports of chromosomal abnormalities involving deletion of the long arm of chromosome 8 (Weidmer-Mikhail et al. 1998); duplication of chromosome 15 (Cook et al. 1997; Gurrieri et al. 1999); and XYY syndrome (Weidmer-Mikhail et al. 1998).

Gillberg and Coleman (1996) reported that the overall prevalence of medical disorders in atypical autism was similar to that found in typical autism (about 24%). Volkmar et al. (1988) concluded that 25% of the atypical autism group had some evidence of organicity.

In the study by Burd et al. (1987), 19% of the atypical PDD group had seizure disorders, and 71% had associated medical conditions. About 4.2% of the children with childhood-onset PDD (Dahl et al. 1986) had evidence of neurological disturbance (i.e., congenital central nervous system malformation). For more than two-thirds of the children in the study conducted by Levine and Demb (1987), the mothers had histories of medically complicated pregnancies and/or perinatal complications. About 44% of the children had neurological signs, including increased reflexes, lax ligaments, positive Babinski reflex, hypotonia, poor cerebellar functioning, cataracts, macrocephaly, decreased strength, and drooling.

Children with PDDNOS were noted to be deficient in theory of mind ability, as determined by performance on the brain function task and the false belief task tests (Sicotte and Stemberger 1999).

Available information appears to indicate that atypical autism has a great heterogeneity in terms of etiology. Thus, it is expected that numerous etiological factors will be identified in future research in this area.

■ Treatment

The treatment of patients with PDDNOS, including atypical autism, is similar to that for those with autistic disorder or Asperger's disorder. For example, Brodkin et al. (1997) reported that 6 (55%) of 11 patients with PDDNOS were considered to be responsive to clomipramine treatment; Zuddas et al. (2000) reported, on the basis of behavioral rating scales in patients with PDDNOS, that risperidone was effective.

However, special-education systems in most U.S. states do not have an educational category specifically for students with PDDNOS/atypical autism. Many students with such a diagnosis are placed in programs for students with other disorders, such as mental retardation, emotional disturbance, or behavior disorder. Hence, these students with PDDNOS/atypical autism do not receive any programming that attends to their unique educational needs. It is important for the psychiatrist to work closely with school personnel to ensure that students with PDDNOS/atypical autism receive necessary educational services.

■ Clinical Course and Prognosis

The age of recognition of atypical PDD was somewhat later than that of autistic disorder. At present, limited information is available on the prognosis and outcome for individuals with atypical PDD. Gillberg and Steffenburg (1987) found that most of the children with atypical PDD, when reevaluated at puberty, tended to have poor outcomes. Sparrow et al. (1986) reported a 7-year follow-up study of 11 preschool-age children with atypical development, and the results indicated that the impairment in reciprocal social interaction was quite stable. Demb and Weintraub (1989) reported on the outcome for 12 children with atypical PDD reevaluated at a mean age of 11 years 3 months. Ten children received a diagnosis of PDD, 1 had schizotypal personality disorder, and 1 had attention problems. Many of these children had symptoms of anxiety and depression.

It is not clear whether these individuals would show significant improvement with longer educational and other treatments. More prolonged follow-up is needed to determine the final outcome for these individuals.

■ Research Issues

Patients with atypical autism may be more common but less frequently studied than those with autistic disorder. The validity of this diagnostic entity and its relationship to autistic disorder and other PDDs are unclear. In a comparison study of 205 autistic subjects, 80 PDDNOS patients, and 174 individuals with other non-PDD disorders, Buitelaar et al. (1999) found that only a limited number of items from the ICD-10 and DSM-IV-TR systems for autistic disorder significantly discriminated the PDDNOS group from those with other disorders. It is not evident whether PDDNOS (including atypical autism) as it is currently defined in DSM-IV-TR can be considered a distinct diagnostic subgroup of PDDs. Existing data indicate great heterogeneity, and the need to divide it further into smaller groups may arise in the future. Hence, the development of more explicit and well-validated diagnostic criteria is an important topic of future research.

References

Allen DA, Steinberg M, Dunn M, et al: Autistic disorder versus other pervasive developmental disorder in young children: same or different? Eur Child Adolesc Psychiatry 10:67–78, 2001

Amano K, Nomura Y, Segawa M, et al: Mutational analysis of the *MECP2* gene in Japanese patients with Rett syndrome. J Hum Genet 45:231–236, 2000

American Psychiatric Association: Diagnostic and Statistical Manual of Mental Disorders, 3rd Edition. Washington, DC, American Psychiatric Association, 1980

American Psychiatric Association: Diagnostic and Statistical Manual of Mental Disorders, 3rd Edition, Revised. Washington, DC, American Psychiatric Association, 1987

American Psychiatric Association: Diagnostic and Statistical Manual of Mental Disorders, 4th Edition. Washington, DC, American Psychiatric Association, 1994

American Psychiatric Association: Diagnostic and Statistical Manual of Mental Disorders, 4th Edition, Text Revision. Washington, DC, American Psychiatric Association, 2000

Amir RE, Zoghbi HY: Rett syndrome: methyl-CpG-binding protein 2 mutations and phenotype-genotype correlations. Am J Med Genet 97:147–152, 2000

Amir RE, Van den Veyver IB, Wan M, et al: Rett syndrome is caused by mutation in X-linked *MECP2*, encoding methyl-CpG-binding protein 2. Nat Genet 23:185–188, 1999

Amir RE, Van den Veyver IB, Schultz R, et al: Influence of mutation type and X-chromosome inactivation on Rett syndrome phenotypes. Ann Neurol 47:670–679, 2000

Armstrong D: The neuropathology of Rett syndrome. Brain Dev 14 (suppl):S89–S98, 1992

Armstrong D, Dunn JK, Antalffy B, et al: Selective dendritic alterations in the cortex of Rett syndrome. J Neuropathol Exp Neurol 54:195–201, 1995

Armstrong D, Dunn JK, Antalffy B: Decreased dendritic branching in frontal, motor and limbic cortex in Rett syndrome compared with trisomy 21. J Neuropathol Exp Neurol 57:1013–1017, 1998

Aron M: The use and effectiveness of elbow splints in the Rett syndrome. Brain Dev 12:162–163, 1990

Asperger H: Die autistischen psychopathen im kindesalter. Archiv for Psychiatrie und Nervenkrankheiten 117:76–136, 1944 ["Autistic psychopathy" in childhood, in Autism and Asperger Syndrome. Translated and edited by Frith U. Cambridge, MA, Cambridge University Press, 1991, pp 37–92]

Auranen M, Vanhala R, Vosman M, et al: MECP2 gene analysis in classical Rett syndrome and in patients with Rett-like features. Neurology 56:611–617, 2001

Bader GG, Witt-Engerström I, Hagberg B: Neurophysiological findings in the Rett syndrome, II: visual and auditory brainstem, middle and late evoked responses. Brain Dev 11:110–114, 1989

Baron-Cohen S, Jolliffe T, Mortimore C, et al: Another advanced test of theory of mind: evidence from very high functioning adults with autism or Asperger syndrome. J Child Psychol Psychiatry 38:813–822, 1997

Baron-Cohen S, Ring HA, Wheelwright S, et al: Social intelligence in the normal and autistic brain: an fMRI study. Eur J Neurosci 11:1891–1898, 1999

Bauman ML, Kemper TL, Arin DM: Microscopic observations of the brain in Rett syndrome. Neuropediatrics 26:105–108, 1995

Belichenko PV, Hagberg B, Dahlstrom A: Morphological study of neocortical areas in Rett syndrome. Acta Neuropathol 93:50–61, 1997

Berthier ML, Starkstein SE, Leiguarda R: Developmental cortical anomalies in Asperger's syndrome: neuroradiological findings in two patients. J Neuropsychiatry Clin Neurosci 2:197–201, 1990

Berthier ML, Bayes A, Tolosa ES: Magnetic resonance imaging in patients with concurrent Tourette's disorder and Asperger's syndrome. J Am Acad Child Adolesc Psychiatry 32:633–639, 1993

Bettison S: The long-term effects of auditory training on children with autism. J Autism Dev Disord 26:361–374, 1996

Bienvenu T, Carrie A, de Roux N, et al: MECP2 mutations account for most cases of typical forms of Rett syndrome. Hum Mol Genet 9:1377–1384, 2000

Bjure J, Uvebrant P, Vestergren E, et al: Regional cerebral blood flow abnormalities in Rett syndrome. Eur Child Adolesc Psychiatry 6 (suppl 1):64–66, 1997

Blue ME, Naidu S, Johnston MV: Altered development of glutamate and GABA receptors in the basal ganglia of girls with Rett syndrome. Exp Neurol 156:345–352, 1999

Bolton PF, Griffiths PD: Association of tuberous sclerosis of temporal lobes with autism and atypical autism. Lancet 349:392–395, 1997

Bourdon V, Philippe C, Labrune O, et al: A detailed analysis of the MECP2 gene: prevalence of recurrent mutations and gross DNA rearrangement in Rett syndrome patients. Hum Genet 108:43–50, 2001

Bowler DM, Gardiner JM, Grice SJ: Episodic memory and remembering in adults with Asperger syndrome. J Autism Dev Disord 30:295–304, 2000

Brase DA, Myer EC, Dewey WL: Minireview: possible hyperendorphinergic pathophysiology of the Rett syndrome. Life Sci 45:359–366, 1989

Brodkin ES, McDougle CJ, Naylor ST, et al: Clomipramine in adults with pervasive developmental disorders: a prospective open-label investigation. J Child Adolesc Psychopharmacol 7:109–121, 1997

Buhler EM, Malik NJ, Alkan M: Another model for the inheritance of Rett syndrome. Am J Med Genet 36:126–131, 1990

Buitelaar JK, van der Gaag R, Klin A, et al: Exploring the boundaries of pervasive developmental disorder not otherwise specified: analyses of data from the DSM-IV Autistic Disorder Field Trial. J Autism Dev Disord 29:33–43, 1999

Burd L, Fisher W, Kerbeshian J: A prevalence study of pervasive developmental disorders in North Dakota. J Am Acad Child Psychiatry 26:700–703, 1987

Burd L, Fisher W, Kerbeshian J: Pervasive disintegrative disorder: are Rett syndrome and Heller dementia infantilis subtypes? Dev Med Child Neurol 31:609–616, 1989

Burd L, Ivey M, Barth A, et al: Two males with childhood disintegrative disorder: a prospective 14-year outcome study. Dev Med Child Neurol 40:702–707, 1998

Burroni L, Aucone AM, Volterrani D, et al: A qualitative and quantitative SPECT study with 99Tc(m)-ECD. Nucl Med Commun 18:527–534, 1997

Buyse IM, Fang P, Hoon KT, et al: Diagnostic testing for Rett syndrome by DHPLC and direct sequencing analysis of the MECP2 gene: identification of several novel mutations and polymorphisms. Am J Hum Genet 67:1482–1436, 2000

Chatterjee S, Ghosh N, Goh KM, et al: Glycosphingolipids in patients with the Rett syndrome. Brain Dev 12:85–87, 1990

Cheadle JP, Gill H, Fleming N, et al: Long-read sequence analysis of the MECP2 gene in Rett syndrome patients: correlation of disease severity with mutation type and location. Hum Mol Genet 9:1119–1129, 2000

Chiron C, Bulteau C, Loc'h C, et al: Dopaminergic D_2 receptor SPECT imaging in Rett syndrome: increase of specific binding in striatum. J Nucl Med 34:1717–1721, 1993

Christen HJ, Hanefeld F: Male Rett variant. Neuropediatrics 26:81–82, 1995

Clayton-Smith J, Watson P, Ramsden S, et al: Somatic mutation in MECP2 as a non-fatal neurodevelopmental disorder in males. Lancet 356:830–832, 2000

Coleman M: Is classical Rett syndrome ever present in males? Brain Dev 12:31–32, 1990

Cook EH Jr, Lindgren V, Leventhal BL, et al: Autism or atypical autism in maternally but not paternally derived proximal 15q duplication. Am J Hum Genet 60:928–934, 1997

Cooke DW, Naidu S, Plotnick L, et al: Abnormalities of thyroid function and glucose control in subjects with Rett syndrome. Horm Res 43:273–278, 1995

Cooper RA, Kerr AM, Amos PM: Rett syndrome: critical examination of clinical features, serial EEG and video-monitoring in understanding and management. Eur J Paediatr Neurol 2:127–135, 1998

Craig L, Baron-Cohen S: Creativity and imagination in autism and Asperger syndrome. J Autism Dev Disord 29:319–326, 1999

Craig L, Baron-Cohen S: Story-telling in children with autism or Asperger syndrome: a window into the imagination. Isr J Psychiatry Relat Sci 37:64–70, 2000

Creak EM: Childhood psychosis: a review of 100 cases. Br J Psychiatry 109:84–89, 1963

Critchley HD, Daly EM, Bullmore ET, et al: The functional neuroanatomy of social behaviour: changes in cerebral blood flow when people with autistic disorder process facial expressions. Brain 123(pt 11):2203–2212, 2000

Dahl EK, Cohen DJ, Provence S: Clinical and multivariate approaches to the nosology of pervasive developmental disorders. J Am Acad Child Psychiatry 25:170–180, 1986

De Bona C, Zappella M, Hayek G, et al: Preserved speech variant is allelic of classic Rett syndrome. Eur J Hum Genet 8:325–330, 2000

Deguchi K, Antalffy BA, Twohill LJ, et al: Substance P immunoreactivity in Rett syndrome. Pediatr Neurol 22:259–266, 2000

Demb HB, Weintraub AG: A five-year follow-up of preschool children diagnosed as having an atypical pervasive developmental disorder. J Dev Behav Pediatr 10:292–298, 1989

Egger J, Hofacker N, Schiel W, et al: Magnesium for hyperventilation in Rett's syndrome. Lancet 340:621–622, 1992

Ehlers S, Gillberg C: The epidemiology of Asperger syndrome: a total population study. J Child Psychol Psychiatry 34:1327–1350, 1993

Ehlers S, Nyden A, Gillberg C, et al: Asperger syndrome, autism and attention disorder: a comparative study of cognitive profiles of 120 children. J Child Psychol Psychiatry 38:207–217, 1997

Elian M, de M Rudolf N: Observations on hand movements in Rett syndrome: a pilot study. Acta Neurol Scand 94:212–214, 1996

Ellaway C, Sholler G, Leonard H, et al: Prolonged QT interval in Rett syndrome. Arch Dis Child 80:470–472, 1999a

Ellaway C, Williams K, Leonard H, et al: Rett syndrome: randomized controlled trial of L-carnitine. J Child Neurol 14:162–167, 1999b

Engerström IW: Rett syndrome: the late infantile regression period—a retrospective analysis of 91 cases. Acta Paediatr 81:167–172, 1992

Evans-Jones LG, Rosenbloom L: Disintegrative psychosis in childhood. Dev Med Child Neurol 20:462–470, 1978

Fiumara A, Sciotto A, Barone R, et al: Peripheral lymphocyte subset and other immune aspects in Rett syndrome. Pediatr Neurol 21:619–621, 1999

Galbraith GC, Philipart M, Stephen LM: Brainstem frequency-following responses in Rett syndrome. Pediatr Neurol 15:26–31, 1996

Ghaziuddin M, Butler E: Clumsiness in autism and Asperger syndrome: a further report. J Intellect Disabil Res 42(pt 1):43–48, 1998

Ghaziuddin M, Gerstein L: Pedantic speaking style differentiates Asperger syndrome from high-functioning autism. J Autism Dev Disord 26:585–595, 1996

Ghaziuddin M, Tsai L, Ghaziuddin N: Brief report: violence in Asperger syndrome, a critique. J Autism Dev Disord 21:349–354, 1991

Ghaziuddin M, Butler E, Tsai L, et al: Is clumsiness a marker for Asperger syndrome? J Intellect Disabil Res 38:519–527, 1994

Ghaziuddin M, Leininger L, Tsai L: Brief report: thought disorder in Asperger syndrome: comparison with high-functioning autism. J Autism Dev Disord 25:311–317, 1995a

Ghaziuddin M, Shakal J, Tsai L: Obstetric factors in Asperger syndrome: comparison with high-functioning autism. J Intellect Disabil Res 39(pt 6):538–543, 1995b

Ghaziuddin M, Weidmer-Mikhail E, Ghaziuddin N: Comorbidity of Asperger syndrome: a preliminary report. J Intellect Disabil Res 42(pt 4):279–283, 1998

Gillberg C: Autistic syndrome in Rett syndrome: the first two years according to mother reports. Brain Dev 9:499–501, 1987

Gillberg C: Asperger syndrome in 23 Swedish children. Dev Med Child Neurol 31:520–531, 1989

Gillberg C: Outcome in autism and autistic-like conditions. J Am Acad Child Adolesc Psychiatry 30:375–382, 1991

Gillberg C, Coleman M: Autism and medical disorders: a review of literature. Dev Med Child Neurol 38:191–202, 1996

Gillberg IC, Gillberg C: Asperger syndrome: some epidemiological considerations—a research note. J Child Psychol Psychiatry 30:631–638, 1989

Gillberg C, Steffenburg S: Outcome and prognostic factors in infantile autism and similar conditions: a population-based study of 46 cases followed through puberty. J Autism Dev Disord 17:273–288, 1987

Gillberg C, Nordin V, Ehlers S: Early detection of autism. Diagnostic instruments for clinicians. Eur Child Adolesc Psychiatry 5:67–74, 1996

Girard M, Couvert P, Carrie A, et al: Parental origin of de novo MECP2 mutations in Rett syndrome. Eur J Hum Genet 9:231–236, 2001

Glaze DG, Schultz RJ, Frost JD: Rett syndrome: characterization of seizures versus non-seizures. Electroencephalogr Clin Neurophysiol 106:79–83, 1998

Godbout R, Bergeron C, Limoges E, et al: A laboratory study of sleep in Asperger's syndrome. Neuroreport 11:127–130, 2000

Goutieres F, Aicardi J: Atypical forms of Rett syndrome. Am J Med Genet 24:184–194, 1986

Goutieres F, Aicardi J: New experience with Rett syndrome in France: the problem of atypical cases. Brain Dev 9:502–505, 1987

Green J, Gilchrist A, Burton D, et al: Social and psychiatric functioning in adolescents with Asperger syndrome compared with conduct disorder. J Autism Dev Disord 30:279–293, 2000

Grossman JB, Klin A, Carter AS, et al: Verbal bias in recognition of facial emotions in children with Asperger syndrome. J Child Psychol Psychiatry 41:369–379, 2000

Guerrini R, Bonanni P, Parmeggiani, et al: Cortical reflex myoclonus in Rett syndrome. Ann Neurol 43:472–479, 1998

Guideri F, Acampa M, Hayek G, et al: Reduced heart rate variability in patients affected with Rett syndrome: a possible explanation for sudden death. Neuropediatrics 30:146–148, 1999

Gurrieri F, Battaglia A, Torris L, et al: Pervasive developmental disorder and epilepsy due to maternally derived duplication of 15q11–q13. Neurology 52:1694–1697, 1999

Haas RH: The history and challenge of Rett syndrome. J Child Neurol 3(suppl):S3–S5, 1988

Haas RH, Rice MA, Trauner DA, et al: Therapeutic effects of a ketogenic diet in Rett syndrome. Am J Med Genet 24(suppl 1):225–246, 1986

Haas RH, Dixon SD, Sartoris DJ, et al: Osteopenia in Rett syndrome. J Pediatr 131:771–774, 1997

Hagberg BA: Rett syndrome: clinical peculiarities, diagnostic approach, and possible cause. Pediatr Neurol 5:75–83, 1989

Hagberg BA, Witt-Engerström I: Rett syndrome: a suggested staging system for describing impairment profile with increasing age toward adolescence. Am J Med Genet 24:47–59, 1986

Hagberg BA, Witt-Engerström I: Rett syndrome: epidemiology and nosology—progress in knowledge 1986: a conference communication. Brain Dev 9:451–457, 1987

Hagberg BA, Witt-Engerström I: Early stages of the Rett syndrome and infantile neuronal ceroid lipofuscinosis: a difficult differential diagnosis. Brain Dev 12:20–22, 1990

Hagberg BA, Aicardi J, Dias K, et al: A progressive syndrome of autism, dementia, ataxia, and loss of purposeful hand use in girls: Rett's syndrome: report of 35 cases. Ann Neurol 14:471–479, 1983

Hagberg BA, Goutieres F, Hanefeld F, et al: Rett syndrome: criteria for inclusion and exclusion. Brain Dev 7:372–373, 1985

Hagberg G, Stenbom Y, Witt-Engerström I: Head growth in Rett syndrome. Acta Paediatrica 89:198–202, 2000

Hamberger A, Gillberg C, Palm A, et al: Elevated CSF glutamate in Rett syndrome. Neuropediatrics 23:212–213, 1992

Hanks SB: The role of therapy in Rett syndrome. Am J Med Genet 24(suppl 1):247–252, 1986

Happe E, Ehlers S, Fletcher P, et al: Theory of mind in the brain: evidence from a PET scan study of Asperger syndrome. Neuroreport 8:197–201, 1996

Harrison DJ, Webb PJ: Scoliosis in the Rett syndrome: natural history and treatment. Brain Dev 12:154–156, 1990

Hebebrand J, Henninghausen K, Nau S, et al: Low body weight in male children and adolescents with schizoid personality disorder or Asperger's disorder. Acta Psychiatr Scand 96:64–67, 1997

Heller T: Uber Dementia infantalis. Zeitschrift fur Kinderforschung 37:661–667, 1930 [Reprinted in Howells JG (ed): Modern Perspectives in International Child Psychiatry. Edinburgh, Scotland, Oliver and Boyd, 1979]

Hill AE, Rosenbloom L: Disintegrative psychosis of childhood: teenage follow-up. Dev Med Child Neurol 28:34–40, 1986

Hoffbuhr K, Devaney JM, LaFleur B, et al: *MeCP2* mutations in children with and without the phenotype of Rett syndrome. Neurology 56:1486–1495, 2001

Holm VA, King HA: Scoliosis in the Rett syndrome. Brain Dev 12:151–153, 1990

Horska A, Naidu S, Herskovits EH, et al: Quantitative ^{1}H spectroscopic imaging in early Rett syndrome. Neurology 54:715–722, 2000

Howlin P, Asgharian A: The diagnosis of autism and Asperger syndrome: findings from a survey of 770 families. Dev Med Child Neurol 41:834–839, 1999

Huang TJ, Lubicky JP, Hammerberg KW: Scoliosis in Rett syndrome. Orthopaedic Review 23:931–937, 1994

Hunter K: Rett syndrome: parents' views about specific symptoms. Brain Dev 9:535–538, 1987

Huppke P, Laccone F, Kramer N, et al: Rett syndrome: analysis of *MECP2* and clinical characterization of 31 patients. Hum Mol Genet 9:1369–1395, 2000

Inui K, Akagi M, Ono J, et al: Mutation analysis of *MECP2* in Japanese patients with atypical Rett syndrome. Brain Dev 23:212–215, 2001

Ishizaki A: Electroencephalographical study of the Rett syndrome with special reference to the monorhythmic theta activities in adult patients. Brain Dev 14(suppl):S31–S36, 1992

Ishizaki A, Inoue Y, Sasaki H, et al: Longitudinal observation of electroencephalograms in the Rett syndrome. Brain Dev 11:407–412, 1989

Jan MM, Dooley JM, Gordon KE: Male Rett syndrome variant: application of diagnostic criteria. Pediatr Neurol 20:238–240, 1999

Jellinger K, Armstrong D, Zoghbi HY, et al: Neuropathology of Rett syndrome. Acta Neuropathol (Berl) 76:142–158, 1988

Johnston MV, Hohmann C, Blue ME: Neurobiology of Rett syndrome. Neuropediatrics 26:119–122, 1995

Jolliffe T, Baron-Cohen S: A test of central coherence theory: linguistic processing in high-functioning adults with autism or Asperger syndrome: is local coherence impaired? Cognition 71:149–185, 1999a

Jolliffe T, Baron-Cohen S: The Strange Stories Test: a replication with high-functioning adults with autism or Asperger syndrome. J Autism Dev Disord 29:395–406, 1999b

Jones PB, Kerwin RW: Left temporal lobe damage in Asperger's syndrome. Br J Psychiatry 156:570–572, 1990

Julu PO, Kerr AM, Apartopoulos F, et al: Characterisation of breathing and associated central autonomic dysfunction in the Rett disorder. Arch Dis Child 85:29–37, 2001

Kadesjo B, Gillberg C: Tourette's disorder: epidemiology and comorbidity in primary school children. J Am Acad Child Adolesc Psychiatry 39:548–555, 2000

Kalmanchey R: Evoked potentials in the Rett syndrome. Brain Dev 12:73–76, 1990

Kerr AM, Stephenson JBP: Rett's syndrome in the west of Scotland. BMJ 291:579–582, 1985

Kerr AM, Armstrong DD, Prescott RJ, et al: Rett syndrome: analysis of death in the British survey. Eur Child Adolesc Psychiatry 6(suppl 1):71–74, 1997

Kimura K, Nomura Y, Segawa M: Middle and short latency somatosensory evoked potentials (SEPm, SEPs) in Rett syndrome: chronological changes of cortical and subcortical involvements. Brain Dev 14(suppl):S37–S42, 1992

Kitt CA, Wilcox BJ: Preliminary evidence for neurodegenerative changes in the substantia nigra of Rett syndrome. Neuropediatrics 26:114–118, 1995

Klin A: Attributing social meaning to ambiguous visual stimuli in higher-functioning autism and Asperger syndrome: the Social Attribution Task. J Child Psychol Psychiatry 41:831–846, 2000

Klin A, Volkmar FR, Sparrow SS, et al: Validity and neuropsychological characterization of Asperger syndrome: convergence with nonverbal learning disabilities syndrome. J Child Psychol Psychiatry 36:1127–1140, 1995

Kohn Y, Fahum T, Ratzoni G, et al: Aggression and sexual offense in Asperger's syndrome. Isr J Psychiatry Relat Sci 35:293–299, 1998

Koppenhaver DA, Erickson KA, Harris B, et al: Storybook-based communication intervention for girls with Rett syndrome and their mothers. Disabil Rehabil 23:149–159, 2001

Kozinetz CA, Skender ML, McNaughton N, et al: Epidemiology of Rett syndrome: a population-based registry. Pediatrics 91:445–450, 1993

Kumandas S, Caksen H, Ciftci A: Lamotrigine in two cases of Rett syndrome. Brain Dev 23:240–242, 2001

Kurita H: The concept and nosology of Heller's syndrome: review of article and report of two cases. Jpn J Psychiatry Neurol 42:785–793, 1988

Kurita H: Specificity and developmental consequences of speech loss in children with pervasive developmental disorders. Psychiatry Clin Neurosci 50:181–184, 1996

Kurita H: A comparative study of Asperger syndrome with high-functioning atypical autism. Psychiatry Clin Neurosci 51:67–70, 1997

Kurita H, Kita M, Miyake Y: A comparative study of development and symptoms among disintegrative psychosis and infantile autism with and without speech loss. J Autism Dev Disord 22:175–188, 1992

Laccone F, Huppke P, Henefeld F, et al: Mutation spectrum in patients with Rett syndrome in the German population: evidence of hot spot region. Hum Mutat 17:183–190, 2001

Lappalainen R, Riikonen RS: High level of cerebrospinal fluid glutamate in Rett syndrome. Pediatr Neurol 15:213–216, 1996

Lappalainen R, Lindholm D, Riikonen RS: Low level of nerve growth factor in cerebrospinal fluid of children with Rett syndrome. J Child Neurol 11:296–300, 1996

Lappalainen R, Liewendahl K, Sainio K, et al: Brain perfusion SPECT and EEG findings in Rett syndrome. Acta Neurol Scand 95:44–50, 1997

Larsen FW, Mouridsen SE: The outcome in children with childhood autism and Asperger syndrome originally diagnosed as psychotic: a 30-year follow-up study of subjects hospitalized as children. Eur Child Adolesc Psychiatry 6:181–190, 1997

Leckman A, Hagberg B, Svennerholm LT: Altered cerebellar ganglioside pattern in Rett syndrome. Neurochem Int 19:505–509, 1991

Leckman A, Hagberg B, Svennerholm LT: Cerebrospinal fluid gangliosides in patients with Rett syndrome and infantile neuronal ceroid lipofuscinosis. Eur J Paediatr Neurol 3:119–123, 1999

Leonard H, Bower C, English D: The prevalence and incidence of Rett syndrome. Eur Child Adolesc Psychiatry 6(suppl 1):8–10, 1997

Leontovich TA, Mukhina JK, Fedorov AA, et al: Morphological study of the entorhinal cortex, hippocampal formation, and basal ganglia in Rett syndrome patients. Neurobiol Dis 6:77–91, 1999

Levine JM, Demb HB: Characteristics of preschool children diagnosed as having an atypical pervasive developmental disorder. J Dev Behav Pediatr 8:77–82, 1987

Lidstrom J, Stockland E, Hagberg B: Scoliosis in Rett syndrome: clinical and biological aspects. Spine 19:1632–1635, 1994

Lieb-Lundell C: The therapist's role in the management of girls with Rett syndrome. J Child Neurol 3(suppl):S31–S34, 1988

Lipani JD, Bhattacharjee MB, Corey DM, et al: Reduced nerve growth factor in Rett syndrome postmortem brain tissue. J Neuropathol Exp Neurol 59:889–895, 2000

Loder RT, Lee CL, Richards BS: Orthopedic aspects of Rett syndrome: a multicenter review. J Pediatr Orthop 9:557–562, 1989

Lotter V: Epidemiology of autistic conditions in young children, I: prevalence. Soc Psychiatry 1:124–137, 1966

Mahoney WJ, Szatmari P, MacLean JE, et al: Reliability and accuracy of differentiating pervasive developmental disorder subtypes. J Am Acad Child Adolesc Psychiatry 37:278–285, 1998

Malamud N: Heller's disease and childhood schizophrenia. Am J Psychiatry 116:215–218, 1959

Manjiviona J, Prior M: Comparison of Asperger syndrome and high-functioning autistic children on a test of motor impairment. J Autism Dev Disord 25:23–39, 1995

Marcus CL, Carroll JL, McColley SA, et al: Polysomnographic characteristic of patients with Rett syndrome. J Pediatr 125:218–224, 1994

Marriage K, Miles T, Stokes D, et al: Clinical and research implication of the co-occurrence of Asperger's and Tourette syndromes. Aust N Z J Psychiatry 27:666–672, 1993

Matsuishi T, Nagamitsu S, Yamashita Y, et al: Decreased cerebrospinal fluid levels of substance P in patients with Rett syndrome. Ann Neurol 42:978–981, 1997

Mayes SD, Calhoun SL, Crites DL: Does DSM-IV Asperger's disorder exist? J Abnorm Child Psychol 29:263–271, 2001

McArthur AJ, Budden SS: Sleep dysfunction in Rett syndrome: a trial of exogenous melatonin treatment. Dev Med Child Neurol 40:186–192, 1998

Meloni I, Bruttini M, Longo I, et al: A mutation in the Rett syndrome gene, MECP2, causes X-linked mental retardation and progressive spasticity in males. Am J Hum Genet 67:982–985, 2000

Messahel S, Pheasant AE, Pall H, et al: Abnormalities in urinary pterin levels in Rett syndrome. Eur J Paediatr Neurol 4:211–217, 2000

Miller JN, Ozonoff S: Did Asperger's cases have Asperger disorder? A research note. J Child Psychol Psychiatry 38:247–251, 1997

Millichap JG: Rett syndrome: a variant of Heller's dementia? (letter) Lancet 1:440, 1987

Miyamoto A, Oki J, Takahashi S, et al: Serum melatonin kinetics and long-term melatonin treatment for sleep disorder in Rett syndrome. Brain Dev 21:59–62, 1999

Morris RG, Rowe A, Fox N, et al: Spatial working memory in Asperger's syndrome and in patients with focal frontal and temporal lobe lesions. Brain Cogn 41:9–26, 1999

Morton RE, Bonas R, Minford J, et al: Feeding ability in Rett syndrome. Dev Med Child Neurol 39:331–335, 1997

Motil KJ, Schultz RJ, Browning K, et al: Oropharyngeal dysfunction and gastroesophageal dysmotility are present in girls and women with Rett syndrome. J Pediatr Gastroenterol Nutr 29:31–37, 1999

Mouridsen SE, Rich B, Isager T: Validity of childhood disintegrative psychosis: general findings of a long-term follow-up study. Br J Psychiatry 172:263–267, 1998

Mouridsen SE, Rich B, Isager T: Epilepsy in disintegrative psychosis and infantile autism: a long-term validation study. Dev Med Child Neurol 41:110–114, 1999a

Mouridsen SE, Rich B, Isager T: Psychiatric morbidity in disintegrative psychosis and infantile autism: a long-term follow-up study. Psychopathology 32:177–183, 1999b

Mouridsen SE, Rich B, Isager T: A comparative study of genetic and neurobiological findings in disintegrative psychosis and infantile autism. Psychiatry Clin Neurosci 54:441–446, 2000

Murakami JW, Courchesne E, Haas RH: Cerebellar and cerebral abnormalities in Rett syndrome: a quantitative MR analysis. AJR Am J Roentgenol 159:177–183, 1992

Myer EC, Tripathi HL, Brase DA, et al: Elevated CSF beta-endorphin immunoreactivity in Rett's syndrome: report of 158 cases and comparison with leukemic children. Neurology 42:357–360, 1992

Myhr G: Autism and other pervasive developmental disorders: exploring the dimensional view. Can J Psychiatry 43:589–595, 1998

Nagamitsu S, Matsushi T, Kisa T, et al: CSF beta-endorphin levels in patients with infantile autism. J Autism Dev Disord 27:155–163, 1997

Naidu S, Wong DF, Kitt C, et al: Positron emission tomography in the Rett syndrome: clinical, biochemical and pathological correlates. Brain Dev 14(suppl):S75–S79, 1992

Niedermeyer E, Naidu SB, Plate C: Unusual EEG theta rhythms over central region in Rett syndrome: considerations of the underlying dysfunction. Clin Electroencephalogr 28:36–43, 1997

Nielsen JB, Friberg L, Lou H, et al: Immature pattern of brain activity in Rett syndrome. Arch Neurol 47:982–986, 1990

Nielsen JB, Henriksen KF, Hansen C, et al: MECP2 mutations in Danish patients with Rett syndrome: high frequency of mutations but no consistent correlations with clinical severity or with the X chromosome inactivation pattern. Eur J Hum Genetic 9:178–184, 2001

Nihei K, Naitoh H: Cranial computed tomographic and magnetic resonance imaging studies on the Rett syndrome. Brain Dev 12:101–105, 1990

Njardvik U, Matson JL, Cherry KE: A comparison of social skills in adults with autistic disorder, pervasive developmental disorder not otherwise specified, and mental retardation. J Autism Dev Disord 29:287–295, 1999

Nomura Y, Segawa M, Hasegawa M: Rett syndrome: clinical studies and pathophysiological consideration. Brain Dev 6:475–486, 1984

Nomura Y, Kimura A, Arai H, et al: Involvement of the autonomic nervous system in the pathophysiology of Rett syndrome. Eur Child Adolesc Psychiatry 6(suppl 1):42–46, 1997

Nyden A, Billstedt E, Hjelmquist E, et al: Neurocognitive stability in Asperger syndrome, ADHD, and reading and writing disorder: a pilot study. Dev Med Child Neurol 43:165–171, 2001

Oktem F, Diren B, Karaagaoglu E, et al: Functional magnetic resonance imaging in children with Asperger's syndrome. J Child Neurol 16:253–256, 2001

Oldfors A, Hagberg B, Nordgren H, et al: Rett syndrome: spinal cord pathology. Pediatr Neurol 4:172–174, 1988

Oldfors A, Sourander P, Armstrong DL, et al: Rett syndrome: cerebellar pathology. Pediatr Neurol 6:310–314, 1990

Olsson B, Rett A: Behavioral observations concerning differential diagnosis between the Rett syndrome and autism. Brain Dev 7:281–289, 1985

Olsson B, Rett A: A review of the Rett syndrome with a theory of autism. Brain Dev 12:11–15, 1990

Orrico A, Lam C, Galli L, et al: *MECP2* mutation in male patients with non-specific X-linked mental retardation. FEBS Lett 481:285–288, 2000

Ozbayrak KR, Kapucu O, Erdem E, et al: Left occipital hypoperfusion in a case with the Asperger syndrome. Brain Dev 13:454–456, 1991

Percy AK: The Rett syndrome: the recent advances in genetic studies in the USA. Brain Dev 14(suppl):S104–S105, 1992

Percy AK: Meeting report: second International Rett Syndrome Workshop and Symposium. J Child Neurol 8:97–100, 1993

Percy AK: Genetics of Rett syndrome: properties of the newly discovered gene and pathology of the disorder. Curr Opin Pediatr 12:589–595, 2000

Percy AK, Hagberg B: Therapy in Rett syndrome: drug trials and failures, in Rett Syndrome: Clinical and Biological Aspects. Edited by Hagberg B. London, Mac Keith Press, 1993, pp 108–110

Percy AK, Zoghbi HY, Lewis KR, et al: Rett syndrome: qualitative and quantitative differentiation from autism. J Child Neurol 3(suppl):S65–S67, 1988

Percy AK, Glaze DG, Schultz RJ, et al: Rett syndrome: controlled study of an oral opiate antagonist, naltrexone. Ann Neurol 35:464–470, 1994

Perry AK, Sarlo-McGarvey N, Factor DC: Stress and family functioning in parents of girls with Rett syndrome. J Autism Dev Disord 22:235–248, 1992

Philippart M: The Rett syndrome in males. Brain Dev 12:33–36, 1990

Piazza CC, Fisher W, Kiesewetter K, et al: Aberrant sleep patterns in children with the Rett syndrome. Brain Dev 12:488–493, 1990

Piazza CC, Anderson C, Fisher W: Teaching self-feeding skills to patients with Rett syndrome. Dev Med Child Neurol 35:991–996, 1993

Pini G, Milan M, Zappella M: Rett syndrome in northern Tuscany (Italy): family tree studies. Clin Genet 50:486–490, 1996

Piven J, Palmer P, Jacobi D, et al: Broader autism phenotype: evidence from a family history study of multiple-incidence autism families. Am J Psychiatry 154:185–190, 1997

Prior M, Eisenmajer R, Leekam S, et al: Are there subgroups wihin the autistic spectrum? A cluster analysis of a group of children with autistic spectrum disorders. J Child Psychol Psychiatry 39:893–902, 1998

Ramberg C, Ehlers S, Nyden A, et al: Language and pragmatic functions in school-age children on the autism spectrum. Eur J Disord Commun 31:387–413, 1996

Reiss AL, Faruque F, Naidu S, et al: Neuroanatomy of Rett syndrome: a volumetric imaging study. Ann Neurol 34:227–234, 1993

Rescorla L: Cluster analytic identification of autistic preschoolers. J Autism Dev Disord 18:475–492, 1988

Rett A: Über ein zerebral-atrophisches Syndrom bei Hyperammoniämie. Vienna, Broder Hollinek, 1966 [A cerebral atrophy associated with hyperammonaemia, in Handbook of Clinical Neurology. Edited by Vinken PJ, Bruyn GW. Amsterdam, North-Holland, 1977]

Ribeiro RA, Romano AR, Birman EG, et al: Oral manifestations in Rett syndrome: a study of 17 cases. Pediatr Dent 19:349–352, 1997

Riikonen R, Vanhala R: Levels of cerebrospinal fluid nerve-growth factor differ in infantile autism and Rett syndrome. Dev Med Child Neurol 41:148–152, 1999

Ringman JM, Jankovic J: Occurrence of tics in Asperger's syndrome and autistic disorder. J Child Neurol 15:394–400, 2000

Roane HS, Piazza CC, Sgro GM, et al: Analysis of aberrant behavior associated with Rett syndrome. Disabil Rehabil 23:139–148, 2001

Rocchigiani M, Sestina S, Micheli V, et al: Purine and pyridine nucleotide metabolism in the erythrocytes of patients with Rett syndrome. Neuropediatrics 26:288–292, 1995

Rutter M: Infantile autism and other pervasive developmental disorders, in Child and Adolescent Psychiatry. Edited by Rutter M, Hersov L. London, Blackwell, 1985, pp 545–566

Rutter M, Lebovici S, Eisenberg L, et al: A triaxial classification of mental disorder in childhood. J Child Psychol Psychiatry 10:41–61, 1969

Sansom D, Krishnan VH, Corbett J, et al: Emotional and behavioral aspects of Rett syndrome. Dev Med Child Neurol 35:340–345, 1993

Satoi M, Matsuishi T, Yamada S, et al: Decreased cerebrospinal fluid levels of beta-phenylethylamine in patients with Rett syndrome. Ann Neurol 47:801–803, 2000

Schanen NC, Kurczynski TW, Brunelle D, et al: Neonatal encephalopathy in two boys in families with recurrent Rett syndrome. J Child Neurol 13:229–231, 1998

Schultz RT, Gauthier I, Klin A, et al: Abnormal ventral temporal cortical activity during face discrimination among individuals with autism and Asperger syndrome. Arch Gen Psychiatry 57:331–340, 2000

Scragg P, Shah A: Prevalence of Asperger's syndrome in a secure hospital. Br J Psychiatry 165:679–682, 1994

Searcy E, Burd L, Kerbeshian J, et al: Asperger's syndrome, X-linked mental retardation (*MRX23*), and chronic vocal tic disorder. J Child Neurol 15:699–702, 2000

Segawa M: Possible lesions of the Rett syndrome: opinions of contributors. Brain Dev 14(suppl):S149–S150, 1992

Segawa M, Nomura Y: Polysomnography in the Rett syndrome. Brain Dev 14(suppl):S46–S54, 1992

Sekul EA, Moak JP, Schultz RJ, et al: Electrocardiographic findings in Rett syndrome: an explanation for sudden death? J Pediatr 125:80–82, 1994

Serra M, Minderaa RB, van Geert PL, et al: Social-cognitive abilities in children with lesser variants of autism: skill deficits or failure to apply skills? Eur Child Adolesc Psychiatry 8:301–311, 1999

Shahbazian MD, Zoghbi HY: Molecular genetics of Rett syndrome and clinical spectrum of *MECP2* mutations. Curr Opin Neurol 14:171–176, 2001

Sharpe PA: Comparative effects of bilateral hand splints and an elbow orthosis on stereotypic hand movements and toy play in two children with Rett syndrome. Am J Occup Ther 46:134–140, 1992

Sicotte C, Stemberger RM: Do children with PDDNOS have a theory of mind? J Autism Dev Disord 29:225–233, 1999

Skjeldal OH, von Tetzchner S, Aspelund F, et al: Rett syndrome: geographic variation in prevalence in Norway. Brain Dev 19:258–261, 1997

Sobanski E, Marcus A, Hennighausen K, et al: Further evidence for a low body weight in male children and adolescents with Asperger's disorder. Eur Child Adolesc Psychiatry 8:312–314, 1999

Sparrow SS, Rescorla LA, Provence S, et al: Follow-up of "atypical" children: a brief report. J Am Acad Child Psychiatry 25:181–185, 1986

Stach BA, Stoner WR, Smith SL, et al: Auditory evoked potentials in Rett syndrome. J Am Acad Audiol 5:226–230, 1994

Steffenburg S, Gillberg C: Autism and autistic-like conditions in Swedish rural and urban area: a population study. Br J Psychiatry 149:81–87, 1986

Steffenburg U, Hagberg G, Hagberg B: Epilepsy in a representative series of Rett syndrome. Acta Paediatr 90:34–39, 2001

Stella J, Mundy P, Tuchman R: Social and nonsocial factors in the Childhood Autism Rating Scale. J Autism Dev Disord 29:307–317, 1999

Stenbom Y, Engerstrom IW, Hagberg G: Gross motor disability and head growth in Rett syndrome: a preliminary report. Neuropediatrics 26:85–86, 1995

Stenbom Y, Tonnby B, Hagberg B: Lamotrigine in Rett syndrome: treatment experience from a pilot study. Eur Child Adolesc Psychiatry 7:49–52, 1998

Subramaniam B, Naidu S, Reiss AL: Neuroanatomy in Rett syndrome: cerebral cortex and posterior fossa. Neurology 48:399–407, 1997

Szatmari P, Streiner DL: The effect of selection criteria on outcome studies of children with pervasive developmental disorder (PDD). Eur Child Adolesc Psychiatry 5:179–184, 1996

Szatmari P, Bremner R, Nagy J: Asperger's syndrome: a review of clinical features. Can J Psychiatry 34:554–560, 1989

Szatmari P, Tuff L, Finlayson MAJ, et al: Asperger's syndrome and autism: neurocognitive aspects. J Am Acad Child Adolesc Psychiatry 29:130–136, 1990

Szatmari P, Archer L, Fisman S, et al: Asperger's syndrome and autism: difference in behavior, cognition, and adaptive functioning. J Am Acad Child Adolesc Psychiatry 34:1662–1671, 1995

Szatmari P, Bryson, Streiner DL, et al: Two-year outcome of preschool children with autism or Asperger's syndrome. Am J Psychiatry 157:1980–1987, 2000a

Szatmari P, MacLean JE, Jones MB, et al: The familial aggregation of lesser variant in biological and nonbiological relatives of PDD probands: a family history study. J Child Psychol Psychiatry 41:579–586, 2000b

Tantam D: Asperger's syndrome. J Child Psychol Psychiatry 29:245–255, 1988

Tantam D: Asperger syndrome in adulthood, in Autism and Asperger Syndrome. Edited by Frith U. Cambridge, UK, Cambridge University Press, 1991, pp 147–183

Thommessen M, Kase BF, Heiberg A: Growth and nutrition in 10 girls with Rett syndrome. Acta Paediatr 81:686–690, 1992

Trappe R, Laccone F, Cobilanschi J, et al: *MECP2* mutations in sporadic cases of Rett syndrome are almost exclusively of paternal origin. Am J Hum Genet 68:1093–1101, 2001

Trevathan E, Moser HW: Diagnostic criteria for Rett syndrome. Ann Neurol 23:425–428, 1988

Trevathan E, Naidu S: The clinical recognition and differential diagnosis of Rett syndrome. J Child Neurol 3(suppl):S6–S16, 1988

Tsai LY: High-functioning autistic disorder: diagnostic issue, in High-Functioning Individuals With Autism. Edited by Schopler E, Mesibov GB. New York, Plenum, 1992, pp 11–40

Tsai LY: Rett syndrome. Child and Adolescent Psychiatric Clinics of North America 3:105–118, 1994

Tsai LY: Asperger syndrome: effective intervention, in Geneva Centre 1996 Autism Conference Proceedings. Toronto, Ontario, Canada, Geneva Centre for Autism, 1996, pp 55–68

Tsai LY: Children with autism spectrum disorder: medicine today and in the new millennium. Focus on Autism and Other Developmental Disabilities 15:138–145, 2000

Vacca M, Filippini F, Budillon A, et al: Mutation analysis of *MECP2* gene in British and Italian Rett syndrome females. J Mol Med 78:648–655, 2001

Van den Veyver IB, Zoghbi HY: Methyl-CpG-binding protein 2 mutations in Rett syndrome. Curr Opin Genet Dev 10:274–279, 2000

Vanhala R, Korhonen L, Mikelsaar M, et al: Neurotrophic factors in cerebrospinal fluid and serum of patients with Rett syndrome. J Child Neurol 13:429–433, 1998

Vanhanen SL, Raininko R, Santavuori P: Early differential diagnosis of infantile neuronal ceroid lipofuscinosis, Rett syndrome, and Krabbe disease by CT and MR. AJNR Am J Neuroradiol 15:1443–1453, 1994

Villard L, Kpebe A, Cardoso C, et al: Two affected boys in a Rett syndrome family: clinical and molecular findings. Neurology 55:1188–1193, 2000

Volkmar FR: Childhood disintegrative disorder: issues for DSM-IV. J Autism Dev Disord 22:625–642, 1992

Volkmar FR: Childhood disintegrative disorder. Child Adolesc Psychiatr Clin N Am 3:119–129, 1994

Volkmar FR, Cohen DJ: Disintegrative disorder or "late onset" autism. J Child Psychol Psychiatry 30:717–724, 1989

Volkmar FR, Rutter M: Childhood disintegrative disorder: results of DSM-IV autism field trial. J Am Acad Child Adolesc Psychiatry 34:1092–1095, 1995

Volkmar FR, Cohen DJ, Hoshino Y, et al: Phenomenology and classification of the childhood psychoses. Psychol Med 18:191–201, 1988

von Tetzchner S: Communication skills among females with Rett syndrome. Eur Child Adolesc Psychiatry 6(suppl 1):33–37, 1997

Vourc'h P, Bienvenu T, Beldjord C, et al: No mutations in coding region of the Rett syndrome gene MECP2 in 59 autistic patients. Eur J Hum Genet 9:556–558, 2001

Wan M, Lee SS, Zhang X, et al: Rett syndrome and beyond: recurrent spontaneous and familial MECP2 mutations at CpG hotspots. Am J Hum Genet 65:1520–1529, 1999

Weidmer-Mikhail E, Sheldon S, Ghaziuddin M: Chromosomes in autism and related pervasive developmental disorders: a cytogenetic study. J Intellect Disabil Res 42(pt 1):8–12, 1998

Weisz CL: Family social problems in the Rett syndrome. Brain Dev 12:173–175, 1990

Wenk GL: Alterations in dopaminergic function in Rett syndrome. Neuropediatrics 26:123–125, 1995

Wenk GL: Rett syndrome: evidence for normal dopaminergic function. Neuropediatrics 27:256–259, 1996

Wenk GL, Hauss-Wegrzyniak B: Altered cholinergic function in the basal forebrain of girls with Rett syndrome. Neuropediatrics 30:125–129, 1999

Wenk GL, O'Leary M, Nemeroff CB, et al: Neurochemical alterations in Rett syndrome. Brain Res Dev Brain Res 74:67–72, 1993

Wing L: Asperger's syndrome: a clinical account. Psychol Med 11:115–129, 1981

Wing L, Gould J: Severe impairments of social interaction and association abnormalities in children: epidemiology and classification. J Autism Dev Disord 9:11–30, 1979

Witt-Engerström I, Gillberg C: Rett syndrome in Sweden. J Autism Dev Disord 17:149–150, 1987

Witt-Engerström I, Hagberg B: The Rett syndrome: gross motor disability and neural impairment in adults. Brain Dev 12:23–26, 1990

Woodyatt G, Ozanne A: Communication abilities and Rett syndrome. J Autism Dev Disord 22:155–173, 1992

Woodyatt G, Ozanne A: A longitudinal study of cognitive skills and communication behaviors in children with Rett syndrome. J Intellect Disabil Res 37:419–435, 1993

Woodyatt G, Ozanne A: Rett syndrome (RS) and profound intellectual disability: cognitive and communicative similarities and differences. Eur Child Adolesc Psychiatry 6(suppl 1):31–32, 1997

World Health Organization: International Classification of Diseases, 9th Revision. Geneva, World Health Organization, 1977

World Health Organization: International Statistical Classification of Diseases and Related Health Problems, 10th Revision. Geneva, World Health Organization, 1992

Xiang F, Buervenich S, Nicolao P, et al: Mutation screening in Rett syndrome patients. J Med Genet 37:250–255, 2000

Yano S, Yamashita Y, Matsuishi T, et al: Four adult Rett patients at an institution for the handicapped. Pediatr Neurol 7:289–292, 1991

Yoshikawa H, Fueki N, Suzuki H, et al: Cerebral blood flow and oxygen metabolism in the Rett syndrome. Brain Dev 14(suppl):S69–S74, 1990

Zappella M: Motivational conflicts in Rett syndrome. Am J Med Genet 24(suppl 1):143–151, 1986

Zappella M, Genazzani A, Facchinetti F, et al: Bromocriptine in the Rett syndrome. Brain Dev 12:221–225, 1990

Zappella M, Gillberg C, Ehlers S: The preserved speech variant: a subgroup of the Rett complex: a clinical report of 30 cases. J Autism Dev Disord 28:519–526, 1998

Ziatas K, Durkin K, Pratt C: Belief term development in children with autism, Asperger syndrome, specific language impairment, and normal development: links to theory of mind development. J Child Psychol Psychiatry 39:755–763, 1998

Zuddas A, Di Martino A, Muglia P, et al: Long-term risperidone for pervasive developmental disorder: efficacy, tolerability, and discontinuation. J Child Adolesc Psychopharmacol 10:79–90, 2000

Zwaigenbaum L, Szatmari P, Mahoney W, et al: High functioning autism and childhood disintegrative disorder in half brothers. J Autism Dev Disord 30:121–126, 2000

Developmental Disorders of Learning, Motor Skills, and Communication

Carl Feinstein, M.D.

Jennifer M. Phillips, Ph.D.

DSM-IV-TR (American Psychiatric Association 2000) includes the broad diagnostic categories of developmental disorders of learning, motor skills, and communication separately, with subclassifications within each area. The types of learning disorders (formerly academic skills disorders) include reading disorder, mathematics disorder, disorder of written expression, and learning disorder not otherwise specified. Developmental coordination disorder is classified as a motor skills disorder in DSM-IV-TR. Communication disorders (formerly language disorders) are divided into expressive language disorder, mixed receptive-expressive language disorder, phonological disorder (formerly developmental articulation disorder), stuttering, and communication disorder not otherwise specified. Throughout this chapter, we use the terms *communication disorder* and *language disorder* more or less interchangeably. All of these disorders were coded in DSM-III-R (American Psychiatric Association 1987) as developmental disorders on Axis II but are now coded on Axis I in DSM-IV (American Psychiatric Association 1994) and DSM-IV-TR (American Psychiatric Association 2000).

Learning, communication, and motor skills disorders are common developmental impairments with significant implications for both children's mental health and their ability to function successfully at school and in other psychosocial contexts. The relation of these disorders to other DSM disorders is complex. They stand apart from the other Axis I disorders of childhood, which describe emotional or behavioral abnormalities. Thus, when they occur in isolation, they usually do not come to the attention of the child psychiatrist. However, they are very common as comorbid conditions in children with psychiatric disorders (Osman 2000). Conversely, many children with these disorders have significant psychiatric disorders and are, unfortunately, never referred for treatment of their mental health problems. Many children and adolescents who are delinquent or who have found their way into the juvenile justice system may also have these developmental disorders.

Communication disorders and motor skills disorders are distinct from learning disorders, in that they may occur in children who are performing relatively poorly but "getting by" in school. They are, however, closely associated with and often co-occur with learning disorders. There is, in fact, considerable evidence that developmental reading disorder (dyslexia) is closely associated with and related to developmental language disorder (American Speech-Language-Hearing Association 2002; Hummel and Feinstein 1997; Lovett 1992). Follow-up assessment of preschool children with diagnosed language disorders reveals that many receive a diagnosis of learning disability during the school-age years (American Academy of Child and Adolescent Psychiatry 1998; Aram and Hall 1989; Baker and Cantwell 1987; Silva 1987; Stevenson et al. 1985). Conversely, many school-age children who receive a diagnosis of learning disability are found to have an underlying communication disorder (Schoenbrodt et al. 1997; Silva 1987; Stevenson and Richman

1978). There is also a reported higher rate of occurrence of developmental coordination disorder with both communication and learning disorders (American Psychiatric Association 2000). Finally, numerous specific cognitive deficits occur in various combinations in children with both learning disability and communication disorders (Cohen 2001; Hummel and Feinstein 1997; Morris et al. 1986; Nussbaum et al. 1986).

A considerable body of clinical and epidemiological research points to a strong association between attention-deficit/hyperactivity disorder (ADHD) and overlapping learning, language, and motor disorders (Tannock 2000). The co-occurrence of these symptoms and impairments is increasingly referred to by the acronym DAMP (deficits in attention, motor control, and perception) and is recognized in several countries as a distinct neurodevelopmental phenotype (Kadesjo and Gillberg 1999).

Unlike mental retardation, an Axis II disorder, the learning, communication, and motor skills disorders do not have deficient intellectual functioning as a diagnostic feature, and these disorders are most commonly not associated with deficient overall intelligence. However, they are highly associated with lower social and adaptive competence, poor school achievement, and lower vocational attainment—outcomes that not infrequently overlap with those seen in people with borderline cognitive functioning and mild retardation. In fact, a large body of research has repeatedly confirmed that these disorders are among the most problematic risk factors yet identified for psychiatric disorders, delinquency, a variety of adverse psychosocial outcomes in late adolescence and adulthood, early school dropout, and poor academic achievement in children and adolescents (American Academy of Child and Adolescent Psychiatry 1998; Beitchman et al. 1986; Cantwell and Baker 1987, 1991; Rutter and Lord 1987).

Furthermore, the high prevalence and multiple adverse consequences of these disabilities constitute a major public health and public policy concern. In 1995, the U.S. Department of Education reported that 5.3% of all students in public schools in the United States had had a learning disability diagnosed and were receiving educational services. It was reported that 2.3% of students had had a language disorder diagnosed and were receiving services under this classification. The U.S. Interagency Committee on Learning Disabilities estimated the actual prevalence rate of learning disabilities in U.S. students to be 5%–10% (Silver 1989), with estimates ranging from 1% to 10% in other studies (American Academy of Child and Adolescent Psychiatry 1998; American Psychiatric Association 2000). The prevalence rate for language disorders is similar, ranging from 1% to 15%, depending on the age of the population and the specific disorder (American Academy of Child and Adolescent Psychiatry 1998; American Psychiatric Association 2000; Beitchman et al. 1986; Castrogiovanni 2002; Silva 1987). In total, it is thought that anywhere from 10% to 20% of children and adolescents have communication and/or learning disorders (Beitchman et al. 1986; Beitchman and Young 1997). About 50% of these children have a comorbid psychiatric disorder (American Academy of Child and Adolescent Psychiatry 1998).

According to DSM-IV-TR, both communication and learning disorders generally occur more frequently in boys than in girls (American Psychiatric Association 2000). However, in girls who have these problems, the impairment and psychosocial consequences are at least as serious as they are in boys (Baker and Cantwell 1987). One of the suspected contributing factors in the number of children found to have communication and learning problems is subtle central nervous system sequelae in some high-risk infants and children with serious childhood illnesses whose lives have been spared by advances in medical technology (Bernbaum and Batshaw 1997; Gamis and Nesbit 1991; Hill et al. 1997; Sullivan 1995; Waber 1989).

The psychiatrist treating children and adolescents plays a critical role in the assessment and treatment of children with communication, motor skills, and learning disorders. Effective treatment of children with these issues, as well as secondary prevention of psychiatric disorders, requires a coordinated multidisciplinary intervention (Silver and Hagin 1989). This includes cognitive and educational remediation, psychotherapeutic approaches, and measures to strengthen the family's ability to support the child's optimal development. Effective participation by the psychiatrist in this multidisciplinary setting requires a working familiarity with the concepts and procedures of pediatric neurology, speech and language pathology, neuropsychological assessment, and special-education programming. Yet, despite the involvement of these many disciplines, major gaps exist in current knowledge regarding phenomenology, classification, pathogenesis, and natural history of these disorders. The various causal relationships between these disabilities and psychiatric disorders are difficult to elucidate, and the outcome of different intervention programs is unclear and insufficiently documented.

Learning Disorders

■ Definition

The National Joint Committee on Learning Disabilities defines learning disorders as "a heterogeneous group of disorders manifested by significant difficulties in the acquisition and use of listening, speaking, reading, writing, reasoning, or mathematical skills" (National Joint Committee on Learning Disabilities 1997). In DSM-IV-TR, learning disorders (termed *academic skills disorders* in DSM-III-R) are defined as impairments in an academic area (i.e., reading, mathematics, or written expression) such that scores on individually administered standardized tests of achievement are substantially below those expected for age, schooling, and intelligence. Each of the learning disorders defined in DSM has the same general definition, based on a discrepancy in standardized test scores, and differs only in the specific capacity that is deficient. The DSM criteria for each learning disorder are presented in Tables 22–1 to 22–4. A significant change in the definition and diagnosis of learning disorders in DSM-IV-TR from DSM-III-R allows the presence of a cognitive or sensory deficit (i.e., visual, linguistic, attention, memory) but requires the learning difficulty to be in excess of the difficulty usually associated with this deficit. In addition, it is possible for a person with mental retardation also to meet criteria for a learning disorder when the academic deficit is significantly greater than can be accounted for by the degree of intellectual deficit.

The Education for All Handicapped Children Act of 1975 (U.S. Public Law 94–142; U.S. Congress 1975), and the more recent version, the Individuals with Disabilities Education Act (IDEA; U.S. Congress 1997), are national mandates for special education in the United States that have profoundly affected referrals and programming for children with disabilities. These laws provide for "free appropriate public education" for children meeting any of the following disability categories: impairment of hearing, speech-language, or vision; mental retardation; emotional disturbance; autism; traumatic brain injury; orthopedic impairment, other health impairments; and specific learning disabilities. Under IDEA, "specific learning disabilities" are defined in the following way:

Table 22–1. DSM-IV-TR diagnostic criteria for reading disorder

A. Reading achievement, as measured by individually administered standardized tests of reading accuracy or comprehension, is substantially below that expected given the person's chronological age, measured intelligence, and age-appropriate education.

B. The disturbance in Criterion A significantly interferes with academic achievement or activities of daily living that require reading skills.

C. If a sensory deficit is present, the reading difficulties are in excess of those usually associated with it.

Coding note: If a general medical (e.g., neurological) condition or sensory deficit is present, code the condition on Axis III.

Source. Reprinted from the *Diagnostic and Statistical Manual of Mental Disorders,* 4th Edition, Text Revision. Washington, DC, American Psychiatric Association, 2000. Copyright 2000, American Psychiatric Association. Used with permission.

Table 22–2. DSM-IV-TR diagnostic criteria for mathematics disorder

A. Mathematical ability, as measured by individually administered standardized tests, is substantially below that expected given the person's chronological age, measured intelligence, and age-appropriate education.

B. The disturbance in Criterion A significantly interferes with academic achievement or activities of daily living that require mathematical ability.

C. If a sensory deficit is present, the difficulties in mathematical ability are in excess of those usually associated with it.

Coding note: If a general medical (e.g., neurological) condition or sensory deficit is present, code the condition on Axis III.

Source. Reprinted from the *Diagnostic and Statistical Manual of Mental Disorders,* 4th Edition, Text Revision. Washington, DC, American Psychiatric Association, 2000. Copyright 2000, American Psychiatric Association. Used with permission.

The term "specific learning disability" means a disorder in one or more of the basic psychological processes involved in understanding or in using language, spoken or written, which disorder may manifest itself in imperfect ability to listen, think, speak, read, write, spell, or do mathematical calculations. Such term includes such conditions as perceptual disabilities, brain injury, minimal brain dysfunction, dyslexia, and developmental aphasia. Such term does not include a learning problem that is primarily the result of visual, hearing, or motor disabilities, of mental retardation, of emotional disturbances,

Table 22–3. DSM-IV-TR diagnostic criteria for disorder of written expression

A. Writing skills, as measured by individually administered standardized tests (or functional assessments of writing skills), are substantially below those expected given the person's chronological age, measured intelligence, and age-appropriate education.

B. The disturbance in Criterion A significantly interferes with academic achievement or activities of daily living that require the composition of written texts (e.g., writing grammatically correct sentences and organized paragraphs).

C. If a sensory deficit is present, the difficulties in writing skills are in excess of those usually associated with it.

Coding note: If a general medical (e.g., neurological) condition or sensory deficit is present, code the condition on Axis III.

Source. Reprinted from the *Diagnostic and Statistical Manual of Mental Disorders*, 4th Edition, Text Revision. Washington, DC, American Psychiatric Association, 2000. Copyright 2000, American Psychiatric Association. Used with permission.

Table 22–4. DSM-IV-TR diagnostic criteria for learning disorder not otherwise specified

This category is for disorders in learning that do not meet criteria for any specific learning disorder. This category might include problems in all three areas (reading, mathematics, written expression) that together significantly interfere with academic achievement even though performance on tests measuring each individual skill is not substantially below that expected given the person's chronological age, measured intelligence, and age-appropriate education.

Source. Reprinted from the *Diagnostic and Statistical Manual of Mental Disorders*, 4th Edition, Text Revision. Washington, DC, American Psychiatric Association, 2000. Copyright 2000, American Psychiatric Association. Used with permission.

or of environmental, cultural, or economic disadvantage. (U.S. Congress 1997)

The DSM-IV-TR definition and IDEA differ in that IDEA includes only children of normal intelligence, whereas DSM allows for mentally retarded children with uneven cognitive profiles to have a diagnosed learning disorder. The DSM definition no longer excludes children whose learning problem is due to a neurological disorder; likewise, IDEA encompasses brain injury and dysfunction.

■ History

Case studies of children with learning disabilities appeared as early as 1896 (Morgan 1896). An early theoretical explanation for learning disabilities was offered by Orton (1937), who proposed that the problem was a failure to establish cerebral dominance during development. Orton later divided developmental disorders into alexia, agraphia, word deafness, motor aphasia, apraxia, and stuttering, thus including language and motor disabilities in the same framework as reading disorder (Doris 1993). In the 1950s, Cruickshank (1967) studied a group of children with perceptual disabilities, attention deficit, poor motor coordination, and impulsivity. Because of their behavioral similarity to brain-damaged children, these children were described as having "minimal brain damage," despite the absence of any clear evidence of frank neurological problems.

By the early 1960s, the concept of brain damage gave way to the notion of brain dysfunction or immaturity. Clements and Peters (1962) coined the term *minimal brain dysfunction* to describe a syndrome with a variety of features, including specific learning deficits, perceptual-motor problems, poor coordination, hyperkinesis, impulsivity, equivocal neurological signs, and abnormal electroencephalographic findings. Concurrently, the term *specific learning disability* was applied to describe the same population of children (Farnham-Diggory 1978).

During the 1970s, the focus was on the attentional deficits in children thought to have minimal brain dysfunction. However, it became increasingly clear that use of stimulant medication significantly reduced hyperactivity and improved attention but had no effect on specific learning problems (Gittelman 1983; Silver 1986). Recent research confirms this disassociation (Tannock 2000). Neurologists became increasingly involved with these children, who were believed to have underlying brain dysfunction. However, sensorimotor neurological examinations did not adequately address the higher cortical functions presumed to be impaired in learning disorders (Kinsbourne 1973). The inability to identify "hard" neurological signs in most children continues to impede progress in establishing the role of the central nervous system in learning disorders. Recently, functional magnetic resonance imaging, coupled with neuropsychological and linguistic tests, is illuminating the brain mechanisms underlying these conditions (Shaywitz et al. 2000).

■ Clinical Presentation

Clinically, children with learning disorders present with poor academic achievement relative to their intelligence. Symptoms vary with level of intellectual functioning, measured by scores on standardized measures of intelligence (IQ scores); children with higher IQs show fewer neurological signs and fewer symptoms of motor skills and language disorders (Shepherd et al. 1989). In general, many children with learning disorders have difficulty with active information processing (American Academy of Child and Adolescent Psychiatry 1998; Torgeson 1982), which may manifest as difficulty in developing strategies for organizing, prioritizing, rehearsing, or presenting information, especially when it is linguistically based. In many cases, by the time of referral for evaluation, the child not only has poor academic performance but also lacks the basic learning skills that are necessary for comprehending or mastering the more advanced material they are currently confronting in school.

According to the DSM-IV-TR (American Psychiatric Association 2000), children with reading disorder have poor reading ability (including rate, accuracy, and comprehension), often combined with spelling problems, poor writing, speech delay, or dyspraxia. Reading disorder (often referred to as dyslexia) is thought to occur in 2%–10% of children, accounting for 80% of all children with a diagnosed learning disorder (Lerner 1989; Shaywitz et al. 2000). Some research shows that approximately 80% of those affected are boys (American Psychiatric Association 2000), although this is contradicted by recent epidemiological research, which fails to find a true sex difference (Flynn and Rahbar 1994; Shaywitz et al. 1990; Wenar and Kerig 2000).

Mathematics disorder, which is less well studied, is characterized by difficulty in mathematical calculation or reasoning, which can be manifest in a variety of difficulties, including problems with the linguistic, perceptual, attention, and mathematical skills needed to understand mathematical concepts. This disorder is reported to occur in 1%–6% of school-age children, with higher rates in girls than boys (American Academy of Child and Adolescent Psychiatry 1998).

In disorder of written expression, the essential impairment is in writing ability, as demonstrated by the use of grammar and punctuation, organization, spelling, and handwriting. Disorder of written expression has been suggested to occur in 2%–8% of children, is more common in boys than girls, and is usually reported in combination with other learning disorders (American Academy of Child and Adolescent Psychiatry 1998; American Psychiatric Association 2000).

Often, a negative emotional cycle develops in which poor self-esteem, anxiety, depression, deficits in social competence, alienation, or rebellion further interfere with the child's ability to participate effectively in school (Beitchman and Young 1997; Bryan 1991). As with communication disorders, the rate of concurrent Axis I psychopathology is as high as 50% in children and adolescents with learning disorders, and the combination of having both a learning and a language disorder may further increase the likelihood of an Axis I diagnosis (American Academy of Child and Adolescent Psychiatry 1998; Beitchman et al 1986; Glosser and Koppell 1987; Hunt and Cohen 1984; McConaughy and Ritter 1986). Attention-deficit disorders are reported to occur in 20% or more of the population with learning disabilities (Halperin et al. 1984; Hinshaw 1992; Shaywitz and Shaywitz 1989). DSM-IV-TR (American Psychiatric Association 2000) reports that 10%–25% of children diagnosed with a disruptive behavior disorder (conduct disorder, oppositional-defiant disorder, ADHD) or depressive disorders (major depressive disorder, dysthymic disorder) have comorbid learning disorders. In fact, children who ultimately receive a diagnosis of a learning disorder often present initially with emotional or behavioral problems. Conversely, many children who initially present with a learning disorder are found to meet criteria for a psychiatric disorder later in childhood (American Academy of Child and Adolescent Psychiatry 1998). Relative or absolute failure in school, a major developmental arena for the child and adolescent, is likely to be a major risk factor for psychiatric disorder (Offord and Waters 1983; Rutter and Giller 1983). There is also significant evidence that in adolescence, there is a significant relationship between conduct problems and learning disorders (Klein and Mannuzza 2000), with up to 85% of juvenile delinquents reportedly receiving a diagnosis of a learning disorder (Moffitt 1995; Tallal 2000). A significant related risk is for the development of a substance use disorder. Karacostas and Fisher (1993) looked at a group of adolescents with and without learning disabilities and found that 70% of a group of adolescents who screened positive for a substance use disorder were found to have a learning disorder. Of students identified as having a learning disorder, 23.9% were found to have a substance use disorder, whereas only 8.9% of the students who did not have a learning disorder reported a substance use disorder.

■ Diagnosis

From the point of view of the public education system (as outlined in IDEA), a psychiatric evaluation is indicated only when the exclusionary criteria of emotional disturbance must be addressed as a causative factor in poor academic achievement. However, in view of the high rate of comorbidity between learning disorders and psychiatric disorders, the psychiatrist treating children and adolescents must always be vigilant to the substantial possibility that those referred for psychiatric evaluation of emotional or behavioral problems may also have an undetected learning disability.

The first step in making the diagnosis of a learning disorder involves establishing a discrepancy between the academic skill or skills in question and the child's intelligence, and then eliminating all other explanations for the discrepancy. To establish this discrepancy, a psychoeducational evaluation is typically performed by a qualified psychologist, using scores on standardized academic achievement tests as compared with standardized intelligence test scores. Although intelligence tests usually are composed of verbal and nonverbal components, consideration of the use of a nonverbal intelligence test may be appropriate when a child is already known to have a communication disorder. The Leiter International Performance Scale—Revised (LIPS-R; Roid and Miller 1996) is one such test. Table 22–5 briefly describes some of the most commonly used intelligence, achievement, and linguistic tests. A significant difference between scores is frequently defined as a 1- to 2-SD (standard deviation) discrepancy, with achievement level lower than IQ.

Although this discrepancy model for identification of learning disorders is used in DSM and IDEA, it should be noted that much research has suggested that using IQ–achievement discrepancy to diagnose learning disorders is not an empirically validated approach and may result in underdiagnosis for children of average or low average IQ, as well as for children with socioeconomic deprivation and/or minority status (Fletcher et al. 1994, 1998). As yet, however, the scientific community has not agreed on a more appropriate method of identification (American Academy of Child and Adolescent Psychiatry 1998). One suggested strategy involves evaluation of achievement in specific academic domains, with comparison to abilities that are matched with the specific skill areas (Fletcher et al. 1998; Zigmond 1993). In addition, use of multidisciplinary evaluations may prove useful. For example, a speech-language pathologist may be helpful in the assessment process by providing information about a child's phonological awareness skills, a key component thought to underlie reading disorder and disorder of written expression. In addition, information on speech and language skills may prove useful in the diagnostic process (American Speech-Language-Hearing Association 2002).

The second part of the diagnostic procedure for learning disorders involves differential diagnosis. Other conditions often resulting in poor academic performance and associated with learning disorders include mental retardation, neurological damage or disease, and psychiatric disturbance. In addition, factors such as sensory impairment, inadequate schooling, cultural factors, nonnative English-speaking, and environmental deprivation should also be differentiated from learning disorders. A learning disorder should not be the diagnosis in these situations if the academic difficulties are due primarily to these factors, unless the difficulties seen are greater than would be expected given these conditions alone. The child suspected of having a learning disorder should always have a vision and hearing screen, to check for impairments that could be contributing to poor academic performance.

■ Etiology and Pathogenesis

The etiology of learning disorders is unknown but presumed to include a variety of neurocognitive deficits or dysfunction resulting in disruptions of cognitive processing. It is likely that each subtype of learning disorder is associated with its own specific neuropathology (Hynd et al. 1988; Lyon 1983; Morris 1988; Nussbaum et al. 1986). Most advances in understanding the neural basis for learning disorders have been based on the study of reading disorder. There is considerable overlap in findings with those from research in the language disorders, because problems in language processing are strongly associated with deficits in components of language processing (Beitchman and Young 1997).

There are numerous causes for poor reading, including both hereditary and environmental factors. Environmental factors with known associations to reading delays in children include prematurity, major

Table 22–5. Tests and measures

Test	Age range (age expressed as year-month)
General intelligence tests	
Wechsler Preschool and Primary Scale of Intelligence—3rd Edition (WPPSI-III; Wechsler 2002)	3–0 to 7–3
Wechsler Intelligence Scale for Children—3rd Edition (WISC-III; Wechsler 1991)	6–0 to 16–11
Stanford-Binet Intelligence Scale—5th Edition (SB5; Roid 2003)	2–0 to 23–11
Leiter International Performance Scale—Revised (LIPS-R; Roid and Miller 1996)	2–0 to 18–11
Kaufman Assessment Battery for Children (K-ABC; Kaufman and Kaufman 1983)	2–6 to 12–5
Educational achievement tests	
Wide Range Achievement Test—3rd Edition (WRAT-3; Wilkinson 1993)	5–0 to 75–0
Peabody Individual Achievement Test—Revised (PIAT-R; Markwardt 1989)	K–12
Wechsler Individual Achievement Test (WIAT; Psychological Corporation 1992)	5–0 to 19–11
Woodcock-Johnson Psychoeducational Battery—3rd Edition (WJ-III; Woodcock et al. 2001)	3–0 to adult
Kaufman Test of Educational Achievement (K-TEA; Kaufman and Kaufman 1985)	6–0 to 18–11
KeyMath Diagnostic Arithmetic Test (Connolly et al. 1971)	Grades 1–6
Language tests	
Batteries	
Sequenced Inventory of Communication Development—Revised (SICD-R; Hedrick et al. 1984)	0–4 to 4–0
Test of Early Language Development, 2nd Edition (TELD-2; Hresko et al. 1991)	2–0 to 7–11
Test of Language Development, 2nd Edition (TOLD-2), Versions 2P and 2I (Newcomer and Hammill 1988)	2P: 4–0 to 8–11 2I: 8–6 to 12–11
Test of Adolescent and Adult Language—3rd Edition (TAAL-3; Hammill et al. 1994)	11–0 to 24–0
Clinical Evaluation of Language Fundamentals—Preschool (CELF–P; Wiig et al. 1992)	3–0 to 6–11
Clinical Evaluation of Language Fundamentals—3rd Edition (CELF–3; Semel et al. 1995)	5–0 to 21–0
Preschool Language Scale—3rd Edition (PLS-3; Zimmerman et al. 1992)	0–1 to 6–11
Tests of specific functions	
Peabody Picture Vocabulary Test—3rd Edition (PPVT-III; Dunn et al. 1997)	2–6 to 90+
Token Test for Children (DiSimoni 1978)	3–0 to 12–5
Goldman-Fristoe Test of Articulation (G-FTA; Goldman and Fristoe 1986)	2–0 to 16+
Goldman-Fristoe-Woodcock Test of Auditory Discrimination (Goldman et al. 1970)	3–0 to adult
Expressive One-Word Picture Vocabulary Test—Revised (EOWPVT-R; Gardner 1990)	2–0 to 11–11
Arizona Articulation Proficiency Scale—2nd Edition (Fudala and Reynolds 1986)	3–0 to 11–0
Test of Language Competence—Expanded Edition (TLC; Wiig and Secord 1989)	Level 1: 5–0 to 9–11 Level 2: 9–0 to 18–11
MacArthur Communicative Development Inventory (MCDI; Fensen et al. 1993)	0–8 to 2–6
Test of Pragmatic Language (TOPL; Phelps-Terasaki and Phelps-Gunn 1992)	5–0 to 13–11
Communication and Symbolic Behavior Scales (CSBS; Wetherby and Prizant 1993)	0–9 to 6–11
Comprehensive Receptive and Expressive Vocabulary Test (CREVT; Wallace and Hammill 1994)	5–0 to 17–11
Test of Auditory Comprehension of Language—Revised (TACL-R; Carrow-Woolfolk 1985)	3–0 to 9–11
Comprehensive Test of Phonological Processing (CTOPP; Wagner et al. 1999)	5–0 to 24–11
Neuropsychological tests	
Batteries	
Halstead-Reitan Neuropsychological Test Battery for Older Children (HRNB; Reitan and Wolfson 1985)	9–0 to 14–11
Reitan-Indiana Neuropsychological Test Battery for Children (Reitan and Wolfson 1985)	5–0 to 8–11
Luria-Nebraska Neuropsychological Battery: Children's Revision (Golden 1987)	8–0 to 12–11

Table 22–5. Tests and measures *(continued)*

Test	Age range (age expressed as year-month)
Tests of specific functions	
Developmental Test of Visual Motor Integration (VMI; Beery and Buktenica 1989)	3–0 to 18–11
Raven's Progressive Matrices (Raven et al. 1976)	6–5 to adult
Wisconsin Card Sorting Test (WCST; Berg 1948)	8–0 to adult
Adaptive behavior tests	
Vineland Adaptive Behavior Scales (VABS; Sparrow et al. 1984)	0–1 to 18–11; low-functioning adults

perinatal adversity, poverty, malnutrition, poor schooling, early abuse and neglect, and parental substance abuse. However, it is becoming evident, with the accumulation of genetic studies, that hereditary factors also play an important role. The familial risk for reading disorder in first-degree relatives of children with reading disorder is between 35% and 45% (Pennington 1995; Shepherd and Uhry 1993). There is also considerable evidence for a link between reading disability and ADHD on a hereditary basis (Beitchman and Young 1997). For example, Light et al. (1995) found that 70% of the covariance between reading disability and ADHD is heritable. Stevenson et al. (1993) found that 75% of the comorbidity of spelling disability and ADHD is heritable.

Genetic loci on chromosomes 6 and 15 have been identified as linked to some familial cases of reading disability (Grigorenko et al. 1997). A gene locus on chromosome 6 is linked to deficits in phonological awareness, which impair the rapid association of written material with speech sounds that is essential for efficient reading. The chromosome 15 locus seems more related to deficits in reading single whole words. An abnormality of the *FOX P2* gene on chromosome 7 has recently been identified as causal to both deficits in phonological processing and grammatical usage (Lai et al. 2001).

Although single-gene causes are associated with some forms of familial reading impairment, many genes influence the various neurobiological processes underlying reading ability. Unfavorable variants of these numerous genes, in multiple combinations, constitute cumulative hereditary risk factors for the majority of hereditary reading problems. Thus, although a relatively small number of severe familial reading disorders might be due to single abnormal genes, most inherited variations in reading ability are due to polygenic influences. This perspective is supported by the findings of Shaywitz et al. (1996). These researchers used an epidemiological approach to establish that children's reading abilities were spread along a continuum rather than splitting at categorical break points between normal and abnormal reading. This finding supports a polygenic, multiple-risk model for variations in reading ability, rather than a causal mode that emphasizes categorical differences between normal and deficient readers. It is likely that there are no categorical differences between children at the lower end of the normal spectrum of reading disability and those classified as reading disordered (Shaywitz et al. 1992).

Considerable recent progress has been made in elucidating the functional neuroanatomical correlates of poor reading. These findings use functional neuroimaging and neurophysiological techniques to support and extend previously established findings (Galaburda et al. 1985; Rumsey et al. 1987) regarding the importance of the temporoparietal region of the left brain. Deficits in phonological processing, primarily a left-hemisphere function, are the most common neurocognitive impairments responsible for reading disorders, although they do not account for all cases or types of reading disorder (Merzenich et al. 1996; Shaywitz et al. 2000; Tallal et al. 1996). Functional neuroimaging and electrophysiological techniques have succeeded in clarifying the brain pathways by which the various left-brain regions involved in reading decode and translate both written and auditory language (orthographic and phonetic units of information) from one modality to the other and then interface with brain centers more concerned with meaning (semantics). This involves pathways from the occipital lobe to the posterior superior temporal, middle temporal, supramarginal and angular gyri, and the inferior frontal region (Broca's area; Pugh et al. 1997; Simos et al.

2000, 2001). Extrastriate and basal temporal areas are also involved in the processing of visually presented written words into their component graphemes (Pugh et al. 1996).

■ Treatment

A wide variety of therapies has been used for children who have learning disorders, but only a few of these therapies have been subjected to well-controlled efficacy studies. Direct treatment approaches to dyslexia have addressed underlying perceptual or visuomotor deficits, or underlying phonetic deficits (Merzenich et al. 1996; Tallal et al. 1996). Other treatments focus on presenting information multimodally, using multiple sensory formats, such as presenting material in a visual format in addition to an auditory format (American Academy of Child and Adolescent Psychiatry 1998). Enhancing the child's attention and motivation for academic tasks is another method used, with attentional enhancement primarily addressed pharmacologically, and motivational enhancement addressed with behavioral techniques. Other educational and behavioral strategies include remediation of deficits through direct and specific instruction in areas of weakness, and use of behavioral techniques to address academic issues (Wenar and Kerig 2000).

By law (IDEA; U.S. Congress 1997), children who qualify for special education are entitled to a "free appropriate public education" from birth to age 21. Each child must have an individualized education program (IEP) and must receive specialized instruction in the least restrictive setting. For some children with learning disorders, this translates into resource-room placement for a portion of the school day, spending the rest of the day in a regular education classroom. For others, this could entail placement in special classroom settings (American Academy of Child and Adolescent Psychiatry 1998). Specialized tutorial help is also a common modality. During the IEP process, yearly goals are written for areas of concern, and these are then targeted in the classroom with specific objectives for how to meet the goal and methods for evaluating progress. Goals are revisited each year in the IEP meeting, and every 3 years a formal reevaluation of achievement should occur (National Joint Committee on Learning Disabilities 1997).

In addition to treating the learning disorder, treatment of any comorbid psychiatric conditions should take the limitations imposed by the learning disorder itself into consideration. Thus, a child or adolescent with marked deficits in receptive and expressive language might not be an ideal candidate for verbally based psychotherapy, unless great care is taken to ensure that the communicative modalities are truly effective. This includes individual, family, group, and milieu-based psychotherapy. With evidence that up to 75% of children with learning disorders have significant social skills deficits (Kavale and Forness 1996), another important treatment consideration is social skills training. Developing a social skills treatment approach that is matched to the specific deficits seen in children with learning disorders is important for maximum effectiveness (Sheehan 2001).

There has been increasing interest in creating a new diagnostic category within learning disabilities: *nonverbal learning disability* (Rourke and Del Dotto 2001; Torgeson 1993). This disability is postulated to result from right-hemisphere deficits and is associated with mathematics disorder, handwriting difficulties, deficits in spatial reasoning, visuomotor integration problems, and social skills deficits (American Academy of Child and Adolescent Psychiatry 1998; Rourke and Del Dotto 2001).

■ Prognosis and Natural History

U.S. Public Law 94–142, which mandated individualized education programming, has had a considerable effect on the education of children with learning disorders; therefore, it is difficult to distinguish between the natural longitudinal course of learning disorders and the effects of educational intervention. Few longitudinal studies have been done on children with mathematics disorder or disorder of written expression; more work has been done in the area of reading disorder. One early study (Watson et al. 1982) found that 25% of children with mild reading disorders and 5% of those with severe disorders early in elementary school read at grade level by the end of high school. Learning disorders may continue to be present into a person's adulthood and can lead to problems such as school dropout, problems with employment, and poor socialization (American Psychiatric Association 2000; Klein and Mannuzza 2000). When a diagnosis is made early, however, a child has a better chance of remediation of problem areas. In terms of long-term psychiatric disorder diagnosis, Klein and Mannuzza (2000) reported that even children with uncomplicated reading disorder (i.e., no concurrent psychiatric disorder) go on to have a greater prevalence of mood and substance use disorders at 16-year follow-up assessment.

Motor Skills Disorder

■ Definition and History

Historically, motor delays and coordination problems not meeting criteria for disorders such as cerebral palsy have been identified in the literature for many years. Terms used have included *clumsiness syndrome, dyspraxia syndrome, poor coordination of developmental onset,* and *specific motor developmental disorder* (Denckla and Roeltgen 1992). Currently, developmental coordination disorder is identified in DSM-IV-TR as a motor skills disorder and is defined as a significant impairment in either gross or fine motor coordination, as evidenced by delays in developmental motor milestones or difficulty with other expected motor tasks during development. Diagnostic criteria for developmental coordination disorder are listed in Table 22–6. This disorder is distinct in DSM-IV-TR from medical conditions that cause motor difficulties, as well as other conditions with a common motor skills delay component, such as pervasive developmental disorders (PDDs; American Psychiatric Association 2000).

■ Clinical Presentation

In addition to delays and deficits in motor skills, children with developmental coordination disorder often have associated delays of other developmental milestones, such as language. Other disorders commonly observed include learning and communication disorders (American Psychiatric Association 2000; Sugden and Wright 1998). The clumsiness associated with this disorder can lead to peer teasing that can have a harmful emotional impact on these children, leading to psychosocial sequelae such as social withdrawal, low self-esteem, and feelings of incompetence and low self-efficacy. In addition, comorbid conditions such as ADHD are frequently seen (Denckla and Roeltgen 1992; Tannock 2000).

DSM-IV-TR estimates prevalence of developmental coordination disorder at up to 6% in children ages 5–11 years. Typically, it is first diagnosed when parents notice a delay in development of specific motor skills or difficulty with skills once attempted. Although these deficits can be remediated, in some cases problems continue throughout life.

Table 22–6. DSM-IV-TR diagnostic criteria for developmental coordination disorder

A. Performance in daily activities that require motor coordination is substantially below that expected given the person's chronological age and measured intelligence. This may be manifested by marked delays in achieving motor milestones (e.g., walking, crawling, sitting), dropping things, "clumsiness," poor performance in sports, or poor handwriting.
B. The disturbance in Criterion A significantly interferes with academic achievement or activities of daily living.
C. The disturbance is not due to a general medical condition (e.g., cerebral palsy, hemiplegia, or muscular dystrophy) and does not meet criteria for a pervasive developmental disorder.
D. If mental retardation is present, the motor difficulties are in excess of those usually associated with it.

Coding note: If a general medical (e.g., neurological) condition or sensory deficit is present, code the condition on Axis III.

Source. Reprinted from the *Diagnostic and Statistical Manual of Mental Disorders,* 4th Edition, Text Revision. Washington, DC, American Psychiatric Association, 2000. Copyright 2000, American Psychiatric Association. Used with permission.

■ Diagnosis and Treatment

In addition to a medical evaluation to rule out medical causes of the motor impairment, a thorough history is necessary, in addition to standardized procedures and a child observation. An evaluation by an occupational therapist can also inform the diagnosis. History information collected should include developmental motor milestones, as well as other early motor behaviors seen in infancy and toddlerhood, such as sucking, swallowing, crying, tracking, grasping, toileting, feeding, dressing, drawing, and others (Denckla and Roeltgen 1992).

Other conditions often resulting in motor difficulties that should be ruled out before a diagnosis of developmental coordination disorder is made include neurological conditions that affect motor coordination and PDDs. It is possible for a child to have this disorder if mental retardation is also present. However, it must be demonstrated that the motor deficits present are above what would be expected, given the diagnosis of mental retardation.

Treatment approaches used fall into the broad categories of being either task-oriented or process-oriented. Process-oriented treatment is based on the underlying assumption that there is a deficit that needs to be addressed before functional skills can be taught, whereas task-oriented treatment approaches focus on teaching functional skills (Sugden and Wright 1998). The primary treatment modality for motor skills disorder is occupational therapy. In the educational setting, this typically translates to a regular education classroom setting with pull-out occupational therapy sessions either in an individual or group format. As with learning disorders, if a child meets criteria for special education in the public school system, an IEP with annual goals for improvement will be implemented.

Communication Disorders

■ Definition

Communication may be defined as the imparting, receiving, and interchange of information, whether it be facts; situational, relational, or sociocultural context; thoughts; requests; intentionality; or feelings. *Language* may be defined as the means of transmission: the symbol system, associated behaviors, techniques, and modes for delivering the communication (Bloom and Lahey 1978).

The ability to exchange information through language is at the heart of human social processes and culture and permeates every aspect of human activity. The effective and developmentally appropriate use of language to communicate is critical to the adaptive competence of every person. For children, speech and language development has a profound influence on many other aspects of development, including general cognition, play, educational achievement, peer relations, and both emotional and behavioral development (Cantwell and Baker 1987, 1991; Cohen 2001). Impairments in communicative function impede adaptation and, even in relatively mild forms, are highly associated with a variety of adverse psychosocial outcomes and with increased risk of psychiatric disorders (Beitchman and Young 1997; Cantwell and Baker 1977, 1987, 1991), as well as affecting long-term social, emotional, and vocational functioning (Cohen 2001).

The American Speech-Language-Hearing Association (1993) defines *communication disorder* as "an impairment in the ability to receive, send, process, and comprehend concepts or verbal, nonverbal and graphic symbol systems" (p. 40). The association further divides communication disorder into speech disorder and language disorder. *Speech disorders* involve problems with articulation, fluency, or voice. Articulation disorder (equivalent to phonological disorder in DSM-IV-TR) involves impairment in the intelligibility of speech resulting from difficulty with correct production of the sounds used in speech. This disorder may involve sound omissions, additions, or distortions. With fluency disorder (stuttering), a child has difficulty maintaining the flow of speech, with difficulties noted in terms of rate and rhythm, as well as repetitions of speech parts (e.g., sounds, words). Voice disorder involves age- or sex-inappropriate abnormalities in voice characteristics, such as quality, pitch, volume, resonance, and duration. *Language disorder* is defined as "the impaired comprehension and/or use of spoken, written, and/or other symbol systems" (American Speech-Language-Hearing Association 1993, p. 40). It can involve the form, context, and/or function of language. The form of language includes phonology, morphology, and syntax; the context of language includes semantics; and the function of language includes pragmatics (American Speech-Language-Hearing Association 1993). The definitions of these components of language are included in Table 22–7.

Table 22–7. Components of language

Form of language	
Phonology	A language's sound system and accompanying rules governing the combination of sounds; phonemes are the basic sound components of speech
Morphology	The system that governs the structure and formation of words in a language; morphemes are the smallest meaningful linguistic units
Syntax	The system that governs the order and combination of words to form sentences, clauses, and phrases, and the relationships among elements of a sentence
Context of language	
Semantics	The system that governs the meaning of words and sentences
Function of language	
Pragmatics	The system that combines the above language components into functional and socially appropriate communication

The DSM-IV-TR classification of communication disorders (Tables 22–8 to 22–12) focuses primarily on disorders of speech production and content and on comprehension of spoken language. Although impairment of these functions in alternative modes of communication such as sign language (presumably to include hearing-impaired individuals) is included, it is not discussed in any detail. Disorders of reading and written expression are classified under learning disorders, although they are clearly associated with language and communication, and there is a clear comorbidity between these diagnoses. In fact, some professionals in the field prefer the term *language-based learning disabilities* when discussing reading and written expression disorders, acknowledging the relationship between spoken and written language, and the frequent comorbidity of communication problems in these children (American Speech-Language-Hearing Association 2002).

As with learning disorders, communication disorders are also included under IDEA, as preschool speech-language delay and speech/language impairment (U.S. Congress 1997). Children meeting such criteria are eligible by law for remediation services through the school system. Such services can include placement in communication-handicapped classroom settings for all or part of the day, or pull-out speech therapy services with inclusion in a regular education classroom.

■ History

The concept of *developmental language disorder* (DLD) has evolved, starting in the twentieth century, as the result of contributions from many disciplines, including speech and language pathology, neurology, psychiatry, educators of the deaf and of children with developmental disabilities, and neuropsychology. Starting in the 1930s, increasing attention was focused on the distinction between the acquired aphasias of adulthood and the congenital or developmental language impairments of childhood. The term *developmental dysphasia* came into use to describe the deficient, delayed, and/or partial acquisition of language, as distinguished from acquired aphasias caused by focal lesions of the brain (Benton 1978; Rapin and Allen 1988; Zangwill 1987). Investigators attempted to devise empirical classifications of DLD by studying large numbers of children with language problems on a range of linguistic and other cognitive and neurological variables and

Table 22–8. DSM-IV-TR diagnostic criteria for expressive language disorder

A. The scores obtained from standardized individually administered measures of expressive language development are substantially below those obtained from standardized measures of both nonverbal intellectual capacity and receptive language development. The disturbance may be manifest clinically by symptoms that include having a markedly limited vocabulary, making errors in tense, or having difficulty recalling words or producing sentences with developmentally appropriate length or complexity.

B. The difficulties with expressive language interfere with academic or occupational achievement or with social communication.

C. Criteria are not met for mixed receptive-expressive language disorder or a pervasive developmental disorder.

D. If mental retardation, a speech-motor or sensory deficit, or environmental deprivation is present, the language difficulties are in excess of those usually associated with these problems.

Coding note: If a speech-motor or sensory deficit or a neurological condition is present, code the condition on Axis III.

Source. Reprinted from the *Diagnostic and Statistical Manual of Mental Disorders*, 4th Edition, Text Revision. Washington, DC, American Psychiatric Association, 2000. Copyright 2000, American Psychiatric Association. Used with permission.

applying statistical techniques to classify them into clinically significant subgroups (Aram and Nation 1975; Aram et al. 1984). More recently, techniques such as functional magnetic resonance imaging are being used to identify neurological markers for language disorders (Paul 2001). Although disorders of the pragmatics of language for communication are not yet represented in DSM, they have attracted considerable clinical and research attention, particularly because they are correlated with a variety of psychiatric disorders in children and adults (Andreasen 1986; Baltaxe and Simmons 1988).

■ Clinical Presentation

Children suspected to have communication disorders are generally referred first for a speech-language or cognitive psychological evaluation. The linguistic phenomena that lead to these referrals are quite variable, depending on the type of deficit and the age of the child. For toddlers and preschoolers, primary consid-

Table 22–9. DSM-IV-TR diagnostic criteria for mixed receptive-expressive language disorder

A. The scores obtained from a battery of standardized individually administered measures of both receptive and expressive language development are substantially below those obtained from standardized measures of nonverbal intellectual capacity. Symptoms include those for expressive language disorder as well as difficulty understanding words, sentences, or specific types of words, such as spatial terms.

B. The difficulties with receptive and expressive language significantly interfere with academic or occupational achievement or with social communication.

C. Criteria are not met for a pervasive developmental disorder.

D. If mental retardation, a speech-motor or sensory deficit, or environmental deprivation is present, the language difficulties are in excess of those usually associated with these problems.

Coding note: If a speech-motor or sensory deficit or a neurological condition is present, code the condition on Axis III.

Source. Reprinted from the *Diagnostic and Statistical Manual of Mental Disorders*, 4th Edition, Text Revision. Washington, DC, American Psychiatric Association, 2000. Copyright 2000, American Psychiatric Association. Used with permission.

Table 22–10. DSM-IV-TR diagnostic criteria for phonological disorder

A. Failure to use developmentally expected speech sounds that are appropriate for age and dialect (e.g., errors in sound production, use, representation, or organization such as, but not limited to, substitutions of one sound for another [use of /t/ for target /k/ sound] or omissions of sounds such as final consonants).

B. The difficulties in speech sound production interfere with academic or occupational achievement or with social communication.

C. If mental retardation, a speech-motor or sensory deficit, or environmental deprivation is present, the speech difficulties are in excess of those usually associated with these problems.

Coding note: If a speech-motor or sensory deficit or a neurological condition is present, code the condition on Axis III.

Source. Reprinted from the *Diagnostic and Statistical Manual of Mental Disorders*, 4th Edition, Text Revision. Washington, DC, American Psychiatric Association, 2000. Copyright 2000, American Psychiatric Association. Used with permission.

erations include whether the child speaks at all, how many words are in the child's spoken vocabulary and

Table 22–11. DSM-IV-TR diagnostic criteria for stuttering

A. Disturbance in the normal fluency and time patterning of speech (inappropriate for the individual's age), characterized by frequent occurrences of one or more of the following:
   (1) sound and syllable repetitions
   (2) sound prolongations
   (3) interjections
   (4) broken words (e.g., pauses within a word)
   (5) audible or silent blocking (filled or unfilled pauses in speech)
   (6) circumlocutions (word substitutions to avoid problematic words)
   (7) words produced with an excess of physical tension
   (8) monosyllabic whole-word repetitions (e.g., "I-I-I-I see him")

B. The disturbance in fluency interferes with academic or occupational achievement or with social communication.

C. If a speech-motor or sensory deficit is present, the speech difficulties are in excess of those usually associated with these problems.

Coding note: If a speech-motor or sensory deficit or a neurological condition is present, code the condition on Axis III.

Source. Reprinted from the *Diagnostic and Statistical Manual of Mental Disorders*, 4th Edition, Text Revision. Washington, DC, American Psychiatric Association, 2000. Copyright 2000, American Psychiatric Association. Used with permission.

Table 22–12. DSM-IV-TR diagnostic criteria for communication disorder not otherwise specified

This category is for disorders in communication that do not meet criteria for any specific communication disorder; for example, a voice disorder (i.e., an abnormality of vocal pitch, loudness, quality, tone, or resonance).

Source. Reprinted from the *Diagnostic and Statistical Manual of Mental Disorders*, 4th Edition, Text Revision. Washington, DC, American Psychiatric Association, 2000. Copyright 2000, American Psychiatric Association. Used with permission.

their intelligibility, whether the child understands simple directions, and whether the child is able to name objects. For school-age children, problems in the comprehension, formulation, and spoken expression of the syntactically and semantically more complex material required to function successfully at school are more common causes of referral. For teenagers, the issue is more likely to be the ability to formulate or comprehend abstract ideas, complex instructions, or metaphoric expressions in spoken or written language (Cohen 2001; Hummel and Feinstein 1997). Because of the dramatic changes in language capacities over time and the greatly increased complexity of the phenomena being evaluated, it is not surprising that nonspecialist clinicians are more likely to suspect a language disorder in the very young child than in the older child, unless the deficits in the older child are profound.

Children with expressive language disorder generally have good understanding of language but have difficulty using it to communicate. Very young children with this disorder may have no speech at all. Other children tend to use developmentally immature forms of language, to speak in shorter, more telegraphic sentences, and to rely heavily on contextual cues and nonverbal communication. These children tend to make syntactic or semantic errors in sentence construction. Word retrieval difficulties may result in circumlocutions, reliance on jargon, or word substitutions (Richardson 1989). These problems result in speech that appears awkward, incoherent, or unintelligible. Adolescents with DLD may have special difficulty with the pragmatic uses of language. For example, they may fail to tailor their communication to the listener's needs and status by not providing adequate contextual information. Expressive language delays are most common in children under age 3, with prevalence in this group being between 10% and 15%. These numbers decrease with age, and by school age, only 3%–7% of children present with this disorder. Developmental expressive language disorder is more common than the acquired form and more often occurs in boys than girls, although this finding may be reflective of a referral bias (American Psychiatric Association 2000; Beitchman and Young 1997). Associated findings may include phonological disorder, erratic rate and rhythm of speech, learning disorders (particularly of written expression), developmental coordination disorder, enuresis, and neurological abnormalities (American Academy of Child and Adolescent Psychiatry 1998; American Psychiatric Association 2000).

Children with mixed receptive-expressive language disorder manifest deficits in expression as well as in comprehension of language. As a result, this form of communication disorder is more socially and academically disabling. Mixed receptive-expressive language disorder is not as prevalent as expressive language disorder, with approximately 5% of preschoolers and 3% of school-age children affected (American Psychiatric Association 2000). As with expressive language disorder, more boys than girls are thought to have this disorder, but this may again be an artifact of referral bias rather than a true discrepancy. Associated findings may include auditory processing problems, phonological disorder, speech perception deficits, memory problems, learning disabilities, developmental coordination disorder, enuresis, and neurological abnormalities (American Psychiatric Association 2000).

Phonological disorder describes the failure to use age-appropriate and expected speech sounds. Accordingly, the diagnosis is made by considering articulatory proficiency relative to age as well as the consistency of any deficit. The primary clinical finding in a child who has phonological disorder is decreased intelligibility of speech production in the context of normal sentence production and comprehension. Typically, the child's speech sounds immature. There is wide variation in the degree of intelligibility in children with this disorder. Moderate to severe phonological disorder is estimated to affect 2% of early school-age children in whom other organic causes are not identified, and a somewhat higher rate is seen in the milder form of the disorder, with estimates of up to 20% reported (American Academy of Child and Adolescent Psychiatry 1998; American Psychiatric Association 2000). The disorder is more common in boys than in girls (American Psychiatric Association 2000). Many children with phonological disorder have associated nonlinguistic findings, including neurological soft signs, enuresis, developmental coordination disorder, and learning disorders (Cantwell and Baker 1987). Anywhere from 50% to 70% of children with phonological disorder are reported to also have general academic problems throughout school, and children with this disorder are at risk for later learning disorders (Castrogiovanni 2002).

Stuttering is essentially a disturbance in the age-appropriate fluency and patterning of speech, including characteristics such as repetitions, prolongations, blocking, and substitutions. Stuttering begins early in life, usually between ages 2 and 7, and is often exacerbated by stress or anxiety. The prevalence of stuttering is 1% in young children, with more males affected than females, by a ratio of about 3:1 (American Psychiatric Association 2000; National Institute on Deafness and Other Communication Disorders 1997). Phonological disorder and expressive language disorder are seen more frequently in children who stutter than in the general population (American Psychiatric Association 2000), with as many as 44% of children who stutter having one or both of these other communication disorders as well (Arndt and Healey 2001). Some investigators have distinguished between "remediable" and "chronic perseverative" stuttering, noting that children with remediable stuttering are able to learn and use techniques to overcome this problem, whereas chronic perseverative stuttering involves problems that extend beyond developmental disfluency and are less amenable to treatment. Approximately two-thirds of children who stutter have the remediable form, whereas 1 in 5 people who stutter have the chronic perseverative form (Cooper 1993, 1987).

■ Relation to Psychiatric Disorder

A wide range of emotional and behavioral disorders has been described in children and adolescents with communication disorders. These may be emotional reactions to the linguistic deficit, symptoms of concomitant psychiatric disorders, or manifestations of a common underlying neurological substrate. Signs of impulsivity, inattentiveness, aggressiveness, lack of self-confidence, low self-esteem, social withdrawal, low frustration tolerance, anxiety, and social immaturity have been noted in younger children with communication disorders (American Psychiatric Association 2000; Cantwell and Baker 1987; Cohen 2001; Love and Thompson 1988). Emotional problems also are common in adolescents with communication disorders. Symptoms may include anxiety, compulsiveness, withdrawal, aggressiveness, and rigidity (Beitchman et al. 1996; Bergman 1987; Cohen 2001; Shapiro 1985).

Research suggests that about half of all children with language disorders seen in speech and language clinics are also found to have an Axis I psychiatric disorder, and particular associations have been found with ADHD, disruptive behavior disorders, and anxiety disorders (Baker and Cantwell 1982, 1985; Barkley 1997; Beitchman et al. 1986; Cantwell and Baker 1987, 1991; Paul 2001). Specifically, Cantwell and Baker (1991) found that a group of children who had a diagnosed communication disorder had a comorbid disruptive behavior disorder 26% of the time, with ADHD most common (19%), followed by oppositional defiant disorder and conduct disorder in 7% of children seen. Anxiety disorders were found in 10% of the children. Children with mixed receptive-expressive language disorder are the most likely to have comorbid psychiatric disorders, and language disorders overall are more likely than speech disorders (phonological disorder or stuttering) to be associated with comorbid psychiatric conditions (Cantwell and Baker 1991; Stevenson 1996). Longitudinal data suggest that language problems at age 5 are risk factors for a variety of psychiatric disorders, including ADHD and antisocial personality disorder, as well as criminal behavior and substance use disorders, by age 19 (Beitchman et al. 1996, 1999). A thorough assessment of the presence of substance use disorders would be important in adolescents with language disorders, as these are often comorbid with conduct disorder, ADHD, and anxiety disorders (Kandel et al. 1999; Riggs and Whitmore 1999; Zeitlin 1999).

Several well-designed research studies suggest that up to two-thirds of children seen in psychiatric settings have language disorders that are often too subtle to be detected without specialized evaluations (as cited in Cohen et al. 1989; Paul 2001; Stevenson 1996). Approximately 30% of these children have communication problems that are previously undiagnosed (Cohen et al. 1993). In a psychiatric setting, language disorder can be especially difficult to detect when expressive abilities are less than profoundly impaired. Cohen et al. (1993) found that in a group of children from outpatient child psychiatry clinics who were identified as having language disorders, those whose disorder had been previously undiagnosed had less difficulty with expressive sentence formation, milder language difficulties overall, and higher rates of externalizing problems, such as delinquency, than those whose disorder had been previously diagnosed.

■ Diagnosis

Psychiatric Language Assessment

In view of the high comorbidity of language deficits and psychiatric disorders, the child psychiatrist should routinely take a careful history of language development and assess the current level of linguistic functioning. A useful preliminary evaluation can be done in the context of the clinical interview and mental status examination before any referral for specialized language evaluations. Specific areas that the clinician should observe include inner language, comprehension, production, phonation, and pragmatics (Rutter 1987).

Inner language refers to the use of symbolization in the child's thought and can be evaluated most easily in younger children by observing play behavior for evidence of symbolic play (Rutter 1987). Language *comprehension* should be evaluated in terms of the child's ability to follow commands without gestures, to answer questions both relevant to the situation and out of context, to follow conversation, to understand abstract language, and to draw inferences. Language *production* involves an assessment of the amount of speech produced, fluency, and intelligibility. Additionally, specific components of the content to be evaluated are morphology (use of inflectional endings and function words), syntax (word order, use of pronouns, and verb tense), and semantics (range of vocabulary). *Phonation* refers to the quality of the child's voice and includes pitch, volume, intonation, and prosody (melody of speech). *Pragmatic language* involves the child's ability to use language for effective communication. This is evaluated by observing the child's ability to take into account the perspective of his or her conversational partner. It includes the child's adherence to social conventions for eye contact, gestures, and both verbal and nonverbal cues. It further involves the child's ability to sustain conversation, maintain a shared topic, and take turns in a dialogue. Finally, the age-appropriate comprehension and use of idiomatic expressions and metaphoric language should be assessed.

Formal Cognitive and Linguistic Assessment

For both expressive and mixed receptive-expressive language disorder, diagnosis, as defined in DSM-IV-TR, is predicated on demonstration of a significant difference between nonverbal cognitive functioning and language development. The assessment of cognitive and linguistic abilities requires psychometric testing, which should not be limited to merely comparing verbal and nonverbal dimensions on an intelligence test. Although an overall measure of intelligence (and a specific measure of nonverbal intelligence) is essential, it will provide neither the specificity nor sensitivity to detect or delineate many linguistic deficits. Standardized measures of linguistic functioning are necessary to determine a child's expressive and receptive language abilities. Table 22–5 provides a list of commonly used linguistic and psychological tests. Typically, such testing requires referral to a psychologist and speech-language pathologist. Of importance is the consideration of a child's cultural context in determining the most appropriate measures of functioning, including bilingualism. In addition to linguistic and psychological testing, hearing evaluation is an important part of the assessment.

It should be noted that the DSM requirement of a discrepancy between cognitive and language functioning is a controversial one, with little empirical evidence to support it. It has been suggested, instead, that a more appropriate means of identification involves simply targeting all children with language skills that are below expected for age (American Academy of Child and Adolescent Psychiatry 1998; Paul 2001). Additionally, diagnosis in infants and toddlers is difficult using this narrow model of diagnosis. Diagnosis in younger children has been increasingly realized as critical to implementation of appropriate treatment, but assessment measures for this younger population are inadequate because the discrepancy model fails to provide authentic assessment of young children's language development (Wetherby and Prizant 1997). The Communication and Symbolic Behavior Scales (CSBS) is one recently developed measure to correct for this problem; it assesses communication, social/affective, and symbolic abilities of infants and toddlers (Weatherby and Prizant 1993).

Differential Diagnosis

The diagnostic reasoning process, using DSM-IV-TR criteria, involves two steps. First, a discrepancy between language skills and intelligence must be established. Second, because language disorders share symptoms with a number of other disorders, there must be a differential diagnosis, considering hearing impairment, mental retardation, autism or other PDD, and selective mutism. Traditionally, children with low scores on both verbal and nonverbal intelligence tests have been labeled mentally retarded. However, research suggests that language disorders can and do occur in mentally retarded individuals (Cohen et al. 1986; Rondal 1987). Both disorders should be diagnosed in these children if language function is impaired beyond what can be accounted for by the retardation.

Autism, a disorder that has as one of its key diagnostic features impairment in communication, must be differentiated from communication disorder by assessment of reciprocal social interaction and repetitive patterns of behavior (American Psychiatric Association 2000). Although children with communication disorders can also present with social deficits, they show greater awareness of affect and engage more in reciprocal social interaction and symbolic play than do children with autism (Allen et al. 1988). Children with autism present with more global impairment in development and frequently show evidence of impaired imaginative and creative play, repetitive behaviors, sensory over- or understimulation, and impaired social cognition. In addition, the quality of speech in children with language disorders differs from the quality of speech in children with autism, with the latter characterized by echolalia, perseveration, pragmatic deficits, and lack of emotional inflection (Paul 2001). Moreover, the child with autism shows deficits in intentional communication and may fail to compensate for language delays with nonverbal communication (Paul 2001). Selective mutism can mimic expressive and mixed receptive-expressive language disorder, but the diminished expressive language seen in these children is present in some settings but not others (American Psychiatric Association 2000).

■ Etiology and Pathogenesis

The etiology of communication disorders is primarily biological, but family environment and sociological factors also clearly play a role (Cantwell and Baker 1991; Wetherby and Prizant 1997). Biological factors that have been demonstrated to affect the development of language include prenatal risk factors (including exposure to intrauterine teratogens such as alcohol, drugs, or environmental toxins such as lead), perinatal risk factors (anoxia, asphyxia, low birth weight), early childhood risk factors (such as recurrent persistent otitis media or childhood illnesses), and genetic and metabolic disorders (Aram 1988; Paul 2001; Wetherby and Prizant 1997). Important environmental risk factors include poverty, abuse or neglect, and psychiatric disorders in caregivers (Wetherby and Prizant 1997). Although individual risk factors may not play roles as statistically important as etiological factors in language disorders (Browman et al. 1987), a more important predictor is the accumulation of multiple risk factors, both biological and environmental (Wetherby and Prizant 1997).

Because there is no empirical validation for the current discrepancy-based method of classifying language disorders, the boundary between categorical language disorder and simply poor skills on a continuum of language ability is uncertain. Nevertheless, there is considerable evidence that hereditary factors are a prominent cause of language disorder, particularly expressive language disorder (American Academy of Child and Adolescent Psychiatry 1998; Bishop et al. 1995; Tomblin and Buckwalter 1994). Early language delay (as measured by vocabulary at age 2 years) is under strong hereditary influence, as documented by Dale et al. (1998) in a study of 3,000 twin pairs. Group differences in heritability for those children with the lowest 5% of vocabulary scores was 73%. Shared environment was only a quarter as important for the language-delayed sample as for the entire sample. Twin research also documents an association between motor immaturity and specific language impairment in children (Bishop 2002). Much of the evidence for the role of specific genetic factors in language dysfunction (particularly regarding genes on chromosomes 6, 7, and 15) is reviewed in the section of this chapter on reading disorders (see *reading disorder* under "Learning Disorders" above).

In the case of phonological disorder, the etiology appears to be genetic, with evidence of heritability noted in several studies (Lewis 1992; Lewis and Thompson 1992). In stuttering, there also appears to be a familial pattern, with strong evidence of a genetic factor in the etiology. It is estimated that half of people who stutter have other family members who also stutter (Felsenfeld 1998). Stuttering is over three times more common in first-degree relatives of people who stutter than in the general population, and a family history of other communication disorders increases the risk of stuttering. In families in which fathers stuttered, approximately 10% of daughters and 20% of sons also stutter (American Psychiatric Association 2000).

As with the phonological processing deficit models of reading disorder, there is considerable evidence that the very rapid neural processing of speech sounds required to decode and comprehend spoken language is impaired in children with receptive language problems (Fitch et al. 1997). It is likely, however, that there are other neurological dysfunctions involved in language disorder that are not due to phonological deficits. Working verbal memory deficits appear to be a factor in phonological and semantic information processing for some children with receptive language disorder (Johnson 1994).

■ Treatment

The goals of intervention vary from child to child and may include elimination of the deficit (if possible), teaching specific strategies to change the deficit and increase skills, teaching compensatory coping strategies, or changing the child's environment (Paul 2001). Intervention approaches may include clinician-directed approaches (drill, drill play, and modeling), which follow a formal, behavioral approach to treatment; child-centered approaches (indirect language stimulation or facilitative play, and whole language), which are appropriate for children who are unassertive or refuse to participate in a clinician-directed approach; and hybrid approaches (focused stimulation, vertical structuring, milieu teaching, and script therapy), which combine aspects of the previous two approaches (Paul 2001).

Two commonly used methods for treating language impairments are imitation-based and modeling therapies, which have been shown to improve more than the specific targeted aspects of language taught (Leonard 1998). Language therapy is increasingly designed to take place in relevant social environments where the focus is on functional language in transactional contexts (Schiefelbusch and Lloyd 1988; Weatherby and Prizant 1997). In addition, assisting caregivers to develop appropriate styles of communication with their children that encourage successful interactions and thus target language delay in this manner is also an important identified treatment approach (Weatherby and Prizant 1997).

Fast ForWord is a computer-assisted intervention program developed by the Scientific Learning Corporation (Oakland, CA) for children with language impairments that claims to improve a child's temporal auditory processing abilities. It is based on the notion that deficits in temporal processing are one causative factor in language disorders. The makers have suggested that it can lead to a 1.5- to 3-year gain in language in 6 weeks (Loeb et al. 2001), and significant gains in speech and nonspeech discrimination and language comprehension (Merzenich et al. 1996; Tallal et al. 1996). However, although subsequent studies have noted gains in oral and written language and pragmatics, those gains have been more modest, with dramatic gains in spontaneous language less common or not sustained over time (Friel-Patti et al. 2001; Gillam et al. 2001; Loeb et al. 2001; Thibodeau et al. 2001). A separate study found that children receiving Fast ForWord training showed improvements in phonemic awareness, speaking, and syntax, but not in word identification or attack (Hook et al. 2001). Other treatment programs are also available and have been shown to be effective. For example, Laureate Learning Systems has been proven equally effective in improving language in children with communication disorders, although the two programs take different approaches to language learning (Gillam et al. 2001). In addition, train-ing in the Orton-Gillingham approach to language use has been shown to lead to improvements in phonemic awareness and word attack (Hook et al. 2001).

A recent treatment program developed for stuttering, the Lidcombe Program, involves operant conditioning principles. Parents are taught how to use these principles on a day-to-day basis in natural contexts with their children, providing verbal contingencies in the form of praise for nonstuttered speech and occasional corrections for stuttering. Research suggests that this is a promising treatment method, leading to alleviation of symptoms in preschool children and low rates of relapse (Onslow et al. 2001; Woods et al. 2002).

If a child meets criteria under IDEA for special-education services in the school because of a speech-language impairment, then an IEP, with a set of annual goals for progress in identified areas of concern, is developed. These goals include specific methods of intervention and ways of tracking improvement. Treatment of communication disorders typically involves individual or group speech therapy, offered as a pull-out service in addition to participation in a regular education classroom. Alternatively, placement in a classroom for communication-handicapped students may be recommended.

As with learning disorders, when treating any comorbid psychiatric conditions, the language disorder should be taken into consideration. This includes prevention programs, which are typically verbally mediated and thus may be less effective for this population of children. In addition, children and adolescents with language disorders who are in treatment programs for psychiatric disorders, particularly in group formats, are likely to have difficulty understanding the information presented to them. It is likely that deficits in expressive and receptive language impede treatment response in verbally based psychotherapy. Consideration of the impact of language disorders on any verbally based psychiatric treatment, including individual, group, and family therapies, should be carefully made. Care should be taken not to misinterpret language impairment as oppositionality, when the observed behavior may actually be the result of the child's or adolescent's not understanding information or knowing how to respond.

■ Prognosis and Natural History

Most children with DLD speak by the time they are of school age and have normal language abilities by late adolescence. However, subtler but highly significant language and learning deficits persist for up to half of these children, particularly those with more severe initial impairment (Cantwell and Baker 1987; Shapiro and Rich 1999). A 10-year systematic prospective study of children with DLD as preschoolers (Aram et al. 1984) found that only 30% of these children had a normal academic course. The remainder had either repeated a grade or were in special-education classes. Follow-up language testing of these children revealed that 62% had language scores significantly below average. Research has consistently shown that children with DLD are at a heightened risk for the development of learning, emotional, and behavioral disorders (Baker and Cantwell 1987; Wetherby and Prizant 1997). Children with mixed receptive-expressive language disorder have a poorer prognosis than those with an expressive language disorder, with fewer children improving over time and a higher rate of learning disorders and psychiatric diagnoses (Cantwell and Baker 1987, 1991). Continuing language impairment can lead to academic failure, which can affect adult achievement in areas such as occupational and social functioning. In addition, decreased self-esteem, depression, and learned helplessness are risks, as well as insufficient social learning, leading to later social difficulties (Settle and Milich 1999; Weinberg et al. 1999). Children with language and learning disabilities have a 50% greater than average rate of school dropout (U.S. Department of Education 1995).

Spontaneous recovery of mild to moderate phonological disorder not due to a medical condition occurs by age 6 years in approximately 75% of cases and may be hastened by appropriate therapy. The prevalence by age 17 years is 0.5% (American Psychiatric Association 2000). Poorer prognoses are mostly seen in children with co-occurring problems, such as stuttering or hypernasality (Johnson 1980). Stuttering often resolves spontaneously by midadolescence, with a prevalence rate of 0.8% at that point. In anywhere between 20% and 80% of cases, stuttering is reported to remit (American Psychiatric Association 2000). Children with remediable stuttering will be more likely to experience an alleviation of symptoms, whereas those with chronic perseverative stuttering will be more likely to continue to have symptoms (Cooper 1993, 1987).

■ Research Issues

Although significant progress has been made, current concepts require further study to determine their validity and usefulness. In particular, major operational problems persist in making the diagnosis of DLD by simply identifying a discrepancy between measures of nonverbal intelligence and measures of language functioning (Fletcher et al. 1998). This discrepancy is typically based on test scores, but there is a lack of agreement about which tests to use for this purpose and how large this discrepancy must be for diagnosis. Although 1 SD has been used traditionally, this informal clinical practice has not been empirically validated. Also, no consensus exists about which aspects of language are essential to the diagnosis and about how many linguistic capacities must be deficient and to what degree (Aram and Morris 1992). An important issue in test score interpretation is whether poor performance on language tasks represents a developmental delay as opposed to deviant or deficient language mechanisms. Although considerable individual variation exists in the attainment of language milestones, guidelines are unclear about how large a delay is pathological. If language delay is part of a broader picture of developmental immaturity, it becomes particularly difficult to distinguish "normal variability" from neurologically based pathology (Beitchman 1985; Paul 2001).

A major unresolved controversy in defining language disorders that has attracted considerable attention concerns the validity of the assumption that language functioning is sufficiently independent of other aspects of cognitive functioning to provide a basis for using discrepancy between language test scores and nonverbal IQ as a core diagnostic criterion (Aram et al. 1994; Fletcher and Morris 1986; Paul 2001). Although this approach is widely used and is reflected in DSM-IV-TR, many theoretical, practical, and methodological questions are unanswered. "Nonverbal" and "verbal" psychometric measures frequently are correlated and may indeed include mixed cognitive functions or reasoning strategies. Discrepancy-based approaches do not address the issue of whether important functional or etiological differences exist between children whose language functioning is low but who do not have substantially higher nonverbal cognitive scores and children who meet the discrepancy criteria. Also unaddressed is the problem of how to classify children who meet nonverbal–verbal discrepancy criteria but whose scores on language tests do not fall in the deficient range. Technical problems also remain in determining the degree of discrepancy sufficient to establish the diagnosis.

In addition to the presently identified language disorders, researchers have proposed other specific subtypes of language disorders. For example, it has long been noted that some children with language disorder also have a deficit in understanding the context and function of language and appear socially impaired (Cantwell and Baker 1991). These children miss the cues involved in reciprocal conversation. They fail to attend to the listener with respect to what that person is interested in and to whether the person wants to hear about a particular topic. They have difficulty interpreting the social cues involved in communication with others and may tend to interrupt or intrude on others during conversation. Although these language impairments are frequently described in PDDs, several investigators have suggested that this disorder also exists separate from PDDs (Cohen 2001; Toppelberg and Shapiro 2000).

Conclusion

Learning, motor skills, and communication disorders are a heterogeneous set of neurocognitive deficits seen in significant numbers of children and adolescents. They constitute a major vulnerability factor for psychiatric disorder and are comorbid conditions in many youngsters with psychiatric disorder. Because of these considerations, learning and language skills should be carefully assessed during all psychiatric evaluations of children and adolescents. Treatment planning must address these deficits in academic and communication skills as well as any other Axis I disorder and associated family problems. Untreated problems in these important domains of a child's development are likely to undermine both therapeutic efforts and ongoing successful psychosocial adaptation.

References

Allen DA, Rapin I, Wiznitzer M: Communication disorders of preschool children: the physician's responsibility. J Dev Behav Pediatr 9:164–170, 1988

American Academy of Child and Adolescent Psychiatry: Practice parameters for the assessment and treatment of children and adolescents with language and learning disorders. J Am Acad Child Adolesc Psychiatry 37:46S–62S, 1998

American Psychiatric Association: Diagnostic and Statistical Manual of Mental Disorders, 3rd Edition, Revised. Washington, DC, American Psychiatric Association, 1987

American Psychiatric Association: Diagnostic and Statistical Manual of Mental Disorders, 4th Edition, Washington, DC, American Psychiatric Association, 1994

American Psychiatric Association: Diagnostic and Statistical Manual of Mental Disorders, 4th Edition, Text Revision, Washington, DC, American Psychiatric Association, 2000

American Speech-Language-Hearing Association (Ad Hoc Committee on Service Delivery in the Schools): Definitions of communication disorders and variations. ASHA 35 (suppl 10):40–41, 1993

American Speech-Language-Hearing Association: Language-based learning disabilities. Rockville, MD, American Speech-Language-Hearing Association, 2002. Available at: http://www.asha.org/speech/disabilities/Language-Based-Learning-Disabilities.cfm. Accessed May 24, 2003

Andreasen N: Scale for Assessment of Thought, Language, and Communication. Schizophr Bull 12:473–481, 1986

Aram D: Language sequelae of unilateral brain lesions in children, in Language, Communication, and the Brain. Edited by Plum F. New York, Plenum, 1988, pp 171–197

Aram DM, Hall NE: Longitudinal follow-up of children with pre-school communication disorders: treatment implications. School Psychology Review 18:487–501, 1989

Aram DM, Morris R: Validity of discrepancy criteria for identifying children with developmental language disorder. J Learn Disabil 25:549–554, 1992

Aram DM, Nation JE: Patterns of language behavior in children with developmental language disorders. J Speech Hear Res 18:229–241, 1975

Aram DM, Ekelman BL, Nation JE: Preschoolers with language disorders: 10 years later. J Speech Hear Res 27:232–244, 1984

Aram D, Morris R, Hall N, et al: Clinical and research congruence in identifying children with specific language impairment. J Speech Hear Res 37:824–830, 1994

Arndt J, Healey EC: Concomitant disorders in school-age children who stutter. Language, Speech, and Hearing Services in School (special issue) 32:68–78, 2001

Baker L, Cantwell D: Psychiatric disorder in children with different types of communication disorders. J Commun Disord 15:113–126, 1982

Baker L, Cantwell D: Psychiatric and learning disorders in children with speech and language disorders: a critical review. Advances in Learning and Behavior Disorders 4:1–28, 1985

Baker L, Cantwell DP: A prospective psychiatric follow-up of children with speech/language disorders. J Am Acad Child Adolesc Psychiatry 26:546–553, 1987

Baltaxe C, Simmons J: Pragmatic deficits in emotionally disturbed children and adolescents, in Language Perspectives: Acquisition, Retardation and Intervention. Edited by Schiefelbusch R, Loyd L. Austin, TX, Pro-Ed, 1988

Barkley RA: ADHD and the Nature of Self-Control. New York, Guilford, 1997

Beery KE, Buktenica NA: Developmental Test of Visual-Motor Integration. Odessa, FL, Psychological Assessment Resources, 1989

Beitchman JH: Speech and language impairment and psychiatric risk: toward a model of neurodevelopmental immaturity. Psychiatr Clin North Am 8:721–725, 1985

Beitchman JH, Young A: Learning disorders with a special emphasis on reading disorders: a review of the past 10 years. J Am Acad Child Adolesc Psychiatry 36:1020–1032, 1997

Beitchman JH, Nair R, Clegg M, et al: Prevalence of psychiatric disorders in children with speech and language disorders. J Am Acad Child Adolesc Psychiatry 25:528–535, 1986

Beitchman JH, Wilson B, Brownlie EB, et al: Long-term consistency in speech/language profiles, I: developmental and academic outcomes. J Am Acad Child Adolesc Psychiatry 35:804–814, 1996

Beitchman JH, Douglas L, Wilson B, et al: Adolescent substance use disorders: findings from a 14-year follow-up of speech/language-impaired and control children. J Clin Child Psychol 28:312–321, 1999

Benton AL: The cognitive functioning of children with developmental dysphasia, in Developmental Dysphasia. Edited by Wyke MA. London, Academic Press, 1978

Berg EA: A simple objective treatment for measuring flexibility in thinking. J Gen Psychol 39:15–22, 1948

Bergman MM: Social grace or disgrace: adolescent social skills and learning disability subtypes. Reading, Writing, and Learning Disorders 3:161–166, 1987

Bernbaum J, Batshaw M: Born too soon, born too small, in Children with Disabilities. Edited by Batshaw MI. Baltimore, MD, Paul H Brooks, 1997, pp 115–142

Bishop DV: Motor immaturity and specific speech and language impairment: evidence for a common genetic basis. Am J Med Genet 114:56–63, 2002

Bishop DVM, North T, Donlan C: Genetic basis of specific language impairments: evidence from a twin study. Dev Med Child Neurol 37:56–71, 1995

Bloom L, Lahey M: Language development and language disorders. New York, Wiley, 1978

Browman S, Nichol PL, Shaughnessy P, et al: Retardation in Young Children: A Developmental Study of Cognitive Deficit. Hillsdale, NJ, Lawrence Erlbaum, 1987

Bryan T: Social problems and learning disabilities, in Learning About Learning Disabilities. Edited by Wong BY. San Diego, CA, Academic Press, 1991, pp 195–229

Cantwell DP, Baker L: Psychiatric disorder in children with speech and language retardation: a critical review. Arch Gen Psychiatry 34:583–591, 1977

Cantwell D, Baker L: Developmental Speech and Language Disorders. New York, Guilford, 1987

Cantwell DP, Baker L: Psychiatric and Developmental Disorders in Children with Communication Disorder. Washington, DC, American Psychiatric Press, 1991

Carrow-Woolfolk, E: Test for Auditory Comprehension of Language—Revised. Allen, TX, DLM Teaching Resources, 1985

Castrogiovanni A: Communication Facts: Incidence and Prevalence of Communication Disorders and Hearing Loss in Children—2002 Edition. American Speech-Language-Hearing Association. Available at: http://professional.asha.org/resources/factsheets/children.cfm. Accessed May 24, 2003

Clements S, Peters J: Minimal brain dysfunctions in the school-age child. Arch Gen Psychiatry 6:185–197, 1962

Cohen D, Paul R, Volkmar FR: Issues in the classification of pervasive and other developmental disorders: toward DSM-IV. J Am Acad Child Adolesc Psychiatry 25:213–220, 1986

Cohen NJ: Language impairment and psychopathology in infants, children, and adolescents, in Developmental Clinical Psychology and Psychiatry, Vol 45. Thousand Oaks, CA, Sage Publications, 2001, pp 1–38

Cohen NJ, Davine M, Meloche-Kelly M: Prevalence of unsuspected language disorders in a child psychiatric population. J Am Acad Child Adolesc Psychiatry 28:107–111, 1989

Cohen NJ, Davine M, Horodesky N, et al: Unsuspected language impairment in psychiatrically disturbed children: relevance and language and behavioral characteristics. J Am Acad Child Adolesc Psychiatry 32:595–603, 1993

Connolly AJ, Nachtman W, Pritchett EM: The KeyMath Diagnostic Arithmetic Test. Circle Pines, MN, American Guidance Service, 1971

Cooper EB: The chronic perseverative stuttering syndrome: incurable stuttering. J Fluency Disord 12:381–388, 1987

Cooper EB: Chronic perseverative stuttering syndrome: a harmful or helpful construct? American Journal of Speech-Language Pathology 3:11–22, 1993

Cruickshank WM: The Brain-Injured Child in Home, School, and Community. Syracuse, NY, Syracuse University Press, 1967

Dale PS, Simonoff E, Bishop DV, et al: Genetic influence on language delay in two-year-old children. Nat Neurosci 1:324–328, 1998

Denckla MB, Roeltgen DP: Disorders of motor function and control, in Handbook of Neuropsychology, Vol 6. Edited by Rapin I, Segalowitz SJ. Amsterdam, Elsevier, 1992, pp 455–476

DiSimoni F: Token Test for Children. Allen, TX, DLM Teaching Resources, 1978

Doris JL: Defining learning disabilities: a history of the search for consensus, in Better Understanding Learning Disabilities: New Views from Research and Their Implications for Education and Public Policies. Edited by Lyon GR, Gray DB, Kavanagh, JF, et al. Baltimore, MD, Paul H Brookes, 1993, pp 97–115

Dunn LlM, Dunn LM, Williams TK: Peabody Picture Vocabulary Test—III. Circle Pines, MN, American Guidance Service, 1997

Farnham-Diggory S: Learning Disabilities. Cambridge, MA, Harvard University Press, 1978, pp 1–27

Felsenfeld S: What can genetic research tell us about stuttering treatment issues?, in Treatment Efficacy for Stuttering: A Search for Empirical Bases. Edited by Cordes AK, Ingham RJ. San Diego, CA, Singular Publishing Group, 1998, pp 51–65

Fensen L, Dale PS, Reznick JS, et al: MacArthur Communicative Development Inventory. San Antonio, TX, Psychological Corporation, 1993

Fitch RH, Miller S, Tallal P: Neurobiology of speech perception. Ann Rev Neurosci 20:331–353, 1997

Fletcher J, Morris R: Classification of disabled learners: beyond exclusionary definitions, in Handbook of Cognitive, Social, and Neuropsychological Aspects of Learning Disabilities. Edited by Ceci S. Hillsdale, NJ, Lawrence Erlbaum, 1986, pp 55–80

Fletcher JM, Shaywitz S, Shankweiler D, et al: Cognitive profiles of reading disability: comparison of discrepancy and low achievement definitions. Journal of Educational Psychology 86:6–23, 1994

Fletcher JM, Francis DJ, Shaywitz SE, et al: Intelligence testing and the discrepancy model for children with learning disabilities. Learning Disabilities Research and Practice 13:186–203, 1998

Flynn JM, Rahbar MH: Prevalence of reading failure in boys compared to girls. Psychology in the Schools 31:66–71, 1994

Friel-Patti S, DesBarres K, Thibodeau L: Case studies of children using Fast ForWord. Am J Speech-Lang Pathology 10:203–215, 2001

Fudala JB, Reynolds WM: Arizona Articulation Proficiency Scale—2nd Edition. Los Angeles, CA, Western Psychological Services, 1986

Galaburda AM, Sherman GR, Rosen GD, et al: Developmental dyslexia: four consecutive patients with cortical anomalies. Ann Neurol 18:222–233, 1985

Gamis AS, Nesbit ME: Neuropsychologic (cognitive) disabilities in long-term survivors of childhood cancer. Pediatrician 18:11–19, 1991

Gardner MF: Expressive One-Word Picture Vocabulary Test—revised. Novato, CA, Academic Therapy Publications, 1990

Gillam RB, Crofford JA, Gale MA, et al: Language change following computer-assisted language instruction with Fast ForWord or Laureate Learning Systems software. Am J Speech-Lang Pathology (Special Forum on Fast ForWord) 10:231–247, 2001

Gittelman R: Treatment of reading disorders, in Developmental Neuropsychiatry. Edited by Rutter M. New York, Guilford, 1983, pp 520–541

Glosser B, Koppell S: Emotional-behavioral patterns in children with learning disabilities: lateralized hemispheric differences. J Learn Disabil 20:365–369, 1987

Golden CJ: Luria-Nebraska Neuropsychological Battery: Children's Revision. Los Angeles, CA, Western Psychological Services, 1987

Goldman R, Fristoe M: Goldman-Fristoe Test of Articulation (G-FTA). Circle Pines, MN, American Guidance Service, 1986

Goldman R, Fristoe M, Woodcock RW: Goldman-Fristoe-Woodcock Test of Auditory Discrimination. Circle Pines, MN, American Guidance Service, 1970

Grigorenko EL, Wood FB, Meyer MS, et al: Susceptibility loci for distinct components of developmental dyslexia on chromosomes 6 and 15. Am J Hum Genet 60:27–39, 1997

Halperin JM, Gittelman R, Klein DF, et al: Reading-disabled hyperactive children: a distinct subgroup of attention deficit disorder with hyperactivity? J Abnorm Child Psychol 12:1–14, 1984

Hammill DD, Brown VL, Larsen SC, et al: Test of Adolescent and Adult Language—3rd Edition. Austin, TX, ProEd Inc, 1994

Hedrick DL, Prather EM, Tobin AR: Sequenced Inventory of Communication Development—Revised. Seattle, WA, University of Washington Press, 1984

Hill DE, Ciesielski KT, Sethre-Hofstad L, et al: Visual and verbal short-term memory deficits in childhood leukemia survivors after intrathecal chemotherapy. J Pediatr Psychol 22:861–870, 1997

Hinshaw SP: Externalizing behavior problems and academic underachievement in childhood and adolescence: causal relationships and underlying mechanisms. Psychol Bull 111:127–155, 1992

Hook PE, Macaruso P, Jones S: Efficacy of Fast ForWord training on facilitating acquisition of reading skills by children with reading difficulties—a longitudinal study. Annals of Dyslexia 51:75–96, 2001

Hresko WP, Reid DK, Hammill DD: Test of Early Language Development—2nd edition. Austin, TX, ProEd Inc, 1991

Hummel L, Feinstein C: Developmental language disorders in school-age children, in Handbook of Child and Adolescent Psychiatry, Vol 2: The Grade-School Child: Development and Syndromes. Edited by Kernberg PF, Bemporad JR (Noshpitz JD, editor-in-chief). New York, Wiley, 1997, pp 420–435

Hunt RD, Cohen DJ: Psychiatric aspects of learning disabilities. Pediatr Clin North Am 31:471–497, 1984

Hynd GW, Connor RT, Nieves N: Learning disability subtypes: perspectives and methodological issues in clinical assessment, in Assessment Issues in Child Neuropsychology. Edited by Tramontana MG, Hooper SR. New York, Plenum, 1988, pp 281–312

Johnson J: Cognitive abilities of children with language impairment, in Specific Language Impairments in Children. Edited by Watkins R, Rice M. Baltimore, MD, Paul H Brookes, 1994, pp 107–121

Johnson JP: Nature and Treatment of Articulation Disorders. Springfield, IL, Charles C Thomas, 1980

Kadesjo B, Gillberg C: Developmental coordination disorder in Swedish 7-year-old children. J Am Acad Child Adolesc Psychiatry 38:820–828, 1999

Kandel DB, Johnson JG, Bird HR, et al: Psychiatric comorbidity among adolescents with substance use disorders: findings from the MECA study. J Am Acad Child Adolesc Psychiatry 38:693–699, 1999

Karacostas DD, Fisher GL: Chemical dependency in students with and without learning disabilities. J Learn Disabil 26:213–219, 1993

Kaufman AS, Kaufman NL: K-ABC: Kaufman Assessment Battery for Children. Circle Pines, MN, American Guidance Service, 1983

Kaufman AS, Kaufman NL: Kaufman Test of Educational Achievement. Circle Pines, MN, American Guidance Service, 1985

Kavale KA, Forness SR: Social skill deficits and learning disabilities: a meta-analysis. J Learn Disabil 29:226–237, 1996

Kinsbourne M: School problems. Pediatrics 52:697–710, 1973

Klein RG, Mannuzza S: Children with uncomplicated reading disorders grown up: a prospective follow-up into adulthood, in Learning Disabilities: Implications for Psychiatric Treatment. Edited by Greenhill LL (Review of Psychiatry Series; Oldham JO and Riba MB, series eds.). Washington, DC, American Psychiatric Press, 2000, pp 1–31

Lai CSL, Fisher SE, Hurst JA, et al: A forkhead-domain gene is mutated in a severe speech and language disorder. Nature 413:519–523, 2001

Leonard LB: Children With Specific Language Impairment. Cambridge, MA, MIT Press, 1998

Lerner JW: Educational interventions in learning disabilities. J Am Acad Child Adolesc Psychiatry 28:326–331, 1989

Lewis BA: Pedigree analysis of children with phonology disorders. J Learn Disabil 25:586–597, 1992

Lewis BA, Thompson LA: A study of developmental speech and language disorders in twins. J Speech Hear Res 35:1086–1094, 1992

Light JG, Pennington BF, Gilger JW, et al: Reading disability and hyperactivity disorder; evidence for a common genetic etiology. Devel Neuropsychol 11:323–335, 1995

Loeb DF, Stoke C, Fey ME: Language changes associated with Fast ForWord-Language: evidence from case studies. Am J Speech-Lang Pathology 10:216–230, 2001

Love AJ, Thompson MGG: Language disorders and attention deficit disorders in young children referred for psychiatric services: analysis of prevalence and a conceptual synthesis. Am J Orthopsychiatry 58:52–64, 1988

Lovett MW: Developmental dyslexia, in Handbook of Neuropsychology, Vol 7. Edited by Segalowitz SJ, Rapin I. Amsterdam, Elsevier, 1992, pp 163–185

Lyon GR: Learning disabled readers: identification of subgroups, in Progress in Learning Disabilities. Edited by Myklebust HR. New York, Grune & Stratton, 1983

Markwardt FC: The Peabody Individual Achievement Test—Revised. Circle Pines, MN, American Guidance Service, 1989

McConaughy SH, Ritter DR: Social competence and behavioral problems of learning-disabled boys aged 6–11. J Learn Disabil 19:39–45, 1986

Merzenich MM, Jenkins WM, Johnston P, et al: Temporal processing deficits of language-learning impaired children ameliorated by training. Science 271:77–81, 1996

Moffitt TE: The neuropsychology of conduct disorder. Dev Psychopathol 5:135–151, 1995

Morgan WP: A case of congenital word-blindness. BMJ 2:1378, 1896

Morris RD: Classification of learning disabilities: old problems and new approaches. J Consult Clin Psychol 56:789–794, 1988

Morris R, Blashfield R, Satz P: Developmental classification of reading-disabled children. J Clin Exp Neuropsychol 8:371–392, 1986

National Institute on Deafness and Other Communication Disorders: NIDCD facts sheet: Stuttering. NIH Publication No. 97–4232. Bethesda, MD, 1997

National Joint Committee on Learning Disabilities: Operationalizing the NJCLD definition of learning disabilities for ongoing assessment in schools. February 1, 1997. Available at: http://www.ldonline.org/njcld/operationalizing.html. Accessed May 24, 2003

Newcomer P, Hammill DD: Test of Language Development P and I (TOLD-2P and TOLD-2I). Austin, TX, Pro-Ed, 1988

Nussbaum NL, Bigler ED, Koch W: Neuropsychologically derived subgroups of learning-disabled children: personality/behavioral dimensions. Journal of Research and Development in Education 19:57–67, 1986

Offord DR, Waters BG: Socialization and its failure, in Developmental-Behavioral Pediatrics. Edited by Levine MD, Carey WB, Crocker AC, et al. Philadelphia, PA, WB Saunders, 1983

Onslow M, Menzies RG, Packman A: An operant intervention for early stuttering: the development of the Lidcombe program. Behav Modif 25:116–139, 2001

Orton ST: Reading, Writing and Speech Problems in Children. New York, WW Norton, 1937

Osman B: Learning disabilities and the risk of psychiatric disorders in children and adolescents, in Learning Disabilities: Implications for Psychiatric Treatment. Edited by Greenhill L (Review of Psychiatry Series; Oldham JM and Riba MB, series eds.). Washington, DC, American Psychiatric Press, 2000, pp 33–58

Paul R: Language Disorders from Infancy Through Adolescence: Assessment and Intervention, 2nd Edition. St. Louis, MO, Mosby, 2001, pp 1–20, 62–115, 135, 140–147, 208–210

Pennington BF: Genetics of learning disabilities. J Child Neurol 10 (suppl 1): S69–S77, 1995

Phelps-Terasaki D, Phelps-Gunn T: Test of Pragmatic Language. Austin, TX, ProEd Inc, 1992

Psychological Corporation: Wechsler Individual Achievement Test (WIAT). San Antonio, TX, Harcourt Brace Jovanovich, 1992

Pugh KR, Shaywitz BA, Shaywitz SE, et al: Cerebral organization of component processes in reading. Brain 119:1221–1238, 1996

Pugh KR, Shaywitz BA, Shaywitz SE, et al: Predicting reading performance from neuroimaging profiles: the cerebral basis of phonological effects in printed word identification. J Exp Psychol Hum Percept Perform 23:299–318, 1997

Rapin I, Allen DA: Syndromes in developmental dysphasia and adult aphasia, in Language, Communication, and the Brain. Edited by Plum F. New York, Plenum, 1988, pp 57–75

Raven JC, Court JH, Raven J: Manual for Raven's Progressive Matrices. London, HK Lewis, 1976

Reitan RM, Wolfson D: The Halstead-Reitan Neuropsychological Test Battery. Tucson, AZ, Neuropsychology Press, 1985

Richardson SO: Developmental language disorder, in Comprehensive Textbook of Psychiatry, 5th Edition, Vol 2. Edited by Kaplan HI, Sadock BJ. Baltimore, MD, Williams & Wilkins, 1989, pp 1812–1817

Riggs PD, Whitmore EA: Substance use disorders and disruptive behavior disorders, in Disruptive Behavior Disorders in Children and Adolescents. Washington, DC, American Psychiatric Press, 1999, pp 133–173

Roid GH: Stanford-Binet Intelligence Scales, 5th Edition. Itasca, IL, Riverside Publishing, 2003

Roid GH, Miller L: The Leiter International Performance Scale—Revised. Wood Dale, IL, Stoelting, 1996

Rondal J: Language development and mental retardation, in Language Development and Disorders. Edited by Yule W, Rutter M. Philadelphia, PA, JB Lippincott, 1987

Rourke BP, Del Dotto JE: Learning disabilities: a neuropsychological perspective, in Handbook of Clinical Child Psychology, 3rd Edition. Edited by Walker CE, Roberts MC. New York, Wiley, 2001, pp 576–602

Rumsey JM, Berman KF, Denckla MB, et al: Regional cerebral blood flow in severe developmental dyslexia. Arch Neurol 44:1144–1150, 1987

Rutter M: Assessment objectives and principles, in Language Development and Disorders. Edited by Yule W, Rutter M. Philadelphia, PA, JB Lippincott, 1987, pp 295–311

Rutter M, Giller H: Juvenile Delinquency: Trends and Perspectives. New York, Penguin, 1983

Rutter M, Lord C: Language disorders associated with psychiatric disturbance, in Language Development and Disorders. Edited by Yule W, Rutter M. Philadelphia, PA, JB Lippincott, 1987

Schiefelbusch RL, Lloyd LL: Language Perspectives: Acquisition, Retardation and Intervention. Austin, TX, Pro-Ed, 1988

Schoenbrodt L, Kumin L, Sloan J: Learning disabilities existing concomitantly with communication disorder. J Learn Disabil 30:264–281, 1997

Semel E, Wiig EH, Secord WA: Clinical Evaluation of Language Fundamentals, 3rd Edition (CELF-3). San Antonio, TX, Psychological Corporation, 1995

Settle SA, Milich R: Social persistence following failure in boys and girls with LD. J Learn Disabil 32:201–212, 1999

Shapiro T: Adolescent language: its use for diagnosis, group identity, values, and treatment. Paper presented at the annual meeting of the American Society for Adolescent Psychiatry, Evanston, IL, March 1985

Shapiro J, Rich R: Facing learning disabilities in the adult years. New York, Oxford Press, 1999

Shaywitz BA, Shaywitz SE: Learning disabilities and attention disorders, in Pediatric Neurology, Vol 2. Edited by Swaimar KF. St. Louis, MO, CV Mosby, 1989

Shaywitz BA, Pugh KR, Fletcher JM, et al: What cognitive and neurobiological studies have taught us about dyslexia, in Learning Disabilities: Implications for Psychiatric Treatment. Edited by Greenhill L (Review of Psychiatry Series; Oldham JM and Riba MB, series eds.). Washington, DC, American Psychiatric Press, 2000, pp 59–96

Shaywitz SE, Shaywitz BA, Fletcher JM, et al: Prevalence of reading disability in boys and girls: results of the Connecticut Longitudinal Study. JAMA 264:998–1002, 1990

Shaywitz SE, Escobar MD, Shaywitz BA, et al: Evidence that dyslexia may represent the lower tail of a normal distribution of reading ability. N Engl J Med 326:145–150, 1992

Shaywitz SE, Fletcher JM, Shaywitz BA: A conceptual model and definition of dyslexia, findings emerging from the Connecticut Longitudinal Study, in Language, Learning, and Behavior Disorders: Developmental, Biological and Clinical Perspectives. Edited by Beitchman J, Cohen N, Konstantareas M, et al. New York, Cambridge University Press, 1996, pp 199–223

Sheehan JA: Social skills training with children and adolescents: an overview and guidelines. Unpublished doctoral dissertation, West Hartford, CT, University of Hartford, 2001 [Dissertation Abstracts International 62:2078, 2001]

Shepherd MJ, Uhry JK: Reading disorder. Child Adolesc Psychiatr Clin N Am 2:193–208, 1993

Shepherd MJ, Charnow DA, Silver LB: Developmental reading disorder, in Comprehensive Textbook of Psychiatry, 5th Edition, Vol 2. Edited by Kaplan HI, Sadock BJ. Baltimore, MD, Williams & Wilkins, 1989, pp 1790–1796

Silva PA: Epidemiology, longitudinal course and some associated factors: an update, in Language Development and Disorders. Edited by Yule W, Rutter M. Philadelphia, PA, JB Lippincott, 1987, pp 1–15

Silver AA, Hagin RA: Prevention of learning disorders, in Prevention of Mental Disorders, Alcohol and Other Drug Use in Children and Adolescents. Edited by Shaffer D, Silverman M, Anthony V. Washington, DC, Office of Substance Abuse Prevention (Monogr No 2), U.S. Department of Health and Human Services, 1989, pp 413–442

Silver LB: The "magic cure": a review of the current controversial approaches for treating learning disabilities. American Journal of the Disabled Child 140:1045–1052, 1986

Silver LB: Learning disabilities: introduction. J Am Acad Child Adolesc Psychiatry 28:309–313, 1989

Simos PG, Breier JI, Wheless JW, et al: Brain mechanisms for reading: the role of the superior temporal gyrus in word and pseudoword naming. Neuroreport 11:2443–2447, 2000

Simos PG, Breier JI, Fletcher JM, et al: Age-related changes in regional brain activation during phonological decoding and printed word recognition. Dev Neuropsychol 19:191–210, 2001

Sparrow SS, Balla DA, Cicchetti DV: Vineland Adaptive Behavior Scales. Circle Pines, MN, American Guidance Service, 1984

Stevenson J: Developmental changes in the mechanisms linking language disabilities and behavior disorders, in Language, Learning, and Behavior Disorders: Developmental, Biological, and Clinical Perspectives. Edited by Beitchman JH, Cohen NJ, Konstantareas MM, et al. New York, Cambridge University Press, 1996, pp 78–99

Stevenson J, Richman N: Behavior, language and development in three-year-old children. Journal of Autism and Childhood Schizophrenia 8:299–313, 1978

Stevenson J, Richman N, Graham P: Behavior problems and language abilities at three years and behavioral deviance at eight years. J Child Psychol Psychiatry 26:215–230, 1985

Stevenson J, Pennington BF, Gilger JW, et al: Hyperactivity and spelling disability: testing for shared genetic aetiology. J Child Psychol Psychiat 34:1137–1152, 1993

Sugden DA, Wright HC: Motor coordination disorders in children, in Developmental Clinical Psychology and Psychiatry, Vol 39. Thousand Oaks, CA, Sage Publications, 1998

Sullivan NA: Educational implications of surviving acute lymphoblastic leukemia and its treatment regimes: perspectives and reflections of long-term survivors. Unpublished doctoral dissertation, Pittsburgh, PA, University of Pittsburgh, 1995 [Dissertation Abstracts International 56:1737, 1995]

Tallal P: The science of literacy: From the laboratory to the classroom. Proc Natl Acad Sci USA 97:2402–2404, 2000

Tallal P, Miller SL, Bedi G, et al: Language comprehension in language-learning impaired children improved with acoustically modified speech. Science 271:81–84, 1996

Tannock R: Language, reading, and motor control problems in ADHD: a potential behavioral phenotype, in Learning Disabilities: Implications for Psychiatric Treatment. Edited by Greenhill L (Review of Psychiatry Series; Oldham JM and Riba MB, series eds.). Washington, DC, American Psychiatric Press, 2000, pp 129–168

Thibodeau LM, Friel-Patti S, Britt L: Psychoacoustic performance in children completing Fast ForWord training. Am J Speech-Lang Pathology 10:248–257, 2001

Tomblin JB, Buckwalter PR: Studies of the genetics of specific language impairment, in Specific Language Impairments in Children. Edited by Watkins R, Rice M. Baltimore, MD, Paul H Brookes, 1994, pp 7–34

Toppelberg CO, Shapiro T: Language disorders: a 10-year research update review. J Am Acad Child Adolesc Psychiatry 39:143–152, 2000

Torgesen JK: The learning disabled child as an inactive learner: educational implications. Topics in Learning Disabilities 2:45–52, 1982

Torgesen JK: Variations on theory in learning disabilities, in Better Understanding Learning Disabilities: New Views From Research and Their Implications for Education and Public Policies. Edited by Lyon GR, Gray DB, Kavanagh JF, et al. Baltimore, MD, Paul H. Brooks, 1993

U.S. Congress: Public Law 94–142, "Education for All Handicapped Children Act of 1975." Washington, DC, U.S. Government Printing Office, 1975

U.S. Congress: Amendments to the Individuals with Disabilities Education Act. Washington, DC, U.S. Government Printing Office, 1997

U.S. Department of Education: Seventeenth Annual Report to Congress on the Implementation of the Individuals With Disabilities Education Act. Washington, DC, U.S. Office of Special Education Programs, 1995

Waber D: Learning disabilities in children with cancer. Paper presented at educators' symposium, Dana Farber Cancer Institute, Boston, MA, 1989

Wagner R, Torgesen J, Rashotte C: Comprehensive Test of Phonological Processing (CTOPP). Austin, TX, ProEd, 1999

Wallace G, Hammill DD: Comprehensive Receptive and Expressive Vocabulary Test. Austin, TX, ProEd, 1994

Watson BU, Watson CS, Fredd R: Follow-up studies of specific reading disability. J Am Acad Child Psychiatry 21:376–382, 1982

Wechsler D: Wechsler Intelligence Scale for Children—Third Edition. San Antonio, TX, Psychological Corporation, 1991

Wechsler D: Wechsler Preschool and Primary Scale of Intelligence—3rd Edition. San Antonio, TX, Psychological Corporation, 2002

Weinberg WA, Gallagher LS, Harper CR, et al: The impact of school on academic achievement. Child Adolesc Psychiatr Clin N Am 6:593–606, 1999

Wenar C, Kerig P: Developmental Psychopathology: From Infancy Through Adolescence, 4th Edition. Boston, MA, McGraw-Hill, 2000, pp 131–141

Wetherby AM, Prizant BM: Communication and Symbolic Behavior Scales. Itasca, IL, Riverside Publishing, 1993

Wetherby AM, Prizant BM: Speech, language, and communication disorders in young children, in Handbook of Child and Adolescent Psychiatry, Vol 1: Infants and Preschoolers: Development and Syndromes. Edited by Greenspan S, Wieder S, Osofsky J (Noshpitz JD, editor-in-chief). New York, Wiley, 1997, pp 473–491

Wiig EH, Secord WA: Test of Language Competence—Expanded Edition. San Antonio, TX, Psychological Corporation, 1989

Wiig EH, Secord WA, Semel E: Clinical Evaluation of Language Fundamentals—Preschool. San Antonio, TX, Psychological Corporation, 1992

Wilkinson GS: Wide Range Achievement Test, 3rd Edition. Wilmington, DE, Jastak Associates, 1993

Woodcock RW, McGrew KS, Mather N: Woodcock-Johnson III Tests of Achievement. Itasca, IL, Riverside Publishing, 2001

Woods S, Shearsby J, Onslow M, et al: Psychological impact of the Lidcombe Program of early stuttering intervention. Int J Lang Commun Disord 37:31–40, 2002

Zangwill OL: The concept of developmental dysphasia, in Developmental Dysphasia. Edited by Wyke MA. London, Academic Press, 1987

Zeitlin H: Psychiatric comorbidity with substance misuse in children and teenagers. Drug Alcohol Depend 55:225–234, 1999

Zigmond N: Learning disabilities from an educational perspective, in Better Understanding Learning Disabilities: New Views from Research and Their Implications for Education and Public Policies. Edited by Lyon GR, Gray DB, Kavanagh JF, et al. Baltimore, MD, Paul H Brookes, 1993, pp 251–272

Zimmerman IL, Steiner VG, Pond RE: Preschool Language Scale—3rd Edition. San Antonio, TX, Psychological Corporation, 1992

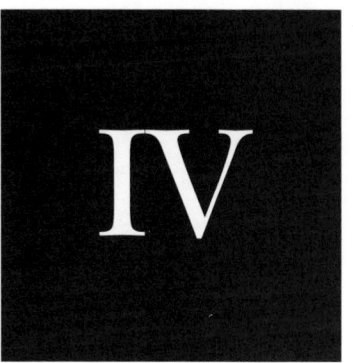

Schizophrenia, Other Psychotic Disorders, and Mood Disorders

Schizophrenia and Other Psychotic Disorders

Luke Y. Tsai, M.D.
Donna J. Champine, M.D.

Historical Background

The term *schizophrenic syndrome of childhood* (or its synonym *childhood schizophrenia*) has a different meaning from the term *schizophrenia in childhood*. The former term, proposed by the British Working Party (Creak et al. 1961) and later adopted in DSM-II (American Psychiatric Association 1968), was intended to apply to a wide spectrum of patients, including those with autism, schizophrenia, disintegrative psychosis, and other childhood psychoses. Thus, it is clear that data derived from studies (mostly conducted before 1980) that used the diagnostic criteria for childhood schizophrenia are not very meaningful because they failed to make any distinction between autism and schizophrenia in childhood and because they had methodological flaws (e.g., standardized, well-defined diagnostic criteria were not used, and diagnostic criteria used for children were less restrictive than those applied to adult schizophrenic patients).

In DSM-III (American Psychiatric Association 1980) the term *schizophrenia in childhood and adolescence* was introduced to apply to children and adolescents in whom clear schizophrenic symptoms, as found in adult schizophrenia, are present.

For the purposes of this chapter, the definition and diagnostic criteria for schizophrenia in childhood are the same as those described in DSM-IV-TR (American Psychiatric Association 2000) for adult schizophrenia. There are at least three good reasons to use the adult criteria. First, there is now convincing evidence supporting the view that infantile autism and schizophre-

nia in childhood are two distinct disorders. Second, it is clear that schizophrenia, as described in the adult literature, can begin in childhood. Third, according to DSM-IV-TR, children and adolescents display the same symptoms as do adults diagnosed with schizophrenia.

Current Diagnostic Criteria for Schizophrenia

The diagnosis of schizophrenia in children and adolescents is currently made by using the criteria outlined in DSM-IV-TR (Table 23–1). According to DSM-IV-TR, the active phase of the illness is characterized by the presence of at least two of the following symptoms, each present for a significant portion of time during a 1-month period: 1) delusions, 2) hallucinations, 3) disorganized speech, 4) grossly disorganized or catatonic behavior, and 5) negative symptoms (e.g., affective flattening, alogia, avolition). Only one symptom is needed, however, if the delusions are bizarre or if the hallucinations involve either a voice giving a running commentary on the person's behavior or thinking or two or more voices conversing. If treatment results in a resolution of the symptoms, then the duration of acute-phase symptoms can be less than 1 month.

In addition to the symptoms described above, there must also be a marked deterioration in social or occupational functioning present for a significant amount of time since the onset of the disturbance. This requirement is modified in child and adolescent schizophrenia, for which the criterion is "failure to achieve expected level of interpersonal, academic, or occupational achievement" (American Psychiatric Association 2000, p. 312).

Also included in DSM-IV-TR is the requirement that signs of the disturbance be present for at least 6 months, with at least 1 month of active-phase symptoms (fewer if successfully treated). The 6-month duration may include periods of prodromal or residual symptoms.

In making a diagnosis of schizophrenia, mood disorders and schizoaffective disorders must be ruled out. Because adolescents with bipolar disorder often present at onset with manic episodes with psychosis, this distinction becomes especially important in making a diagnosis in adolescents (American Academy of Child and Adolescent Psychiatry 2001; Carlson 1990; McClellan et al. 1993; McGlashan 1988; Werry et al. 1991). Psychosis due to a general medical condition, medication, or illicit drug use should also be ruled out.

Diagnostic Criteria for Other Psychotic Disorders

DSM-IV-TR diagnostic criteria for the other psychotic disorders, including schizophreniform disorder, schizoaffective disorder, delusional disorder, brief psychotic disorder, shared psychotic disorder, psychotic disorder due to a general medical condition, substance-induced psychotic disorder, and psychotic disorder not otherwise specified, are listed in Tables 23–2 to 23–9. These disorders are discussed below under "Differential Diagnosis."

Epidemiology

■ Prevalence

The true incidence of schizophrenia in childhood is unknown. Karno and Norquist (1989) suggested that the prevalence of schizophrenia with onset in childhood was 50 times less than that of schizophrenia with onset in adulthood. Population studies have suggested that the prevalence may be less than 1 in 1,000 (reviewed by Werry 1979). Makita (1966) found that only 3 of the 32 schizophrenia patients in his study had onset before age 13 (2 at age 10 and 1 at 11). Kydd and

Werry (1982) reviewed schizophrenic children admitted as inpatients to a child psychiatric unit in Auckland, New Zealand. They found only 15 cases over a period of 10 years. (The at-risk population served by the unit was approximately 130,000.) Similar findings have been reported by Loranger's (1984) study of the age at first treatment of 100 males and 100 females with a DSM-III diagnosis of schizophrenia. Loranger found that 18% of male and 11% of female schizophrenia patients were first treated before age 15 years. In a study of prevalence in children between ages 2 and 12 in North Dakota (population 110,723 at time of the study), no patients with schizophrenia were found. However, within the next year, 2 of the children were reevaluated by the investigators and met DSM-III criteria for schizophrenia. Thus, point prevalence in North Dakota was 0.19 in 10,000 for this age group (Burd and Kerbeshian 1987). In the study in Dunedin, New Zealand (a prospective longitudinal study in which each subject was evaluated with a variety of measures, including the Diagnostic Interview Schedule for Children), no cases of schizophrenia were reported in a sample of 792 children (Anderson et al. 1987).

■ Sex Ratio

Kydd and Werry (1982) noted a nearly equal sex ratio (8 boys and 7 girls), and Eggers (1978) found a slight female preponderance (25 boys and 32 girls) in their respective samples. Green and Padron-Gayol (1986) reported a male-to-female ratio of 4.3:1 in a sample of 16 schizophrenic children. Spencer and Campbell (1994) noted a male-to-female ratio of 3.8:1 in a sample of 24 children.

It appears that age may determine the sex ratio in schizophrenia occurring in childhood. Although most studies have shown a higher male-to-female ratio, as age increases, the ratio tends to even out. Adult studies have suggested that the onset of schizophrenia is 5 years earlier in males than in females (American Academy of Child and Adolescent Psychiatry 2001; Loranger 1984). Therefore the reported male predominance in early-onset schizophrenia may be a cross-sectional effect (American Academy of Child and Adolescent Psychiatry 2001).

■ Socioeconomic Status

Although Kydd and Werry (1982) found that the social class distribution of the families of schizophrenic chil-

Table 23–1. DSM-IV-TR diagnostic criteria for schizophrenia

A. *Characteristic symptoms:* Two (or more) of the following, each present for a significant portion of time during a 1-month period (or less if successfully treated):

    (1) delusions

    (2) hallucinations

    (3) disorganized speech (e.g., frequent derailment or incoherence)

    (4) grossly disorganized or catatonic behavior

    (5) negative symptoms, i.e., affective flattening, alogia, or avolition

    Note: Only one Criterion A symptom is required if delusions are bizarre or hallucinations consist of a voice keeping up a running commentary on the person's behavior or thoughts, or two or more voices conversing with each other.

B. *Social/occupational dysfunction:* For a significant portion of the time since the onset of the disturbance, one or more major areas of functioning such as work, interpersonal relations, or self-care are markedly below the level achieved prior to the onset (or when the onset is in childhood or adolescence, failure to achieve expected level of interpersonal, academic, or occupational achievement).

C. *Duration:* Continuous signs of the disturbance persist for at least 6 months. This 6-month period must include at least 1 month of symptoms (or less if successfully treated) that meet Criterion A (i.e., active-phase symptoms) and may include periods of prodromal or residual symptoms. During these prodromal or residual periods, the signs of the disturbance may be manifested by only negative symptoms or two or more symptoms listed in Criterion A present in an attenuated form (e.g., odd beliefs, unusual perceptual experiences).

D. *Schizoaffective and mood disorder exclusion:* Schizoaffective disorder and mood disorder with psychotic features have been ruled out because either (1) no major depressive, manic, or mixed episodes have occurred concurrently with the active-phase symptoms; or (2) if mood episodes have occurred during active-phase symptoms, their total duration has been brief relative to the duration of the active and residual periods.

E. *Substance/general medical condition exclusion:* The disturbance is not due to the direct physiological effects of a substance (e.g., a drug of abuse, a medication) or a general medical condition.

F. *Relationship to a pervasive developmental disorder:* If there is a history of autistic disorder or another pervasive developmental disorder, the additional diagnosis of schizophrenia is made only if prominent delusions or hallucinations are also present for at least a month (or less if successfully treated).

Classification of longitudinal course (can be applied only after at least 1 year has elapsed since the initial onset of active-phase symptoms):

    Episodic With Interepisode Residual Symptoms (episodes are defined by the reemergence of prominent psychotic symptoms); *also specify if:* **With Prominent Negative Symptoms**

    Episodic With No Interepisode Residual Symptoms

    Continuous (prominent psychotic symptoms are present throughout the period of observation); *also specify if:* **With Prominent Negative Symptoms**

    Single Episode In Partial Remission; *also specify if:* **With Prominent Negative Symptoms**

    Single Episode In Full Remission

    Other or Unspecified Pattern

Source. From American Psychiatric Association: *Diagnostic and Statistical Manual of Mental Disorders,* 4th Edition, Text Revision. Washington, DC, American Psychiatric Association, 2000. Copyright 2000, American Psychiatric Association. Used with permission.

dren resembles that of the base population, schizophrenic children probably tend to come from families of lower social class, just as adults with schizophrenia do (Green et al. 1984; Kolvin et al. 1971b; Rutter 1972). An exception to these findings is a study by Russell and associates (1989), in which 54% of the subjects came from families in the top two categories of socioeconomic status (Hollingshead 1965). However, most available studies have a selection bias toward inpatient samples (American Academy of Child and Adolescent Psychiatry 2001).

■ **Premorbid Functioning**

Many studies have reported that the majority of patients with childhood-onset schizophrenia have premorbid abnormalities. A variety of general, nonspecific behavioral symptoms, social problems, cognitive

Table 23–2. DSM-IV-TR diagnostic criteria for schizophreniform disorder

A. Criteria A, D, and E of schizophrenia are met.
B. An episode of the disorder (including prodromal, active, and residual phases) lasts at least 1 month but less than 6 months. (When the diagnosis must be made without waiting for recovery, it should be qualified as "Provisional.")

Specify if:

Without Good Prognostic Features
With Good Prognostic Features: as evidenced by two (or more) of the following:

(1) onset of prominent psychotic symptoms within 4 weeks of the first noticeable change in usual behavior or functioning
(2) confusion or perplexity at the height of the psychotic episode
(3) good premorbid social and occupational functioning
(4) absence of blunted or flat affect

Source. From American Psychiatric Association: *Diagnostic and Statistical Manual of Mental Disorders*, 4th Edition, Text Revision. Washington, DC, American Psychiatric Association, 2000. Copyright 2000, American Psychiatric Association. Used with permission.

Table 23–3. DSM-IV-TR diagnostic criteria for schizoaffective disorder

A. An uninterrupted period of illness during which, at some time, there is either a major depressive episode, a manic episode, or a mixed episode concurrent with symptoms that meet Criterion A for Schizophrenia.

Note: The major depressive episode must include Criterion A1: depressed mood.

B. During the same period of illness, there have been delusions or hallucinations for at least 2 weeks in the absence of prominent mood symptoms.
C. Symptoms that meet criteria for a mood episode are present for a substantial portion of the total duration of the active and residual periods of the illness.
D. The disturbance is not due to the direct physiological effects of a substance (e.g., a drug of abuse, a medication) or a general medical condition.

Specify type:

Bipolar Type: if the disturbance includes a manic or a mixed episode (or a manic or a mixed episode and major depressive episodes)
Depressive Type: if the disturbance only includes major depressive episodes

Source. From American Psychiatric Association: *Diagnostic and Statistical Manual of Mental Disorders*, 4th Edition, Text Revision. Washington, DC, American Psychiatric Association, 2000. Copyright 2000, American Psychiatric Association. Used with permission.

and academic difficulties, speech and language problems, developmental delays, and specific diagnoses of other mental disorders before the onset of schizophrenia have been described (Alaghband-Rad et al. 1995; Asarnow and Ben-Meir 1988; Eggers 1978; Green and Padron-Gayol 1986; Kolvin 1971a; McClellan and McCurry 1999; Mednick and Schulsinger 1968; Offord and Cross 1969; Parnas et al. 1982; Spencer and Campbell 1994; Watkins et al. 1988; Werry et al. 1991).

A significant number of children who meet criteria for adult schizophrenia receive a diagnosis of pervasive developmental disorder, particularly autistic disorder, at preschool age (Cantor et al. 1982; Petty et al. 1984; Watkins et al. 1988). However, some investigators have disagreed with this conclusion (Green et al. 1984; Volkmar et al. 1988). Even though in a great percentage of patients schizophrenia can be preceded by a variety of developmental delays and symptoms, these symptoms usually do not meet DSM-IV-TR criteria for autism.

Clinical and neurobiological characterization of children with childhood-onset schizophrenia is ongoing at the National Institute of Mental Health (NIMH) (Alaghband-Rad et al. 1995; Frazier et al. 1994; Gordon et al. 1994; McKenna et al. 1994a, 1994b). Alagh-

band-Rad et al. (1995) reviewed premorbid histories of 23 children with onset of schizophrenia before age 12 (all of whom met DSM-III criteria) and compared the results with childhood data of subjects with adult-onset schizophrenia. Specific developmental disabilities and transient early symptoms of autism, especially motor stereotypies, were common. Compared with childhood characteristics of subjects with adult-onset schizophrenia, the subjects with childhood onset showed greater delay in language development, more premorbid speech and language disorders, disruptive behavior disorders, and learning disorders. Although they acknowledged the selection and ascertainment bias present in their sample, the authors concluded that childhood-onset schizophrenia might represent a more malignant form of the disorder.

■ Age at Onset

It long has been known that schizophrenia seldom becomes apparent in children before age 9 years

Table 23–4. DSM-IV-TR diagnostic criteria for delusional disorder

A. Nonbizarre delusions (i.e., involving situations that occur in real life, such as being followed, poisoned, infected, loved at a distance, or deceived by spouse or lover, or having a disease) of at least 1 month's duration.

B. Criterion A for schizophrenia has never been met. **Note:** Tactile and olfactory hallucinations may be present in delusional disorder if they are related to the delusional theme.

C. Apart from the impact of the delusion(s) or its ramifications, functioning is not markedly impaired and behavior is not obviously odd or bizarre.

D. If mood episodes have occurred concurrently with delusions, their total duration has been brief relative to the duration of the delusional periods.

E. The disturbance is not due to the direct physiological effects of a substance (e.g., a drug of abuse, a medication) or a general medical condition.

Specify type (the following types are assigned based on the predominant delusional theme):

    Erotomanic Type: delusions that another person, usually of higher status, is in love with the individual

    Grandiose Type: delusions of inflated worth, power, knowledge, identity, or special relationship to a deity or famous person

    Jealous Type: delusions that the individual's sexual partner is unfaithful

    Persecutory Type: delusions that the person (or someone to whom the person is close) is being malevolently treated in some way

    Somatic Type: delusions that the person has some physical defect or general medical condition

    Mixed Type: delusions characteristic of more than one of the above types but no one theme predominates

    Unspecified Type

Source. From American Psychiatric Association: *Diagnostic and Statistical Manual of Mental Disorders*, 4th Edition, Text Revision. Washington, DC, American Psychiatric Association, 2000. Copyright 2000, American Psychiatric Association. Used with permission.

Table 23–5. DSM-IV-TR diagnostic criteria for brief psychotic disorder

A. Presence of one (or more) of the following symptoms:

    (1) delusions

    (2) hallucinations

    (3) disorganized speech (e.g., frequent derailment or incoherence)

    (4) grossly disorganized or catatonic behavior

    Note: Do not include a symptom if it is a culturally sanctioned response pattern.

B. Duration of an episode of the disturbance is at least 1 day but less than 1 month, with eventual full return to premorbid level of functioning.

C. The disturbance is not better accounted for by a mood disorder with psychotic features, schizoaffective disorder, or schizophrenia and is not due to the direct physiological effects of a substance (e.g., a drug of abuse, a medication) or a general medical condition.

Specify if:

    With Marked Stressor(s) (brief reactive psychosis): if symptoms occur shortly after and apparently in response to events that, singly or together, would be markedly stressful to almost anyone in similar circumstances in the person's culture

    Without Marked Stressor(s): if psychotic symptoms do *not* occur shortly after, or are not apparently in response to events that, singly or together, would be markedly stressful to almost anyone in similar circumstances in the person's culture

    With Postpartum Onset: if onset within 4 weeks postpartum

Source. From American Psychiatric Association: *Diagnostic and Statistical Manual of Mental Disorders*, 4th Edition, Text Revision. Washington, DC, American Psychiatric Association, 2000. Copyright 2000, American Psychiatric Association. Used with permission.

Table 23–6. DSM-IV-TR diagnostic criteria for shared psychotic disorder

A. A delusion develops in an individual in the context of a close relationship with another person(s), who has an already-established delusion.

B. The delusion is similar in content to that of the person who already has the established delusion.

C. The disturbance is not better accounted for by another psychotic disorder (e.g., schizophrenia) or a mood disorder with psychotic features and is not due to the direct physiological effects of a substance (e.g., a drug of abuse, a medication) or a general medical condition.

Source. From American Psychiatric Association: *Diagnostic and Statistical Manual of Mental Disorders,* 4th Edition, Text Revision. Washington, DC, American Psychiatric Association, 2000. Copyright 2000, American Psychiatric Association. Used with permission.

Table 23–7. DSM-IV-TR diagnostic criteria for psychotic disorder due to a general medical condition

A. Prominent hallucinations or delusions.

B. There is evidence from the history, physical examination, or laboratory findings that the disturbance is the direct physiological consequence of a general medical condition.

C. The disturbance is not better accounted for by another mental disorder.

D. The disturbance does not occur exclusively during the course of a delirium.

Code based on predominant symptom:

.81 **With Delusions:** if delusions are the predominant symptom

.82 **With Hallucinations:** if hallucinations are the predominant symptom

Coding note: Include the name of the general medical condition on Axis I, e.g., 293.81 psychotic disorder due to malignant lung neoplasm, with delusions; also code the general medical condition on Axis III (see DSM-IV-TR Appendix G for codes).

Coding note: If delusions are part of vascular dementia, indicate the delusions by coding the appropriate subtype, e.g., 290.42 vascular dementia, with delusions.

Source. From American Psychiatric Association: *Diagnostic and Statistical Manual of Mental Disorders,* 4th Edition, Text Revision. Washington, DC, American Psychiatric Association, 2000. Copyright 2000, American Psychiatric Association. Used with permission.

(E. Bleuler 1950; Green et al. 1984; Kraepelin 1899/ 1919; Makita 1966; Russell et al. 1989; Thomsen 1996). Green and Padron-Gayol (1986) reported that the youngest schizophrenic child admitted to a large municipal acute-care hospital during an 8-year period was age 5.7 years. In another sample of 35 schizophrenic children (Russell et al. 1989), a 4.9-year-old was the youngest child diagnosed with schizophrenia, whereas the earliest age of symptom onset was reported to be 3 years. In a study of 312 youths in Denmark who were hospitalized for schizophrenia over a 13-year period, Thomsen (1996) found only 28 children younger than age 15 and only 4 children younger than age 13.

Adult literature on schizophrenia suggests that the average age at onset in males is 5 years earlier than in females. Loranger (1984) examined consecutive discharges from a hospital (100 adult men and 100 adult women) to determine if men had an earlier age at onset than women. Records were examined to determine age at first treatment, age at first hospitalization, and age at first psychotic symptoms (by family's report). It was found that 39% of the men had their first psychotic symptoms by age 19, whereas 23% of women had their first psychotic symptoms by age 19. However, in a follow-up study of childhood-onset schizophrenia, Eggers and Bunk (1997) did not find an earlier age at onset for males among prepubertal patients.

■ Type of Onset

The onset of the condition in childhood-onset schizophrenia is usually insidious, with acute onset observed in perhaps 25% of cases (Werry 1992). In a sample of 24 children younger than 12 years, 23 had insidious onset of schizophrenia, whereas only 1 had subacute onset (Spencer et al. 1994). Of 33 patients studied by Kolvin (1971b), 22 had insidious onset, 7 had insidious onset with acute exacerbation, and 4 had acute onset of schizophrenia. Of 17 hospitalized schizophrenic subjects, ages 7–13 years, studied by Asarnow and Ben-Meir (1988), 8 had insidious onset, 8 had chronic onset, and 1 had acute onset. Gordon et al. (1994) reported similar figures. Thus, acute mode of onset is relatively rare in childhood. In a study of 29 children and adolescents who met DSM-III criteria for schizophrenia with onset before age 12, Alaghband-Rad et al. (1997) found that males were more likely to have had an insidious onset than females.

Table 23–8. DSM-IV-TR diagnostic criteria for substance-induced psychotic disorder

A. Prominent hallucinations or delusions. **Note:** Do not include hallucinations if the person has insight that they are substance induced.

B. There is evidence from the history, physical examination, or laboratory findings of either (1) or (2):
  (1) the symptoms in Criterion A developed during, or within a month of, substance intoxication or withdrawal
  (2) medication use is etiologically related to the disturbance

C. The disturbance is not better accounted for by a psychotic disorder that is not substance induced. Evidence that the symptoms are better accounted for by a psychotic disorder that is not substance induced might include the following: the symptoms precede the onset of the substance use (or medication use); the symptoms persist for a substantial period of time (e.g., about a month) after the cessation of acute withdrawal or severe intoxication, or are substantially in excess of what would be expected given the type or amount of the substance used or the duration of use; or there is other evidence that suggests the existence of an independent non-substance-induced psychotic disorder (e.g., a history of recurrent non-substance-related episodes).

D. The disturbance does not occur exclusively during the course of a delirium.

Note: This diagnosis should be made instead of a diagnosis of substance intoxication or substance withdrawal only when the symptoms are in excess of those usually associated with the intoxication or withdrawal syndrome and when the symptoms are sufficiently severe to warrant independent clinical attention.

Code [specific substance]–induced psychotic disorder:

(291.5 alcohol, with delusions; 291.3 alcohol, with hallucinations; 292.11 amphetamine [or amphetamine-like substance], with delusions; 292.12 amphetamine [or amphetamine-like substance], with hallucinations; 292.11 cannabis, with delusions; 292.12 cannabis, with hallucinations; 292.11 cocaine, with delusions; 292.12 cocaine, with hallucinations; 292.11 hallucinogen, with delusions; 292.12 hallucinogen, with hallucinations; 292.11 inhalant, with delusions; 292.12 inhalant, with hallucinations; 292.11 opioid, with delusions; 292.12 opioid, with hallucinations; 292.11 phencyclidine [or phencyclidine-like substance], with delusions; 292.12 phencyclidine [or phencyclidine-like substance], with hallucinations; 292.11 sedative, hypnotic, or anxiolytic, with delusions; 292.12 sedative, hypnotic, or anxiolytic, with hallucinations; 292.11 other [or unknown] substance, with delusions; 292.12 other [or unknown] substance, with hallucinations)

Specify if:

  With Onset During Intoxication: if criteria are met for intoxication with the substance and the symptoms develop during the intoxication syndrome
  With Onset During Withdrawal: if criteria are met for withdrawal from the substance and the symptoms develop during, or shortly after, a withdrawal syndrome

Source. From American Psychiatric Association: *Diagnostic and Statistical Manual of Mental Disorders*, 4th Edition, Text Revision. Washington, DC, American Psychiatric Association, 2000. Copyright 2000, American Psychiatric Association. Used with permission.

■ Deterioration in Functioning

For adults, one of the DSM-IV-TR diagnostic criteria for schizophrenia is marked deterioration in functioning in the areas of work, social relationships, and self-care (see Table 23–1). However, the equivalent criterion for children and adolescents is failure to reach the expected level of interpersonal, academic, or social achievement. Russell et al. (1989) reported that all 35 subjects with schizophrenia in their sample (ages 4–13 years) exhibited a marked deterioration from a previous level of functioning, which was verified by parents: the child either required psychiatric hospitalization or showed severe deterioration in behavior in school. Green et al. (1984) reported a clear-cut deterioration

in behavior with the onset of schizophrenia in all 24 of their subjects. All children in the study by Spencer et al. (1994) were inpatients who had required psychiatric hospitalization because of the severity of their presenting complaints.

Clinical Symptoms

A review of studies of the phenomenology of psychotic illnesses in children and adolescents reveals that for both childhood-onset and adolescent-onset schizophrenia, the same symptoms that have been noted in adults are present. Schizophrenia has been described

---

Table 23–9. DSM-IV-TR diagnostic criteria for psychotic disorder not otherwise specified

---

This category includes psychotic symptomatology (i.e., delusions, hallucinations, disorganized speech, grossly disorganized or catatonic behavior) about which there is inadequate information to make a specific diagnosis or about which there is contradictory information, or disorders with psychotic symptoms that do not meet the criteria for any specific Psychotic Disorder.

Examples include

1. Postpartum psychosis that does not meet criteria for mood disorder with psychotic features, brief psychotic disorder, psychotic disorder due to a general medical condition, or substance-induced psychotic disorder
2. Psychotic symptoms that have lasted for less than 1 month but that have not yet remitted, so that the criteria for brief psychotic disorder are not met
3. Persistent auditory hallucinations in the absence of any other features
4. Persistent nonbizarre delusions with periods of overlapping mood episodes that have been present for a substantial portion of the delusional disturbance
5. Situations in which the clinician has concluded that a psychotic disorder is present, but is unable to determine whether it is primary, due to a general medical condition, or substance induced

---

Source. From American Psychiatric Association: *Diagnostic and Statistical Manual of Mental Disorders*, 4th Edition, Text Revision. Washington, DC, American Psychiatric Association, 2000. Copyright 2000, American Psychiatric Association. Used with permission.

---

as having two broad sets of symptom clusters, positive and negative, both of which also are described in children and adolescents. Positive symptoms include hallucinations, delusions, and thought disorder. Negative symptoms are deficit symptoms, such as flattened affect, amotivation, and alogia (American Psychiatric Association 1997).

■ Hallucinations

Hallucinations are the most frequently reported positive symptoms. Russell et al. (1989) reported that auditory hallucinations were present in about 80% of patients. Other investigators reported hallucinations in up to 100% of children with schizophrenia who were age 13 years or younger (Spencer and Campbell 1994; Spencer et al. 1994). Visual hallucinations were reported in between 30.3% (Kolvin et al. 1971a) and 50% (Green and Padron-Gayol 1986) of patients and were usually accompanied by auditory hallucinations. A small percentage of children with schizophrenia reported tactile hallucinations (Green and Padron-Gayol 1986; Green et al. 1984; Russell et al. 1989; Spencer and Campbell 1994; Spencer et al. 1994).

■ Delusions

Werry et al. (1991, 1994) and Russell (1994) reported that children with schizophrenia had fewer delusions than did adults with schizophrenia. Other studies reported frequencies of delusions ranging from 43.8%

(Green and Padron-Gayol 1986) to 100% (Spencer and Campbell 1994; Spencer et al. 1994). Although the types of delusions were not always specified, Russell et al. (1989) found that persecutory and somatic delusions were most common (about 20% each), whereas thought control and religious delusions were rare (3%) in children ages 4–13 years. Russell et al. (1989) noted that the delusions of older children were more complex than those of younger children.

■ Affective Disturbances

Werry et al. (1991) and Watkins et al. (1988) reported that affective disturbance was common in children with schizophrenia. Affective disturbance was also reported by Green et al. (1984) in 83.3%, by Russell et al. (1989) in 74%, by Volkmar et al. (1988) in 70.7%, and by Spencer et al. (1994) in 87.5% of children with schizophrenia. Flattened affect, a negative symptom, has also been consistently reported in early-onset schizophrenia, although catatonic symptoms may be less frequent (Green et al. 1992; Russell et al. 1989; Werry 1992).

■ Thought Disorder

Thought disorder has been reported to be present in between 40% (Russell et al. 1989) and 100% (Green et al. 1984; Watkins et al. 1988) of children with schizophrenia under age 13. Various investigators (Arboleda and Holzman 1985; Caplan 1994b; Caplan et al. 1989) have discussed problems of assessing thought disorder in children. Caplan and associates (1989, 1990) developed the Kiddie Formal Thought Disorder Rating Scale, an instrument that operationalized the four DSM-III criteria of formal thought disorder (illogical thinking, loose associations, incoherence, and poverty of content of speech) for use with children. Two of the measures, illogical thinking and loose associations, were reliable in differentiating 14 schizophrenic and 3 schizotypal children from 15 psychiatrically healthy children matched by gender and mental age (Caplan et al. 1989). In a later study, Caplan et al. (1992) showed that compared with psychiatrically healthy children, children with schizophrenia used fewer linguistic cohesive devices to connect ideas within and across sentences. Poverty of content of speech, however, was not noted in children with early-onset schizophrenia, either in the studies cited above or in a subsequent study (Caplan et al. 2000), and therefore this does not appear to be a formal thought-disorder sign characteristic of childhood schizophrenia. More recently, Caplan et al. (2001) compared thought disorder and associated cognitive variables in 115 children with attention-deficit/hyperactivity disorder (ADHD), 88 children with schizophrenia, and 190 psychiatrically healthy children. Compared with the healthy children, the subjects in both the ADHD and the schizophrenic groups exhibited thought disorder, although the subjects with ADHD had a narrower range of less severe thought disorder than did the schizophrenic children. The authors concluded that thought disorder in childhood was not specific to schizophrenia and reflected impaired development of communication skills.

■ Cognitive Functioning

Most schizophrenic children function in the low average to average range of intelligence. Mean IQ scores in four studies reviewed by Volkmar (1996) ranged from 82 (SD=12.5) to 94 (SD=10.5). In a brief review of studies and a discussion of cognitive delays in early-onset schizophrenia, it is noted that 10%–20% of children with early-onset schizophrenia have IQs in the borderline to mentally retarded range (American Academy of Child and Adolescent Psychiatry 2001). Determining whether delays are due to the impact of illness on cognitive functioning or whether they existed premorbidly is difficult because premorbid test results are often not available. McClellan and McCurry

(1998) suggested that the finding of low IQ might represent a general risk for psychopathology and psychosis rather than a specific risk for early-onset schizophrenia. Nevertheless, schizophrenia is associated with cognitive deficits that produce functional impairment (American Academy of Child and Adolescent Psychiatry 2001). Bedwell et al. (1999) investigated postpsychotic decline in Full-Scale IQ during adolescence for 31 patients with childhood-onset schizophrenia to determine whether the decline noted was due to a dementing process or failure to acquire new information and skills. Subjects had significant declines in scores on three postpsychotic subtest scales, including picture arrangement, information, and block design. However, there was no decline in the raw scores (which are not age corrected) for any subtest. The authors concluded that the decline during adolescence in full-scale IQ of patients with childhood-onset schizophrenia reflected an inability to acquire new information and abilities rather than dementia.

■ Language, Communication, and Information Processing

Language and communication deficits are described widely in the literature (Baltaxe and Simmons 1995; Caplan 1994a; Caplan et al. 1996, 2000). Information-processing problems in children with schizophrenia have been observed (Asarnow et al. 1994).

■ Neurobiological Deficits

Deficits in smooth-pursuit eye movements and autonomic responsiveness have been described in addition to abnormal neuroimaging findings (Frazier et al. 1996; Gordon et al. 1994; Jacobsen and Rapoport 1998; Jacobsen et al. 1997b; Zahn et al. 1997). Briefly, neuroimaging studies have shown a progressive increase in ventricular size in subjects over 2 years (Rapoport et al. 1997); a decrease in cortical gray matter during adolescence, especially in the frontal and temporal regions (Rapoport et al. 1999); correlation of smaller total cerebral volumes with negative symptoms (Alaghband-Rad et al. 1997); and frontal lobe dysfunction consistent with that noted in adults (Thomas et al. 1998). These findings are described in more detail below under "Neuroanatomical Factors." It should be noted, however, that none of the findings described above are diagnostic for schizophrenia at this time. Therefore, the primary role for laboratory tests and neuroimaging studies in the assessment and diagnosis of childhood-onset schizophrenia is to rule out other medical disorders (American Academy of Child and Adolescent Psychiatry 2001).

Course and Outcome

DSM-IV-TR diagnostic criteria—like those in DSM-III-R (American Psychiatric Association 1987) and DSM-III—require continuous signs of disorder for a 6-month period, during which there is at least 1 month of active-phase symptoms. Schizophrenia is considered to be a phasic disorder in which there can be much individual variation. It is important for clinicians to be cognizant of the various phases of schizophrenia when making diagnostic or treatment decisions. The phases are as follows (American Academy of Child and Adolescent Psychiatry 2001):

- *Prodrome.* Before the onset of psychotic symptoms, most patients experience some degree of functional deterioration. There may be unusual behaviors, bizarre preoccupations, social withdrawal and isolation, poor academic performance, dysphoria, or problems with sleep and appetite (American Academy of Child and Adolescent Psychiatry 2001). Substance abuse, sometimes comorbid with an emerging psychosis in adolescents, may confuse the diagnostic picture. The length of the prodromal phase may be days to weeks or months to years (Werry and Taylor 1994). Distinguishing premorbid personality characteristics or cognitive/developmental deficits from the onset of symptoms may be difficult.

- *Acute phase.* During this phase, positive symptoms (i.e., hallucinations, delusions, thought disorder, and disorganized behavior) are predominant. This phase usually lasts 1–6 months, sometimes longer, and the length is affected by treatment response. Symptoms may shift from positive to negative during the course of treatment.

- *Recovery phase.* After the remission of acute-phase symptoms, there is often a continuing period (lasting several months) of impairment that is frequently characterized by negative symptoms of flattened affect, apathy, anergia, and social withdrawal (Remschmidt et al. 1991). Postpsychotic depressive disorder of schizophrenia may be seen in some patients and is characterized by dysphoria and flat affect.

Positive symptoms may still be present to some degree.

- *Residual phase.* As recovery continues, patients may experience periods of several months or more between acute phases during which there are few positive symptoms but some degree of persisting impairment due to negative symptoms

- *Chronically ill patients.* Some patients remain chronically symptomatic over several years despite appropriate treatment (Asarnow et al. 1994; Eggers and Bunk 1997; Maziade et al. 1996; McClellan et al. 1993; Werry et al. 1991). The availability of atypical antipsychotic medications offers some hope; clozapine has been effective in some cases of treatment-resistant schizophrenia (Sporn and Rapoport 2001).

Some youths with schizophrenia experience only one cycle of these phases, although most have more (Asarnow et al. 1994; Eggers 1978; McClellan et al. 1993; Werry et al. 1991). Werry and Taylor (1994) noted that recovery was incomplete in 80% of cases in which youths had had more than one episode.

Schulz et al. (1998) reviewed outcome studies in childhood-onset and adolescent-onset schizophrenia. They cited a study conducted in Germany with a large population of adolescent-onset patients who were assessed 5–11 years after onset of illness (Krausz and Muller-Thomsen 1993). Many were judged to have continuous illness and required ongoing care. Anxiety and suicidality were issues of comorbidity at follow-up. Females in this study had a better overall outcome than males.

Eggers (1978, 1989) studied a group of 57 patients with childhood schizophrenia for a mean follow-up period of 16 years. The age at onset of illness in the children was 7–13 years. In terms of outcome, 20% had complete remission, 30% had good to satisfying social adaptation, and 50% remained significantly impaired (Eggers 1978). Diagnostically, 28% were identified as having schizoaffective disorder according to ICD-9 criteria (World Health Organization 1977). Eggers and Bunk (1997) reported on a 42-year follow-up of a subset of the cohort described above, consisting of 44 subjects. Overall, the outcome for patients with childhood onset was poor, with 50% judged to be poorly remitted. However, 25% had complete remission. Insidious onset and onset before age 12 were associated with a poorer outcome, and none of the patients with insidious onset had a full remission.

Maziade et al. (1996) conducted a study designed to verify the presence and stability across life of the positive and negative symptom distinction in childhood-onset schizophrenia and to identify factors predictive of long-term outcome for childhood-onset schizophrenia. Across a 14.8-year follow-up period, two separate factors corresponding to the positive and negative symptom dimensions were identified. The best childhood predictors of adult outcome were premorbid functioning and severity of positive and negative symptoms during acute episodes. However, the presence of premorbid developmental problems and premorbid nonpsychotic behavioral disturbances was not related to severity of outcome.

Symptom dimensions of childhood-onset schizophrenia were described by Bunk et al. (1999) in a study focusing on the clinical features of 44 patients at onset of illness during their first episode and at follow-up assessment 42 years after onset. All of the subjects were rediagnosed by using DSM-IV criteria (American Psychiatric Association 1994), and symptomatology evaluated with the Positive and Negative Syndrome Scale for Schizophrenia (PANSS) (Kay et al. 1987) at onset and at follow-up. Factor analysis revealed five symptom dimensions (factors) at the onset of psychosis: cognitive symptoms, social withdrawal, antisocial behavior, excitement, and reality distortion. At follow-up, a five-factor solution was also found, but the dimensions differed from those identified at onset; the follow-up factors were positive, negative, excitement, cognitive, and anxiety/depression components. The first psychotic episode of childhood-onset schizophrenia was accompanied by symptoms that were less specific, such as social withdrawal and antisocial behavior, whereas in later stages the symptom dimensions changed to those recognized in adult-onset schizophrenia. In general, positive and global symptoms decreased over the course of the illness, but the frequency of negative symptoms did not change.

Diagnostic Issues

The diagnosis of schizophrenia in younger children or in children with developmental disabilities is challenging for a number of reasons. Difficulties in communication, developmental changes in thought processes, changing conceptions of reality, and the nature of expression of symptoms in younger children may compli-cate the diagnostic picture. In general, diagnosis should be made only after any possible organic causes have been ruled out. Appropriate studies to rule out endocrinologic, metabolic, neurological, infectious, or toxic causes of psychosis, as well as genetic studies, may be needed. Evaluation over several sessions, using information from multiple informants (including family and collaborative sources), in addition to direct mental status examination of the child, may be necessary in making the diagnosis. Psychotic manifestations in young patients are influenced by the developmental stage, and eliciting target symptoms requires the ability to understand and communicate with the child (Tolbert 1996).

Misdiagnosis of children and adolescents is a significant problem, as suggested by the observation that a number of youths first diagnosed with schizophrenia have other disorders at follow-up, including bipolar disorder (Werry et al. 1991) and personality disorders (Thomsen 1996). Of 215 patients referred to and interviewed at NIMH for possible participation in an ongoing study of childhood-onset schizophrenia, only 64 actually met DSM-III or DSM-IV criteria for the disorder (McKenna et al. 1994a; Nicolson and Rapoport 1999). Of the remaining 151 patients, 27% were ultimately diagnosed with a primary mood disorder (12% had major depressive disorder with psychotic features and 15.2% had bipolar disorder), and 4.6% had prominent mood episodes and chronic hallucinations and were diagnosed as having schizoaffective disorder.

It is important to note that hallucinations in children are not necessarily a sign of schizophrenia but can also be seen in a variety of other conditions in healthy children (Pilowsky and Chambers 1986). In preschool children, hallucinations must be distinguished from sleep-related phenomena and from other developmental phenomena such as imaginary friends or fantasy figures (Volkmar 1996). Rothstein (1981) noted that at times of stress and anxiety, transient hallucinations in preschool children might be observed. Often, these hallucinations are visual or tactile and have their onset at night, although they can also occur when the child is fully awake (Volkmar 1996). Prognostically, such hallucinations are generally benign. However, in school-age children, hallucinations may be more persistent and are often associated with more serious disorders (Carlson and Kashani 1988; Del Beccaro et al. 1988; Russell et al. 1989; Volkmar et al. 1988). In this age group, the content of hallucinations and delusions frequently reflects developmental concerns (Volkmar 1996). Hallucinations may involve monsters, pets, or toys. Delusions often involve aspects of identity and are not as systematic or complex as those in adults (Garralda 1985; Russell et al. 1989; Volkmar et al. 1988).

Cultural and religious factors need to be considered when diagnosing schizophrenia because cultural and religious beliefs, taken out of context, may be misconstrued as psychotic symptoms. Clinician biases may also influence diagnostic decisions. Kilgus et al. (1995) found that African American youths were less likely to receive mood, anxiety, or substance abuse diagnoses and were more likely to be described as having either an organic or a psychotic illness.

When a patient with treatment-refractory schizophrenia is being assessed, a medication-free period for the child as an inpatient may be clinically useful. Kumra et al. (1999) evaluated risks and benefits of a medication-free trial in 31 children and adolescents who were admitted with a diagnosis of treatment-resistant childhood-onset schizophrenia. At the completion of the 4-week drug-free period, 7 of the patients (23%) were diagnosed with another disorder on the basis of information gathered from the drug-free period and a lack of schizophrenic symptoms. Revised diagnoses were posttraumatic stress disorder in 1 subject, an atypical psychosis labeled "multidimensional impairment" in 4 subjects, and personality disorder in 2 subjects.

Differential Diagnosis

■ Autistic Disorder

The relationship between autistic disorder (see also Chapter 20, "Austistic Disorder," in this volume) and schizophrenia has long been the subject of controversy. There are isolated reports of children originally diagnosed as having autism who later exhibited schizophrenic symptomatology (Howells and Guirguis 1984; Petty et al. 1984). However, a study by Howells and Guirguis (1984) demonstrated that whether an autistic child develops schizophrenia in adulthood was dependent on which set of diagnostic criteria was used. Rutter and Schopler (1987) also questioned what weight to attach to these reports. They suspected that the "supposed autism-to-schizophrenia change reflects a broader concept of autism or of schizophrenia or a difference in the interpretation of the odd thinking that is quite common in older autistic individuals" (p. 176).

Most individuals with autism do manifest prodromal or residual symptoms similar to those seen in schizophrenia, such as social isolation, impairment in role functioning or grooming, and inappropriate affect. Many higher-functioning autistic people exhibit illogical thinking, incoherence, and poverty in content of speech. Their lack of nonverbal communication may be seen as blunt affect. Inappropriate laughing or weeping in autism, due to inability to comprehend the meaning of events, may be interpreted as labile or abnormal affect. Some higher-functioning verbal autistic persons have strange beliefs (e.g., believing there is no air in other states), idiosyncratic interests (e.g., spending an enormous amount of time studying dinosaurs), or sensory experiences (e.g., seeing other people's faces in the air when alone in the room) bordering on delusions or hallucinations. These symptoms, however, are qualitatively different from those seen in schizophrenic patients. These "schizophrenic symptoms" seen in autism may be caused by underdevelopment of cognitive and language/speech functions in autistic individuals, whereas the schizophrenic symptoms in schizophrenic patients are a deviance in previously relative normal cognitive and language/speech development. Autistic persons tend to answer "yes" to questions they do not quite understand or tend to interpret meanings of words literally. Often an autistic person may talk or laugh to himself or herself while looking at something the observer cannot identify or while having funny thoughts that he or she does not know how to share with the observer. This tends to be interpreted as listening to voices or seeing visions. Some autistic adolescents or adults continue to have childlike fantasies of being an inanimate object, an animal, or a character of a fairy tale, which may be mistaken for delusions, whereas the tendency of others to make irrelevant remarks or to talk excessively on their favorite topics may lead to a mistaken diagnosis of thought disorder.

However, individuals with schizophrenia can be differentiated from higher-functioning autistic people on the basis of such factors as age at onset, developmental history, clinical features, and family history. Almost all persons with autism have an onset before age 5 years, whereas most often the onset of schizophrenia in childhood is during the preadolescent or adolescent period. Eggers (1978) reported that the early development in about half of the schizophrenic children was unremarkable. Although there is no evidence that schizophrenic children diagnosed by DSM-IV-TR criteria manifest severe developmental deficits, all autistic people, including those with a higher-functioning disorder, have a clear history of pervasive developmental disorder.

There is increased incidence of schizophrenia, but not of autistic disorder, in the families of children with schizophrenia (Kolvin et al. 1971c). Moreover, in a study of patterns involving intellectual functioning (as measured by factor scores on the Wechsler Intelligence Scale for Children—Revised), Asarnow and colleagues (1987) found that schizophrenic and autistic children did not significantly differ on the verbal and perceptual organization factors but that the schizophrenic children had significantly lower scores on the freedom from distraction factor (including attention, short-term memory, visuomotor coordination, speed of responding, and mental arithmetic) than the nonretarded (higher-functioning) autistic children. The only subtest on which the autistic children scored significantly lower than the schizophrenic children was the comprehension subtest.

■ Schizophreniform Disorder, Brief Psychotic Disorder, Psychotic Disorder Not Otherwise Specified

Children presenting with schizophreniform disorder (Table 23–2), brief psychotic disorder (Table 23–5), and psychotic disorder not otherwise specified (Table 23–9) may appear to have schizophrenia but do not meet DSM-IV-TR criteria for schizophrenia. Children with schizophreniform disorder have duration of illness less than 6 months, and with time they may receive a diagnosis of schizophrenia. Also, diagnosis of schizophreniform disorder does not require a decline in functioning (American Psychiatric Association 2000).

Children with a diagnosis of brief psychotic disorder experience psychotic symptoms for at least 1 day but usually less than 1 month; these symptoms often follow a severe precipitating stress. The children subsequently return to their premorbid level of functioning. It is emphasized, however, that the onset of psychosis in schizophrenic children may also be in response to stress.

Psychotic patients whose symptoms do not meet specified DSM-IV-TR diagnostic criteria are classified as having psychotic disorder not otherwise specified, a relatively common diagnosis in hospitalized adolescents (Armenteros et al. 1995a; Kafantaris et al.

1992). This diagnosis may be used when there is insufficient information to decide between a diagnosis of schizophrenia and other psychotic disorders, or when the presenting symptoms may possibly be substance induced or the result of a general medical condition that has not yet been determined. This type of uncertainty is more likely early in the course of a disorder.

■ Multidimensional Impairment

In the NIMH study of schizophrenia in children (McKenna et al. 1994a), a subsample of subjects whose hallucinations did not meet DSM-III-R criteria were given the diagnosis of multidimensional impairment. Approximately 85% of these children also met criteria for ADHD (McKenna et al. 1994a). The validity of the diagnostic criteria for this subgroup of children designated as multidimensionally impaired was examined by Kumra et al. (1998b). Nineteen children displayed poor affect control, poor attention and impulse control, and psychotic symptoms in the form of visual hallucinations (42.9%), auditory hallucinations (76.2%), and delusions (33.3%). These children were compared with a group of 29 children with schizophrenia (based on DSM-III-R criteria) and a group of 19 children with ADHD. Results showed that the children with multidimensionally impaired syndrome and the patients with very-early-onset schizophrenia shared a similar pattern of early transient autistic features, postpsychotic cognitive decline, and an increased risk of schizophrenia-spectrum disorders among their first-degree relatives, a pattern that was not seen in the ADHD group. The researchers concluded that there was support for making a distinction between multidimensional impairment and other psychiatric disorders. It was suggested that the disorder be considered to be within the schizophrenia spectrum.

■ Personality Disorders

Children and adolescents who later develop schizotypal, borderline, schizoid, and paranoid personality disorders (see also Chapter 42, "Personality Disorders," in this volume) may exhibit transient psychotic symptoms. Comprehensive evaluation of these children and adolescents should focus on clarifying whether schizophrenic symptomatology and deterioration of daily functioning are present.

■ Affective Disorders

It is important to distinguish between schizophrenia and mood disorders with psychotic features (see also Chapter 24, "Mood Disorders in Prepubertal Children," and Chapter 25, "Mood Disorders in Adolescents," in this volume) when diagnosing children and adolescents. Psychotic depressive disorders may present with mood-congruent or mood-incongruent psychotic features in the form of hallucinations or delusions (American Academy of Child and Adolescent Psychiatry 1998a). Chambers et al. (1982) found that about 48% of prepubertal children with major depressive disorder had hallucinations of any type and that 36% reported complex auditory hallucinations. Delusions, however, were described as rare in major depressive disorder with onset in childhood (Puig-Antich et al. 1985).

At times it may be difficult to distinguish bipolar affective disorder from schizophrenia in adolescence (Carlson and Strober 1978; Taylor et al. 1974; Werry et al. 1994). A study by McKenna et al. (1994a), described above under "Diagnostic Issues," delineates subsequent diagnoses in a group of patients thought to have childhood-onset schizophrenia upon referral to NIMH for an ongoing study. On subsequent evaluation, 27% were diagnosed with a primary mood disorder.

Making an accurate diagnosis of schizoaffective disorder can be difficult. Although retrospective evaluation of a temporal relationship between mood episodes and psychotic symptoms can be a problem, overlap of the two is what distinguishes schizoaffective disorder from bipolar disorder in DSM-IV-TR (Calderoni et al. 2001). The presence of psychotic symptoms in the presence of mood symptoms is a criterion for diagnosis of schizoaffective disorder. If mood symptoms are depressive and resemble the negative symptoms of schizophrenia, then the diagnosis of schizoaffective disorder could be missed. Likewise, it can be difficult to distinguish the activation of mania from the agitation and disorganization of schizophrenia (Carlson et al. 2000).

■ Organic Syndromes

Patients presenting with psychotic symptoms should also receive a thorough medical evaluation, including a neurological examination, to rule out an organic etiology. Although the list of potential etiological organic conditions and neuropsychiatric conditions that could cause or contribute to a psychotic presentation is very long, the following, among other conditions, have been associated with psychotic symptoms and should be routinely considered: 1) seizure disorders; 2) delirium; 3) central nervous system lesions, including brain tumors, vascular lesions, congenital malformations, and head trauma; 4) metabolic and endocrine disorders (e.g., hypothyroidism, Wilson's disease); 5) neurodegenerative disorders (Huntington's disease, lipid storage disorders); 6) developmental disorders; 7) toxic encephalopathies (including those caused by abuse of substances such as amphetamines, cocaine, hallucinogens, phencyclidine, alcohol, and cannabis; those caused by solvents, heavy metals, and environmental toxins; and those caused by medications such as stimulants, corticosteroids, and anticholinergic agents); 8) infectious diseases (such as human immunodeficiency virus infection, encephalitis, and meningitis); and 9) autoimmune disorders (e.g., systemic lupus erythematosus).

■ Substance Abuse

The issue of substance abuse (see also Chapter 43, "Substance Abuse Disorders," in this volume) warrants careful consideration when considering early-onset schizophrenia. There is a significant rate of comorbid substance abuse in adolescents with schizophrenia, as much as 50% in some studies (McClellan and McCurry 1998; McClellan et al. 1993). Diagnosis is sometimes complicated by the presence of active substance use or abuse at the first onset of psychiatric symptoms. Many different types of substance-related disorders may produce symptoms similar to those of schizophrenia. Sustained amphetamine or cocaine use may produce hallucinations or delusions (American Psychiatric Association 2000). Phencyclidine use may produce a mixture of both positive and negative symptoms. 3,4-Methylenedioxymethamphetamine (MDMA), also known as ecstasy, has been associated with neurotoxicity. One case report describes a 19-year-old woman with overlapping symptoms of neuroleptic malignant syndrome and serotonin syndrome after a single exposure to MDMA (Demirkiran et al. 1996). Hall and Degenhardt (2000) examine the relationship between cannabis use and psychosis. It is known that cannabis use can potentially exacerbate the symptoms of schizophrenia. However, it is unclear whether cannabis use can precipitate schizophrenia or whether the association is due to the use of other drugs (e.g., amphetamines, cocaine) that heavy cannabis users may be more likely to use (Hall and Degenhardt 2000).

Ideally, it is recommended that the clinician try to observe the individual during a sustained period (at least 4 weeks) of abstinence, although this is often difficult to accomplish (American Psychiatric Association 2000). Therefore, the clinician may need to rely on other evidence, such as whether psychotic symptoms appear to be exacerbated by the substance use and diminished when it has been discontinued; level of functioning before the onset of substance use; and severity of psychotic symptoms in relation to the amount and duration of substance use. A thorough knowledge of characteristic symptoms produced by particular substances is also needed if the clinician is to distinguish the effects of substance use from psychotic symptoms (American Psychiatric Association 2000).

■ Other Nonpsychotic Conditions

Youths with conduct disorder and other emotional disorders that are nonpsychotic may report psychotic-like symptoms and may therefore be misdiagnosed as having a primary psychotic disorder such as schizophrenia (Del Beccaro et al. 1988; Garralda 1984a, 1984b; Hornstein and Putnam 1992; McClellan and McCurry 1999; Walters and McClellan 1998). However, compared with psychotic youths, this group has lower rates of negative symptoms, thought disorder, and bizarre behavior (Garralda 1985; McClellan and McCurry 1999).

■ Anxiety Disorders

Famularo et al. (1992) reported significantly higher rates of psychotic symptoms in children with posttraumatic stress disorder than in control subjects. Children with posttraumatic stress disorder who report psychotic-like symptoms may be describing dissociative or anxiety phenomena such as intrusive thoughts or worries, depersonalization, or derealization (Altman et al. 1997; Hornstein and Putnam 1992; McClellan and McCurry 1999). It is important to keep in mind that children with schizophrenia also may have been maltreated, so the diagnosis of schizophrenia should not be ruled out just on the basis of an abuse history (McClellan and McCurry 1999).

Children and adolescents with obsessive-compulsive disorder (see also Chapter 30, "Obsessive-Compulsive Disorder," in this volume) may experience intrusive thoughts and ritualistic behaviors that at times are difficult to distinguish from psychosis. For example, fears related to contamination by germs or toxic chemicals may be a paranoid delusion, an obsessive symptom, or even a realistic response to threat of biochemical warfare, depending on the circumstances. Generally, patients with obsessive-compulsive disorder recognize their symptoms as being products of their own obsessive thinking or as being unreasonable (American Academy of Child and Adolescent Psychiatry 1998b). However, in children, insight into the nature of symptoms is not always apparent, and lack of insight does not preclude a diagnosis of obsessive-compulsive disorder.

Etiology

The etiology of schizophrenia is unknown, and the relative roles of genetic, neurobiological, and environmental and psychosocial influences remain controversial.

■ Genetic Factors

Cytogenetic Abnormalities

Specific cytogenetic abnormalities have recently been examined in a cohort from the ongoing NIMH study of childhood-onset schizophrenia (Nicolson et al. 1999). Five of 47 patients with childhood-onset schizophrenia were found to have cytogenetic abnormalities, including a girl with Turner's syndrome, a boy with a balanced translocation of chromosomes 1 and 7 (Yan et al. 2000), and two girls and a boy with velocardiofacial syndrome (22q11 deletion). Other genetic studies reported in the literature (Moriniere et al. 1999) have focused on the potential role of polyglutamine expansion, which is encoded by a CAG repeat, as a candidate for schizophrenia and have searched for polyglutamine expansion in nuclear families in which a member is affected by childhood-onset schizophrenia. Burgess et al. (1998) reported on an association between trinucleotide expansions and childhood-onset schizophrenia. Kumra et al. (1998c) reported that out of 66 pediatric patients who were nonresponsive to neuroleptic medications, 4 (6.1%) were found to have sex chromosome anomalies. Three patients were characterized as multidimensionally impaired, whereas one had a diagnosis of childhood-onset schizophrenia.

Kumra et al. (1998c) suggested that karyotyping of children with psychotic disorders should be routinely carried out. Other studies have investigated a dopamine D_4 receptor polymorphism in association with catatonic schizophrenia (Kaiser et al. 2000); a neurotrophin gene polymorphism in relation to hippocampal volume in psychoses (Kunugi et al. 1999); and 22q11 deletions in adults with schizophrenia (Bassett et al. 1998; Murphy et al. 1999; Usiskin et al. 1999).

Familial Patterns

Several studies reported an increased family history of schizophrenia and schizophrenia-spectrum disorders—including schizoaffective, schizotypal, and paranoid personality disorders—in patients diagnosed with childhood-onset schizophrenia (Asarnow et al. 2001; Eggers 1978; Green et al. 1992; Kendler et al. 1993a, 1993b, 1993c; Kolvin et al. 1971c; McClellan and McCurry 1998; McClellan et al. 1993; Nicolson and Rapoport 1999; Werry et al. 1991). Kolvin et al. (1971c) described an increased rate of isolated personalities among the parents of children with childhood-onset schizophrenia, suggesting the possibility of a greater genetic diathesis. Other, earlier studies had shown increased prevalence of schizophrenia in family members, as demonstrated in offspring (M. Bleuler 1978; Gottesman et al. 1982, 1987; Mirsky et al. 1985) and in siblings (Gottesman and Shields 1972), as well as in adoption studies (Heston 1966; Kety et al. 1975, 1994) and twin studies (Gottesman and Shields 1972; Gottesman et al. 1982, 1987). Whereas the risk of developing schizophrenia is not greater than 1% in the general population, it is 10%–15% if one parent has schizophrenia (Gottesman et al. 1982; Kendler and Diehl 1993).

Nicolson et al. (2000) reported the results of a recent screening of first-degree relatives of the NIMH cohort. Nineteen relatives under age 18 years were given the Diagnostic Interview Schedule for Children and Adolescents, and 105 relatives over age 17 years were administered the Schedule for Affective Disorders and Schizophrenia and the Structured Clinical Interview for DSM-IV Personality Disorders. Two first-degree relatives were determined to have schizophrenia, and one was determined to have schizoaffective disorder. Approximately 25.7% of the first-degree relatives assessed had either paranoid or schizotypal personality disorder; 42.6% of the probands had at least one relative with a schizophrenia-spectrum disorder. Asarnow et al. (2001) determined that there was an increased lifetime

morbid risk for schizophrenia (4.95%±2.16%) and schizotypal personality disorder (4.2%±2.06%) in parents of probands with childhood schizophrenia compared with the parents of subjects with ADHD and community control subjects. There is remarkable similarity in the disorders that do and do not aggregate in the parents of adult-onset schizophrenia and in the parents of probands with childhood-onset schizophrenia, a finding that provides support for the hypothesis of etiological continuity between adult-onset and childhood-onset schizophrenia.

In a study of Danish identical and fraternal discordant twins, the risk of schizophrenia in the offspring of the nonschizophrenic co-twins of identical twins was the same as in the offspring of the schizophrenic twin. In contrast, the offspring of the nonschizophrenic co-twins of fraternal twins had a risk for schizophrenia much below the risk in the offspring of the schizophrenic twin (Gottesman and Bertelsen 1989). These results suggest that environmental events may trigger the development of schizophrenia. They may also explain the etiology for childhood-onset schizophrenia: in an individual who has the genetic predisposition, an environmental trigger—such as birth trauma, prematurity, low birth weight, or viral illness in utero or even in the first few years of life—may initiate the onset of schizophrenia in childhood. Further research in this area may clarify the genetic contributions to childhood-onset schizophrenia and better elucidate the biological/environmental (including psychosocial) risk factors and their interaction with genetics as they affect ongoing neurodevelopment.

■ Risk Factors

Several risk factors have been examined in childhood schizophrenia for evidence of greater predominance and severity. These risk factors include obstetrical complications, gender, pubertal development, medical conditions, and neurological signs.

Obstetrical Complications

A number of studies have noted an excess of prenatal and perinatal complications in patients with schizophrenia (Nicolson et al. 2000). Patients with adult-onset schizophrenia have been reported to have higher rates of obstetrical complications compared with their siblings or healthy control subjects (Eagles et al. 1990; Gunther-Genta et al. 1994; O'Callaghan et al. 1993), although results are not consistent (Done et al. 1991). A reanalysis of original data from a number of studies has suggested that birth complications were greater in patients with an earlier onset of illness (Verdoux et al. 1997); however, others have found no differences in obstetrical complications between patients with childhood-onset schizophrenia and sibling control subjects (Nicolson et al. 2000). Therefore, although obstetrical complications may play a role in some patients in the development of schizophrenia, they may not be more salient in childhood-onset cases (Lewis et al. 1989; Nicolson et al. 2000).

Gender

Males are overrepresented in many clinical studies of childhood-onset schizophrenia. However, in the NIMH childhood-onset schizophrenia cohort, an equal sex ratio is observed. As noted by Jacobsen and Rapoport (1998), this is consistent with analyses of epidemiological data related to first psychiatric admissions for schizophrenia and paranoia in children and adolescents in France and England, which showed an equal sex ratio for patients below age 15 years (Galdos et al. 1993; Lewine 1994).

Pubertal Development

In many neurodevelopmental theories of schizophrenia, a brain change at puberty that triggers the onset of schizophrenia is proposed (Feinberg 1982–1983; Keshavan et al. 1994; Weinberger 1987). A prediction of this model is that in childhood-onset schizophrenia there would be some physical or endocrine manifestation of early puberty or an acceleration of developmental brain changes (Jacobsen and Rapoport 1998). Most prospective studies of childhood-onset schizophrenia have not mentioned pubertal status of the samples (Green et al. 1992; Russell 1994; Spencer and Campbell 1994; Werry et al. 1994). The NIMH study looked at the onset of psychosis in relation to the development of secondary sex characteristics and menarche in 28 adolescents with childhood-onset schizophrenia (Frazier et al. 1997). Males and females developed psychotic symptoms at a similar age. There was no significant correlation between the development of psychosis and menarche. The age at development of secondary sex characteristics was associated with onset of psychoses for girls, but this finding was driven by one outlier. Therefore, there was no clear relationship between onset of psychosis and indices of sexual development for childhood-onset schizophrenia.

Medical Conditions

Kolvin et al. (1971a) reported that 2 of 33 children with onset of psychosis between ages 5 and 12 also had temporal lobe epilepsy. One long-term follow-up study of 100 children with temporal lobe epilepsy found that 10% developed schizophrenia in adulthood (Lindsay et al. 1979). Caplan et al. (1992, 1993) noted that children with complex partial seizure disorders had significantly more illogical thinking and used fewer linguistic cohesive devices, findings similar to those noted in children with childhood-onset schizophrenia.

Neurological Signs

Several studies have documented a variety of neurological soft signs or motor dysfunctions in subjects at high risk for schizophrenia; impaired fine motor coordination is among the signs most frequently reported (Erlenmeyer-Kimling and Cornblatt 1987; Hanson et al. 1976; Marcus 1974; Marcus et al. 1985; Rieder and Nichols 1979). Jacobsen and Rapoport (1998) noted a higher frequency of neurological dysfunction— including movement disorders, poor sensory integration, and impaired coordination—in the NIMH childhood-onset schizophrenia cohort. Karp et al. (2001) reported that neurological signs decreased with age in control subjects but did not decrease in children with schizophrenia. The researchers concluded that this finding suggested a delay in or failure of normal brain maturation in the children with schizophrenia.

■ Neuroanatomical Factors

Computed Tomographic Studies

Benes et al. (1982) studied the computed tomographic scans of 11 adolescents and young adults with schizophrenia and found that they did not differ from those of matched control subjects. Schulz et al. (1983) used computed tomography to study ventricular enlargement in adolescents with schizophrenia and in medical control subjects and patients with personality disorder. The adolescent schizophrenic patients (average age, 16 years), who had been ill for less than 2 years, had greater ventricular brain ratios compared with both of the other groups. In the schizophrenic teenagers, ventricular brain ratio was not related to length of illness. Jennings et al. (1985) found that ventricular brain ratio in psychotic adolescents was inversely correlated with the dopamine metabolite homovanillic acid and with the serotonin metabolite 5-hydroxyindoleacetic acid.

Magnetic Resonance Imaging Studies

Researchers are using magnetic resonance imaging (MRI) with increasing frequency to study the schizophrenic population. In a comprehensive review of neuroimaging findings in child and adolescent psychiatric disorders, including childhood-onset schizophrenia, Hendren and colleagues (2000) summarized MRI findings and suggested that brain changes in childhood-onset schizophrenia appeared to occur in two waves: 1) early in neurodevelopment, with asymmetries, basal ganglia reductions, and nonspecific reductions in overall brain size associated with negative symptoms; and 2) in adolescence, with reductions in frontal and temporal structures and ventricular enlargement associated with positive symptoms. Some of the MRI studies supporting these conclusions are briefly reviewed below.

Cerebellum. Jacobsen and colleagues (1997b) studied 24 schizophrenic adolescents and 52 matched control subjects. Volumes of the cerebellar vermis, midsagittal area, and inferior posterior lobe were significantly smaller in subjects with schizophrenia, and no correlation with neuroleptic exposure was found.

Cerebral hemispheres and ventricles. Several studies have found smaller total cerebral volume in children with childhood-onset schizophrenia (Frazier et al. 1996; Jacobsen et al. 1997b; Rapoport et al. 1997, 1999). Rapoport and colleagues, in a 1997 study (replicated in 1999), scanned subjects (mean age at first scan, 14.8 years) at initial admission and again 2 years later, using identical equipment and measurement methods. Children with childhood-onset schizophrenia showed a significantly greater decrease in total cerebral volume and increase in ventricular volume than did control subjects. Jacobsen and colleagues (1998a) also found decreased total cerebral volume in 10 schizophrenic adolescents with childhood onset compared with control subjects at 2-year follow-up (Frazier et al. 1996; Rapoport et al. 1997). Cerebral asymmetry, with right hemisphere larger than the left, across groups was also noted. In contrast to the studies cited above (the NIMH group), Hendren et al. (1995) and Yeo et al. (1997) found no differences in the childhood-onset schizophrenia group in overall brain volume, total ventricular volume, or frontal area. They found a reversal of normal asymmetry in the childhood-onset schizophrenia-spectrum group. However,

the group studied by Hendren et al. (1995) was younger and had less severe symptoms than the NIMH group.

Temporal lobe structures. Jacobsen et al. (1996a) found that children with childhood-onset schizophrenia had larger volumes of the superior temporal lobe gyrus and its posterior segment and that they displayed a trend toward larger temporal lobe volumes compared with control subjects. The researchers concluded that these areas might be spared in whatever process decreased the size of other brain areas in these patients. In 1998, Jacobsen and associates published data after rescanning part of the original group and control subjects. The researchers found that the schizophrenic subjects had significantly greater decreases in volume in the right temporal lobe, bilateral superior temporal gyrus, posterior superior temporal gyrus, right anterior superior temporal gyrus, and left hippocampus (Jacobsen et al. 1998a). Greater decreases in hippocampal volume over the follow-up interval were associated with greater negative symptoms at baseline and greater delusions at follow-up. In a longitudinal study of 15 original subjects from the same cohort, Rapoport et al. (1999) noted decreases in frontal and parietal lobe gray matter volumes, with greater decreases in children with schizophrenia. The schizophrenic subjects also showed a decrease in temporal gray matter. Hendren et al. (1995) and Yeo et al. (1997) found smaller amygdala and reduced temporal cortex volumes in children with schizophrenia-spectrum disorder. Findling et al. (1996) found no differences in hippocampal volume between adolescents with childhood-onset schizophrenia and control subjects.

Thalamic area. Frazier et al. (1996) reported a smaller midsagittal thalamic area in children with schizophrenia than in control subjects. Rapoport et al. (1997) noted a significant decrease on the rescanned midsagittal thalamic area among the schizophrenic group but no change in control subjects.

Corpus callosum. The only two studies of the corpus callosum in childhood-onset schizophrenia had conflicting results. Jacobsen et al. (1997d) reported larger corpus callosum areas in 25 adolescents with childhood-onset schizophrenia, whereas Yeo et al. (1997) reported reduced corpus callosum areas in younger children (mean age, 11 years) with schizophrenia-spectrum disorders.

Cavum septi pellucidi. In a study by Nopoulos et al. (1998), there was a significantly higher frequency of enlarged cavum septi pellucidi in adolescents with childhood-onset schizophrenia than in matched control subjects.

Magnetic Resonance Spectroscopy Studies

Several magnetic resonance spectroscopy studies have reported abnormalities in the frontal lobes in childhood-onset schizophrenia groups, with lower *N*-acetylaspartate/creatine ratios (Bertolino et al. 1998; Brooks et al. 1998). The role of *N*-acetylaspartate has not yet been firmly established.

Positron Emission Tomographic Studies

In a positron emission tomographic study, Gordon et al. (1994) found decreased right parietal metabolism in children with schizophrenia compared with control subjects on an auditory continuous-performance task, possibly secondary to poor attentional performance. Jacobsen and colleagues (1997e) used positron emission tomography with an auditory continuous-performance task to study 16 adolescents with childhood-onset schizophrenia and 26 matched control subjects and found no hypofrontality in either group.

Summary of Neuroanatomical Factors

In general, results from neuroimaging studies indicate consistency in the structures found to be abnormal but some inconsistencies in the nature of the abnormalities (Hendren et al. 2000).

■ Infectious Disease and Immunological Factors

Infectious Diseases

Some investigators had reported findings of association between maternal infections (particularly influenza) during pregnancy and the development of childhood-onset schizophrenia (Mednick et al. 1988; O'Callaghan et al. 1991). However, other studies reported that maternal influenza was not associated with increased risk for the development of schizophrenia (Erlenmeyer-Kimling et al. 1994; Kendell and Kemp 1989; Morgan et al. 1997; Selten et al. 1999; Susser et al. 1994). More recent studies have also focused on the hypothesis that maternal infections during pregnancy are associated with the subsequent development of schizophrenia and other psychoses in adulthood. Buka et al. (2001) found that offspring of mothers with elevated levels of total IgG and IgM immunoglobulins and antibodies to herpes simplex virus type 2 are at increased risk for the development of schizophrenia and other psychotic illnesses in adulthood. Brown et al. (2001)—having previously demonstrated that a birth cohort that was clinically and serologically documented with prenatal rubella evidenced a marked increase in the risk of developing nonaffective psychosis—examined whether rubella-exposed subjects who would later develop schizophrenia or schizophrenia-spectrum disorders had greater impairment in premorbid functioning. Compared with rubella-exposed control subjects, rubella-exposed subjects who developed a schizophrenia-spectrum psychosis demonstrated a decline in IQ from childhood to adolescence and increased premorbid neuromotor and behavioral abnormalities.

Autoimmune Diseases

Evidence of immune system abnormalities in adult schizophrenia has prompted studies of the human leukocyte antigen (HLA) system. In an investigation of the immune system in childhood-onset schizophrenia, Jacobsen et al. (1998b) compared 8 schizophrenic children and 51 ethnically matched control subjects for frequencies of HLAs that were previously reported to be associated with schizophrenia or autoimmune disorders. Results showed no significant differences between schizophrenic and healthy subjects in the frequency of any of the antigens tested, thus failing to support HLA-associated pathology in childhood-onset schizophrenia. Mittleman et al. (1997) studied levels of cytokines relevant to cell-mediated (type 1) and humoral-mediated (type 2) immunity in groups of children with childhood-onset schizophrenia, obsessive-compulsive disorder, and ADHD. The results of this study showed that there was a lack of involvement of either cell-mediated or humoral immunity in schizophrenia.

■ Neurophysiological Factors

Event-Related Potential Studies

Studies of event-related potentials and neurophysiological tests in schizophrenic children suggest some dysfunction in the prefrontal cortex (Asarnow et al. 1986).

Eye Tracking Studies

Abnormalities of smooth-pursuit eye movements in adults with schizophrenia have been well described in the literature (Levy et al. 1993). A study of eye tracking in adolescents with schizophrenia reported significantly greater catch-up saccade amplitude and a trend for lower gain in this population (Friedman et al. 1993). Jacobsen et al. (1996b) examined smooth-pursuit eye movements in schizophrenic children compared with psychiatrically healthy subjects and subjects with ADHD. The purpose of the study was to determine if there was correspondence in eye movement dysfunction between child-onset and adult-onset forms of schizophrenia. Schizophrenic children exhibited significantly greater impairments in smooth-pursuit eye movements than either subjects with ADHD or healthy control subjects, and the pattern of abnormalities in smooth-pursuit movements was similar to that seen in adult-onset schizophrenia.

Autonomic Function Studies

Abnormalities in peripheral measures of autonomic activity, such as skin conductance and heart rate, have been reported in adult schizophrenia. Autonomic function was studied in 21 subjects (mean age, 14.1 years) with childhood-onset schizophrenia and in 54 age-matched control subjects. The study showed that abnormalities in autonomic functioning in the patients with childhood-onset schizophrenia included high levels of resting activity, impaired response to novel stimuli, and failure to stop responding to familiar stimuli (Zahn et al. 1997). This pattern is also seen in adults with chronic schizophrenia, thus providing support for the hypothesis of continuity between child and adult forms of the disorder.

■ Neurochemical Factors

Studies of Cerebrospinal Fluid Metabolites

Although no specific cerebrospinal fluid monoamine profile has been consistently associated with schizophrenia, treatment response has been associated with changes in monoamine concentrations (Jacobsen et al. 1997a). In the study by Jacobsen et al. (1997a), concentrations and ratios of homovanillic acid to 5-hydroxyindoleacetic acid, and ratios of homovanillic acid to 3-methoxy-4-hydroxyphenylglycol (a norepinephrine metabolite) did not change significantly with 6 weeks' treatment with either haloperidol or clozapine, despite reduction in both positive and negative symptoms with both medications. However, reduction of homovanillic acid concentration in patients taking clozapine was associated with reduction in positive psychotic symptoms. A similar result was noted in adults taking clozapine, suggesting continuity between adult-onset and child-onset schizophrenia.

■ Neuropsychological Factors

In assessing neuropsychological functioning in childhood-onset schizophrenia, Asarnow and colleagues (1994) found that children with schizophrenia perform poorly on tasks involving fine motor speed or tasks requiring attention or short-term memory. They do not, however, exhibit impairment in rote language skills and simple perceptual processing tasks. In studies using the Span of Apprehension Task, children with schizophrenia had delayed initiation of serial search or carried out the serial search more slowly than did nonschizophrenic children. Data from a study of adolescents with schizophrenia suggested deficits in attention, short-term memory, and recent long-term memory (Friedman et al. 1996). Karatekin and Asarnow (1998) investigated both verbal and spatial working memory in children with childhood-onset schizophrenia, children with ADHD, and age-matched healthy control subjects. Both children with schizophrenia and children with ADHD showed deficits in verbal and spatial working memory. The results suggest that in both disorders the capacity of sensory buffers may be diminished or the availability or allocation of resources to the central executive may be limited.

Jacobsen and Rapoport (1998) reported that children with schizophrenia showed a significant deterioration in intellectual functioning during the time between the premorbid period and after the onset of psychosis. Furthermore, the subjects' IQ scores continued to decline 24–48 months after the onset of psychosis. This pattern is different from that noted in adults with schizophrenia. This pattern of intellectual decline and insidious onset seems to suggest that there may be an ongoing pathological process that continually erodes brain function in childhood-onset schizophrenia, in contrast to a fixed lesion that may underlie the adult-onset disorder (Breslin and Weinberger 1991; Weinberger 1987).

■ Neurolinguistic Factors

Baltaxe and Simmons (1995) examined communication characteristics and specific language deficits in 47 children diagnosed with childhood-onset schizophrenia using DSM-III-R criteria. Standardized tests and formal measures were used to assess impairment in specific areas, including pragmatics, receptive and expressive vocabulary and syntax, abstract language, auditory processing, and speech production. Results showed that pragmatics, prosody, auditory processing, and abstract language had the greatest impairment. Communication deficits in the group with childhood-onset schizophrenia were found to be similar to the phenomenology reported in studies of the communication characteristics of adult-onset schizophrenia.

■ Psychological and Social Factors

No evidence exists that psychological or social factors cause schizophrenia. However, environmental risks are thought to interact with biological and genetic risk factors and thus affect the timing, severity, and course of the illness. Psychosocial stressors, including expressed emotion within the family environment, are believed to affect the onset or worsening of acute episodes and may influence relapse rates (American Psychiatric Association 1997). In general, interactions between psychological, social, and illness factors are thought to be complex and "bidirectional" (American Academy of Child and Adolescent Psychiatry 2001).

■ Summary of Etiology

Neurodevelopmental theory can be conceptualized in at least three ways. One theory is that in a normally developing brain, some insult, such as birth trauma or viral infection, occurs during the critical period of brain development. This insult may change the brain structure, with the subsequent development of schizophrenic behaviors. The second theory is that the actual development of the fetal brain is defective in a way that may not be apparent in the earlier years and that certain stresses during maturation may trigger the onset of the schizophrenic behavior. The third theory is that there is a genetic predisposition to schizophrenia that is expressed as a disruption of fetal brain areas undergoing rapid development in the second trimester of intrauterine life. These disruptions in neural development can result in an increased vulnerability to certain complications of pregnancy and delivery, and the combination of these factors may produce periventricular damage. Data from recent genetic research; neuroimaging studies; studies of familial associations and risk factors; and studies of vulnerability, protective factors, and stressful life events as well as their interactions continue to add to a growing body of evidence supporting a neurodevelopmental perspective and a genetic–environment interaction model for the development of childhood-onset schizophrenia.

Treatment

There is little research available regarding the effectiveness of various treatments for children and adolescents with schizophrenia. However, given the strong evidence for continuity between the childhood-onset and adult-onset forms of the disorder, it is assumed by many that the treatments used in adults will also apply to children, provided that modifications are made that take into account age, developmental stage, and other individual circumstances. In clinical practice, careful assessment of a child's strengths, weaknesses, and environmental resources is critical in treatment planning. Combined modalities for an individual patient will likely be required and may include psychoeducation of patient and family, individual therapy, group therapy, parent counseling, family therapy, special education services, community support services, case management, vocational training, and psychopharmacology as deemed appropriate. Within the school setting, services offered may include teacher consultant services, resource room services, self-contained classroom services, speech and language therapy, occupational therapy, physical therapy, and social work services. Vocational training during secondary years may also need to be considered. Individualized educational plans will need to be developed for each child in accordance with his or her specific needs as assessed by a multidisciplinary evaluation team.

■ Nonpharmacological Therapies

Psychoeducational interventions aimed at family functioning, problem-solving and communication skills, and relapse prevention have been shown to decrease relapse rates in adults with schizophrenia (Hogarty et al. 1986). Social skills training has been reported to be helpful in enhancing socialization and vocational skills (Heinssen et al. 2000). In terms of individual therapy, supportive psychotherapy may be of benefit to some children (Cantor and Kestenbaum 1986). Behavior modification procedures may also be useful in reducing levels of maladaptive behavior. More recently, cognitive-behavioral therapy techniques have been shown to be efficacious in the care of patients with chronic psychiatric illnesses (Buckley et al. 2000). This approach was noted to be helpful in the management of suicidality in young people with a first episode of schizophrenia (Buckley et al. 2000). In a literature review, McClellan and Werry (1994) noted that certain combined treatments that are effective in adult patients might also be effective in younger schizophrenic patients. These treatments are family treatment programs combined with administration of psychoactive agents (Falloon 1992; Goldstein 1989) and family therapy and pharmacotherapy combined with social skills training (Falloon 1992; Hogarty et al. 1986).

■ Psychopharmacotherapy

Conventional Antipsychotics

There have been very few controlled trials using antipsychotic medications in children and adolescents with schizophrenia. Poole et al. (1976) conducted a randomized, double-blind, placebo-controlled study of haloperidol and loxapine in 75 adolescents (ages 13–18 years) with schizophrenia. Results supported a modest but significant superiority of these medications over placebo, but high rates of sedation and extrapyramidal side effects were noted in the active medication groups. Only one double-blind, placebo-controlled study has involved prepubertal schizophrenic patients (Spencer and Campbell 1994). In this study, 16 hospitalized children (ages 5.5–11.75 years) had a good response to haloperidol: 12 showed marked improvement, and 4 showed mild or moderate improvement as measured by the Global Clinical Judgments consensus scale (Spencer and Campbell 1994). Persecutory ideation and delusions, hallucinations, ideas of reference, and other thinking disorders, as measured by the Child Psychiatric Rating Scale, were significantly reduced in patients who received haloperidol in dosages ranging from 0.5 to 3.5 mg/day (mean, 1.9 mg/day). The most common side effects were sedation, acute dystonia, and extrapyramidal symptoms. Older children, children with higher IQs,

and those with later onset of schizophrenia showed greater response to haloperidol (Spencer and Campbell 1994). These findings were confirmed when the sample was enlarged to 24 children (Spencer et al. 1994).

Atypical Antipsychotics

Recently, an increasing number of new-generation atypical antipsychotics have been developed, the prototype of which is clozapine. Since their development, these agents have been widely used in the treatment of children and adolescents with schizophrenia. A recently published comprehensive review of all identified published and unpublished studies of the use of antipsychotic medications in children and adolescents from 1996 onward addresses efficacy and tolerability (Bryden et al. 2001). Most of the studies reported reasonable treatment response, but problems with excessive weight gain, sedation, and some degree of extrapyramidal side effects are noted with many of these medications. Studies involving the use of clozapine, risperidone, olanzapine, and quetiapine in children and adolescents are briefly discussed below.

Clozapine. Although some of the newer atypical neuroleptics may have more benign side-effect profiles, clozapine is often the drug of choice in nonresponders or partial responders (Sporn and Rapoport 2001). In general, data from adult studies have shown clozapine to be beneficial in as many as 30% of patients who have not responded to multiple trials of other neuroleptics, both typical and atypical (Sporn and Rapoport 2001). Kumra et al. (1996) report on a 6-week double-blind, parallel randomized study of haloperidol and clozapine in 21 patients with treatment-refractory childhood-onset schizophrenia. Clozapine was superior to haloperidol for treatment of both positive and negative symptoms. However, clozapine was associated with severe side effects, including blood dyscrasias, seizures, excessive weight gain, and a significant increase in liver enzymes, necessitating discontinuation in several patients. Turetz et al. (1997) conducted an open trial of clozapine (mean dosage, 227 mg/day) in 11 children ages 9–13 years with treatment-refractory schizophrenia and noted significant improvements in both positive and negative symptoms as measured by the Brief Psychiatric Rating Scale (BPRS) (Overall and Gorham 1962) and the PANSS (Kay et al. 1987). Adverse effects, including sedation, sialorrhea, and weight gain, were noted in both of the studies mentioned above (Kumra et al. 1996; Turetz et al. 1997). Tolerability of clozapine may be enhanced by administering it at low initial dosages with subsequent slow dosage increases (Bryden et al. 2001).

There are several other reports of open studies or case reports of the use of clozapine (Birmaher et al. 1992; Blanz and Schmidt 1993; Frazier et al. 1994; Kumra et al. 1996; Remschmidt et al. 1992, 1994). The role of clozapine in the treatment of children and adolescents with schizophrenia and its long-term efficacy and safety in this age group remain to be determined in large samples of patients under adequately controlled, double-blind conditions.

Risperidone.   An atypical antipsychotic approved by the U.S. Food and Drug Administration (FDA) in 1993, risperidone has a profile similar to that of clozapine and is reported to exert therapeutic effects on both positive and negative symptoms in adults with schizophrenia (Chouinard et al. 1993; Marder and Meibach 1994). Several reports, mainly open trials and case reports, suggest that risperidone may also be efficacious in the treatment of children and adolescents. In 3 patients ages 11–17 years with schizophrenia, Simeon et al. (1995) reported marked improvement associated with administration of risperidone at dosages ranging from 2 to 6 mg/day (taken in two divided doses). Paranoid ideation, impulsivity, and aggressive behavior were among the symptoms most responsive to risperidone. The patients did not experience untoward effects. In another study of a diagnostically heterogeneous group of 10 patients, all improved clinically with risperidone (2–6 mg/day), but untoward effects were noted in 8 patients and extrapyramidal symptoms were observed in 6 (Mandoki 1995). Two of the 10 patients, ages 10 and 17 years, had a diagnosis of schizophrenia. In a letter to the editor, Cozza and Edison (1994) reported significant improvement in 2 adolescents within 1 week of treatment with risperidone. Extrapyramidal side effects associated with risperidone seem to be dose related (Cozza and Edison 1994; Fras and Major 1995).

Armenteros et al. (1997), in an open pilot study, treated 10 youths (ages 12–18 years) with acute schizophrenia for a 6-week period with dosages of risperidone ranging from 4 to 10 mg/day. Significant reduction in both positive and negative symptoms as assessed by the PANSS, BPRS, and Clinical Global Impression (CGI) Scale were noted. Side effects included weight gain (8 subjects with a mean weight increase of 4.5 kg), mild somnolence (in 8 subjects), dystonic reaction (in 2 sub-

jects), parkinsonism (in 3 subjects), blurred vision (in 1 subject), and poor concentration (in 1 subject). Extrapyramidal signs were noted to be minimal at smaller doses and increased at doses greater than 6 mg. Quintana and Keshavan (1995) reported on 4 children (ages 12–17 years) who received risperidone treatment. Of the 4 subjects, 3 responded well to risperidone at dosages of 4–5 mg/day with improvement in positive and negative symptoms. Relatively few side effects were reported. In a retrospective review of 16 children with schizophrenia or schizoaffective disorder, many of whom had previously undergone failed trials of typical agents, Grcevich and colleagues (1996) reported that 15 had a significant reduction in BPRS scores.

Olanzapine.   Another atypical antipsychotic medication, olanzapine, was approved by the FDA in 1996. Sholevar and colleagues (2000) described the use of olanzapine in 15 hospitalized schizophrenic children ages 6–13 years. The majority of patients improved with olanzapine treatment. It was noted that age was inversely correlated with positive response to olanzapine, and patients with no history of antipsychotic use did better than those who had previously undergone a failed medication trial. Kumra et al. (1998a) studied 8 children diagnosed with schizophrenia and compared sequential trials of clozapine and olanzapine. Olanzapine led to a 17% reduction in BPRS scores and a 27% improvement in negative symptoms. However, at 8 weeks with olanzapine treatment, effect size was smaller than the effect size at 6 weeks with clozapine treatment.

Quetiapine.   Quetiapine was introduced in 1997. It has not yet been studied much in children and adolescents with schizophrenia. McConville et al. (2000) studied quetiapine at doses of 100 mg given twice daily and 400 mg given twice daily in 10 children with psychoses, ages 12.3–15.9 years. Improvement in both positive and negative symptoms was observed. Adverse events included postural tachycardia and insomnia, but there were no extrapyramidal symptoms and no increase in prolactin levels.

Ziprasidone.   In February 2001, the newest of the atypical neuroleptics, ziprasidone, was approved by the FDA. It had been studied in pediatric patients before its release. Sallee and colleagues (2000), reporting on a pilot study of 28 children with Tourette's disorder, noted side effects of mild somnolence, but no weight gain or extrapyramidal symptoms (other than akathisia in 1 patient).

Side Effects of Atypical Neuroleptic Treatment. In general, sedation and anticholinergic effects are frequently noted with use of the atypical antipsychotic medications. Extrapyramidal symptoms and neuroleptic malignant syndrome are rare, but they do occur. Buck (2001) notes that each agent in the atypical class can potentially cause serious adverse side effects. Clozapine has been associated with agranulocytosis and seizures, and frequent regular blood sampling is needed if this medication is used. Risperidone and ziprasidone have been associated with prolonged QT interval, which can increase the risk of cardiac arrhythmia and sudden death. Quetiapine has been associated with elevations in liver enzyme levels. The atypical antipsychotics in general have been associated with increased prolactin levels, weight gain, hyperglycemia, and new-onset or worsening diabetes. There is increasing clinical evidence suggesting that diabetes occurs at higher-than-expected rates in patients with schizophrenia who are treated with atypical antipsychotics. The most evidence exists for clozapine, followed by olanzapine. There have been numerous case reports of patients treated with clozapine or olanzapine developing diabetic ketoacidosis—which significantly increases the risk of death—shortly after initiation of treatment (Henderson 2002). Patients treated with atypical antipsychotics should be routinely screened for diabetes and other metabolic disorders. Close monitoring of blood glucose levels, lipid profiles, blood pressure, and changes in body weight is highly recommended in patients treated with atypical antipsychotics.

Research Issues

The current understanding of the etiology and treatment of childhood-onset and adolescence-onset schizophrenia is still quite limited because it is a relatively rare disorder. It is critical to have a multidisciplinary collaborative study at many major research institutions. Such a multicenter study should also include centers from other countries of various racial or ethnic groups. Such a study should examine the similarities and differences between childhood-onset and late adolescence–onset schizophrenia in terms of phenomenology, risk factors, and neurobiological and psychosocial factors. Such studies will provide answers to the question of whether childhood-onset schizophrenia is the same or different from adult-onset schizophrenia. Prospective longitudinal studies of subjects with childhood-onset schizophrenia will provide further data to answer this question. Family and genetic studies based on molecular genetic technologies should also be actively pursued so that effective treatment or prevention of childhood-onset schizophrenia can become possible soon.

In the meantime, carefully designed studies are critically needed to examine the treatment efficacy of the newly developed atypical neuroleptics because there are opponents of medication treatment of schizophrenia who constantly challenge the practice of using medications in individuals with schizophrenia. The medication studies should include short-term and long-term assessment of both treatment efficacy and adverse effects of these new neuroleptics.

References

Alaghband-Rad J, McKenna K, Gordon CT: Childhood-onset schizophrenia: the severity of premorbid course. J Am Acad Child Adolesc Psychiatry 34:1273–1283, 1995

Alaghband-Rad J, Hamburger SD, Giedd JN, et al: Childhood-onset schizophrenia: biological markers in relation to clinical characteristics. Am J Psychiatry 154:64–68, 1997

Altman H, Collins M, Mundy P: Subclinical hallucinations and delusions in nonpsychotic adolescents. J Child Psychol Psychiatry 38:413–420, 1997

American Academy of Child and Adolescent Psychiatry: Practice parameters for the assessment and treatment of children and adolescents with depressive disorders. J Am Acad Child Adolesc Psychiatry 37 (suppl):63S–83S, 1998a

American Academy of Child and Adolescent Psychiatry: Practice parameters for the assessment and treatment of children and adolescents with obsessive-compulsive disorder. J Am Acad Child Adolesc Psychiatry 37 (suppl):27S–45S, 1998b

American Academy of Child and Adolescent Psychiatry: Practice parameters for the assessment and treatment of children and adolescents with schizophrenia. J Am Acad Child Adolesc Psychiatry 40 (suppl):4S–23S, 2001

American Psychiatric Association: Diagnostic and Statistical Manual of Mental Disorders, 2nd Edition. Washington, DC, American Psychiatric Association, 1968

American Psychiatric Association: Diagnostic and Statistical Manual of Mental Disorders, 3rd Edition. Washington, DC, American Psychiatric Association, 1980

American Psychiatric Association: Diagnostic and Statistical Manual of Mental Disorders, 3rd Edition, Revised. Washington, DC, American Psychiatric Association, 1987

American Psychiatric Association: Diagnostic and Statistical Manual of Mental Disorders, 4th Edition. Washington, DC, American Psychiatric Association, 1994

American Psychiatric Association: Practice guidelines for the treatment of patients with schizophrenia. Am J Psychiatry 154(suppl):1–63, 1997

American Psychiatric Association: Diagnostic and Statistical Manual of Mental Disorders, 4th Edition, Text Revision. Washington DC, American Psychiatric Association, 2000

Anderson JC, Williams S, McGee R, et al: DSM-III disorders in preadolescent children. Arch Gen Psychiatry 44:69–76, 1987

Arboleda C, Holzman PS: Thought disorder in children at risk for psychosis. Arch Gen Psychiatry 42:1004–1013, 1985

Armenteros JL, Fennelly BW, Hallin A, et al: Schizophrenia in hospitalized adolescents: clinical diagnosis, DSM-III-R, DSM-IV and ICD-10 criteria. Psychopharmacol Bull 31:383–387, 1995

Armenteros JL, Whitaker AH, Welikson M, et al: Risperidone in adolescents with schizophrenia: an open pilot study. J Am Acad Child Adolesc Psychiatry 36:694–700, 1997

Asarnow JR, Ben-Meir S: Children with schizophrenia spectrum and depressive disorders: a comparative study of premorbid adjustment, onset pattern and severity of impairment. J Child Psychol Psychiatry 29:477–488, 1988

Asarnow R, Sherman T, Strandburg R: The search for the psychobiological substrate of childhood-onset schizophrenia. J Am Acad Child Psychiatry 26:601–614, 1986

Asarnow RF, Tanguay PE, Bott L, et al: Patterns of intellectual functioning in non-retarded autistic and schizophrenic children. J Child Psychol Psychiatry 28:273–280, 1987

Asarnow RF, Asamen J, Granholm E, et al: Cognitive/neuropsychological studies of children with a schizophrenic disorder. Schizophr Bull 20:647–669, 1994

Asarnow RF, Nuechterlein KH, Fogelson D, et al: Schizophrenia and schizophrenia-spectrum personality disorders in the first-degree relatives of children with schizophrenia: the UCLA family study. Arch Gen Psychiatry 58:581–588, 2001

Baltaxe CA, Simmons JQ 3rd: Speech and language disorders in children and adolescents with schizophrenia. Schizophr Bull 21:677–692, 1995

Bassett AS, Hodgkinson K, Chow EW, et al: 22q11 deletion syndrome in adults with schizophrenia. Am J Med Genet 81:328–337, 1998

Bedwell JS, Keller B, Smith AK, et al: Why does postpsychotic IQ decline in childhood-onset schizophrenia? Am J Psychiatry 156:1996–1997, 1999

Benes F, Sunderland P, Jones BD, et al: Normal ventricles in young schizophrenics. Br J Psychiatry 141:90–93, 1982

Bertolino A, Kumra S, Callicott JH, et al: Common pattern of cortical pathology in childhood-onset and adult-onset schizophrenia as identified by proton magnetic resonance spectroscopic imaging. Am J Psychiatry 155:1376–1383, 1998

Birmaher B, Baker R, Kapur S, et al: Clozapine for the treatment of adolescents with schizophrenia. J Am Acad Child Adolesc Psychiatry 31:160–164, 1992

Blanz B, Schmidt MH: Clozapine for schizophrenia (letter). J Am Acad Child Adolesc Psychiatry 32:223–224, 1993

Bleuler E: Dementia Praecox or the Group of Schizophrenias (1911). Translated by Zinkin J. New York, International Universities Press, 1950

Bleuler M: The Schizophrenic Disorders: Long-Term Patient and Family Studies. New Haven, CT, Yale University Press, 1978

Breslin NA, Weinberger DR: Neurodevelopmental implications of findings from brain imaging studies of schizophrenia, in Fetal Neural Development and Adult Schizophrenia. Edited by Mednick SA, Cannon TD, Barr CE, et al. New York, Cambridge University Press, 1991, pp 199–215

Brooks WM, Hodde-Vargas J, Vargas LA, et al: Frontal lobe of children with schizophrenia spectrum disorders: a proton magnetic resonance spectroscopic study. Biol Psychiatry 43:263–269, 1998

Brown AS, Cohen P, Harkavy-Friedman J, et al: A.E. Bennett Research Award. Prenatal rubella, premorbid abnormalities and adult schizophrenia. Biol Psychiatry 49:473–486, 2001

Bryden K, Carrey N, Kutcher S: Update and recommendations for the use of antipsychotics in early onset psychoses. J Child Adolesc Psychopharmacol 11:113–130, 2001

Buck ML: Using the atypical antipsychotic agents in children and adolescents. Pediatric Pharmacotherapy 7(8):1–5, 2001

Buckley PF, Buchanan RW, Tamminga CA, et al: Schizophrenia research: a progress report, summarizing proceedings of the 1999 International Congress on Schizophrenia Research. Schizophr Bull 26:411–419, 2000

Buka SL, Tsuang MT, Torrey EF, et al: Maternal infections and subsequent psychosis among offspring. Arch Gen Psychiatry 58:1032–1037, 2001

Bunk D, Eggers C, Klapal M: Symptom dimensions in the course of childhood-onset schizophrenia. Eur Child Adolesc Psychiatry 8 (suppl 1):129–135, 1999

Burd L, Kerbeshian J: A North Dakota prevalence study of schizophrenia presenting in childhood. J Am Acad Child Adolesc Psychiatry 26:347–350, 1987

Burgess CE, Lindblad K, Sidransky E, et al: Large CAG/CTG repeats are associated with childhood-onset schizophrenia. Mol Psychiatry 3:321–327, 1998

Calderoni D, Wudarsky M, Bhangoo R, et al: Differentiating childhood-onset schizophrenia from psychotic mood disorders. J Am Acad Child Adolesc Psychiatry 40:1190–1196, 2001

Campbell M, Spencer EK, Kowalik SC, et al: Schizophrenia and psychotic disorders, in Textbook of Child and Adolescent Psychiatry, 2nd Edition. Edited by Wiener JM. Washington, DC, American Psychiatric Press, 1997, pp 223–239

Cantor S, Kestenbaum C: Psychotherapy with schizophrenic children. J Am Acad Child Psychiatry 25:623–630, 1986

Cantor S, Evans J, Pearce J, et al: Childhood schizophrenia: present but not accounted for. Am J Psychiatry 139:758–762, 1982

Caplan R: Communication deficits in children with schizophrenia spectrum disorders. Schizophr Bull 20:671–684, 1994a

Caplan R: Thought disorder in childhood. J Am Acad Child Adolesc Psychiatry 33:605–615, 1994b

Caplan R, Guthrie D, Fish B, et al: The Kiddie Formal Thought Disorder Rating Scale: clinical assessment, reliability, and validity. J Am Acad Child Adolesc Psychiatry 28:408–416, 1989

Caplan R, Perdue S, Tanguay PE, et al: Formal thought disorder in childhood-onset schizophrenia and schizotypal personality disorder. J Child Psychol Psychiatry 31:169–177, 1990

Caplan R, Guthrie D, Foy JG: Communication deficits and formal thought disorder in schizophrenic children. J Am Acad Child Adolesc Psychiatry 31:151–159, 1992

Caplan R, Guthrie D, Shields WD, et al: Communication deficits in children undergoing temporal lobectomy. J Am Acad Child Adolesc Psychiatry 32:604–611, 1993

Caplan R, Guthrie D, Komo S: Conversational repair in schizophrenic and normal children. J Am Acad Child Adolesc Psychiatry 35:950–958, 1996

Caplan R, Guthrie D, Tang B, et al: Thought disorder in childhood schizophrenia: replication and update of concept. J Am Acad Child Adolesc Psychiatry 39:771–778, 2000

Caplan R, Guthrie D, Tang B, et al: Thought disorder in attention-deficit hyperactivity disorder. J Am Acad Child Adolesc Psychiatry 40:965–912, 2001

Carlson GA: Child and adolescent mania: diagnostic considerations. J Child Psychol Psychiatry 31:331–342, 1990

Carlson GA, Kashani JH: Phenomenology of major depression from childhood through adulthood: analysis of three studies. Am J Psychiatry 145:1222–1225, 1988

Carlson GA, Strober M: Manic-depressive illness in early adolescence. J Am Acad Child Psychiatry 17:138–153, 1978

Carlson GA, Bromert EJ, Sievers S: Phenomenology and outcome of subjects with early and adult-onset psychotic mania. Am J Psychiatry 157:213–219, 2000

Chambers WJ, Puig-Antich J, Tabrizi MA, et al: Psychotic symptoms in pre-pubertal major depressive disorder. Arch Gen Psychiatry 39:921–927, 1982

Chouinard G, Jones B, Remington G, et al: A Canadian multicenter placebo-controlled study of fixed doses of risperidone and haloperidol in the treatment of chronic schizophrenic patients. J Clin Psychopharmacol 13:25–40, 1993

Cozza SJ, Edison DL: Risperidone in adolescents (letter). J Am Acad Child Adolesc Psychiatry 33:1211, 1994

Creak M, Cameron K, Cowie V, et al: Schizophrenic syndrome in childhood. Br Med J 2:889–890, 1961

Del Beccaro MA, Burke P, McCauley E: Hallucinations in children: a follow-up study. J Am Acad Child Adolesc Psychiatry 27:462–465, 1988

Demirkiran M, Jankovic J, Dean JM: Ecstasy intoxication: an overlap between serotonin syndrome and neuroleptic malignant syndrome. Clin Neuropharmacol 19:157–164, 1996

Done DJ, Johnstone EC, Frith CD, et al: Complications of pregnancy and delivery in relation to psychosis in adult life: data from the British perinatal mortality survey sample. BMJ 302:1576–1580, 1991

Eagles JM, Gibson I, Bremner MH, et al: Obstetric complications in DSM-III schizophrenics and their siblings. Lancet 335:1139–1141, 1990

Eggers C: Course and prognosis of childhood schizophrenia. J Autism Child Schizophr 8:21–36, 1978

Eggers C: Schizoaffective psychosis in childhood: a follow-up study. J Autism Dev Disord 19:327–334, 1989

Eggers C, Bunk D: The long-term course of childhood-onset schizophrenia: a 42-year follow-up. Schizophr Bull 23:105–117, 1997

Erlenmeyer-Kimling L, Cornblatt B: High-risk research in schizophrenia: a summary of what has been learned. J Psychiatr Res 21:401–411, 1987

Erlenmeyer-Kimling L, Folgenovic Z, Hrabak-Zerjavic V, et al: Schizophrenia and prenatal exposure to the 1957 A2 influenza epidemic in Croatia. Am J Psychiatry 151:1496–1498, 1994

Falloon IRH: Psychotherapy for schizophrenic disorders: a review. Br J Hosp Med 48:164–170, 1992

Famularo R, Kinscherff R, Fenton T: Psychiatric diagnoses of maltreated children: preliminary finding. J Am Acad Child Adolesc Psychiatry 31:863–867, 1992

Feinberg I: Schizophrenia: caused by a fault in programmed synaptic elimination during adolescence? J Psychiatr Res 17:319–334, 1982–1983

Findling RL, Friedman L, Henny JT, et al: Hippocampal volume in adolescent schizophrenia. Schizophr Res 18:185–188, 1996

Fras I, Major LF: Clinical experience with risperidone (letter). J Am Acad Child Adolesc Psychiatry 34:833, 1995

Frazier JA, Gordon CT, McKenna K, et al: An open trial of clozapine in 11 adolescents with childhood-onset schizophrenia. J Am Acad Child Adolesc Psychiatry 33:658–663, 1994

Frazier JA, Giedd JA, Hamburger SD, et al: Brain anatomic magnetic resonance imaging in childhood-onset schizophrenia. Arch Gen Psychiatry 53:617–624, 1996

Frazier JA, Alaghband-Rad J, Jacobsen L, et al: Pubertal development and onset of psychosis in childhood-onset schizophrenia. Psychiatry Res 70:1–7, 1997

Friedman L, Schulz SC, Jesberger JA: Smooth pursuit eye movement performance in adolescent-onset psychosis. Schizophr Res 9:157, 1993

Friedman L, Findling RL, Buch J, et al. Structural MRI and neuropsychological assessments in adolescent patients with either schizophrenia or affective disorders. Schizophr Res 18:189–190, 1996

Galdos PM, Van Os J, Murray RM: Puberty and onset of psychosis. Schizophr Res 10:7–14, 1993

Garralda ME: Hallucinations in children with conduct and emotional disorders, I: the clinical phenomena. Psychol Med 14:589–596, 1984a

Garralda ME: Hallucinations in children with conduct and emotional disorders, II: the follow-up study. Psychol Med 14:597–604, 1984b

Garralda ME: Characteristics of the psychoses of late onset in children and adolescents (a comparative study of hallucinating children). J Adolesc 8:195–207, 1985

Goldstein MJ: Psychosocial treatment of schizophrenia, in Schizophrenia: Scientific Progress. Edited by Schulz SC, Tamminga CA. New York, Oxford University Press, 1989, pp 318–324

Gordon CT, Frazier JA, McKenna K, et al: Childhood-onset schizophrenia: an NIMH study in progress. Schizophr Bull 20:697–712, 1994

Gottesman II, Bertelsen A: Confirming unexpressed genotypes for schizophrenia: risks in the offspring of Fischer's Danish identical and fraternal discordant twins. Arch Gen Psychiatry 46:867–872, 1989

Gottesman II, Shields J: Schizophrenia and Genetics: A Twin Study Vantage Point. New York, Academic Press, 1972

Gottesman II, Shields J, Hanson DR: Schizophrenia: The Epigenetic Puzzle. New York, Cambridge University Press, 1982

Gottesman II, McGuffin P, Farmer AE: Clinical genetics as clues to the "real" genetics of schizophrenia: a decade of modest gains while playing for time. Schizophr Bull 13:23–47, 1987

Grcevich SJ, Findling RL, Rowane WA, et al: Risperidone in the treatment of children and adolescents with schizophrenia: a retrospective study. J Child Adolesc Psychopharmacol 6:251–257, 1996

Green WH, Padron-Gayol M: Schizophrenic disorder in childhood: its relationship to DSM-III criteria, in Biological Psychiatry 1985. Edited by Shagass C, Josiassen RC, Bridger WH, et al. New York, Elsevier, 1986, pp 1484–1486

Green WH, Campbell M, Hardesty AS, et al: A comparison of schizophrenic and autistic children. J Am Acad Child Psychiatry 23:399–409, 1984

Green WH, Pardon-Gayol M, Hardesty AS, et al: Schizophrenia with childhood-onset: a phenomenological study of 38 cases. J Am Acad Child Adolesc Psychiatry 31:968–976, 1992

Gunther-Genta F, Bovet P, Hohlfeld P: Obstetric complications and schizophrenia: a case-control study. Br J Psychiatry 164:165–170, 1994

Hall W, Degenhardt L: Cannabis use and psychosis: a review of clinical and epidemiological evidence. Aust N Z J Psychiatry 34:26–34, 2000

Hanson DR, Gottesman II, Heston LL: Some possible childhood indicators of adult schizophrenia inferred from children of schizophrenics. Br J Psychiatry 129:142–154, 1976

Heinssen RK, Liberman RP, Kopelowicz A: Psychosocial skills training for schizophrenia: lessons from the laboratory. Schizophr Bull 26:21–46, 2000

Henderson DC: Atypical antipsychotic-induced diabetes mellitus. CNS Drugs 16(2):77–89, 2002

Hendren RL, Hodde-Varges J, Yeo RA, et al: Neuropsychophysiological study of children at risk for schizophrenia: a preliminary report. J Am Acad Child Adolesc Psychiatry 34:1284–1291, 1995

Hendren RL, De Backer I, Pandina GJ: Review of neuroimaging studies of child and adolescent psychiatric disorders from the past 10 years. J Am Acad Child Adolesc Psychiatry 39:815–827, 2000

Heston LL: Psychiatric disorders in foster home reared children of schizophrenic mothers. Br J Psychiatry 112:819–825, 1966

Hogarty GE, Anderson CM, Reiss DJ, et al: Family psychoeducation, social skills training, and maintenance chemotherapy in the aftercare treatment of schizophrenia, I: one-year effects of a controlled study on relapse and expressed emotion. Arch Gen Psychiatry 43:633–642, 1986

Hollingshead AB: Two Factor Index of Social Position. New Haven, CT, privately printed, 1965

Hornstein JL, Putnam FW: Clinical phenomenology of child and adolescent dissociative disorders. J Am Acad Child Adolesc Psychiatry 31:1077–1085, 1992

Howells JG, Guirguis WR: Childhood schizophrenia 20 years later. Arch Gen Psychiatry 41:123–128, 1984

Jacobsen LK, Rapoport J: Research update: childhood-onset schizophrenia: implications of clinical and neurobiological research. J Child Psychol Psychiatry 39:101–113, 1998

Jacobsen LK, Giedd JN, Vaituzis AC, et al: Temporal lobe morphology in childhood-onset schizophrenia. Am J Psychiatry 153:355–361, 1996a

Jacobsen LK, Hong WL, Hommer DW, et al: Smooth pursuit eye movements in childhood-onset schizophrenia: comparison with attention-deficit hyperactivity disorder and normal controls. Biol Psychiatry 40:1144–1154, 1996b

Jacobsen LK, Frazier JA, Malhotra AK, et al: Cerebrospinal fluid monoamine metabolites in childhood-onset schizophrenia. Am J Psychiatry 154:69–74, 1997a

Jacobsen LK, Giedd JN, Berquin PC, et al: Quantitative morphology of the cerebellum and fourth ventricle in childhood-onset schizophrenia. Am J Psychiatry 154:1663–1669, 1997b

Jacobsen LK, Giedd JN, Tanrikut C, et al: Three-dimensional cortical morphometry of the planum temporale in childhood-onset schizophrenia. Am J Psychiatry 154:685–687, 1997c

Jacobsen LK, Giedd JN, Vaituzis AC, et al: Quantitative magnetic resonance imaging of the corpus callosum in childhood-onset schizophrenia. Psychiatry Res 68:77–86, 1997d

Jacobsen LK, Hamburger SD, Van Horn JD, et al: Cerebral glucose metabolism in childhood-onset schizophrenia. Psychiatry Res 75:131–144, 1997e

Jacobsen LK, Giedd JN, Castellanos FX, et al: Progressive reduction of temporal lobe structures in childhood-onset schizophrenia. Am J Psychiatry 155:678–685, 1998a

Jacobsen LK, Mittleman BB, Kumra S, et al: HLA antigens in childhood-onset schizophrenia. Psychiatry Res 78:123–132, 1998b

Jennings WS, Schulz SC, Narasimhachari N, et al: Brain ventricular size and CSF monoamine metabolites in an adolescent inpatient population. Psychiatry Res 16:87–94, 1985

Kafantaris V, Ernst M, Samuel R, et al: Psychotic disorders in hospitalized adolescents: diagnostic issues (abstract), in Scientific Proceedings, 39th Annual Meeting of the American Academy of Child and Adolescent Psychiatry, Washington, DC, October 20–25, 1992. Washington, DC, American Academy of Child and Adolescent Psychiatry, 1992, p 63

Kaiser R, Konneker M, Henneken M, et al: Dopamine D_4 receptor 48-bp repeat polymorphism: no association with response to antipsychotic treatment, but association with catatonic schizophrenia. Mol Psychiatry 5:418–424, 2000

Karatekin C, Asarnow RF: Working memory in childhood-onset schizophrenia and attention-deficit/hyperactivity disorder. Psychiatry Res 17:165–176, 1998

Karno M, Norquist GS: Schizophrenia: epidemiology, in Comprehensive Textbook of Psychiatry, 5th Edition, Vol 1. Edited by Kaplan HI, Sadock BJ. Baltimore, MD, Williams & Wilkins, 1989, pp 699–705

Karp BI, Garvey M, Jacobsen LK, et al: Abnormal neurologic maturation in adolescents with early onset schizophrenia. Am J Psychiatry 158:118–122, 2001

Kay SR, Fishbein A, Opier LA: The positive and negative syndrome scale (PANSS) for schizophrenia. Schizophr Bull 13:261–276, 1987

Kendell RE, Kemp JW: Maternal influenza in the etiology of schizophrenia. Arch Gen Psychiatry 46:878–882, 1989

Kendler KS, Diehl SR: The genetics of schizophrenia: a current, genetic-epidemiologic perspective, in Special Report: Schizophrenia 1993 (NIMH Publ No 93-3499). Edited by Shore D. Rockville, MD, U.S. Department of Health and Human Services, 1993, pp 87–111

Kendler KS, McGuire M, Gruenberg AM, et al: The Roscommon Family Study, I: methods, diagnosis of probands, and risk of schizophrenia in relatives. Arch Gen Psychiatry 50:527–540, 1993a

Kendler KS, McGuire M, Gruenberg AM, et al: The Roscommon Family Study, II: the risk of nonschizophrenic nonaffective psychoses in relatives. Arch Gen Psychiatry 50:645–652, 1993b

Kendler KS, McGuire, Gruenberg AM, et al: The Roscommon Family Study, III: schizophrenia-related personality disorders in relatives. Arch Gen Psychiatry 50:781–788, 1993c

Keshavan MS, Anderson S, Pettegrew JW: Is schizophrenia due to excessive synaptic pruning in the prefrontal cortex? The Feinberg hypothesis revisited. J Psychiatr Res 28:239–265, 1994

Kety SS, Rosenthal D, Wender PH, et al: Mental illness in the biological and adoptive families of adopted individuals who have become schizophrenic, in Genetic Research in Psychiatry. Edited by Fieve RR, Rosenthal D, Brill H. Baltimore, MD, Johns Hopkins University Press, 1975, pp 147–165

Kety SS, Wender PH, Jacobsen B, et al: Mental illness in the biological and adoptive relatives of schizophrenic adoptees: replication of the Copenhagen study in the rest of Denmark. Arch Gen Psychiatry 51:442–455, 1994

Kilgus MD, Pumariega AJ, Cuffe SP: Influence of race on diagnosis in adolescent psychiatric inpatients. J Am Acad Child Adolesc Psychiatry 34:67–72, 1995

Kolvin I: Psychoses in childhood: a comparative study, in Infantile Autism: Concepts, Characteristics and Treatment. Edited by Rutter M. Edinburgh, Churchill Livingstone, 1971a, pp 7–26

Kolvin I: Studies in the childhood psychoses, I: diagnostic criteria and classification. Br J Psychiatry 118:381–384, 1971b

Kolvin I, Ounsted C, Humphrey M, et al: Studies in the childhood psychoses, II: the phenomenology of childhood psychoses. Br J Psychiatry 118:385–395, 1971a

Kolvin I, Ounsted C, Richardson LM, et al: Studies in the childhood psychoses, III: the family and social background in childhood psychoses. Br J Psychiatry 118:396–402, 1971b

Kolvin I, Garside RF, Kidd JS: Studies in the childhood psychoses, IV: parental personality and attitude and childhood psychoses. Br J Psychiatry 118:403–406, 1971c

Kraepelin E: Dementia Praecox and Paraphrenia (1899). Translated by Barclay RM from the 8th German edition of the Textbook of Psychiatry. Edinburgh, Livingstone, 1919

Krausz M, Muller-Thomsen T: Schizophrenia with onset in adolescence: an 11-year followup. Schizophr Bull 19:831–841, 1993

Kumra S, Frazier JA, Jacobsen LK, et al: Childhood-onset schizophrenia: a double-blind clozapine-haloperidol comparison. Arch Gen Psychiatry 53:1090–1097, 1996

Kumra S, Jacobsen LK, Lenane M, et al: Childhood-onset schizophrenia: an open label study of olanzapine in adolescents. J Am Acad Child Adolesc Psychiatry 37:377–385, 1998a

Kumra S, Jacobsen LK, Lenane M, et al: "Multidimensionally impaired disorder": is it a variant of very early onset schizophrenia? J Am Acad Child Adolesc Psychiatry 37:91–99, 1998b

Kumra S, Wiggs E, Krasnewich D, et al: Brief report: association of sex chromosome anomalies with childhood-onset psychotic disorder. J Am Acad Child Adolesc Psychiatry 37:292–296, 1998c

Kumra S, Briguglio C, Lenane M, et al: Including children and adolescents with schizophrenia in medication-free research. Am J Psychiatry 156:1065–1068, 1999

Kunugi H, Hattori M, Nanko S, et al: Dinucleotide repeat polymorphism in the neurotrophin-3 gene and hippocampal volume in psychoses. Schizophr Res 37:271–273, 1999

Kydd RR, Werry JS: Schizophrenia in children under 16 years. J Autism Dev Disord 12:343–357, 1982

Levy DL, Holzman PS, Matthysse S, et al: Eye tracking dysfunction and schizophrenia: a critical perspective. Schizophr Bull 19:461–536, 1993

Lewine RRJ: Comments on "Puberty and the onset of psychosis" by P.M. Galdos et al. Schizophr Res 13:81–83, 1994

Lewis SW, MJ Owen, Murray RM: Obstetric complications and schizophrenia: methodology and mechanisms, in Schizophrenia: Scientific Progress. Edited by Schulz SC, Tamminga CA. New York, Oxford University Press, 1989, pp 56–68

Lindsay J, Ounsted C, Richards P: Long-term outcome in children with temporal lobe seizures, II: marriage, parenthood, and sexual indifference. Dev Med Child Neurol 21:433–440, 1979

Loranger AW: Sex difference in age at onset of schizophrenia. Arch Gen Psychiatry 41:157–161, 1984

Makita K: The age of onset of childhood schizophrenia. Folia Psychiatr Neurol Jpn 20:111–121, 1966

Mandoki MW: Risperidone treatment of children and adolescents: increased risk of extrapyramidal side effects? J Child Adolesc Psychopharmacol 5:49–67, 1995

Marcus J: Cerebral functioning in offspring of schizophrenics: a possible genetic factor. Int J Ment Health 3:57–73, 1974

Marcus J, Hans SL, Lewow E, et al: Neurological findings in high-risk children: childhood assessment and 5-year follow-up. Schizophr Bull 11:85–100, 1985

Marder SR, Meibach RC: Risperidone in the treatment of schizophrenia. Am J Psychiatry 151:825–835, 1994

Maziade M, Bouchard S, Gingras N, et al: Long-term stability of diagnosis and symptom dimensions in a systematic sample of patients with onset of schizophrenia in childhood and early adolescence, II: postnegative distinction and childhood predictors of adult outcome. Br J Psychiatry 169:371–378, 1996

McClellan J, McCurry C: Neurocognitive pathways in development of schizophrenia. Semin Clin Neuropsychiatry 3:320–332, 1998

McClellan J, McCurry C: Early onset psychotic disorders: diagnostic stability and clinical characteristics. Eur Child Adolesc Psychiatry 8 (suppl 2):1S–7S, 1999

McClellan J, Werry J: Practice parameters for the assessment and treatment of children and adolescents with schizophrenia. J Am Acad Child Adolesc Psychiatry 33:616–635, 1994

McClellan JM, Werry S, Ham M: A follow-up study of early onset psychosis: comparison between outcome diagnoses of schizophrenia, mood disorder and personality disorders. J Autism Dev Disord 23:243–262, 1993

McConville B, Arvanitis L, Thyrum PT, et al: Pharmacokinetics, tolerability and clinical effectiveness of quetiapine fumarate in adolescents with selected psychotic disorders. J Clin Psychiatry 61:252–260, 2000

McGlashan TH: Adolescent versus adult onset of mania. Am J Psychiatry 145:221–223, 1988

McKenna K, Gordon CT, Lenane M, et al: Looking for childhood-onset schizophrenia: the first 71 cases screened. J Am Acad Child Adolesc Psychiatry 33:636–644, 1994a

McKenna K, Gordon CT, Rapoport JL: Childhood-onset schizophrenia: timely neurobiological research. J Am Acad Child Adolesc Psychiatry 33:771–781, 1994b

Mednick S, Schulsinger F: Some premorbid characteristics related to breakdown in children with schizophrenic mothers, in The Transmission of Schizophrenia: Proceedings of the Second Research Conference of the Foundations' Fund for Research in Psychiatry, Dorado, Puerto Rico, 26 June to 1 July 1967. Edited by Rosenthal D, Kety SS. New York, Pergamon, 1968, pp 267–291

Mednick SA, Machon RA, Huttunen MO, et al: Adult schizophrenia following prenatal exposure to an influenza epidemic. Arch Gen Psychiatry 45:189–192, 1988

Mirsky AF, Silberman EK, Latz A, et al: Adult outcomes of high-risk children: differential effects of town and kibbutz rearing. Schizophr Bull 11:150–154, 1985

Mittleman BB, Castellanos FX, Jacobsen LK, et al: Cerebrospinal fluid cytokines in pediatric neuropsychiatric disease. J Immunol 159:2994–2999, 1997

Morgan V, Castle D, Page A, et al: Influenza epidemics and incidence of schizophrenia, affective disorder and mental retardation in Western Australia: no evidence of a major effect. Schizophr Res 26:25–39, 1997

Moriniere S, Saada C, Holbert S, et al: Detection of polyglutamine expansion in a new acidic protein: a candidate for childhood-onset schizophrenia? Mol Psychiatry 4:58–63, 1999

Murphy KC, Jones LA, Owen MJ: High rates of schizophrenia in adults with velo-cardio-facial syndrome. Arch Gen Psychiatry 56:940–945, 1999

Nicolson R, Rapoport JL: Childhood-onset schizophrenia: rare but worth studying. Biol Psychiatry 46:1418–1428, 1999

Nicolson R, Giedd J, Lenane M, et al: Clinical and neurobiological correlates of cytogenetic abnormalities in childhood-onset schizophrenia. Am J Psychiatry 156:1575–1579, 1999

Nicolson R, Lenane M, Singaracharlu S, et al: Premorbid speech and language impairments in childhood-onset schizophrenia: association with risk factors. Am J Psychiatry 157:794–800, 2000

Nopoulos PC, Giedd JN, Andreasen NC, et al: Frequency and severity of enlarged cavum septi pellucidi in childhood-onset schizophrenia. Am J Psychiatry 155:1074–1079, 1998

O'Callaghan E, Sham P, Takei N, et al: Schizophrenia after prenatal exposure to 1958 A$_2$ influenza epidemic. Lancet 337:1248–1250, 1991

O'Callaghan, Gibson T, Colohan HA, et al: Risk of schizophrenia in adults born after obstetric complications and their association with early onset of illness: a controlled study. BMJ 305:1256–1259, 1993

Offord DR, Cross LA: Behavioral antecedents of adult schizophrenia: a review. Arch Gen Psychiatry 21:267–283, 1969

Overall JE, Gorham DR: The Brief Psychiatric Rating Scale. Psychol Rep 10:799–812, 1962

Parnas J, Schulsinger F, Schulsinger H, et al: Behavioral precursors of schizophrenia spectrum. Arch Gen Psychiatry 39:658–664, 1982

Petty LK, Ornitz EM, Michelman JD, et al: Autistic children who become schizophrenic. Arch Gen Psychiatry 41:129–135, 1984

Pilowsky D, Chambers WJ (eds): Hallucinations in Childhood. Washington, DC, American Psychiatric Press, 1986

Poole D, Bloom W, Mielke DH, et al: A controlled evaluation of Loxitane in seventy-five adolescent schizophrenic patients. Curr Ther Res Clin Exp 19:99–104, 1976

Puig-Antich J, Ryan N, Rabinovich H: Affective disorders in childhood and adolescence, in Diagnosis and Psychopharmacology of Childhood and Adolescent Disorders. Edited by Wiener J. New York, Wiley, 1985, pp 113–150

Quintana H, Keshavan M: Case study: risperidone in children and adolescents with schizophrenia. J Am Acad Child Adolesc Psychiatry 34:1292–1296, 1995

Rapoport JL, Giedd J, Kumra S, et al: Childhood-onset schizophrenia. Progressive ventricular change during adolescence. Arch Gen Psychiatry 54:897–903, 1997

Rapoport JL, Giedd JN, Blumenthal J: Progressive cortical change during adolescence in childhood-onset schizophrenia: a longitudinal magnetic resonance imaging study. Arch Gen Psychiatry 56:649–654, 1999

Remschmidt H, Martin M, Schulz E, et al: The concept of positive and negative schizophrenia in child and adolescent psychiatry, in Negative Versus Positive Schizophrenia. Edited by Marneros A, Andreasen NC, Tsuang MT. New York, Springer-Verlag, 1991, pp 219–242

Remschmidt H, Schulz E, Martin M: Die Behandlung schizophrener Psychosen in der Adoleszenz mit Clozapin (Leponex) [The treatment of schizophrenic psychoses in adolescence with clozapine (Leponex)], in Clozapin, Pharmakologie und Klinik eines atypischen Neuroleptikums. Eine kritische Bestands-aufnahme [Clozapine, Pharmacology and Clinical Properties of an Atypical Neuroleptic]. Edited by Naber D, Müller-Spahn F. Stuttgart, Schattauer, 1992, pp 99–119

Remschmidt HE, Schulz E, Martin M: An open trial of clozapine in thirty-six adolescents with schizophrenia. J Child Adolesc Psychopharmacol 4:31–41, 1994

Rieder RO, Nichols PL: Offspring of schizophrenics, III. Arch Gen Psychiatry 36:665–674, 1979

Rothstein A: Hallucinatory phenomena in childhood: a critique of the literature. J Am Acad Child Psychiatry 20:623–635, 1981

Russell AT: The clinical presentation of childhood-onset schizophrenia. Schizophr Bull 20:631–646, 1994

Russell AT, Bott L, Sammons C: The phenomenology of schizophrenia occurring in childhood. J Am Acad Child Adolesc Psychiatry 28:399–407, 1989

Rutter M: Childhood schizophrenia reconsidered. J Autism Child Schizophr 2:315–337, 1972

Rutter M, Schopler E: Autism and pervasive developmental disorders: concept and diagnostic issues. J Autism Dev Disord 17:159–186, 1987

Sallee FR, Kurlan R, Goetz CG, et al: Ziprasidone treatment of children and adolescents with Tourette's syndrome: a pilot study. J Am Acad Child Adolesc Psychiatry 39:292–299, 2000

Schulz SC, Koller MM, Kishore PR, et al: Ventricular enlargement in teenage patients with schizophrenia spectrum disorder. Am J Psychiatry 140:1592–1595, 1983

Schulz SC, Findling RL, Wise A, et al: Child and adolescent schizophrenia. Psychiatr Clin North Am 21:43–56, 1998

Selten JP, Brown AS, Moons KG, et al: Prenatal exposure to the 1957 influenza pandemic and non-affective psychosis in the Netherlands. Schizophr Res 38:85–91, 1999

Sholevar EH, Baron DA, Hardie TL: Treatment of childhood-onset schizophrenia with olanzapine. J Child Adolesc Psychopharmacol 10:69–78, 2000

Simeon JG, Carrey NJ, Wiggins DM, et al: Risperidone effects in treatment-resistant adolescents: preliminary case reports. J Child Adolesc Psychopharmacol 5:69–79, 1995

Spencer EK, Campbell M: Children with schizophrenia: diagnosis, phenomenology, and pharmacotherapy. Schizophr Bull 20:713–725, 1994

Spencer EK, Alpert M, Pouget ER, et al: Baseline characteristics and side-effect profile as predictors of haloperidol treatment outcome in schizophrenic children. Paper presented at National Institute of Mental Health New Clinical Drug Evaluation Unit 34th annual meeting, Marco Island, FL, May–June 1994

Sporn A, Rapoport J: Childhood-onset schizophrenia. Child and Adolescent Psychopharmacology News 2:1–6, 2001

Susser E, Lin S, Brown A, et al: No increase in schizophrenia after prenatal exposure to influenza. Am J Psychiatry 151:922–924, 1994

Taylor MA, Gaztanaga P, Abrams R: Manic-depressive illness and acute schizophrenia: a clinical, family history and treatment-response study. Am J Psychiatry 131:678–682, 1974

Thomas MA, Ke Y, Levitt J: Preliminary study of frontal lobe ^{1}H MR spectroscopy in childhood-onset schizophrenia. J Magn Reson Imaging 8:841–846, 1998

Thomsen PS: Schizophrenia with childhood and adolescent onset: a nationwide register-based study. Acta Psychiatr Scand 94:187–193, 1996

Tolbert HA: Psychoses in children and adolescents: a review. J Clin Psychiatry 57 (suppl 3):4–8, 1996

Turetz M, Mozes T, Toren P, et al: An open trial of clozapine in neuroleptic-resistant childhood-onset schizophrenia. Br J Psychiatry 170:507–510, 1997

Usiskin SI, Nicolson R, Krasnewich DM, et al: Velocardiofacial syndrome in childhood-onset schizophrenia. J Am Acad Child Adolesc Psychiatry 38:1536–1543, 1999

Verdoux H, Geddes JR, Takei N, et al: Obstetric complications and age at onset in schizophrenia: an international collaborative meta-analysis of individual patient data. Am J Psychiatry 154:1220–1227, 1997

Volkmar FR: Childhood schizophrenia, in Child and Adolescent Psychiatry, A Comprehensive Textbook. Edited by Lewis M. Baltimore, MD, Williams & Wilkins, 1996, pp 629–635

Volkmar FR, Cohen DJ, Hoshino Y, et al: Phenomenology and classification of the childhood psychoses. Psychol Med 18:191–201, 1988

Walters V, McClellan J: Psychotic symptoms in seriously mentally ill youth. Poster presented at the annual meeting of the American Academy of Child and Adolescent Psychiatry, Anaheim, CA, October 27–November 1, 1998

Watkins JM, Asarnow RF, Tanguay PE: Symptom development in childhood-onset schizophrenia. J Child Psychol Psychiatry 29:865–878, 1988

Weinberger DR: Implications of normal brain development for the pathogenesis of schizophrenia. Arch Gen Psychiatry 44:660–669, 1987

Werry JS: The childhood psychoses, in Psychopathological Disorders of Childhood, 2nd Edition. Edited by Quay HC, Werry JS. New York, Wiley, 1979, pp 41–89

Werry JS: Child and adolescent (early onset) schizophrenia: a review in light of DSM-III-R. J Autism Dev Disord 22:601–624, 1992

Werry JS, Taylor E: Schizophrenia and allied disorders, in Child and Adolescent Psychiatry: Modern Approaches, 3rd Edition. Edited by Rutter M, Taylor EA, Hersov LA. Boston, MA, Blackwell Scientific, 1994, pp 594–615

Werry JS, McClellan JM, Chard L: Childhood and adolescent schizophrenic, bipolar, and schizoaffective disorders: a clinical and outcome study. J Am Acad Child Adolesc Psychiatry 30:457–465, 1991

Werry JS, McClellan JM, Andrews LK, et al: Clinical features and outcome of child and adolescent schizophrenia. Schizophr Bull 20:619–630, 1994

World Health Organization: International Classification of Diseases, 9th Revision. Geneva, World Health Organization, 1977

Yan WL, Guan XY, Green ED, et al: Childhood-onset schizophrenia/autistic disorder and t(1;7) reciprocal translocation: identification of a BAC contig spanning the translocation breakpoint at 7q21. Am J Med Genet 96:749–753, 2000

Yeo RA, Hodde-Vargas J, Hendren RL, et al: Brain abnormalities in schizophrenia-spectrum children: implications for a neurodevelopmental perspective. Psychiatr Res 76:1–13, 1997

Zahn TP, Jacobsen LK, Gordon CT, et al: Autonomic nervous system markers of psychopathology in childhood-onset schizophrenia. Arch Gen Psychiatry 54:904–912, 1997

Mood Disorders in Prepubertal Children

Elizabeth B. Weller, M.D.

Ronald A. Weller, M.D.

Arman K. Danielyan, M.D.

Early-onset mood disorders are chronic and recurrent conditions that have a high likelihood of persisting into adulthood. Despite their potentially debilitating effects on growth and development—including school failure, school dropout (Weinberg and Rehmet 1983), and the risk of suicide attempts and completed suicide—mood disorders in prepubertal children have received little attention until recently. Childhood depression was not officially recognized in the United States until the 1975 National Institute of Mental Health (NIMH) Conference on Depression in Childhood (Schulterbrandt and Raskin 1977), at which it was concluded that adult criteria could be used to diagnose depression in children if appropriate modifications were made to accommodate for age and stage of development. Recognition of depression in children and adolescents in Europe had taken place in 1971, when the Union of European Pedopsychiatrists officially recognized and addressed the needs of depressed children and adolescents by declaring that depression is an important illness that constitutes a significant proportion of mental disorders in children and adolescents.

In the past, childhood mood disorders were underdiagnosed and misdiagnosed (E.B. Weller et al. 1995). Affective disorders in prepubertal children are now receiving much more attention but continue to present difficult diagnostic problems. Underdiagnosis of childhood bipolar disorder has been noted by several authors—a high prevalence of underdiagnosis on inpatient services (Gammon et al. 1983; Isaac 1995) and a high prevalence of undiagnosed cases on chart reviews (R.A. Weller et al. 1986). This tendency toward underdiagnosis has been partly due to the belief that a child's immature superego and personality structure do not permit the development or experience of a mood disorder (Koran 1975). Another factor is that many children lack the capacity to express their emotions verbally and thus tend to present with somatic symptoms and complaints of "not feeling well," which in turn is seen by pediatricians as evidence of physical illness. As to the difficulties of diagnosing mania in children, Ziehen (1902) wrote, "The behavior of a normal child resembles closely hypomanic activity and any slight variations are not apt to be noticed." Another source of underdiagnosis of early-onset mood disorders is that parents who are bipolar—and therefore at increased risk of having bipolar offspring—themselves remain underdiagnosed (Geller 1996). These parents may not recognize the pathological implications of manic behaviors in their children.

Difficulties in diagnosing mania and depression in children also may be due to the fact that language does not begin to be used as a main source for communicating information appropriately until about age 7 years. Unfortunately, it has become common practice to use quick checklists or to talk only to parents about the child rather than to carefully evaluate the child directly and to listen to what the child has to say. Without a direct evaluation of the child, the core symptoms of mood disorders (feeling sad, having low self-esteem, feeling inadequate, having suicidal thoughts) may be missed and only symptoms that motivate parents to bring their children for treatment (irritability, getting in fights, and other disruptive behaviors) may be detected (Cantwell and Carlson 1983; E.B. Weller and Weller 1984). Another problem is that the clinical presentation of bipolar disorder in children very often shows similarities with externalizing disorders, such as attention-deficit/hyperactivity disorder (ADHD) and conduct disorder. It is now well established that bipolar disorder in prepubertal children is frequently comorbid with externalizing disorders and can present in a rapid-cycling or "mixed" picture (Bowring and Kovacs 1992; Kovacs and Pollock 1995; Milberger et al. 1995). Previously, children and adolescents with mood disorders were often diagnosed with adjustment disorder, conduct disorder, ADHD, and schizophrenia (Akiskal and Weller 1989). Clinical descriptions in case reports and case series suggest that both a developmentally different presentation of bipolar disorder in young children (Carlson 1984; Weinberg and Brumback 1976; R.A. Weller et al. 1986) and symptom overlap with ADHD (Carlson 1984; Potter 1983; Poznanski et al. 1984; Reiss 1985) make it difficult to diagnose bipolar disorder in children.

History of Childhood Mood Disorders

Kraepelin (1921) believed that mania existed in prepubertal children and that the occurrence of mania increased with the onset of puberty. Of 900 manic patients he studied, 0.4% had the onset of mania before age 10 years. Kraepelin also presented the case of a 5-year-old boy with mania. Kasanin (1931) also believed that mood disorders can originate at a young age, and, along with Homburger (1926), he believed there was a tendency to classify mood disturbances that occurred in children as childhood schizophrenia. In a review of bipolar disorder in children, E.B. Weller et al. (1995) found descriptions of mania in preschool children more than 150 years ago by Esquirol (1845), as well as reports by Barrett (1931), Bleuler (1934), Olsen (1961), and Campbell (1952).

Despite this long clinical tradition, some (Kanner 1937) doubted the existence of mania in children. Anthony and Scott (1960) presented narrow criteria for the diagnosis of manic-depressive illness in childhood and doubted that the condition existed in this age

group. In reviewing 28 papers published between 1884 and 1954, they reported that only 3 (5%) of 60 reported cases of childhood mania actually met their criteria for bipolar disorder. However, careful evaluation of this article showed that these findings occurred partly as a result of the very strict diagnostic criteria the authors applied, most of which are not part of the current DSM. Despite the presence of all these questions and controversies, Akiskal (1995) reasserted the existence of bipolar disorder in juvenile subjects based on the analysis of a number of scientific reports. In his work Akiskal referred to the studies of Annell (1969) and DeLong (1978), who reported lithium-responsive behavioral disturbances in children; Weinberg and Brumback (1976), who noted how frequently childhood mania coexisted with depressive symptomatology; and Carlson and Strober (1978), who described in depth the phenomenology of mania in early adolescence. Finally, Akiskal et al. (1977, 1979) reported on 50 cyclothymic probands, who had a biphasic illness that in most cases started in adolescence or earlier and later switched into more intense hypomanic or manic episodes.

Although recognition, assessment, and diagnosis of bipolar disorder have improved, they still remain difficult tasks for many clinicians. In a retrospective review of more than 200 articles published between 1809 and 1982, R.A. Weller et al. (1986) focused on case reports of children with severe psychiatric symptomatology (excluding developmental disorders and ADHD). These authors found that approximately one-half of the children diagnosed in their review as manic, according to DSM-III (American Psychiatric Association 1980) criteria, had originally received another diagnosis. Juvenile manic-depressive patients are also often misdiagnosed as neurotic, medical-neurological, or schizophrenic (Campbell 1953).

Assessment

A longitudinal history that includes psychiatric symptoms, treatment, response to treatment, and psychosocial stressors should be obtained during the interview. The child should be interviewed alone and with the family. Family members should also be interviewed separately. A factor that complicates diagnosing mood disorders in children is that parents often have ongoing psychopathology. Therefore, it is critical to determine that the parents are reporting their child's symptoms and not their own. It is often necessary to obtain input from teachers and other school personnel to confirm that parents are accurately reporting the child's symptoms. Most teachers can provide an objective assessment that compares the identified child with age-matched children in the classroom and demonstrates the child's behavior in a setting with different task demands than are present at home (e.g., to sit still and focus attention in a group setting). Before initiating treatment of a child with a mood disorder, a complete physical examination and appropriate laboratory tests are needed to rule out medical conditions that mimic depression or mania and to monitor treatment. These tests should include a complete blood cell count with differential, electrolyte concentrations, liver function tests, thyroid function tests, blood urea nitrogen and creatinine levels, urinalysis, and electrocardiogram. If they are clinically indicated, electroencephalography and computerized tomographic or magnetic resonance imaging should be performed to assess the presence of epileptic discharge or other organicity.

Currently a noticeable emphasis is placed on the use of structured and semistructured diagnostic instruments in the process of assessment of children (see Chapter 9, "The Clinical Interview of the Adolescent," and Chapter 13, "Rating Scales," in this volume). An advantage of structured interviews is that they can be satisfactorily performed by trained psychometricians. Semistructured instruments usually require an experienced clinician to be the interviewer. All of these diagnostic tools provide thorough coverage of DSM-defined disorders. Widely used structured interviews include the Diagnostic Interview for Children and Adolescents–Revised (Reich 2000; Welner et al. 1987), the Diagnostic Interview Schedule for Children (Costello et al. 1982; Shaffer et al. 2000), and the Children's Interview for Psychiatric Syndromes (E.B. Weller et al. 1999). Semistructured interviews include the Schedule for Affective Disorders and Schizophrenia for School-Age Children (K-SADS; Puig-Antich and Chambers 1978), the Washington University Kiddie and Young Adult Schedule for Affective Disorders and Schizophrenia–Lifetime and Present Episode Version for DSM-IV (Geller et al. 1998a), the Interview Schedule for Children (Kovacs 1978, 1985), and the Children's Assessment Schedule (Hodges et al. 1982).

During treatment, clinical rating scales can be used to document severity and track changes in target symptoms. The Mania Rating Scale (Young et al. 1978) has acceptable validity and reliability. It can distinguish between manic and hyperactive children (Fristad et al. 1992, 1995), whereas the Conners Teacher and Parent Scales did not distinguish these two groups (Fristad et al. 1992). The Child Behavior Checklist has also been reported to distinguish manic children from those with ADHD (Biederman et al. 1995; Geller et al. 1998a). However, it is not a diagnostically derived instrument, and it has not been validated in bipolar disorder. Differences in scores may reflect severity of illness rather than diagnostic differences.

Two instruments for rating the severity of depression, the Children's Depression Inventory (Kovacs 1985) and the Children's Depression Rating Scale—Revised (Poznanski et al. 1985), both have excellent psychometric properties.

Clinical Presentation

■ Major Depressive Disorder

Although the essential features of major depression are similar in children, adolescents, and adults, there are noticeable differences in phenomenology. Somatic complaints, psychomotor agitation, and mood-congruent hallucinations are considered to be more prevalent among prepubertal children. Comorbid anxiety disorders are also common (Kovacs et al. 1989). Among adolescents, antisocial behavior, substance use, restlessness, grouchiness, aggression, withdrawal, problems with family and school, and feelings of wanting to leave home or of not being understood and approved of are more frequent.

Several authors have noted that many children with childhood depression have atypical features that can make it difficult to diagnose the depression. Williamson et al. (2000) assessed 1,046 youths, ages 6–19 years, who met DSM-III-R (American Psychiatric Association 1987) criteria for major depressive disorder. A diagnosis of atypical depression required mood reactivity and at least one of the following symptoms: hypersomnia, increased appetite, weight gain, or psychomotor retardation, derived from the K-SADS. The frequency of atypical symptoms in the overall sample of 1,046 depressed youths was as follows: mood reactivity, 40.9%; increased appetite, 13.6%; weight gain, 11.6%; hypersomnia, 21.8%; and psychomotor retardation, 10.7%. In total, 162 (15.5%) of the depressed youths met criteria for atypical depression, suggesting that atypical features commonly occur in depressed children and adolescents. Birmaher et al. (1996) discuss developmental differences in major depression in different age groups. The authors state that symptoms of "endogenicity"—melancholia, psychosis, suicide attempts, lethality of suicide attempt, and impairment of functioning—increase with age. However, separation anxiety, phobias, somatic complaints, and behavioral problems may occur more frequently in children (Carlson and Kashani 1988a; Kolvin et al. 1991; Mitchell et al. 1988; Ryan et al. 1987). In psychotic depressed children, auditory hallucinations appear to be more common than delusions; the latter are more common in adolescents and adults. This may be related to the lack of cognitive maturation in children (Ryan et al. 1987).

The long-term prognosis of childhood-onset depressive disorders is of great concern. Although the likelihood of recovery from first-episode depression is good, Kovacs et al. (1997) found that episodes are long, run their own course, and show little variability as a function of many clinical and demographic characteristics.

Age at onset of major depressive disorder affects the duration of the illness in adolescents (McCauley et al. 1993) but has no appreciable impact on recovery. Kovacs et al. (1984b) studied 42 children and found that younger age at onset of major depression was associated with longer episodes. Among youths in the community (Lewinsohn et al. 1994) and nonreferred but at-risk children (Warner et al. 1992), younger age at onset was also associated with a more protracted course of major depression. These studies suggest that earlier onset of depressive illness is associated with greater severity of illness and with less individual resiliency.

Recovery from major depression in children and adolescents does not seem to be influenced by sex; social class; depression severity defined by symptom; or endogenous, melancholic, or psychotic subtype (Lewinsohn et al. 1994; McCauley et al. 1993; Strober et al. 1993; Warner et al. 1992). However, some of these variables (e.g., gender) have been shown to influence onset or recurrence of major depression and mania (Coryell et al. 1992; Lewinsohn et al. 1994). Mean time to recovery in children ages 8–14 years with major depressive disorder was studied by Kovacs et al. (1984a, 1984b, 1989). These studies found that 74% of children with major depressive disorder had remission within 1 year; however, 33% experienced recurrence

within 2 years, and 72% had recurrence within 5 years. In addition, predictors of duration of depression were different from predictors of recurrence of depression. Children with an early age at onset of major depressive disorder and those receiving more outpatient treatment had a longer duration of illness. Children with combined major depressive disorder and dysthymic disorder and older age at onset had higher recurrence rates. Similar findings were reported by Harrington et al. (1991). They followed up 80 depressed children and adolescents as adults. Forty percent of subjects had another episode of depression within 5 years of the index episode (age less than 21 years). There was a 0.6 cumulative probability of recurrence for the entire follow-up period, which was much higher than for nondepressed psychiatric control subjects. In a 1-year follow-up study of depressed children ages 7–17 years, Goodyer et al. (1991) found that 50% had remission during the follow-up period. Remission was predicted by low exposure to adverse life events and improvement in the maternal relationship.

■ Bipolar Disorder

In contrast to a relatively large body of literature on childhood depression, little is yet known about childhood bipolar disorder. One of the main issues in bipolar disorder in childhood is how to properly diagnose the disorder. Fifteen years after Anthony and Scott's (1960) paper, discussed above in the section "History of Childhood Mood Disorders," Weinberg and Brumback (1976), based on the criteria of Feighner et al. (1972), proposed a second set of criteria to diagnose mania in children. These criteria included euphoria or irritable mood and three or more of the following symptoms, which must constitute a change from the child's normal behavior: 1) hyperactivity, 2) push of speech, 3) flight of ideas, 4) grandiosity, 5) sleep disturbance, and 6) distractibility. Symptom duration of at least 1 month was required to diagnose mania in children.

In 1979, Davis proposed that mania in children be diagnosed using broader and softer criteria than those proposed for adults, a concept somewhat comparable to the idea of "depressive equivalents," used at one time in the diagnosis of depression in childhood. To diagnose mania in childhood required all of the following primary criteria: 1) affective storms, 2) positive family history for mania, 3) hyperactivity, 4) chronically disturbed personal relationships, and

5) absence of psychotic thought disorder. One or more of the following secondary criteria were also required: 1) sleep disturbance, 2) minimal brain dysfunction, 3) an abnormal electroencephalogram, 4) enuresis, and 5) neuropathology.

In every DSM revision published since DSM-III in 1980, adult criteria are applied to the diagnosis of mania in children, but with some modifications for differences in age and developmental stage. However, even after these improvements in diagnostic criteria, mania in childhood is still frequently underdiagnosed or misdiagnosed (R.A. Weller et al. 1986). Its sometimes atypical clinical picture is one of the main reasons for this diagnostic confusion surrounding childhood bipolar disorder.

It is now generally accepted that the clinical presentation of mania in childhood may be atypical by adult standards (Bowring and Kovacs 1992). Most notable is that clear differentiation between episodes of mania and episodes of depression is often lacking (Carlson 1984). In contrast to manic adults, manic children are seldom characterized by euphoric mood (Carlson 1983, 1984). Instead, the mania in young children usually presents as irritability, with affective storms or prolonged and aggressive temper outbursts (Davis 1979), worsening of disruptive behavior, moodiness, difficulty sleeping at night, impulsivity, hyperactivity, inability to concentrate, explosive anger followed by guilt, depression, and poor school performance (E.B. Weller et al. 1995). Mixed features, rapid-cycling features, psychotic features, high rates of comorbidity (especially with externalizing disorders), and significant psychosocial impairment are common. In preschool children, pathologically prolonged states of emotional arousal in response to minimal stimuli and episodic violent activity with minor symptoms of depression have both been described by Carlson (1983). There are case reports of model children who dramatically change and become "wild" (Carlson 1990). McGlashan (1988) reported that juvenile-onset mania may be particularly explosive and disorganized and that children with mania have more trouble with the law and more "psychotic assaultiveness" than do adults with mania. Explosive and unmanageable temper tantrums, sexual joking, and nightmares with violent imagery have been described by Popper (1984). Aggressive temper outbursts—which often include threatening and attacking behavior toward family members, other children, adults, and teachers—have also been reported (Davis 1979).

The clinical picture of mania is considered to be more atypical in children than in adolescents (McElroy et al. 1997). At very early ages (1–8 years), symptoms of a mood disorder are very nonspecific and include irritability and emotional lability. These two symptoms are more common in manic children who are younger than age 9 years (Carlson 1983), but euphoria, elation, paranoia, and grandiose delusions are more typical in children older than age 9 years. In a study of 10 prepubertal children 6–12 years old who were diagnosed with bipolar disorder according to DSM-III-R criteria, 5 reported a primarily elated mood and 5 reported a primarily irritable mood. All were restless; 9 reported decreased need for sleep; 7 reported visual hallucinations and persecutory delusions; 6 reported increased sexual activity, pressured speech, and racing thoughts; 5 reported increased talkativeness, increased distractibility, flight of ideas, and auditory hallucinations. Grandiose delusions were reported only by 2 (Varanka et al. 1988).

The prodromal symptoms most frequently reported by the families in the initial admission histories of 58 subjects later diagnosed with bipolar disorder (Egeland et al. 2000) were depressed mood (53%), increased energy (47%), decreased energy and tiredness (38%), anger dyscontrol or quick temper and argumentativeness (38%), and irritable mood (33%). Other symptoms included bold or intrusive behaviors, excessive behaviors, and conduct problems (28%–29%); decreased sleep and crying (26%); and oversensitivity (24%). Mood changes, irritability, anger, and the vegetative symptoms of energy and sleep were the most frequently reported symptoms marking the onset of bipolar disorder.

Several authors have postulated that mania in childhood may be a more serious form of the adult illness and that mania in prepubertal children resembles the treatment-resistant mania seen in chronically ill adults (Geller and Luby 1997; Wozniak et al. 1995).

The course of childhood-onset bipolar disorder tends to be chronic and continuous rather than episodic and acute (Carlson 1983, 1984; Feinstein and Wolpert 1973; McGlashan 1988). According to Klein et al. (1998), the differences in phenomenology between childhood bipolar disorder and classic adult bipolar I disorder are not in the symptoms of childhood hypomanic and manic states but in the atypical longitudinal course of childhood manic symptoms, including the short durations of acute manic symptoms and the frequent interepisode persistence of less severe manic symptoms. Childhood-onset mania is characterized by a nonepisodic, chronic course and by rapid cycling with mixed manic states (Geller and Luby 1997). Carlson et al. (2000) reported that patients with early-onset mania were more likely to have comorbid behavior disorders in childhood and had fewer episodes of remission in a 2-year period than did those with adult-onset mania.

Community studies have demonstrated substantial persistence of childhood depressive symptoms and disorders into adolescence and the overlapping of major depressive disorder with other disorders. For instance, McGee and Williams (1988) reported that 40 nine-year-olds with major depressive disorder were more likely to have depressive symptoms at ages 11 and 13 years than were 81 nondepressed comparison children. Depressed boys had higher rates of persistent antisocial behavior than girls or nondepressed boys. Fleming et al. (1993) found that adolescents with a pure "major depressive syndrome" were at increased risk for major depressive disorder, anxiety disorder, and substance use disorder at 4-year follow-up than were subjects with no disorder.

As many as one-third of children with major depressive episodes may show signs of bipolar disorder by adolescence (Geller et al. 1994). Akiskal et al. (1983) studied 41 patients with major depression who converted to bipolarity throughout adulthood over an observation period up to 25 years. All patients whose first depressive episodes had occurred before age 18 years were among the converters. High rates of mood disorders in adults with prepubertal major depressive disorder were also reported by Weissman et al. (1999). Irritability, insomnia, and agitation characteristic of childhood depression were found to change to lethargic hypersomnia and retardation postpubertally (Carlson and Kashani 1988b). In two independent studies (Akiskal et al. 1983; Strober and Carlson 1982), bipolar outcome in postpubertal depression was associated with early pubertal age at onset of first depression, acute onset of depression, hypersomnic-retarded phenomenology, psychotic features, tricyclic-induced hypomania, bipolar family history, and a pedigree loaded with mood disorders in consecutive generations. Akiskal (1995) raised the possibility that many, if not most, depressive episodes in children and adolescents might represent precursors of adult bipolar disorders. Akiskal based his postulation on longitudinal observations that depression—emerging acutely or evolving more insidiously before age 20—presents a very high

risk for eventual transformation to bipolar disorder (Akiskal et al. 1977, 1983, 1985). Geller et al. (2001b) reported that subjects with prepubertal major depressive disorder had significantly higher rates in adulthood of the following disorders than members of a comparison group with no history of depression: bipolar I disorder (33.3% versus 0.0%), any bipolar diagnosis (48.6% versus 7.1%), major depressive disorder (36.1% versus 14.3%), substance use disorders (30.6% versus 10.7%), and suicidality (22.2% versus 3.6%).

Bipolar disorder may originate in early childhood and continue through the life span and is often atypical by adult criteria. Therefore, there is a question whether prepubertal bipolar disorder is a distinct subtype of later-onset bipolar disorder or simply an earlier manifestation of the same disease. Schurhoff et al. (2000) suggested early- and late-onset bipolar disorder differ in clinical expression and familial risk and may therefore be considered to be different subforms of manic-depressive illness. They reported that in a sample of 210 bipolar patients, the early-onset group had the most severe form of bipolar disorder with more psychotic features, more mixed episodes, greater comorbidity with panic disorder, and poorer prophylaxis with lithium. Geller et al. (1998a) also described some characteristic features of children with prepubertal versus postpubertal onset of bipolar disorder. The prevalence of vegetative symptoms was lower among prepubertal subjects. The prevalence of rapid, ultrarapid, and ultradian cycling was higher than in adult patients with bipolar disorder. Biederman et al. (2000) postulated that pediatric mania may represent a developmental subtype of bipolar disorder, which differs in its presentation, correlates, and treatment from the adult form. Thus, there are varying opinions about the phenomenology of bipolar disorder.

■ Infants

Literature on the clinical presentation of mood disorders in infants is very limited. Anaclictic depression (Spitz 1946) was described in this age group and appeared phenomenologically similar to depression in adults. Spitz (1946) and Bowlby (1951) described the mood of children who had been separated from their primary caretakers at an early age. These children look depressed, cry a lot, react slowly to stimuli, exhibit retarded movements, and may have sleep and appetite disturbances. In institutionalized infants and toddlers, this clinical picture has been called hospitalism. Mania has been described in an 11.5-month-old child, and there is mention of embryonic mania in the literature (Thompson and Schindler 1976).

■ Preschool-Age Children

In preschool children, pathologically prolonged states of emotional arousal in response to minimal stimuli and episodic frenzied activity with minor symptoms of depression have been described by Carlson (1983). Explosive and unmanageable temper tantrums, sexual joking, and nightmares with violent imagery have been described by Popper (1984) in prepubertal manic children. Preschoolers with depression look very sad, have limited verbal communication, appear slowed down, and lack a twinkle in their eyes.

■ School-Age Children

School-age children are able to describe symptoms such as poor mood ("low, down in the dumps" or "wanting to be nothing when I grow up"), trouble concentrating, poor performance in school, irritability, crying, and suicidal thoughts that are often unknown to their parents. Because of the myth that children do not attempt suicide, it is not uncommon for children who have attempted suicide to have the attempt go unrecognized or be mistakenly characterized by their physicians as an accident. Clear-cut suicides in children younger than age 10 years have almost always been labeled accidental deaths by the coroner. Somatic symptoms may coexist with depressive symptoms in children. The most common are headaches and abdominal pain and discomfort. Such depressed children are often seen by the pediatrician or family physician, who conducts an extensive and expensive laboratory workup. At the end of this evaluation, the parents and child are told that nothing is wrong or "it's all in the head," with no recognition of or suggestion for treatment of the depression.

Mania in school-age children is characterized by pressured speech, which is difficult or impossible to interrupt. Racing thoughts are frequently described by children and adolescents in very concrete terms. For example, children state that they are not able to get anything done because their thoughts keep interrupting. Increased motor activity and goal-directed behavior, involvement in pleasurable activities with a high level of danger, hypersexuality, disordered sleep pattern with high activity levels in the bedroom before sleep, and many other symptoms are typical for manic school-age children.

Differential Diagnosis and Comorbidity

Comorbid diagnoses in children and adolescents with mood disorders are the rule rather than the exception. Clinical and community studies have shown that initial episodes of major depression, especially in children, often present with a range of coexisting symptoms of anxiety and behavior disorders (Kovacs et al. 1984a, 1988, 1994; Lewinsohn et al. 1993; Mitchell et al. 1988; Ryan et al. 1987). Kovacs et al. (1997) reported that of 87 children between ages 8 and 13 at initial presentation of the first episode of major depressive disorder, 30 (34.5%) had underlying dysthymic disorder, 44 (50.6%) had anxiety disorder, and 23 (26.4%) had an externalizing disorder.

The differential diagnosis of mood disorders includes both medical and psychiatric conditions. Symptoms of mania can result from a variety of medical conditions, including prescription drug use (e.g., steroids, antidepressants, stimulants), neurological disorders (e.g., head trauma, multiple sclerosis, temporal lobe seizures), systemic disorders (e.g., hyperthyroidism, porphyria), and substances of abuse (e.g., amphetamines, cocaine). Symptoms of depression may arise from medical conditions such as cancer and diabetes; from neurological disorders such as multiple sclerosis; from systemic disorders such as hypothyroidism; and from medications such as steroids.

■ Attention-Deficit/Hyperactivity Disorder

A leading source of diagnostic confusion in prepubertal mania is the symptom overlap with ADHD. Because distractibility, impulsivity, hyperactivity, and emotional lability can be present in both ADHD and bipolar disorder, the differential diagnosis can be difficult (Carlson 1984). Although ADHD and mania should be considered in the differential diagnosis of both disorders, they can and frequently do coexist, which adds to the diagnostic confusion (Biederman et al. 1996). A child with both mania and ADHD may be regarded as having severe ADHD by ADHD experts, or severe mania by mood disorder experts. Considering the history of skepticism surrounding the existence of mania in children (Carlson 1995; R.A. Weller et al. 1986), experts are concerned that the diagnosis of mania may be ignored by child and adolescent psychiatrists. A missed diagnosis of bipolar disorder may lead to a chronic course and treatment resistance (Post et al. 1986).

ADHD differs from mania in several respects. The onset of ADHD is typically in the preschool age when the child starts to walk or early elementary school years (i.e., before age 7), whereas the onset of mania is more common after puberty. The sleep disturbance and overactivation associated with ADHD are chronic and are part of the child's baseline behavior. The sleep disturbance in mania is associated with the onset of the mood disturbance and is often described as a diminished need for sleep instead of inability to sleep. ADHD is not associated with psychosis, flight of ideas, euphoria, or grandiosity, which are common symptoms in mania. Children with ADHD usually display low self-esteem. The overactivity of a manic child is goal directed, whereas that of a child with ADHD is often disorganized and haphazard. Ongoing research should provide additional information on the differences between these two disorders.

■ Conduct Disorder

Conduct disorder should also be considered in the differential diagnosis. Kovacs and Pollock (1995) reported a 69% prevalence of conduct disorder in a referred sample of youths with mania. Kutcher et al. (1989) found that 42% of hospitalized youths with mania had comorbid conduct disorder, and Wozniak et al. (1995) reported that preadolescent children satisfying structured interview criteria for mania often had comorbid conduct disorder. Lewinsohn and colleagues (1995b) also found high rates of comorbidity between bipolar disorder and disruptive behavior.

The difficulty in differentiating childhood mania from conduct disorder is not surprising because juvenile mania is frequently mixed (dysphoric). It also can be associated with affective storms, or prolonged and aggressive temper outbursts (Carlson 1983, 1984; Davis 1979), which can include threatening or attacking behavior toward family members, children, adults, and teachers. Children with conduct disorder and children with mania often become involved in dangerous acts with painful consequences. However, children with mania are mischievous rather than vindictive and calculating. Their conflicts with authority usually result from poor judgment and grandiosity.

■ Dysthymia

Kovacs et al. (1984a) first reported the association between major depressive disorder and dysthymia in children. Among a group of referred 8- to 13-year-old children, 38% of children with major depressive disorder had underlying dysthymia, and 57% of those with dysthymia had concurrent major depressive disorder. A number of papers point to similarities between major depressive disorder and dysthymia. For example, boys and girls are equally represented in both disorders (Ferro et al. 1994; Kovacs et al. 1994). In addition, groups with pure major depressive disorder do not differ from those with pure dysthymia with regard to age, parents' marital status, socioeconomic status, child's IQ, history of school suspension, or school failure (Ferro et al. 1994; Kovacs et al. 1994).

Studies of community samples have not found significant differences between children with pure major depressive disorder and those with pure dysthymia. For example, Lewinsohn et al. (1991) found no differences in age, gender, ethnicity, parents' marital status, or history of treatment for depression. Neither Garrison et al. (1992) nor Lewinsohn et al. (1991) found differences in rates of other psychiatric disorders. Goodman et al. (2000) compared sociodemographics, clinical course and characteristics, family and life events, and competence and functional impairment in a community sample of children and adolescents with pure forms of major depressive disorder and dysthymia. They found no differences in sociodemographics, clinical course, and clinical characteristics. The one exception was age at onset, which was older for those with major depressive disorder. With respect to family and life events, the major depressive disorder and dysthymia groups differed only in frequency of harsh physical punishment. The parents of children in the pure dysthymia group more often reported the use of more harsh physical punishment. On indicators of competence and impairment, there were no significant differences between those with major depressive disorder and those with dysthymia. For both disorders, early onset predicts poor rate of recovery (Kovacs et al. 1984a).

These consistent correlations, along with high rates of comorbidity between these two disorders, suggest that major depressive disorder and dysthymic disorder may not be two totally separate disorders.

Schizophrenia

Because of greater perceptual distortions seen in bipolar illness during adolescence, schizophrenia is a major differential diagnosis (Carlson et al. 1994; Horowitz 1975). Diagnosis is greatly aided by a family history of mania, which is more probable for bipolar than for schizophrenic adolescents (Strober et al. 1988). Sometimes the schizophrenic prodrome in children starts with affective symptoms. A positive family history of schizophrenia should alert the physician to this possibility. If the clinician is unsure whether to diagnose schizophrenia or a mood disorder, because there has been no long-term follow-up or history of prior episodes, the condition can be termed undiagnosed and then treated initially as a mood disorder, because mood disorders have a better prognosis than schizophrenic disorders (Akiskal and Weller 1989).

Substance Abuse

Substance abuse begins to be an important comorbid condition during the teenage years and is important in the differential diagnosis (Horowitz 1975, 1977; Lewinsohn et al. 1995a; Merikangas et al. 1996). For example, laughing fits due to smoking marijuana may mimic the laughing fits that occur during childhood and adolescence as a manifestation of elation. Furthermore, very rapid cycling, which can occur in child and adolescent bipolar disorder (Geller et al. 1995), can easily be mimicked by amphetamine highs followed by withdrawal crashes. Effects of hallucinogens can mimic bipolar perceptual distortions (Horowitz 1975, 1977; Lewinsohn et al. 1995a; Merikangas et al. 1996).

Anxiety Disorders

Just as comorbid anxiety conditions can be seen with major depressive disorder, bipolar patients also manifest multiple comorbid anxiety conditions. This was found in approximately 33% of prepubertal bipolar patients and 12% of adolescent bipolar patients (Geller et al. 1995).

Adjustment Disorder

In the school-age child, adjustment disorder with depressed mood in response to a circumscribed noxious event in a child's life (e.g., parents' divorce or sibling's birth) must be considered in the differential diagnosis of depression. Children with adjustment disorder with depressed mood do not satisfy criteria for a major depressive episode but may have a few depressive symptoms. Normal bereavement should also be in the differential diagnosis because 37% of children who experience the death of a parent satisfy criteria for major depression in the 3 months after the death of the parent (E.B. Weller and R.A. Weller 1990).

Other

Infants or toddlers who look sad, seem depressed or apathetic, and are not gaining weight should be evaluated for organic failure to thrive. The differential diagnosis would include central nervous system, hormonal, metabolic, and gastrointestinal disorders. In the absence of organic reasons for failure to thrive, etiologies such as neglect, abuse, and Munchausen syndrome by proxy should be considered. Hospitalization may be helpful in clarifying the diagnosis because children whose failure to thrive is nonorganic quickly improve their affect and gain weight under the care of nurturing professionals. The clinician also must carefully assess these children's primary caretakers (usually mothers), who often have undiagnosed depression, so that they can be treated and thus be better able to care effectively and safely for their children. Similarly, in the depressed preschool child, a malignancy or neglect and abuse (both physical and sexual) must be ruled out when considering the diagnosis of depression (E.B. Weller and R.A. Weller 1990).

Sexual abuse is especially important as a differential diagnosis during the childhood years because manic hypersexuality is often manifested in children by self-stimulatory behaviors, including frequent masturbation. Therefore, it is essential to obtain a careful history of whether the child could have been abused sexually or exposed to adult sexual behaviors.

Epidemiology

According to some studies, depressive disorders affect 0.3% of preschoolers, 1%–2% of elementary school–age children, and 5% of adolescents (Anderson et al. 1987; Bird et al. 1988). However, no large epidemiological studies have been done on the prevalence of major depressive disorder in prepubertal children.

Kashani et al. (1983) reported that 2% of a sample

of 9-year-old children from the general population were depressed. Fewer than 1% of 1,000 preschoolers on a child development unit were depressed (Kashani and Carlson 1987). Depression was reported in 7% of children admitted to pediatric hospitals for medical reasons (Kashani et al. 1981) and in 40% of children in pediatric neurology clinics presenting with headaches (Ling et al. 1970).

Current data on the prevalence of bipolar disorder in childhood are also based on relatively small community surveys or retrospective data. In a retrospective study involving 200 adult patients with well-established diagnoses of bipolar disorder, 0.5% reported the age at onset of their illness to have been between 5 and 9 years; 7.5% reported onset between ages 10 and 14 years (Loranger and Levine 1978). However, in another study of adults with bipolar disorder, a childhood onset was reported by 59% of subjects (Lish et al. 1994). Furthermore, an increasingly earlier onset of bipolar disorder in more recently born cohorts has been suggested (Gershon et al. 1987). Joyce (1984) estimated that 20%–40% of adults report the onset of their illness during childhood. In a review of 898 cases from 1977 to 1985, Goodwin and Jamison (1990) found that 3 (0.3%) patients had onset of illness before age 10 years. In a recent study, Geller et al. (1998b) reported that the mean age at onset of bipolar disorder in the children they studied was 8.1±3.5 years. Burke et al. (1990) noted that for the patients with bipolar disorder they examined, most had an onset between ages 15 and 19. Bipolar disorder has even been reported in an 11.5-month-old boy (LaGrone 1981).

Epidemiological studies of mood disorders done in various countries have reported different rates. This may be attributed to several factors, such as different procedures for recruiting subjects as well as varying methodologies of assessment instruments. The first epidemiological study of childhood depression in Spain reported the prevalence of major depression in children age 9 to be 1.8% (Polaino and Domenech 1993). Billy et al. (1992) reported the prevalence of major depressive disorder in French students ages 14–23 years to be 4.4%. This is similar to figures in the articles reviewed by Birmaher et al. (1996). Later, Canals et al. (1997) used a two-stage design and DSM-III-R criteria to prospectively investigate epidemiological characteristics of depression in 500 Spanish adolescents from the general population. An increase in the estimated prevalence of major depressive disorder in girls

according to age was reported (2.2% at age 11, 2.7% at age 12, and 4.1% at age 13), but in boys this trend was not observed. No association between pubertal development stages and depression was found in boys. When the same sample was followed up at age 18, the estimated point-prevalence rates of major depressive disorder were 3.3% in females and 1.4% in males (Canals et al. 1997). Goodyer and Cooper (1993) estimated a rate of 3.5% of current major depression in a community sample of 1,068 girls ages 11–16 years.

The male-to-female ratio of bipolar disorders in children has been addressed in several studies. Although bipolar disorder in adulthood affects both sexes equally, reports of mania in childhood suggest that prepubertal-onset mania may be more common in boys than in girls (Geller et al. 1998b; Varanka et al. 1988). Major depressive disorder occurs at approximately the same rate in girls as in boys, whereas in adolescents, the female-to-male ratio is estimated to be approximately 2:1, similar to the ratio reported in adults (Fleming and Offord 1990; Kessler et al. 1994; Lewinsohn et al. 1994).

Etiology

■ Genetic Studies

Support for a genetic component in depression has been provided by twin studies, which show the concordance rates for depression to be higher in adult monozygotic twins than in dizygotic twins (McGuffin and Katz 1989). Studies of the biological and adoptive parents of adults with depression show higher rates of depression in the biological parents than in the adoptive parents. The same is true for adults with mania.

Strober et al. (1988) noted that significantly increased aggregation of bipolar I disorder in first-degree relatives and decreased antimanic response to lithium carbonate were two variables distinguishing adolescent probands with childhood-onset psychiatric illness from probands who had no prepubertal psychiatric disorders. As a general principle, it is assumed that early age at onset predicts a higher familial loading in bipolar affective disorder (Strober 1992).

■ Biochemical Factors

Several neurotransmitter systems have been implicated in depression. These include the noradrenergic, serotonergic, cholinergic, and dopaminergic systems. In particular, monoamine systems (serotonin, norepinephrine, and dopamine) are reported to play important roles in the pathophysiology of adult major depressive disorder and are involved in the regulation of neuroendocrine systems (Goodwin and Jamison 1990).

Cortisol has been postulated to have some role in the etiology of depression. Some studies (Casat and Powell 1988; Dahl et al. 1989; Puig-Antich et al. 1989a) have shown that severely depressed and suicidal children and adolescents may manifest cortisol hypersecretion (Dahl et al. 1991; Pfeffer et al. 1991). In a study of 38 medically healthy children with prepubertal major depression and 28 medically and psychiatrically healthy control children (who had very low rates of depression in their families), De Bellis et al. (1996) reported that prepubertal children with depression had lower cortisol secretion during the first 4 hours after sleep onset.

Growth hormone has also been suggested to have a role in the pathogenesis of depression. Ryan et al. (1992a, 1994) found significant group differences between prepubertal children with major depressive disorder and control subjects in both provocative growth hormone testing and a serotonergic challenge. Higher nocturnal concentrations of basal growth hormone were found in depressed adolescents compared with matched control subjects (Kutcher et al. 1988, 1991) and in depressed children compared with nondepressed psychiatrically ill children (Puig-Antich et al. 1984). However, another study found that there were no overall group differences in nocturnal growth hormone secretion in adolescents with major depressive disorder compared with control subjects (Dahl et al. 1992). In this latter study, when those with major depressive disorder were divided into suicidal and nonsuicidal groups, the presence of suicidality revealed a significant blunting of nocturnal growth hormone secretion compared with the nonsuicidal group.

Although there has been some speculation on the role of prolactin secretion in the mechanism of manifestation of mood disorders, a study by Waterman et al. (1994) did not find a significant difference in basal 24-hour prolactin concentrations in adolescents with major depressive disorder compared with control subjects.

Secretion of adrenocorticotropin, prolactin, and growth hormone did not differ between depressed and nondepressed groups in the study by De Bellis et al. (1996). Their examination of clinical characteristics in depressed children revealed lower nocturnal adrenocorticotropin concentrations in depressed inpatients versus depressed outpatients and in depressed sexually abused versus depressed nonabused children. A significant sex-by-diagnosis effect revealed lower growth hormone secretion in depressed females compared with depressed males. The authors concluded that in contrast to neuroendocrine challenge studies in these same subjects, nocturnal neuroendocrine measures did not reveal any of the expected group differences. These results emphasize the contrasts between unstimulated (resting state) and challenge studies of neuroendocrine secretion and of the importance of considering clinical characteristics and maturation influences in biological studies of prepubertal depression.

■ Environmental Factors

Environmental factors, such as loss or stress, may also be important etiological variables. Because depression runs in families, depressed children are often living with and being cared for by a depressed parent (most often the mother). Depressed mothers' interactions with their children can be negative. When depressed adults are asked about their childhood, they often report having had very negative interactions with their parents.

Early-onset depression is generally associated with increased familial aggregation. Evidence from some studies (Kovacs and Gatsonis 1994; Ryan et al. 1992b) of early-onset depression indicates that it is unlikely that genetics alone could account for increasing rates of depression, because it is improbable that the population frequency of even a single gene allele could increase rapidly enough to account for the observed trend. In a family study of prepubertal-onset depression by Puig-Antich et al. (1989b), the non-age-adjusted rate for depression was approximately two times higher in both the first-degree relatives (34% versus 16%) and second-degree relatives (8% versus 4%) of depressed children than in healthy control subjects. In addition, Puig-Antich and colleagues (1989b), using the Family History–Research Diagnostic Criteria, found that "other" psychiatric disorders (mostly anxiety) were significantly increased in both the first- and second-degree relatives of depressed children. Lifetime rates of alcoholism were significantly elevated in the second-degree relatives of the depressed children compared with the relatives of healthy control subjects.

In a study by Todd et al. (1993), major depressive disorder was found to be aggregated in the first-degree (46%) and second-degree relatives (25%) of prepubertal depressed children. However, statistical comparisons with relatives of healthy control subjects were not possible because of the selection criteria for control subjects (subjects were excluded if they had a parent or sibling with an ongoing or recurrent affective disorder).

Brain Imaging

Magnetic resonance imaging studies of older adults with major depressive disorder have documented decreases in frontal lobe volume relative to age- and sex-matched comparison subjects (Coffey et al. 1993). Because the frontal lobe continues to undergo substantial maturational changes during adolescence (Jernigan et al. 1991), several authors have questioned if and when decreases in frontal lobe volume occur in early-onset depression. Steingard et al. (1996) measured frontal lobe and lateral ventricular volume in 125 children and adolescents (ages 6–17 years) who were hospitalized for a depressive disorder. Hospitalized psychiatric control subjects without depressive symptoms served as a comparison group. There was a decrease in frontal lobe volume and an increase in ventricular volume in the depressed children compared with nondepressed children. These results are consistent with magnetic resonance imaging findings of reduced frontal lobe volume in adults with major depression (Coffey et al. 1993) and reduced volume of structures adjacent to the lateral ventricles, such as the putamen (Husain et al. 1991) and caudate nucleus (Krishnan et al. 1992). In addition, a significant inverse relationship was found between age and frontal lobe volume that was consistent with previous observations (Jernigan et al. 1991).

Treatment

Mood disorders in children and adolescents cause substantial morbidity and mortality; therefore, medications have been used extensively to treat these disorders. For example, from 1996 to 1997, children between ages 6 and 18 years received 792,000 prescriptions for selective serotonin reuptake inhibitors (SSRIs) to treat depression (Hoar 1998). During this same period, the number of children age 5 and younger taking SSRIs jumped 500%, from 8,000 to 40,000 (Hughes et al. 1999). However, despite the phenomenological literature about juvenile-onset bipolar disorder, rather little has been published about pharmacotherapy for this disorder. Scientific studies on lithium efficacy and safety for treatment of juvenile-onset bipolar disorder remain few (Kafantaris 1995). Although valproate appears to be relatively well tolerated by children and young adolescents, scientific studies demonstrating its efficacy are lacking. A report of adverse effects associated with its long-term use in the treatment of seizure disorder in mentally retarded children and its possible association with polycystic ovaries are of concern (Isojarvi et al. 1996). Carbamazepine has been shown to be effective in adults in the treatment of acute manic episodes (Keck and McElroy 1996). However, scientific studies in children are again lacking.

■ Psychotherapy

It has been suggested that play therapy or psychotherapy (including family therapy) may be effective in preschoolers. If psychotherapy is used for a depressed child, the clinician should take an active role. It becomes "depressing" to sit and wait for a depressed child to talk. Engaging games such as the Talking, Feeling, and Doing Game and mutual storytelling are helpful. Supportive therapy with the child and the family can be very productive, especially when accompanied by education about the illness. The clinician must not blame the child or the family for having caused the depression. Many families are eager to cooperate when the depression is described in terms of an illness model. As the acute phase of the illness abates, patients and families are often more open to work on family interactions that might be perceived as being stressful by the depressed child and the family. See Chapters 51–54 in this volume for detailed discussions of psychotherapy for children and adolescents.

■ Pharmacotherapy

Major Depressive Disorder

Antidepressants are widely used to treat major depressive disorder in children and adolescents. Because of the significant morbidity of the disorder, such treatment seems appropriate despite the relative absence of evidence from controlled studies indicating efficacy of antidepressants in youth. The suggested pharmacological approaches for children and adolescents with depressive disorders are based primarily on data available from adult studies as well as anecdotal, clinical, and research experience. The child psychiatry literature provides some evidence that juvenile mood disorders may be more refractory to pharmacological intervention than adult mood disorders (Ambrosini et al. 1993). Another problem in evaluating the efficacy of treatment is the fact that the average length of a depressive episode in community samples is 6 months (in clinical samples the average length is 8 months) (Kovacs 1996; Lewinsohn et al. 1994). However, the majority of clinical trials on either pharmacological or psychosocial treatments of depression in children and adolescents have been of 8–16 weeks in duration. This is probably too brief a time to completely treat a depressive episode. As a result, there are relatively low response rates (50%–60%) with the briefer psychosocial or pharmacological treatments, as well as a relatively high rate of relapse on follow-up (Brent et al. 1998; Emslie et al. 1998; Vostanis et al. 1996; Wood et al. 1996).

Selective serotonin reuptake inhibitors. SSRIs are considered to be the first-line pharmacologic treatment (DeVane and Sallee 1996; Kutcher 1997; Leonard et al. 1997) for depression because of their favorable side-effect profile, ease of use, suitability for long-term maintenance, low lethality after overdose, and studies supporting their efficacy. Such studies include double-blind placebo-conrolled trials with fluoxetine for children and adolescents (Emslie et al. 1997) and paroxetine for adolescents (Keller et al. 1998). Sertraline (Ambrosini et al. 1999) and fluoxetine (Strober et al. 1999), in open trials, have been safe and helpful.

Fluoxetine. Emslie et al. (1997) conducted the first double-blind, placebo-controlled study of fluoxetine in children and adolescents. Ninety-six outpatients (ages 7–17 years) with nonpsychotic major depressive disorder were randomized (stratified for age and sex) to 20 mg of fluoxetine or placebo and were seen weekly for 8 consecutive weeks. Three evaluation visits that included structured diagnostic interviews during the first 2 weeks, and a 1-week single-blind placebo run-in preceded randomization. Primary outcome measures were global improvement on the Clinical Global Impression (CGI) Scale and the Children's Depression

Rating Scale–Revised (CDRS-R), a measure of the severity of depressive symptoms. Twenty-seven (56%) of those receiving fluoxetine and 16 (33%) receiving placebo were rated "much" or "very much" improved on the CGI scale at the end of the study. Significant differences were also noted in weekly ratings of the CDRS-R after 5 weeks of treatment. However, complete symptom remission (CDRS-R score of 28 or less) occurred in only 15 (31%) of the fluoxetine-treated patients and 11 (23%) of the placebo patients. This was the first study to show that fluoxetine was superior to placebo in the acute-phase treatment of major depressive disorder in child and adolescent outpatients.

Paroxetine. Paroxetine is an SSRI that has been proposed as a possible first-line treatment for severe depression in adolescent patients (Harrington 1995). To date, it has been used in the treatment of depressed adolescent patients and in children with depressive symptoms associated with other psychiatric disorders, such as attention-deficit disorder, Tourette's syndrome, obsessive-compulsive disorder (Budman et al. 1995; Telegdy et al. 1984), and self-injurious behavior (Snead et al. 1994). Rey-Sanchez and Gutierrez-Casares (1997) evaluated the efficacy, tolerability, and safety of paroxetine in an open-label treatment of 54 children younger than age 14 with major depressive disorder.

In a more recent double-blind, placebo-controlled study, Keller et al. (2001) compared paroxetine and imipramine (a tricyclic antidepressant) in adolescents with major depression. This was an 8-week, multicenter, double-blind, randomized, parallel-design comparison of paroxetine with placebo and imipramine with placebo in 275 adolescents with major depression. Subjects included males and females, ages 12–18, who fulfilled DSM-IV (American Psychiatric Association 1994) criteria for a current episode of major depression at least 8 weeks in duration. Major depression was diagnosed by a systematic clinical interview that used the Schedule for Affective Disorders and Schizophrenia for Adolescents–Lifetime version (K-SADS-L) rating scale (Endicott and Spitzer 1978). In addition to fulfilling DSM-IV criteria for major depression, subjects were required to have a score of at least 12 on the 17-item Hamilton Rating Scale for Depression (Ham-D), a score less than 60 on the Children's Global Assessment Scale, and a score of at least 80 on the Peabody Picture Vocabulary Test. After a 7- to 14-day screening phase, subjects were randomly assigned to an 8-week course of treatment with paroxetine (20–

40 mg), imipramine (gradual upward titration to 200–300 mg), or placebo in a 1:1:1 ratio.

The mean duration of the current depressive episode was more than 1 year, with a mean baseline Ham-D total score between 18 and 19. Sixty-three percent of paroxetine subjects, 50% of imipramine subjects, and 46% of placebo subjects achieved a Ham-D total score of 8 or less at the endpoint of the study. Among patients who completed 8 weeks of treatment, 76.1% of paroxetine subjects, 64.3% of imipramine subjects, and 57.6% of placebo subjects achieved a mean Ham-D total score of 8 or less. In the paroxetine group, 65.6% of patients were rated as very much or much improved on the CGI. Improvement rates for the imipramine and placebo groups were 52.1% and 48.3%, respectively. Paroxetine was significantly more effective than placebo as determined by Ham-D total score of 8 or less, CGI score of 1 (very much improved) or 2 (much improved), and improvements in the depressed mood items of the Ham-D and the K-SADS-L. Paroxetine was not statistically different from placebo for K-SADS-L depression subscore, mean CGI score, or Ham-D total score. Based on these results, the authors suggested that paroxetine is well tolerated and effective for major depression in adolescents.

Sertraline. Sertraline is an SSRI that has been effective in dosages ranging from 50 to 200 mg/day for treatment of both depression and obsessive-compulsive disorder. Its pharmacokinetic profile is well established in adults (Chouinard et al. 1990; Cohn et al. 1990; Greist et al. 1995a, 1995b; Murdoch and McTavish 1992). Alderman et al. (1998) studied the single- and multiple-dose pharmacokinetics of sertraline and its major metabolite, desmethylsertraline, in children (ages 6–12 years) and adolescents (ages 13–17 years) with depression or obsessive-compulsive disorder or both. A dosage range of 25–200 mg/day was used to evaluate the safety and efficacy of sertraline in these subjects. Children (n=29) and adolescents (n=32) with major depression, obsessive-compulsive disorder, or both received a single dose of 50 mg of sertraline followed 1 week later by 35 days of sertraline treatment as follows: 1) either a starting dose of 25 mg/day titrated to 200 mg/day in 25-mg increments or 2) a starting dose of 50 mg/day titrated to 200 mg/day in 50-mg increments. Sertraline and desmethylsertraline pharmacokinetics were determined weekly, and efficacy measures were assessed before drug administration and at the end of treatment. In this study the pharmacokinetic profiles of sertraline and its major metabolite in pediatric patients were similar to the profiles previously established in adults. The authors suggested that sertraline is safe and likely to be effective in the treatment of pediatric patients with either major depression or obsessive-compulsive disorder. A maximum dose of 200 mg, and upward titration in weekly 50-mg increments, was believed suitable for patients between ages 6 and 17 years.

Tricyclic antidepressants. In the past, tricyclic antidepressants (TCAs) were considered the first line of treatment of depressive disorders. However, after the introduction of SSRIs and following reports of sudden death associated with the use of TCAs, their use in psychiatric practice has greatly decreased.

Open pharmacological trials in depressed children have found that 60%–80% respond to TCAs (Geller et al. 1986; Preskorn et al. 1982; Puig-Antich et al. 1979). However, with the exception of the study by Preskorn et al. (1987), who found a statistically significant but clinically small antidepressant effect in one of the outcome measurements, all of the controlled double-blind trials reported no significant differences between placebo and TCAs (Geller et al. 1989; Hughes et al. 1990; Kashani et al. 1984; Puig-Antich et al. 1987). Furthermore, except for the study by Geller and colleagues (1989), who found 31% response to nortriptyline and 17% to placebo in a sample of children with chronic depression, most trials have found approximately a 50% response rate to both TCAs and placebo.

The first double-blind, placebo-controlled study of TCAs for childhood depression was reported in 1987 by Puig-Antich and associates. In this study, the effectiveness of imipramine (up to 5 mg/kg/day) was investigated in 53 prepubertal children with major depressive disorder. Fifteen of the 16 children randomly assigned to active drug in the first study also participated in the second. Response rates in the double-blind study were similar in both groups (imipramine, 56%; placebo, 68%). In the plasma-level study, total maintenance plasma level (imipramine plus desipramine) was found to positively and linearly predict clinical response. Weight-corrected imipramine dosage did not predict either clinical response or plasma level in individual subjects. No predictors of response were found in the placebo group. These results suggested that the mean imipramine dosage was too low and that future double-blind, placebo-controlled studies of imipramine in prepubertal major depression should include plasma-level titration to above 150 ng/mL and an initial placebo washout period.

In another study, Preskorn et al. (1987) treated hospitalized depressed prepubertal children with imipramine and adjusted plasma levels to be between 125 and 250 ng/mL. The depressed children who showed nonsuppression on the dexamethasone suppression test responded to imipramine but not to placebo. Children who showed suppression on the dexamethasone suppression test responded equally well to imipramine and placebo. Children with comorbid anxiety responded better to imipramine, whereas children with comorbid conduct disorder had no difference in response to imipramine or placebo.

Other double-blind studies using amitriptyline, desipramine, and nortriptyline have also been conducted, but in general none found TCAs to be superior to placebo in the treatment of depression in prepubertal children or adolescents.

It should be remembered that fewer than 300 children and adolescents have been studied in well-designed double-blind, placebo-controlled studies of antidepressants, whereas thousands of adults have been treated in such controlled trials.

Bipolar Disorder

The treatment of childhood bipolar disorder remains an understudied area despite increasing knowledge and experience on the subject (Botteron et al. 1995; Fetner and Geller 1992; Kafantaris 1995; Youngerman and Canino 1978). Therefore, unless there is an expectation that childhood bipolar disorder completely and exactly mimics adult bipolar disorder, specific studies in children are warranted. Compelling arguments against the identical treatment of bipolar disorder across age groups can be derived by analogy to treatment differences between children and adults with major depressive disorder (Geller et al. 1996). Because there are still almost no published double-blind, placebo-controlled medication studies on mania in children or adolescents (Geller and Luby 1997), the clinician will be tempted to extrapolate from studies of adults. However, extrapolation from treatment of major depressive disorder in adults to children has not always been useful. For example, TCAs have not been proved to be better than placebo in depressed children and adolescents.

Lithium. Lithium carbonate has been recommended in the treatment of bipolar illness in children (Youngerman and Canino 1978). Although lithium has been effective in adults (Schou 1968) and in some adolescents with mania (Strober et al. 1990), only a few studies have examined the efficacy of lithium in prepubertal children (DeLong and Aldershof 1987). Lithium is approved by the U.S. Food and Drug Administration for treatment of bipolar disorder in adolescents who are age 12 years and older. However, it has been used in younger children with bipolar disorder. Lithium is reported to have a shorter half-life in children than in adults (Vitiello et al. 1988). The literature on lithium suggests that it can be given to children with the same safety precautions used in adults, such as monitoring renal, thyroid, calcium, and phosphorus indices at 6-month intervals (Fetner and Geller 1992; Khandelwal et al. 1984). However, a double-blind, placebo-controlled study of the use of lithium in aggressive children found that some children can develop cognitive impairment at low plasma levels (Silva et al. 1992). This also was noted in a double-blind, placebo-controlled study of lithium usage in depressed children who had risk factors for developing bipolar disorder (Geller et al. 1994).

Because of the chronic course of childhood bipolar disorder and the rapid-cycling, mixed features that predict poor response in older populations (Geller et al. 1995; Himmelhoch and Garfinkel 1986; Hsu 1986; Keller et al. 1993), the optimal duration of antimanic treatments has not been settled. Furthermore, some adult literature suggests that intermittent lithium therapy leads to a worse outcome than uninterrupted therapy. Furthermore, it can be difficult to restabilize patients on lithium after interruptions in treatment (Ahrens et al. 1995; Muller-Oerlinghausen et al. 1992, 1994; Schou 1995; Schou et al. 1989).

Strober et al. (1990) kept adolescents on antimanic treatments throughout the teenage years. The same authors (Strober et al. 1995) also published an open, uncontrolled naturalistic follow-up study of adolescents taking lithium. Those data strongly support long-term maintenance with lithium, because subjects who discontinued lithium had a significantly higher relapse rate.

Numerous case reports and case series of lithium treatment for bipolar disorder in children and adolescents have suggested that lithium is efficacious (R.A. Weller et al. 1986). In prepubertal children, open trials of lithium treatment for bipolar disorder appear to give response rates similar to those seen in adults (DeLong and Aldershof 1987; Varanka et al. 1988). DeLong and Aldershof (1987) studied long-term treatment of bipolar outpatients under age 14 years; 39

(66%) of the 59 bipolar children who continued to take lithium for more than 2 months were treated successfully. Varanka et al. (1988) reported that lithium alone was effective in an open study of 10 prepubertal children with psychotic bipolar disorder. In addition, positive effects of lithium treatment were reported in 82% of depressed children with neurovegetative and other episodic symptoms (DeLong and Aldershof 1987).

Two main approaches have been described to calculate lithium dosage for children and adolescents with bipolar disorder: weight-based calculation (E.B. Weller et al. 1986) and the kinetics-based method (Geller and Fetner 1989).

E.B. Weller et al. (1986) reported that a dosage of 30 mg/kg/day in three divided doses will produce a lithium level between 0.6 and 1.2 mEq/L within 5 days in a 6- to 12-year-old child. Lithium levels as high as 1.4 mEq/L have been reported with minimal side effects. Because children are often phobic about blood drawing, the authors reported that lithium levels could be monitored safely using saliva (E.B. Weller et al. 1986).

Geller and Fetner (1989) proposed a kinetics-based method to adjust dosage based on a 24-hour serum level determined after administration of a single 600-mg dose. This method has shown good predictive values for serum lithium level in children.

Anticonvulsants. There are a few open, uncontrolled studies of anticonvulsant treatment of bipolar disorder. In an open, randomized 6-week trial of mood-stabilizing agents, 42 children and adolescents (mean age, 11.4 years) with type I and type II bipolar disorder, with mixed or classic manic episodes, were treated with valproate, lithium, and carbamazepine (Kowatch et al. 2000). The response rates were 46% for valproate, 34% for lithium, and 34% for carbamazepine. The authors pointed out that in some patients treated with valproate sodium there was an increase in bipolar symptoms after 3 weeks of treatment that would typically resolve the following week. A similar phenomenon has not been observed among adult bipolar patients treated with valproate, which, according to the authors, suggests a transitory difference between adults and children in their neurochemical response to valproate.

Carbamazepine is used extensively in younger patients with bipolar disorder. However, the majority of carbamazepine reports are of children and adolescents with ADHD or conduct disorder, some of whom also had neurological disorders. Carbamazepine was reported to be effective in seven manic adolescents who were nonresponsive to lithium (Hsu 1986), and it appeared to be a safe and effective treatment for acute mania and long-term maintenance treatment in three cases of juvenile-onset bipolar I disorder (Woolston 1999). Carbamazepine should be started with a low dose (100 mg twice a day for children under age 8) (Ballenger 1988). The usual maintenance dose for children is 10–20 mg/kg daily (200–600 mg/day), administered in divided doses. Because of its effect on hepatic cytochrome P450, carbamazepine can induce its own metabolism as well as that of other hepatically metabolized medications, resulting in lower than expected blood levels.

Valproate has been used successfully in treating mania in adults (Bowden et al. 1996), and there are some promising results of its use in children and adolescents (Papatheodorou and Kutcher 1993). Isojarvi et al. (1993) reported the development of polycystic ovarian disease in 89% of young women receiving valproic acid for epilepsy compared with 27% of epileptic women who were not taking valproic acid. In a more recent article, Isojarvi et al. (1996) noted that valproate use was associated with the onset of obesity and masculinization in more than half of the women, and polycystic ovarian disease developed in these individuals as well. Obviously, these would be prohibitive side effects for most female children with bipolar disorder. Further work is needed on whether or not this serious side effect appears only when the medication is given for epilepsy.

Prognosis

Recurrence of depression is common in children (Kovacs et al. 1984a). In addition, dysthymic children have developed major depression (Kovacs et al. 1984b). Approximately 80% of hospitalized depressed children are rehospitalized within 2 years of discharge (Asarnow et al. 1988).

Geller et al. (2001a) reported the 1-year recovery rate of 89 bipolar subjects (mean age, 10.9 years) to be 37.1%. The 1-year relapse rate for the same group was 38.3%. The low recovery and high relapse rates in this study supported a hypothesis of risk factors for poor outcomes that was based on similarities between the characteristics of the prepubertal and early adolescent bipolar disorder phenotype (long episode duration and high prevalence of mixed mania, psychosis, and rapid cycling) and those of severe bipolar disorder in adults.

Some have suggested that children with prepubertal major depressive disorder in fact have bipolar major depressive disorder but have not yet had their first manic episode (Geller et al. 1992, 1994). This hypothesis was supported by Geller et al. (1994) at the 2- to 5-year follow-up of subjects in their nortriptyline study. Of subjects diagnosed with prepubertal major depressive disorder, 31.6% had their diagnoses changed to bipolar disorder.

Geller et al. (2001b) followed up subjects who had participated in an earlier study of nortriptyline treatment for childhood depression (Geller et al. 1992). In the original study, the mean age of the children was 10.3 years. At follow-up, the mean age was 20.7 years. The follow-up study group consisted of 100 (90.9%) of the original 110 subjects and included 72 subjects who had a prepubertal diagnosis of major depressive disorder and 28 nondepressed comparison subjects. At follow-up, significantly more of the subjects who had a prepubertal diagnosis of major depressive disorder had bipolar I disorder (33.3%) than did comparison subjects (0%). Subjects who had prepubertal diagnoses of major depressive disorder also had significantly higher rates of any bipolar disorder (48.6% versus 7.1%), major depressive disorder (36.1% versus 14.3%), substance use disorder (30.6% versus 10.7%), and suicidality (22.2% versus 3.6%) than did comparison subjects. A history of mania in parents and grandparents predicted bipolar I disorder in the child.

Puig-Antich et al. (1985a, 1985b) reported impaired psychosocial functioning in subjects who had prepubertal major depressive disorder. More recently, Geller et al. (2000) found impaired psychosocial functioning in a sample of subjects with prepubertal and early adolescent bipolar disorder phenotype.

Anecdotal reports suggest that children with mania do not "grow out of it" (Poznanski 1993; Poznanski et al. 1993). The only naturalistic prospective follow-up study involved 54 adolescents with bipolar disorder. All but 2 recovered from their initial episode over a 5-year period (Strober et al. 1995). Of the 54 adolescents, 24 (44%) had a relapsing course and 11 (20%) experienced two or more episodes during the 5-year follow-up. Furthermore, rate of recovery was influenced by the polarity of the index episode. Subjects with an index depressive episode took longer to recover (median, 26 weeks) than did subjects with cycling (median, 15 weeks), mixed (median, 11 weeks), or pure manic (median, 9 weeks) episodes.

Research Issues

Mood disorders have been understudied in preschool-age and school-age children. In particular, there is little research on treatment. Despite this, clinicians are using antidepressants, mood stabilizers, and anticonvulsants in an effort to treat this population. More double-blind, placebo-controlled studies are needed in this age group to document the beneficial effects of these medications. There is also a need to refine diagnostic instruments to make accurate diagnosis and to monitor the course of mania and depression. Children at high risk for developing mood disorders should be carefully studied; these high-risk individuals include children with prepubertal depression or dysthymia, children of parents with mood disorders, and children with a family history of depression or mania. Predictors of depression and bipolar disorder in children should be more precisely identified; such predictors might include family history, family environment and supports, and stressful life events. Biological markers of mood disorder need to be identified. Finally, with the advances in molecular genetics, every study of mood disorders in children and adolescents should attempt to enhance our knowledge of the genetic contribution to these disorders of high morbidity and mortality.

References

Ahrens B, Grof P, Moller HJ, et al: Extended survival of patients on long-term lithium treatment. Can J Psychiatry 40:241–246, 1995

Akiskal HS: Developmental pathways to bipolarity: are juvenile-onset depressions pre-bipolar? J Am Acad Child Adolesc Psychiatry 34:754–763, 1995

Akiskal HS, Weller EB: Mood disorders and suicide in children and adolescents, in Comprehensive Textbook of Psychiatry. Edited by Kaplan HI, Sadock BJ. Baltimore, MD, Williams & Wilkins, 1989, pp 1981–1994

Akiskal HS, Djenderedjian AM, Rosenthal RH, et al: Cyclothymic disorder: validating criteria for inclusion in the bipolar affective group. Am J Psychiatry 134:1227–1233, 1977

Akiskal H, Khani M, Scott-Strauss A: Cyclothymic temperamental disorders. Psychiatr Clin North Am 2:527–554, 1979

Akiskal HS, Walker P, Puzantian VR, et al: Bipolar outcome in the course of depressive illness. Phenomenologic, familial, and pharmacologic predictors. J Affect Disord 5:115–128, 1983

Akiskal HS, Downs J, Jordan P, et al: Affective disorders in referred children and younger siblings of manic-depressives. Mode of onset and prospective course. Arch Gen Psychiatry 42:996–1003, 1985

Alderman J, Wolkow R, Chung M, et al: Sertraline treatment of children and adolescents with obsessive-compulsive disorder or depression: pharmacokinetics, tolerability, and efficacy (comments). J Am Acad Child Adolesc Psychiatry 37:386–394, 1998

Ambrosini PJ, Bianchi MD, Rabinovich H, et al: Antidepressant treatments in children and adolescents, I: affective disorders. J Am Acad Child Adolesc Psychiatry 32:1–6, 1993

Ambrosini PJ, Wagner KD, Biederman J, et al: Multicenter open-label sertraline study in adolescent outpatients with major depression. J Am Acad Child Adolesc Psychiatry 38:566–572, 1999

American Psychiatric Association: Diagnostic and Statistical Manual of Mental Disorders, 3rd Edition. Washington, DC, American Psychiatric Association, 1980

American Psychiatric Association: Diagnostic and Statistical Manual of Mental Disorders, 3rd Edition, Revised. Washington, DC, American Psychiatric Association, 1987

American Psychiatric Association: Diagnostic and Statistical Manual of Mental Disorders, 4th Edition. Washington, DC, American Psychiatric Association, 1994

Anderson JC, Williams S, McGee R, et al: DSM-III disorders in preadolescent children: prevalence in a large sample from the general population. Arch Gen Psychiatry 44:69–76, 1987

Annell A: Lithium in the treatment of children and adolescents. Acta Psychiatr Scand Suppl 207:19–30, 1969

Anthony J, Scott P: Manic-depressive psychosis in childhood. Child Psychology and Psychiatry 4:53–72, 1960

Asarnow JR, Goldstein MJ, Carlson GA, et al: Childhood-onset depressive disorders: a follow-up study of rates of rehospitalization and out-of-home placement among child psychiatric inpatients. J Affect Disord 15:245–253, 1988

Ballenger JC: The use of anticonvulsants in manic-depressive illness. J Clin Psychiatry 49:21–25, 1988

Barrett A: Manic-depressive psychosis in childhood. Int Clin 3:205–217, 1931

Biederman J, Wozniak J, Kiely K, et al: CBCL clinical scales discriminate prepubertal children with structured interview-derived diagnosis of mania from those with ADHD. J Am Acad Child Adolesc Psychiatry 34:464–471, 1995

Biederman J, Faraone S, Mick E, et al: Attention-deficit hyperactivity disorder and juvenile mania: an overlooked comorbidity? J Am Acad Child Adolesc Psychiatry 35:997–1008, 1996

Biederman J, Mick E, Faraone SV, et al: Pediatric mania: a developmental subtype of bipolar disorder? Biol Psychiatry 48:458–466, 2000

Billy D, Beuscart R, Collinet C, et al: Sex differences in the manifestations of depression in young people: a study of French high school students, part I: prevalence and clinical data. Eur Child Adolesc Psychiatry 1:135–145, 1992

Bird HR, Canino G, Rubio-Stipec M, et al: Estimates of the prevalence of childhood maladjustment in a community survey in Puerto Rico: the use of combined measures. Arch Gen Psychiatry 45:1120–1126, 1988

Birmaher B, Ryan ND, Williamson DE, et al: Childhood and adolescent depression: a review of the past 10 years, part II. J Am Acad Child Adolesc Psychiatry 35:1575–1583, 1996

Bleuler E: Textbook of Psychiatry. New York, Macmillan, 1934

Botteron KN, Vannier MW, Geller B, et al: Preliminary study of magnetic resonance imaging characteristics in 8- to 16-year-olds with mania. J Am Acad Child Adolesc Psychiatry 34:742–749, 1995

Bowden CL, Janicak PG, Orsulak P, et al: Relation of serum valproate concentration to response in mania. Am J Psychiatry 153:765–770, 1996

Bowlby J: Maternal Care and Mental Health, 2nd Edition. Geneva, World Health Organization, 1951

Bowring MA, Kovacs M: Difficulties in diagnosing manic disorders among children and adolescents. J Am Acad Child Adolesc Psychiatry 31:611–614, 1992

Brent DA, Kolko DJ, Birmaher B, et al: Predictors of treatment efficacy in a clinical trial of three psychosocial treatments for adolescent depression. J Am Acad Child Adolesc Psychiatry 37:906–914, 1998

Brumback RA, Weinberg WA: Mania in childhood, II: therapeutic trial of lithium carbonate and further description of manic-depressive illness in children. Am J Dis Child 131:1122–1126, 1977

Budman CL, Sherling M, Bruun RD: Combined pharmacotherapy risk. J Am Acad Child Adolesc Psychiatry 34:263–264, 1995

Burke KC, Burke JD, Regier DA, et al: Age at onset of selected mental disorders in five community populations. Arch Gen Psychiatry 47:511–518, 1990

Campbell J: Manic-depressive psychoses in children. J Nerv Ment Dis 116:424–439, 1952

Campbell JD: Manic-Depressive Disease: Clinical and Psychiatric Significance. Philadelphia, PA, JB Lippincott, 1953

Canals J, Domenech E, Carbajo G, et al: Prevalence of DSM-III-R and ICD-10 psychiatric disorders in a Spanish population of 18-year-olds. Acta Psychiatr Scand 96:287–294, 1997

Cantwell DP, Carlson GA: Affective Disorders in Childhood and Adolescence: An Update. Child Behavior and Development Series. New York, Spectrum, 1983

Carlson GA: Bipolar affective disorders in childhood and adolescence, in Affective Disorders in Childhood and Adolescence. Edited by Cantwell DP, Carlson GA. New York, Spectrum, 1983, pp 61–83

Carlson GA: Classification issues of bipolar disorders in childhood. Psychiatr Dev 2:273–285, 1984

Carlson GA: Child and adolescent mania: diagnostic considerations. J Child Psychol Psychiatry 31:331–341, 1990

Carlson GA: Identifying prepubertal mania. J Am Acad Child Adolesc Psychiatry 34:750–753, 1995

Carlson GA, Kashani JH: Manic symptoms in a non-referred adolescent population. J Affect Disord 15:219–226, 1988a

Carlson GA, Kashani JH: Phenomenology of major depression from childhood through adulthood: analysis of three studies. Am J Psychiatry 145:1222–1225, 1988b

Carlson G, Strober M: Manic-depressive illness in early adolescence: a study of clinical and diagnostic characteristics in six cases. J Am Acad Child Adolesc Psychiatry 17:138–153, 1978

Carlson GA, Fennig S, Bromet EJ: The confusion between bipolar disorder and schizophrenia in youth: where does it stand in the 1990s? J Am Acad Child Adolesc Psychiatry 33:453–460, 1994

Carlson GA, Bromet EJ, Sievers S: Phenomenology and outcome of subjects with early and adult-onset psychotic mania. Am J Psychiatry 157:213–219, 2000

Casat CD, Powell K: The dexamethasone suppression test in children and adolescents with major depressive disorder: a review. J Clin Psychiatry 49:390–393, 1988

Chouinard G, Goodman W, Greist J, et al: Results of a double-blind placebo controlled trial of a new serotonin uptake inhibitor, sertraline, in the treatment of obsessive-compulsive disorder. Psychopharmacol Bull 26:279–284, 1990

Coffey CE, Wilkinson WE, Weiner RD, et al: Quantitative cerebral anatomy in depression: a controlled magnetic resonance imaging study. Arch Gen Psychiatry 50:7–16, 1993

Cohn CK, Shrivastava R, Mendels J, et al: Double-blind, multicenter comparison of sertraline and amitriptyline in elderly depressed patients. J Clin Psychiatry 51 (suppl B):28–33, 1990

Coryell W, Endicott J, Keller M: Major depression in a non-clinical sample: demographic and clinical risk factors for first onset. Arch Gen Psychiatry 49:117–125, 1992

Costello A, Edelbrook C, Kalas R, et al: The NIMH Diagnostic Interview Schedule for Children (DISC). Pittsburgh, PA, Pergamon, 1982

Dahl R, Puig-Antich J, Ryan N, et al: Cortisol secretion in adolescents with major depressive disorder. Acta Psychiatr Scand 80:18–26, 1989

Dahl RE, Ryan ND, Puig-Antich J, et al: 24-Hour cortisol measures in adolescents with major depression: a controlled study. Biol Psychiatry 30:25–36, 1991

Dahl RE, Ryan ND, Williamson DE, et al: Regulation of sleep and growth hormone in adolescent depression. J Am Acad Child Adolesc Psychiatry 31:615–621, 1992

Davis RE: Manic-depressive variant syndrome in childhood: a preliminary report. Am J Psychiatry 136:702–706, 1979

De Bellis MD, Dahl RE, Perel JM, et al: Nocturnal ACTH, cortisol, growth hormone, and prolactin secretion in prepubertal depression. J Am Acad Child Adolesc Psychiatry 35:1130–1138, 1996

DeLong GR: Lithium carbonate treatment of select behavior disorders in children suggesting manic-depressive illness. J Pediatr 93:689–694, 1978

DeLong GR, Aldershof AL: Long-term experience with lithium treatment in childhood: correlation with clinical diagnosis. J Am Acad Child Adolesc Psychiatry 26:389–394, 1987

DeVane CL, Sallee FR: Serotonin selective reuptake inhibitors in child and adolescent psychopharmacology: a review of published experience. J Clin Psychiatry 57:55–66, 1996

Egeland JA, Hostetter AM, Pauls DL, et al: Prodromal symptoms before onset of manic-depressive disorder suggested by first hospital admission histories. J Am Acad Child Adolesc Psychiatry 39:1245–1252, 2000

Emslie GJ, Rush AJ, Weinberg WA, et al: A double-blind, randomized, placebo-controlled trial of fluoxetine in children and adolescents with depression. Arch Gen Psychiatry 54:1031–1037, 1997

Emslie GJ, Rush AJ, Weinberg WA, et al: Fluoxetine in child and adolescent depression: acute and maintenance treatment. Depress Anxiety 7:32–39, 1998

Endicott J, Spitzer RL: A diagnostic interview: the Schedule for Affective Disorders and Schizophrenia. Arch Gen Psychiatry 35:837–844, 1978

Esquirol E: Mental Maladies: A Treatise on Insanity. Philadelphia, PA, Lea & Blanchard, 1845

Feighner JP, Robins E, Guze SB, et al: Diagnostic criteria for use in psychiatric research. Arch Gen Psychiatry 26:57–63, 1972

Feinstein SC, Wolpert EA: Juvenile manic-depressive illness: clinical and therapeutic considerations. J Am Acad Child Psychiatry 12:123–136, 1973

Ferro T, Carlson GA, Grayson P, et al: Depressive disorders: distinctions in children. J Am Acad Child Adolesc Psychiatry 33:664–670, 1994

Fetner HH, Geller B: Lithium and tricyclic antidepressants. Psychiatr Clin North Am 15:223–224, 1992

Fleming JE, Offord DR: Epidemiology of childhood depressive disorders: a critical review. J Am Acad Child Adolesc Psychiatry 29:571–580, 1990

Fleming JE, Boyle MH, Offord DR: The outcome of adolescent depression in the Ontario Child Health Study follow-up. J Am Acad Child Adolesc Psychiatry 32:28–33, 1993

Fristad MA, Weller EB, Weller RA: The Mania Rating Scale: can it be used in children? A preliminary report. J Am Acad Child Adolesc Psychiatry 31:252–257, 1992

Fristad MA, Weller RA, Weller EB: The Mania Rating Scale (MRS): further reliability and validity studies with children. Ann Clin Psychiatry 7:127–132, 1995

Gammon GD, John K, Rothblum ED, et al: Use of a structured diagnostic interview to identify bipolar disorder in adolescent inpatients: frequency and manifestations of the disorder. Am J Psychiatry 140:543–547, 1983

Garrison CZ, Addy CL, Jackson KL, et al: Major depressive disorder and dysthymia in young adolescents. Am J Epidemiol 135:792–802, 1992

Geller B: The high prevalence of bipolar parents among prepubertal mood-disordered children necessitates appropriate questions to establish bipolarity. Curr Opin Psychiatry 9:239–240, 1996

Geller B, Fetner HH: Children's 24-hour serum lithium level after a single dose predicts initial dose and steady-state plasma level (letter). J Clin Psychopharmacol 9:155, 1989

Geller B, Luby J: Child and adolescent bipolar disorder: a review of the past 10 years. J Am Acad Child Adolesc Psychiatry 36:1168–1176, 1997. (Published erratum appears in J Am Child Adolesc Psychiatry 36:1642, 1997.)

Geller B, Cooper TB, Chestnut EC, et al: Preliminary data on the relationship between nortriptyline plasma level and response in depressed children. Am J Psychiatry 143:1283–1286, 1986

Geller B, Cooper TB, McCombs HG, et al: Double-blind, placebo-controlled study of nortriptyline in depressed children using a "fixed plasma level" design. Psychopharmacol Bull 25:101–108, 1989

Geller B, Cooper TB, Graham DL, et al: Pharmacokinetically designed double-blind placebo-controlled study of nortriptyline in 6- to 12-year-olds with major depressive disorder. J Am Acad Child Adolesc Psychiatry 31:34–44, 1992

Geller B, Fox LW, Clark KA: Rate and predictors of prepubertal bipolarity during follow-up of 6- to 12-year-old depressed children. J Am Acad Child Adolesc Psychiatry 33:461–468, 1994

Geller B, Sun K, Zimerman B, et al: Complex and rapid-cycling in bipolar children and adolescents: a preliminary study. J Affect Disord 34:259–268, 1995

Geller B, Todd RD, Luby J, et al: Treatment-resistant depression in children and adolescents. Psychiatr Clin North Am 19:253–267, 1996

Geller B, Warner K, Williams M, et al: Prepubertal and young adolescent bipolarity versus ADHD: assessment and validity using the WASH-U-KSADS, CBCL and TRF. J Affect Disord 51:93–100, 1998a

Geller B, Williams M, Zimerman B, et al: Prepubertal and early adolescent bipolarity differentiate from ADHD by manic symptoms, grandiose delusions, ultra-rapid or ultradian cycling. J Affect Disord 51:81–91, 1998b

Geller B, Bolhofner K, Craney JL, et al: Psychosocial functioning in a prepubertal and early adolescent bipolar disorder phenotype. J Am Acad Child Adolesc Psychiatry 39:1543–1548, 2000

Geller B, Craney JL, Bolhofner K, et al: One-year recovery and relapse rates of children with a prepubertal and early adolescent bipolar disorder phenotype. Am J Psychiatry 158:303–305, 2001a

Geller B, Zimerman B, Williams M, et al: Bipolar disorder at prospective follow-up of adults who had prepubertal major depressive disorder. Am J Psychiatry 158:125–127, 2001b

Gershon ES, Hamovit JH, Guroff JJ, et al: Birth-cohort changes in manic and depressive disorders in relatives of bipolar and schizoaffective patients. Arch Gen Psychiatry 44:314–319, 1987

Goodman SH, Schwab-Stone M, Lahey BB, et al: Major depression and dysthymia in children and adolescents: discriminant validity and differential consequences in a community sample. J Am Acad Child Adolesc Psychiatry 39:761–770, 2000

Goodwin F, Jamison K: Manic-Depressive Illness. New York, Oxford University Press, 1990

Goodyer I, Cooper PJ: A community study of depression in adolescent girls, II: the clinical features of identified disorder. Br J Psychiatry 163:374–380, 1993

Goodyer I, Germany E, Gowrusankur J, et al: Social influences on the course of anxious and depressive disorders in school-age children. Br J Psychiatry 158:676–684, 1991

Greist J, Chouinard G, DuBoff E, et al: Double-blind parallel comparison of three dosages of sertraline and placebo in outpatients with obsessive-compulsive disorder. Arch Gen Psychiatry 52:289–295, 1995a

Greist JH, Jefferson JW, Kobak KA, et al: A 1-year double-blind placebo-controlled fixed dose study of sertraline in the treatment of obsessive-compulsive disorder. Int Clin Psychopharmacol 10:57–65, 1995b

Harrington R: Depressive disorder in adolescence. Arch Dis Child 72:193–195, 1995

Harrington R, Fudge H, Rutter M, et al: Adult outcomes of childhood and adolescent depression, II: links with antisocial disorders. J Am Acad Child Adolesc Psychiatry 30:434–439, 1991

Himmelhoch JM, Garfinkel ME: Soources of lithium resistance in mixed mania. Psychopharmacol Bull 22:613–620, 1986

Hoar W: Prozac Rx for children jumps 500%. Mental Health News Alert, September 29, 1998, p 13

Hodges KK, Kline J, Stern L: The development of a child assessment interview for research and clinical use. J Abnorm Psychol 10:173–189, 1982

Homburger A: Lectures on the Psychopathology of Childhood. Berlin, Springer, 1926, p 852

Horowitz HA: The use of lithium in the treatment of the drug-induced psychotic reaction. Dis Nerv Syst 36:159–163, 1975

Horowitz HA: Lithium and the treatment of adolescent manic depressive illness. Dis Nerv Syst 38:480–483, 1977

Hsu LK: Lithium-resistant adolescent mania. J Am Acad Child Psychiatry 25:280–283, 1986

Hughes CW, Preskorn SH, Weller E, et al: The effect of concomitant disorders in childhood depression on predicting treatment response. Psychopharmacol Bull 26:235–238, 1990

Hughes CW, Emslie GJ, Crismon ML, et al: The Texas Children's Medication Algorithm Project: report of the Texas Consensus Conference Panel on Medication Treatment of Childhood Major Depressive Disorder. J Am Acad Child Adolesc Psychiatry 38:1442–1454, 1999

Husain MM, McDonald WM, Doraiswamy PM, et al: A magnetic resonance imaging study of putamen nuclei in major depression. Psychiatry Res 40:95–99, 1991

Isaac G: Is bipolar disorder the most common diagnostic entity in hospitalized adolescents and children? Adolescence 30:273–276, 1995

Isojarvi JI, Laatikainen TJ, Pakarinen AJ, et al: Polycystic ovaries and hyperandrogenism in women taking valproate for epilepsy. N Engl J Med 329:1383–1388, 1993

Isojarvi JI, Laatikainen TJ, Knip M, et al: Obesity and endocrine disorders in women taking valproate for epilepsy (comments). Ann Neurol 39:579–584, 1996

Jernigan TL, Trauner DA, Hesselink JR, et al: Maturation of human cerebrum observed in vivo during adolescence. Brain 114(pt 5):2037–2049, 1991

Joyce PR: Age of onset in bipolar affective disorder and misdiagnosis as schizophrenia. Psychol Med 14:145–149, 1984

Kafantaris V: Treatment of bipolar disorder in children and adolescents. J Am Acad Child Adolesc Psychiatry 34:732–741, 1995

Kanner L: The development and present status of psychiatry in pediatrics. J Pediatr 11:418–435, 1937

Kasanin J: The affective psychoses in children. Am J Psychiatry 10:897–926, 1931

Kashani JH, Carlson GA: Seriously depressed preschoolers. Am J Psychiatry 144:348–350, 1987

Kashani JH, Barbero GJ, Bolander FD: Depression in hospitalized pediatric patients. J Am Acad Child Psychiatry 20:123–134, 1981

Kashani JH, McGee RO, Clarkson SE, et al: Depression in a sample of 9-year-old children: prevalence and associated characteristics. Arch Gen Psychiatry 40:1217–1223, 1983

Kashani JH, Shekim WO, Reid JC: Amitriptyline in children with major depressive disorder: a double-blind crossover pilot study. J Am Acad Child Psychiatry 23:348–351, 1984

Keck PE Jr, McElroy SL: Outcome in the pharmacologic treatment of bipolar disorder. J Clin Psychopharmacol 16:15S–23S, 1996

Keller MB, Lavori PW, Coryell W, et al: Bipolar I: a five-year prospective follow-up. J Nerv Ment Dis 181:238–245, 1993

Keller MB, Ryan ND, Strober M, et al: Efficacy of paroxetine in the treatment of adolescent major depression: a randomized, controlled trial. J Am Acad Child Adolesc Psychiatry 40:762–772, 2001

Kessler RC, McGonagle KA, Zhao S, et al: Lifetime and 12-month prevalence of DSM-III-R psychiatric disorders in the United States: results from the National Comorbidity Survey. Arch Gen Psychiatry 51:8–19, 1994

Khandelwal SK, Varma VK, Srinivasa Murthy R: Renal function in children receiving long-term lithium prophylaxis. Am J Psychiatry 141:278–279, 1984

Klein DN, Norden KA, Ferro T, et al: Thirty-month naturalistic follow-up study of early onset dysthymic disorder: course, diagnostic stability, and prediction of outcome. J Abnorm Psychol 107:338–348, 1998

Kolvin I, Barrett ML, Bhate SR, et al: The Newcastle Child Depression Project: diagnosis and classification of depression. Br J Psychiatry Suppl Jul (11):9–21, 1991

Koran LM: The reliability of clinical methods, data and judgments (first of two parts). N Engl J Med 293:642–646, 1975

Kovacs M: The Interview Schedule for Children. Psychopharmacol Bull 21:991–994, 1978

Kovacs M: The Children's Depression Inventory (CDI). Psychopharmacol Bull 21:995–998, 1985

Kovacs M: Presentation and course of major depressive disorder during childhood and later years of the life span. J Am Acad Child Adolesc Psychiatry 35:705–715, 1996

Kovacs M, Gatsonis C: Secular trends in age at onset of major depressive disorder in a clinical sample of children. J Psychiatr Res 28:319–329, 1994

Kovacs M, Pollock M: Bipolar disorder and comorbid conduct disorder in childhood and adolescence. J Am Acad Child Adolesc Psychiatry 34:715–723, 1995

Kovacs M, Feinberg TL, Crouse-Novak MA, et al: Depressive disorders in childhood, I: a longitudinal prospective study of characteristics and recovery. Arch Gen Psychiatry 41:229–237, 1984a

Kovacs M, Feinberg TL, Crouse-Novak M, et al: Depressive disorders in childhood, II: a longitudinal study of the risk for a subsequent major depression. Arch Gen Psychiatry 41:643–649, 1984b

Kovacs M, Paulauskas S, Gatsonis C, et al: Depressive disorders in childhood, III: a longitudinal study of comorbidity with and risk for conduct disorders. J Affect Disord 15:205–217, 1988

Kovacs M, Gatsonis C, Paulauskas SL, et al: Depressive disorders in childhood, IV: a longitudinal study of comorbidity with and risk for anxiety disorders. Arch Gen Psychiatry 46:776–782, 1989

Kovacs M, Akiskal HS, Gatsonis C, et al: Childhood-onset dysthymic disorder. Clinical features and prospective naturalistic outcome. Arch Gen Psychiatry 51:365–374, 1994

Kovacs M, Obrosky DS, Gatsonis C, et al: First-episode major depressive and dysthymic disorder in childhood: clinical and sociodemographic factors in recovery. J Am Acad Child Adolesc Psychiatry 36:777–784, 1997

Kowatch RA, Suppes T, Carmody TJ, et al: Effect size of lithium, divalproex sodium, and carbamazepine in children and adolescents with bipolar disorder. J Am Acad Child Adolesc Psychiatry 39:713–720, 2000

Kraepelin E: Manic-Depressive Insanity and Paranoia. Edinburgh, Scotland, Livingstone, 1921

Krishnan KR, McDonald WM, Escalona PR, et al: Magnetic resonance imaging of the caudate nuclei in depression: preliminary observations. Arch Gen Psychiatry 49:553–557, 1992

Kutcher SP: Child and Adolescent Psychopharmacology. Philadelphia, PA, WB Saunders, 1997

Kutcher SP, Williamson P, Silverberg J, et al: Nocturnal growth hormone secretion in depressed older adolescents. J Am Acad Child Adolesc Psychiatry 27:751–754, 1988

Kutcher SP, Marton P, Korenblum M: Relationship between psychiatric illness and conduct disorder in adolescents. Can J Psychiatry 34:526–529, 1989

Kutcher S, Malkin D, Silverberg J, et al: Nocturnal cortisol, thyroid stimulating hormone, and growth hormone secretory profiles in depressed adolescents. J Am Acad Child Adolesc Psychiatry 30:407–414, 1991

LaGrone DM: Manic-depressive illness in early childhood: the case of Christopher. South Med J 74:479–481, 1981

Leonard HL, March J, Rickler KC, et al: Review of the pharmacology of the selective serotonin reuptake inhibitors in children and adolescents. J Am Acad Child Adolesc Psychiatry 36:725–736, 1997

Lewinsohn PM, Rohde P, Seeley JR, et al: Comorbidity of unipolar depression, I: major depression with dysthymia. J Abnorm Psychol 100:205–213, 1991

Lewinsohn PM, Hops H, Roberts RE, et al: Adolescent psychopathology, I: prevalence and incidence of depression and other DSM-III-R disorders in high school students. J Abnorm Psychol 102:133–144, 1993

Lewinsohn PM, Clarke GN, Seeley JR, et al: Major depression in community adolescents: age at onset, episode duration, and time to recurrence. J Am Acad Child Adolesc Psychiatry 33:809–818, 1994

Lewinsohn PM, Gotlib IH, Seeley JR: Adolescent psychopathology, IV: specificity of psychosocial risk factors for depression and substance abuse in older adolescents. J Am Acad Child Adolesc Psychiatry 34:1221–1229, 1995a

Lewinsohn PM, Klein DN, Seeley JR: Bipolar disorders in a community sample of older adolescents: prevalence, phenomenology, comorbidity, and course. J Am Acad Child Adolesc Psychiatry 34:454–463, 1995b

Ling W, Oftedal G, Weinberg W: Depressive illness in childhood presenting as severe headache. Am J Dis Child 120:122–124, 1970

Lish JD, Dime-Meenan S, Whybrow PC, et al: The National Depressive and Manic-Depressive Association (DMDA) survey of bipolar members. J Affect Disord 31:281–294, 1994

Loranger AW, Levine PM: Age at onset of bipolar affective illness. Arch Gen Psychiatry 35:1345–1348, 1978

McCauley E, Myers K, Mitchell J, et al: Depression in young people: initial presentation and clinical course. J Am Acad Child Adolesc Psychiatry 32:714–722, 1993

McElroy SL, Strakowski SM, West SA, et al: Phenomenology of adolescent and adult mania in hospitalized patients with bipolar disorder. Am J Psychiatry 154:44–49, 1997

McGee R, Williams S: A longitudinal study of depression in nine-year-old children. J Am Acad Child Adolesc Psychiatry 27:342–348, 1988

McGlashan TH: Adolescent versus adult onset of mania. Am J Psychiatry 145:221–223, 1988

McGuffin P, Katz R: The genetics of depression and manic-depressive disorder. Br J Psychiatry 155:294–304, 1989

Merikangas KR, Angst J, Eaton W: Comorbidity and boundaries of affective disorders with anxiety disorders and substance misuse: results of an international task force. Br J Psychiatry Suppl 30:58–67, 1996

Milberger S, Biederman J, Faraone SV, et al: Attention deficit hyperactivity disorder and comorbid disorders: issues of overlapping symptoms. Am J Psychiatry 152:1793–1799, 1995

Mitchell J, McCauley E, Burke PM, et al: Phenomenology of depression in children and adolescents. J Am Acad Child Adolesc Psychiatry 27:12–20, 1988

Muller-Oerlinghausen B, Ahrens B, Grof E, et al: The effect of long-term lithium treatment on the mortality of patients with manic-depressive and schizoaffective illness. Acta Psychiatr Scand 86:218–222, 1992

Muller-Oerlinghausen B, Wolf T, Ahrens B, et al: Mortality during initial and during later lithium treatment. A collaborative study by the International Group for the Study of Lithium-treated Patients. Acta Psychiatr Scand 90:295–297, 1994

Murdoch D, McTavish D: Sertraline: a review of its pharmacodynamic and pharmacokinetic properties, and therapeutic potential in depression and obsessive-compulsive disorder. Drugs 44:604–624, 1992

Olsen T: Follow-up study of manic-depressive patients whose first attack occurred before the age of 19. Acta Psychiatr Scand Suppl 162:45–51, 1961

Papatheodorou G, Kutcher SP: Divalproex sodium treatment in late adolescent and young adult acute mania. Psychopharmacol Bull 29:213–219, 1993

Pfeffer CR, Stokes P, Shindledecker R: Suicidal behavior and hypothalamic-pituitary-adrenocortical axis indices in child psychiatric inpatients. Biol Psychiatry 29:909–917, 1991

Polaino A, Domenech E: Prevalence of childhood depression: results of the first study in Spain. Journal of Child Psychology 34:1007–1017, 1993

Popper C: Biological cyclicity in two preschool children. Conference proceedings, American Academy of Child and Adolescent Psychiatry, Los Angeles, CA, 1984

Post RM, Rubinow DR, Ballenger JC: Conditioning and sensitisation in the longitudinal course of affective illness. Br J Psychiatry 149:191–201, 1986

Potter RL: Manic-depressive variant syndrome of childhood. Diagnostic and therapeutic considerations. Clin Pediatr (Phila) 22:495–499, 1983

Poznanski EO, Freeman LN, Mokros H: Violent events reported by normal urban school-aged children: characteristics and depression correlate. J Am Acad Child Adolesc Psychiatry 32:419–423, 1993

Poznanski EO, Grossman JA, Buchsbaum Y, et al: Preliminary studies of the reliability and validity of the Children's Depression Rating Scale. J Am Acad Child Psychiatry 23:191–197, 1984

Poznanski EO, Freman LN, Mokros HB: Children's Depression Rating Scale—Revised. Psychopharmacol Bull 21:979–989, 1985

Poznanski EO: Mania in preschool children with case vignette and videotape: questions and answers. Conference proceedings, American Academy of Child and Adolescent Psychiatry, San Francisco, CA, 1993

Preskorn SH, Weller EB, Weller RA: Depression in children: relationship between plasma imipramine levels and response. J Clin Psychiatry 43:450–453, 1982

Preskorn SH, Weller EB, Hughes CW, et al: Depression in prepubertal children: dexamethasone nonsuppression predicts differential response to imipramine vs. placebo. Psychopharmacol Bull 23:128–133, 1987

Puig-Antich J, Chambers W: The Schedule for Affective Disorders and Schizophrenia for School-Age Children (Kiddie-SADS). New York, New York State Psychiatric Institute, 1978

Puig-Antich J, Perel JM, Lupatkin W, et al: Plasma levels of imipramine (IMI) and desmethylimipramine (DMI) and clinical response in prepubertal major depressive disorder: a preliminary report. J Am Acad Child Psychiatry 18:616–627, 1979

Puig-Antich J, Goetz R, Davies M, et al: Growth hormone secretion in prepubertal children with major depression, II: sleep-related plasma concentrations during a depressive episode. Arch Gen Psychiatry 41:463–466, 1984

Puig-Antich J, Lukens E, Davies M, et al: Psychosocial functioning in prepubertal major depressive disorders, I: interpersonal relationships during the depressive episode. Arch Gen Psychiatry 42:500–507, 1985a

Puig-Antich J, Lukens E, Davies M, et al: Psychosocial functioning in prepubertal major depressive disorders, II: interpersonal relationships after sustained recovery from affective episode. Arch Gen Psychiatry 42:511–517, 1985b

Puig-Antich J, Perel JM, Lupatkin W, et al: Imipramine in prepubertal major depressive disorders. Arch Gen Psychiatry 44:81–89, 1987

Puig-Antich J, Dahl R, Ryan N, et al: Cortisol secretion in prepubertal children with major depressive disorder: episode and recovery. Arch Gen Psychiatry 46:801–809, 1989a

Puig-Antich J, Goetz D, Davies M, et al: A controlled family history study of prepubertal major depressive disorder. Arch Gen Psychiatry 46:406–418, 1989b

Reich W: Diagnostic Interview for Children and Adolescents (DICA). J Am Acad Child Adolesc Psychiatry 39:59–66, 2000

Reiss AL: Developmental manifestations in a boy with prepubertal bipolar disorder. J Clin Psychiatry 46:441–443, 1985

Rey F, Gutierrez-Casares JR: Paroxetine in children with major depressive disorder: an open trial. J Am Acad Child Adolesc Psychiatry 36:1443–1447, 1997

Ryan ND, Puig-Antich J, Ambrosini P, et al: The clinical picture of major depression in children and adolescents. Arch Gen Psychiatry 44:854–861, 1987

Ryan ND, Birmaher B, Perel JM, et al: Neuroendocrine response to L-5-hydroxytryptophan challenge in prepubertal major depression: depressed vs normal children. Arch Gen Psychiatry 49:843–851, 1992a

Ryan ND, Williamson DE, Iyengar S, et al: A secular increase in child and adolescent onset affective disorder. J Am Acad Child Adolesc Psychiatry 31:600–605, 1992b

Ryan ND, Dahl RE, Birmaher B, et al: Stimulatory tests of growth hormone secretion in prepubertal major depression: depressed versus normal children. J Am Acad Child Adolesc Psychiatry 33:824–833, 1994

Schou M: Lithium in psychiatric therapy and prophylaxis. J Psychiatr Res 6:67–95, 1968

Schou M: Prophylactic lithium treatment of unipolar and bipolar manic-depressive illness. Psychopathology 28:81–85, 1995

Schou M, Hansen HE, Thomsen K, et al: Lithium treatment in Aarhus, 2: risk of renal failure and of intoxication. Pharmacopsychiatry 22:101–103, 1989

Schulterbrandt JG, Raskin A: Depression in Childhood: Diagnosis, Treatment, and Conceptual Models. New York, Raven, 1977

Schurhoff F, Bellivier F, Jouvent R, et al: Early and late onset bipolar disorders: two different forms of manic-depressive illness? J Affect Disord 58:215–221, 2000

Shaffer D, Fisher P, Lucas CP, et al: NIMH Diagnostic Interview Schedule for Children Version IV (NIMH DISC-IV): description, differences from previous versions, and reliability of some common diagnoses. J Am Acad Child Adolesc Psychiatry 39:28–38, 2000

Silva RR, Campbell M, Golden RR, et al: Side effects associated with lithium and placebo administration in aggressive children. Psychopharmacol Bull 28:319–326, 1992

Snead RW, Boon F, Presberg J: Paroxetine for self-injurious behavior. J Am Acad Child Adolesc Psychiatry 33:909–910, 1994

Spitz R: Anaclitic depression. Psychoanal Study Child 2:113–117, 1946

Steingard RJ, Renshaw PF, Yurgelun-Todd D, et al: Structural abnormalities in brain magnetic resonance images of depressed children. J Am Acad Child Adolesc Psychiatry 35:307–311, 1996

Strober M: Relevance of early age-of-onset in genetic studies of bipolar affective disorder. J Am Acad Child Adolesc Psychiatry 31:606–610, 1992

Strober M, Carlson G: Bipolar illness in adolescents with major depression: clinical, genetic, and psychopharmacologic predictors in a three- to four-year prospective follow-up investigation. Arch Gen Psychiatry 39:549–555, 1982

Strober M, Morrell W, Burroughs J, et al: A family study of bipolar I disorder in adolescence: early onset of symptoms linked to increased familial loading and lithium resistance. J Affect Disord 15:255–268, 1988

Strober M, Morrell W, Lampert C, et al: Relapse following discontinuation of lithium maintenance therapy in adolescents with bipolar I illness: a naturalistic study. Am J Psychiatry 147:457–461, 1990

Strober M, Lampert C, Schmidt S, et al: The course of major depressive disorder in adolescents, I: recovery and risk of manic switching in a follow-up of psychotic and nonpsychotic subtypes. J Am Acad Child Adolesc Psychiatry 32:34–42, 1993

Strober M, Schmidt-Lackner S, Freeman R, et al: Recovery and relapse in adolescents with bipolar affective illness: a five-year naturalistic, prospective follow-up. J Am Acad Child Adolesc Psychiatry 34:724–731, 1995

Strober M, DeAntonio M, Schmidt-Lackner S, et al: The pharmacotherapy of depressive illness in adolescents: an open-label comparison of fluoxetine with imipramine-treated historical controls. J Clin Psychiatry 60:164–169, 1999

Telegdy L, Kovacs M, Bodor G, et al: [Diagnostic problems of paraquat poisoning] (Hungarian). Orv Hetil 125:2057–2061, 1984

Thompson RJ Jr, Schindler FH: Embryonic mania. Child Psychiatry Hum Dev 6:149–154, 1976

Todd RD, Neuman R, Geller B, et al: Genetic studies of affective disorders: should we be starting with childhood onset probands? J Am Acad Child Adolesc Psychiatry 32:1164–1171, 1993

Varanka TM, Weller RA, Weller EB, et al: Lithium treatment of manic episodes with psychotic features in prepubertal children. Am J Psychiatry 145:1557–1559, 1988

Vitiello B, Behar D, Malone R, et al: Pharmacokinetics of lithium carbonate in children. J Clin Psychopharmacol 8:355–359, 1988

Vostanis P, Feehan C, Grattan E, et al: A randomised controlled out-patient trial of cognitive-behavioural treatment for children and adolescents with depression: 9-month follow-up. J Affect Disord 40:105–116, 1996

Warner V, Weissman MM, Fendrich M, et al: The course of major depression in the offspring of depressed patients: incidence, recurrence, and recovery. Arch Gen Psychiatry 49:795–801, 1992

Waterman GS, Dahl RE, Birmaher B, et al: The 24-hour pattern of prolactin secretion in depressed and normal adolescents. Biol Psychiatry 35:440–445, 1994

Weinberg WA, Brumback RA: Mania in childhood: case studies and literature review. Am J Dis Child 130:380–385, 1976

Weinberg WA, Rehmet A: Childhood affective disorder and school problems, in Affective Disorders in Childhood and Adolescence: An Update. Edited by Cantwell DP, Carlson GA. Jamaica, NY, Spectrum, 1983, pp 109–128

Weissman MM, Wolk S, Wickramaratne P, et al: Children with prepubertal-onset major depressive disorder and anxiety grown up. Arch Gen Psychiatry 56:794–801, 1999

Weller EB, Weller RA: Current Perspectives on Major Depressive Disorders. Washington, DC, American Psychiatric Press, 1984

Weller EB, Weller RA: Grief in children and adolescents, in Psychiatric Disorders in Children and Adolescents. Edited by Garfinkel B, Carlson G, Weller EB. Philadelphia, PA, W.B. Saunders, 1990, pp 37–47

Weller EB, Weller RA, Fristad MA: Lithium dosage guide for prepubertal children: a preliminary report. J Am Acad Child Psychiatry 25:92–95, 1986

Weller EB, Weller RA, Fristad MA: Bipolar disorder in children: misdiagnosis, underdiagnosis, and future directions. J Am Acad Child Adolesc Psychiatry 34:709–714, 1995

Weller EB, Weller RA, Fristad MA, et al: Children's Interview for Psychiatric Syndromes (ChIPS). Washington, DC, American Psychiatric Press, 1999

Weller RA, Weller EB, Tucker SG, et al: Mania in prepubertal children: has it been underdiagnosed? J Affect Disord 11:151–154, 1986

Welner Z, Reich W, Herjanic B, et al: Reliability, validity, and parent-child agreement studies of the Diagnostic Interview for Children and Adolescents (DICA). J Am Acad Child Adolesc Psychiatry 26:649–653, 1987

Williamson DE, Birmaher B, Brent DA, et al: Atypical symptoms of depression in a sample of depressed child and adolescent outpatients. J Am Acad Child Adolesc Psychiatry 39:1253–1259, 2000

Wood A, Harrington R, Moore A: Controlled trial of a brief cognitive-behavioural intervention in adolescent patients with depressive disorders. J Child Psychol Psychiatry 37:737–746, 1996

Woolston JL: Case study: carbamazepine treatment of juvenile-onset bipolar disorder. J Am Acad Child Adolesc Psychiatry 38:335–338, 1999

Wozniak J, Biederman J, Kiely K, et al: Mania-like symptoms suggestive of childhood-onset bipolar disorder in clinically referred children (comments). J Am Acad Child Adolesc Psychiatry 34:867–876, 1995

Young RC, Biggs JT, Ziegler VE, et al: A rating scale for mania: reliability, validity and sensitivity. Br J Psychiatry 133:429–435, 1978

Youngerman J, Canino IA: Lithium carbonate use in children and adolescents: a survey of the literature. Arch Gen Psychiatry 35:216–224, 1978

Ziehen T: Psychiatrie fur Arzte und Studierende. Leipzig, Germany, S Hirzel, 1902

Mood Disorders in Adolescents

Elizabeth B. Weller, M.D.

Ronald A. Weller, M.D.

Arman K. Danielyan, M.D.

Mood disorders are among the most debilitating illnesses in our society, exerting a major impact on social, emotional, and occupational functioning. Early-onset major depressive disorders, bipolar disorders, and dysthymic disorders are associated with significant morbidity and mortality, lengthy course, and risk for recurrence. Usually these disorders persist into adulthood (Birmaher et al. 1996b; Emslie et al. 1997; Fleming and Offord 1990; Fleming et al. 1993; Kovacs et al. 1984a, 1984b, 1993; Lewinsohn et al. 1994b; McCauley et al. 1993; Rao et al. 1993; Strober and Carlson 1982; Strober et al. 1993). They also contribute to significant psychosocial morbidity, including impairment in family and peer relationships and poor school performance (Fleming and Offord 1990; Kashani et al. 1987b; Kolvin et al. 1991; Puig-Antich et al. 1985b, 1993; Rutter et al. 1976; Weinberg et al. 1973). Afflicted adolescents are at increased risk for suicide and attempted suicide (Brent 1987; Garfinkel et al. 1982; Kovacs et al. 1993; Pfeffer et al. 1991; Rao et al. 1993; Shaffer 1974). More than 90% of youths who commit suicide have an associated psychiatric illness, most commonly a mood disorder. This fact highlights the importance of preventive measures aimed at the detection of mood disorders as early as possible (Bhatara 1992). In addition, early-onset depression predicts future depressive episodes during adolescence (Kovacs et al. 1984b) and adulthood (Harrington et al. 1990) and is associated with poor prognosis (E.B. Weller and Weller 1991).

Diagnostic Criteria and Clinical Presentations

■ Major Depressive Disorder

Major depressive disorder appears to occur in older adolescents at rates comparable to its occurrence in adults. Point prevalence rates have been reported to be between 2% and 5% (Kashani et al. 1987b; Lewinsohn et al. 1993a; Verhulst et al. 1997). In light of its relatively high prevalence, it is important to consider the clinical presentations, course, and outcome of major depressive disorder in adolescents.

In DSM-IV-TR (American Psychiatric Association 2000), major depressive episode is characterized by five or more of the following symptoms that have been present during the same 2-week period and represent a change from previous functioning: 1) depressed mood most of the day (can be irritable mood in children and adolescents), 2) markedly diminished interest or pleasure in all (or almost all) activities, 3) changes in appetite or weight, 4) insomnia or hypersomnia, 5) psychomotor agitation or retardation, 6) fatigue or loss of energy, 7) feelings of worthlessness or excessive or inappropriate guilt, 8) diminished ability to think or concentrate, 9) recurrent thoughts of death. The only distinction between adult and adolescent criteria is the allowance of either irritable or depressed mood in adolescents compared with depressed mood only in adults (American Psychiatric Association 2000, p. 356).

The symptoms listed above should represent a change from the individual's previous level of functioning and should cause distress or impairment. The symptoms must not be due to the effects of medication, alcohol or drug abuse, or a general medical condition. Uncomplicated bereavement is also specifically excluded from the diagnosis of major depressive disorder. The duration of a major depressive episode varies. An episode is considered to have ended when the symptoms have diminished below the threshold for diagnosis or have been resolved completely for at least 2 consecutive months. DSM-IV-TR allows for specification of the current or most recent episode as mild, moderate, severe without psychotic features, severe with psychotic features, in partial remission, in full remission, chronic, with catatonic features, with melancholic features, with atypical features, and with postpartum onset. The longitudinal course may be specified as a single episode, recurrent with full interepisode recovery, recurrent without full interepisode recovery, and with seasonal pattern.

In adolescents, major depression and dysthymic disorder are frequent, recurrent, and often familial disorders that tend to continue into adulthood. They are frequently associated with other psychiatric conditions, poor psychosocial and academic outcome, and increased risk of substance abuse, bipolar disorder, and suicide. The clinical picture of major depression in different age groups varies, and each has its own characteristics. Kashani et al. (1989) studied three groups of children—ages 8, 12, and 17 years—drawn from the general population ($N=210$). The youngest group (age 8 years) experienced symptoms related to withdrawal and negative outlook. The middle group (age 12 years) reported depressive symptoms related to pessimism about the future and general somatic complaints. The oldest group (age 17 years) was more likely to be careless about their own safety, to report feeling guilty about the occurrence of bad events, and to experience suicidal ideation. Other studies of the phenomenology of depression at different ages showed equal rates of depressed mood, impaired concentration, insomnia, and suicidal ideation in all groups. With increasing age, the occurrence of somatic complaints and depressed appearance declined, and the occurrence of anhedonia, diurnal variation, hopelessness, psychomotor retardation, and delusions increased (Carlson and Kashani 1988b). Ryan et al.

(1987) found that anhedonia, hopelessness, hypersomnia, weight change, and drug abuse were more common in adolescents than in children. Although there was no significant difference in the severity of suicidal ideation between depressed adolescents and children, adolescents chose significantly more lethal methods.

Often the presenting problem in a depressed adolescent is an overt behavior problem, and the accompanying depression may not be detected. An early study of the phenomenology associated with depressed mood in adolescents found that most looked sad only when discussing their depression (Inamdar et al. 1979). Teenagers usually desire to be with their friends and be involved in many extracurricular activities. When adolescents become depressed, their symptoms often evolve into boredom, apathy, and lack of attention to their usual friends and interests. They may become socially withdrawn and often report feeling lonely and unloved (Inamdar et al. 1979). Adolescents with major depressive disorder tend to have few friends, poor peer relationships (Goodyer et al. 1989; Puig-Antich et al. 1985a, 1985b), and negative self-esteem (Asarnow 1988). There is some evidence that the social skills deficits and psychological morbidity associated with major depressive disorder in adolescence may persist after recovery from the depressive episode (Rao et al. 1995).

Adolescents with major depressive disorder may be at increased risk for developing bipolar disorder. Follow-up studies have found that 20%–40% of adolescents with major depressive disorder develop bipolar I disorder within a period of 5 years after the onset of depression (Geller et al. 1994; Kovacs et al. 1989; Rao et al. 1995; Strober and Carlson 1982; Strober et al. 1993). Rao et al. (1995) studied 28 depressed adolescents and 35 matched control subjects and found the rate of switching to bipolar disorder was substantially higher (19%) than rates reported in adult subjects (5%–10%). Clinical characteristics associated with an increased risk of developing bipolar I disorder in adolescents with major depressive disorder include early-onset depression, depression accompanied by psychomotor retardation or psychotic features, family history of bipolar disorder or heavy familial loading for mood disorders, and the occurrence of pharmacologically induced hypomania (Akiskal et al. 1995; Geller et al. 1994; Strober and Carlson 1982). In depressed adolescents, the conversion to bipolar II disorder has been associated with early-onset depression, atypical depression, seasonal affective disorder, protracted depressive episodes, mood lability, comorbid substance abuse, and high rates of psychosocial problems (Akiskal et al. 1995; Brent et al. 1988, 1993; Lewinsohn et al. 1995). The presence of bipolar II disorder in adolescents may be missed because its clinical presentation may be easily misdiagnosed as a disruptive disorder or a personality disorder, particularly borderline personality disorder.

A large proportion of adolescents exhibit depressive symptoms that are subthreshold for a diagnosis. Studies among adults suggest that such subclinical syndromes carry a high risk for full-blown episodes of major depression (Horwath et al. 1992). Based on the study of an epidemiologically selected cohort of 776 adolescents, Pine et al. (1999) reported that there was a predictive relationship between subclinical depressive symptoms in adolescence and major depression in adulthood.

Poor school performance, a change in grades, or academic failure may be important markers of adolescent depression related to impaired concentration, fatigue, and withdrawal. Conduct disorders, promiscuous sexual behavior, and substance abuse are also common among depressed adolescents and often complicate the clinical picture. Drug abuse is the presenting symptom in approximately 20% of adolescents with a mood disorder (E.B. Weller and Weller 1990). There is some evidence for sex-related differences in how adolescents experience emotional disturbance and manifest various depressive symptoms. Girls tend to report more inwardly directed symptoms of depression and anxiety. Boys report more acting-out behaviors, such as running away, theft, or substance abuse (Ostrov et al. 1989).

As with adults, the course of major depression in adolescents is often characterized by protracted episodes; frequent recurrence; impairment in work, family, and social lives; and high rate of suicide attempts. Suicide is the third leading cause of death in adolescents (Kovacs et al. 1993; Rao et al. 1995; Weissman et al. 1999). Although several longitudinal studies with depressed adolescents have been conducted, few have followed participants into adulthood. As a result, little is known about the long-term course of adolescent major depressive disorder and its continuity with adult major depressive disorder. Of the few studies that have followed adolescents with major depressive disorder in both clinical samples (Garber et al. 1988; Harrington et al. 1990; Kovacs et al. 1984b) and community samples (Cohen et al. 1993; Garrison et al. 1990; Kandel and Davies 1982; Reinherz et al. 1993b) into adulthood, most report relatively high rates of mood disorders in these individuals as young adults.

In general, studies suggest that

1. The rate of mood disorders in adulthood is significantly higher among individuals diagnosed with major depressive disorder during childhood and adolescence than among those with nonaffective disorders during childhood and adolescence (Garber et al. 1988; Harrington 1990) and psychiatrically healthy control subjects (Rao et al. 1995).

2. Most children and adolescents recover from the index major depressive episode (Kovacs 1996; Lewinsohn et al. 1994b).

3. The relapse/recurrence rate of juvenile major depressive disorder is substantial (Kovacs et al. 1984a; Lewinsohn et al. 1994b; McCauley et al. 1993; Rao et al. 1995).

4. A minority of children and adolescents with major depressive disorder develop manic or hypomanic episodes (Geller et al. 1994; Lewinsohn et al. 1995; Strober et al. 1993).

5. The course of major depressive disorder in adolescents appears to be similar for males and females (Kovacs et al. 1984a), although one study suggested that females may have a higher rate of recurrence (McCauley et al. 1993).

6. Comorbid nonaffective disorders predict a more severe course of depression (Sanford et al. 1995), but one study found that comorbid externalizing disorders are associated with lower rates of depression at follow-up (Harrington et al. 1991).

7. The rate of anxiety disorders in adulthood among individuals diagnosed with major depressive disorder in childhood and adolescence is higher than that among those without a psychiatric diagnosis in childhood or adolescence (Rao et al. 1995).

The risk for children and adolescents with a history of major depressive disorder to develop major depressive disorder in adulthood was further studied by Lewinsohn et al. (1999). They examined children and adolescents with a history of major depressive disorder and determined their risk for new episodes of major depressive disorder and other affective and nonaffective psychiatric disorders as adults. Subjects with a history of major depressive disorder in childhood or adolescence were compared with 1) subjects with a history of adjustment disorder with depressed mood before age 19 years, 2) subjects with other nonaffective disorders before age 19 (primarily anxiety, substance use, and disruptive behavior disorders), and 3) subjects with no history of psychiatric disorder before age 19. Subjects were 261 participants with major depressive disorder, 73 with adjustment disorder, 133 with nonaffective disorder, and 272 with no disorder through age 18. Results of the study showed that major depressive disorder in young adulthood was significantly more common in the adolescent major depressive disorder group than in the nonaffective disorder and no-disorder groups. The average annual rates of major depressive disorder were 9.0% for the major depressive disorder group, 5.6% for the nonaffective disorder group, and 3.7% for the no-disorder group. Adolescents with major depressive disorder also had a high rate of nonaffective disorders in young adulthood but did not differ from adolescents with nonaffective disorder. The authors concluded that adolescent major depressive disorder confers a high degree of risk for recurrence of major depressive disorder in young adulthood as well as an increased probability of future nonaffective disorders (predominantly substance use disorders) and Axis II pathology.

In a separate study by Lewinsohn et al. (2000), the authors identified factors related to the recurrence of major depressive disorder during young adulthood (ages 19–23 years) in a community sample of formerly depressed adolescents. A total of 274 subjects with adolescent-onset major depressive disorder were assessed twice during adolescence and again after their 24th birthday. Low levels of excessive emotional reliance, a single episode of major depressive disorder in adolescence, a low proportion of family members with recurrent major depressive disorder, low levels of antisocial and borderline personality disorder symptoms, and a positive attributional style (males only) independently predicted which formerly depressed adolescents would remain free of future psychopathology. Female gender; multiple, more severe depressive episodes (e.g., longer episode duration, multiple episodes, greater number of symptoms, history of suicide attempts) in adolescence; higher proportion of family members with recurrent major depressive disorder; increased borderline personality disorder symptoms; and conflict with parents (females only) each predicted recurrent major depressive disorder. Comorbid anxiety and substance use disorders in adolescence and increased antisocial personality disorder symptoms independently distinguished adolescents who developed recurrent major depressive disorder comorbid with nonmood disorder from those who developed pure major depressive disorder. The authors suggested that clinical characteristics, both of the proband and of the first-degree relatives, are among the strongest predictors of recurrence of major depressive disorder. In contrast to some previous reports, they found no evidence that adolescent comorbidity acted as a risk factor for pure major depressive disorder in young adulthood. The presence of nonmood disorders in adolescence predicted nonmood disorders in young adulthood, which were often comorbid with recurrent major depressive disorder. Comorbid dysthymia also failed to predict recurrence of major depressive disorder. Unlike previous research on the impact of double depression, adolescent major depressive disorder and dysthymia in this study occurred largely at different time periods.

The rate of recurrence of major depression in adolescents and the factors that may predict recurrence have been studied. McCauley et al. (1993) studied 65 depressed adolescents over a 3-year period and reported that 80% experienced remission by 1 year (mean duration of the initial episode was 9 months) and 54% had recurrence of major depressive disorder during follow-up. Longer duration of the index episode was associated with greater severity of depression, female gender, and length of therapeutic intervention. Higher socioeconomic status, greater length of initial episode, and endogenicity were all associated with shorter time to recurrence. A more stressful family environment predicted poor overall social competence at follow-up.

In another study, Sanford et al. (1995) examined 67 adolescents, ages 13–19 years, with major depression who were drawn from consecutive referrals to psychiatric clinics in a defined geographic catchment area. The subjects were evaluated to determine whether specific clinical variables independently predicted major depressive disorder remission or persistence. At 1-year follow-up, major depression was in remission in 66% of subjects. Approximately one-third of those with major depressive disorder had anxiety disorder (especially agoraphobia and avoidant disorder), one-third had substance use disorder, and one-fifth had dysthymic disorder. Comorbid substance use disorder, comorbid anxiety disorder, older age at interview, low involvement with father, and poor response to mother's discipline were predictors of persistence of major depressive disorder. In contrast to some earlier studies (Kovacs et al. 1984a), comorbid anxiety disorder predicted persistence of major depressive disorder in this study.

The role of gender in clinical presentation, course, and prognosis of major depressive disorder in adolescents has also been a focus of discussion. Epidemiological studies have documented gender differences in the prevalence of depressed mood, depressive syndromes, and depressive disorders. However, gender was not believed to affect recovery from major depression (Kovacs et al. 1984a, 1997; McCauley et al. 1993) or its recurrence (Kovacs et al. 1984b; Rao et al. 1995). Although studies of clinical adolescent samples have not reported compelling gender effects on depression as a disorder, gender was reported to have an impact on symptom presentation. Specifically, in epidemiological, community, and some clinical samples, girls have been found to report higher levels of depressive symptoms than boys (Allgood-Merten et al. 1990; Avison and Mcalpine 1992) and were more likely than boys to complain of depressed mood (Compas et al. 1997). Girls with depressive disorders have more mood symptoms related to feeling sad, whereas depressed boys may have higher rates of irritability. In community samples, girls had lower self-worth or poorer self-esteem than boys (Avison and Mcalpine 1992). Lewinsohn et al. (1999) reported that females were more likely to develop major depressive disorder and adjustment disorder in young adulthood, whereas males were more likely to develop nonaffective Axis I disorders and Axis II psychopathology. However, there was no significant interaction between gender and adolescent diagnostic group in predicting psychopathology in young adulthood.

Kovacs (2001) reported that there were no compelling gender effects on salient presenting features and adolescent outcomes of major depressive disorder in clinically referred youth. She explored possible gender differences in the various features of major depressive disorder from late childhood to late adolescence among psychiatrically referred youngsters. Ninety-two subjects were studied longitudinally with repeated standardized psychiatric evaluations. Similarities between boys and girls in the features of depression up to late adolescence (during an average follow-up of about 6 years) were more prominent than were differences. The background and initial clinical characteristics of depressed boys and girls at the average age of 11 years were generally indistinguishable.

Although gender differences have been documented in epidemiological and community samples with respect to rates and correlates of depressed mood and some features of depressive disorders, results of various studies are conflicting. Additional work is needed to determine whether gender effects are detectable on other clinical parameters of major depressive disorder during adolescence or further along in development.

In summary, major depressive disorder may have a variable clinical presentation in adolescents but is recognizable by the core features of depressed or irritable mood, loss of interest, poor concentration, feelings of guilt or worthlessness, neurovegetative symptoms, and suicidal thoughts. Adolescents with major depression have a twofold to fourfold greater risk for depression as young adults (Pine et al. 1998). Adolescent major depressive disorder can co-occur with conduct, anxiety, and substance use disorders both at inception and at follow-up, and the rates of these comorbid disorders may be high in patients with severe major depressive disorder, potentially confounding disorder severity with comorbidity. Aside from two studies (Goodyer et al. 1991; McCauley et al. 1993), there has been relatively little investigation of the influence of social functioning on outcome despite the fact that children with major depressive disorder have persistent social functioning deficits in comparison with psychiatrically healthy children (Joffe and Singer 1990; Puig-Antich et al. 1985b).

■ Dysthymic Disorder

Diagnostic criteria for dysthymic disorder in adolescents require the presence of a persistent depressed or irritable mood that occurs for most of the day, for more days than not, for at least 1 year. In adults the duration of the mood disturbance must be at least 2 years. As with major depressive disorder, the symptoms must result in clinically significant distress or impairment in functioning or require markedly increased effort to maintain a previous level of functioning. During the initial 1-year interval, a major depressive episode must not be present (American Psychiatric Association 2000, pp. 380–381). After the initial year, major depressive episodes may be superimposed on the dysthymic disorder. This circumstance is called double depression.

Early-onset dysthymic disorder has a protracted course (mean episode length of 4 years) and is associated with increased risk for subsequent major depressive disorder (70%), bipolar disorder (13%), and substance abuse (15%) (Keller et al. 1988; Kovacs et al. 1984a, 1984b, 1994; Lewinsohn et al. 1991). Children with dysthymic disorder usually have their first episode of major depressive disorder 2–3 years after the onset of dysthymia. Kovacs et al. (1994) theorized that dysthymic disorder is one of the "gateways" to the development of recurrent mood disorders. They conducted a longitudinal prospective study of 55 school-age clinically referred youngsters whose first mood disorder was dysthymic disorder, and a comparison group of 60 youngsters whose first affective episode was major depressive disorder. Dysthymic disorder had an earlier age of onset than major depressive disorder. Dysthymia also had frequent symptoms of affective dysregulation, low rates of anhedonia and neurovegetative symptoms, and greater overall risk of any subsequent affective disorder. Children with dysthymic disorder developed first-episode major depressive disorder (76%) and bipolar disorder (13%). After the first episode of major depressive disorder, the clinical course of the initially dysthymic youths was similar to the course of the comparison patients with regard to rates of recurrent major depression, bipolar disorder, and certain nonaffective disorders. The authors concluded that childhood-onset dysthymic disorder is an early marker of recurrent affective illness, and dysthymic children who have subsequent mood disorders are most likely to first have an episode of major depressive disorder. These findings agree with those of Lewinsohn et al. (1991), who reported that dysthymic disorder, especially of early onset, was much more likely to precede than follow major depressive disorder in community-based samples.

Teenagers with dysthymic disorder may have significant academic, social, and psychological deficits, including hopelessness and low self-esteem (Kashani et al. 1989). The interval between the onset of dysthymia and the first major depression provides a good window of opportunity for intervention and possible prevention of later episodes (Kovacs et al. 1994).

■ Bipolar Disorder

Bipolar disorder is a chronic and recurrent condition. It often originates in childhood and is associated with marked impairment in family, social, and occupational functioning. Compared with adults, adolescents with bipolar disorder may have a more prolonged early course and be less responsive to treatment (McGlas-

han 1988; Strober et al. 1995).

Bipolar I disorder requires the existence of a manic or mixed episode. A manic episode is defined in DSM-IV-TR as a distinct period of "abnormally and persistently elevated, expansive, or irritable mood" (American Psychiatric Association 2000, p. 357). A mixed episode is characterized by "rapidly alternating moods…accompanied by symptoms of a manic episode and a major depressive episode" (p. 362). The duration of the mood disturbance should be at least 1 week. The episode should be severe enough to require hospitalization, cause marked impairment in functioning, or have psychotic features. During the period of mood disturbance, at least three (or four if the mood is irritable rather than elevated or expansive) of the following symptoms must be present: 1) inflated self-esteem or grandiosity, 2) decreased need for sleep, 3) more talkativeness than usual or pressure to keep talking, 4) flight of ideas or racing thoughts, 5) distractibility, 6) increased goal-directed activity or psychomotor agitation, and 7) excessive involvement in pleasurable activities that have a high potential for painful consequences (p. 362).

Bipolar II disorder is characterized by one or more major depressive episodes accompanied by at least one hypomanic episode, which is defined as "a distinct period during which there is an abnormally and persistently elevated, expansive, or irritable mood that lasts at least 4 days" (American Psychiatric Association 2000, p. 365). It should be accompanied by a minimum of three (if the mood is elevated or expansive) or four (if the mood is irritable) of the above-mentioned seven manic symptoms. A hypomanic episode, in contrast to a manic episode, is not severe enough to require hospitalization and does not cause a marked impairment in social or other important areas of functioning. The switch rate from bipolar II disorder to bipolar I disorder in adults has been estimated by Coryell et al. (1998) to be similar to the rate (31.7%) reported by Geller et al. (1994) for prepubertal subjects to switch from major depressive disorder to bipolar I disorder during the prepubertal period. However, it is still possible that bipolar II disorder in children and adolescents may be an age-specific, developmental precursor to bipolar I disorder (Geller et al. 1994).

Cyclothymic disorder is also a chronic and fluctuating mood disorder that usually begins in adolescence or early adult life. It is characterized by "numerous periods of hypomanic symptoms and numerous periods of depressive symptoms" (American Psychiatric Association 2000, p. 398). Both the hypomanic and depressive symptoms must be insufficient in number, severity, duration, and pervasiveness to meet full criteria for a manic or depressive episode. In adolescents, symptoms must be present for an initial period of at least 1 year without the presence of manic, major depressive, or mixed episodes and without a symptom-free interval longer than 2 months. As with dysthymic disorder, cyclothymic disorder is characterized as a chronic but less severe mood disorder. It was initially considered in the spectrum of personality disorders. Unlike dysthymic disorder, cyclothymic disorder is not frequently diagnosed in clinical settings.

In a retrospective evaluation of 200 adult bipolar patients, Loranger and Levine (1978) found that first symptoms of the disorder had occurred between ages 5 and 9 years in only 1 (0.5%) of these patients; 15 (7.5%) of these patients reported onset between ages 10 and 14 years. Joyce (1984) estimated that 20%–40% of adults report the onset of their illness during childhood. Lish et al. (1994) found that 59% of adults with bipolar disorder recalled having their first affective symptoms as children or adolescents. Burke et al. (1990) noted that for most of their bipolar patients, the disorder started between ages 15 and 19.

Diagnosing bipolar disorder in adolescents can be a difficult task because of several factors. First, when manic symptoms initially appear in adolescence, they may build up gradually or be less severe and thus not receive clinical attention. The first episode of a mood disorder in adolescents with bipolar disorder is often not a manic episode. Of the 18 adolescents with bipolar disorder in a community sample of 1,709 adolescents, the condition first started with a manic or hypomanic episode in only 1 (5.5%); it started with a major or minor depressive episode in 11 (61.1%); and in 6 (33.3%) the first episode could not be determined (Lewinsohn et al. 1995).

Second, an atypical clinical presentation of mania in children and adolescents is quite common. In general, psychotic symptoms, suicidal attempts, inappropriate sexual behavior, and a "stormy" first year of illness were reported by E.B. Weller et al. (1995) as typical symptoms of adolescent mania. Kovacs and Pollock (1995) reported that some youngsters with mania show serious acting-out behaviors, including burglary, stealing, vandalism, and a history of school suspensions. Behavioral symptoms that masked bipolar disorder were reported by Isaac (1992). In his study of 12 adolescents (ages 13–19 years) with behavioral disor-

ders, 8 later turned out to have the characteristics of bipolar disorder. Akiskal and collaborators (1985) described 68 young family members of patients with bipolar disorder, who were referred for a variety of behavioral problems. McGlashan (1988) noted that a delay of up to 5 years often occurs between the onset of symptoms during adolescence and an episode of sufficient severity to require hospitalization or treatment.

Carlson et al. (1994) and Carlson and Kashani (1988a) observed that although full-blown bipolar disorder may be rare in adolescence, manic symptoms are common. Developmental issues and symptom overlap with more frequent childhood psychiatric disorders pose additional challenges in diagnosis (Bowring and Kovacs 1992). Irritability and an unpredictable and labile mood are more common than euphoria. Mixed or dysphoric episodes (McElroy et al. 1992a) and psychotic features (Ballenger et al. 1982) are also common among the more severely ill teenagers with bipolar disorder.

Patients who have early onset may have higher rates of psychotic features than those who are older at onset (Ballenger et al. 1982; Joyce 1984; McElroy et al. 1997; McGlashan 1988; Rosen et al. 1983). Early onset often indicates a more severe course of the illness.

Carlson et al. (2000) used data from an epidemiologically derived sample to assess similarities and differences in psychopathology in subjects with early-onset bipolar disorder (i.e., hospitalized with a first episode of psychotic mania between ages 15 and 20) and those with adult onset (i.e., age over 30 when hospitalized with a first episode). The two groups were compared with regard to demographic characteristics, psychotic and depressive symptoms, childhood behavior problems and school functioning, substance or alcohol use disorders, and episode recurrence. Male subjects predominated in the early-onset group (69.6% versus 26.6%). Subjects with early-onset psychotic mania were significantly more likely to have had a clinically significant behavior disorder in childhood. Poor school performance was noted more often in the early-onset subjects (50% versus 20.0%). The early-onset subjects were significantly more likely to have a substance use disorder before age 16 that clearly antedated the onset of mood disorder. Early-onset subjects were also more likely than adult-onset subjects to have substance use disorder present at the onset of their mood disorder. Although high lifetime rates of heavy substance use (70%) or abuse (30%) were seen in the adult-onset subjects, most had stopped this behavior by the time they developed their index manic episode. Early-onset subjects were significantly more likely than adult-onset subjects to report paranoid (100% versus 80%) and grandiose (73.9% versus 40%) delusions but not mood-incongruent psychotic symptoms, formal thought disorder, or hallucinations. More early-onset than adult-onset subjects experienced either partial or no remissions during the follow-up period (40.9% versus 10.3%). Conversely, more adult-onset than early-onset subjects experienced either a single episode (44.8% versus 22.7%) or more than one episode but with complete remission between episodes (44.8% versus 36.4%). Early-onset subjects spent significantly more time in the hospital during the 24-month follow-up period than adult-onset subjects (6.8 weeks versus 3.7 weeks). Manic episodes recurred more frequently in early-onset subjects (64.7% versus 12.5%), and depressive episodes recurred more frequently in adult-onset subjects (62.5% versus 17.6%). Equal numbers of subjects experienced both types of episodes. The early-onset and adult-onset subjects had similar rates of mania according to baseline consensus research diagnoses (56.5% and 73.3%) and discharge diagnoses (56.5% and 67.9%). At the 6-month research consensus diagnosis conference, 100% of the adult-onset subjects but only 81.8% of the early-onset group were identified as having bipolar disorder. Mixed episodes were much more likely to be experienced by early-onset subjects (26.1% versus 3.3%). Mixed episodes were the most difficult to diagnose. They were often initially diagnosed as psychosis not otherwise specified, drug-induced psychosis, or schizoaffective disorder.

Adolescents with bipolar disorder may have a more prolonged early course and be less responsive to treatment than adults (McGlashan 1988; Strober et al. 1995). This may be due to the fact that adolescents with bipolar disorder frequently present with either mixed features, psychotic symptoms, or comorbid behavior or substance abuse, all of which predict a more refractory response to lithium. In a 5-year naturalistic prospective follow-up study of 54 adolescents with bipolar disorder, 2 never achieved complete remission (Strober et al. 1995). Of the remaining patients, 44% had a relapsing course (either major depression or mania), and 21% had two or more additional episodes. Recovery from the index episode took longer for patients with depression (median time to recovery, 26 weeks) than for patients with either mania (median recovery time, 9 weeks) or mixed episodes (median recovery time, 11 weeks).

Long-term studies of hospitalized manic patients suggest that short-term course is not necessarily predictive of ultimate functioning, especially in young people (Carlson et al. 1977; McGlashan 1988). Longer follow-up is therefore needed.

Disturbed psychosocial functioning is a severe consequence of bipolar illness. Geller et al. (2001) compared the adult psychosocial functioning of subjects with prepubertal major depressive disorder (mean age, 10.3±1.5 years) to that of a psychiatrically healthy comparison group (mean age, 20.7±2.0 years) after follow-up into adulthood. The time between baseline and follow-up was 9.9±1.5 years. In the prepubertal major depressive disorder group, subjects with major depressive disorder, bipolar disorder, or substance use disorders during the previous 5 years had significantly worse psychosocial functioning than the healthy comparison group subjects at follow-up. Impairment in psychosocial functioning included significantly worse relationships with parents, siblings, and friends; significantly worse functioning in home, school, and work settings; and poorer overall quality of life and global social adjustment.

Comorbidity and Differential Diagnosis

Comorbid diagnoses are common in adolescents with mood disorders. In general, comorbid diagnoses appear to influence the risk for recurrent depression, duration of the depressive episode, suicide attempts or suicidal behavior, functional outcome, response to treatment, and utilization of mental health services (Brent et al. 1988, 1993; Kovacs et al. 1993; Kutcher et al. 1989; Lewinsohn et al. 1993a, 1994c, 1995; Rohde et al. 1991; Sanford et al. 1995).

■ Major Depressive Disorder

Clinical (Kovacs et al. 1984a, 1984b; Ryan et al. 1986, 1987) and epidemiological investigations (Angold and Costello 1993; Bird et al. 1988; Kashani et al. 1987a, 1987b; Rohde et al. 1991) have revealed that 40%–70% of depressed children and adolescents have comorbid psychiatric disorders. At least 20%–50% have two or more comorbid diagnoses. The most frequent comorbid diagnoses are dysthymic disorder (30%–80%) and anxiety disorders (30%–80%), disruptive disorders (10%–80%), and substance abuse (20%–30%). Major depressive disorder is more likely to occur after the onset of other psychiatric disorders (except substance abuse) (Biederman et al. 1995; Kovacs et al. 1989; Reinherz et al. 1993a). However, conduct problems may develop as a complication of the depression and may persist after the depression remits (Kovacs et al. 1988).

In a community sample of adolescents (ages 14–18), 33% of those with major depressive disorder also had a diagnosis of dysthymic disorder, but only 7% of those with dysthymic disorder also had major depressive disorder (Lewinsohn et al. 1991). These figures are higher than have been reported in adults (Keller and Shapiro 1982). In particular, youths with double depression (major depressive disorder and dysthymic disorder) have been found to have more severe and longer depressive episodes, a higher rate of comorbid disorders, more suicidality, and worse social impairment than youths with either major depressive disorder or dysthymic disorder alone (Ferro et al. 1994; Kovacs et al. 1994; Lewinsohn et al. 1991).

Kovacs et al. (1994) found that approximately 70% of patients with early-onset dysthymic disorder have a superimposed major depressive disorder and 50% have other preexisting psychiatric disorders, including anxiety disorders (40%), conduct disorder (30%), attention-deficit/hyperactivity disorder (ADHD) (24%), and enuresis or encopresis (15%), with 15% having two or more comorbid disorders.

The comorbidity of depression and anxiety may also have clinical implications, as evidenced by studies showing an increased severity and duration of depressive symptoms, increased risk for substance abuse, increased suicidality, poor response to psychotherapy, and more psychosocial problems (Brent et al. 1988, 1993; Kendall et al. 1992; Kovacs et al. 1989).

More than 60% of depressed adolescents have comorbid personality disorders, with borderline personality disorder accounting for 30% of all comorbid personality disorders (Kutcher et al. 1989). After the depression has remitted, however, personality disorder symptoms are often no longer evident. This indicates the value of giving only provisional or no personality disorder diagnoses during acute depressive episodes.

Depressive and externalizing disorders often are comorbid and may represent more serious psychopathology than either condition alone. In clinical samples, from 36% to 80% of depressed juveniles meet criteria for conduct disorder (Ferro et al. 1994; Kovacs et

al. 1988). In an epidemiological study, more than 50% of youths with affective disorder also had conduct disorder or oppositional defiant disorder (Bird et al. 1988). Youths with both depressive and conduct disorders have been reported to be at increased risk for suicide (Brent et al. 1988) and to have less favorable short-term clinical outcomes (Harrington et al. 1991). According to Asarnow (1988), child psychiatric inpatients with these comorbid diagnoses had worse peer relationships than the ones with depression but no conduct disorder. Rejected schoolchildren were reported to have high levels of both antisocial and depressive symptoms (Cole and Carpentieri 1990). Young adults who had depression and conduct problems in childhood reported greater social dysfunction in adulthood than those who had depression only (Harrington et al. 1991). Depressed patients with comorbid disruptive disorders were reported to have worse short-term outcome, fewer melancholic symptoms, fewer recurrences of depression, a lower familial aggregation of mood disorders, a higher incidence of adult criminality, more suicide attempts, higher levels of family criticism, and a higher response to placebo than patients with major depressive disorder who did not have disruptive disorders (Harrington et al. 1990, 1991; Hughes et al. 1990; Kutcher et al. 1989; Puig-Antich et al. 1989). These findings suggest that depressed children with disruptive disorders may constitute a distinct subgroup.

Substance use disorder is often comorbid with depressive disorders in adolescents. Rao et al. (1995) presented data on the rates of substance use disorders in adolescents with unipolar major depressive disorder. They also examined demographic, clinical, and biological factors associated with the development of substance use disorders. Twenty-eight adolescents (mean age, 15.4±1.3 years) with unipolar major depression and no history of substance use disorders and 35 group-matched psychologically healthy control subjects who had participated in a cross-sectional sleep polysomnography and neuroendocrine study were reassessed clinically 7 years later. The risk for substance use disorders was high in both groups (34.6% in the depressed group and 24.2% in the control group). Depressed adolescents had earlier onset of substance use disorders than control subjects. Depressed adolescents who developed substance use disorders had more significant psychosocial impairment than depressed adolescents who did not develop substance use disorders.

Substance-induced mood disorder with depressive

features is diagnosed when the depressed mood is determined to be due to the physiological effects of a medication, a drug of abuse, exposure to a toxin, or other somatic treatment. A substance-induced mood disorder with depressive features is distinguished from a major depressive disorder or other depressive disorders by considering the onset, course, and clinical presentation. Substance-induced mood disorder with depressive features arises only in association with the states of withdrawal or intoxication, whereas primary depressive disorders may precede the onset of substance use or may occur during times of sustained abstinence. Because the use of alcohol and illegal drugs is widespread among adolescents, this factor must always be considered in the differential diagnosis. Medically or psychiatrically ill youngsters are most likely to be taking medications. It is crucial to examine the patient's list of medications (including over-the-counter medications) and dosages to rule out drug–drug interactions, toxicity, and pharmacologically induced depressive symptoms.

Many medical illnesses—including malignancy, brain injury, infection, endocrine disorders, metabolic abnormalities, acquired immunodeficiency syndrome (AIDS), multiple sclerosis, and chronic fatigue syndrome—can produce symptoms of depression. Migraine headaches (which frequently begin during adolescence) may be associated with shifts in mood, depression, and irritability. Seizure disorders should be considered in the differential diagnosis of depressive disorders because focal seizures in individuals with brain damage may present as sudden fluctuations in mood. Adolescents with intracranial tumors may develop not only seizures but also increased intracranial pressure, which may present initially as a change in mood. Apathy, bradykinesia, and anhedonia are most commonly seen in individuals with right-hemisphere disease, frontal-lobe damage, or disorders of dopaminergic transmission. Patients who are 25% above or below ideal body weight or have other clinical indicators should be tested for thyroid and adrenal dysfunctions. Testing for mononucleosis is also recommended for depressed adolescents. Adolescents in high-risk groups should be tested for human immunodeficiency virus (HIV).

When there is a history of psychotic symptoms (such as delusions, hallucinations, or disorganized speech or behavior), their severity, scope, duration, and prominence in relation to mood symptoms must be determined. This is necessary to differentiate among a mood disorder with psychotic features, schizoaffective disorder, schizophreniform disorder, schizophrenia, brief psychotic disorder, delusional disorder, and psychotic disorder not otherwise specified. If the patient's symptoms are limited to the depressive spectrum, it must be determined whether the disturbance is in response to an identifiable stressor. The severity and duration of the symptoms should be evaluated to discriminate among major depressive disorder, dysthymia, depressive disorder not otherwise specified, and adjustment disorder with depressed mood.

The excessive weight loss and emaciated appearance of an anorexic adolescent combined with a history of intense fear of gaining weight and disturbance in body image help to differentiate anorexia from a depressive disorder. Hyperphagia may be present in both bulimia nervosa and major depressive disorder. However, the inappropriate compensatory behaviors (vomiting, excessive exercise, or use of purgatives) and characteristic preoccupation with body shape and weight are not typically seen in patients with depressive disorders.

■ Bipolar Disorder

Manic episodes and bipolar disorders have been reported to occur after traumatic brain injury. However, their occurrence is less frequent than that of depressive episodes after brain injury. Factors that appear to predispose to the development of mania after brain injury include damage to the basal region of the right temporal lobe and right orbitofrontal cortex in patients with a family history of bipolar disorder.

Use of various medications and illicit substances is associated with manic symptoms and should be considered in the differential diagnosis of adolescent mania. The classic example is that of euphoric mood, decreased need for sleep, decreased appetite, grandiosity, and increased goal-directed activity, which are associated with cocaine intoxication. In the intoxicated state, the symptoms are indistinguishable from those of acute mania. However, without repeated administration of cocaine, the euphoric effects are short-lived and are followed by symptoms of dysphoria referred to as the "crash." Antidepressant-induced mania is well described in the adult literature and has also been reported in adolescents (Achamallah and Decker 1991; Rosenberg et al. 1992).

Adolescents with bipolar disorder are frequently misdiagnosed as having schizophrenia. Mood-incongruent hallucinations, paranoia, and thought disorders have been reported. In contrast to bipolar disorder, children with schizophrenia usually have an insidious onset of illness, lack the engaging quality associated with mania, and are less likely to have a family history of mania. In the past, psychotic mood disorders in youths were frequently misdiagnosed as schizophrenia (Ferro et al. 1994; R.A. Weller et al. 1986). Some clinicians have argued that, if in doubt, one should diagnose a mood disorder rather than schizophrenia, which is generally believed to have a less favorable prognosis and poorer response to treatment (E.B. Weller and Weller 1990). In their review, Carlson et al. (1994) concluded that although bipolar disorder is still underdiagnosed in youths compared with adults, frank schizophrenia is no longer the alternative diagnosis. Instead, a range of other diagnoses such as psychosis not otherwise specified, schizophreniform psychosis, and brief reactive psychosis were given. The authors noted equal frequencies of bipolar disorder and schizophrenia in youths (ages 15–20) with their first psychiatric admissions for psychosis.

Because bipolar disorder and mania in childhood and adolescence are often associated with an atypical presentation and a confusing clinical history and because they may include disruptive, unmanageable, and explosive behaviors (Ballenger et al. 1982; Isaac 1992; McGlashan 1988), they can be confused with externalizing disorders. Systematic studies of children and adolescents found rates of ADHD ranging from 57% to 98% in bipolar patients (Geller et al. 1995; West et al. 1995; Wozniak et al. 1995) and a 22% rate of bipolar disorder in inpatients with ADHD (Butler et al. 1995). The disruptive or externalizing behavior disorders of childhood may present with volatile and irritable behavior, impulsive risk taking, hyperactivity, talkativeness, distractibility, intrusiveness, poor judgment, and irregular sleep habits. Adolescents with hyperactivity and conduct disorder may brag and tell exaggerated tales, which can make them appear grandiose as well. In a review of child and adolescent mania, Carlson (1990) noted that the major symptomatic difference between youths with bipolar disorder and a group with disruptive behavior disorders (ADHD or conduct disorder) was that those with behavior disorders had a chronic course with an age at onset usually before 6 or 7 years, whereas those with mania had an episodic course that usually began at a later age. In addition, an elevated mood is usually absent in ADHD. However, in the absence of clear-cut episodes, such as the overlapping symptoms seen in mixed states, the diagnosis becomes more difficult.

Isaac (1992) reevaluated the diagnoses of 12 highly problematic adolescents in a special educational day school and found that 8 clearly had bipolar disorder but had been misdiagnosed with ADHD or conduct disorder. Three other adolescents received a diagnosis of conduct disorder that was thought to be related to an emerging bipolar disorder. Isaac argued that adolescent bipolar disorder may be marked by incomplete remissions with waxing and waning symptoms and dysphoric, mixed, and atypical features rather than euphoric symptoms. Accurate diagnosis may require a prolonged period of observation along with structured and semistructured interviews. Wozniak et al. (1995) noted that juvenile mania is often comorbid with ADHD and recommended 1) examining overlapping symptoms to determine the robust quality of the diagnosis and 2) using family history data and other external validators such as the Achenbach Child Behavior Checklist. Kovacs and Pollock (1995) evaluated clinically referred subjects, ages 8–13 years, in a longitudinal investigation of childhood-onset psychiatric disorders. There was a 69% rate of lifetime comorbidity and 54% rate of episode comorbidity with conduct disorder. Youngsters without conduct disorder comorbidity had a higher rate of primary affective illness, a somewhat greater number of bipolar episodes, and slightly better overall clinical course. The researchers concluded that comorbid conduct disorder may exist in a large portion of young patients with bipolar disorder, which may confuse the clinical presentation of bipolar disorder and may possibly account for some of the failure to detect it.

The role of comorbid personality disorders in determining the prognosis and course of adolescent bipolar disorder remains poorly studied. The importance of this issue is suggested by the report of impaired personality traits in adults with bipolar disorder (Solomon et al. 1996). Johnson et al. (1995) reported that cluster II personality disorders were more prominent among adolescents with bipolar disorder.

Adolescents with bipolar disorder may be at increased risk for suicide compared with adolescents with other psychiatric diagnoses (Brent et al. 1988, 1993). In addition, comorbidity of mood and substance use disorders has been correlated with higher suicide risk in older adolescents and young adults (Rich et al. 1986, 1990). The well-known high rate of comorbidity of substance dependency and bipolar disorder in adults is important to note because "secondary" substance use may be more amenable to treatment and have a better prognosis (Geller and Luby 1997; Winokur et al. 1995).

In summary, in the differential diagnosis for both depressive disorders and bipolar disorders, all of the following should be considered: medical illnesses; exposure to prescription medications, illegal drugs, or alcohol; and other psychiatric disorders. Psychological, social, and environmental factors may also be contributing to presenting symptoms.

Epidemiology

In the United States, 1.3 million young people between ages 15 and 19 have depression each year (Angold et al. 1998). Population studies have found prevalence rates of depression ranging between 0.4% and 8.3% in adolescents (Fleming et al. 1989; Kashani et al. 1987a, 1987b; Lewinsohn et al. 1993a, 1994b). The lifetime prevalence rate of major depressive disorder in adolescents, which has been estimated to range from 15% to 20%, is comparable with the lifetime rate of major depressive disorder in adults; this suggests that depression in adults may actually begin in adolescence (Kessler et al. 1994; Lewinsohn et al. 1986, 1993a, 1993b). Data from 1,769 adolescents and young adults in the National Comorbidity Survey (Kessler and Walters 1998) showed a lifetime prevalence rate of 15.3% for major depression, which is comparable with the 17% lifetime prevalence of depression observed in adults (Kessler et al. 1994). In a cross-sectional community survey of 2,852 children ages 6–16 years, the prevalence rate of a "DSM-III-like" major depressive syndrome was 1.8% for adolescents (Fleming et al. 1989).

Several studies have determined the prevalence of major depressive disorder in adolescents. Kashani et al. (1987b) used a structured interview to assess a community sample of 150 adolescents. The prevalence was 4.7% for major depressive disorder and 3.3% for dysthymic disorder. Epidemiological studies on dysthymic disorder have reported point prevalence rates from 1.6% to 8.0% in adolescents (Kashani et al. 1987a, 1987b; Lewinsohn et al. 1993a, 1994b). In the study by Lewinsohn et al. (1993a) on point and lifetime prevalence, 1-year incidence, and comorbidity of depression with other disorders in a randomly selected sample of 1,710 high school students, 9.6% met criteria for a current disorder, more than 33% had experienced a disorder over their lifetimes, and 31.7% of the latter had experienced a second disorder. However, the prevalence of depression in adolescents is much higher in clinical populations (18.7%–27.0%) than in community samples (Robbins et al. 1982; Strober et al. 1981).

There are some interesting findings on the male–female ratio of mood disorders. Lewinsohn et al. (1993a) reported a 1-year first incidence of major depression of 5.26%, including 7.14% for female adolescents and 4.35% for males, in a sample of 112 high school students ages 14–18 years. For dysthymia the rates were 0.13% for females and 0% for males. Kashani et al. (1987b) also agreed with these findings and showed that among depressed adolescents ages 14–16 years, girls outnumbered boys by a ratio of 5:1. Whitaker et al. (1990) studied a sample of high-school students and also found depressive disorders to be more common in girls. The combined lifetime prevalence rates for both sexes in this study were 4.0% for major depression and 4.9% for dysthymia. These researchers also found that the pattern of sex distribution of depression observed in adults (i.e., depression is significantly more common in women than in men) does not appear until puberty, when the rate of depression quadruples in girls and doubles in boys. They postulated that the youngsters with an earlier onset of depression appear to have a first major depressive episode of longer duration and of greater severity than those with later onset (Clarke et al. 1995; Garland and Weiss 1995; Lewinsohn et al. 1994b). Interestingly, the incidence of major depressive disorder in adolescents observed in several studies was significantly higher than that reported in many adult studies. For example, in adolescents annual incidence rates of 1.1% for males and 2.0% for females were reported in the Epidemiologic Catchment Area program (Eaton et al. 1989; Marangell et al. 1997). These compare to annual incidences of 0.43% for men and 0.76% for women in the Lunby study (Rorsman et al. 1990) and 0.21% for men and 0.25% for women in the Stirling County study conducted in eastern Canada (Murphy et al. 1988).

Despite the somewhat diverse findings of different authors, the following general conclusions can be drawn. First, there is a tendency for major depressive disorder to have higher incidence among adolescents than among preschool children (Kashani et al. 1987a). Discrepancies between the prevalence and incidence rates of major depression in adolescents and adults can be explained by the use of different methodologies. For example, the study by Rorsman et al. (1990) did not use a standardized, structured diagnostic interview or a modern definition of depression but relied on the retrospective report of illness over a 15-year period. The Stirling County study used a structured interview designed in the 1950s and relied on the retrospective report of illness over 16 years (Murphy et al. 1988). Furthermore, the Epidemiologic Catchment Area program (Eaton et al. 1989) used lay interviewers to administer the Diagnostic Interview Schedule, which may underestimate depressive disorders. However, it should be noted that it is possible that adolescents may have a lower threshold for reporting depressive symptoms, or the incidence of depression may be increasing.

There are reports indicating that the incidence of depression is greater among those from lower socioeconomic classes. Some researchers have also found significant associations between the incidence of depression and major life events such as health problems, family disorder, conflict with parents, or death of a parent (Lewinsohn et al. 1994c; Reinherz et al. 1993b). Reinherz et al. (1993b) reported that remarriage of a parent for males and death of a parent for females significantly increased the risk of developing major depressive disorder. However, Lewinsohn et al. (1994c) found that the death of a parent or living with fewer than two biological parents did not increase risk for depression in adolescents. Therefore, it is currently unclear if undesirable life events or family structure are always associated with incidence of major depressive disorder.

Available data on bipolar disorder in childhood and adolescence are mostly derived from patient samples. In comparison to major depressive disorder, bipolar disorder is much less common in the general population, with lifetime prevalence estimates of 0.4%–1.6% among adults. Lewinsohn et al. (1995) conducted an epidemiological study of community samples of adolescents with bipolar disorder. Their subjects, randomly selected Oregon high school students, were assessed with a structured diagnostic interview—the Schedule for Affective Disorders and Schizophrenia for School-Age Children (K-SADS)—at two different times: at initial assessment ($N=1{,}709$) and at follow-up assessment approximately 1 year later ($N=1{,}507$). Bipolar disorder was diagnosed in 18 patients after the two evaluations, which translated to a combined lifetime prevalence of bipolar disorder of approximately 1%. Of the 18 patients with bipolar disorder, 2 met full DSM-III-R (American Psychiatric Association 1987) criteria for a lifetime manic episode (bipolar I disorder), 11 met criteria for bipolar II disorder, and 5 received a diagnosis of cyclothymia. An additional 5.7% of the sample reported having experienced a distinct period of abnormally and persistently elevated, expansive, or irritable mood even though they never met criteria for bipolar disorder. These rates were much lower than those reported by Carlson and Kashani (1988a). They found that of 150 adolescents in a community sample, 20 (13.3%) reported periods of at least 2 days during which they experienced four or more manic symptoms. Although none of these adolescents exhibited sufficient impairment to meet criteria for a manic episode, 3 (1.5%) appeared to qualify for a diagnosis of bipolar II disorder or cyclothymia.

Krasa and Tolbert (1994) found a 3.4% incidence rate of bipolar disorder in a sample of adolescent inpatients. The authors identified more girls (60.5%) than boys (39.5%) with bipolar disorder. Psychotic symptoms were found in 50%, and half of the sample also had presented at some point with a mixed episode.

Etiology and Pathogenesis

■ Biological Factors

Growth Hormone

The role of growth hormone in the etiology and pathogenesis of depression has been studied. Nevertheless, different studies have produced varying—sometimes even opposite—results. Depressed children and adolescents have been shown to have hyposecretion of growth hormone after various challenges, including insulin-induced hypoglycemia and oral administration of clonidine, levodopa, desmethylimipramine, and growth hormone–releasing hormone (Jensen and Garfinkel 1990; Ryan et al. 1994). Ryan et al. (1994) found that depressed adolescents had a blunted growth hormone response to an intramuscular injection of the antidepressant desipramine compared with nondepressed control subjects. The largest group differences were among the subgroup of suicidal depressed adolescents. Furthermore, blunted growth hormone response to insulin-induced hypoglycemia has been reported to persist after remission of a major depressive episode. This finding might be a "trait" or "scar" marker for major depressive disorder (Ryan et al. 1994). These authors also suggested that dysregulation in growth hormone secretion in depression may reflect changes in the central noradrenergic receptors or may be secondary to changes in other neurotransmitters such as somatomedin and somatostatin, which have been reported to be altered in some depressed patients.

The secretion of growth hormone during sleep has also been studied, but results have been contradictory. Although studies of children (Puig-Antich et al. 1984a) and adolescents (Kutcher et al. 1988, 1991) suggested that there may be a relative hypersecretion of growth hormone during sleep, a more recent study by De Bellis et al. (1996) failed to replicate this finding. In another study comparing 44 adolescents with major depressive disorder and 37 matched nondepressed control subjects, no differences in growth hormone secretion during the night were found between depressed subjects and nondepressed control subjects. However, splitting the major depressive disorder group on the basis of suicidal versus nonsuicidal depressed adolescent inpatients showed decreased nocturnal growth hormone secretion in the former (Dahl et al. 1992b). A reexamination of nocturnal growth hormone secretion in depressed children (Puig-Antich et al. 1984b) suggested that stressful life events may have contributed to increased nocturnal growth hormone secretion (Williamson et al. 1996).

Cortisol and ACTH

Several studies of adults with major depressive disorder have suggested that dysregulation of the central serotonergic function may be a vulnerability factor for the development of depression (Maes et al. 1995). However, dysregulation of the hypothalamic-pituitary-adrenal axis in depressed children and adolescents has not been studied systematically. Some investigators found no significant differences in baseline plasma cortisol secretion (24-hour or nocturnal sampling) between depressed outpatients and nondepressed child and adolescent control subjects (Birmaher et al. 1992a, 1992b; Dahl et al. 1989, 1991b; Kutcher et al. 1991). However, Ryan et al. (1992) found that children with early-onset major depressive disorder had significantly lower cortisol levels than nondepressed children after infusion of L-5-hydroxytryptophan. Therefore, it is possible that depressed individuals have an

abnormality in cortisol regulatory mechanisms, with a tendency to hypersecrete corticotropin-releasing hormone (CRH) or cortisol in response to stressful stimuli. In a study by Birmaher et al. (1996a), no significant differences were found between prepubertal children with major depressive disorder and nondepressed control subjects in baseline or post-CRH stimulation values of either cortisol or adrenocorticotropic hormone (ACTH). However, the depressed inpatients and the subjects in melancholic subgroups were found to secrete significantly less overall ACTH. Abnormalities in ACTH secretion in response to CRH have also been observed in abused children, with the nature of the ACTH disturbances being affected by both past history of abuse and current stressors (De Bellis et al. 1994). However, further studies in children and adolescents are clearly needed.

The dexamethasone suppression test (DST) is designed to test the sensitivity of the hypothalamic-pituitary-adrenal axis to feedback inhibition. The DST has been the most extensively studied biological marker in juvenile depression. A positive (abnormal) DST result indicates that exogenous dexamethasone has failed to suppress cortisol secretion. The DST has been postulated to be a nonspecific state marker for depression.

Several studies of the DST in depressed children and adolescents (Casat et al. 1989; Dahl et al. 1992a) found that 1) sensitivity of the DST was higher in inpatients than in outpatients (61% versus 29%); 2) sensitivity was somewhat better in depressed children than in depressed adolescents (58% versus 44%); 3) specificity was greater in adolescent samples than in preadolescent samples (84% versus 74%); 4) specificity was greater in inpatient than in outpatient settings (61% versus 29%); and 5) specificity for child inpatients was less than for adolescent inpatients (60% versus 85%). In adolescent inpatients, approximately 16% of all psychiatric control subjects, regardless of diagnosis, had a positive DST. A number of factors may explain the variance of findings across studies. These include suicidality, differences in dexamethasone metabolism, and variations in the stress of subjects (such as venipunctures for blood samples and hospitalization) (Birmaher et al. 1992a, 1992b; Dahl et al. 1992a).

The studies mentioned above have led some to suggest that the DST has little value as a diagnostic screening test for depression. However, a positive DST may prove useful when following up on treatment response.

Thyroid Hormones

Thyroid hormones have long been considered to be involved in the etiology and pathogenesis of mood disorders. Different studies, however, provide conflicting evidence regarding this issue. Some studies of depressed adults found increased concentrations of total thyroxine (T_4) (Hatotani et al. 1977; Kirkegaard and Faber 1981; Linnoila et al. 1979) in patients with major depressive disorder. In some depressed adults administration of exogenous thyroid hormone was shown to potentiate the effect of antidepressants (Joffe and Singer 1990) or to cause nonresponders to antidepressants to become responders (Wehr et al. 1982). Yet, other studies found thyroid hormone was an ineffective adjunctive treatment in antidepressant-resistant depression (Thase et al. 1989). Brambilla et al. (1989) also reported that the thyroid-stimulating hormone (TSH) response to stimulation with thyrotropin-releasing hormone in children and adolescents with dysthymia did not differ from the response in children and adolescents without dysthymia. Conversely, Khan (1988) reported a blunting of the TSH response to thyrotropin-releasing hormone in 36.6% of children and adolescents with major depression, 20.8% of those with conduct disorder, 17% of those with adjustment disorders, and 43% of those with substance abuse. No blunting of the response was found in those with ADHD or dysthymia. In another study of depressed adolescents, TSH level was elevated at only one point during serial sampling throughout the day (Kutcher et al. 1991). In a retrospective chart review, T_4 level was elevated in depressed adolescents and manic adolescents compared with control subjects without depression or mania (Sokolov et al. 1993).

Dorn et al. (1996) examined thyroid hormone concentrations and their influence on mood and behavior in adolescents with depression. Subjects were 21 depressed adolescents (11 girls, 10 boys) and 20 healthy control subjects (11 girls, 9 boys) who were pair-matched by age, gender, race, and socioeconomic status. Ages ranged from 12.7 years to 16.9 years, with mean ages of 15.2 years for the depressed group and 15.1 years for the control group. Blood was drawn to measure TSH, free thyroxine (FT_4), thyroxine, and triiodothyronine (T_3). Symptom scores for major depression, attention deficit, and obsessive-compulsive behavior were abstracted from the Diagnostic Interview Schedule for Children. Total behavior problem scores from the Youth Self-Report were also obtained. There were no significant group or gender differences or group-by-gender interactions for TSH, T_4, or T_3. TSH did not significantly correlate with any of the psychological measures. In the depressed group there were negative correlations (although not always significant) between FT_4 and total behavior problems and symptom scores for major depression, attention-deficit spectrum, and obsessive-compulsive spectrum. The authors concluded that FT_4 concentrations were lowered in depressed adolescents, which suggested a relationship between negative behaviors and dysfunction of the hypothalamic-pituitary-thyroid axis in adolescents with depression. The same study also revealed a trend (although not significant) for concentrations of immunoreactive morning TSH to be lower in the depressed group.

Melatonin

Several studies of melatonin in depressed adults found a decrease in the nocturnal serum or urine levels or a phase shift in the melatonin peak (R.P. Brown et al. 1985, 1987; Kennedy et al. 1989; Lewy et al. 1980). A few studies showed no difference in these measures (Jimerson et al. 1977; Mendlewicz et al. 1979; C. Thompson et al. 1988). Two studies showed an increase in melatonin (Rubin et al. 1992; Sitholey 1999). In healthy individuals, nocturnal serum melatonin levels begin to increase 2 hours before bedtime but surge a half hour after lights-out during sleep. Most melatonin is secreted during the dark cycle of the night, from 11:00 P.M. to 3:00 A.M., with a peak at 2:00 A.M. There are only a few studies on melatonin levels in major depression in youths. Cavallo et al. (1987) found that nocturnal serum melatonin levels were lower in 9 depressed boys ages 7–13 years than in a control group of 10 boys who were of normal height, were genetically short, or had delayed pubescence. Shafii et al. (1988) measured bedtime and overnight urine melatonin levels in 96 psychiatric inpatients ages 6–16 years. Patients with primary major depression had overnight urine melatonin levels that were significantly higher than those of patients with secondary depression or nondepressed psychiatric control subjects. However, Waterman et al. (1992) reported no difference between the level of 6-hydroxymelatonin sulfate in the overnight urine of youths with major depression and the level measured in control subjects. In this study (unlike in the two studies mentioned above), the metabolite of melatonin, rather than melatonin itself, was measured.

Also, urine was collected 12 hours after the administration of insulin as part of a growth hormone challenge study, which might have affected results.

Shafii et al. (1990) examined pineal gland function by measuring nocturnal serum melatonin levels during wakefulness and sleep in depressed children and adolescents. Twenty-two youths ages 8–17 years with major depressive disorder were compared with 19 control subjects. Blood samples were drawn every half hour from 6:00 P.M. to 7:00 A.M. Serum melatonin levels were determined by radioimmunoassay. The overall nocturnal serum melatonin profile from 6:00 P.M. to 7:00 A.M. was significantly higher in the depressed group than in the control group. In dim light, when subjects were awake, there were no differences between the two groups. After lights-out, from 10:00 P.M. to 7:00 A.M., melatonin levels rose in both groups. However, the depressed subjects had significantly higher increases than the control subjects. Melatonin levels were significantly higher in depressed subjects without psychosis ($n=15$) than in depressed subjects with psychosis ($n=7$) or control subjects. The authors concluded that determining the overall nocturnal serum melatonin profile during darkness may help differentiate between children and adolescents with major depression but without psychosis, those with psychosis, and those who are psychiatrically healthy.

Carlson and Abbott (1995) compared adolescents and children with primary major depressive disorder to those with comorbid major depressive disorder and to a control group of youngsters who had only behavioral disorders. Only the group with primary depression had significantly abnormal melatonin secretion.

Neurotransmitters

Major depressive disorder. Norepinephrine and serotonin are the biogenic amines that are believed to play an important role in the regulation of mood, and consequently in the pathophysiology of depression. The major classes of antidepressants—which include monoamine oxidase inhibitors (MAOIs), tricyclic antidepressants (TCAs), and selective serotonin reuptake inhibitors (SSRIs)—appear to function by restoring regulation of the dysregulated neurotransmitter system in the brain (Ryan 1990; Thase et al. 1995). A possible relationship between dopamine and serotonin and mood disorders has been demonstrated in adults. It has also been postulated that high levels of sex hormones during puberty may decrease the effectiveness of TCAs (Kutcher et al. 1994).

Acetylcholine is another important neurotransmitter that may be involved in mood disorders. Drugs that increase acetylcholine levels have been reported to induce depressive symptoms in adult control subjects and to exacerbate depression in depressed patients (Green et al. 1995).

Bipolar disorder. In bipolar disorder, the Na^+-K^+-ATPase hypothesis (el Mallakh and Li 1993) proposes that the manic symptoms of flight of ideas, irritability, distractibility, and high energy are related to a decrease in the activity of the Na^+-K^+-ATPase pump, which results in an increase in neuronal excitability. Bipolar depression is hypothesized to be secondary to a larger decrease in pump activity and a subsequent decrease in neurotransmitter release.

Guanine nucleotide binding proteins (Tappia et al. 1997) have also been postulated to play an important role in the molecular etiology of bipolar disorder (Schreiber and Avissar 1991). This hypothesis is based on the finding that lithium attenuates the functioning of G-protein and damps the oscillatory system, thereby resulting in a more stable state.

Neurobiological studies include a single case study of a hypomanic child who had a significantly different urinary methoxyhydroxyphenyl glycol level from that of healthy control subjects (McKnew et al. 1974). Enlarged ventricles and increased numbers of hyperintensities were found in a small open pilot study of bipolar children and adolescents (Botteron et al. 1995).

Sleep abnormalities. Depressed children and adolescents frequently describe disturbed sleep (Goetz et al. 1987). However, electroencephalographic studies have not demonstrated consistent sleep changes paralleling those observed in adults with major depressive disorder. Studies in adults with major depression have found increased rapid eye movement (REM) density in early REM periods, decreased delta (slow-wave) sleep, disturbed sleep continuity, and shortened REM latency (Yaylayan et al. 1990). There are several studies of depressed children and adolescents, but the results have been inconsistent. Among studies of depressed children (Dahl et al. 1991a; Emslie et al. 1990; Puig-Antich et al. 1982; Young et al. 1982), only one study found decreased REM latency and increased sleep latency in an inpatient sample (Emslie et al. 1990). Among studies of depressed adolescents (Boulos et al. 1992; Dahl et al. 1990, 1996; Emslie et al. 1994; Goetz et al. 1987; Lahmeyer et al. 1983), five studies reported prolonged sleep latency, four studies found reduced REM latency, and three studies reported decreased sleep. The same studies observed greater rates of sleep changes in inpatient adolescent samples and also in association with psychosis, suicidality, and endogenous major depressive disorder subtypes (Boulos et al. 1992; Dahl et al. 1990; Emslie et al. 1994; Naylor et al. 1990).

■ Genetic Factors

Major Depressive Disorder

Twin studies provide support for a genetic factor in the etiology of depression. Concordance rates for depression are much higher in monozygotic twins (54%) (McGuffin and Katz 1989) than in dizygotic twins (24%) (Carlson and Abbott 1995). Adult twin studies also indicate that mood disorders are strongly heritable, with a much stronger genetic component for bipolar disorder than for major depressive disorder. A German study by Zerbin-Rudin (1969) reviewed the pattern of inheritance of mood disorders by polarity in twin studies. The researchers also noted a strong degree of specificity of transmission, which was again much greater for bipolar disorder than for unipolar disorder. For the twin of an individual with unipolar depression, the relative risk of having unipolar depression was estimated to be 2.4 (43% concordance for monozygotic twins and 18% concordance for dizygotic twins) and the relative risk of bipolar depression was 1.8 (11% concordance for monozygotic twins and 6% concordance for dizygotic twins).

Several reports (Kutcher and Marton 1991; Mitchell et al. 1989) indicate that early-onset depression is associated with increased familial aggregation. Lifetime prevalence rates in the first-degree relatives of depressed youths have ranged from 17% (Strober 1984) to 46% (Mitchell et al. 1989; Todd et al. 1993). The lifetime rates of affective disorders in the first-degree relatives of depressed inpatient adolescents were significantly higher than expected rates in the general population (Strober 1984).

Weissman et al. (1984a) assessed the lifetime prevalence rates of psychopathology in the first-degree (n=228) and second-degree (n=736) relatives of 76 adolescents with major depressive disorder and the first-degree (n=107) and second-degree (n=323) relatives of 34 psychiatrically healthy control adolescents in a case-control family history study. The relatives of depressed adolescents had significantly higher lifetime rates of major depressive disorder than the first-degree relatives of healthy control subjects (25% versus 13%) and also had higher lifetime rates of "any" of the Family History–Research Diagnostic Criteria psychiatric disorders (53% versus 36%). A lifetime rate of depression of 20% in the first-degree relatives of depressed adolescents was reported by Kutcher and Marton (1991). Using the family history method, these researchers assessed 259 first-degree relatives of 23 adolescents with bipolar depression (81 relatives), of 26 adolescents with unipolar depression (95 relatives), and of 24 psychiatrically healthy control subjects (83 relatives) to determine the presence of affective disorders. The relatives of healthy control adolescents in this study had considerably lower lifetime rates of depression (4%) compared with the relatives of healthy control adolescents in the study by Weissman et al. (1984a) (13%). The second-degree relatives of adolescents with major depressive disorder also had significantly higher lifetime rates of other psychiatric disorders (5%) than did the relatives of healthy control subjects (6%). The first-degree relatives of depressed adolescents who were also suicidal had increased lifetime rates of suicidal behavior, which significantly cosegregated with major depressive disorder.

Overall, family studies have consistently reported a twofold to threefold increase in the lifetime rates of depressive disorders in the relatives of depressed subjects compared with healthy control subjects (Gershon et al. 1982; Weissman et al. 1982, 1984b, 1984c). Some of these studies also reported that late-onset depression (at age 60 years or later) was associated with the least risk for depression in family members and that early-onset depression (at age 20 years or before) was associated with the greatest risk for depression in family members (Puig-Antich et al. 1989; Weissman et al. 1984c, 1988).

The lifetime risk for major depressive disorder in children of depressed parents has been estimated to range from 15% (Orvaschel et al. 1988) to 45% (Hammen et al. 1990). Factors in the depressed parent such as early onset and recurrence of depression appear to contribute to the highest risk for major depressive disorder in their children (Orvaschel 1990; Warner et al. 1995; Weissman et al. 1987, 1988). The risk for depression was also increased when both parents had a mood disorder. Several studies report that children of depressed parents are not only at high risk to develop depression but are also at increased risk to have other psychopathology, including anxiety and disruptive disorders (Hammen et al. 1990; Keller et al. 1988; Orvaschel et al. 1988; Warner et al. 1995; Weissman et al. 1987, 1988).

The occurrence of familial aggregation of depression suggests a family genetic component for depression. However, it is postulated that a vulnerability to depression and anxiety is what is actually inherited. Thus, certain environmental stressors may be required for one of these disorders to be manifested (Kendler 1995; Warner et al. 1995).

Bipolar Disorder

Bipolar disorder may have the strongest genetic component of any mental disorder. The concordance rate is much higher in monozygotic twins (65%) than in dizygotic twins (14%) (Nurnberger and Gershon 1982). Family studies of adolescent-onset bipolar disorder have shown increased rates of bipolar disorder among relatives. Furthermore, early onset predicted higher prevalence of illness in family members (Rice et al. 1987; Strober 1992; Strober et al. 1988). Todd et al. (1993) found elevated rates of mood disorders and increased severity of mood disorders in relatives of children with bipolar affective disorder and major depressive disorder. These were manifested by earlier onset and increased numbers of suicide attempts. Kutcher and Marton (1991) studied adolescents between ages 13 and 19 years and found a significantly higher prevalence rate of bipolar illness in their first-degree relatives. The relatives of the bipolar probands had significantly higher rates of bipolar disorder than the relatives of the unipolar probands. Rates of unipolar illness or other psychiatric disorders were not increased. The rate of bipolar illness in the first-degree relatives of adolescent probands was approximately 15%. These data suggest a strong genetic component in early-onset bipolar disorder.

Genetic studies have also suggested that environmental factors—particularly nonshared intrafamilial and extrafamilial environmental experiences—have an important impact. These factors include differences in how individual parents treat each of their children (Kendler 1995; Plomin 1994). Individuals at high genetic risk appear to be more sensitive to the effects of adverse environment than individuals at low genetic risk (Kendler 1995). It has also been suggested that environmental effects may be, at least in part, under genetic influence (Plomin 1994).

■ Structural Brain Abnormalities

New brain imaging techniques allow the identification of structural brain abnormalities in patients with mood disorders. However, the number of studies on brain imaging in bipolar adolescents is very limited.

Botteron et al. (1995) suggested that there are structural differences in the central nervous system between young manic individuals and healthy subjects. The authors assessed a sample of consecutively referred 8- to 16-year-old manic ($n=10$) and psychiatrically healthy ($n=5$) subjects with the Schedule for Affective Disorders and Schizophrenia for School-Age Children—Present Episode Version; the Children's Global Assessment Scale; and the Family History–Research Diagnostic Criteria. Magnetic resonance scans of four manic subjects and one control subject showed ventricular or white matter abnormalities. There were significant positive correlations between increasing age and both right and left ventricular volumes. Two of eight manic subjects and no control subjects had confluent subcortical hyperintensities. Subjective review of scans and the structured ratings suggested that there are neuromorphometric differences between children and adolescents with bipolar disorder and healthy children and adolescents.

A magnetic resonance imaging scan of a 15-year-old girl who developed bipolar disorder after a mild head injury showed small lesions caudal to the right amygdala, the right putamen, and the right side of the pituitary gland (Sayal et al. 2000). It was unclear whether these lesions represented hematomas secondary to the head injury or whether spontaneous bleeding had led to the head injury.

■ Psychological Theories

There are several psychological theories of depression. Although all of them contain useful and important elements, none provides a full explanation of the etiology and pathogenesis of this severe illness.

Psychoanalytic Model

Psychoanalytic theory suggests that depression results from aggression turned inward after the loss of an ambivalently loved object. Freud likened serious melancholic depressive states to normal grief but with some differences. Gabbard (1995) identified four key points to the psychodynamic understanding of depression:

1) disruption of the early infant-mother relationship during the oral phase increases an individual's vulnerability to depression in later life; 2) depression can be related to either real or imagined loss; 3) introjection, a defense mechanism in which the person internalizes the lost object, is used to cope with the distress connected to the loss of the departed object; 4) because of mixed feelings of love, hatred, and anger toward the lost object, feelings of anger are directed inward toward the self.

Although there is widespread belief in this model, there is little scientific data to support it. A transition from grief to pathological depression occurs in no more than 10%–15% of children and 2%–5% of adults (Akiskal 1995).

Cognitive-Behavioral Models

Beck's (1967) cognitive model represents an important paradigm shift (L.M. Thompson et al. 1992) from the psychoanalytical tradition. In Beck's model, distorted, negative thoughts characteristic of depressed individuals are seen as underlying depression. The cognitive model redefines depression in terms of the cognitive triad, which consists of pessimistic, deprecatory thoughts about oneself, one's experiences, and one's future. Research with children and adolescents supports the validity and clinical utility of this model in youths (Brent et al. 1997; Deal and Williams 1988; Kashani et al. 1989). This model led to the development of treatment strategies aimed at modifying maladaptive cognitive patterns, which have proved to be a major advance in the treatment of depression.

Studies of depressed children and adolescents revealed that they had maladaptive attributional styles (Asarnow and Bates 1988; Seligman et al. 1984; Summerville et al. 1992), cognitive distortions (Kendall et al. 1990), and negative self-concept (Hammen 1988; Lewinsohn et al. 1994d), as well as social skills deficits, impaired problem solving, and passive or avoidant coping strategies (Adams and Adams 1991). Although these factors may not be specific to depression, they are important because they typically serve as the targets of treatment in cognitive-behavioral therapy (CBT).

Learned Helplessness Model

The learned helplessness model (Seligman and Peterson 1986) connects depression to the experience of uncontrollable life events. In relation to depression, the learned helplessness model describes deficits in all areas of human responsiveness—cognitive, emotional, and motivational.

Self-Control Model

Rehm's (1977) self-control model proposes that persons with depression have deficiencies in self-monitoring, self-evaluation, and self-reinforcement that result in cognitive distortions that lead to depression. The depressed individual's misperceptions create selective attention to negative events and misattribution of personal success and failure. These result in maladaptive behavioral styles such as focusing attention on short-term rather than long-term consequences, setting unrealistic goals, engaging in excessive self-punishment, and applying inadequate positive self-reinforcement.

■ Social and Environmental Factors

Major Depressive Disorder

Studies of depressed adults, offspring of depressed parents, and depressed youths have found a modest but significant relationship between stressful life events and depression in both clinical and community samples. The family interactions in these patients were characterized by more conflict, more rejection, more problems with communication, less expression of affect, less support, and more abuse than the family interactions of nondepressed control subjects (Kaufman 1991; Williamson et al. 1995a).

The mechanisms by which abnormal family interactions might lead to depression in children are not clear. Abnormal early interactions between mother and child may cause children to develop patterns of handling stress that predispose them to depression. Family conflicts are also thought to be one of the triggers of depression in individuals susceptible to it. Other factors such as lack of affect, irritability directed toward the child, and abuse may also contribute to increased vulnerability to depression or other psychopathology in children (Adrian and Hammen 1993). Finally, depressed children may also generate conflicts that contribute to the maintenance of their parents' and their own depression or create conflicts in an otherwise normally functioning family.

Several studies of children (Banez and Compas 1990; Mullins et al. 1985) and adolescents (Swearingen and Cohen 1985) examine the relationship between stressful life events and symptoms of depression. Overall, these studies have found life events to be positively correlated with symptoms of depression, which suggests that life events may play a causal role in the development of depressive symptoms. Similarly, studies of clinically depressed youths have found stressful life events to be increased in depressed adolescents (Williamson et al. 1995a). A few studies specifically show that stressful life events were significantly more frequent before the onset of a depressive episode. Specific events—including loss, divorce, bereavement, and exposure to suicide—individually or in combination with other risk factors (e.g., lack of support) have been associated with the onset of depression (Brent et al. 1993; Reinherz et al. 1993b; E.B. Weller and Weller 1991). For example, women who lost a parent before age 17 and had poor parental care were at risk for having poor self-esteem, getting married early, and having children at an earlier age. Furthermore, these women were at increased risk of developing depression when exposed to stressful life events, but depression could be prevented by having a supportive spouse (G.W. Brown and Harris 1993).

Exposure to suicide has been described as a severe, stressful event that is associated with a threefold increase in acute and recurrent major depressive disorder in friends, siblings, and mothers of the suicide victims (Brent et al. 1988, 1993). The risk of developing depression was proportional to the individual's closeness to the victim and the intensity of the exposure. Factors such as history of additional interpersonal losses, additional stressors, family psychiatric history, and prior psychopathology (including depression) also increased the risk for depression.

Gore et al. (1992) examined the relationship between life stress and depressive symptoms in 1,208 randomly selected high-school students ($N=1,208$). There were statistically significant associations of moderate to high magnitude between depressed mood and all stress indicators. Higher levels of depressed mood were positively correlated with higher levels of stress and negatively correlated with higher levels of social support.

Lewinsohn et al. (1994c) examined psychosocial risk factors thought to be associated with depression in a community sample of 1,508 adolescents. Depressed teenagers were more likely to have a history of current or past mental illness (especially anxiety and substance use disorders), to have made a suicide attempt, to show greater pessimism and person-

al attributions for failure, to have a more negative body image, to have lower self-esteem, to be overly emotionally dependent on others, to be more self-conscious, to use less effective coping skills, to report less social support from family and friends, and to be more likely to smoke more cigarettes than nondepressed peers. Factors that were not associated with being depressed but that were predictive of subsequent depression included conflict with parents, dissatisfaction with grades, and failure to do homework. Neither major life events nor "daily hassles" appeared to act as triggers for future depression. The authors concluded that stressful events were characteristically present in depressed individuals before, during, and after an episode of depression.

Williamson et al. (1998) examined acute life events and ongoing difficulties in adolescents with a recent major depressive disorder. Twenty-six adolescents (ages 13–18 years) with a recent episode of DSM-III-R major depressive disorder and 15 psychiatrically healthy control subjects without any Axis I lifetime psychiatric disorders were assessed using the investigator-based Life Events and Difficulties Schedule in this study. More than twice as many depressed adolescents reported having had a traditionally defined severe event occur in the year before the onset of depression (Friedman et al. 1999) than did healthy control adolescents (20%). However, this difference failed to reach statistical significance. Compared with healthy control adolescents, depressed adolescents had significantly more major difficulties and a significantly higher average number of defined severe events in the year before the onset of the illness.

A major limitation of the research on stressful life events in early-onset depression is the fact that much of the research has focused on cross-sectional correlational data obtained from self-report checklists. Therefore, it is difficult to establish a causal relationship because events could be either a cause or a result of the depression. Studies using an adaptation of the adult Life Event and Difficulty Schedule Interview (G.W. Brown and Harris 1989) for use in children and adolescents found significantly more severe and nonsevere stressful life events (especially in the areas of romantic relationships, education, relationships with friends or parents, work, and health) in depressed youths 12 months before the onset of depression compared with psychiatrically healthy control subjects (Goodyer et al. 1985, 1988).

Bipolar Disorder

Although biological factors figure more prominently in the etiology of bipolar disorder, psychological and environmental influences are also important and may be involved in precipitating manic episodes. Psychodynamic theories of bipolar illness have focused primarily on mania as a defensive reaction to depression (Gabbard 1995). Other explanations of mania include the view that manic euphoria is a compensatory reaction to profound depression or an unconscious wish fulfillment of narcissistic aspirations. The grandiose and expansive style of a manic individual is viewed as a compensatory reaction to true feelings of extremely low self-esteem.

In summary, even less is speculated about the etiology of early-onset bipolar disorder than about the etiology of juvenile depression. Most research has focused on biological mechanisms, but psychological, social, and environmental factors are also thought to play a role in precipitating episodes of mania and depression. Advances in molecular biology and neuroimaging have opened the door to further study in these areas and will certainly contribute to the future understanding of this illness. It must be emphasized that all of these theories contribute to the understanding of the etiology of depression and serve as some of the components of the biopsychosocial model of mood disorders.

Treatment

The earlier the treatment is initiated, the better the outcome is. Depressive symptomatology, even at a subsyndromal level, may predict the eventual development of a full-blown depressive episode (Clarke et al. 1995; Prien and Kupfer 1986). Therefore, targeting subsyndromal depressive symptomatology may prevent relapse in adolescents in remission and prevent the need for more extensive treatment (Clarke et al. 1995; Kroll et al. 1996). Treatment may be divided into acute treatment, continuation treatment, and maintenance treatment. The setting for care is generally selected as the least restrictive environment. However, the safety and psychosocial circumstances of the adolescent are also important considerations. Hospitalization should be considered when the adolescent is actively suicidal, frankly psychotic, volatile, aggressive, or at risk for ongoing abuse or neglect if returned to the home environment. In addition, hospitalization may be appropriate when adolescents require medication trials but adequate observation or supervision is not possible because of either the psychosocial situation or complicated general medical conditions. Aggression, deterioration in symptomatic and functional status, and family discord are the main predictors or correlates of inpatient hospitalization for children and adolescents (Costello et al. 1991; Gutterman et al. 1993). Treatment is currently oriented more to outpatient models.

The first step in treating an adolescent is to establish rapport and to develop a therapeutic alliance. The youth and his or her family should always be informed and educated about the diagnosis and possible treatment modalities.

■ Major Depressive Disorder

Biological and Pharmacological Treatments

Despite insufficient evidence of effectiveness from randomized controlled trials, antidepressant medications continue to be widely prescribed in adolescents. Arguments supporting the practice of prescribing antidepressants to adolescents with depression include 1) the well-studied efficacy of antidepressants in treating depression in adults, 2) the evidence for continuity between adolescent and adult depression (Harrington et al. 1990), and 3) the significant morbidity and mortality rates of adolescent depression (Kye and Ryan 1995).

Controlled studies of antidepressants in adolescents are gradually occurring. One study demonstrated the superiority of fluoxetine over placebo in both children and adolescents with major depressive disorder (Emslie et al. 1997). There have been attempts to explain the weak response to antidepressants among youths with major depressive disorder. Methodological critiques have suggested that dosing may have been inadequate and that too few patients were studied. The changing hormonal status of children and adolescents compared with adults was postulated to account for the poor response to TCAs, but there has been no convincing evidence that sex hormones can consistently augment antidepressant response.

Selective serotonin reuptake inhibitors. SSRIs, a comparatively new class of antidepressants, were shown to be more effective than TCAs in a preliminary study. SSRIs have fewer side effects, lower toxicity in overdose, and a potentially broader range of clinical indications. SSRIs have been used to treat a variety of conditions, including affective disorders, obsessive-compulsive disorder, and other anxiety disorders (Emslie et al. 1999).

Published studies of SSRIs. Even though the SSRIs have been available for more than a decade, there are currently only two published placebo-controlled trials of the efficacy and safety of SSRIs in children and adolescents: 1) a double-blind, randomized, placebo-controlled trial of fluoxetine (Emslie et al. 1997) and 2) a randomized, controlled study of the efficacy of paroxetine and its placebo-controlled comparison with a TCA, imipramine (Keller et al. 2001).

Emslie and colleagues (1997) evaluated the comparative efficacy, safety, and tolerability of fluoxetine treatment compared with placebo in child and adolescent outpatients with nonpsychotic major depressive disorder. Ninety-six child and adolescent outpatients (ages 7–17 years), who were self-referred or were referred by other practitioners and met DSM-III-R criteria for nonpsychotic major depressive disorder, were studied. Subjects were randomized to 20 mg of fluoxetine or placebo and were seen weekly for 8 consecutive weeks. Randomization was preceded by three evaluation visits that included structured diagnostic interviews during 2 weeks, followed a week later by a 1-week single-blind placebo run-in. Primary outcome measurements were the Global Improvement subscale of the Clinical Global Impressions (CGI) Scale and the Children's Depression Rating Scale–Revised (CDRS-R), a measure of the severity depressive symptoms. Forty-eight patients were randomized to fluoxetine treatment and 48 to placebo. Using the intent-to-treat model, 27 (56%) of those receiving fluoxetine and 16 (33%) receiving placebo were rated "much" or "very much" improved on the CGI Scale at study exit. Significant differences were also noted in weekly ratings of the CDRS-R after 5 weeks of treatment (using last observation carried forward). Equivalent response rates were found for patients ages 12 years and younger (n=48) and those ages 13 years and older (n=48). However, complete symptom remission (CDRS-R score of 28 or below) occurred in only 31% of the patients treated with fluoxetine and in 23% of the patients treated with placebo.

In summary, fluoxetine treatment was superior to placebo in relieving depressive symptoms. The difference between fluoxetine treatment and placebo was evident in clinician assessment of clinical global improvement (the CGI scale) and in weekly clinician ratings of depressive symptom severity (the CDRS-R). Differences between fluoxetine treatment and placebo became statistically significant after 5 weeks.

Keller et al. (2001) conducted a multicenter double-blind, randomized, parallel-design comparison of paroxetine with placebo and imipramine with placebo in adolescents with major depression. Two hundred seventy-five subjects were randomly assigned to one of the three arms of treatment. Subjects included males and females, ages 12–18 years, who met the DSM-IV (American Psychiatric Association 1994) criteria for a current episode of major depression of at least 8 weeks' duration. Major depression was diagnosed by a systematic clinical interview that used the juvenile version of the Schedule for Affective Disorders and Schizophrenia for Adolescents–Lifetime Version (K-SADS-L; Endicott and Spitzer 1978). In addition to fulfilling DSM-IV criteria for major depression, subjects were required to have a total score of at least 12 on the 17-item Hamilton Rating Scale for Depression (Ham-D), a score of less than 60 on the Children's Global Assessment Scale, and a score of at least 80 on the Peabody Picture Vocabulary Test. After a 7- to 14-day screening phase, subjects were randomly assigned to an 8-week course of treatment with paroxetine (20–40 mg), imipramine (gradual upward titration to 200–300 mg), or placebo in a 1:1:1 ratio. The mean duration of the current depressive episode was more than 1 year, with a mean baseline Ham-D total score between 18 and 19. Paroxetine was significantly more effective than placebo with regard to achievement of a Ham-D total score of 8 or less, a CGI score of 1 (very much improved) or 2 (much improved), and improvements in the depressed mood items of the Ham-D and the K-SADS-L. Paroxetine did not differ statistically from placebo for K-SADS-L depression subscale score, mean CGI score, or Ham-D total score. The response to imipramine was not significantly different from placebo for any measure.

Another study in children and adolescents with obsessive-compulsive disorder or depression showed that the pharmacokinetics of sertraline in patients ages 6–17 years was similar to that reported for adults (Alderman et al. 1998).

Ambrosini et al. (1999) conducted a prospective multicenter trial of sertraline in 53 adolescent outpatients with major depressive disorder. The subjects were treated in a 10-week open-label acute-phase trial with sertraline; if subjects responded, they were treated for an additional 12-week continuation phase. Diagnostic and response assessments included the K-SADS, a 17-item K-SADS–derived depression severity score, the Ham-D, the Beck Depression Inventory, and the CGI Scale. The protocol design consisted of a 2-week single-blind placebo assessment period followed by a 10-week open-label acute treatment phase with sertraline. The mean duration of the index depressive episode was substantial (78 ± 79 weeks), as was the degree of psychosocial impairment at baseline (mean Children's Global Assessment Scale score, 48.6 ± 8.5). When analyzed as continuous variables, all severity scores showed significant differences from baseline by 2 weeks. This pattern persisted through 10 weeks, with a significantly greater response occurring when treatment went from 6 to 10 weeks. Both clinician- and patient-rated improvement were maintained during continuation treatment. Sertraline was generally well tolerated and did not induce manic symptoms. This open-label study suggested that sertraline was a safe and well-tolerated antidepressant for use in adolescent major depressive disorder in doses up to 200 mg/day. However, the lack of a placebo comparison group limits the study.

In summary, despite insufficient double-blind controlled trials of the efficacy of SSRIs for depressed youths, preliminary data suggest that serotonergic agents may be beneficial for depressive states in youths and that treatment should be maintained for at least 8–10 weeks.

SSRI pharmacokinetics. Fluoxetine is a phenylpropylamine, paroxetine is a phenylpiperidine, and sertraline is a naphthaleneamine. In vitro, sertraline and paroxetine are more potent inhibitors of serotonin uptake than is fluoxetine. None of the SSRIs appreciably inhibit noradrenaline uptake in vitro. Sertraline appears to inhibit dopamine uptake to a greater extent than other SSRIs. Whether these relative differences have any clinical significance is unknown. Paroxetine, fluvoxamine, and sertraline have inactive metabolites, but the primary metabolite of fluoxetine, norfluoxetine, is reported to be four times more potent than fluoxetine in inhibiting serotonin reuptake.

Fluoxetine, paroxetine, and sertraline are more than 90% plasma protein bound. The half-life of fluoxetine is 2 days after a single dose and 8 days after repeated dosing. Norfluoxetine, its active metabolite, has a half-life of 7–19 days. The half-lives of other SSRIs range from 12 to 36 hours. Although there is substantial individual variability in steady-state levels, the

SSRIs appear to have a wide therapeutic range, so steady-state levels are thought to have little clinical significance in adults. Whether children and adolescents are different in this regard is not known.

The SSRIs are metabolized in the liver by the cytochrome P450 isoenzyme system. The SSRIs differentially inhibit the cytochrome P450 isoenzymes, which can lead to drug-drug interactions with drugs that are metabolized by the same isoenzyme (DeVane 1994).

In children and adolescents, little information on the impact of age on absorption, metabolism, therapeutic levels, or possible drug interactions is available. However, to achieve the same serum levels in children compared with adults, it is expected that the relative dosage (milligrams per kilogram) would need to be higher.

Other nontricyclic antidepressants. Bupropion, venlafaxine, trazodone, and nefazodone all have different modes of action but—similar to the SSRIs—have relatively few side effects. Bupropion (an aminoketone) undergoes extensive biotransformation to three metabolites that are pharmacologically active. Increased incidence of side effects may be associated with increased levels of the metabolite hydroxybupropion. Side effects may worsen if bupropion is combined with fluoxetine. Bupropion is primarily noradrenergic and anticholinergic. Antihistamine and orthostatic hypotensive effects are negligible. Concerns about seizures in bulimic adults have limited the use of bupropion. However, seizures are rare in adults if divided doses are used and dosages are below 450 mg/day. Bupropion has a half-life in adults of 10–21 hours, and it is quickly absorbed. Pharmacological data are not available for children and adolescents, but it is expected that multiple daily doses would be even more important in children than in adults because the half-life would be expected to be shorter. Dosages used in studies of ADHD range from 1.5 to 6.0 mg/kg per day.

Venlafaxine (a phenylethylamine) inhibits reuptake of both serotonin and norepinephrine. Similar to the SSRIs, venlafaxine has no significant affinity for muscarinic, cholinergic, histaminic, or α_1-adrenergic receptors. It has a relatively short half-life in adults (3–7 hours) and is given in divided doses. Venlafaxine is a much less potent inhibitor of cytochrome P450 2D6 isoenzymes than SSRIs in vitro (Conde Lopez et al. 1997). Venlafaxine is one of the few newer antidepressants to have pharmacokinetic data for children and adolescents (Derivan et al. 1995). Double-blind, placebo-controlled study results for depression are pending.

Nefazodone (a phenylpiperazine) is in the same chemical class as trazodone. The antidepressant activity of nefazodone is presumed to be linked to the potentiation of serotonergic activity. Nefazodone works at both sites of the serotonin (5-hydroxytryptamine [5-HT]) receptors. It blocks the 5-HT$_2$ receptor (postsynaptic) and inhibits serotonin reuptake (presynaptic). Nefazodone has no significant affinity for α_2-adrenergic, β-adrenergic, histaminergic, dopaminergic, or cholinergic receptors and has weak α_1-adrenergic blocking activity.

Findling et al. (2000) conducted an 8-week open-label trial of nefazodone in depressed children and adolescents. Twenty-eight depressed children and adolescents ages 7–17 years participated in the study. Nefazodone was relatively well tolerated by subjects. The incidence and magnitude of nefazodone-associated side effects were modest. Discontinuation of drug therapy was necessary in only one patient who developed a skin rash. Moreover, nefazodone administration was associated with a marked reduction in depressive symptoms.

Wilens et al. (1997) also reported improvement in seven children and adolescents (mean age±SD, 12.4±3.1) with treatment-refractory and highly comorbid juvenile mood disorders who were treated with nefazodone for 13 (±8) weeks at a mean daily dosage of 357±151 mg (3.4 mg/kg). Fifty-six percent of children and adolescents who were previously unresponsive to multiple medication trials were assessed as much to very much improved as measured by the CGI. Two of four children with bipolar depression responded well to treatment, but the other two had mild manic activation. Overall, nefazodone was well tolerated, with adverse effects reported in only three subjects.

Tricyclic antidepressants. Studies of TCAs in adults with major depressive disorder have established their efficacy in acute (Morris and Beck 1974) and maintenance treatment (Frank et al. 1990). However, literature reviews (Ambrosini et al. 1993; Kye and Ryan 1995) and a meta-analysis of 12 randomized controlled trials of TCAs in patients ages 6–18 years (Hazell et al. 1995) showed that TCAs were no more effective than placebo in the treatment of depression in children and adolescents.

Despite widespread clinical use of the TCAs, concerns about their possible cardiovascular risk have arisen after published reports of sudden death in five children associated with their use.

To identify relevant studies that evaluated cardiovascular effects of TCAs, Wilens et al. (1996) performed a systematic search of the literature from 1967 to 1996. Twenty-four studies involving 730 children and adolescents given imipramine, amitriptyline, desipramine, or nortriptyline were found. TCA treatment was associated with minor increases in systolic and diastolic blood pressure; in heart rate; and in the electrocardiographic conduction parameters PR, QRS, and QT$_c$. Holter electrocardiographic monitoring and exercise testing also revealed minor treatment effects. Some electrocardiographic changes related to specific TCAs emerged. Few age-related electrocardiographic differences in TCA-treated children, adolescents, or adults were detected. Electrocardiographic abnormalities were associated with relatively higher serum TCA levels. The authors interpreted those data as suggesting a fatality rate of 1% associated with TCA overdose, primarily due to cardiovascular and central nervous system events. There was a statistically significant higher relative risk of fatality reported with desipramine compared with the other TCAs in adults (Kapur et al. 1992). In addition, further concerns have been raised that the occurrence of sudden death may be underreported or erroneously attributed to overdose in some cases.

Monoamine oxidase inhibitors. In adults, MAOIs are more effective than TCAs for depression with atypical features (Thase et al. 1995). MAOIs have several limitations, including drug–diet and drug–drug interactions, inability to monitor adequately in public health settings, and lack of established data demonstrating efficacy in children and adolescents.

There are only a few studies on the use of MAOIs in adolescents. Ryan et al. (1988) reported the efficacy of irreversible mixed MAOIs from a chart review of 23 depressed adolescents, 21 of whom had not responded to treatment with heterocyclic antidepressants. Treatment with MAOIs alone or in combination with heterocyclic antidepressants resulted in 70% having "good" or "fair" response. Dietary noncompliance was a significant problem in 80% during the study. Because of the relatively high risk of noncompliance with the tyramine-free diet in a population with high impulsivity and potential substance use, Ryan et al. (1988) estimated that the risks of MAOI treatment outweighed the potential therapeutic benefits in unreliable patients or families.

The selective reversible MAOIs have advantages over the classic MAOIs in terms of dangerousness, side effects, drug interactions, and cognitive effects. Furthermore, the absence of detrimental effects on cognitive function of moclobemide in young adults (Hindmarch and Kerr 1992) is a significant advantage for children, whose main task is to learn.

However, the potentially very serious drug interactions, toxic effects, and dietary restrictions significantly limit the usefulness of MAOIs in the treatment of adolescent depression. These agents are reserved for use only in the most responsible adolescents with the most treatment-resistant depression.

Psychological and Social/Environmental Treatments

Psychosocial treatments for adolescent depression may be divided into five general types (McCracken and Cantwell 1992): cognitive, behavioral, psychodynamic, group, and family therapies.

Cognitive and behavioral therapies. Cognitive therapies for depression were initially derived from the works of Beck and colleagues (1979) and Ellis and Bernard (1983). Cognitive therapy is an active, problem-oriented treatment that seeks to identify and change maladaptive beliefs, attitudes, and behaviors that contribute to emotional distress. Cognitive models propose that a number of processes—including negativistic expectancies, dysfunctional attitudes or beliefs, biased attentional processes, cognitive distortions, problem-solving deficits, social skills deficits, and negativistic attributional style—may play a role in the development and maintenance of depressive disorders among adults.

Behavior therapies for adolescent depression focus on the principles of operant conditioning and learning theory. According to behavioral theory, a depressed adolescent may be subject to the following types of influences, either singly or in combination: 1) an environment with a paucity of positive reinforcers, 2) an environment with an excess number of aversive contingencies, 3) a lack of skills to elicit positive reinforcement from others, and 4) involvement in behaviors that offend others (Lewinsohn et al. 1994a). The goal of behavior therapy is to teach skills and modify contingencies that will change the quality of the teenager's interaction with the environment.

Only a few well-designed investigations in nonpharmacological interventions such as cognitive-behavioral therapy (CBT) in children and adolescents with major depressive disorder have been published. CBT was reported to be effective in the treatment of depressed adolescents with dysphoric features. In a critical review of

CBT with depressed and dysphoric adolescents, Reinecke et al. (1998) conducted a meta-analysis of published studies on the effectiveness of CBT. The authors found that CBT may be useful for reducing dysphoria among adolescents and that treatment gains are maintained over time. Reynolds and Coats (1986) investigated the efficacy of CBT for the treatment of depressive symptoms among adolescents. They randomly assigned 30 moderately dysphoric adolescents to either CBT, relaxation, or a waiting list. The CBT and relaxation groups were superior to the waiting-list group with regard to reduction of dysphoria at both post-test evaluation and 5-week follow-up.

Stark et al. (1987) compared self-control therapy and a behavioral problem-solving therapy for treating dysphoric adolescents. Twenty-nine subjects were randomly assigned to either a self-control, a behavioral problem-solving, or a waiting-list condition. Adolescents in both active treatments reported significant reductions in depressive symptoms relative to control subjects. These gains were maintained over an 8-week follow-up period.

CBT produced improvements in both depressive symptoms and depressive disorders in both clinical and nonclinical samples (Kahn et al. 1990; Lewinsohn et al. 1990; Reynolds and Coats 1986; Stark et al. 1987; Wood et al. 1996). It also had some advantages over other psychotherapeutic techniques. For example, preliminary findings from a large controlled study comparing 12–16 weeks of individual CBT, nondirective supportive psychotherapy, and systemic behavior family therapy showed that 70% of adolescents with major depressive disorder responded to each of the three treatments. CBT had the most rapid reduction in self-reported depression and achieved the greatest increases in parent- and child-rated treatment credibility (Johnson et al. 1995). Lewinsohn et al. (1990) investigated the efficacy of two versions of a cognitive-behavioral intervention for treating depression. Fifty-nine high school students who met DSM-III and research diagnostic criteria for depression were randomly assigned to one of three conditions: adolescent-and-parent therapy, adolescent-only therapy, and waiting-list control. Adolescents in both treatment groups improved significantly more than the control subjects on self-report measures of dysphoria. These gains were maintained at 2 years posttreatment.

Brent et al. (1997) also reported that CBT resulted in more rapid and complete symptomatic relief of depression than either systemic-behavioral family therapy or nondirective supportive therapy. In another study, Brent et al. (1998) extended data from the previous study. They found that CBT given individually to adolescent outpatients with depressive disorders showed a clear advantage over relaxation training at the posttreatment assessment on measures of depression and overall outcome. Kahn et al. (1990) investigated the efficacy of short-term CBT, relaxation, and self-modeling interventions for treating depressive symptoms in middle-school students ages 10–14 years. Subjects were randomly assigned to one of three active treatments or a waiting-list control group. All three treatments resulted in a significant reduction in dysphoria compared with control subjects.

Finally, Wood et al. (1996) studied the effectiveness of brief individual CBT and relaxation training for treating clinically depressed adolescent outpatients. A combination of cognitive, social problem-solving, and symptom-focused interventions was associated with significant reductions in dysphoria and improved general adjustment. Patients who had received CBT were more likely to experience remission from their depressive disorder than patients in the control condition.

Findings from community studies of children and adolescents designated as "at risk" as a result of having depressive symptoms have been encouraging. Researchers found that short-term CBT is associated with a reduced risk of subsequent depression (Clarke et al. 1995; Jaycox et al. 1994). Studies on long-term results are needed given the high risk of relapse that occurs in both the short term and the long term (Harrington et al. 1990; Kovacs et al. 1984b; Rao et al. 1995; Wood et al. 1996). Available data indicate that the relapse rate after the conclusion of CBT is very high, especially in clinical samples. Wood and colleagues (1996) found that more than 40% of adolescent patients who responded to CBT had relapsed within 6 months of remission. Brent et al. (1997) reported that approximately one-third of subjects admitted to a comparative trial of three psychosocial treatments (one of which was CBT) had a recurrence during the follow-up period. Moreover, data from other studies suggest that even after acute symptoms have remitted, social impairment persists (Puig-Antich et al. 1985b), often into adulthood (Rao et al. 1995).

As a result of these reports, Kroll et al. (1996) conducted a pilot study of continuation cognitive-behavioral therapy (CBT-C) for adolescents who had experienced remission from major depressive disorder. The aims of the study were to establish whether CBT-C is

feasible and to compare the risk of relapse in depressed adolescents treated with CBT-C with that found in a historical control group of depressed adolescents who had been treated with CBT during the acute episode but who had then had only routine clinical follow-up. Seventeen patients who had CBT-C for 6 months after remission from major depressive disorder were compared with a historical control group of 12 patients who had had no further treatment after remission. The average number of treatment sessions was 7 (range, 5 to 12). There were fewer relapses in the group who had CBT-C than in the historical control group. Differences between the groups were particularly striking during the first 3 months, when there was just one relapse in the CBT-C group compared with six relapses in the historical control group (1 of 17 versus 6 of 12).

Continuity of CBT in depressed adolescents was further assessed in the study by Brent et al. (1999). One hundred seven adolescents ages 13–18 years, who met DSM-III-R criteria for major depression and had a Beck Depression Inventory score of at least 13, were randomly assigned to either CBT, systemic behavioral family therapy, or nondirective supportive therapy for 12–16 weeks of acute treatment. Subjects were followed up periodically for 24 months after the end of acute treatment. More than half of the 107 randomized adolescents (57, or 53.3%) received additional treatment beyond that provided in the clinical trial. Median time to additional treatment from intake was 7.2 months. The rates of additional treatment and the times to additional treatment were similar in the three treatment groups despite the superior efficacy of CBT in the acute phase. The severity of the index depressive episode and comorbid dysthymia were predictors of additional treatment in the acute phase. In the follow-up period, the severity of depressive symptoms, the presence of disruptive disorders, and family problems predicted additional treatment. The authors emphasized the need to consider the treatment of an adolescent depressive episode in two phases: acute and continuation.

Prevention of depression in children and adolescents at high risk of developing depression—such as the offspring of depressed parents (Beardslee et al. 1993) and children with depressive symptomatology but not full-blown clinical depression (e.g., Dohrenwend et al. 1980; Weissman et al. 1992)—is of prime importance. Studies of high-school students (Clarke et al. 1995) and schoolchildren (Jaycox et al. 1994) with subclinical symptoms of depression showed that cognitive interventions reduced depressive symptoms and lowered the risk for developing depression up to 2 years after the intervention.

Some other techniques were reported to be effective in the treatment of adolescent depression. Lerner and Clum (1990) evaluated the efficacy of social problem-solving therapy and supportive psychotherapy for treating suicidal adolescents. Problem-solving therapy was more effective than supportive therapy for reducing dysphoria, hopelessness, and loneliness at posttreatment and at a 3-month follow-up.

As described above, cognitive and behavioral techniques have been useful in adolescents with depression. However, further investigations with more controlled studies are needed.

Psychodynamic psychotherapy. Psychodynamic psychotherapy for adolescent depression emphasizes the importance of object loss and self-critical internal representations. The objectives of psychoanalytical therapy include a reduction in the use of maladaptive defense mechanisms, resolution of past psychological trauma, and greater acceptance of the realistic limitations of one's family and one's own abilities. The aim of psychodynamic psychotherapy is not only to relieve the symptoms of depression but also to ensure maintenance of improvement and prevention of relapse through modification of the individual's adaptive style and personality organization. Outcome research on the efficacy of psychodynamic psychotherapy in the treatment of adolescent depression is currently limited to case studies (Bemporad 1988; Kestenbaum and Kron 1987).

Interpersonal psychotherapy is an important new form of psychodynamic therapy for depression in adolescents. This is a brief treatment directed toward the relief of symptoms through the resolution of interpersonal problems associated with the onset of depression. It differs significantly from traditional psychoanalytical psychotherapy in that it is a short-term treatment focused on the individual's present social adaptation. Four interpersonal problem areas are interpersonal deficits, interpersonal role conflicts, abnormal grief, and difficult role transitions (Klerman et al. 1984). The technique has been subsequently modified for use in depressed adolescents (Mufson et al. 1994). The most significant modifications were the addition of a fifth problem area (single-parent families) and the involvement of the parents in all phases of therapy. Feedback from the school was also incorpo-

rated to ensure school attendance and to monitor performance. The duration of treatment was decreased from 16 to 12 weeks. Brief telephone sessions were allowed when the adolescent was unable to keep an appointment. Mufson et al. (1994) found that depressive symptoms significantly decreased over the course of treatment. Depression was measured by scores on the Beck Depression Inventory and the Milton Rating Scale for Depression. The most dramatic decline in symptoms occurred between weeks 8 and 12. Although the results of this study were encouraging, no control group was used, the sample size was small, and only one therapist performed the therapy.

In another study (Mufson and Fairbanks 1996) a sample of depressed adolescents who received 12 weeks of modified interpersonal psychotherapy in an open clinical trial was followed up. The 14 depressed adolescents were contacted approximately 1 year after completion of 3 months of interpersonal psychotherapy to participate in an evaluation of depressive symptomatology, social functioning, and life events. Both self-report and clinician-rated measures were administered. Of the 10 adolescents who participated in the follow-up evaluation, only 1 met criteria for an affective disorder. The majority reported few depressive symptoms and had maintained improvement in social functioning since completion of treatment for depression. The life events survey suggested that they had experienced a significant number of negative life events. There were no reported hospitalizations, pregnancies, or suicide attempts since the completion of treatment. All were attending school regularly. Improvements that occurred during the course of the 12-week open clinical trial were maintained for the year immediately after completion of treatment.

The results of these studies indicate that further study of interpersonal psychotherapy in adolescents appears to be warranted.

Group therapy. Some consider group therapy to be the treatment of choice for adolescent depression (Scheidlinger 1985) because the developmental tasks of adolescence include emotional separation and individuation from parents and identification with a peer group. Fine et al. (1991) compared two forms of short-term group therapy for depressed adolescents: a therapeutic support group (TSG) and a social skills group (SSG). Subjects were referred throughout the 3-year duration of the project. Groups were run alternately, each for 12 weeks. Individuals were assigned to whichever group was meeting closest to their referral date. Subjects in the TSG shared common problems, developed new ways to cope with stressful situations, and provided mutual support. SSG subjects focused on learning a variety of specific skills such as assertiveness, conversational skills, recognizing feelings, giving and receiving positive and negative feedback, social problem solving, and negotiating to resolve conflict; one session was devoted to each target skill. The authors hypothesized that the SSG would be more effective in reducing depressive symptoms. However, they found that the subjects in the TSG improved significantly more than those in the SSG, as measured by a number of instruments. Adolescents treated with TSG therapy had significantly greater reductions in their depressive symptoms and increases in self-concept immediately after treatment. However, these group differences were no longer evident at 9-month follow-up. Adolescents in the TSG maintained improvement, whereas those in the SSG caught up. Again, this study is limited by the lack of a control group. Another potentially confounding factor was that some subjects received other forms of therapy concurrently.

Another group intervention for depressed adolescents is the Adolescent Coping With Depression course (Clarke et al. 1990; Lewinsohn et al. 1994a). This course is conducted as sixteen 2-hour didactic sessions over an 8-week period. Group leaders teach adolescents methods of controlling their depressed mood through a variety of skills. In addition, a separate treatment format has been developed for the parents of depressed teenagers (Lewinsohn et al. 1991). The authors reported an 80% response rate, with no relapse over 2 years, when maintenance therapy was used.

Family therapy. Family therapy is an important part of the treatment of depressed adolescents. There are a number of schools of family therapy. The structural family therapy approach focuses on the relationship between family dysfunction and adolescent psychopathology. This approach emphasizes the understanding of the meaning or function of an adolescent's symptom within the context of the family unit (Minuchin 1974). Minuchin described enmeshed parent–child relationships that may perpetuate a chronic dysphoric mood in the child. Treatment in the family systems approach concentrates on the various aspects of the system that support or reinforce the depression. So far, the research on family systems treatment has been limited.

■ Bipolar Disorder

Bipolar disorder is a chronic and recurrent condition that is associated with high rates of morbidity and with impairment in family, school, and social environment. Therefore, early and appropriate treatment is needed to provide the best chance to help adolescents with this disorder.

Biological and Pharmacological Treatments

Treatment of childhood bipolar disorder remains a remarkably understudied area despite an increasing body of literature documenting its occurrence (Botteron and Geller 1995; Fetner and Geller 1992; Kafantaris 1995; Youngerman and Canino 1978). In general, clinicians have made pharmacological treatment decisions based on the studies of adults and their own clinical experience. A variety of mood stabilizers have been used to treat bipolar disorders in adolescents and adults.

Lithium. Lithium is approved by the U.S. Food and Drug Administration for treatment of bipolar disorder in adolescents ages 12 years or older. Current literature on lithium suggests that it can be given to adolescents using the same safety precautions as in adults with monitoring at 6-month intervals for renal, thyroid, calcium, and phosphorus indices (Fetner and Geller 1992; Khandelwal et al. 1984). Furthermore, a double-blind, placebo-controlled study of lithium for aggressive children suggested that some children develop cognitive impairment at low plasma levels (Silva et al. 1992).

Open trials of lithium for bipolar disorder in adolescents appear to demonstrate response rates similar to those in adults (DeLong and Aldershof 1987; Youngerman and Canino 1978).

Strober et al. (1988) studied 50 hospitalized acutely manic bipolar probands ages 13–17. Only 40% of those with prepubertal onset of psychopathology responded to lithium, compared with 80% of those with no prepubertal psychopathology. Although other psychoactive medications, including carbamazepine and neuroleptics, were administered concurrently with lithium in some patients, 34 (68%) of the 50 subjects had a good response after 6 weeks of lithium treatment, with blood levels between 0.9 and 1.5 mmol/L.

Strober et al. (1990) examined lithium prophylaxis in a naturalistic study of 37 bipolar adolescents. The relapse rate of noncompliant subjects (92.3%) was significantly higher than the relapse rate for subjects who remained compliant with lithium treatment (37.5%).

There is only one double-blind, randomized, placebo-controlled prospective study of lithium. DSM-IV criteria were used for diagnosis. Subjects were 25 adolescents with bipolar disorder and a secondary substance dependency disorder (alcohol and marijuana dependence) (Geller et al. 1998). Diagnosis of bipolar disorder preceded the substance abuse by several years. A 2-week single-blind placebo washout phase was followed by a 10-week placebo-controlled, double-blind short-term treatment. In 6 weeks, those randomly assigned to lithium had a significant decrease in their substance abuse compared with those randomly assigned to placebo. The authors postulated that lithium may be efficacious in the treatment of bipolar disorder in adolescents with comorbid substance abuse.

The distribution and elimination of lithium have been systematically studied in children and adolescents. Findings parallel observations in adults. However, there is evidence of a shorter elimination half-life and higher total clearance in children. Available side effects data are from case reports, small case series, and systematic reporting of side effects in small, controlled efficacy studies. Common lithium side effects in children include nausea, diarrhea, tremor, enuresis, fatigue, ataxia (Silva et al. 1992), leukocytosis, and malaise; less common are renal, ocular, thyroid, neurological, dermatological, and cardiovascular effects. Changes in weight and growth, diabetes, and hair loss are also seen (Rosenberg et al. 1994). Children younger than age 6 may experience neurological effects relatively frequently (Hagino et al. 1995). In general younger children seem to experience more side effects than older children (Campbell et al. 1984). Few details are available regarding the negative effects of lithium in adolescents. Khandelwal et al. (1984) reported no impairment in renal function in four adolescents who received lithium for 3–5 years. A concern with lithium therapy in sexually active adolescents is its potential teratogenic effects. Lithium has been reported to be associated with a variety of congenital abnormalities, specifically Ebstein's anomaly. However, a prospective study by Jacobson et al. (1992) found that the risk for Ebstein's anomaly and other birth defects may be lower than was previously thought. As with adult patients, a medical evaluation and baseline laboratory studies should be performed before initiating lithium therapy in adolescents. Lithium levels, serum electrolytes, and thyroid and renal functions should be monitored periodically. The patient and family should be educated about how changes in diet and use of other medications may affect lithium levels. Female patients should be advised to avoid pregnancy and breastfeeding while taking lithium.

The therapeutic blood level of lithium is considered to be between 0.6 and 1.2 mEq/L, based on adult data. This is usually achieved within five half-lives, but it ultimately depends on the individual's lithium excretion rate. The narrow therapeutic range of lithium and the potential for significant toxicity must always be considered.

Two approaches have been published to calculate the dosage for lithium in children and adolescents with bipolar disorder: a weight-based method (E.B. Weller et al. 1986) and a kinetics-based method (Geller and Fetner 1989). According to E.B. Weller et al. (1986), in a 6- to 12-year-old child, a dosage of 30 mg/kg per day in three divided doses will produce a lithium level of 0.6–1.2 mEq/L within 5 days. Lithium levels as high as 1.4 mEq/L have been reported with minimal side effects. Because children are often phobic of blood draws, the authors suggested that lithium levels can be safely monitored using saliva. Geller and Fetner (1989) proposed a single-dose, kinetics-based method that used a single lithium dose of 600 mg. This method has shown good predictive values for serum lithium in children and is used to adjust dosage based on a 24-hour serum level drawn after the single 600-mg dose.

Anticonvulsants. Anticonvulsants also play a role in the acute and prophylactic treatment of bipolar disorder in children and adolescents. They are reported to be most useful in the management of mixed states and rapid-cycling bipolar disorder (Keck and McElroy 1996; Post et al. 1990). Although both carbamazepine and valproate are used extensively in children and adolescents with bipolar disorder, controlled studies of these medications in this age group are still lacking.

Carbamazepine. Carbamazepine is approved for the treatment of simple and complex absence seizures and trigeminal neuralgia in adults in the United States and for the treatment of bipolar disorder in Canada (Ketter et al. 1992). It is not yet approved for the treatment of any psychiatric disorders in children in the United States. No controlled studies have been published on the use of carbamazepine in children and adolescents with mood disorders. Nevertheless, it is frequently used in younger patients with bipolar disorder, especially when there are contraindications to lithium or intolerance to lithium.

In adults, approximately 20 nonblinded and 5 double-blind, placebo-controlled studies showed the efficacy of carbamazepine in acute mania (Post et al. 1996). In adults it was also found to be superior to lithium alone in "mixed" or rapid-cycling mania (Solomon et al. 1996). In addition, the combination of lithium and carbamazepine has been suggested to be superior to lithium therapy alone (Calabrese et al. 1996).

Carbamazepine was reported to be effective in seven manic adolescents who were nonresponsive to lithium (Hsu 1986). It also appeared to be a safe and effective treatment for acute mania and long-term maintenance treatment in three cases of juvenile-onset bipolar I disorder (Woolston 1999).

Treatment with carbamazepine is usually started with a low dose (100 mg twice a day), and the dosage is adjusted upward based on side effects to achieve a blood level of 6–12 μL/mL (Ballenger 1988; Post et al. 1987). The maintenance dosage for adolescents may go as high as 1,200 mg/day or more (Pedley et al. 1995; Viesselman et al. 1993). Plasma levels should be checked 2–4 days after achieving steady-state plasma concentration. A baseline complete blood cell count should be obtained, and differential platelet and reticulocyte counts should be obtained periodically.

In addition to common side effects—such as drowsiness, loss of coordination, and vertigo—other potential side effects—such as hematological, dermatological, hepatic, and pancreatic effects—have been described. Twenty-seven cases of aplastic anemia and 10 cases of agranulocytosis (Ryan et al. 1999) have been reported with the use of carbamazepine. Symptoms such as weakness, headache, nausea, edema, and lethargy in children taking carbamazepine may be associated with the syndrome of inappropriate antidiuretic hormone secretion. Water retention and hyponatremia may result.

In children with seizure disorders, cognitive and behavioral effects such as impaired performance in learning and memory tasks, irritability, agitation, insomnia, and emotional lability have been reported (Carpenter and Vining 1993). However, Stores and colleagues (1992) found no significant cognitive or behavior effects after 1 year of therapy with either carbamazepine or valproate.

Increased incidence of congenital anomalies, including neural tube defects, in the offspring of women who took carbamazepine during pregnancy has been reported (Jones et al. 1989; Rosa 1991).

Valproic acid. Valproic acid is approved for treatment of adults with simple and complex absence seizures (Guay 1995). However, it has been efficacious in acute and maintenance treatment of bipolar disorder, including pure mania, mixed mania, and rapid cycling (Bowden et al. 1994; Calabrese et al. 1993a, 1993b; Delucchi and Calabrese 1989; Emrich et al. 1985; McElroy et al. 1988, 1992b). In a retrospective comparison with lithium (Strober 1977), valproic acid was equally effective in the treatment of classic mania but was more effective than lithium in the treatment of mixed mania in adults. A review of adult studies of the acute treatment of mania with valproic acid (Janicak 1993) showed an average response rate of 56%.

There are no placebo-controlled studies of valproic acid in the treatment of bipolar disorder in adolescents. Several single case reports and small open series suggest that valproic acid is an effective mood stabilizer in adolescents. In three open studies, the addition of valproate to previously ineffective psychotropic treatments in hospitalized adolescents resulted in symptomatic improvement (Papatheodorou and Kutcher 1993; West et al. 1994; Whittier et al. 1995). Strober (1977) examined the clinical course of the mixed manic state treated with valproate compared with a historical control group treated with lithium who were otherwise similar. Valproic acid was superior to lithium for the mixed form of mania, but there was no difference in efficacy for classic mania.

All 10 adolescents with chronic temper outbursts and mood lability improved in an open, naturalistic study of valproic acid (Donovan et al. 1997). Discontinuation of medication led to relapse, with subsequent improvement after restarting medication in 5 of 6 subjects.

Good control of manic symptoms, psychotic symptoms, agitation, and aggression with only a few side effects was reported with valproic acid treatment in a naturalistic study of 20 Swedish adolescent inpatients with bipolar disorder. Sixteen subjects had a mixed form of bipolar disorder (Deltito et al. 1998). Whittier et al. (1995) described an instance in which valproic acid was effective in treating a 13-year-old girl with dysphoric mania and mild retardation.

The common side effects of valproate include sedation, nausea, vomiting, appetite and weight gain, tremor, hepatic toxicity, hyperammonemia, blood dyscrasias, alopecia, decreased serum carnitine, neural tube defects, pancreatitis, hyperglycemia, and menstrual changes (Rosenberg et al. 1994). Hepatic toxicity (which may lead to death) appears to occur almost exclusively in young children, especially those younger than 2 years, who have been treated with a combination of medications (Bryant and Dreifuss 1996; Silberstein and Wilmore 1996).

A recent concern regarding valproic acid is that it may induce a metabolic syndrome characterized by obesity, hyperinsulinemia, lipid abnormalities, polycystic ovaries, and hyperandrogenism, particularly in younger women. In a cohort of Finnish women taking valproic acid for seizures, 80% of the women who began valproate before age 20 years had polycystic ovaries compared with 43% of all women taking valproate (Isojarvi et al. 1993). When valproate was replaced with lamotrigine in 16 women, Isojarvi et al. (1998) found that the severity of this metabolic syndrome was reduced (suggesting a partial reversibility). The generalizability of these findings to psychiatric populations is unknown because reports of this syndrome, so far, are confined to this single cohort with epilepsy.

Other anticonvulsants. Lamotrigine, gabapentin, and topiramate have been approved for the treatment of epilepsy in adults. Both lamotrigine and gabapentin were reported to have moderate to marked mood-stabilizing effects in adults with bipolar disorder (Fatemi et al. 1997; Knoll et al. 1998). Kusumakar and Yatham (1997) studied 22 adolescents with bipolar disorder that was refractory to treatment with a combination of valproic acid and another mood stabilizer and an antidepressant. When lamotrigine was combined with valproic acid in a 6-week open trial, 72% had a positive response by week 4. There is one report that a 13-year-old boy with bipolar disorder responded to a combination of gabapentin and carbamazepine (Soutullo et al. 1998).

Antipsychotics. Although there are no controlled studies of antipsychotics in juvenile bipolar disorder, many antipsychotics have been used in children and adolescents with mania. Clozapine was reported to be effective in an adolescent with bipolar disorder (Fuchs 1994) and in five children and adolescents with mixed mania who did not respond to treatment with other neuroleptics (Kowatch et al. 1995). Based on a retrospective chart review of 28 outpatients (mean age ±SD, 10.4±3.8 years) with bipolar disorder treated with risperidone, Frazier et al. (1999) suggested that risperi-

done may be effective in treating the dysphoric aggression displayed by manic children. Soutullo et al. (1999) reported moderate to marked improvement in 5 of 7 manic adolescents (mean age, 12–17 years) who were treated with olanzapine.

Other pharmacological treatments and electroconvulsive therapy. Other medications used in the treatment of adult bipolar disorder—such as calcium channel blockers, clonidine, and L-thyroxine—have not been systematically studied in adolescents. Electroconvulsive therapy (ECT) has been an effective treatment for acute mania in adults (Lish et al. 1994; Prien and Potter 1990). ECT has been underutilized, largely because of stigma and campaigns by groups with a bias against the treatment. Campbell (1952) reported favorable results in adolescents treated with ECT. More recently Schneekloth et al. (1993) also reported remission of bipolar symptoms in adolescents after ECT. Potential side effects of ECT include mild cognitive impairment, transient effects on short-term memory, anxiety reactions, disinhibitions, and altered seizure threshold (Bertagnoli and Borchardt 1990).

Psychological and Social/Environmental Treatments

The practice guidelines for treatment of adult patients with bipolar disorder (Lish et al. 1994) list eight specific interventions essential for psychiatric management of bipolar disorder: 1) developing and maintaining rapport; 2) monitoring the patient's mood and behavior; 3) providing information and education about bipolar disorder; 4) enhancing compliance with medication and other treatments; 5) promoting regular patterns of sleep and daily activities; 6) promoting integration and adaptation to the psychosocial effects of bipolar disorder; 7) recognizing new episodes early; 8) minimizing the morbidity and academic, social, and interpersonal consequences of bipolar disorder.

The same principles may be applied to treatment of bipolar disorder in adolescents, but developmental considerations should be taken into account. Involvement of the family in treatment is also essential. Although medication treatment is considered to be essential for managing acute episodes and maintenance, psychosocial treatments are a mainstay of therapy between acute episodes and are aimed at reducing morbidity and preventing relapse. An additional factor to be considered in treatment is the fact that bipolar disorder is often comorbid with other problems such as disruptive behavior disorders, substance abuse, and learning disabilities. Each of these additional problems requires specifically targeted psychosocial interventions.

Prognosis

The assessment and treatment of adolescent mood disorders requires a comprehensive approach. The specific elements of treatment include pharmacotherapy, various types of psychotherapy, and environmental interventions. Involvement of the family in treatment is also important. Although much has been learned about the phenomenology and natural history of adolescent mood disorders during the past decade, treatment studies have lagged behind. However, efforts are under way to develop practice parameters for the assessment and treatment of bipolar and depressive disorders in children and adolescents similar to those published for adults.

Major depressive disorder in children and adolescents causes significant morbidity and mortality (Fleming and Offord 1990; McCracken and Cantwell 1992). Depression is a major factor in adolescent suicide (Brent 1987; Kovacs et al. 1993; Pfeffer et al. 1991; Rao et al. 1993) and is a common cause of school failure and school dropout (Weinberg et al. 1973). Adolescents with bipolar disorder are at increased risk for suicide relative to children with other psychiatric illnesses (Brent et al. 1988, 1993). Depression in children and adolescents is also associated with an increased risk of suicidal behaviors, homicidal ideation, tobacco use, and abuse of alcohol and other substances during later adolescence (Deykin et al. 1992; Kandel et al. 1986) and adulthood (Rao et al. 1995). Eleven of 54 bipolar adolescents made suicide attempts that required medical attention during 5-year follow-up (Strober et al. 1995).

Early-onset depressive disorders are believed to have a stronger genetic predisposition and poorer prognosis than adult-onset depressive disorders and are less responsive to treatment (McGlashan 1988; Strober et al. 1995). Longitudinal studies have shown that adolescent depression is associated with a high risk of recurrent illness and an increased risk of the development of bipolar disorder. However, the long-term outcome is reported to be similar to that for adult-onset bipolar disorder. Approximately half of affected persons are significantly impaired compared with

their premorbid state (McGlashan 1988; Werry et al. 1991). In a study of a community sample of 1,709 adolescents ages 14–18, Lewinsohn et al. (1995) reported that the bipolar subjects had significantly lower ratings on the Global Assessment of Functioning scale than did the core positive group (these subjects experienced a distinct period of abnormally and persistently elevated, expansive, or irritable mood even though they never met criteria for bipolar disorder), both currently and during the previous year.

During an episode of depression, children and adolescents frequently experience impairment in school performance and relationships with others (Asarnow and Ben Meir 1988; Asarnow et al. 1987; Hammen et al. 1990; Puig-Antich et al. 1985b, 1993; Rao et al. 1995; Strober et al. 1993; Williamson et al. 1995b). However, these psychosocial disturbances do not appear to be specific for depression in children and adolescents because they have been observed in youths with other psychopathology (Puig-Antich et al. 1985a).

Prospective studies have also demonstrated that after recovery children and adolescents may continue to show subclinical symptoms of depression, negative attributions, impairment in interpersonal relationships, increased smoking, impairment in global functioning, early pregnancy, and increased physical problems (Kandel and Davies 1986; Puig-Antich et al. 1985a, 1985b, 1993; Rao et al. 1995; Rohde et al. 1994; Strober et al. 1993). Adolescents with two or more depressive episodes appear to have poorer functioning, whereas adolescents with nonrecurrent major depressive disorder may have good psychosocial outcomes similar to nondepressed control subjects (Rao et al. 1995; Warner et al. 1995).

Kovacs et al. (1984b) have conducted the largest follow-up study to date of a clinically referred sample. They found that 26% of the adolescents relapsed within a year, and 40% within 2 years of their initial depressive episode. Two-thirds of subjects with major depression and dysthymic disorder had a subsequent episode by 5 years. A significant number of the adolescents also had school-related problems, including academic failure and peer relationship problems, suggesting that the recurrence rate and recovery rate have significantly hampered successful development in several areas. Several other follow-up studies found a generally poor prognosis for depressed adolescents. There was a high risk for future episodes of affective illness and chronic psychosocial problems (Garber et al. 1988; Kandel and Davies 1986). Follow-up studies on hospitalized depressed adolescents also report chronicity and recurrence of depression (Welner et al. 1979).

Research Issues

Noticeable progress has been made during the past 15 years in the field of mood disorders in adolescents. The reconsideration of diagnostic criteria, better description of the clinical picture (particularly with regard to atypical features), the development of diagnostic instruments, improved knowledge on short- and long-term prognosis, and the beginning of controlled treatment studies on adolescent mood disorders are all important developments. However, much work remains to be done. There needs to be more emphasis on research in the etiopathogenesis of both depressive disorder and bipolar disorder. The interconnections between major depressive disorder and bipolar disorder also need further study.

Psychosocial and pharmacological treatments are vital to improving the acute and long-term course of mood disorders in adolescents. However, further research is needed to refine treatment strategies with an emphasis on prevention of recurrences. The high incidence of parental mental health problems indicates the need for further research on concurrent treatment of parents and youths with mood disorders. Also, more research is needed on the treatment of dysthymia, double depression, psychotic depression, and refractory depression (Birmaher et al. 1996b).

References

Achamallah NS, Decker DH: Mania induced by fluoxetine in an adolescent patient. Am J Psychiatry 148:1404–1405, 1991

Adams M, Adams J: Life events, depression, and perceived problem solving alternatives in adolescents. J Child Psychol Psychiatry 32:811–820, 1991

Adrian C, Hammen C: Stress exposure and stress generation in children of depressed mothers. J Consult Clin Psychol 61:354–359, 1993

Akiskal HS: Mood disorders: introduction and overview, in Comprehensive Textbook of Psychiatry, 4th Edition. Edited by Kaplan HI, Sadock BJ. Baltimore, MD, Williams & Wilkins, 1995, pp 1067–1069

Akiskal HS, Downs J, Jordan P, et al: Affective disorders in referred children and younger siblings of manic-depressives: mode of onset and prospective course. Arch Gen Psychiatry 42:996–1003, 1985

Akiskal HS, Maser JD, Zeller PJ, et al: Switching from "unipolar" to bipolar II: an 11-year prospective study of clinical and temperamental predictors in 559 patients. Arch Gen Psychiatry 52:114–123, 1995

Alderman J, Wolkow R, Chung M, et al: Sertraline treatment of children and adolescents with obsessive-compulsive disorder or depression: pharmacokinetics, tolerability, and efficacy. J Am Acad Child Adolesc Psychiatry 37:386–394, 1998

Allgood-Merten B, Lewinsohn PM, Hops H: Sex differences and adolescent depression. J Abnorm Psychol 99:55–63, 1990

Ambrosini PJ, Bianchi MD, Rabinovich H, et al: Antidepressant treatments in children and adolescents, I: affective disorders. J Am Acad Child Adolesc Psychiatry 32:1–6, 1993

Ambrosini PJ, Wagner KD, Biederman J, et al: Multicenter open-label sertraline study in adolescent outpatients with major depression. J Am Acad Child Adolesc Psychiatry 38:566–572, 1999

American Psychiatric Association: Diagnostic and Statistical Manual of Mental Disorders, 3rd Edition, Revised. Washington, DC, American Psychiatric Association, 1987

American Psychiatric Association: Diagnostic and Statistical Manual of Mental Disorders, 4th Edition. Washington, DC, American Psychiatric Association, 1994

American Psychiatric Association: Diagnostic and Statistical Manual of Mental Disorders, 4th Edition, Text Revision. Washington, DC, American Psychiatric Association, 2000

Angold A, Costello EJ: Depressive comorbidity in children and adolescents: empirical, theoretical, and methodological issues. Am J Psychiatry 150:1779–1791, 1993

Angold A, Costello EJ, Worthman CM: Puberty and depression: the roles of age, pubertal status and pubertal timing. Psychol Med 28:51–61, 1998

Asarnow JR: Peer status and social competence in child psychiatric inpatients: a comparison of children with depressive, externalizing, and concurrent depressive and externalizing disorders. J Abnorm Child Psychol 16:151–162, 1988

Asarnow JR, Bates S: Depression in child psychiatric inpatients: cognitive and attributional patterns. J Abnorm Child Psychol 16:601–615, 1988

Asarnow JR, Ben Meir S: Children with schizophrenia spectrum and depressive disorders: a comparative study of premorbid adjustment, onset pattern and severity of impairment. J Child Psychol Psychiatry 29:477–488, 1988

Asarnow JR, Carlson GA, Guthrie D: Coping strategies, self-perceptions, hopelessness, and perceived family environments in depressed and suicidal children. J Consult Clin Psychol 55:361–366, 1987

Avison WR, Mcalpine DD: Gender differences in symptoms of depression among adolescents. J Health Soc Behav 33:77–96, 1992

Ballenger JC: The use of anticonvulsants in manic-depressive illness. J Clin Psychiatry 49:21–25, 1988

Ballenger JC, Reus VI, Post RM: The "atypical" clinical picture of adolescent mania. Am J Psychiatry 139:602–606, 1982

Banez GA, Compas BE: Children's and parents' daily stressful events and psychological symptoms. J Abnorm Child Psychol 18:591–605, 1990

Beardslee WR, Salt P, Porterfield K, et al: Comparison of preventive interventions for families with parental affective disorder. J Am Acad Child Adolesc Psychiatry 32:254–263, 1993

Beck AT: Depression: Clinical, Experimental and Theoretical Aspects. New York, Harper, 1967

Beck AT, Rush AJ, Shaw B, et al: Cognitive States of Depression. New York, Guilford, 1979

Bemporad JR: Psychodynamic treatment of depressed adolescents. J Clin Psychiatry 49 (suppl):26–31, 1988

Bertagnoli MW, Borchardt CM: A review of ECT for children and adolescents. J Am Acad Child Adolesc Psychiatry 29:302–307, 1990

Bhatara VS: Early detection of adolescent mood disorders. S D J Med 45:75–78, 1992

Biederman J, Faraone S, Mick E, et al: Psychiatric comorbidity among referred juveniles with major depression: fact or artifact? J Am Acad Child Adolesc Psychiatry 34:579–590, 1995

Bird HR, Canino G, Rubio-Stipec M, et al: Estimates of the prevalence of childhood maladjustment in a community survey in Puerto Rico: the use of combined measures. Arch Gen Psychiatry 45:1120–1126, 1988

Birmaher B, Dahl RE, Ryan ND, et al: The dexamethasone suppression test in adolescent outpatients with major depressive disorder. Am J Psychiatry 149:1040–1045, 1992a

Birmaher B, Ryan ND, Dahl R, et al: Dexamethasone suppression test in children with major depressive disorder. J Am Acad Child Adolesc Psychiatry 31:291–297, 1992b

Birmaher B, Dahl RE, Perel J, et al: Corticotropin-releasing hormone challenge in prepubertal major depression. Biol Psychiatry 39:267–277, 1996a

Birmaher B, Ryan ND, Williamson DE, et al: Childhood and adolescent depression: a review of the past 10 years. Part II. J Am Acad Child Adolesc Psychiatry 35:1575–1583, 1996b

Botteron KN, Geller B: Pharmacologic treatment of childhood and adolescent mania. Child Adolesc Psychiatr Clin N Am 4:283–304, 1995

Botteron KN, Vannier MW, Geller B, et al: Preliminary study of magnetic resonance imaging characteristics in 8- to 16-year-olds with mania. J Am Acad Child Adolesc Psychiatry 34:742–749, 1995

Boulos C, Kutcher S, Gardner D, et al: An open naturalistic trial of fluoxetine in adolescents and young adults with treatment-resistant major depression. J Child Adolesc Psychopharmacol 2:103–111, 1992

Bowden CL, Brugger AM, Swann AC, et al: Efficacy of divalproex vs lithium and placebo in the treatment of mania. The Depakote Mania Study Group [published erratum appears in JAMA 271:1830, 1994]. JAMA 271:918–924, 1994

Bowring MA, Kovacs M: Difficulties in diagnosing manic disorders among children and adolescents. J Am Acad Child Adolesc Psychiatry 31:611–614, 1992

Brambilla F, Musetti C, Tacchini C, et al: Neuroendocrine investigation in children and adolescents with dysthymic disorders: the DST, TRH and clonidine tests. J Affect Disord 17:279–284, 1989

Brent DA: Correlates of the medical lethality of suicide attempts in children and adolescents. J Am Acad Child Adolesc Psychiatry 26:87–91, 1987

Brent DA, Perper JA, Goldstein CE, et al: Risk factors for adolescent suicide: a comparison of adolescent suicide victims with suicidal inpatients. Arch Gen Psychiatry 45:581–588, 1988

Brent DA, Perper JA, Moritz G, et al: Psychiatric risk factors for adolescent suicide: a case-control study. J Am Acad Child Adolesc Psychiatry 32:521–529, 1993

Brent DA, Holder D, Kolko D, et al: A clinical psychotherapy trial for adolescent depression comparing cognitive, family, and supportive therapy. Arch Gen Psychiatry 54:877–885, 1997

Brent DA, Kolko DJ, Birmaher B, et al: Predictors of treatment efficacy in a clinical trial of three psychosocial treatments for adolescent depression. J Am Acad Child Adolesc Psychiatry 37:906–914, 1998

Brent DA, Kolko DJ, Birmaher B, et al: A clinical trial for adolescent depression: predictors of additional treatment in the acute and follow-up phases of the trial. J Am Acad Child Adolesc Psychiatry 38:263–270, 1999

Brown GW, Harris TO: Life Events and Illness. New York, Guilford, 1989

Brown GW, Harris TO: Aetiology of anxiety and depressive disorders in an inner-city population, I: early adversity. Psychol Med 23:143–154, 1993

Brown RP, Caroff S, Kocsis JH, et al: Nocturnal serum melatonin in major depressive disorder before and after desmethylimipramine treatment. Psychopharmacol Bull 21:579–581, 1985

Brown RP, Kocsis JH, Caroff S, et al: Depressed mood and reality disturbance correlate with decreased nocturnal melatonin in depressed patients. Acta Psychiatr Scand 76:272–275, 1987

Bryant AE 3rd, Dreifuss FE: Valproic acid hepatic fatalities, III: U.S. experience since 1986. Neurology 46:465–469, 1996

Burke KC, Burke JD, Regier DA, et al: Age at onset of selected mental disorders in five community populations. Arch Gen Psychiatry 47:511–518, 1990

Butler SF, Arredondo DE, McCloskey V: Affective comorbidity in children and adolescents with attention deficit hyperactivity disorder. Ann Clin Psychiatry 7:51–55, 1995

Calabrese JR, Rapport DJ, Kimmel SE, et al: Rapid cycling bipolar disorder and its treatment with valproate. Can J Psychiatry 38:57–61, 1993a

Calabrese JR, Woyshville MJ, Kimmel SE, et al: Predictors of valproate response in bipolar rapid cycling. J Clin Psychopharmacol 13:280–283, 1993b

Calabrese JR, Fatemi SH, Kujawa M, et al: Predictors of response to mood stabilizers. J Clin Psychopharmacol 16:24S–31S, 1996

Campbell J: Manic-depressive psychoses in children. J Nerv Ment Dis 116:424–439, 1952

Carlson GA: Child and adolescent mania—diagnostic considerations. J Child Psychol Psychiatry 31:331–341, 1990

Carlson GA, Abbott SF: Mood disorders and suicide, in Comprehensive Textbook of Psychiatry, 4th Edition. Edited by Kaplan HI, Sadock BJ. Baltimore, MD, Williams & Wilkins, 1995, pp 2367–2391

Carlson GA, Kashani JH: Manic symptoms in a non-referred adolescent population. J Affect Disord 15:219–226, 1988a

Carlson GA, Kashani JH: Phenomenology of major depression from childhood through adulthood: analysis of three studies. Am J Psychiatry 145:1222–1225, 1988b

Carlson GA, Davenport YB, Jamison K: A comparison of outcome in adolescent- and later-onset bipolar manic-depressive illness. Am J Psychiatry 134:919–922, 1977

Carlson GA, Fennig S, Bromet EJ: The confusion between bipolar disorder and schizophrenia in youth: where does it stand in the 1990s? J Am Acad Child Adolesc Psychiatry 33:453–460, 1994

Carlson GA, Bromet EJ, Sievers S: Phenomenology and outcome of subjects with early and adult-onset psychotic mania. Am J Psychiatry 157:213–219, 2000

Carpenter RO, Vining EPG: Antiepileptics (anticonvulsants), in Practitioner's Guide to Psychoactive Drugs for Children and Adolescents. Edited by Werry JS, Aman MG. New York, Plenum, 1993, pp 321–346

Casat CD, Arana GW, Powell K: The DST in children and adolescents with major depressive disorder. Am J Psychiatry 146:503–507, 1989

Cavallo A, Holt KG, Hejazi MS, et al: Melatonin circadian rhythm in childhood depression. J Am Acad Child Adolesc Psychiatry 26:395–399, 1987

Clarke GN, Lewinsohn PM, Hops H: Instructive Manual for the Adolescent Coping With Depression Course. Eugene, OR, Castalia, 1990

Clarke GN, Hawkins W, Murphy M, et al: Targeted prevention of unipolar depressive disorder in an at-risk sample of high school adolescents: a randomized trial of a group cognitive intervention. J Am Acad Child Adolesc Psychiatry 34:312–321, 1995

Cohen P, Cohen J, Brook J: An epidemiological study of disorders in late childhood and adolescence, II: persistence of disorders. J Child Psychol Psychiatry 34:869–877, 1993

Cole DA, Carpentieri S: Social status and the comorbidity of child depression and conduct disorder. J Consult Clin Psychol 58:748–757, 1990

Compas BE, Oppedisano G, Connor JK, et al: Gender differences in depressive symptoms in adolescence: comparison of national samples of clinically referred and nonreferred youths. J Consult Clin Psychol 65:617–626, 1997

Conde Lopez VJ, Ballesteros Alcalde MC, Franco Martin MA, et al: [Critical evaluation of the use of antidepressives in childhood] (Spanish). Actas Luso Esp Neurol Psiquiatr Cienc Afines 25:105–117, 1997

Coryell W, Turvey C, Endicott J, et al: Bipolar I affective disorder: predictors of outcome after 15 years. J Affect Disord 50:109–116, 1998

Costello AJ, Dulcan MK, Kalas R: A checklist of hospitalization criteria for use with children. Hosp Community Psychiatry 42:823–828, 1991

Dahl R, Puig-Antich J, Ryan N, et al: Cortisol secretion in adolescents with major depressive disorder. Acta Psychiatr Scand 80:18–26, 1989

Dahl RE, Puig-Antich J, Ryan ND, et al: EEG sleep in adolescents with major depression: the role of suicidality and inpatient status. J Affect Disord 19:63–75, 1990

Dahl RE, Ryan ND, Birmaher B, et al: Electroencephalographic sleep measures in prepubertal depression. Psychiatry Res 38:201–214, 1991a

Dahl RE, Ryan ND, Puig-Antich J, et al: 24-Hour cortisol measures in adolescents with major depression: a controlled study. Biol Psychiatry 30:25–36, 1991b

Dahl RE, Kaufman J, Ryan ND, et al: The dexamethasone suppression test in children and adolescents: a review and a controlled study. Biol Psychiatry 32:109–126, 1992a

Dahl RE, Ryan ND, Williamson DE, et al: Regulation of sleep and growth hormone in adolescent depression. J Am Acad Child Adolesc Psychiatry 31:615–621, 1992b

Dahl RE, Ryan ND, Matty MK, et al: Sleep onset abnormalities in depressed adolescents. Biol Psychiatry 39:400–410, 1996

Deal SL, Williams JE: Cognitive distortions as mediators between life stress and depression in adolescents. Adolescence 23:477–490, 1988

De Bellis MD, Chrousos GP, Dorn LD, et al: Hypothalamic-pituitary-adrenal axis dysregulation in sexually abused girls. J Clin Endocrinol Metab 78:249–255, 1994

De Bellis MD, Dahl RE, Perel JM, et al: Nocturnal ACTH, cortisol, growth hormone, and prolactin secretion in prepubertal depression. J Am Acad Child Adolesc Psychiatry 35:1130–1138, 1996

DeLong GR, Aldershof AL: Long-term experience with lithium treatment in childhood: correlation with clinical diagnosis. J Am Acad Child Adolesc Psychiatry 26:389–394, 1987

Deltito JA, Levitan J, Damore J, et al: Naturalistic experience with the use of divalproex sodium on an in-patient unit for adolescent psychiatric patients. Acta Psychiatr Scand 97:236–240, 1998

Delucchi GA, Calabrese JR: Anticonvulsants for treatment of manic depression. Cleve Clin J Med 56:756–761, 1989

Derivan A, Entsuah AR, Kikta D: Venlafaxine: measuring the onset of antidepressant action. Psychopharmacol Bull 31:439–447, 1995

DeVane CL: Pharmacokinetics of the newer antidepressants: clinical relevance. Am J Med 97:13S–23S, 1994

Deykin EY, Buka SL, Zeena TH: Depressive illness among chemically dependent adolescents. Am J Psychiatry 149:1341–1347, 1992

Dohrenwend BP, Shrout PE, Egri G, et al: Nonspecific psychological distress and other dimensions of psychopathology. Measures for use in the general population. Arch Gen Psychiatry 37:1229–1236, 1980

Donovan SJ, Susser ES, Nunes EV, et al: Divalproex treatment of disruptive adolescents: a report of 10 cases. J Clin Psychiatry 58:12–15, 1997

Dorn LD, Burgess ES, Dichek HL, et al: Thyroid hormone concentrations in depressed and nondepressed adolescents: group differences and behavioral relations. J Am Acad Child Adolesc Psychiatry 35:299–306, 1996

Eaton WW, Dryman A, Sorenson A, et al: DSM-III major depressive disorder in the community: a latent class analysis of data from the NIMH epidemiologic catchment area programme. Br J Psychiatry 155:48–54, 1989

Ellis A, Bernard M: Rational-Emotive Approaches to the Problems of Childhood. New York, Plenum, 1983

el Mallakh RS, Li R: Is the Na(+)-K(+)-ATPase the link between phosphoinositide metabolism and bipolar disorder? J Neuropsychiatry Clin Neurosci 5:361–368, 1993

Emrich HM, Dose M, von Zerssen D: The use of sodium valproate, carbamazepine and oxcarbazepine in patients with affective disorders. J Affect Disord 8:243–250, 1985

Emslie GJ, Rush AJ, Weinberg WA, et al: Children with major depression show reduced rapid eye movement latencies. Arch Gen Psychiatry 47:119–124, 1990

Emslie GJ, Rush AJ, Weinberg WA, et al: Sleep EEG features of adolescents with major depression. Biol Psychiatry 36:573–581, 1994

Emslie GJ, Rush AJ, Weinberg WA, et al: A double-blind, randomized, placebo-controlled trial of fluoxetine in children and adolescents with depression. Arch Gen Psychiatry 54:1031–1037, 1997

Emslie GJ, Walkup JT, Pliszka SR, et al: Nontricyclic antidepressants: current trends in children and adolescents. J Am Acad Child Adolesc Psychiatry 38:517–528, 1999

Endicott J, Spitzer RL: A diagnostic interview: the schedule for affective disorders and schizophrenia. Arch Gen Psychiatry 35:837–844, 1978

Fatemi SH, Rapport DJ, Calabrese JR, et al: Lamotrigine in rapid-cycling bipolar disorder. J Clin Psychiatry 58:522–527, 1997

Ferro T, Carlson GA, Grayson P, et al: Depressive disorders: distinctions in children. J Am Acad Child Adolesc Psychiatry 33:664–670, 1994

Fetner HH, Geller B: Lithium and tricyclic antidepressants. Psychiatr Clin North Am 15:223–224, 1992

Findling RL, Preskorn SH, Marcus RN, et al: Nefazodone pharmacokinetics in depressed children and adolescents. J Am Acad Child Adolesc Psychiatry 39:1008–1016, 2000

Fine S, Forth A, Gilbert M, et al: Group therapy for adolescent depressive disorder: a comparison of social skills and therapeutic support. J Am Acad Child Adolesc Psychiatry 30:79–85, 1991

Fleming JE, Offord DR: Epidemiology of childhood depressive disorders: a critical review. J Am Acad Child Adolesc Psychiatry 29:571–580, 1990

Fleming JE, Offord DR, Boyle MH: Prevalence of childhood and adolescent depression in the community. Ontario Child Health Study. Br J Psychiatry 155:647–654, 1989

Fleming JE, Boyle MH, Offord DR: The outcome of adolescent depression in the Ontario Child Health Study follow-up. J Am Acad Child Adolesc Psychiatry 32:28–33, 1993

Frank E, Kupfer DJ, Perel JM, et al: Three-year outcomes for maintenance therapies in recurrent depression. Arch Gen Psychiatry 47:1093–1099, 1990

Frazier JA, Meyer MC, Biederman J, et al: Risperidone treatment for juvenile bipolar disorder: a retrospective chart review. J Am Acad Child Adolesc Psychiatry 38:960–965, 1999

Friedman L, Findling RL, Kenny JT, et al: An MRI study of adolescent patients with either schizophrenia or bipolar disorder as compared to healthy control subjects [published erratum appears in Biol Psychiatry 46(4):following 584, 1999]. Biol Psychiatry 46:78–88, 1999

Fuchs DC: Clozapine treatment of bipolar disorder in a young adolescent. J Am Acad Child Adolesc Psychiatry 33:1299–1302, 1994

Gabbard GO: Mood disorders: psychodynamic etiology, in Comprehensive Textbook of Psychiatry, 6th Edition. Edited Kaplan HI, Sadock BJ. Baltimore, MD, Williams & Wilkins, 1995, pp 1116–1123

Garber J, Kriss MR, Koch M, et al: Recurrent depression in adolescents: a follow-up study. J Am Acad Child Adolesc Psychiatry 27:49–54, 1988

Garfinkel BD, Froese A, Hood J: Suicide attempts in children and adolescents. Am J Psychiatry 139:1257–1261, 1982

Garland EJ, Weiss M: Subgroups of adolescent depression. J Am Acad Child Adolesc Psychiatry 34:831–833, 1995

Garrison CZ, Jackson KL, Marsteller F, et al: A longitudinal study of depressive symptomatology in young adolescents. J Am Acad Child Adolesc Psychiatry 29:581–585, 1990

Geller B, Fetner HH: Children's 24-hour serum lithium level after a single dose predicts initial dose and steady-state plasma level (letter). J Clin Psychopharmacol 9:155, 1989

Geller B, Luby J: Child and adolescent bipolar disorder: a review of the past 10 years [published erratum appears in J Am Acad Child Adolesc Psychiatry 36(11):1642, 1997]. J Am Acad Child Adolesc Psychiatry 36:1168–1176, 1997

Geller B, Fox LW, Clark KA: Rate and predictors of prepubertal bipolarity during follow-up of 6- to 12-year-old depressed children. J Am Acad Child Adolesc Psychiatry 33:461–468, 1994

Geller B, Sun K, Zimerman B, et al: Complex and rapid-cycling in bipolar children and adolescents: a preliminary study. J Affect Disord 34:259–268, 1995

Geller B, Warner K, Williams M, et al: Prepubertal and young adolescent bipolarity versus ADHD: assessment and validity using the WASH-U-KSADS, CBCL and TRF. J Affect Disord 51:93–100, 1998

Geller B, Zimerman B, Williams M, et al: Adult psychosocial outcome of prepubertal major depressive disorder. J Am Acad Child Adolesc Psychiatry 40:673–677, 2001

Gershon ES, Hamovit J, Guroff JJ, et al: A family study of schizoaffective, bipolar I, bipolar II, unipolar, and normal control probands. Arch Gen Psychiatry 39:1157–1167, 1982

Goetz RR, Puig-Antich J, Ryan N, et al: Electroencephalographic sleep of adolescents with major depression and normal controls. Arch Gen Psychiatry 44:61–68, 1987

Goodyer I, Kolvin I, Gatzanis S: Recent undesirable life events and psychiatric disorder in childhood and adolescence. Br J Psychiatry 147:517–523, 1985

Goodyer IM, Wright C, Altham PM: Maternal adversity and recent stressful life events in anxious and depressed children. J Child Psychol Psychiatry 29:651–667, 1988

Goodyer IM, Wright C, Altham PM: Recent friendships in anxious and depressed school age children. Psychol Med 19:165–174, 1989

Goodyer I, Germany E, Gowrusankur J, et al: Social influences on the course of anxious and depressive disorders in school-age children. Br J Psychiatry 158:676–684, 1991

Gore S, Aseltine RH Jr, Colton ME: Social structure, life stress and depressive symptoms in a high school-aged population. J Health Soc Behav 33:97–113, 1992

Green AI, Mooney JJ, Posemer JA, et al: Mood disorders: biochemical aspects, in Comprehensive Textbook of Psychiatry, 4th Edition. Edited by Kaplan HI, Sadock BJ. Baltimore, MD, Williams & Wilkins, 1995, pp 1089–1102

Guay DR: The emerging role of valproate in bipolar disorder and other psychiatric disorders. Pharmacotherapy 15:631–647, 1995

Gutterman EM, Markowitz JS, LoConte JS, et al: Determinants for hospitalization from an emergency mental health service. J Am Acad Child Adolesc Psychiatry 32:114–122, 1993

Hagino OR, Weller EB, Weller RA, et al: Untoward effects of lithium treatment in children aged four through six years. J Am Acad Child Adolesc Psychiatry 34:1584–1590, 1995

Hammen C: Self-cognitions, stressful events, and the prediction of depression in children of depressed mothers. J Abnorm Child Psychol 16:347–360, 1988

Hammen C, Burge D, Burney E, et al: Longitudinal study of diagnoses in children of women with unipolar and bipolar affective disorder. Arch Gen Psychiatry 47:1112–1117, 1990

Harrington RC: Depressive disorder in children and adolescents. Br J Hosp Med 43:108, 110, 112, 1990

Harrington R, Fudge H, Rutter M, et al: Adult outcomes of childhood and adolescent depression, I: psychiatric status. Arch Gen Psychiatry 47:465–473, 1990

Harrington R, Fudge H, Rutter M, et al: Adult outcomes of childhood and adolescent depression, II: links with antisocial disorders. J Am Acad Child Adolesc Psychiatry 30:434–439, 1991

Hatotani N, Nomura J, Yamaguchi T, et al: Clinical and experimental studies on the pathogenesis of depression. Psychoneuroendocrinology 2:115–130, 1977

Hazell P, O'Connell D, Heathcote D, et al: Efficacy of tricyclic drugs in treating child and adolescent depression: a meta-analysis. BMJ 310:897–901, 1995

Hindmarch I, Kerr J: Behavioural toxicity of antidepressants with particular reference to moclobemide. Psychopharmacology (Berl) 106 (suppl): S49–S55, 1992

Horwath E, Johnson J, Klerman GL, et al: Depressive symptoms as relative and attributable risk factors for first-onset major depression. Arch Gen Psychiatry 49:817–823, 1992

Hsu LK: Lithium-resistant adolescent mania. J Am Acad Child Psychiatry 25:280–283, 1986

Hughes CW, Preskorn SH, Weller E, et al: The effect of concomitant disorders in childhood depression on predicting treatment response. Psychopharmacol Bull 26:235–238, 1990

Inamdar SC, Siomopoulos G, Osborn M, et al: Phenomenology associated with depressed moods in adolescents. Am J Psychiatry 136:156–159, 1979

Isaac G: Misdiagnosed bipolar disorder in adolescents in a special educational school and treatment program. J Clin Psychiatry 53:133–136, 1992

Isojarvi JI, Laatikainen TJ, Pakarinen AJ, et al: Polycystic ovaries and hyperandrogenism in women taking valproate for epilepsy. N Engl J Med 329:1383–1388, 1993

Isojarvi JI, Rattya J, Myllyla VV, et al: Valproate, lamotrigine, and insulin-mediated risks in women with epilepsy. Ann Neurol 43:446–451, 1998

Jacobson SJ, Jones K, Johnson K, et al: Prospective multicentre study of pregnancy outcome after lithium exposure during first trimester. Lancet 339:530–533, 1992

Janicak PG: The relevance of clinical pharmacokinetics and therapeutic drug monitoring: anticonvulsant mood stabilizers and antipsychotics. J Clin Psychiatry 54:35–41, 1993

Jaycox LH, Reivich KJ, Gillham J, et al: Prevention of depressive symptoms in school children. Behav Res Ther 32:801–816, 1994

Jensen JB, Garfinkel BD: Growth hormone dysregulation in children with major depressive disorder. J Am Acad Child Adolesc Psychiatry 29:295–301, 1990

Jimerson DC, Lynch HJ, Post RM, et al: Urinary melatonin rhythms during sleep deprivation in depressed patients and normals. Life Sci 20:1501–1508, 1977

Joffe RT, Singer W: A comparison of triiodothyronine and thyroxine in the potentiation of tricyclic antidepressants. Psychiatry Res 32:241–251, 1990

Johnson BA, Brent DA, Connolly J, et al: Familial aggregation of adolescent personality disorders. J Am Acad Child Adolesc Psychiatry 34:798–804, 1995

Jones KL, Lacro RV, Johnson KA, et al: Pattern of malformations in the children of women treated with carbamazepine during pregnancy. N Engl J Med 320:1661–1666, 1989

Joyce PR: Age of onset in bipolar affective disorder and misdiagnosis as schizophrenia. Psychol Med 14:145–149, 1984

Kafantaris V: Treatment of bipolar disorder in children and adolescents. J Am Acad Child Adolesc Psychiatry 34:732–741, 1995

Kahn J, Kehle T, Enson W, et al: Comparison of cognitive-behavioral, relaxation, and self-modeling interventions for depression among middle-school students. School Psychology Review 9:196–211, 1990

Kandel DB, Davies M: Epidemiology of depressive mood in adolescents: an empirical study. Arch Gen Psychiatry 39:1205–1212, 1982

Kandel DB, Davies M: Adult sequelae of adolescent depressive symptoms. Arch Gen Psychiatry 43:255–262, 1986

Kandel DB, Davies M, Karus D, et al: The consequences in young adulthood of adolescent drug involvement: an overview. Arch Gen Psychiatry 43:746–754, 1986

Kapur S, Mieczkowski T, Mann JJ: Antidepressant medications and the relative risk of suicide attempt and suicide. JAMA 268:3441–3445, 1992

Kashani JH, Beck NC, Hoeper EW, et al: Psychiatric disorders in a community sample of adolescents. Am J Psychiatry 144:584–589, 1987a

Kashani JH, Carlson GA, Beck NC, et al: Depression, depressive symptoms, and depressed mood among a community sample of adolescents. Am J Psychiatry 144:931–934, 1987b

Kashani JH, Reid JC, Rosenberg TK: Levels of hopelessness in children and adolescents: a developmental perspective. J Consult Clin Psychol 57:496–499, 1989

Kaufman J: Depressive disorders in maltreated children. J Am Acad Child Adolesc Psychiatry 30:257–265, 1991

Keck PE Jr, McElroy SL: Outcome in the pharmacologic treatment of bipolar disorder. J Clin Psychopharmacol 16:15S–23S, 1996

Keller MB, Shapiro RW: "Double depression": superimposition of acute depressive episodes on chronic depressive disorders. Am J Psychiatry 139:438–442, 1982

Keller MB, Beardslee W, Lavori PW, et al: Course of major depression in non-referred adolescents: a retrospective study. J Affect Disord 15:235–243, 1988

Keller MB, Ryan ND, Strober M, et al: Efficacy of paroxetine in the treatment of adolescent major depression: a randomized, controlled trial. J Am Acad Child Adolesc Psychiatry 40:762–772, 2001

Kendall PC, Stark KD, Adam T: Cognitive deficit or cognitive distortion in childhood depression. J Abnorm Child Psychol 18:255–270, 1990

Kendall PC, Kortlander E, Chansky TE, et al: Comorbidity of anxiety and depression in youth: treatment implications. J Consult Clin Psychol 60:869–880, 1992

Kendler KS: Is seeking treatment for depression predicted by a history of depression in relatives? Implications for family studies of affective disorder. Psychol Med 25:807–814, 1995

Kennedy SH, Garfinkel PE, Parienti V, et al: Changes in melatonin levels but not cortisol levels are associated with depression in patients with eating disorders. Arch Gen Psychiatry 46:73–78, 1989

Kessler RC, Walters EE: Epidemiology of DSM-III-R major depression and minor depression among adolescents and young adults in the National Comorbidity Survey. Depress Anxiety 7:3–14, 1998

Kessler RC, McGonagle KA, Zhao S, et al: Lifetime and 12-month prevalence of DSM-III-R psychiatric disorders in the United States. Results from the National Comorbidity Survey. Arch Gen Psychiatry 51:8–19, 1994

Kestenbaum CJ, Kron L: Psychoanalytic intervention with children and adolescents with affective disorders: a combined treatment approach. J Am Acad Psychoanal 15:153–174, 1987

Ketter TA, Pazzaglia PJ, Post RM: Synergy of carbamazepine and valproic acid in affective illness: case report and review of the literature. J Clin Psychopharmacol 12:276–281, 1992

Khan AU: Sensitivity and specificity of TRH stimulation test in depressed and nondepressed adolescents. Psychiatry Res 25:11–17, 1988

Khandelwal SK, Varma VK, Srinivasa Murthy R: Renal function in children receiving long-term lithium prophylaxis. Am J Psychiatry 141:278–279, 1984

Kirkegaard C, Faber J: Altered serum levels of thyroxine, triiodothyronines and diiodothyronines in endogenous depression. Acta Endocrinol (Copenh) 96:199–207, 1981

Klerman GL, Weissman MM, Rounsaville BJ, et al: Interpersonal Therapies of Depression. New York, Basic Books, 1984

Knoll J, Stegman K, Suppes T: Clinical experience using gabapentin adjunctively in patients with a history of mania or hypomania. J Affect Disord 49:229–233, 1998

Kolvin I, Barrett ML, Bhate SR, et al: The Newcastle Child Depression Project. Diagnosis and classification of depression. Br J Psychiatry Suppl 9–21, 1991

Kovacs M: Presentation and course of major depressive disorder during childhood and later years of the life span. J Am Acad Child Adolesc Psychiatry 35:705–715, 1996

Kovacs M: Gender and the course of major depressive disorder through adolescence in clinically referred youngsters. J Am Acad Child Adolesc Psychiatry 40:1079–1085, 2001

Kovacs M, Pollock M: Bipolar disorder and comorbid conduct disorder in childhood and adolescence. J Am Acad Child Adolesc Psychiatry 34:715–723, 1995

Kovacs M, Feinberg TL, Crouse-Novak MA, et al: Depressive disorders in childhood, I: a longitudinal prospective study of characteristics and recovery. Arch Gen Psychiatry 41:229–237, 1984a

Kovacs M, Feinberg TL, Crouse-Novak M, et al: Depressive disorders in childhood, II: a longitudinal study of the risk for a subsequent major depression. Arch Gen Psychiatry 41:643–649, 1984b

Kovacs M, Paulauskas S, Gatsonis C, et al: Depressive disorders in childhood, III: a longitudinal study of comorbidity with and risk for conduct disorders. J Affect Disord 15:205–217, 1988

Kovacs M, Gatsonis C, Paulauskas SL, et al: Depressive disorders in childhood, IV: a longitudinal study of comorbidity with and risk for anxiety disorders. Arch Gen Psychiatry 46:776–782, 1989

Kovacs M, Goldston D, Gatsonis C: Suicidal behaviors and childhood-onset depressive disorders: a longitudinal investigation. J Am Acad Child Adolesc Psychiatry 32:8–20, 1993

Kovacs M, Akiskal HS, Gatsonis C, et al: Childhood-onset dysthymic disorder. Clinical features and prospective naturalistic outcome. Arch Gen Psychiatry 51:365–374, 1994

Kovacs M, Obrosky DS, Gatsonis C, et al: First-episode major depressive and dysthymic disorder in childhood: clinical and sociodemographic factors in recovery. J Am Acad Child Adolesc Psychiatry 36:777–784, 1997

Kowatch RA, Suppes T, Gilfillan SK, et al: Clozapine treatment of children and adolescents with bipolar disorder and schizophrenia: a clinical case series. J Child Adolesc Psychopharmacol 5:241–253, 1995

Krasa NR, Tolbert HA: Adolescent bipolar disorder: a nine-year experience. J Affect Disord 30:175–184, 1994

Kroll L, Harrington R, Jayson D, et al: Pilot study of continuation cognitive-behavioral therapy for major depression in adolescent psychiatric patients. J Am Acad Child Adolesc Psychiatry 35:1156–1161, 1996

Kusumakar V, Yatham LN: Lamotrigine treatment of rapid cycling bipolar disorder (letter; comment). Am J Psychiatry 154:1171–1172, 1997

Kutcher S, Marton P: Affective disorders in first-degree relatives of adolescent onset bipolars, unipolars, and normal controls. J Am Acad Child Adolesc Psychiatry 30:75–78, 1991

Kutcher SP, Williamson P, Silverberg J, et al: Nocturnal growth hormone secretion in depressed older adolescents. J Am Acad Child Adolesc Psychiatry 27:751–754, 1988

Kutcher SP, Marton P, Korenblum M: Relationship between psychiatric illness and conduct disorder in adolescents. Can J Psychiatry 34:526–529, 1989

Kutcher S, Malkin D, Silverberg J, et al: Nocturnal cortisol, thyroid stimulating hormone, and growth hormone secretory profiles in depressed adolescents. J Am Acad Child Adolesc Psychiatry 30:407–414, 1991

Kutcher S, Boulos C, Ward B, et al: Response to desipramine treatment in adolescent depression: a fixed-dose, placebo-controlled trial. J Am Acad Child Adolesc Psychiatry 33:686–694, 1994

Kye CH, Ryan ND: Pharmacologic treatment of child and adolescent depression. Child Adolesc Psychiatr Clin N Am 4:261–281, 1995

Lahmeyer HW, Poznanski EO, Bellur SN: EEG sleep in depressed adolescents. Am J Psychiatry 140:1150–1153, 1983

Lerner M, Clum G: Treatment of suicide ideators: a problem-solving approach. Behavioral Therapy 21:403–411, 1990

Lewinsohn PM, Duncan EM, Stanton AK, et al: Age at first onset for nonbipolar depression. J Abnorm Psychol 95:378–383, 1986

Lewinsohn PM, Clarke GN, Hops H, et al: Cognitive-behavioral treatment for depressed adolescents. Behavioral Therapy 21:385–401, 1990

Lewinsohn PM, Rohde P, Seeley JR, et al: Comorbidity of unipolar depression, I: major depression with dysthymia. J Abnorm Psychol 100:205–213, 1991

Lewinsohn PM, Hops H, Roberts RE, et al: Adolescent psychopathology, I: prevalence and incidence of depression and other DSM-III-R disorders in high school students. J Abnorm Psychol 102:133–144, 1993a

Lewinsohn PM, Rohde P, Seeley JR, et al: Age-cohort changes in the lifetime occurrence of depression and other mental disorders. J Abnorm Psychol 102:110–120, 1993b

Lewinsohn PM, Clarke GN, Rohde P: Psychological approaches to the treatment of depression in adolescents, in Handbook of Depression in Children and Adolescents. Edited by Reynolds WM, Johnston HF. New York, Plenum, 1994a, pp 309–344

Lewinsohn PM, Clarke GN, Seeley JR, et al: Major depression in community adolescents: age at onset, episode duration, and time to recurrence. J Am Acad Child Adolesc Psychiatry 33:809–818, 1994b

Lewinsohn PM, Roberts RE, Seeley JR, et al: Adolescent psychopathology, II: psychosocial risk factors for depression. J Abnorm Psychol 103:302–315, 1994c

Lewinsohn PM, Rohde P, Seeley JR: Psychosocial risk factors for future adolescent suicide attempts. J Consult Clin Psychol 62:297–305, 1994d

Lewinsohn PM, Klein DN, Seeley JR: Bipolar disorders in a community sample of older adolescents: prevalence, phenomenology, comorbidity, and course. J Am Acad Child Adolesc Psychiatry 34:454–463, 1995

Lewinsohn PM, Rohde P, Klein DN, et al: Natural course of adolescent major depressive disorder, I: continuity into young adulthood. J Am Acad Child Adolesc Psychiatry 38:56–63, 1999

Lewinsohn PM, Rohde P, Seeley JR, et al: Natural course of adolescent major depressive disorder in a community sample: predictors of recurrence in young adults. Am J Psychiatry 157:1584–1591, 2000

Lewy AJ, Wehr TA, Goodwin FK, et al: Light suppresses melatonin secretion in humans. Science 210:1267–1269, 1980

Linnoila M, Lamberg BA, Rosberg G, et al: Thyroid hormones and TSH, prolactin and LH responses to repeated TRH and LRH injections in depressed patients. Acta Psychiatr Scand 59:536–544, 1979

Lish JD, Dime-Meenan S, Whybrow PC, et al: The National Depressive and Manic-Depressive Association (DMDA) survey of bipolar members. J Affect Disord 31:281–294, 1994

Loranger AW, Levine PM: Age at onset of bipolar affective illness. Arch Gen Psychiatry 35:1345–1348, 1978

Maes M, Meltzer HY, D'Hondt P, et al: Effects of serotonin precursors on the negative feedback effects of glucocorticoids on hypothalamic-pituitary-adrenal axis function in depression. Psychoneuroendocrinology 20:149–167, 1995

Marangell LB, George MS, Callahan AM, et al: Effects of intrathecal thyrotropin-releasing hormone (protirelin) in refractory depressed patients. Arch Gen Psychiatry 54:214–222, 1997

McCauley E, Myers K, Mitchell J, et al: Depression in young people: initial presentation and clinical course. J Am Acad Child Adolesc Psychiatry 32:714–722, 1993

McCracken J, Cantwell DP: Management of child and adolescent mood disorder. Child Adolesc Psychiatr Clin N Am 1:229–255, 1992

McElroy SL, Keck PE Jr, Pope HG Jr, et al: Valproate in the treatment of rapid-cycling bipolar disorder. J Clin Psychopharmacol 8:275–279, 1988

McElroy SL, Keck PE Jr, Pope HG Jr, et al: Clinical and research implications of the diagnosis of dysphoric or mixed mania or hypomania. Am J Psychiatry 149:1633–1644, 1992a

McElroy SL, Keck PE Jr, Pope HG Jr, et al: Valproate in the treatment of bipolar disorder: literature review and clinical guidelines. J Clin Psychopharmacol 12:42S–52S, 1992b

McElroy SL, Strakowski SM, West SA, et al: Phenomenology of adolescent and adult mania in hospitalized patients with bipolar disorder. Am J Psychiatry 154:44–49, 1997

McGlashan TH: Adolescent versus adult onset of mania. Am J Psychiatry 145:221–223, 1988

McGuffin P, Katz R: The genetics of depression and manic-depressive disorder. Br J Psychiatry 155:294–304, 1989

McKnew DH Jr, Cytryn L, White I: Clinical and biochemical correlates of hypomania in a child. J Am Acad Child Psychiatry 13:576–585, 1974

Mendlewicz J, Linkowski P, Branchey L, et al: Abnormal 24 hour pattern of melatonin secretion in depression (letter). Lancet 2:1362, 1979

Minuchin S: Families and Family Therapy. Cambridge, MA, Harvard University Press, 1974

Mitchell J, McCauley E, Burke P, et al: Psychopathology in parents of depressed children and adolescents. J Am Acad Child Adolesc Psychiatry 28:352–357, 1989

Morris JB, Beck AT: The efficacy of antidepressant drugs: a review of research (1958–1972). Arch Gen Psychiatry 30:667–674, 1974

Mufson L, Fairbanks J: Interpersonal psychotherapy for depressed adolescents: a one-year naturalistic follow-up study. J Am Acad Child Adolesc Psychiatry 35:1145–1155, 1996

Mufson L, Moreau D, Weissman MM, et al: Modification of interpersonal psychotherapy with depressed adolescents (IPT-A): phase I and II studies. J Am Acad Child Adolesc Psychiatry 33:695–705, 1994

Mullins LL, Siegel LJ, Hodges K: Cognitive problem-solving and life event correlates of depressive symptoms in children. J Abnorm Child Psychol 13:305–314, 1985

Murphy JM, Olivier DC, Monson RR, et al: Incidence of depression and anxiety: the Stirling County Study. Am J Public Health 78:534–540, 1988

Naylor MW, Shain BN, Shipley JE: REM latency in psychotically depressed adolescents. Biol Psychiatry 28:161–164, 1990

Nurnberger JI, Gershon E: Genetics, in Handbook of Effective Disorders. Edited by Pakel ES. Edinburgh, Scotland, Churchill-Livingstone, 1982, pp 126–145

Orvaschel H: Early onset psychiatric disorder in high risk children and increased familial morbidity. J Am Acad Child Adolesc Psychiatry 29:184–188, 1990

Orvaschel H, Walsh-Allis G, Ye WJ: Psychopathology in children of parents with recurrent depression. J Abnorm Child Psychol 16:17–28, 1988

Ostrov E, Offer D, Howard KI: Gender differences in adolescent symptomatology: a normative study. J Am Acad Child Adolesc Psychiatry 28:394–398, 1989

Papatheodorou G, Kutcher SP: Divalproex sodium treatment in late adolescent and young adult acute mania. Psychopharmacol Bull 29:213–219, 1993

Pedley TA, Scheuer ML, Walczak TS: Epilepsy, in Merritt's Textbook of Neurology. Edited by Rowland LP. Baltimore, MD, Williams & Wilkins, 1995, pp 845–869

Pfeffer CR, Klerman GL, Hurt SW, et al: Suicidal children grow up: demographic and clinical risk factors for adolescent suicide attempts. J Am Acad Child Adolesc Psychiatry 30:609–616, 1991

Pine DS, Cohen P, Gurley D, et al: The risk for early adulthood anxiety and depressive disorders in adolescents with anxiety and depressive disorders. Arch Gen Psychiatry 55:56–64, 1998

Pine DS, Cohen E, Cohen P, et al: Adolescent depressive symptoms as predictors of adult depression: moodiness or mood disorder? Am J Psychiatry 156:133–135, 1999

Plomin R: The Emanuel Miller Memorial Lecture 1993. Genetic research and identification of environmental influences. J Child Psychol Psychiatry 35:817–834, 1994

Post RM, Uhde TW, Roy-Byrne PP, et al: Correlates of antimanic response to carbamazepine. Psychiatry Res 21:71–83, 1987

Post RM, Kramlinger KG, Altshuler LL, et al: Treatment of rapid cycling bipolar illness. Psychopharmacol Bull 26:37–47, 1990

Post RM, Ketter TA, Denicoff K, et al: The place of anticonvulsant therapy in bipolar illness. Psychopharmacology 128:115–129, 1996

Prien RF, Kupfer DJ: Continuation drug therapy for major depressive episodes: how long should it be maintained? Am J Psychiatry 143:18–23, 1986

Prien RF, Potter WZ: NIMH workshop report on treatment of bipolar disorder. Psychopharmacol Bull 26:409–427, 1990

Puig-Antich J, Goetz R, Hanlon C, et al: Sleep architecture and REM sleep measures in prepubertal children with major depression: a controlled study. Arch Gen Psychiatry 39:932–939, 1982

Puig-Antich J, Goetz R, Davies M, et al: Growth hormone secretion in prepubertal children with major depression, II: sleep-related plasma concentrations during a depressive episode. Arch Gen Psychiatry 41:463–466, 1984a

Puig-Antich J, Goetz R, Davies M, et al: Growth hormone secretion in prepubertal children with major depression, IV: sleep-related plasma concentrations in a drug-free, fully recovered clinical state. Arch Gen Psychiatry 41:479–483, 1984b

Puig-Antich J, Lukens E, Davies M, et al: Psychosocial functioning in prepubertal major depressive disorders, I: interpersonal relationships during the depressive episode. Arch Gen Psychiatry 42:500–507, 1985a

Puig-Antich J, Lukens E, Davies M, et al: Psychosocial functioning in prepubertal major depressive disorders, II: interpersonal relationships after sustained recovery from affective episode. Arch Gen Psychiatry 42:511–517, 1985b

Puig-Antich J, Goetz D, Davies M, et al: A controlled family history study of prepubertal major depressive disorder. Arch Gen Psychiatry 46:406–418, 1989

Puig-Antich J, Kaufman J, Ryan ND, et al: The psychosocial functioning and family environment of depressed adolescents. J Am Acad Child Adolesc Psychiatry 32:244–253, 1993

Rao U, Weissman MM, Martin JA, et al: Childhood depression and risk of suicide: a preliminary report of a longitudinal study. J Am Acad Child Adolesc Psychiatry 32:21–27, 1993

Rao U, Ryan ND, Birmaher B, et al: Unipolar depression in adolescents: clinical outcome in adulthood. J Am Acad Child Adolesc Psychiatry 34:566–578, 1995

Rehm LP: A self-control model of depression. Behavior Therapy 8:787–804, 1977

Reinecke MA, Ryan NE, DuBois DL: Cognitive-behavioral therapy of depression and depressive symptoms during adolescence: a review and meta-analysis. J Am Acad Child Adolesc Psychiatry 37:26–34, 1998

Reinherz HZ, Giaconia RM, Lefkowitz ES, et al: Prevalence of psychiatric disorders in a community population of older adolescents. J Am Acad Child Adolesc Psychiatry 32:369–377, 1993a

Reinherz HZ, Giaconia RM, Pakiz B, et al: Psychosocial risks for major depression in late adolescence: a longitudinal community study. J Am Acad Child Adolesc Psychiatry 32:1155–1163, 1993b

Reynolds WM, Coats KI: A comparison of cognitive-behavioral therapy and relaxation training for the treatment of depression in adolescents. J Consult Clin Psychol 54:653–660, 1986

Rice J, Reich T, Andreasen NC, et al: The familial transmission of bipolar illness. Arch Gen Psychiatry 44:441–447, 1987

Rich CL, Young D, Fowler RC: San Diego suicide study, I: young vs old subjects. Arch Gen Psychiatry 43:577–582, 1986

Rich CL, Sherman M, Fowler RC: San Diego Suicide Study: the adolescents. Adolescence 25:855–865, 1990

Robbins DR, Alessi NE, Cook SC, et al: The use of the Research Diagnostic Criteria (RDC) for depression in adolescent psychiatric inpatients. J Am Acad Child Psychiatry 21:251–255, 1982

Rohde P, Lewinsohn PM, Seeley JR: Comorbidity of unipolar depression, II: comorbidity with other mental disorders in adolescents and adults. J Abnorm Psychol 100:214–222, 1991

Rohde P, Lewinsohn PM, Seeley JR: Are adolescents changed by an episode of major depression? J Am Acad Child Adolesc Psychiatry 33:1289–1298, 1994

Rorsman B, Grasbeck A, Hagnell O, et al: A prospective study of first-incidence depression: the Lundby study, 1957–72. Br J Psychiatry 156:336–342, 1990

Rosa FW: Spina bifida in infants of women treated with carbamazepine during pregnancy. N Engl J Med 324:674–677, 1991

Rosen LN, Rosenthal NE, Van Dusen PH, et al: Age at onset and number of psychotic symptoms in bipolar I and schizoaffective disorder. Am J Psychiatry 140:1523–1524, 1983

Rosenberg DR, Johnson K, Sahl R: Evolving mania in an adolescent treated with low-dose fluoxetine. J Child Adolesc Psychopharmacol 2:299–306, 1992

Rosenberg DR, Holttum J, Gershon S: Textbook of Pharmacotherapy for Child and Adolescent Psychiatric Disorders. New York, Brunner/Mazel, 1994

Rubin RT, Heist EK, McGeoy SS, et al: Neuroendocrine aspects of primary endogenous depression, XI: serum melatonin measures in patients and matched control subjects. Arch Gen Psychiatry 49:558–567, 1992

Rutter M, Grahm D, Chadwick OF, et al; Adolescent turmoil: fact or fiction? J Child Psychol Psychiatry 17:35–36, 1976

Ryan ND: Pharmacotherapy of adolescent major depression: beyond TCAs. Psychopharmacol Bull 26:75–79, 1990

Ryan ND, Puig-Antich J, Cooper T, et al: Imipramine in adolescent major depression: plasma level and clinical response. Acta Psychiatr Scand 73:275–288, 1986

Ryan ND, Puig-Antich J, Ambrosini P, et al: The clinical picture of major depression in children and adolescents. Arch Gen Psychiatry 44:854–861, 1987

Ryan ND, Puig-Antich J, Rabinovich H, et al: MAOIs in adolescent major depression unresponsive to tricyclic antidepressants. J Am Acad Child Adolesc Psychiatry 27:755–758, 1988

Ryan ND, Birmaher B, Perel JM, et al: Neuroendocrine response to L-5-hydroxytryptophan challenge in prepubertal major depression: depressed vs normal children. Arch Gen Psychiatry 49:843–851, 1992

Ryan ND, Dahl RE, Birmaher B, et al: Stimulatory tests of growth hormone secretion in prepubertal major depression: depressed versus normal children. J Am Acad Child Adolesc Psychiatry 33:824–833, 1994

Ryan ND, Bhatara VS, Perel JM: Mood stabilizers in children and adolescents. J Am Acad Child Adolesc Psychiatry 38:529–536, 1999

Sanford M, Szatmari P, Spinner M, et al: Predicting the one-year course of adolescent major depression. J Am Acad Child Adolesc Psychiatry 34:1618–1628, 1995

Sayal K, Ford T, Pipe R: Case study: bipolar disorder after head injury. J Am Acad Child Adolesc Psychiatry 39:525–528, 2000

Scheidlinger S: Group treatment of adolescents: an overview. Am J Orthopsychiatry 55:102–111, 1985

Schneekloth TD, Rummans TA, Logan KM: Electroconvulsive therapy in adolescents. Convuls Ther 9:158–166, 1993

Schreiber G, Avissar S: Lithium sensitive G protein hyperfunction: a dynamic model for the pathogenesis of bipolar affective disorder. Med Hypotheses 35:237–243, 1991

Seligman ME, Peterson C: A learned helplessness perspective on child depression: theory and research, in Depression in Young People. Edited by Rutter M, Izard CE, Read PB. New York, Guilford, 1986, pp 223–249

Seligman ME, Peterson C, Kaslow NJ, et al: Attributional style and depressive symptoms among children. J Abnorm Psychol 93:235–238, 1984

Shaffer D: Suicide in childhood and early adolescence. J Child Psychol Psychiatry 15:275–291, 1974

Shafii M, Foster MB, Greenberg RA, et al: Urinary melatonin in depressed children and adolescents, in Syllabus and Proceedings Summary, American Psychiatric Association 141st Annual Meeting, Montreal, QE, Canada, May 7–12, 1988. Washington, DC, American Psychiatric Association, 1988

Shafii M, Foster MB, Greenberg RA, et al: The pineal gland and depressive disorders in children and adolescents, in Biological Rhythms, Mood Disorders, Light Therapy, and the Pineal Gland. Edited by Shafii M, Shafii SL. Washington, DC, American Psychiatric Press, 1990, pp 97–116

Silberstein SD, Wilmore LJ: Divalproex sodium: migraine treatment and monitoring. Headache 36:239–242, 1996

Silva RR, Campbell M, Golden RR, et al: Side effects associated with lithium and placebo administration in aggressive children. Psychopharmacol Bull 28:319–326, 1992

Sitholey P: Pediatric depression and psychopharmacology. Indian J Pediatr 66:613–620, 1999

Solomon DA, Keitner GI, Ryan CE, et al: Polypharmacy in bipolar I disorder. Psychopharmacol Bull 32:579–587, 1996

Soutullo CA, Casuto LS, Keck PE Jr: Gabapentin in the treatment of adolescent mania: a case report. J Child Adolesc Psychopharmacol 8:81–85, 1998

Soutullo CA, Sorter MT, Foster KD, et al: Olanzapine in the treatment of adolescent acute mania: a report of seven cases. J Affect Disord 53:279–283, 1999

Stark KD, Reynolds WM, Kaslow NJ: A comparison of the relative efficacy of self-control therapy and a behavioral problem-solving therapy for depression in children. J Abnorm Child Psychol 15:91–113, 1987

Stores G, Williams PL, Styles E, et al: Psychological effects of sodium valproate and carbamazepine in epilepsy. Arch Dis Child 67:1330–1337, 1992

Strober M: Familial aspects of depressive disorders in early adolescence, in An Update of Childhood Depression. Edited by Weller EB, Weller RA. Washington, DC, American Psychiatric Association, 1984, pp 38–48

Strober M: Relevance of early age-of-onset in genetic studies of bipolar affective disorder. J Am Acad Child Adolesc Psychiatry 31:606–610, 1992

Strober M, Carlson G: Bipolar illness in adolescents with major depression: clinical, genetic, and psychopharmacologic predictors in a three- to four-year prospective follow-up investigation. Arch Gen Psychiatry 39:549–555, 1982

Strober M, Green J, Carlson G: Phenomenology and subtypes of major depressive disorder in adolescence. J Affect Disord 3:281–290, 1981

Strober M, Morrell W, Burroughs J, et al: A family study of bipolar I disorder in adolescence. Early onset of symptoms linked to increased familial loading and lithium resistance. J Affect Disord 15:255–268, 1988

Strober M, Morrell W, Lampert C, et al: Relapse following discontinuation of lithium maintenance therapy in adolescents with bipolar I illness: a naturalistic study. Am J Psychiatry 147:457–461, 1990

Strober M, Lampert C, Schmidt S, et al: The course of major depressive disorder in adolescents, I: recovery and risk of manic switching in a follow-up of psychotic and nonpsychotic subtypes. J Am Acad Child Adolesc Psychiatry 32:34–42, 1993

Strober M, Schmidt-Lackner S, Freeman R, et al: Recovery and relapse in adolescents with bipolar affective illness: a five-year naturalistic, prospective follow-up. J Am Acad Child Adolesc Psychiatry 34:724–731, 1995

Summerville MB, Abbate MF, Siegel AM, et al: Psychopathology in urban female minority adolescents with suicide attempts. J Am Acad Child Adolesc Psychiatry 31:663–668, 1992

Swearingen EM, Cohen LH: Measurement of adolescents' life events: the junior high life experiences survey. Am J Community Psychol 13:69–85, 1985

Tappia PS, Ladha S, Clark DC, et al: The influence of membrane fluidity, TNF receptor binding, cAMP production and GTPase activity on macrophage cytokine production in rats fed a variety of fat diets. Mol Cell Biochem 166:135–143, 1997

Thase ME, Kupfer DJ, Jarrett DB: Treatment of imipramine-resistant recurrent depression, I: an open clinical trial of adjunctive L-triiodothyronine. J Clin Psychiatry 50:385–388, 1989

Thase ME, Trivedi MH, Rush AJ: MAOIs in the contemporary treatment of depression. Neuropsychopharmacology 12:185–219, 1995

Thompson C, Franey C, Arendt J, et al: A comparison of melatonin secretion in depressed patients and normal subjects. Br J Psychiatry 152:260–265, 1988

Thompson LM, Rubin RT, McCracken JT: Neuroendocrine aspects of primary endogenous depression, XII: receiver operating characteristic and kappa analyses of serum and urine cortisol measures in patients and matched controls. Psychoneuroendocrinology 17:507–515, 1992

Todd RD, Neuman R, Geller B, et al: Genetic studies of affective disorders: should we be starting with childhood onset probands? J Am Acad Child Adolesc Psychiatry 32:1164–1171, 1993

Verhulst FC, van der EJ, Ferdinand RF, et al: The prevalence of DSM-III-R diagnoses in a national sample of Dutch adolescents. Arch Gen Psychiatry 54:329–336, 1997

Viesselman JO, Yaylayan S, Weller EB, et al: Antidysthymic drugs (antidepressants and antimanics), in Practitioner's Guide to Psychoactive Drugs for Children and Adolescents. Edited by Werry JS, Aman MG. New York, Plenum, 1993, pp 239–268

Warner V, Mufson L, Weissman MM: Offspring at high and low risk for depression and anxiety: mechanisms of psychiatric disorder. J Am Acad Child Adolesc Psychiatry 34:786–797, 1995

Waterman GS, Ryan ND, Perel JM, et al: Nocturnal urinary excretion of 6-hydroxymelatonin sulfate in prepubertal major depressive disorder. Biol Psychiatry 31:582–590, 1992

Wehr TA, Goodwin FK, Wirz-Justice A, et al: 48-hour sleep-wake cycles in manic-depressive illness: naturalistic observations and sleep deprivation experiments. Arch Gen Psychiatry 39:559–565, 1982

Weinberg WA, Rutman J, Sullivan L, et al: Depression in children referred to an educational diagnostic center: diagnosis and treatment—preliminary report. J Pediatr 83:1065–1072, 1973

Weissman MM, Kidd KK, Prusoff BA: Variability in rates of affective disorders in relatives of depressed and normal probands. Arch Gen Psychiatry 39:1397–1403, 1982

Weissman MM, Gershon ES, Kidd KK, et al: Psychiatric disorders in the relatives of probands with affective disorders: the Yale University–National Institute of Mental Health Collaborative Study. Arch Gen Psychiatry 41:13–21, 1984a

Weissman MM, Leckman JF, Merikangas KR, et al: Depression and anxiety disorders in parents and children: results from the Yale family study. Arch Gen Psychiatry 41:845–852, 1984b

Weissman MM, Wickramaratne P, Merikangas KR, et al: Onset of major depression in early adulthood: increased familial loading and specificity. Arch Gen Psychiatry 41:1136–1143, 1984c

Weissman MM, Gammon GD, John K, et al: Children of depressed parents: increased psychopathology and early onset of major depression. Arch Gen Psychiatry 44:847–853, 1987

Weissman MM, Leaf PJ, Tischler GL, et al: Affective disorders in five United States communities [published erratum appears in Psychol Med 18(3):following 792, 1988]. Psychol Med 18:141–153, 1988

Weissman MM, Fendrich M, Warner V, et al: Incidence of psychiatric disorder in offspring at high and low risk for depression. J Am Acad Child Adolesc Psychiatry 31:640–648, 1992

Weissman MM, Wolk S, Wickramaratne P, et al: Children with prepubertal-onset major depressive disorder and anxiety grown up. Arch Gen Psychiatry 56:794–801, 1999

Weller EB, Weller RA: Depressive disorders in children and adolescents, in Psychiatric Disorders in Children and Adolescents. Edited by Garfinkel BD. Philadelphia, PA, WB Saunders, 1990, pp 3–20

Weller EB, Weller RA: Mood disorders in prepubertal children, in Textbook of Child and Adolescent Psychiatry. Edited by Wiener JM. Washington, DC, American Academy of Child and Adolescent Psychiatry, 1991, pp 333–342

Weller EB, Weller RA, Fristad MA: Lithium dosage guide for prepubertal children: a preliminary report. J Am Acad Child Psychiatry 25:92–95, 1986

Weller EB, Weller RA, Fristad MA: Bipolar disorder in children: misdiagnosis, underdiagnosis, and future directions. J Am Acad Child Adolesc Psychiatry 34:709–714, 1995

Weller RA, Weller EB, Tucker SG, et al: Mania in prepubertal children: has it been underdiagnosed? J Affect Disord 11:151–154, 1986

Welner A, Welner Z, Fishman R: Psychiatric adolescent inpatients: eight- to ten-year follow-up. Arch Gen Psychiatry 36:698–700, 1979

Werry JS, McClellan JM, Chard L: Childhood and adolescent schizophrenic, bipolar, and schizoaffective disorders: a clinical and outcome study. J Am Acad Child Adolesc Psychiatry 30:457–465, 1991

West SA, Keck PE, McElroy SL, et al: Open trial of valproate in the treatment of adolescent mania. J Child Adolesc Psychopharmacol 4:263–267, 1994

West SA, McElroy SL, Strakowski SM, et al: Attention deficit hyperactivity disorder in adolescent mania. Am J Psychiatry 152:271–273, 1995

Whitaker A, Johnson J, Shaffer D, et al: Uncommon troubles in young people: prevalence estimates of selected psychiatric disorders in a nonreferred adolescent population. Arch Gen Psychiatry 47:487–496, 1990

Whittier MC, West SA, Galli VB, et al: Valproic acid for dysphoric mania in a mentally retarded adolescent (letter). J Clin Psychiatry 56:590–591, 1995

Wilens TE, Biederman J, Baldessarini RJ, et al: Cardiovascular effects of therapeutic doses of tricyclic antidepressants in children and adolescents. J Am Acad Child Adolesc Psychiatry 35:1491–1501, 1996

Wilens TE, Spencer TJ, Biederman J, et al: Case study: nefazodone for juvenile mood disorders. J Am Acad Child Adolesc Psychiatry 36:481–485, 1997

Williamson DE, Birmaher B, Anderson BP, et al: Stressful life events in depressed adolescents: the role of dependent events during the depressive episode. J Am Acad Child Adolesc Psychiatry 34:591–598, 1995a

Williamson DE, Ryan ND, Birmaher B, et al: A case-control family history study of depression in adolescents. J Am Acad Child Adolesc Psychiatry 34:1596–1607, 1995b

Williamson DE, Birmaher B, Dahl RE, et al: Stressful life events influence nocturnal growth hormone secretion in depressed children. Biol Psychiatry 40:1176–1180, 1996

Williamson DE, Birmaher B, Frank E, et al: Nature of life events and difficulties in depressed adolescents. J Am Acad Child Adolesc Psychiatry 37:1049–1057, 1998

Winokur G, Coryell W, Akiskal HS, et al: Alcoholism in manic-depressive (bipolar) illness: familial illness, course of illness, and the primary-secondary distinction. Am J Psychiatry 152:365–372, 1995

Wood A, Harrington R, Moore A: Controlled trial of a brief cognitive-behavioural intervention in adolescent patients with depressive disorders. J Child Psychol Psychiatry 37:737–746, 1996

Woolston JL: Case study: carbamazepine treatment of juvenile-onset bipolar disorder. J Am Acad Child Adolesc Psychiatry 38:335–338, 1999

Wozniak J, Biederman J, Kiely K, et al: Mania-like symptoms suggestive of childhood-onset bipolar disorder in clinically referred children. J Am Acad Child Adolesc Psychiatry 34:867–876, 1995

Yaylayan SA, Weller EB, Weller RA: Biology of depression in children and adolescents. J Child Adolesc Psychopharmacol 1:215–227, 1990

Young W, Knowles JB, MacLean AW, et al: The sleep of childhood depressives: comparison with age-matched controls. Biol Psychiatry 17:1163–1168, 1982

Youngerman J, Canino IA: Lithium carbonate use in children and adolescents: a survey of the literature. Arch Gen Psychiatry 35:216–224, 197

Zerbin-Rudin E: [Genetics in medicine] (German). Wien Med Wochenschr 119:759–764, 1969

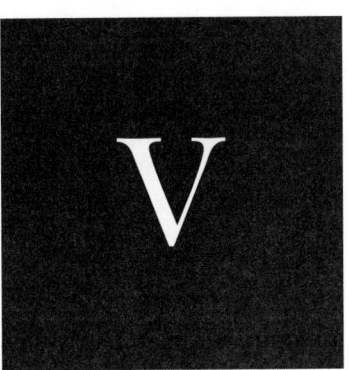

Attention-Deficit and Disruptive Behavior Disorders

Attention-Deficit/Hyperactivity Disorder

Bruce Waslick, M.D.

Laurence L. Greenhill, M.D.

Disruptive behavior continues to be one of the most common reasons for referral of a child or adolescent to a child psychiatrist. It has long been recognized, clinically and in research studies, that not all disruptive behavior in children is the same. The core symptoms of attention-deficit/hyperactivity disorder (ADHD) (Table 26–1)—inability to maintain focused attention, lack of control over impulsive behavior, and generalized behavioral overactivity—have long been recognized and reported on by mental health specialists dealing with children and adolescents. It also has been recognized that not all children with ADHD display other types of disruptive behavior such as aggression, intentional rule-breaking, or willful violation of social norms.

Nevertheless, the diagnosis of ADHD continues to be controversial. In 1998 the National Institutes of Health convened a special consensus development conference to address the degree of controversy related to the disorder. Issues concerning the validity of the diagnosis and the diagnostic process associated with practice, as well as the issues regarding using psychostimulants as a mainstay of treatment in the disorder, led to the inclusion of the following sentences in the conference summary statement: "The diverse and conflicting opinions about ADHD have resulted in confusion for families, care providers, educators, and policymakers. The controversy raises questions concerning the literal existence of the disorder, whether it can be reliably diagnosed, and, if treated, what interventions are the most effective" (National Institutes of Health 2000, p. 5).

In this chapter we review research on ADHD, emphasizing the new knowledge that has emerged in the past few decades and addressing some of the confusion and controversies. ADHD remains one of the most intensively researched areas in child psychiatry, and the literature on this disorder is expanding in terms of recognizing and understanding adolescent and adult presentations of the disorder. Although the shift toward more interest in the biological basis of mental disorders is certainly evident in new research on ADHD—as seen by studies examining molecular, genetic, neurochemical, and neuroimaging correlates of the disorder—more information also continues to be gathered on the psychological manifestations of the disorder and the effect of psychological interventions. In this chapter we summarize current clinical and research understandings of ADHD and present biological, psychological, and social perspectives that contribute to the evolving definition of this complex psychiatric disorder.

Diagnostic Considerations

In the DSM-IV-TR (American Psychiatric Association 2000) definition of ADHD, three core symptom clusters are identified; subtyping of the disorder is based on the presence or absence of these key clusters (Table 26–1). Each of the symptom clusters is described more extensively below under "Clinical Description."

In addition to the symptom clusters, certain other important diagnostic features of the disorder are highlighted in DSM-IV-TR. These include the following:

Table 26–1. DSM-IV-TR diagnostic criteria for attention-deficit/hyperactivity disorder

---

A. Either (1) or (2):

(1) six (or more) of the following symptoms of **inattention** have persisted for at least 6 months to a degree that is maladaptive and inconsistent with developmental level:

Inattention

(a) often fails to give close attention to details or makes careless mistakes in schoolwork, work, or other activities

(b) often has difficulty sustaining attention in tasks or play activities

(c) often does not seem to listen when spoken to directly

(d) often does not follow through on instructions and fails to finish schoolwork, chores, or duties in the workplace (not due to oppositional behavior or failure to understand instructions)

(e) often has difficulty organizing tasks and activities

(f) often avoids, dislikes, or is reluctant to engage in tasks that require sustained mental effort (such as schoolwork or homework)

(g) often loses things necessary for tasks or activities (e.g., toys, school assignments, pencils, books, or tools)

(h) is often easily distracted by extraneous stimuli

(i) is often forgetful in daily activities

(2) six (or more) of the following symptoms of **hyperactivity-impulsivity** have persisted for at least 6 months to a degree that is maladaptive and inconsistent with developmental level:

Hyperactivity

(a) often fidgets with hands or feet or squirms in seat

(b) often leaves seat in classroom or in other situations in which remaining seated is expected

(c) often runs about or climbs excessively in situations in which it is inappropriate (in adolescents or adults, may be limited to subjective feelings of restlessness)

(d) often has difficulty playing or engaging in leisure activities quietly

(e) is often "on the go" or often acts as if "driven by a motor"

(f) often talks excessively

Impulsivity

(g) often blurts out answers before questions have been completed

(h) often has difficulty awaiting turn

(i) often interrupts or intrudes on others (e.g., butts into conversations or games)

B. Some hyperactive-impulsive or inattentive symptoms that caused impairment were present before age 7 years.

C. Some impairment from the symptoms is present in two or more settings (e.g., at school [or work] and at home).

D. There must be clear evidence of clinically significant impairment in social, academic, or occupational functioning.

E. The symptoms do not occur exclusively during the course of a pervasive developmental disorder, schizophrenia, or other psychotic disorder and are not better accounted for by another mental disorder (e.g., mood disorder, anxiety disorder, dissociative disorder, or a personality disorder).

Code based on type:

314.01 Attention-Deficit/Hyperactivity Disorder, Combined Type: if both Criteria A1 and A2 are met for the past 6 months

314.00 Attention-Deficit/Hyperactivity Disorder, Predominantly Inattentive Type: if Criterion A1 is met but Criterion A2 is not met for the past 6 months

314.01 Attention-Deficit/Hyperactivity Disorder, Predominantly Hyperactive-Impulsive Type: if Criterion A2 is met but Criterion A1 is not met for the past 6 months

Coding note: For individuals (especially adolescents and adults) who currently have symptoms that no longer meet full criteria, "In Partial Remission" should be specified.

Source. Reprinted from the *Diagnostic and Statistical Manual of Mental Disorders*, 4th Edition, Text Revision. Washington, DC, American Psychiatric Association, 2000. Copyright 2000, American Psychiatric Association. Used with permission.

- *Discriminant validity of ADHD*—ADHD is one disorder in the disruptive behavior disorders category, which also includes oppositional defiant disorder (see Chapter 27, "Conduct Disorder and Oppositional Defiant Disorder," and Chapter 28, "Conduct and Antisocial Disorders in Adolescence," in this volume). Although it is recognized that the different disorders are highly associated, the distinction between these different behavior disorders is supported by empirical evidence (Fergusson et al. 1994; Halperin et al. 1993).
- *Early onset*—some symptoms must be present before age 7 years.
- *Duration of symptoms*—the symptoms must be present for at least 6 months.
- *Pervasiveness of symptoms*—the symptoms must be evident in at least two different environments, typically (in children) at school and at home.
- *Abnormality of the symptoms*—the symptoms are clearly inappropriate for the child's developmental age and are maladaptive in terms of functioning.

Also, a criterion requiring that the individual manifest "clinically significant impairment" in social, academic, or occupational functioning was added, eliminating persons who have appropriate symptoms, but no impairment, from receiving this diagnosis. DSM-IV-TR represents the most recent attempt by the American Psychiatric Association to classify children with behavioral problems into separate, at least partially homogeneous, diagnostic categories; it should be noted that other diagnosis-based and dimensionally based systems exist (Werry 1992).

The diagnosis of mental disorders in children, however, continues to present challenges in both research studies and clinical application. Establishing a diagnosis in child psychiatry requires that information from multiple sources be synthesized, which can be a problem when contradictory information is presented to the diagnostician. Often, the information reported by adults (e.g., parents, teachers) of a child's behavioral problems and the individual child's self-report are significantly different (Bird et al. 1992). This discrepancy can be found in both emotional and behavior disorders. Children with behavior disorders report symptoms of their disruptive behavior with less frequency than do the adults around them, and self-reports of symptoms from young children (i.e., between ages 6 and 11 years) are not reliable (Schwab-Stone et al. 1994).

In general, teachers and parents tend to agree on the identification of a child with a behavior disorder, even though the correlation between their reports of individual symptoms is quite low (Biederman et al. 1993), possibly because of the differing contexts of the observations available to each informant (Pelham et al. 1992). Although it is probably not the case with more emotionally based symptoms and problems, it appears that the diagnosis of disruptive behavior disorder tends to be more valid if it is based on adult reports than on the child's self-report (Pelham et al. 1992). Further complicating the diagnostic assessment is the suggestion that individual parental psychopathology may influence the parent's reporting of the child's behavior—for example, the tendency of depressed mothers to report increased numbers of symptoms (Fergusson et al. 1993). Adults' reports of symptoms of ADHD may also be affected by the presence of comorbid conduct disturbance in the child (Abikoff et al. 1993) as well as by cultural factors (Mann et al. 1992).

Dimensional scales (e.g., the Child Behavior Checklist and Conners' Teacher Rating Scale) have been applied to the study of attentional and hyperactive disorders of childhood in an attempt to identify cases of disorder on the basis of cutoff points representing significant deviation from normality on the respective symptom scales (Achenbach and Edelbrock 1983; Goyette et al. 1978). Highly structured interviews (e.g., the Diagnostic Interview Schedule for Children [Shaffer et al. 2000]), corresponding to specific diagnostic classification systems such as DSM, also are used for research purposes. There is significant correlation between structured diagnostic interviews and well-established dimensional scales for the identification of behavior disorders in children (Jensen et al. 1993a). There is active research focusing on attempts to move from diagnoses based on subjective human reports toward the use of more objective neuropsychological tests and laboratory assessments (such as the Continuous Performance Test, described under "Inattention" below). However, these types of assessments currently represent at best research tools and sources of supplementary clinical information (Barkley et al. 1991).

Although there are increasing numbers of research reports documenting the presence of ADHD in adults, no separate definition of the adult type of the disorder currently exists in DSM-IV-TR. To meet criteria for ADHD, the adult presentation must conform to the diagnostic criteria for the childhood presentation.

These include a 6-month duration of symptoms, evidence of impairment in at least two settings, and the onset of symptoms before age 7 years. A residual type of ADHD has been demonstrated to exist in adolescents and adults and may be an increasingly recognized and important clinical entity. Recent research reports of children with ADHD observed prospectively in longitudinal studies demonstrate the relative decrease in symptoms of behavioral overactivity and the relative persistence of striking attentional mechanism problems (Biederman et al. 2000; Denckla 1991; Shaffer 1994). There is also increasing evidence demonstrating that in some cases ADHD can present with an onset of symptoms after age 7, especially in patients with the inattentive subtype (Applegate et al. 1997; Barkley and Biederman 1997; Willoughby et al. 2000).

In summary, ADHD can in some ways be viewed as a developmental disorder with somewhat varying symptom presentations appearing at different life phases. There is increasing recognition that the different developmental phases of the disorder are not captured well in the present diagnostic classification systems and that this should be clarified in the future.

Clinical Description

Establishing the diagnosis of ADHD depends more on taking a good behavioral history and less on a direct mental status examination of the child in the office. Under direct questioning, the child will often deny being symptomatic and will not complain about any problem. The clinician must rely on reports from parents and teachers and should use direct observations of the patient's behavior only if it is conducted in a social situation, such as a classroom. Even after gathering a classic history of ADHD, little chaos and mayhem may be seen in the first one-to-one exchange with the child. How can the clinician make a diagnosis if the disorder cannot be validated by direct observation in the interview?

The diagnostic decision and choice of treatment depend on the clinician's experience in working with other children with ADHD and common-sense clinical judgment. In addition, psychological reports can help by revealing attentional lapses during tedious repetitive tasks, such as the coding task of the Wechsler Intelligence Scale for Children–Revised (Wechsler 1974). One clinical rule of thumb, now made explicit in DSM-IV-TR, is that the signs of the disorder must be present to a moderate degree in at least two of three settings (e.g., home, school, and clinician's office). The clinical descriptions of ADHD and its functional impairment vary across settings.

Despite changes in the DSM classification system over the past 20 years, the diagnosis of ADHD has retained three key elements: 1) a developmentally inappropriate level of motor hyperactivity, 2) inattention at school, and 3) impulsivity with regard to rule-governed behavior (Barkley 1982; Carlson et al. 1986). The clinician's history-taking approach works best when the inquiry focuses on the positive signs of the disorder, exclusion criteria, severity measures, associated conditions, and family history. Such information is best collected from both parents together, if possible.

The behavioral traits in a child with ADHD often seem to be exaggerations of normal childhood activities. Signs of inattention and overactivity unpredictably interact with the environmental setting and are age dependent. The younger the child, the more pervasive is the motor drivenness, and its appearance is less dependent on the setting. The preschool-age child with ADHD rapidly moves about the room and is stimulus driven to touch everything and manipulate each object in a haphazard manner. He or she climbs, jumps, and runs as if "driven by a motor" out of control. Birthday parties and peer-group get-togethers are quickly derailed by the child with ADHD, who becomes wild, overactive, noisy, and unmanageable if the occasion is unstructured.

The school-age child may show a narrower range of impulsive and overactive behaviors, with large group settings required to bring out the most severe disturbances. In class, the inattentiveness predominates; the child with ADHD appears to be daydreaming or preoccupied. The child squirms and moves restlessly about when seated. The inattentiveness seriously interferes with academic performance, as revealed in the child's sloppy handwriting, careless errors, and messy papers. At home, parents find that the child with ADHD does not listen, does not follow through on even the most simple requests, and is unable to complete homework.

Children with ADHD may have a history of longstanding difficulties with impulse control, high levels of motor activity, and disruptiveness in groups. Activity levels in children with ADHD are generally higher, even during sleep (Porrino et al. 1983). In physical education class, activity levels may be lower because children with ADHD have trouble modulating their behavior downward (in academic class) or upward (during a soccer game) as the social setting demands. On the playground during recess, these children may seem to be just as active as their playmates, yet other children often find that impulsivity and inattentiveness make them poor teammates (Porrino et al. 1983; Whalen et al. 1979, 1987). Situations involving self-paced work exert the greatest stress (Whalen et al. 1979).

In the following sections, we discuss the three cardinal features of the disorder in detail.

■ Hyperactivity

Although developmentally inappropriate levels of hyperactivity have been both emphasized and deemphasized over the past decades (Carlson et al. 1986), the importance of the high activity level in children with ADHD has been supported by research in the past decades. Children with ADHD, compared with control children, display higher activity levels, particularly when carrying out structured, in-seat activities (Abikoff and Gittelman 1985a; Conners and Werry 1979). Naturalistic studies employing small, solid-state memory-activity monitors mounted on the belt or vest have also shown that children with ADHD manifest significantly higher levels of activity in the classroom, at home, and while sleeping at night than do children without ADHD (Porrino et al. 1983). Monitored activity levels fall to normal when stimulants are given to children with ADHD. The high levels of sleep activity in children with ADHD and the normalization of activity with stimulant treatment strengthen the concurrent validity of the syndrome.

The higher-than-usual level of motility makes the child with ADHD appear to be driven, restless, and never tiring. Although some degree of hyperactivity is found ordinarily in school-age boys (Lapouse and Monk 1953), the diagnosis of ADHD should be limited to a developmentally inappropriate degree of gross motor activity in the school and/or home setting. The child with ADHD seems to have the same difficulty sitting as does the patient with neuroleptic-induced akathisia. Therefore, sedentary activities—such as sitting in school or church, riding in the car, or even going to a movie—lead to high levels of noncompliance and restlessness. In the classroom—where children are asked to sit still, remain quiet, and work independently—children with ADHD squirm in their chairs, hum, make noises, and tap on their desks. This activity disturbs other children. Hyperactive children also enjoy climbing; for example, they will climb along kitchen counters when their peers choose to walk on the floor.

■ Inattention

To date, no standardized office procedure is established to validly measure specific attentional abnormalities in children. The inattention component is best determined by history. The clinician inquires about attentional problems by asking the parents or teacher if the child has a short attention span, difficulty concentrating, an inability to modulate attention in response to externally imposed demands, a problem in initiating tasks, or trouble selectively attending to relevant stimuli while filtering out unnecessary noise (Carlson et al. 1986). Distractibility may reflect not a breakdown in filtering out unwanted input but rather an active seeking out of more stimuli when the activity requiring attention produces boredom (Zentall and Meyer 1987).

Inattentive children have difficulty processing classwork. They cannot complete goal-directed work without frequent refocusing from another person. They spend more time off the task and out of their seat than do children with more normal attentional abilities. These children are typically oversolicitous with the teacher (calling out more often or trying to answer questions that are not understood). Whereas other children complete their assignment sheets, tests, and workbook drills, children with ADHD produce very little "product," even if they are the brightest in the class. Teachers become frustrated when one of their brighter students produces scanty, poor-quality work.

At home, school-age children with ADHD often have trouble listening to adults. These children look away and do not make eye contact when speaking with an adult. In doing chores, they forget what they were asked to do and have difficulty carrying out multicommission commands. Following written instructions for constructing a model airplane requires effortful redirecting and maintenance of attention, from the instruction sheet to the model and back again. Faced with a multistep instruction sheet, children with ADHD may decide to slap together the model, based on only the picture on the box. As a result, important pieces are ignored or left out. In just such a manner, ADHD children always seem to be rushed, too busy, or "on the way in a hurry" to some other activity. In other instances, they may start several activities at once and finish none of them.

Laboratory-based research studies have used a number of procedures to monitor the task performance of children with ADHD and have claimed that these laboratory measures detect attentional difficulties that otherwise would be seen only in a classroom. The best known of such tests is the Continuous Performance Test (CPT), which measures sustained attention (Cornblatt et al. 1988; Sykes et al. 1972; Weingartner et al. 1980). This test requires the child to watch a computer screen continuously for 10–15 minutes. The child is instructed to pick out the correct target among a group of nontarget letters that flash on the screen and to press a key as soon as the correct letter or combination of letters is seen. A wide range of modifications have been employed to avoid floor and ceiling effects (Cornblatt et al. 1988), including visually degrading the stimuli on the screen, playing movie soundtracks over earphones during the visual task, and even varying the time between stimuli, depending on the performance of the child. The CPT has been shown to be sensitive to drug effects (Garfinkel et al. 1986) and to dose of drug (Cornblatt et al. 1987; Rapport et al. 1985).

However, laboratory-based measures of attention do not always correlate with classroom performance (DuPaul et al. 1992). Any laboratory tool used in a 1-to-1 (1 researcher with 1 child) situation cannot easily recreate the demand set of the 1-to-30 environment found in a classroom (1 teacher to 30 students). Douglas (1983) wisely pointed out that sustained attention, which is tracked by the CPT, does not tap other important attentional functions required in complex tasks, such as self-regulation, the extent to which attention is self-directed and organized, the amount of effort that is invested, or whether the approach to a task involves a search strategy or is just simple exploration. In addition, research has downplayed the role of a sustained attention deficit as the sole cognitive deficit in ADHD (Corkum and Siegel 1993; Solanto and Wender 1989; Swanson and Cantwell 1989).

Other laboratory measures have been used in research, and some find their way into a marketplace for practitioners. None of these tasks has been widely accepted for clinical work. One simple device tests motor steadiness; one group has been able to correlate diminishing error rates and the plasma levels of methylphenidate (Birmaher et al. 1989). A rugged, portable CPT has been marketed with normative data to support its utility as a screening device (Gordon and Mettelman 1988). The Paired-Associates Learning Task measures short-term memory and is also medication sensitive, showing significant correlations with stimulant blood levels (Kupietz et al. 1982). The quality of performance on this test at various dosages of methylphenidate, for example, has been used as an argument for choosing lower doses to optimize cognitive performance in the classroom (Sprague and Sleator 1977).

These laboratory measures are not diagnostically specific. Werry et al. (1987) reported no differences among children with ADHD, conduct disorder, or anxiety disorder in CPT results, suggesting that attentional dysfunction (as measured by CPT) is a nonspecific correlate of child psychopathology in general (Barkley 1991; Werry et al. 1987).

■ Impulsivity

Impulsivity means that the child acts without forethought of the consequences, appearing to be unaware of danger or the relationship between cause and effect. The child with ADHD is willing to "take dares" that other children would not.

Complex academic tasks—which require individual initiation, self-monitoring, organization, and self-pacing—may best reveal the impulsivity in children with ADHD. In particular, behavior during homework may be the most distressing of the child's "invisible handicaps." Even bright children with ADHD report the rapid onset of boredom during homework and a strong feeling that "I work in school, so why should I have to continue this stuff at home?" In addition, teachers may insist that the child with ADHD finish uncompleted classwork at home, which further burdens the child with the very tasks that he or she finds most difficult. Secondary behavior patterns often develop during the homework struggle, particularly avoidance routines, such as "forgetting" assignments, leaving important books at school, and even rushing through the homework without concern for errors. When such a child is unsupervised, he or she will start three other activities and not finish either the schoolwork or the other projects. Parents quickly become discouraged after spending much of their leisure time hovering over their child while he or she struggles with homework.

During the early years, the impulsivity of the child with ADHD may take the form of "stimulus drivenness," a robotlike behavior in which the child must pick up, touch, or manipulate every object in the room. This pressure drives toddlers from one toy to the next, disrupting all objects in their path. During school-age years, these children constantly interrupt others and refuse to wait their turn in games. The thoughtless, unpremeditated quality of the hyperkinetic child's rule breaking often leads such children into situations where they get caught "holding the bag," while the real instigators are long gone. As a result, the child with ADHD can land in trouble and be included with children who have long histories of conduct problems.

Research studies have had the challenge of operationalizing an "impulsivity" dimension, a concept that is inferential at best. Measures have been developed using a number of approaches, including direct observations of a child's self-control during interactions with adults and peers, inhibition of behavior (e.g., a "draw-a-line-slowly" task), and cognitive problem-solving measures (e.g., the Matching Familiar Figures Test) (Carlson et al. 1986). Direct observation studies have been most successful in tapping this impulsive dimension. These studies show that the child with ADHD interrupts others often, does not wait for his or her turn in games, and is disliked by potential peers.

Comorbidity

Comorbid disorders occurring with ADHD have become an area of intense clinical and research concern. Developmental, medical, educational, and psychiatric conditions have all been recognized to contribute to the presentation, longitudinal course, and prognosis of ADHD. In some cases, the comorbidity may be suspected to result from a genetic relationship; in other cases, the comorbidity may be associated with environmental correlates; and in still others, the comorbidity is not clearly accounted for by a known or suspected causative factor.

A number of psychiatric disorders have been commonly associated with ADHD in children and adults. Other disruptive behavior disorders, such as oppositional defiant disorder and conduct disorder, occur with a high frequency in children with ADHD, with as many as 30%–50% of children affected (Biederman et al. 1991). Anxiety and mood disorders co-occur with ADHD in some children and may affect the child's overall degree of impairment, the course of the disorder, and the necessary treatment plan (Jensen et al. 1993b). A high proportion of children with tic disorders also manifest symptoms of ADHD as well as other disorders, leading some to conclude that a genetic relationship may exist (Comings and Comings 1990). ADHD is being increasingly recognized in other populations of children with special needs such as those with mental retardation (Aman et al. 1991). In adolescents, residual symptoms of ADHD may be associated with conduct problems, substance abuse, and mood and anxiety disorders (Klein and Mannuzza 1991). Patterns of comorbidity in adults with ADHD may approximate those seen in the childhood disorder, which lends support to the validity of the diagnosis in adulthood (Biederman et al. 1993). A significant number of adults who abuse cocaine and seek treatment have histories of childhood ADHD, as well as other co-occurring present and past diagnoses (Hoegerman et al. 1993; Rounsaville et al. 1991).

Specific learning disorders have been associated with the diagnosis of ADHD in a subgroup of children (Cantwell and Baker 1991). In general and as a group, children with ADHD perform more poorly in educational settings than nonaffected children, even if they do not have a specific learning disorder (Faraone et al. 1993). However, an unrecognized learning disorder that is inappropriately attributed to the behavioral disturbance and left untreated, leading to unnecessary school failure, can have a detrimental effect on the child's overall functioning and self-esteem.

Evidence of minor neurological dysfunction is present in a subgroup of children with ADHD, which reinforces the concept that the disturbance represents subtle organic insults to the child's brain that impair psychological development and behavioral control (Mayes et al. 1994). Some studies support, and others refute, the association between ADHD and allergy-related disorders such as asthma, eczema, and hay fever, and the issue is currently unresolved (McGee et al. 1993; Roth et al. 1991).

Evaluation and Differential Diagnosis

Children with ADHD should receive a complete medical evaluation and examination. On occasion, a standard physical examination may reveal neurological problems that completely explain the child's inattentiveness, restlessness, and impulsivity; for example, in the sensory area, children with partial deafness or very poor vision may appear inattentive and restless to a teacher. Nonspecific signs found during a careful neurological evaluation, on the other hand, probably contribute little to the evaluation of children with ADHD. These nonspecific signs, including minor physical anomalies, have been referred to as *soft neurological signs* (Shaffer and Greenhill 1979). Soft signs present as asymmetries in reflex findings, minor choreoathetoid movements, an inability to carry out rapid alternating movements, and generally poor coordination. They are subject to intertest and interrater reliability problems. Their presence does not aid in making the diagnosis of ADHD (Shaffer and Greenhill 1979). In fact, an epidemiological study showed that these soft signs predict persistence of a higher-than-normal prevalence of anxiety disorders, not ADHD (Shaffer et al. 1985).

Some medical problems may lead to overactive and inattentive behavior. Language disorders will produce aberrant behavior and at times are associated with motor hyperactivity and severe inattentiveness. Dermatological conditions, such as eczema and even pinworms, may produce restlessness and disruptiveness in grade-school children and to the teacher may appear to be a pure behavior disorder. Even more rare, Sydenham's chorea generates intense restlessness in children and requires careful workup and treatment. Finally, as many as 50%–60% of patients ages 6–18 years with Tourette's disorder also may have ADHD (Cohen and Leckman 1989). Stimulants, which cause a release of catecholamines in the central nervous system, can exacerbate motor tics in these patients (Lowe et al. 1982), possibly by further intensifying the putative hyperdopaminergic state found in Tourette's disorder.

The child's height and weight should be measured before any treatment—particularly if the child will be given stimulant medication, which may cause a temporary delay in weight gain. Other tests, such as computed tomography or magnetic resonance imaging, have no current role in routine clinical evaluation.

Age-appropriate hyperactivity may occur in children who show no impulsive or attentional problems. The high level of activity found in ADHD differs from that of other clinical states by its intense, non–goal-directed quality. Children who have a comorbid Axis I diagnosis of conduct disorder will have all the features of ADHD, but their high propensity for aggressivity differs from the more typical behavior in a child with ADHD. The impulsivity of a child with conduct disorder has more of a calculating, premeditated

quality not found in the reactive and impulsive misbehaviors of the hyperactive child.

Children with other psychiatric disorders (such as severe and profound mental retardation, schizophrenia, and mania)—who may display impulsivity, hyperactivity, and inattentiveness—may display the chaotic, stimulus-bound motor drivenness of children with ADHD, but because the symptoms are secondary to the primary diagnosis, these children are not diagnosed with ADHD.

Epidemiology

Epidemiological surveys of disruptive behavior in children have produced somewhat confusing and conflicting information over the years. Most of the confusion is due to the nature of the diagnostic process used in the survey, as well as the varied samples studied. The most frequently cited epidemiological studies use different methodologies and examine somewhat different populations (see Scahill and Schwab-Stone 2000 for a comprehensive review). Disorder is variably defined by cutoffs on certain rating scales or by a categorical diagnosis based on structured or semistructured interviews of parents or teachers. These studies may or may not include information from children in the sample, depending on the age range. Because epidemiological literature has not yet been published on the DSM-IV-TR definition of the ADHD diagnosis, the closest approximation of this information is in studies that have attempted to diagnose the disorder based on earlier DSM definitions by using objective criteria elicited from multiple sources.

Based on published studies in which investigators have attempted to diagnose ADHD by DSM criteria, the prevalence rate ranges from 1.9% to 14.4% (Scahill and Schwab-Stone 2000). The prevalence reported in DSM-IV-TR is the frequently cited estimate of 3%–7% of school-age children. It is commonly accepted that the disorder is more common in boys than in girls, at a ratio ranging from 2.5:1 to 5.6:1. ADHD is most common in school-age children, and prevalence rates are lower in studies of older populations (McGee et al. 1990). Rates of the disorder may vary in different cultures and countries (Verhulst et al. 1993) and depending on whether the sample studied is urban, suburban, or rural (Shen et al. 1985; Zahner et al. 1993).

Etiology

No clear etiological variable appears to lead to all, or even most, cases of ADHD. The precise cause of the disorder is unknown. A number of biological and environmental correlates have been implicated as being important in individual cases and groups of children with ADHD.

■ Genetics

ADHD is certainly a familial disorder and is likely to have a genetic component. Gene knockout strategies (i.e., eliminating the gene coding for the dopamine transport protein) have produced mice strains with high levels of behavioral hyperactivity (Gainetdinov and Caron 2001), suggesting a role for behavioral genetics in understanding important features of the disorder. Symptoms of the disorder are more highly correlated in identical than in fraternal twin pairs (Goodman and Stevenson 1989). Adoption studies have confirmed that ADHD tends to occur more frequently in first-degree biological relatives of adopted probands than in families in which adopted probands cohabitate (Hechtman 1994). Several studies have reported that relatives of proband children with ADHD have a higher likelihood to have the disorder than do relatives of comparison children without ADHD (Biederman et al. 1990), and this appears to be true for girls as well as boys (Faraone et al. 1991). Offspring of adults who have a history of childhood-onset ADHD are at high risk for the development of the disorder (Biederman et al. 1995). Increasing interest in genes expressing gene products related to the functioning of dopamine in the central nervous system has been stimulated by reports supporting the association of the 7-repeat allele of the D_4 dopamine receptor with the ADHD diagnosis in some but not all studies (Faraone et al. 2001). Some authors (Sprich-Buckminster et al. 1993) have suggested that familial and nonfamilial subtypes of ADHD exist, with the familial subtype being accounted for by mostly genetic mechanisms and the nonfamilial subtype caused by environmentally induced circumstances, such as perinatal complications. In summary, abnormalities in genes coding for proteins involved in central nervous system dopamine function have been implicated in a preliminary fashion in the etiology of ADHD, but definitive replications are currently lacking. Identifying genetic polymorphisms that convey an elevated risk for ADHD in children remains an area of intense research interest.

■ Perinatal Complications

The concept that perinatal complications may have an etiological role in ADHD comes from two main areas of investigation. In animal-model studies of infant rats (Speiser et al. 1983) and monkeys (Sechzer et al. 1973) asphyxiated at or near birth, overactivity and attentional problems in exposed organisms were reported, but the correlation with human behavior is speculative. Retrospective human studies that compared individuals with a diagnosis of ADHD with children without such a diagnosis found that perinatal complications (e.g., antepartum hemorrhage, prolonged maternal labor, low Apgar scores at 1 minute) had occurred more frequently in affected than in nonaffected subjects (Chandola et al. 1992). Maternal smoking during pregnancy appears to be a risk factor for the development of ADHD in offspring (Milberger et al. 1997). Infants with low birth weight and manifesting evidence of white matter injury may be at increased risk for the development of ADHD over time as well (Whitaker et al. 1997).

■ Neurological Illness

Investigators have continued to study the role of neurological problems in the etiology of ADHD, including soft signs of neurological illness (Vitiello et al. 1990), poor motor coordination, and subtle signs of abnormal brain function (Ornoy et al. 1993). The term formerly used to describe this disorder, *minimal brain dysfunction*, seemed to derive from this particular aspect in these children. Recent reports of the onset of ADHD syndromes after closed head trauma support the role of organic factors in the etiology of the disorder. An uncontrolled, prospective follow-up study of children who had been afflicted with septic meningitis found that a high percentage of children had developed ADHD (Alon et al. 1979), lending support to the idea that early insult to the central nervous system may increase the risk for ADHD. Recent anatomical neuroimaging studies have supported the concept that the brains of children with ADHD are different, if perhaps in subtle ways, from those of children without ADHD and that the structural abnormalities may be correlated to neuropsychological deficits (Casey et al. 1997; Castellanos et al. 2001; Semrud-Clikeman et al. 2000). Loss of the normal asymmetry of the caudate nucleus and regional abnormalities in the architecture of the corpus callosum have been identified (Castellanos et al. 1994; Giedd et al. 1994; Hynd et al. 1993) and may serve as markers of the disorder in at least a subgroup of children. Functional neuroimaging studies, using functional magnetic resonance imaging and positron emission tomography, have been performed in adults (Matochik et al. 1993), adolescents (Ernst et al. 1997; Rubia et al. 1999; Zametkin et al. 1993) and children (Ernst et al. 1999) with ADHD. Although the results have been equivocal, findings have suggested that subjects with ADHD may show abnormalities in prefrontal cortex function (Rubia et al. 1999) and disturbed central nervous system dopaminergic activity (Ernst et al. 1999). Animal models of neuronal hypoplasia, induced generally by exposure to chemical agents or locally by focal X-irradiation (Diaz-Granados et al. 1994; Mercugliano et al. 1990; Shaywitz et al. 1976), have produced individual organisms that manifest many behavioral similarities to human hyperactivity and inattentiveness (Altman 1987).

Diet

The role of diet in the onset or exacerbation of hyperactivity and behavioral problems remains somewhat controversial, because evidence exists both to support and to refute the effects of different dietary agents (Barling and Bullen 1985; Egger et al. 1992; Rowe and Rowe 1994). The studies that support the notion that diet influences behavioral problems have focused on the roles of sugar, preservatives, and artificial dyes and on food allergies. Despite the fact that dietary factors most likely do not play a role in the vast majority of children with ADHD, evidence indicates that teachers frequently believe that diet influences children with behavior disorders and will counsel parents to restrict suspected offending agents as a means of helping their child (DiBattista and Shepherd 1993).

Allergy

The idea that children with allergies or allergic-type illnesses (e.g., asthma, eczema) are at greater risk for developing ADHD does not appear to be supported by current evidence (Biederman et al. 1994; McGee et al. 1993; Roth et al. 1991).

Environmental Toxins

The role of exposure to toxins (e.g., heavy metals, illicit drugs, alcohol) prenatally or postnatally is currently speculative, although children and animals exposed to lead toxicity (Minder et al. 1994; Sobotka and Cook 1974) or prenatal alcohol use by mothers (Streissguth et al. 1994) can manifest many symptoms of hyperactivity and attentional problems during development.

Other Pediatric Illnesses

Although a study reporting on the increased incidence of ADHD in individuals with a genetically transmitted, generalized resistance to thyroid hormone may be describing a highly biologically determined subtype of the disorder (Hauser et al. 1993), the rate of thyroid abnormalities in clinically referred children with ADHD is very low (Elia et al. 1994). Routine screening with thyroid function tests of children with ADHD is not currently recommended in the absence of other indicators of thyroid disease. The symptoms of ADHD may be increased in children with histories of other medical illnesses, such as recurrent early childhood ear infections (Adesman et al. 1990; Arcia and Roberts 1993; Hagerman and Falkenstein 1987) and acquired sensorineural hearing loss (Kelly et al. 1993).

Natural History

We discuss three factors in the natural history of ADHD: the age at onset, the clinical presentation, and the duration of the disorder. We discuss long-term outcome of the disorder at the end of this chapter. It should be noted that data are limited in each of these domains.

Age at Onset

Estimates of the age at onset in any individual case are often difficult to determine in a research study or a clinical assessment (see Barkley and Biederman 1997 for a thorough discussion of this issue). Most studies of clinical populations (Sullivan et al. 1990), as well as prevalence-focused epidemiological studies (McGee et al. 1992), can provide only estimates of age at onset based on retrospective reports of the child or parent, and studies may or may not attempt to validate this estimate by collecting information from different sources, such as physician records or school reports. Large-scale prospective epidemiological studies of the general population can provide more accurate estimates of age at onset of the disorder if observations of children begin at a very early age and if diagnostic assessments are repeated at regularly spaced intervals. Parents' reports of the onset of their child's behavioral problems appear to be stable over time and may have good reliability (Green et al. 1991). Children have little capacity to provide reasonable estimates of the onset of the disorder, although retrospective assessments of the patients' own behavior may be the clinical standard for diagnosing ADHD in adults (Ward et al. 1993). It is generally understood that the roots of the disorder (according to the DSM-IV-TR definition) begin in early childhood, with at least some symptoms being present before age 7 years, but this may be more true in children with prominent hyperactivity as opposed to the inattentive subtype of the disorder (Applegate et al. 1997). With the increased use of preschool and day-care services for children, the behavior disorders of this age group may be attracting more clinical attention, and treatment of disruptive behavior disorders in this age group has become a focus of additional research (DuPaul et al. 2001; Lahey et al. 1998; McGee et al. 1991; Palfrey et al. 1985; Strayhorn and Weidman 1989).

■ Clinical Presentation

The typical clinical referral comes to the attention of mental health providers as a result of disruptive behavior at home or in a structured setting, such as school, or because of academic failure. It is clear that not all persons in the general population who meet criteria for ADHD come to clinical attention and that those who do present for clinical attention may be different from community cases in the population at large (Bird et al. 1993). Often before eventual referral to a mental health specialist, parents of children with ADHD may seek intervention for their child from their pediatrician, from their family doctor, from personnel at the child's school, or from clergy members. There is evidence that stimulant therapy in the United States is routinely prescribed by primary care physicians and pediatricians as well as by child psychiatrists (Hoagwood et al. 2000). It is likely that patients presenting to mental health clinicians may have ADHD that has particularly severe symptoms, is more highly associated with comorbid clinical conditions, or is more refractory to conventional therapies than ADHD that is described in community-based epidemiological studies.

■ Duration of Disorder

In general, several studies suggest that some symptoms of ADHD—particularly hyperactivity—tend toward re-

mission over time but that inattention problems are remarkably persistent and intractable (for example, see Biederman et al. 2000). The disorder generally is not thought to be episodic but rather chronic and enduring (Keller et al. 1992) and has been likened to other developmental disorders with their onset in childhood. Prospective studies of clinical samples report that at least some impairment from the disorder is present in most adolescents who had been referred for clinical treatment as school-age children (Barkley et al. 1991; Gittelman et al. 1985). Follow-up studies of referred cohorts (and control subjects) into adulthood report that impairment persists in a sizable percentage of patients and that complications of the disorder include lower academic and professional achievement and an increased risk for developing antisocial behavior and possibly substance abuse (Klein and Mannuzza 1991). Some studies suggest that there may be different outcomes for the different symptom cores: that inattention-spectrum symptoms tend to predict problems with educational achievement, but prominent hyperactivity and impulsivity symptoms may place a child at greater risk for the development of antisocial outcomes (for example, see Babinski et al. 1999). Sufficient evidence does not yet exist to suggest that treatment interventions unequivocally aid in preventing adverse long-term outcomes.

Treatment

The body of research literature devoted to the treatment of ADHD in children exceeds that of any other diagnosis in child psychiatry. With the recent publication of the main intent-to-treat results of the National Institute of Mental Health–funded multisite Multimodal Treatment of ADHD (MTA) study (MTA Cooperative Group 1999), clearer guidelines about the central role of medication treatment are now available. Less clear is the role of psychotherapy and other psychosocial interventions as components of treatment plans for individual children with the disorder.

■ Medication

Psychostimulants

The psychostimulants are the first-line agents of choice for symptom suppression. Methylphenidate, amphetamine preparations, and magnesium pemoline have all demonstrated efficacy in double-blind, placebo-controlled studies of children with ADHD, and the literature reporting the efficacy of the use of these agents in children and adults is expanding (Greenhill et al. 1999; Spencer et al. 1996). Methylphenidate tends to be the most popular drug of first choice, although whether it has greater efficacy or safety compared with other stimulants has not been proved.

Methylphenidate is a short-acting agent that, in its unmodified form, generally requires multiple daily dosing. The duration of symptom suppression in responsive children ranges from 1 to 4 hours, with an average of 2 or 3 hours (Srinivas et al. 1992). Delivery of the medication on a daily basis is generally timed to match the child's schedule when peak demands are placed on behavioral control and ability to pay attention, which, for a child, is during school hours. Administering the medication shortly after breakfast, after lunch, and during the late afternoon often provides good coverage of symptoms and minimizes the most common side effects of appetite suppression and insomnia. Because the medication is rapidly eliminated by the body's metabolizing capacity, "rebound" periods of exacerbation of symptoms before the next dose are possible. At times, this exacerbation of symptoms is problematic and requires more frequent dosing or the use of long-acting methylphenidate preparations (Birmaher et al. 1989). In children of normal weight, it is usually recommended to begin the medication at a dosage of 5 mg two or three times a day and to increase the dosage every 3 days until therapeutic effects are sufficient. The limiting factor related to maximal dosage is generally untoward side effects, although the *Physicians' Desk Reference* (2001) recommends that doses greater than 60 mg/day not be exceeded in children. Longer-acting preparations are also available that have incorporated a variety of drug delivery systems to maintain effective drug dosing and symptom control throughout the course of a day.

Dextroamphetamine is the amphetamine agent that until recently was most often used in the treatment of ADHD. Currently short-acting and longer-acting preparations of Adderall, which consists of a mixture of amphetamine salts, are also available for use with patients with ADHD. Short-acting amphetamine preparations probably have a somewhat longer half-life and duration of action than short-acting methylphenidate in children with ADHD, but multiple daily dosing remains essential for all short-acting stimulant

preparations. The efficacy rates and side-effect profile reported by most research studies are generally equivalent to those seen in studies of methylphenidate (Greenhill et al. 1999). The starting dosage is generally 2.5–5 mg twice a day, and the dosage is gradually increased until the desired clinical effects are obtained. The medication is approved for children as young as 3 years. Dosages exceeding 40 mg/day are rarely needed. As is the case with methylphenidate, longer-acting preparations of dextroamphetamine and Adderall are available for clinical use and may eliminate the need to administer an in-school dose for many children.

Magnesium pemoline has been less well studied than the other two more frequently used stimulants, but it appears to be effective in children with symptoms of ADHD (Conners and Taylor 1980) and can be used in patients whose conditions do not respond to other stimulants. It has been known to cause liver toxicity rarely (Pratt and Dubois 1990), and routine assessment of liver function tests before and during treatment is necessary. It has been clinically recognized that the onset of therapeutic effect may be delayed for a few weeks after initiation of pemoline therapy, which is unlike treatment with the other stimulants; however, this finding has been challenged in a pharmacokinetic/pharmacodynamic study (Sallee et al. 1992). Pemoline is a longer-acting agent and may need to reach a steady-state serum level for maximum effects. It can be given once a day, with a usual starting dose of 37.5 mg, advancing in increments of 18.75 mg every 3–5 days until the desired clinical benefit is observed.

Side effects of stimulant medications include appetite suppression, weight loss, sleep problems, irritability, headache, stomach ache, skin picking, rash, and occasional association with the development (or exacerbation) of tics. Although psychostimulants may lead to time-limited delay of growth in some children, no long-term adverse effects on growth or achievement of final adult height are apparent (Klein and Mannuzza 1988). Children treated with psychostimulants generally achieve their predicted adult size if they are followed up into adulthood. However, it is common in children treated with stimulants to allow drug holidays during vacations or weekends if the behavioral problems tend to be more severe and compromising in a school setting and the parents feel that a temporary drug-free state will not adversely affect the child or the family. Weekend drug holidays can free the child from the appetite-suppressant effects of the stimulants and can lead to increased calorie consumption on weekends, which prevents unwanted weight loss or delayed weight gain. Holidays from drugs in the summer or during vacations can also help the clinician to assess the degree of persistence of the symptoms by observing a drug-free state and can provide useful information about the need for continuing treatment with medication.

In general, based on the results of numerous controlled trials, approximately 70%–75% of children with ADHD are expected to benefit from initiation of treatment with stimulant medication (Greenhill et al. 1999). When treatment with one stimulant results in insufficient benefit, treatment with the other stimulants should be attempted before changing to a different class of medication. It has been reported that as many as 90% of children will respond to treatment with either methylphenidate or dextroamphetamine (Elia et al. 1991). Nevertheless, because of the high prevalence of ADHD in the population, many children with ADHD will require other treatments.

Tricyclic Antidepressants

Tricyclic antidepressants are considered a second-line agent in the treatment of ADHD. Of the tricyclics, research supports the effectiveness of two agents in particular—imipramine and desipramine (Biederman et al. 1989a; Cox 1982; Gross 1973; Pliszka 1987)—and suggests the usefulness of a third—nortriptyline (Wilens et al. 1993a)—in treatment of the disorder. Tricyclics have been tested in patients who previously have not been offered medication treatment as well as in individuals who have responded poorly to psychostimulant trials (Biederman et al. 1989a). In general, tricyclic antidepressants appear to be well tolerated by most children and adolescents who take them for ADHD and other indications (enuresis, depression), although benign effects on heart rate and blood pressure have been seen in some groups of children (Biederman et al. 1989b; Wilens et al. 1993b). There has been concern about the safety of the use of desipramine in children, based on the occurrence of sudden death associated with treatment in a small number of children (Riddle et al. 1993). The exact nature of the association is currently unclear. Explanations that have been proposed range from chance occurrence to a heightened cardiotoxicity of the medication to the hearts of young patients (Walsh et al. 1994). In any event, caution is warranted in patients who develop

significant cardiovascular symptoms or changes in electrocardiographic parameters during the course of treatment. Younger patients appear to metabolize these agents more efficiently than do adults and may require twice- or three-times-a-day dosing to achieve maximal clinical benefit, as opposed to the once-a-day dosing that is often effective in adults.

Other Medications

Alpha-adrenergic agonists.   The use of clonidine (and the related agent guanfacine) for symptoms of ADHD has some scientific support, but because of the lack of replicated double-blind, placebo-controlled trials, α-adrenergic agonists are currently considered third-line agents. Alpha-adrenergic agents have been used in patients with ADHD alone or as an adjunct to stimulants for associated aggression or stimulant-induced sleep disturbance (Connor et al. 1999; Prince et al. 1996). They also appear to have efficacy in treating the symptoms of ADHD and tics in children with the comorbid diagnosis of Tourette's disorder (Scahill et al. 2001; Steingard et al. 1993). The most notable side effects include drowsiness and drug-induced hypotension. Clonidine should be slowly tapered during discontinuation because rebound hypertension may occur if it is suddenly discontinued in patients who have been taking significant doses for a prolonged time.

Other antidepressants.   Bupropion has shown some promise in the treatment of ADHD in children and adults (Barrickman et al. 1995; Conners et al. 1996; Wender and Reimherr 1990; Wilens et al. 2001), although it may worsen tics in children with tic disorder (Spencer et al. 1993). Fluoxetine may be effective in some patients with treatment-refractory ADHD, although placebo-controlled trials are lacking (Barrickman et al. 1991). The role of monoamine oxidase inhibitors has scientific support (Zametkin et al. 1985), but their use also carries the risk of hypertensive crisis if dietary compliance cannot be guaranteed by the parents of the child.

Caffeine.   Caffeine appears to effectively reduce some symptoms of ADHD, but its role in the management of clinical cases, as opposed to its effectiveness in research studies, is unclear (Arnold et al. 1978; Garfinkel et al. 1975; Schechter and Timmons 1985).

Antipsychotics.   Antipsychotics appear to be effective in controlling some manifestations of ADHD in children, but the risk of neurological side effects with long-term treatment precludes the use of these medications except in severely ill patients who have not responded to other interventions.

■ Psychosocial Interventions

Psychosocial treatments are also commonly used in the treatment of ADHD. Three main modalities of treatment are individual psychotherapeutic interventions with the child who has the disorder, strategic educational interventions, and family approaches to altering the child's disruptive behavior pattern.

Individual Psychotherapy

Targeting the child as the focus of attention through psychological intervention has some support from scientific studies (Whalen and Henker 1991). There have been empirical trials of behavior therapy and cognitive therapy (Abikoff and Gittelman 1984; Brown et al. 1986; Fehlings et al. 1991). In general, behavior therapy techniques seem to have a higher success rate than do cognitive interventions in the reduction of symptoms of ADHD. Controlled trials of psychodynamic psychotherapy are not available, although one series of studies reported that insight-oriented psychotherapy appears to be less effective as a treatment for children and adolescents with disruptive behavior disorders than for those with more emotionally based symptoms (Fonagy and Target 1994).

Behavior therapy attempts to deliver consistent targeted behavioral contingencies that reinforce desired positive behaviors and extinguish negative unwanted behaviors. Positive reinforcement is delivered when the child is attending appropriately, is keeping on task, and is maintaining some degree of control over hyperactivity and impulsivity. Some therapists recommend the judicious and consistent use of "response cost" and punishment techniques, including "time-out" and loss of positive reinforcements, as necessary to reduce ingrained disruptive behaviors, such as aggression and oppositional defiance. Behavior therapy techniques have been used both in children taking medication and in those not taking medication. One problem with applying behavioral techniques in an individual psychotherapy format is that the therapist generally will not be present in the contexts where the problematic behavior is most likely to occur—namely, at home or at school. Therefore, attempts have been made to edu-

cate teachers and parents to use behavior management with the child directly in the environment of the classroom and at home. In effect, the parent and teacher may become surrogate behavior therapists. The role of the professional psychotherapist in this situation is to teach and supervise the use of the techniques by the teacher and parent and to monitor the efficacy of the therapy in helping the child.

Educational Interventions

The academic risk for the child with ADHD is significant (Frick et al. 1991). School performance and achievement in children with ADHD are generally significantly worse than in nonaffected children (Faraone et al. 1993). Behavioral problems may cause poor academic performance and recurrent conflicts with teachers and school administrators. Learning disabilities also appear to co-occur with ADHD at an increased rate compared with children without ADHD (Semrud-Clikeman et al. 1992). Psychological testing can be beneficial in determining learning potential and cognitive strengths, as well as in identifying specific learning disorders. With appropriate intervention, children with uncomplicated forms of ADHD can usually be educated in regular mainstream classrooms. Appropriate medication treatment may occasionally normalize the child's behavior to such a degree that no supplementary educational intervention may be necessary (Abikoff and Gittelman 1985b). Classroom behavior management techniques may be of additional benefit with children who have persistent symptoms, children who are not taking medications, or children who have comorbid oppositional behavior or conduct disturbances. Some children who cannot be educated in classrooms with a large student-to-teacher ratio may require special classrooms.

Intensive summer treatment programs (essentially summer day camps for children with ADHD) have been promoted as beneficial therapeutic interventions whereby focused treatment strategies can be applied over several weeks to modify the child's behavior (Pelham et al. 1993). Usually, these programs incorporate classroom time and structured recreational activities to create a school-like atmosphere in which the efficacy of the introduction of a behavior management program can be monitored and measured. The benefits of such a summer treatment program can presumably be enhanced if program personnel can directly link therapeutic strategies established in the summer to the child's educational setting in the following fall. In some programs, this is accomplished by having counselors from the summer program work directly in the classroom for a period during the following school year to help educational staff members work with the individual child in a therapeutic fashion.

Family Interventions

The parental relationships with children with ADHD are often negative and permeated with frustrations (Befera and Barkley 1985). This does not necessarily mean that the adults lack parenting skills, because their relationships with siblings who do not have ADHD may be more appropriate and positive (Tarver-Behring et al. 1985). Children with ADHD may require more specialized parenting skills than do nonaffected children. Although different family interventions have been used in the treatment of ADHD in children, parent training is the most common approach and, until the recent findings of the MTA study were made available, had received increasing support from the scientific literature (Anastopoulos et al. 1993) as an effective approach to intervention. Essentially, the parents are taught the techniques of sophisticated behavior therapy to be used with their children (Strayhorn and Weidman 1989). The therapist arranges individual or group meetings with the parents, supplemented by readings and homework. Treatment plans are developed with child-oriented positive reinforcements and response cost contingencies.

■ Multimodality Treatment and the NIMH MTA Study

Although it would seem logical that combined treatments would improve the treatment plan of the child with ADHD (Whalen and Henker 1991), this is not necessarily supported by the scientific literature. It appears that a subgroup of children treated with medication may actually normalize in terms of their observable behavior and functioning (Abikoff and Gittelman 1985b), and the additional benefit provided by psychosocial interventions with these children is minimal. Multimodality treatment has been theorized to be of particular benefit for children who do not normalize with medication or who have comorbid disorders.

The MTA study randomly assigned children ages 7–9 years with DSM-IV ADHD (combined subtype), with and without comorbid disorders, to either

1) algorithmic medication treatment (mainly relying on psychostimulants), 2) a comprehensive psychosocial treatment package (parent training, intensive summer treatment program, and school consultation), 3) the combined psychosocial package and algorithmic medication treatment, or 4) community referral as a control group. Treatments in the four study arms were delivered over the course of 14 months. Children randomized to the medication treatment arms overall had significantly improved outcomes compared with children receiving psychosocial treatment alone or those referred out for community care. The role of psychosocial interventions delivered in combination with medication treatment may be of questionable benefit, since the results of this study also suggest that subjects receiving the combination medication and psychosocial treatment fared little better in general than subjects receiving medication treatment alone. In secondary analyses of the MTA data, there was some evidence suggesting that using alternative definitions of treatment response may support a statistically significant better response to combination therapy than relying solely on medication treatment strategies (Conners et al. 2001; Swanson et al. 2001), but overall the advantage of combination therapy over medication treatment alone was small. This historic study provides important evidence of the strong treatment effect of well-delivered pharmacotherapy and some evidence that combination treatment may benefit some patients. The study refutes any ideas that an intensive psychosocial treatment package provides therapeutic effects equivalent to medication treatment for children with the combined subtype of ADHD and suggests that medication treatment should be considered first-line therapy in these children.

■ General Rules for Successful Management

Practice parameters for children and adolescents with ADHD are currently available (American Academy of Child and Adolescent Psychiatry 1997). The best management of the many needs of children with ADHD is through the assembly of a multidisciplinary team, consisting of the child, the parents, a medical doctor, a psychologist, a social worker, and an educational specialist. The professionals on the team may be practitioners in separate offices, with referrals alternating among colleagues, or in group practice settings.

The use of medication intervention strategies for all patients with ADHD should be seriously considered as a first-line intervention and should be discussed with parents. If medications are incorporated into the treatment plan, then certain approaches can be helpful. On completion of the evaluation of the child, it is often best to set a meeting with parents to present the results of the evaluation and for psychoeducational counseling. An open discussion of the benefits and risks of the various treatment options, including medication strategies, should be included. If a medication trial is recommended and is agreed to by the parents, it is optimal to plan a trial that will allow for an eventual once-a-day dosing regimen. Regular contact with school personnel is absolutely essential to collect information about the child's behavior and academic progress as well as the evaluation by the school personnel of the child's response to the medication trial. Once a satisfactory acute response is obtained, medication treatment is best maintained as tolerated for several months to allow the child to consolidate gains made in terms of behavioral control and academic achievement. Intermittent drug holidays can be used once or twice a year to evaluate the need for continued medication treatment. Tutoring may be necessary to teach compensatory skills to children with learning difficulties. Clinicians should see children on a once-weekly (during titration) to once-monthly (during maintenance) schedule during treatment. The use of psychosocial interventions—such as parent training, school interventions, intensive summer treatment programs, and individual therapy—above and beyond common-sense parenting advice and communication with the educational system may best be held in reserve pending the outcome of the medication trial and may be of more benefit for children with comorbid externalizing or internalizing disorders.

Long-Term Outcome

The outcome studies available are, for the most part, based on follow-up of clinically referred samples, generally males, who may have a particularly severe form of the disorder and may have more associated comorbid conditions. Multiple studies have found that the disorder persists into adolescence and adulthood in a substantial proportion of patients, and conduct disorder develops in 25%–50% (Babinski et al. 1999; Barkley et al. 1991; Biederman et al. 1996; Gittelman et al. 1985; Hechtman 1991; Lie 1992; Mannuzza et al. 1998;

McGee et al. 1991). Compared with control subjects without ADHD, children with ADHD followed up into adulthood show higher rates of antisocial behavior and residual symptoms of ADHD, although the percentage of patients meeting full criteria for ADHD may be low. An increased risk of substance use disorders has been reported in some studies, and the substance use will generally follow (not precede) the onset of antisocial behavior (Gittelman et al. 1985).

It can be expected that in a minority of children, after clinical referral and proper diagnosis, the disorder will remit by adolescence, but the majority of cases will remit at least partially by adulthood. As a group, children with ADHD can be expected to have a more negative outcome as they grow up than children without the disorder, showing higher rates of criminal activity, incarceration, and substance abuse, particularly in the subgroup who develop antisocial personality disorder (Mannuzza et al. 1993). On an individual basis, however, it is difficult to forecast the future for a child with ADHD. Clear predictors of negative outcome in children with the disorder, other than the onset of conduct disorder or antisocial personality disorder (Satterfield et al. 1994), have not been identified (Fischer et al. 1993). Little information about the course of the disorder specifically in females is available.

Conclusion

ADHD maintains its central position in psychiatry as a leading cause of problems for children and adolescents. It is a complex syndrome that is best understood, researched, and treated within a biopsychosocial model. Underlying biological abnormalities appear to exist at least in a subgroup of these patients, and with the application of more sophisticated functional neuroimaging and other technologies, the biology of the disorder likely will be better understood in the years to come. The psychological manifestations of the disorder cause major problems for patients and lead to difficulties with interpersonal relationships and academic and vocational performance and often a loss of self-worth and self-esteem. Socially, these children are often stigmatized by the symptoms of the disorder and ostracized by peers and family members. However, clinical and research experience with these patients continues to grow. A clinician can confidently state to a parent and the patient that effective treatments are now available. At this point, medication treatment is clearly established as effective in terms of suppressing the core symptoms of the disorder in the short and the middle term, and in general it appears that psychostimulant medication is safe and well tolerated by the majority of patients. What is necessary in the future is to better understand subgroups of patients, distinguished by associated conditions or various etiological subtypes of the disorder, and to learn to predict how these patients differ in terms of the natural history of their symptoms and associated morbidity. Eventually it may be possible to understand the role of treatment interventions in affecting the long-term outcomes of large numbers of patients.

References

Abikoff H, Gittelman R: Does behavior therapy normalize the classroom behavior of hyperactive children? Arch Gen Psychiatry 41:449–454, 1984

Abikoff H, Gittelman R: Hyperactive children treated with stimulants: is cognitive training a useful adjunct? Arch Gen Psychiatry 42:953–961, 1985a

Abikoff H, Gittelman R: The normalizing effects of methylphenidate on the classroom behavior of ADHD children. J Abnorm Child Psychol 13:33–44, 1985b

Abikoff H, Courtney M, Pelham WEJ, et al: Teachers' ratings of disruptive behaviors: the influence of halo effects. J Abnorm Child Psychol 21:519–533, 1993

Achenbach TM: Manual for the Child Behavior Checklist/4–18 and 1991 Profile. Burlington, VT, University of Vermont Department of Psychiatry, 1991

Achenbach TM, Edelbrock CS: Manual of the Child Behavior Checklist and Revised Child Behavior Profile. Burlington, VT, University of Vermont, Department of Psychiatry, 1983

Adesman AR, Altshuler LA, Lipkin PH, et al: Otitis media in children with learning disabilities and in children with attention deficit disorder with hyperactivity. Pediatrics 85:442–446, 1990

Alon U, Naveh Y, Gardos M, et al: Neurological sequelae of septic meningitis: a follow-up study of 65 children. Isr J Med Sci 15:512–517, 1979

Altman J: Morphological and behavioral markers of environmentally induced retardation of brain development: an animal model. Environ Health Perspect 74:153–168, 1987

Aman MG, Marks RE, Turbott SH, et al: Clinical effects of methylphenidate and thioridazine in intellectually subaverage children. J Am Acad Child Adolesc Psychiatry 30:246–256, 1991

American Psychiatric Association: Diagnostic and Statistical Manual of Mental Disorders, 4th Edition, Text Revision. Washington, DC, American Psychiatric Association, 2000

Anastopoulos AD, Shelton TL, DuPaul GJ, et al: Parent training for attention-deficit hyperactivity disorder: its impact on parent functioning. J Abnorm Child Psychol 21:581–596, 1993

Applegate B, Lahey BB, Hart EL, et al: Validity of the age-of-onset criterion for ADHD: a report from the DSM-IV field trials. J Am Acad Child Adolesc Psychiatry 36:1211–1221, 1997

Arcia E, Roberts JE: Otitis media in early childhood and its association with sustained attention in structured situations. J Dev Behav Pediatr 14:181–183, 1993

Arnold LE, Christopher J, Huestis R, et al: Methylphenidate vs dextroamphetamine vs caffeine in minimal brain dysfunction: controlled comparison by placebo washout design with Bayes' analysis. Arch Gen Psychiatry 35:463–473, 1978

Babinski LM, Hartsough CS, Lambert NM: Childhood conduct problems, hyperactivity-impulsivity, and inattention as predictors of adult criminal activity. J Child Psychol Psychiatry 40:347–355, 1999

Barkley RA: Hyperactive Children: A Handbook for Diagnosis and Treatment. New York, Guilford, 1982

Barkley RA: The ecological validity of laboratory and analogue assessment methods of ADHD symptoms. J Abnorm Child Psychol 19:149–178, 1991

Barkley RA, Biederman J: Toward a broader definition of the age-of-onset criterion for attention-deficit hyperactivity disorder. J Am Acad Child Adolesc Psychiatry 36:1204–1210, 1997

Barkley RA, Fischer M, Edelbrock C, et al: The adolescent outcome of hyperactive children diagnosed by research criteria, III: mother-child interactions, family conflicts and maternal psychopathology. J Child Psychol Psychiatry 32:233–255, 1991

Barling J, Bullen G: Dietary factors and hyperactivity: a failure to replicate. J Genet Psychol 146:117–123, 1985

Barrickman L, Noyes R, Kuperman S, et al: Treatment of ADHD with fluoxetine: a preliminary trial. J Am Acad Child Adolesc Psychiatry 30:762–767, 1991

Barrickman LL, Perry PJ, Allen AJ, et al: Bupropion versus methylphenidate in the treatment of attention-deficit hyperactivity disorder. J Am Acad Child Adolesc Psychiatry 34:649–657, 1995

Befera MS, Barkley RA: Hyperactive and normal girls and boys: mother-child interaction, parent psychiatric status and child psychopathology. J Child Psychol Psychiatry 26:439–452, 1985

Biederman J, Baldessarini RJ, Wright V, et al: A double-blind placebo controlled study of desipramine in the treatment of ADD, I: efficacy. J Am Acad Child Adolesc Psychiatry 28:777–784, 1989a

Biederman J, Baldessarini RJ, Wright V, et al: A double-blind placebo controlled study of desipramine in the treatment of ADD, II: serum drug levels and cardiovascular findings. J Am Acad Child Adolesc Psychiatry 28:903–911, 1989b

Biederman J, Faraone SV, Keenan K, et al: Family genetic and psychosocial risk factors in DSM-III attention deficit disorder. J Am Acad Child Adolesc Psychiatry 29:526–533, 1990

Biederman J, Newcorn J, Sprich S: Comorbidity of attention deficit hyperactivity disorder with conduct, depressive, anxiety, and other disorders. Am J Psychiatry 148:564–577, 1991

Biederman J, Faraone SV, Milberger S, et al: Diagnoses of attention-deficit hyperactivity disorder from parent reports predict diagnoses based on teacher reports. J Am Acad Child Adolesc Psychiatry 32:315–317, 1993

Biederman J, Milberger S, Faraone SV, et al: Associations between childhood asthma and ADHD: issues of psychiatric comorbidity and familiality. J Am Acad Child Adolesc Psychiatry 33:842–848, 1994

Biederman J, Faraone SV, Mick E, et al: High risk for attention deficit hyperactivity disorder among children of parents with childhood onset of the disorder: a pilot study. Am J Psychiatry 152:431–435, 1995

Biederman J, Faraone S, Milberger S, et al: A prospective 4-year follow-up study of attention-deficit hyperactivity and related disorders. Arch Gen Psychiatry 53:437–446, 1996

Biederman J, Mick E, Faraone SV: Age-dependent decline of symptoms of attention deficit hyperactivity disorder: impact of remission definition and symptom type. Am J Psychiatry 157:816–818, 2000

Bird HR, Gould MS, Staghezza B: Aggregating data from multiple informants in child psychiatry epidemiological research. J Am Acad Child Adolesc Psychiatry 31:78–85, 1992

Bird HR, Gould MS, Staghezza BM: Patterns of diagnostic comorbidity in a community sample of children aged 9 through 16 years. J Am Acad Child Adolesc Psychiatry 32:361–368, 1993

Birmaher B, Greenhill LL, Cooper TB, et al: Sustained release methylphenidate: pharmacokinetic studies in ADHD males. J Am Acad Child Adolesc Psychiatry 28:768–772, 1989

Brown RT, Wynne ME, Borden KA, et al: Methylphenidate and cognitive therapy in children with attention deficit disorder: a double-blind trial. J Dev Behav Pediatr 7:163–174, 1986

Cantwell DP, Baker L: Association between attention deficit–hyperactivity disorder and learning disorders. J Learn Disabil 24:88–95, 1991

Carlson C, Lahey BB, Neeper R: Direct assessment of the cognitive correlates of attention deficit disorders with and without hyperactivity. Journal of Psychopathology and Behavioral Assessment 8:69–86, 1986

Casey BJ, Castellanos FX, Giedd JN, et al: Implication of right frontostriatal circuitry in response inhibition and attention-deficit/hyperactivity disorder. J Am Acad Child Adolesc Psychiatry 36:374–383, 1997

Castellanos FX, Giedd JN, Eckburg P, et al: Quantitative morphology of the caudate nucleus in attention deficit hyperactivity disorder. Am J Psychiatry 151:1791–1796, 1994

Castellanos FX, Giedd JN, Berquin PC, et al: Quantitative brain magnetic resonance imaging in girls with attention-deficit/hyperactivity disorder. Arch Gen Psychiatry 58:289–295, 2001

Chandola CA, Robling MR, Peters TJ, et al: Pre- and perinatal factors and the risk of subsequent referral for hyperactivity. J Child Psychol Psychiatry 33:1077–1090, 1992

Cohen DJ, Leckman JF: Commentary. J Am Acad Child Adolesc Psychiatry 28:580–582, 1989

Comings DE, Comings BG: A controlled family history study of Tourette's syndrome, I: attention-deficit hyperactivity disorder and learning disorders. J Clin Psychiatry 51:275–280, 1990

Conners CK, Taylor E: Pemoline, methylphenidate, and placebo in children with minimal brain dysfunction. Arch Gen Psychiatry 37:922–930, 1980

Conners CK, Werry JL: Pharmacotherapy of psychopathology in children, in Psychopathological Disorders of Childhood, 2nd Edition. Edited by Quay H, Werry JL. New York, Wiley, 1979, pp 336–386

Conners CK, Casat CD, Gualtieri CT, et al: Bupropion hydrochloride in attention deficit disorder with hyperactivity. J Am Acad Child Adolesc Psychiatry 35:1314–1321, 1996

Conners CK, Sitarenios G, Parker JD, et al: The revised Conners' Parent Rating Scale (CPRS-R): factor structure, reliability, and criterion validity. J Abnorm Child Psychol 26:257–268, 1998

Conners CK, Epstein JN, March JS, et al: Multimodal treatment of ADHD in the MTA: an alternative outcome analysis. J Am Acad Child Adolesc Psychiatry 40:159–167, 2001

Connor DF, Fletcher KE, Swanson JM: A meta-analysis of clonidine for symptoms of attention-deficit hyperactivity disorder. J Am Acad Child Adolesc Psychiatry 38:1551–1559, 1999

Corkum PV, Siegel LS: Is the Continuous Performance Test a valuable research tool for use with children with attention-deficit-hyperactivity disorder? J Child Psychol Psychiatry 34:1217–1239, 1993

Cornblatt BA, Winters L, Maminski B, et al: Methylphenidate-SR: effect on sustained attention in ADHD males (abstract). Proceedings of the American Academy of Child and Adolescent Psychiatry 3:47, 1987

Cornblatt BA, Risch JJ, Faris G, et al: The Continuous Performance Test, Identical Pairs Version (CPT-IP), I: new findings about sustained attention in normal families. Psychiatry Res 26:223–238, 1988

Cox WHJ: An indication for use of imipramine in attention deficit disorder. Am J Psychiatry 139:1059–1060, 1982

Denckla MB: Attention deficit hyperactivity disorder—residual type. J Child Neurol 6 (suppl):S44–S50, 1991

Diaz-Granados JL, Greene PL, Amsel A: Selective activity enhancement and persistence in weanling rats after hippocampal X-irradiation in infancy: possible relevance for ADHD. Behav Neural Biol 61:251–259, 1994

DiBattista D, Shepherd ML: Primary school teachers' beliefs and advice to parents concerning sugar consumption and activity in children. Psychol Rep 72:47–55, 1993

Douglas VI: Attentional and cognitive problems, in Developmental Neuropsychiatry. Edited by Rutter M. New York, Guilford, 1983, pp 280–329

DuPaul GJ, Anastopoulos AD, Shelton TL, et al: Multimethod assessment of attention-deficit hyperactivity disorder: the diagnostic utility of clinic-based tests. J Clin Child Psychol 21:394–402, 1992

DuPaul GJ, McGoey KE, Eckert TL, et al: Preschool children with attention-deficit/hyperactivity disorder: impairments in behavioral, social, and school functioning. J Am Acad Child Adolesc Psychiatry 40:508–515, 2001

Egger J, Stolla A, McEwen LM: Controlled trial of hyposensitisation in children with food-induced hyperkinetic syndrome. Lancet 339:1150–1153, 1992

Elia J, Borcherding BG, Rapoport JL, et al: Methylphenidate and dextroamphetamine treatments of hyperactivity: are there true nonresponders? Psychiatry Res 36:141–155, 1991

Elia J, Gulotta C, Rose SR, et al: Thyroid function and attention-deficit hyperactivity disorder. J Am Acad Child Adolesc Psychiatry 33:169–172, 1994

Ernst M, Cohen RM, Liebenauer LL, et al: Cerebral glucose metabolism in adolescent girls with attention-deficit/hyperactivity disorder. J Am Acad Child Adolesc Psychiatry 36:1399–1406, 1997

Ernst M, Zametkin AJ, Matochik JA, et al: High midbrain [^{18}F]DOPA accumulation in children with attention deficit hyperactivity disorder. Am J Psychiatry 156:1209–1215, 1999

Faraone SV, Biederman J, Keenan K, et al: A family genetic study of girls with DSM-III attention deficit disorder. Am J Psychiatry 148:112–117, 1991

Faraone SV, Biederman J, Lehman BK, et al: Intellectual performance and school failure in children with attention deficit hyperactivity disorder and in their siblings. J Abnorm Psychol 102:616–623, 1993

Faraone SV, Biederman J, Monuteaux MC: Toward guidelines for pedigree selection in genetic studies of attention deficit hyperactivity disorder. Genet Epidemiol 18:1–16, 2000

Faraone SV, Doyle AE, Mick E, et al: Meta-analysis of the association between the 7-repeat allele of the dopamine D(4) receptor gene and attention deficit hyperactivity disorder. Am J Psychiatry 158:1052–1057, 2001

Fehlings DL, Roberts W, Humphries T, et al: Attention deficit hyperactivity disorder: does cognitive behavioral therapy improve home behavior? J Dev Behav Pediatr 12:223–228, 1991

Fergusson DM, Lynskey MT, Horwood LJ: The effect of maternal depression on maternal ratings of child behavior. J Abnorm Child Psychol 21:245–269, 1993

Fergusson DM, Horwood LJ, Lynskey MT: Structure of DSM-III-R criteria for disruptive childhood behaviors: confirmatory factor models. J Am Acad Child Adolesc Psychiatry 33:1145–1157, 1994

Fischer M, Barkley RA, Fletcher KE, et al: The adolescent outcome of hyperactive children: predictors of psychiatric, academic, social, and emotional adjustment. J Am Acad Child Adolesc Psychiatry 32:324–332, 1993

Fonagy P, Target M: The efficacy of psychoanalysis for children with disruptive disorders. J Am Acad Child Adolesc Psychiatry 33:45–55, 1994

Frick PJ, Kamphaus RW, Lahey BB, et al: Academic underachievement and the disruptive behavior disorders. J Consult Clin Psychol 59:289–294, 1991

Gainetdinov RR, Caron MG: Genetics of childhood disorders: XXIV. ADHD, part 8: hyperdopaminergic mice as an animal model of ADHD. J Am Acad Child Adolesc Psychiatry 40:380–382, 2001

Gainetdinov RR, Wetsel WC, Jones SR, et al: Role of serotonin in the paradoxical calming effect of psychostimulants on hyperactivity. Science 283:397–401, 1999

Garfinkel BD, Webster CD, Sloman L: Individual responses to methylphenidate and caffeine in children with minimal brain dysfunction. Can Med Assoc J 113:729–732, 1975

Garfinkel BD, Brown WA, Klee SH, et al: Neuroendocrine and cognitive responses to amphetamine in adolescents with a history of attention deficit disorder. J Am Acad Child Adolesc Psychiatry 25:503–510, 1986

Giedd JN, Castellanos FX, Casey BJ, et al: Quantitative morphology of the corpus callosum in attention deficit hyperactivity disorder. Am J Psychiatry 151:665–669, 1994

Gittelman R, Mannuzza S, Shenker R, et al: Hyperactive boys almost grown up, I: psychiatric status. Arch Gen Psychiatry 42:937–947, 1985

Goodman R, Stevenson J: A twin study of hyperactivity, II: the aetiological role of genes, family relationships and perinatal adversity. J Child Psychol Psychiatry 30:691–709, 1989

Gordon M, Mettelman BB: The assessment of attention, I: standardization and reliability of a behavior-based measure. J Clin Psychol 44:682–690, 1988

Goyette CH, Conners CK, Ulrich RF: Normative data on Revised Conners' Parent and Teacher Rating Scales. J Abnorm Child Psychol 6:221–236, 1978

Green SM, Loeber R, Lahey BB: Stability of mothers' recall of the age of onset of their child's attention and hyperactivity problems. J Am Acad Child Adolesc Psychiatry 30:135–137, 1991

Greenhill LL, Halperin JM, Abikoff H: Stimulant medications. J Am Acad Child Adolesc Psychiatry 38:503–512, 1999

Gross MD: Imipramine in the treatment of minimal brain dysfunction in children. Psychosomatics 14:283–285, 1973

Hagerman RJ, Falkenstein AR: An association between recurrent otitis media in infancy and later hyperactivity. Clin Pediatr (Phila) 26:253–257, 1987

Halperin JM, Newcorn JH, Matier K, et al: Discriminant validity of attention-deficit hyperactivity disorder. J Am Acad Child Psychiatry 32:1038–1043, 1993

Hauser P, Zametkin AJ, Martinez P, et al: Attention deficit–hyperactivity disorder in people with generalized resistance to thyroid hormone. N Engl J Med 328:997–1001, 1993

Hechtman L: Resilience and vulnerability in long-term outcome of attention deficit hyperactive disorder. Can J Psychiatry 36:415–421, 1991

Hechtman L: Genetic and neurobiological aspects of attention deficit hyperactive disorder: a review. J Psychiatry Neurosci 19:193–201, 1994

Hoagwood K, Kelleher KJ, Feil M, et al: Treatment services for children with ADHD: a national perspective. J Am Acad Child Adolesc Psychiatry 39:198–206, 2000

Hoegerman GS, Resnick RJ, Schnoll SH: Attention deficits in newly abstinent substance abusers: childhood recollections and attention performance in thirty-nine subjects. J Addict Dis 12:37–53, 1993

Hynd GW, Hern KL, Novey ES, et al: Attention deficit–hyperactivity disorder and asymmetry of the caudate nucleus. J Child Neurol 8:339–347, 1993

Jensen PS, Salzberg AD, Richters JE, et al: Scales, diagnoses, and child psychopathology, I: CBCL and DISC relationships. J Am Acad Child Adolesc Psychiatry 32:397–406, 1993a

Jensen PS, Shervette RE, Xenakis SN, et al: Anxiety and depressive disorders in attention deficit disorder with hyperactivity: new findings. Am J Psychiatry 150:1203–1209, 1993b

Keller MB, Lavori PW, Beardslee WR, et al: The disruptive behavioral disorder in children and adolescents: comorbidity and clinical course. J Am Acad Child Adolesc Psychiatry 31:204–209, 1992

Kelly DP, Kelly BJ, Jones ML, et al: Attention deficits in children and adolescents with hearing loss: a survey. Am J Dis Child 147:737–741, 1993

Klein RG, Mannuzza S: Hyperactive boys almost grown up, III: methylphenidate effects on ultimate height. Arch Gen Psychiatry 45:1131–1134, 1988

Klein RG, Mannuzza S: Long-term outcome of hyperactive children: a review. J Am Acad Child Adolesc Psychiatry 30:383–387, 1991

Kupietz SS, Winsberg BG, Sverd J: Learning ability and methylphenidate (Ritalin) plasma concentration in hyperkinetic children. J Am Acad Child Psychiatry 21:27–30, 1982

Lahey BB, Pelham WE, Stein MA, et al: Validity of DSM-IV attention-deficit/hyperactivity disorder for younger children. J Am Acad Child Adolesc Psychiatry 37:695–702, 1998

Lapouse R, Monk M: An epidemiologic study of behavioral characteristics in children. Am J Public Health 48:1134–1144, 1953

Lie N: Follow-ups of children with attention deficit hyperactivity disorder (ADHD): review of literature. Acta Psychiatr Scand Suppl 368:1–40, 1992

Lowe TL, Cohen DJ, Detlor J, et al: Stimulant medications precipitate Tourette's syndrome. JAMA 247:1729–1731, 1982

Mann EM, Ikeda Y, Mueller CW, et al: Cross-cultural differences in rating hyperactive-disruptive behaviors in children. Am J Psychiatry 149:1539–1542, 1992

Mannuzza S, Klein RG, Bessler A, et al: Adult outcome of hyperactive boys: educational achievement, occupational rank, and psychiatric status. Arch Gen Psychiatry 50:565–576, 1993

Mannuzza S, Klein RG, Bessler A, et al: Adult psychiatric status of hyperactive boys grown up. Am J Psychiatry 155:493–498, 1998

Matochik JA, Nordahl TE, Gross M, et al: Effects of acute stimulant medication on cerebral metabolism in adults with hyperactivity. Neuropsychopharmacology 8:377–386, 1993

Mayes SD, Crites DL, Bixler EO, et al: Methylphenidate and ADHD: influence of age, IQ and neurodevelopmental status. Dev Med Child Neurol 36:1099–1107, 1994

McGee R, Feehan M, Williams S, et al: DSM-III disorders in a large sample of adolescents. J Am Acad Child Adolesc Psychiatry 29:611–619, 1990

McGee R, Partridge F, Williams S, et al: A twelve-year follow-up of preschool hyperactive children. J Am Acad Child Adolesc Psychiatry 30:224–232, 1991

McGee R, Williams S, Feehan M: Attention deficit disorder and age of onset of problem behaviors. J Abnorm Child Psychol 20:487–502, 1992

McGee R, Stanton WR, Sears MR: Allergic disorders and attention deficit disorder in children. J Abnorm Child Psychol 21:79–88, 1993

Mercugliano M, Hyman SL, Batshaw ML: Behavioral deficits in rats with minimal cortical hypoplasia induced by methylazoxymethanol acetate. Pediatrics 85:432–436, 1990

Milberger S, Biederman J, Faraone SV, et al: ADHD is associated with early initiation of cigarette smoking in children and adolescents. J Am Acad Child Adolesc Psychiatry 36:37–44, 1997

Minder B, Das-Smaal EA, Brand EFJM, et al: Exposure to lead and specific attentional problems in schoolchildren. J Learn Disabil 27:393–399, 1994

MTA Cooperative Group: A 14-month randomized clinical trial of treatment strategies for attention-deficit/hyperactivity disorder: the MTA Cooperative Group. Multimodal Treatment Study of Children with ADHD. Arch Gen Psychiatry 56:1073–1086, 1999

National Institutes of Health Consensus Development Conference Statement: diagnosis and treatment of attention-deficit/hyperactivity disorder (ADHD). J Am Acad Child Adolesc Psychiatry 39:182–193, 2000

Ornoy A, Uriel L, Tennenbaum A: Inattention, hyperactivity and speech delay at 2–4 years of age as a predictor for ADD-ADHD syndrome. Isr J Psychiatry Relat Sci 30:155–163, 1993

Palfrey JS, Levine MD, Walker DK, et al: The emergence of attention deficits in early childhood: a prospective study. J Dev Behav Pediatr 6:339–348, 1985

Pelham WEJ, Gnagy EM, Greenslade KE, et al: Teacher ratings of DSM-III-R symptoms for the disruptive behavior disorders. J Am Acad Child Adolesc Psychiatry 31:210–218, 1992

Pelham WEJ, Carlson C, Sams SE, et al: Separate and combined effects of methylphenidate and behavior modification on boys with attention deficit-hyperactivity disorder in the classroom. J Consult Clin Psychol 61:506–515, 1993

Physicians' Desk Reference, 55th Edition. Montvale, NJ, Medical Economics, 2001

Pliszka SR: Tricyclic antidepressants in the treatment of children with attention deficit disorder. J Am Acad Child Adolesc Psychiatry 26:127–132, 1987

Porrino LJ, Rapoport JL, Behar D, et al: A naturalistic assessment of the motor activity of hyperactive boys, I: comparison with normal controls. Arch Gen Psychiatry 40:681–687, 1983

Pratt DS, Dubois RS: Hepatotoxicity due to pemoline (Cylert): a report of two cases. J Pediatr Gastroenterol Nutr 10:239–241, 1990

Prince JB, Wilens TE, Biederman J, et al: Clonidine for sleep disturbances associated with attention-deficit hyperactivity disorder: a systematic chart review of 62 cases. J Am Acad Child Adolesc Psychiatry 35:599–605, 1996

Rapport MD, Stoner G, DuPaul GJ, et al: Methylphenidate in hyperactive children: differential effects of dose on academic, learning, and social behavior. J Abnorm Child Psychol 13:227–243, 1985

Riddle MA, Geller B, Ryan N: Another sudden death in a child treated with desipramine. J Am Acad Child Adolesc Psychiatry 32:792–797, 1993

Roth N, Beyreiss J, Schlenzka K, et al: Coincidence of attention deficit disorder and atopic disorders in children: empirical findings and hypothetical background. J Abnorm Child Psychol 19:1–13, 1991

Rounsaville BJ, Anton SF, Carroll K, et al: Psychiatric diagnoses of treatment-seeking cocaine abusers. Arch Gen Psychiatry 48:43–51, 1991

Rowe KS, Rowe KJ: Synthetic food coloring and behavior: a dose response effect in a double-blind, placebo-controlled, repeated-measures study. J Pediatr 125:691–698, 1994

Rubia K, Overmeyer S, Taylor E, et al: Hypofrontality in attention deficit hyperactivity disorder during higher-order motor control: a study with functional MRI. Am J Psychiatry 156:891–896, 1999

Sallee FR, Stiller RL, Perel JM: Pharmacodynamics of pemoline in attention-deficit disorder with hyperactivity. J Am Acad Child Adolesc Psychiatry 31:244–251, 1992

Satterfield J, Swanson J, Schell A, et al: Prediction of antisocial behavior in attention-deficit hyperactivity disorder boys from aggression/defiance scores. J Am Acad Child Adolesc Psychiatry 33:185–190, 1994

Scahill L, Schwab-Stone M: Epidemiology of ADHD in school-age children. Child Adolesc Psychiatr Clin N Am 9:541–555, 2000

Scahill L, Chappell PB, Kim YS, et al: A placebo-controlled study of guanfacine in the treatment of children with tic disorders and attention deficit hyperactivity disorder. Am J Psychiatry 158:1067–1074, 2001

Schechter MD, Timmons GD: Objectively measured hyperactivity, II: caffeine and amphetamine effects. J Clin Pharmacol 25:276–280, 1985

Schwab-Stone M, Fallon T, Briggs M, et al: Reliability of diagnostic reporting for children aged 6–11 years: a test-retest study of the Diagnostic Interview Schedule for Children–Revised. Am J Psychiatry 151:1048–1054, 1994

Sechzer JA, Faro MD, Windle WF: Studies of monkeys asphyxiated at birth: implications for minimal cerebral dysfunction. Semin Psychiatry 5:19–34, 1973

Semrud-Clikeman M, Biederman J, Sprich-Buckminster S, et al: Comorbidity between ADDH and learning disability: a review and report in a clinically referred sample. J Am Acad Child Adolesc Psychiatry 31:439–448, 1992

Semrud-Clikeman M, Steingard RJ, Filipek P, et al: Using MRI to examine brain-behavior relationships in males with attention deficit disorder with hyperactivity. J Am Acad Child Adolesc Psychiatry 39:477–484, 2000

Shaffer D: Attention deficit hyperactivity disorder in adults (editorial). Am J Psychiatry 151:633–688, 1994

Shaffer D, Greenhill LL: A critical note on the predictive validity of the hyperactive syndrome. J Child Psychol Psychiatry 20:61–72, 1979

Shaffer D, Schoenfeld I, O'Conner P, et al: Neurological soft signs. Arch Gen Psychiatry 42:329–335, 1985

Shaffer D, Fisher P, Lucas CP, et al: NIMH Diagnostic Interview Schedule for Children Version IV (NIMH DISC-IV): description, differences from previous versions, and reliability of some common diagnoses. J Am Acad Child Adolesc Psychiatry 39:28–38, 2000

Shaywitz BA, Yager RD, Klopper JH: Selective brain dopamine depletion in developing rats: an experimental model of minimal brain dysfunction. Science 191:305–308, 1976

Shen YC, Wang YF, Yang XL: An epidemiological investigation of minimal brain dysfunction in six elementary schools in Beijing. J Child Psychol Psychiatry 26:777–787, 1985

Sobotka TJ, Cook MP: Postnatal lead acetate exposure in rats: possible relationship to minimal brain dysfunction. Am J Ment Defic 79:5–9, 1974

Solanto MV, Wender EH: Does methylphenidate constrict cognitive functioning? J Am Acad Child Adolesc Psychiatry 28:897–902, 1989

Speiser Z, Korczyn AD, Teplitzky I, et al: Hyperactivity in rats following postnatal anoxia. Behav Brain Res 7:379–382, 1983

Spencer TJ, Biederman J, Steingard R, et al: Bupropion exacerbates tics in children with attention-deficit hyperactivity disorder and Tourette's syndrome. J Am Acad Child Adolesc Psychiatry 32:211–214, 1993

Spencer T, Biederman J, Wilens T, et al: Pharmacotherapy of attention-deficit hyperactivity disorder across the life cycle. J Am Acad Child Adolesc Psychiatry 35:409–432, 1996

Sprague RL, Sleator EK: Methylphenidate in hyperkinetic children: differences in dose effects on learning and social behavior. Science 198:1274–1276, 1977

Sprich-Buckminster S, Biederman J, Milberger S, et al: Are perinatal complications relevant to the manifestation of ADD? issues of comorbidity and familiality. J Am Acad Child Adolesc Psychiatry 32:1032–1037, 1993

Srinivas NR, Hubbard JW, Quinn D, et al: Enantioselective pharmacokinetics and pharmacodynamics of dl-threo-methylphenidate in children with attention deficit hyperactivity disorder. Clin Pharmacol Ther 52:561–568, 1992

Steingard R, Biederman J, Spencer T, et al: Comparison of clonidine response in the treatment of attention-deficit hyperactivity disorder with and without comorbid tic disorders. J Am Acad Child Adolesc Psychiatry 32:350–353, 1993

Strayhorn JM, Weidman CS: Reduction of attention deficit and internalizing symptoms in preschoolers through parent-child interaction training. J Am Acad Child Adolesc Psychiatry 28:888–896, 1989

Streissguth AP, Barr HM, Sampson PD, et al: Prenatal alcohol and offspring development: the first fourteen years. Drug Alcohol Depend 36:89–99, 1994

Sullivan A, Kelso J, Stewart M: Mothers' views on the ages of onset for four childhood disorders. Child Psychiatry Hum Dev 20:269–278, 1990

Swanson J, Cantwell D: Cognitive toxicity of methylphenidate: evidence from reaction times study of memory scanning. Proceedings of the Annual Meeting of the American Academy of Child and Adolescent Psychiatry 5:49–50, 1989

Swanson JM, Kraemer HC, Hinshaw SP, et al: Clinical relevance of the primary findings of the MTA: success rates based on severity of ADHD and ODD symptoms at the end of treatment. J Am Acad Child Adolesc Psychiatry 40:168–179, 2001

Sykes DH, Douglas VI, Morgenstern G: The effect of methylphenidate (Ritalin) on sustained attention in hyperactive children. Psychopharmacologia 25:262–274, 1972

Tarver-Behring S, Barkley RA, Karlsson J: The mother-child interactions of hyperactive boys and their normal siblings. Am J Orthopsychiatry 55:202–209, 1985

Verhulst FC, Achenbach TM, Ferdinand RF, et al: Epidemiological comparisons of American and Dutch adolescents' self-reports. J Am Acad Child Adolesc Psychiatry 32:1135–1144, 1993

Vitiello B, Stoff D, Atkins M, et al: Soft neurological signs and impulsivity in children. J Dev Behav Pediatr 11:112–115, 1990

Walsh BT, Giardina EG, Sloan RP, et al: Effects of desipramine on autonomic control of the heart. J Am Acad Child Adolesc Psychiatry 33:191–197, 1994

Ward MF, Wender PH, Reimherr FW: The Wender Utah Rating Scale: an aid in the retrospective diagnosis of childhood attention deficit hyperactivity disorder. Am J Psychiatry 150:885–890, 1993

Wechsler J: Wechsler Intelligence Scale for Children–Revised. New York, Psychological Corporation, 1974

Weingartner H, Rapoport JL, Buchsbaum MS, et al: Cognitive processes in normal and hyperactive children and their response to amphetamine treatment. J Abnorm Psychol 89:25–35, 1980

Wender PH, Reimherr FW: Bupropion treatment of attention-deficit hyperactivity disorder in adults. Am J Psychiatry 147:1018–1020, 1990

Werry JS: Child psychiatric disorders: are they classifiable? Br J Psychiatry 161:472–480, 1992

Werry JS, Elkind GS, Reeves JC: Attention deficit, conduct, oppositional, and anxiety disorders in children, III: laboratory differences. J Abnorm Child Psychol 15:409–428, 1987

Whalen CK, Henker B: Therapies for hyperactive children: comparisons, combinations, and compromises. J Consult Clin Psychol 59:126–137, 1991

Whalen CK, Henker B, Collins BE, et al: A social ecology of hyperactive boys: medication effects in structured classroom environments. J Appl Behav Anal 12:65–81, 1979

Whalen CK, Henker B, Castro J, et al: Peer perception of hyperactivity and medication effects. Child Dev 58:816–828, 1987

Whitaker AH, Van Rossem R, Feldman JF, et al: Psychiatric outcomes in low-birth-weight children at age 6 years: relation to neonatal cranial ultrasound abnormalities. Arch Gen Psychiatry 54:847–856, 1997

Wilens TE, Biederman J, Geist DE, et al: Nortriptyline in the treatment of ADHD: a chart review of 58 cases. J Am Acad Child Adolesc Psychiatry 32:343–349, 1993a

Wilens TE, Biederman J, Spencer T, et al: A retrospective study of serum levels and electrocardiographic effects of nortriptyline in children and adolescents. J Am Acad Child Adolesc Psychiatry 32:270–277, 1993b

Wilens TE, Spencer TJ, Biederman J, et al: A controlled clinical trial of bupropion for attention deficit hyperactivity disorder in adults. Am J Psychiatry 158:282–288, 2001

Willoughby MT, Curran PJ, Costello EJ, et al: Implications of early versus late onset of attention-deficit/hyperactivity disorder symptoms. J Am Acad Child Adolesc Psychiatry 39:1512–1519, 2000

Zahner GE, Jacobs JH, Freeman DHJ, et al: Rural-urban child psychopathology in a Northeastern U.S. state: 1986–1989. J Am Acad Child Adolesc Psychiatry 32:378–387, 1993

Zametkin A, Rapoport JL, Murphy DL, et al: Treatment of hyperactive children with monoamine oxidase inhibitors, I: clinical efficacy. Arch Gen Psychiatry 42:962–966, 1985

Zametkin AJ, Liebenauer LL, Fitzgerald GA, et al: Brain metabolism in teenagers with attention-deficit hyperactivity disorder. Arch Gen Psychiatry 50:333–340, 1993

Zentall SS, Meyer MJ: Self-regulation of stimulation of ADD-H children during reading and vigilance task performance. J Abnorm Child Psychol 15:519–536, 1987

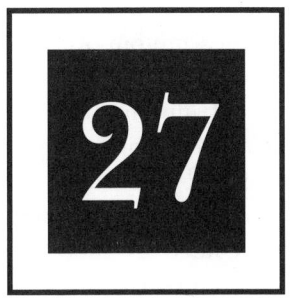

Conduct Disorder and Oppositional Defiant Disorder

Robert L. Hendren, D.O.

David J. Mullen, M.D.

Children with conduct disorder and oppositional defiant disorder (ODD) are a varied group because of the myriad manifestations of antisocial behavior and the numerous and complex factors that contribute to the evolution of antisocial behavior. First, the classification of conduct disorder is a controversial and unsettled issue in mental health (Cantwell and Baker 1988; Frick et al. 1994), and the relationship between conduct disorder and ODD remains unclear. Depending on the constellation of symptoms, conduct disorder might be diagnosed based predominantly on irresponsible, delinquent behaviors such as truancy and running away; covert violations of the rights of others such as nonconfrontative theft; or overt physical aggression such as assault or rape. These behaviors share an antisocial quality but differ significantly in other respects. In addition, the specific antisocial behaviors involved tend to vary significantly with development. For example, oppositional defiant behaviors tend to precede more serious violations of age-appropriate behavioral norms. Second, the etiology of conduct disorder is manifold, with biological, psychological, and social factors having various degrees of significance. Some children may have a prominent family history of criminality, whereas in others histories of abuse and neglect or social chaos and the presence of neighborhood youth gangs may be more prominent. Or, not uncommonly, all of these and other factors may be present. In addition, children with conduct disorder and ODD frequently manifest other psychiatric symptoms, and many (if not most) will meet criteria for another psychiatric disorder, further complicating issues of assessment, diagnosis, and treatment. It is clear that a comprehensive assessment and treatment program depends not only on the knowledge of developmental signs and symptoms but also on a thorough exploration of the underlying biopsychosocial factors. Finally, as with many other psychiatric syndromes, conduct disorder and ODD may be conceptualized as stemming at least in part from disturbances in the self-regulation of affect and behavior. In the case of conduct disorder and ODD, problems with the regulation of anger and impulsivity may be the principal self-regulatory defects observed, and these defects may be initiated and maintained by a broad range of underlying biological, psychological, and social factors (Bradley 2000; Moeller et al. 2001).

Prevalence

The prevalence of conduct disorder is difficult to estimate because of the different definitions that have been used and the variations that occur in different age groups and between the sexes. In DSM-IV (American Psychiatric Association 1994) the prevalence of conduct disorder is estimated as approximately 9% for males and 2% for females younger than 18 years. In DSM-IV-TR (American Psychiatric Association 2000) the prevalence is estimated to be between 1% and 16%. The childhood-onset type of the disorder, defined by the presence of at least one criterion characteristic of conduct disorder before age 10 years, is clearly much more common in males; physical aggression is frequently displayed toward others, peer relationships are typically disturbed, and criteria for ODD are often met during early childhood. Individuals with childhood-onset conduct disorder appear to be more likely to develop adult antisocial personality disorder than are young people with onset of conduct disorder in adolescence. The preponderance of males also appears to be less prominent in the adolescent-onset type.

ODD occurs at a prevalence ranging from 2% to 16% according to both DSM-IV and DSM-IV-TR and is approximately twice as common in males as in females.

Diagnostic Classification

■ DSM-IV-TR Criteria

The essential feature of conduct disorder, according to DSM-IV-TR, is a persistent pattern of behavior that violates the basic rights of others and major age-appropriate social norms or rules. Diagnostic criteria are divided into four basic categories: 1) aggression to people and animals, which includes behaviors ranging from bullying or intimidating others to physical cruelty and forcing someone into sexual activity; 2) destruction of property, which includes fire setting or other deliberate property destruction; 3) deceitfulness or theft, which includes more surreptitious or covert antisocial behaviors such as lying or nonconfrontative theft; and 4) serious violations of rules, which includes truancy or socially irresponsible behaviors. Three or more of these criteria must have been present within 12 months of the assessment, with at least one criterion occurring within 6 months. Because the diagnosis is based on a broad range of behavioral criteria without reference to etiology, individuals who meet criteria for conduct disorder may have significantly different underlying psychopathology. Furthermore, the impact of social context may result in diagnostic variation (Angold and Costello 1996). Thus, individuals with a diagnosis of conduct disorder are a very heterogeneous group (Lavigne et al. 2001).

ODD is characterized by a pattern of hostile, negativistic, defiant, and disobedient attitudes and behaviors, especially toward authority figures, that is associated with impairment. This pattern is frequently seen in young people who meet the criteria for conduct disorder, and there is some controversy regarding the validity of ODD as a separate diagnosis. In DSM-IV-TR, conduct disorder and ODD are not allowed to be diagnosed together, given the extent of symptom overlap. However, the current consensus supports the idea that there is a valid distinction between symptoms of ODD and some of the symptoms of conduct disorder, especially the covert variety. In DSM-IV-TR it is also recognized that in many children increased negativity and hostility may occur as part of the course of a mood or psychotic disorder, and the diagnosis of ODD is not allowed when the symptoms occur exclusively during the course of a psychotic or mood disorder.

■ Subtypes of Conduct Disorder

Several approaches have been used in the classification of conduct disorder. In DSM-IV-TR two diagnostic subtypes—a childhood-onset type and an adolescent-onset type—are recognized. The value of this subtyping is clearly related to the prognostic significance of age at onset, with early onset being more ominous. However, some have questioned the clinical usefulness of this classification, citing problems in retrospective recall of age at onset by informants (Sanford et al. 1999).

In a cluster analysis of the symptoms of disturbed children, Wolff (1971) found two groups of children with behavioral disturbance: aggressive-overactive and antisocial. Hospitalized children with conduct disorder and aggressive and destructive behavior have a particularly poor prognosis (Gabel and Shindledecker 1991).

Subtyping aggressive behavior into predatory and affective categories is another useful distinction (Blair 2001; Vitiello et al. 1990). Predatory aggression is goal directed, with minimal associated autonomic arousal. Affective aggression is characterized by the presence of high levels of autonomic and emotional arousal with little apparent instrumental gain. Vitaro et al. (1998) found that children who manifested proactive aggression (similar conceptually to predatory aggression) were more delinquent than those whose problems with aggression tended to be more reactive (and affective) in nature.

In a review of the literature on delinquency, Rutter and Giller (1984) found that the categories of socialized and undersocialized conduct disorder were the most valid, with the socialized group having the better prognosis. However, at least one study found that group involvement is common in delinquent conduct and that no category of offense is predominantly solitary (Emler et al. 1987). Adolescent girls were especially likely to commit offenses in the company of others. In a 4-year follow-up study, Cantwell and Baker (1989) found that the conduct disorder diagnoses were not stable. At follow-up, many children with an initial diagnosis of conduct disorder had other diagnoses, and a few had no disorders. Thus, the research literature suggests that age at onset, degree of aggressivity, and extent of socialization are important variables to consider in conduct disorder; however, no system of subclassification is completely validated.

■ Other Approaches

Other approaches to classification attempt to identify salient symptoms that yield reliable and clinically meaningful subgroups of children with antisocial behavior (Kazdin 1987). Patterson (1982) found two symptom clusters in children: a primary problem of aggression and a significant problem of theft. Family structure and treatment responsiveness differed between the two groups; the group who stole had the poorer prognosis. Children with both types of characteristics were likely to have been abused.

Recently, some attempt has been made to subtype youths with conduct disorder by the presence or absence of the trait of callousness—a central feature of the concept of psychopathy. The presence of this trait was indeed found to correlate with more police contacts and a greater number and variety of conduct problems (Christian et al. 1997; Frick and Ellis 1999). Interestingly, in these studies, children and adolescents with high levels of callousness tended to have higher IQs than other children with conduct disorder.

Another classification method for antisocial behavior is based on the distinction between overt and covert behavior (Loeber and Schmaling 1985). Overt behaviors, such as physical and verbal aggression, are more direct and obvious. Covert behaviors, such as stealing and fire setting, are not as openly confrontational. Cluster analyses support the validity of these distinctions. Children with a mixture of the two types appear to be at greater risk for future dysfunction.

The 10th revision of the *International Classification of Diseases* (World Health Organization 1992) presents yet another method for the classification of conduct disorder, which includes a number of "combination categories" that represent commonly co-occurring conditions. For example, categories exist for depressive conduct disorder and hyperkinetic conduct disorder. Subdivisions of conduct disorder include conduct disorder confined to the family context, unsocialized conduct disorder, socialized conduct disorder, and conduct disorder not otherwise specified. In a study examining the symptom patterns and correlates of the depressive conduct disorder subtype, Simic and Fombonne (2001) found that patients with the depressive subtype of conduct disorder had fewer biological depressive features, fewer anxiety symptoms, less guilt, and less overall depressive severity than patients with depressive disorder and less overt aggression and violence than patients with simple conduct disorder. The results of the study were believed to tentatively support the depressive conduct disorder construct.

All the classification systems proposed for antisocial behavior in childhood and adolescence contain some commonalities. Each approach identifies certain symptom clusters, such as aggression and delinquency, or the time course of symptoms as important subcategories. However, neither the category of conduct disorder nor the subcategories have been fully validated as to their developmental and predictive significance.

The principal subdivision to be made in ODD is between the variety that appears to progress to conduct disorder and the variety that does not. Greater severity and early onset of oppositional behavior, frequent physical fighting, parental substance abuse, and low socioeconomic status appear to increase the risk of progression to the more severe antisocial behaviors observed in conduct disorder (Loeber et al. 1995).

Comorbidity

Many children and adolescents who meet the criteria for a diagnosis of conduct disorder or ODD have coexisting psychiatric disorders that may have led to their antisocial behavior and will influence their responsiveness to treatment and their long-term prognosis (Woolston et al. 1989). For instance, depression-like symptoms have been noted in some patients with conduct disorder (Harrington et al. 1991; Kovacs et al. 1988). Puig-Antich (1982) reported that symptoms of conduct disorder may start and stop with the onset of and recovery from affective illness. Conduct disorder that is comorbid with depression is found to have a variable course, and conduct disorder may or may not abate as the depression diminishes (Kovacs et al. 1988). Lavigne et al. (2001) found ODD in preschool children to be a moderate to highly stable diagnosis and that it displayed a pattern of increasing comorbidity with attention-deficit/hyperactivity disorder (ADHD), anxiety, or mood disorders over time.

Children and adolescents with bipolar mood disorder may also meet criteria for a comorbid conduct disorder. Some authors have considered the possibility that the combination presents a unique subtype of conduct disorder (Wozniak et al. 2001). Conceptually, the poor judgment, irritability, increased activity level, and impaired impulse control associated with mania might easily lead to repeated instances of antisocial behavior such that the criteria for conduct disorder are met.

Children and adolescents with conduct disorder or ODD frequently also have coexisting ADHD. Reeves et al. (1987) found that children with ADHD plus conduct disorder or ODD had many demographic and clinical variables that were very similar to those of children with ADHD alone. The combination of ADHD and conduct disorder is associated with more severe physical aggression and antisocial behavior than is conduct disorder alone (Walker et al. 1987). In addition, a significant number of children who are first given a diagnosis of conduct disorder are found to have ADHD at follow-up (Cantwell and Baker 1989). Although it is clear that the comorbidity is common, the relationship between the conditions requires further clarification. Some studies suggest that children with ADHD are more likely to subsequently develop conduct disorder; others have found no evidence that children initially diagnosed with ADHD alone were more likely to develop antisocial behavior (Loeber et al. 2000). However, as noted above, when the two are found together, the severity of the conduct disorder is often worse.

One notable difference between American and British psychiatry is that British clinicians are more likely to diagnose conduct disorder in patients whom American clinicians are likely to diagnose with ADHD. Clearly, ADHD is closely linked conceptually to problems with behavioral self-regulation and impulsivity, features that seem to play a central role in the development of conduct disorders.

Some children and adolescents may exhibit antisocial and aggressive behavior in the years preceding the onset of schizophrenia that could lead to a diagnosis of conduct disorder (Offord and Cross 1969; Watt et al. 1983). A clear familial link exists between antisocial behavior and schizophrenia (Silverton et al. 1988). The basis of this linkage is not clear, although para-

noid ideation and other cognitive distortions in psychotic patients could well contribute to antisocial behavior.

Disturbances in conduct are also found in children with Tourette's syndrome. In fact, associated behavioral disturbances often contribute substantially to the overall impairment observed in patients with Tourette's syndrome. Of note, the basal ganglia are likely involved in the etiology of tics as well as obsessive-compulsive disorder, and this brain region also appears to be involved in impulse regulation (D.L. Clark and Boutros 1999)—as noted above, a common prominent area of impairment in children with conduct disorder. One study estimated that in children who are not economically disadvantaged, 10%–30% of cases of conduct disorder may be due to the presence of a Tourette's syndrome gene (Comings and Comings 1987).

Substance use frequently co-occurs with conduct disorder. One study reported that more than 50% of youths with conduct disorder also met criteria for substance use disorder (Reebye et al. 1995). The comorbidity was higher in the younger (ages 10–13) group. Childhood aggression is a predictor of adolescent drug use and delinquency, and delinquency predicts later drug use (Brook et al. 1992). Substance abuse likely reflects the presence of temperamental risk factors—novelty seeking and impulsivity—but is also likely to directly promote antisocial behavior through adversely affecting judgment, further decreasing impulse control, and—in the presence of marked psychological or physiological dependence—leading to strenuous and illegal efforts to obtain the substance. Of course, antisocial behavior may be indirectly promoted through increasing affiliation with antisocial peers.

Although the majority of the literature on conduct disorder has focused on males, due to a previous assumption that the disorder is rare in females, an increasing recognition that the disorder is common among girls has led to a growing literature regarding the disorder in females. Relative to males, females may be more likely to develop internalizing disorders as comorbid conditions (Keenan et al. 1999). Females also appear less likely to engage in overt physical aggression and are more inclined to use verbal and relational aggression such as alienation and character defamation (Loeber et al. 2000).

This diagnostic comorbidity found in children and adolescents who meet criteria for conduct disorder or ODD demonstrates the heterogeneity of this patient group. Clinicians and researchers working with these young people must carefully examine all of the symptoms and background information to accurately identify factors to classify each child and adolescent.

Etiology

Conduct disorder and ODD have complex and multifactorial etiologies. Biological, psychological, social, and developmental factors each contribute in differing degrees to the development and clinical course of the disorders (Lewis et al. 1987). We delineate some of the known biopsychosocial factors, but it is the interaction of these variables that leads to a complete understanding of the etiology of the disorder. For instance, the presence of birth complications combined with early maternal rejection at age 1 year is associated with violent crime at age 18 years. This effect was specific to violence and was not associated with either risk factor alone (Raine et al. 1994). As noted above, numerous factors are likely to contribute to the observed impairments in affective and behavioral regulation in conduct disorder and ODD. Some factors may contribute through direct alterations in brain structure and function stemming from the actions of gene products; others, through adverse effects on intrauterine development; and still others, through postnatal damage impinging through mechanical, toxic, or psychological injury. Other factors are likely to relate to deviant learning acquired though exposure to chaotic and destructive family and peer environments.

■ Biological Factors

Genetics

The role of genetic vulnerability in developing conduct disorder has yet to be fully elucidated, although it is likely that genetic factors play at least some role either directly or through a mediating factor such as temperament. Genetic factors have been identified in a number of traits that are believed to contribute to conduct disorder, including inattention, hyperactivity, aggressiveness, and novelty seeking. The role of genetics in adult antisocial personality is fairly robust. It is likely that psychosocial factors play a stronger role in child and adolescent conduct disorder because children, unlike adults, are less able to self-select the social contexts in which they must live and develop. Most

studies involving youths with disruptive behavior disorders suggest a significant role for psychosocial and environmental factors that, acting in concert with genetic factors, substantially increase the risk of psychopathology (Burt et al. 2001; Steiner and Wilson 1999).

Characteristics of childhood temperament are considered to be genetic or constitutional in origin and to show some consistency across time (Thomas and Chess 1977). Children characterized as possessing a difficult temperament are more likely to show or develop behavioral problems (Rutter et al. 1964). When familial genetic factors predispose a child to conduct disorder and delinquency, it is also more likely that at least one parent is antisocial (Lahey et al. 1988b; Mednick et al. 1984; Moffitt 1987). Children with a difficult temperament may interact with their family and environment in such a way that the initial behavioral disturbance becomes even more problematic. For instance, self-regulation at age 4 years could be predicted by maternal ratings of the child's impulsivity and attention span, an objective measure of delay ability, and maternal negativity at age 24 months (Silverman and Ragusa 1993). In a study using the Junior Temperament and Character Inventory, adolescents who showed elevations in novelty seeking and reduced harm avoidance demonstrated increased rates of aggressive and delinquent behavior (Schmeck and Poustka 2001).

There have been some interesting findings of specific gene frequencies and genetic polymorphisms found to be associated with conduct disturbances. Enhanced rates of expression of the L/L variant of the serotonin transporter gene, the presence of which effectively increases the function of the serotonin transporter, were found in a sample of hyperactive children and adolescents both with and without conduct disorder (Seeger et al. 2001). In a multivariate regression analysis of 20 genes, Comings et al. (2000) found that adrenergic genes were strongly implicated in ADHD and that these same genes were often shared with patients with conduct disorder and ODD.

Hormonal Factors

It is commonly believed that hormonal changes have a direct influence on adolescent behavior. However, there are few scientific studies that demonstrate this influence as a direct effect. A few studies have found that hormone levels correlate with emotional and aggressive attributes in boys. Olweus and colleagues (1988) found that high levels of testosterone caused boys to be more impatient and irritable, resulting in an increased propensity to engage in aggressive-destructive behavior. Susman et al. (1987) found that higher levels of androstenedione were related to higher levels of acting-out problems in boys. Dmitrieva et al. (2001) found dehydroepiandrosterone (DHEAS) and corticotropin levels to be elevated in boys with conduct disorder. van Goozen et al. (2000) found similar elevations in DHEAS in boys with ODD.

There is also some evidence of diminished salivary cortisol levels in aggressive boys. This finding was most robust, and was more indicative of persistent aggression, when a restricted range of cortisol levels was found on repeated measures than when a low concentration was identified at any particular point in time (McBurnett et al. 2000). Decreased plasma cortisol levels were also found in girls with conduct disorder (Pajer et al. 2001).

Neurotransmitter Dysfunction

Evidence of potential monoamine neurotransmitter dysfunction or deviation has been identified in numerous studies of antisocial and aggressive adults, children, and adolescents. The systems studied have also been heavily implicated in expression and regulation of affect and in impulse control. Disturbed serotonergic function has been implicated in episodic aggression and appears to be related to the capacity for behavioral inhibition. The role of serotonin is likely to be that of a neuromodulator ensuring that the motivational systems do not "overshoot" their targets through modifying the "signal-to-noise ratio" (Spoont 1992). Male monkeys with low cerebrospinal fluid levels of 5-hydroxyindoleacetic acid (5-HIAA) are at risk for violent, aggressive behavior and loss of impulse control (Mehlman et al. 1994) and have less social competence and sociality (Mehlman et al. 1995). Cloninger (1987) described a central role of serotonin in affecting the trait of harm avoidance—a characteristic observed to be low in antisocial patients. Measures of cerebrospinal fluid 5-HIAA have been found to be low in adult samples with violent suicidal behavior and early-onset alcoholism (Steiner and Wilson 1999). Platelet serotonin measures have been found to be abnormal in adolescents with conduct disorder (Unis and Cook 1997). There is a strong suggestion that cerebrospinal fluid levels of 5-HIAA and homovanillic acid and autonomic measures can be used to predict risk for future problems (Kruesi et al. 1992). Disturbed platelet monoamine oxidase levels have been reported in disruptive behavior disorders (Stoff et al. 1989). Decreased levels of methoxyhydroxyphenyl glycol have been identified in aggressive patients (Steiner and Wilson 1999). van Goozen et al. (1999) found plasma 5-HIAA and homovanillic acid to be inversely related to aggression in a sample of boys with ODD.

Neurological and Autonomic Findings

Minor neurological abnormalities are found in some children and adolescents with delinquency (Lewis et al. 1987). In adolescents with conduct disorder, the frontal P300 event-related potential shows reduced amplitude in association with deficits in executive function and inhibition (Kim et al. 2001). Bauer and Hesselbrock (2001) also found abnormalities in the frontal P300 event-related potential in a sample of adolescents with conduct disorder, suggesting frontal cortex dysfunction. However, it is not clear whether these abnormalities are related to conduct disorder per se or to comorbid ADHD-like symptoms and executive dysfunction. For example, Satterfield et al. (1987) followed up hyperactive children into adolescence and found that the nondelinquent hyperactive subjects had abnormal auditory evoked-response potentials, whereas the delinquent hyperactive subjects had normal maturational changes in these same measures. In addition, because delinquent children are known to have had more head and face trauma (Lewis et al. 1979), early neurological signs may be the result of abuse or risk-taking behavior rather than constitutional abnormalities (Kazdin 1987).

Neuropsychological deficit is clearly associated with delinquency. A consistent association is found between low IQ and delinquency that persists when assessed prospectively and is independent of social class (Moffitt et al. 1981). Studies routinely cite impaired verbal and executive functions (attention, concentration, abstraction, planning, inhibition of inappropriate responses, and sequencing) (Moffitt and Silva 1988).

Young people with conduct disorder also may possess a degree of autonomic hypoactivity, which results in the individual being slow to respond to stressful stimuli with anticipatory anxiety (Mednick 1981). These individuals then tend to recover slowly once aroused. Such a pattern may result in impairment in the person's ability to learn to escape harm or punishment through passive avoidance. Higher levels of arousal may be protective. Fifteen-year-old males with antisocial behavior who had higher electrodermal and cardiovascular arousal were less likely to have engaged in criminal behavior by age 29 than the group with lower arousal (Raine et al. 1995). Some recent work by Beauchaine and colleagues (2001) suggests that patients with conduct disorder may be differentiated from patients with ADHD by differential patterns of autonomic responsiveness. However, the relationship between anxiety and conduct disorder needs further refining because some data suggest that the presence of anxiety may protect against the development of conduct disorder, whereas other data suggest an increased likelihood of developing anxiety symptoms after the establishment of conduct disorder. One possible issue may be a confounding of the concepts of trait anxiety with behavioral inhibition—features that may have a low correlation (Frick et al. 1999).

Prenatal Toxin Exposures

Wakschlag et al. (1997) demonstrated that maternal smoking during pregnancy is associated with a significant increase in the rate of conduct disorder even after controlling for previously identified risk factors. However, it is unclear if the effect is due to direct impact on the developing fetus or if maternal smoking is a marker for an unidentified maternal characteristic of etiologic significance for the development of conduct disorder. Children with fetal alcohol exposure are frequently noted to manifest disruptive behavior disorders characterized by substantial inattention and hyperactivity as well as poor social judgment (Kelly et al. 2000).

Children and adolescents with chronic medical illness, especially illnesses affecting the nervous system, also appear to have substantially increased risk of conduct disorder (Rutter 1988).

Evolutionary Biology

A perspective derived from evolutionary biology suggests that antisocial behavior in some individuals belonging to a strongly prosocial but behaviorally flexible species is likely to persist at a relatively stable equilibrium given a substantial potential for a Darwinian advantage to be gained through cheating to obtain resources from more trusting persons. This model suggests that at least some antisocial individuals are likely to be present in any population, and their problems

with self-regulation are most likely to be perceived as problems from the perspective of the victims, whereas the perpetrators themselves may be quite satisfied with themselves and their behavior. These individuals may be conceived as primary antisocials, whereas another group, who appear to adopt antisocial strategies secondary to difficulties achieving a more prosocial adaptation or in reaction to environmental constraints, may be described as secondary antisocials (Mealy 1997). In this model, the primary antisocials are likely to develop along the lines of the concept of psychopathy with high levels of callousness associated with low anxiety and minimal mood disturbances, whereas the secondary antisocials are likely to manifest more internalizing comorbidity and other evidence of adaptive dysfunction.

■ Psychological Factors

Cognitive Factors

Delinquent and aggressive children have distinctive cognitive and psychological profiles compared with children with other psychiatric disorders and control subjects. A group of delinquent males in a correctional facility displayed more immature modes of role taking, logical cognition, and moral reasoning (Lee and Prentice 1988). Compared with low-aggressive boys, high-aggressive boys 1) defined social problems based on the perception that others are hostilely motivated adversaries, 2) found fewer and less effective solutions, and 3) were less likely to get into trouble for exhibiting aggression (Guerra and Slaby 1989). Webster-Stratton and Lindsay (1999) found that boys with conduct disorder or ODD had significantly fewer social problem-solving strategies, more negative conflict management strategies, and delayed play skills relative to their peers without these disorders.

In addition, high-aggressive delinquent children were less able to perceive the viewpoints of other people than were low-aggressive delinquent children (Short and Simeonsson 1986). Aggressive children pay greater attention to aggressive environmental cues than do nonaggressive children and often misperceive cues. They quickly and impulsively think of nonverbal, action-oriented solutions to social situations (Kendall 1993). In a large longitudinal study that explored Cloninger's suggestion that boys who were high in impulsivity, low in anxiety (harm avoidance), and low in reward dependence would be at greater risk for delinquency, Tremblay et al. (1994)

demonstrated that boys in kindergarten with this combination of traits were more likely to develop a stable pattern of antisocial behavior. Increased reward dependence decreased delinquency.

Although some studies have identified the presence of executive dysfunction in patients with conduct disorder, the extent to which executive function impairments are related to conduct disorder per se versus comorbid conditions such as ADHD remains unclear. In one study examining the issue specifically, marked impairments in executive function seemed to be principally related to the presence of comorbid ADHD rather than primarily associated with conduct disorder or ODD (C. Clark et al. 2000).

Steiner and co-workers identified different patterns of antisocial behavior related to the extent of psychic distress reported by a group of delinquent youths compared with their respective levels of restraint (Steiner and Wilson 1999; Steiner et al. 1997). Those characterized by low restraint had longer courses of antisocial behavior. However, adolescents who appeared to be overcontrolled (high restraint) often presented with short but dramatic criminal careers. A particularly interesting finding here is that restraint, typically considered to be a protective factor in conduct disorder, may under some circumstances be associated with episodes of severe antisocial behavior. This suggests that significant potential variability in specific delinquency presentation may be generated by the interaction between issues related to subjective affective distress and degree of inhibition. It also suggests that the relationship between inhibition and acting out is not a simple one.

Familial Factors

Parental psychopathology and seriously disadvantaged, dysfunctional, and disorganized home environments are common in children who have or who eventually develop conduct disorder (Fergusson et al. 1994). Antisocial personality disorder, criminal behavior, and alcoholism—particularly in the father—are the stronger and more consistently reported familial factors that increase the child's risk for conduct disorder (Robins 1966; Rutter and Giller 1984). In addition, mothers of children with a diagnosis of conduct disorder often have antisocial personality, somatization, or alcohol abuse (Lahey et al. 1988b). Lahey and colleagues (1988b) found evidence of parental psychopathology among children with conduct disorder

but not among children with ADHD.

An accepted theory is that children who are aggressive have parents who are also aggressive, especially toward the children. However, a critical review of the studies supporting this association (Widom 1989) concluded that convincing evidence is lacking that this linkage is simple or direct. Further refinement of the study of the association between parental and child violence reveals that certain processes transmit aggressiveness to children (McCord 1988). Such processes include messages that expressive behavior (including injurious actions) is normal and justified and that egocentrism is both normal and virtuous.

Learning theorists have posited that oppositional defiant behaviors may be promoted through a negative reinforcement model. In this model the child learns to escape unpleasant tasks such as chores by becoming hostile and negativistic. Repeated parental requests for compliance are met with escalating negativity until the parent eventually relents and the child escapes the demand situation. Failure of parental follow-through with consequences is also a factor in this model. However, what is not addressed is, of course, why some children seem willing very early to escalate hostility and negativity to a marked extent despite frequently very negative relationship repercussions (Forehand et al. 1975; Wells and Egan 1988).

Familial, peer, and attentional variables interact to predict delinquency (Hoge et al. 1994). Family interactions that are characterized as unsupportive and lacking in the ability to cope with transitions and stress may lead to delinquency (Tolan 1988). The families of delinquent children also tend to emphasize personal growth dimensions, such as achievement, and cultural and ethical interests less than families of nondelinquent children (LeFlore 1988). In addition, the mother–child dyad is characterized by more conflict when adolescents have behavioral problems (Forehand et al. 1987).

Families of children and adolescents with conduct disorder have several other characteristics in common that have emerged from descriptive studies. Parental divorce is correlated with the development of conduct disorder in the children (Rutter 1971). However, this association is found between parental antisocial personality disorder, divorce, and conduct disorder but not directly between divorce and conduct disorder (Lahey et al. 1988a). Also, it appears that regardless of whether the parents are separated, it is the extent of the parental discord that is associated with the high risk for childhood dysfunction (Hetherington and

Stanley-Hagan 1999). Other family variables related to offspring with conduct disorder include large family size and greater risk for conduct disorder in the middle child, especially when separated by several years from older brothers (Wadsworth 1979). The absence of the biological father has also been identified as a risk factor for antisocial behavior in any family member (Pfiffner et al. 2001). This absence was not mitigated by the presence of stepfathers and was not accounted for by lower socioeconomic status.

■ Social Factors

The contribution of general social factors is another unsettled issue in the literature on disruptive behavior disorders. Loeber and colleagues (1995) found low socioeconomic status to be a risk factor for the progression of ODD to conduct disorder, and others have also found associations between low socioeconomic status and conduct disorder (Rutter and Giller 1984). However, when factors associated with social class—such as family size, overcrowding, and supervision—are controlled for, social class shows very little relation to antisocial behavior (Wadsworth 1979). These data suggest that the influence of low socioeconomic status on the risk of conduct disorder and ODD is primarily indirect and is mediated by a variety of other factors. Early antisocial behavior and peer group rejection are important factors that have been found to precede delinquent behavior (Snyder et al. 1986). However, the ability for deviant peer affiliation to predict delinquent outcome is related to the amount of parental supervision. Cultural variables are also associated with antisocial behavior. Culturally derived beliefs—such as acceptance of aggression, respect for authority, role of the parent, and the value of independence—are noted to be significant factors in the expression of aggression and antisocial behaviors (Ekblad 1988). It also appears that minority children are more likely to be incarcerated—and thereby identified as delinquent—than are nonminority youths, given a similar degree of disturbance (R. Cohen et al. 1990).

Assessment

The assessment of the signs, symptoms, and risk factors of conduct disorder in children should include information from multiple sources. This information should focus on current behavior as well as developmental signs and symptoms. Diagnostic interviews, rating scales, and a review of pertinent records from the school and clinics (health care, mental health, juvenile court) are useful ways to gather information.

The assessment is guided by knowledge of the biopsychosocial model of etiology. This model includes information about cognitive style, family structure and functioning, and physical signs and symptoms. This information should include the presence or absence of symptoms necessary to make a DSM-IV-TR diagnosis. However, as discussed above, the symptoms are not specific to one particular disorder and do not guide treatment or predict outcome. Additional biopsychosocial and developmental information may help determine treatment and prognosis.

A number of rating scales are available to help identify disturbed behavior. The Child Behavior Checklist (Achenbach 1991a, 1991b, 1991c, 1992) is designed for teachers and parents to complete and yields a scale score on symptom clusters such as delinquency, aggression, hyperactivity, and depression. Self-report measures have proved effective in identifying antisocial behavior, especially in adolescents. Specific scales for rating aggression include the Iowa Conners Aggression Factor (Loney and Milich 1985), derived from the Conners Teacher Questionnaire (Conners 1969), and the Modified Overt Aggression Scale (Kay et al. 1988). Peer and teacher ratings of behavior and likeability in elementary school are significant predictive factors for delinquent behavior in adolescence (Tremblay et al. 1988).

One of the most important factors in the assessment of antisocial behavior in children and adolescents is the attitude of the clinician making the assessment. Clinical judgment is significantly affected by contextual factors such as resource availability and agency setting in the assessment of amenability to treatment (Mulvey and Reppucci 1988). The setting in which one works, as well as one's own biases, can in part determine the adequacy of the assessment and treatment recommendations. For this reason, the clinician must know the etiology, treatment approaches, resources, and outcome variables to assess antisocial behavior in a youth.

Working with an impulsive patient requires regular monitoring and management of feelings aroused in the therapist by the patient. Some of these feelings are expected reactions to undependable behavior such as missed appointments, dangerous risk-taking behavior, impulsive and thoughtless comments, and potential legal issues raised in working with these high-risk patients. At times, these patients also may arouse countertransference feelings in the therapist. These feelings might range from envy and vicarious pleasure derived from exciting, unrestricted behavior to anger, revulsion, indignation, and even hatred for thoughtless, destructive acts with consequences that go far beyond the patient and the therapist. The first and most important step is for the therapist to recognize and acknowledge these feelings, which often prevents the feelings from becoming counterproductive or destructive. When the feelings significantly interfere with the therapy or the well-being of the patient or therapist, outside consultation should be sought.

Treatment

Treatment of youths with conduct disorder takes place in a variety of settings, including short- and long-term inpatient psychiatric units, residential and day treatment centers, correctional facilities, and outpatient settings. Treatment approaches also differ greatly. Behavior therapy, family therapy, individual and group therapy, parent management training, cognitive therapy, systems theory–based approaches, and pharmacotherapy are all used to a greater or lesser extent, depending on the treatment setting and the clinician's orientation. One of the major problems facing researchers in this area is the nonspecificity of the diagnosis of conduct disorder. In addition, clinicians may approach this group of children with a sense of therapeutic nihilism that clearly does not promote therapeutic success. Fortunately there are now a number of empirically well-supported approaches to the treatment of these often challenging patients and families. In general, the effective treatment of conduct disorder requires a multimodal approach that addresses multiple areas of impairment and continues over an extensive period of time (Steiner 1997).

As discussed above, children and adolescents with antisocial behavior have extremely varied psychopathology. Some may have depression, some may have psychosis, and others may have ADHD. Others may not have any psychiatric disorder other than conduct disorder. Their behavior may be the result of their culture or a history of abuse or neglect. Most treatment studies do not differentiate the associated psychopathology. As a result, an approach believed to be suc-

cessful for certain patients with conduct disorder in a particular setting cannot be generalized to all children and adolescents with a diagnosis of conduct disorder. Keeping this caveat in mind, we briefly describe the more successful approaches. Further descriptions of treatment modalities can be found in Chapters 50–56 in this volume.

■ Problem-Solving Skills Training

Cognitive-behavioral approaches with youths who have conduct disorder focus on modifying cognitive deficiencies (e.g., communication skills, problem-solving skills, impulse control, and anger management) that are believed to underlie antisocial behavior (Faulstich et al. 1988). Generally, these are step-by-step approaches to interpersonal situations that use modeling, rehearsal, role playing, and development of an internal dialogue for self-evaluation (Kazdin 1987). Most studies of this approach provide anecdotal evidence attesting to its success (Englander-Golden et al. 1989; Haggerty et al. 1989; Hains and Hains 1987). In a controlled study, Kazdin et al. (1989) randomly assigned 112 children with severe behavior disorder to one of three treatments: problem-solving skills training, problem-solving skills training with therapeutic practice activities, or client-centered relationship therapy. Both problem-solving skills training interventions showed significantly greater reductions in antisocial behavior and greater increases in prosocial behavior than did relationship therapy. These effects were evident at the end of treatment and at 1-year follow-up.

■ Family-Focused Treatments

Dysfunctional family structure and interactions have an important role in the development of antisocial behavior. Family therapy, using a wide variety of techniques, attempts to alter the family system. Many studies of the efficacy of family therapy in alleviating antisocial behavior in children rely on weak or questionable methodologies. However, in a review of the extensive literature, Tolan et al. (1986) found consistently positive results from family therapy. In many cases, family therapy was more effective than other therapeutic modalities. Behavioral, structural, strategic, and communication techniques appeared to be the most effective. Future research needs to delineate the family systems variables that are associated with childhood antisocial behavior, verify which techniques are effective with particular family dysfunctions, and evaluate the long-term effectiveness of family therapy compared with other treatment modalities. Functional family therapy (Alexander and Parsons 1982) is a family-based technique that has clear empirical support for its effectiveness (Kazdin 1998). The main goals of this treatment approach are to increase reciprocity and positive reinforcement among family members, improve communication, promote effective negotiation, and improve interpersonal problem solving.

Parent management training attempts to alter coercive parent–child interactions that foster antisocial behavior in the child (Patterson 1982). The major intervention is the direct training of parents to interact differently with their child, so that prosocial behavior is rewarded. Outcome studies of this technique demonstrate consistently positive results (Kazdin 1987; Kazdin et al. 1992). Outcome is affected by the duration of treatment, the severity of family dysfunction, and social supports outside the home. Preliminary evidence suggests that parent management training is more effective with aggressive children with conduct disorder than with nonaggressive youths with conduct disorder (Patterson 1982). Further research is needed to delineate parent and child characteristics that respond best to parent management training. Nevertheless, parent management training is currently one of the best-researched and most promising treatment interventions for children and adolescents with conduct disorder.

Multisystemic therapy is another empirically well-supported treatment methodology that uses a systems theory perspective. This approach assumes that antisocial behavior becomes embedded within the life space of the patient such that the individual has been increasingly rewarded for engaging in antisocial conduct at the expense of more prosocial behaviors. The treatment involves extensive contact between the therapist and the multiple actual living contexts of the patient, especially those of the family and peer group. More individually focused elements may be used as appropriate to target specific issues (e.g., depression), but the majority of the treatment focuses on enabling the family to more successfully and positively shape the behavior of the child (Henggeller et al. 1998).

■ Peer Relationship and School-Based Interventions

Although disturbed parent–child interactions are clearly implicated in the developmental etiology of conduct disorder, problematic peer relationships and poor school performance are also significant factors, particularly in middle childhood (Offord and Bennett 1994). Peer rejection has been correlated with aggression, and school failure has been correlated with the development of behavioral problems. A variety of interventions have targeted these two areas. Social skills training programs have aimed to improve the peer relationships of children at high risk for antisocial behavior (Bierman and Furman 1984), and specific academic skills programs have sought to reduce rates of school failure (Kellam et al. 1991). Preliminary data are promising, but further study is indicated.

■ Pharmacotherapy

Because the range of psychopathology in conduct disorder is extensive and comorbidity is likely the rule rather than the exception, if another psychiatric syndrome is identified clearly, aggressive pharmacotherapy is probably warranted and may significantly diminish the behavioral morbidity. Psychotropic drugs have not yet shown specific effectiveness in the treatment of conduct disorder. However, several drugs are used to treat symptoms associated with conduct disorder, especially aggression.

Antipsychotic drugs have been extensively used in the treatment of acute and chronic aggression in a variety of clinical populations. For instance, haloperidol was effective in reducing aggressiveness, temper tantrums, and explosiveness in children with behavior disorder (Werry and Aman 1975). However, concerns about the potential for serious side effects associated with traditional antipsychotic agents have increasingly limited their use. With the advent of atypical antipsychotics and their greater tolerability and reduced liability for producing extrapyramidal side effects and tardive dyskinesia, these drugs may be used more frequently for the treatment of serious aggression. Risperidone was shown to be superior to placebo for the treatment of aggression in a small double-blind study of youths with conduct disorder (Findling et al. 2000).

Psychostimulants have also been used to treat conduct disorder, but the results do not provide definite conclusions about effectiveness because of equivocal findings or methodological problems. In a recent meta-analysis, Connor et al. (2002) found psychostimulants to be as effective for aggressive symptoms within the context of ADHD as they are for the core symptoms of inattention, impulsivity, and hyperactivity. However, the effect sizes for overt aggression were noted to diminish in the presence of conduct disorder.

The number of studies examining the efficacy of antidepressants in the treatment of conduct disorder is surprisingly small, considering the degree of comorbidity with depression. Puig-Antich (1982) found that conduct disorder symptoms abated after imipramine treatment in a group of boys with comorbid major depressive disorder and conduct disorder. In a small open trial, trazodone was found to be effective for the treatment of aggressive children (Ghaziuddin and Alessi 1992). In boys with chronic conduct disorder and attention-deficit disorder, treatment with bupropion resulted in improvements in behavior, affect, and anxiety (Simeon et al. 1986). An open-label trial of bupropion was positive in a sample of adolescents with ADHD and substance use plus conduct disorder (Riggs et al. 1998). Theoretically, selective serotonin reuptake inhibitors (SSRIs) may be of benefit in conduct disorder given the evidence of serotonergic dysfunction in disorders of impulse control, and several adult studies have suggested that the SSRIs may have antiaggressive effects. However, in an open trial of SSRIs for aggression in hospitalized adolescents, no beneficial effects were demonstrated and the SSRIs may have contributed to an observed increase in verbal aggression (Constantino et al. 1997). Methodologically sound studies are necessary to delineate the subgroup of youths with conduct disorder who respond to antidepressants.

When comorbid bipolar disorder is suspected, trials of lithium or anticonvulsants are indicated (Arredondo and Butler 1994). Lithium was also effective in reducing aggressive and explosive behavior in a subgroup of children with behavior disorder who had symptoms of an affective disorder (DeLong and Aldershof 1987). In the same study, another subgroup of children who had behavior disorder and neurological and medical disease also had decreased rage and aggressive outbursts after lithium treatment. Both haloperidol and lithium carbonate have been found to be effective in decreasing behavioral symptoms in hospitalized children with treatment-resistant conduct disorder (Campbell et al. 1984, 1995). In blind trials, carbamazepine has also been shown to be useful in the treatment of aggressive behavior (Kafantaris et al. 1992; Rosenberg et al. 1994). However, in a double-blind, placebo-controlled study in children with conduct disorder, carbamazepine was found not to be

superior to placebo in reducing aggressive behavior, and untoward effects were common (Cueva et al. 1996). Valproate was shown to be efficacious in a double-blind, placebo-controlled crossover study of youths with explosive temper and mood lability, supporting previous open-label trials (Donovan et al. 2000).

A small randomized, blind-group comparison study of methylphenidate and clonidine both alone and in combination suggested that clonidine had potential efficacy for aggression in ADHD comorbid with either ODD or conduct disorder (Connor et al. 2000). Propranolol has been proved to be effective in the treatment of aggressive behavior in children and adolescents with chronic brain dysfunction and in a few youths with conduct disorder that was refractory to other pharmacological approaches (Kuperman and Stewart 1987). Additional studies are needed to delineate effective psychotropic medications for youths with severe behavior disorders.

Prognosis

The clinical course of conduct disorder in children is variable: mild forms show improvement over time, whereas more severe forms tend to be chronic (American Psychiatric Association 1994). The difficulty in developing a definite subclassification system of conduct disorder has hindered outcome research, and researchers have developed their own subtypes to classify outcome. Aggressive conduct disorder is a commonly used subtype and has a worse prognosis. Outcome studies of aggressive boys with conduct disorder found that about half continued to have conduct disorder at follow-up 2 years later (Stewart and Kelso 1987). Persistence of conduct disorder was predicted by various antisocial and aggressive symptoms, fire setting, early age at onset, family deviance, and inattention (Kelso and Stewart 1986). Data are mixed regarding the stability of symptoms in males versus females; some studies suggest that externalizing symptoms are more stable in males (McGee et al. 1992), whereas others suggest an approximately equal degree of stability in both sexes (Tremblay et al. 1992). In either case, severity of symptoms tends to be positively correlated with persistence of symptoms (P. Cohen et al. 1993). However, girls with conduct disorder may subsequently develop more internalizing disorders, as noted above, and may have more general health problems as adults than males (Bardone et al. 1998). Clearly, issues of early pregnancy and parenting often present significant issues in females with severe behavioral disorders.

It appears that children's neuropsychological problems interact cumulatively with their environment across development to determine the outcome of early antisocial behavior (Moffitt 1993). Lewis et al. (1989) found that the interaction of intrinsic vulnerabilities such as cognitive, psychiatric, and neurological impairment and a history of abuse or family violence was a better predictor of adult violent crime than was a history of violence. Longer-term outcome studies (Robins and Ratcliff 1979) found that 23%–41% of highly antisocial children became antisocial adults, 17%–28% did not become clearly antisocial, and the remainder did not fall clearly into either group. Factors that predicted adult antisocial behavior included a variety of antisocial behaviors in childhood, drug use before age 15, placement out of the home, and growing up in extreme poverty (Robins and Ratcliff 1979). When young people with antisocial behavior were followed up, the most frequent explanations for death were found to be uncertain causes and suicides (Rydelius 1988).

Early age at onset is the factor most consistently found to be associated with poor outcome (Tolan and Lorion 1988). Tolan (1987) found that a combination of demographic, individual, school, and family variables predicted age at onset. In a longitudinal study of high-risk children in Hawaii, certain factors were frequently found in adult men with a criminal record (Werner 1989). These factors included 1) having a younger sibling born less than 2 years after the subject, 2) being raised by an unmarried mother, 3) not having a father present during infancy and early childhood, 4) experiencing prolonged disruptions in family life, and 5) having a working mother without suitable caregivers during the first year of life.

Not all children with antisocial behavior become antisocial adults. Results of the long-term follow-up study in Hawaii found that "resilient" high-risk children who did not develop serious behavior disorders were more likely to be first-born children with high intelligence from smaller families with low discord (Werner 1989). In a longitudinal study of children from families judged to be at high risk for producing a delinquent child, it was found that boys who were characterized as neurotic at age 10, had few or no friends at age 8, and did not spend leisure time with their fathers demonstrated satisfactory social adjustment as men (Farrington et al. 1988). Shyness appeared to act as a protective factor for nonaggressive boys, but it was found to be an aggravating factor for aggressive boys.

In summary, the most consistent factors that predict poor prognosis for children with antisocial behavior are early age at onset; high rates of antisocial behavior; antisocial acts across multiple settings, such as the home, school, and community; and diverse antisocial behaviors (Rutter and Giller 1984). Further research is needed to identify prognostic factors associated with disorders comorbid with conduct disorder, such as ADHD, psychosis, and depression.

Prevention

Conduct disorder and the eventual outcome of this disorder appear to have a developmental etiology. Identifying children at neurodevelopmental risk and intervening early may therefore be helpful (Moffitt and Caspi 2001). Symptoms such as impaired executive function, poor impulse control, and autonomic underreactivity suggest increased risk. Patterson et al. (1989) proposed that a reliable developmental sequence of experiences leads to antisocial behavior. This sequence starts with ineffective parenting practices and is followed by academic failure and peer rejection, which lead to depressed mood and involvement in a deviant peer group. Prevention efforts that intervene early in this sequence have greater success than those that intervene later. Parent training interventions have been successful when applied to younger antisocial children (Kazdin 1987). As noted above in the section "Peer-Related and School-Based Interventions," academic skills training has also shown promise as an intervention with predelinquent children (Johnson and Brekenridge 1982), especially when a learning disability is associated (Grande 1988; Meltzer et al. 1986). School-based interventions with the parent, teacher, and child have significantly decreased short- and long-term behavioral problems at school and in the community (Bry 1982). Finally, community-based interventions that involve activity and skill training programs have shown some promise (Offord and Jones 1983), although they have not yet demonstrated broad-based and long-lasting results.

Research Issues

It is clear that additional and better quality research is necessary. More specific diagnostic criteria will help to delineate subcategories within the currently heterogeneous group of children with conduct disorders. Research should focus on comorbidity and etiological factors, such as family dysfunction and cognitive and neurological dysfunction, as well as cultural and environmental influences. Neuroimaging and neuropsychobiological testing will advance the understanding of the biological basis of impulse-control disorders and may help distinguish subcategories of conduct disorder. Outcome studies will be more meaningful when a specific subclassification system delineates particular aspects of the disorder that make an individual more vulnerable or resilient. Greater diagnostic specificity will also help to assess the effectiveness of various treatment interventions with particular symptom constellations. This exciting area for research has far-reaching implications not only for the prevention and treatment of serious mental disorders but also for the healthy functioning of society.

References

Achenbach TM: Manual for the Child Behavior Checklist/4–18 and 1991 Profile. Burlington, VT, University of Vermont, 1991a

Achenbach TM: Manual for the Teacher's Report Form and 1991 Profile. Burlington, VT, University of Vermont, 1991b

Achenbach TM: Manual for the Youth Self-Report and 1991 Profile. Burlington, VT, University of Vermont, 1991c

Achenbach TM: Manual for the Child Behavior Checklist/2–3 and 1992 Profile. Burlington, VT, University of Vermont, 1992

Alexander JF, Parsons BV: Functional Family Therapy. Monterey, CA, Brooks/Cole, 1982

American Psychiatric Association: Diagnostic and Statistical Manual of Mental Disorders, 4th Edition. Washington, DC, American Psychiatric Association, 1994

American Psychiatric Association: Diagnostic and Statistical Manual of Mental Disorders, 4th Edition, Text Revision. Washington, DC, American Psychiatric Association, 2000

Angold A, Costello EJ: Toward establishing an empirical basis for the diagnosis of oppositional defiant disorder. J Am Acad Child Adolesc Psychiatry 35:1205–1212, 1996

Arredondo DE, Butler SF: Affective comorbidity in psychiatrically hospitalized adolescents with conduct disorder or oppositional defiant disorder: should conduct disorder be treated with mood stabilizers? J Child Adolesc Psychopharmacol 4:151–158, 1994

Bardone AM, Moffitt TE, Caspi A, et al: Adult physical health outcomes of adolescent girls with conduct disorder, depression, and anxiety. J Am Acad Child Adolesc Psychiatry 37:594–601, 1998

Bauer LO, Hesselbrock VM: CSD/BEM localization of P300 sources in adolescents "at-risk": evidence of frontal cortex dysfunction in conduct disorder. Biol Psychiatry 50:600–608, 2001

Beauchaine TP, Katkin ES, Strassburg Z, et al: Disinhibitory psychopathology in male adolescents discriminating conduct disorder from attention deficit/hyperactivity disorder through assessment of multiple autonomic states. J Abnorm Psychol 110:610–624, 2001

Bierman KL, Furman W: The effects of social skills training and peer involvement on the social adjustment of pre-adolescents, in Primary Prevention of Psychopathology, Vol 10: Prevention of Delinquent Behavior. Edited by Burchard JD, Burchard SN. Newbury Park, CA, Sage, 1984, pp 220–240

Blair RJ: Neurocognitive models of aggression, the antisocial personality, and psychopathy. J Neurol Neurosurg Psychiatry 71:727–731, 2001

Bradley S: Affect Regulation and the Development of Psychopathology. New York, Guilford, 2000

Brook JS, Whiteman NM, Finch S: Childhood aggression, adolescent delinquency, and drug use: a longitudinal study. J Genet Psychol 153:369–383, 1992

Bry BH: Reducing the incidence of adolescent problems through preventive intervention: one- and five-year follow-up. Am J Community Psychol 10:265–276, 1982

Burt SA, Krueger RF, McGue M, et al: Sources of covariation among attention deficit/hyperactivity disorder, oppositional defiant disorder, and conduct disorder: the importance of shared environment. J Abnorm Psychol 110:516–525, 2001

Campbell M, Small AM, Green WH, et al: Behavioral efficacy of haloperidol and lithium carbonate. Arch Gen Psychiatry 41:650–656, 1984

Campbell M, Adams PB, Small AM, et al: Lithium in hospitalized aggressive children with conduct disorder: a double-blind and placebo-controlled study. J Am Acad Child Adolesc Psychiatry 34:445–453, 1995

Cantwell DP, Baker L: Issues in the classification of child and adolescent psychopathology. J Am Acad Child Adolesc Psychiatry 27:521–533, 1988

Cantwell DP, Baker L: Stability and natural history of DSM-III childhood diagnoses. J Am Acad Child Adolesc Psychiatry 28:691–700, 1989

Christian RE, Frick PJ, Hill NL, et al: Psychopathy and conduct problems in children, II: implications for subtyping children with conduct problems. J Am Acad Child Adolesc Psychiatry 36:233–241, 1997

Clark C, Prior M, Kinsella GJ: Do executive function deficits differentiate between adolescents with AD/HD and oppositional defiant/conduct disorder? A neuropsychological study using the Six Elements Test and Hayling Sentence Completion Test. J Abnorm Psychol 28:403–414, 2000

Clark DL, Boutros NN: The Brain and Behavior: An Introduction to Behavioral Neuroanatomy. Malden, MA, Blackwell Science, 1999

Cloninger CR: A systematic method for clinical description and classification of personality variants: a proposal. Arch Gen Psychiatry 44:573–588, 1987

Cohen P, Cohen J, Brook J: An epidemiological study of disorder in late childhood and adolescence, II: persistence of disorders. J Child Psychol Psychiatry 34:869–877, 1993

Cohen R, Parmelee DX, Irwin L, et al: Characteristics of children and adolescents in a psychiatric hospital and a corrections facility. J Am Acad Child Adolesc Psychiatry 29:909–913, 1990

Comings DE, Comings BG: A controlled study of Tourette syndrome, II: conduct. Am J Hum Genet 41:742–760, 1987

Comings DE, Gade-Andavolu R, Gonzales N, et al: Comparison of the role of dopamine, serotonin, and noradrenaline genes in ADHD, ODD and conduct disorder: multivariate regression analysis of 20 genes. Clin Genet 57:178–196, 2000

Conners CK: A teacher rating scale for use in drug studies with children. Am J Psychiatry 126:884–888, 1969

Connor DF, Barkley RA, Davis HT: A pilot study of methylphenidate, clonidine, or the combination in ADHD comorbid with aggressive oppositional defiant or conduct disorder. Clin Pediatr (Phila) 39:15–25, 2000

Connor DF, Glatt SJ, Lopez ID, et al: Psychopharmacology and aggression, I: a meta-analysis of stimulant effects on overt/covert aggression—related behaviors in ADHD. J Am Acad Child Adolesc Psychiatry 41:253–261, 2002

Constantino JN, Liberman M, Kincaid M: Effects of serotonin reuptake inhibitors on aggressive behavior in psychiatrically hospitalized adolescents: results of an open trial. J Child Adolesc Psychopharmacol 7:31–44, 1997

Cueva JE, Overall JE, Small AM, et al: Carbamazepine in aggressive children with conduct disorder: a double blind and placebo-controlled study. J Am Acad Child Adolesc Psychiatry 35:480–490, 1996

DeLong GR, Aldershof AL: Long-term experience with lithium treatment in childhood: correlation with clinical diagnosis. J Am Acad Child Adolesc Psychiatry 26:389–394, 1987

Dmitrieva TN, Oades RD, Hauffa BP, et al: Dehydroepiandrosterone sulphate and corticotropin levels are high in young male patients with conduct disorder: comparisons for growth factors, thyroid, and gonadal hormones. Neuropsychobiology 43:134–140, 2001

Donovan SJ, Stewart JW, Nunes EV, et al: Divalproex treatment for youth with explosive temper and mood lability: a double-blind, placebo-controlled crossover design. Am J Psychiatry 157:818–820, 2000

Ekblad S: Influence of child-rearing on aggressive behavior in a transcultural perspective. Acta Psychiatr Scand Suppl 344:133–139, 1988

Emler N, Reicher S, Ross A: The social context of delinquent conduct. J Child Psychol Psychiatry 28:99–109, 1987

Englander-Golden P, Jackson JE, Crane K, et al: Communication skills and self-esteem in prevention of destructive behaviors. Adolescence 24:481–502, 1989

Farrington DP, Gallagher B, Morley L, et al: Are there any successful men from criminogenic backgrounds? Psychiatry 51:116–130, 1988

Faulstich ME, Moore JR, Roberts RW, et al: A behavioral perspective on conduct disorders. Psychiatry 51:398–416, 1988

Fergusson DM, Horwood LJ, Lynskey M: The childhoods of multiple problem adolescents: a 15-year longitudinal study. J Child Psychol Psychiatry 35:1123–1140, 1994

Findling RL, McNamara WK, Branicky MA, et al: Pilot study of risperidone in the treatment of conduct disorder. J Am Acad Child Adolesc Psychiatry 39:509–516, 2000

Forehand R, King H, Peed S, et al: Mother-child interactions: comparison of a non-compliant clinic group and a non-clinic group. Behav Res Ther 13:79–84, 1975

Forehand R, Long N, Hedrick M: Family characteristics of adolescents who display overt and covert behavior problems. J Behav Ther Exp Psychiatry 18:325–328, 1987

Frick PJ, Ellis M: Callous-unemotional traits and subtypes of conduct disorder. Clin Child Fam Psychol Rev 2:149–168, 1999

Frick PJ, Lahey BB, Applegate B, et al: DSM-IV field trials for the disruptive behavior disorders: symptom utility estimates. J Am Acad Child Adolesc Psychiatry 33:529–539, 1994

Frick PJ, Lilienfeld SO, Loney B, et al: The association between anxiety and psychopathy dimensions in children. J Abnorm Child Psychol 27:383–392, 1999

Gabel S, Shindledecker R: Aggressive behavior in youth: characteristics, outcome, and psychiatric diagnoses. J Am Acad Child Adolesc Psychiatry 30:982–988, 1991

Ghaziuddin N, Alessi N: An open clinical trial of trazodone in aggressive children. J Child Adolesc Psychopharmacol 2:291–297, 1992

Grande CG: Delinquency: the learning disabled student's reaction to academic school failure? Adolescence 23:209–219, 1988

Guerra NG, Slaby RG: Evaluative factors in social problem solving by aggressive boys. J Abnorm Child Psychol 17:277–289, 1989

Haggerty KP, Wells EA, Jenson JM, et al: Delinquents and drug use: a model program for community reintegration. Adolescence 24:439–456, 1989

Hains AA, Hains AH: The effects of a cognitive strategy intervention on the problem-solving abilities of delinquent youths. J Adolesc 10:399–413, 1987

Harrington R, Fudge H, Rutter M, et al: Adult outcomes of childhood and adolescent depression, II: links with antisocial disorders. J Am Acad Child Adolesc Psychiatry 30:434–439, 1991

Henggeller SW, Schoenwald SK, Borduin CM, et al: Multi-systemic Treatment of Anti-social Behavior in Children and Adolescents. New York, Guilford, 1998

Hetherington EM, Stanley-Hagan M: The adjustment of children with divorced parents: a risk and resiliency perspective. J Child Psychol Psychiatry 40:129–140, 1999

Hoge RD, Andrews DA, Leschied AW: Tests of three hypotheses regarding the predictors of delinquency. J Abnorm Child Psychol 22:547–559, 1994

Johnson DL, Brekenridge JN: The Houston Parent-Child Development Center and the primary prevention of behavior problems in young children. Am J Community Psychol 10:305–316, 1982

Kafantaris V, Campbell M, Padron-Gayol MV, et al: Carbamazepine in hospitalized aggressive conduct disorder children: an open pilot study. Psychopharmacol Bull 28:193–199, 1992

Kay SR, Wolkenfield F, Murrill LM: Profiles of aggression among psychiatric patients, I: nature and prevalence. J Nerv Ment Dis 176:539–546, 1988

Kazdin AE: Conduct Disorders in Childhood and Adolescence (Developmental Clinical Psychology and Psychiatry Series, Vol 9). Newbury Park, CA, Sage, 1987

Kazdin AE: Psychosocial treatments for conduct disorder in children, in Treatments That Work. Edited by Nathan PE, Gorman JM. New York, Oxford University Press, 1998, pp 85–91

Kazdin AE, Bass D, Siegel T, et al: Cognitive-behavior therapy and relationship therapy in the treatment of children referred for antisocial behavior. J Consult Clin Psychol 57:522–535, 1989

Kazdin AE, Siegel TC, Bass D: Cognitive problem-solving skills training and parent management training in the treatment of antisocial behavior in children. J Consult Clin Psychol 60:733–747, 1992

Keenan K, Loeber R, Green S: Conduct disorder in girls: a review of the literature. Clin Child Fam Psychol Rev 2:3–19, 1999

Kellam SG, Werthamer-Larsson L, Dolan LF, et al: Developmental epidemiologically based preventative trials: baseline modeling of early target behaviors and depressive symptoms. Am J Community Psychol 4:563–584, 1991

Kelly SJ, Day N, Streissguth AP: Effects of pre-natal alcohol exposure on social behavior in humans and other species. Neurotoxicol Teratol 22:143–149, 2000

Kelso J, Stewart MA: Factors which predict the persistence of aggressive conduct disorder. J Child Psychol Psychiatry 27:77–86, 1986

Kendall PC: Cognitive-behavioral therapies with youth: guiding theory, current status, and emerging development. J Consult Clin Psychol 61:235–247, 1993

Kim MS, Kim JJ, Kwon JS: Frontal P300 decrement and executive dysfunction in adolescents with conduct problems. Child Psychiatry Hum Dev 32:93–106, 2001

Kovacs M, Paulauskas S, Gatsonis C, et al: Depressive disorders in childhood, III: a longitudinal study of comorbidity with and risk for conduct disorders. J Affect Disord 15:205–217, 1988

Kruesi MJP, Hibbs ED, Zahn TP, et al: A 2-year prospective follow-up of children and adolescents with disruptive behavior disorders. Arch Gen Psychiatry 49:429–435, 1992

Kuperman S, Stewart M: Use of propranolol to decrease aggressive outbursts in younger patients. Psychosomatics 28:315–319, 1987

Lahey BB, Hartdagen SE, Frick PJ, et al: Conduct disorder: parsing the confounded relation to parental divorce and antisocial personality. J Abnorm Psychol 97:334–337, 1988a

Lahey BB, Piacentini JC, McBurnett K, et al: Psychopathology in the parents of children with conduct disorder and hyperactivity. J Am Acad Child Adolesc Psychiatry 27:163–170, 1988b

Lavigne JV, Cicchetti C, Gibbons RD, et al: Oppositional defiant disorder with onset in preschool years: longitudinal stability and pathways to other disorders. J Am Acad Child Adolesc Psychiatry 40:1393–1400, 2001

Lee M, Prentice NM: Interrelations of empathy, cognition, and moral reasoning with dimensions of juvenile delinquency. J Abnorm Child Psychol 16:127–139, 1988

LeFlore L: Delinquent youths and family. Adolescence 23:629–642, 1988

Lewis DO, Shanok SS, Balla DA: Perinatal difficulties, head and face trauma, and child abuse in the medical histories of seriously delinquent children. Am J Psychiatry 136:419–423, 1979

Lewis DO, Pincus JH, Lovely R, et al: Biopsychosocial characteristics of matched samples of delinquents and nondelinquents. J Am Acad Child Adolesc Psychiatry 26:744–752, 1987

Lewis DO, Lovely R, Yeager C, et al: Toward a theory of the genesis of violence: a follow-up study of delinquents. J Am Acad Child Adolesc Psychiatry 28:431–436, 1989

Loeber R, Schmaling KB: Empirical evidence for overt and covert patterns of antisocial conduct problems: a meta-analysis. J Abnorm Child Psychol 13:315–335, 1985

Loeber R, Green SM, Keenan K, et al: Which boys will fare worse? Early predictors for the onset of conduct disorder in a six-year longitudinal study. J Am Acad Child Adolesc Psychiatry 34:499–509, 1995

Loeber R, Burke JD, Lahey BB, et al: Oppositional defiant disorder and conduct disorder: a review of the last 10 years, part I. J Am Acad Child Adolesc Psychiatry 39:1468–1484, 2000

Loney J, Milich R: Hyperactivity, aggression, and inattention in clinical practice, in Advances in Developmental and Behavioral Pediatrics. Edited by Wollrach M, Routh D. New York, JAI Press, pp 113–147, 1985

McBurnett K, Lahey BB, Rathouz PJ, et al: Low salivary cortisol and persistent aggression in boys referred for disruptive behavior. Arch Gen Psychiatry 57:38–43, 2000

McCord J: Parental behavior in the cycle of aggression. Psychiatry 51:14–23, 1988

McGee R, Williams S, Feehan M: Attention deficit disorder and age of onset of problem behaviors. J Abnorm Child Psychol 20:487–502, 1992

Mealy L: The sociobiology of sociopathy: an integrated evolutionary model, in The Maladapted Mind: Classic Readings in Evolutionary Psychopathology. Edited by Baron-Cohen S. Sussex, United Kingdom, Psychology Press, 1997, pp 133–173

Mednick SA: The learning of morality: biosocial bases, in Vulnerabilities to Delinquency. Edited by Lewis DO. New York, Spectrum, 1981, pp 187–204

Mednick SA, Gabrielli WF, Hutchings B: Genetic factors in criminal behavior: evidence from an adoption cohort. Science 224:891–893, 1984

Mehlman PT, Higley JD, Faucher I, et al: Low CSF 5-HIAA concentrations and severe aggression and impaired impulse control in nonhuman primates. Am J Psychiatry 151:1485–1491, 1994

Mehlman PT, Higley JD, Faucher I, et al: Correlation of CSF 5-HIAA concentration with sociality and the timing of emigration in free-ranging primates. Am J Psychiatry 152:907–913, 1995

Meltzer LJ, Roditi BN, Fenton T: Cognitive and learning profiles of delinquent and disabled adolescents. Adolescence 21:581–591, 1986

Moeller FG, Barratt ES, Dougherty, et al: Psychiatric aspects of impulsivity. Am J Psychiatry 158:1783–1793, 2001

Moffitt TE: Parental mental disorder and offspring criminal behavior: an adoption study. Psychiatry 50:346–360, 1987

Moffitt TE: Adolescence-limited and life-course-persistent antisocial behavior: a developmental taxonomy. Psychol Rev 100:674–701, 1993

Moffitt TE, Caspi A: Childhood predictors differentiate life-course persistent and adolescence-limited antisocial pathways among males and females. Dev Psychopathol 13:355–375, 2001

Moffitt TE, Silva PA: Neuropsychological deficit and self-reported delinquency in an unselected birth cohort. J Am Acad Child Adolesc Psychiatry 27:233–240, 1988

Moffitt TE, Gabrielli WF, Mednick SA: Socioeconomic status, IQ, and delinquency. J Abnorm Psychol 90:152–156, 1981

Mulvey EP, Reppucci ND: The context of clinical judgement: the effect of resource availability on judgements of amenability to treatment in juvenile offenders. Am J Community Psychol 16:525–545, 1988

Offord DR, Bennett KJ: Conduct disorder: long-term outcomes and intervention effectiveness. J Am Acad Child Adolesc Psychiatry 33:1069–1078, 1994

Offord DR, Cross LA: Behavioral antecedents of adult schizophrenia. Arch Gen Psychiatry 21:267–283, 1969

Olweus D, Mattsson A, Schalling D, et al: Circulating testosterone levels and aggression in adolescent males: a causal analysis. Psychosom Med 50:261–272, 1988

Pajer K, Gardner W, Rubin RT, et al: Decreased salivary cortisol levels in adolescent girls with conduct disorder. Arch Gen Psychiatry 58:297–302, 2001

Patterson GR: Coercive Family Process. Eugene, OR, Castalia, 1982

Patterson GR, DeBaryshe BD, Ramsey E: A developmental perspective on antisocial behavior. Am Psychol 44:329–355, 1989

Pfiffner LJ, McBurnett K, Rathouz PJ: Father absence and familial anti-social characteristics. J Abnorm Psychol 29:347–367, 2001

Puig-Antich J: Major depression and conduct disorder in prepuberty. J Am Acad Child Psychiatry 2:118–128, 1982

Raine A, Brennan P, Sarnoff A, et al: Birth complications combined with early maternal rejection at age 1 year predispose to violent crime at age 18 years. Arch Gen Psychiatry 51:984–988, 1994

Raine A, Venables PH, Williams M: High autonomic arousal and electrodermal orienting at age 15 years as protective factors against criminal behavior at age 29 years. Am J Psychiatry 152:1595–1600, 1995

Reebye P, Moretti MM, Lessard JC: Conduct disorder and substance use disorder: comorbidity in a clinical sample of preadolescents and adolescents. Can J Psychiatry 40:313–319, 1995

Reeves JC, Werry JS, Elkind GS, et al: Attention deficit, conduct oppositional, and anxiety disorders in children, II: clinical characteristics. J Am Acad Child Adolesc Psychiatry 26:144–155, 1987

Riggs PD, Leon SL, Mikulich SK, et al: An open label trial of bupropion for ADHD in adolescents with substance use disorders and conduct disorder. J Am Acad Child Adolesc Psychiatry 37:1271–1278, 1998

Robins LN: Deviant Children Grown Up. Baltimore, MD, Williams & Wilkins, 1966

Robins LN, Ratcliff KS: Risk factors in the continuation of childhood antisocial behavior into adulthood. Int J Ment Health 7:96–111, 1979

Rosenberg D, Holltum J, Gershon S: Textbook of Child and Adolescent Psychiatric Disorders. New York, Brunner/Mazel, 1994

Rutter M: Parent-child separation: psychological effects on the child. J Child Psychol Psychiatry 12:233–260, 1971

Rutter M: Studies of Psychosocial Risk: The Power of Longitudinal Data. New York, Cambridge University Press, 1988

Rutter M, Giller H: Juvenile Delinquency: Trends and Perspectives. New York, Penguin, 1984

Rutter M, Birch HG, Thomas A, et al: Temperamental characteristics in infancy and the later development of behavior disorders. Br J Psychiatry 110:651–661, 1964

Rydelius A: The development of antisocial behavior and sudden violent death. Acta Psychiatr Scand 77:398–403, 1988

Sanford M, Boyle MH, Szatmari P, et al: Age-of-onset of conduct disorder: reliability and validity in a prospective cohort study. J Am Acad Child Adolesc Psychiatry 38:992–999, 1999

Satterfield JH, Schell AM, Backs RW: Longitudinal study of AERP's in hyperactive and normal children: relationship to antisocial behavior. Electroencephalogr Clin Neurophysiol 67:531–536, 1987

Schmeck K, Poustka F: Temperament and disruptive behavior disorders. Psychopathology 34:159–163, 2001

Seeger G, Schloss P, Schmidt MH: Functional polymorphism within the promoter of the serotonin transporter gene is associated with severe hyperkinetic disorders. Mol Psychiatry 6:235–238, 2001

Short RJ, Simeonsson RJ: Social cognition and aggression in delinquent adolescent males. Adolescence 21:159–176, 1986

Silverman IW, Ragusa DM: A short-term longitudinal study of the early development of self-regulation. J Abnorm Psychol 20:415–435, 1993

Silverton L, Harrington ME, Mednick SA: Motor impairment and antisocial behavior in adolescent males at high risk for schizophrenia. J Abnorm Child Psychol 16:177–186, 1988

Simeon JG, Ferguson HB, Fleet JVW: Bupropion effects in attention deficit and conduct disorders. Can J Psychiatry 31:581–585, 1986

Simic M, Fombonne E: Depressive conduct disorder: symptom patterns and correlates in referred children and adolescents. J Affect Disord 62:175–185, 2001

Snyder JJ, Dishian TJ, Petterson GR: Determinants and consequences of associating with deviant peers during preadolescence. Journal of Early Adolescence 61:20–43, 1986

Spoont MR: Modulatory role of serotonin in neural information processing: implications for human psychopathology. Psychol Bull 112:330–350, 1992

Steiner H: Practice parameters for the assessment and treatment of children and adolescents with conduct disorder. J Am Acad Child Adolesc Psychiatry 36:122S–139S, 1997

Steiner H, Wilson J: Conduct disorder, in Disruptive Behavior Disorders in Children and Adolescents. Edited by Hendren RL. Washington, DC, American Psychiatric Press, 1999, pp 47–92

Steiner H, Garcia IG, Matthews Z: Posttraumatic stress disorder in incarcerated juvenile delinquents. J Am Acad Child Adolesc Psychiatry 36:357–365, 1997

Stewart M, Kelso J: A two-year follow-up of boys with aggressive conduct. Psychopathology 20:296–304, 1987

Stoff DM, Friedman E, Pollack L, et al: Elevated platelet MAO is related to impulsivity in disruptive behavior disorders. J Am Acad Child Adolesc Psychiatry 28:754–760, 1989

Susman EJ, Inoff-Germain G, Nottelmann ED, et al: Hormones, emotional dispositions and aggressive attributes in young adolescents. Child Dev 58:1114–1134, 1987

Thomas A, Chess S: Temperament and Development. New York, Brunner/Mazel, 1977

Tolan PH: Implications of age of onset for delinquency risk. J Abnorm Child Psychol 15:45–63, 1987

Tolan PH: Socioeconomic, family, and social stress correlates of adolescent antisocial and delinquent behavior. J Abnorm Child Psychol 16:317–331, 1988

Tolan PH, Lorion RP: Multivariate approaches to the identification of delinquency proneness in adolescent males. Am J Community Psychol 16:547–561, 1988

Tolan PH, Cromwell RE, Brasswell M: Family therapy with delinquents: a critical review of the literature. Fam Process 25:619–650, 1986

Tremblay RE, LeBlanc M, Schwartzman AE: The pediatric power of first-grade peer and teacher ratings of behavior: sex differences in antisocial behavior and personality at adolescence. J Abnorm Child Psychol 16:571–583, 1988

Tremblay RE, Masse B, Perron D, et al: Early disruptive behavior, poor school achievement, delinquent behavior, and delinquent personality: longitudinal analyses. J Consult Clin Psychol 60:64–72, 1992

Tremblay RE, Pihl RO, Vitaro F, et al: Predicting early onset of male antisocial behavior from preschool behavior. Arch Gen Psychiatry 51:732–739, 1994

Unis AS, Cook EH, Vincent JG, et al: Platelet serotonin measures in adolescents with conduct disorder. Biol Psychiatry 42:553–559, 1997

van Goozen SH, Matthys W, Cohen-Kettenis PT, et al: Plasma monoamine metabolites and aggression: two studies of normal and oppositional defiant disorder children. Eur Neuropsychopharmacol 9:141–147, 1999 van Goozen SH, van den Ban E, Matthys W, et al: Increased adrenal androgen functioning in children with oppositional defiant disorder: a comparison with psychiatric and normal controls. J Am Acad Child Adolesc Psychiatry 39:1446–1451, 2000

Vitaro F, Gendreau PL, Tremblay RE, et al: Reactive and proactive aggression differentially predict later conduct problems. J Child Psychol Psychiatry 39:377–385, 1998

Vitiello B, Behar D, Hunt J, et al: Subtyping aggression in children and adolescents. J Neuropsychiatry Clin Neurosci 2:189–192, 1990

Wadsworth MEJ: Roots of Delinquency: Infancy, Adolescence, and Crime. New York, Barnes & Noble Books, 1979

Wakschlag LS, Lahey B, Loeber R, et al: Maternal smoking during pregnancy and the risk of conduct disorder in boys. Arch Gen Psychiatry 54:670–676, 1997

Walker JL, Lahey BB, Hynd GW, et al: Comparison of specific patterns of antisocial behavior in children with conduct disorder with or without coexisting hyperactivity. J Consult Clin Psychol 55:910–913, 1987

Watt NF, Grup TW, Erlenmeyer-Kimling L: Social, emotional, and intellectual behavior at school among children at high risk for schizophrenia. J Consult Clin Psychol 50:171–181, 1983

Webster-Stratton LC, Lindsay DW: Social competence and conduct disorder problems in young children: issues in assessment. J Clin Child Psychol 28:25–43, 1999

Wells KC, Egan J: Social learning and systems family therapy for childhood oppositional disorder: comparative treatment outcome. Compr Psychiatry 29:138–146, 1988

Werner EE: High risk children in young adulthood: a longitudinal study from birth to 32 years. Am J Orthopsychiatry 59:72–81, 1989

Werry JS, Aman MG: Methylphenidate and haloperidol in children: effects on attention, memory and activity. Arch Gen Psychiatry 32:790–795, 1975

Widom CSA: Does violence beget violence? a critical examination of the literature. Psychol Bull 106:3–28, 1989

Wolff S: Dimensions and clusters of symptoms in disturbed children. Br J Psychiatry 118:421–427, 1971

Woolston JL, Rosenthal SL, Riddle MA, et al: Childhood comorbidity of anxiety/affective disorders and behavior disorders. J Am Acad Child Adolesc Psychiatry 28:707–713, 1989

World Health Organization: The ICD-10 Classification of Mental and Behavioural Disorders: Clinical Descriptions and Diagnostic Guidelines. Geneva, World Health Organization, 1992

Wozniak J, Biederman J, Faraone SV, et al: Heterogeneity of childhood conduct disorder: further evidence of a subtype of conduct disorder linked to bipolar disorder. J Affect Disord 64:121–131, 2001

Conduct and Antisocial Disorders in Adolescence

Dorothy Otnow Lewis, M.D.

Definition and Diagnostic Criteria

The diagnostic category of conduct disorder is so inclusive that it covers a multitude of sins as well as a multitude of biopsychosocial vulnerabilities. As Kazdin (2001) observes, "conduct disorder represents an array of child, parent, family and contextual conditions." (p. 408). The category is so broad and encompasses so many different kinds of behaviors that it requires more sophistication to avoid the diagnosis than to make it. Because the definition is so broad, it is one of the most—if not *the* most—frequently made diagnoses in child psychiatry (McDermott 1996). Experienced clinicians, however, know that almost all other psychiatric conditions of childhood and adolescence can, at one time or another, manifest themselves in disruptive, obnoxious, aggressive behaviors. In fact, conduct disorder is one of the most serious, incapacitating chronic conditions encountered in child psychiatry.

In a recently published analysis of the nature of the disorder, Lambert and colleagues (2001) studied the clinical characteristics, degrees of impairment, chronicity, cost of treatment, and response to treatment for 984 children ages 5–17 years treated in comprehensive continuum-of-care programs at three different sites. Multiple-informant mental health measurements were used at intake and periodically thereafter during a 5-year follow-up. Assessments regarding the presence or absence of DSM-III-R (American Psychiatric Association 1987) diagnoses as well as the number and nature of symptoms were determined. In addition, externalizing and internalizing behaviors and symptoms were documented using the Child Behavior Checklist (Achenbach 1992; Achenbach and Edelbrock 1988). An index of overall functional impairment that correlated significantly with the amount of services required and the cost of interventions was also employed. The researchers found that children with conduct disorder compared with those having other diagnoses were older, were likely to have more serious emotional disturbance, required longer and more intensive outpatient treatment, and had higher rates of psychiatric hospitalization. The cost of treating these children for the first 6 months was 278% that of treating the children with other diagnoses. Children with a diagnosis of conduct disorder had the highest numbers of problems. When children diagnosed with conduct disorder were compared with those in 10 other diagnostic categories, they were found to be the most impaired.

In addition to the alarming findings described above, children with conduct disorder averaged 2.2 primary diagnoses, compared with 1.3 primary diagnoses for children in other diagnostic categories. It was not surprising to find that the sample with conduct disorder had significantly higher pathological externalizing scores on the Child Behavior Checklist. What came as a surprise was the finding that children with conduct disorders also had more serious internalizing symptoms. They were significantly more withdrawn and had more somatic problems, more anxiety, more depression, and more thought problems. By DSM-III-R criteria, they had more symptoms of major depression, dysthymia, and overanxious disorder. In short, children with conduct disorder had more psychiatric problems in nearly every dimension than children carrying other diagnoses.

The findings described above are consistent with

529

our own findings regarding previously unrecognized severe neuropsychiatric symptoms and cognitive dysfunction in samples of violent, delinquent youths compared with their less violent peers (Lewis et al. 1979b, 1988a, 1989, 1991, 1994) and compared with demographically similar nondelinquents (Lewis et al. 1987). The findings are also consistent with our findings of similarities in the nature and severity of psychopathology between adolescents sent to a correctional institution and those sent to the adolescent ward of a state hospital (Lewis et al. 1980).

Given the facts that most adolescents with severe conduct disorder have a multitude of other kinds of neuropsychiatric and cognitive vulnerabilities, that many have symptoms consistent with other diagnoses, and that most of these other disorders have more specific treatment implications and better prognoses than conduct disorder, the clinician is medically and ethically obliged to rule out these other conditions before simply settling for a diagnosis of conduct disorder.

The current definition of conduct disorder must be understood in the context of its history as a diagnostic category. In DSM-II (American Psychiatric Association 1968), the diagnosis of antisocial personality could be applied to children and adolescents as well as to adults. Individuals so designated were described as being "incapable of significant loyalty to individuals, groups or social values" and of being "grossly selfish, callous, irresponsible, impulsive, and unable to feel guilt or to learn from experience and punishment" (p. 45). These unfortunate attributes were considered "life-long patterns, often recognizable by the time of adolescence or earlier" (p. 41).

Because of the apparent immutability of this condition, an alternative diagnosis—unsocialized aggressive reaction of childhood (or adolescence)—was instituted in DSM-II for children and adolescents whose characterological traits were not so firmly established as to preclude all change. Of note, the nouns and adjectives used to delineate youngsters with antisocial personality and unsocialized aggressive reaction in DSM-II were more judgmental than scientific and clearly reflected the attitude of many clinicians toward behaviorally disturbed children and adolescents.

In DSM-III (American Psychiatric Association 1980) a new category was introduced: conduct disorder. Like its predecessor, unsocialized aggressive reaction, conduct disorder was used to designate behaviors ranging from relatively minor infractions of rules to violent acts. Heavily influenced by the work of Jenkins

and Hewitt (1944), Robins (1966), and Quay (1964a, 1964b, 1975) on delinquency, the DSM-III definition of conduct disorder was divided into four different categories: aggressive or nonaggressive, and socialized or undersocialized. Patients classified as undersocialized and aggressive were described as lacking normal empathy and affection. How to measure empathy and affection was left to the wisdom of each clinician.

In an effort to eliminate clinical criteria based on moral judgments or unconscious attitudes, DSM-III-R (American Psychiatric Association 1987) presented exclusively behavioral criteria for the diagnosis of conduct disorder. In this revision of DSM, the syndrome was defined as a disturbance of behavior lasting at least 6 months in which the basic rights of others and the major age-appropriate norms and rules of society are violated. To receive the diagnosis, a child or adolescent had to manifest at least 3 of 13 problematic behaviors, ranging in severity from truancy and running away to rape and assault. There was no lower age limit, and the upper age limit was vague (e.g., a person age 18 years or older who does not meet criteria for antisocial personality may receive a diagnosis of conduct disorder). The categories of aggressive/nonaggressive and socialized/undersocialized were replaced by solitary aggressive, group, and undifferentiated subtypes. The severity of the disorder was rated on a three-point scale—mild, moderate, and severe.

The DSM-IV (American Psychiatric Association 1994) definition of conduct disorder is similar to that found in DSM-III-R. In this DSM version, conduct disorder is defined as "a repetitive and persistent pattern of behavior in which the basic rights of others or major age-appropriate societal norms or rules are violated, as manifested by the presence of three or more of the following criteria in the past 12 months, with at least one criterion present in the past 6 months" (p. 90). A list of 15 undesirable behaviors follows, which are grouped into four categories: 1) aggression to people and animals, 2) destruction of property, 3) deceitfulness or theft, and 4) serious violations of rules. Two behaviors were added to the 13 undesirable behaviors listed in DSM-III-R: bullying or intimidating and staying out late despite parental prohibitions. The criteria for making the diagnosis have remained the same in DSM-IV-TR (American Psychiatric Association 2000).

As can be seen in this newest definition, the types of undesirable behaviors that qualify a child or adolescent for the diagnosis of conduct disorder are so different qualitatively from one another that the teenager who steals makeup from cosmetic counters, repeatedly lies about her grades, and stays out until 2:00 A.M. when she has a midnight curfew could receive the same diagnosis as the adolescent who sets fire to cats, sexually molests small children, and pistol whips math teachers. The severity rating scale of mild to moderate to severe is intended to help clinicians distinguish shoplifters from potential murderers. This rating scale differs from scales for other disorders such as depression in that severity for conduct disorder can be used to indicate very different kinds of behaviors rather than degrees of the same symptomatology.

A study of youths from four U.S. communities documented a strong association between very early behavior problems, subsequent serious aggressive behaviors, and psychiatric problems (Lahey et al. 1999). In one of the longest longitudinal studies of children and adolescents with disruptive behaviors, Loeber et al. (2003) also found that adolescent serious offenders tended to have manifested behavioral problems in childhood and that by age 14 years, the vast majority had settled into a pattern of habitual serious offending. Because of these kinds of findings, DSM-IV and DSM-IV-TR distinguish two types of conduct disorder based on age at onset. *Childhood-onset* type is defined by 3 or more of the 15 listed behaviors, at least one of which has occurred before age 10 years. *Adolescent-onset* type is defined by an absence of any of these behaviors before age 10 years. The distinction between these types is made because of the generally poor prognosis for children whose maladaptive behaviors begin early in life.

Because the DSM-IV-TR criteria for conduct disorder are signs, not symptoms, the clinician cannot just look at behaviors but must distinguish among adolescents who frequently fight because they are paranoid and feel threatened, those who fight because of impulsivity and emotional lability secondary to organic impairment, and those who fight in response to teasing. Similarly, those who stay away from school because voices tell them to must be differentiated from those who are truant because of frustration caused by a learning disability and those whose families keep them home to baby-sit younger siblings. In flamboyantly psychotic adolescents, the cause of disruptive behavior is obvious. In many repeatedly aggressive adolescents, however, paranoid ideation is a subtle phenomenon that is identified only if suspected by the clinician.

In fact, all 15 of the behaviors defining conduct disorder and combinations thereof occur as part of many other diagnoses, the common manifestations of which may be some form of antisocial behavior. Underlying or co-occurring disorders include mental retardation, mood disorders, organic syndromes, attentional disorders, pathological dissociation, and the different forms of psychotic disorders currently categorized as schizophrenia. The clinician must therefore take care to identify the underlying neuropsychiatric disorders that present as behavior problems. The more sophisticated the clinician, the less frequently he or she will simply diagnose conduct disorder.

Clinical Findings

■ Psychiatric Vulnerabilities

Because the behavioral characteristics of conduct disorder can be manifestations of so many different kinds of neuropsychiatric conditions, the first job of the clinician is to try to identify the intrinsic vulnerabilities and environmental stressors of the adolescent that may underlie or give rise to the offensive behaviors. The environmental factors contributing to the behaviors are usually blatant (e.g., impoverished households, high-crime neighborhoods, broken homes, household violence, parental psychopathology). In contrast, the psychopathology of the adolescents themselves is rarely obvious. Rather, their psychiatric signs and symptoms often teeter on the borders of several other neuropsychiatric diagnoses.

When subtle indications of psychotic, affective, organic, and dissociative symptoms fail to meet full criteria for diagnoses other than conduct disorder, there is a temptation to ignore them. Because the behaviors of such adolescents usually meet the criteria for conduct disorder, these multiply handicapped, behaviorally disturbed teenagers tend to receive that diagnosis based exclusively on the nature and timing of their antisocial acts. When, on the other hand, the clinician confronted with a disruptive adolescent looks on the patient's aberrant behaviors as a diagnostic puzzle, calling on every aspect of the clinician's training and experience to be solved, the work becomes a fascinating challenge. Now it is up to the clinician to discern the potentially remediable psychiatric, neurological, medical, cognitive, and environmental problems contributing to the adolescent's undesirable behaviors.

■ Attention-Deficit/Hyperactivity Disorder

Attention-deficit/hyperactivity disorder (ADHD) is probably the most common previous or comorbid diagnosis of delinquent children, violent and nonviolent. It is characterized by impulsiveness, short attention span, disinhibition, overactivity, socially inappropriate behavior, poor judgment, and school difficulties—the very same characteristics as those observed in children diagnosed with conduct disorder (Barkley 1997). However, the relationship between the two diagnoses is unclear. Longitudinal studies indicate that ADHD alone in childhood, although associated to some degree with subsequent adolescent antisocial behavior (August et al. 1983; Lambert et al. 1987; Mannuzza et al. 1989), is nowhere near as predictive of poor outcome as is childhood ADHD coupled with early conduct problems (Dalteg and Levander 1998; Farrington et al. 1990; Foley et al. 1996).

ADHD, like conduct disorder, seems to be an impairment of self-regulation (Costellanos 1999). Like children with conduct disorders, children with ADHD have problems with executive functions as well as with other aspects of cognitive functioning. These frontal-lobe functions include foresight, judgment, and control of impulses. Notably, recent studies comparing evoked potentials in adolescents with and without conduct disorders during different kinds of mental tasks revealed diminished right and left prefrontal activity in the sample with conduct disorder compared with the sample without conduct disorder. Localization of the diminished functioning depended on the nature of the cognitive task (Bauer and Hesselbrock 2001).

A word of caution: inattention, overactivity, impulsiveness, and poor judgment are characteristic not only of ADHD and conduct disorder but also of numerous other neuropsychiatric disorders (e.g., bipolar disorders and dissociative disorders), all of which must be part of the differential diagnosis.

■ Mood Disorders

Clinicians have long been aware of the association between depression, suicidal behavior, and adolescent behavior disorders (White et al. 2001; Zoccolillo 1992). The irritability and rage that often accompany adolescent depression, especially when aggravated by alcohol or drug abuse, can masquerade as aggressive conduct disorder. It has been well established that alcohol and drug abuse are frequent concomitants of se-

rious delinquency and of violence in adolescents and adults (Huizinga et al. 2000). It is of special note that persistent internalizing problems have been found to be characteristic of delinquent children and adolescents with substance abuse (Loeber et al. 1999a)—another suggestion of the linkage among depression, substance abuse, and behavioral disturbance.

Less well recognized is the relationship of bipolar mood disorders—especially mania and hypomania—to delinquent, often violent behaviors. Mania and hypomania in adolescence may present as episodic destructive behavior or sporadic sprees of robbery and burglary. In a recent study, Pliszka and colleagues (2000) found that of 50 incarcerated youths, 10 (20%) met diagnostic criteria for mania.

The tendency for manic adolescents to indulge in dangerous behavior and stay up all night risks being dismissed as part of normal adolescence. Clinicians must keep in mind that normal adolescent turmoil is not the flamboyant, rebellious condition it was once thought to be. Mania in adolescence can mimic ADHD, oppositional defiant disorder, and conduct disorder and does not necessarily have the classic adult presentation (Carlson 1996).

Unfortunately, manic youngsters, with their grandiosity and boastfulness, are especially likely to alienate their examiners. Their heedlessness of the consequences of their acts and their apparent lack of empathy cause unsophisticated clinicians to dismiss them as simply narcissistic and sociopathic. A careful mood history and documentation of the periodicity of their obnoxious, destructive behaviors (not to mention a careful family history) will often bring to light a hitherto unrecognized bipolar disorder.

■ Psychotic Symptomatology

Most adolescents with conduct disorder do not appear to be mentally ill—at least not if they can help it. They would rather be thought "bad" than "crazy." They strive to deny or minimize their symptoms. Although few at the time of evaluation in court clinics or detention facilities seem to have schizophrenia, sensitive interviewing will often enable some of the most repetitively violent youngsters to reveal their delusional beliefs and hallucinatory experiences. Bender (1959) observed that many children who had been diagnosed as psychotic in adolescence appeared to be simply antisocial. It is likely that the psychotically disturbed delinquent teenager's desire to appear normal (i.e., just bad) and the examining clinician's tolerance for aberrant behavior in sullen or grandiose delinquents conspire to obfuscate serious psychopathology.

However, studies of adult psychiatric patients (Volavka 1995) as well as studies of psychopathology in violent delinquent adolescents (Lewis et al. 1979b, 1988a, 1988b, 1989, 1994; Myers et al. 1995; Steiner et al. 1997) indicate that violence and serious psychopathology often go hand in hand. In a sophisticated study of representative community samples, Swanson (1994) reported that major mental illness (e.g., the schizophrenia spectrum and affective disorders) was associated with violence even after controlling for the effects of demographics and institutionalization. Robins (1966) reported that 19% of antisocial children seen at a clinic but not referred to court as delinquent were subsequently diagnosed as schizophrenic. Stueve and Link (1997) reported that the most common psychiatric symptoms associated with violent behavior were delusions of thought control, thought insertion, and persecution. In our own studies of seriously delinquent youths, the most common symptom associated with recurrent violence was paranoid ideation (Lewis et al. 1979b, 1988a, 1988b). Our finding of an association between paranoid thinking and violence has been confirmed by others (Dodge et al. 1990; Myers et al. 1995; Ulzen and Hamilton 1998).

In our own studies, we found that almost 60% of the first group of violent adolescents committed to a newly established secure unit at the only juvenile correctional facility in Connecticut had been treated in psychiatric hospitals and residential treatment centers for a variety of diagnoses other than conduct disorder before their secure incarcerations (Lewis and Shanok 1980). We have noted that many aggressive children with a behavior disorder who, early on, were diagnosed with psychotic or organic disorders and were treated in residential settings were discharged in early adolescence and eventually wound up in the juvenile correctional system. Their signs and symptoms and aggressive behaviors went unchanged; however, they had grown and were more intimidating and dangerous. Paranoid adolescents—with their tendency to misperceive cues, feel threatened, and lash out—frighten clinicians and treatment staff. When this happens their symptoms and behaviors tend to be reinterpreted as signs of character pathology. Having been evicted from psychiatric facilities, many seriously disturbed adolescents, unable to cope in society at large, find themselves in juvenile correctional institutions, a stepping stone to adult prison. With the closure of so many state hospitals, it is not surprising that prisons are forced to accept more and more psychiatrically impaired inmates. We have found, however, that the more violent and bizarre the adolescent's behaviors, the more likely the existence of underlying psychotic symptoms.

■ Dissociative Disorders

The literature on conduct disorder, delinquency, and aggression by and large ignores the very existence of dissociative disorders, not to mention their role in many violent acts of children, adolescents, and adults. Our own work illustrates the point. From the mid-1970s through the better part of the 1980s the thought that dissociative phenomena might explain some of the puzzling symptoms and bizarre behavior of some of the violent adolescents we evaluated never crossed our minds. It literally took us years to recognize that many of the symptoms and behaviors we had attributed to complex partial seizures, psychosis, mood disorders, or just plain orneriness were sometimes manifestations of pathological dissociation. Over time we came to recognize that during dissociative episodes children may scream obscenities, take the belongings of others, set fires, and even attack others, then deny their acts because they do not recall their actions. Such denials are usually regarded by clinicians as lying.

The signs, symptoms, and behaviors of children and adolescents with dissociative disorders mimic those of other neuropsychiatric disorders. For example, their lapses of attention, staring spells, impaired memory for actions, and dreamlike states are also characteristic of complex partial seizures; their auditory hallucinations of voices arguing in their heads or telling them to hurt others or themselves are characteristic of schizophrenia or other psychotic states; and their rapid changes of mood and demeanor are often mistaken for bipolar disorders. Finally, their erratic school performances, distractibility, episodic aggression, and denial of destructive acts that others may have actually witnessed cause many such children and adolescents to be diagnosed with ADHD and conduct disorder. Some of the most common externalizing or antisocial behaviors of children and adolescents with dissociative disorders that cause them to be misdiagnosed as having conduct disorder are episodic aggression, inappropriate sexual behaviors, leaving school or home for hours to days, and having in their possession the property of others but denying having taken it.

In our experience, children and adolescents with dissociative disorders have almost always been severely abused physically or sexually. They often do not recall the abuse, and therefore information from other sources may be vital to making the diagnosis. Sometimes their medical histories of injuries, urinary tract infections, and rectal problems, or the scars on their backs, chests, arms, legs, and feet, attest to the maltreatment they cannot recall. When the clinician fails to consider this diagnosis, the child or adolescent risks being dismissed as a bully, a liar, and a thief.

■ Substance Abuse

According to regional surveys in the United States, somewhere between 40% and 60% of arrested male juveniles have drugs or alcohol in their bloodstreams (Arrestee Drug Abuse Monitoring Program 1999). Estimates of the prevalence of multiproblem youths (i.e., those suffering from substance abuse, emotional problems, and violent behavior) have varied widely, from 4% to 20% (Dryfoos 1990; Ellickson et al. 1997; Elliot et al. 1989). Unfortunately, by the time the clinician is apprised of misbehavior and substance abuse, the child has usually reached adolescence, and it is hard to recognize retrospectively what other kinds of biopsychosocial vulnerabilities may have led to the substance abuse and behavioral problems.

The effects of most substances depend in great measure on the psychological and physiological state of the user/abuser and on the situational context. Only a few substances are believed to cause violence in and of themselves. They include crack cocaine (Honer et al. 1987; Taylor 1990), phencyclidine (PCP) (Fauman and Fauman 1982), and the amphetamines (King and Ellinwood 1992). In the recent past, we have evaluated several homicidal methamphetamine users, one an adolescent who committed murder while in a paranoid state secondary to methamphetamine withdrawal. In low doses, benzodiazepines and barbiturates cause relaxation; however, high doses have been associated with aggressive behaviors (Cherek 1990; Taylor 1990). Although marijuana, the substance most commonly used by teenagers in the United States, usually causes relaxation and euphoria, it can cause panicky states and paranoia, leading to violence. Probably the greatest danger for teenagers who use marijuana is the fact that it may be laced with violence-inducing drugs such as PCP (Hall and Solowij 1998).

Some teenagers, particularly boys, try to enhance their athletic performance or their appearance with anabolic steroids. Unbeknownst to them, these kinds of substances can promote irritability, hostility, and even violence (Bahrke et al. 1990a, 1990b). Some nonsteroidal substances promoted by manufacturers to body builders have been known to promote aggression. We evaluated a previously nonviolent young man who—under the influence of a natural remedy containing ephedrine, caffeine, and chromium picolinate—went on a violent rampage. This particular person also had a predisposition to mania, which probably increased his vulnerability to the violence-inducing effects of that combination of substances. (Notably, bipolar disorder has been shown to be an especially strong risk factor for alcohol and substance abuse [Biederman et al. 2000].)

Comorbidity

A reflection of the many conditions that may manifest as conduct disorder is the burgeoning literature on comorbidity. As Newcorn and Halperin (1994) accurately observed, "Comorbidity among disruptive disorders is the rule rather than the exception" (p. 227). For example, ADHD has been reported to coexist in most cases of early-onset conduct disorder (Hinshaw et al. 1993). Conversely, between 50% and 80% of children with ADHD also manifest evidence of oppositional defiant disorder or conduct disorder, depending on the sample studied (Newcorn and Halperin 1994). Conduct disorders have been reported to coexist with depressive disorders (Zoccolillo 1992), anxiety disorders (Zoccolillo 1992), borderline and psychotic disorders (Andrulonis et al. 1982; Bellak 1985; Lewis 1976), and even Tourette's disorder (Comings and Comings 1987; Pauls et al. 1986). Newcorn and Halperin (1994) summarized the diagnostic confusion regarding the diagnosis of conduct disorder: "Comorbidity could also be artifactually increased if a diagnostic category does not include certain information required for accurate differential diagnosis, thereby making it difficult to distinguish between disorders that are related although distinct" (p. 229).

■ Neurological Vulnerabilities

Few adolescents with conduct disorders have obvious signs of neurological impairment. Furthermore, although some have histories of severe trauma to the head, many repeatedly aggressive adolescents have histories of multiple different kinds of head trauma, each of which by itself may not have seemed serious (Lewis and Shanok 1977, 1979; Lewis et al. 1979a). However, it is now known that the effects of a series of apparently minor injuries such as mild concussions can have cumulative adverse effects (McCrea et al. 1997; Pearl 1998). Especially vulnerable are the temporal and frontal poles of the brain (Varney 1999). Damage to the frontal lobes—the regions of the brain that are involved with judgment, foresight, impulse control, and the recognition of interpersonal cues—can contribute not only to behavior problems but also to violence itself. Frontal lobe dysfunction has been shown to be characteristic of aggressive adult offenders (Raine et al. 1994, 1997b, 2000). Our own clinical evaluations of delinquent adolescents have shown that the more aggressive teenagers tend to have more "soft" neurological signs indicative of frontal lobe dysfunction (Lewis et al. 1979a, 1979b, 1989).

For years researchers have noted apparent parasympathetic unresponsiveness in delinquent adolescents (Aniskiewicz 1979; Siddle et al. 1976) and, based on that, have hypothesized an innate predisposition to conduct disorder. More recently, Damasio (1998) documented the association between injury to the ventromedial parts of the frontal lobes and diminished autonomic responsivity. Studies of patients with such damage have shown them to have an impaired physiological responsiveness to emotionally charged material. Recent research on emotionally and behaviorally disturbed boys (Blair et al. 2001a, 2001b) suggests that both orbitofrontal and amygdaloid dysfunction may underlie diminished emotional responsivity to charged stimuli. However, these findings must be regarded with caution because data were not collected concerning the presence of neuropsychiatric disorders and histories of child abuse—both of which could account for apparent "callous and unemotional traits" (Blair et al. 2001a, p. 493). It may be that a combination of frontal and amygdaloid dysfunction and an upbringing in a violent, abusive household together create diminished autonomic and emotional responsivity and the appearance of callousness or lack of empathy. Furthermore, although early studies (e.g., Mednick et al. 1984) implied that such autonomic unresponsiveness was hereditary, given the horrendous medical histories of children with behavioral disorders it is equally likely that the neurophysiological dysfunction

resulted from environmental factors.

Unfortunately, the kinds of neuroimaging studies of frontal lobe function that might shed light on the neurological roots of conduct disorder are problematic because, at this time, they require the use of radioactive substances. However, a recent clinical report of two young children who experienced early damage to the orbitofrontal region indicate that, although both had normal developmental milestones, over time they exhibited signs of social maladaptation that included difficulty following rules, an apparent lack of empathy, lying, stealing, an inability to make normal friendships, and aggression (Anderson et al. 1999).

■ Epilepsy

Few adolescents with conduct disorder have epilepsy, although some evidence suggests that psychomotor seizures (complex partial seizures) are more common in violent delinquent individuals than in the general population (Lewis and Pincus 1989; Lewis et al. 1982a). Psychomotor symptoms—such as impaired memory for nonviolent and violent behavior, olfactory hallucinations, and vivid recurrent episodes of déjà vu—are fairly common in the aggressive delinquent population (Lewis et al. 1982a). Many seriously delinquent children (and many incarcerated adults) will be found to have equivocal or diffusely abnormal electroencephalograms. These kinds of signs and symptoms suggest that in some youngsters with conduct disorder, abnormal electrical activity in the brain, possibly in the limbic system, may contribute to behavioral problems.

■ Acute Confusional Migraine

One of the least often recognized but most interesting conditions causing episodic serious behavior problems is the acute confusional state that is sometimes associated with migraine headaches. Children who experience the auras associated with migraine sometimes have episodic, uncontrollable tantrums (Ehyai and Fenichel 1978; Pietrini et al. 1987). Migraine headaches are now recognized as abnormal electrical activity originating in the brainstem, spreading through the cortex and affecting the vasculature of the brain (Goadsby et al. 2002). In children, auras may occur years before the onset of migraine headaches themselves. Auras can occur before, during, after, or between headaches. When they do happen, some children and adolescents may hallucinate, feel as though things are unreal, become paranoid, and even go on rampages, destroying objects and hurting others. Their memory for this behavior is often impaired. The symptoms are similar to those of complex partial seizures.

Thus, as in the case of the psychoses, the signs and symptoms of children with conduct disorder place them on the border of several different neurological diagnoses.

■ Cognitive Vulnerabilities

Although few adolescents with conduct disorder have severe retardation, their low-normal scores on standard intelligence tests (Hirschi and Hinderlang 1977; Lynam et al. 1993; Rutter and Giller 1984; Schonfeld et al. 1988; West 1982; Wilson and Herrnstein 1986) again place them on the border of a diagnosis with potential treatment implications. The association of behavioral problems and low test scores often occurs as early as age 3 years and is thought not to be a result of school failure (Richman et al. 1982). Because so many delinquent youngsters come from minority and socioeconomically disadvantaged backgrounds, clinicians tend to dismiss low scores as merely evidence of cultural deprivation rather than as an indication for remediation. Whether cognitive problems reflect intrinsic limitations or environmental adversity, they do affect functioning and require attention. Poor judgment, impaired abstract reasoning, and difficulty planning ahead and anticipating consequences all contribute to behavioral problems.

In adolescents with conduct disorder, learning disabilities are important manifestations of cognitive dysfunction (Poremba 1975; Virkkunen and Nuutila 1976). Deficits in verbal skills are especially characteristic of this population and account in great measure for low IQ scores (Wilson and Herrnstein 1986). In a recent study, reading problems and delinquency were found to be related to attentional problems (Maguin and Loeber 1996). However, it would be a mistake to interpret these findings necessarily as evidence of an inherent verbal deficit. Many severely behaviorally disturbed children have been raised in dysfunctional, often violent households, in which verbal stimulation is insufficient (Cicchetti and Carlson 1989). In these homes, actions tend to speak louder than words.

The language and reading problems characteristic of many delinquent youths impair their ability to put their thoughts, feelings, and attitudes into words rather than actions. For these children, school becomes a place of frustration rather than of gratification and learning (Lynam et al. 1993). Without proper assistance, such children often drop out of school early. When adolescents are left to their own devices on the streets, relatively minor behavioral problems often evolve into delinquent acts. Because children with conduct disorder are often on the border of organic impairment and mental retardation, they are rarely afforded the attention reserved for the severely intellectually impaired and the intellectually gifted.

When one considers the myriad signs of central nervous system dysfunction in many repetitively delinquent aggressive adolescents—their mild intellectual limitations, their reading difficulties, their attentional problems, and their misinterpretations of the motivations of others—it becomes clear that no single deficit accounts for their adaptational problems. Learning difficulties, hyperactivity, and attentional problems seem to be the most obvious indicators of a more pervasive problem with executive functioning. Recent studies of frontal lobe functioning, using evoked potentials, have shown youths with conduct disorders to have less right and left frontal activation than their peers without conduct disorders, depending on the nature of the stimulus task (Bauer and Hesselbrock 1999, 2001). Frontal lobe dysfunction impairs memory, abstract reasoning, concentration, and the ability to process social cues and respond appropriately. Thus, it compromises all facets of the adolescent's life.

In summary, children and adolescents with conduct disorder have a clinical picture of a multiplicity of neuropsychiatric and cognitive vulnerabilities that place them on the border of other diagnoses. Unfortunately, none of these vulnerabilities is obvious. However, if recognized, each has implications for treatment.

Differential Diagnosis

Conduct disorder is a common expression of numerous different conditions. Children and adolescents are limited in their abilities both to conceptualize and to convey in words how they are feeling, what they are thinking, and why they are acting as they are. Any condition or combination of conditions that diminishes impulse control, jeopardizes reality testing, increases suspiciousness, and impairs judgment is likely to result in a conduct disorder. At some stage in the evolution of neuropsychiatric conditions ranging from schizophrenia to encephalitis, antisocial or even aggressive behaviors may occur. Therefore, the differential diagnosis of conduct disorder is almost as broad as the field of child and adolescent psychiatry itself. Various disorders—ADHD, learning disabilities, mood disorders, dissociative disorders, seizures and other kinds of central nervous system (CNS) dysfunction, and schizophreniform disorders—may present as a behavior disorder. A careful evaluation will usually reveal a multiplicity of neuropsychiatric and psychosocial vulnerabilities, each of which must be identified and addressed.

Often, conduct disorder is a transitional designation used when underlying causes for aberrant behaviors have not yet been identified. Therefore, the diagnosis of conduct disorder in psychiatry, at this point in our understanding, is analogous to the diagnosis of fever of unknown origin in internal medicine.

Epidemiology and Stages of Development

The incidence and prevalence of conduct disorder are not known with certainty because diagnostic criteria vary according to time and place, data are not uniform in different studies, and manifestations differ according to developmental stage. Therefore, widely varying prevalence estimates have been reported (Bauermeister et al. 1994). Esser et al. (1990), using ICD-9 (World Health Organization 1977) criteria, reported a prevalence less than 1% among German 8-year-olds. In contrast, using DSM-III criteria, Kashani et al. (1987) found a prevalence of 8.7% in Missouri teenagers. In DSM-IV, prevalence rates of 6%–16% in males and 2%–9% in females are suggested.

In an elegant review of the literature, Bauermeister and colleagues (1994) concluded that preschool behavioral problems were a strong indicator of risk for future disruptive disorders. Lefkowitz et al. (1977) reported that aggressive behaviors at age 8 years were good predictors of aggression during adolescence. Similarly, West and Farrington (1973) found that 27% of 8- and 10-year-old children who (according to teachers and peers) had behavioral problems later developed repeatedly delinquent behaviors in adolescence. In contrast, fewer than 1% of nontroublesome 8- and 10-year-olds became recidivist delinquents. Several fol-

low-up studies of children and adolescents have reported a greater prevalence of conduct disorder during adolescence than during preadolescence (Esser et al. 1990; McGee et al. 1992; Offord et al. 1992). McGee and colleagues (1992) called attention to an increase in nonaggressive behavioral problems, such as drug abuse, during adolescence. In DSM-IV-TR, two subtypes of conduct disorder are defined: an aggressive type with childhood onset and a nonaggressive type starting in preadolescence or adolescence. A study of 20,000 adults age 18 years or older in the United States reported that conduct problems in childhood were predictive of adult antisocial behavior (Robins 1991; Robins and Price 1991; Robins and Regier 1991). This association was greater in males than in females. Whatever the actual prevalence of conduct disorders, statistics from the United States and western European countries suggest that violent crime by juveniles has increased substantially over the past half century (Angold and Costello 2001).

Despite these findings, it is fortunate that most behaviorally disturbed children do not become sociopathic adults (Robins 1966; Rutter and Giller 1984). Moreover, although in certain areas more than 30% of adolescents may come in conflict with the law, only about 5% of this group will become recidivists (Wolfgang et al. 1972). Although longitudinal studies indicate that the onset of minor aggression tends to be followed by more and more serious forms of aggression (e.g., from bullying to physical fighting to violence) (Loeber et al. 1999b), most seriously delinquent boys do not go on to become violent adult offenders.

Less well recognized is the fact that "conduct disorders tend to be followed by a wide range of emotional, social and relationship problems in addition to antisocial behavior" (Rutter and Giller 1984, p. 60). Furthermore, even children with behavior disorders who are later given a diagnosis of sociopathy have a multitude of other unrecognized nonsociopathic psychiatric symptoms (Lewis et al. 1988a, 1989, 1991, 1994; Robins 1966). In DSM-IV-TR it is acknowledged that individuals with conduct disorder are at risk for subsequent mood disorders, somatoform disorders, anxiety disorders, and substance abuse. Our studies of violent adolescents and adults indicate that psychoses, organic syndromes, and dissociative disorders should be added to this list. Our follow-up studies of formerly incarcerated boys and girls (Lewis et al. 1991, 1994) are consistent with the recent observations of Hechtman and Offord (1994) that in addition to adult criminality and mental illness, early disorders of conduct also are associated with subsequent "widespread social malfunction, as seen in high rates of divorce and separation, poor work history, and unsatisfactory social relationships" (p. 382). A relationship also appears to exist in delinquent youths among degrees of early neuropsychiatric impairment, family dysfunction, and the severity of adult violent behaviors (Lewis et al. 1989). Our follow-up studies of incarcerated violent, delinquent boys showed that although early aggression was associated with later violence, it alone was not the best predictor (Lewis et al. 1989, 1994). Rather, the combination of neuropsychiatric and cognitive vulnerabilities with an upbringing in a violent, abusive household was most highly correlated with adult violent criminality. Thus, data from various sources indicate strong linkages among early, serious conduct problems; a variety of neuropsychiatric signs, symptoms, and disorders; and ongoing major problems in social adaptation.

Although males in society—whether children, adolescents, or adults—are far more physically violent than females, a word should be said about girls with conduct disorders. Several researchers have reported that although girls are less overtly aggressive than boys, they indulge in more relational aggression (e.g., damaging the reputation of other girls through gossip and rumor) (Crick and Grotpeter 1995; Tiet et al. 2001). Tiet et al. (2001) actually suggested broadening the conduct disorder category to include relational aggression, thus making the diagnosis "more gender neutral" (p. 182). Our follow-up of seriously delinquent girls revealed that although many were aggressive during adolescence, few became violent adult criminals. However, the majority of these girls cohabited with violent, abusive men, and most who gave birth to children from these couplings were unable to care for them (Lewis et al. 1991). This study provided a window into a mechanism for the intergenerational transmission of violence.

Etiology

An important relationship undeniably exists between the sociocultural environment in which a child is raised and the development of behavioral problems. Clearly, more violent crime occurs in the United States than in Great Britain. As well, violence is more common in socioeconomically disadvantaged inner-city neighborhoods than in suburban and rural settings.

Sociologists once suggested that crime was primarily the result of attempts of disadvantaged persons to achieve status and material wealth through the only means available to them (Merton 1938, 1957). Others theorized that certain antisocial behaviors were not abnormal; rather, they were thought to reflect the values promulgated within delinquent subcultures (Cohen 1955). The influence of peers on the development of antisocial behavior has also been emphasized. However, evidence suggests that the disruptive behavior of adolescents in delinquent groups may be more a reflection of the kind of youngster who tries to join the group than the effect of the group on the adolescent. Wilson and Herrnstein (1986) observed that the onset of antisocial behavior almost always precedes gang membership. In fact, Friedman et al. (1975) found that the most powerful predictor of gang membership was a youngster's violent behavior *before* joining a gang. Therefore, the importance of peer influences and the notion of a subculture of violence require careful reexamination. Notably, evidence exists that would-be therapeutic peer interactive groups often have the opposite effect, encouraging misbehavior in previously less disruptive adolescents (Dishion et al. 1999).

To what extent does family instability, social disorganization, poor physical health, and a disproportionate prevalence of mental illness in certain socioeconomically disadvantaged neighborhoods contribute to adaptational problems? To what extent do especially vulnerable individuals gravitate to these kinds of environments? The questions remain to be answered. Nevertheless, it is clear that seriously antisocial behavior cannot be regarded simply as the reflection of a characterological flaw or as a consciously chosen alternative lifestyle.

■ Genetics, Neurotransmitters, and Hormones

Conduct disorder is associated with so many other neuropsychiatric and environmental vulnerabilities that it is extremely hard to measure the genetic predisposition to conduct disorder alone (if indeed there is such a specific predisposition). Conduct disorder is associated with ADHD, bipolar and unipolar mood disorders, anxiety disorders, dissociative disorders, phobias, learning disabilities, and psychoses (Bender 1959; Lewis et al. 1979b, 1988a, 1988b; Myers et al. 1995; Simonoff 2001). A multiplicity of adverse environmental factors are also closely associated with conduct disorder, including poverty (Currie 2000), social disorganization (Currie 1985), parental mental illness (Lewis et al. 1981, 1988a, 1988b; Yeager and Lewis 1996), parental criminality (Hutchings and Mednick 1974), and the influence of deviant peer groups (Elliott and Menard 1996). Furthermore, the criteria for the diagnosis are so diverse as to raise the question of whether or not there really is a single diagnosis with characteristic signs and symptoms that can be tracked genetically.

Reports from the 1960s and 1970s that suggested an association between certain chromosomal anomalies (e.g., 47 XYY constellation) and antisocial behaviors (Casey et al. 1966; Nielson 1968) have been reassessed. Few prisoners have the 47 XYY complement of chromosomes, and most individuals who carry that anomaly are not incarcerated (Gerald 1976). On the other hand, a variety of different kinds of chromosomal anomalies may produce special vulnerabilities to environmental stressors, which, in certain circumstances, may be manifested by aggression (Owen 1972; Robinson and de la Chapelle 1990). Clinical descriptions of XYY children report hyperactivity, distractibility, and temper tantrums, but these behavioral problems may be a reflection of concomitant intellectual limitations and learning disabilities (Gotz et al. 1999). In her extensive review of heritability studies, Simonoff (2001) noted that "heritability estimates are enormously variable across studies" and that "even within the same study, using the same measures, responses from different informants produce wide variability in heritability estimates." (p. 357).

In one of the early studies exploring genetics and antisocial behavior, Hutchings and Mednick (1974) reported that the adopted-away children of criminal fathers were more likely to become antisocial than were the adopted-away children of noncriminals. The children at greatest risk for antisocial behavior were those whose fathers were criminal and who were adopted into criminal adoptive families. These kinds of studies, which rely on registered criminality, must be interpreted with caution because they do not consider the likelihood that parental criminality may be the most obvious and well-documented sign of maladaptation, obfuscating other kinds of potentially heritable psychopathology. There is, after all, strong evidence that the children of parents who have a wide variety of psychopathology are more likely to have behavioral problems than are the children of healthy parents (Moffitt 1987; Wilson and Herrnstein 1986). Similarly, delinquents are more likely to have psychiatrically disturbed parents than are nondelinquents (Lewis et al. 1981, 1988a, 1988b).

Of course, one cannot assume that the child of mentally ill parents has necessarily inherited a predisposition to maladaptation. Life is more complicated than that. Mentally ill parents are more likely than stable parents to behave in erratic, neglectful, or aggressive ways toward their children, thereby contributing to the children's behavior problems. Contrariwise, behaviorally disturbed adoptive children who are the offspring of antisocial parents often elicit harsh discipline from their adoptive parents (Ge et al. 1996), which in turn exacerbates behavior problems in the children.

The study of the genetics of antisocial behavior does little to clarify the influence of nature versus nurture in the development of antisocial maladapation. To quote Alsobrook and Pauls (2000), "Studying the genetics of behavior and psychiatric disorders is a particularly difficult endeavor since they are complex traits.... Genetic variables may be independent single genes (loci) or, as is more likely to be the case, multiple loci functioning within a larger context of numerous environmental influences" (p. 766). Thus, behaviors that appear to be genetically engendered may not be.

Because conduct disorder encompasses so many different kinds of behaviors, from lying to murder, it does not lend itself easily to genetic studies. On the other hand, when researchers have focused on more discrete behaviors such as attachment and aggressiveness, they have had greater success identifying potential genetic and biochemical influences on behavior. For example, animal studies have shown that neurotransmitters such as serotonin (Sahakian 1981), dopamine (McKenzie 1971), norepinephrine (Stolk et al. 1984), vasopressin, and oxytocin (Coccaro et al. 1998; Ferguson et al. 2001; Insel 1997) and many of the glucocorticoids and sex hormones affect nurturant as well as aggressive behaviors.

In many instances the genes controlling the manufacture and breakdown of specific neurotransmitters have been identified. Brunner and colleagues (1993) described a family in the Netherlands in which a mutation of the gene regulating monoamine oxidase A was associated with aggressive, impulsive behavior. The gene regulating the production of catechol O-methyltransferase has also been identified.

A number of studies have reported associations between low cerebrospinal fluid levels of 5-hydroxyindoleacetic acid, a serotonin metabolite, and impulsiveness and aggression (Brown et al. 1979; Linnoila et al. 1983; Virkkunen et al. 1989). Bjork and colleagues (1999) recently reported increased aggressiveness in men depleted of tryptophan, a serotonin precursor. However, a study of aggressive boys, ages 7–11 years, with ADHD showed increased prolactin responsivity to fenfluramine, a measure of serotonin system function. Other studies have found increased blood serotonin levels in aggressive adolescents (Halperin et al. 1996; Unis et al. 1997).

The study of conduct disorders and neurotransmitters or biological markers is fraught with difficulty because of the numerous environmental variables that influence biology and behavior. For example, a recent study by Matthews et al. (2000) documented the relationship between low socioeconomic status, low prolactin response to fenfluramine, and aggression. In short, conduct disorder is influenced by myriad biopsychosocial factors and is unlikely ever to be explained simply genetically or neurochemically. An organism may possess a particular gene or constellation of genes, but whether or not those genes are activated depends on a variety of conditions.

Animal studies have shown the importance of oxytocin and vasopressin for normal bonding to occur in certain rodents. In prairie voles, one of the few monogamous mammals on the planet, the female requires adequate central nervous system oxytocin to form a bond with her mate, whereas the male prairie vole requires vasopressin to bond with a female (Insel 1997). To date, the neurophysiological role of oxytocin and vasopressin in human bonding behavior has not yet been elucidated; however, some data exist on the roles of oxytocin and vasopressin in primate bonding (Winslow and Insel 1991).

The importance of human mother–child bonding to normal psychosocial development and adaptation is known, however. Many children and adolescents with conduct disorders have had less than optimal nurturing, and the most violent have usually been the victims of parental abuse. Studies of laboratory rats and mice have revealed the important role of oxytocin in maternal bonding. Whereas injection of oxytocin into the CNS of estrogen-primed nulliparous female rats induces maternal behaviors, the blockade of oxytocin transmission by central injection of an antagonist inhibits maternal behavior. Notably, an oxytocin antagonist given before the onset of maternal behavior inhibits it, whereas once the mother rat has bonded with her pups, oxytocin antagonists do not interrupt maternal behaviors (Pederson and Prange 1979).

Oxytocin has been found to be important in numerous social behaviors (e.g., maternal care, social attachment) in a variety of different animals from rats to sheep (Insel 1997). Its role in human parent-child bonding and in the subsequent ability of children to develop empathy remains to be explored. The apparent lack of empathy frequently described in abused children and adolescents with conduct disorders may well be partly a result of early compromise to the limbic-hypothalamic-pituitary-adrenal system and of the biochemical effects of poor nurturing on the developing brain. Researchers are just beginning to identify some of the genes and neurotransmitters that influence human temperament, behavior, and aggression. It is already known that certain genes affect the manufacture and breakdown of hormones and neurotransmitters. Whether or not specific genes will be activated or suppressed is influenced by environment and nurturance.

Although no abnormal constellation of chromosomes has yet been identified that is associated specifically with violence, a normal condition, the XY syndrome, has been shown time and again to be related to aggressiveness. Male human beings (including children, adolescents, and adults) are more violent than females. These differences have been found in societies as different from each other as Ethiopia and Switzerland, and, in the United States, men are approximately 9 times as likely to commit violent crimes as women. Men also commit many more nonviolent crimes. Maltreatment of women by men is reported the world over (Heise et al. 1994; Levinson 1989). Although one may wish to believe that male aggressiveness is primarily influenced by culture, such is not the case. Overwhelming evidence exists that male and female brains develop differently in utero and that gonadal hormones play important roles in fetal development, affecting sexually dimorphic areas of the brain. Ironically, although male brains are larger than female brains and the male cerebrum is about 8% larger than that of the female, these alleged repositories of reason and judgment do not seem to curtail male aggression to the extent that one might hope. The relationship of the masculinization of the fetal brain to the production of neurotransmitters and receptors is not yet well understood (Reznikov et al. 1999). The effects on behavior of sex differences in the CNS are complex. For the past quarter century, researchers have been exploring the relationship of testosterone levels to degrees of aggression in males and females. Some studies have reported that girls born with adrenogenital syndrome are more energetic than those subjected in utero to lower levels of androgens (Ehrhardt 1975). Others have called these findings into question (Hines 1982). Although some researchers have reported positive correlations between aggression and plasma testosterone levels, other have failed to replicate the findings (Meyer-Bahlburg et al. 1974; Monti et al. 1977). Virkkunen et al. (1994) reported elevated CSF testosterone levels in impulsive, assaultive, alcoholic men. Constantino and colleagues (1993) found no differences in serum testosterone levels between aggressive and nonaggressive prepubertal boys. And Mattsson and colleagues (1980), in one of the few studies of male adolescents, found incarcerated delinquent males to have somewhat higher serum testosterone levels than nondelinquent male adolescents. In short, the jury is still out regarding the role of testosterone (after birth) in the development of aggression. Perhaps the most convincing evidence of the possible role of androgens in aggression comes from the case studies of individuals who, under the influence of anabolic steroids, behave in uncharacteristically aggressive ways (Choi et al. 1990; Uzych 1992).

■ Quality of Nurturing

Nurturing affects temperament, which in turn affects behavior. Mice bred to be gentle, if cross-fostered by adult female mice of an aggressive strain, will become more aggressive than littermates raised by nonaggressive mothers (Southwick 1968). Isolation during critical developmental periods can also engender aggressiveness in otherwise gentle animals (Goldsmith et al. 1976; Luciano and Lore 1975). Just as very early experiences have powerful and enduring effects on animals, so too are human infants affected, not only by prenatal and perinatal events (e.g., maternal stress; maternal viral infections; traumatic delivery) but also by the way they are treated during the first months and years of life. There is strong evidence that the ways that mothers and infants interact during the first weeks and months of life affect subsequent childhood aggression (Lyons-Ruth 1996). Adequate mothers sense their infants' needs and respond reassuringly. Infants so nurtured attach securely to their mothers and turn to them unambivalently at times of stress. Mothers lacking appropriate responsiveness to their infants seem to engender insecure, avoidant attachment in their children. Some of the most disturbed mothers—those with psychiatric illness and those who themselves have been abused and abandoned—engender a kind of disturbed, disorganized attachment in their children. These kinds of pathological, insecure, and disorganized attachments are often associated with children's subsequent aggressiveness (Lyons-Ruth and Block 1993; Main and Solomon 1990; Renken et al. 1989). Poor mothering takes its toll intellectually as well as emotionally, and the combination of disorganized attachment and cognitive developmental lags have together been associated with aggressiveness at age 7 years (Lyons-Ruth 1996).

During the first two years of life, an enormous proliferation of brain cells, axons, dendrites, and synapses occurs. Which connections or pathways survive and which will be pruned and disappear depends on experience (Singer 1995). Certain types of mothering experiences must occur for the infant brain to develop normally. During these crucial periods, infants cannot modulate their own arousal states and require a responsive caregiver to reduce stress and restore a sense of safety. It is likely that these early lessons in affect and impulse control affect brain function and structure and thus affect adaptation throughout life (Sroufe et al. 1999). It may be that the apparent lack of empathy in certain children and adolescents with conduct disorders, as well as their aggressiveness and poor impulse control, have their biological roots in the deficient early nurturing they received and the way in which inadequate caretaking affected brain function and structure.

■ Abuse, Parental Violence, and Behavior Problems

Although psychiatric, neurological, genetic, hormonal, and neurophysiological factors influence the development of conduct disorder, in the end the most important influences on behavior problems and violence are environmental. Violence may not invariably beget violence, but there is ample evidence of an association between early maltreatment and the development of aggressive coping styles. Our own clinical studies (Lewis et al. 1979b, 1988a, 1988b, 1989, 2001) as well as larger epidemiological studies (Malinosky-Rummel and Hansen 1993; Widom 1989) have confirmed the devastating effects of child maltreatment on social adaptation. As Farrington and Loeber (2000) observe,

"Among the most important family risk factors for juvenile violence are parental criminality, parental child rearing techniques (physical discipline, poor supervision, low attachment), child maltreatment, parental conflict, large family size and family poverty." (p. 738)

Abuse begets violence in a variety of ways: first, parental violence becomes a model for behavior; second, it often leads to CNS injury, which in turn compromises impulse control, intellectual functioning, judgment, and the ability to accurately read the emotional cues of others. By disrupting the limbic-hypothalamic-pituitary-adrenal axis, the stress itself of life within a violent household can increase production of corticotropin-releasing hormone and cortisol and cause damage to the hippocampus (Bremner et al. 1997; Brunson et al. 2001). Of note, people with posttraumatic stress disorder resulting from early sexual abuse often have a plethora of neurodevelopmental problems and subtle signs of brain dysfunction (Gurvits et al. 2000). Our own clinical and follow-up studies (Lewis et al. 1979b, 1988a, 1988b, 1989, 1991, 1994, 2001) and the work of Raine and colleagues (1996, 1997a) document some of the ways in which early deprivation, abuse, and brain dysfunction predispose children to maladaptive, aggressive behaviors. Furthermore, studies of children who witness household violence have documented their cognitive, developmental, and psychiatric problems and their aggressive behaviors (Edleson 1999; Henning et al. 1996; Song et al. 1998; Spaccarelli et al. 1995). Finally, abuse and witnessing abuse engender rage, which is rarely expressed toward the abuser himself or herself but rather is displaced onto others in the child's world such as teachers, peers, and strangers.

Diagnostic Evaluation

Because of the numerous different kinds of neuropsychiatric disorders that present as behavioral problems, a comprehensive neuropsychiatric evaluation must be conducted and potentially treatable vulnerabilities must be identified before the clinician relegates any adolescent simply to the diagnostic category of conduct disorder. The more sullen, boastful, condescending, aggressive, or just plain obnoxious the adolescent, the more important it is to become aware of one's own negative feelings and not permit them to interfere with the thoroughness of the evaluation.

A plethora of rating scales for behaviors exist (e.g., the Conners Rating Scales [Rosenberg and Beck 1986], the Child Behavior Checklist [Achenbach and Edelbrock 1983], and the Revised Behavior Problems Checklist [Quay and Peterson 1987]). Unfortunately, these focus primarily on conduct, inattention, and hyperactivity and do not help parents, teachers, and children share other kinds of data relevant to diagnosis. Therefore, some of the semistructured diagnostic interviews such as the National Institute of Mental Health Diagnostic Interview Schedule for Children—Revised (Schaffer et al. 1996) or the Schedule for Affective Disorders and Schizophrenia for School-Age Children (Ambrosini and Dixon 1996) may be more useful. Nothing can substitute for detailed, comprehensive, systematic clinical interviews with adolescents and family members and sometimes with friends and others.

■ Behaviors

The nature, onset and frequency of problematic behaviors as well as their precipitants and the adolescent's ability to control them must be explored. Does the adolescent know beforehand that an aggressive act will occur? Can he or she prevent it or stop it in its midst? How does the teenager feel afterward? Does he or she always recall saying or doing things, or is memory ever clouded or absent? After an assaultive act, paranoid adolescents often insist they are glad because the victim deserved what he or she got. Children with dissociative disorders, complex partial seizures, and acute confusional migraine may feel groggy or as if things were unreal, or they may have partial, distorted, or no memory at all for some of their acts.

■ Medical Histories

Adolescents with conduct disorders tend to have lengthy medical histories (Lewis and Shanok 1977, 1979; Lewis et al. 1979a, 1982b). Often one finds that the more aggressive the adolescent, the greater the number and nature of accidents, injuries, and illnesses. The history taker must avoid questions with yes or no answers and must pursue answers to their fullest. After learning of a particular injury, the interviewer must be prepared to ask, "And what other injuries have you had? How about a bike accident? A car? Ever been knocked out? Knocked dizzy? Any blackouts? Headaches?" and so on.

In the context of the medical history, the interviewer can inquire about scars. After looking at the adolescent's face, head, arms, and legs and asking the origin of scars, depending on the setting, the interviewer may ask to see the adolescent's back or may later request that a pediatrician examine the youngster's body for signs of other injuries or abuse. Many delinquent youngsters have scars on their thighs and buttocks from beatings. We once evaluated a teenager whose medical history mentioned a scar on his penis. When we were able to examine him in the privacy of a jail infirmary, we discovered a scar beneath his penis that ran from the glans down the shaft and onto the right scrotal skin. We also saw evidence of an amateurish attempt to sew up the wound.

■ Mental Status

Even the most disturbed adolescents are unlikely to reveal hallucinations or delusions if they can avoid doing so. We have found that an excellent way of inquiring about visual and auditory hallucinations is in the context of the medical history (e.g., Have you ever had an earache? How was it treated? Have your ears ever played tricks on you? Have you ever thought you heard someone say something bad about you or your mom, and you turned around, ready to fight, but the kid hadn't said anything?). In this context, many repeatedly aggressive, paranoid youngsters often are able to describe numerous times that such misperceptions caused fights.

Many clinicians fail to inquire about dissociative phenomena. This omission is especially unfortunate when examining aggressive adolescents and children, many of whom have been severely abused. Still in the context of the medical history, the interviewer can comment, "Many kids who have been through a lot can space out and go somewhere in their heads so they get away from it all. Can/could you ever do that?" Similarly, most severely dissociative youngsters hear voices in their heads arguing with each other. The interviewer may say, "Many kids who have had a tough time have been able to talk with someone in their heads. Could you ever do that?" It is as much an art as a science to enable such traumatized children and adolescents to open up and reveal what goes on in their minds.

■ Sexual and Physical Abuse

Some of the most traumatized children and adolescents will not speak of abuse because they do not recall it. Others try to protect their abusers. Questions about being touched in private places often lead nowhere. We have found that asking, "Who taught you about sex? Have you ever had sex with someone a lot older than you?" is a more acceptable way of opening up the topic. Again, using the medical history to ask about pain or bleeding while urinating or defecating is an excellent way of beginning to explore what is a difficult topic for examiner and patient. Children are reluctant to reveal parental physical abuse. They often say they deserved whatever they got. Therefore, we say, "We know of times when you've given your mom a hard time. Did she ever go further than she meant to?" Space precludes a detailed description of the diagnostic evaluation, but a more comprehensive discussion can be found in Lewis (1996).

■ Neurological, Neuropsychological, and Educational Assessment

A careful behavioral, medical, and educational history and mental status examination will frequently provide information suggesting the need for neurological, neuropsychological, and educational evaluations. The clinician must make each referral thoughtfully, providing colleagues with all of the information gathered that suggests the need for specialized examinations (e.g., this adolescent had head trauma from a severe bicycle accident, has since then complained of headaches, and has olfactory auras and memory distortions for behaviors). It should be made clear that what is being requested is not a routine examination. The consultant should be made curious enough to perform a sophisticated evaluation.

The diagnostician must keep in mind the fact that the neurological and cognitive deficits of most children and adolescents with conduct disorders are subtle. Children with clear evidence of brain dysfunction on neuropsychological testing will usually have normal electroencephalograms and magnetic resonance imaging scans. Neuropsychological testing is often a more sensitive measure of neurological impairment than more high-technology diagnostic tools. Furthermore, children with complex partial seizures—even those with grand mal seizures—can have normal electroencephalograms. It is the evaluator's job to acquire as much clinical data as possible and then attempt to treat the identified vulnerabilities.

Treatment

Conduct disorder encompasses such a heterogeneous group of signs, symptoms, and behaviors that no single psychotherapeutic, social, educational, or pharmacological intervention or combination of interventions is likely to be helpful, much less curative, for the majority of adolescents with the diagnosis. It is unlikely that the treatment protocol designed to help a paranoid 15-year-old boy with a learning disability, a history of ADHD, and a tendency to lash out in response to imagined provocations will be of much use to a sexually promiscuous 13-year-old girl who stays away from home because her father abuses her and who turns tricks to make enough money to eat. In other words, for a treatment to be effective it must address the individual biopsychosocial vulnerabilities and needs of the individual adolescent.

As discussed above, children whose behaviors are caught within the wide conduct disorder net are likely to have other psychiatric problems, to have learning disabilities, to have difficulty recognizing the moods and feelings of others, and therefore to have poor interpersonal skills. In addition, they live in households with disturbed, often violent parents who, from the start, had difficulty caring for themselves, much less nurturing their children. Further exacerbating the disorder, children with conduct disorders usually come from socioeconomically deprived and crime-ridden communities. No single type of intervention can possibly address all of these adversities.

■ Validated Treatment Modalities

Although many different kinds of treatment have been tried, from pharmacotherapy to community-based programs, few have been evaluated systematically (Kazdin 2001). Of those that have been studied, according to Kazdin, only four have been validated—that is, shown to produce positive behavioral change. They are described below.

Parent Management Training

Parent management training teaches the parents of children with conduct disorders techniques for interacting with their offspring to encourage appropriate behavior and diminish oppositional, aggressive behaviors. In brief, its premise is that many parents of behav-iorally disturbed children have increased if not engendered these behaviors through harsh punishments for infractions and through failure to acknowledge good behaviors. Therapists teach parents methods for positive reinforcement of children's desirable behaviors, the use of mild, nonphysical punishment for infractions, and communication techniques for negotiating with their offspring. In their review of treatment modalities, Brestan and Eyberg (1998) singled out parent management training as the only well-established, effective treatment for conduct disorder.

Effective as this method may be for participants, its major drawback is that often the most behaviorally disturbed children come from the most chaotic households, in which a parent or parents will have the greatest difficulty cooperating with treatment.

Cognitive Problem-Solving Skills Training

Cognitive problem-solving skills training is based on the premise that children with conduct disorder do not know how to make use of their potential cognitive abilities to identify problems, anticipate consequences, and consider alternative ways of understanding and coping with difficult situations. In essence, it tries to help children and adolescents make use of their frontal lobes to evaluate situations rather than simply react to them impulsively. Older children reportedly respond better than younger children to this modality (Durlak et al. 1991), which is not surprising given the increasing myelinization of the frontal lobes during adolescence and beyond. Problem-solving skills training has been less successful with children who have other neuropsychiatric disorders in addition to conduct disorder. It has also been less successful with children whose households are especially chaotic. This is not surprising given that the burden of treatment is entirely on the child or adolescent who, even provided with the best of cognitive skills, may still come home to an overwhelming set of problems with which he or she cannot be expected to cope.

Multisystemic Therapy

Multisystemic therapy is based on the fact that the child with conduct disorder interacts with and is part of a variety of different systems: the family, the peer group, the school, and the neighborhood or community at large. Treatment focuses on problems a given child may be experiencing interacting with others in any or all of these systems. Treatment will differ depending on the nature of the child's problems. A major focus of this modality is the family: identifying problems, improving communication, and diminishing negative interactions between parents themselves as well as between parents and children. Depending on the needs of the family, multisystemic treatment may make use of parent management training, problem-solving skills training for the child, or marital counseling. Its greatest advantages are its ability to address individual needs and vulnerabilities, as well as intrapersonal and interpersonal issues, and its ability to make use of a wide variety of interventions. With multisystemic treatment, one size does not fit all. It is therefore customized for each child and family. As such, it has been more successful than the usual probation or individual counseling afforded to children and adolescents with conduct disorder (Henggeler et al. 1998). However, this customization of treatment poses replication problems (Kazdin 2001).

Functional Family Therapy

Functional family therapy is based on conceptualizing the presenting clinical problem from the standpoint of the functions it serves within the family as well as its function for the individual. What is it within the family that permits the problematic behaviors to continue? Who gets what out of the resultant interactions? Are there alternative ways of interacting that would be more gratifying and more productive? How do family members communicate their needs, wishes, and feelings, and are there more constructive ways of interacting and meeting their own and each other's needs? Our own studies (Lewis et al. 1979b, 1987, 1988b) as well as those of others (Dodge et al. 1990) indicate a tendency for aggressive delinquents to think in paranoid ways. Alexander and colleagues (1989) found that the parents of delinquents tend to be more defensive and blaming of others than the parents of nondelinquents. A major goal of functional family therapy is to help family members correct misattributions and develop more reality-based and mutually supportive ways of communicating and interacting. Those who developed this treatment modality have also tried to evaluate its outcome. They have reported benefits not only in terms of better family communications but also in terms of lower recidivism rates for adolescent delinquents (Alexander et al. 1994).

A point to note is that three of the four apparently successful treatment modalities focus on helping the parents of delinquents with their interactions with each other and with their children. Unfortunately, most delinquents, especially the most violent and recidivistic, come from dysfunctional homes in which parents are mentally ill or violent and are unlikely to be able to take advantage of the cognitively based therapies that rely so strongly on interpersonal verbal communication.

■ Pharmacotherapy

Because conduct disorder encompasses so many different neuropsychiatric conditions and combinations thereof, no single medication or type of medication is especially useful. Stimulants, antidepressants, antipsychotics, mood stabilizers, antiepileptics, and even beta-blockers have been tried. Except for the use of stimulants for clearly defined attentional problems and hyperactivity, results have been inconsistent and equivocal (Karper and Krystal 1997; Werry 1994). On the other hand, we have found clinically that judicious use of medication, based on the nature of well-defined and documented symptoms and signs (e.g., the slow titration of antipsychotic medication to therapeutic levels for paranoid adolescents; the use of stimulant medication for adolescents with conduct disorder and severe attentional problems), can mean the difference between an adolescent's ability to make use of a therapeutic environment and his sabotaging his placement.

Prognosis

Numerous studies indicate that the diagnosis of conduct disorder has a grim prognosis (Hechtman and Offord 1994). As mentioned earlier in this chapter, follow-up studies of children and adolescents with conduct disorder suggest that a minority go on to commit aggressive antisocial acts in adulthood. However, the overall adult adjustment of seriously behaviorally disordered adolescents is often poor, as reflected in unstable marriages, unsatisfactory job histories, and many symptoms of maladaptation other than antisocial behaviors. Suicide and other forms of violent death are common outcomes (Yeager and Lewis 1990). Strategies that focus on the early prevention of behavioral problems in preschool children hold more promise than late treatment strategies (Zigler et al. 1992).

On the other hand, one can expect remarkably positive behavioral responses to individually tailored therapeutic interventions. As Kazdin (1987) observed, "The breadth of dysfunctions of antisocial youths and their families makes the task of developing effective treatments demanding, if not close to impossible" (p. 95).

Clinical experience suggests that a treatment program can be expected to be successful only when it identifies and addresses each vulnerability and need of the child with behavioral disturbance. In addition, because the vulnerabilities and needs are chronic, programs must recognize the need for ongoing support systems and continuity of care throughout adolescence for such multiply handicapped youngsters to adapt appropriately to society (Kazdin 2001).

Research Issues

Considering the extraordinary cost to society of antisocial behavior, remarkably little research has focused on its causes, treatment, or prevention. The research budget of the U.S. Office of Juvenile Justice is unusually small compared with other government agencies. The reason that so little scientific investigation has addressed the phenomenon of juvenile violence is in itself an important question to be explored.

Because violent acts take such a great toll on society, the study of violent antisocial behavior deserves special emphasis. Research is needed to better understand the types of intrinsic vulnerabilities that decrease impulse control, intensify feeling states, and impair judgment and reality testing. These kinds of investigations should be conducted on different levels, from the molecular and biochemical to the clinical. Because the intrinsic vulnerabilities contributing to antisocial behavior are so varied, research that increases the understanding of the etiology and treatment of most other psychiatric conditions (e.g., mood disorders, psychoses) will also be relevant to understanding violent behavior in many children and adolescents

Research strategies that focus only on individual biochemical and genetic factors are unlikely to diminish antisocial behavior. It is extremely unusual for a single biological vulnerability, in and of itself, to cause antisocial behavior. Although reports of the onset of violent behavior secondary to the growth of specific hypothalamic brain tumors have appeared occasionally in the literature, the ways in which biological vulnerabilities will manifest themselves behaviorally typically depend on the individual's upbringing and on immediate environmental stressors or precipitants. Therefore, research on aggression must focus on environmental and experiential issues as well as on intrinsic biological vulnerabilities. Experience influences biology. These kinds of environmental studies should focus not only on individual family characteristics but also on social conditions and personal and cultural values.

To begin to understand the causes of violence and to diminish its impact, multidisciplinary collaborative research is clearly needed. It is not enough to recognize the different factors associated with violent behavior; rather, it is necessary to elucidate the ways in which these biopsychosocial phenomena interact with one another to produce violence.

Finally, it should be noted that both large epidemiological studies and smaller clinical studies are needed. Although large studies facilitate certain kinds of statistical analyses, their methodology (e.g., use of questionnaires, interviews by paraprofessionals) precludes the kinds of observations and insights made possible when well-trained, experienced clinicians from different disciplines collaborate in conducting careful, systematic, sophisticated evaluations. Hence, a balance must be struck between support for large epidemiological studies and smaller, controlled, comprehensive clinical studies. As understanding of the underlying factors contributing to behavioral problems increases, the diagnosis of conduct disorder will likely resolve into more discrete clinical entities amenable to specific treatments. The diagnosis itself may even disappear.

References

Achenbach TM: Manual for the Child Behavior Checklist/2–3 and 1992 Profile. Burlington, University of Vermont, 1992

Achenbach TM, Edelbrock C: Manual for the Child Behavior Checklist and Revised Child Behavior Profile. Burlington, VT, TM Achenbach, 1983

Alexander JF, Waldron HB, Barton C, et al: The minimizing of blaming attributions and behaviors in delinquent families. J Consult Clin Psychol 57:19–24, 1989

Alexander JF, Holtzworth-Munroe A, Jameson PB: The process and outcome of marital and family therapy research: review and evaluation, in Handbook of Psychotherapy and Behavior Change, 4th Edition. Edited by Bergin AE, Garfield SL. New York, Wiley, 1994, pp 595–630

Alsobrook JP 2nd, Pauls DL: Genetics and violence. Child Adolesc Psychiatr Clin N Am 9:765–776, 2000

Ambrosini P, Dixon M: The Schedule for Affective Disorders and Schizophrenia for School-Age Children, 4th Edition. Philadelphia, PA, Allegheny University of Health Sciences, 1996

American Psychiatric Association: Diagnostic and Statistical Manual of Mental Disorders, 2nd Edition. Washington, DC, American Psychiatric Association, 1968

American Psychiatric Association: Diagnostic and Statistical Manual of Mental Disorders, 3rd Edition. Washington, DC, American Psychiatric Association, 1980

American Psychiatric Association: Diagnostic and Statistical Manual of Mental Disorders, 3rd Edition, Revised. Washington, DC, American Psychiatric Association, 1987

American Psychiatric Association: Diagnostic and Statistical Manual of Mental Disorders, 4th Edition. Washington, DC, American Psychiatric Association, 1994

American Psychiatric Association: Diagnostic and Statistical Manual of Mental Disorders, 4th Edition, Text Revision. Washington, DC, American Psychiatric Association, 2000

Anderson S, Bechara A, Damasio H, et al: Impairment of social and moral behavior related to early damage in human prefrontal cortex. Nat Neurosci 2:1032–1037, 1999

Andrulonis PA, Glueck BC, Stroebel CR, et al: Borderline personality subcategories. J Nerv Ment Dis 170:670–679, 1982

Angold A, Costello EJ: The epidemiology of disorders of conduct: nosological issues and comorbidity, in Conduct Disorders in Childhood and Adolescence. Edited by Hill J, Maughan B. New York, Cambridge University Press, 2001

Aniskiewicz AS: Autonomic components of vicarious conditioning and psychopathy. J Clin Psychol 35:60–67, 1979

Arrestee Drug Abuse Monitoring Program (ADAM): 1998 Annual Report on Drug Use Among Adult and Juvenile Arrestees. Washington, DC, National Institute of Justice, 1999

August GJ, Stewart MA, Holmes CS: A four year follow-up of hyperactive boys with and without conduct disorder. Br J Psychiatry 143:192–198, 1983

Bahrke MS, Wright JE, O'Connor JS, et al: Selected psychological characteristics of anabolic-androgenic steroid users. N Engl J Med 323:834–835, 1990a

Bahrke MS, Yesalis CE, Wright JE: Psychological and behavioral efforts of endogenous testosterone level and anabolic-androgenic steroids among males: a review. Sports Med 10:303–337, 1990b

Barkley RA: Behavioral inhibition, sustained attention, and executive functions: constructing a unifying theory of ADHD. Psychol Bull 121:65–94, 1997

Bauer LO, Hesselbrock VM: P300 decrements in teenagers with conduct problems: implications for substance abuse risk and brain development. Biol Psychiatry 46:263–272, 1999

Bauer LO, Hesselbrock VM: CSD/BEM localization of P300 sources in adolescents "at-risk": evidence of frontal cortex dysfunction in conduct disorder. Biol Psychiatry 50:600–608, 2001

Bauermeister JJ, Canino G, Bird H: Epidemiology of disruptive behavior disorders. Child Adolesc Psychiatr Clin N Am 3:177–194, 1994

Bellak L: ADD psychosis as a separate entity. Schizophr Bull 11:523–527, 1985

Bender L: The concept of pseudopsychopathic schizophrenia in adolescents. Am J Orthopsychiatry 29:491–509, 1959

Biederman J, Faraone SV, Wozniak J, et al: Parsing the association between bipolar, conduct, and substance use disorders: a familial risk analysis. Biol Psychiatry 48:1037–1044, 2000

Bjork JM, Dougherty DM, Moeller FG, et al: The effects of tryptophan depletion and loading on laboratory aggression in men: time course and a food-restricted control. Psychopharmacology (Berl) 142:24–30, 1999

Blair RJ, Colledge E, Murray L, et al: A selective impairment in the processing of sad and fearful expressions in children with psychopathic tendencies. J Abnorm Child Psychol 29:491–498, 2001a

Blair RJ, Colledge E, Mitchell DG: Somatic markers and response reversal: is there orbitofrontal cortex dysfunction in boys with psychopathic tendencies? J Abnorm Child Psychol 29:499–511, 2001b

Bremner JD, Randall PR, Vermetten E, et al: MRI-based measurement of hippocampal volume in posttraumatic stress disorder related to childhood physical and sexual abuse: a preliminary report. Biol Psychiatry 41:23–32, 1997

Brestan EV, Eyberg SM: Effective psychosocial treatment of conduct-disordered children and adolescents: 29 years, 82 studies, 5275 children. J Clin Child Psychol 27:180–189, 1998

Brown GL, Goodwin FK, Ballenger JC, et al: Aggression in humans correlates with cerebrospinal fluid amine metabolites. Psychiatry Res 1:131–139, 1979

Brunner HG, Nelen M, Breakefield XO, et al: Abnormal behavior associated with a point mutation in the structural gene for monoamine oxidase-A. Science 262:578–580, 1993

Brunson KL, Eghbal-Ahmadi M, Bender R, et al: Long-term, progressive hippocampal cell loss and dysfunction induced by early life administration of corticotropin-releasing hormone reproduce the effects of early life stress. Proc Natl Acad Sci U S A 98:8856–8861, 2001

Carlson GA: Clinical features and pathogenesis of child and adolescent mania, in Mood Disorders Across the Life Span. Edited by Shulman KI, Tohen M, Kutcher SP. New York, Wiley-Liss, 1996, pp 127–147

Casey LJ, Segall DR, Street K, et al: Sex chromosomes abnormalities in two state hospitals for patients requiring special security. Nature 209:641–642, 1966

Cherek DR: Laboratory studies of aggression and drugs. Paper presented at the annual meeting of the American Psychological Association, Boston, MA, 1990

Choi PY, Parrott AC, Cowan D: High dose anabolic steroids in strength athletics: effects upon hostility and aggression. Hum Psychopharmacol 5:349–356, 1990

Cicchetti D, Carlson V: Child Maltreatment: Theory and Research on the Causes and Consequences of Child Abuse and Neglect. New York, Cambridge University Press, 1989

Coccaro EF, Kavoussi RJ, Hauger RL, et al: Cerebrospinal fluid vasopressin levels: correlates with aggression and serotonin function in personality-disordered subjects. Arch Gen Psychiatry 55:708–714, 1998

Cohen AK: The origin and nature of the delinquent subculture, in Delinquent Boys: The Culture of the Gang. New York, Free Press, 1955

Comings DE, Comings BG: A controlled study of Tourette's syndrome in attention deficit disorder, learning disorders, and school problems. Am J Hum Genet 41:701–741, 1987

Constantino JN, Grosz D, Sainger P, et al: Testosterone and aggression in children. J Am Acad Child Adolesc Psychiatry 32:1217–1222, 1993

Costellanos FX: The psychology of attention-deficit/hyperactivity disorder, in Handbook of Disruptive Behavior Disorders. Edited by Quay HC, Hogan AD. New York, Kluwer Academic/Plenum, 1999, pp 179–198

Crick NR, Grotpeter JK: Relational aggression, gender and social-psychological adjustment. Child Dev 66:710–722, 1995

Currie E: Confronting Crime: An American Challenge. New York, Pantheon, 1985

Currie E: Sociologic perspectives on juvenile violence. Child Adolesc Psychiatr Clin N Am 9:749–763, 2000

Dalteg A, Levander S: Twelve thousand crimes by 75 boys: a 20 year follow-up study of childhood hyperactivity. Journal of Forensic Psychiatry 9:39–57, 1998

Damasio AR: The somatic marker hypothesis and the possible functions of the prefrontal cortex, in The Prefrontal Cortex: Executive and Cognitive Functions. Edited by Roberts AC, Robbins TW, Weiskrantz L. New York, Oxford University Press, 1998, pp 36–51

Dishion TJ, McCord J, Poulin F: When interventions harm: peer groups and problem behavior. Am Psychol 54:755–764, 1999

Dodge KA, Price JM, Bachorowski JA, et al: Hostile attributional biases in severely aggressive adolescents. J Abnorm Psychol 99:385–392, 1990

Dryfoos JG: Adolescents at Risk: Prevalence and Prevention. New York, Oxford University Press, 1990

Durlak JA, Fuhrman T, Lampman C: Effectiveness of cognitive-behavioral therapy for maladapting children: a meta-analysis. Psychol Bull 110:204–214, 1991

Edleson JL: The overlap between child maltreatment and woman battering. Violence Against Women 14:839–870, 1999

Ellickson P, Saner H, McGuigan K: Profiles of violent youth: substance use and other concurrent problems. Am J Public Health 87:985–991, 1997

Elliott DS, Menard S: Delinquent friends and delinquent behavior: temporal and developmental patterns, in Delinquency and Crime: Current Theories. Edited by Hawkins JD. Cambridge, UK, Cambridge University Press, 1996, pp 28–67

Elliot DS, Huzinga D, Menard S: Multiple Problem Youth: Delinquency, Substance Use and Mental Health Problems. New York, Springer-Verlag, 1989

Ehrhardt AA: Prenatal hormonal exposure and psychosexual differentiation, in Topics in Psychoendocrinology. Edited by Sachar EJ. New York, Grune & Stratton, 1975, pp 67–82

Ehyai A, Fenichel GM: The natural history of acute confusional migraine. Arch Neurol 35:368–369, 1978

Esser G, Schmidt MH, Woermer W: Epidemiology and course of psychiatric disorders in school-age children: results of a longitudinal study. J Child Psychol Psychiatry 31:243–263, 1990

Farrington DP, Loeber R: Epidemiology of juvenile violence. Child Adolesc Psychiatr Clin N Am 9:733–748, 2000

Farrington DP, Loeber R, Van Kammen WB: Long-term criminal outcomes of hyperactivity-impulsivity-attention deficit and conduct problems in childhood, in Straight and Devious Pathways From Childhood to Adulthood. Edited by Robins L, Rutter M. New York, Cambridge University Press, 1990, pp 62–81

Fauman BJ, Fauman MA: Phencyclidine, abuse and crime: a psychiatric perspective. Bull Am Acad Psychiatry Law 10:171–176, 1982

Ferguson JN, Alday JM, Insel TR, et al: Oxytocin in the medial amygdala is essential for social recognition in the mouse. J Neurosci 21:8278–8285, 2001

Foley HA, Carlton CO, Howell RJ: The relationship of attention deficit hyperactivity disorder and conduct disorder to juvenile delinquency: legal implications. Bull Am Acad Psychiatry Law 24:333–345, 1996

Friedman CJ, Mann F, Friedman AS: A profile of juvenile street gang members. Adolescence 40:563–607, 1975

Ge XR, Conger RD, Cadoret RJ, et al: The developmental interface between nature and nurture: a mutual influence model of child antisocial behavior and parent behaviors. Dev Psychol 32:574–589, 1996

Gerald PS: Sex chromosome disorders. N Engl J Med 294:706–708, 1976

Goadsby PJ, Lipton RB, Ferrari MD: Migraine: current understanding and treatment. N Engl J Med 346:257–270, 2002

Goldsmith JF, Brain PF, Benton D: Effects of age at differential housing and the duration of individual housing/grouping on intermale fighting behavior and adrenocortical activity in TO strain mice. Aggress Behav 2:307–323, 1976

Gotz MJ, Johnstone EC, Radcliffe SG: Criminality and antisocial behaviour in unselected men with sex chromosome abnormalities. Psychol Med 29:953–962, 1999

Gurvits TV, Gilbertson MW, Lasko MB, et al: Neurologic soft signs in posttraumatic stress disorder. Arch Gen Psychiatry 57:181–186, 2000

Hall W, Solowij N: Adverse effects of cannabis. Lancet 352:1611–1616, 1998

Halperin JM, Newcorn JH, Schwartz ST, et al: Age-related changes in the association between serotonergic function and aggression in boys with ADHD. Biol Psychiatry 41:682–689, 1996

Hechtman L, Offord DR: Long-term outcome of disruptive disorders. Child Adolesc Psychiatr Clin N Am 3:379–403, 1994

Heise L, Pitanguy J, Germain A: Violence Against Women: The Hidden Health Burden (World Bank Discussion Paper No. 255). Washington, DC, World Bank, 1994

Henggeler SW, Schoenwald SK, Borduin CM, et al: Multisystemic Treatment of Antisocial Behavior in Children and Adolescents. New York, Guilford, 1998

Henning K, Leitenber H, Coffey P, et al: Long term psychological and social impact of witnessing physical conflict between parents. J Interpers Violence 11:35–51, 1996

Hines M: Prenatal gonadal hormones and sex differences in human behavior. Psychol Bull 92:56–80, 1982

Hinshaw SP, Lahey BB, Hart EL: Issues of taxonomy and comorbidity in the development of conduct disorder. Dev Psychopathol 5:31, 1993, pp 31–49

Hirschi T, Hinderlang MJ: Intelligence and delinquency: a revisionist view. Am Sociol Rev 42:571–587, 1977

Honer WG, Gewertz G, Turey M: Psychosis and violence in cocaine smokers. Lancet 2:451–452, 1987

Huizinga D, Loeber R, Thornberry T, et al: Co-occurrence of delinquency and other problem behaviors (Juvenile Justice Bulletin, November). Washington, DC, Office of Juvenile Justice and Delinquency Prevention, 2000

Hutchings B, Mednick SA: Registered criminality in the adoptive and biological parents of registered male criminal adoptees, in Genetics, Environment and Psychopathology. Edited by Mednick SA, Schulsinger F, Higgins J, et al. New York, Elsevier, 1974, pp 215–227

Insel TR: The neurobiological basis of social attachment. Am J Psychiatry 154:726–735, 1997

Jenkins RL, Hewitt L: Types of personality structure encountered in child guidance clinics. Am J Orthopsychiatry 14:84–94, 1944

Karper LP, Krystal JH: Pharmacotherapy of violent behavior, in Handbook of Antisocial Behavior. Edited by Stoff DM, Breiling J, Maser JD. New York, Wiley, 1997, pp 36–44

Kashani JH, Beck NC, Hoeper EW, et al: Psychiatric disorders in a community sample of adolescents. Am J Psychiatry 144:584–589, 1987

Kazdin AE: Conduct Disorders in Childhood and Adolescence (Developmental Clinical Psychology and Psychiatry Series, Vol 9). Newbury Park, CA, Sage, 1987

Kazdin AE: Treatment of conduct disorders, in Conduct Disorders in Childhood and Adolescence (Cambridge Child and Adolescent Psychiatry Series). Edited by Hill J, Maughan B. New York, Cambridge University Press, 2001, pp 408–448

King GR, Ellinwood EH: Amphetamines and other stimulants, in Substance Abuse: A Comprehensive Textbook. Edited by Lowinson JH, Ruiz P, Millman RB, et al. Baltimore, MD, Williams & Wilkins, 1992, pp 247–270

Lahey BB, Goodman SH, Waldman ID, et al: Relation of age of onset to the type and severity of child and adolescent conduct problems. J Abnorm Child Psychol 27:247–260, 1999

Lambert N, Hartsaugh C, Sassone D: Persistence of hyperactivity symptoms from childhood to adolescence. Am J Orthopsychiatry 57:22–31, 1987

Lambert N, Wahler RG, Andrade AR, et al: Looking for the disorder in conduct disorder. J Abnorm Psychol 110:110–123, 2001

Lefkowitz MM, Eron LD, Walder LO, et al: Growing Up to Be Violent: A Longitudinal Study of Aggression. Oxford, UK, Pergamon, 1977

Levinson D: Family Violence in Cross-Cultural Perspective. Thousand Oaks, CA, Sage, 1989

Lewis DO: Delinquency, psychomotor epileptic symptoms, and paranoid ideation: a triad. Am J Psychiatry 133:1395–1398, 1976

Lewis DO: Diagnostic evaluation of the child with dissociative identity disorder/multiple personality disorder. Child Adolesc Psychiatr Clin N Am 5:303–332, 1996

Lewis DO, Pincus JH: Epilepsy and violence: evidence for a neuropsychotic-aggressive syndrome. J Neuropsychiatry Clin Neurosci 1:413–418, 1989

Lewis DO, Shanok S: Medical histories of delinquent and nondelinquent children: an epidemiological study. Am J Psychiatry 134:527–533, 1977

Lewis DO, Shanok S: A comparison of the medical histories of incarcerated delinquent children and a matched sample of nondelinquent children. Child Psychiatry Hum Dev 9:210–214, 1979

Lewis DO, Shanok S: The use of a correctional setting for follow-up care of psychiatrically disturbed adolescents. Am J Psychiatry 137:953–955, 1980

Lewis DO, Shanok S, Balla D: Perinatal difficulties, head and face trauma and child abuse in the medical histories of seriously delinquent children. Am J Psychiatry 136:419–423, 1979a

Lewis DO, Shanok S, Pincus J, et al: Violent juvenile delinquents: psychiatric, neurological, psychological and abuse factors. J Am Acad Child Psychiatry 18:307–319, 1979b

Lewis DO, Shanok S, Cohen RJ, et al: Race bias in the diagnosis and disposition of violent adolescents. Am J Psychiatry 137:1211–1216, 1980

Lewis DO, Shanok S, Balla D: Parents of delinquents, in Vulnerabilities to Delinquency. Edited by Lewis DO. New York, Spectrum, 1981, pp 265–292

Lewis DO, Pincus JH, Shanok SS, et al: Psychomotor epilepsy and violence in a group of incarcerated adolescent boys. Am J Psychiatry 139:882–887, 1982a

Lewis DO, Shanok S, Pincus JH, et al: The medical assessment of seriously delinquent boys: a comparison of pediatric, psychiatric, neurologic, and hospital record data. J Adolesc Health Care 3:160–164, 1982b

Lewis DO, Pincus JH, Lovely R, et al: Biopsychosocial characteristics of matched samples of delinquents and nondelinquents. J Am Acad Child Adolesc Psychiatry 26:744–752, 1987

Lewis DO, Lovely R, Yeager C, et al: Intrinsic and environmental characteristics of juvenile murderers. J Am Acad Child Adolesc Psychiatry 27:582–587, 1988a

Lewis DO, Pincus JA, Bard B, et al: Neuropsychiatric, psychoeducational and family characteristics of 14 juveniles condemned to death in the United States. Am J Psychiatry 145:584–589, 1988b

Lewis DO, Lovely R, Yeager C, et al: Toward a theory of the genesis of violence: a follow-up study of delinquents. J Am Acad Child Adolesc Psychiatry 28:431–436, 1989

Lewis DO, Yeager CA, Cobham-Porterreal CS, et al: A follow-up of female delinquents: maternal contributions to the perpetuation of deviance. J Am Acad Child Adolesc Psychiatry 30:197–201, 1991

Lewis DO, Yeager CA, Lovely R: A clinical follow-up of delinquent males: ignored vulnerabilities, unmet needs, and the perpetuation of violence. J Am Acad Child Adolesc Psychiatry 33:518–528, 1994

Lewis DO, Yeager CA, Gidlow B, et al: Six adoptees who murdered: neuropsychiatric vulnerabilities and characteristics of biological and adoptive parents. J Am Acad Psychiatr Law 29:387–397, 2001

Linnoila M, Virkkunen M, Scheinin M, et al: Low cerebrospinal fluid 5-hydroxyindoleactic acid concentration differentiates impulsive from nonimpulsive violent behavior. Life Sci 33:2609–2614, 1983

Loeber R, Stouthamer-Loeber M, White HR: Developmental aspects of delinquency and internalizing problems and their association with persistent juvenile substance use between ages 7 and 18. J Clin Child Psychol 28:322–332, 1999a

Loeber R, Wei E, Stouthamer-Loeber M, et al: Behavioral antecedents to serious and violent juvenile offending: joint analyses from the Denver Youth Survey, Pittsburgh Youth Study, and the Rochester Development Study. Studies in Crime and Crime Prevention 8:245–263, 1999b

Loeber R, Farrington DP, Stouthamer-Loeber M, et al: The development of male offending: key findings from 14 years of the Pittsburgh Youth Study, in Taking Stock of Delinquency: An Overview of Findings From Contemporary Longitudinal Studies (Longitudinal Research in the Social and Behavioral Sciences Series). Edited by Thornberry TH, Krohn M. New York, Kluwer/Plenum Press, 2003

Luciano D, Lore R: Aggression and social experience in domesticated rats. J Comp Physiol 88:917–923, 1975

Lynam DR, Moffitt TE, Stouthamer-Loeber M: Explaining the relation between IQ and delinquency: class, race, test motivation, school failure, or self-control? J Abnorm Psychol 102:187–196, 1993

Lyons-Ruth K: Attachment relationships among children with aggressive behavior problems: the role of disorganized early attachment patterns. J Consult Clin Psychol 64:64–73, 1996

Lyons-Ruth K, Block D: The disturbed caregiving system: conceptualizing the impact of childhood trauma on maternal caregiving behavior during infancy. Presented at the biennial meeting of the Society for Research in Child Development, New Orleans, LA, 1993

Maguin E, Loeber R: Academic performance and delinquency. Crime and Justice 20:145–264, 1996

Main M, Soloman J: Procedures for identifying infants as disorganized/disoriented during the Ainsworth Strange Situation, in Attachment in the Preschool Years: Theory, Research, and Intervention. Edited by Greenberg M, Cicchetti D, Cummings EM. Chicago, University of Illinois Press, 1990, pp 121–160

Malinosky-Rummel R, Hansen D: Long-term consequences of childhood physical abuse. Psychol Bull 114:68–79, 1993

Mannuzza S, Gittelman-Klein R, Horowitz-Konig P, et al: Hyperactive boys almost grown up, IV: criminality and its relationship to psychiatric status. Arch Gen Psychiatry 46:1073–1079, 1989

Matthews K, Flory J, Mudoon MF, et al: Does socioeconomic status relate to central serotonergic responsivity in healthy adults? Psychosom Med 62:231–237, 2000

Mattsson A, Schalling D, Olweus D, et al: Plasma testosterone, aggressive behavior, and personality dimensions in young male delinquents. J Am Acad Child Psychiatry 19:476–491, 1980

McCrea M, Kelly JP, Kluge J, et al: Standardized assessment of concussion in football players. Neurology 48:586–588, 1997

McDermott PA: A nationwide study of developmental and gender prevalence for psychopathology in childhood and adolescence. J Abnorm Child Psychol 24:53, 1996

McGee R, Feehan M, Williams S, et al: DSM-III disorders from age 11 to age 15 years. J Am Acad Child Adolesc Psychiatry 31:50–59, 1992

McKenzie GM: Apomorphine-induced aggression in the rat. Brain Res 34:323–330, 1971

Mednick SA, Gabrielli WF, Hutchings B: Genetic influences in criminal convictions: evidence from an adoption cohort. Science 224:891–894, 1984

Merton RK: Social structure and anomie. American Sociological Review 3:672–682, 1938

Merton RK: Social Theory and Social Structure, Revised Edition. New York, Free Press, 1957

Meyer-Bahlburg HFL, Nat R, Boon DA, et al: Aggressiveness and testosterone measures in man. Psychosom Med 36:269–274, 1974

Moffitt T: Parental mental disorders and offspring criminal behavior: an adoption study. Psychiatry 50:346–360, 1987

Monti PM, Brown WA, Corriveau MA: Testosterone and components of aggressive and sexual behavior in man. Am J Psychiatry 134:692–694, 1977

Myers WC, Scott K, Burgess AW, et al: Psychopathology, biopsychosocial factors, crime characteristics, and classification of 25 homicidal youths. J Am Acad Child Adolesc Psychiatry 34:1483–1489, 1995

Newcorn JH, Halperin JM: Comorbidity among disruptive behavior disorder: impact on severity, impairment, and response to treatment. Child Adolesc Psychiatr Clin N Am 3:227–252, 1994

Nielson J: The XXY syndrome in a mental hospital. British Journal of Criminology 8:186–203, 1968

Offord DR, Boyle MH, Racine YA, et al: Outcome, prognosis, and risk in a longitudinal follow-up study. J Am Acad Child Adolesc Psychiatry 31:916–923, 1992

Owen DR: The 47XYY male: a review. Psychol Bull 79:209–233, 1972

Pauls DL, Hurst CR, Kruger SD, et al: Gilles de la Tourette's syndrome and attention deficit disorder with hyperactivity: evidence against a genetic relationship. Arch Gen Psychiatry 43:1177–1179, 1986

Pearl GS: Traumatic neuropathology. Clin Lab Med 18:39–64, 1998

Pederson CA, Prange AJ: Induction of maternal behavior in virgin rats after intracerebroventricular administration of oxytocin. Proc Natl Acad Sci U S A 76:6661–6665, 1979

Pietrini V, Terzano MG, D'Andrea G, et al: Acute confusional migraine: clinical and electroencephalographic aspects. Cephalgia 7:29–37, 1987

Pliszka SR, Sherman JO, Barrow MV, et al: Affective disorders in juvenile offenders: a preliminary study. Am J Psychiatry 157:130–132, 2000

Poremba C: Learning disabilities, youth and delinquency: programs for intervention, in Progress in Learning Disabilities, Vol 3. Edited by Myklebust HR. New York, Grune & Stratton, 1975, pp 123–149

Quay HC: Dimensions of personality in delinquent boys as inferred from the factor analysis of case history data. Child Dev 35:479–484, 1964a

Quay HC: Personality dimensions in delinquent males as inferred from the factor analysis of behavior ratings. Journal of Research in Crime and Delinquency 1:33–37, 1964b

Quay HC: Classification in the treatment of delinquency and antisocial behavior, in Issues on the Classification of Children, Vol 1. Edited by Hobbs N. San Francisco, CA, Jossey-Bass, 1975, pp 377–392

Quay HC, Peterson DR: Manual for the Revised Behavior Problem Checklist. Coral Gables, FL, University of Miami, 1987

Raine A, Buchsbaum M, Stanley J, et al: Selective reductions in prefrontal glucose metabolism assessed with positron emission tomography in accused murderers pleading not guilty by reason of insanity. Biol Psychiatry 36:365–373, 1994

Raine A, Brennen P, Mednick S, et al: High rates of violence, crime, academic problems, and behavioral problems in males with both early neuromotor deficits and unstable family environments. Arch Gen Psychiatry 53:544–549, 1996

Raine A, Brennen P, Mednick S: Interaction between early maternal rejection in predisposing individuals to adult violence: specificity to serious, early onset violence. Am J Psychiatry 154:1265–1271, 1997a

Raine A, Buchsbaum M, LaCasse L: Brain abnormalities in murderers indicated by positron emission tomography. Biol Psychiatry 42:495–508, 1997b

Raine A, Lencz T, Bihrle S, et al: Reduced prefrontal gray matter volume and reduced autonomic activity in antisocial personality disorder. Arch Gen Psychiatry 57:119–127, 2000

Renken B, Egeland B, Marvinney D, et al. Early childhood antecedents of aggression and passive withdrawal in early elementary school. J Pers 57:257–281, 1989

Reznikov AG, Nosenko ND, Tarasenko LV: Prenatal stress and glucocortical effects on the developing, gender-related brain. J Steroid Biochem Mol Biol 69:109–115, 1999

Richman N, Stevenson J, Graham PJ: Pre-school to School: A Behavioural Study. London, Academic Press, 1982

Robins LN: Deviant Children Grown-Up. Baltimore, MD, Williams & Wilkins, 1966

Robins LN: Conduct disorder. J Child Psychol Psychiatry 32:193–212, 1991

Robins LN, Price RK: Adult disorders predicted by childhood conduct problems: results from the NIMH Epidemiologic Catchment Area project. Psychiatry 54:116–132, 1991

Robins LN, Regier DA (eds): Psychiatric Disorders in America: The Epidemiologic Catchment Area Study. New York, Free Press, 1991

Robinson A, de la Chapelle A: Sex chromosome anomalies, in Principles and Practice of Medical Genetics, 3rd Edition. Edited by Rimoin D, Connor JM, Pyritz RE. Edinburgh UK, Churchill Livingstone, 1990, pp 973–999

Rosenberg RP, Beck S: Preferred assessment methods and treatment modalities for hyperactive children among clinical child and school psychologists. J Clin Child Psychol 15:142–147, 1986

Rutter M, Giller H: Juvenile Delinquency: Trends and Perspectives. New York, Guilford, 1984

Sahakian BJ: The neurochemical basis of hyperactivity and aggression induced by social deprivation, in Vulnerabilities to Delinquency. Edited by Lewis DO. New York: Spectrum, 1981, pp 173–186

Schaffer D, Fisher P, Dulcan FM, et al: The NIMH Diagnostic Interview Schedule for Children, Version 2.3: description, acceptability, prevalence rates, and performance in the MECA study. J Am Acad Child Adolesc Psychiatry 35:865–877, 1996

Schonfeld IS, Shaffer D, O'Connor P, et al: Conduct disorder and cognitive functioning: testing three causal hypotheses. Child Dev 59:993–1007, 1988

Siddle DA, Mednick SA, Nicol AR: Skin conductance recovery in antisocial adolescents. Br J Soc Clin Psychol 15:425–428, 1976

Simonoff E: Gene-environment interplay in oppositional defiant and conduct disorder. Child Adolesc Psychiatr Clin N Am 10:351–374, 2001

Singer W: Development and plasticity of cortical processing architectures. Science 270:758–764, 1995

Song L, Singer M, Anglin T: Violence exposure and emotional trauma as contributors to adolescents' violent behaviors. Arch Pediatr Adolesc Med 152:531–536, 1998

Southwick CH: Effect of maternal environment on aggressive behavior of inbred mice. Commun Behav Biol 1:129–132, 1968

Spaccarelli S, Coatsworth JD, Bowden BS: Exposure to serious family violence among incarcerated boys: its association with violent offending and potential mediating variables. Violence Vict 10:163–182, 1995

Sroufe LA, Carlson EB, Levy AK, et al: Implications of attachment theory for developmental psychopathology. Dev Psychopathol 11:1–13, 1999

Steiner H, Garcia I, Matthews Z: Posttraumatic stress disorder in incarcerated juvenile delinquents. J Am Acad Child Adolesc Psychiatry 36:357–365, 1997

Stolk JM, Conner RL, Levine S, et al: Brain norepinephrine metabolism and shock-induced fighting behavior in rats: differential effects of shocks and fighting on the neurochemical response to a foot shock stimulus. J Pharmacol Exp Ther 190:193–209, 1984

Stueve A, Link BG: Violence and psychiatric disorders: results from an epidemiological study of young adults in Israel. Psychiatr Q 68:327–342, 1997

Swanson JW: Mental disorder, substance abuse, and community violence: an epidemiological approach, in Violence and Mental Disorder: Developments in Risk Assessment. Edited by Monahan J, Steadman HJ. Chicago, IL, University of Chicago Press, 1994, pp 101–136

Taylor SP: Alcohol, drugs and human aggressive behavior. Paper presented at the 98th American Psychological Association Convention, Boston, MA, 1990

Tiet QQ, Wasserman GA, Loeber R, et al: Development and sex differences in types of conduct problems. Journal of Child and Family Studies 10:181–197, 2001

Ulzen TP, Hamilton H: The nature and characteristics of psychiatric comorbidity in incarcerated adolescents. Can J Psychiatry 43:57–63, 1998

Unis AS, Cook EH, Vincent JG, et al: Platelet serotonin measures in adolescents with conduct disorder. Biol Psychiatry 42:553–559, 1997

Uzych L: Anabolic-androgenic steroids and psychiatric-related effects: a review. Can J Psychiatry 37:23–28, 1992

Varney NR: Posttraumatic anosmia and orbital frontal injury, in The Evaluation and Treatment of Mild Traumatic Brain Injury. Edited by Varney NR, Roberts RJ. Mahwah, NJ, Lawrence Erlbaum, 1999, pp 115–132

Virkkunen M, Nuutila A: Specific reading retardation, hyperactive child syndrome and juvenile delinquency. Acta Psychiatr Scand 54:25–28, 1976

Virkkunen M, DeJong J, Bartko J, et al: Relationship of psychobiological variables to recidivism in violent offenders and impulsive fire setters: a follow-up study. Arch Gen Psychiatry 46:600–603, 1989

Virkkunen M, Rawlings R, Tokola R, et al: CSF biochemistries, glucose metabolism and diurnal activity rhythms in alcoholic, violent offenders, fire setters, and healthy volunteers. Arch Gen Psychiatry 50:20–27, 1994

Volavka J: Neurobiology of Violence. Washington, DC, American Psychiatric Press, 1995

Werry JS: Pharmacotherapy of disruptive behavior disorders. Child Adolesc Psychiatr Clin N Am 3:321–341, 1994

West DJ: Delinquency: Its Roots, Careers and Prospects. Cambridge, MA, Harvard University Press, 1982

West DJ, Farrington DP: Who Becomes Delinquent? London, Heinemann Educational, 1973

White HR, Xie M, Thompson W, et al: Psychopathology as a predictor of adolescent drug use trajectories. Psychol Addict Behav 15:210–218, 2001

Widom CS: The cycle of violence. Science 244:160–166, 1989

Wilson JQ, Herrnstein RJ: Crime and Human Nature. New York, Simon & Schuster, 1986

Winslow JT, Insel TR: Social status in pairs of male squirrel monkeys determines response to central oxytocin administration. Neuroscience 11:2032–2038, 1991

Wolfgang ME, Figlio RM, Sellin T: Delinquency in a Birth Cohort: Studies in Crime and Justice. Chicago, IL, University of Chicago Press, 1972

World Health Organization: International Classification of Diseases, 9th Revision. Geneva, World Health Organization, 1977

Yeager CA, Lewis DO: Mortality in a group of formerly incarcerated juvenile delinquents. Am J Psychiatry 147:612–614, 1990

Yeager CA, Lewis DO: The intergenerational transmission of violence and dissociation. Child Adolesc Psychiatr Clin N Am 5:393–430, 1996

Zigler E, Taussig C, Black K: Early childhood intervention: a promising preventive for juvenile delinquency. Am Psychol 47:997–1006, 1992

Zoccolillo M: Co-occurrence of conduct disorder and its adult outcomes with depressive and anxiety disorders: a review. J Am Acad Child Adolesc Psychiatry 31:547–556, 1992

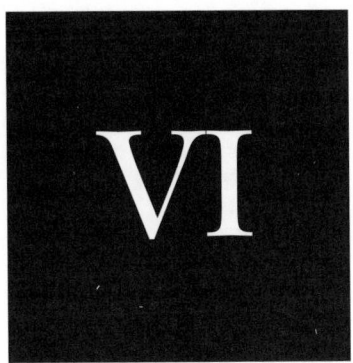

Anxiety Disorders

Separation Anxiety Disorder and Generalized Anxiety Disorder

Gail A. Bernstein, M.D.

Ann E. Layne, Ph.D.

In DSM-IV-TR (American Psychiatric Association 2000), separation anxiety disorder (SAD) is characterized by developmentally inappropriate and excessive anxiety about being apart from the individuals to whom a child is most attached. Frequently, the individual worries excessively that harm may come to either a parent (or attachment figure) or himself or herself, which would result in their separation.

Generalized anxiety disorder (GAD) is characterized by marked worry and anxiety that the individual finds difficult to control. The worry causes impairment in functioning. Before the publication of DSM-IV (American Psychiatric Association 1994), children with excessive worry were diagnosed with overanxious disorder (OAD) rather than GAD. Reasons for the change from OAD to GAD included concern that the criteria for OAD were vague and nonspecific and a recognition that the symptoms overlapped with those of other disorders, including social phobia (Beidel 1991; Werry 1991). Because the previous research on children with generalized anxiety was done using DSM-III-R criteria for OAD, some data on OAD are included in this chapter.

Diagnostic Criteria

Separation anxiety is a normative part of development, typically beginning around 6 or 7 months, peaking around 18 months, and decreasing after 30 months.

Features of separation anxiety may persist into childhood and early adolescence while remaining subclinical in nature. In a study of 62 children without any psychiatric diagnoses, isolated subclinical SAD symptoms were reasonably common (Bell-Dolan et al. 1990). For example, fear of harm to attachment figures was present at a subclinical level in 16.1% of the sample, and fear of harm to self was endorsed at a subclinical level in 9.7% of the sample. Each of these symptoms was present at a clinical level in 1.6% of the sample. However, when separation anxiety develops outside these normative parameters, is persistent and excessive, and is associated with significant distress or impairment, a diagnosis of SAD should be considered. The child must have three of the eight symptoms listed in Table 29–1 to meet DSM-IV-TR diagnostic criteria. The individual must have the symptoms for at least 4 weeks and an onset before age 18 years.

Worry, like separation anxiety, can also be a normative part of development. Muris et. al. (1998) found that 69% of children and adolescents worry every now and then. Unlike normative worry, GAD is characterized by excessive and uncontrollable worry that results in significant impairment or distress. In addition, the worry is associated with feelings of restlessness, fatigability, difficulty concentrating, irritability, muscle tension, and sleep disturbance. Three of these six symptoms are required for adults; only one is needed in children. Symptoms must be present for at least 6 months. DSM-IV-TR diagnostic criteria for GAD are presented in Table 29–2.

Table 29–1. DSM-IV-TR criteria for separation anxiety disorder

A. Developmentally inappropriate and excessive anxiety concerning separation from home or from those to whom the individual is attached, as evidenced by three (or more) of the following:

    (1) recurrent excessive distress when separation from home or major attachment figures occurs or is anticipated

    (2) persistent and excessive worry about losing, or about possible harm befalling, major attachment figures

    (3) persistent and excessive worry that an untoward event will lead to separation from a major attachment figure (e.g., getting lost or being kidnapped)

    (4) persistent reluctance or refusal to go to school or elsewhere because of fear of separation

    (5) persistently and excessively fearful or reluctant to be alone or without major attachment figures at home or without significant adults in other settings

    (6) persistent reluctance or refusal to go to sleep without being near a major attachment figure or to sleep away from home

    (7) repeated nightmares involving the theme of separation

    (8) repeated complaints of physical symptoms (such as headaches, stomachaches, nausea, or vomiting) when separation from major attachment figures occurs or is anticipated

B. The duration of the disturbance is at least 4 weeks.

C. The onset is before age 18 years.

D. The disturbance causes clinically significant distress or impairment in social, academic (occupational), or other important areas of functioning.

E. The disturbance does not occur exclusively during the course of a pervasive developmental disorder, schizophrenia, or other psychotic disorder and, in adolescents and adults, is not better accounted for by panic disorder with agoraphobia.

Specify if:

    Early Onset: if onset occurs before age 6 years

Source.   Reprinted from American Psychiatric Association: *Diagnostic and Statistical Manual of Mental Disorders,* 4th Edition, Text Revision. Washington, DC, American Psychiatric Association, 2000. Copyright 2000, American Psychiatric Association. Used with permission.

Clinical Findings

■ Separation Anxiety Disorder

In SAD, there is an overwhelming fear of losing or becoming separated from a parent. Typically, the child fears that separation or loss will occur as the result of a catastrophic event such as death, kidnapping, or serious accident (Albano et al. 1996). Frequently the manifestations of the underlying fear of separation include the reluctance to be apart or nightmares about separation. Thus, children with SAD display a range of avoidance behaviors from procrastination during the morning routine before school to refusing to leave the side of their parent (e.g., refusing to attend school or to sleep alone). Individuals with SAD often have multiple somatic complaints (e.g., stomachaches, headaches). These complaints can be the result of anxiety or can be designed to support the individual's avoidance of separation (e.g., complaining of a stomachache so that he or she can stay home from school).

SAD can interfere with normative development in a number of ways. Children and adolescents with SAD often have difficulty attending school, participating in extracurricular activities, and attending sleepovers. As a result, academic achievement, peer relationships, and overall maturation are often compromised. School refusal, although not a separate DSM-IV-TR diagnosis, is a childhood symptom commonly presumed to be the behavioral manifestation of SAD. However, "not all children with school refusal or fear of school suffer from SAD, and not all children with SAD manifest school refusal" (Black 1995, p. 217). School refusal can be associated with many different diagnoses, including SAD, specific phobia of school, and depression.

The prevalence of SAD decreases with increasing age (Anderson et al. 1987; McGee et al. 1990). In a recent study of community (*n*=2,384) and clinical (*n*=217) samples, Compton and colleagues (2000) found that preadolescents were significantly more likely than adolescents to endorse symptoms of separation anxiety on the Multidimensional Anxiety Scale for Children (March et al. 1997). Results also indicated that females were more likely to endorse symptoms of

Table 29–2. DSM-IV-TR criteria for generalized anxiety disorder

A. Excessive anxiety and worry (apprehensive expectation), occurring more days than not for at least 6 months, about a number of events or activities (such as work or school performance).

B. The person finds it difficult to control the worry.

C. The anxiety and worry are associated with three (or more) of the following six symptoms (with at least some symptoms present for more days than not for the past 6 months).   **Note:** Only one item is required in children.

  (1) restlessness or feeling keyed up or on edge

  (2) being easily fatigued

  (3) difficulty concentrating or mind going blank

  (4) irritability

  (5) muscle tension

  (6) sleep disturbance (difficulty falling or staying asleep, or restless unsatisfying sleep)

D. The focus of the anxiety and worry is not confined to features of an Axis I disorder, e.g., the anxiety or worry is not about having a panic attack (as in panic disorder), being embarrassed in public (as in social phobia), being contaminated (as in obsessive-compulsive disorder), being away from home or close relatives (as in separation anxiety disorder), gaining weight (as in anorexia nervosa), having multiple physical complaints (as in somatization disorder), or having a serious illness (as in hypochondriasis), and the anxiety and worry do not occur exclusively during posttraumatic stress disorder.

E. The anxiety, worry, or physical symptoms cause clinically significant distress or impairment in social, occupational, or other important areas of functioning.

F. The disturbance is not due to the direct physiological effects of a substance (e.g., a drug of abuse, a medication) or a general medical condition (e.g., hyperthyroidism) and does not occur exclusively during a mood disorder, a psychotic disorder, or a pervasive developmental disorder.

Source. Reprinted from American Psychiatric Association: *Diagnostic and Statistical Manual of Mental Disorders,* 4th Edition, Text Revision. Washington, DC, American Psychiatric Association, 2000. Copyright 2000, American Psychiatric Association. Used with permission.

separation anxiety than were males. Sociodemographic assessment of a large clinic sample (*N*=188) of children with anxiety disorders showed that those with SAD had the earliest age at onset (7.5 years) and the earliest age at intake (10.3 years) (Last et al. 1992). The gender ratio of those with SAD was approximately equal. Children with SAD were more likely to be from single-parent homes than were children with other anxiety disorders.

■ Generalized Anxiety Disorder

The primary symptom of GAD is excessive worry for at least 6 months. Children with GAD worry a great deal about things such as future events, peer relationships, social acceptability, competency, and pleasing others. Unlike children with social phobia, SAD, or specific phobia, children with GAD have numerous and diffuse worries that are not limited to a specific stimulus or environment. They are often described by their parents as "worry warts" and as overly conscientious. Children with GAD tend to overestimate the likelihood of negative consequences, predict catastrophic outcomes for future events, and underestimate their ability to cope

with unfavorable situations (Albano et al. 1996).

As mentioned above, worry and anxiety can be a normative part of development and are experienced throughout life. Fears, worries, and scary dreams are common in healthy children, occurring at rates of 76%, 68%, 81%, respectively (*N*=190) (Muris et al. 2000). Normative anxiety in children without an anxiety diagnosis can be differentiated from worry associated with GAD on a number of levels. Muris and colleagues (1998) compared patterns of worry associated with OAD and GAD with patterns of worry in children and adolescents not meeting criteria for an anxiety disorder. Results indicated that children with OAD or GAD reported, on average, six specific worries whereas control children identified, on average, one topic of worry. Children with OAD or GAD endorsed a higher frequency of their main worry, stronger interference associated with their worry, more anxiety linked to their worry, and increased difficulty controlling their worry. Although 31% of the control children reported that their worry had some positive aspects, none of the children with OAD or GAD identified their worry as having positive aspects. Finally, children with OAD or GAD less frequently engaged in activities that distracted them from their worried thoughts and more frequently discussed their worries with others.

Masi and colleagues (1999) investigated the symptoms most commonly associated with GAD in 58 children and adolescents. Results indicated that feelings of tension (98%), apprehension (95%), the need for reassurance (83%), irritability (81%), negative self-image (74%), and physical complaints (72%) were the most common symptoms co-occurring with GAD. Less common symptoms included psychomotor agitation (31%), fear of sleeping alone (34%), and fear of being alone (36%).

A number of studies have demonstrated that girls tend to worry more and have more numerous worries than boys (e.g., Muris et al. 1998; Silverman et al. 1995). Therefore, it is not surprising that higher prevalence rates for GAD have been reported for females (9%) than for males (3.8%) (N=193) (Muris et al. 1998). Among those diagnosed with GAD, the total number of symptoms associated with GAD did not differ based on age or gender (Masi et al. 1999). However, some symptoms were more common in different age groups. Brooding (i.e., ruminating) was found to be significantly more common in adolescents, whereas the need for reassurance was more common in children.

Comorbidity

Children and adolescents with anxiety disorders often present with comorbid disorders. In a recent study of children and adolescents ages 7–18 with GAD, only 13% had GAD as a unique disorder (Masi et al. 1999). More than half of the sample had a comorbid depressive disorder (62%). SAD was commonly comorbid among the child participants (42%) but was less common among adolescents (10%). Twenty-nine percent of the sample had comorbid specific phobia and 10% had comorbid obsessive-compulsive disorder. Comorbid externalizing disorders were present in 9%. Another study showed that attention-deficit/hyperactivity disorder was present in 25%–30% of children with anxiety disorders (Biederman et al. 1991). In addition, children with anxiety disorders are at risk for developing alcohol abuse in adolescence (Manassis and Monga 2001).

A poorer prognosis has been found in children with anxiety disorders and comorbid behavioral problems (Manassis and Hood 1998), comorbid depression (Last et al. 1997; Masi et al. 1999), and comorbid anxiety disorders (Woodward and Fergusson 2001) than in children with anxiety disorders without comorbid disorders. Manassis and Hood (1998) found that of a number of significant predictors (child depression, maternal phobic anxiety, developmental problems, and psychosocial adversity), maternal reporting of child conduct problems was most predictive of functional impairment in children with a primary anxiety disorder. Woodward and Fergusson (2001) conducted a 21-year longitudinal study of 1,265 New Zealand children. They found that among those with anxiety disorders there existed a significant association between a greater number of anxiety disorders reported in adolescence and later risks of additional anxiety disorders, major depression, illicit drug dependence, and failure to attend college. Finally, studies have reported that children and adolescents with comorbid anxiety and depressive disorders present with greater symptom severity (Bernstein 1991; Last et al. 1996), have a poorer response to treatment (Berman et al. 2000; Brent et al. 1998; Clarke et al. 1992), and have more anxiety disorders (Masi et al. 1999).

Kendall and colleagues (2001) investigated the relationship between comorbidity in childhood anxiety disorders and treatment outcome. In their sample, 79% of children with a primary diagnosis of an anxiety disorder had at least one comorbid diagnosis. Because only 4% of the sample had comorbid depression, those participants were not included in the group analysis. The most frequent comorbid diagnoses were simple phobia (46%), social phobia (34%), and GAD (29%). The study found that participants with comorbid diagnoses displayed more severe internalizing symptoms than participants with only a single anxiety disorder. However, the results of the treatment outcome indicated that comorbid diagnoses (i.e., anxiety and externalizing behavior disorders) did not affect treatment outcome; children with comorbid diagnoses at pretreatment were not significantly less likely to respond to treatment, as evidenced by remission of the primary diagnoses.

Differential Diagnosis

Because anxiety disorders share some common features, to make accurate diagnoses the primary focus of the anxiety must be carefully delineated. In GAD, the anxiety is generalized and is not specifically focused on separation (as in SAD) and not specifically focused on social situations (as in social phobia). In panic disorder, the anxiety is focused on the fear of having a panic attack rather than on actually being separated from parental figures (as in SAD) and is not diffuse (as in GAD). Furthermore, whereas children with SAD and GAD may become extremely anxious and have accompanying sympathetic arousal (i.e., sweating, shaking, racing heart) when faced with separation or a focus of their worry (e.g., taking a test), panic attacks associated with panic disorder are most often out of the blue and in situations in which escape would be difficult. In obsessive-compulsive disorder, the child has specific, recurrent, intrusive thoughts that he or she attempts to ignore or neutralize with another thought or action. Although children with GAD describe their worry as difficult to control and may be ruminative, these worries can be differentiated from obsessions related to obsessive-compulsive disorder based on the content of the worry (i.e., they are usually related to daily stressors rather than a specific domain such as contamination) and because of the absence of rituals. All the symptoms of an adjustment disorder with anxiety would be related to the onset of a *specific* psychosocial stressor and occur within 3 months of the onset of the stressor. After the stressor remits, the anxiety symptoms in an adjustment disorder do not continue for longer than 6 months.

Epidemiology

The Great Smoky Mountains Study sampled 4,500 children ages 9, 11, and 13 years and produced the following 3-month prevalence rates for SAD and GAD: females with SAD, 4.3%; males with SAD, 2.7%; total with SAD, 3.5%; females with GAD, 2.4%; males with GAD, 1%; and total with GAD, 1.7% (Costello et al. 1996). Higher rates for GAD in a sample of 8- to 13-year-olds were reported by Muris et al. (1998), with 3.8% of males and 9% of females meeting criteria for GAD. A similar rate for SAD (3.6%) was recently reported based on children ages 5–9 ($N=1,886$) presenting in pediatric care settings (Briggs-Gowan et al. 2000).

Rates of SAD and GAD vary by age, with SAD being more prevalent among younger children and OAD/ GAD being more prevalent among older children and adolescents (Last et al. 1987; Masi et al. 1999). Although rates of SAD decrease with age, rates of OAD/ GAD increase with age (Anderson et al. 1987; McGee et al. 1990). Westenberg and colleagues (1999) found that participants with SAD (mean age, 10.3) were significantly younger than those with OAD (mean age, 14.5). Interestingly, the results indicate that the difference in prevalence could be attributed to differences in psychosocial maturity. The study found that level of ego development was the strongest predictor of having either SAD or OAD and that adding age, gender, IQ, or socioeconomic status did not improve the regression equation. The results also indicated that even within the same age cohort, the presence of SAD or OAD could be attributed to psychosocial maturity. These findings suggest that changes in the prevalence rates associated with SAD and OAD may represent changes in developmental maturity rather than age.

Etiology

The development of anxiety disorders in children is the result of interactions between a variety of factors, including genetics, child characteristics, and environment. There are generally five domains recognized as being the most significant for consideration in the etiology of childhood anxiety disorders: genetics/temperament, attachment to caregivers, parental anxiety, parenting style, and life experiences (e.g., traumatic events, negative experiences).

■ Temperament

Temperament of the child is an important factor in the development of anxiety symptoms in children and adolescents. It has been found that approximately 20% of healthy infants are born with temperamental traits that predispose them to being highly reactive in novel or unfamiliar situations (Kagan and Snidman 1999). It appears that the crying and vigorous motor activity seen in highly reactive infants may be continuous with shy and fearful reactions in toddlers and with cautious, introverted, and avoidant behavior in school-age children in response to new situations (Kagan 1994; Kagan and Snidman 1999). The opposite of shy, inhibited, introverted children are those who are sociable, uninhibited, outgoing, extroverted, or fearless in response to unfamiliar people, objects, or events (Rosenbaum et al. 1988). Kagan (1994) described the temperamental characteristic of behavioral inhibition as a child's tendency to approach unfamiliar or novel situations with distress, restraint, and avoidance. Behavioral inhibition has been measured in the laboratory beginning at age 9 months (Kagan 1994). This area of study is of interest because temperament characteristics, such as behavioral inhibition, are thought to have a genetic basis (Daniels and Plomin 1985; Goldsmith 1983; Robinson et al. 1992).

Two independent samples of children identified as being either behaviorally inhibited or uninhibited at 21 or 31 months have been studied prospectively by Kagan and colleagues (1988). It was found that the tendency to approach or avoid new situations is often an enduring temperamental trait. Children with behavioral inhibition are differentiated from those without behavioral inhibition based on neurophysiological markers, including increased, less variable heart rates; elevated urinary catecholamine levels; increased salivary cortisol levels; and increased tension in the larynx and vocal cords (Kagan et al. 1988).

A 3-year follow-up study of children with behavioral inhibition showed increased rates of avoidant disorder, SAD, agoraphobia, and two or more anxiety disorders per child (Biederman et al. 1993). Subsequently it was found that behavioral inhibition was linked specifically to an increased risk of social phobia in adolescence, with about one-third of the inhibited toddlers showing symptoms of social phobia as adolescents (Kagan and Snidman 1999). In a review by Biederman and colleagues (1995), it was emphasized that the increased risk for anxiety disorders was primarily in children with a history of persistent shyness and inhibition from 21 months to 7.5 years. Furthermore, risk for developing anxiety disorders was greater if the parents had anxiety disorders (Biederman et al. 1995).

A large community sample of children in Australia ($N=2,443$) was studied from infancy to adolescence to evaluate the role of shy-inhibited temperament in the development of anxiety disorders (Prior et al. 2000). Children were assessed every 18 months with parent, teacher, and self-report ratings from questionnaires based on the models of temperament developed by Thomas and Chess (1977). No observational data were obtained. Logistic regression analyses showed that shy temperament was associated with increased risk of later anxiety symptoms, especially at ages 9–10 years and 12–13 years. Children who were rated as shy at multiple time points were at greater risk for anxiety symptoms compared with children who were described as never shy or only occasionally rated as shy. Highly reactive temperament, in combination with shy temperament, did not confer additional risk for developing anxiety symptoms. It is also important to note that many very shy children did not develop anxiety problems.

■ Attachment

An insecure attachment pattern between mother and child appears to be another factor contributing to the development of childhood anxiety disorders. Attachment theory suggests that a tendency toward anxiety can be exacerbated or alleviated in the context of the child's interactions with primary attachment figures (Manassis and Bradley 1994). A study evaluated attachment patterns of 18 mothers with anxiety disorders and their 20 preschool children (Manassis et al. 1994). All mothers were classified as insecure in their current and past relationships. Similarly, 80% of the preschoolers were identified as having insecure attachments with their mothers. Of the 3 children with a diagnosis of an anxiety disorder (2 with SAD and 1 with avoidant disorder), all were classified as insecurely attached.

Infants with anxious-resistant attachment (i.e., type of insecure attachment) are at risk for anxiety disorders in childhood and adolescence compared with securely attached infants (Warren et al. 1997). In the longitudinal study by Warren et al. (1997), beginning in the third trimester of pregnancy, mothers and their offspring were studied prospectively. At 12 months, attachment was assessed with Ainsworth's Strange Situation Procedure, and at age 17.5 years anxiety disorders were evaluated with a semistructured psychiatric interview. It was found that anxious-resistant attachment significantly predicted anxiety disorders in adolescence. In the regression analyses, this finding accounted for a larger percentage of the variance than the role of maternal anxiety and the role of the child's temperament in predicting the later onset of anxiety disorders.

■ Parental Anxiety

It has long been recognized that children of parents with anxiety disorders are at greater risk for developing anxiety disorders themselves (Turner et al. 1987; Weissman et al. 1984). Biederman and colleagues (2001) reported that children of parents with major depression or panic disorder were at increased risk for developing SAD. In a study of children with anxiety-based school refusal, Martin and colleagues (1999) found that 81% of the parents had a history of psychiatric illness, with anxiety and depressive disorders being most common. Merikangas and colleagues (1998) examined psychopathology among offspring (ages 7–18) of parents with substance abuse or anxiety disorders. Results indicated that maternal anxiety disorders were significantly associated with anxiety disorders among offspring. The study showed that there was a twofold increased risk of anxiety disorders among offspring of parents with anxiety disorders compared with offspring of substance abusers or control subjects. SAD and GAD/OAD were the most common diagnoses, both occurring in 12% of the children of parents with anxiety disorders. Beidel and Turner (1997) examined the risk for anxiety among children of a parent with an anxiety disorder ($n=28$), major depressive disorder ($n=24$), comorbid anxiety and depressive disorders ($n=29$), and children of psychiatrically healthy control subjects ($n=48$). Anxiety disorders were significantly more common among children of parents with anxiety or depression (33%). The offspring of parents with anxiety disorders primarily had anxiety disorders, whereas the offspring of parents with depression and both anxiety and depression had many different disorders. Merikangas and colleagues (1999) found that children with one parent with an anxiety disorder had a threefold increased risk of OAD and an additional threefold risk when both parents had an anxiety disorder. Donovan and Spence (2000) state that parental anxiety is a risk factor that is not independently causal but is mediated or moderated through another mechanism (e.g., parenting style).

■ Parenting Style

In the domain of parenting style, two main factors have emerged as most relevant to the development of anxiety disorders: parental warmth/rejection and parental control (Rapee 1997). Parental warmth/rejection is conceptualized as the degrees of positive (warm) versus negative (hostile) feelings the parent has toward the child. Parental control refers to the degree to which parental behaviors are designed to protect the child from possible harm. Siqueland and colleagues (1996) observed 17 families of children with SAD and OAD (and 27 control families) during discussion of issues of disagreement. The parents of children

with anxiety disorders were rated by the independent observers as less granting of autonomy than the parents of control children, and children with anxiety disorders rated their mothers and fathers as significantly less accepting than did control children.

Similar results were found by Hudson and Rapee (2001) in an observational study in which children were asked to complete two difficult cognitive tasks while their mothers were told to sit nearby and provide support. The study found that mothers of anxious children were more involved, more intrusive, and more negative than mothers of control children. In discussing ambiguous hypothetical situations, parents of anxious children have also been significantly more likely to agree with and encourage their child's avoidance than were parents of control or aggressive children (Dadds et al. 1996). In addition to research on children with anxiety disorders, Muris and colleagues (1998) found anxious parenting style and parental control to be significantly correlated with GAD and SAD symptomatology occurring in a population of psychiatrically healthy school children. Based on a review of the literature, Rapee (1997) comments that excessive parental control and overprotection may suggest to the child that the world is a dangerous place and may interfere with the child's ability to learn otherwise.

■ Life Experiences

Anxiety in children can be related to exposure to negative life events (Dadds and Barrett 2001). Furthermore, these events need not be traumatic to play a role in the development of anxiety disorders. In a study of the development of worries and fears in healthy children, Muris and colleagues (2000) found that 54% of children attributed the origin of their main worry to a conditioning experience (e.g., the death of a grandmother), 33% reported an information pathway (e.g., the evening news), and 13% reported a modeling experience (e.g., seeing parents worried). The authors concluded that these experiences contribute to common anxiety phenomena in children. However, Muris and colleagues (1998) reported that threatening or aversive life events were *not* critical in the development of worry in children with OAD/GAD. They reported that only 7.7% of children with GAD/OAD recalled their worry as being related to a negative conditioning experience.

Poulton and colleagues (2001) conducted a longitudinal study of the relationship between separation experiences and the development of separation anxiety at ages 3, 11, and 18 years. The results failed to provide strong evidence for a relationship between environmental events (e.g., separation experiences) and separation anxiety at any of the ages. The variable most strongly related to separation anxiety in 11-year-old children was mother's fear of going out alone. The results regarding the development of GAD and SAD are consistent with the following conclusion: "On their own, stressful life events do not provide a full explanation for the development of anxiety disorders" (Dadds and Barrett 2001, p. 1001).

Manassis and Bradley (1994) presented an integrated model for the development of childhood anxiety disorders. In this model, temperament, attachment, social systems (e.g., access to other family members, peers, and community support systems) and the interplay between them are incorporated as important factors contributing to anxiety disorders. The literature reviewed in this chapter supports the notion that temperament, attachment, parental anxiety, and parenting style all play a part in the development of anxiety in children and adolescents.

Treatment

A complete diagnostic assessment of the child with an anxiety disorder would include interviewing the child and parents, both individually and together, and considering whether other important adults and siblings in the child's life should also be included. Reports from the school, previous or current psychotherapists, and the pediatrician may be important. In addition to collecting a complete description of the current symptoms, the clinician should review the developmental, medical, and family psychiatric history. It is important to conduct an assessment of the family to evaluate possible problems such as family discord, marital difficulties, difficulties of an individual family member, inappropriate roles or boundaries, and emotional or physical abuse. In general, a multimodal approach is often designed to integrate psychosocial and psychopharmacological treatments for the child (Bernstein and Shaw 1993).

■ Psychopharmacological

Several classes of psychopharmacological medication have been used in the treatment of childhood anxiety disorders (see reviews by Allen et al. 1995; Kutcher et al. 1995, Velosa and Riddle 2000). The first-line choice is a selective serotonin reuptake inhibitor (SSRI), and a second choice is a tricyclic antidepressant (TCA). Benzodiazepines can be considered on a short-term basis, alone or in combination with an SSRI or a TCA while waiting for the SSRI or TCA to reach therapeutic level.

Selective Serotonin Reuptake Inhibitors

The first choice for the pharmacological treatment of SAD or GAD is an SSRI. This approach is supported by open-label (Birmaher et al. 1994, Fairbanks et al. 1997) and controlled studies (Research Unit on Pediatric Psychopharmacology 2001; Rynn et al. 2001) that demonstrate the efficacy and short-term safety of SSRIs for children and adolescents with anxiety disorders.

In an open-label study of fluoxetine, 21 children with SAD, OAD, or social phobia showed improvement while taking the drug (Birmaher et al. 1994). The children had been unresponsive to other psychotherapeutic and psychopharmacological interventions. After a 10-week trial at a mean dosage of 25.7 mg/day, 17 (81%) showed moderate to marked improvement in anxiety symptoms on the Clinical Global Impressions (CGI) scale (Guy 1976). In general, side effects were mild and short-lived. Subsequently, Fairbanks and colleagues (1997) completed a 9-week open-label study of fluoxetine in 16 participants ages 9–18 years with mixed anxiety disorders. Mean dosages were 24 mg of fluoxetine in children and 40 mg in adolescents. On the CGI scale, all participants showed improvement on the drug. Average time to improvement was 5 weeks, and side effects were transient.

Recently three randomized, controlled trials have added solid support to the efficacy of the SSRIs in treating childhood anxiety disorders. A relatively large multicenter treatment study compared fluvoxamine with pill placebo for 128 youths with GAD, SAD, or social phobia (Research Unit on Pediatric Psychopharmacology 2001). All participants had had no response to 3 weeks of psychosocial intervention for their anxiety symptoms before being randomized to 8 weeks of fluvoxamine or placebo. Medication was given in combination with supportive psychotherapy. Primary outcome measures included the Pediatric Anxiety Rating Scale (PARS) (Research Units on Pediatric Psychopharmacology 2002a) and the CGI improvement scale. After 8 weeks, children in the active medication group showed a significant decrease in clinician-rated anxiety on the PARS compared with the placebo group. In addition, 76% (48 of 63) of the fluvoxamine group versus 29% (19 of 65) in the placebo group were rated at or above "improved" on the CGI. The medication was generally well tolerated, with only 5 children receiving fluvoxamine and 1 child receiving placebo discontinuing due to side effects. With respect to specific side effects, significantly more children in the fluvoxamine group reported stomach aches, and more children receiving fluvoxamine experienced increased motor activity.

Rynn and colleagues (2001) studied sertraline in the treatment of 22 children and adolescents with a primary diagnosis of GAD. A 2–3 week assessment period was followed by random assignment to 9 weeks of sertraline (up to 50 mg/day) or placebo. At the end of treatment, youths receiving sertraline showed significant improvement on the Hamilton Anxiety Scale (Hamilton 1959), a clinician rating scale, compared with those taking placebo. Self-report measures also showed significant decreases in anxiety symptoms for participants in the active medication group versus the placebo group. Significant differences in anxiety between conditions were noted initially at 4 weeks. The anxiolytic effect was independent of the antidepressant effect of the medication. Of note, there was minimal response to placebo. Side effects were mild and not substantially different between groups.

In a controlled study of 74 children and adolescents with GAD, SAD, and/or social phobia, participants were randomly assigned to fluoxetine 20 mg/day or placebo (Birmaher et al. 2003). After 12 weeks of treatment, 61% of the children who received fluoxetine versus 35% of those on placebo were rated as much improved or very much improved on the CGI improvement scale. Other outcome measures also supported the benefit of fluoxetine in decreasing anxiety symptoms and enhancing functioning. Side effects of fluoxetine included transient stomachaches and headaches in the first 2 weeks. Abdominal pain was the only adverse effect that was more common throughout the study in the active medication group compared with the placebo group. With these studies, child and adolescent psychiatrists have scientific evidence that SSRIs are beneficial for targeting anxiety symptoms in youth.

A 6-month open-label extension of the Research Units on Pediatric Psychopharmacology fluvoxamine study was recently published (Research Units on Pediatric Psychopharmacology 2002b). Participants who had been treated in the 8-week study were offered the opportunity to enter an open-label phase. Subjects who responded to fluvoxamine were maintained on the same medication; placebo nonresponders were given fluvoxamine; and participants who did not respond to fluvoxamine were changed to fluoxetine. During the open-label treatment, 94% (33 of 35) of the original fluvoxamine responders continued to show low levels of anxiety symptoms. Of those who were switched to fluoxetine, 71% (10 of 14) showed significant improvement in their anxiety symptoms. In the placebo nonresponders, 56% (27 of 48) had a significant improvement in anxiety symptoms with fluvoxamine. Thus, it appears that beneficial response to fluvoxamine in a short-term trial is likely to be maintained with continuation of treatment, that some fluvoxamine nonresponders will respond to a different SSRI (fluoxetine), and that placebo nonresponders have a reasonable likelihood of responding to fluvoxamine.

In a review of studies employing SSRIs in the short-term treatment of children and adolescents with anxiety disorders or major depression, it was suggested that after remission of target symptoms, a drug-free trial should be considered (Pine 2002). It was further recommended that the medication-free trial should occur during the first period of low stress, after a year of SSRI treatment. If a youth relapses during the period without medication, the SSRI should be restarted (Pine 2002).

Tricyclic Antidepressants

Five controlled studies of TCA trials for SAD or school refusal have reported contrasting findings. Gittelman-Klein and Klein (1971, 1973) reported that imipramine, 100–200 mg/day (mean, 159 mg/day), was superior to placebo in a 6-week study of 35 children with SAD. The imipramine group was significantly more successful in returning to school (81% taking imipramine returned to school versus 47% taking placebo). Furthermore, those taking imipramine were rated by mothers, clinicians, and self-report as having a significant decrease in somatic and anxiety symptoms compared with those taking placebo. Berney et al. (1981) reported that low-dose clomipramine (ranging from 40 mg/day for 9-year-olds to 75 mg/day for 15-year-olds) was not superior to placebo in a 12-week double-blind trial for school refusers. The study included 51 anxious children and adolescents; 44% had comorbid depression. A shortcoming of this study was the low dosage of medication, which was probably subtherapeutic.

Bernstein et al. (1990) compared imipramine, alprazolam, and placebo in an 8-week double-blind trial of 24 school refusers (ages 7–17 years). Mean dosages were 164.3 mg/day for imipramine and 1.8 mg/day for alprazolam. Concurrent treatments consisted of individual psychotherapy and returning the child to school. Trends suggested that the active medications were superior to placebo, but it was unclear whether the trends were due to medication effects or baseline difference in severity of symptoms among groups. Klein and colleagues (1992) reported on a 6-week double-blind study of imipramine compared with placebo in 20 children with SAD (ages 6–15 years). All subjects had had no response to a 1-month trial of behavior therapy. The mean dosage of imipramine was 153 mg/day. At the end of the treatment, no differences were found between the imipramine and placebo groups, with 50% in each group showing improvement. Therefore, this study did not replicate the earlier findings of Gittelman-Klein and Klein (1971, 1973).

Bernstein and colleagues (2000) compared 8 weeks of imipramine versus placebo, each in combination with cognitive-behavioral therapy (CBT) for 63 school-refusing teenagers with comorbid anxiety and major depressive disorders. This sample was a severely symptomatic group of school refusers with an average attendance rate of 31% before entering the study. The mean dosage of imipramine at the end of the study was 182.3 mg/day. School attendance improved significantly for the imipramine plus CBT group but not for the placebo plus CBT group. At the end of 8 weeks, the imipramine group was attending 70% of the time and the placebo group was attending only 28% of the time. In addition, the imipramine group showed a faster rate of improvement in clinician-rated symptoms of depression. Overall, the study demonstrated the efficacy of imipramine in combination with CBT for treating anxious and depressed adolescent school refusers. The findings support a multimodal approach in the treatment of severe school refusal in adolescents.

One of these studies supports the use of TCAs to treat SAD with or without school refusal (Gittelman-Klein and Klein 1971, 1973), and another of the studies supports combining a TCA with CBT for anxious-depressed teenagers with severe, refractory symptoms (Bernstein et al. 2000). The other three studies are hampered by either small sample sizes (Bernstein et al. 1990; Klein et al. 1992) or low medication dosage (Berney et al. 1981). Overall, these studies suggest that a TCA may be considered for targeting anxiety symptoms in children and adolescents. However, the first choice is an SSRI due to the low side-effect profile, safety in overdose, and recent controlled clinical trials that demonstrate the efficacy of SSRIs in children with anxiety disorders (Research Unit on Pediatric Psychopharmacology 2001; Rynn et al. 2001).

Benzodiazepines

There are limited data on the efficacy of benzodiazepines in the treatment of GAD or SAD in children and adolescents. The existing studies are limited by small sample sizes and short duration of treatment. In a 4-week double-blind, placebo-controlled study of 30 children with OAD ($n=21$) or avoidant disorder ($n=9$), participants in the alprazolam group (0.5–3.5 mg/day) showed no significant difference on global ratings of improvement compared with the placebo group (Simeon et al. 1992). A double-blind crossover study of 15 children with anxiety disorders (primarily SAD) evaluated 4 weeks of clonazepam (0.5–2.0 mg/day) versus 4 weeks of placebo (Graae et al. 1994). There was no significant difference in improvement between the two treatment conditions.

Benzodiazepines have also been evaluated for use in children before painful procedures. Pfefferbaum et al. (1987) found alprazolam to be safe and effective when used in an open-label trial for anticipatory and acute anxiety in 13 pediatric cancer patients undergoing bone marrow biopsies and lumbar punctures. In a double-blind placebo-controlled study of 55 preschool children, oral midazolam was beneficial in decreasing anxiety during laceration repair in the emergency room (Hennes et al. 1990). Midazolam, a high-potency benzodiazepine with a short duration of action, is available as a parenteral injection solution.

Thus far, side effects of the benzodiazepines in clinical trials with children and adolescents have been minimal (Pfefferbaum et al. 1987; Simeon et al. 1992). Side effects may include sedation, incoordination, slurred speech, and tremor (Kutcher et al. 1992). Behavioral disinhibition has been reported in children and adolescents taking clonazepam (Graae et al. 1994; Reiter and Kutcher 1991). Physical and psychological dependence after long-term use in adults is of substantial concern (Salzman 1989). The risk of tolerance and dependence in children has not been adequately studied (Velosa and Riddle 2000). However, because of the theoretical potential for dependence in youth (Riddle et al. 1999), trials in children and adolescents should be short. Furthermore, it is recommended that physicians avoid prescribing benzodiazepines to children and adolescents with a history of chemical dependence.

Further studies are needed to evaluate the role of benzodiazepines in children with GAD or SAD. One consideration may be using a benzodiazepine in a highly anxious child on a short-term basis, alone or in combination with an SSRI or a TCA while waiting for the antidepressant to reach therapeutic dosage.

■ Cognitive-Behavioral Therapy

Although a number of psychosocial approaches exist for treating anxiety disorders in children (e.g., CBT, psychodynamic psychotherapy, play therapy, supportive therapy), CBT is the only one whose efficacy is supported by data from randomized controlled studies (Labellarte et al. 1999). Barrios and O'Dell (1998) list major groupings of treatment components common to CBT interventions for anxious children: desensitization, prolonged exposure, modeling, contingency management, and self-management/cognitive strategies. In the past 10 years, a number of treatment programs have been developed and evaluated for use in individual, group, and family therapy that include various combinations of these components. The resulting research has demonstrated the superiority of both individual and group CBT to waiting-list control condition (i.e., no treatment) (Flannery-Schroeder and Kendall 2000; Kendall 1994; Kendall et al. 1997).

Kendall (1994) compared a 16-week cognitive-behavioral treatment package with a waiting-list control group for 47 children ages 9–13 years with anxiety disorders. Of the subjects, 30 had a primary diagnosis of OAD, 8 had SAD, and 9 had avoidant disorder; in addition, 32% of the subjects had comorbid depressive disorder. The treatment program used was based on *The Coping Cat* (Kendall 1990). The CBT included cognitive components of recognizing anxious feelings and thoughts, identifying somatic reactions to anxiety, and developing a plan to cope with these symptoms. Behavioral techniques included modeling, exposure, role playing, relaxation training, and reinforcement. At the end of treatment, subjects who received the cognitive-behavioral package showed significant reductions in anxiety and depressive symptoms compared with those on the waiting list. Of the subjects who received the CBT, 64% no longer met criteria for anxiety disorder after the intervention, whereas only 1 participant in the waiting-list condition no longer met criteria after the wait period. Furthermore, at 1-year follow-up and 3-year follow-up, treatment gains were maintained (Kendall and Southam-Gerow 1996).

Kendall and colleagues (1997) conducted a second randomized trial with 94 participants with OAD (*n*=55), SAD (*n*=22), or avoidant disorder (*n*=17). Treatment was the same as that described above. Results indicated that 50% of the treated patients were free of their primary anxiety disorder compared with 6% in the waiting-list control group when evaluated at posttreatment. Furthermore, those who continued to have an anxiety disorder had significant decreases in ratings of severity. Maintenance of treatment gains was demonstrated at 1-year follow-up.

Flannery-Schroeder and Kendall (2000) compared the efficacy of individual CBT and group CBT based on *The Coping Cat* treatment protocol (Kendall 1990) to waiting-list control condition. Treatment consisted of 18 weeks of 50- to 60-minute sessions for the individual treatment (*n*=13) and 18 weeks of 90-minute sessions for the group treatment (*n*=12). Results indicated that after treatment, 73% of children who had received individual CBT and 50% of children who had received group CBT no longer met diagnostic criteria for their primary anxiety disorder, whereas only 8% of children in the waiting-list control group no longer met criteria. Results indicate that the treatment gains associated with individual CBT versus group CBT were not significantly different. Treatment gains were maintained at 3-month follow-up. Berman and colleagues (2000) also reported no significant difference between treatment outcome for anxious children treated with individual versus group CBT.

Silverman and colleagues (1999) conducted a randomized clinical trial (*N*=56) to evaluate the benefits of group CBT versus a waiting-list control condition for treating anxious children. In this study, children and parents met in separate, concurrent groups. Results supported the superiority of group CBT over waiting-list control condition: 64% of children receiving treatment no longer met criteria for their primary diagnosis compared with only 13% of the children in the waiting-list control group.

Studies have also been conducted to evaluate the role of parental involvement in the treatment of child anxiety disorders (e.g., Barrett 1998; Barrett et al. 1996; Cobham et al. 1998; Mendlowitz et al. 1999). Barrett and colleagues (1996) found that significantly more children who participated in a CBT intervention that included a family therapy component were free of their anxiety diagnosis at posttreatment and at 12-month follow-up than children who participated in CBT that did not include parental involvement. However, at 6-year follow-up the superiority of the CBT plus family therapy was no longer present (Barrett et al. 2001). Mendlowitz and colleagues (1999) reported that child-only group CBT, parent-only group CBT, and child-plus-parent group CBT all resulted in a significant decrease in anxiety and depression symptoms. However, children in the child-plus-parent intervention used coping strategies that had been taught in therapy more often than children in the other treatment groups. In addition, parents in the child-plus-parent intervention rated their children as significantly more improved than did parents of children in the other two treatment conditions. Cobham and colleagues (1998) compared the efficacy of child-focused CBT and child-focused CBT plus parental anxiety management for children with anxiety disorders. Results indicated that the parental anxiety management component increased the efficacy of the CBT component only for children with at least one anxious parent.

Dadds and colleagues (1997, 1999) evaluated the potential benefits of prevention and early intervention with children demonstrating symptoms of anxiety. Almost 2,000 Australian children ages 7–14 years were screened for anxiety symptoms in their classrooms. After screening and diagnostic interviewing, 128 children were selected for inclusion. Children selected for inclusion either had subclinical features of an anxiety disorder or met criteria but had low severity ratings. Participants were assigned to either a 10-week child and parent intervention or a monitoring group. After 10 weeks, both groups showed improvement. At 6-month follow-up, the benefit was maintained in the treatment group only, with a decrease in number of baseline anxiety diagnoses and a lower rate of new anxiety disorders. Only 16% of children who received the preventive intervention developed a new anxiety disorder compared with 54% in the monitoring condition. At 2-year follow-up, only the treatment group showed gains with a durable reduction in anxiety symptoms and decreased likelihood of developing new anxiety disorders (Dadds et al. 1999).

CBT for children with anxiety offers clinicians a time-limited and structured approach to treatment. The results to date support the efficacy of CBT for children with anxiety disorders. Both individual CBT and group CBT appear equally efficacious. Findings also suggest that for children with anxiety who also have a parent with anxiety, parental involvement in therapy may improve treatment outcome.

Prognosis

Studies published in the past 10 years have allowed for insight into the course of anxiety disorders over time and the relationship between anxiety disorders in childhood and adolescence and later functioning in adulthood. Last and colleagues (1996) evaluated children with anxiety disorders every 12 months for 3–4 years. The results suggest a "generally favorable course and outcome" for children with anxiety disorders (Last et al. 1996, p. 1508). The vast majority of primary anxiety disorders (82%) had remitted by the end of the follow-up period, with only 8% experiencing relapse after initial remission. SAD and OAD both had high rates of recovery: 96% for SAD and 80% for OAD. Over the course of follow-up, one-third of participants developed new psychiatric disorders. Children with OAD had the highest rate of new disorders during follow-up. The authors concluded that children with OAD are at increased risk for developing additional psychiatric disorders over time. Cohen and colleagues (1993) found that greater severity of OAD symptoms at baseline interview predicted greater likelihood of continuation of the disorder. At follow-up 2.5 years later, OAD was still present in almost half of the patients with severe symptoms at baseline.

Last and colleagues (1997) also conducted an 8-year follow-up study with young adults who had been evaluated as children and adolescents (see Last et al. 1996 sample described above). The participants had a history of either anxiety and depressive disorders, anxiety disorder only, or no psychiatric illness. The results indicated that participants with anxiety disorders were functioning similarly to control subjects with one exception: young adults with a childhood history of an anxiety disorder (without comorbid depression) were less likely than control subjects to be living independently. The outcome was less positive for young adults with a history of anxiety and comorbid depression. These individuals were 1) less likely than control subjects to be employed or in school, 2) more likely than purely anxious participants to utilize mental health services, and 3) more likely than both groups to report psychological problems (e.g., difficulty with depression, anxiety, drugs, or alcohol).

Pine and colleagues (1998) conducted a prospective epidemiological study of 776 children and adolescents with follow-ups 2 and 9 years later. At initial assessment, 111 participants had OAD or GAD; at the 9-year follow-up (*N*=716) only 36 participants met criteria. However, the study found that having OAD/GAD at initial assessment was significantly predictive of having social phobia, major depression, GAD, or panic disorder at the 9-year follow-up. These results are consistent with the finding reported by Last and colleagues (1996) that children with OAD are especially at risk for new disorders over time. The overall findings indicate that most adolescent disorders are no longer present in adulthood; however, most adult disorders are preceded by an internalizing disorder in adolescence.

Compelling questions pertain to which childhood anxiety disorders are the "equivalents" of or precursors to those of adults. It has been suggested that SAD may be a precursor to panic disorder in adulthood. Manicavasagar and colleagues (1998), using adults' retrospective recall of symptoms of SAD in childhood, found that participants with panic disorder with agoraphobia were likely to be associated with high levels of SAD symptomatology in childhood. However, half of adult participants with panic disorder with agoraphobia did not report heightened levels of early separation anxiety. Furthermore, when studied prospectively over time, children with SAD were not significantly more likely to develop panic disorder (Pine et al. 1998). Therefore, additional research is needed to determine whether a significant relationship exists between SAD in childhood and panic disorder in adulthood.

Research Issues

There are solid data supporting the short-term efficacy of CBT (e.g., Kendall et al. 1997) and SSRIs (Birmaher et al. 2003; Research Unit on Pediatric Psychopharmacology 2001; Rynn et al. 2001) for children and adolescents with anxiety disorders. Direct comparison of CBT, SSRI, CBT plus SSRI, and pill placebo is in

progress through the National Institute of Mental Health (i.e., Child/Adolescent Anxiety Multimodal Treatment Study Collaborative Group). In practice, combined treatments are commonly used for children and adolescents with severe impairing anxiety disorders. Therefore, it is important to delineate whether combined treatments provide additional benefit above and beyond CBT alone or medication alone. Analyses of mediators and moderators of treatment response will help identify which participants are more likely to benefit from a multimodal intervention versus single treatment.

Future research should determine the optimal duration of acute psychosocial and pharmacological treatments. In addition, studies should be designed to evaluate the type, duration, and safety of maintenance treatments. For example, studies are needed to assess the duration of SSRI treatment after anxiety symptoms are in remission. With the increasing use of pharmacotherapy, the long-term safety of SSRIs needs to be studied. Assessing the potential benefit of booster sessions for maintenance of CBT efficacy is also an important goal.

Treatment research needs to progress from efficacy to effectiveness treatment trials (National Advisory Mental Health Council 2001). Future research should include study participants from diverse socioeconomic, ethnic, and racial backgrounds and those with comorbid conditions so that the results can be generalizable to the broad population of youths with anxiety disorders. In addition, the evaluation of treatments in community settings such as schools, pediatric offices, or community mental health clinics will be fruitful. This will facilitate later transfer of the study findings and treatment protocols to community practitioners and to children and families in need.

The interaction of temperament, attachment, parental anxiety, and parenting style in contributing to the onset of anxiety disorders is a fertile area of research to pursue. For example, parenting characteristics (e.g., high maternal expressed emotion) may moderate the child's temperament in determining risk for anxiety disorders (Hirshfeld et al. 1997; Spence 2001). Similarly, attachment pattern may interact with temperament in establishing risk for later onset of anxiety (Spence 2001) The examination of the interplay of multiple risk and protective factors will help identify which children will develop anxiety disorders (Kazdin and Kagan 1994).

Another important avenue for research is early intervention. Early identification and intervention for children with subthreshold anxiety symptoms may serve to prevent the onset of full-criteria anxiety disorders, and for children with mild to moderate anxiety disorders it appears to decrease the likelihood of continuing to manifest an anxiety disorder (Dadds et al. 1999). It is likely that early intervention will help to avert negative outcomes associated with untreated anxiety disorders. Longitudinal follow-up of treated and untreated children will support or refute this prediction.

References

Albano AN, Chorpita BF, Barlow DH: Childhood anxiety disorders, in Child Psychopathology. Edited by Mash EJ, Barkley RA. New York, Guilford, 1996, pp 196–241

Allen AJ, Leonard H, Swedo SE: Current knowledge of medications for the treatment of childhood anxiety disorders. J Am Acad Child Adolesc Psychiatry 34:976–986, 1995

American Psychiatric Association: Diagnostic and Statistical Manual of Mental Disorders, 4th Edition. Washington, DC, American Psychiatric Association, 1994

American Psychiatric Association: Diagnostic and Statistical Manual of Mental Disorders, 4th Edition, Text Revision. Washington, DC, American Psychiatric Association, 2000

Anderson JC, Williams S, McGee R, et al: DSM-III disorders in preadolescent children. Arch Gen Psychiatry 44:69–76, 1987

Barrett PM: Evaluation of cognitive-behavioral group treatments for childhood anxiety disorders. J Clin Child Psychol 27:459–468, 1998

Barrett PM, Dadds MR, Rapee RM: Family treatment of childhood anxiety: a controlled trial. J Consult Clin Psychol 64:333–342, 1996

Barrett PM, Duffy AL, Dadds MR, et al: Cognitive-behavioral treatment of anxiety disorders in children: long-term (6-year) follow-up. J Consult Clin Psychol 69:135–141, 2001

Barrios BA, O'Dell SL: Fears and anxieties, in Treatment of Childhood Disorders, 2nd Edition. Edited by Mash EJ, Barkley RA. New York, Guilford, 1998, pp 249–337

Beidel DC: Social phobia and overanxious disorder in school-age children. J Am Acad Child Adolesc Psychiatry 30:545–552, 1991

Beidel DC, Turner SM: At risk for anxiety, I: psychopathology in the offspring of anxious parents. J Am Acad Child Adolesc Psychiatry 36:918–924, 1997

Bell-Dolan DJ, Last CG, Strauss CC: Symptoms of anxiety disorders in normal children. J Am Acad Child Adolesc Psychiatry 29:759–765, 1990

Berman SL, Weems CF, Silverman WK, et al: Predictors of outcome in exposure-based cognitive and behavioral treatments for phobic and anxiety disorders in children. Behav Ther 31:713–731, 2000

Berney T, Kolvin I, Bhate SR, et al: School phobia: a therapeutic trial with clomipramine and short-term outcome. Br J Psychiatry 138:110–118, 1981

Bernstein GA: Comorbidity and severity of anxiety and depressive disorders in a clinic sample. J Am Acad Child Adolesc Psychiatry 30:43–50, 1991

Bernstein GA, Shaw K: Practice parameters for the assessment and treatment of anxiety disorders. American Academy of Child and Adolescent Psychiatry. J Am Acad Child Adolesc Psychiatry 32:1089–1098, 1993

Bernstein GA, Garfinkel BD, Borchardt CM: Comparative studies of pharmacotherapy for school refusal. J Am Acad Child Adolesc Psychiatry 29:773–781, 1990

Bernstein GA, Borchardt CM, Perwien AR, et al: Imipramine plus cognitive-behavioral therapy in the treatment of school refusal. J Am Acad Child Adolesc Psychiatry 39:276–283, 2000

Biederman J, Newcorn J, Sprich S: Comorbidity of attention deficit hyperactivity disorder with conduct, depressive, anxiety, and other disorders. Am J Psychiatry 148:564–577, 1991

Biederman J, Rosenbaum JF, Bolduc-Murphy EA, et al: A 3-year follow-up of children with and without behavioral inhibition. J Am Acad Child Adolesc Psychiatry 32:814–821, 1993

Biederman J, Rosenbaum JF, Chaloff J, et al: Behavioral inhibition as a risk factor for anxiety disorders, in Anxiety Disorders in Children and Adolescents. Edited by March JS. New York, Guilford, 1995, pp 61–81

Biederman J, Faraone SV, Hirshfeld-Becker DR, et al: Patterns of psychopathology and dysfunction in high-risk children of parents with panic disorder and major depression. Am J Psychiatry 158:49–57, 2001

Birmaher B, Waterman GS, Ryan N, et al: Fluoxetine for childhood anxiety disorders. J Am Acad Child Adolesc Psychiatry 33:993–999, 1994

Birmaher B, Axelson DA, Monk K, et al; Fluoxetine for the treatment of childhood anxiety disorders. J Am Acad Child Adolesc Psychiatry 42:415–423, 2003

Black B: Separation anxiety disorder and panic disorder, in Anxiety Disorders in Children and Adolescents. Edited by March JS. New York, Guilford, 1995, pp 212–234

Brent DA, Kolko DJ, Birmaher B, et al: Predictors of treatment efficacy in a clinical trial of three psychosocial treatments for adolescent depression. J Am Acad Child Adolesc Psychiatry 37:906–914, 1998

Briggs-Gowan MJ, Horwitz SM, Schwab-Stone ME, et al: Mental health in pediatric settings: distribution of disorders and factors related to service use. J Am Acad Child Adolesc Psychiatry 39:841–849, 2000

Clarke G, Hops H, Lewinsohn PM: Cognitive-behavioral group treatment of adolescent depression: prediction of outcome. Behav Ther 23:341–354, 1992

Cobham VE, Dadds MR, Spence SH: The role of parental anxiety in the treatment of childhood anxiety. J Consult Clin Psychol 66:893–905, 1998

Cohen P, Cohen J, Brook J: An epidemiological study of disorders in late childhood and adolescence, II: persistence of disorders. J Child Psychol Psychiatry 34:869–877, 1993

Compton SN, Nelson AH, March JS: Social phobia and separation anxiety symptoms in community and clinical samples of children and adolescents. J Am Acad Child Adolesc Psychiatry 39:1040–1046, 2000

Costello EJ, Angold A, Burns BJ, et al: The Great Smoky Mountains study of youth: goals, design, methods, and the prevalence of DSM-III-R disorders. Arch Gen Psychiatry 53:1129–1136, 1996

Dadds MR, Barrett PM: Practitioner review: psychological management of anxiety disorders in childhood. J Child Psychol Psychiatry 42:999–1011, 2001

Dadds MR, Barrett PM, Rapee RM: Family process and child anxiety and aggression: an observational analysis. J Abnorm Child Psychol 24:715–734, 1996

Dadds MR, Spence SH, Holland DE, et al: Prevention and early intervention for anxiety disorders: a controlled trial. J Consul Clin Psychol 65:627–635, 1997

Dadds MR, Holland DE, Spence SH, et al: Early intervention and prevention of anxiety disorders in children: results at 2-year follow-up. J Consult Clin Psychol 67:145–150, 1999

Daniels D, Plomin RL: Origins of individual differences in shyness. Dev Psychol 21:118–121, 1985

Donovan CL, Spence SH: Prevention of childhood anxiety disorders. Clin Psychol Rev 20:509–531, 2000

Fairbanks JM, Pine DS, Tancer NK, et al: Open fluoxetine treatment of mixed anxiety disorders in children and adolescents. J Child Adolesc Psychopharmacol 7:17–29, 1997

Flannery-Schroeder EC, Kendall PC: Group and individual cognitive-behavioral treatments for youth with anxiety disorders: a randomized clinical trial. Cognit Ther Res 24:251–278, 2000

Gittelman-Klein R, Klein DF: Controlled imipramine treatment of school phobia. Arch Gen Psychiatry 25:204–207, 1971

Gittelman-Klein R, Klein DF: School phobia: diagnostic considerations in the light of imipramine effects. J Nerv Ment Dis 156:199–215, 1973

Goldsmith JJ: Genetic influences on personality from infancy to childhood. Child Dev 54:331–355, 1983

Graae F, Milner J, Rizzotto L, et al: Clonazepam in childhood anxiety disorders. J Am Acad Child Adolesc Psychiatry 33:372–376, 1994

Guy W: ECDEU Assessment Manual for Psychopharmacology (DHEW Publ No ADM 76-338). Rockville, MD, National Institute of Mental Health, Psychopharmacology Research Branch, 1976

Hamilton M: The assessment of anxiety states by rating. Br J Med Psychol 32:50–55, 1959

Hennes HM, Wagner V, Bonadio WA, et al: The effect of oral midazolam on anxiety of preschool children during laceration repair. Ann Emerg Med 19:1006–1009, 1990

Hirshfeld DR, Biederman J, Brody L, et al: Associations between expressed emotion and child behavioral inhibition and psychopathology: a pilot study. J Am Acad Child Adolesc Psychiatry 36:205–213, 1997

Hudson JL, Rapee RM: Parent-child interactions and anxiety disorders: an observational study. Behav Res Ther 39:1411–1427, 2001

Kagan J: Galen's Prophecy. New York, Basic Books, 1994

Kagan J, Reznick JS, Snidman N: Biological bases of childhood shyness. Science 240:167–171, 1988

Kagan J, Snidman N: Early childhood predictors of adult anxiety disorders. Biol Psychiatry 46:1536–1541, 1999

Kazdin AE, Kagan J: Models of dysfunction in developmental psychopathology. Clinical Psychology Science and Practice 1:35–52, 1994

Kendall PC: Coping Cat Workbook. Ardmore, PA, Workbook Publishing, 1990

Kendall PC: Treating anxiety disorders in children: results of a randomized clinical trial. J Consult Clin Psychol 62:100–110, 1994

Kendall PC, Southam-Gerow MA: Long-term follow-up of a cognitive-behavioral therapy for anxiety-disordered youth. J Consult Clin Psychol 64:724–730, 1996

Kendall PC, Flannery-Schroeder E, Panichelli-Mindel SM, et al: Therapy for youths with anxiety disorders: a second randomized clinical trial. J Consult Clin Psychol 65:366–380, 1997

Kendall PC, Brady EU, Verduin TL: Comorbidity in childhood anxiety disorders and treatment outcome. J Am Acad Child Adolesc Psychiatry 40:787–794, 2001

Klein RG, Koplewicz HS, Kanner A: Imipramine treatment of children with separation anxiety disorder. J Am Acad Child Adolesc Psychiatry 31:21–28, 1992

Kutcher S, Reiter S, Gardner D: Pharmacotherapy: approaches and applications, in Anxiety Disorders in Children and Adolescents. Edited by March JS. New York, Guilford, 1995, pp 341–385

Kutcher SP, Reiter S, Gardner DM, et al: The pharmacotherapy of anxiety disorders in children and adolescents. Psychiatr Clin North Am 15:41–67, 1992

Labellarte MJ, Ginsburg GS, Walkup JT: The treatment of anxiety disorders in children and adolescents. Biol Psychiatry 46:1567–1578, 1999

Last CG, Hersen M, Kazdin AE, et al: Comparison of DSM-III separation anxiety and overanxious disorders: demographic characteristics and patterns of comorbidity. J Am Acad Child Adolesc Psychiatry 26:527–531, 1987

Last CG, Perrin S, Hersen M, et al: DSM-III-R anxiety disorders in children: sociodemographic and clinical characteristics. J Am Acad Child Adolesc Psychiatry 31:1070–1076, 1992

Last CG, Perrin S, Hersen M, et al: A prospective study of childhood anxiety disorders. J Am Acad Child Adolesc Psychiatry 35:1502–1510, 1996

Last CG, Hansen C, Franco N: Anxious children in adulthood: a prospective study of adjustment. J Am Acad Child Adolesc Psychiatry 36:645–652, 1997

Manassis K, Bradley S: The development of childhood anxiety disorders: toward an integrated model. J Appl Dev Psychol 15:345–366, 1994

Manassis K, Hood J: Individual and familial predictors of impairment in childhood anxiety disorders. J Am Acad Child Adolesc Psychiatry 37:428–434, 1998

Manassis K, Monga S: A therapeutic approach to children and adolescents with anxiety disorders and associated comorbid conditions. J Am Acad Child Adolesc Psychiatry 40:115–117, 2001

Manassis K, Bradley S, Goldberg S, et al: Attachment in mothers with anxiety disorders and their children. J Am Acad Child Adolesc Psychiatry 33:1106–1113, 1994

Manicavasagar V, Silove D, Hadzi-Pavlovic D: Subpopulations of early separation anxiety: relevance to risk of adult anxiety disorders. J Affect Disord 48:181–190, 1998

March JS, Parker JDA, Sullivan K: The Multidimensional Anxiety Scale for Children (MASC): factor structure, reliability, and validity. J Am Acad Child Adolesc Psychiatry 36:554–565, 1997

Martin C, Cabrol S, Bouvard MP, et al: Anxiety and depressive disorders in fathers and mothers of anxious school-refusing children. J Am Acad Child Adolesc Psychiatry 38:916–922, 1999

Masi G, Mucci M, Favilla L, et al: Symptomatology and comorbidity of generalized anxiety disorder in children and adolescents. Compr Psychiatry 40:210–215, 1999

McGee R, Feehan M, Williams S, et al: DSM-III disorders in a large sample of adolescents. J Am Acad Child Adolesc Psychiatry 29:611–619, 1990

Mendlowitz SL, Manassis K, Bradley S, et al: Cognitive-behavioral group treatments in childhood anxiety disorders: the role of parental involvement. J Am Acad Child Adolesc Psychiatry 38:1223–1229, 1999

Merikangas KR, Dierker LC, Szatmari P: Psychopathology among offspring of parents with substance abuse and/or anxiety disorders: a high-risk study. J Child Psychol Psychiatry 39:711–720, 1998

Merikangas KR, Avenevoli S, Dierker L, et al: Vulnerability factors among children at risk for anxiety disorders. Biol Psychiatry 46:1523–1535, 1999

Muris P, Meesters C, Merckelbach H, et al: Worry in normal children. J Am Acad Child Adolesc Psychiatry 37:703–720, 1998

Muris P, Merckelbach H, Gadet B, et al: Fears, worries, and scary dreams in 4- to 12-year-old children: their content, developmental pattern, and origins. J Clin Child Psychol 29:43–52, 2000

National Advisory Mental Health Council Workgroup on Child and Adolescent Mental Health Intervention Development and Deployment: Blueprint for Change: Research on Child and Adolescent Mental Health. Washington DC, National Institute of Mental Health, 2001

Pfefferbaum B, Overall JE, Boren HA, et al: Alprazolam in the treatment of anticipatory and acute situational anxiety in children with cancer. J Am Acad Child Adolesc Psychiatry 26:532–535, 1987

Pine DS: Treating children and adolescents with selective serotonin reuptake inhibitors: how long is appropriate? J Child Adolesc Psychopharmacol 12:189–203, 2002

Pine DS, Cohen P, Gurley D, et al: The risk for early adulthood anxiety and depressive disorders in adolescents with anxiety and depressive disorders. Arch Gen Psychiatry 55:56–64, 1998

Poulton R, Milne BJ, Craske MG, et al: A longitudinal study of the etiology of separation anxiety. Behav Res Ther 39:1395–1410, 2001

Prior M, Smart D, Sanson A, et al: Does shy-inhibited temperament in childhood lead to anxiety problems in adolescence? J Am Acad Child Adolesc Psychiatry 39:461–468, 2000

Rapee RM: Potential role of childrearing practices in the development of anxiety and depression. Clin Psychol Rev 17:47–67, 1997

Reiter S, Kutcher S: Disinhibition and anger outbursts in adolescents treated with clonazepam (letter). J Clin Psychopharmacol 11:268, 1991

Research Unit on Pediatric Psychopharmacology Anxiety Study Group: Fluvoxamine for the treatment of anxiety disorders in children and adolescents. N Engl J Med 344:1279–1285, 2001

Research Units on Pediatric Psychopharmacology Anxiety Study Group: The Pediatric Anxiety Rating Scale (PARS): development and psychometric properties. J Am Acad Child Adolesc Psychiatry 41:1061–1069, 2002a

Research Units on Pediatric Psychopharmacology Anxiety Study Group: Treatment of pediatric anxiety disorders: an open-label extension of the research units on pediatric psychopharmacology anxiety study. J Child Adolesc Psychopharmacol 12:175–188, 2002b

Riddle MA, Bernstein GA, Cook EH, et al: Anxiolytics, adrenergic agents, and naltrexone. J Am Acad Child Adolesc Psychiatry 38:546–556, 1999

Robinson JL, Kagan J, Reznick JS, et al: The heritability of inhibited and uninhibited behavior: a twin study. Dev Psychol 28:1030–1037, 1992

Rosenbaum JF, Biederman J, Gersten M, et al: Behavioral inhibition in children of parents with panic disorder and agoraphobia. Arch Gen Psychiatry 45:463–470, 1988

Rynn MA, Sigueland L, Rickels K: Placebo-controlled trial of sertraline in the treatment of children with generalized anxiety disorder. Am J Psychiatry 158:2008–2014, 2001

Salzman C: Treatment with antianxiety agents, in Treatments of Psychiatric Disorders: A Task Force Report of the American Psychiatric Association, Vol 3. Washington, DC, American Psychiatric Association, 1989, pp 2036–2052

Silverman WK, La Greca AM, Wasserstein S: What do children worry about? Worries and their relation to anxiety. Child Dev 66:671–686, 1995

Silverman WK, Kurtines WM, Ginsburg GS, et al: Treating anxiety disorders in children with group cognitive-behavioral therapy: a randomized clinical trial. J Consult Clin Psychol 67:995–1003, 1999

Simeon JG, Ferguson HB, Knott V, et al: Clinical, cognitive, and neurophysiological effects of alprazolam in children and adolescents with overanxious and avoidant disorders. J Am Acad Child Adolesc Psychiatry 31:29–33, 1992

Sigueland L, Kendall PC, Steinberg L: Anxiety in children: perceived family environments and observed family interaction. J Clin Child Psychol 25:225–237, 1996

Spence SH: Prevention strategies, in The Developmental Psychopathology of Anxiety. Edited by Vasey M, Dadds MR. New York, Oxford University Press, 2001, pp 325–351

Thomas A, Chess S: Temperament and Development. New York, Brunner/Mazel, 1977

Turner SM, Beidel DC, Costello A: Psychopathology in offspring of anxiety disorders patients. J Consult Clin Psychol 55:229–235, 1987

Velosa JF, Riddle MA: Pharmacologic treatment of anxiety disorders in children and adolescents. Child Adolesc Psychiatr Clin N Am 9:119–133, 2000

Warren SL, Huston L, Egeland B, et al: Child and adolescent anxiety disorders and early attachment. J Am Acad Child Adolesc Psychiatry 36:637–644, 1997

Weissman MM, Leckman JE, Merikangas KR, et al: Depression and anxiety disorders in parents and children: results from the Yale Family Study. Arch Gen Psychiatry 41:845–852, 1984

Werry JS: Overanxious disorder: a review of its taxonomic properties. J Am Acad Child Adolesc Psychiatry 30:533–544, 1991

Westenberg PM, Siebelink BM, Warmenhoven NJC, et al: Separation anxiety and overanxious disorders: relations to age and level of psychosocial maturity. J Am Acad Child Adolesc Psychiatry 38:1000–1007, 1999

Woodward LJ, Fergusson DM: Life course outcomes of young people with anxiety disorders in adolescence. J Am Acad Child Adolesc Psychiatry 40:1086–1093, 2001

Obsessive-Compulsive Disorder

Jennifer B. Freeman, Ph.D.

Abbe M. Garcia, Ph.D.

Susan E. Swedo, M.D.

Judith L. Rapoport, M.D.

Christina M. Fucci, B.A.

Henrietta L. Leonard, M.D.

Obsessive-compulsive disorder (OCD) is characterized in DSM-IV-TR (American Psychiatric Association 2000) by recurrent obsessions or compulsions that are severe enough to cause distress or to interfere in one's life. *Obsessions* are defined as persistent thoughts, images, or impulses that are ego-dystonic, intrusive, and, for the most part, senseless. *Compulsions* are "repetitive behaviors … or mental acts … that the person feels driven to perform in response to an obsession" (American Psychiatric Association 2000, p. 462). A change in the diagnostic criteria from DSM-III-R (American Psychiatric Association 1987) to DSM-IV (American Psychiatric Association 1994) and DSM-IV-TR was that younger children do not always recognize their obsessions and compulsions as being excessive or unreasonable.

Diagnostic Criteria

A person with OCD may have either obsessions or compulsions, or both (Table 30–1). An individual typically attempts to ignore, suppress, or neutralize the intrusive obsessive thoughts. The specific content of the obsession should not be related to another Axis I diagnosis, such as thoughts about food resulting from an eating disorder or guilty thoughts (ruminations) from depression. Generally, compulsions are performed to dispel anxiety or in response to an obses-

sion (e.g., to ward off harm to someone). An adult recognizes that the behavior is excessive or unreasonable, although this may not always hold true for young children. Obsessions and compulsions must be severe enough to "cause marked distress" or to "significantly interfere with the person's normal routine" (American Psychiatric Association 2000, p. 463).

Clinical Findings

In the first report in the literature of childhood OCD, Janet (1903, p. 17) described a 5-year-old's obsessions as an "arduous rethinking of the obvious." He suggested that obsessional thoughts are like "mental tics." In his child psychiatry textbook originally published in 1935, Kanner (1962) reviewed the German literature and reported that children with OCD were raised with an "overdose of parental perfectionism." Berman (1942) reported several cases of OCD in children and commented on their similarity to OCD in adults. Despert's (1955) study of 68 patients with "obsessive-compulsive neurosis" reported that, despite the distress caused by the symptoms, the patients were surprisingly secretive about their obsessions and compulsions. In a thorough description of a series of 49 pediatric patients, Adams (1973) noted the preponderance of boys and, in some cases, a very early age at onset. Interest-

Table 30–1.   DSM-IV-TR diagnostic criteria for obsessive-compulsive disorder

A. Either obsessions or compulsions:

Obsessions as defined by (1), (2), (3), and (4):

    (1) recurrent and persistent thoughts, impulses, or images that are experienced, at some time during the disturbance, as intrusive and inappropriate and that cause marked anxiety or distress

    (2) the thoughts, impulses, or images are not simply excessive worries about real-life problems

    (3) the person attempts to ignore or suppress such thoughts, impulses, or images, or to neutralize them with some other thought or action

    (4) the person recognizes that the obsessional thoughts, impulses, or images are a product of his or her own mind (not imposed from without as in thought insertion)

Compulsions as defined by (1) and (2):

    (1) repetitive behaviors (e.g., hand washing, ordering, checking) or mental acts (e.g., praying, counting, repeating words silently) that the person feels driven to perform in response to an obsession, or according to rules that must be applied rigidly

    (2) the behaviors or mental acts are aimed at preventing or reducing distress or preventing some dreaded event or situation; however, these behaviors or mental acts either are not connected in a realistic way with what they are designed to neutralize or prevent or are clearly excessive

B. At some point during the course of the disorder, the person has recognized that the obsessions or compulsions are excessive or unreasonable.   **Note:** This does not apply to children.

C. The obsessions or compulsions cause marked distress, are time consuming (take more than 1 hour a day), or significantly interfere with the person's normal routine, occupational (or academic) functioning, or usual social activities or relationships.

D. If another Axis I disorder is present, the content of the obsessions or compulsions is not restricted to it (e.g., preoccupation with food in the presence of an eating disorder; hair pulling in the presence of trichotillomania; concern with appearance in the presence of body dysmorphic disorder; preoccupation with drugs in the presence of a substance use disorder; preoccupation with having a serious illness in the presence of hypochondriasis; preoccupation with sexual urges or fantasies in the presence of a paraphilia; or guilty ruminations in the presence of major depressive disorder).

E. The disturbance is not due to the direct physiological effects of a substance (e.g., a drug of abuse, a medication) or a general medical condition.

    Specify if:

        With Poor Insight: if, for most of the time during the current episode, the person does not recognize that the obsessions and compulsions are excessive or unreasonable

Source.   From American Psychiatric Association: *Diagnostic and Statistical Manual of Mental Disorders,* 4th Edition, Text Revision. Washington, DC, American Psychiatric Association, 2000. Copyright 2000, American Psychiatric Association. Used with permission.

ingly, all these early reports described salient features of what is now called OCD. These were the early reports of OCD in children, and it was not until the mid-1980s that OCD was systematically studied in children.

At the National Institute of Mental Health (NIMH), 70 consecutive child and adolescent patients were prospectively examined (Swedo et al. 1989b). These 47 boys and 23 girls met diagnostic criteria for primary severe OCD and had a mean age at onset of 10 years. Seven of the patients had had the onset of their illness before age 7 years. Boys tended to have an earlier (prepubertal) age at onset, around age 9, whereas girls were more likely to have an onset around puberty, such as age 11. The children with early-onset OCD

were more likely to be male and to have a family member with OCD or a tic disorder. Subsequent studies have noted the male predominance in young children (3:2), and in adolescence the gender distribution becomes more equal (Geller et al. 1998).

The clinical presentation of OCD in children is generally similar to that in adults (Hanna 1995; Rapoport 1986). The most commonly reported ritual in the study by Swedo and colleagues (1989b) was excessive cleaning (hand washing, showering, bathing, or tooth brushing), which was experienced at some point by 85% of the patients. Repeating rituals, such as going in and out of doors, getting up and down from chairs, restating phrases, and rereading, were reported by 51%.

Checking behaviors, such as making sure that doors and windows were locked, that appliances were turned off, or that homework was done "right" were reported in 46%. Other common rituals included counting, ordering/arranging, and hoarding. More unusual obsessions included scrupulosity, the preoccupying fear that one might harm oneself or others, and having a tune in the head (Swedo et al. 1989b). Some of the obsessions and rituals involved an internal sense that "it didn't feel right" until the thought or action was completed. For example, a boy might have to retrace his steps from the car into the house in a very elaborate and specific manner (two steps forward, look to the sky, three steps backward, glance to the left, and think a good thought) until it "felt right."

Most patients had both obsessions and compulsions (Swedo et al. 1989b). Some of the younger children acknowledged their ritualistic behaviors but were unable to attribute them to any obsessive thought. In young children, compulsions without obsessions are common (Geller et al. 1998). Although their symptoms still met DSM-IV diagnostic criteria, some of the very young children denied any anxiety or distress in association with their rituals. Children often disguised their rituals until they became so extreme as to be discovered. Interestingly, almost all patients reported that their principal symptom changed over time, and retrospective analysis revealed that most had experienced a wide variety of obsessions and compulsions without any clear pattern of progression (Rettew et al. 1992). Therefore, the specific symptom content (e.g., obsessions versus rituals or washing versus checking) seems unlikely to provide clues into pediatric subgroups of OCD.

The less severely ill patients, and those attempting to hide their symptoms, may be difficult to recognize. Behaviors that suggest a diagnosis of OCD include spending long, unproductive hours doing homework; erasing test papers and homework excessively (until there are holes in the paper); retracing over letters or words; and rereading paragraphs. For example, a child might be unable to complete an assignment because he or she could never get beyond the first question as a result of redoing it many times. A dramatic increase in laundry volume, an insistence on wearing clothes or using a towel only once, or toilets becoming clogged from the use of too much paper may indicate an obsession about germs. Other suspicious behaviors include long, rigid bedtime rituals; an exaggerated need for reassurance; requests for family members to repeat phrases; a preoccupying fear of harm coming to oneself or others; and a persistent fear that one has an illness. Hoarding of useless objects—such as empty juice cans, magazine subscription coupons, or garbage from the street—should be differentiated from normal childhood collecting of rocks, sticks, or sentimental treasures. The reader is referred to the practice parameters of the American Academy of Child and Adolescent Psychiatry (1998) as a general guideline for the assessment of children with OCD. The Children's Yale-Brown Obsessive Compulsive Scale (CY-BOCS) (Scahill et al. 1997b) symptom checklist is a particularly useful tool for detecting baseline symptoms and studying them over time.

Subtypes

Current research focuses on whether early-onset or juvenile OCD is a unique subtype of the disorder. Some proposed subtypes, which are neither necessarily distinct nor mutually exclusive, include early-onset, tic-related, and streptococcal-precipitated OCD. Early-onset OCD was associated with male preponderance, comorbidity with attention-deficit/hyperactivity disorder (ADHD) and other disorders, frequent absence of insight, and increased family loading for OCD (Geller et al. 1998). The ADHD-like symptoms in youths with OCD likely reflect a true comorbid state of OCD with ADHD, and the ADHD syndrome may be independent of OCD in comorbid youths (Geller et al. 2002). Age at onset may help identify meaningful developmental subtypes of the disorder beyond chronological age (Geller et al. 2001a). Patients with onset of OCD before age 9 are more likely to have the familial subtype of OCD and also are likely to have related tic disorders (Pauls et al. 1995). Adult patients with early onset of symptoms (before age 10) had a higher rate of tic-like compulsions and comorbid tic disorders than did adults with onset of OCD after age 17, suggesting that age at onset may be an important factor in subtyping OCD and that the phenotypical differences were not restricted to childhood (Rosario-Campos et al. 2001).

Some have proposed that the combination of OCD and comorbid tics may prove to be a subtype. Patients with OCD and a comorbid tic disorder may be more likely to have compulsions with more sensory phenomena and may need to perform the compulsions until they are "just right" (Leckman et al. 1994).

A subgroup of children with pediatric onset of either OCD or a tic disorder have been described as having pediatric autoimmune neuropsychiatric disorders associated with streptococcal infection (PANDAS). These children have an abrupt onset of symptoms after becoming infected with group A β-hemolytic streptococcus (GABHS), and their course of illness is characterized by dramatic acute worsening of symptoms with periods of remission. These children have a prepubertal onset and have neurological signs (e.g., choreiform movements, tics). Heterogeneity of pediatric OCD has been previously noted, and a large phenomenological study noted that some children have abrupt onset, some have a dramatic and episodic course, and some have coexisting choreiform movements (Swedo et al. 1989b). Only in recent years with parallel studies of neuropsychiatric symptoms in Sydenham's chorea (Allen et al. 1995; Swedo et al. 1989a, 1993, 1994) was this OCD subgroup noted to have onset of symptoms after infection with GABHS (Swedo 1994).

The PANDAS subgroup is defined by five clinical characteristics: 1) the presence of OCD or a tic disorder (or both); 2) prepubertal symptom onset; 3) dramatic onset and acute exacerbations with an episodic course of symptom severity; 4) temporal association between symptom exacerbations and GABHS infections; and 5) associated neurological abnormalities (Swedo et al. 1998). Fifty children meeting these PANDAS criteria were systematically evaluated at the NIMH (Swedo et al. 1998). They had an early onset of symptoms (mean age, 6 years for tics and 7 years for OCD) with a male predominance (2.6:1). Interestingly, half of the children (24) had a primary diagnosis of OCD and half (26) had a primary diagnosis of tic disorder, but 80% (40) had both tics and obsessive-compulsive symptoms. The children with PANDAS had high rates of other comorbid disorders, with 40% (20) having ADHD or oppositional defiant disorder, 36% (18) having major depression, 28% (14) having overanxious disorder, and 20% (10) having separation anxiety. The ADHD and separation anxiety symptoms worsened and improved with the course of the OCD and tic symptoms. In addition, the exacerbations of OCD and tic symptoms were frequently accompanied by emotional lability and irritability, tactile and sensory defensiveness, motoric hyperactivity, deterioration in handwriting, and separation anxiety. This finding was extended by Murphy and Pichichero (2002), who prospectively studied 12 school-age children at the time of appearance of their OCD. A notable feature of the tonsillopharyngitis episode was the lack of severity (sore throats were mild), and none of the patients displayed the typical features of classic severe GABHS tonsillopharyngitis. In follow-up, when recurrence of behavioral symptoms occurred, this sometimes preceded a positive throat culture by 3 days (when there was a high suspicion, patients were asked to return in 3 days for reculture, and at that time cultures were positive).

Delineation of the subtype is important because these children require a different assessment and treatment (Leonard and Swedo 2001). When a child has acute onset of OCD or tics or has had a dramatic deterioration, medical illnesses (including seemingly benign upper-respiratory infections) in the previous months should be carefully considered. Obtaining a throat culture, antistreptolysin O titer, anti-DNase B streptococcal titer, and an antinuclear antibody test (which may be nonspecifically positive) may help to diagnose such an infection.

Differential Diagnosis

Disorders of depression and anxiety (social phobia and generalized anxiety disorder) with obsessional features may initially resemble OCD. Obsessive ruminating and brooding may be seen in major depressive disorder, although the thoughts are likely to be more content specific and not seen as senseless. The fear of harm coming to oneself or others can be typical of separation anxiety disorder, but in OCD the specific thought usually results in the performance of compulsive rituals. The excessive and unrealistic worry of generalized anxiety disorder typically would not be accompanied by classic compulsive rituals. In the avoidance seen secondary to a simple phobia, it would be uncommon for germs to be the primary object avoided. In addition, the phobic person's fear usually decreases when he or she is not confronted with the stimuli, unlike that of patients with OCD.

The repetitive stereotypies seen in children with autism, mental retardation, pervasive developmental disorders, or organic brain damage syndromes may superficially resemble rituals in children with OCD; however, unlike stereotypies, the OCD rituals are well organized, complex, and ego-dystonic. In addition, the clinical picture and the accompanying symptoms can help to differentiate between stereotypies and compulsive rituals.

The patient with anorexia or bulimia may have an "obsessive" interest in calories, exercise, and food and may exhibit "compulsive" avoidance, measuring, and monitoring of food. This behavior may resemble that of OCD, but when considered in context, the foci of the "obsessions" and "compulsions" in the eating disorders are all related to food and body image. There is no disturbance of body image in OCD.

Patients with Tourette's disorder may have associated obsessive-compulsive symptoms or a diagnosis of OCD (Cohen and Leckman 1994; Frankel et al. 1986; Leckman et al. 1993; Leonard et al. 1992). Sometimes it is difficult to categorize a behavior as a ritual or as a tic. Generally, if an action is preceded by a specific cognition, then it is considered to be a compulsive ritual; however, some complex motor tics may be preceded by a sensation or "urge." Sensory tics are usually not accompanied by anxiety. It may be impossible to distinguish a complex motor tic from a compulsive ritual, especially in patients with both OCD and Tourette's disorder. For example, behaviors of tapping, touching, skipping, or spitting may be either a tic or a ritual. However, it is important to attempt to make the distinction, because each responds to different treatments. For a more detailed discussion, refer to Leckman and colleagues (1993).

Epidemiology

Initial estimates of the incidence of childhood OCD were based on psychiatric clinic populations. Berman (1942) reported "obsessive-compulsive phenomena" in 6 of 2,800 patients (0.2%). Hollingsworth et al. (1980) found 17 cases of OCD in 8,367 records of child and adolescent inpatients and outpatients (0.2%). Judd's (1965) retrospective chart review found 5 cases in 425 pediatric records (1.2%).

The Isle of Wight study, the first epidemiological study, reported "mixed obsessional/anxiety disorders" in 7 (0.3%) of 2,199 10- and 11-year-old children surveyed (Rutter et al. 1970). In a whole-population adolescent epidemiological study of OCD, Flament and colleagues (1988) reported a (weighted point) prevalence rate of 0.8% and lifetime prevalence of 1.9%. These figures suggest that OCD is a relatively common psychiatric disorder in adolescents, perhaps as common as 3% (lifetime) in late adolescence (Zohar et al. 1992). This rate is compatible with the estimated prevalence in the general popula-

tion (Karno et al. 1988) and with the finding that at least one-third to one-half of adults with OCD had onset during childhood (Black 1974).

In a cross-sectional and longitudinal epidemiological study, Peterson and colleagues (2001) studied the association among tics, OCD, and ADHD. Tics and ADHD symptoms were associated with OCD symptoms in late adolescence and early adulthood. In prospective analyses, tics in childhood and early adolescence predicted an increase in OCD in late adolescence and early adulthood. Thus, tics and OCD were significantly associated in this sample, as were OCD and ADHD.

Etiology

The etiology of OCD is unknown, but several lines of research suggest that it may be the result of a frontal lobe–limbic–basal ganglia dysfunction (Insel 1992; Wise and Rapoport 1989). Neurotransmitter dysregulation, genetic susceptibility, and environmental triggers appear to play a role in developing illness. The serotonin hypothesis of OCD is primarily based on the results of treatment studies, which report that the serotonin reuptake inhibitors (SRIs) are specifically efficacious for the treatment of OCD. It is unlikely that the neurotransmitter dysregulation can be attributed to just one system, and others (e.g., dopamine) have also been implicated.

Evidence supporting neurobiological etiologies include neuroanatomical, neurophysiological, and neuroimmunological associations and metabolic abnormalities. Numerous brain insults that result in basal ganglia damage (e.g., head injury, brain tumors, and carbon monoxide poisoning) have been reported to be related to the onset of OCD. Patients with known basal ganglia illnesses, including postencephalitic Parkinson's disease (Von Economo 1931) and Huntington's chorea (Cummings and Cunningham 1992), also have an increased rate of OCD. Neuroimaging studies reveal that adult patients with OCD who have a history of childhood onset of their illness have decreased size of the caudate nucleus (a principal structure in the basal ganglia) on computed tomographic scans (Luxenberg et al. 1988) and have abnormal patterns of regional glucose metabolism on positron emission tomographic scans compared with a group of control subjects without OCD (Swedo et al. 1989c, 1992). Brain imaging has dramatically advanced the examination of brain circuitry; for a recent review the reader is directed to Rauch and colleagues (2001).

Perhaps the most exciting work in the field of OCD has been that describing the relationship between OCD and Sydenham's chorea (the neurological variant of rheumatic fever). The incidence of OCD is increased in pediatric patients with Sydenham's chorea. Sydenham's chorea is an autoimmune response in the basal ganglia region caused by misdirected antibodies from a streptococcal infection (Swedo et al. 1989a, 1993). Children with PANDAS may have an underlying pathophysiology similar to that of Sydenham's chorea, although they do not have Sydenham's chorea and the diagnoses are mutually exclusive. This group of children with PANDAS likely represents a genetic vulnerability different from that of later-onset OCD.

A genetic susceptibility for OCD is suggested by the familial links between Tourette's disorder and OCD, initially reported by Pauls et al. (1986). These researchers hypothesized that the two illnesses may be different manifestations of the same gene or genes. More recently, a mixed model of inheritance has been proposed (Walkup et al. 1995). Family studies of OCD probands have reported that 20% of personally interviewed first-degree relatives (i.e., parents and siblings) of the OCD probands met diagnostic criteria for OCD (Lenane et al. 1990). Interestingly, the primary OCD symptom in the affected family member was usually different from that of the proband, which argues against modeling. In a family study, Pauls and colleagues (1995) described OCD as a heterogeneous disorder, with some cases being genetically mediated. Interestingly, they noted that children with an onset between ages 5 and 9 years had a much higher rate of family members with tics (suggesting a genetic association). Subsequent family studies have been consistent and report that tic disorders constitute an alternate expression of the familial OCD phenotype (Grados et al. 2001). Integrating these neuroanatomical and neurophysiological hypotheses with those of genetic susceptibility and environmental stressors remains an important research direction.

Treatment

■ Selection of Treatment

The choice of a treatment plan will depend on the individual symptoms and issues of the child and his or her family. Issues of comorbidity and psychosocial stressors will need to be considered. The expert consensus guidelines (March et al. 1997) and the practice parameters of the American Academy of Child and Adolescent Psychiatry (1998) provide an excellent framework from which to develop the treatment intervention. In general, both guidelines favor cognitive-behavioral therapy (CBT) as the initial treatment, particularly for younger children and for those with milder OCD symptoms and no significant comorbidity. CBT may have more durability than other treatments (although this premise has not been tested in systematic studies), and obviously it does not have the risks associated with medication. Some suggest that pharmacotherapy could be selected as the initial treatment because of severity of illness, the child's inability to participate in CBT, or the absence of skilled CBT therapists. At this point, the treatment guidelines mentioned above are used, and treatment is often individualized. Clearly, large systematic studies to address the relative efficacy of CBT, medication, and their combination are needed.

■ Behavioral Treatment

Cognitive-behavioral treatments are used clinically with much success, although efficacy is predominantly based on empirically supported uncontrolled and open trials (March 1995). Early pediatric case reports suggested that the techniques used with adults (Marks 1987) appeared to be appropriate for children (March et al. 1994; Wolfe and Wolfe 1991). For an excellent review of CBT see Piacentini (1999). Exposure with response prevention (ERP) is the most frequently implemented treatment and may be used in addition to other specific behavioral treatment techniques (e.g., anxiety management training) (March et al. 1994). Habit reversal may play a role in the treatment of the more repetitive complex tic-like rituals (Vitulano et al. 1992).

In one of the first single pediatric behavioral studies reported, Bolton et al. (1983) used response prevention for 15 obsessive adolescents; good treatment results were achieved in 11 (73%). A structured treatment protocol for children with OCD has been developed as a manual, "How I Ran OCD Off My Land: A Cognitive-Behavioral Program for the Treatment of Obsessive Compulsive Disorder in Children and Adolescents" (March and Mulle 1998; March et al. 1994); this protocol appears to be practical to implement and effective for treatment. Behavior modification therapy may be less successful for patients who have obsessions only (as opposed to both obsessions and compulsions), who are very young, and who are uncooperative.

Scahill and colleagues (1996) treated seven children (ages 8–16) with the ERP form of CBT. There was a mean improvement of 61% at the end of treatment and of 51% at 3-month follow-up. Franklin and colleagues (1998) reported that 14 children and adolescents had a mean symptom improvement of 67% at end of treatment and 62% at follow-up. The researchers found no difference in response when the CBT was administered daily rather than weekly.

Although the body of literature is increasing, there are no published large controlled trials of CBT in children and adolescents. It appears that behavioral treatment for children with OCD is appropriate and should be considered as one of the treatments of choice.

■ Pharmacological Treatment

An increasing body of literature supports the short-term efficacy of the SRI clomipramine and of the selective serotonin reuptake inhibitors (SSRIs) in the treatment of children and adolescents with OCD. Clomipramine, which is a tricyclic and an SRI, was the first medication systematically studied in the pediatric OCD population. In those early studies, Flament and colleagues (1985) and Leonard and colleagues (1989) reported that children with OCD responded to clomipramine. In the report by Flament and colleagues (1985), 23 pediatric patients participated in a 10-week double-blind, placebo-controlled crossover study. Clomipramine (in doses of 3 mg/kg) was significantly more effective than placebo in decreasing OCD symptoms at week 5, and a reduction in symptoms was occasionally seen by 3 weeks. Of the 19 children who completed the trial, 14 (74%) had moderate to marked improvement, reporting a significant decrease in time spent in obsessive-compulsive activities as well as in distress experienced. Similarly, in the large multicenter trial, DeVeaugh-Geiss and colleagues (1992) reported that clomipramine was superior to placebo for the treatment of OCD in adolescents, and this finding led to the first approval by the U.S. Food and Drug Administration (FDA) of an SRI in pediatric OCD (in children age 10 years and older).

To address whether the specificity of the medication was important, a double-blind crossover compari-son of clomipramine and desipramine (a selective noradrenergic reuptake blocker) was completed in 48 children and adolescents with OCD (Leonard et al. 1989). Clomipramine was significantly better than desipramine in ameliorating the OCD symptoms at week 5. Desipramine was no more effective in reducing OCD symptoms than placebo had been in the study by Flament et al. (1985). In fact, when desipramine was given in the second phase as the active medication, some of the patients' symptoms that had disappeared during the clomipramine treatment phase returned. Both clomipramine and desipramine were well tolerated at 3 mg/kg/day, and the side-effect profiles for the two drugs were generally similar and consistent with their antihistaminic and anticholinergic effects.

Clomipramine has not been directly compared with an SSRI, and therefore it is not known whether it is more effective than any of the SSRIs. Electrocardiograms are obtained during ongoing clinical care because of concerns about tachycardia and prolongation of the QTc interval. Expert consensus guidelines and clinical experience suggest that clomipramine may be more cost-effective, although it may have a higher rate of discontinuation based on side effects and necessitates periodic administration of electrocardiograms during treatment. It is sometimes used for patients with more treatment-refractory OCD (March et al. 1997, 1998).

With the development and availability of the SSRIs (citalopram, escitalopram, fluoxetine, fluvoxamine, paroxetine, and sertraline), these agents have become popular because of their more tolerable side-effect profile (fewer anticholinergic effects), their relative safety profile in overdoses (in comparison to the tricyclic antidepressants), and the fact that electrocardiographic monitoring is not required. In large multicenter trials, fluvoxamine, fluoxetine, and sertraline have each been shown to be superior to placebo for children and adolescents with OCD (Geller et al. 2001b; March et al. 1998; Riddle et al. 2001). Sertraline has an FDA-approved indication for the treatment of OCD in children ages 6 years and older, fluoxetine in children ages 7 and older, and fluvoxamine has such approval for children ages 8 years and older. The SSRIs have had only limited pharmacokinetic study in the pediatric age group. A study of sertraline (Alderman et al. 1998) and another study of paroxetine (Findling et al. 1999) found wide intraindividual and interindividual pharmacokinetic variability but generally similar results as those reported in adults.

March and colleagues (1998) reported on 187 children and adolescents (ages 6–17 years) with OCD in a randomized, double-blind, placebo-controlled trial of sertraline. Dosages of sertraline were adjusted to a maximum of 200 mg/day during the first 4 weeks, and the drug was then continued at the adjusted dosage for 8 more weeks. Clinically significant differences between the two groups were seen at week 3 and continued for the duration of study. Patients receiving sertraline showed significantly greater improvement than did those receiving placebo as measured by the CY-BOCS, the NIMH Obsessive Compulsive Scale, and the Clinical Global Impression Scale.

Riddle and colleagues (2001) reported the safety and efficacy of fluvoxamine in a randomized, controlled trial of 120 patients ages 8–17 years with OCD. After a single-blind placebo lead-in period, patients were assigned to either fluvoxamine (50–200 mg/day) or placebo for 10 weeks. Those in the fluvoxamine group had a significant improvement (as measured by the CY-BOCS) over those in the placebo group, and the difference emerged as early as the first week. There were significantly more responders (defined as a 25% decrease in CY-BOCS score) in the group treated with fluvoxamine (42%) compared with those in the placebo group (26%).

Geller and colleagues (2001b) reported on 103 children and adolescents (ages 7–17) in a 13-week randomized, double-blind, controlled trial of fluoxetine versus placebo (2:1). Fluoxetine was started at 10 mg/day for 2 weeks and was then increased to 20 mg/day. At week 4 and at week 7, the dosage could be increased to a maximum of 60 mg/day. Intent-to-treat analyses showed that fluoxetine was associated with significantly greater improvement on the CY-BOCS than was placebo. The authors concluded that fluoxetine 20–60 mg/day was effective and well tolerated in this pediatric group. Fluoxetine appears to improve the OCD symptoms without worsening the tic symptoms in those with comorbid tic disorders (Scahill et al. 1997a). Open studies support the use of citalopram and paroxetine (Rosenberg et al. 1999; Thomsen 1997).

Fluoxetine and other SSRIs have fewer anticholinergic side effects than the tricyclic antidepressants; however, activation (or agitation) and insomnia may be more common. Generally, the most common side effects seen with the SSRIs include sedation, nausea, diarrhea, insomnia, anorexia, tremor, sexual dysfunction, and hyperstimulation (March et al. 1998; Riddle et al. 2001). It is not known whether children may be more vulnerable to agitation or activation while taking an SSRI than are adults.

The pediatric treatment literature reveals results similar to those reported in adults. In general, a 30%–40% reduction in OCD symptoms, which corresponds to an average decrease in CY-BOCS score of six points, is reported in the active treatment arm of the controlled studies of SSRIs (March 1999). There is little or no placebo effect detected in the studies. Clinical effects sometimes begin as early as 3 weeks and generally plateau at 10–12 weeks. Most patients achieve maximum benefit with average SSRI dosages, with only a few patients requiring high dosages (March 1999).

Generally, a 12-week trial of an SSRI with adequate dosage is considered necessary. Many patients do not have symptom relief until 6–12 weeks after a trial begins. Evidence has shown that an individual who does not respond to one SRI may respond to another, although a decreasing rate of success with successive trials has been described in the adult literature (March 1999). Most experts would recommend clomipramine after two or three failed SSRI trials (March et al. 1997)

For patients who partially respond to an SSRI, augmentation strategies may be considered. CBT would be a logical choice for augmentation if the patient has not already undergone such treatment, although availability is limited in certain areas, and some children are too sick or not motivated to participate. In considering medication augmentation, clonazepam is occasionally added, but disinhibition, dependence, and tolerance to the medication limit its use (Leonard et al. 1994). An increasing adult literature supports the role of augmentation with a neuroleptic in patients who do not respond or have partial response to SRIs (McDougle et al. 1994). A controlled trial of SRI augmentation using risperidone versus placebo demonstrated that the addition of risperidone was superior in reducing OCD symptoms. Interestingly (unlike in earlier studies), no differences in response were found between patients with and without comorbid tic or schizotypal personality disorders (McDougle et al. 2000). In one case series, children who did not respond to SRI therapy improved significantly after risperidone was added, and the authors called for controlled trials in this age group (Fitzgerald et al. 1999).

How long should patients who respond to medication continue to take it? Although periodically decreasing the dosage should be considered, many patients require long-term maintenance therapy.

A double-blind study of desipramine substitution in adolescents taking long-term clomipramine therapy found that 8 of 9 patients relapsed when switched to desipramine compared with 2 of 11 who continued taking clomipramine (Leonard et al. 1991). The limited durability of pharmacotherapy, although not well studied, argues for the role of CBT in the treatment of children with OCD.

■ Combined Treatments

March and colleagues (1994) reported that patients treated with both medications and CBT seemed to have greater improvement and lower relapse rates (based on small trials). Unfortunately, no large controlled studies have been published that compare CBT, medication, and their combination in children and adolescents. This makes it very difficult to compare the relative efficacies and durability of these treatment modalities. In a study of a small group (22 patients), de Haan and colleagues (1998) compared ERP CBT to clomipramine and found that both treatments had benefit but CBT was more effective in reducing symptom severity and response rate. A large systematic trial of combined treatment (medication versus CBT versus medication plus CBT) is ongoing (Franklin et al. 2003), and that study will inform the field on relative efficacy of treatment options. In clinical practice, CBT and pharmacotherapy work well together for many children.

■ Psychodynamic and Psychosocial Treatments

Jenike (1990) reviewed the psychotherapeutic interventions that are available for the treatment of OCD and concluded that "traditional psychodynamic psychotherapy is not an effective treatment for obsessions or rituals in patients meeting criteria for OCD as defined in the DSM-III-R; there are no reports in the modern psychiatric literature of patients who stopped ritualizing when treated with this method alone" (p. 295). Psychodynamic psychotherapy can play an important role by addressing both general and specific issues in the patient's life—such as how OCD affects the individual's self-esteem, personal relationships, and outlook—and by encouraging compliance with the behavior or psychopharmacological therapies that focus more directly on the OCD symptoms. OCD clearly cannot be understood out of context of an individu-

al's feelings, relationships, and past and current experiences. Character styles consistent with "obsessional defenses" and obsessive-compulsive personality are amenable to psychotherapy (for reviews see Jenike 1990).

Family therapy is an important treatment for pediatric patients with OCD. Family discord, parental marital difficulties, problems of a specific family member, and inappropriate roles or boundaries will interfere with the family's and each member's successful functioning and, ultimately, with the long-term outcome of the identified patient (Hafner et al. 1981; Hoover and Insel 1984; Lenane 1991). A complete family assessment is a necessary part of the initial diagnostic evaluation of every child who has OCD. Lenane (1989) described the goals of family therapy as 1) involving the whole family in treatment, 2) getting all behaviors out in the open, 3) obtaining full and accurate understanding of how everyone participates in the OCD behavior, and 4) reframing of less-than-positive behavior. By dealing with the specific family dynamic issues, the family can participate in the OCD treatment plan of the identified patient in constructive and positive ways. A family-based treatment manual for young children with OCD is currently under development.

■ Investigational Treatments

Children with PANDAS merit a careful assessment of recent medical illnesses, including upper-respiratory infections. To determine whether penicillin prophylaxis would decrease the OCD and tic symptoms in children with PANDAS, an 8-month double-blind, placebo-controlled crossover study of oral penicillin V (250 mg twice a day) was conducted in 37 children (Garvey et al. 1999). The researchers found that there were no significant differences in severity of OCD or tic symptoms in the penicillin versus the placebo phase; however, oral penicillin did not provide adequate prophylaxis, and 14 of 35 GABHS infections were diagnosed during active penicillin treatment. The authors concluded that the study did not provide justification for penicillin prophylaxis in children with PANDAS, but they noted that because prophylaxis was not achieved, no conclusion about the efficacy of penicillin prophylaxis for PANDAS could be drawn. Further studies are needed.

Children with the most severe cases of PANDAS were randomly assigned to plasma exchange (5 single-volume exchanges over 2 weeks), intravenous immunoglobulin (IVIG) (1 g/kg per day on 2 days) or placebo (administered in the same fashion as IVIG) (Perlmutter et al. 1999). Both plasma exchange and IVIG were effective in decreasing the symptom severity for these children. The authors cautioned that these are investigations and should be considered only in severely ill children with clear evidence of immune dysfunction and in the context of an institutional review board–approved research protocol. Further study of immune dysfunction may help clarify the role of these novel investigational treatments.

Prognosis

In the only follow-up study of an epidemiological sample, Berg et al. (1989) reported that of the 16 adolescents with an initial diagnosis of OCD, 5 (31%) still met criteria at 2-year follow-up, and 4 (25%) had "subclinical" OCD. Interestingly, 2 (13%) of the original patients who had OCD no longer met criteria for OCD but did meet criteria for obsessive-compulsive personality disorder. The investigators speculated that some children and adolescents with early-onset OCD might develop obsessive-compulsive personalities as means of coping with the disorder. The relationship between OCD and obsessive-compulsive personality disorder definitely requires additional study.

Follow-up studies of pediatric patients with OCD indicated that at least half of the patients remained symptomatic as adults (Berman 1942; Hollingsworth et al. 1980; Warren 1965). Flament et al. (1990) found that of 25 patients seen 2–7 years after initial presentation, 17 (68%) still met diagnostic criteria for OCD, and 12 (48%) had an additional diagnosis (most often depression or anxiety); only 7 (28%) no longer met DSM-III (American Psychiatric Association 1980) diagnostic criteria for any disorder. Surprisingly, neither baseline measures nor a positive response to clomipramine treatment could predict long-term outcome. These poor results could be explained in part by the fact that this group had not been actively treated during the 2- to 5-year interim period, and only 12 subjects had been taking clomipramine for more than a few months.

The largest and most recent systematic follow-up study of children with OCD took place when the patients had access to the SRIs and to behavior therapy.

The 2- to 7-year follow-up study by Leonard et al. (1993) of 54 consecutively admitted children and adolescents with OCD reported that this group seemed to have a somewhat more improved outcome than did the group studied by Flament et al. (1990). Of the 54 subjects, 38 (70%) were taking psychoactive medication at follow-up; 23 patients (43%) still met diagnostic criteria for OCD, and 43 (80%) were improved from baseline. Of the 6 patients (11%) who were totally asymptomatic, 3 were taking medication at the time of reevaluation; thus, only 3 could be considered to be in true remission. This study suggests that most patients can expect improvement with the new treatments available, but a small group of patients continue to have a chronic and debilitating course.

Research Issues

Several research issues for childhood-onset OCD are important. It is unknown which children respond better to behavioral treatment (CBT) and which respond to drug treatment. It is presumed, but not yet proven, that the availability of these two treatment modalities may improve the long-term prognosis. A systematic efficacy study and a long-term comparison are needed to determine relative efficacy and long-term durability.

Identification of a new subtype of pediatric-onset OCD with abrupt onset and dramatic exacerbations (PANDAS group) may lead to new assessment and treatment techniques. It is unknown what percentage of children with OCD may be part of this subgroup. One treatment trial of penicillin prophylaxis for those with exacerbations of GABHS infection has been completed, and large controlled studies are needed. It will be important to determine the percentage of cases of pediatric-onset OCD that are precipitated by streptococcal infection.

The identification, through genetic or biological studies, of children who are at risk for developing OCD also is a research priority. If a true subtype is validated, new avenues for genetic studies will emerge.

References

Adams PL: Obsessive Children. New York, Penguin Books, 1973

Alderman J, Wolkow R, Chung M, et al: Sertraline treatment of children and adolescents with obsessive compulsive disorder or depression: pharmacokinetics, tolerability, and efficacy. J Am Acad Child Adolesc Psychiatry 37:386–394, 1998

Allen AJ, Leonard HL, Swedo SE: Case study: a new infection-triggered, autoimmune subtype of pediatric OCD and Tourette's syndrome. J Am Acad Child Adolesc Psychiatry 34:307–311, 1995

American Academy of Child and Adolescent Psychiatry: Practice parameters for the assessment and treatment of children and adolescents with obsessive-compulsive disorder. J Am Acad Child Adolesc Psychiatry 37(10, suppl):27S–45S, 1998

American Psychiatric Association: Diagnostic and Statistical Manual of Mental Disorders, 3rd Edition. Washington, DC, American Psychiatric Association, 1980

American Psychiatric Association: Diagnostic and Statistical Manual of Mental Disorders, 3rd Edition, Revised. Washington, DC, American Psychiatric Association, 1987

American Psychiatric Association: Diagnostic and Statistical Manual of Mental Disorders, 4th Edition. Washington, DC, American Psychiatric Association, 1994

American Psychiatric Association: Diagnostic and Statistical Manual of Mental Disorders, 4th Edition, Text Revision. Washington, DC, American Psychiatric Association, 2000

Berg CZ, Rapoport JL, Whitaker A, et al: Childhood obsessive-compulsive disorder: a two-year prospective follow-up of a community sample. J Am Acad Child Adolesc Psychiatry 28:528–533, 1989

Berman L: Obsessive-compulsive neurosis in children. J Nerv Ment Dis 95:26–39, 1942

Black A: The natural history of obsessional neurosis, in Obsessional States. Edited by Beech HR. London, Methuen, 1974, pp 1–23

Bolton D, Collins S, Steinberg D: The treatment of obsessive-compulsive disorder in adolescence: a report of fifteen cases. Br J Psychiatry 142:456–464, 1983

Cohen DJ, Leckman JF: Developmental psychopathology and neurobiology of Tourette's syndrome. J Am Acad Child Adolesc Psychiatry 33:2–15, 1994

Cummings JL, Cunningham K: Obsessive-compulsive disorder in Huntington's disease. Biol Psychiatry 31:263–270, 1992

de Haan E, Hoogduin KA, Buitelaar JK, et al: Behavior therapy versus clomipramine for the treatment of obsessive-compulsive disorder. J Am Acad Child Adolesc Psychiatry 37:1022–1029, 1998

Despert L: Differential diagnosis between obsessive-compulsive neurosis and schizophrenia in children, in Psychopathology of Childhood. Edited by Hoch PH, Zubin J. New York, Grune & Stratton, 1955, pp 240–253

DeVeaugh-Geiss J, Moroz G, Biederman J, et al: Clomipramine hydrochloride in childhood and adolescent obsessive-compulsive disorder: a multicenter trial. J Am Acad Child Adolesc Psychiatry 31:45–49, 1992

Findling RL, Reed MD, Myers C, et al: Paroxetine pharmacokinetics in depressed children and adolescents. J Am Acad Child Adolesc Psychiatry 38:952–959, 1999

Fitzgerald KD, Stewart CM, Tawile V, et al: Risperidone augmentation of serotonin reuptake inhibitor treatment of pediatric obsessive compulsive disorder. J Child Adolesc Psychopharmacol 9:115–23, 1999

Flament MF, Rapoport JL, Berg CJ, et al: Clomipramine treatment of childhood obsessive-compulsive disorder. Arch Gen Psychiatry 42:977–983, 1985

Flament MF, Whitaker A, Rapoport JL, et al: Obsessive compulsive disorder in adolescence: an epidemiological study. J Am Acad Child Adolesc Psychiatry 27:764–771, 1988

Flament MF, Koby E, Rapoport JL, et al: Childhood obsessive compulsive disorder: a prospective follow-up study. J Child Psychol Psychiatry 31:363–380, 1990

Frankel M, Cummings JL, Robertson MM, et al: Obsessions and compulsions in Gilles de la Tourette's syndrome. Neurology 36:378–382, 1986

Franklin ME, Kozak MJ, Cashman LA, et al: Cognitive-behavioral treatment of pediatric obsessive-compulsive disorder: an open clinical trial. J Am Acad Child Adolesc Psychiatry 37:412–419, 1998

Franklin ME, Foa EB, March JS: The Pediatric OCD Treatment Study (POTS): rationale, design and methods. J Child Adolesc Psychopharmacol 13(suppl):39–52, 2003

Garvey MA, Perlmutter SJ, Allen AJ, et al: A pilot study of penicillin prophylaxis for neuropsychiatric exacerbations triggered by streptococcal infections. Biol Psychiatry 45:1564–1571, 1999

Geller DA, Biederman J, Jones J, et al: Is juvenile obsessive-compulsive disorder a developmental subtype of the disorder? A review of the pediatric literature. J Am Acad Child Adolesc Psychiatry 37:420–427, 1998

Geller DA, Biederman J, Faraone SV, et al: Disentagling chronological age from age of onset in children and adolescents with obsessive-compulsive disorder. Int J Neuropsychopharmacol 4:169–178, 2001a

Geller DA, Hoog SL, Heiligenstein JH, et al: Fluoxetine treatment for obsessive-compulsive disorder in children and adolescents: a placebo-controlled clinical trial. J Am Acad Child Adolesc Psychiatry 40:773–779, 2001b

Geller DA, Biederman J, Faraone SV, et al: Attention-deficit/hyperactivity disorder in children and adolescents with obsessive-compulsive disorder: fact or artifact? J Am Acad Child Adolesc Psychiatry 41:52–58, 2002

Grados MA, Riddle MA, Samuels JF, et al: The familial phenotype of obsessive-compulsive disorder in relation to tic disorders: the Hopkins OCD family study. Biol Psychiatry 50:559–565, 2001

Hafner RJ, Gilchrist P, Bowling J, et al: The treatment of obsessional neurosis in a family setting. Aust N Z J Psychiatry 15:145–151, 1981

Hanna GL: Demographic and clinical features of obsessive-compulsive disorder in children and adolescents. J Am Acad Child Adolesc Psychiatry 34:19–27, 1995

Hollingsworth CE, Tanguey PE, Grossman L, et al: Long-term outcome of obsessive compulsive disorder in children. J Am Acad Child Psychiatry 19:134–144, 1980

Hoover CF, Insel TR: Families of origin in obsessive compulsive disorder. J Nerv Ment Dis 172:207–215, 1984

Insel TR: Toward a neuroanatomy of obsessive-compulsive disorder. Arch Gen Psychiatry 49:739–744, 1992

Janet P: Les Obsessions et la Psychasthenie [Obsessions and Psychasthenia], Vol 1. Paris, Felix Alan, 1903

Jenike MA: Psychotherapy of obsessive-compulsive personality disorder, in Obsessive-Compulsive Disorders: Theory and Management. Edited by Jenicke MA, Baer L, Minichiello WE. Chicago, IL, Year Book Medical, 1990, pp 295–305

Judd LL: Obsessive compulsive neurosis in children. Arch Gen Psychiatry 12:136–143, 1965

Kanner L: Child Psychiatry, 3rd Edition. Springfield, IL, Charles C Thomas, 1962

Karno B, Golding J, Sorenson S, et al: The epidemiology of obsessive compulsive disorder in five U.S. communities. Arch Gen Psychiatry 45:1094–1099, 1988

Leckman JF, Walker DE, Cohen DJ: Premonitory urges in Tourette's syndrome. Am J Psychiatry 150:98–102, 1993

Leckman JF, Walker DE, Goodman WK, et al: "Just right" perceptions associated with compulsive behavior in Tourette's syndrome. Am J Psychiatry 151:675–680, 1994

Lenane M: Families and obsessive-compulsive disorder, in Obsessive-Compulsive Disorder in Children and Adolescents. Edited by Rapoport JL. Washington, DC, American Psychiatric Press, 1989, pp 237–249

Lenane M: Family therapy for children with obsessive compulsive disorder, in Current Treatments of Obsessive-Compulsive Disorder. Edited by Pato MT, Zohar M. Washington, DC, American Psychiatric Press, 1991, pp 103–113

Lenane MC, Swedo SE, Leonard HL, et al: Psychiatric disorders in first degree relatives of children and adolescents with obsessive compulsive disorder. J Am Acad Child Adolesc Psychiatry 29:407–412, 1990

Leonard HL, Swedo SE: Paediatric autoimmune neuropsychiatric disorders associated with streptococcal infection (PANDAS). Int J Neuropsychopharmacol 4:191–198, 2001

Leonard HL, Swedo S, Rapoport JL, et al: Treatment of obsessive compulsive disorder with clomipramine and desipramine in children and adolescents: a double-blind crossover comparison. Arch Gen Psychiatry 46:1088–1092, 1989

Leonard HL, Swedo SE, Lenane MC, et al: A double-blind desipramine substitution during long-term clomipramine treatment in children and adolescents with obsessive compulsive disorder. Arch Gen Psychiatry 48:922–926, 1991

Leonard HL, Lenane MC, Swedo SE, et al: Tics and Tourette's syndrome: a 2- to 7-year follow-up of 54 obsessive compulsive children. Am J Psychiatry 149:1244–1251, 1992

Leonard HL, Swedo SE, Lenane MC, et al: A 2- to 7-year follow-up study of 54 obsessive compulsive children and adolescents. Arch Gen Psychiatry 50:429–439, 1993

Leonard HL, Topol D, Bukstein O, et al: Clonazepam as an augmenting agent in the treatment of childhood onset obsessive compulsive disorder. J Am Acad Child Adolesc Psychiatry 33:792–794, 1994

Luxenberg JS, Swedo SE, Flament MF, et al: Neuroanatomical abnormalities in obsessive-compulsive disorder detected with quantitative X-ray computed tomography. Am J Psychiatry 145:1089–1093, 1988

March J: Cognitive-behavioral psychotherapy for children and adolescents with obsessive-compulsive disorder: a review and recommendations for treatment. J Am Acad Child Adolesc Psychiatry 1:7–18, 1995

March J: Current status of pharmacotherapy for pediatric anxiety disorders, in Treating Anxiety Disorders in Youth: Current Problems and Future Solutions (ADAA/NIMH). Edited by Beidel D. Washington, DC, Anxiety Disorders Association of America, 1999, pp 42–62

March JS, Mulle K: OCD in Children and Adolescents: A Cognitive-Behavioral Treatment Manual. New York, Guilford, 1998

March J, Mulle K, Herbel B: Behavioral psychotherapy for children and adolescents with obsessive-compulsive disorder: an open trial of a new protocol driven treatment package. J Am Acad Child Adolesc Psychiatry 33:333–341, 1994

March J, Frances A, Kahn D, et al: Expert consensus guidelines: treatment of obsessive-compulsive disorder. J Clin Psychiatry 58(suppl 4):1–72, 1997

March JS, Biederman J, Wolkow R, et al: Sertraline in children and adolescents with obsessive-compulsive disorder: a multicenter randomized controlled trial. JAMA 280:1752–1756, 1998

Marks IM: Fears, Phobias and Rituals: Panic Anxiety and Their Disorders. New York, Oxford University Press, 1987

McDougle C, Goodman W, Leckman J, et al: Haloperidol addition in fluvoxamine-refractory obsessive-compulsive disorder: a double-blind, placebo-controlled study in patients with and without tics. Arch Gen Psychiatry 5:302–308, 1994

McDougle CJ, Naylor ST, Cohen CJ, et al; A double-blind, placebo-controlled study of risperidone addition to serotonin reuptake inhibitor-refractory obsessive-compulsive disorder. Arch Gen Psychiatry 57:794–801, 2000

Murphy ML, Pichichero ME: Prospective identification and treatment of children with pediatric autoimmune neuropsychiatric disorder associated with group A streptococcal infection (PANDAS). Arch Pediatr Adolesc Med 156:356–361, 2002

Pauls DL, Towbin K, Leckman J, et al: Gilles de la Tourette syndrome and obsessive compulsive disorder: evidence supporting a genetic relationship. Arch Gen Psychiatry 43:1180–1182, 1986

Pauls DL, Alsobrook JP, Goodman W, et al: A family study of obsessive compulsive disorder. Am J Psychiatry 1:76–84, 1995

Perlmutter SJ, Leitman SF, Garvey MA, et al: Therapeutic plasma exchange and intravenous immunoglobulin for obsessive compulsive disorder and tic disorders in childhood. Lancet 354:1153–1158, 1999

Peterson BS, Pine DS, Cohen P, et al: Prospective, longitudinal study of tic, obsessive-compulsive, and attention-deficit/hyperactivity disorders in an epidemiological sample. J Am Acad Child Adolesc Psychiatry 40:685–695, 2001

Piacentini J: Cognitive behavioral therapy of childhood OCD. Child Adolesc Psychiatr Clin N Am 8:599–616, 1999

Rapoport JL: Annotation, child obsessive-compulsive disorder. J Child Psychol Psychiatry 27:285–289, 1986

Rauch SL, Whalen PJ, Curran T, et al: Probing striato-thalamic function in obsessive-compulsive disorder and Tourette syndrome using neuroimaging methods. Adv Neurol 85:207–224, 2001

Rettew DC, Swedo SE, Leonard HL, et al: Obsessions and compulsions across time in 79 children and adolescents with obsessive-compulsive disorder. J Am Acad Child Adolesc Psychiatry 31:1050–1056, 1992

Riddle M, Reeve E, Yaryura-Tobias J, et al: Fluvoxamine for children and adolescents with obsessive compulsive disorder: a randomized controlled multicenter trial. J Am Acad Child Adolesc Psychiatry, 40:222–229, 2001

Rosario-Campos MC, Leckman JF, Mercadante MT, et al: Adults with early onset obsessive-compulsive disorder. Am J Psychiatry 158:1899–1903, 2001

Rosenberg DR, Stewart CM, Fitzgerald KD, et al: Paroxetine open-label treatment of pediatric outpatients with obsessive-compulsive disorder. J Am Acad Child Adolesc Psychiatry 38:1180–1185, 1999

Rutter M, Tizard J, Whitmore K: Education, Health and Behavior. London, Longmans, 1970

Scahill L, Vitulano LA, Brenner EM, et al: Behavioral therapy in children and adolescents with obsessive-compulsive disorder: a pilot study. J Child Adolesc Psychopharmacol 6:191–202, 1996

Scahill L, Riddle MA, King RA, et al: Fluoxetine has no marked effect on tic symptoms in patients with Tourette's syndrome: a double-blind placebo controlled study. J Child Adolesc Psychopharmcol 7:75–85, 1997a

Scahill L, Riddle MA, McSwiggin-Hardin M, et al: Children's Yale-Brown Obsessive Compulsive Scale: reliability and validity. J Am Acad Child Adolesc Psychiatry 36:844–852, 1997b

Swedo SE: Sydenham's chorea: a model for childhood autoimmune neuropsychiatric disorders. JAMA 272: 1788–1791, 1994

Swedo SE, Rapoport JL, Cheslow DL, et al: High prevalence of obsessive-compulsive symptoms in patients with Sydenham's chorea. Am J Psychiatry 146:246–249, 1989a

Swedo S, Rapoport JL, Leonard HL, et al: Obsessive-compulsive disorder in children and adolescents: clinical phenomenology of 70 consecutive cases. Arch Gen Psychiatry 46:335–341, 1989b

Swedo SE, Schapiro MB, Grady CL, et al: Cerebral glucose metabolism in childhood-onset obsessive compulsive disorder. Arch Gen Psychiatry 46:518–523, 1989c

Swedo SE, Pietrini P, Leonard HL, et al: Cerebral glucose metabolism in childhood-onset obsessive compulsive disorder: revisualization during pharmacotherapy. Arch Gen Psychiatry 49:690–694, 1992

Swedo SE, Leonard HL, Schapiro MB, et al: Sydenham's chorea: physical and psychological symptoms of St. Vitus's dance. Pediatrics 91:706–713, 1993

Swedo SE, Leonard HL, Kiessling LS: Speculations on antineuronal antibody-mediated neuropsychiatric disorders of childhood: commentaries. Pediatrics 93:323–326, 1994

Swedo SE, Leonard HL, Garvey M, et al: Pediatric autoimmune neuropsychiatric disorders associated with streptococcal infections: clinical description of the first 50 cases. Am J Psychiatry 155:264–271, 1998

Thomsen PH: Child and adolescent obsessive-compulsive disorder treated with citalopram: findings from an open trial of 23 cases. J Child Adolesc Psychopharmacol 7:157–166, 1997

Vitulano LA, King RA, Scahill L, et al: Behavioral treatment of children and adolescents with trichotillomania. J Am Acad Child Adolesc Psychiatry 31:139–146, 1992

Von Economo C: Encephalitis Lethargica: Its Sequelae and Treatment. Translated by Neuman KO. New York, Oxford University Press, 1931

Walkup JT, LaBuda MJ, Hurko O, et al: Evidence for a mixed model of inheritance in Tourette's syndrome. Paper presented at the 42nd annual meeting of the American Academy of Child and Adolescent Psychiatry, New Orleans, LA, October 21, 1995

Warren W: A study of adolescent psychiatric inpatients and the outcome six or more years later. J Child Psychol Psychiatry 6:141–160, 1965

Wise SP, Rapoport JL: Obsessive-compulsive disorder: is it basal ganglia dysfunction? in Obsessive-Compulsive Disorder in Children and Adolescents. Edited by Rapoport JL. Washington, DC, American Psychiatric Press, 1989, pp 327–344

Wolfe RP, Wolfe LS: Assessment and treatment of obsessive compulsive disorder in children. Behav Modif 15:372–393, 1991

Zohar AH, Ratzoni G, Pauls DL, et al: An epidemiological study of obsessive-compulsive disorder and related disorders in Israeli adolescents. J Am Acad Child Adolesc Psychiatry 31:1057–1061, 1992

Specific Phobia, Panic Disorder, Social Phobia, and Selective Mutism

Bruce Black, M.D.

Abbe M. Garcia, Ph.D.

Jennifer B. Freeman, Ph.D.

Mai Karitani, A.B.

Henrietta L. Leonard, M.D.

Definitions

According to DSM-IV-TR (American Psychiatric Association 2000), specific phobia is a marked and persistent fear of circumscribed objects or situations (phobic stimuli), such as animals, blood, heights, closed spaces, or flying. The fear is excessive or unreasonable. Exposure to the phobic stimuli provokes an immediate anxiety response.

Panic disorder is characterized by recurrent, unexpected panic attacks, which are discrete periods of "intense fear or discomfort" accompanied by specific somatic symptoms and associated with characteristic sequelae such as fear and worry (American Psychiatric Association 2000).

Social phobia (or social anxiety disorder) is a persistent fear of one or more social situations in which a person is exposed to unfamiliar persons or to scrutiny by others. Exposure to the feared social situations provokes marked anxiety (American Psychiatric Association 2000).

Selective mutism is characterized by persistent failure to speak in one or more major social situations in which speaking is expected, despite speaking in other situations. Although selective mutism is not classified as an anxiety disorder in DSM-IV-TR, a growing body of research has demonstrated that it is primarily a manifestation of social anxiety.

Diagnostic Criteria

Specific phobia is a "marked and persistent fear that is excessive or unreasonable, cued by the presence or anticipation of a specific object or situation" (American Psychiatric Association 2000, p. 449) that provokes immediate anxiety. The anxiety response may be accompanied by a variety of somatic symptoms or, in children, may be expressed by crying, tantrums, freezing, or clinging. To meet DSM-IV-TR criteria (Table 31–1), the avoidance, anxious anticipation, or distress in the feared situation must interfere with a person's normal routine, social relationships, or academic (or occupational) functioning, or there must be marked distress about having the fear. The stimulus is either avoided or endured with intense anxiety. By definition, adults recognize that the fear is excessive or unreasonable, although children may not.

To meet the DSM-IV-TR criteria for *panic disorder* (Tables 31–2 and 31–3), an individual must have re-

Table 31–1. DSM-IV-TR diagnostic criteria for specific phobia

A. Marked and persistent fear that is excessive or unreasonable, cued by the presence or anticipation of a specific object or situation (e.g., flying, heights, animals, receiving an injection, seeing blood).

B. Exposure to the phobic stimulus almost invariably provokes an immediate anxiety response, which may take the form of a situationally bound or situationally predisposed panic attack. **Note:** In children, the anxiety may be expressed by crying, tantrums, freezing, or clinging.

C. The person recognizes that the fear is excessive or unreasonable. **Note:** In children, this feature may be absent.

D. The phobic situation(s) is avoided or else is endured with intense anxiety or distress.

E. The avoidance, anxious anticipation, or distress in the feared situation(s) interferes significantly with the person's normal routine, occupational (or academic) functioning, or social activities or relationships, or there is marked distress about having the phobia.

F. In individuals under age 18 years, the duration is at least 6 months.

G. The anxiety, panic attacks, or phobic avoidance associated with the specific object or situation are not better accounted for by another mental disorder, such as obsessive-compulsive disorder (e.g., fear of dirt in someone with an obsession about contamination), posttraumatic stress disorder (e.g., avoidance of stimuli associated with a severe stressor), separation anxiety disorder (e.g., avoidance of school), social phobia (e.g., avoidance of social situations because of fear of embarrassment), panic disorder with agoraphobia, or agoraphobia without history of panic disorder.

Specify type:

> **Animal Type**
> **Natural Environment Type** (e.g., heights, storms, water)
> **Blood-Injection-Injury Type**
> **Situational Type** (e.g., airplanes, elevators, enclosed places)
> **Other Type** (e.g., fear of choking, vomiting, or contracting an illness; in children, fear of loud sounds or costumed characters)

Source.   From American Psychiatric Association: *Diagnostic and Statistical Manual of Mental Disorders*, 4th Edition, Text Revision. Washington, DC, American Psychiatric Association, 2000. Copyright 2000, American Psychiatric Association. Used with permission.

current, unexpected panic attacks (Table 31–4), as well as at least a month of persistent concern about having additional attacks, worry about the implications of the attacks (e.g., somatic preoccupations), or other behavioral changes related to the attacks.

Panic attacks are the hallmark of panic disorder, but they are also associated with other anxiety disorders (including specific phobia, social phobia, obsessive-compulsive disorder, and posttraumatic stress disorder). Panic attacks are discrete periods of fear or discomfort that develop abruptly and reach a peak rapidly and are associated with specific somatic and psychic symptoms (Table 31–4). Panic attacks may be unexpected or uncued, situationally bound (cued), or situationally predisposed. Unexpected panic attacks are required for the diagnosis of panic disorder. Situationally bound panic attacks are more characteristic of specific phobia and social phobia. Situationally predisposed panic attacks are common in panic disorder but also occur in individuals with specific phobia and social phobia.

Panic disorder may occur either with or without agoraphobia (Tables 31–2 and 31–3). Agoraphobia (Table 31–5) is characterized by "anxiety about being in places or situations from which escape might be difficult (or embarrassing) or in which help may not be available in the event of having a panic attack or panic-like symptoms" (American Psychiatric Association 2000, p. 432), as well as pervasive avoidance of the feared situations. Agoraphobia may also occur without a history of panic disorder (Table 31–6).

To meet DSM-IV-TR diagnostic criteria for *social phobia* (Table 31–7), the feared social situation or situations must elicit marked anxiety, resulting in interference with functioning or marked distress about experiencing the fear. Commonly feared situations include speaking in front of others, attending social gatherings, dealing with authority figures, performing in public, and speaking to strangers. As with specific phobia, adults recognize that the fear is excessive or unreasonable, but children may not.

Selective mutism (Table 31–8) is diagnosed in children who fail to speak in specific social situations for at least 1 month (not limited to the first month of school) and when the disturbance significantly interferes with educational or social functioning.

Table 31–2. DSM-IV-TR diagnostic criteria for panic disorder without agoraphobia

A. Both (1) and (2):

  (1) recurrent unexpected panic attacks

  (2) at least one of the attacks has been followed by 1 month (or more) of one (or more) of the following:

    (a) persistent concern about having additional attacks

    (b) worry about the implications of the attack or its consequences (e.g., losing control, having a heart attack, "going crazy")

    (c) a significant change in behavior related to the attacks

B. Absence of agoraphobia

C. The panic attacks are not due to the direct physiological effects of a substance (e.g., a drug of abuse, a medication) or a general medical condition (e.g., hyperthyroidism).

D. The panic attacks are not better accounted for by another mental disorder, such as social phobia (e.g., occurring on exposure to feared social situations), specific phobia (e.g., on exposure to a specific phobic situation), obsessive-compulsive disorder (e.g., on exposure to dirt in someone with an obsession about contamination), posttraumatic stress disorder (e.g., in response to stimuli associated with a severe stressor), or separation anxiety disorder (e.g., in response to being away from home or close relatives).

Source. From American Psychiatric Association: *Diagnostic and Statistical Manual of Mental Disorders,* 4th Edition, Text Revision. Washington, DC, American Psychiatric Association, 2000. Copyright 2000, American Psychiatric Association. Used with permission.

Table 31–3. DSM-IV-TR diagnostic criteria for panic disorder with agoraphobia

A. Both (1) and (2):

  (1) recurrent unexpected panic attacks

  (2) at least one of the attacks has been followed by 1 month (or more) of one (or more) of the following:

    (a) persistent concern about having additional attacks

    (b) worry about the implications of the attack or its consequences (e.g., losing control, having a heart attack, "going crazy")

    (c) a significant change in behavior related to the attacks

B. The presence of agoraphobia

C. The panic attacks are not due to the direct physiological effects of a substance (e.g., a drug of abuse, a medication) or a general medical condition (e.g., hyperthyroidism).

D. The panic attacks are not better accounted for by another mental disorder, such as social phobia (e.g., occurring on exposure to feared social situations), specific phobia (e.g., on exposure to a specific phobic situation), obsessive-compulsive disorder (e.g., on exposure to dirt in someone with an obsession about contamination), posttraumatic stress disorder (e.g., in response to stimuli associated with a severe stressor), or separation anxiety disorder (e.g., in response to being away from home or close relatives).

Source. From American Psychiatric Association: *Diagnostic and Statistical Manual of Mental Disorders,* 4th Edition, Text Revision. Washington, DC, American Psychiatric Association, 2000. Copyright 2000, American Psychiatric Association. Used with permission.

Clinical Findings

■ Specific Phobia

Many children have fears and anxieties; determining at what point the anxiety becomes "clinical" can be a fine distinction. Lapouse and Monk (1959) reported that 43% of interviewed mothers acknowledged that their children had seven or more fears. Ollendick (1983) reported that in 217 children, ages 3–11 years, the average number of extreme fears ranged from 9 to 13. The numerous general fears and anxieties of children decrease with age, and the specific focus of the fears changes (Evans et al. 1997; Graziano et al. 1979; Gullone 2000).

In examining the fears of children and adoles-

cents, it is important to maintain a developmental perspective, because some fears are common and appropriate at young ages. (An excellent review of the development of fears in children and adolescents is available in Marks 1987.) Infants' fears diminish during the preschool years. Preschool children are typically afraid of strangers, the dark, animals, or imaginary creatures. Children of elementary school age are more likely to be afraid of animals, darkness, threats to their own safety, or thunder and lightning. Older children are more concerned with health, social, and school fears. Adolescent fears may focus more on failure, sex, or agoraphobia (Marks 1987). If the fears persist into older ages or if there is significant and persistent distress or functional impairment, then clinical evaluation is indicated.

Specified in DSM-IV-TR are five subtypes of specific

Table 31–4.   DSM-IV-TR criteria for panic attack

Note: A panic attack is not a codable disorder. Code the specific diagnosis in which the panic attack occurs (e.g., 300.21 panic disorder with agoraphobia).

A discrete period of intense fear or discomfort, in which four (or more) of the following symptoms developed abruptly and reached a peak within 10 minutes:

    (1) palpitations, pounding heart, or accelerated heart rate
    (2) sweating
    (3) trembling or shaking
    (4) sensations of shortness of breath or smothering
    (5) feeling of choking
    (6) chest pain or discomfort
    (7) nausea or abdominal distress
    (8) feeling dizzy, unsteady, lightheaded, or faint
    (9) derealization (feelings of unreality) or depersonalization (being detached from oneself)
    (10) fear of losing control or going crazy
    (11) fear of dying
    (12) paresthesias (numbness or tingling sensations)
    (13) chills or hot flushes

Source.   From American Psychiatric Association: *Diagnostic and Statistical Manual of Mental Disorders,* 4th Edition, Text Revision. Washington, DC, American Psychiatric Association, 2000. Copyright 2000, American Psychiatric Association. Used with permission.

Table 31–5.   DSM-IV-TR criteria for agoraphobia

Note: Agoraphobia is not a codable disorder. Code the specific disorder in which the agoraphobia occurs (e.g., 300.21 panic disorder with agoraphobia or 300.22 agoraphobia without history of panic disorder).

A. Anxiety about being in places or situations from which escape might be difficult (or embarrassing) or in which help may not be available in the event of having an unexpected or situationally predisposed panic attack or panic-like symptoms. Agoraphobic fears typically involve characteristic clusters of situations that include being outside the home alone; being in a crowd or standing in a line; being on a bridge; and traveling in a bus, train, or automobile.

   Note: Consider the diagnosis of specific phobia if the avoidance is limited to one or only a few specific situations, or social phobia if the avoidance is limited to social situations.

B. The situations are avoided (e.g., travel is restricted) or else are endured with marked distress or with anxiety about having a panic attack or panic-like symptoms, or require the presence of a companion.
C. The anxiety or phobic avoidance is not better accounted for by another mental disorder, such as social phobia (e.g., avoidance limited to social situations because of fear of embarrassment), specific phobia (e.g., avoidance limited to a single situation like elevators), obsessive-compulsive disorder (e.g., avoidance of dirt in someone with an obsession about contamination), posttraumatic stress disorder (e.g., avoidance of stimuli associated with a severe stressor), or separation anxiety disorder (e.g., avoidance of leaving home or relatives).

Source.   From American Psychiatric Association: *Diagnostic and Statistical Manual of Mental Disorders,* 4th Edition, Text Revision. Washington, DC, American Psychiatric Association, 2000. Copyright 2000, American Psychiatric Association. Used with permission.

phobia: 1) animal type, 2) natural environment type (e.g., fears of storms, heights, or water), 3) blood-injection-injury type, 4) situational type (fear cued by specific situations such as tunnels, bridges, flying, or driving), and 5) other type. Animal type, natural environment type, and blood-injection-injury type all usually begin in childhood. Situational type has a bimodal onset, with one peak in childhood and another in early adulthood. Situational type appears to be closely related to panic disorder with agoraphobia (Verburg et al. 1994).

School phobia is sometimes used broadly with reference to children who refuse or resist going to school for any reason. In fact, children may resist going to school for a variety of reasons, including specific phobia, another anxiety disorder, depression, conduct dis-

Table 31–6. DSM-IV-TR diagnostic criteria for agoraphobia without history of panic disorder

A. The presence of agoraphobia related to fear of developing panic-like symptoms (e.g., dizziness or diarrhea).

B. Criteria have never been met for panic disorder.

C. The disturbance is not due to the direct physiological effects of a substance (e.g., a drug of abuse, a medication) or a general medical condition.

D. If an associated general medical condition is present, the fear described in Criterion A is clearly in excess of that usually associated with the condition.

Source. From American Psychiatric Association: *Diagnostic and Statistical Manual of Mental Disorders,* 4th Edition, Text Revision. Washington, DC, American Psychiatric Association, 2000. Copyright 2000, American Psychiatric Association. Used with permission.

order (truancy), substance abuse, or family psychopathology. A more precise use of the term *school phobia* would be restricted to describing a child's fear of something specific about the school situation, such as a specific teacher or peer, taking a shower after physical education class, or something encountered on the way to school (Black 1995).

■ Panic Disorder

Panic disorder with or without agoraphobia most often begins in adolescence or early adult life but may develop at any age (Abelson and Alessi 1992; Nelles and Barlow 1988). Many cases of both prepubertal and adolescent-onset panic disorder have now been described in the clinical literature (Biederman et al. 1997; Black 1995; Black and Robbins 1990; Black et al. 1990; King et al. 1993, 1997; Moreau and Weissman 1992). Likewise, several studies of adults with panic disorder have reported that many patients recalled the onset to be in childhood or adolescence (Thyer et al. 1985; von Korff et al. 1985).

The symptoms, course, and associated complications and comorbid conditions (agoraphobia, depression) in children and adolescents with panic disorder appear to be very similar to those observed in adults with panic disorder. The most commonly reported symptoms among adolescents with panic attacks are trembling, dizziness or faintness, pounding heart, nausea, shortness of breath, and sweating (Kearney et al. 1997). Cognitive symptoms are reported less frequently than somatic ones (King et al. 1997).

An important and common feature in children and adolescents is comorbid separation anxiety disorder (Black 1995). It is not uncommon for individuals with panic disorder at any age to fear and avoid separation from attachment figures. For adults, these attachment figures are most commonly spouses, parents, or close friends, whereas for children the figure is usually a parent. As suggested by Black et al. (1990), symptoms of separation anxiety disorder may develop in response to panic attacks and may be viewed as "manifestations of agoraphobia, with specific features (e.g., fear of school, fear of not being able to contact a parent *in the event of a panic attack*) that one might expect to see in an agoraphobic child" (p. 835). In fact, it is difficult to imagine how a child could experience recurrent panic attacks and not develop full-blown symptoms of separation anxiety disorder. The extreme distress that the child manifests when separation is threatened or imminent may be seen as a situationally predisposed panic attack.

Children with early development of separation anxiety disorder are at increased risk for later development of panic disorder (Biederman et al. 1993b). Most children described in the clinical literature with prepubertal onset of panic disorder—as well as many adolescents with panic disorder—also manifest symptoms of separation anxiety disorder, which are commonly the primary presenting symptoms (Black 1995). An association between adult-onset panic disorder and childhood anxiety, specifically separation anxiety disorder, has also been noted (Gittelman and Klein 1984). Klein (1964) stated that half of a sample of female adult patients with panic and agoraphobia had a history of separation anxiety or school phobia. The agoraphobic adults with a history of school phobia had an earlier age at onset for the agoraphobia than did those without this history. Offspring of parents with panic disorder have a more than threefold increased risk for separation anxiety disorder (Leckman et al. 1985; Weissman et al. 1984).

The exact explanation for the relationship between panic disorder and separation anxiety disorder is not clear. The childhood anxiety and avoidance symptoms might represent early manifestations of the same disorder, might predispose the adult to develop agoraphobia, or might reflect some more common anxiety symptomatology (Klein 1964). Several investigators have suggested that panic disorder and separation anxiety disorder may be different clinical manifestations of a common underlying disorder (Abelson

Table 31–7. DSM-IV-TR diagnostic criteria for social phobia

A. A marked and persistent fear of one or more social or performance situations in which the person is exposed to unfamiliar people or to possible scrutiny by others. The individual fears that he or she will act in a way (or show anxiety symptoms) that will be humiliating or embarrassing. **Note:** In children, there must be evidence of the capacity for age-appropriate social relationships with familiar people and the anxiety must occur in peer settings, not just in interactions with adults.

B. Exposure to the feared social situation almost invariably provokes anxiety, which may take the form of a situationally bound or situationally predisposed panic attack. **Note:** In children, the anxiety may be expressed by crying, tantrums, freezing, or shrinking from social situations with unfamiliar people.

C. The person recognizes that the fear is excessive or unreasonable. **Note:** In children, this feature may be absent.

D. The feared social or performance situations are avoided or else are endured with intense anxiety or distress.

E. The avoidance, anxious anticipation, or distress in the feared social or performance situation(s) interferes significantly with the person's normal routine, occupational (academic) functioning, or social activities or relationships, or there is marked distress about having the phobia.

F. In individuals under age 18 years, the duration is at least 6 months.

G. The fear or avoidance is not due to the direct physiological effects of a substance (e.g., a drug of abuse, a medication) or a general medical condition and is not better accounted for by another mental disorder (e.g., panic disorder with or without agoraphobia, separation anxiety disorder, body dysmorphic disorder, a pervasive developmental disorder, or schizoid personality disorder).

H. If a general medical condition or another mental disorder is present, the fear in Criterion A is unrelated to it, e.g., the fear is not of stuttering, trembling in Parkinson's disease, or exhibiting abnormal eating behavior in anorexia nervosa or bulimia nervosa.

Specify if:

  Generalized: if the fears include most social situations (also consider the additional diagnosis of avoidant personality disorder)

Source. From American Psychiatric Association: *Diagnostic and Statistical Manual of Mental Disorders,* 4th Edition, Text Revision. Washington, DC, American Psychiatric Association, 2000. Copyright 2000, American Psychiatric Association. Used with permission.

Table 31–8. DSM-IV-TR diagnostic criteria for selective mutism

A. Consistent failure to speak in specific social situations (in which there is an expectation for speaking, e.g., at school) despite speaking in other situations.

B. The disturbance interferes with educational or occupational achievement or with social communication.

C. The duration of the disturbance is at least 1 month (not limited to the first month of school).

D. The failure to speak is not due to a lack of knowledge of, or comfort with, the spoken language required in the social situation.

E. The disturbance is not better accounted for by a communication disorder (e.g., stuttering) and does not occur exclusively during the course of a pervasive developmental disorder, schizophrenia, or other psychotic disorder.

Source. From American Psychiatric Association: *Diagnostic and Statistical Manual of Mental Disorders,* 4th Edition, Text Revision. Washington, DC, American Psychiatric Association, 2000. Copyright 2000, American Psychiatric Association. Used with permission.

and Alessi 1992; Black and Robbins 1990; Klein 1981). For individuals with childhood separation anxiety disorder, the vulnerability to develop excessive distress when attachments are disrupted or threatened may be a stable personality trait throughout childhood and adolescence and into adulthood (Black 1995). Both anxiety symptoms (as manifested by separation anxiety and panic attacks) and depressive symptoms are expressed only when the separation or threat of separation actually occurs. Several studies have found an increased incidence of death or severe illness of a loved one preceding the onset of panic disorder in adults (Roy-Byrne et al. 1986) and adolescents (Black and Robbins 1990; Bradley and Hood 1993), as well as in children with separation anxiety disorder (Costello 1989). A heightened vulnerability to behavioral manifestations of separation distress has also been shown to be a relatively stable trait in nonhuman primates (Suomi et al. 1981). Recent work using a carbon dioxide inhalation procedure with children and adolescents suggests that child anxiety disorders in general and separation anxiety disorder in particular may share pathophysiological features with adult panic disorder (Pine et al. 2000).

■ Social Phobia

The primary features of social phobia are fearful apprehension, distress, and somatic symptoms in social situations in which the individual must interact with new or unfamiliar persons; fears of being evaluated or of being the center of attention; or fears that he or she might be embarrassed in some way. Individuals with social phobia commonly fear that others will find some fault with them; that others will consider them weird, unattractive, or stupid; or that they will do or say something foolish or embarrassing. Somatic symptoms are common and include racing heart, sweating, blushing, tremulousness, light-headedness, and diarrhea. These symptoms may be indistinguishable from a full-blown panic attack. Individuals with social phobia may fear that others will notice the somatic manifestations of their anxiety—such as tremulousness, sweating, or blushing—and that this will cause further embarrassment or ridicule.

Individuals with social phobia may fear one, several, or a wide variety of specific social situations. The most commonly feared situations are public speaking or performing, attending social gatherings, dealing with authority figures, and social interactions such as speaking to strangers or asking directions. Although some individuals with social phobia have very circumscribed fears, such as eating or writing in public or using public restrooms, most fear or avoid many different types of social situations. This clinical finding is part of the rationale that underlies the current trend in the field to refer to this set of symptoms as social anxiety disorder rather than as social phobia (Liebowitz et al. 2000).

Avoidant personality disorder is a closely related diagnostic category that is characterized by "a pervasive pattern of social inhibition, feelings of inadequacy, and hypersensitivity to negative evaluation" (American Psychiatric Association 2000, p. 721). There have been fewer empirical studies of avoidant personality disorder, and the validity of avoidant personality disorder as a distinct diagnostic category has been debated (Turner et al. 1992). The DSM-IV-TR diagnostic criteria for avoidant personality disorder include a pattern of enduring personality characteristics, whereas the DSM-IV-TR criteria for social phobia are more symptom focused. Empirical studies have shown considerable overlap between the two disorders; that is, many individuals meet criteria for both disorders.

An increasing number of studies are documenting the characteristics of children and adolescents with social phobia (Beidel 1991; Beidel et al. 1999; Black 1996; Francis et al. 1992; Last et al. 1987, 1992; Spence et al. 1999; Strauss and Last 1993). These studies have found that the disorder is valid, is not uncommon in clinic populations, and is associated with significant impairment. Significant comorbidity with other anxiety disorders and a high incidence of fear and avoidance of school have also been reported. More in-depth coverage of these issues can be found in the excellent review of the literature on the phenomenology, etiology, and treatment of social anxiety disorder in children and adolescents by Kashdan and Herbert (2001).

Young children with social phobia may cry, have a tantrum, or cling to or hide behind their mothers when confronted with a feared social situation, and they may be reluctant to attend school. Adolescents with social phobia may have great difficulty with dating or establishing any relationships with members of the opposite sex. Children and adolescents with social phobia may avoid participation in classroom activities, avoid class presentations, do poorly on tests or in presentations, and avoid physical education class. Generalized anxiety, multiple specific fears, somatization, school avoidance, and minor obsessive-compulsive symptoms are not uncommon (Beidel and Morris 1995; Black 1996; Francis et al. 1992). Children and adolescents with social phobia have significantly poorer social skills than psychiatrically healthy children (Beidel et al. 1999). Adolescents and young adults with social phobia may drop out of school or college or avoid classes in which classroom participation or presentation would be required. Occupational development may be impaired because of an inability to tolerate or to do well in job interviews or in social interactions at work. Individuals with social phobia have an increased incidence of alcohol abuse in adolescence and early adulthood, more suicidal ideation and suicide attempts, more physical and mental health problems, and greater use of health services than do individuals without social phobia (DeWit et al. 1999; Schneier et al. 1992; Uhde et al. 1991). Alcohol abuse seems to develop after the youth with social phobia discovers (accurately) that alcohol greatly reduces anxiety and facilitates peer interactions such as dating and attending parties (Clark et al. 1995).

■ Selective Mutism

The defining feature of selective mutism is the absence of speech (or an extreme reluctance to speak) in specific social situations in a child who is able to and does so in other situations (Dow et al. 1995). However, social situations are not easily dichotomized into mute and non-mute situations. Rather, the severity of mutism varies across a spectrum from situations in which speech is completely avoided to situations in which speech is completely uninhibited, not unlike the spectrum of social anxiety reported by persons with social phobia.

In a study of 30 school-referred children with selective mutism, Black and Uhde (1995) found that the severity of mutism varies among different types of social interactions, ranging from no reluctance to speak to siblings in the home to an almost complete avoidance of speech with unfamiliar adults at school. The children studied were significantly more reluctant to speak when away from home than at home (and most reluctant to speak at school), were more reluctant to speak to adults than to children, were more reluctant to speak to familiar nonfamily persons than to immediate family members, and were most reluctant to speak to unfamiliar nonfamily individuals. Although most children with selective mutism are markedly reluctant to speak with clinicians, the severity of mutism shown by the child in the clinician's office is not an accurate measure of the child's mutism severity in other settings or of his or her degree of improvement during the course of treatment (Black and Uhde 1995).

Some children with selective mutism will not communicate at all in their mute situations, whereas others may use gestures, head nodding or shaking, or whispering (Steinhausen and Juzi 1996). As children with selective mutism improve, many progress through stages, from virtually no social communication, to communicative facial gestures (e.g., communicative smiling), to gestures such as head-nodding, to limited whispering to more widespread whispering, and finally to normal social speech. Others make more abrupt jumps. Because social communication is intrinsically rewarding, once a mute, noncommunicative child starts to communicate more, his or her improvement is strongly reinforced. Therefore, it is not uncommon that a child will make no progress or very limited progress for very extended periods and then progress to normal social speech in a matter of days, as if a dam had finally broken.

Shyness, fear of embarrassment, and social withdrawal have been commonly mentioned as characteristics of children with selective mutism (Black and Uhde 1992; Kolvin and Fundudis 1981; Tancer 1992). Systematic assessment of children with selective mutism has revealed that nearly every child with selective mutism also meets criteria for either social phobia or avoidant disorder (Black and Uhde 1995; Dummit et al. 1997). In these investigations, social anxiety was the only behavioral feature (other than failure to speak) that stood out as an abnormal behavioral characteristic of the group as a whole. Social anxiety and selective mutism were generally reported to have developed at the same early age. Both parent and teacher behavioral ratings showed that social anxiety symptoms were significantly greater than all other symptom clusters and that only anxiety ratings (anxiety, separation anxiety, and social/performance anxiety) were significantly correlated with mutism severity, suggesting that the severity of the child's anxiety is a key factor determining the severity of mutism. Black and Uhde (1995) concluded that "the failure to speak in specific situations, which is the defining symptom of selective mutism, is a symptom of excessive social anxiety, specifically a fear of public speaking" and that "selective mutism is more appropriately viewed as a symptom or subtype of social phobia in children rather than as a distinct psychiatric disorder" (p. 854).

It has been widely suggested that early trauma is common among children with selective mutism and that selective mutism is often a posttraumatic disorder (Hayden 1980). However, empirical studies have failed to support this concept (Black and Uhde 1995). It has also been reported that children with selective mutism often demonstrate oppositional, stubborn, and negative personality traits and that their refusal to speak is primarily a manifestation of this oppositional and stubborn behavior (i.e., a struggle for control between the child and adults). Other reports have suggested that children with selective mutism often have a history of delayed speech and language development and high incidence rates of enuresis, encopresis, depression, and separation anxiety (Tancer 1992). However, none of these reported associations has been empirically validated, and the data reported by Black and Uhde (1995) did not confirm these associations.

Differential Diagnosis

There is considerable overlap among the different anxiety disorders in children and adolescents, as well as comorbidity with other anxiety disorders, depression, attention-deficit/hyperactivity disorder, and substance abuse (Clark et al. 1995; Curry and Murphy 1995). Anxious children seen in clinical settings often have multiple anxiety symptoms, including generalized anxiety and worry, somatic preoccupations, social anxiety, current or past separation anxiety, specific fears, mild obsessions or compulsions, and spontaneous panic attacks (often developing during early adolescence). The task of differentiating among the anxiety disorders and between anxiety symptoms and other disorders is often complicated in children because they are not yet able to report on the motivation behind their behaviors due to developmental differences in metacognitive awareness (Kashdan and Herbert 2001).

As noted above under "Clinical Findings," various anxiety disorders may cause panic attacks. When at least some of the attacks are uncued or spontaneous, the diagnosis of *panic disorder* is likely to be appropriate. Situationally bound or situationally predisposed panic attacks are common in specific phobia, social phobia, obsessive-compulsive disorder, and posttraumatic stress disorder, but they may also occur in panic disorder. *Specific phobia* is differentiated from posttraumatic stress disorder because the avoidance in posttraumatic stress disorder is directly related to the traumatic event. The avoidance in obsessive-compulsive disorder is related to the content of an obsession—for example, avoiding dirt or germs. Anxiety that is related primarily to separation from mother or father should be classified as *separation anxiety disorder*. When generalized anxiety or panic attacks are related to another medical condition (such as pheochromocytoma, hyperthyroidism, asthma, or encephalitis), the diagnosis of *anxiety disorder due to a general medical condition* should be made. *Substance-induced anxiety disorder* is diagnosed when anxiety or panic attacks occur in association with substance intoxication (e.g., caffeine or cocaine) or withdrawal (e.g., alcohol or sedative-hypnotics).

Epidemiology

■ Prevalence

Prevalence estimates for anxiety disorders vary widely among studies and are influenced by differences in diagnostic ascertainment, survey methodology, and sample characteristics (Costello and Angold 1995). Epidemiological studies have generally reported that anxiety disorders are common at all ages (Anderson et al. 1987; Bird et al. 1989; Kessler et al. 1994; Regier et al. 1988). Estimates of the prevalence of any anxiety disorder in studies with exclusively child and adolescent subjects range from 7.5% to nearly 26% (Anderson et al. 1987; Bird et al. 1989; Costello et al. 1988; Kashani and Orvaschel 1988, 1990).

For simple (specific) phobia, reported prevalence rates range from less than 1% to as high as 9.2%, and rates for social phobia range from 0% to 1.4%. Only one study has reported a prevalence estimate for panic disorder in young people. Whitaker and colleagues (1990) surveyed a large community sample of 14- to 17-year-olds and estimated the prevalence of panic disorder to be 0.6%. The incidence of panic attacks is much higher than the incidence of full-blown panic disorder and increases greatly with the onset of puberty (Hayward et al. 1992).

Social phobia has been estimated to occur in approximately 1% of children and adolescents (Anderson et al. 1987; Costello et al. 1988; Kashani and Orvaschel 1988, 1990). However, studies of the prevalence of social phobia among adults have reported rates from as low as 1.9% to as high as 18.7% (Schneier et al. 1992; Stein et al. 1994) depending on the cutoff criteria used to determine when an individual who reports significant social anxiety qualifies for a diagnosis of social phobia. Other studies have shown that up to 50%–60% of the population consider themselves to be shy or more anxious than others in social performance situations (Stein et al. 1994; Zimbardo 1977). These studies clearly indicate that social anxiety and the perception that one is more socially anxious than others are very common and that it is difficult to determine valid cutoff criteria for a disorder with common and continuously distributed traits. Recent research with adolescents suggests that lifetime prevalence rates for this age group are between 5% and 15% in the United States (Heimberg et al. 2000; Lewinsohn et al. 1993) and in Germany (Wittchen et al. 1999). Based on these figures and the reported early onset of social phobia in adults, it seems likely that the prevalence of 1% reported for social phobia in children may be a significant underestimate.

For selective mutism, two large-scale community-based epidemiological studies have reported prevalence rates. The Newcastle Epidemiologic Study reported a prevalence of 0.8 per 1,000 in a cohort of

7-year-old children (Fundudis et al. 1979). Brown and Lloyd (1975) reported the prevalence of selective mutism in young children: 8 weeks after the beginning of school the rate was 7 per 1,000, and 64 weeks after the beginning of school the rate was 0.17 per 1,000 (1 of 6,000). Thus, many more children appear to manifest selective mutism transiently after starting school rather than having more persistent selective mutism. More recently, two studies from Scandinavia reported higher prevalence rates among slightly older populations of children: 20 per 1,000 among second-graders in Finland (Kumpulainen et al. 1998), and 1.8 per 1,000 among school-age children (ages 7–15 years) in Sweden (Kopp and Gillberg 1997). A survey of teachers of kindergarten, first grade, and second grade in a Los Angeles school district revealed a prevalence of 7.1 per 1,000 (Bergman et al. 2002). Thus, prevalence estimates range from 0.03% to 2%. The variability in these estimates may be a function of the age of the children sampled, differences in the applications of the diagnostic criteria (i.e., differences in the threshold for considering a child mute), and vagueness of the DSM criteria in terms of the degree of impairment required.

■ Age at Onset

Solyom et al. (1986) compared 47 adults with social phobia, 80 adults with agoraphobia, and 72 adults with simple phobia. The subjects with social phobia experienced their first phobic symptoms earlier than the subjects with agoraphobia but later than those with simple phobia. The patients with simple phobia recalled the age at onset of their first symptoms to be 12.8 years on average, with onset of illness at 16.0 years; the patients with social phobia reported their age at onset to be 16.6 years for symptoms and 23.5 years for illness on average. Patients with agoraphobia had the latest age at onset at 24.5 years for symptoms and 26.0 years for illness on average.

The prevalence of panic attacks and panic disorder before puberty is unknown. However, numerous case reports have verified that the disorder does occur before puberty (Black and Robbins 1990; Black et al. 1990; Moreau and Weissman 1992), whereas retrospective studies of adults with panic disorder have shown that onset during adolescence is common. In 3,000 adults questioned retrospectively regarding age at onset of their panic disorder, the peak age at onset was between 15 and 20 years (von Korff et al. 1985). In a retrospective chart review of 62 adult patients with panic disorder without agoraphobia, the mean age at onset was 26.6 years, with 39% of patients reporting onset of symptoms before age 20 and 13% before age 10 years (Thyer et al. 1985). Among 95 patients with panic disorder with agoraphobia, the mean age at onset was 26.3 years, with 29% of these patients having onset before age 20 and 4% before age 10. In another study, 30 of 100 patients with panic disorder with agoraphobia reported that their first panic attack occurred before age 20, and 6 reported onset before age 10 (Sheehan et al. 1981b).

Social phobia has generally been shown to have an early age at onset, with a mean of 15 years and a bimodal distribution with peaks before age 5 years and at about age 13 years (Schneier et al. 1992). Of adult subjects with social phobia, 77% reported onset before age 20.

Onset for selective mutism is often insidious, with parents reporting that the child has "always been this way" (Leonard and Topol 1993). Data from recent studies document age at onset as early as 2.7–4.13 years (Black and Uhde 1995; Dummit et al. 1997; Kristensen 2000; Steinhausen and Juzi 1996).

Etiology

It has long been understood that specific phobias originate with a fright from the first encounter with the phobic stimulus, which results in a classical conditioning paradigm. However, the development of phobias to specific objects or situations clearly is not random among either humans or animals. Rather, both humans and animals are predisposed to develop phobias of specific objects or situations. Controversy has existed regarding whether learning or conditioning is necessary or whether specific phobias may develop in some genetically predisposed individuals without learning ever taking place (Gray 1982; Marks 1987). Research suggests that both genetic (innate) and environmental factors play a role (Kendler et al. 1992).

Family genetic studies have provided substantial evidence that risk for development of an anxiety disorder is strongly influenced by genetic factors. These studies include the following types:

- *Top-down* studies evaluating the prevalence of anxiety disorders in the offspring of adult probands
- *Bottom-up* studies evaluating the prevalence of anxiety disorders in adult relatives of child and adolescent probands

- *High-risk* longitudinal studies examining young offspring of adult probands with anxiety disorders
- *Twin* studies comparing rates of co-occurrence of anxiety disorders in monozygotic and dizygotic twin pairs (Last and Beidel 1991)

Lifetime morbidity risk for first-degree relatives of individuals with specific phobia, panic disorder, and social phobia is threefold to sixfold higher than for first-degree relatives of control subjects without anxiety disorders (Fyer et al. 1990, 1993; Last and Beidel 1991). Twin studies have found significantly greater proband-wise concordance rates among monozygotic twins than among dizygotic twins for specific phobias, panic disorder, and social phobia (Kendler et al. 1992). Black and Uhde (1995) found a high familial prevalence of selective mutism and social phobia among first-degree relatives of subjects with selective mutism. Because the prevalence of social phobia among family members was actually much higher than that of selective mutism, the researchers concluded that social phobia is transmitted familially to children with selective mutism and that selective mutism is merely a symptomatic expression of social phobia. One study, examining age at onset of panic disorder in families with multiple affected individuals in different generations, found a significant decrease in the time before the first episode of panic and onset of panic disorder in the younger generation relative to the older generation (Battaglia et al. 1998).

Although very little work has been done with children or adolescents, neurobiological and neurochemical abnormalities have been detected in individuals with anxiety disorders (see Pine 2002 for a comprehensive review of this literature). For example, panic attacks can be provoked in individuals with panic disorder by administering chemical agents, including sodium lactate, caffeine, cholecystokinin, and carbon dioxide (through inhalation). These responses are specific to patients with panic disorder. Control subjects without anxiety disorder and patients with other anxiety disorders do not have the same responses, and patients with panic disorder do not have panic attacks in response to placebo infusions. Pretreatment with specific pharmacological agents before chemical challenge blocks induction of anxiety symptoms. The differences in responses of individuals with and without panic disorder suggest that the neurobiological mechanisms controlling anxiety are abnormal in the individuals with panic disorder. Recent work examining

the pathophysiological mechanism underlying carbon dioxide–induced panic attacks suggests that spontaneous panic is different from anticipatory anxiety because the hypothalamic–pituitary axis is not activated in the former condition, whereas it is in the latter (Sinha et al. 1999). This work has been replicated in children and adolescents (Coplan et al. 2002). Unique associations with respiratory dysregulation have also been found in patients with panic disorder and their asymptomatic first-degree relatives (Klein 1994; Papp et al. 1989; Pine et al. 1998). Asymptomatic first-degree relatives of patients with panic disorder have also demonstrated heightened sensitivity to carbon dioxide inhalation (Coryell et al. 2001).

Neurochemically, regulatory dysfunction in brain monamine and γ-aminobutyric acid systems have been implicated in anxiety disorders (Crestani et al. 1999; Malizia et al. 1998; Roy-Byrne et al. 1996). In adults with panic disorder and social phobia, neuroendocrine abnormalities have been found, including a hyporesponsive hypothalamic growth hormone axis, as indicated by blunted growth hormone responses to pharmacological or physiological challenge (Uhde et al. 1992).

Conditioning or learning models postulate that anxiety is a learned response to noxious stimuli and that the acquisition of anxious or fearful reactions occurs as a result of conditioning or the linking of a previously benign conditioned stimulus to a noxious unconditioned stimulus. Biological and conditioning models are increasingly being integrated; the biological models illustrate how some individuals are either more or less predisposed or vulnerable to the development of anxiety disorders, whereas conditioning models illustrate how environmental or psychological factors may precipitate the development of an anxiety disorder in a vulnerable individual and can influence the course of the disorder and the development of complications (Barlow 1988). Recent evidence suggests that fear learning may be different in adults with anxiety disorders and in their children compared with unaffected individuals (Grillon et al. 1991, 1997a, 1997b, 1998a, 1998b; Merikangas et al. 1999; Pine and Grun 1999).

Children with panic disorder, social phobia, and selective mutism may have much in common with behaviorally inhibited children. *Behavioral inhibition* refers to an enduring temperamental trait characterized by quiet, withdrawing, and timid behavior; reluctance to speak; and a state of neurophysiological arousal in response to novel situations, including interaction with unfamiliar adults (Biederman et al. 1993a; Kagan et al. 1987). Defined laboratory paradigms have been developed to classify young children as either more or less behaviorally inhibited. Longitudinal studies assessing the stability of behavioral inhibition and risk for development of psychiatric disorder have found that children identified as behaviorally inhibited during early childhood remain inhibited at follow-up in middle childhood, are markedly reluctant to speak to unfamiliar persons in unfamiliar environments, and are at increased risk for the development of anxiety disorders (Biederman et al. 1993b). Schwartz et al. (1999) reported some specificity in terms of the risk conveyed by behavioral inhibition. They reported that 13-year-olds who had been classified as behaviorally inhibited when they were toddlers were more likely to have generalized social anxiety compared with their uninhibited peers. In this study, 34% of the adolescents who were originally classified as behaviorally inhibited met criteria for social phobia at age 13. Family studies have shown a high familial prevalence of social phobia and childhood anxiety disorders among first-degree relatives of inhibited children. Likewise, studies of offspring of adults with panic disorder with agoraphobia have found that 85% are behaviorally inhibited compared with 15% of the offspring of psychiatrically healthy control parents (Rosenbaum et al. 1988).

Treatment

■ Specific Phobia

The most successful treatment approach for children with specific phobia appears to be graduated in vivo exposure in combination with contingency management and self-control strategies (Morris and Kratochwill 1998; Silverman et al. 1999a). In vivo exposure involves gradually bringing the child into contact with progressively more distressful variations on phobic stimuli. Habituation and teaching the child to cope with the anxious feelings are the two primary principles that underlie this approach. Contingency management techniques entail using differential reinforcement to shape the phobic child's behavior. Desired behaviors (e.g., approaching phobic stimuli) are rewarded, and maladaptive behaviors (e.g., avoidance behaviors) are not. Self-control strategies use the cognitive tools of self-evaluation and self-reward to ac-

complish the same ends. Excellent reviews of the behavioral treatments of phobias are available elsewhere (Drobes and Strauss 1993; Marks 1987).

Although pharmacological treatments have not been shown to be effective for specific phobias, many children with specific phobias also have generalized anxiety or other anxiety disorders and may benefit from pharmacotherapy. Please refer to Fyer (1987) for a review of the pharmacological treatment of phobic disorders and to Riddle and colleagues (1999) and Velosa and Riddle (2000) for excellent comprehensive reviews of pharmacological treatment of pediatric anxiety disorders.

■ Panic Disorder

Adult studies have reported the efficacy of tricyclic antidepressants, monoamine oxidase inhibitors, selective serotonin reuptake inhibitors (SSRIs), and benzodiazepines for panic disorder (Schneier et al. 1990; Sheehan et al. 1981a; Spier et al. 1986). Although no controlled studies of the psychopharmacological treatment of panic disorder have been done in children, case reports suggest that childhood-onset panic disorder may be similar in its pharmacological response to that seen in adults (Biederman 1987; Black and Robbins 1990; Kutcher and MacKenzie 1988). Although no systematic treatment trials of SSRIs in children have been conducted, SSRIs are emerging in clinical practice as the first-line medication treatment of choice. Preliminary evidence in support of the use of paroxetine is provided by the 83% response rate reported in a recent open-label study of 18 children and adolescents with panic disorder (Masi et al. 2001). More systematic studies are necessary. Likewise, cognitive and behavioral treatments have proved effective in the treatment of adults with panic disorder (Barlow and Cerney 1988), and preliminary evidence suggests that they are also effective in children and adolescents (Drobes and Strauss 1993; Hoffman and Mattis 2000; Ollendick 1995).

■ Social Phobia

Results of a large-scale systematic study of fluvoxamine in children and adolescents with social phobia, separation anxiety disorder, or generalized anxiety disorder provide the first solid evidence of effective pharmacotherapy for social phobia in children and adolescents (Research Unit on Pediatric Psychopharmacology

Anxiety Study Group 2001). In this study 128 children and adolescents (ages 6–17) were assigned to either fluvoxamine or placebo for 8 weeks. Seventy-six percent of the children in the fluvoxamine group showed significant improvement on the Clinical Global Impression Scale, as opposed to only 29% of children in the placebo group. Similarly, Birmaher et al. (1994) reported that the open treatment with fluoxetine of a mixed group of 21 children and adolescents with anxiety disorders (social phobia, overanxious disorder, or separation anxiety disorder) had generally favorable outcomes. The SSRIs should be considered the pharmacological treatments of choice. Phenelzine may be effective in patients who do not respond to SSRI treatment, but this agent should be used with great caution in adolescents and never in preadolescent children. In general, pharmacotherapy should not be used as the sole intervention for children with social phobia, although it may play an important role in a multimodal treatment plan that includes intensive behavioral intervention (Freeman et al. 2002).

To date, there have been 12 published studies demonstrating the efficacy of cognitive-behavioral treatment approaches for children or adolescents with social phobia. The treatment approaches used in 8 of these 12 studies were designed to treat child anxiety disorders in general (Barrett et al. 1996; Flannery-Schroeder and Kendall 2000; Kendall 1994; Kendall et al. 1997; Lumpkin et al. 2002; Silverman et al. 1999a, 1999b; Manassis et al. 2002). Although these studies did not focus on social phobia, children with social phobia were included in the trials. However, the strength of the treatment effect for social phobia cannot be measured directly from results of these more generalized anxiety treatment studies. Three studies have reported positive results for group treatments designed specifically to target social phobia in children or adolescents (Albano et al. 1995; Beidel et al. 2000; Hayward et al. 2000). To date, one study (Spence et al. 2000) has reported positive effects of two cognitive-behavioral interventions (individual CBT and CBT plus parental involvement) that specifically targeted social phobia in children and adolescents. Although the formats have differed somewhat across studies (e.g., group versus individual versus family; specific focus on social phobia versus anxiety disorders in general), four treatment components were present in all of the interventions: psychoeducation, exposure, skill building (e.g., relaxation training, cognitive restructuring, social skills, problem-solving skills), and home-

work assignments (Kashdan and Herbert 2001). Pilot work investigating the school-based provision of cognitive-behavioral treatment to affected adolescents is also promising (Masia et al. 2001). Clearly, combined treatment trials are needed to study the relative efficacy of medication, cognitive-behavioral treatment, and their combination.

■ Selective Mutism

The evidence-based treatment literature on pharmacotherapy for selective mutism is limited. To date, the majority of this work has been single case studies using monoamine oxidase inhibitors or SSRIs (Black and Uhde 1992; Carlson et al. 1999; Golwyn and Sevlie 1999; Golwyn and Weinstock 1990; Harvey and Milne 1998; Thomsen et al. 1999; Wright et al. 1995). There have also been two more systematic studies using fluoxetine, one an open treatment trial (Dummit et al. 1996) and one a small, double-blind, placebo-controlled trial (Black and Uhde 1994). In the double-blind, placebo-controlled study of 16 children, fluoxetine was shown to be superior to placebo (Black and Uhde 1994). Subjects treated with fluoxetine were significantly more improved on parents' ratings of mutism change and global change at 12 weeks. Parents rated 4 of 6 fluoxetine-treated subjects but only 1 of 9 placebo-treated subjects as significantly improved after 12 weeks. Interestingly, of the 4 fluoxetine responders at 12 weeks, none had responded after 4 weeks of treatment, and only 1 had responded after 8 weeks of treatment. Clinician and teacher ratings did not indicate significant differences between treatment groups. Although improvement occurred, most subjects in both treatment groups remained very symptomatic at the end of the study period.

A sizable body of literature exists on empirical but uncontrolled studies regarding the behavioral treatment of selective mutism. The details of these studies are provided in several comprehensive reviews of this literature (Anstendig 1998; Cline and Baldwin 1994; Kratchowill 1981). Contingency management, exposure-based techniques, and self-modeling are the techniques most frequently employed. Although these studies have some methodological limitations, taken together they suggest that behavioral treatment approaches are often effective in the treatment of selective mutism.

Individual psychodynamically oriented therapy, play therapy, and family therapy are all very commonly used for children with selective mutism. However, the evidence base for these types of treatment is limited, and many methodological issues impede drawing conclusions about their efficacy. In the largest published studies of psychodynamic psychotherapy for selective mutism, Browne and colleagues (1963) and Wergeland (1979) concluded that the treatment was lengthy and the outcome poor.

Prognosis

Little is known about the outcome of children with specific phobia later in life. In a 5-year follow-up study of an epidemiological sample, Agras et al. (1972) found that of 10 children with diagnoses of phobias, all had either improved or recovered. Hampe et al. (1973) saw phobic children at 2-year follow-up and found that 80% were symptom free but that 7% had "serious fear reactions." Because specific phobias are amenable to behavioral treatment, one might hypothesize that treated patients would have a better long-term outcome.

Because panic disorder, social phobia, and selective mutism diagnoses have only recently received attention in children, the long-term outcome of these children is unknown. However, longitudinal studies with adults indicate that panic disorder and social phobia are often chronic disorders, and clinical experience suggests that this also tends to be the case for those with onset in childhood or adolescence (Black 1995, 1996).

Selective mutism, diagnosed according to DSM-IV-TR criteria, almost always resolves during childhood, with or without treatment. However, if selective mutism is viewed instead as a symptom of social phobia, the prognosis is poorer, because most children with selective mutism probably continue to have social phobia even after the selective mutism resolves (Black 1996).

Research Issues

None of the disorders described in this chapter have yet been adequately characterized. Specific phobia is the best described of these disorders, but few studies distinguish between exaggerated fears and the clinical cases. Longitudinal and outcome studies, family studies, and studies assessing the interaction of environmental and genetic factors in determining the risk for the development of these disorders are needed. Although the treatment literature has grown in the last decade, there is still a need for controlled treatment studies to systematically assess the effectiveness of disorder-specific pharmacological and psychosocial treatments, particularly when applied in combination.

References

Abelson JL, Alessi NE: Discussion of child panic revisited. J Am Acad Child Adolesc Psychiatry 31:114–116, 1992

Agras WS, Chapin HN, Oliveau DC: The natural history of phobia. Arch Gen Psychiatry 26:315–317, 1972

Albano AM, Marten PA, Holt CS, et al: Cognitive-behavioral group treatment for social phobia in adolescents: a preliminary study. J Nerv Ment Dis 183:649–656, 1995

American Psychiatric Association: Diagnostic and Statistical Manual of Mental Disorders, 4th Edition, Text Revision. Washington, DC, American Psychiatric Association, 2000

Anderson JC, Williams S, McGee R, et al: DSM-III disorders in preadolescent children. Arch Gen Psychiatry 44:69–76, 1987

Anstendig K: Selective mutism: a review of the treatment literature by modality from 1980–1996. Psychotherapy 35:381–391, 1998

Barlow DH: Current models of panic disorder and a view from emotion theory, in American Psychiatric Press Review of Psychiatry, Vol 7. Edited by Frances AJ, Hales RE. Washington, DC, American Psychiatric Press, 1988, pp 10–28

Barlow DH, Cerney JA: Psychological Treatment of Panic. New York, Guilford, 1988

Barrett PB, Dadds MR, Rapee RM: Family treatment of childhood anxiety: a controlled trial. J Consult Clin Psychol 64:333–342, 1996

Battaglia M, Bertella S, Bajo S, et al: Anticipation of age at onset in panic disorder. Am J Psychiatry 155:590–595, 1998

Beidel DC: Social phobia and overanxious disorder in school-age children. J Am Acad Child Adolesc Psychiatry 30:545–552, 1991

Beidel DC, Morris TL: Social phobia, in Anxiety Disorders in Children and Adolescents. Edited by March JS. New York, Guilford, 1995, pp 181–211

Beidel DC, Turner SM, Morris TL: Psychopathology of childhood social phobia. J Am Acad Child Adolesc Psychiatry 38:643–650, 1999

Beidel DC, Turner SM, Morris TL: Behavioral treatment of childhood social phobia. J Consult Clin Psychol 68:1072–1080, 2000

Bergman RL, Piacentini J, McCracken JT: Prevalence and description of selective mutism in a school-based sample. J Am Acad Child Adolesc Psychiatry 41:938–946, 2002

Biederman J: Clonazepam in the treatment of prepubertal children with panic-like symptoms. J Clin Psychiatry 48:38–41, 1987

Biederman J, Rosenbaum JF, Bolduc-Murphy EA, et al: Behavioral inhibition as a temperamental risk factor for anxiety disorders. Child Adolesc Psychiatr Clin N Am 2:667–684, 1993a

Biederman J, Rosenbaum JF, Bolduc-Murphy EA, et al: A 3-year follow-up of children with and without behavioral inhibition. J Am Acad Child Adolesc Psychiatry 32:814–821, 1993b

Biederman J, Faraone SV, Marrs A, et al: Panic disorder and agoraphobia in consecutively referred children and adolescents. J Am Acad Child Adolesc Psychiatry 36:214–223, 1997

Bird HR, Gould MS, Yager T, et al: Risk factors for maladjustment in Puerto Rican children. J Am Acad Child Adolesc Psychiatry 28:847–850, 1989

Birmaher B, Waterman GS, Ryan N, et al: Fluoxetine for childhood anxiety disorders. J Am Acad Child Adolesc Psychiatry 33:993–999, 1994

Black B: Separation anxiety disorder and panic disorder, in Anxiety Disorders in Children and Adolescents. Edited by March JS. New York, Guilford, 1995, pp 212–234

Black B: Social anxiety and selective mutism, in American Psychiatric Press Review of Psychiatry, Vol 15. Edited by Dickstein LJ, Riba MB, Oldham JM. Washington, DC, American Psychiatric Press, 1996, pp 469–495

Black B, Robbins DR: Panic disorder in children and adolescents. J Am Acad Child Adolesc Psychiatry 29:36–44, 1990

Black B, Uhde TW: Elective mutism as a variant of social phobia. J Am Acad Child Adolesc Psychiatry 31:1090–1094, 1992

Black B, Uhde TW: Treatment of elective mutism with fluoxetine: a double-blind, placebo-controlled study. J Am Acad Child Adolesc Psychiatry 33:1000–1006, 1994

Black B, Uhde TW: Psychiatric characteristics of children with selective mutism: a pilot study. J Am Acad Child Adolesc Psychiatry 34:847–856, 1995

Black B, Uhde TW, Robbins DR: Reply to Klein DF, Klein RG: Does panic disorder exist in childhood? (letter). J Am Acad Child Adolesc Psychiatry 29:834–835, 1990

Bradley SJ, Hood J: Psychiatrically referred adolescents with panic attacks: presenting symptoms, stressors, and comorbidity. J Am Acad Child Adolesc Psychiatry 32:826–829, 1993

Brown JB, Lloyd H: A controlled study of children not speaking at school. Journal of the Association of Workers With Maladjusted Children 3:49–63, 1975

Browne E, Wilson V, Laybourne PC: Diagnosis and treatment of elective mutism in children. J Am Acad Child Adolesc Psychiatry 2:605–617, 1963

Carlson JS, Kratochwill TR, Johnson HF: Sertraline treatment of 5 children diagnosed with selective mutism: a single-case research trial. J Child Adolesc Psychopharmacol 9:293–306, 1999

Clark DB, Bukstein OG, Smith MG, et al: Identifying anxiety disorders in adolescents hospitalized for alcohol abuse or dependence. Psychiatr Serv 46:618–620, 1995

Cline T, Baldwin S: Selective Mutism in Children. San Diego, CA, Singular, 1994

Coplan JD, Moreau D, Chaput F, et al: Salivary cortisol concentrations before and after carbon-dioxide inhalations in children. Biol Psychiatry 51:326–333, 2002

Coryell W, Fyer A, Pine D, et al: Aberrant respiratory sensitivity to CO_2 as a trait of familial panic disorder. Biol Psychiatry 49:582–587, 2001

Costello EJ: Child psychiatric disorders and their correlates: a primary care pediatric sample. J Am Acad Child Adolesc Psychiatry 28:851–855, 1989

Costello EJ, Angold A: Epidemiology, in Anxiety Disorders in Children and Adolescents. Edited by March JS. New York, Guilford, 1995, pp 109–124

Costello EJ, Costello AJ, Edelbrock C, et al: Psychiatric disorders in pediatric primary care: prevalence and risk factors. Arch Gen Psychiatry 45:1107–1116, 1988

Crestani F, Lorez M, Baer K, et al: Decreased GABA-receptor clustering results in enhanced anxiety and a bias for threat cues. Nat Neurosci 2:833–839, 1999

Curry JF, Murphy LB: Comorbidity of anxiety disorders, in Anxiety Disorders in Children and Adolescents. Edited by March JS. New York, Guilford, 1995, pp 301–320

DeWit DJ, MacDonald K, Offord DR: Childhood stress and symptoms of drug dependence in adolescents and early adulthood: social phobia as a mediator. Am J Orthopsychiatry 69:61–71, 1999

Dow SP, Sonies BC, Scheib D, et al: Practical guidelines for the assessment and treatment of selective mutism. J Am Acad Child Adolesc Psychiatry 34:836–846, 1995

Drobes DJ, Strauss CC: Behavioral treatment of childhood anxiety disorders. Child Adolesc Psychiatr Clin N Am 2:779–794, 1993

Dummit ES 3rd, Klein RG, Tancer NK, et al: Fluoxetine treatment of children with selective mutism: an open trial. J Am Acad Child Adolesc Psychiatry 35:615–621, 1996

Dummit ES 3rd, Klein RG, Tancer NK, et al: Systematic assessment of 50 children with selective mutism. J Am Acad Child Adolesc Psychiatry 36:653–660, 1997

Evans DW, Leckman JF, Carter A, et al: Ritual, habit, and perfectionism: the prevalence and development of compulsive-like behavior in normal young children. Child Dev 68:58–68, 1997

Flannery-Schroeder E, Kendall PC: Group and individual cognitive-behavioral treatments for youth with anxiety disorders: a randomized clinical trial. Cognit Ther Res 24:251–278, 2000

Francis G, Last CG, Strauss CC: Avoidant disorder and social phobia in children and adolescents. J Am Acad Child Adolesc Psychiatry 31:1086–1089, 1992

Freeman JB, Garcia AM, Leonard HL: Anxiety disorders, in Child and Adolescent Psychiatry: A Comprehensive Textbook, 3rd Edition. Edited by Lewis M. Baltimore, MD, Williams and Wilkins, 2002, pp 821–834

Fundudis T, Kolvin I, Garside RF: Speech Retarded and Deaf Children: Their Psychological Development. London, Academic Press, 1979

Fyer AJ: Simple phobia. Mod Probl Pharmacopsychiatry 22:174–192, 1987

Fyer AJ, Mannuzza S, Gallops MS, et al: Familial transmission of simple phobia and fears: a preliminary report. Arch Gen Psychiatry 47:252–256, 1990

Fyer AJ, Mannuzza S, Chapman TF, et al: A direct interview family study of social phobia. Arch Gen Psychiatry 50:286–293, 1993

Gittelman R, Klein DF: Relationship between separation anxiety and panic and agoraphobic disorders. Psychopathology 17 (suppl 1):56–65, 1984

Golwyn DH, Sevlie CP: Phenelzine treatment of selective mutism in four prepubertal children. J Child Adolesc Psychopharmacol 9:109–113, 1999

Golwyn DH, Weinstock RC: Phenelzine treatment of elective mutism. J Clin Psychiatry 51:384–385, 1990

Gray JA: The Neuropsychology of Anxiety. New York, Oxford University Press, 1982

Graziano AM, DeGiovanni IS, Garcia K: Behavioral treatment of children's fears: a review. Psychol Bull 86:804–830, 1979

Grillon C, Ameli R, Woods SW, et al: Fear-potentiated startle in humans: effects of anticipatory anxiety on the acoustic blink reflex. Psychophysiology 28:588–595, 1991

Grillon C, Dierker L, Merikangas K: Startle modulation in children at risk for anxiety disorders and/or alcoholism. J Am Acad Child Adolesc Psychiatry 36:925–932, 1997a

Grillon C, Pellowski M, Merikangas K, et al: Darkness facilitates the acoustic startle reflex in humans. Biol Psychiatry 42:453–460, 1997b

Grillon C, Dierker L, Merikangas K: Fear potentiated startle in adolescent offspring of parents with anxiety disorders. Biol Psychiatry 44:990–997, 1998a

Grillon C, Morgan CA, Davis M, et al: Effect of darkness on acoustic startle in Vietnam veterans with PTSD. Am J Psychiatry 155:812–817, 1998b

Gullone E: The development of normal fear: a century of research. Clin Psychol Rev 20:429–451, 2000

Hampe E, Noble H, Miller LC, et al: Phobic children one and two years posttreatment. J Abnorm Psychol 82:446–453, 1973

Harvey BH, Milne M: Pharmacotherapy of selective mutism: two case studies of severe entrenched mutism responsive to adjunctive treatment with fluoxetine. South African Journal of Child and Adolescent Mental Health 10:59–66, 1998

Hayden TL: Classification of elective mutism. J Am Acad Child Psychiatry 19:118–133, 1980

Hayward C, Killen JD, Hammer LD, et al: Pubertal stage and panic attack history in sixth- and seventh-grade girls. Am J Psychiatry 149:1239–1243, 1992

Hayward C, Varady S, Albano AM, et al: Cognitive-behavioral group therapy for social phobia in female adolescents: results of a pilot study. J Am Acad Child Adolesc Psychiatry 39:721–726, 2000

Heimberg RG, Stein MB, Hiripi E: Trends in the prevalence of social phobia in the United States: a cohort analysis of changes over four decades. Eur Psychiatry 15:29–37, 2000

Hoffman EC, Mattis SG: A developmental adaptation of panic control treatment for panic disorder in adolescence. Cognitive and Behavioral Practice 7:253–261, 2000

Kagan J, Reznick JS, Snidman N: The physiology and psychology of behavioral inhibition in young children. Child Dev 58:1459–1473, 1987

Kashani JH, Orvaschel H: Anxiety disorders in mid-adolescence: a community sample. Am J Psychiatry 145:960–964, 1988

Kashani JH, Orvaschel H: A community study of anxiety in children and adolescents. Am J Psychiatry 147:313–318, 1990

Kashdan TB, Herbert JD: Social anxiety disorder in childhood and adolescence: current status and future directions. Clin Child Fam Psychol Rev 4:37–61, 2001

Kearney CA, Albano AM, Eisen AR, et al: The phenomenology of panic disorder in youngsters: an empirical study of a clinical sample. J Anxiety Disord 11:49–62, 1997

Kendall PC: Treating anxiety disorders in youth: results of a randomized clinical trial. J Consult Clin Psychol 62:100–110, 1994

Kendall PC, Flannery-Schroeder E, Panichelli-Mindel SM, et al: Therapy for youths with anxiety disorders: a second randomized clinical trial. J Consult Clin Psychol 65:366–380, 1997

Kendler KS, Neale MC, Kessler RC, et al: The genetic epidemiology of phobias in women: the interrelationship of agoraphobia, social phobia, situational phobia, and simple phobia. Arch Gen Psychiatry 49:273–281, 1992

Kessler RC, McGonagle KA, Zhao S, et al: Lifetime and 12-month prevalence of DSM-III-R psychiatric disorders in the United States: results from the National Comorbidity Survey. Arch Gen Psychiatry 51:8–19, 1994

King NJ, Gullone E, Tonge BJ, et al: Self-reports of panic attacks and manifest anxiety in adolescents. Behav Res Ther 31:111–116, 1993

King NJ, Ollendick TH, Mattis SG, et al: New clinical panic attacks in adolescents: prevalence, symptomatology, and associated features. Behav Change 13:171–183, 1997

Klein DF: Delineation of two drug-responsive anxiety syndromes. Psychopharmacologia 5:397–408, 1964

Klein DF: Anxiety reconceptualized, in Anxiety: New Research and Changing Concepts. Edited by Klein DF, Rabkin J. New York, Raven, 1981, pp 235–263

Klein DF: Testing the suffocation false alarm theory of panic disorder. Anxiety 1:144–148, 1994

Kolvin I, Fundudis T: Elective mute children: psychological development and background factors. J Child Psychol Psychiatry 22:219–232, 1981

Kopp S, Gillberg C: Selective mutism: a population-based study: a research note. J Child Psychol Psychiatry 38:257–262, 1997

Kratchowill TR: Selective Mutism: Implications for Research and Treatment. Hillsdale, NJ, Erlbaum, 1981

Kristensen H: Selective mutism and comorbidity with developmental disorder/delay, anxiety disorder, and elimination disorder. J Am Acad Child Adolesc Psychiatry 39:249–256, 2000

Kumpulainen K, Rasanen E, Raaska H, et al: Selective mutism among second-graders in elementary school. Eur Child Adolesc Psychiatry 7:24–29, 1998

Kutcher SP, MacKenzie S: Successful clonazepam treatment of adolescents with panic disorder. J Clin Psychopharmacol 8:299–300, 1988

Lapouse R, Monk MA: Fears and worries in a representative sample of children. Am J Orthopsychiatry 29:223–248, 1959

Last CG, Beidel DC: Anxiety, in Child and Adolescent Psychiatry: A Comprehensive Textbook. Edited by Lewis M. Baltimore, MD, Williams & Wilkins, 1991, pp 281–292

Last CG, Strauss CG, Francis G: Comorbidity among childhood anxiety disorders. J Nerv Ment Dis 175:726–730, 1987

Last CG, Perrin S, Hersen M, et al: DSM-III-R anxiety disorders in children: sociodemographic and clinical characteristics. J Am Acad Child Adolesc Psychiatry 31:1070–1076, 1992

Leckman JF, Weissman MM, Merikangas KR, et al: Major depression and panic disorder. Psychopharmacol Bull 21:543–545, 1985

Leonard HL, Topol DA: Elective mutism, in Anxiety Disorders, Vol 2. Philadelphia, WB Saunders, 1993, pp 695–707

Lewinsohn PM, Hops H, Roberts RE, et al: Adolescent psychopathology: I. Prevalence and incidence of depression and other DSM-III-R disorders in high school students. J Abnorm Psychol 102:133–144, 1993

Liebowitz MR, Heimberg RG, Fresco DM: Social phobia or social anxiety disorder: what's in a name? (letter). Arch Gen Psychiatry 57:191–192, 2000

Lumpkin PW, Silverman WK, Weems CF, et al: Treating a heterogeneous set of anxiety disorders in youths with group cognitive behavioral therapy: a partially nonconcurrent multiple-baseline evaluation. Behav Ther 33:163–177, 2002

Malizia AL, Cunningham VJ, Bell CJ, et al: Decreased brain GABA(A)-benzodiazepine receptor binding in panic disorder: preliminary results from a quantitative PET study. Arch Gen Psychiatry 55:715–720, 1998

Manassis K, Mendlowitz SL, Scapillato D, et al: Group and individual cognitive-behavioral therapy for childhood anxiety disorders: a randomized trial. J Am Acad Child Adolesc Psychiatry 41:1423–1430, 2002

Marks IM: Fears, Phobias, and Rituals. New York, Oxford University Press, 1987

Masi G, Toni C, Mucci M, et al: Paroxetine in child and adolescent outpatients with panic disorder. J Child Adolesc Psychopharmacol 11:151–157, 2001

Masia CL, Klein RG, Storch EA, et al: School-based behavioral treatment for social anxiety disorder in adolescents: results of a pilot study. J Am Acad Child Adolesc Psychiatry 40:780–786, 2001

Merikangas KR, Avenevoli S, Dierker L, et al: Vulnerability factors among children at risk for anxiety disorders. Biol Psychiatry 46:1523–1535, 1999

Moreau D, Weissman MM: Panic disorder in children and adolescents: a review. Am J Psychiatry 149:1306–1314, 1992

Morris RJ, Kratochwill TR: Childhood fears and phobias, in The Practice of Child Therapy, 3rd Edition. Edited by Kratochwill TR, Morris RJ. Needham Heights, MA, Allyn & Bacon, 1998, pp 91–131

Nelles WB, Barlow DH: Do children panic? Clin Psychol Rev 8:359–372, 1988

Ollendick TH: Reliability and validity of the Revised Fear Surgery Schedule for Children (FSSC-R). Behav Res Ther 21:685–692, 1983

Ollendick TH: Cognitive-behavioral treatment of panic disorder with agoraphobia in adolescents: a multiple baseline design analysis. Behav Ther 26:517–531, 1995

Papp LA, Goetz R, Cole R, et al: Hypersensitivity to carbon dioxide in panic disorder. Am J Psychiatry 146:779–781, 1989

Pine DS: Development of the symptom of anxiety, in Child and Adolescent Psychiatry, 3rd Edition. Edited by Lewis M. Philadelphia, PA, Lippincott Williams & Wilkins, 2002, pp 343–351

Pine DS, Grun J: Research on pediatric anxiety: integrating affective neuroscience and developmental psychopathology. J Child Adolesc Psychopharmacol 9:1–12, 1999

Pine DS, Coplan JD, Papp LA, et al: Ventilatory physiology of children and adolescents with anxiety disorders. Arch Gen Psychiatry 55:123–129, 1998

Pine DS, Klein RG, Coplan JD, et al: Differential carbon dioxide sensitivity in childhood anxiety disorders and non-ill comparison group. Arch Gen Psychiatry 57:960–967, 2000

Regier DA, Boyd JH, Burke JD, et al: One month of mental disorders in the United States based on five Epidemiologic Catchment Area sites. Arch Gen Psychiatry 45:977–986, 1988

Research Unit on Pediatric Psychopharmacology Anxiety Study Group: Fluvoxamine for the treatment of anxiety disorders in children and adolescents. N Engl J Med 344:1279–1285, 2001

Riddle MA, Bernstein GA, Cook EH, et al: Anxiolytics, adrenergic agents, and naltrexone. J Am Acad Child Adolesc Psychiatry 38:546–556, 1999

Rosenbaum JF, Biederman J, Gersten M, et al: Behavioral inhibition in children of parents with panic disorder and agoraphobia. Arch Gen Psychiatry 45:463–470, 1988

Roy-Byrne P, Geraci M, Uhde TW: Life events and the onset of panic disorder. Am J Psychiatry 143:1424–1427, 1986

Roy-Byrne P, Wingerson DK, Radant A, et al: Reduced benzodiazepine sensitivity in patients with panic disorder: comparison with patients with obsessive-compulsive disorder and normal subjects. Am J Psychiatry 153:1444–1449, 1996

Schneier FR, Liebowitz MR, Davies SO, et al: Fluoxetine in panic disorder. J Clin Psychopharmacol 10:119–121, 1990

Schneier FR, Johnson J, Hornig CD, et al: Social phobia: comorbidity and morbidity in an epidemiological sample. Arch Gen Psychiatry 49:282–289, 1992

Schwartz CE, Snidman N, Kagan J: Adolescent social anxiety as an outcome of inhibited temperament in childhood. J Am Acad Child Adolesc Psychiatry 38:1008–1015, 1999

Sheehan DV, Ballenger J, Jacobson G: Relative efficacy of monoamine oxidase inhibitors and tricyclic antidepressants in the treatment of endogenous anxiety, in Anxiety: New Research and Changing Concepts. Edited by Klein DF, Rabkin J. New York, Raven, 1981a, pp 47–67

Silverman WK, Kurtines WM, Ginsburg GS, et al: Contingency management, self-control, and education support in the treatment of childhood phobic disorders: a randomized clinical trial. J Consult Clin Psychol 67:675–687, 1999a

Silverman WK, Kurtines WM, Ginsburg GS, et al: Treating anxiety disorders in children with group cognitive-behavioral therapy: a randomized clinical trial. J Consult Clin Psychol 67:995–1003, 1999b

Sinha SS, Coplan JD, Gorman JM, et al: Panic induced by carbon dioxide inhalation and lack of hypothalamic-pituitary-adrenal axis activation. Psychiatry Res 86:93–98, 1999

Solyom L, Ledwidge B, Solyom C: Delineating social phobia. Br J Psychiatry 149:464–470, 1986

Spence SH, Donovan C, Brechman-Toussaint M: Social skills, social outcomes, and cognitive features of childhood social phobia. J Abnorm Psychol 108:211–221, 1999

Spence SH, Donovan C, Brechman-Toussaint M: The treatment of childhood social phobia: the effectiveness of a social skills training-based, cognitive-behavioural intervention, with and without parental involvement. J Child Psychol Psychiatry 41:713–726, 2000

Spier SA, Tesar GE, Rosenbaum JF, et al: Treatment of panic disorder and agoraphobia with clonazepam. J Clin Psychiatry 47:238–242, 1986

Stein MB, Walker JR, Forde DR: Setting diagnostic thresholds for social phobia: considerations from a community survey of social anxiety. Am J Psychiatry 151:408–412, 1994

Steinhausen HC, Juzi C: Elective mutism: an analysis of 100 cases. J Am Acad Child Adolesc Psychiatry 35:606–614, 1996

Strauss CC, Last CG: Social and simple phobias in children. J Anxiety Disord 7:141–152, 1993

Suomi SJ, Kraemer GW, Baysinger CM, et al: Inherited and experiential factors associated with individual differences in anxious behavior displayed by rhesus monkeys, in Anxiety: New Research and Changing Concepts. Edited by Klein DF, Rabkin J. New York, Raven, 1981, pp 179–199

Tancer NK: Elective mutism: a review of the literature, in Advances in Clinical Child Psychology, Vol 14. Edited by Lahey BB, Kazdin AE. New York, Plenum, 1992, pp 265–288

Thomsen PH, Rasmussen G, Anderson CB: Elective mutism: a 17-year-old girl treated successfully with citalopram. Nord J Psychiatry 53:427–429, 1999

Thyer BA, Parrish RT, Curtis GC, et al: Ages of onset of DSM-III anxiety disorders. Compr Psychiatry 26:113–122, 1985

Turner SM, Beidel DC, Townsley RM: Social phobia: a comparison of specific and generalized subtypes and avoidant personality disorder. J Abnorm Psychol 101:326–331, 1992

Uhde TW, Tancer ME, Black B, et al: Phenomenology and neurobiology of social phobia: comparison with panic disorder. J Clin Psychiatry 52 (11, suppl):31–40, 1991

Uhde TW, Tancer ME, Rubinow DR, et al: Evidence for hypothalamo-growth hormone dysfunction in panic disorder: profile of growth hormone responses to clonidine, yohimbine, caffeine, glucose, GRF, and TRH in panic disorder patients versus healthy volunteers. Neuropsychopharmacology 6:101–118, 1992

Velosa JF, Riddle MA: Pharmacologic treatment of anxiety disorders in children and adolescents. Child Adolesc Psychiatr Clin N Am 9:119–133, 2000

Verburg C, Griez E, Meijer J: A 35% carbon dioxide challenge in simple phobias. Acta Psychiatr Scand 90:420–423, 1994 von Korff MR, Eaton WW, Keyl PM: The epidemiology of panic attacks and panic disorder. Am J Epidemiol 122:970–981, 1985

Weissman MM, Leckman JE, Merikangas KR, et al: Depression and anxiety disorders in parents and children. Arch Gen Psychiatry 41:845–852, 1984

Wergland H: Elective mutism. Acta Psychiatr Scand 59:218–228, 1979

Whitaker A, Johnson J, Shaffer D, et al: Uncommon troubles in young people: prevalence estimates of selected psychiatric disorders in a nonreferred adolescent population. Arch Gen Psychiatry 47:487–496, 1990

Wittchen HU, Stein MB, Kessler RC: Social fears and social phobia in a community sample of adolescents and young adults: prevalence, risk factors, and co-morbidity. Psychol Med 29:309–323, 1999

Wright HH, Cuccaro ML, Leonhardt TV, et al: Case study: fluoxetine in the multimodal treatment of a preschool child with selective mutism. J Am Acad Child Adolesc Psychiatry 34:857–862, 1995

Zimbardo PG: Shyness: What It Is and What to Do About It. New York, Addison-Wesley, 1977

Pediatric Posttraumatic Stress Disorder

Craig L. Donnelly, M.D., M.A.

John S. March, M.D., M.P.H.

Lisa Amaya-Jackson, M.D., M.P.H.

Historical Overview

It has long been recognized that the experience of extreme stress can exert profound and lasting changes on human cognition, emotion, and behavior. The early literature on stress and trauma dates from the time of the Civil War and evolved over subsequent wars, when terms such as *battle fatigue, shell shock,* and *nervous breakdown* were used to describe the mental and behavioral syndromes of men who experienced extreme battlefield stress. Historically, children's responses to stress and trauma have been less well characterized and studied than have reactions in adults. It was not until the 1970s that researchers began to systematically examine trauma in childhood. Earlier reports in the literature were chiefly theoretical, descriptive, or speculative treatises primarily in the tradition of psychoanalytic case reports. Sigmund Freud (1926/1959), concerning himself with adult stress reactions in the aftermath of World War I, identified a key component of the psychological reaction to extreme stress as originating in a sense of utter helplessness. Freud's conceptualization of pathological stress processes involved the sudden breaching of a person's usual protective barriers of coping tactics and defense mechanisms, a conceptualization that has relevance and practical utility even today.

In the 1940s and 1950s descriptions of traumatic stress reactions in childhood tended to focus on the quality of the mother-child dyad, with parental loss and parental coping being viewed as the major determinants of children's responses. Anna Freud's group at Hampstead, in particular, made important contributions to the relational aspects of children's responses to trauma in their descriptive studies of children who had experienced the blitz in London, German concentration camps, and maternal separation (A. Freud and Burlingham 1943/1967; A. Freud and Dann 1951). In the post–World War II period the literature on childhood trauma overemphasized parental reporting of children's traumatic responses. Failing to sample specific reports from children about their own symptoms, many of these authors imputed causation and resiliency factors primarily to parental functioning while de-emphasizing factors intrinsic to the child—nervous mothers engender nervous children, and calm mothers engender calm children (Bloch et al. 1956; Carey-Trefzger 1949). In the 1960s and 1970s, focus shifted to the description of resiliency factors, defense mechanisms, and coping strategies used by children in response to traumatic experience. Factors intrinsic both to the child (such as intelligence and a sense of humor) and to the immediate environment of the child (such as solid relationships and good schools) were identified as serving important protective functions against the ill effects of stress (Garmezy 1987; Rutter et al. 1979). In the late 1970s and 1980s, childhood stress and trauma began to receive systematic and detailed empirical examination. The sophistication of the childhood trauma field emerged with the simultaneous development of a specific diagnostic nomenclature for stress disorders in adults and the publication of studies of children who experienced horrendous single-incident traumas. In one such incident, 26 children in Chowchilla, California, were kidnapped in a school bus and held in an underground bunker for 17 hours before escaping. Terr's (1979, 1981a, 1983a, 1983b, 1988) pioneering studies of these children, who were observed prospectively and individually, established many of the key manifestations of childhood posttraumatic stress disorder (PTSD).

PTSD entered the modern psychiatric nomenclature with the publication of DSM-III in 1980 (American Psychiatric Association 1980). Since then a multitude of studies have shown that exposure to life-threatening stressors may lead to serious and often debilitating PTSD in young persons just as in adults (March 1990, 1993; Pynoos 1994). The establishment of specific and defined diagnostic criteria for PTSD has numerous direct benefits. Such criteria improve recognition of the extent to which children are exposed to traumatic situations and increase appreciation of the severity of their acute distress. Specific criteria allow for better characterization of the potentially serious long-term sequelae and provide the opportunity for systematic empirical investigation of the effects of traumatic events and their posttraumatic ramifications within a developmental framework (Pynoos et al. 1995).

In this chapter we present a comprehensive review of pediatric PTSD from the standpoint of basic knowledge expected of child and adolescent psychiatrists. Interested readers may pursue more in-depth treatments of developmental approaches to PTSD (Pynoos 1994; Pynoos et al. 1995), assessment (McNally 1991), diagnosis and comorbidity (Amaya-Jackson and March 1995a, 1995b; March and Amaya-Jackson 1994), pharmacological treatment (Donnelly et al. 1999), psychosocial interventions (Pynoos and Nader 1993; Saigh 1992; Yule and Canterbury 1994), neurobiology (De Bellis 1999a, 1999b), current recommended practice parameters for assessment and treatment (Cohen 1998), and other reviews of PTSD in childhood and adolescence (Perrin et al. 2000; Pfefferbaum 1997; Seedat et al. 2000; Terr 1996; Yule 1994).

Diagnostic Criteria and Clinical Findings

The diagnostic criteria for PTSD in children are the same as those used in adults. Four criteria must be sat-

isfied to establish a DSM-IV-TR (American Psychiatric Association 2000) diagnosis of PTSD (Table 32–1). First, the individual must have been exposed to a stressor of significant magnitude. There must follow the development of a triad of symptom clusters: subsequent reexperiencing of the event, avoidance of stimuli or numbing of general responsiveness, and persistent increased arousal. The stressor criterion defines the primary risk factor for PTSD and the essential feature of the diagnosis, namely, establishing exposure to a life-threatening event. The time course of the disorder can be variable, and PTSD may develop months or even years after the index trauma exposure. Symptoms must be debilitating and must be present for more than 1 month to meet the diagnostic criteria. Children who meet the symptom criteria but who do not meet the time criteria of symptom expression lasting for 1 month or more are considered under the category of acute stress disorder (Table 32–2).

◼ Exposure to a Stressor

Objectively, PTSD stressors are characterized by threat to life, potential for physical injury, and an element of grotesqueness or horror that demarcates these events from less traumatic experiences, such as the expected death of a loved one from a serious illness or a highly embarrassing or humiliating personal event. Not surprisingly, children and adolescents generally react acutely to traumatic events with surprise, terror, and a sense of helplessness; these characterize the subjective features of the DSM-IV-TR PTSD stressor criterion. Table 32–3 lists characteristic stressors associated with PTSD in the pediatric population (e.g., kidnapping; serious animal bites; or severe injury due to burns, accidental shootings, or hit-and-run accidents). Children are at special risk for PTSD from witnessing violence to a family member (e.g., rape or murder, suicide behavior, and spousal or sibling abuse). Also, as Saigh (1991) and others have pointed out, PTSD can result either from direct, witnessed, or verbal exposure or from "contaminant" effects of trauma indirectly experienced from a distance (Green 1995; Pfefferbaum et al. 2000).

Stressors and traumas are by nature environmentally determined events that, if sufficiently intense, can traumatize any child (Pynoos et al. 1987a). In making the diagnosis of PTSD it is imperative that clinicians establish what might at first appear to be self-evident: that the traumatic event truly occurred and that the

Table 32–1. DSM-IV-TR diagnostic criteria for posttraumatic stress disorder

A. The person has been exposed to a traumatic event in which both of the following were present:

  (1) the person experienced, witnessed, or was confronted with an event or events that involved actual or threatened death or serious injury, or a threat to the physical integrity of self or others

  (2) the person's response involved intense fear, helplessness, or horror.   **Note:** In children, this may be expressed instead by disorganized or agitated behavior

B. The traumatic event is persistently reexperienced in one (or more) of the following ways:

  (1) recurrent and intrusive distressing recollections of the event, including images, thoughts, or perceptions.   **Note:** In young children, repetitive play may occur in which themes or aspects of the trauma are expressed.

  (2) recurrent distressing dreams of the event.   **Note:** In children, there may be frightening dreams without recognizable content.

  (3) acting or feeling as if the traumatic event were recurring (includes a sense of reliving the experience, illusions, hallucinations, and dissociative flashback episodes, including those that occur on awakening or when intoxicated).   **Note:** In young children, trauma-specific reenactment may occur.

  (4) intense psychological distress at exposure to internal or external cues that symbolize or resemble an aspect of the traumatic event

  (5) physiological reactivity on exposure to internal or external cues that symbolize or resemble an aspect of the traumatic event

C. Persistent avoidance of stimuli associated with the trauma and numbing of general responsiveness (not present before the trauma), as indicated by three (or more) of the following:

  (1) efforts to avoid thoughts, feelings, or conversations associated with the trauma

  (2) efforts to avoid activities, places, or people that arouse recollections of the trauma

  (3) inability to recall an important aspect of the trauma

  (4) markedly diminished interest or participation in significant activities

  (5) feeling of detachment or estrangement from others

  (6) restricted range of affect (e.g., unable to have loving feelings)

  (7) sense of a foreshortened future (e.g., does not expect to have a career, marriage, children, or a normal life span)

D. Persistent symptoms of increased arousal (not present before the trauma), as indicated by two (or more) of the following:

  (1) difficulty falling or staying asleep

  (2) irritability or outbursts of anger

  (3) difficulty concentrating

  (4) hypervigilance

  (5) exaggerated startle response

E. Duration of the disturbance (symptoms in Criteria B, C, and D) is more than 1 month.

F. The disturbance causes clinically significant distress or impairment in social, occupational, or other important areas of functioning.

  Specify if:

   Acute: if duration of symptoms is less than 3 months
   Chronic: if duration of symptoms is 3 months or more

  Specify if:

   With Delayed Onset: if onset of symptoms is at least 6 months after the stressor

Source.   Reprinted from American Psychiatric Association: *Diagnostic and Statistical Manual of Mental Disorders*, 4th Edition, Text Revision. Washington, DC, American Psychiatric Association, 2000. Copyright 2000 American Psychiatric Association. Used with permission.

child was in fact exposed to it. Vague, secondhand, or unsubstantiated reports have no place in making the diagnosis of PTSD. It is known that PTSD is far more likely to occur after direct trauma exposure than after indirect exposure; however, it can occur in persons indirectly affected, such as those who have witnessed a violent injury to another or who have learned that a loved one was involved in a trauma (Green 1995). Nev-

---

Table 32–2. DSM-IV-TR diagnostic criteria for acute stress disorder

---

A. The person has been exposed to a traumatic event in which both of the following were present:

  (1) the person experienced, witnessed, or was confronted with an event or events that involved actual or threatened death or serious injury, or a threat to the physical integrity of self or others

  (2) the person's response involved intense fear, helplessness, or horror

B. Either while experiencing or after experiencing the distressing event, the individual has three (or more) of the following dissociative symptoms:

  (1) a subjective sense of numbing, detachment, or absence of emotional responsiveness

  (2) a reduction in awareness of his or her surroundings (e.g., "being in a daze")

  (3) derealization

  (4) depersonalization

  (5) dissociative amnesia (i.e., inability to recall an important aspect of the trauma)

C. The traumatic event is persistently reexperienced in at least one of the following ways: recurrent images, thoughts, dreams, illusions, flashback episodes, or a sense of reliving the experience; or distress on exposure to reminders of the traumatic event.

D. Marked avoidance of stimuli that arouse recollections of the trauma (e.g., thoughts, feelings, conversations, activities, places, people).

E. Marked symptoms of anxiety or increased arousal (e.g., difficulty sleeping, irritability, poor concentration, hypervigilance, exaggerated startle response, motor restlessness).

F. The disturbance causes clinically significant distress or impairment in social, occupational, or other important areas of functioning or impairs the individual's ability to pursue some necessary task, such as obtaining necessary assistance or mobilizing personal resources by telling family members about the traumatic experience.

G. The disturbance lasts for a minimum of 2 days and a maximum of 4 weeks and occurs within 4 weeks of the traumatic event.

H. The disturbance is not due to the direct physiological effects of a substance (e.g., a drug of abuse, a medication) or a general medical condition, is not better accounted for by brief psychotic disorder, and is not merely an exacerbation of a preexisting Axis I or Axis II disorder.

Source.   Reprinted from American Psychiatric Association: *Diagnostic and Statistical Manual of Mental Disorders*, 4th Edition, Text Revision. Washington, DC, American Psychiatric Association, 2000. Copyright 2000 American Psychiatric Association. Used with permission.

---

ertheless, caution is advised when attempting to delineate the traumatic exposure. Children's self-reports of trauma cannot be taken uncritically and automatically at face value, because it is known that even children with bona fide trauma histories often retain false details of their recollections of these real exposures (Terr 1979, 1981a, 1981b; also see Bremner et al. 2000). Memory is fluid and malleable, and children's recollections can be influenced both inadvertently and purposefully. Therefore, a neutral questioning stance on the part of the clinician is imperative. Both internal and external confirmations are often necessary to establish traumatic exposure in children. Child self-reports as gleaned in the clinical interview must be supplemented by parental histories and potentially important collateral information taken from other sources, including eyewitnesses, child protective teams, hospital records, and police documents. Aspects of the symptom picture vary with stressor-specific factors (Famularo et al. 1990; Kendall-Tackett et al. 1993; Nader

et al. 1991); therefore, careful attention to the nature of the stressor is mandatory (Table 32–3). Thoroughness in sampling for traumatic experiences and attention to symptoms that relate even to subthreshold trauma exposure are important considerations in the assessment of stressors. For example, physically abused boys may be at greater risk for developing externalizing behavior and conduct disorder that may hide or mask the presence of PTSD, and the diagnosis may be missed in the absence of a thorough assessment of trauma exposure (Pelcowitz et al. 1994). Also, even though many sexually abused children do not meet strict diagnostic criteria for PTSD (Kendall-Tackett et al. 1993), clinicians must not underestimate the level of psychological impairment in this population, since the effects of sexual abuse on the level of symptoms and on long-term personality functioning are often profound (Cahill et al. 1991).

Societal conditions also influence the types of traumatic events to which children are likely to be exposed

Table 32–3. Stressors causing posttraumatic stress disorder

Objective features

Experiencing a serious threat to life or physical integrity

Witnessing serious threat, harm, or grotesque death

In some cases, learning about violent threat or harm to a close friend or relative

Sudden destruction of home or community

Salient subjective responses

Intense fear, terror

Horror

Coercion

Helplessness

Magnitude

High intensity, duration, suddenness, or personal impact

Sufficient to be markedly distressing to almost anyone

Range of stressors reported in children

Kidnapping and hostage situations

Exposure to violence, including terrorism, gang violence, sniper attacks, war atrocities

Witnessing rape, murder, or suicide behavior

Sexual or physical abuse

Severe accidental injury, including burns, hit-and-run accidents, animal bites, toxic exposures

Life-threatening illness or life-endangering medical procedures

Severe automobile, railroad, airplane, ship, or boating accidents

Natural or human disasters

(Garbarino et al. 1991; Yehuda 2002). Large-scale disasters like the Oklahoma City bombing of the Murrah Federal Building and the September 11th attack on the World Trade Center may constitute an amalgam of traumatic experiences—including interpersonal violence, technological disaster, injury, loss of life, and displacement—as well as secondary traumatic phenomena. Changing family patterns in contemporary culture may contribute to increased rates of intrafamilial sexual molestation and physical abuse. Incidents around the world lead to significant exposure of children and adolescents to extrafamilial violence, as seen with inner-city violence and gang warfare, civil war atrocities, torture, and religious fundamentalist or state-sponsored terrorism. In cases of natural or technological disasters (e.g., an earthquake or a building collapse), the effect of trauma varies, depending not only on the severity of the disaster but also on the location, context, evacuation and recovery methods, advanced communication, popular media coverage, and disaster relief efforts.

Secondary adversities commonly befall children after tragedies—including displacement, relocation, attendance at a new school, separation from siblings, involuntary unemployment of a parent, and increased financial difficulties (Goenjian et al. 1994)—as well as changes in lifestyle and daily routines, which may be disruptive in and of themselves. Globally, the public health consequences of adversity secondary to trauma are immense. It is estimated that in the world today there are more than 14 million refugees and displaced persons, three-fourths of whom are women and children (Berman 2001). Medical procedures and rehabilitation may be ongoing for physical injuries and disability, and reintegration into school may be difficult. Children exposed to war atrocities may also experience malnutrition, deprivation, family disruption, loss, immigration, and resettlement. When the violence or disaster results in the death of a family member or a friend, an important interplay occurs between trauma and grief reactions, including continued preoccupation with the circumstances of the death and psychological upheavals among family members with different degrees of exposure (Pynoos et al. 1987b). Grief reactions and secondary depression in particular may complicate the reaction to a traumatic event.

Nevertheless, although the various environmental events that may produce PTSD differ somewhat with age and life circumstances, recent literature confirms that the objective magnitude of the stressor is directly proportional to the risk of developing PTSD (March 1993; McNally 1993). For example, in studies of the aftermath of a schoolyard sniper attack, Pynoos and Nader (1989a) and Pynoos et al. (1987b) showed that degree of exposure (proximity) was linearly related to the risk for PTSD symptoms and that children's memory disturbances, indicating distorted cognitive processing during the event, closely followed the extent of exposure. Thus, clinicians working with severely traumatized children and adolescents must remember that the PTSD symptom picture is most easily understood in the context of a precise understanding of the traumatic event itself, its quality, intensity, controllability, predictability, duration of exposure, and perceived degree of threat.

A variety of factors may intensify the magnitude of the direct stressor exposure. Events that involve interpersonal violence or threat appear to be more likely to cause PTSD than technological or natural disasters (Yehuda 2002). PTSD occurs more frequently in those who experience rape and physical or sexual molestation than in those who are involved in accidents or natural disasters or who hear about traumatic events happening to others (Breslau et al. 1998). Traumas that are unpredictable or uncontrollable; that are perceived as lethal; or that lead to injury or exposure to pain, heat, or cold are more likely to invoke an intense response (Holbrook et al. 2001; Schreiber and Galai-Gat 1993).

■ Reexperiencing

Recall of traumatic exposure involves intense perceptual experiences and internal appraisals of the threat (Eth and Pynoos 1985). Children and adolescents with PTSD typically reexperience traumatic events in distressing intrusive thoughts or memories, in dreams, and (less commonly) in flashbacks. Reexperiencing may occur spontaneously or in response to traumatic reminders, called trauma triggers, that are linked to traumatic moments within the event itself. The nature of this symptom complex recapitulates parts of the actual traumatic event. Recurrent intrusive and distressing images, sounds, smells, or impressions often focus on moments of extreme horror or helplessness during the event—for example, the impact from a flying object, the sight of the stabbing, the eyes of the rapist, or the appearance of the motionless, blood-covered body. In addition, children mentally return to their experience, searching for ways to offset traumatic helplessness or to alter the outcome in thought and fantasy. Intrusive images may incorporate mental modifications that minimize or protect the child from the full horror of the experience—for example, by altering their proximity to the immediate danger or by freezing the action before irreversible injury occurs. In young children whose trauma exposure may have occurred preverbally before a narrative account and clear memory could be established, reexperiencing may take the form of fear reactions; reenactment; violent, odd, or repetitive posttraumatic actions; or distressing dreams and night terrors.

Children's traumatic dreams include repetitions of aspects of the experience; depiction of other life-threatening dangers; or, over time, more general fearful dreams (e.g., in young children, being pursued by monsters) (Terr 1988). These dreams depict direct personal threat, even death, or threat of harm to others, especially family members, and they renew emotions associated with the experience. For example, a boy who was wounded in a massacre dreamed that his family died in earthquakes; recall of the dreams 2 years later produced persistent distress.

Traumatic play refers to the repetitive dramatization in play of elements or themes of the event (Terr 1990). Children may involve siblings or peers in their traumatic play (Terr 1988). As with traumatic images, this play may recur because the child alters the action—for instance, by compulsively catching the bullet before it strikes. With time, the incorporation of traumatic elements may impede the normative uses of play (Pynoos and Nader 1990). Traumatic play may go unnoticed by parents unless it is overtly distressing, dangerous, violent, suicidal, or sexually precocious, or unless children appear overly stuck on a particular enactment. The qualities of a persistent noxious theme, intensity, and repetitiveness that characterize traumatic play are in contrast to the usual fluidity, flexibility, and spontaneity that characterizes normal childhood play.

Reenactment behavior refers to conscious or unconscious replication of some aspect of the traumatic experience (Saylor et al. 1992; Terr 1990). In younger children, the behavior may derive from an "action memory." For example, a preschool child who was trapped in a well began to squeeze herself into small spaces. Terr (1991) describes the compelling case of a 13-month-old girl whose baby sister was found mutilated, bitten, and shaken to death. After removal from her home and entering into therapy this child subsequently engaged in biting herself, biting others, and attacking young babies. Adolescents especially may seek out opportunities to engage in reenactment behavior or thrill seeking and thus attempt to master or take command of the situation. The reenactment behavior of adolescents can be dangerous because teenagers often have access to guns, automobiles, and drugs. Traumatic reminders may elicit acting out or dysfunctional behavior. For example, when one adolescent boy felt helpless in meeting a personal demand or confrontation, he would lie down on the floor in the way he had during a hostage taking.

Traumatic reminders—which may be technically defined as conditioned stimuli that provoke conditioned responses directly or indirectly related to the traumatic event itself—include the external circumstances of the event and the internal emotional and physical reactions of the child. The role of these reminders is in triggering physiological and psychological reactions and accounts for much of the phasic nature of the disorder. The unexpectedness of reminders may reevoke a sense of vulnerability and lack of control. Common reminders include the following:

- Circumstances (e.g., location, time, preceding activity, clothes worn)
- Precipitating conditions (e.g., noises, high winds after experiencing a tornado, arguing)
- Other signs of danger (e.g., staring eyes, blaring horns, flashing lights)
- Endangering objects (e.g., trees, broken glass, weapons, belts)
- Situations presenting a sense of helplessness (e.g., cries for help, crying, fast heartbeat, a sinking feeling, ineffectualness, or moments of aloneness)

Normal school procedures and academic exercises may serve as reminders. For example, a fire drill may re-evoke a sense of a prior emergency; harsh words from a teacher may trigger reminders of an abusive parent; or a civics class discussion of judicial proceedings may kindle fear and rage about the trial of a father's murderer.

■ Avoidance of Stimuli or Numbing of General Responsiveness

Children with PTSD invariably make conscious attempts to avoid traumatic reminders—namely, the thoughts, feelings, or activities that precipitate distressing recollections of the event. Cognitive suppression, distraction, and behavioral avoidance are particularly common, as is a frank refusal to talk about or discuss the trauma. However, children pay a high price for these survival strategies, because they inevitably affect other areas of functioning. For example, child survivors of trauma may show markedly diminished interest in usually significant activities or increased somatic and autonomic symptoms. The loss of previously acquired skills may cause a child to be less verbal or to regress to behaviors such as thumb sucking or enuresis. Rather than reporting feeling "numb," younger children report not wanting to know how they feel, tell of feeling alone with their subjective experience, or describe efforts to keep an emotion from emerging (e.g., by going to sit alone). Children who are engaged in avoidance may appear deconcentrated and aloof. Parents are not always aware of the sense of aloneness or isolation, because the child may continue to cling or to seek comfort. Other features of avoidance or numbing include periods of blank stares or looking dazed, withdrawal from social contact, and the appearance of being shut down. It is worth pointing out that a child's refusal to acknowledge or to talk about a potential traumatic experience does not, de facto, imply that the child is demonstrating the avoidance criterion of PTSD. The absence of evidence is not necessarily, in this case, evidence for diagnosis. When attempting to validate the diagnosis of PTSD, clinicians need to exert caution in this regard. Children will often refuse to directly discuss traumatic events whether or not they meet criteria for a diagnosis of PTSD. Close clinical scrutiny usually reveals other stigmata of avoidance of traumatic stimuli or numbing of responsiveness in addition to simple refusal to discuss the trauma.

Children may avoid specific thoughts, locations, objects, themes in their play, and behaviors that remind them of the incident. They may discontinue pleasurable activities to avoid excitement or fear. Traumatic avoidance may selectively restrict daily activity or generalize to more phobic behavior. Diminished activity may represent a preoccupation with intrusive phenomena, a depressive reaction, an avoidance of affect-laden states or of traumatic reminders, or an effort to reduce the risk of further trauma. Active behaviors, such as disruptions in the classroom, may be attempts to divert intrusive thoughts or anxieties (e.g., yelling out bad words when high winds appear after having experienced a tornado or hurricane disaster). Astute clinicians will be wary of automatically interpreting such symptom manifestations as derivatives of PTSD in the absence of other evidence that they truly represent trauma-related avoidance.

Although earlier observations suggested a relative absence of major amnesia in children, more recent studies have reported a variety of memory disturbances (Pynoos and Nader 1989a). These disturbances may be introduced during recall rather than during perception or storage. Children may omit moments of extreme threat to life (at times screened by detailed recounting of other fearful moments); may distort proximity, duration, or sequencing; may introduce premonitions; and may minimize their life threat in other ways. Dissociative memory disturbances may also occur, especially in response to physical coercion, molestation, or abuse (Putnam and Trickett 1993).

■ Increased States of Arousal

Sleep disturbances, irritability, difficulty concentrating, hypervigilance, exaggerated startle responses, and outbursts of aggression represent a state of increased physiological arousal (Perry 1994; Perry and Pate 1994). Somatic symptoms of autonomic hyperactivity or increased arousal may reflect both tonic and phasic physiological activity and tend to reinforce the disorder. Phasic symptoms occur more often when the child encounters traumatic reminders. The child is seen as being "on alert," hypervigilant, scanning, and ready to respond to any environmental threat (Ornitz and Pynoos 1989). Especially in school-age children, physiological reactivity may include somatic symptoms as a form of hyperarousal. Sleep disturbance may be severe and persistent; changes seen in sleep architecture have been noted in adult studies (Pitman 1993). Difficulty falling asleep, sleepwalking, and night terrors are common. These sleep problems can further decrease the child's ability to concentrate and attend to important tasks and thus also may adversely affect mood states, learning, and behavior in school.

Hypervigilance and exaggerated startle responses may lead to ongoing efforts to ensure personal security or the safety of others (Ornitz and Pynoos 1989). These recurrent bouts of fear may seriously change a child's sense of competence and negatively alter emerging self-concept and self-confidence. Incident-specific fears commonly occur in children. Fears are particularly evident during times of vulnerability (in the bathroom, at bedtime, or when alone) or in response to specific reminders.

Lastly, temporary or chronic difficulty in modulating aggression can make children act more irritable and easy to anger, resulting in a reduced tolerance for the normal behaviors, demands, and slights of peers and family members and in unusual acts of aggression or social withdrawal (Yule and Canterbury 1994). Often the externalizing behaviors, hyperreactivity, and irritability can be the most manifest of the symptom triad in children and adolescents with PTSD and may further complicate the diagnosis by masking other less obvious symptoms.

PTSD Complexity: From Individual Diagnosis to Population Frequency

Childhood and adolescent PTSD is a complex disorder with a myriad of symptom presentations. For example, there are at least 1,750 different symptom combinations possible in the diagnosis of PTSD (i.e., one of five symptoms for criterion B, plus three of five symptoms for criterion C, plus two of five symptoms for criterion D yields 1,750 possible symptom combinations; see

Table 32–1). Stated differently, there are 1,750 ways a child can "look" symptomatically, using only the minimum criteria to meet diagnostic threshold for the disorder. Establishing the diagnosis itself is thus fraught with complexity. In addition, like adults, children often present with multiple overlapping comorbid conditions adding still further layers of symptom complexity. Owing to its complexity, PTSD is commonly misdiagnosed due to the failure of adequate trauma-history taking on the part of some clinicians and due to the ease with which other clinicians make the diagnosis based simply on a history of trauma exposure in the midst of psychiatric symptoms. Therefore PTSD in childhood has high rates of both false negative and false positive diagnoses.

Although the events that cause PTSD are common (Eth 1990; Reiss et al. 1993), there are no large-scale epidemiological studies that look specifically at the general-population incidence or prevalence of PTSD in children and adolescents. Existing data suggest variability in prevalence ranging from 10% (Breslau et al. 1991) to as much as 40% (Richters 1993; Richters and Martinez 1993) in children and youths from violence-ridden neighborhoods. However, rates of PTSD vary widely depending on the nature of the trauma and the population studied—perhaps so widely, in fact, as to render large-population measures of incidence and prevalence relatively uninformative. In Terr's (1981b) cohort, for example, 100% of children developed PTSD, whereas rates of PTSD development in natural disasters are in the range of 3%–5% (Kessler et al. 1995). Despite the lack of large epidemiological studies in childhood and the wide-ranging rates of PTSD reported in the literature, several generalizations can be made about rates of PTSD by trauma type, based on smaller-scale community samples and on data gleaned from adult studies.

The diverse traumatic events that have been reported to result in PTSD include criminal assault (Pynoos and Eth 1985; Pynoos and Nader 1988a; Pynoos et al. 1987a); hostage taking (Schwarz and Kowalski 1991; Terr 1981b); combat (Clarke et al. 1993); bone marrow transplantation (Stuber et al. 1991); severe burns (Stoddard et al. 1989); general injury (McHugo et al. 2000); and transportation accidents, such as naval disaster in the sinking of the cruise ship *Jupiter* (Yule 1992; Yule and Williams 1990; Yule et al. 1990) and motor vehicle accidents (Stallard and Law 1993). Studies across a variety of natural disasters also show elevated rates of posttraumatic stress in child victims

(Burke et al. 1986; Goenjian et al. 1994; Green et al. 1991; Lonigan et al. 1994; McFarlane 1987; Shannon et al. 1994). It appears that children are more sensitive to the effects of trauma than adults, given the same trauma exposure, and consequently may exhibit higher rates of PTSD development.

Rates of PTSD are clearly high in youths exposed to life-threatening events. Homicide is the leading cause of death among minority adolescent males in many inner-city areas (Foy and Goguen 1998), and motor vehicle accidents are the leading health threat among youths in America (de Vries et al. 1999). A study of children exposed to a schoolyard sniper attack revealed that almost 60% of exposed children continued to meet full criteria for PTSD 1 year after the incident (Pynoos et al. 1987a). Terr's (1981b) report of the Chowchilla school bus kidnapping indicated that all 26 children involved had moderate to severe PTSD regardless of their developmental or psychiatric history, parental relationships, or past trauma. In a study of adolescent Cambodian refugees who survived the atrocities of the Pol Pot regime, 50% were found to have PTSD, with persistent symptoms noted 3 years later, not only for PTSD but also for depression and anxiety (Clarke et al. 1993).

Once established, PTSD in children is often both chronic and debilitating (March and Amaya-Jackson 1994; Nader et al. 1990; Terr 1983a), although the clinical course of PTSD in a given child can be highly variable. Factors responsible for the variability in course of illness include circumstantial ones (the nature of the stressor); attributes intrinsic to the child such as preexisting psychopathology, quality of attachment, and coping and resiliency strengths; and extrinsic influences that govern the nature of the recovery environment such as poverty or family support. In general, the more severe the stressor—in terms of intensity, duration, suddenness, and personal impact—the more prolonged the course. For those with mild exposure and minimum interpersonal impact, the symptoms of the trauma usually diminish within days or weeks of the event. For adults, the trajectory of acute PTSD appears to sort in two directions: either tending to resolve within 3–4 months or tending to follow a chronic course (Rothbaum et al. 1992). Chronicity may be expected when a child has been exposed to multiple incidents of trauma, sexual abuse, trauma involving personal injury and/or mutilation, experiencing or witnessing numerous losses of life and massive destruction. Multiple adversities in the child's environ-ment significantly add to the risk of comorbidity, and therefore to the chronicity and seriousness of the clinical condition.

For a variety of reasons, stress reactions in young people are increasingly common in clinical settings. The opportunities for trauma exposure in modern life are numerous. In our studies of PTSD in a rural North Carolina community, the median number of PTSD-magnitude stressors in children with posttraumatic symptomatology was five (March et al. 1995a). A Chicago study of more than 1,000 middle- and high school students found that 35% had witnessed a stabbing, 39% had seen a shooting, and almost 25% had seen someone being killed (Breslau et al. 1991). Nearly half of the victims were friends, family, classmates, or neighbors. In addition, 46% reported that they had personally been a victim of at least one highly violent crime, such as armed robbery, rape, or being shot or stabbed. The prevalence of childhood sexual abuse is substantial (Ernst et al. 1993), with more than 2 million children in the United States each year being abused or neglected. Contemporary society thus sets the stage for children to be exposed to a great variety of technological and interpersonal traumas on a scale that is perhaps unprecedented (e.g., the extensive media coverage of the September 11th attack on the World Trade Center). Given the great diversity of possible types of traumatic exposure, there is likely to be heuristic, research, clinical outcome, or treatment utility in characterizing trauma by type. Apart from the qualitative distinctions made between different kinds of trauma (e.g., combat-related and interpersonal trauma, child sexual abuse, and natural and technological disasters), Terr (1991) provided a useful distinction between different traumatic processes: type I traumas (sudden and unpredictable, with a single-incident stressor) and type II traumas (chronic, expected, with a repeated stressor, typical of childhood physical and sexual abuse).

The scope of child and adolescent trauma is wide-ranging, from the standpoint of both symptom presentations in individual children and the larger public health concerns regarding the substantial numbers of children and adolescents who are in need of treatment (Amaya-Jackson and March 1993). Important questions for the field of child and adolescent psychiatry include the following: How do acute, single-incident traumatic experiences differ from chronic, ongoing trauma (Terr's type I and type II traumas) in their relationship to the development, severity, and prognosis of PTSD? What is the impact of single-incident versus multiple-incident trauma on the development of co-morbid conditions? How does the nature of the trauma—whether natural disaster, technological, or interpersonal—relate to the risk, development, severity, treatment, and prognosis of PTSD? What are the common comorbid conditions found with PTSD, and how do these differ by developmental phase, nature of the trauma, and the timing of the index trauma exposure? What are the important gender differences that relate to risk for PTSD and responsiveness to treatment? What are the important risk, resiliency, and protective factors, both intrinsic to the child and more broadly in the child's developmental milieu? What are the roles of the family and the primary adult caretaker in childhood PTSD? What specific neurobiological systems are dysregulated in traumatic experiences and how do they lead to the development of PTSD and associated disorders? What are the essential ingredients in effective psychotherapy for childhood PTSD, and what are the best ways to deliver them? What medications are effective in ameliorating the symptoms of PTSD in children?

Developmental Considerations

The developmental stage exerts important influence over children's registration of danger, appraisals of threat, attribution of meaning, emotional and cognitive means of coping, toleration of their reactions, expectations about recovery, and effectiveness in addressing life changes (Pynoos 1994; Pynoos et al. 1995). Particularly problematic is the assessment of PTSD in infants and toddlers, in whom the lack of language development makes diagnosis difficult. Therefore, clinicians and researchers must synthesize current knowledge about child and adolescent exposure to traumatic stress and must be cognizant of markers distinguishing between disrupted and normal development. The criteria set as evolved in DSM-IV-TR is not particularly sensitive to PTSD symptoms in infants and toddlers. Alternative criteria have been proposed that are more behaviorally anchored and are more sensitive to the likely manifestations of trauma in this early age group (Scheeringa et al. 1995; Zero to Three 1994).

Loss of acquired skills or failure to acquire new skills may manifest differently according to age. For ex-

ample, younger children may become less verbal or may even experience mutism, enuresis, or thumb sucking in response to trauma. School-age children may show more inconsistency in behavior and mood, report forgetting recently acquired knowledge, and perform household chores as they did when they were younger. Adolescents may report becoming confused, similar to a younger child, when asked too many questions at once and then may cry or appear to have a tantrum. Decisions made by adolescents after trauma may reflect feelings of increased dependence or helplessness—for example, deciding not to leave home or pursue college, or making premature efforts to enter adulthood.

Perhaps as a result of constitution, temperament, or experiential factors, children differ in the degree of general or specific avoidant behavior and cognitive discrimination between reminders and the original traumatic stimulus. Younger or temperamentally anxious children may overgeneralize threat and danger or be more socially reticent. Depressed children may have undue guilt. Impulsive children may increase their hyperreactivity, explosiveness, and other problematic behaviors. Children may experience a renewal of symptoms or concerns due to prior stressful events (trauma reactivation), and, in the case of prior trauma, these reactions may significantly prolong recovery from the current traumatic episode.

Pynoos and colleagues (Pynoos 1994; Pynoos et al. 1995), in a developmental approach, assign a prominent role to trauma-related expectations because these are expressed in the thoughts, emotions, behavior, and biology of the developing child. They include skewed expectations about the world, the safety and security of interpersonal life, and the child's sense of personal integrity. In this sense, traumatic experiences often unfavorably alter a child's inner plans and outer expectations of the world and catastrophically shape concepts of self and others. These internal schemas exert a forecasting effect about the future that have a powerful and negative influence on both current and future outlook and behavior. After traumatic exposures, these altered expectations place the child at risk for proximal and distal developmental disturbances. Such a developmental approach focusing on trauma-related expectations applies to the entire spectrum of child and adolescent traumatic stress. It may help explain the increased risk of future exposure and the construction and evolution of enduring traumatic memory, personal narrative, and sense of self as victim.

The presence of PTSD in childhood or adolescence has a ripple effect throughout development. At present it is unknown whether it is incurable and remains as a lasting scar, as some researchers view it (Terr 1991), or whether it introduces an altered yet recoverable developmental trajectory that can be compensated for with appropriate interventions.

Comorbidity and Differential Diagnosis

Traumatized children frequently have symptoms of disorders other than PTSD, and children with other disorders often have PTSD as a comorbid diagnosis (Famularo et al. 1992; Ford et al. 2000; Goldman et al. 1992; Pynoos et al. 1987a; Wozniak et al. 1999). There is reason to believe that comorbidities become more complicated with time; epidemiological studies sampling adults with child trauma histories indicate that serious and multiple comorbid conditions aggregate with PTSD (Breslau et al. 1998; Kessler et al. 1995; Muller et al. 2000). In traumatized children a wide variety of social behaviors have been reported to be abnormal, with problematic social behaviors serving both as a risk factor for and an outcome of traumatic experiences (Conaway and Hansen 1989).

In addition to true comorbidity, spurious comorbidity with PTSD results from overlap between criteria sets (e.g., affective constriction in PTSD overlaps with anhedonia in depression; symptoms of hypervigilance may mimic symptoms of generalized anxiety) and confounding similar symptoms of other diagnoses with those of PTSD (e.g., the inattention, impulsivity, and reactive defiance of attention-deficit/hyperactivity disorder and oppositional defiant disorder appear like the hyperarousal symptoms of PTSD). To clarify the diagnostic picture, careful questioning of parents, teachers, and especially the child vis-à-vis his or her internal experiences is necessary. Because of the high prevalence of dimensional and transitional symptoms in children with PTSD, treatment outcome studies must include non-PTSD symptoms as targets for treatment and as predictors of treatment response. On the other hand, although multiple diagnoses should be made (when appropriate) to facilitate treatment planning, it is important to focus on the traumatic event when considering the overall symptom picture.

Traumatic experiences have an inherent potential to induce a variety of anxiety symptoms (Lonigan et al. 1994; March et al. 1995a). Many children experience increased attachment behaviors such as clinging, seeking reassurance, and worrying about the safety of family members or friends. Some children may be genetically prone to separation anxiety; others may have separation anxiety because of prior threats to important attachment bonds. However, most children respond directly to a traumatic event by activating attachment behaviors. A diagnosis of separation anxiety disorder is warranted when symptoms of separation anxiety interfere with the child's daily life, but the clinician must remember the reasonableness of the originating threat. Thus, reconstituting a safe environment must always precede otherwise premature attempts to enforce or encourage separation. The establishment of safety and assurance that basic needs are met must take place for a thorough and accurate differential diagnosis to be made and should certainly take place before any treatment is undertaken (Scheeringa 1999). Children who do not meet full criteria for PTSD often manifest symptoms of generalized anxiety disorder. It is important to remember the traumatic origin of the child's anxiety when designing a treatment plan for such children, who may otherwise be at risk for delayed-onset PTSD.

Other children display somatic rather than cognitive anxiety symptoms as a form of traumatic reenactment. These symptoms can resemble limited-symptom panic attacks, and without adequate treatment they may progress to panic disorder or to PTSD. When panic disorder is present, specific panic treatments are warranted (Black 1995). Children may exhibit diffuse physical complaints derived from anxiety that may be related to the trauma, such as headache, stomach ache, genital pain, or pain on urination.

Trauma-specific phobias are relatively easy to distinguish from PTSD in that they are more isolated, lack tonic arousal, do not readily generalize to new situations, and result in less psychosocial dysfunction than does PTSD.

Intrusive thoughts, urges, and images—not all of them pathological (Terr 1983b)—are found in several childhood psychiatric disorders other than PTSD. Intrusive phenomena following a traumatic event can often be distinguished from nontraumatic intrusions by the presence of trauma-specific contents, a subjective link made by the child with the trauma, or by contextual features. Obsessive-compulsive disorder is distinguished from PTSD in that obsessive-compulsive disorder usually lacks a PTSD-magnitude precipitant and trauma-specific intrusions. Rarely, obsessive-compulsive disorder may develop in the context of PTSD by secondary generalization. For example, children who have been sexually assaulted commonly develop obsessional thoughts of contamination and may handle the anxiety associated with these thoughts through washing rituals. Checking rituals in response to obsessional concerns about safety issues also occur.

Depressive-spectrum conditions—ranging from simple demoralization to adjustment reactions to chronic low-level mood (dysthymia) to more serious melancholic major depression—are among the most common secondary comorbidities in PTSD and often constitute an important treatment focus (Yule 1992; Yule and Canterbury 1994). Depression can sometimes be distinguished from PTSD by the self-punitive nature of the child's thoughts, by a more pervasive anhedonia than is usually seen with phobically driven affective constriction, or by the presence of bereavement or other life adversities. A full depressive syndrome is frequently a normal reaction to the loss of a loved one (Pynoos et al. 1987b). However, the trauma response often significantly interferes with the normal grief process. For example, reminiscing, an essential part of the bereavement process, can be drastically inhibited because the intrusive recollections of the traumatic event interfere with the child's effort to recall pleasant memories of the deceased (Pynoos et al. 1987b). Children appear to be especially vulnerable to what Eth and Pynoos (1985) refer to as the dual demands of trauma mastery and grief work. Therefore, the struggle with the child's traumatic responses must be addressed so that the process of mourning may be completed without the encumbrance of PTSD symptoms.

Schizophrenia, the delusional disorders, and brief reactive psychoses are readily differentiated from PTSD based on dissimilarities between psychotic intrusive thoughts and PTSD reexperiencing and the presence of otherwise intact reality testing in PTSD. Flashbacks, dissociative and hyperarousal symptoms, and isolated quasi-psychotic symptoms (e.g., seeing the face of the perpetrator around sleep onset) may transiently be present in the PTSD symptom presentation. However, it is the pervasiveness of psychotic symptoms and the odd, aberrant behavior that accompanies them that sets true psychosis apart from PTSD.

Self-mutilation, sexual or highly aggressive play, and suicidal behaviors may represent traumatic reenactments in children who have experienced sexual or physical abuse or who have been tortured, and these behaviors should always prompt a search for traumatic antecedents (Albach and Everaerd 1992). When children who have experienced repeated victimization demonstrate contradictory behaviors across different contexts, the diagnosis of a dissociative identity disorder, though rare, should be considered.

As noted above, trauma can exacerbate, and PTSD can mimic, disruptive behavior disorders. Indeed, there appears to be an associated risk in children who have attention-deficit/hyperactivity disorder (ADHD) and oppositional defiant disorder for developing PTSD (Ford et al. 2000). A study of children after the Hamlet, North Carolina, fire showed that the development of PTSD exacerbated or led to disruptive behavior disorders (March et al. 1995a). Similar results have been noted in studies of children after Hurricane Hugo in Florida (Lonigan et al. 1994; Shannon et al. 1994) and in studies of children who have been chronically maltreated (Famularo et al. 1992). Traumatic events can also exaggerate preexisting learning disorders, making it more difficult for the child to process traumatic experiences. Reciprocal exacerbation may be especially characteristic of youths who use drugs as a maladaptive coping strategy; that is, the substance abuse and associated behaviors actually increase the risk for future traumatic exposure and exacerbation of PTSD symptoms. However, before diagnosing oppositional defiant disorder, conduct disorder, or ADHD in a child who has experienced abuse or a life-threatening event, the clinician must rule out PTSD as the cause of the child's deteriorating school performance, inattention, irritability, or aggression. Substance abuse can complicate clinical presentations in adolescence, especially in teenagers who have trauma or abuse histories. Diagnoses such as conduct disorder and substance abuse should be addressed in their own right, even if the primary clinical focus is on PTSD. Treatment attention should of course be given to each symptom, once a thorough differential diagnosis has been considered, and it should not be assumed that collateral conditions will simply improve once PTSD is addressed.

Finally, it is important to recognize that not all reactions to traumatic events are necessarily pathological. This is especially true during the initial days and weeks following a traumatic event (Famularo et al. 1990; March 1991). When the stressor is modest in severity, partial PTSD may be present, or when symptoms interfere with the child's daily functioning, an adjustment disorder diagnosis is appropriate (Forster 1992). If full syndrome criteria are present for less than 1 month, the diagnosis of acute stress disorder should be given. In children with subsyndromal PTSD symptoms lasting longer than 6 months, the diagnosis becomes mood or anxiety disorder not otherwise specified, depending on the clinician's preference. The more important points are that clinicians should not overlook the traumatic origin of and need for intervention in subsyndromal symptoms when formulating a treatment plan, and conversely that they should not assume that PTSD is present simply on the basis of trauma exposure.

Etiology and Pathogenesis

The interplay between an environmental event (i.e., the stressor) and a complex neurobiological system characterizes the pathogenesis of PTSD. With this cardinal fact in mind, the current conceptual framework for understanding psychological trauma has evolved primarily from three theoretical perspectives: psychoanalytic theory, social learning theory, and more recently, neurobiology.

■ Psychoanalytic Theory

In 1920, Freud noted that psychic trauma results when a traumatic stimulus overwhelms the ego and renders it helpless (S. Freud 1920/1955). Along with Pierre Janet (van der Kolk and van der Hart 1989), Freud believed that the essential element in the pathogenesis of the traumatic response was the energy the trauma victim needed to utilize in warding off unbearable traumatic affects:

> An external trauma is bound to provoke a disturbance on a large scale in the functioning of the organism's energy and to set in motion every possible defensive measure. An anticathexis on a large scale is set up, for whose benefit all other psychical systems are impoverished, so that the remaining psychical functions are extensively paralyzed or reduced. (S. Freud 1920/1955)

Freud also described the patient's "repetition compulsion" as an attempt to achieve mastery over the event by repeating themes of the trauma in actions of everyday life, leading to fixation on the trauma. Other psychodynamically defined defense mechanisms that are important in trauma work are suppression, repression, denial, dissociation, projection, doing-undoing, and identification with the aggressor. As the traumatic event proceeds, most children imagine doing something to stop the trauma or to get rescued; others imagine punishing the "cause" of the trauma. Pynoos and Nader (1993) refer to these intraevent cognitive attempts to stave off helplessness as *intervention fantasies,* and the exploration of these fantasies is often critical to the identification and resolution of specific traumatic moments within the traumatic event.

■ Social Learning Theory

In contrast to psychoanalytic theory, a two-factor conditioning model derived from social learning theory frames PTSD as a stimulus-driven anxiety disorder in which both classical (factor 1) and instrumental or operant (factor 2) conditioning play important roles (Foa and Riggs 1995; Jones and Barlow 1990). In classical conditioning, the stressor or traumatic event acts as an unconditioned stimulus that elicits an unconditioned (reflexive) response characterized by physiological activation (fight-flight-freeze), extreme fear, and the cognitive perception of helplessness in the child. Cognitive, affective, physiological, and environmental cues accompanying the traumatic event then constitute conditioned stimuli, which, as mentioned earlier, are often called *traumatic reminders* or *trauma triggers.* Traumatic reminders, via stimulus generalization, become capable of eliciting a conditioned response in the form of PTSD symptoms. In instrumental conditioning, children quickly learn by trial and error how to reduce PTSD symptoms through cognitive and behavioral avoidance and sometimes anxiety-damping rituals. It is unfortunate that these behaviors also preclude the extinction of trauma-based anxiety and foster stimulus generalization. Avoidance strategies and behaviors are partially effective in the short run and are therefore self-reinforcing, although in the long run they essentially reinforce the continued aversive nature of the trauma reminders and thus continue maladaptive responses.

Like psychoanalytic theories, cognitive-behavioral theories regarding the genesis of PTSD acknowledge that both perceived and actual threat determine an individual's response. Foa and colleagues (1989) summarized the literature on cognitive information processing in PTSD, hypothesizing that persons who have PTSD develop "fear structures" that are conditioned by both the event and the PTSD symptom picture. Fear structures are exceptionally sensitive to activation by internal and external cues reminiscent of the initiating trauma, including thoughts and affects incorporated during and after the event. Moreover, they contain automatic stimulus-response elements and verbal, somatic, and behavioral cues that attach to the meaning of the event. For example, a female adolescent victimized by rape and the experience of extreme violation may lose her sense that the world is a just or a safe place. Symptoms may be maintained through the altered and inaccurate threat assessment that children with PTSD have established, whereby neutral stimuli are continuously being misappraised and perceived as threatening.

■ Neurobiology

Although neurobiology is conceptually separate from social learning theory, it is not difficult to imagine that fear structures are also represented at the neurobiological level (Perry 1994; Perry and Pate 1994). The literature on the neurobiology of PTSD in children and adolescents has begun to develop only in the past decade (De Bellis et al. 1994a, 1994b; Perry 1994; Perry and Pate 1994). Little is known about the specific neurobiological effects of early trauma on human growth and development. De Bellis and colleagues (1999a, 1999b) have extensively reviewed the psychobiology of pediatric PTSD.

It appears that early life trauma has an effect, not surprisingly, on a variety of central nervous system functions and anatomy as well as on neuroendocrine and immunological regulation (De Bellis et al. 1999a, 1999b; Heim et al. 2001; Heit et al. 1999; Wilson et al. 1999; Yehuda et al. 2001). Theoretical models, largely based on dysregulation in the neurophysiological and neuroanatomical systems regulating the stress response, are gradually becoming more sophisticated (Ornitz and Pynoos 1989; Putnam and Trickett 1993) although the child and adolescent literature remains quite unsystematic and lags considerably behind adult research. Neurotransmitters implicated in traumatic stress include norepinephrine, serotonin, dopamine, γ-aminobutyric acid (GABA), excitatory amino acids, corticosteroids and their modulators, and endogenous opioids (De Bellis et al. 1994a, 1994b). Not surprisingly, these neurotransmitter systems ramify through a variety of neuroanatomical regions implicated in PTSD, including brain stem arousal mechanisms, diencephalic modulatory centers of sensory and emotional information, and cortical and limbic structures of memory and motivation (including areas mediating selective appraisal of threat). De Bellis and colleagues (1999a, 1999b, 2001) showed that, compared with control children, maltreated children had smaller intracranial and cerebral volumes (but not hippocampal volumes tracked over 2 years of development). Maltreated children were also shown to exhibit more suicidal ideation and behavior, greater depression, overall rates of psychopathology (based on parent reports), and increased frequency of dissociation. Dysregulation in the hypothalamic-pituitary-adrenal axis and in secretion of cortisol (a "stress" hormone) is known to be present in both adults and children with PTSD (Cicchetti and Rogosch 2001; Yehuda 1998; Yehuda et al. 2001), although the specific abnormality tends to be variable. Studies in adults—especially those involving individuals with rape trauma or early childhood sexual abuse—have shown that adults with PTSD, unlike those with depression, have low cortisol levels and that these individuals may be supersuppressors of cortisol secretion when challenged with dexamethasone—again unlike in depression, where there is a failure to suppress with dexamethasone challenge. King et al. (2001) demonstrated that girls age 5–7 years exposed to recent sexual abuse exhibited significantly lower salivary cortisol levels than age-matched control subjects. Although these findings are intriguing, the precise developmental implications for early-life dysregulation in hypothalamic-pituitary axis function have yet to be worked out. Future studies of the neurobiology of PTSD in children and adolescents will seek to be more systematic in cross-correlating clinical symptoms, functional and anatomical neuroimaging, relevant neuroendocrine findings, and neuropsychiatric assessment.

Assessment

As in all psychiatric disorders, the first step in establishing a treatment program is a careful, thorough assessment that, in the case of PTSD, is stressor focused (Nader et al. 1991). Although semistructured interviews are useful for assessing psychiatric problems in children and adolescents, reliability and validity data for PTSD instruments have been slow to emerge (March and Albano 1996), and no structured instrument can replace a well-conducted series of clinical interviews in this most complex disorder. The most commonly used instrument—the Pynoos-Nader version of the Stress-Reaction Index—shows modest empirical support as a semistructured interview (R. Pynoos, personal communication, September 1995); it has been used as a self-report measure (Lonigan et al. 1991; March et al. 1995a) but does not adequately capture the DSM-IV criteria (American Psychiatric Association 1994), nor does it yield a DSM-IV diagnosis. With the support of the National Center for PTSD, Nader and colleagues (1994) developed the Clinician-Administered PTSD Scale—Child and Adolescent Version (CAPS-C). The CAPS-C allows for current and lifetime diagnoses and dimensional assessment of DSM-IV PTSD symptoms and collateral psychopathology. It is time consuming and demanding on the clinician to conduct and is probably best reserved for clinical-research settings. The CAPS-C is undergoing psychometric evaluation in diverse populations, and it has become the consensus choice for diagnostic and treatment outcome studies in PTSD (M. Friedman, National Center for PTSD, personal communication, March 2002). Table 32–4 presents a template of domains, symptoms, and associated factors of coping, social support, and other features intrinsic to the child and environment that should be considered in assessing PTSD in this age group.

With the caveat that parents are generally better at evaluating children's externalizing symptoms than evaluating their internalizing symptoms (Costello 1989), a multimethod, multimodal evaluation is preferable, including information from multiple sources (Amaya-Jackson and March 1993). In children younger than 48 months the most important trauma-variable predictor appears to be whether a caregiver was threatened, and therefore caregiver reports are crucial sources of clinical information (Scheeringa 1999). Parent-teacher measures, such as the Conners Parent and Teacher Rating Scales (Conners et al. 1995) and the SNAP IV (Swanson 1992) are efficient adjuncts for assessing collateral externalizing symptoms. Self-report measures, such as the Children's Depression Inventory (Kovacs 1985) and the Multidimensional Anxiety Scale for Children (March et al. 1995b), can be used to assess internalizing comorbidities. Table 32–4 summarizes important domains of assessment in pediatric PTSD.

Finally, the assessment of PTSD in children and adolescents must be embedded within developmental and social contexts. To some extent, because the DSM-IV-TR nosology is less sensitive to evaluation of early-life trauma and because it underemphasizes both developmental differences and social contextual factors, it is less than adequate for evaluating childhood-onset PTSD. For example, some aspects of the PTSD symptom complex may best be reported by the affected child, others by parents, and still others by teachers or other observers. Moreover, because the child's social matrix—neighborhood, family, peer, and school environments—may strongly affect the risk of PTSD and corollary symptoms, it is important to consider variables such as loss, secondary adversities, family functioning, and attachment-related symptoms when evaluating a child for PTSD. Because posttraumatic sequelae vary with the nature of the stressor (e.g., chronic abuse versus sudden trauma), the ability to map the events onto a developmental framework depends on a precise characterization of the stressor and accompanying secondary adversities and comorbid conditions identified in thorough diagnostic evaluation.

Treatment

■ Psychotherapy and Psychosocial Management

Other than case reports, few published treatment studies specifically focus on PTSD in children. However, researchers and clinicians have reported a variety of techniques that have proved valuable in clinical trauma work (Yule and Canterbury 1994). The adult PTSD literature points to tactics that may prove beneficial to children as well. In general, a "prevention-intervention" model—which incorporates triage for children exposed to stressors, support and strengthening of coping skills for anticipated grief and trauma responses, treatment of other disorders that may develop or become exacerbated in the context of PTSD, and treatment of acute PTSD symptoms—is recommended (Amaya-Jackson and March 1995a, 1995b; Pynoos and Nader 1993). The horrific effects of trauma may never be fully undone, and therefore "cure" may not be the appropriate treatment goal, but trauma victims can become well-functioning survivors if appropriate treatment is given and facilitation of healing takes place.

Solomon et al. (1992) reviewed empirical studies of psychotherapeutic, cognitive-behavioral, and drug treatments for PTSD. They correctly noted that the literature provides greater support for cognitive-behavioral treatment than for other treatments. However, considering the substantial literature on PTSD, the

Table 32–4. Assessment of posttraumatic stress disorder

Domain	Subdomains
Diagnosis	DSM-IV-TR
Criterion A1: objective	Multiple events
	Stressor dimensions
Criterion A2: subjective	Emotions (e.g., feeling terrified)
	Appraisal (e.g., life threat)
	Attribution (e.g., helplessness)
	Beliefs (e.g., "can't be happening to me")
	Peridissociation (e.g., temporal or spatial distortions)
	Parental response
Life events	Pre-event
	Post-event
	Secondary adversities
Traumatic reminders	Mapped from stressor
PTSD symptoms	Cluster B, C, D
PTSD corollary symptoms	Guilt
	Anger
	Event-specific new fears
Functioning	Global
	Academic (behavioral and pedagogic arenas)
	Family
	Peer
Loss/grief	Family and friends
Comorbidity	Affective disorder
	Anxiety disorders
	Disruptive behavior disorders
	Anger and aggression
	Substance abuse
	Dissociation
	Somatization
	Learning disorders and problems
	Eating disorders
	Sleep disorders
	Enuresis
Child intrinsic factors	Demographics
	IQ
	Medical history
	Family genetic history
	Temperament
	Psychiatric history
	Attachment
Coping behaviors	General
	To traumatic reminders

Table 32–4. Assessment of posttraumatic stress disorder (*continued*)

Domain	Subdomains
Social support	Socioeconomic status
	Parenting style
	Family functioning
	Expressed emotion
	Marital function
	Relationship with siblings
	Peers
	Neighborhood
Parent psychopathology	PTSD
	Grief
	Other
Social cognition	Self-efficacy
	Locus of control
	Trauma-specific attributions
Social skills	General
	Peers
	Trauma-specific
Mental and physical health services	Psychiatric
	Medical
	Other

dearth of treatment outcome studies, especially in the area of drug treatment, is quite striking (Richters 1993). It is interesting to note that, despite the lack of randomized controlled trials, the majority of child psychiatric clinicians questioned about their treatment strategies for PTSD utilized pharmacotherapy as a primary treatment element (Cohen et al. 2001). Treatment providers to children and adolescents are inevitably forced to operate from clinical consensus, uncontrolled trials, and downward extrapolation from adult studies. Treatment options are considered within a combined pharmacological, psychodynamic, and cognitive-behavioral framework—a reasonable consensus is that these approaches are best used adjunctively with one another.

The mainstay of treatment is usually an admixture of cognitive-behavioral, family-supportive, and psychodynamically informed psychotherapy, spread over several phases: brief preventive or initial therapy, long-term therapy, and pulsed intervention. Additional interventions include formal group and family therapy. Early preventive and initial therapy interventions are especially important in the setting of acute trauma, catching a window of opportunity when the youngster's symptoms are most prominent and the sealing over of affect has not had a chance to occur. Central to almost all treatment strategies is an emphasis on re-exposing the individual to traumatic cues under safe conditions, incorporating reparative and mastery elements in a structured, supportive manner. An important point concerning psychotherapy for children with PTSD is that poorly conducted therapy at best can be a waste of precious time in the life of a child and at worst can be harmful and can inadvertently lead to retraumatization. Long-term therapy, especially in young children, can easily devolve into unfocused, repetitive sessions of "fiddling around." Therapists need to be diligent about continually rethinking the symptom picture, keeping focused on current dysfunction, and directing the therapy to specifically facilitate higher levels of adaptation and coping. Good intentions and an empathic stance on the part of child therapists are necessary but are no substitute for clinical skills in cognitive-behavioral therapy (CBT), detailed knowledge of child development, and supervised experience in conducting psychotherapy with children.

■ Initial Interventions

Critical incident stress debriefing and psychological first aid are techniques that are particularly applicable in crisis centers and in classrooms (Pynoos and Nader 1988b, 1989b). Applications of these techniques typically involve groups of children gathering together in a specific setting. School settings in particular serve as an optimum site for immediate crisis intervention, ventilation, information processing, and screening of children who may need further evaluation (Motta 1994; Pynoos and Nader 1989b). Debriefing interviews with teachers and parents can help to identify, clarify, and normalize adults' and children's reactions to a traumatic event. Adults may need assistance around resurfacing of their own prior losses or guilt and helplessness over not being able to prevent what happened. During classroom discussions, children describe the traumatic event on a moment-to-moment basis, allowing clarification of traumatic and grief reactions as they affect current functioning.

In both individual therapy and group settings, free-form or semistructured projective play techniques such as spontaneous drawing, Winnicott's (1971) squiggle game, or Levy's (1939) preset play can be used as a means to express feelings, clarify confusion, and identify needs. Although it is often underestimat-

ed, simply allowing the time and a format for the basic human need to put experience into words and thus share traumatic events with others can be a potent early-phase intervention. Reparative drawings or role-playing vignettes are important components in the early treatment phase: tornado-ravaged houses can be rebuilt, injuries can be healed, and children whose last view of a dying friend was tarnished by blood can find some relief by drawing their friend whole from the memory of the last time they played or as they would like to imagine them to be "up in heaven." Children identified as highly exposed or having difficulty adjusting may be referred for further treatment. Additional interventions may be needed and can be done through the schools, including support-counseling groups for parents or children and consultation-liaison with guidance staff and teachers. Amaya-Jackson et al. (2002) described a protocol-based cognitive-behavioral treatment for PTSD designed to be used in groups of children as a school-based treatment intervention. This may be especially useful in situations where there are high rates of shared trauma exposure among populations of children in definable geographic regions such as neighborhoods or school districts. Saltzman et al. (in press) described a screening- and school-based group treatment package wherein there is a relatively seamless flow in the process of identifying symptomatic children and then treating them—all in the safe, familiar, and easily accessible environment of school.

The initial evaluation of children can incorporate many other interview techniques and goals that lead naturally into therapeutic intervention. Through the use of play, drawings, puppets, and role-playing, the child's experience as well as subjective meaning and attributions can be strategically explored. Clinicians must pay close attention to their own countertransference and rescue fantasies, the tendency to shy away from particularly upsetting aspects of the child's experiences, and well-intended but misguided attempts to spare the child distress when asking precise questions about the trauma. That the therapist can endure the recounting of the event and the affect involved is crucial to the child's ability to utilize the treatment in general and to tolerate exposure in particular. Children's reactions can at times be normalized, intervention fantasies can be acknowledged, traumatic reminders can be identified, and confusion and distortions can be clarified. The psychotherapeutic evaluation period should not be rushed, because it may take several sessions, especially in younger children, to develop a working therapeutic alliance and to detect emergent trauma themes in play assessment encounters.

An important but often neglected element of all types of therapy for pediatric PTSD is the initial didactic explanation to parents and children of the components of PTSD and the specific rationale for therapy, collectively referred to as psychoeducation. Children as well as adolescents need to understand the nature of their disorder and how their therapy relates to the bad things that have happened to them. Parents especially need to understand the rationale and basic behavioral principles of CBT, because by its very nature it requires some amount of discomfort during the course of treatment. Explanations by way of therapeutic metaphors are often useful in play-based therapies for younger children. Without a clear understanding of the connection between therapeutic tactics and symptom relief, parents and children are more likely to withdraw from treatment.

■ Brief Therapy

Trauma work frequently involves brief psychotherapy. Because controlled reexposure to traumatic cues is an essential aspect of treatment, traumatic memories and associated specific reminders must be worked through in their entirety, both in therapy and in real-life activities. A key treatment concept necessary for successful "working through" is to approach the trauma as a series of traumatic moments, that is, sequential vivid memories of distress linked by less distressing narrative content (Pynoos and Nader 1988b). Specific moments are frequently linked to intervention fantasies (described above under "Etiology and Pathogenesis"). Often the worst moment occurs at the time of real or fantasized helplessness. Children commonly wish to rush through the most difficult aspects in an attempt to avoid the intense affects that accompany reexperiencing. Systematically strategizing recall in a moment-by-moment fashion minimizes cognitive and behavioral avoidance and thus promotes exposure and habituation of anxiety. Brief therapies may be most appropriate in situations where a child is seen soon after a traumatic exposure, in situations of single-incident trauma and when the target symptoms and goals of treatment are clearly defined and of a limited scope.

■ Cognitive-Behavioral Therapy

PTSD is the quintessential threat-induced anxiety disorder (March 1991; March and Amaya-Jackson 1994).

As with other anxiety disorders, some clinicians believe that cognitive-behavioral therapy (CBT) optimized for the PTSD symptom picture may be the treatment of choice for PTSD symptoms per se (Foa et al. 1989) and may be delivered both to individual children and in group-based therapeutic formats (Amaya-Jackson et al. 2002). Saigh (1992) made a persuasive case for the efficacy of CBT as a treatment of single-incident trauma in young persons. Deblinger and colleagues (1990, 1999) showed that CBT benefits children with PTSD caused by sexual abuse and that the benefits of therapy are durable until the 2-year follow-up, not only for core PTSD symptoms but also for associated depressive symptoms and externalizing behavior problems.

Theoretical Model Underlying PTSD and Its Treatment with CBT

Earlier behavioral theories of PTSD conceptualized PTSD within two-factor conditioning theory in which both classical conditioning (factor 1) and instrumental conditioning (factor 2) played important roles (Dollard and Miller 1950). In the first (classical conditioning) stage, the traumatic event is thought to act as an unconditioned stimulus that elicits fear, the unconditioned response. Cognitive, affective, physiological, and environmental cues accompanying the traumatic event constitute conditioned stimuli, which, as noted earlier, are often called *traumatic reminders*. In turn, traumatic reminders become capable of eliciting fear (the conditioned response), which should decrease with prolonged, repeated exposure (habituation), assuming the absence of real threat. In the second (instrumental conditioning) stage, the individual learns to reduce trauma-related distress through cognitive and behavioral avoidance. These operant anxiety-reducing behaviors preclude the extinction of trauma-relevant anxiety and therefore are customarily targeted in exposure-based interventions.

Recognizing the limitations of nonmediational (i.e., strictly behavioral) accounts for anxiety such as two-factor theory, cognitive-behavioral theorists proposed that the interpretation of events and their resultant emotional reactions mediate psychiatric symptoms and pathological behaviors (e.g., Beck 1985; Foa and Kozak 1985a, 1985b). Influenced by information-processing theories of behavior change (O'Donohue and Kransner 1998), these conceptualizations rest on the assumption that knowledge acquired throughout life is represented in memory in the form of abstract, generic knowledge structures, referred to as *schemas*. Accordingly, Foa and colleagues (e.g., Foa and Riggs 1995; Foa and Rothbaum 1998) proposed that two sets of dysfunctional cognitions (i.e., schemas) underlie the development of this disorder: the world is indiscriminately dangerous and oneself (the victim) is extremely incompetent.

Typically, CBT for children with PTSD targets specific features of the PTSD symptom picture, using anxiety-management training, anger-coping, and exposure-based interventions. Numerous studies have shown that these interventions effectively reduce target symptoms in anxious children (Kendall 1991; Thyer 1991). By promoting habituation, exposure—encountering contact with the phobic stimulus until anxiety diminishes substantially—probably forms the core intervention in PTSD (Foa and Riggs 1995; Foa et al. 1989). When necessary, response prevention facilitates exposure by blocking rituals and avoidance behaviors, thereby undoing the reinforcing effects of avoidance. Anxiety-management training–which includes relaxation, breathing training, and cognitive restructuring—facilitates exposure, promotes provision of cognitive and behavioral corrective information, and enhances positive coping (Foa and Rothbaum 1992).

In addition to phobic anxiety to traumatic stimuli, PTSD presents other treatment targets for CBT, including generalized anxiety (such as worry and tension), mood symptoms (such as irritability and hostility), and disruption in social functioning (such as peer or academic problems). Clinically, some youngsters with PTSD feel chronically angry and are prone to aggressive behavior; treatment for such children with PTSD would be incomplete without addressing these symptoms. CBT effectively targets these unskilled behaviors and associated cognitions to reduce the frequency of inappropriate behaviors, emphasizing both the external environment (i.e., teachers, parents) and the internal thoughts and feelings of the child (Feindler 1991; Lochman et al. 1987). Anger-coping groups have been particularly successful in addressing maladaptive aggressive behavior (Lochman et al. 1987). Treatment of externalizing symptoms also involves the use of contingency management strategies, including reinforcement of appropriate behavior, withdrawal of reinforcement for inappropriate behavior (referred to as *extinction*), and use of "time-out" when problematic behavior is displayed. At the outset of treatment, it is often necessary to incorporate tangible rewards for appropriate behavior into the contingency management plan, with these rewards gradually phased out as the child internalizes reinforcement for appropriate behavior. In all cases, CBT for these target symptoms must be integrated into the total treatment picture so that the trauma-relevant meaning of the symptoms to the child can be placed in an appropriate therapeutic context.

■ Group and Family-Based Therapy

Group and family therapy are additional interventions that can play an important role in treatment. Family therapy is particularly helpful in addressing the needs of children who are not receiving necessary emotional support within the family. Family members may have difficulty facing the child's distress or may lack necessary (but still teachable) skills to meet the child's needs adequately. Parents may be preoccupied with their own reactions and may not be aware of the child's symptoms. Families can be taught coping strategies, such as how to recognize and deal with traumatic reminders. In designing treatment interventions for young children, Scheeringa (1999) designed an eight-component package that places primary emphasis on parent-based interventions and on simply keeping the parent coming and engaged in therapy. CBT has been successfully applied with physically and sexually abused children and their offending and nonoffending parents with good outcomes reported at 1 year (Cohen and Mannerino 1997; Deblinger and Heflin 2000; Kolko 1996). Direct inclusion of parents in the treatment process may be especially important in situations involving intense interpersonal trauma such as in cases of intrafamilial physical or sexual abuse. Inclusion of parents and the use of group formats may also be useful in community shared trauma exposure such as Stubenbort et al. (2001) report in their use of CBT group therapy for children and adults after an air disaster. In traumatic situations with multiple victims, such as after a natural disaster or mass violence, group psychotherapy can be of tremendous benefit following (or concomitant with) individual treatment. Layperson support groups help provide emotional sustenance to deal with traumatic symptoms and can facilitate exposure therapy through shared successes in resisting the urge to avoid traumatic reminders.

■ Long-Term Treatment and Pulsed Intervention

A subgroup of children require long-term treatment. Exposure to massive violence, intrafamilial homicide or suicide, prolonged abuse, or repetitively distressing events suggests that brief trauma work may be insufficient. The presence of preexisting psychopathology in the child or a parent, a history of abuse, multiple foster placements, or ongoing exposure to a disruptive living situation also suggest a need for more intensive, longer-term intervention. Long-term treatment can occur weekly or as pulsed intervention (i.e., on a recurrent as-needed basis) based on the child's developmental phase, capacity for response, and clinical issues. Pulsed intervention is based on the assumption that brief therapy is suspended (rather than terminated) until further treatment becomes necessary, such as during developmental transitions, changes in living situation, formation of intimate relationships, and marriage. "Pulsing" the treatment helps to prevent ongoing helplessness by minimizing dependence on the therapist as "the only one who really understands." Severe PTSD requires arduous and critical dedication to treatment on the part of the patient and therapist. Longer-term therapy may also be necessary when issues related to character formation and the capacity to form meaningful relationships are present.

■ Medication Management

Although PTSD has an exogenous origin and requires psychological treatments, it is nevertheless, using Kardiner's (1941) term, a true *physioneurosis*, and psychotropic medication often proves helpful in allowing psychological treatment to progress. Unfortunately, few data exist to guide the use of medication in children and adolescents with PTSD (for review, see Donnelly et al. 1999; Maletic et al. 1994). Yet, in a large sampling of treatment providers Cohen et al. (2001) found that 95% of medical practitioners who treat pediatric PTSD use pharmacotherapy, in combination with psychodynamic or cognitive-behavioral therapies. Medication use in children and adolescents with PTSD should be based on a stepwise approach in which broad-spectrum agents are considered first, followed by attention to comorbid diagnoses that are likely to be amenable to pharmacological intervention. Medication algorithms have been developed for such a stepwise approach in both adults and children (Donnelly and Amaya-Jackson 2002; Friedman et al. 2000).

Ideally, medications should decrease intrusions, avoidance, and anxious arousal; minimize impulsivity; improve sleep; treat secondary disorders; facilitate cognitive-behavioral psychotherapies; and improve functioning in daily life. It should be borne in mind that effective treatment of even one symptom in children with PTSD (e.g., improvement of sleep-onset disturbance) can have a positive ripple effect across multiple domains of functioning. In adults, many case reports, uncontrolled trials, and newly emerging randomized controlled trials suggest that the benefits of conventional drug treatments in PTSD are modest to significant (Friedman 2000; Friedman et al. 2000; Hidalgo and Davidson 2000). Two selective serotonin reuptake inhibitors (SSRIs), paroxetine and sertraline, have recently received U.S. Food and Drug Administration (FDA) approval for the treatment of PTSD in adults (Beebe 2001; Brady et al. 2000; Marshall et al. 2001). Although much more limited than for adults, clinical experience is similar for children and adolescents.

Table 32–5 lists the published studies examining medication effects in the treatment of children and adolescents with PTSD. The decision to use medication is based primarily on the types of target symptoms present that are likely to be responsive to medication (both core PTSD symptoms and comorbid condition symptoms), their severity, and the degree of disability that they cause. Although no medication currently has an FDA label indication for the treatment of PTSD in childhood, data from adult studies and clinical experience with other disorders in childhood provide guidance in selecting pharmacological agents. Pharmacotherapy may be an important component in the multimodal treatment of PTSD because it may offer relief from highly debilitating symptoms and buffer children against intense symptoms, allowing for easier confrontation of traumatic material in therapy and better functioning in life activities.

The SSRIs have received perhaps the most attention and are likely first-line choices in childhood owing to their broad-spectrum activity in anxiety, mood, and obsessive-compulsive spectrum disorders and the fact that they have demonstrated effectiveness in adult populations (Brady et al. 2000; Hidalgo and Davidson 2000; Marshall et al. 2001; van der Kolk et al. 1994) and are being actively investigated in childhood. Seedat et al. (2001) report the effectiveness of citalopram in a 12-week open-label trial in eight adolescents with moderate to severe PTSD. Subjects in their trial exhibited a 38% reduction in PTSD symptoms at the end of treatment (however, curiously, self-reported depressive symptoms failed to improve). The SSRIs can be effective in reducing trauma-associated reexperiencing,

Table 32–5. Pediatric posttraumatic stress disorder pharmacotherapy studies

Study	Medication	Design	Subjects	Results	Adverse effects/comments
Domon and Andersen (2000)	Nefazodone Avg, 200 mg/d Range, 200–600 mg/d	Open-label case report ? Time frame	Adolescents	Improvement in hyperarousal, aggression, insomnia	Nausea, vomiting, morning somnolence
Famularo et al. (1988)	Propranolol 0.8 mg/kg/d tid–2.5 mg/kg/d tid	Off-on-off open label 4-wk tx phase	N=11 Mean age, 8.5 yr Physical/sexual abuse	Significantly fewer PTSD symptoms when taking med; improved hyperarousal, agitation	Three subjects did not tolerate dosage escalation
Harmon and Riggs (1996)	Clonidine 0.1 mg hs– 0.05 mg bid and 0.1 mg hs po; also TTS patch	Open label 3–4 wks	N=7 3–6-year-old preschoolers	Moderate to great improvement in aggression, hyperarousal, insomnia	Sedation, patch skin irritation, rebound hypertension
Horrigan (1996)	Clonidine 0.05 mg hs, guanfacine 0.5 mg hs	Single-subject case report	N=1 7-year-old female	Clonidine improved nightmares for 4 wks, lost effect; switch to guanfacine resumed improvement	None reported
Looff et al. (1995)	Carbamazepine 300–1,200 mg/d; levels 10–11.5	Open label 17–92 days	N=28 12 females 16 males	22 of 28 patients asymptomatic, remaining 6 "improved"	No adverse effects reported; multiple meds/multiple comorbidities in tx patients
Perry (1994)	Clonidine 0.05–0.1 mg bid	Open label	N=17	Improvement in anxiety, arousal, concentration, mood, impulsivity	
Robert et al. (1999)	Imipramine 1 mg/kg hs vs. chloral hydrate 25 mg/kg, max 500 mg	Prospective, randomized, double-blind 7 days	N=25 burn patients 11 females 14 males 2–19 y.o. Acute stress disorder	All acute stress disorder symptoms improved in 10/12 patients treated with imipramine 80% experienced remission of hyperarousal/intrusive re-experiencing. 5/13 responded to chloral hydrate	None reported
Seedat et al. (2001)	Citalopram 20 mg/d fixed dose	Open label	N=8 adolescents	All symptom clusters showed response on CAPS-C, 38% reduction in scores; self-report depression scores did not improve	Benign adverse events, generally well tolerated

Note. CAPS-C=Clinician-Administered PTSD Scale—Child and Adolescent Version; TTS=transdermal therapeutic system (skin patch); tx=trial.

anxiety, and collateral mood symptoms, although they may be less effective in avoidance or numbing symptoms. They are generally safe and well tolerated and tend to be the agents of first choice.

Nefazodone, a serotonergic antagonist antidepressant, has been reported to be helpful in PTSD and associated irritability and disruptive behavior in adolescents in an uncontrolled case series reported by Domon and Andersen (2000). Mirtazapine, an antidepressant with serotonin and norepinephrine activity, has shown promise—either alone or in combination with an SSRI—for the treatment of PTSD (Conner et al. 1999; Good and Petersen 2001).

Adrenergic agents such as the α_2-adrenergic agonists clonidine and guanfacine and the β-adrenergic antagonist propranolol reduce sympathetic tone and may be effective in the symptoms of hyperarousal, impulsivity, activation, sleep problems, and nightmares seen in PTSD (De Bellis 1994b; Horrigan 1996; Marmar et al. 1993). Clonidine in particular has been shown to decrease startle responses and may target other symptoms of physiological lability, as measured by autonomic arousal (Ornitz and Pynoos 1989). In an open-label trial involving 17 children with PTSD, Perry et al. (1994) found significant improvement in anxiety arousal, concentration, mood, and behavioral impulsivity using relatively low doses of clonidine. Harmon and Riggs (1996) reported the effectiveness of the transdermal clonidine patch in reducing PTSD symptoms in all 7 patients in their open-label trial. Horrigan (1996) in a single case study reported the effectiveness of guanfacine in reducing PTSD-associated nightmares in a 7-year-old. There is evidence that if tolerance develops to one agent (e.g., clonidine), replacement with guanfacine can provide renewed symptomatic response (Horrigan and Barnhill 1996). Propranolol has also been shown to reduce arousal symptoms in survivors of childhood sexual abuse, presumably by blocking sympathetic nervous system hyperreactivity, although central effects may also play a role (Famularo et al. 1988). Adrenergic agents deserve consideration in managing the hyperarousal, activation, motor hyperactivity, and sleep-onset problems often associated with PTSD in childhood.

The benzodiazepines have been used to treat anxiety disorders in children and adults, although there are few if any data to support their effectiveness in the core symptoms of PTSD (Friedman 1998). These agents (e.g., clonazepam, lorazepam) may have a minor role to play in reducing acute and intense symptoms of anxiety or agitation, or as a short-term adjunctive treatment to facilitate exposure tasks in psychotherapy. However, they should be used with caution in children and adolescents owing to their propensity to cause paradoxical disinhibition and their abuse potential. The benzodiazepines cannot be recommended as first- or second-line therapy at present.

The mood stabilizers may have a role to play in the treatment of childhood PTSD, especially in cases of severe affective instability. Lithium, valproate, and carbamazepine may reduce extreme mood lability and anger dyscontrol. Carbamazepine has received the most attention and has been shown to markedly reduce flashbacks, traumatic nightmares, intrusive recollections, and sleep disturbance in adults (Lipper et al. 1986). Looff et al. (1995) found carbamazepine to be highly effective in treating core PTSD symptoms in 22 of 28 patients with sexual abuse histories who had high rates of comorbidity with other disorders of children and adolescents.

Atypical neuroleptics such as risperidone, olanzapine, quetiapine, and ziprasidone may have a limited role to play in childhood PTSD but should be reserved for cases in which psychotic symptoms, severe aggression, or self-injurious behaviors are complicating management and first-line treatments are not containing these symptoms.

Tricyclic antidepressants such as imipramine and desipramine have been largely supplanted in child and adolescent psychiatry by the newer antidepressant agents owing to unwanted side effects and potential cardiotoxicity. These agents may have a second-line utility in childhood PTSD when comorbid conditions such as ADHD, enuresis, or sleep disorders are present. Robert et al. (1999) found that low-dose imipramine was effective in treating sleep disturbances in burn patients soon after their injury and may have reduced the frequency of development of full-blown PTSD compared with children treated with chloral hydrate.

Cyproheptadine, a histaminergic agent with serotonin partial agonist/antagonist activity, is a safe agent that is commonly used in clinical practice for sleep-onset problems and traumatic nightmares. There is little in the way of controlled evidence for its efficacy; however, some investigators report benefits, and it carries few risks in the child and adolescent age group (Brophy 1991).

In summary, the state of knowledge regarding medication treatments for children and adolescents is in the earliest stages of development. There are no well-conducted randomized clinical trials to guide practitioners. Medication may have an important role in reducing debilitating symptoms of PTSD and providing a buffer for children while they confront difficult material in therapy and may also help to improve their general day-to-day functioning. A reasonable approach is to begin with a broad-spectrum agent such as an SSRI, which should target anxiety, mood, and reexperiencing symptoms. Adrenergic agents such as clonidine, either used alone or in combination with an SSRI, may be useful when symptoms of hyperarousal and impulsivity are problematic. Supplementing with a mood stabilizer may be necessary in severe affective dyscontrol. Similarly, introduction of an atypical neuroleptic may be necessary in cases of severe self-injurious behavior, dissociation, psychosis, or aggression. Comorbid conditions such as ADHD should of course be targeted with pharmacotherapy known to be effective, such as the psychostimulants.

Conclusion

PTSD is a common cause of psychiatric morbidity in children and adolescents. The disorder in youth is similar to that in adulthood, with differences primarily stemming from divergent stressors, the differential impact across stages of development, developmental themes, and family considerations. Children appear to be more sensitive to the effects of trauma, and early-life trauma exposure may set into play a complex sequence of events leading to development of multiple psychiatric disorders in adulthood. Treatment of PTSD in childhood involves debriefing and ventilation, psychoeducation of parent and child, brief psychotherapy, and pulsed long-term intervention using an admixture of psychodynamic, cognitive-behavioral, and pharmacological treatments.

References

Albach F, Everaerd W: Posttraumatic stress symptoms in victims of childhood incest. Psychother Psychosom 57:143–151, 1992

Amaya-Jackson L, March J: Post-traumatic stress disorder in children and adolescents, in Child Psychiatric Clinics of North America: Anxiety Disorders, Vol 2. Edited by Leonard HL. New York, WB Saunders, 1993, pp 639–654

Amaya-Jackson L, March J: Posttraumatic stress disorder, in Anxiety Disorders in Children and Adolescents. Edited by March J. New York, Guilford, 1995a, pp 276–300

Amaya-Jackson L, March J: Post-traumatic stress disorder in adolescents. Adolesc Med 6:251–270, 1995b

Amaya-Jackson L, Reynolds V, Murray MC, et al: Cognitive-behavioral treatment for pediatric posttraumatic stress disorder: protocol and application in school and community settings. Cognitive and Behavioral Practice 10(3), 2003

American Psychiatric Association: Diagnostic and Statistical Manual of Mental Disorders, 3rd Edition. Washington, DC, American Psychiatric Association, 1980

American Psychiatric Association: Diagnostic and Statistical Manual of Mental Disorders, 4th Edition. Washington, DC, American Psychiatric Association, 1994

American Psychiatric Association: Diagnostic and Statistical Manual of Mental Disorders, 4th Edition, Text Revision. Washington, DC, American Psychiatric Association, 2000

Beck AT: Theoretical perspectives on clinical anxiety, in Anxiety and the Anxiety Disorders. Edited by Tuma AH, Maser JD. Hillsdale, NJ, Erlbaum, 1985, pp 183–196

Beebe KL: Paroxetine in the treatment of PTSD: a 12-week, placebo-controlled, multicenter study. GlaxoSmithKline, 2001

Berman H: Children and war: current understandings and future directions. Public Health Nurs 18:243–252, 2001

Black B: Separation anxiety disorder and panic disorder, in Anxiety Disorders in Children and Adolescents. Edited by March J. New York, Guilford, 1995, pp 212–234

Bloch DA, Silber E, Perry SE: Some factors in the emotional reactions of children to disaster. Am J Psychiatry 113:416–422, 1956

Brady K, Pearlstein T, Asnis GM, et al: Efficacy and safety of sertraline treatment of posttraumatic stress disorder: a randomized controlled trial. JAMA 283:1837–1844, 2000

Bremner JD, Shobe KK, Kihlstrom JF: False memories in women with self-reported childhood sexual abuse: an empirical study. Psychol Sci 11:333–337, 2000

Breslau N, Davis GC, Andreski P, et al: Traumatic events and posttraumatic stress disorder in an urban population of young adults. Arch Gen Psychiatry 48:216–222, 1991

Breslau N, Kessler RC, Chilcoat-Schultz LR, et al: Trauma and posttraumatic stress disorder in the community: the 1996 Detroit Area Survey of Trauma. Arch Gen Psychiatry 55:626–632, 1998

Brophy MH: Cyproheptadine for combat nightmares in posttraumatic stress disorder and dream anxiety disorder. Mil Med 156:100–101, 1991

Burke JD, Moccia P, Borus JF, et al: Emotional distress in fifth-grade children ten months after a natural disaster. J Am Acad Child Psychiatry 25:536–541, 1986

Cahill C, Llewelyn SP, Pearson C: Long-term effects of sexual abuse which occurred in childhood: a review. Br J Clin Psychol 30:117–130, 1991

Carey-Trefzger C: The results of a clinical study of war damaged children who attended the Child Guidance Clinic, The Hospital for Sick Children, Great Ormand Street, London. Journal of Mental Science 95:535–559, 1949

Cicchetti D, Rogosch FA: Diverse patterns of neuroendocrine activity in maltreated children. Dev Psychopathol 13:677–693, 2001

Clarke G, Sack WH, Goff B: Three forms of stress in Cambodian adolescent refugees. J Abnorm Child Psychol 21:65–77, 1993

Cohen JA: Practice parameters for the assessment and treatment of children and adolescents with posttraumatic stress disorder. J Am Acad Child Adolesc Psychiatry 37 (10, suppl):4S–26S, 1998

Cohen JA, Mannerino AP: A treatment study of sexually abused preschool children: outcome during a one-year follow-up. J Am Acad Child Adolesc Psychiatry 35:42–50, 1997

Cohen JA, Mannarino AP, Rogal S: Treatment practices for childhood posttraumatic stress disorder. Child Abuse Negl 25:123–135, 2001

Conaway LP, Hansen DJ: Social behavior of physically abused and neglected children: a critical review. Clin Psychol Rev 9:627–652, 1989

Conner KM, Davidson JR, Weisler RH, et al: A pilot study of mirtazapine in post-traumatic stress disorder. Int Clin Psychopharmacol 14:29–31, 1999

Conners C, March J, Erhardt D, et al: Assessment of attention-deficit disorders. Journal of Psychoeducational Assessment 28:186–205, 1995

Costello E: Developments in child psychiatric epidemiology. J Am Acad Child Adolesc Psychiatry 28:836–841, 1989

De Bellis MD, Chrousos GP, Dorn LD, et al: Hypothalamic-pituitary-adrenal axis dysregulation in sexually abused girls [see comments]. J Clin Endocrinol Metab 78:249–255, 1994a

De Bellis MD, Lefter L, Trickett PK, et al: Urinary catecholamine excretion in sexually abused girls. J Am Acad Child Adolesc Psychiatry 33:320–327, 1994b

De Bellis MD, Baum AS, Birmaher B, et al: A.E. Bennett Research Award. Developmental traumatology, I: biological stress systems. Biol Psychiatry 45:1259–1270, 1999a

De Bellis MD, Keshavan MS, Clark DB, et al: A.E. Bennett Research Award. Developmental traumatology, II: brain development. Biol Psychiatry 45:1271–1284, 1999b

De Bellis MD, Hall J, Boring AM, et al: A pilot longitudinal study of hippocampal volumes in pediatric maltreatment-related posttraumatic stress disorder. Biol Psychiatry 50:305–309, 2001

Deblinger E, Heflin AH: Treating sexually abused children and their nonoffending parents: a cognitive behavioral approach. Thousand Oaks, CA, Sage, 2000

Deblinger E, McLeer SV, Henry D: Cognitive behavioral treatment for sexually abused children suffering post-traumatic stress: preliminary findings. J Am Acad Child Adolesc Psychiatry 29:747–752, 1990

Deblinger E, Steer RA, Lippmann J: Two-year follow-up study of cognitive behavioral therapy for sexually abused children suffering post-traumatic stress symptoms. Child Abuse Negl 23:1371–1378, 1999

de Vries AP, Kassam-Adams N, Cnaan A, et al: Looking beyond the physical injury: posttraumatic stress disorder in children and parents after pediatric traffic injury. Pediatrics 104:1293–1299, 1999

Dollard J, Miller NE: Personality and Psychotherapy: An Analysis in Terms of Learning, Thinking, and Culture. New York, McGraw-Hill, 1950

Domon SE, Andersen MS: Nefazodone for PTSD. J Am Acad Child Adolesc Psychiatry 39:942–943, 2000

Donnelly CL, Amaya-Jackson L: Post-traumatic stress disorder in children and adolescents: epidemiology, diagnosis, and treatment options. Paediatr Drugs 4:159–170, 2002

Donnelly CL, Amaya-Jackson L, March JS: Psychopharmacology of pediatric posttraumatic stress disorder. J Child Adolesc Psychopharmacol 9:203–220, 1999

Ernst C, Angst J, Foldenyi M: The Zurich Study, XVII: sexual abuse in childhood: frequency and relevance for adult morbidity data of a longitudinal epidemiological study. Eur Arch Psychiatry Clin Neurosci 242:293–300, 1993

Eth S: Post-Traumatic Stress Disorder in Childhood. New York, Pergamon, 1990

Eth S, Pynoos RS: Post-Traumatic Stress Disorder in Children. Washington, DC, American Psychiatric Press, 1985

Famularo R, Kinscherff R, Fenton T: Propranolol treatment for childhood posttraumatic stress disorder, acute type. Am J Dis Child 142:1244–1247, 1988

Famularo R, Kinscherff R, Fenton T: Symptom differences in acute and chronic presentation of childhood post-traumatic stress disorder. Child Abuse Negl 14:439–444, 1990

Famularo R, Kinscherff R, Fenton T: Psychiatric diagnoses of maltreated children: preliminary findings. J Am Acad Child Adolesc Psychiatry 31:863–867, 1992

Feindler E: Cognitive strategies in anger control interventions for children and adolescents, in Child and Adolescent Therapy. Edited by Kendall P. New York, Guilford, 1991, pp 66–97

Foa EB, Kozak MJ: Emotional processing and treatment of anxiety disorders: implications for psychopathology, in Anxiety and the Anxiety Disorders. Edited by Tuma AH, Maser JD. Hillsdale, NJ, Erlbaum, 1985a

Foa EB, Kozak M: Treatment of anxiety disorders: implications for psychopathology, in Anxiety and the Anxiety Disorders. Edited by Tuma AH, Maser JD. Hillsdale, NJ, Erlbaum, 1985b, pp 421–452

Foa EB, Riggs DS: Posttraumatic stress disorder following assault: theoretical considerations and empirical findings. Current Directions in Psychological Science 4(2):61–65, 1995

Foa E, Rothbaum E: Cognitive-behavioral treatment of post-traumatic stress disorder, in Post-Traumatic Stress Disorder: A Behavioral Approach to Diagnosis and Treatment. Edited by Saigh P. Needham Heights, MA, Allyn & Bacon, 1992, pp 85–110

Foa EB, Rothbaum BO: Treating the Trauma of Rape. New York, Guilford, 1998

Foa E, Steketee G, Rothbaum B: Behavioral/cognitive conceptualizations of post-traumatic stress disorder. Behav Ther 20:155–176, 1989

Ford JD, Racusin R, Ellis CG, et al: Child maltreatment, other trauma exposure, and posttraumatic symptomatology among children with oppositional defiant and attention deficit hyperactivity disorders. Child Maltreat 5:205–217, 2000

Forster P: Nature and Treatment of Acute Stress Reactions. Washington, DC, American Psychiatric Press, 1992

Foy DW, Goguen CA: Community violence-related PTSD in children and adolescents. PTSD Research Quarterly 9:1–3, 1998

Freud A, Burlingham D: Infants without families (1943), in The Writings of Anna Freud, Vol 3. New York, International Universities Press, 1967

Freud A, Dann S: An experiment in group upbringing. Psychoanal Study Child 6:127–168, 1951

Freud S: Beyond the pleasure principle (1920), in The Standard Edition of the Complete Psychological Works of Sigmund Freud, Vol 18. Translated and edited by Strachey J. London, Hogarth Press, 1955, pp 7–64

Freud S: Inhibitions, symptoms and anxiety (1926), in The Standard Edition of the Complete Psychological Works of Sigmund Freud, Vol 20. Translated and edited by Strachey J. London, Hogarth Press, 1959, pp 77–175

Friedman MJ: Current and future drug treatment for post-traumatic stress disorder patients. Psychiatr Ann 28:461–468, 1998

Friedman MJ: A guide to the literature on pharmacotherapy for PTSD. PTSD Research Quarterly 11:1–3, 2000

Friedman M, Davidson JR, Mellman TA, et al: Guidelines for pharmacotherapy and position paper on practice guidelines, in Effective Treatments for PTSD: Practice Guidelines From the International Society for Traumatic Stress Studies. Edited by Foa EB, Keane TM, Friedman MJ. New York, Guilford, 2000, pp 84–105

Garbarino J, Kostelny K, Dubrow N: What children can tell us about living in danger. Am Psychol 46:376–383, 1991

Garmezy N: Stress, competence and development. Am J Orthopsychiatry 57:159–174, 1987

Goenjian AK, Najarian LM, Pynoos RS, et al: Posttraumatic stress disorder in elderly and younger adults after the 1988 earthquake in Armenia. Am J Psychiatry 151:895–901, 1994

Goldman SJ, D'Angelo EJ, DeMaso DR, et al: Physical and sexual abuse histories among children with borderline personality disorder. Am J Psychiatry 149:1723–1726, 1992

Good C, Petersen C: SSRI and mirtazapine in PTSD. J Am Acad Child Adolesc Psychiatry 40:263–264, 2001

Green BL: Defining trauma: terminology and generic stressors dimensions. J Appl Soc Psychol 20:1632–1642, 1995

Green BL, Korol M, Grace MC, et al: Children and disaster: age, gender, and parental effects on PTSD symptoms. J Am Acad Child Adolesc Psychiatry 30:945–951, 1991

Harmon RJ, Riggs PD: Clinical perspectives: clonidine for posttraumatic stress disorder in preschool children. J Am Acad Child Adolesc Psychiatry 35:1247–1249, 1996

Heim C, Newport DJ, Bonsall R, et al: Altered pituitary-adrenal axis responses to provocative challenge tests in adult survivors of childhood abuse. Am J Psychiatry 158:575–581, 2001

Heit S, Graham Y, Nemeroff CB: Neurobiological effects of early trauma. Harv Ment Health Lett 16:4–6, 1999

Hidalgo RB, Davidson JR: Selective serotonin reuptake inhibitors in post-traumatic stress disorder. J Psychopharmacol 14:70–76, 2000

Holbrook TL, Hoyt DB, Stein MB, et al: Perceived threat to life predicts posttraumatic stress disorder after major trauma: risk factors and functional outcome. J Trauma 51:287–292, 2001

Horrigan JP: Guanfacine for posttraumatic stress disorder nightmares (letter). J Am Acad Child Adolesc Psychiatry 35:975–976, 1996

Horrigan JP, Barnhill LJ: The suppression of nightmares with guanfacine (letter). J Clin Psychiatry 57:371, 1996

Jones JC, Barlow DH: The etiology of posttraumatic stress disorder. Clin Psychol Rev 10:299–328, 1990

Kardiner A: The Traumatic Neurosis of War. New York, Paul B Hoeber, 1941

Kendall P (ed): Child and Adolescent Therapy. New York, Guilford, 1991

Kendall-Tackett KA, Williams LM, Finkelhor D: Impact of sexual abuse on children: a review and synthesis of recent empirical studies. Psychol Bull 113:164–180, 1993

Kessler RC, Sonnega A, Bromet E, et al: Posttraumatic stress disorder in the National Comorbidity Survey. Arch Gen Psychiatry 52:1048–1060, 1995

King JA, Mandansky D, King S, et al: Early sexual abuse and low cortisol. Psychiatry Clin Neurosci 55:71–74, 2001

Kolko DJ: Individual cognitive-behavioral therapy and family therapy for physically abused children and their offending parents: a comparison of clinical outcomes. Child Maltreat 1:322–342, 1996

Kovacs M: The Children's Depression Inventory (CDI). Psychopharmacol Bull 21:995–998, 1985

Levy D: Release therapy. Am J Orthopsychiatry 9:713–736, 1939

Lipper S, Davidson JR, Grady TA, et al: Preliminary study of carbamazepine in post-traumatic stress disorder. Psychosomatics 27:849–854, 1986

Lochman J, Lampron L, Gemmer T, et al: Anger coping intervention with aggressive children: a guide to implementation in school settings, in Innovations in Clinical Practice: A Source Book, Vol 6. Edited by Keller P, Heyman S. Sarasota, FL, Professional Resource Exchange, 1987, pp 339–356

Lonigan CJ, Shannon MP, Finch AJ, et al: Children's reactions to a natural disaster: symptom severity and degree of exposure. Advances in Behavior Research and Therapy 13(3):135–154, 1991

Lonigan CJ, Shannon MP, Taylor CM, et al: Children exposed to disaster, II: risk factors for the development of post-traumatic symptomatology. J Am Acad Child Adolesc Psychiatry 33:94–105, 1994

Looff D, Grimley P, Kuller F, et al: Carbemazepine for PTSD. J Am Acad Child Adolesc Psychiatry 34:703–704, 1995

Maletic V, March J, Johnston H: Child and adolescent psychopharmacology, in Psychiatric Clinics of North America: Annual of Drug Therapy, Vol 1. Edited by Jefferson J, Greist J. Philadelphia, PA, WB Saunders, 1994, pp 101–124

March J: The nosology of post-traumatic stress disorder. J Anxiety Disord 4:61–82, 1990

March J: Post-traumatic stress in the emergency setting. Emergency Care Quarterly 7(1):74–81, 1991

March JS: What constitutes a stressor? The "Criterion A" issue, in Posttraumatic Stress Disorder: DSM-IV and Beyond. Edited by Davidson JRT, Foa EB. Washington, DC, American Psychiatric Press, 1993, pp 37–54

March JS, Albano AM: Assessment of anxiety in children and adolescents, in American Psychiatric Press Annual Review of Psychiatry, Vol 15. Edited by Dickstein LJ, Riba MB, Oldham JM. Washington, DC, American Psychiatric Press, 1996, pp 405–427

March JS, Amaya-Jackson L: Post-traumatic stress disorder in children and adolescents. PTSD Research Quarterly 4(4):1–7, 1994

March JS, Amaya-Jackson L, Costanzo P, et al: Post-traumatic stress in children and adolescents after an industrial fire. Paper presented at the annual meeting of the Anxiety Disorders Association of America, Pittsburgh, PA, April 1995a

March JS, Stallings P, Parker J, et al: The Multidimensional Anxiety Scale for Children (MASC): development and factor structure. Paper presented at the annual meeting of the Anxiety Disorders Association of America, Pittsburgh, PA, April 1995b

Marmar CR, Foy D, Kagan B, et al: An integrated approach for treating post-traumatic stress, in Post-Traumatic Stress Disorder: A Clinical Review. Edited by Pynoos RS. Lutherville, MD, Sidran Press, 1993

Marshall RD, Beebe KL, Oldham M, et al: Efficacy and safety of paroxetine treatment for chronic PTSD: a fixed-dose, placebo-controlled study. Am J Psychiatry 158:1982–1988, 2001

McFarlane AC: Posttraumatic phenomena in a longitudinal study of children following a natural disaster. J Am Acad Child Adolesc Psychiatry 26:764–769, 1987

McHugo G, Mooney D, Racusin R, et al: Predicting posttraumatic stress after hospitalization for pediatric injury. J Am Acad Child Adolesc Psychiatry 39:576–583, 2000

McNally RJ: Assessment of posttraumatic stress disorder in children. Psychol Assess 3:531–537, 1991

McNally RJ: Stressors that produce posttraumatic stress disorder in children, in Posttraumatic Stress Disorder: DSM-IV and Beyond. Edited by Davidson JRT, Foa EB. Washington, DC, American Psychiatric Press, 1993, pp 57–74

Motta RW: Identification of characteristics and causes of childhood posttraumatic stress disorder. Psychol Sch 31:49–56, 1994

Muller RT, Sicoli LA, Lemieux KE: Relationship between attachment style and posttraumatic stress symptomatology among adults who report the experience of childhood abuse. J Trauma Stress 13:321–332, 2000

Nader K, Pynoos RS, Fairbanks L, et al: Childhood PTSD reactions one year after a sniper attack. Am J Psychiatry 147:1526–1530, 1990

Nader K, Stuber M, Pynoos RS: Posttraumatic stress reactions in preschool children with catastrophic illness: assessment needs. Comprehensive Mental Health Care 1:223–239, 1991

Nader K, Blake D, Kriegler J, et al: Clinician Administered PTSD Scale for Children (CAPS-C), Current and Lifetime Diagnosis Version, and Instruction Manual. Los Angeles, CA, UCLA Neuropsychiatric Institute and National Center for PTSD, 1994

O'Donohue W, Kransner L: Theories of Behavior Therapy: Exploring Behavior Change. Washington, DC, American Psychological Association, 1998

Ornitz E, Pynoos R: Startle modulation in children with post-traumatic stress disorder. Am J Psychiatry 146:866–870, 1989

Pelcowitz D, Kaplan S, Goldenberg B, et al: Posttraumatic stress disorder in physically abused adolescents. J Am Acad Child Adolesc Psychiatry 33:305–312, 1994

Perrin S, Smith P, Yule W: Practitioner review: the assessment and treatment of post-traumatic stress disorder in children and adolescents. J Child Psychol Psychiatry 41:277–289, 2000

Perry BD: Neurobiological sequelae of childhood trauma: posttraumatic stress disorders in children, in Catecholamine Function in Posttraumatic Stress Disorder: Emerging Concepts. Edited by Murburg M. Washington, DC, American Psychiatric Press, 1985, pp 233–255

Perry BD, Pate JE: Neurodevelopment and the Psychobiological Roots of Post-Traumatic Stress Disorder. Springfield, IL, Charles C Thomas, 1994

Pfefferbaum B: Posttraumatic stress disorder in children: a review of the past 10 years. J Am Acad Child Adolesc Psychiatry 36:1503–1511, 1997

Pfefferbaum B, Seale TW, McDonald NB, et al: Posttraumatic stress two years after the Oklahoma City bombing in youths geographically distant from the explosion. Psychiatry 63:358–370, 2000

Pitman RK: Biological findings in posttraumatic stress disorder: implications for DSM-IV classification, in Posttraumatic Stress Disorder: DSM-IV and Beyond. Edited by Davidson JRT, Foa EB. Washington, DC, American Psychiatric Press, 1993, pp 173–189

Putnam FW, Trickett PK: Child sexual abuse: a model of chronic trauma. Psychiatry 56:82–95, 1993

Pynoos RS: Traumatic Stress and Developmental Psychopathology in Children and Adolescents. Lutherville, MD, Sidran Press, 1994

Pynoos RS, Eth S: Children traumatized by witnessing acts of personal violence: homicide, rape, or suicide behavior, in Post-Traumatic Stress Disorder in Children. Edited by Eth S, Pynoos RS. Washington, DC, American Psychiatric Press, 1985, pp 17–43

Pynoos RS, Nader K: Children who witness the sexual assaults of their mothers. J Am Acad Child Adolesc Psychiatry 27:567–572, 1988a

Pynoos RS, Nader K: Psychological first aid and treatment approach to children exposed to community violence: research implications. J Trauma Stress 1:445–473, 1988b

Pynoos RS, Nader K: Children's memory and proximity to violence. J Am Acad Child Adolesc Psychiatry 28:236–241, 1989a

Pynoos RS, Nader K: Prevention of Psychiatric Morbidity in Children After Disaster. Washington, DC, U.S. Government Printing Office, 1989b

Pynoos RS, Nader K: Children's exposure to violence and traumatic death. Psychiatr Ann 20:334–344, 1990

Pynoos RS, Nader K: Issues in the treatment of posttraumatic stress in children and adolescents, in International Handbook of Traumatic Stress Syndromes. Edited by Wilson JP, Raphael B. New York, Plenum, 1993, pp 535–549

Pynoos RS, Frederick CJ, Nader K, et al: Life threat and posttraumatic stress in school-age children. Arch Gen Psychiatry 44:1057–1063, 1987a

Pynoos RS, Nader K, Frederick CJ, et al: Grief reactions in school age children following a sniper attack at school. Isr J Psychiatry Relat Sci 24:53–63, 1987b

Pynoos RS, Steinberg AM, Wraith R: A Developmental Model of Childhood Traumatic Stress. New York, Wiley, 1995, pp 72–95

Reiss D, Richters J, Radke-Yarrow M, et al: Children and Violence. New York, Guilford, 1993

Richters J: Community violence and children's development: toward a research agenda for the 1990s. Psychiatry 56:3–6, 1993

Richters J, Martinez P: The NIMH Community Violence Project, I: children as victims and witnesses to violence. Psychiatry 56:7–21, 1993

Robert R, Blakeney PE, Villarreal C, et al: Imipramine treatment in pediatric burn patients with symptoms of acute stress disorder: a pilot study. J Am Acad Child Adolesc Psychiatry 38:873–882, 1999

Rothbaum BO, Foa EB, Murdock T, et al: A prospective examination of post-traumatic stress disorder in rape victims. J Trauma Stress 5:455–475, 1992

Rutter M, Maugham B, Mortimore P, et al: Fifteen Thousand Hours: Secondary Schools and Their Effect on Children. London, Open Books, 1979

Saigh PA: The development of posttraumatic stress disorder following four different types of traumatization. Behav Res Ther 29:213–216, 1991

Saigh PA: The behavioral treatment of child and adolescent posttraumatic stress disorder. Advances in Behaviour Research and Therapy 14:247–275, 1992

Saltzman WR, Pynoos RS, Layne CM, et al: Trauma/grief focused intervention for adolescents exposed to community violence: results of a school-based screening and group treatment protocol. Group Dynamics: Theory, Research and Practice, in press

Saylor CF, Swenson CC, Powell P: Hurricane Hugo blows down the broccoli: preschoolers' post-disaster play and adjustment. Child Psychiatry Hum Dev 22:139–149, 1992

Scheeringa MS: Treatment for posttraumatic stress disorder in infants and toddlers. Journal of Systemic Therapies 18:21–31, 1999

Scheeringa MS, Zeanah CH, Drell MJ, et al: Two approaches to the diagnosis of posttraumatic stress disorder in infancy and early childhood. J Am Acad Child Adolesc Psychiatry 34:191–200, 1995

Schreiber S, Galai-Gat T: Uncontrolled pain following physical injury as the core-trauma in post-traumatic stress disorder. Pain 54:107–110, 1993

Schwarz ED, Kowalski JM: Malignant memories: PTSD in children and adults after a school shooting. J Am Acad Child Adolesc Psychiatry 30:936–944, 1991

Seedat S, Kaminer D, Lockhat R, et al: An overview of posttraumatic stress disorder in children and adolescents. Primary Care Psychiatry 6:43–48, 2000

Seedat S, Lockhat R, Kaminer D, et al: An open trial of citalopram in adolescents with post-traumatic stress disorder. Int Clin Psychopharmacol 16:21–25, 2001

Shannon MP, Lonigan CJ, Finch AJ, et al: Children exposed to disaster, I: epidemiology of post-traumatic symptoms and symptom profiles. J Am Acad Child Adolesc Psychiatry 33:80–93, 1994

Solomon SD, Gerrity ET, Muff AM: Efficacy of treatments for posttraumatic stress disorder: an empirical review. JAMA 268:633–638, 1992

Stallard P, Law F: Screening and psychological debriefing of adolescent survivors of life-threatening events. Br J Psychiatry 163:660–665, 1993

Stoddard FJ, Norman DK, Murphy JM: A diagnostic outcome study of children and adolescents with severe burns. J Trauma 29:471–477, 1989

Stubenbort K, Donnelly GA, Cohen JA: Cognitive-behavioral group therapy for bereaved adults and children following an air disaster. Group Dyn 5:261–276, 2001

Stuber ML, Nader K, Yasuda P, et al: Stress responses after pediatric bone marrow transplantation: preliminary results of a prospective longitudinal study. J Am Acad Child Adolesc Psychiatry 30:952–957, 1991

Swanson JM: School-Based Assessments and Interventions for ADD Students. Irvine, CA, KC Publications, 1992

Terr LC: Children of Chowchilla. Psychoanal Study Child 34:547–623, 1979

Terr LC: "Forbidden games": post-traumatic child's play. J Am Acad Child Adolesc Psychiatry 20:740–759, 1981a

Terr LC: Psychic trauma in children: observations following the Chowchilla school-bus kidnapping. Am J Psychiatry 138:14–19, 1981b

Terr LC: Chowchilla revisited: the effects of psychic trauma four years after a school-bus kidnapping. Am J Psychiatry 140:1543–1550, 1983a

Terr LC: Life attitudes, dreams, and psychic trauma in a group of "normal" children. J Am Acad Child Psychiatry 22:221–230, 1983b

Terr L: What happens to early memories of trauma? A study of twenty children under age five at the time of documented traumatic events. J Am Acad Child Adolesc Psychiatry 27:96–104, 1988

Terr LC: Too Scared to Cry: Psychic Trauma in Childhood. New York, Harper & Row, 1990

Terr LC: Childhood traumas: an outline and overview. Am J Psychiatry 148:10–20, 1991

Terr LC: Acute responses to external events and posttraumatic stress disorder, in Child and Adolescent Psychiatry: A Comprehensive Textbook, 2nd Edition. Edited by Lewis M. Baltimore, MD, Williams & Wilkins, 1996, pp 753–763

Thyer BA: Diagnosis and treatment of child and adolescent anxiety disorders. Behav Modif 15:310–325, 1991

van der Kolk B, van der Hart O: Pierre Janet and the breakdown of adaptation in psychological trauma. Am J Psychiatry 146:1530–1540, 1989

van der Kolk BA, Dreyfuss D, Michaels M, et al: Fluoxetine in posttraumatic stress disorder. J Clin Psychiatry 55:517–522, 1994

Wilson SN, van der Kolk B, Burbridge J, et al: Phenotype of blood lymphocytes in PTSD suggest chronic immune activation. Psychosomatics 40:222–225, 1999

Winnicott DW: Therapeutic Consultation in Child Psychiatry. New York, Basic Books, 1971

Wozniak J, Crawford MH, Biederman J, et al: Antecedents and complications of trauma in boys with ADHD: findings from a longitudinal study. J Am Acad Child Adolesc Psychiatry 38:48–56, 1999

Yehuda R: Recent developments in the neuroendocrinology of posttraumatic stress disorder. CNS Spectr 2 (suppl):22–29, 1998

Yehuda R: Post-traumatic stress disorder. N Engl J Med 346:108–114, 2002

Yehuda R, Hallig SL, Grossman R: Childhood trauma and risk for PTSD: relationship to intergenerational effects of trauma, parental PTSD and cortisol excretion. Dev Psychopathol 13:733–753, 2001

Yule W: Post-traumatic stress disorder in child survivors of shipping disasters: the sinking of the 'Jupiter.' Psychother Psychosom 57:200–205, 1992

Yule W: Posttraumatic stress disorders, in Child and Adolescent Psychiatry: Modern Approaches, 3rd Edition. Edited by Rutter M, Taylor E, Hersov L. Cambridge, MA, Blackwell Science, 1994, pp 392–406

Yule W, Canterbury R: The treatment of post traumatic stress disorder in children and adolescents. Int Rev Psychiatry 6:141–151, 1994

Yule W, Williams RM: Post-traumatic stress reaction in children. J Trauma Stress 3:279–295, 1990

Yule W, Udwin O, Murdoch K: The 'Jupiter' sinking: effects on children's fears, depression and anxiety. J Child Psychol Psychiatry 31:1051–1061, 1990

Zero to Three: Diagnostic classification: 0–3: Diagnostic Classification of Mental Health and Developmental Disorders of Infancy and Early Childhood. Arlington, VA, Zero to Three, 1994

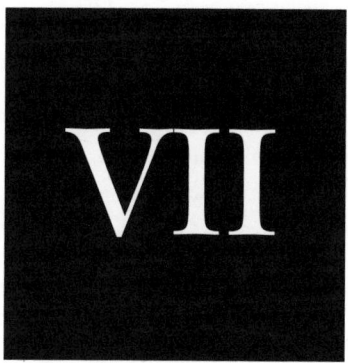

Eating Disorders

Feeding and Eating Disorders of Infancy and Early Childhood

Irene Chatoor, M.D.

It is estimated that up to 25% of otherwise healthy infants and young children and up to 80% of those with developmental handicaps have feeding problems (Lindberg et al. 1991; Reilly et al. 1999; Richman 1981). These common feeding difficulties include eating too little or too much, food refusal, restricted food preferences, objectionable mealtime behaviors, and bizarre food habits (Satter 1990). Severe feeding problems such as refusal to eat or vomiting, which are associated with poor weight gain, have been reported to occur in 1%–2% of infants younger than age 1 year (Dahl and Sundelin 1986).

Very few studies have followed the natural history of feeding problems. Dahl and Sundelin (1992) reported that infants who had been identified with refusal to eat in the first year of life had significantly more problems in eating patterns, behavior, and growth at age 2 years; and 70% of these children continued to exhibit serious eating problems at ages 4 and 6 years (Dahl and Sundelin 1992; Dahl et al. 1994). Marchi and Cohen (1990) followed up a sample of 800 children from early childhood to late childhood and adolescence and reported that feeding problems in young children were stable over time. They linked gastrointestinal symptoms and picky eating in early childhood to anorectic behavior during adolescence. Problem behaviors during mealtime and pica early in life were linked to bulimia nervosa during adolescence.

In the literature, the term *feeding disorder* generally encompasses a variety of conditions ranging from problem behaviors during feeding, food refusal, food selectivity, and vomiting to rumination and pica (Benoit 1993). The term *feeding disorder* is generally used to emphasize the dyadic nature of eating problems in infants and young children.

In addition to feeding disorders, the literature has focused on *failure to thrive* as a diagnostic label. Failure to thrive is a common problem in pediatrics. The term is used to describe infants and young children who have failure in physical growth. The diagnosis is made when the child's decelerated or arrested growth results in weight and height measurements that fall below the fifth percentile on the Boston Growth Standards or that have a persistent deviation below the established growth curve across two major percentiles over time (Woolston 1985).

After Chapin (1908) alerted pediatricians to the failure of growth and development associated with poverty and institutional care of infants and young children, research focused on an awkward and not useful dichotomy: the differentiation between organic and nonorganic failure to thrive. Spitz (1945) gave new importance to Chapin's observations of nonorganic failure to thrive by reporting that infants raised in institutions had severe retardation of growth and development. He called this syndrome *hospitalism*. Spitz (1946) also demonstrated that failure to thrive and "anaclitic depression" occurred in infants whose mothers were abruptly withdrawn when the infant was between ages 6 and 12 months.

Over the years, there has been an appreciation of the many organic diseases that can lead to failure to thrive, and nonorganic failure to thrive has been seen as resulting from the relative absence of adequate maternal care and warmth. This is reflected in the various labels that have been used to describe nonorganic failure to thrive: *environmental failure to thrive* (Barbero and Shaheen 1967), *psychosocial deprivation* (Caldwell

1971), *maternal deprivation* (Patton and Gardner 1962), *deprivation dwarfism* (Silver and Finkelstein 1967), and *psychosocial dwarfism* (Reinhart 1979). More recently, several authors suggested a third category of failure to thrive; these patients have a combination of organic and nonorganic factors in the etiology of their growth disturbance (Casey et al. 1984; Homer and Ludwig 1981).

The terms *feeding disorder* and *failure to thrive* have been used interchangeably by some authors, although other authors have pointed out that not all infants with feeding disorders fail to thrive and not all infants with failure to thrive have feeding problems (Benoit 1993; Chatoor 1997). In more recent years, the use of failure to thrive as a diagnostic category has been sharply criticized. Goldbloom (1987) has pointed out that failure to thrive is a purely descriptive term for growth failure rather than a diagnosis. Others have also argued that failure to thrive represents a symptom rather than a diagnostic category (Benoit 1993; Kessler 1999). However, there was no consensus definition of what constitutes a feeding disorder until the publication of DSM-IV (American Psychiatric Association 1994), which included a definition of feeding disorder of infancy or early childhood (Table 33–1). This general definition is a first step toward delineating feeding disorders. However, it does not take into consideration the heterogeneity of feeding disorders and the need for different treatments for different disorders.

Because of the diverse feeding disorders associated with failure to thrive, a developmental classification of feeding disorders associated with failure to thrive was first suggested by Chatoor and colleagues in 1984 and 1985. This classification incorporates a multifactorial etiology, including various organic and nonorganic factors that can create, exacerbate, or be sequelae of the infant's feeding and growth problems. The developmental classification of feeding disorders drew from Greenspan and Lourie's (1981) stages of early infant development and from Mahler and colleagues' (1975) concept of separation and individuation. Chatoor and colleagues (1984, 1985) classified three stages of feeding development in which adaptive and maladaptive behaviors in both the infant and the mother can be identified: homeostasis, attachment, and separation. As described later in this chapter, feeding disorders can develop during each of these stages. Until 2001, these three developmental feeding disorders were described by Chatoor and colleagues as feeding disorder of homeostasis, feeding disorder of attachment, and

feeding disorder of separation (infantile anorexia). However, in collaboration with the Task Force on Research Diagnostic Criteria: Infancy and Preschool (in press), supported by the American Academy of Child and Adolescent Psychiatry, feeding disorder of homeostasis was renamed feeding disorder of state regulation, and feeding disorder of attachment was renamed feeding disorder of caregiver–infant reciprocity.

Table 33–1. DSM-IV-TR diagnostic criteria for feeding disorder of infancy or early childhood

A. Feeding disturbance as manifested by persistent failure to eat adequately with significant failure to gain weight or significant loss of weight over at least 1 month.
B. The disturbance is not due to an associated gastrointestinal or other general medical condition (e.g., esophageal reflux).
C. The disturbance is not better accounted for by another mental disorder (e.g., rumination disorder) or by lack of available food.
D. The onset is before age 6 years.

Source. Reprinted from American Psychiatric Association: *Diagnostic and Statistical Manual of Mental Disorders*, 4th Edition, Text Revision. Washington, DC, American Psychiatric Association, 2000. Copyright 2000 American Psychiatric Association. Used with permission.

In this chapter I describe the three developmental feeding disorders mentioned above, as well as the three feeding disorders that can occur independently of the child's developmental stage. I conclude with a discussion of pica.

Feeding Disorder of State Regulation

The diagnostic criteria for feeding disorder of state regulation are presented in Table 33–2.

■ Differential Diagnosis

Organic problems (e.g., prematurity, cardiac or pulmonary disease, and functional or structural abnormalities of the oropharynx or gastrointestinal tract) may contribute to, but do not fully explain, the feeding difficulties.

Table 33–2.   Diagnostic criteria for feeding disorder of state regulation

A. The infant has difficulty reaching and maintaining a calm state of alertness for feeding; is either too sleepy or too agitated and/or distressed to feed.
B. The feeding difficulties start in the newborn period.
C. The infant shows significant failure to gain weight or exhibits weight loss.

Source.   Task Force on Research Diagnostic Criteria: Infancy and Preschool (in press).

■ Description and Etiology

In the first few months of life, the infant's task is to achieve regulation of state. The infant must form basic cycles and rhythms of sleep and wakefulness, feeding, and elimination. To feed successfully, the infant must signal hunger and fullness to the caregiver and achieve a state of calm alertness for feeding. This also requires a sensitive caregiver who can interpret the infant's cues and facilitate the infant's regulation of sleep and feedings. Infants with this feeding disorder typically exhibit state regulation problems. They have difficulties reaching and maintaining a state of calm alertness and are too sleepy, too excited, or too distressed to feed.

Feeding problems at this stage of development can stem from constitutional characteristics or medical difficulties. For example, infants with a labile autonomic nervous system are easily overstimulated and are commonly referred to as being "colicky." A sensitive and patient caregiver is needed to regulate the stimulation for these infants in a way that allows them to settle down to be able to eat or sleep. On the other hand, some infants are so passive or tire so quickly during feedings that the caregiver must wake them up or stimulate them to feed adequately. In particular, infants who have cardiac or respiratory diseases that cause compromised breathing and infants with immature oral-motor development tire easily during feedings.

These feeding difficulties frequently generate anxiety or depression in the mother. Mothers experience a sense of inadequacy because of their tendency to measure their competence as mothers by their ability to feed their infants. Anxiety and depression, in turn, make it more difficult for these mothers to read their infants' cues and to optimize their feedings. Mother and infant become caught in a vicious cycle that frequently leads to the infant's growth failure and generates frustration, anxiety, and depression in the mother.

As demonstrated in the study by Dowling (1977), early regulation of feeding has a significant effect on the overall development, motivation, and drive of the infant. Successful self-regulation of the infant lays the foundation for the next stage of development. Experiences of feeding difficulties early in life frequently leave infant and mother vulnerable to problems during the subsequent stages of development.

■ Treatment

Treatment of infants with feeding disorder of state regulation depends on the findings of the diagnostic assessment; treatment may be primarily directed toward the infant, toward the mother, or toward interactions between the mother and infant. In infants with severe growth failure, temporary nasogastric tube feedings may be necessary until the infant grows stronger and is able to feed more effectively.

An inexperienced or fatigued mother may benefit from having an experienced caretaker or nurse temporarily take over feedings. The mother can then learn problem-solving skills to facilitate a feeding environment that provides the optimal amount of stimulation for her vulnerable infant. For example, infants who are very reactive to environmental stimuli can benefit from being placed in a quiet room of the house when siblings come home from school and the noise level in the house is high. On the other hand, the intervention might need to be directed primarily toward the mother to treat her anxiety or depression so that she can be more effective in feeding her infant.

It can be very helpful for a therapist to videotape the feeding and later observe the tape with the mother to augment her ability to read the infant's cues. This can facilitate a discussion of how to respond to the infant's cues most effectively. Because a complexity of factors may contribute to feeding disorders of state regulation, the therapist must consider both partners in the feeding relationship and use a flexible approach that fosters reciprocity between the mother and her infant.

Feeding Disorder of Caregiver–Infant Reciprocity

The diagnostic criteria for feeding disorder of caregiver–infant reciprocity are presented in Table 33–3.

Table 33–3. Diagnostic criteria for feeding disorder of caregiver–infant reciprocity

A. The infant shows a lack of developmentally appropriate signs of social reciprocity (e.g., visual engagement, smiling, or babbling) with the primary caregiver during feeding.
B. The infant shows significant growth deficiency.
C. The growth deficiency and lack of relatedness are not due solely to a physical disorder or a pervasive developmental disorder.

Source. Task Force on Research Diagnostic Criteria: Infancy and Preschool (in press).

■ Differential Diagnosis

Feeding disorder of caregiver–infant reciprocity must be differentiated from organic conditions, such as heart or lung disease, that have led to the infant's growth failure. However, infants with organic conditions usually show better engagement with their mothers. In addition, the infant's lack of engagement may be due to a pervasive developmental disorder. However, these infants are not socially responsive despite the caregivers' appropriate engaging behaviors.

■ Description and Etiology

Most infants with this feeding disorder present in the first year of life and are detected when they become acutely ill and require emergency treatment. The infants appear weak and malnourished, have disturbed body tone (such as being floppy or rigid), feed poorly, avoid eye contact, and are usually developmentally delayed. When these infants are picked up, they are unable to cuddle and mold to the caregiver's body. Frequently, the mothers are distrustful, difficult to engage, elusive, and avoidant of any contact with professionals. When asked about their infants' feeding and growth, they cannot explain the onset of the growth failure and seem unaware that the infant has a feeding problem. Some mothers admit that their infants sleep

for long periods of time without being fed and that to save time they prop bottles to feed their infants.

Feeding disorder of reciprocity was classified in DSM-III-R (American Psychiatric Association 1987) as reactive attachment disorder of infancy or early childhood. However, in DSM-IV the definition of reactive attachment disorder was changed to encompass problems primarily of relatedness without special attention being directed to the child's feeding and growth. In the pediatric literature this feeding disorder has been referred to as *nonorganic failure to thrive,* whereas in the psychiatric literature it has been described as *maternal deprivation* (Patton and Gardner 1963), *deprivation dwarfism* (Silver and Finkelstein 1967), and *psychosocial deprivation* (Caldwell 1971).

Because many of the infant's interactions with the caregiver during the first 6 months of life occur around feedings, regulation of food intake is closely linked to the infant's affective engagement with the caregiver. Consequently, a lack of meaningful engagement is usually marked by impaired physical, cognitive, and emotional growth and development. As Spitz (1945, 1946) pointed out in his early studies on hospitalism and anaclitic depression, the lack of a primary caregiver or the sudden withdrawal of the mother in the first year of life leads to loss of appetite, depressed affect, drop in developmental quotient, and failure to thrive.

Much has been written about mothers whose infants show early growth failure. Fishhoff and colleagues (1971) found that 10 of 12 mothers of infants with failure to thrive had character disorders, whereas 2 were considered to have psychoneurosis. Evans and colleagues (1972) distinguished three groups of parents of infants with failure to thrive and classified them along a continuous spectrum of psychopathology. The first group of mothers had acute depression after experiencing the loss of an important person. The second group of mothers had experienced repeated losses, lived in deprived conditions, demonstrated severe depression, and appeared helpless and overwhelmed. The third group of mothers had the most severe psychopathology; they were openly hostile and very angry in their interactions with the infants.

Fraiberg and colleagues (1975) pointed out that the lack of nurturing in the mother's own infancy and childhood and the lack of a satisfying relationship with another emotionally supportive person lead to the mother's inability to nurture her infant. Drotar and Sturm (1987) postulated that the manner in which traumatic or deprived experiences in childhood influence the mother–infant relationship is mediated by the mother's current family relationships, especially with her spouse.

Some studies of family relations established that the mothers of infants with failure to thrive have increased rates of abuse by their partners or parents compared with mothers of well-thriving infants (Crittenden 1987; Stewart 1973; Weston and Colloton 1993). In addition, poverty and unemployment have been observed to be more prevalent in families with infants with failure to thrive (Altemeier et al. 1985).

Several studies have reported that between 45% and 93% of infants with failure to thrive were insecurely attached to their mothers compared with a significantly lower percentage of well-thriving control infants (Gordon and Jameson 1979; Valenzuela 1990). Benoit and colleagues (1989) studied the attachment relationships between mothers of infants with failure to thrive and the mothers' own parents and found that these mothers were more likely to be classified as insecurely attached than were the mothers in the control group. A study by Main and Goldwyn (1984) systematically explored the mother's attachment behaviors from her childhood into her adult life. These researchers reported that the mother's experience of her own mother as rejecting was related to specific distortions in her cognitive processes, to the rejection of her infant, and to the infant's avoidant insecure attachment as observed in the laboratory. These studies indicate a transgenerational pattern of insecure attachment that appears to be at the root of the mother's difficulty in engaging and nurturing her infant physically and emotionally.

■ Treatment

Because the issues involved are complex, a multidisciplinary team composed of a pediatrician, a nutritionist, a physical or occupational therapist, a social worker, and a child psychiatrist is generally required. Because of the large number of personnel involved, the seriousness of the disorder, and the degree of malnutrition, hospitalization is frequently necessary for a thorough assessment and initiation of nutritional rehabilitation.

During the hospitalization, a number of specialized infant-directed interventions can be undertaken, including nutritional rehabilitation, developmental stimulation, and emotional nurturance. It is important to facilitate as much as possible a special relationship between the primary caregivers and the infant. Improvement in the infant's health and affective availability can then be used to motivate the mother to become involved in the treatment process and to form an alliance for treatment after discharge. Harris (1982) pointed out that "changes in growth and cognition are frequently rapid; changes in personality and behavior are much slower. Recovery from growth failure does not indicate that the parent child relationship is adequate; it is only a first step" (pp. 240–241).

The mothers frequently have a variety of social and psychological disturbances, which must be explored while treating the infant. As pointed out earlier in this chapter, many of the mothers have experienced deprivation or losses during their own childhood and avoid engaging in any therapeutic relationship. It is important to identify any positive behavior a mother demonstrates toward her infant to use as a building block to bolster her competence as a mother. Nurturance of the mother is the first critical step in the treatment to facilitate her potential to nurture the infant. However, some mothers are too impaired to move beyond their distrust and avoidance of those who want to help. The hospitalization of the infant provides a critical time to assess whether the mother can be engaged in a therapeutic relationship or whether the infant needs to be placed in alternative care.

A critical period follows the hospitalization of the infant. Fraiberg and colleagues (1975) emphasized the importance of the parent–infant work to facilitate attachment. They highlighted the need to address the mother's painful past experiences and the "ghosts" from the mother's childhood to free her from repeating those same experiences. Addressing her past experiences will thereby allow her to become a different mother to her infant. Not only the mother, but also the family in relation to the mother–infant pair, must be considered in the treatment process. Drotar and colleagues (1979) discussed the role of the family as a stress-buffering or stress-producing system. Sturm and Drotar (1989) compared three treatment approaches (short-term assistance with social and economic problems, family-centered intervention, and parent intervention) and found that none of the treatments was more effective than the other. In a controlled prospective study of infants with failure to thrive by Black and coworkers (1994), infants were randomly assigned to treatment in a multidisciplinary feeding and nutrition clinic or to a home-based intervention by trained visitors. Although both interventions improved the children's growth patterns, the mothers in the home-based intervention created a more child-focused home environment for their children.

Because of the complexity of the problems involved, multiple case-specific interventions may be required. However, Schmitt and Mauro (1989) warn that an outpatient approach may be safe in cases of mild neglect only if the infant is older than 12 months and if the parents have a support system and have sought medical care for previous sickness. These authors recommend immediate hospitalization of infants if the failure to thrive is associated with nonaccidental trauma, if there is serious hygiene neglect, if the mother is severely disturbed, if the mother is abusing alcohol or drugs, if the mother lives a chaotic lifestyle and appears overwhelmed with stresses, or if the mother–infant interactions appear angry and uncaring. In these cases, placement of the infant in alternative care may have to be considered.

Infantile Anorexia

The diagnostic criteria for infantile anorexia are presented in Table 33–4.

■ Differential Diagnosis

Infantile anorexia needs to be differentiated from other feeding disorders that are characterized by food refusal, including sensory food aversions, posttraumatic feeding disorder, and feeding disorder associated with concurrent medical condition. The central symptom of infantile anorexia is the lack of hunger and the lack of interest in food in general. On the other hand, children with sensory food aversions reject specific foods but eat well as long as they are given their favorite foods. Children with a posttraumatic feeding disorder demonstrate fear of having food put in their mouths and fear of swallowing food, and children with a feeding disorder associated with a concurrent medical condition may start feeding without difficulty but stop feeding when they experience distress.

■ Description and Etiology

Infantile anorexia usually begins during the developmental period described by Mahler and colleagues (1975) as the period of separation and individuation,

Table 33–4. Diagnostic criteria for infantile anorexia

A. Refusal to eat adequate amounts of food for at least 1 month.
B. Onset of the food refusal under age 3 years, most commonly during the transition to spoon feeding and self-feeding.
C. The infant does not communicate hunger signals and lacks interest in food but shows strong interest in exploration and/or interaction with caregiver.
D. The infant shows significant growth deficiency.
E. The food refusal did not follow a traumatic event.
F. The food refusal is not due to an underlying medical illness.

Source. Task Force on Research Diagnostic Criteria: Infancy and Preschool (in press).

when infants and their caretakers need to negotiate issues of autonomy and dependency. This is played out daily in the feeding situation when the mother and her infant need to negotiate who is going to place the spoon in the infant's mouth. Infantile anorexia is characterized by conflict and struggles for control between infants and caretakers over the infants' food intake. Consequently, in a clinical report of nine patients, infantile anorexia was first described as a feeding disorder of separation (Chatoor and Egan 1983). Later, because of the similarities with anorexia nervosa in the child's struggle for control and food refusal, the disorder was called *infantile anorexia nervosa* (Chatoor 1989; Chatoor et al. 1988b), but eventually, to mark the early onset of the feeding disorder and the lack of hunger in these children, it was called *infantile anorexia* (Chatoor et al. 1992, 1998).

Usually, the parents describe the infant's lack of hunger cues, food refusal, and undereating despite all their efforts to increase the infant's food intake. Some parents report feeding difficulties from birth, but most commonly the food refusal becomes a concern between ages 9 and 18 months, when infants are making the transition to self-feeding. The food refusal of the infant may vary from meal to meal as well as with different caretakers. The parents perceive the infant as having a poor appetite and as being bright and demanding of attention but as being difficult and stubborn during feedings. Frequently, the parents are frightened that the infant may die as a result of starvation. The parental anxiety and frustration about the infant's poor food intake frequently lead to coaxing the infant to eat more; to distracting the infant with toys, games, or television; to feeding the infant around the clock; and to force-feeding when the parents feel desperate.

The poor food intake leads to growth failure, which initially manifests as a lack of appropriate weight gain. It then leads to stunting of linear growth and eventually in very slow overall growth. These children appear proportionately small, and at age 4 might be the same size as a 2½-year-old child. The growth failure is also manifested in a delayed bone age but, interestingly, does not seem to affect brain growth. Despite poor overall growth, the child's head size is normal and the child has average or even superior cognitive development.

However, the struggle between the parent and the infant over the infant's food intake interferes with the infant's learning of somatopsychological differentiation. That is, the process of learning to distinguish somatic sensations (such as hunger and satiety) from emotional feelings (such as affection, anger, or frustration) is clouded by efforts of the parents to feed the infant at all times. As a result, the infant's eating is controlled externally by emotional experiences with the caretaker rather than by physiological needs experienced as hunger and satiety.

In a series of studies, Chatoor and colleagues explored mother–infant interactional patterns, as well as infant and parent characteristics, that are associated with infantile anorexia. A study of 42 toddlers with infantile anorexia and 30 control subjects matched by age, sex, and race revealed significant differences in mother–infant interactions between the two groups (Chatoor et al. 1988b). The group of children with infantile anorexia demonstrated less dyadic reciprocity, less maternal contingency, more dyadic conflict, and more struggle for control. This group's play was also characterized by less dyadic reciprocity, more dyadic conflict, less maternal responsiveness to the infant's needs, and more maternal intrusiveness. These findings were replicated in a later study by Chatoor and colleagues (1998).

Chatoor and colleagues postulated a transactional model to understand the conflict and struggle for control between infants with this feeding disorder and their mothers. According to this model, certain characteristics of the infant combine with certain vulnerabilities in the mother to bring out negative responses and conflict in their interactions. In a study of infant temperament and parent characteristics, Chatoor and colleagues (2000) found that toddlers with infantile anorexia were rated by their mothers to be more difficult, more irregular in feeding and sleeping patterns, more negative in mood, more dependent, and more unstoppable than toddlers without feeding problems. The mothers of the toddlers with infantile anorexia were found to demonstrate more attachment insecurity to their own parents than the mothers of the control group. The toddlers' temperament characteristics described above, the mothers' insecure attachment history, and the mothers' drive for thinness correlated significantly with mother–toddler conflict during feeding. Finally, conflict during feeding and the toddlers' temperament characteristics correlated negatively with the toddlers' weight. The more conflict was displayed by mothers and toddlers during feeding, the more malnourished the toddlers were (Chatoor et al. 2000).

■ Treatment

The psychotherapeutic intervention for infantile anorexia is based on the transactional developmental model described above (Chatoor 1997). The major goal of the intervention is to remove the conflict from the mother–infant relationship and to facilitate internal regulation of eating by the infant. This intervention consists of three components:

1. *Assessing and reframing the infant's temperament characteristics.* It is helpful for the parents to understand that the infant is special in the way that he or she is intensely curious and interpersonally sensitive. This drive to interact and to explore appears to lead to intense emotional arousal and seems to make it difficult for the infant to relax and to tune in to his or her physiological signals of hunger. Consequently, these infants need special parenting to increase their awareness of hunger and fullness. In addition, most of these infants are very strong-willed and determined to be in control. Because it is not effective to have a "2-year-old executive" in the house, the therapist helps the parents to realize that these infants require firm limit setting.

2. *Exploring the mother's upbringing to understand its effect on her own development and the relationship with her infant.* It is very important for the therapist to establish a therapeutic alliance with the mother and to understand her background before any work on limit setting can begin. The therapist must understand how the mother feels about setting limits

compared with nurturing her infant, because many mothers struggle with conflicts over control. If the mother feels that the therapist understands and supports her, she will be in a better position to work with the therapist on setting limits on her infant's inappropriate feeding behaviors.

3. *Providing the parents with specific feeding guidelines and instructions for limit setting for inappropriate behaviors that interfere with feeding.* Helping the parents to develop mealtime routines facilitates the infant's awareness of hunger and leads to internal regulation of eating, improved food intake, and growth. This last step involves setting limits on the infant's demanding and provocative behaviors, which interfere with feeding. Because this is best accomplished if both parents work together, the therapist should make every effort to include the father and should explain the infant's special temperament and developmental conflict over autonomy and dependency to both parents. The therapist also needs to fully explain how the child uses food refusal to express this conflict. Then the parents are given "feeding guidelines" and special instructions on how to use time-out to set limits to the infant's inappropriate behaviors and to facilitate self-calming when the infant gets frustrated.

The feeding guidelines include a feeding schedule of regular meal and snack times, spaced at least 3 to 4 hours apart, and a recommendation not to feed the infant between meals so that the infant can experience hunger. The parents are encouraged to separate mealtimes from playtimes to help the infant distinguish physiological hunger for food from emotional hunger for attention. They are asked to deal with the infant's food intake in a neutral manner, by neither playing games to distract the infant so that they can sneak a bite into the infant's mouth nor exaggerating their approval for every mouthful the infant swallows. Parents are also encouraged to withhold expressions of disapproval and frustration if the infant eats little or nothing. The therapist can reassure them that experiencing hunger is the only way to induce the infant to eat. In this way, the infant's attention can be focused on his or her inner state of hunger or satiety rather than on his or her interactions with parents. Parents are encouraged to introduce a playtime after the meal to appropriately provide the attention they previously showered on the infant when persuading him or her to eat.

Parents who are able to support each other can apply this approach and can successfully change the infant's eating patterns. Some children will experience the change within a few days or weeks, but with other children the change can be seen only after several months of consistent management (Chatoor et al. 1997b). However, parents who are in conflict with each other, or mothers who continue to struggle with unresolved issues of control stemming from their own childhoods, may not be able to follow through with these behavioral instructions. In these cases, treatment may have to extend to couples therapy to address disagreements in child rearing, or the mother may require individual psychotherapy to deal with her struggle over control by bringing out the "ghosts" from her childhood, as saliently described by Fraiberg et al. (1975).

■ Prognosis

At present, only one treatment study is available (Chatoor et al. 1997b). In an open clinical trial, 20 anorexic toddlers who received treatment as described above and 20 control children (who were matched by age, sex, race, and socioeconomic background) were evaluated before the intervention and 6 months to 2 years later. Before the treatment, mother–infant interactions during feeding were rated with the Chatoor Feeding Scale (Chatoor et al. 1997a) and revealed significantly more conflict and struggle for control and less dyadic reciprocity between the anorexic infants and their mothers compared with the control group. After treatment, 17 of the 20 mother–infant pairs with infantile anorexia appeared indistinguishable from the control subjects, and as a group, the children had moved from 82.7% of ideal weight for height before the intervention to 89.4% of ideal weight for height after the intervention. However, 3 children continued to have intense conflict with their mothers. In each case the mother had been unable to follow through with the feeding guidelines. The children who responded to the treatment were described by their parents as having developed good awareness of hunger and fullness. They generally ate well, but if they were excited due to social circumstance (e.g., a birthday party, the presence of house guests, or traveling), they did not seem to feel hungry. However, when the excitement was over, they seemed to compensate by eating more.

No systematic data about the natural course of this disorder are available. Anecdotal data from individual case reports suggest different outcomes. Some adults who recalled struggling with their parents about eating and being very small and thin as children reported that they ate more when they moved away from home but continued to struggle with eating as adults. They stated that they ate too much when they were bored but forgot to eat when they were busy. They were still unable to eat when they were stressed, angry, or upset. Children who presented with a history of food refusal, poor food intake, and poor growth since infancy were usually small and thin and had delayed bone age. However, there appears to be a different course of infantile anorexia for girls and boys. A few girls who presented with classic symptoms of anorexia nervosa during childhood or early adolescence had a history of food refusal and poor growth dating back to infancy. These girls were afraid of fatness, purposely restricted their food intake, and had severe body image distortion. They saw themselves as having a "fat stomach and fat thighs" despite their small size and thin appearance. However, some older boys whose food refusal began in infancy were very worried about their small body size because they were teased by their peers and called names, such as "shrimp" or "peanut." These boys would admit to not eating their lunch at school because "they did not have enough time" or "lunch time was the only time to talk to their friends." They clearly had very little awareness of hunger and would easily forgo eating to do other more interesting things. However, these boys could be motivated to pay more attention to their body signals of hunger and fullness, and they experienced catch-up growth once they started to eat more.

Sensory Food Aversions

The diagnostic criteria for sensory food aversions are presented in Table 33–5.

■ Differential Diagnosis

Sensory food aversions need to be differentiated from infantile anorexia and posttraumatic feeding disorder, which are also characterized by food refusal. Toddlers with infantile anorexia refuse to eat regardless of what food they are offered, whereas children with sensory food aversions have consistent food choices and are selective about which foods they are willing to eat and which foods they refuse. Infants and children with a

posttraumatic feeding disorder are afraid of choking, gagging, pain, or vomiting during feeding. Their food refusal involves foods of a specific consistency, either milk or solid food, depending on what food the infant associates with trauma experienced during feeding.

Table 33–5. Diagnostic criteria for sensory food aversions

A. The child consistently refuses to eat specific foods with specific tastes, textures, and/or smells.

B. Onset of the food refusal is during the introduction of a different type of food (e.g., the child may drink one type of milk but refuse another; may eat carrots but refuse green beans; may eat baby foods but refuse chewy meats).

C. The child eats without difficulty when offered preferred foods.

D. The food refusal has resulted in specific nutritional deficiencies and/or delay of oral motor development.

Source. Task Force on Research Diagnostic Criteria: Infancy and Preschool (in press).

■ Description and Etiology

Sensory food aversions occur along a spectrum of severity. Some children refuse to eat only a few types of food, and the parents accommodate the child's food preferences without any conflict over the child's eating. Others may refuse whole food groups (e.g., all fruits, vegetables, or meats), causing the parents to have serious concerns about the adequacy of the child's diet and leading to intense struggles with the child to eat more variety. The diagnosis of a feeding disorder should be made only if the child's food selectivity results in nutritional deficiencies or has led to oral motor delay.

This feeding disorder becomes apparent during infancy or early childhood during the introduction of various baby foods or table foods. However, some infants already may have difficulty switching from one type of formula or milk to another. The food refusal is related to the taste, texture, or smell of particular foods. When specific foods are placed in the infant's mouth, the infant's aversive reactions range from grimacing and spitting out the food to gagging and vomiting. After an initial aversive reaction, infants usually refuse to finish eating that particular food, cry, and refuse to open their mouths if the food is offered again. Some infants generalize their reluctance to eat one food to other foods that may look or smell like the first food that they did not like. This may result, for example, in an infant refusing all green vegetables or all meats. In addition, some children become so particular that they may refuse to eat a preferred food if it has touched another food on the plate. In some cases, the children accept a preferred food only if it was prepared by a specific restaurant or company.

If whole food groups are refused, such limited diets can lead to nutritional deficiencies, for example, vitamin deficiencies or deficiencies in zinc, iron, or protein. In addition, if foods that require a significant amount of chewing (e.g., hard vegetables or meats) are refused, oral motor development and expressive speech may be delayed.

In addition to their sensory aversions to certain foods, many of these children experience hypersensitivities in other sensory areas as well, such as touching food or being touched, walking on grass or sand, wearing shoes or certain types of clothing, or the feel of labels in their clothing. Also, some children are very sensitive to odors and loud sounds. Once these children reach school age and engage in more social activities that involve eating, e.g., birthday parties, sleepovers, or school lunchtime, some experience social anxiety because of their limitations in what they can eat. Their social anxiety may cause them to avoid these situations altogether.

Other terms used to refer to this feeding disorder include *food selectivity* (Shore et al. 1998; Timimi et al. 1997), *food neophobia* (Birch 1999; Pliner and Lowen 1997), *food aversion* (Archer and Szatmari 1990), and descriptors such as "picky eaters" (Marchi and Cohen 1990) or "choosy eaters" (Rydell et al. 1995). I chose the term *sensory food aversions* because these children experience certain foods as being strongly aversive in taste, texture, or smell, and they may also have other sensory difficulties as described above.

Some studies have explored whether taste sensitivities are heritable or learned. It has been suggested that there are various models of genetic transmission, which range from incomplete penetrance (Das 1958) to multilocus and multiallele models (Morton et al. 1981) to a two-locus model (Olson et al. 1989). Other authors (Birch and Marlin 1982; Birch et al. 1990) have postulated that the child's eating environment can also have a strong influence on food preferences. Limited exposure to certain foods because of the parents' own food selectivity can augment the toddler's food selectivity (Birch and Marlin 1982; Harper and Sanders 1975), and parents' efforts to induce children to eat certain foods by coupling their eating with certain consequences (Birch et al. 1982) seems to backfire and make those foods even less desirable.

◼ Treatment

Limited research is available regarding the treatment of this feeding disorder. The work by Birch and her colleagues (Birch and Marlin 1982; Birch et al. 1982, 1990, 1998) indicates that infants in the first year of life are more willing to accept new foods after one exposure only, whereas toddlers require repeated exposure before they become comfortable with new foods. Consequently, following developmental stages, the parents can be given the following guidelines. It is useful to expose infants in the first year of life to a variety of new foods by offering a small amount of a new food and waiting for the infant's reaction. If the infant indicates a dislike for a new food, it is helpful to offer a familiar food and hold off with the next exposure to the new food for another day. At the next exposure, it is best to give the new food in small amounts. This should be done until the infant accepts the new food without any difficulty. On the other hand, if the infant gags or vomits when given a new food, it is best not to offer this food again for a while. Frequent exposure becomes more difficult with toddlers and young children who have learned to self-feed. However, because toddlers love to imitate and are very curious about what their parents eat, an effective way to peak the toddlers' curiosity is for the parents to model eating new foods.

Some toddlers and young children get locked into very restrictive eating patterns and refuse to try any new foods. These children may not eat adequate amounts of vegetables or fruits and require supplementation with vitamins. Others may refuse to eat any meat and—because of inadequate intake of zinc, iron, or protein—may require supplementation of these nutrients to prevent nutritional complications of their feeding disorder. Toddlers who refuse to eat any chewy foods and have fallen behind in their oral motor development may benefit from oral-motor therapy by an occupational therapist. During school age, some children have a strong desire to be able to eat the kind of food they see their peers eating. At that point, a gradual desensitization program with the introduction of one food at a time, and behavioral reinforcement for "courage" when trying a new food seem to be helpful. However, more research is needed to help children and their families with this feeding disorder.

Posttraumatic Feeding Disorder

The diagnostic criteria for posttraumatic feeding disorder are presented in Table 33–6.

■ Differential Diagnosis

Posttraumatic feeding disorder must be differentiated from the other feeding disorders previously discussed that are associated with food refusal, and from feeding disorder associated with concurrent medical condition. Infants who refuse certain foods because of sensory food aversions usually accept other types of food with the same texture (e.g., an infant may refuse to eat green vegetables but may eat fruits). Infantile anorexia and posttraumatic feeding disorder can be differentiated by the infant's affective expressions when approached with food and the intensity of feeding resistance during feeding. An infant with a posttraumatic feeding disorder will display fear and distress when approached with food and will intensely resist swallowing any textured food placed in his or her mouth (Chatoor et al. 2001). Anorexic infants usually take a few bites of food without resistance but quickly lose interest in feeding. They show neutral or cheerful affect during feeding unless they are angered and distressed by being asked to eat when they want to play. Infants with a feeding disorder associated with a concurrent medical condition usually begin to feed without resistance but stop feeding when they experience pain or distress secondary to their medical illness.

■ Description and Etiology

Posttraumatic feeding disorder can be observed at any stage of development from infancy to adulthood. It is characterized by the sudden onset of total or partial food refusal. Parents may report that their infants refused to eat any solid food after an incident of choking, after one or more episodes of severe gagging, or after severe vomiting. Some parents have observed that the food refusal followed intubation, the insertion of nasogastric feeding tubes, or major surgery requiring vigorous suctioning (Chatoor et al. 2001). Depending on the mode of feeding that the infants appear to associate with the traumatic experience, some infants may refuse to eat solids but will continue to drink from the bottle, whereas other infants may refuse to drink from the bottle but are willing to eat solids (e.g., an in-

Table 33–6. Diagnostic criteria for posttraumatic feeding disorder

A. Food refusal follows a traumatic event or repeated traumatic insults to the oropharynx or gastrointestinal tract (e.g., choking, severe vomiting, reflux, insertion of nasogastric or endotracheal tubes, suctioning) that trigger intense distress in the infant.

B. Consistent refusal to eat manifests in one of the following ways:
1. The infant refuses to drink from the bottle but may accept food offered by spoon (although he or she consistently refuses to drink from the bottle when awake, the infant may drink from the bottle when sleepy or asleep).
2. The infant refuses solid food but may accept the bottle.
3. The infant refuses all oral feedings.

C. Reminders of the traumatic events cause distress as manifested by one or more of the following:
1. The infant shows anticipatory distress when positioned for feeding.
2. The infant shows intense resistance when approached with the bottle or food.
3. The infant shows intense resistance to swallow food placed in his or her mouth.

D. The food refusal poses an acute or long-term threat to the child's nutrition.

Source. Task Force on Research Diagnostic Criteria: Infancy and Preschool (in press).

fant who choked on a piece of cereal may refuse to eat solids but will drink from the bottle, and an infant who experienced painful reflux or severe vomiting while drinking from the bottle may refuse the bottle but will continue to eat from the spoon).

Feeding appears to be associated with pain or distress, causing anticipatory fear, as demonstrated by crying, gagging, or vomiting at the sight of objects associated with feeding (e.g., the bottle, food, the high chair, the bib) or when positioned for feeding. The infants resist feeding by crying, arching, refusing to open their mouths, gagging or vomiting, letting the food drop out of their mouths, or actively spitting it out. Some infants may resist swallowing the food by storing it in their cheeks and spitting it out later. The fear of eating seems to override any awareness of hunger, and infants who refuse all food—liquids and solids—are in acute danger of dehydration and starvation.

The infant's food refusal frequently leads to parental anxiety and frustration. The parents try to coax or distract the infant with toys, television, or games to induce the infant to eat. Some infants accept the bottle when sleepy or asleep but refuse it when awake. Therefore, it is not uncommon that some parents attempt to feed the infant throughout the day and the night. Some parents become desperate and attempt to force-feed the infant, which frequently intensifies the anticipatory anxiety and leads to more severe food refusal by the infant.

Other terms for this feeding disorder include *feeding resistance* (Geertsma et al. 1985), *food aversion* (Siegel 1982), *food phobia* (Singer et al. 1992), and *food refusal* (Linscheid et al. 1987; Ramsay and Zelazo 1988). Chatoor et al. (1988a) first described the posttraumatic eating disorder in latency-age children. In these children, one incident of choking or severe gagging was sufficient to cause severe fear of choking and dying. These children had many symptoms of a posttraumatic stress disorder. They were preoccupied with the fear of choking and dying, dreamed of choking or dying, and avoided any activity that could be associated with choking.

It is difficult to determine the inner experience of a young nonverbal infant. However, an infant's affective expressions do provide a window to his or her inner life. The behavior of these infants clearly indicates that they are frightened and that the fear is associated with the anticipation of eating. If the infant is forced to open his or her mouth or is fed forcefully, severe distress is triggered and the infant becomes even more fearful the next time.

Over time, secondary complications of this feeding disorder develop. In severe and persistent cases of food refusal, the infant does not practice sucking, chewing, and swallowing, leading to a delay of oral motor development. The infant does not learn how to move his or her tongue in the side of the mouth and to move food effectively to the pharynx to be swallowed. When the infant finally relaxes enough and puts food in his or her mouth, he or she frequently does not know what to do with the food, and gags and chokes. This evokes old fears, and the infant again refuses to accept food. Consequently, the oral motor assessment is an important part of the evaluation of this feeding disorder.

As the infant becomes more aware of cause and effect in interactions with caregivers, certain emotional responses and behaviors in the caregivers are anticipated. The food refusal usually arouses such intense feelings of anxiety, anger, or frustration in the parents that they try anything to motivate the infant to eat, including coaxing, cajoling, bargaining, pleading, distracting, or forcing food into the infant's mouth. Because nothing seems to work, feeding time becomes a highly charged emotional experience for both the infant and the parent. The infant learns to associate feeding with intense emotional experiences instead of feelings of hunger and satiety. These secondary complications—the delay of oral-motor development and the inability to differentiate emotional experiences from feelings of hunger and satiety—perpetuate the posttraumatic feeding disorder.

■ Treatment

All of the aforementioned factors (i.e., fear of eating and lack of development of oropharyngeal coordination and of somato-psychological differentiation) must be considered for effective treatment. Although several authors have suggested treating food refusal by manipulating consequences (positive reinforcement and punishment), there are only two reports from a controlled research study that have demonstrated that behavioral therapy (extinction) is effective for young children with a posttraumatic feeding disorder (Benoit and Coolbear 1998; Benoit et al. 2000). This intervention requires trained therapists and parents who can walk the fine line between being firm and reassuring to the frightened infant versus being too forceful and causing the infant to become even more frightened of feeding.

Another more gradual desensitization approach has been used by me clinically but has not been tested in a research study. This treatment of an infant with a posttraumatic feeding disorder involves three steps:

1. *Desensitization.* The infant must be desensitized to the fear of eating. This requires a thorough exploration of what seems to trigger the infant's anticipatory anxiety about eating, such as for example the sight of the bottle or being placed in the high chair. These objects should be presented without association to feeding until the infant is comfortable and can tolerate exposure to them. If the infant fears being touched around the mouth, the mother should engage in playful touching until the infant is comfortable with mouth opening, mouthing a toy, or taking a spoon without fear. Because mothers are frequently so upset that it is difficult for them to break the old patterns, a professional

might need to initiate the desensitization process and model it for the mother. Once the infant is able to mouth toys without fear, food can be introduced.

2. *Introduction of food.* It is important to begin the introduction of food with water to avoid the association of feeding with milk. Also, the infant is less likely to gag or choke when drinking water. Once the infant is comfortable with drinking water, juices and then milk can be introduced. A professional must assess the infant's oral-motor coordination and work with the infant directly on chewing and swallowing semisolids that dissolve in the mouth before any type of food that can lead to choking is introduced. Again, a hierarchy of solid food should be followed. During this stage, the emphasis is on teaching the infant oral-motor skills. Because many infants like to imitate, parental modeling of placing food in the mouth and chewing and swallowing is very helpful. While the infant works on desensitization and oral-motor coordination, the amount of food taken in should not be emphasized, and positive reinforcement should be liberally given for newly acquired skills (e.g., "You opened your mouth nicely; that was good chewing and good swallowing.").

3. *Regulation of food intake.* Once the infant has acquired fairly good eating skills, the experience of hunger becomes an important new goal. Many infants with a posttraumatic feeding disorder require tube feedings to prevent starvation. The tube feedings further interfere with the infant's awareness of hunger, and the regulation of these tube feedings is the first step to enhance the infant's awareness of hunger. Continuous infusion at night and fewer bolus feedings during the day should be considered to make the infant hungry at feeding time. The parents must not exert pressure on the infant to eat more and must allow the infant to learn how to regulate intake according to physiological needs. This regulation requires time and patience.

Feeding Disorder Associated With Concurrent Medical Condition

The diagnostic criteria for feeding disorder associated with concurrent medical condition are presented in Table 33–7.

Table 33–7. Diagnostic criteria for feeding disorder associated with concurrent medical condition

A. The infant readily initiates feeding but shows distress over the course of feeding and refuses to continue feeding.

B. The infant has a concurrent medical condition that is believed to cause the distress.

C. Medical management improves but does not fully alleviate the feeding problem.

D. The infant fails to gain adequate weight or loses weight.

Source. Task Force on Research Diagnostic Criteria: Infancy and Preschool (in press).

■ Differential Diagnosis

Typically, infants with this feeding disorder are well engaged with their caregivers and begin feeding without difficulty. However, they interrupt feeding and show signs of distress that seem to be triggered internally and to be unrelated to the interactions with the caregivers. This differentiates these infants from anorexic infants who only become distressed when in conflict with the caregivers. This behavior also is different from the behavior of infants with sensory food aversions, whose distress is triggered by certain foods that they do not want to eat, and from the behavior of infants with a posttraumatic feeding disorder, who show distress in anticipation of feeding.

■ Description and Etiology

Originally feeding disorders, referred to as failure to thrive, were believed to be caused by either organic diseases or by nonorganic problems (e.g., maternal deprivation) until Homer and Ludwig (1981) described a third category of failure to thrive that was caused by a combination of various organic and psychosocial problems. Since that time it has been accepted that various organic diseases can lead to or be associated with various psychological stresses for the child and the caregiver and can lead to severe feeding difficulties. In some medical conditions, food refusal may be the leading symptom. For example, food allergies are not easily diagnosed in young infants, and silent reflux is frequently overlooked by pediatricians because the infant does not vomit, which is usually considered the leading symptom of reflux.

Often, infants with gastroesophageal reflux can initiate feeding and can drink an ounce or two without difficulty until the reflux becomes activated; they then become agitated and interrupt the feeding. If the caregiver becomes anxious and insists on continuing the feeding, the infant becomes increasingly distressed, but if the caregiver remains calm and resumes feeding when the infant seems comfortable, some infants can continue feeding until another episode of internal distress occurs. A similar pattern can be observed in infants with cardiac or pulmonary disease associated with respiratory distress.

These infant feeding difficulties and growth problems generate severe anxiety in parents, who frequently try to compensate for the infant's feeding difficulties by feeding the infant frequently during the day and at night. In some infants, the food refusal is so severe that the parents cannot get adequate amounts of calories into the infant, and the infant's poor oral intake is being supplemented with tube feedings (Dellert et al. 1993). Lemons and Dodge (1998) reported that in some cases, even after successful surgery of gastroesophageal reflux, the severe feeding difficulties and growth failure continued.

■ Treatment

As the case reports indicate, this feeding disorder is most challenging to treat, requiring a multidisciplinary team to deal with the various aspects of the disorder. Psychiatric treatment begins with the observation of the mother and her infant during feeding to assess how much distress the infant experiences during feeding and how the mother deals with the infant's distress. It is helpful to videotape the feeding and to observe the videotape together with the mother. By observing the feeding with the therapist, the mother can be helped to better understand her infant's distress, and the therapist can explore techniques with the mother that will help to calm the infant before resuming feeding.

In situations in which the medical intervention cannot control the medical illness and the mother is too exhausted to continue the frequent and lengthy feedings, and the caloric intake of the infant is limited, supplemental nutrition through nasogastric or gastrostomy tubes needs to be considered. The therapist can help the parents deal with this difficult decision and can work with them to maintain the infant's oral feeding skills, while most of the nutrition is given via tube feedings. This requires a sensitive approach to the infant's tolerance of oral feedings and limit setting for inappropriate behaviors (throwing of food or feeding utensils) that interfere with the infant's feeding even though they are unrelated to the infant's medical condition. In summary, these cases require individualized interventions by an experienced multidisciplinary team.

Pica

The diagnostic criteria for pica are presented in Table 33–8.

Table 33–8. DSM-IV-TR diagnostic criteria for pica

A. Persistent eating of nonnutritive substances for a period of at least 1 month.
B. The eating of nonnutritive substances is inappropriate to the developmental level.
C. The eating behavior is not part of a culturally sanctioned practice.
D. If the eating behavior occurs exclusively during the course of another mental disorder (e.g., mental retardation, pervasive developmental disorder, schizophrenia), it is sufficiently severe to warrant independent clinical attention.

Source. Reprinted from American Psychiatric Association: *Diagnostic and Statistical Manual of Mental Disorders,* 4th Edition, Text Revision. Washington, DC, American Psychiatric Association, 2000. Copyright 2000 American Psychiatric Association. Used with permission.

■ Differential Diagnosis

Before ages 18–24 months, mouthing and occasionally eating nonnutritive substances are relatively common. Pica should be considered only when the behavior persists for longer than 1 month and is judged inappropriate for the developmental level of the child.

■ Description and Etiology

Infants and young children with pica typically eat paint, plaster, paper, strings, hair, and cloth. Older children may eat insects, animal droppings, sand, pebbles, and dirt. Lead poisoning is the most common complication associated with eating paint and plaster; another complication associated with pica is the development of a bezoar—a ball of hair, plant, or chemical substances that are indigestible in the intestinal tract. Trichobezoars (hair) and phytobezoars (plants) are reported to account for most of the clinical cases (De-Bakey and Ochsner 1938).

The onset of pica usually is during the second year of life. Because infants mouth objects quite commonly, it is difficult to make the diagnosis in young infants. In a survey of 12- to 36-month-old toddlers in a pediatric clinic population representing a broad spectrum of races and socioeconomic backgrounds, Chatoor et al. (1994) reported that 22% of the mothers observed their children putting nonnutritive substances in their mouths. An almost linear decline in this behavior occurred with age. Of the 12-month-old infants, 75% were reported to put nonfood objects in their mouths compared with an average of 15% of 24- to 36-month-old toddlers who engaged in this behavior. In many instances, the disorder is believed to be self-limited and to remit spontaneously after a few months.

Millican et al. (1962) surveyed the prevalence of pica in three groups of children ages 1–6 years and reported that pica occurred in 32% of an African American low-income group, in 10% of a Caucasian middle- and upper-income population, and in 55% of a group of children hospitalized for accidental poisoning. The prevalence of pica declined sharply in both high- and low-income groups after age 3 years. Millican et al. (1968) postulated that the higher incidence of pica in the African American low-income group was partially due to the cultural acceptance of pica. They observed that 63% of mothers who had children with pica had pica themselves. Gutelius et al. (1962) reported that 87% of children with pica had mothers or siblings with pica. Wortis et al. (1962) reported that of 272 premature infants at age 30–33 months, 22% had pica. The prevalence of pica has been reported to range from 10% to 33% among institutionalized mentally retarded individuals (Danford and Huber 1982; McAlpine and Singhi 1986).

Various hypotheses have been proposed to explain the phenomenon of pica. Organic, psychodynamic, socioeconomic, and cultural factors have been implicated in the etiology of pica. There are reports of pica being induced in rats by iron deficiency (Woods and Weisinger 1970) or by a low-calcium diet (Jacobson and Snowdon 1976). Some clinical studies confirmed an association between iron deficiency and pica (Lanzkowsky 1959; Reynolds et al. 1968), whereas in a double-blind study, Gutelius et al. (1962) concluded that intramuscular iron was no more effective than saline injection in reducing pica.

Millican et al. (1979) proposed a multifactorial etiology in which constitutional, developmental, emotional, socioeconomic, and cultural factors interact with one another. They observed that young children with pica had a high degree of other oral activities, such as thumb sucking and nail biting. The researchers interpreted the ingestion of inedible substances as a distorted form of instinctual seeking of gratification and as a defense against the loss of security caused by the lack of parental availability and nurture. They reported that these children experienced frequent separations from one or both parents, followed by replacement with inadequate or rapidly changing caregivers. In addition, these investigators observed that the mothers seemed to encourage oral gratification in response to the child's expression of anxiety or distress. The mothers would offer a pacifier or a bottle with milk in response to the infant's distress as a substitute for their personal involvement in helping the infant cope.

Singhi et al. (1981) reported on the role of psychosocial stress in the families of children with pica and found a strong association with maternal deprivation, child neglect and abuse, poor parent–child interactions, and disorganized family structure. Vermeer and Frate (1979) noted the cultural acceptance of pica, especially in rural families of African lineage.

■ Treatment

Formulating a treatment plan must take into account the various factors that appear to contribute to pica. Lourie (1977) proposed a psychoeducational treatment approach. Mothers must be taught the dangers of pica and how to become more available to their children. These mothers, who may be economically deprived and socially isolated, require social support and may require therapy for depression or other psychopathology. Some investigators have used aversive behavior therapy (Danford and Huber 1982), overcorrection and physical restraint (Singhi and Bakker 1984), and environmental enrichment with group or individual play (Madden et al. 1980) to treat pica.

In addition to treating the symptoms of pica, the clinician must not overlook possible complications of the disorder. The child's nutritional state must be monitored, and any iron deficiency or lead poisoning must be treated.

■ Prognosis

Although pica is often thought to be self-limited, some authors emphasize the seriousness of the disorder. Millican and colleagues (1962) reported on the psychopathology that is associated with pica. As a group, younger children were somewhat retarded in their use of speech and showed conflicts about their dependency needs and aggressive feelings. Half of the adolescents had some degree of depression, and several had personality disorders, primarily passive-dependent type or borderline. Many adolescents continued to engage in other forms of oral activities (e.g., thumb sucking; nail biting; aberrant food habits; and tobacco, alcohol, and drug abuse).

In addition to the concerns raised by Millican about the seriousness of pica, a more recent study by Marchi and Cohen (1990) reported a correlation between pica in early childhood and bulimic behavior during adolescence. These studies indicate that more research should be directed toward the prevention and early treatment of pica.

References

Altemeier WA, O'Connor SM, Sherrod KB, et al: Prospective study of antecedents for nonorganic failure to thrive. J Pediatr 106:360–365, 1985

American Psychiatric Association: Diagnostic and Statistical Manual of Mental Disorders, 3rd Edition, Revised. Washington, DC, American Psychiatric Association, 1987

American Psychiatric Association: Diagnostic and Statistical Manual of Mental Disorders, 4th Edition. Washington, DC, American Psychiatric Association, 1994

American Psychiatric Association: Diagnostic and Statistical Manual of Mental Disorders, 4th Edition, Text Revision. Washington, DC, American Psychiatric Association, 2000

Archer LA, Szatmari P: Assessment and treatment of food aversion in a four-year-old boy: a multidimensional approach. Can J Psychiatry 35:501–505, 1990

Barbero GJ, Shaheen E: Environmental failure to thrive: a clinical review. J Pediatr 71:638–644, 1967

Benoit D: Phenomenology and treatment of failure to thrive. Child Adolesc Psychiatr Clin N Am 2:61–73, 1993

Benoit D, Coolbear J: Post-traumatic feeding disorders in infancy: behaviors predicting treatment outcome. Infant Ment Health J 19:409–421, 1998

Benoit D, Zeanah CH, Barton ML: Maternal attachment disturbances in failure to thrive. Infant Ment Health J 10:185–202, 1989

Benoit D, Wang EE, Zlotkin SH: Discontinuation of enterostomy tube feeding by behavioral treatment in early childhood: a randomized control trial. J Pediatr 137:498–503, 2000

Birch LL: Development of food preferences. Annu Rev Nutr 19:41–62, 1999

Birch LL, Marlin DW: I don't like it; I never tried it: effects of exposure on two-year old children's food preferences. Appetite 3:353–360, 1982

Birch LL, Birch D, Marlin D, et al: Effects of instrumental eating on children's food preferences. Appetite 3:125–134, 1982

Birch LL, Zimmerman SI, Hind H: The influence of social-affective context on the formation of children's food preferences. Child Dev 51:556–561, 1990

Birch LL, Gunder L, Grimm-Thomas K: Infants' consumption of a new food enhances acceptance of similar foods. Appetite 30:283–295, 1998

Black M, Hutcheson J, Dubowitz H, et al: Parenting style and developmental status among children with non-organic failure to thrive. J Pediatr Psychol 19:689–707, 1994

Caldwell BM: The effects of psychosocial deprivation on human development in infancy, in Annual Progress in Child Psychiatry and Child Development. Edited by Chess S, Thomas A. New York, Brunner/Mazel, 1971, pp 3–22

Casey PH, Bradley R, Wortham B: Social and nonsocial home environments and infants with nonorganic failure to thrive. Pediatrics 73:348–353, 1984

Chapin HD: A plan of dealing with atrophic infants and children. Arch Pediatr 25:491–496, 1908

Chatoor I: Infantile anorexia nervosa: a developmental disorder of separation and individuation. J Am Acad Psychoanal 17:43–64, 1989

Chatoor I: Feeding and other disorders of infancy, in Psychiatry. Edited by Tasman A, Kay J, Lieberman J. Philadelphia, PA, WB Saunders, 1997, pp 683–701

Chatoor I, Egan J: Nonorganic failure to thrive and dwarfism due to food refusal: a separation disorder. J Am Acad Child Psychiatry 33:294–301, 1983

Chatoor I, Schaefer S, Dickson L, et al: Nonorganic failure to thrive: a developmental perspective. Pediatr Ann 13:829–843, 1984

Chatoor I, Dickson L, Schaefer S, et al: A developmental classification of feeding disorders associated with failure to thrive: diagnosis and treatment, in New Directions in Failure to Thrive: Research and Clinical Practice. Edited by Drotar D. New York, Plenum, 1985, pp 235–258

Chatoor I, Conley C, Dickson L: Food refusal after an incident of choking: a posttraumatic eating disorder. J Am Acad Child Adolesc Psychiatry 27:105–110, 1988a

Chatoor I, Egan J, Getson P, et al: Mother-infant interactions in infantile anorexia nervosa. J Am Acad Child Adolesc Psychiatry 27:535–540, 1988b

Chatoor I, Kerzner B, Zorc L, et al: Two-year-old twins refuse to eat: a multidisciplinary approach to diagnosis and treatment. Infant Ment Health J 13:252–268, 1992

Chatoor I, Hamburger E, Fullard R, et al: A survey of picky eating and pica behaviors in toddlers, in Scientific Proceedings of the Annual Meeting of the American Academy of Child and Adolescent Psychiatry, Vol 10. Washington, DC, American Academy of Child and Adolescent Psychiatry, 1994, p 50

Chatoor I, Getson P, Menvielle E, et al: A feeding scale for research and clinical practice to assess mother-infant interactions in the first three years of life. Infant Ment Health J 18:76–91, 1997a

Chatoor I, Hirsch R, Persinger M: Facilitating internal regulation of eating: a treatment model for infantile anorexia. Infants Young Child 9:12–22, 1997b

Chatoor I, Hirsch R, Ganiban J, et al: Diagnosing infantile anorexia: the observation of mother-infant interactions. J Am Acad Child Adolesc Psychiatry 37:959–967, 1998

Chatoor I, Ganiban J, Hirsch R, et al: Maternal characteristics and toddler temperament in infantile anorexia. J Am Acad Child Adolesc Psychiatry 39:743–751, 2000

Chatoor I, Ganiban J, Harrison J, et al: Observation of feeding in the diagnosis of posttraumatic feeding disorder of infancy. J Am Acad Child Adolesc Psychiatry 40:595–602, 2001

Crittenden PM: Non-organic failure-to-thrive: deprivation or distortion? Infant Ment Health J 8:51–64, 1987

Dahl M, Sundelin C: Early feeding problems in an affluent society, I: categories and clinical signs. Acta Paediatr Scand 75:370–379, 1986

Dahl M, Sundelin C: Feeding problems in an affluent society: follow-up at four years of age in children with early refusal to eat. Acta Paediatr Scand 81:575–579, 1992

Dahl M, Rydell AM, Sundelin C: Children with early refusal to eat: follow-up during primary school. Acta Paediatr Scand 83:54–58, 1994

Danford DE, Huber AM: Pica among mentally retarded adults. Am J Ment Defic 87:141–146, 1982

Das SR: Inheritance of PTC taste character in man: an analysis of 126 Rarhi Brahmin families in West Bengal. Ann Hum Genet 22:200–212, 1958

DeBakey M, Ochsner A: Bezoars and concretions: comprehensive review of literature with analysis of 303 collected cases and presentation of 8 additional cases. Surgery 4:934–964, 1938

Dellert SF, Hyams JS, Treem WR, et al: Feeding resistance and gastroesophageal reflux in infancy. J Pediatr Gastroenterol Nutr 17:66–71, 1993

Dowling S: Seven infants with esophageal atresia: a developmental study. Psychoanal Study Child 32:215–256, 1977

Drotar D, Sturm LA: Paternal influences in nonorganic failure to thrive: implications for psychosocial management. Infant Ment Health J 8:37–50, 1987

Drotar D, Malone C, Negray J: Psychosocial intervention with families of children who fail to thrive. Child Abuse Negl 3:927–935, 1979

Evans SL, Reinhart JB, Succop RA: Failure to thrive: a study of 45 children and their families. J Am Acad Child Psychiatry 11:440–457, 1972

Fishhoff J, Whitten CF, Pettit MG: A psychiatric study of mothers of infants with growth failure secondary to maternal deprivation. J Pediatr 79:209–215, 1971

Fraiberg S, Anderson E, Shapiro V: Ghosts in the nursery. J Am Acad Child Psychiatry 14:387–421, 1975

Geertsma MA, Hyams J, Pelletier JM, et al: Feeding resistance after parenteral hyperalimentation. Am J Dis Child 139:255–256, 1985

Goldbloom R: Growth failure in infancy. Pediatr Rev 9:57–61, 1987

Gordon AH, Jameson JC: Infant-mother attachment in patients with nonorganic failure to thrive syndrome. J Am Acad Child Psychiatry 18:251–259, 1979

Greenspan SI, Lourie RS: Developmental structuralist approach to classification of adaptive and pathologic personality organizations: infancy and early childhood. Am J Psychiatry 138:725–735, 1981

Gutelius MF, Millican FK, Layman EH, et al: Children with pica: treatment of pica with iron given intramuscularly. Pediatrics 29:1018–1023, 1962

Harper LV, Sanders KM: The effect of adults' eating on young children's acceptance of unfamiliar foods. J Exp Child Psychol 20:206–214, 1975

Harris JC: Nonorganic failure to thrive syndromes, in Failure to Thrive in Infancy and Early Childhood. Edited by Accardo PY. Baltimore, MD, University Park Press, 1982, pp 229–241

Homer C, Ludwig S: Categorization of etiology of failure to thrive. Am J Dis Child 135:848–851, 1981

Jacobson JL, Snowdon CT: Increased lead ingestion in calcium deficient monkeys. Nature 162:51–52, 1976

Kessler D: Failure to thrive and pediatric undernutrition: historical and theoretical context, in Failure to Thrive and Pediatric Undernutrition. Edited by Kessler DB, Dawson P. Baltimore, MD, Paul H Brookes, 1999, pp 3–17

Lanzkowsky P: Investigation into the etiology and treatment of pica. Arch Dis Child 34:140–148, 1959

Lemons PK, Dodge NN: Persistent failure-to-thrive: a case study. J Pediatr Health Care 12:27–32, 1998

Lindberg L, Bohlin G, Hagekull B: Early feeding problems in a normal population. Int J Eat Disord 10:395–405, 1991

Linscheid TR, Tarnowski KJ, Rasnake LK, et al: Behavioral treatment of food refusal in a child with short-gut syndrome. J Pediatr Psychol 12:451–459, 1987

Lourie RS: Pica and lead poisoning. Am J Orthopsychiatry 41:697–699, 1977

Madden NA, Russo DC, Michael FC: Environmental influences on mouthing in children with lead intoxication. J Pediatr Psychol 5:207–216, 1980

Mahler MS, Pine F, Berman A: The Psychological Birth of the Human Infant. New York, Basic Books, 1975

Main M, Goldwyn R: Predicting rejection of her infant from mother's representation of her own experiences: implications for the abused abusing interactional cycle. Child Abuse Negl 8:203–217, 1984

Marchi M, Cohen P: Early childhood eating behaviors and adolescent eating disorders. J Am Acad Child Adolesc Psychiatry 29:112–117, 1990

McAlpine C, Singhi NN: Pica in institutional mentally retarded persons. J Ment Defic Res 30:171–178, 1986

Millican FK, Lourie RS, Layman EM, et al: The prevalence of ingestion and mouthing of nonedible substances by children. Clin Proc Child Hosp Dist Columbia 18:207–214, 1962

Millican FK, Layman EM, Lourie RS, et al: Study of an oral fixation: pica. J Am Acad Child Psychiatry 7:79–107, 1968

Millican FK, Dublin CC, Lourie RS: Pica, in Basic Handbook of Child Psychiatry, Vol 2: Disturbances in Development. Edited by Noshpitz JD. New York, Basic Books, 1979, pp 660–666

Morton CC, Cantor RM, Cory LA, et al: A genetic analysis of taste threshold for phenylthiocarbamide. Acta Genet Med Gemellol (Roma) 30:51–57, 1981

Olson JM, Boehnke M, Neiswanger K, et al: Alternative genetic models for the inheritance of phenylthiocarbamide (PTC) taste deficiency. Genet Epidemiol 6:423–434, 1989

Patton RG, Gardner LI: Influence of family environment on growth: the syndrome of "maternal deprivation." Pediatrics 30:957–962, 1962

Patton RG, Gardner LI: Growth Failure in Maternal Deprivation. Springfield, IL, Charles C Thomas, 1963

Pliner P, Lowen ER: Temperament and food neophobia in children and their mothers. Appetite 28:239–254, 1997

Ramsay M, Zelazo P: Food refusal in failure to thrive infants: nasogastric feeding combined with interactive behavioral treatment. J Pediatr Psychol 13:329–347, 1988

Reilly SM, Skuse DH, Wolke D, et al: Oral-motor dysfunction of children who fail to thrive: organic or non-organic? Dev Med Child Neurol 42:115–122, 1999

Reinhart JB: Failure to thrive, in Basic Handbook of Child Psychiatry, Vol 2: Disturbances in Development. Edited by Noshpitz JD. New York, Basic Books, 1979, pp 593–599

Reynolds RD, Binder HJ, Miller MB, et al: Pagophagia and iron deficiency anemia. Ann Intern Med 69:435–440, 1968

Richman N: A community survey of characteristics of one to two year olds with sleep disturbances. J Am Acad Child Adolesc Psychiatry 20:281–291, 1981

Rydell AM, Dahl M, Sundelin C: Characteristics of school children who are choosy eaters. J Genet Psychol 156:217–229, 1995

Satter E: The feeding relationship: problems and interventions. J Pediatr 12:115–120, 1990

Schmitt B, Mauro R: Nonorganic failure to thrive: an outpatient approach. Child Abuse Negl 13:235–248, 1989

Shore BA, Babbitt RL, Williams KE, et al: Use of texture fading in the treatment of food selectivity. J Appl Behav Anal 31:621–633, 1998

Siegel L: Classical and operant procedures in the treatment of a case of food aversion in a young child. J Clin Child Psychol 11:167–172, 1982

Silver H, Finkelstein M: Deprivation dwarfism. J Pediatr 70:317–324, 1967

Singer L, Ambuel B, Wade S, et al: Cognitive-behavioral treatment of health-impairing food phobias in children. J Am Acad Child Adolesc Psychiatry 31:847–852, 1992

Singhi NN, Bakker LW: Suppression of pica by overcorrection and physical restraint: a comparative analysis. J Autism Dev Disord 14:331–341, 1984

Singhi S, Singhi P, Adwani GB: Role of psychosocial stress in the cause of pica. Clin Pediatr (Phila) 20:783–785, 1981

Spitz R: Hospitalism: an inquiry into the psychiatric conditions of early childhood. Psychoanal Study Child 1:53–74, 1945

Spitz R: Anaclitic depression: an inquiry into the psychiatric conditions of early childhood. Psychoanal Study Child 2:313–342, 1946

Stewart RF: The family that fails to thrive, in Family Health Care. Edited by Hymovich DP, Barnard MU. New York, McGraw-Hill, 1973, pp 341–364

Sturm LA, Drotar D: Prediction of weight for height following intervention in three-year-old children with early histories of nonorganic failure to thrive. Child Abuse Negl 13:19–27, 1989

Task Force on Research Diagnostic Criteria: Infancy and Preschool: Research diagnostic criteria for infants and preschool children: the process and empirical support. J Am Acad Child Adolesc Psychiatary (in press)

Timimi S, Douglas J, Tsiftsopoulou K: Selective eaters: a retrospective case note study. Child Care Health Dev 23:265–278, 1997

Valenzuela M: Attachment in chronically underweight young children. Child Dev 61:1984–1996, 1990

Vermeer DE, Frate DA: Geophagia in rural Mississippi: environmental and cultural contexts and nutritional implications. Am J Clin Nutr 32:2129–2135, 1979

Weston J, Colloton M: A legacy of violence in nonorganic failure to thrive. Child Abuse Negl 17:709–733, 1993

Woods SC, Weisinger RS: Pagophagia in the albino rat. Science 169:1334–1336, 1970

Woolston J: Diagnostic classification: the current challenge in failure to thrive research, in New Directions in Failure to Thrive: Research and Clinical Practice. Edited by Drotar D. New York, Plenum, 1985, pp 225–233

Wortis H, Rue R, Heimer C, et al: Children who eat noxious substances. J Am Acad Child Psychiatry 1:537–547, 1962

Infant and Childhood Obesity

Joseph L. Woolston, M.D.

David Szydlo, M.D., Ph.D.

Considerable attention has been focused on the eating disorders of early childhood that result in growth failure, such as rumination and failure to thrive. In contrast, the eating disorders that result in excessive weight gain have been virtually ignored despite the fact that in most cases, adults with weight problems began their struggles with food in childhood. DSM-IV-TR (American Psychiatric Association 2000) has reinforced this omission by describing obesity only as a physical disorder. As a result of this lack of interest in obesity of early childhood, misconceptions about its etiology, course, and even heterogeneity of subtypes prevail. This state of clinical indifference about the fundamentals of infantile obesity makes a scientific strategy for intervention difficult. The ICD-10 (*International Statistical Classification of Diseases and Related Health Problems*, 10th Revision; World Health Organization 1992) also lists a number of physical conditions that are related to obesity but acknowledges some psychological-familial component in its general description (code 278.00).

The first step in the elucidation of any new field of study is a consensual, operational definition that is phenomenologically accurate. In the study of obesity, an easy, accurate, reliable method to define the clinical condition is necessary. Because obesity denotes being excessively fat, the operational definition must differentiate the condition of having excessive adipose tissue for chronological age from simply being heavy for chronological age. Triceps skin-fold thickness (Garn and Clark 1976) and an obesity index using weight gain, suprailiac skin fold, and waist circumference (Crawford et al. 1974) are two well-standardized measurements that appear to satisfy the requirements for a useful, operational definition of obesity. A sim-

pler, but slightly less valid, measurement of obesity is defined as exceeding 120% of ideal body weight for height (IBWH) for a given age and sex. IBWH is calculated by dividing actual weight by the expected weight for a given age, sex, and height percentile. The American Academy of Child and Adolescent Psychiatry considers a child as obese when his or her weight is at least 10% higher than what is recommended for the height and body type.

Unlike the physical definition of obesity, the etiological hypothesis of obesity has changed markedly since the 1950s, when the psychoanalytic theory was that obesity was related to abnormal personality development (Stunkard 1988). This theoretical base obviously was inadequate to explain infantile obesity. In the mid-1960s, behaviorists argued that obesity was the result of a learned behavior (Stuart 1967), but the validity of this construct was challenged by the poor long-term results of behavioral-based treatments and by data from laboratory animals. By the mid-1990s, physiologists proposed a set-point theory in which weight was tightly regulated by a complex interaction of neural, hormonal, and metabolic factors (Keesey 1986).

Many studies have supported and further refined the set-point theory. First, studies have reported that obesity in adulthood is under substantial genetic control (Bouchard and Perusse 1993; Stunkard et al. 1986a, 1990). Second, body weight in adults is remarkably stable for long periods. In the Framingham Heart Study, the body weight of the average adult increased only 10% over a 20-year period (Belanger et al. 1988). Third, resting metabolic rate has a strong familial component (Bogardus et al. 1986) and is adjusted in response to changes in body weight to maintain a consistent weight (Leibel et al. 1995). Fourth, regulation of

24-hour energy expenditure also has a strong familial element and is a significant risk factor for obesity in adults (Ravussin et al. 1988) and infants (Roberts et al. 1988). A major proportion of the variance in this energy expenditure in both adults and infants is associated with differences in spontaneous physical activity (Ravussin et al. 1986, 1988).

As science has accepted more readily the idea of open systems whose controls and regulations are determined by an enormous variety of phenomena, the flow of information and the treatment of signals have added to the understanding of concepts such as flows of energy and mass. These ideas have been used to describe the stability of body weight. Perhaps the most powerful evidence supporting the set-point theory has been the cloning of the mouse *obese* gene (*ob*) (Zhang et al. 1994) and the finding that its gene product causes animals to lose weight and maintain this weight loss (Campfield et al. 1995; Halaas et al. 1995; Pelleymounter et al. 1995).

These discoveries have led to a complex and sophisticated elaboration of the set-point theory, described as the adipostat theory (Bennett 1995; Frederich et al. 1995). The adipostat hypothesis suggests that circulating hormone concentrations reflect levels of body adiposity that act as a signal to control food intake and reproduction (Schneider et al. 2000). However, despite the increasing evidence for the role of the adipostat in the development and maintenance of adult obesity, its role in obesity of infancy and early childhood has been studied less systematically.

Animal studies have shed some light on a possible mechanism behind human obesity; human research has recently begun to do so through important data relating hormonal functioning to obesity. Leptin has been in the forefront of research topics (Blumberg et al. 1999; Friedman et al. 1998; Greenberg et al. 1999; Soukas et al. 2000), and many studies have established its role as part of the complex brain processes to sense, regulate, and respond to energy status; to control storage capacity; and to maintain energy balance. Most of these studies also link their findings to the set-point theory, suggesting that leptin, in a manner similar to that of insulin and glucose, regulates long-term nervous system responses, which could perpetuate an abnormally high body weight set point (Levin et al. 1996).

The melanocortin system (Cone 1999) has been linked to both normal regulation of energy homeostasis and genetic predisposition to obesity. Ghrelin has been shown to be involved in the regulation of feeding behavior and energy homeostasis: Elevated levels are present in fasting conditions and negative energy balance; levels decrease when positive energy balance is achieved (Ariyasu et al. 2001; Otto et al. 2001; Shiiya et al. 2002).

These studies, along with previous research on the adipostat and the set–point theory, are bringing new understanding of childhood obesity in general. Neuropeptides and hypothalamic function have also been at the center of researchers' attention, given the relevance of findings in these areas to the understanding of the adipostat and obesity in childhood and adolescence (Cowley et al. 1999; Karydis and Tolis 1998; Thorburn and Proietto 1988).

Natural History of Infantile and Childhood-Onset Obesity

■ Developmental Evolution

The study of the natural history of obesity in infancy and early childhood is in its preliminary stages. Data about the typical course of this disorder are contradictory. The most widely held belief is that early-onset obesity is a chronic and steadily progressive disorder with very few remissions. Of infants who exceeded the ninetieth percentile in weight, 36% were reported to be overweight as adults, as opposed to 14% of average or lightweight infants (Charney et al. 1976). Eid (1970) found that infants who gained weight rapidly were four times more likely to be obese by age 8 years than infants who gained weight at a normal rate. This grim prognosis has been buttressed by a network of theory (e.g., adipostat theory) and experimental data about fat-cell proliferation in early childhood and its deleterious effect on appetite and weight gain later in life.

Other investigators (Poskitt 1980; Shapiro et al. 1984) reported that obesity in infancy is a poorer predictor of later-childhood obesity than was believed previously. Poskitt (1980) showed that the relative risk that an overweight infant would become an overweight 5-year-old was about 2.5 times that for a normal-weight infant. Of 203 children, 40% had been overweight (>110% IBWH) or obese (>120% IBWH) as infants. By age 5 years, 13.5% were overweight and 2.5% were obese. Most overweight infants did not become overweight children, but 60% of the 27 overweight 5-year-olds also had been overweight in infancy. Poskitt's findings indicate that obesity in infancy leads to an increased risk for obesity in early childhood, but this risk is less than was thought previously. Shapiro et al. (1984) completed an 8.5-year follow-up study of 450 six-month-old infants. These investigators found that of the 26 children (17 boys and 9 girls) who were obese at age 6 months, fewer and fewer were obese at subsequent annual measurements, until only 1 was obese at age 9 years. In contrast, infants who were not obese at age 6 months but who later became obese at ages 4–8 years were much more likely to be obese at age 9 years. Other studies have supported the premise that genetic factors do not produce stable obesity until age 6 or 7 years (Rolland-Cacherna et al. 1987; Sørensen et al. 1992).

This rather poor correlation between obesity in infancy and obesity in later childhood challenges the notion that relentlessly progressive obesity is triggered by fat-cell proliferation in infancy or early childhood. It is likely the case that the degree and duration of obesity are the major determinants of total number of adipose cells in humans rather than that a critical phase in infancy is responsible for fat-cell proliferation (Kirtland and Gurr 1979; Knittle et al. 1979). Poskitt (1980) reported that adipose cells multiply very infrequently in infancy. The natural increase in size of those adipose cells present at birth accounts for almost all the increase in fat stored in the first year, without an increase in cell number.

■ Epidemiology, Social Factors, and Eating Habits

The incidence and prevalence of obesity in early childhood are not nearly as well studied as those of obesity in adulthood. The few studies that have been conducted indicate that the prevalence of obesity in preschool-age children is 5%–10% (Maloney and Klykylo 1983). Obesity tends to follow throughout life, and according to Whitaker et al. (1997) its presence at any age will increase the risk of persistence at subsequent ages. This means that although most obese infants will not remain so, they have a higher risk of becoming obese children. These children are in turn more likely to be obese adolescents, who could very likely become obese adults. Occasionally, "epidemics" of infantile obesity have been reported, with a prevalence rate of 16.7% for infants younger than 12 months (Shukla et al.

1972). These reports note that in the United States the prevalence of the most severe cases—defined as a body mass index (BMI, expressed as weight/height^2 or kg/m^2) for age over the ninety-fifth percentile—has virtually doubled since 1980, reaching 25%–30%, whereas the prevalence of standard cases (BMI for age over the eighty-fifth percentile) has increased about 50% (Gortmaker et al. 1987; Moran 1999). Furthermore, on the basis of the National Health Examination Survey and the National Health and Nutrition Examination Surveys, the prevalence of obesity was shown to increase by 54% in children 6–11 years old and by 39% in adolescents 12–17 years old. The prevalence of severe obesity jumped 98% and 64% within these groups, respectively. Hispanic, Native American, and black patients tend to be more affected than other populations (Kumanyika 1993). Overweight alone has almost tripled in children (6–19 years old) between 1970 and 1999, according to a report by the Centers for Disease Control and Prevention (2002), putting the proportion of overweight children ages 6–11 years at 13%, and of adolescents ages 12–19 years at 14%.

These epidemics appear to be caused by culturally determined misinformation or fads about infant feeding practices (Dounchis et al. 2001; Shukla et al. 1972; Taitz 1971). The most well publicized and best-documented epidemic occurred in England between 1960 and 1975 (Taitz 1977). At that time, English parents were encouraged to follow the maxim "One cannot overfeed a young baby." Parents commonly used full-cream milk powder with added sucrose as baby formula, and, in many parts of England, mothers were encouraged to begin feeding solids to infants at a very early age. By 1973, the dangers of infantile obesity and hypertonic dehydration were well publicized. Between 1971 and 1976, the rate of 6-week-old infants being fed unmodified milk powder declined from 90% to 0%, and the rate of infants above the fiftieth percentile in weight decreased from 79% to 43% (Taitz 1977). In a similar fashion, nonorganic failure to thrive has been reported to occur as a result of parental misconceptions about diet (Pugliese et al. 1987; Woolston 1983).

In a more classic picture, obesity appears to be related to cultural practices because it covaries with social class. Obesity in females is nine times more common in social classes III and IV than in social classes I and II (Stunkard et al. 1972). The prevalence of obesity is linked to the socioeconomic status of the parents almost as strongly as it is to the subject's own socioeconomic status (Goldblatt et al. 1965). Mei et al. (1998)

reported that between 1983 and 1995, there was a consistent increase in the prevalence of overweight among low-income preschool children in the United States, being the result of a general upward shift of the weight-for-height distribution in the population—the same trend as documented in the U.S. population in preschool children, schoolchildren, adolescents, and adults. Their analysis showed that these trends were observed even before the age of 24 months, suggesting that the entire population in the United States is getting heavier. The increasing prevalence of overweight was also observed for each age, sex, and racial/ethnic group. The study claimed that there is a trend in the relative increases with age, with children ages 48–59 months having the highest relative increase in the prevalence of overweight compared with other age groups, suggesting that the prevalence of overweight increases with age.

The prevalence of overweight was higher for girls than for boys, with a parallel increase in the prevalence of overweight between boys and girls among the low-income preschoolers. Hispanic preschool children had a higher prevalence of overweight than did children of other racial or ethnic groups. It was suggested that the higher prevalence of overweight among Hispanic preschool children could be related partially to dietary, environmental, or genetic factors. An increase in the prevalence of overweight among both urban and rural children was reported, although trends were more marked and consistent in the urban areas. Power et al. (1997) concluded that overweight in children younger than age 3 years is not a predictor of future obesity, unless at least one parent is also obese. After that age, the likelihood that obesity will persist into adulthood increases with age and is higher in children with severe obesity. For example, after age 6 years, the probability that obesity will persist exceeds 50%, and 70%–80% of adolescents who are obese will remain so as adults. These findings indicate that socioeconomic status is linked to obesity in a causal rather than a simple associative manner, perhaps mediated through culturally determined eating habits and dietary misconceptions.

■ Genetic/Familial Factors

A family line analysis of obesity indicated that a strong correlation exists between body weight of parents and that of their children. For example, by age 17 years, the children of obese parents are three times more likely to be obese than are the children of lean parents. If one sibling is overweight, the possibility that a second sibling will be overweight is 40% (Garn and Clark 1976). If two siblings are overweight, the possibility that the third sibling will be overweight is 80% (Garn and Clark 1976). According to the American Academy of Child and Adolescent Psychiatry (1997), if one parent is obese, there is a 50% chance that the children will also be obese, and when both parents are obese, the children have an 80% chance of being obese. These data seem to support a genetic basis for obesity, but one must keep other nongenetic but family-related factors in mind. Garn and Clark (1976) also found that if one spouse is overweight, the likelihood that the other spouse will be overweight is 30%. This finding obviously cannot be explained by genetic factors.

The familial factors related to infantile obesity are less clear. Poskitt (1980) reported no significant difference between the number of overweight and normal-weight infants who had one or two overweight parents. But by age 5 years, 78% of the overweight and only 35% of the normal-weight children had at least one overweight parent. This difference was significant and showed that the relative risk of a child being overweight with at least one overweight parent was more than five times that for a child with two normal-weight parents.

Well-designed genetic studies involving monozygotic and dizygotic concordance (Stunkard et al. 1986a) and adoption samples (Price and Gottesman 1991; Stunkard et al. 1986b, Van Itallie 1988) support a strong genetic contribution to all forms of body habitus, ranging from fatness to thinness. In a more recent study, Proietto and Thorburn (1994) suggested that abnormalities at the fat-cell level could be acquired but could also be genetic. Hirsch et al. (1998) described five different genes that are capable of causing obesity in mice (each with a human homologue).

■ Temperament

Although temperament has become a focus of study in pediatrics and child psychiatry (Thomas and Chess 1977), it has been generally neglected in research on childhood-onset obesity. This lack of investigation is surprising because temperament could be associated with the development and course of obesity in three ways: 1) etiology (e.g., low activity output, sedentary vs. active temperament), 2) correlates or consequences (e.g., social undesirability might result in negative peer interactions and social withdrawal), and 3) management problems (e.g., lack of self-control would interfere with treatment compliance) (Carey et al. 1988). Because temperament has been demonstrated to have a major genetic determination (Wilson and Mathany 1986), it may be one mediating factor for the genetic contribution to obesity. To date, one study has shown an association between eight difficult temperament characteristics and rapid weight gain and obesity in middle childhood (Carey et al. 1988). Chatoor et al. (2000) suggested in their study that maternal characteristics and perceptions of toddlers' temperament characteristics should be addressed in treatment of infantile eating disorders.

■ Organic Factors

A primary focus of clinicians who are studying the etiology of infantile obesity is determining specific organic dysfunctions that produce endogenous obesity. This *endogenous* form of obesity is in contradistinction to *exogenous* obesity, in which no physical dysfunction is present other than an excess caloric intake. Endogenous obesity is caused by discrete genetic, endocrinological, or neurological syndromes. Hormonal causes include hypothyroidism, hypercortisolism, primary hyperinsulinism, pseudohypoparathyroidism, acquired hypothalamic problems (e.g., tumors, infections, traumatic syndromes, vascular lesions). Genetic syndromes include Alström, Bardet-Biedl, Beckwith-Wiedemann, Börjeson-Forssman-Lehmann, Cohen, familial lipodystrophy, Fröhlich's, Kleine-Levin, Klinefelter's, Laurence-Moon, Mauriac, Prader-Willi, and Turner's. Of special research interest is the fact that Prader-Willi syndrome appears to be associated with a microdeletion of the proximal long arm of chromosome 15, band q11.2 (Donlon 1988). This is the first specifically defined gene alteration associated with a syndrome involving obesity, insatiable appetite, mental retardation, hypogonadism, and strabismus. Other genetic associations have also been made to leptin and β_3-adrenergic receptor.

Although clinicians often suspect that these organic syndromes have an etiological role in obesity in early childhood, they occur quite rarely, probably in less than 1% of obese patients. In addition, exogenous and endogenous obesity can be easily distinguished: Children with endogenous obesity usually are below the twenty-fifth percentile in height and have delayed bone age; a family history of obesity is uncommon, and there tend to be associated findings on physical examination. Children with exogenous obesity usually are above the fiftieth percentile in height and have an advanced bone age.

■ Psychogenic Factors

Studies of psychiatric disorders in obese adults have been as contradictory as studies of other aspects of obesity. Although many authors have reported no objective data indicating an increased incidence of psychopathology in obese adolescents and adults (McCance 1961; Shipman and Plesset 1963), other authors such as Bruch (1973) and Stunkard (1975) have reported the opposite. Silverstone (1969) attempted to reconcile these discrepant reports by proposing a new categorization that differentiates between late-onset obesity secondary to a gradual accumulation of fat and early-onset obesity characterized by a sudden increase in weight caused by anxiety-driven overeating. Some authors have attempted to relate obesity to personality disorders (Sansone et al. 2000) or psychiatric pathology (Delvin et al. 2000b), but the results are far from conclusive.

Very little is known about psychopathology in infantile obesity. In one report, Kahn (1973) described a sample of 73 obese children younger than 3 years. He found that 32% of these children had a sudden weight gain after a major, traumatic separation from their primary caretakers. This report alludes to a discrete syndrome related to traumatic separation that results in a sudden onset of obesity.

Another type of psychogenic obesity of infancy and early childhood occurs in the context of a disorganized family in which the child's needs are poorly perceived and even more poorly differentiated (Christoffel and Forsyth 1985). Typically, any sign of distress in the infant or toddler is responded to by feeding and/or neglect. Szydlo (1999) described the three most common psychogenic findings in a group of obese children ages 4–14 years as being 1) early separation from their mothers (before 24 months of age), 2) family dysfunctionality, and 3) exposure to traumatic and/or violent events.

The observed psychosocial characteristics of obesity parallel features of failure to thrive of psychosocial origin (Barbero and Shaheen 1967; Leonard et al. 1966). Children with this form of psychogenic obesity have severely disrupted and disorganized families. Factors that contribute to and are an expression of family dysfunction include separation of the parents, parental abuse of alcohol or drugs, and failure to maintain a stable living environment. The severe family disorganization not only is related to the etiology of obesity but also is a major obstacle to treatment because it frequently results in poor medical care, failure to follow through with management plans, and, sometimes, hostility toward health care professionals. The family members often deny the severity—or even the existence—of the problem.

In one study, the parents of all patients were unable to set limits, which also was evident in other parent–child interactions (Kahn 1973). Some mothers were depressed. Case reports (Boxer and Miller 1987; Woolston and Forsyth 1989) described a high level of parental noncompliance, direct undermining, and lack of parents' participation in the treatment of their child.

Some authors have attributed obesity in adolescence to defensive processes that are related to growing up, sexuality, and intimacy. This hypothesis has been described only in individual accounts from mental health professionals working with this age group. A study based on the defensive element of obesity concluded that for some sexually abused women, obesity may have an adaptive function (Wiederman et al. 1999).

Classification Schema for Infantile Obesity

One of the most obvious explanations for the contradictory results of various studies of infantile obesity is that it is an etiologically heterogeneous syndrome. Many authors (e.g., Maloney and Klykylo 1983; Stunkard 1975, 1980) have identified multiple factors, including emotional, socioeconomic, genetic, developmental, energetic, and neurological factors, that contribute to the development of obesity.

However, virtually no attempts have been made to subdivide forms of juvenile-onset obesity into phenomenologically homogeneous groupings. Although such an attempt might be seen as reductionistic, it is warranted by the evidence of heterogeneity in this syndrome. In this subtyping schema, endogenous and exogenous obesity should be differentiated. Endogenous obesity should be classified according to specific organic etiology. Causes of exogenous obesity should be subdivided into simple excessive caloric intake and genetic/familial, psychogenic, and mixed factors.

■ Obesity of Simple Excessive Caloric Intake

Obesity of simple excessive caloric intake results when a primary caretaker overfeeds the infant because of misinformation or cultural practice. The infant and the caretaker do not have any psychiatric disorders, and the family history for obesity is negative. This form of infantile obesity is relatively responsive to dietary intervention, assuming that the cultural attitudes that influence feeding can be modified. The age at onset can range from the neonatal period to early childhood, and the course may be rapid or gradual.

■ Genetic/Familial Obesity

In genetic/familial obesity, an underlying genetic or familial vulnerability to obesity is presumed. No evidence of psychopathology or nutritional misinformation is seen, but the family history for obesity is positive. In addition, the child may have characteristics associated with a so-called difficult temperament (low rhythm/predictability and low persistence/attention). Although both the age at onset and course are variable, usually the obesity is gradual and progressive, starting by age 5 or 6 years. Intervention has rather poor results, especially if it is introduced after the obesity has been present for several years.

■ Psychogenic Obesity

In psychogenic obesity, the family history for obesity may be negative and no evidence of nutritional misinformation may be found, but the infant and/or primary caretaker has strong evidence of psychopathology. Current data indicate two specific types of psychogenic obesity—one related to a traumatic separation from the primary caretaker and the other related to severe, chronic familial disorganization. The first type of psychogenic obesity has a sudden onset (usually before age 3 years) and can progress rapidly. Intervention must address the psychological and nutritional needs of the child and primary caretaker. Because the etiology is related to psychology more than to genetics, the results of intervention will be more variable than the rather poor prognosis for familial obesity. The second type of psychogenic obesity is associated with severely disorganized families in which the child's developmental needs are either ignored or misperceived. In these families, infants and toddlers are fed at the slightest sign of distress.

■ Obesity of Mixed Etiology

In obesity of mixed etiology, more than one of the previously listed etiologies is found. It is obvious that infants who are overfed, who have a positive family history for obesity, and who have significant psychological disturbances will have a very resistant form of obesity. Each factor acts synergistically to maintain the obesity despite vigorous intervention. A clustering of these three etiological factors is not uncommon.

Complications

Children and adolescents are exposed to a great number of health risks related to being overweight and/or obese. Many of these are preventable, but unfortunately, most studies indicate that there is rising number of children with unhealthy body composition, which in turn has immediate and long-term negative effects on them. Pediatricians and child psychiatrists are finding that diseases typically seen in adults are now increasingly seen in children and adolescents; such diseases include asthma, sleep apnea and other sleep disorders, pickwickian syndrome, hypertension, high cholesterol and dyslipidemia, syndrome X, type 2 diabetes, insulin resistance, hyperandrogenemia, menstrual abnormalities, gallbladder disease, liver steatosis, liver fibrosis and/or cirrhosis, and orthopedic complications such as degenerative arthritis and slipped femoral epiphysis (Bao et al. 1994; Dietz 1998; Freedman et al. 1999; Pinhas-Hamiel et al. 1996).

The negative psychological effects and cognitive complications of these diseases can last a lifetime: neurocognitive deficits; depression and other emotional problems; social difficulties and rejection; stigma; struggles with self-image, self-esteem, and insecurity; and body image distortion. These have been related to increased behavioral problems, learning disabilities, and personality difficulties during adolescence (Szydlo 1999). At times, especially under the effects of media, family, and peer pressure, unplanned and unmanaged radical dieting and heavy exercising take the nutritional dysregulation process to the opposite side of the continuum, resulting in other eating disorders such as anorexia nervosa, bulimia nervosa, and binge eating disorder.

Treatment Approaches

No obesity treatment can claim long-term efficacy, despite the many algorithms that exist to define effective interventions modalities, such as self-help, pharmacological treatment, psychological therapies of all sorts, education, and surgery. A plethora of treatment options based on unproven explanatory models (e.g., the food addiction model) have been proposed in the popular media in an attempt to respond both to the need of patients who buy into the "look slim" mentality and the despair of obese patients who have impaired health and psychosocial dysfunction.

Unfortunately, a model of linear causality is still frequently employed to evaluate and treat infantile and childhood obesity. Typically, the clinician searches for a specific cause, especially organic or endogenous. However, this search usually is futile, because endogenous obesity is quite rare and virtually never occurs in children who are ranked above the twenty-fifth percentile in height. The clinician then often focuses on a very narrow nutritional approach. This focus is closer to the biological underpinnings of the problem—a positive balance between caloric intake and expenditure—but it frequently ignores the powerful biopsychosocial influences that permit or encourage the child to overeat and underexercise. As would be expected, a multidisciplinary team approach is necessary to assess and treat such a multifactorial, chronic disorder (Boxer and Miller 1987; Woolston and Forsyth 1989). An ideal multidisciplinary team consists of a pediatrician, developmental psychologist, child psychiatrist, social worker, nurse, and nutritionist. The team assesses the child's physical, developmental, psychiatric, familial, adaptive, functional, and maturational status. Because childhood obesity is so complex and severe, an inpatient evaluation may be required. The family's involvement is the most important variable in successful treatment. Pharmacological and nonpharmacological management combinations have been tried, with sufficient short-term success (Greenberg et al. 1999).

The clinician must perform a full medical assessment of the child to determine concomitant disorders, sequelae, and possible causes of obesity. Disorders such as slipped femoral epiphysis, diabetes mellitus, hypoxia, papilledema, sleep apnea, hypertension, cardiomegaly, pneumonia, polycythemia, and pickwickian syndrome may result from obesity and must be treated vigorously. This is critical in pickwickian syndrome because the respiratory hypoventilation and daytime hypersomnolence associated with severe obesity have a reported mortality of 40% in children (Boxer and Miller 1987). Prader-Willi syndrome should be aggressively approached because of the behavioral problems in this group, although current therapies do not seem to help in the behavioral manifestations of the disorder (Akefeldt and Gillberg 1999). Because of the apparent correlation between severe familial disorganization and some cases of infantile obesity, the child should be examined for other medical problems associated with neglect, such as inadequate immunization, lead poisoning, iron deficiency, and tuberculosis.

The therapist must carefully assess developmental, cognitive, and emotional status to define various psychological and developmental strengths and weaknesses. If the child is older than 30 months, he or she should be enrolled in an early intervention school program. The child should be examined for specific psychiatric disorders, such as attention-deficit/hyperactivity disorder, anxiety disorders, mood disorders, and oppositional defiant disorder.

In addition to evaluating all aspects of family functioning, the therapist must assess potential mental health and social resources for the family. The overall nutritional state of the child, the caloric intake for weight maintenance, and perhaps the nutritional status of other family members should be determined. The daily functioning of the child and family, including feeding and other mealtime behavior, should be ascertained, and specific behaviors that must be eliminated or strengthened should be identified. In this manner, the team evaluates the overall strengths and weaknesses of the child and family to discover the multiple factors behind the child's excessive caloric intake and inadequate caloric expenditure. As with other severe growth and eating disorders, the child may need to be removed from the home. This most restrictive alternative must be seen as a relatively undesirable intervention because the problem frequently reemerges when the child returns to the home.

The proposed subtyping schema for exogenous obesity helps to guide specific treatment approaches. Infants with simple excessive caloric intake respond well to parental nutritional counseling and the implementation of a more appropriate, balanced diet. Pre-

liminary data contradict conventional wisdom by indicating that children with genetic/familial obesity also may have a relatively good response to brief, family-based behavioral intervention. A study by Epstein et al. (1990) using a prospective, randomized, controlled experimental design reported that an 8-week behavioral intervention program for both the obese child and his or her parents significantly reduced the obesity in the child at the end of the 10-year follow-up period. Unfortunately, this study's results have not been replicated. In the absence of other types of obesity, children with exogenous obesity rarely become morbidly obese and thus rarely develop major medical complications. Levine et al. (2001) showed that a short-term family behavioral program was successful in containing weight gain for most children in their trial, as well as in improving the children's mood and eating disorder symptomatology.

Although pharmacotherapy has not been studied in the treatment of childhood obesity, several medications have been tested extensively for the treatment of adult obesity. Fluoxetine has been reported to cause an acute dose-related weight loss (Levine et al. 1989); however, a 1-year multicenter double-blind, placebo-controlled study found that the therapeutic effect of fluoxetine was not sustained after 1 year (Goldstein et al. 1994). In contrast, a double-blind, placebo-controlled study found that the combination of fenfluramine and phentermine produced significant and sustained weight loss (Weintraub et al. 1984). Delvin et al. (2000a) used phentermine and fluoxetine as an adjunct to cognitive-behavioral therapy, with patients achieving positive results at the end of treatment but unable to sustain their weight loss after 1 year. They concluded that with medication, binge suppression and weight loss was higher than with cognitive-behavioral therapy alone but that weight was regained when medication stopped. Sibutramine has been researched for use both in combination with diet and exercise (Berube-Parent et al. 2001) and on its own, as continuously or intermittently administered (Wirth and Krause 2001). Weight loss in all trials was achieved, but contradictory information exists as to the side effects and risks of using this new drug (Taflinski and Chojnacka 2000). More research is needed on all of these agents and newer ones. New pharmacological treatments developed from the results of the *ob* gene discoveries may become powerful treatments for obesity.

References

Akefeldt A, Gillberg C: Behavior and personality characteristics of children and young adults with Prader-Willi syndrome: a controlled study. J Am Acad Child Adolesc Psychiatry 38:761–769, 1999

American Academy of Child and Adolescent Psychiatry: Obesity in children and teens. Facts for Families Series (79). Washington, DC, American Academy of Child and Adolescent Psychiatry, 1997. Available at: http://www.aacap.org/publications/factsfam/79.htm. Accessed May 4, 2003

American Psychiatric Association: Diagnostic and Statistical Manual of Mental Disorders, 4th Edition, Text Revision. Washington, DC, American Psychiatric Association, 2000

Ariyasu H, Takaya K, Tagami T, et al: Stomach is a major source of circulating ghrelin, and feeding state determines plasma ghrelin-like immunoreactivity levels in humans. J Clin Endocrin Metab 86:4753–4758, 2001

Bao W, Srinivasan SR, Wattigney WA, et al: Persistence of multiple cardiovascular risk clustering related to syndrome X from childhood to young adulthood. Arch Intern Med 154:1842–1847, 1994

Barbero G, Shaheen E: Environmental failure to thrive: a clinical interview. J Pediatr 73:690–698, 1967

Belanger AJ, Cupples LA, D'Agostino RB: Means at each examination and inter-examination: consistency of specified characteristics. Framingham Heart Study: 30-Year Follow-up. Sect 36 in The Framingham Study: An Epidemiological Investigation of Cardiovascular Disease (NIH Publ No 88–2970). Edited by Kannel WB, Wolf PA, Garrison RJ. Washington, DC, U.S. Government Printing Office, 1988, pp 156–172

Bennett WI: Beyond overeating. N Engl J Med 332:673–674, 1995

Berube-Parent S, Prud'homme D, St-Pierre S, et al: Obesity treatment with a progressive clinical tri-therapy combining sibutramine and supervised diet-exercise intervention. Int J Obes Relat Metab Disord 25:1144–1153, 2001

Blumberg MS, Deaver K, Kirby RF: Leptin disinhibits nonshivering thermogenesis in infants after maternal separation. Am J Physiol 276: 606–610, 1999

Bogardus C, Lillioja S, Ravussin E, et al: Familial dependence of resting metabolic rate. N Engl J Med 315:96–100, 1986

Bouchard C, Perusse L: Genetics of obesity. Annu Rev Nutr 13:337–354, 1993

Boxer GH, Miller BD: Treatment of a 7-year-old boy with obesity-hypoventilation (Pickwickian syndrome) on a psychosomatic inpatient unit. J Am Acad Child Adolesc Psychiatry 5:798–805, 1987

Bruch H: Eating Disorders: Obesity, Anorexia Nervosa, and the Person Within. New York, Basic Books, 1973

Campfield LA, Smith F, Guisez Y, et al: Recombinant mouse OB protein: evidence for a peripheral signal linking adiposity and central neural networks. Science 269:546–548, 1995

Carey WB, Heguik RL, McDevitt SC: Temperamental factors associated with rapid weight gain and obesity in middle childhood. J Dev Behav Pediatr 4:194–198, 1988

Centers for Disease Control and Prevention: Prevalence of overweight among children and adolescents: United States, 1999. Hyattsville, MD, National Center for Health Statistics, 2002

Charney E, Chamblee H, McBride M, et al: The childhood antecedents of adult obesity: do chubby infants become obese adults? N Engl J Med 195:6–9, 1976

Chatoor I, Ganiban J, Hirsch R, et al: Maternal characteristics and toddler temperament in infantile anorexia. J Am Acad Child Adolesc Psychiatry 39:743–751, 2000

Christoffel KK, Forsyth BWC: The ineffective parent, childhood obesity syndrome (abstract). Paper presented at the 25th annual meeting of the Ambulatory Pediatric Association, New York, September 1985

Cone RD: The central melanocortin system and its role in energy homeostasis. Ann Endocrinol (Paris) 60:3–9, 1999

Cowley MA, Pronchuk N, Fan W, et al: Integration of NPY, AGRP, and melanocortin signals in the hypothalamic paraventricular nucleus: evidence of a cellular basis of the adipostat. Neuron 24:155–163, 1999

Crawford PB, Keller CA, Hampton MC, et al: An obesity index for six-month-old children. Am J Clin Nutr 27: 706–711, 1974

Delvin MJ, Goldfein JA, Carino JS, et al: Open treatment of overweight eaters with phentermine and fluoxetine as an adjunct to cognitive-behavioral therapy. Int J Eat Disord 28:325–332, 2000a

Delvin MJ, Yanovski SZ, Wilson GT: Obesity: what mental health professionals need to know. Am J Psychiatry 157:854–866, 2000b

Dietz W: Health consequences of obesity in youth: childhood predictors of adult disease. Am J Dis Child Pediatr 101:518–525, 1998

Donlon TA: Similar molecular deletions on chromosome 15q11.2 are encountered in both the Prader-Willi and Angelman syndromes. Hum Genet 80:322–328, 1988

Dounchis JZ, Hayden HA, Wilfley DE: Obesity, body image, and eating disorders in ethnically diverse children and adolescents, in Body Image, Eating Disorders, and Obesity in Youth: Assessment, Prevention, and Treatment. Edited by Thomson JK, Smolak L. Washington, DC, American Psychological Association, 2001, pp 67–98

Eid EE: Follow-up study of physical growth of children who had excessive weight gain in the first six months of life. BMJ 2:72–76, 1970

Epstein LH, Valoski A, Wing RR, et al: Ten-year follow-up of behavioral, family-based treatment for obese children. JAMA 264:2519–2523, 1990

Frederich RC, Lollmann B, Hamann A, et al: Expression of *ob* mRNA and its encoded protein in rodents: impact of nutrition and obesity. J Clin Invest 96:1658–1663, 1995

Freedman DS, Dietz WH, Srinivasan SR, et al: The relation of overweight to cardiovascular risk factors among children and adolescents: the Bogulusa Heart Study. Pediatrics 103:1175–1182, 1999

Friedman JM, Halaas JL: Leptin and the regulation of body weight in mammals. Nature 395:763–770, 1998

Garn SM, Clark DC: Trends in fatness and the origins of obesity: Ad Hoc Committee to Review the Ten-State Nutrition Survey. Pediatrics 57:443–456, 1976

Goldblatt PB, Moore ME, Stunkard AJ: Social factors in obesity. JAMA 192:1039–1044, 1965

Goldstein DJ, Rampsey AH, Enas GG, et al: Fluoxetine: a randomized clinical trial in the treatment of obesity. Int J Obes Relat Metab Disord 18:129–135, 1994

Gortmaker SL, Dietz WH Jr, Sobol AM, Webler CA: Increasing pediatric obesity in the United States. Am J Dis Child 141:535–540, 1987

Greenberg I, Chan S, Blackburn GL: Nonpharmacologic and pharmacologic management of weight gain. J Clin Psychiatry 60:31–36, 1999

Greenberg JA, Boozer CN: The leptin-fat ratio is constant, and leptin may be part of two feedback mechanisms for maintaining the body fat set point in non-obese male Fischer 344 rats. Horm Metab Res 31:525–532, 1999

Halaas JL, Gajiwala KS, Maffei M, et al: Weight-reducing effect of the plasma protein encoded by the *obese* gene. Science 259:543–546, 1995

Hirsch J, Leibel RL: The genetics of obesity. Hosp Pract 33:55–59, 62–65, 69–70, 1998

Kahn EJ: Obesity in children, in The Psychology of Obesity: Dynamics and Treatment. Edited by Kiell N. Springfield, IL, Charles C Thomas, 1973, pp 121–146

Karydis I, Tolis G: Orexis, anorexia and thyrotropin-releasing hormone. Thyroid 8:947–950, 1998

Keesey RE: A set point theory of obesity, in Handbook of Eating Disorders: Physiology, Psychology, and Treatment of Obesity, Anorexia, and Bulimia. Edited by Brownell KB, Foreyt JP. New York, Basic Books, 1986, pp 63–87

Kirtland J, Gurr MI: Adipose tissue hypercellularity: a review, II: the relationship between cellulocity and obesity. Int J Obes Relat Metab Disord 3:15–55, 1979

Knittle JC, Timmers K, Ginsberg-Fellner F, et al: The growth of adipose tissue in children and adolescents. J Clin Invest 63:239–246, 1979

Kumanyika S: Ethnicity and obesity development in children. Ann N Y Acad Sci 699:81–92, 1993

Leibel RL, Rosenbaum M, Hirsch J: Changes in energy expenditure resulting from altered body weight. N Engl J Med 332:621–628, 1995

Leonard M, Rhymes J, Solnit AJ: Failure to thrive in infants. Am J Dis Child 111:600–612, 1966

Levin BE, Routh VH: Role of the brain in energy balance and obesity. Am J Physiol 271:491–500, 1996

Levine LR, Enas GG, Thompson WL, et al: Use of fluoxetine, a selective serotonin-uptake inhibitor, in the treatment of obesity: a dose-response study (with a commentary by Michael Weintraub). Int J Obes Relat Metab Disord 13:635–645, 1989

Levine MD, Ringham RM, Kalarchian MA, et al: Is family-based behavioral weight control appropriate for severe pediatric obesity? Int J Eat Disord 30:318–328, 2001

Maloney MJ, Klykylo WM: An overview of anorexia nervosa, bulimia, and obesity in children and adolescents. J Am Acad Child Psychiatry 22:99–107, 1983

McCance C: Psychiatric factors in obesity. Dissertation for diploma in psychological medicine, University of London, London, England, 1961

Mei Z, Scanlon KS, Grummer-Strawn LM, et al: Increasing prevalence of overweight among US low-income preschool children: the Centers for Disease Control and Prevention pediatric nutrition surveillance, 1983 to 1995 (comment). Pediatrics 101:E12, 1998

Moran R: The evaluation and treatment of childhood obesity. Am Fam Physician 59:859–873, 1999

Otto B, Cuntz U, Fruehauf E, et al: Weight gain decreases elevated plasma ghrelin concentrations of patients with anorexia nervosa. Eur J Endocrinol 145:669–673, 2001

Pelleymounter MA, Cullen MJ, Baker MB, et al: Effects of the *obese* gene product on body weight regulation in *ob/ob* mice. Science 269:540–543, 1995

Pinhas-Hamiel O, Dolan LM, Daniels SR, et al: Increased incidence of non-insulin-dependant diabetes mellitus among adolescents. J Pediatr 128:608–615, 1996

Poskitt EME: Obese from infancy: a re-evaluation. Topics in Pediatrics 2:81–89, 1980

Power C, Lake JK, Cole TJ: Measurement and long-term health risks of child and adolescent fatness. Int J Obes Relat Metab Disord 21:507–526, 1997

Price RA, Gottesman II: Body fat in identical twins reared apart: roles for genes and environment. Behav Genet 21:1–7, 1991

Proietto J, Thorburn AW: Animal models of obesity—theories of aetiology. Baillieres Clin Endocrinol Metabol 8:509–525, 1994

Pugliese MT, Weyman-Daum M, Moses N, et al: Parental health beliefs as a cause of nonorganic failure to thrive. Pediatrics 80:175–182, 1987

Ravussin E, Lillioja S, Anderson TE, et al: Determinants of 24-hour energy expenditure in man: methods and results using a respiratory chamber. J Clin Invest 78:1568–1578, 1986

Ravussin E, Lillioja S, Knowles WC, et al: Reduced rate of energy expenditure as a risk factor for body weight gain. N Engl J Med 318:467–472, 1988

Roberts SB, Savage J, Coward WA, et al: Energy expenditure and intake in infants born to lean and overweight mothers. N Engl J Med 318:461–466, 1988

Rolland-Cacherna MF, Deheger M, Guilloud-Bataille M: Tracking of development of adiposity from one month of age to adulthood. Ann Hum Biol 14:219–229, 1987

Sansone RA, Wiederman MW, Sansone LA: The prevalence of borderline personality disorder among individuals with obesity: a critical review of the literature. Eating Behaviors 1:94–104, 2000

Schneider JE, Blum RM, Wade GN: Metabolic control of food intake and estrous cycles in Syrian hamsters, I: plasma insulin and leptin. Am J Physiol 278:476–485, 2000

Shapiro LR, Crawford PB, Clark MJ: Obesity prognosis: a longitudinal study of children from age six months to nine years. Am J Public Health 74:968–972, 1984

Shiiya T, Nakazato M, Mizuta M, et al: Plasma ghrelin levels in lean and obese humans and the effect of glucose on ghrelin secretion. J Clin Endocrinol Metab 87:240–244, 2002

Shipman MG, Plesset M: Anxiety and depression in obese dieters. Arch Gen Psychiatry 8:530–535, 1963

Shukla A, Forsyth AA, Anderson CM, et al: Infantile overnutrition in the first year of life: a field study in Dudley Worcestershire. BMJ 4:507–515, 1972

Silverstone JT: Psychological factors in obesity, in Obesity: Medical and Scientific Aspects. Edited by Baird IM, Howard AN. London, E and S Livingstone, 1969, pp 45–55

Sørensen TIA, Holst C, Stunkard AJ: Childhood body mass index: genetic and familial environmental influences assessed in a longitudinal adoption study. Int J Obes Relat Metab Disord 15:705–714, 1992

Soukas A, Cohen P, Socci ND, et al: Leptin-specific patterns of gene expression in white adipose tissue. Genes Dev 14:963–980, 2000

Stuart RB: Behavioral control of overeating. Behav Res Ther 5:357–365, 1967

Stunkard AJ: Obesity, in American Handbook of Psychiatry. Edited by Reiser MF. New York, Basic Books, 1975, pp 325–333

Stunkard AJ: Obesity, in Comprehensive Textbook of Psychiatry, 3rd Edition. Edited by Kaplan HI, Freedman AM, Sadock BJ. Baltimore, MD, Williams & Wilkins, 1980, pp 1872–1881

Stunkard AJ: Some perspectives on human obesity: its causes. Bull N Y Acad Med 64:902–923, 1988

Stunkard AJ, d'Aquill E, Fox S, et al: Influence of social class on obesity and thinness in children. JAMA 221:579–584, 1972

Stunkard AJ, Foch TT, Hrubec A: A twin study of human obesity. JAMA 256:51–54, 1986a

Stunkard AJ, Sørensen TIA, Hanis C, et al: An adoption study of human obesity. N Engl J Med 314:193–198, 1986b

Stunkard AJ, Harris JR, Pederson NL, et al: A separated twin study of the Body Mass Index. N Engl J Med 322:1483–1487, 1990

Szydlo D: Psychological and familial determinants of eating disorders: causes and effects. Keynote lecture. National Conference on Psychiatric Disorders. American British Cawdray Hospital, Mexico, October 1999

Taflinski T, Chojnacka J: Sibutramine-associated psychotic episode. Am J Psychiatry 157:2057–2058, 2000

Taitz L: Infantile overnutrition among artificially fed infants in the Sheffield region. BMJ 1:315–316, 1971

Taitz L: Obesity in pediatric practice: infantile obesity. Pediatr Clin North Am 24:107–122, 1977

Thomas A, Chess S: Temperament and Development. New York, Brunner/Mazel, 1977

Thorburn AW, Proietto J: Neuropeptides, the hypothalamus and obesity: insights into the central control of body weight. Pathology 30:229–236, 1988

Van Itallie TB: Obesity, Genetics and ponderal set point. Clinical Neuropharmacology 11 (suppl 1): 1–7, 1988

Weintraub M, Hasday JD, Mushlin AI, et al: A double-blind clinical trial in weight control: use of fenfluramine and phentermine alone and in combination. Arch Intern Med 144:1143–1148, 1984

Whitaker RC, Wright JA, Pepe MS, et al: Predicting obesity in young adulthood from childhood and parental obesity. N Engl J Med 337:869–873, 1997

Wiederman MW, Sansone RA, Sansone LA: Obesity among sexually abused women: an adaptive function for some? Women Health 29:89–100, 1999

Wilson RS, Mathany AP: Behavioral-genetics in infant temperament: the Louisville Twin Study, in The Study of Temperament: Changes, Continuities, and Challenges. Edited by Plomin R, Dunn J. Hillsdale, NJ, Lawrence Erlbaum, 1986, pp 81–97

Wirth A, Krause J: Long-term weight loss with sibutramine: a randomized controlled trial. JAMA 286:1331–1339, 2001

Woolston JL: Eating disorders in infancy and early childhood. J Am Acad Child Psychiatry 22:114–121, 1983

Woolston JL, Forsyth B: Obesity of infancy and early childhood: a diagnostic schema, in Advances in Clinical Child Psychology, Vol 12. Edited by Lahey BB, Kazdin AE. New York, Plenum, 1989, pp 179–192

World Health Organization: International Statistical Classification of Diseases and Related Health Problems, 10th Revision. Geneva, World Health Organization, 1992

Zhang Y, Proenca R, Maffei M, et al: Positional cloning of the mouse obese gene and its human homologue. Nature 372:425–432, 1994

Anorexia Nervosa

David B. Herzog, M.D.

Eugene V. Beresin, M.D.

Valerie E. Charat, Ed.M.

norexia nervosa is an elusive and significant disorder among adolescent and adult females. It is characterized by extreme weight loss, body-image disturbance, and an intense fear of becoming obese. Preoccupation with food is a commonly associated feature.

The medical community has recognized anorexia nervosa as a diagnosis since the turn of the nineteenth century. Medical accounts of the physical manifestations of anorexia nervosa resemble Allbutt's (1910) highly detailed description:

> A young woman thus afflicted, her clothes scarcely hanging together on her anatomy, her pulse slow and slack, her temperature two degrees below the normal mean, her bowels closed, her hair like that of a corpse—dry and lustreless, her face and limbs ashy and cold, her hollow eyes the only vivid thing about her—this wan creature whose daily food intake might lie on a crown piece, will be busy with mother's meetings, with little sister's frocks, with university extension and with what you please else of unselfish effort, yet on what funds God only knows. (p. 398)

The anorexia nervosa of the present day has historical correlates in the religiously inspired cases of "anorexia mirabilis" in female saints, such as Catherine of Siena (1347–1380), in whom fasting denoted female holiness; in the "miraculous maids" of the Reformation period, such as Eva Fleigen in 1599, in whom fasting indicated humility and underscored purity; and in the cases of "fasting girls," such as Sarah Jacob, the "Welsh Fasting Girl," during the Victorian era (1870s), when the transition from fasting as a sign of divine intervention to fasting as a medical and scientifically ex-plainable state began (Brumberg 1988). The investigation of anorexia nervosa in (and since) the twentieth century has focused on the psychological, physiological, psychodynamic, psychosocial, and now the multidimensional factors and biological and genetic vulnerabilities of this population.

In this chapter, we describe the diagnostic criteria, clinical findings, differential diagnoses, epidemiology, etiology, treatment, and prognosis of anorexia nervosa.

Diagnostic Criteria

Anorexia nervosa typically has its onset in an adolescent female who perceives herself to be overweight. Anorexic patients commonly lose weight by restricting their food intake, excessively exercising, inducing vomiting after meals, and abusing laxatives, diuretics, or diet pills. DSM-IV-TR (American Psychiatric Association 2000) criteria for anorexia nervosa are shown in Table 35–1.

Within anorexia nervosa, DSM-IV-TR distinguishes between two subtypes—restricting and binge-eating/purging—on the basis of the presence or absence of bulimic symptoms. When compared with patients with restricting anorexia, those with binge-eating/purging anorexia are more likely to have drug use disorders, receive a diagnosis of borderline personality disorder, display impulse control problems and mood lability, and have a history of suicide attempts (American Psychiatric Association 2000). On the Minnesota Multiphasic Personality Inventory, patients with binge-eat-

Table 35–1. DSM-IV-TR diagnostic criteria for anorexia nervosa

A. Refusal to maintain body weight at or above a minimally normal weight for age and height (e.g., weight loss leading to maintenance of body weight less than 85% of that expected; or failure to make expected weight gain during period of growth, leading to body weight less than 85% of that expected).

B. Intense fear of gaining weight or becoming fat, even though underweight.

C. Disturbance in the way in which one's body weight or shape is experienced, undue influence of body weight or shape on self-evaluation, or denial of the seriousness of the current low body weight.

D. In postmenarcheal females, amenorrhea, i.e., the absence of at least three consecutive menstrual cycles. (A woman is considered to have amenorrhea if her periods occur only following hormone, e.g., estrogen, administration.)

Specify type:

   Restricting Type: during the current episode of anorexia nervosa, the person has not regularly engaged in binge-eating or purging behavior (i.e., self-induced vomiting or the misuse of laxatives, diuretics, or enemas)

   Binge-Eating/Purging Type: during the current episode of anorexia nervosa, the person has regularly engaged in binge-eating or purging behavior (i.e., self-induced vomiting or the misuse of laxatives, diuretics, or enemas)

Source. Reprinted from American Psychiatric Association: *Diagnostic and Statistical Manual of Mental Disorders*, 4th Edition, Text Revision. Washington, DC, American Psychiatric Association, 2000. Copyright 2000 American Psychiatric Association. Used with permission.

ing/purging anorexia scored higher than did patients with restrictive anorexia on the Psychopathic Deviate (impulsivity), Depression, Psychasthenia (anxiety and compulsion), and Schizophrenia (rumination and alienation) scales (Casper et al. 1980; Norman and Herzog 1983). However, it is important to note that the majority of patients with restricting anorexia nervosa develop bulimic symptomatology during the course of the disorder (Bulik et al. 1997; Eddy et al. 2002).

The etiological relationship between bulimia nervosa and anorexia nervosa is unclear at present. It is not uncommon for people with anorexia nervosa to develop bulimia nervosa and for those with bulimia nervosa to develop anorexia nervosa (Bulik et al. 1997). Research suggests the two disorders may have shared etiological factors (Walters and Kendler 1995). However, Lillenfeld et al. (1998) found that subjects with anorexia nervosa had a higher prevalence of obsessive-compulsive disorder, obsessive-compulsive personality disorder, generalized anxiety disorder, and social and simple phobias than did subjects with bulimia nervosa and control subjects. Additionally, they found that the risk of obsessive-compulsive personality disorder was elevated only among first-degree relatives of anorexic patients, with evidence showing the disorders may have shared familial risk factors. Lastly, substance abuse is less likely to occur in women with anorexia than bulimia nervosa, although it is unclear what role age and other comorbid disorders play in this observation (Eddy et al. 2002; Schuckit et al. 1996).

Clinical Features

■ Physical Symptoms

Common physical complaints include cold intolerance, dizziness, constipation, abdominal discomfort, and bloating. Despite having malnutrition, the patient with anorexia is often hyperactive; lethargy is worrisome because it may indicate cardiovascular compromise or severe depression.

■ Physical Examination

Patients with anorexia may wear multiple layers of bulky, oversized clothing. Adolescent anorexic patients tend to appear younger than their chronological age, whereas those with chronic anorexia may look considerably older than their age. Cachexia and breast atrophy are noticeable. The skin is often dry and may be yellow-tinged as a result of carotenemia. Bradycardia, hypotension, hypokalemia, growth of lanugo hair, alopecia, and edema of the lower extremities are common (Becker et al. 1999). Dental enamel erosion and lesions on the dorsal surfaces of the hands—Russell's sign (Russell 1985)—are noted in anorexic patients who vomit.

■ Medical Complications

Medical complications, which can be life-threatening, are present in the cardiovascular, hematological, gastrointestinal, renal, neurological, endocrine, and skeletal systems of the body.

Cardiovascular Complications

Electrocardiographic abnormalities are common among anorexic patients and normalize on refeeding. Low voltage, bradycardia, T-wave inversions, and ST segment depression may be found separately or in conjunction with arrhythmias, such as supraventricular premature beats or ventricular tachycardia (with and without exercise). Prolonged QT intervals and emetine-induced myocardial damage may be life-threatening (Gottdiener et al. 1978). However, anorexic patients commonly have a long-standing bradycardia because of regular exercise. Although it is often not possible to predict which patients will ultimately have life-threatening cardiac consequences, those who vomit or abuse diuretics are at greatest risk for fatal cardiovascular complications because of resulting imbalances in electrolyte levels.

Hematological Changes

Mild anemia and leukopenia are common, and thrombocytopenia is also observed. These abnormalities usually reverse with refeeding.

Gastrointestinal Complications

Decreased gastric motility and delayed gastric emptying are often found in patients with restrictive anorexia (Mitchell 1983). Metoclopramide and edrophonium have been used successfully to increase motility and to decrease dyspeptic flatulence, and weight restoration also results in the dissipation of these symptoms (Buchman et al. 1994). Although pancreatic disease is unusual, pancreatitis has been reported in some patients. Liver enzyme and amylase levels may be elevated but will reverse with refeeding. Acute gastric dilation and rupture and acute vascular compression of the duodenum leading to intestinal obstruction are rare but have a high mortality.

Renal Abnormalities

Dehydration results in increased levels of blood urea nitrogen. Polyuria often develops in this population and may be traced to the decrease in renal concentrating capacity and an abnormality in vasopressin secretion, which may produce a partial diabetes insipidus. Peripheral edema is present in 20% of anorexic patients, usually during refeeding and rehydration. Restoration of weight reverses these symptoms, although vasopressin abnormalities may persist for some time.

Neurological Abnormalities

Neurological abnormalities are rarely found on physical examination. Extensive neurological assessment is usually unwarranted, except in atypical presentations such as prepubertal females, male patients, and patients who do not respond to treatment.

Crisp et al. (1968) noted electroencephalographic abnormalities in 10% of patients with anorexia. Katzman et al. (1996) found that brain magnetic resonance images of anorexic adolescents show enlarged lateral ventricles and cortical sulci, findings that strongly correlated with the degree of weight loss. In weight-recovered patients, magnetic resonance images reveal significantly larger sulcal cerebrospinal fluid (CSF) volumes and smaller gray matter volumes compared with those of control subjects, suggesting anorexia nervosa may have long-lasting effects on the brain (Lambe et al. 1997).

Endocrine Complications

A hallmark of anorexia nervosa is amenorrhea, which most often results from starvation-induced hypogonadism. However, in 20%–30% of anorexic patients, amenorrhea precedes weight loss and often persists despite weight recovery (Becker et al. 1999). Clinical signs of hypothyroidism may be present and are due to decreased levels of triiodothyronine. Primary hypothyroidism is rare because serum thyroxine and thyroid-stimulating hormone levels are usually in the low-normal to normal range. Patients with diabetes mellitus may induce further complications by manipulating insulin intake to regulate their weight (Szmukler 1984). Reduced levels of growth hormone binding protein, insulin-like growth factor, and insulin-like growth factor binding protein-3 have been reported in anorexic patients and may explain the growth retardation seen in anorexia nervosa (Golden et al. 1994). These levels revert to normal after nutritional rehabilitation. Serum leptin levels are also significantly decreased in anorexic subjects and have been found to correlate highly with weight, body fat percentage, and insulin-like growth factor-I (IGF-I) (Grinspoon et al. 1996).

Skeletal Complications

Clinical reports of skeletal fractures in anorexic patients have encouraged bone density studies. Findings show bone mineral density is reduced at several skeletal sites in most women with anorexia nervosa. Grinspoon et al. (2000) found that in a community sample of 130 women with anorexia nervosa, bone mineral density was reduced by at least 1 standard deviation in 92% of patients and by at least 2.5 standard deviations in 38% of patients. Castro et al. (2000) found the following variables to be predictive of osteopenia in adolescents: a diagnosis of anorexia nervosa for at least 1 year, at least 6 months of amenorrhea, a body mass index below 15, low calcium intake (<600 mg/day), and fewer than 3 hours a week of physical activity. Female patients for whom onset of the disorder occurs in adolescence are at greater risk for osteoporosis than those whose onset is later (Biller et al. 1989). This is largely because 90% of adult bone mass is formed during adolescence. Thus, not only does the patient with adolescent-onset anorexia lose bone mass but she also does not form bone mass during a critical phase of development.

When examining the effect of weight recovery on bone density, Bachrach et al. (1991) found weight gain resulted in increased bone mineral density before the resumption of menses. However, the persistence of osteopenia despite recovery from anorexia indicated that loss of bone mineral during adolescence may not be completely reversible. Premenarchal anorexic patients whose disorder remits during adolescence may have better bone mineral density repletion (Jagielska et. al. 2001).

Hypercortisolism and hypoestrogenism are proposed causal mechanisms of the osteopenia and warrant further investigation. Recent studies have also focused on the association between low bone formation and low levels of IGF-I, a nutritionally dependent endogenous bone trophic factor, investigating the potential role of low IGF-I levels in the development of osteopenia (Grinspoon et al. 1996; Soyka et al. 1999). To date no studies have shown estrogen administration to be effective in preventing bone loss, and no other effective drug treatment has been found.

■ Psychological Assessment

Anorexic patients constitute a heterogeneous psychiatric population. Psychopathology can range from mild to profound impairment within the confines of a single eating disorder, with comorbid characterological, mood, anxiety, or psychotic disorders in the more severe cases. Some patients may appear high functioning at the first interview but demonstrate more impairment after a few sessions, or vice versa.

The prototypic anorexic patient manifests severe body-image distortion, interoceptive disturbance, and a pervasive sense of ineffectiveness (Bruch 1973). Personality characteristics of anorexic adolescents include obsessional traits, interpersonal insecurity, minimization of emotional expression, perfectionism, identity confusion, excessive conformity and guilt, rigid control over impulses, underlying low self-esteem, heightened industriousness, competitiveness, envy, and increased sense of responsibility (Crisp et al. 1979; Strober 1980). Some of these features, such as competitiveness and envy, are often fiercely denied. Ambivalence about sexual and emotional maturation, separation anxiety, and fears of being controlled are typical areas of conflict. The most common comorbid Axis I disorders in anorexic patients are mood and anxiety disorders. Several studies have reported that 50%–70% of anorexic patients meet criteria for major depressive disorder (Herzog et al. 1999; Ivarsson et al. 2000), whereas over 50% report a lifetime history of an anxiety disorder (Braun et al. 1994; Bulik et al. 1997). Mood disorders can precede the onset, have a simultaneous onset, or follow the onset of anorexia nervosa, whereas anxiety disorders have been found to most often precede the onset of the eating disorder (Bulik et al. 1997; Deep et al. 1995). Kleptomania, substance abuse (among patients with binge-eating/purging anorexia), obsessive-compulsive disorder, psychosis, and personality disorders are also prevalent comorbid disorders (Herzog et al. 1999; Hudson et al. 1984). In our experience, the most commonly associated personality disorders include avoidant, schizoid, borderline, and narcissistic.

The affective range of expression for anorexic patients is highly variable. On a mental status examination, the anorexic patient may be cheerful and hyperactive, may be in a nearly hypomanic state, or may appear sad and hypoactive, seemingly depressed. Most often, the patient's affect is quite restricted, and depressive features, although not openly acknowledged, may be inferred from the patient's behavior (e.g., neurovegetative signs and symptoms, social isolation, or depressive thought content). The patient may be aloof or withdrawn and irritated about being brought for an evaluation. Suicidal ideation may be present. The patient usually has a very limited capacity for self-observation, psychological mindedness, or personal insight. Cognitive impairments, such as diminished attention, concentration, and short-term memory, or obsessive thinking about food, may be starvation induced.

Differential Diagnoses

Initial medical assessment must address the possibility that organic illness may mimic signs and symptoms of eating disorders (Palla and Litt 1988). Physical disorders that have clinical symptoms in common with anorexia nervosa include diabetes mellitus, Crohn's disease, colitis, thyroid disease, inflammatory bowel disease, acid peptic diseases, Addison's disease, intestinal motility disorders such as achalasia, and brain tumors. Anorexia nervosa may occur concurrently with these disorders. Psychiatric disorders that may manifest weight loss and purging include conversion disorder, schizophrenia, and mood disorders (Garfinkel et al. 1983).

Epidemiology

Lifetime prevalence of anorexia nervosa, according to large-scale population and archival surveys, ranges from 0.1% to 0.7% (Becker et al. 1999; Lucas et al. 1988). Research has also been done with student populations. Crisp et al. (1976) found a 1% incidence of current treated and untreated cases of anorexia in British private secondary school populations. Additionally, concern about weight and shape among young girls is widespread. In a study of children in grades 3–6, 45% wanted to be thinner, 39% had tried to lose weight, and 6.9% scored within the high-risk range on the Eating Attitudes Test (Maloney et al. 1989).

Approximately 90%–95% of patients with anorexia are female. Age at onset ranges from 8 years to mid-30s, with bimodal peaks at ages 13–14 and 17–18 years (Halmi et al. 1979). In regard to ethnicity, in earlier studies patients with anorexia nervosa were typically white and middle to upper-middle class. However, more recent studies indicate anorexia nervosa is prevalent across ethnicity and socioeconomic status. A review article found that minority females at greater risk for eating disorders are those who are younger, weigh more, are well educated, and more closely aligned with "white, middle-class values" (Crago et al. 1996). Additionally a large self-report health survey from a community sample of adolescent girls indicated that although socioeconomic status was significantly correlated with unhealthy dieting behaviors, it was not correlated with clinically significant eating-disordered behaviors (Rogers et al. 1997).

Etiology

■ High-Risk Populations

Populations most likely to be at a greater risk for anorexia because of occupational and recreational environments include ballet dancers, male and female long-distance runners, gymnasts, ice skaters, and female models. Each of these activities requires highly focused attention on weight, appearance, and lean body mass. Other susceptible groups include chronically ill women with diseases such as cystic fibrosis (Pumariega et al. 1986), diabetes (Rodin et al. 1986), and mood disorders, particularly depression (Garfinkel et al. 1987), and women in professions that require high standards of achievement and appearance (Herzog et al. 1987b). Although men constitute a smaller statistical group of anorexic patients, particular subgroups that are more susceptible to anorexia nervosa include athletes (e.g., runners, wrestlers) and male homosexuals (Andersen 1990; Carlat et al. 1997).

Sexual abuse is commonly found among clinical populations of anorexic patients and, more recently, in family (Karwautz et al. 2001) and community-based studies (Romans et al. 2001). In a community-based study of women who experienced childhood sexual abuse, belonging to a younger age group, experiencing menarche at an early age, and high paternal overcontrol independently increased the risk of developing an eating disorder (Romans et al. 2001). Specifically, a low level of maternal care was correlated with the development of anorexia nervosa in women who had experienced childhood sexual abuse. Wonderlich et al. (1997) hypothesized that childhood sexual abuse is a risk factor for bulimic disorders more so than for restricting anorexia, with the binge/purge symptoms perhaps serving as an escape from psychological and physiological memories, fears, and reactions to the past abuse.

■ Pathogenesis

Some investigators theorize that anorexia nervosa results from arrestment at an early developmental stage (Bruch 1973). Others view anorexia nervosa as a family problem in which the anorexic patient is the identified patient. In these families, the anorexic child is viewed by other family members as the "sick" individual rather than being perceived as a member of a dysfunctional family unit that itself is the locus of the problem. Still others view anorexia nervosa as a form of mood disorder. The most comprehensive picture emerging suggests that a combination of genetic, neurochemical, psychodevelopmental, and sociocultural factors are implicated in the onset of the disorder (Becker et al. 1999).

Individual Development

Anorexia nervosa can be understood psychodynamically as a compromise solution in the patient's attempt to solve intrapsychic conflicts. In this framework, eating symptoms are seen as a behavioral manifestation of emotional conflict. Purging behaviors such as exercising and vomiting help the anorexic patient to achieve affective homeostasis by being able to rid herself or himself of painful affect and retain a sense of accomplishment by furthering weight loss (Herzog et al. 1987a).

Early developmental theory hypothesized that the infant's primary sense of trust in others, self-confidence, positive self-esteem, gratification of basic physical and emotional needs, and accurate awareness of his or her affective and interoceptive sensations are dependent on a caretaker, typically the mother, who responds appropriately to her child. The mother's empathic attunement to her child's experience and needs both confirms their validity and, it is hoped, satisfies them, because the infant is virtually totally dependent on the mother.

When a mother imposes her own needs on the child, serious consequences in one or more areas noted above may result. This may be clearly demonstrated in the feeding situation. The mother who responds appropriately to her child's cues of hunger provides biological gratification and nurturance, demonstrates a validation of the child's interoceptive sensation of hunger, and instills a sense of confidence in the child that his or her needs can be recognized, understood, valued, and satisfied by another person. However, when feeding takes place because of the mother's need to quiet the child rather than in response to the child's hunger, the child develops uncertainty about his or her inner states and his or her ability to evoke care from the mother. The child feels drawn to comply with the needs of his or her mother to maintain the

fragile connection between mother and child on which the child's survival depends (Bruch 1982). This very same compliance and primacy of the mother's needs over the child's can occur in many areas other than the feeding situation. When experiences of this kind occur repeatedly, the child feels increasingly controlled, exploited, and devalued, although such feelings are often denied, repressed, or repudiated to protect the mother. The last thing the child wants to do is to alienate the mother on whom he or she depends. Moreover, anorexic mothers are generally caring, devoted women and are not easy targets for scorn or ingratitude.

From an object-relational viewpoint, the child's disturbed relationship with the mother affects the child's ability to integrate his or her own aggression and hostility. Mothers of anorexic patients can be self-sacrificing and almost saintly in their care of others and in denial of their own impulses and appetites. However, the apparent selfless nurturance of others often derives from an inner sense of badness, unworthiness, and insecurity and, as such, is not really attuned to the particular needs of others as much as it is attuned to the needs of the self. Such mothers are always trying to make something right in the effort to elevate their own self-esteem, protect their inner fragility, and mitigate a pervasive fear of loss. They, like their children, are exquisitely sensitive to perceived rejection, hostility, and conflict. This particular mother–child relationship makes it exceedingly difficult for the child to take responsibility for his or her own feelings and impulses and to express aggression toward the mother. The child must disavow or defend against his or her anger, because wielding it could result in loss of the mother either by her destruction or abandonment. Hostility is projected and relegated to the external world, which is then viewed as dangerous and untrustworthy.

The typical profile of fathers poses additional conflicts and burdens on the child. The mother's deferentiality and apparent generosity are matched by a complementary entitlement to this behavior in the father. Many fathers, who tend to be highly successful men, are prone to being autocratic in the family, just as they are in their professional roles. Underneath the professional success and mastery frequently lie serious problems in self-esteem and basic trust that are similar to their wives' issues—a needy, dependent side that is often denied. These men often appear counterdependent and self-sufficient on the surface. Such men usually distrust women and perceive them as powerful in their ability to betray and abandon them. They frequently manage this distrust by attempts to dominate women. They also do not trust their wives' apparent self-sacrifice and nurturance and are quite sensitive to the often underlying hidden anger and resentment.

Thus, relationships in the family may appear fine on the surface, but there lurks a mysterious, dangerous side to male–female relationships as exemplified by the parents. The parents are emotionally isolated from each other; each has grave difficulties in intimacy and trust, yet they remain bound together in a self-sustaining cycle. The father senses that beneath his wife's solicitude is terrible anger and contempt, which is just what he expects from powerful women. The mother's experiences with her husband's entitlement, demands, explosiveness, and misogyny reinforce just the defense she wields. This relationship, usually concealed under a façade of smooth functioning, preserves both parents from the twin dangers of excessive closeness on the one hand and abandonment on the other. The parents' relationship, although not consciously understood by the anorexic child, is perceived as somehow troubled, dangerous, and, at times, terrifying. It certainly does not represent an attainable model of male-female relationships; it is one that the anorexic child consciously and unconsciously avoids, largely through symptoms. The female child is terrified of becoming the woman her mother is and simultaneously is distrustful of relationships with men.

Approval and affection are seen as unreliable states that can quickly become negative and disapproving. Ambivalence is poorly tolerated. Anorexic patients protect themselves from the hostile elements by using ritualistic algorithms of good and bad (Gordon et al. 1989; Kernberg 1975). Although the anorexic patient fiercely defends against aggression, largely by denial and projection, such defenses are rarely capable of keeping angry impulses unconscious. An inadequate defensive structure further contributes to low self-esteem and profound guilt. Aggression is acted out by self-directed punitive attacks (e.g., through self-starvation, deprivation, self-loathing, and deprecation), combined with a passive-aggressive assault on the family (starvation in the face of frantic attempts of others to rescue the patient). Concomitantly, the inner experience is not of aggression but rather of a noble, ascetic, powerful activity that makes the child feel special and misunderstood by the world.

The self psychological perspective views anorexia nervosa as a defensive structure mobilized to cope with a disruption in the parent–child relationship (Geist 1989). Maternal failures of empathy and admiration result in the child's overcompliance with maternal wishes. The anorexic patient turns to the father to satisfy emotional needs of empathy and admiration. The closeness present between father and daughter before sexual maturity is threatened during adolescence (Geist 1984). The underdeveloped physical state of anorexic patients may be understood as an attempt to preserve this preadolescent relationship.

Parental Roles

The family structure of many anorexic patients, with an overly giving mother who is unable to take for herself and a powerful father who demands deference and unquestioned loyalty, compounds the child's sense of ineffectiveness (Gordon et al. 1989). The daughter, faced with the prospect of a submissive and subordinate life in a world of powerful and demanding men, is bound by loyalty to her mother and the father's expectations of outward harmony (Gordon et al. 1989). Sexual maturity represents separation from a dependent mother and attraction toward a man like her father. Anorexia nervosa, then, is a compromise between the Scylla of maternal loyalty and the Charybdis of male dominance.

Family Perspectives

Although anorexia nervosa has not been found conclusively to result from errant family dynamics, family theory and therapy have been useful in providing support and a theoretical context for the anorexic family. Family theorists attempt to understand anorexia nervosa in the context of family interaction in which the family is the unit of dysfunction and treatment. The identified patient is viewed as the symptom-bearer of the larger family unit.

Anorexic families often present a happy, conflict-free exterior that serves to mask feelings of mistrust, lack of intimacy between parents, enmeshment, overprotection, rigidity, and lack of conflict resolution (Minuchin et al. 1978). The role of the anorexic daughter is to divert attention from impending family conflict and marital problems; her symptoms serve as a stabilizing force for the family. As the anorexic daughter becomes increasingly thin, she becomes increasingly dependent on and inseparable from the family (Minuchin 1984).

Empirical work with anorexic families that focused on their dynamic-interactive characteristics has confirmed clinical findings relative to "normal" families. Humphrey (1989) found that parents of anorexic children were both "too nurturant" and "too neglectful." Excessive nurturance seemed to undermine the daughter's efforts at separation; her attempts at genuine self-expression were neglected.

Sociocultural Factors

It is indeed remarkable that anorexia nervosa tends to affect females almost 10 times as frequently as males. It also tends to erupt at times of sexual maturation: menarche, puberty, and during development of a mature female body shape. The reason that anorexia afflicts mostly females is probably associated with femininity and/or the female role in society, but the exact nature of this pattern is currently speculative. Many researchers have attributed this distribution to the greater cultural pressure on women toward thinness. Thinness is commonly portrayed in the media and in the Western cultural value structure as a prerequisite to success and beauty and as evidence of willpower.

Perhaps an even more powerful social force is the difference in socialization between girls and boys. Gilligan (1982) demonstrated that girls are brought up to espouse "feminine" values: service to others, attention to relationships, and empathy for those with whom relationships are formed. Interrelationships are at the center of feminine development. Boys, on the other hand, are trained to be more autonomous, self-directed, and rule oriented in their relationships with others. Modern culture is transforming the traditional models of male and female role definition by encouraging girls to be more autonomous, self-directed, and rule oriented in their relationships with others (a role analogous to the traditional model of male behavior). Hence, girls find themselves in a double bind. The socialization process is frightening and perplexing. Anorexia nervosa, at least for some, may be a response to the pressures of socialization.

Biological Factors

Controlled family studies of anorexic patients have found a familial risk of mood disorders among first- and second-degree relatives of anorexic patients (Hudson et al. 1983; Winokur et al. 1980). Strober et al. (1990) and Biederman et al. (1985) observed that increased morbid risk for mood disorders in first- and second-degree relatives was associated with the depressed anorexic subpopulation.

The presence of comorbid mood disorders in anorexic patients and of familial mood disorders has stimulated neurochemical research in this population. Starvation itself produces extensive changes in hypothalamic and metabolic functioning, although it has been difficult to elicit abnormalities specific to anorexia nervosa. Anorexia nervosa is associated with changes in the noradrenergic, serotonergic, dopaminergic, and opioid neurotransmitter systems and with alterations in neuromodulators such as corticotropin-releasing hormone (Fava et al. 1989). Abnormalities have been noted in the production of CSF levels of 3-methoxy-4-hydroxyphenylglycol (MHPG), 5-hydroxyindoleacetic acid (5-HIAA), homovanillic acid, β-lipotropin, adrenocorticotropic hormone, β-endorphin, N-terminal fragment of pro-opiomelanocortin, thyrotropin-releasing hormone, and cortisol. Differences in prolactin response to L-tryptophan in dieting states have suggested alterations in brain 5-hydroxytryptamine-mediated responses (Goodwin et al. 1987). Nearly all these levels normalize after weight gain. Anorexic patients also have decreased levels of CSF norepinephrine and an elevated ratio of CSF-to-plasma arginine vasopressin for long periods after weight gain (Gold et al. 1983).

Genetic factors in the transmission of anorexia among family members are at the forefront of research on anorexia. Results of population-based twin studies as well as clinical samples suggest significant genetic and nonshared environmental influences on anorexic symptomatology (Klump et al. 2001; Wade et al. 2000). In a review of six family studies on eating disorders, Strober (1995) found that overall, anorexia is several times more common in biological relatives of anorexic patients than in the general population. Analyses of the phenotypic presentation of personality and behavioral characteristics in women with eating disorders suggest that the following factors—trait anxiety, harm avoidance, perfectionism, obsessive-compulsive behaviors, and diminished self-directedness—can effectively differentiate subjects into eating disorder subtypes and may be conceptualized as parts of the same underlying construct among individuals with anorexia nervosa (Anonymous 2001). Strong indications of a genetic component contributing to the expression of anorexia nervosa prompted a recent multisite genetic study, which provided initial evidence for the presence of an anorexia nervosa–susceptibility locus on chromosome 1p (Grice et al. 2002).

Biological research on mechanisms of perception and taste in anorexia nervosa has probed the relation between eating behaviors and taste percepts; an abnormal sensory response to high-calorie foods may be responsible for bingeing behaviors (Sunday et al. 1992). An alternative view, the set-point hypothesis, expects emaciated anorexic patients to show initially elevated taste preferences for calorie-dense foods, followed by decreased levels after nutritional therapy. Drewnowski et al. (1987) found that optimal sugar-to-fat ratios were elevated among both patients with restrictive anorexia and those with bulimic anorexia compared with control subjects. Such differences seem to be consistent despite weight gain. Abnormal taste profiles may be an enduring characteristic in patients with eating disorders.

Lastly, neurochemical research points to growing evidence that hypothalamic epinephrine and serotonin under certain circumstances induce loss of appetite, whereas norepinephrine increases food intake (Stoving et al. 1999). Elevated levels of serotonin found in women with anorexia, both during their illness and after recovery, suggest the chemical may contribute to the development of the disorder (Frank et al. 2001; Kaye 1997; Stoving et al. 1999).

Treatment

Treatment of anorexia nervosa presents unique difficulties to the clinician. Anorexia nervosa is largely an ego-syntonic disorder. Patients are typically resistant to initiating treatment focused on weight gain. Patients may not come to medical attention until they have lost a considerable amount of weight (Maloney and Klykylo 1983). In the face of divisive family issues, family members may attempt to split (i.e., cause disagreements and, at worst, disputes between) treating clinicians on the basis of differing opinions. This often occurs by the communication of different thoughts, feelings, or behaviors to different clinicians. Such behavior is usually an unconscious attempt to undermine coordinated treatment and maintain the status quo. Patients and their families may evoke reactions of anger, stress, and helplessness in medical personnel (Brotman et al. 1984).

Evaluation of the anorexic patient should incorporate a team approach and include medical, psychiatric, family, and nutritional assessments. The first determination in the evaluation of the anorexic patient is often whether inpatient treatment is indicated.

The clinician should be attentive to ways of engaging the reluctant or openly resistant patient. Usually, an initial alliance will draw on some area of acknowledged difficulty, including symptoms such as restlessness, irritability, insomnia, hyperactivity, cold intolerance, poor concentration, family problems, and social isolation. In the absence of an identified problem, the clinician may develop an alliance by empathically understanding the patient's perspective, such as her irritation and indignation that others around her will not leave her alone. Her condition forces others to pay attention and take control when, paradoxically, this is precisely what she fears. This pattern of a literal starvation for attention and caretaking, coupled with stoic isolation and passive, fearful, or, rarely, overtly hostile resistance, is played out in dyadic control struggles, both in the family and with the clinician. Hence, an interplay of sensitivity, empathy, and respect for the anorexic patient, with steadfast adherence to basic bottom lines of physical safety, is necessary for an adequate psychological assessment or treatment plan to proceed. Although many anorexic patients will view limits on safety as evidence of further imposed "control," or an intention to "get me fat," often there is a sense of relief (usually unconscious) that someone is taking over a situation gone out of control (Beresin et al. 1989). Such relief may not be acknowledged until later in the course of treatment. Early on, limits are commonly rejected, repudiated, and treated with disdain.

■ Inpatient

Inpatient treatment of anorexia nervosa is mandated by the severity of the patient's physical and psychological status. Although hospitalization often is indicated, it must be viewed as one phase in long-term treatment that also will include outpatient care.

Criteria suggested by the American Academy of Child and Adolescent Psychiatry for hospitalization of children and adolescents with anorexia are listed in Table 35–2. Body mass index (BMI), a measure of weight (kg) divided by height squared (m^2), is used to indicate the degree of severity of anxorexia nervosa in an individual. A BMI of 17.5 kg/m^2 correlates with a body weight of less than 85% the expected and indi-

Table 35–2. Guidelines for hospitalization of anorexic patients

Justification for admission

A. Presence of severe or persistent medical complications that threaten life or health to the point of producing impairment that renders outpatient treatment management ineffective

Presence of at least one of the major and three of the minor complications, or at least six of the minor complications

Major complications

Weight <75% of ideal body weight (IBW), either emaciated or cathexic

Hypoglycemic syncope or "grayouts"

Severe fluid and electrolyte imbalance

Cardiac arrhythmia

Severe dehydration

Minor complications

Moderate malnutrition, weight <85% of IBW

Recalcitrant vomiting

Bradycardia

Hypotension

Hypothermia

Lanugo

Amenorrhea for three consecutive cycles

Acute starvation

Vasomotor instability

Minor electrolyte imbalance or hypoglycemia

Hypothyroidism

Nutritional anemia

Exercise-induced injury

Impaired renal functioning

Intestinal atony

B. Patient has been stabilized on medical or pediatric inpatient service and is then transferred to child and adolescent psychiatric/eating disorder treatment

C. Failure of 2 months of weekly outpatient medical psychotherapy to produce expected weight and appropriate eating patterns

Source. Adapted from Stevenson 1989.

cates lower than adequate weight. Inpatient treatment should incorporate a comprehensive psychiatric evaluation, a thorough medical examination, appropriate laboratory studies to determine the patient's physiological status, and close observation (Andersen et al. 1985). During the course of hospitalization, a team approach must be used and may include a psychiatrist, nutritionist, family therapist, recreational therapist, educator, and nursing staff trained to treat eating disorders.

The patient may be hospitalized on either a pediatric or a psychiatric ward. Patients with severe depression in the midst of a family crisis or in severe denial can receive more effective treatment on a psychiatric ward; those who primarily need nutritional repletion can often be treated adequately on a medical ward. Those deciding on which ward to hospitalize the pa-

tient must take into consideration the staff's experience and comfort in dealing with anorexic patients.

One innovative treatment design is the pediatric day-care unit (Danziger et al. 1988), where parents are incorporated into the day-to-day interventions of patient care. This approach seeks to eliminate the punitive aspects of patient separation from parents. Parental supervision of patient behavior and meals aids in the restoration of positive patient and parental interaction as well as in the natural hierarchy of the family.

The inpatient treatment program must have a nutritional rehabilitation protocol to which all treating clinicians can agree. The physician must explain the treatment regimen in detail to the patient before hospitalization. The staff, patient, and family must be aware that the administration of a feeding regimen is a life-saving act rather than a punishment. At the time of admission, a target weight for discharge should be established. The American Psychiatric Association suggests as a healthy target weight one "at which normal menstruation and ovulation are restored" or, for premenarchal girls, a weight at which "normal physical and sexual development resumes" (American Psychiatric Association Work Group on Eating Disorders 2000). However, some patients may continue to menstruate at low weights and others may not regain menses with weight gain; therefore, the minimum target weight is often estimated at 90% of ideal weight for height according to standard tables (American Psychiatric Association Work Group on Eating Disorders 2000). Patients need not actually reach ideal body weight during the hospital stay. However, the target weight must be sufficiently high to protect the patient from bordering on a medically precarious state. This target weight should be maintained for a period prior to discharge. Once the patient has reached the target weight, a reasonable range should be established to allow for day-to-day fluctuations. The success of the protocol depends on the ability of the staff to be open, honest, empathic, and firm (but not inflexible) in its implementation. Once weight is increased to a medically stable level, the patient will be more psychologically amenable to other treatment modalities. Favorable outcome from inpatient treatment has been demonstrated. In a 10- to 15-year follow-up study of women with adolescent-onset anorexia who received comprehensive multimodal psychotherapeutic treatment in an inpatient setting, about three-fourths of the patients showed no signs of an eating disorder at follow-up evaluation (Strober et al. 1997). However, median time to recovery, defined by resumption of menses and ideal weight, was 57.4 months, highlighting the protracted length of time it takes for many patients to recover.

Recent limitations in health care coverage have led to reduced lengths of hospital stays. Currently, national data show that the average number of days of inpatient and outpatient treatment for an eating disorder is less than the minimum recommended by standards of care (Striegel-Moore et al. 2000). As a result, many anorexic patients who are still underweight are being discharged. Baran et al. (1995) monitored 22 anorexic patients for a mean of 29 months after discharge from an inpatient unit and found that individuals who were severely underweight when discharged had significantly higher rates of rehospitalization and were more symptomatic than those individuals discharged at normal weight (i.e., those who reached more than 90% of the recommended average body weight).

■ Outpatient

Diverse theoretical orientations all lead to a wide range of therapeutic techniques for anorexia nervosa. Many techniques seem to be effective, but none have been validated or "proved" effective in the long run by prospective, double-blind, empirical inquiry. In most cases, a multimodal approach incorporating several therapeutic techniques is necessary. Because the disorder is complex—severe medical complications may ensue, and the individual and/or the family are typically resistant to treatment—treatment should be based on a biopsychosocial formulation and should be internally consistent, and members of the treatment team must be in close contact with one another.

The core outpatient treatment for anorexic patients should include ongoing medical management as well as individual and family psychotherapy. Additional treatment options include nutritional counseling, group therapy, and pharmacotherapy. The treatment program should be tailored to the needs of the individual. Gowers et al. (1994) reevaluated 20 anorexic patients who participated in outpatient treatment consisting of individual and family psychotherapy. At the 2-year follow-up evaluation, 60% (12) of the individuals were classified as "well" or "nearly well" (i.e., weight within 15% of mean matched population weight, resumption of menses, and normal or mildly disordered eating patterns).

Psychotherapy

The goal of psychotherapy is to help the patient achieve a capacity for self-regulation that is more adaptive than current eating behaviors. Patient and/or family denial of the existence of a problem impedes the formation of a therapeutic alliance. Denial of the illness by the patient or his or her family is an attempt to maintain an existing solution (i.e., the disorder), albeit a costly one, for deeply rooted feelings of despair and inadequacy. Initially, the therapist must establish trust by acknowledging the patient's ongoing pain and recognizing the multiple determinants of the disorder (social, psychopathological, genetic, biological, behavioral, and familial). The patient is often reassured by the therapist's knowledge about eating disorders and relieved to discover that the therapist neither minimizes, is fearful of, nor is repulsed by the patient's symptoms. The patient's physical condition may dictate close attention to medical status. Clinicians should create a "therapeutic envelope" designed to provide a safety net for the patient if weight or vital signs fall below agreed-on minimums (Hamburg et al. 1989). The continuation of outpatient therapy may be contingent on the patient's maintenance of a minimum weight requirement (Bruch 1988). Clear guidelines regarding weight, vital signs, and hospitalization should be established early in treatment and can be formalized as a contract. Only in the context of medical safety can the work of therapy proceed. Over the course of treatment, the therapist may be challenged to respect the psychological need of the patient to be very thin while holding steadfast to protecting the patient's life.

A wide range of psychotherapeutic theoretical orientations and techniques have been advocated in the treatment of anorexic patients, including supportive, psychoeducational, cognitive-behavior, and insight-oriented therapies. Although specific techniques may differ among the schools of psychotherapy, these approaches share common elements that are therapeutic for the anorexic patient. Within the category of insight-oriented therapy, considerable variations are demonstrated in object-relations, ego-psychological, self psychological, or traditional psychoanalytic approaches. Bruch (1973) cautioned that some features of this approach might be harmful to anorexic patients. The anorexic patient often views the silence of traditional psychoanalytic therapy as rejection and interpretations as demands for compliance, thus perpetuating the destructive cycle of constant concessions to the needs of others.

Cognitive-behavioral therapy offers a different approach to therapy. It is a technique designed to identify and change unhealthy thoughts and feelings about body shape and weight, teach normal eating habits in place of food restriction, and provide coping skills to resist binge-eating and purging (Wilson and Fairburn 1993). Cognitive-behavioral therapy has been shown to be moderately effective in treating anorexia nervosa (Fernandez-Aranda et al. 1998; Peterson and Mitchell 1999); however, more research is needed to determine its impact on long-term outcome in adolescents.

Because a fundamental problem for the anorexic patient is thought to lie in the earliest dyadic relationships, the therapist must be aware of the patient's deep distrust of relationships and the motives of others. The therapist, above all, should be empathic and accurately "mirror" the perceived wants, needs, and feelings of the patient. It is important that the therapist be tolerant, undemanding, reliable, consistent, flexible, and able to empathize with the patient, sharing and tolerating affect without denial, resistance, or criticism. An effective therapeutic alliance demonstrates that relationships can sustain anger, conflict, and misunderstanding (Beresin et al. 1989). Empathic failures are inevitable and should be mended promptly. As in all psychotherapy, empathy and caring are perfectly consistent with limit-setting. The therapist must clearly indicate that the success of psychotherapy depends on at least minimal nutritional and physical requirements.

Psychotherapy with the anorexic patient is a slow, difficult process. Transferential anger and devaluation, suspension of therapy, struggles with monetary and time boundaries, critical illness, and hospitalization may occur throughout the course of therapy. Erroneous assumptions are discussed, and conflicts that may be embodied in the eating symptom may be addressed. Over time, the experience of the therapist's consistency in care and boundary maintenance may also facilitate the patient's ability to make effective use of additional forms of treatment such as group therapy or pharmacotherapy. As mentioned previously, a multimodal approach to care is optimal because clinical experience suggests that psychotherapy alone is not adequate to treat patients with anorexia nervosa (American Psychiatric Association Work Group on Eating Disorders 2000).

Group Therapy

Anorexic patients will often express little interest in group treatment because they are socially avoidant and mistrustful. Moreover, their competitiveness can result in substantial weight loss for group members unless at least a few members are well on their way toward recovery. Group therapy evolved from friendships formed by patients on inpatient units, the common feelings of being misunderstood, and the vulnerability of discharged patients in the 6- to 8-week postdischarge period (Rollins and Piazza 1981). The goal of group therapy is to decrease the patient's feelings of isolation by creating a nonthreatening environment in which patients may share thoughts and feelings (Piazza et al. 1983). Patients find it helpful to learn that other people also experience the same feelings and symptoms.

Self-help groups provide information, support,

and encouragement to patients with eating disorders and to their families. Often these groups provide an initial outreach to patients in the community. Outside contact is encouraged among members, and feelings of self-worth and hope are reinforced.

A recent development that practitioners should be aware of is the increasingly common use of online Web sites that offer eating disorder information or host chat rooms and group discussions (American Psychiatric Association Work Group on Eating Disorders 2000). Lack of professional supervision on these sites may have detrimental effects. Patient and family use of the Internet for information and support should therefore be monitored.

Family Therapy

Family therapy may be initially introduced to the family as a means of support for coping with the adolescent's anorexia. It is often not clear that family problems have led to the onset or maintenance of the eating disorder. Nevertheless, families are uniformly affected by anorexia nervosa. A family member with an eating disorder presents a severe challenge to the family. Family therapies use a variety of techniques with anorexic families.

One technique is reformulating the child's "disease" to the "symptom" of the family in distress. The identified patient is empowered to see herself or himself as potentially well, whereas the communication and affective patterns of other family members are addressed and restructured to provide support and tolerable independence to the patient (Minuchin 1984; Minuchin et al. 1978). Indirect interventions may be used to modify the family's rigid beliefs and behavioral patterns. Paradoxical interventions are used when an open approach to the problem is likely to elicit denial or resistance in the family. The patient may be urged not to give up her or his problems too quickly as the consequences of the behavioral change are outlined. In such families, the need for control supersedes the symptomatic behavior of the anorexic child. Paradoxically instructing the child to *maintain* anorexic symptoms results in a shift in the family system in a direction contrary to the therapist's instructions (Schwartz et al. 1985).

A similar strategy is to reframe the "problem" of the patient as the "solution" to the family's multiple dilemmas. The problem then becomes viewed as a larger familial process in which all members play a part rather than as the individual's illness (Selvini-Palazzoli 1978).

Conversely, a manualized family-based treatment developed by Eisler and Dare suggests that the family, instead of being viewed as problematic or "pathological," should be used by the therapist as an important resource to help patients recover (Locke et al. 2001). Long-term benefits from this form of family therapy have been shown to be strongest in patients with early-onset anorexia nervosa who are treated at an early stage in the disorder (Eisler et al. 1997).

Ultimately, family therapy seeks to provide a safe holding environment for the children and the parents. One goal of therapy is to discuss openly and to resolve any issues of incomplete or nonexistent individuation and separation in the family. Issues from a parent's childhood family that are transferred onto the children may be addressed.

Pharmacotherapy

To date, no psychotropic medication has been shown to effectively reverse anorexia nervosa. Although cyproheptadine and amitriptyline have been found to be statistically superior to placebo in short-term inpatient trials (Halmi et al. 1986), clinical efficacy has not yet been demonstrated. Two studies, one a 6-week open-label clinical trial in adolescents (Strober et al. 1999) and the other a 7-week randomized, placebo-controlled, double-blind study in adults (Attia et al. 1998), found that fluoxetine did not significantly improve treatment outcome for anorexic inpatients. Similarly, clomipramine, lithium, thiothixene, pimozide, sulpiride, and naloxone have yielded negative or equivocal results. However, case reports of atypical antipsychotics such as risperidone, olanzapine, and quetiapine suggest that such agents may be useful in the symptomatic treatment of certain aspects of anorexia (e.g., obsessive-compulsive symptoms).

Research examining the efficacy of fluoxetine in treating weight-recovered anorexic patients has shown promise. Gwirtsman et al. (1990) and Kaye et al. (1991) conducted open trials of fluoxetine in weight-recovered anorexic outpatients and found that selective serotonin reuptake inhibitors may help anorexic patients maintain their weight. Double-blind, placebo-controlled studies of fluoxetine in weight-recovered anorexic patients noted a similar response (Hsu 1995; Kaye et al. 2001).

Pharmacotherapy can be a useful adjunct to other

treatments. All comorbid disorders (e.g., obsessive-compulsive disorder, depression, and anxiety disorder) should be treated with the appropriate medication. The administration of antianxiety agents before meals may help the anorexic patient manage the anxiety experienced when consuming a modest amount of food. The use and effects of the medication should be explained carefully to the anorexic patient to avoid misconceptions by the patient and to encourage family support of the treatment. Medication should be monitored very closely. Initially, low dosages are necessary to reduce possible side effects in this low-weight population.

It is important to emphasize that psychotropic medication should be prescribed only in the context of psychotherapy. The following principles are essential in prescribing psychotropics to malnourished, dehydrated, and physically compromised patients who are often resistant to such treatment:

- Educate the patient and family about the use and effects of medication.
- Select the specific target symptoms (e.g., obsessions, depression).
- Start at a low dose and increase slowly.
- Monitor serum levels of the medication, vital signs, and electrocardiograms.

■ Additional Treatment Options

Anorexic patients often have difficulty negotiating the transition between inpatient and outpatient programs. Additional treatment options for this population include residential treatment programs, halfway houses, and day-hospital group treatment programs.

In rare cases, it is unsafe or inappropriate for the anorexic patient to return to the parental home. Options for continued treatment in such circumstances may be residential treatment or, for older adolescents or young adults, a halfway house. In extreme cases, such as when parental contact repeatedly results in additional weight loss for the patient, it may be prudent to instruct or to confront the parents, seek voluntary change of the patient's residence, pursue legal stabilization through parental retention of custody and appointment of a guardian, or facilitate voluntary or involuntary transfer of custody to the state (Harper 1983).

Piran and Kaplan (1989) developed a day-hospital group treatment program that incorporates the closely supervised and highly scheduled environment of an inpatient setting. This treatment program offers an alternative to hospitalization for patients who require a structured environment.

Prognosis

■ Outcome

Outcome for anorexia nervosa can be assessed in terms of mortality, weight gain or loss, eating attitudes and behaviors, menstruation, and psychological functioning. Long-term follow-up studies examining inpatient subjects 10–15 years after intake show rates of chronic anorexia nervosa ranging from 12% to 14% (Eckert et al. 1995; Strober et al. 1997). In a 7.5-year naturalistic follow-up study, 33.7% of anorexic subjects achieved full recovery, of which 40% experienced a relapse (Herzog et al. 1999). Predictors of full recovery included higher body weight at intake and shorter duration of intake episode. There were no significant predictors of relapse.

The mortality rate for anorexia nervosa, 0.56% per year, is more than 12 times as high as that expected for young women in the general population (Becker et al. 1999). At 10-year posthospitalization follow-up evaluation of 76 anorexic women, Eckert et al. (1995) found a mortality of 6% (5 women); none of the women had died by suicide. In a survey of 13 outcome studies, Herzog et al. (1988) found that 24% of the deaths reported were due to suicide. An 11-year follow-up study of women with eating disorders had a mortality rate of 5.1% for the subjects with anorexia nervosa, where three of the seven deaths were due to suicide (Herzog et al. 2000). Factors found to predict death in women with anorexia nervosa include abnormally low serum albumin levels and low weight at intake (Herzog et al. 1997), poor social functioning (Lowe et al. 2001), longer duration of illness, bingeing and purging, comorbid substance abuse, and comorbid affective disorders (Herzog et al. 2000). Although death is commonly due to suicide, it is also frequently ascribed to inanition. However, the exact cause of death is often unclear.

Eckert et al. (1995) found high percentages of psychological problems such as depression (80%), suicide attempts (21%), social and general anxiety (55%), obsessive thinking (66%), compulsive behaviors (70%), perfectionism (87%), and boredom

(69%) at 10-year follow-up evaluation. Underweight women tended to have more psychological problems during the follow-up period ($r=0.05$). Cantwell et al. (1977) found that 33% of the adolescent patients had an affective disorder at a mean follow-up point of 4 years. Similarly, Smith et al. (1993) reported that of 23 adolescents with anorexia, 30% had an affective disorder and 43% had an anxiety disorder at 6-year follow-up evaluation.

In a review of long-term outcome studies, Swift (1982) found conflicting results regarding the correlation between better prognosis and early onset (defined as age 11–15 years) of anorexia nervosa. No clear predictors of outcome are currently available for the anorexic population.

■ Course

The majority of anorexic patients engage in bingeing and purging behaviors during the course of the disorder (Casper et al. 1980; Eckert et al. 1995; Eddy et al. 2002). In our long-term follow-up study of women with eating disorders, we found that 6% of patients with restricting anorexia and 39% of patients with binge-eating/purging anorexia met full criteria for bulimia nervosa over the course of the study, indicating that within a subgroup of those with anorexia nervosa, crossover to bulimia nervosa may be common.

Can anorexic patients ever recover? Beresin et al. (1989) reported on 13 severely ill anorexic patients who had been assessed as recovered on the basis of weight, menses, eating attitudes and behaviors, body image, and psychosocial and psychiatric adjustment. These investigators found that among the factors most helpful in the process of recovery were "therapeutic" relationships with professionals, friends, and family members. The presence of another person who relates to the anorexic patient honestly and who encourages expression of the patient's feelings allows the anorexic patient to escape his or her solitary existence, clarify distortions in perceptions and thought, develop trust in people, and, above all, consolidate a strong sense of self.

Research Issues

Research in anorexia nervosa is advancing. Investigating valid and reliable diagnostic criteria is a priority.

Additional research is necessary to address the subdivision in DSM-IV (and its Text Revision, DSM-IV-TR) of anorexia nervosa into restrictive and bulimic subtypes, to explore the necessity of amenorrhea as a symptom for diagnosis, to investigate risk and protective factors, and to address the relationship between anorexia nervosa and bulimia nervosa.

Family studies of anorexia nervosa will increase our understanding of the etiological role of genetics in this disorder. Prospective longitudinal studies on the naturalistic course of anorexia nervosa will establish base rates of short-interval and long-term recovery, chronicity, and morbidity.

Current research in the areas of cognitive functioning and neuroimaging are helping elucidate patterns of cognitive impairment as well as identifying neural systems implicated in anorexia nervosa. Further research on the neurochemistry (neurotransmitter systems and neuromodulators) of anorexia nervosa and on changes in the central nervous system that precede onset is necessary to increase our understanding of the pathophysiology and to develop more effective pharmacological and cognitive-behavioral treatments (Fava et al. 1989).

Research on the pattern of sensory responsiveness to sweets and fat during childhood or early adolescence may determine early psychobiological markers for eating disorders (Grill 1985). Investigations of osteoporosis, a frequent and severe complication of anorexia nervosa, will elucidate mediating mechanisms and appropriate treatment.

The current financial climate in medical care mandates outcome research on the effects of 1- to 2-week hospitalization on weight maintenance, eating attitudes, and nutritional stabilization. Similarly, because psychotherapy remains the outpatient treatment of choice for anorexia nervosa, the exploration of how psychotherapy works (i.e., comparison of different psychotherapy techniques) is a high priority.

Conclusion

Anorexia nervosa is a life-threatening disorder that has come to the forefront of public attention since the 1970s. The successful collaboration of clinical researchers from all disciplines is necessary to further the understanding of the pathogenesis and treatment of the disorder.

References

Allbutt TC: Neuroses of the stomach and of other parts of the abdomen, in A System of Medicine, Vol III. Edited by Allbutt TC, Rolleston HD. London, Macmillan, 1910

American Psychiatric Association: Diagnostic and Statistical Manual of Mental Disorders, 4th Edition. Washington, DC, American Psychiatric Association, 1994

American Psychiatric Association: Diagnostic and Statistical Manual of Mental Disorders, 4th Edition, Text Revision. Washington, DC, American Psychiatric Association, 2000

American Psychiatric Association Work Group on Eating Disorders: Practice guideline for the treatment of patients with eating disorders (revision). Am J Psychiatry 157 (suppl 1):1–39, 2000

Andersen AE: Diagnosis and treatment of males with eating disorders, in Males With Eating Disorders. Edited by Andersen AE. New York, Brunner/Mazel, 1990, pp 133–162

Andersen AE, Morse CL, Santmyer KS: Inpatient treatment for anorexia nervosa, in Handbook of Psychotherapy for Anorexia Nervosa and Bulimia. Edited by Garner DM, Garfinkel PE. New York, Guilford, 1985, pp 311–343

Anonymous: Deriving behavioural phenotypes in an international, multi-centre study of eating disorders. Psychol Med 31:635–645, 2001

Attia E, Haiman C, Walsh BT, et al: Does fluoxetine augment the inpatient treatment of anorexia nervosa? Am J Psychiatry 155:548–551, 1998

Bachrach LK, Katzman DK, Litt IF, et al: Recovery from osteopenia in adolescent girls with anorexia nervosa. J Clin Endocrinol Metab 72:602–606, 1991

Baran SA, Weltzin TE, Kaye WH: Low discharge weight and outcome in anorexia nervosa. Am J Psychiatry 152:1070–1072, 1995

Becker AE, Grinspoon SK, Klibanski AK, et al: Eating disorders. N Engl J Med 340:1092–1098, 1999

Beresin EV, Gordon C, Herzog DB: The process of recovering from anorexia nervosa, in Psychoanalysis and Eating Disorders. Edited by Bemporad JR, Herzog DB. New York, Guilford, 1989, pp 103–130

Biederman J, Rivinus RM, Kemper K, et al: Depressive disorders in relatives of anorexia nervosa patients with and without a current episode of non-bipolar major depression. Am J Psychiatry 142:1495–1497, 1985

Biller BMK, Saxe V, Herzog DB, et al: Mechanisms of osteoporosis in adult and adolescent women with anorexia nervosa. J Clin Endocrinol Metab 68:548–554, 1989

Braun DL, Sunday SR, Halmi KA: Psychiatric comorbidity in patients with eating disorders. Psychol Med 24:859–867, 1994

Brotman AW, Stern TA, Herzog DB: Emotional reactions of house officers to patients with anorexia nervosa, diabetes, and obesity. Int J Eat Disord 3:71–77, 1984

Bruch H: Eating Disorders. New York, Basic Books, 1973

Bruch H: Anorexia nervosa: therapy and theory. Am J Psychiatry 139:1531–1538, 1982

Bruch H: The task of psychotherapy, in Conversations With Anorexics. Edited by Czyzewski D, Suhr MA. New York, Basic Books, 1988, pp 3–13

Brumberg JJ: Fasting Girls: The Emergence of Anorexia Nervosa as a Modern Disease. Cambridge, MA, Harvard University Press, 1988

Buchman AL, Ament ME, Weiner M, et al: Reversal of megaduodenum and duodenal dysmotility associated with improvement in nutritional status in primary anorexia nervosa. Dig Dis Sci 39:433–440, 1994

Bulik C, Sulliva PF, Fear J, et al: Predictors of the development of bulimia nervosa in women with anorexia nervosa. J Nerv Ment Dis 185:704–707, 1997

Cantwell DP, Sturzenberg S, Burroughs J, et al: Anorexia nervosa: an affective disorder? Arch Gen Psychiatry 33:1039–1044, 1977

Carlat DJ, Camargo CA Jr., Herzog DB: Eating disorders in males: a report on 135 patients. Am J Psychiatry 154:1127–1132, 1997

Casper RC, Elke ED, Halmi KA, et al: Bulimia: its incidence and clinical importance in patients with anorexia nervosa. Arch Gen Psychiatry 37:1030–1040, 1980

Castro J, Lazaro L, Pons F, et al: Predictors of bone mineral density reduction in adolescents with anorexia nervosa. J Am Acad Child Adolesc Psychiatry 39:1365–1370, 2000

Crago M, Shisslak CM, Estes LS: Eating disturbances among American minority groups: a review. Int J Eat Disord 19:239–248, 1996

Crisp AH, Fenton GW, Scotton L: A controlled study of the EEG of anorexia nervosa. Br J Psychiatry 114:1149–1160, 1968

Crisp AH, Palmer RL, Kalucy RS: How common is anorexia nervosa? A prevalence study. Br J Psychiatry 128:549–554, 1976

Crisp AH, Hsu RL, Stonehill L: Personality, body weight and ultimate outcome in anorexia nervosa. Br J Psychiatry 40:335–352, 1979

Danziger Y, Carol CA, Varsano I, et al: Parental involvement in treatment of patients with anorexia nervosa in a pediatric day-care unit. Pediatrics 81:159–162, 1988

Deep A, Nagy L, Weltzin T, et al: Premorbid onset of psychopathology in long-term recovered anorexia nervosa. Int J Eat Disord 17:291–298, 1995

Drewnowski A, Halmi KA, Pierce B, et al: Taste and eating disorders. Am J Clin Nutr 46:442–450, 1987

Eckert ED, Halmi KA, Marchi P, et al: Ten-year follow-up of anorexia nervosa: clinical course and outcome. Psychol Med 25:143–156, 1995

Eddy KT, Keel, PK, Dorer DJ, et al: A longitudinal comparison of anorexia nervosa subtypes. Int J Eat Disord 31:191–201, 2002

Eisler I, Dare C, Russell GFM, et al: Family and individual therapy in anorexia nervosa: a five-year follow-up. Arch Gen Psy 54:1025–1030, 1997

Fava M, Copeland PM, Schweiger U, et al: Neurochemical abnormalities of anorexia nervosa and bulimia nervosa. Am J Psychiatry 146:963–971, 1989

Fernandez-Aranda F, Bel M, Jimenez S, et al: Outpatient group therapy for anorexia nervosa: a preliminary study. Eat Weight Disord 3:1–6, 1998

Frank GK, Kaye WH, Weltzin TE, et al: Altered response to meta-chlorophenylpiperazine in anorexia nervosa: support for a persistent alteration of serotonin activity after short-term weight restoration. Int J Eat Disord 30:57–68, 2001

Garfinkel PE, Garner DM, Kaplan AS: Differential diagnosis of emotional disorders that cause weight loss. Can Med Assoc J 129:939–945, 1983

Garfinkel PE, Garner DM, Goldbloom DS: Eating disorders: implications for the 1990s. Can J Psychiatry 32:624–630, 1987

Geist RA: Psychotherapeutic dilemmas in the treatment of anorexia nervosa: a self-psychological perspective. Contemporary Psychotherapy Review 2:268–288, 1984

Geist RA: Self-psychological reflections on the origins of eating disorders, in Psychoanalysis and Eating Disorders. Edited by Bemporad JR, Herzog DB. New York, Guilford, 1989, pp 5–27

Gilligan C: In a Different Voice: Psychological Theory and Women's Development. Cambridge, MA, Harvard University Press, 1982

Gold PW, Kaye W, Robertson GL, et al: Abnormalities in plasma and cerebrospinal-fluid arginine vasopressin in patients with anorexia nervosa. N Engl J Med 308:1117–1123, 1983

Golden NH, Kreitzer P, Jacobson MS, et al: Disturbances in growth hormone secretion and action in adolescents with anorexia nervosa. J Pediatr 125:655–660, 1994

Goodwin GM, Fairburn CG, Cowen PJ: Dieting changes serotonergic function in women, not men: implications for the aetiology of anorexia nervosa? Psychol Med 17:839–842, 1987

Gordon C, Beresin E, Herzog DB: The parent's relationship and the child's illness in anorexia nervosa. J Am Acad Psychoanal 17:29–42, 1989

Gottdiener JS, Gross HA, Henry WL, et al: Effects of self-induced starvation on cardiac size and function in anorexia nervosa. Circulation 58:426–433, 1978

Gowers S, Norton K, Halek C, et al: Outcome of outpatient psychotherapy in a random allocation treatment study of anorexia nervosa. Int J Eat Disord 15:165–177, 1994

Grice DE, Halmi KA, Fichter MM, et al: Evidence for a susceptibility gene for anorexia nervosa on chromosome 1. Am J Hum Genet 70:787–792, 2002

Grill HJ: Introduction: physiological mechanisms in conditioned taste aversions. Ann N Y Acad Sci 443:67–88, 1985

Grinspoon S, Baum H, Lee K, et al: Effects of short-term recombinant human insulin-like growth factor 1 administration on bone turnover in osteopenic women with anorexia nervosa. J Clin Endocrinol Metab 81:3864–3870, 1996

Grinspoon S, Thomas E, Pitts S, et al: Prevalence and predictive factors for regional osteopenia in women with anorexia nervosa. Ann Intern Med 133:790–794, 2000

Gwirtsman HE, Guze BH, Yager J, et al: Fluoxetine treatment of anorexia nervosa: an open clinical trial. J Clin Psychiatry 51:378–382, 1990

Halmi KA, Casper RC, Eckert ED, et al: Unique features associated with the age of onset of anorexia nervosa. Psychiatry Res 1:209–215, 1979

Halmi KA, Eckert E, LaDu TJ, et al: Anorexia nervosa: treatment efficacy of cyproheptadine and amitriptyline. Arch Gen Psychiatry 43:177–181, 1986

Hamburg P, Herzog DB, Brotman AW, et al: The treatment resistant eating disordered patient. Psychiatr Ann 19:494–499, 1989

Harper G: Varieties of parenting failure in anorexia nervosa: protection and parentectomy, revisited. J Am Acad Child Psychiatry 22:134–139, 1983

Herzog DB, Borus JF, Hamburg P, et al: Substance abuse, eating behaviors, and social impairment of medical students. J Med Educ 62:651–657, 1987a

Herzog DB, Hamburg P, Brotman AW: Psychotherapy and eating disorders: an affirmative view. Int J Eat Disord 6:545–550, 1987b

Herzog DB, Keller MB, Lavori PW: Outcome in anorexia nervosa and bulimia nervosa: a review of the literature. J Nerv Ment Dis 176:131–143, 1988

Herzog W, Deter HC, Fiehn W, et al: Medical findings and predictors of long-term physical outcome in anorexia nervosa: a prospective 12-year follow-up study. Psychol Med 27: 269–279, 1997

Herzog DB, Dorer DJ, Keel PK, et al: Recovery and relapse in anorexia and bulimia nervosa: a 7.5-year follow-up study. J Am Acad Child Adolesc Psychiatry 38:829–837, 1999

Herzog DB, Greenwood DN, Dorer DJ, et al: Mortality in eating disorders: a descriptive study. Int J Eat Disord 28:20–26, 2000

Hsu LK: Psychopharmacology in anorexia nervosa. Symposium presented at the annual meeting of the American Psychiatric Association, Miami, FL, May 1995

Hudson JI, Pope HG, Jonas JM, et al: Family history study of anorexia nervosa and bulimia. Br J Psychiatry 142:428–429, 1983

Hudson JI, Pope HG, Jonas JM: Psychosis in anorexia nervosa and bulimia. Br J Psychiatry 145:420–423, 1984

Humphrey LL: Observed family interactions among subtypes of eating disorders using structural analysis of social behavior. J Consult Clin Psychol 57:206–214, 1989

Ivarsson T, Rastam M, Wentz E, et al: Depressive disorders in teenage-onset anorexia nervosa: a controlled longitudinal partly community-based study. Compr Psychiatry 41:398–403, 2000

Jagielska G, Wolanczyk T, Komender J, et al: Bone mineral content and bone mineral density in adolescent girls with anorexia nervosa: a longitudinal study. Acta Psychiatr Scand 104:131–137, 2001

Karwautz A, Rabe-Hesketh S, Hu X, et al: Individual-specific risk factors for anorexia nervosa: a pilot study using a discordant sister-pair design. Psychol Med 31:317–329, 2001

Katzman DK, Lambe EK, Mikulis DJ, et al: Cerebral gray matter and white matter volume deficits in adolescent girls with anorexia nervosa. J Pediatr 129:794–803, 1996

Kaye WH: Anorexia nervosa, obsessional behavior, and serotonin. Psychopharmacol Bull. 33:335–344, 1997

Kaye WH, Weltzin TE, Hsu LK, et al: An open trial of fluoxetine in patients with anorexia nervosa. J Clin Psychiatry 52:464–471, 1991

Kaye WH, Nagata T, Weltzin TE, et al: Double-blind placebo-controlled administration of fluoxetine in restricting- and restricting-purging-type anorexia nervosa. Biol Psychiatry 49:644–652, 2001

Kernberg O: Borderline Conditions and Pathological Narcissism. Northvale, NJ, Jason Aronson, 1975

Klump KL, Miller K, Keel PK, et al: Genetic and environmental influences on anorexia nervosa syndromes in a population-based twin sample. Psychol Med 31:737–740, 2001

Lambe EK, Katzman DK, Mikulis DJ, et al: Cerebral gray matter volume deficits after weight recovery from anorexia nervosa. Arch Gen Psychiatry 54:537–542, 1997

Lillenfeld LR, Kaye WH, Greeno CG, et al: A controlled family study of anorexia nervosa and bulimia nervosa: psychiatric disorders in first-degree relatives and effects of proband comorbidity. Arch Gen Psychiatry 55:603–610, 1998

Locke J, Le Grange D, Agras WS, Dare C: Treatment Manual for Anorexia Nervosa: A Family-Based Approach. New York, Guilford, 2001

Lowe B, Zipfel S, Buchholz C, et al: Long-term outcome of anorexia nervosa in a prospective 21-year follow-up study. Psychol Med 31:881–890, 2001

Lucas AR, Beard CM, O'Fallon WM, et al: Anorexia nervosa in Rochester, Minnesota: a 45-year study. Mayo Clin Proc 63:433–442, 1988

Maloney M, Klykylo WM: An overview of anorexia nervosa, bulimia, and obesity in children and adolescents. J Am Acad Child Psychiatry 22:99–107, 1983

Maloney M, McGuire J, Daniels SR, et al: Dieting behavior and eating attitudes in children. Pediatrics 84:482–489, 1989

Minuchin S: Family Kaleidoscope. Cambridge, MA, Harvard University Press, 1984

Minuchin S, Rosman BL, Baker L: Psychosomatic Families: Anorexia Nervosa in Context. Cambridge, MA, Harvard University Press, 1978

Mitchell JE: Medical complications of anorexia nervosa and bulimia. Psychiatr Med 1:229–255, 1983

Norman DK, Herzog DB: Bulimia, anorexia nervosa, and anorexia nervosa with bulimia: a comparative analysis of MMPI profiles. Int J Eat Disord 2:43–52, 1983

Palla B, Litt IF: Medical complications of eating disorders in adolescents. Pediatrics 81:613–623, 1988

Peterson CB, Mitchell JE: Psychosocial and pharmacological treatment of eating disorders: a review of research findings. J Clin Psychol 55:685–97, 1999

Piazza E, Carni JD, Kelly J, et al: Group psychotherapy for anorexia nervosa. J Am Acad Child Psychiatry 22:276–278, 1983

Piran N, Kaplan AS (eds): A Day Hospital Group Treatment Program for Anorexia Nervosa and Bulimia Nervosa (Eating Disorders Monogr Ser No 3). New York, Brunner/Mazel, 1989

Pumariega AJ, Pursell J, Spock A, et al: Eating disorders in adolescents with cystic fibrosis. J Am Acad Child Psychiatry 25:269–275, 1986

Rodin G, Daneman D, Johnston L, et al: Anorexia nervosa and bulimia in insulin-dependent diabetes mellitus. Int J Psychiatry Med 16:46–57, 1986

Rogers L, Resnick MD, Mitchell JE, et al: The relationship between socioeconomic status and eating-disordered behaviors in a community sample of adolescent girls. Int J Eat Disord 22:15–23, 1997

Rollins N, Piazza E: Anorexia nervosa: a quantitative approach to follow-up. J Am Acad Child Adolesc Psychiatry 20:167–183, 1981

Romans SE, Gendall KA, Martin JL, et al: Child sexual abuse and later disordered eating: a New Zealand epidemiological study. Int J Eat Disord 29:380–392, 2001

Russell GFM: Anorexia and bulimia nervosa, in Child and Adolescent Psychiatry: Modern Approaches. Edited by Rutter M, Hersor L. Oxford, UK, Blackwell Scientific, 1985, pp 625–637

Schuckit MA, Tipp JE, Anthenelli RM, et al: Anorexia nervosa and bulimia nervosa in alcohol-dependent men and women and their relatives. Am J Psychiatry 153:74–82, 1996

Schwartz R, Barrett MJ, Saba G: Family therapy for bulimia, in Handbook of Psychotherapy for Anorexia Nervosa and Bulimia. Edited by Garner DM, Garfinkel PE. New York, Guilford, 1985, pp 280–307

Selvini-Palazzoli M: Self-Starvation: From Individual to Family Therapy in the Treatment of Anorexia Nervosa. Northvale, NJ, Jason Aronson, 1978

Smith C, Feldman S, Nasserbakht A, et al: Psychological characteristics and DSM-III-R diagnoses at 6-year follow-up of adolescent anorexia nervosa. J Am Acad Child Adolesc Psychiatry 32:1237–1245, 1993

Soyka LA, Grinspoon S, Levitsky LL, et al: The effects of anorexia nervosa on bone metabolism in female adolescents. J Clin Endocrinol Metab 84:4489–4496, 1999

Stevenson K: Guidelines for peer review of child and adolescent psychiatric treatment including substance abuse disorder and eating disorders, in Child and Adolescent Psychiatric Illness: Guidelines for Treatment Resources, Quality Assurance, Peer Review and Reimbursement. Edited by DuPrat MM, Stevenson K. Washington, DC, American Academy of Child and Adolescent Psychiatry, 1989, pp 29–72

Stoving RK, Hangaard J, Hansen-Nord M, et al: A review of endocrine changes in anorexia nervosa. J Psychiatr Res 33:139–152, 1999

Striegel-Moore RH, Leslie D, Petrill SA, et al: One-year use and cost of inpatient and outpatient services among female and male patients with an eating disorder: evidence from a national database of health insurance claims. Int J Eat Disord 27:381–389, 2000

Strober M: Personality and symptomatological features in young, nonchronic anorexia nervosa patients. J Psychosom Res 24:353–359, 1980

Strober M: Family genetic perspectives on anorexia nervosa and bulimia nervosa, in Eating Disorders and Obesity: A Comprehensive Handbook. Edited by Brownell KD, Fairburn CG. New York, Guilford, 1995, pp 212–218

Strober M, Lampert C, Morrell W, et al: A controlled family study of anorexia nervosa: evidence of familial aggregation and lack of shared transmission with affective disorders. Int J Eat Disord 9:239–253, 1990

Strober M, Freeman R, Morrell W: The long-term course of severe anorexia nervosa in adolescents: survival analysis of recovery relapse and outcome predictors over 10–15 years in a prospective study. Int J Eat Disord 22:339–360, 1997

Strober M, Pataki C, Freeman R, et al: No effect if adjunctive fluoxetine on eating behavior or weight phobia during the inpatient treatment of anorexia nervosa: an historical case-control study. J Child Adolesc Psychopharmacol 9:195–201, 1999

Sunday SR, Einhorn A, Halmi KA: Relationship of perceived macronutrient and caloric content to affective conditions about food in eating-disordered, restrained, and unrestrained subjects. Am J Clin Nutr 55:362–371, 1992

Swift WJ: The long-term outcome of early onset anorexia nervosa. J Am Acad Child Adolesc Psychiatry 21:38–46, 1982

Szmukler GI: Anorexia nervosa and bulimia in diabetics. J Psychosom Res 28:365–369, 1984

Wade TD, Bulik CM, Neale M, et al: Anorexia nervosa and major depression: an examination of shared genetic and environmental risk factors. Am J Psychiatry 157:469–471, 2000

Walters E, Kendler K: Anorexia nervosa and anorexic-like syndromes in a population-based female twin sample. Am J Psychiatry 152:64–71, 1995

Wilson GT, Fairburn CG: Cognitive treatments for eating disorders. J Consult Clin Psychol 61:261–269, 1993

Winokur A, March V, Mendels J: Primary affective disorder in relatives of patients with anorexia nervosa. Am J Psychiatry 137:695–698, 1980

Wonderlich SA, Brewerton TD, Jocic Z, et al: Relationship of childhood sexual abuse and eating disorders. J Am Acad Child Adolesc Psychiatry 36:1107–1115, 1997

Bulimia Nervosa

David Szydlo, M.D., Ph.D.

Joseph L. Woolston, M.D.

Bulimia (from the Greek *bous*, meaning "ox," plus *limos*, meaning "hunger") is defined as an abnormal increase in the sense of hunger. Also known as "ravenous appetite," it has been associated with a variety of nosological entities and has been described as behaviors that indicate pathological processes or personality traits. The term *la boulimie* appeared in French literature during the eighteenth century. Bulimia was recognized as a distinct illness in 1979, when Professor Gerald Russell in England officially named it bulimia nervosa. As a *symptom* it has been related to 1) an expected consequence of starvation, 2) a result of cultural attitudes toward food (e.g., the Roman vomitoriums), 3) a condition associated with brain disease, and 4) a trait associated with a major psychiatric syndrome.

Bulimia as a *syndrome* has been included as a diagnosis only since DSM-III (American Psychiatric Association 1980). The earliest mention of bulimia in the ICD (*International Classification of Diseases and Causes of Death*) was in its fourth revision (1938), listed under "other diseases of the nervous system." Given that bulimia nervosa is often a sequel of anorexia nervosa, it is of interest that the term *anorexia, hysterical* was first mentioned in the first revision of the ICD (1902) as "other diseases of the nervous system." Although the first recorded report of the disorder dates back 2,500 years, and there are many historical as well as anecdotic accounts of women with sporadic outbreaks of bingeing and vomiting (Ziolko 1996), bulimia nervosa was defined as a distinct syndrome in 1979 by Russell (Russell 1979).

A problem that in the nineteenth century was present mostly in women of the Western bourgeoisie has now clearly permeated all social classes in both developed and developing countries to such an extent that it is common to find women who report having binged and purged throughout most of their life to control their weight, as well as children who worry about being or becoming fat and who have begun to engage in restricting food intake.

Prevalence and Epidemiology

Eating disorders are serious, sometimes life-threatening conditions that tend to be chronic (Herzog et al. 1999). About 3% of young women have one of the three main eating disorders: anorexia nervosa, bulimia nervosa, or binge-eating disorder (Becker et al. 1999). Johnson et al. (1999) found, in a prevalence study of 1,445 student athletes, that 1.1% of females and 0.01% of males met the criteria for bulimia nervosa; clinically significant problems were identified in 9.2% of the females and 0.01% of the males. Timmerman et al. (1990) found the prevalence to be 2% in high school women and 0% in men. Kaltiala-Heino et al. (1999), in a Scandinavian study of 4,453 girls between ages 14 and 16 years and 4,334 boys of the same age, found the prevalence to be 1.8% for the females and 0.3% for the males. They concluded that bulimia and bulimic eating behavior appear to be more common than was previously thought in middle adolescence. Studies in England (Fairburn et al. 1991) and Canada (Garfinkel et al. 1995) indicated an incidence of less than 2% on the basis of DSM-III-R (American Psychiatric Association 1987) criteria. Whitaker (1990) found a 4% incidence of bulimia nervosa, based on DSM-III-R criteria, in U.S. female adolescents. Killen (1995) found that 5% (40) of 800 sixth- and seventh-grade U.S. children were already restricting intake, bingeing, and purging. Studies from Spain, Japan, Switzerland, and Iran found the prevalence of the disorder in those countries to be either slightly higher or slightly lower than in other Western countries. These differences might be due to real variations in the prevalence rate in these countries, to differences in the referral system, or to variables in the threshold filters used by the systems of care. Other studies that examine both the prevalence of bulimia nervosa in relatives of probands and the probandwise specificity for familial clustering have found the rates for the disorder to be between 3.3% and 4.3%, as opposed to the rate for anorexia nervosa, which is 20.5% (Strober et al. 2001; Woodside et al. 1998). In a study of twins, Kendler et al. (1991) reported a prevalence of 2.8%. Similar prevalence rates were found in selected minority populations such as British Asians (Hill and Bhatti 1995; Hill et al. 1992; Ratan et al. 1998) and Mexican Americans (Lester et al. 1998). Other groups studied the armed forces and sorority women. For example, a study of college women found the incidence of bulimia nervosa to be 4% (Drewnowski et al. 1988).

This rapid growth in the incidence and prevalence of bulimia, primarily but not exclusively in westernized countries, is attributed to the influence and interchange that occurs between countries through television, advertising, cinema, and the Internet; the globalization process has reached virtually every corner of the planet. Female ideals of beauty and thinness are consistently reinforced through all these media. In Latin America, Asia, and the Middle East, as in the United States, strict diet regimens and the use of laxatives and purging methods are in vogue, and eating disorders and their complications are becoming important public health issues (Goleman 1995; Szydlo 2000). Some of the emblematic distinctiveness of bulimia has also changed with time: Although the classic description of patients with the disorder included female sex, high socioeconomic status, and youth, the population affected by this condition is slowly expanding. For example, even if the incidence in women is still higher than in men (0.1%–0.5% for males, which is 10–11 times less common than in females) (Shotte and Stunkard 1987), the assertion that males rarely develop bulimia nervosa no longer holds true. A recent study (Strober et al. 2001) suggested that there is no evidence that familial genetic factors distinguish the occurrence of eating disorders in the two sexes; another study (Olivardia et al. 1995) found similar features in patients of both sexes. An interesting study by Powell and Kahn (1995) analyzed racial differences in women's desires to be thin and found data suggesting that black women are still under less pressure to be thin than white women are.

Subjects for studies of bulimia nervosa usually consist of those individuals who are given a diagnosis of bulimia nervosa (on the basis of a multitude of study-specific diagnostic criteria). There is, however, another group that does not come to the attention of researchers, health care professionals, or mental health care providers but that is nevertheless dieting, often with very low calorie intakes, excessive exercising, or occasional bingeing and purging (Button and Whitehouse 1981). Some of these bulimic patients often avail themselves of health care services for a variety of other complaints, remaining silent about their eating patterns or being treated only for symptoms related to them. Still, it is important to note that bulimic patients tend to seek help and are more willing to talk about their symptoms, feelings, and struggles, than are anorexic patients. Because psychiatric comorbidity is often present (Albert et al. 2001; Ghadirian et al. 1999), bulimia nervosa is frequently diagnosed during routine mental health examinations. Also, patients with anorexia nervosa habitually progress to bulimia nervosa. Studies report that 15% of bulimic patients were previously treated for anorexia nervosa and that 30%–50% of bulimic patients would have met criteria for anorexia nervosa at the onset of their disorder (Fairburn and Cooper 1981; Pyle et al. 1981; Turnbull et al. 1989).

Definition and Diagnostic Criteria

Table 36–1 lists the DSM-IV-TR (American Psychiatric Association 2000) diagnostic criteria for bulimia nervosa. In this definition, there is an attempt to clarify three subjective elements: 1) amount of food consumed ("definitely larger than most individuals would eat…under similar circumstances"), 2) the time span during which the food is ingested (usually less than 2 hours), and 3) "lack of control" during the binge. These subjective definitions match many patients' accounts, which generally stress control difficulties, a compulsion to eat very fast, and variability in calorie consumption, from several hundred to thousands of calories (Rosen et al. 1986; Rossiter and Agras 1990).

The ICD-10 (*International Classification of Diseases and Related Health Problems*, 10th Revision; World

Table 36–1. DSM-IV-TR diagnostic criteria for bulimia nervosa

A. Recurrent episodes of binge eating. An episode of binge eating is characterized by both of the following:

   (1) eating, in a discrete period of time (e.g., within any 2-hour period), an amount of food that is definitely larger than most people would eat during a similar period of time and under similar circumstances

   (2) a sense of lack of control over eating during the episode (e.g., a feeling that one cannot stop eating or control what or how much one is eating)

B. Recurrent inappropriate compensatory behavior in order to prevent weight gain, such as self-induced vomiting; misuse of laxatives, diuretics, enemas, or other medications; fasting; or excessive exercise.

C. The binge eating and inappropriate compensatory behaviors both occur, on average, at least twice a week for 3 months.

D. Self-evaluation is unduly influenced by body shape and weight.

E. The disturbance does not occur exclusively during episodes of anorexia nervosa.

  Specify type:

    Purging Type: during the current episode of bulimia nervosa, the person has regularly engaged in self-induced vomiting or the misuse of laxatives, diuretics, or enemas

    Nonpurging Type: during the current episode of bulimia nervosa, the person has used other inappropriate compensatory behaviors, such as fasting or excessive exercise, but has not regularly engaged in self-induced vomiting or the misuse of laxatives, diuretics, or enemas

Source. Reprinted from American Psychiatric Association: *Diagnostic and Statistical Manual of Mental Disorders*, 4th Edition, Text Revision. Washington, DC, American Psychiatric Association, 2000. Copyright 2000 American Psychiatric Association. Used with permission.

Health Organization 1992), used more in European countries than in the United States, defines bulimia nervosa as a syndrome characterized by repeated bouts of overeating and an excessive preoccupation with the control of body weight, leading the patient to adopt extreme measures so as to mitigate the "fattening" effects of ingested food. The term should be restricted to the form of the disorder that is related to anorexia nervosa by virtue of sharing the same psychopathology. The age and sex distribution is similar to that of anorexia nervosa, but the age of presentation tends to be slightly later. The disorder may be viewed as a sequel to persistent anorexia nervosa (although the reverse sequence may also occur). A previously anorexic patient may first appear to improve as a result of weight gain and possibly a return of menstruation, but a pernicious pattern of overeating and vomiting then becomes established. Repeated vomiting is likely to give rise to disturbances of body electrolytes, physical complications (tetany, epileptic seizures, cardiac arrhythmias, muscular weakness), and further severe loss of weight.

For a definite diagnosis under the ICD-10 classification, all the following are required:

- A persistent preoccupation with eating and an irresistible craving for food; the patient succumbs to episodes of overeating in which large amounts of food are consumed in short periods of time.

- Attempts to counteract the "fattening" effects of food by one or more of the following: self-induced vomiting; purgative abuse, alternating with periods of starvation; use of drugs such as appetite suppressants, thyroid preparations, or diuretics. When bulimia occurs in diabetic patients, they may choose to neglect their insulin treatment.

- Psychopathology consisting of a morbid dread of fatness and setting of a sharply defined weight threshold, well below the premorbid weight that constitutes the optimum or healthy weight in the opinion of the physician. There is often, but not always, a history of an earlier episode of anorexia nervosa, the interval between the two disorders ranging from a few months to several years. This earlier episode may have been fully expressed or may have assumed a minor cryptic form with a moderate weight loss and/or a transient phase of amenorrhea.

Both diagnostic definitions (DSM-IV-TR and ICD-10) seem to indicate that there is a link between anorexia nervosa and bulimia nervosa, a continuum that characterizes either a progression or a mutually interrelated entity. That is why some authors consider these categories more arbitrary than actual (Abraham and Beaumont 1982; Casper et al. 1980). In DSM-IV-TR, for example, the subtypes for bulimia nervosa are similar to those for anorexia nervosa, which is subdivided into restricting and binge-eating/purging types. Therefore, a diagnostic problem may be encountered with lower-weight bulimic patients when we try to classify them as having anorexia nervosa, binge-eating/purging type, or bulimia nervosa, purging type. Some authors (Barber 1997) have suggested that it would be helpful to have a standard, such as body mass index (kg/m^2), to distinguish between these groups. Another important consideration in describing the diagnostic complications is that a number of patients present with characteristics of a new syndrome, binge-eating disorder. These patients can be confused with bulimic patients (nonpurging type), and they typically have no history of anorexia nervosa and no indication of significant psychopathology.

Etiology

There is no one single etiological explanation of bulimia nervosa. A combination of biopsychosocial factors is probably the most plausible explanation for the genesis and the maintenance of this eating disorder. From the pathogenic perspective, it is likely that a variety of triggering factors impinge on a predisposed foundation. Nature and nurture—in the form of preoccupation with weight and body shape, justified dieting, physical stressors, and/or dysfunctional family interactions—prompt genetics, biology, and psychological processes to begin the disorder that we call bulimia nervosa.

■ Biological Hypothesis

There are many studies that have supported a genetic load in patients with eating disorders in general, and with bulimia nervosa in particular. Klump et al. (2001) reviewed family, twin, and molecular genetics studies; their findings suggested a substantial genetic influence in both anorexia nervosa and bulimia nervosa. Kortegaard et al. (2001) found, in a study of 34,142 twins, that the concordance rates between monozygotic and dyzygotic pairs for self-reported eating disorders differed significantly from those in the general population. Bulik et al. (2000) concluded, in an interesting review, that although it was not possible to draw firm conclusions regarding the precise contributions of genetic and environmental factors for anorexia nervosa, twin studies confirmed a familial contribution of additive genetic effects and of unique environmental factors in bulimia nervosa. Another fascinating study (Sullivan et al. 1998) sought to define the relationship of bingeing and induced vomiting from a genetic perspective. The investigators concluded that these two

symptoms are complex traits resulting from multiple gene interactions and environmental influences, but they suggested that genetic influences might be particularly relevant to the etiology of bingeing and vomiting. Nevertheless, Fairburn et al. (1999) concluded that findings from twin studies are inconsistent and difficult to interpret; they suggested that it is best to keep a broad view regarding the etiology of these disorders, looking not only at environmental mechanisms but also at gene–environment interactions and genetic studies.

Many researchers have concentrated their efforts on the control mechanisms of appetite, with studies attempting to define how hormonal secretion is regulated. In the 1990s, animal studies covered almost every area of biological interest. Neurotransmitters (norepinephrine, serotonin, and dopamine), neuropeptides (cholecystokinase, opioids, neuropeptide Y, peptide YY, and hypocretin/orexin), and hormones (cortisol and insulin) were linked to appetite, satiety, food selection, meal size, meal frequency, rate and duration of eating, intermeal intervals, total caloric intake, and body weight (Mitchell and deZwaan 1993; Willie et al. 2001). Neuropeptide Y and peptide YY, which had been linked to the stimulation of eating behavior in laboratory animals, have been shown to have elevated levels in patients with bulimia (Kaye et al. 1990). Cholecystokinin, a hormone that has been shown to have low levels in some women with bulimia, causes laboratory animals to feel full and stop eating (Covasa et al. 2001). Plasma leptin concentration is significantly higher in bulimic patients than it is in those with anorexia nervosa but tends to be lower than normal in healthy control subjects (Kaye et al. 2000). Further research is needed to clarify whether these findings are primarily a cause or a consequence of the eating disorder. Because the concentration of these chemicals is similar in patients with depression, some authors have tried to link both conditions. Future researchers will need to address this question as well.

Certain physical ailments have been thought of as predisposing factors for the development of eating disorders. Patients with insulin-dependent diabetes mellitus, for example, have been considered at high risk for developing bulimia (Peveler 1995).

Clinicians and researchers across the United States have linked eating disorders with substance use and abuse. Biological, genetic, psychological, and social theories have been offered as explanations for the association between these conditions on the basis of their multilevel similarities. Many treatment programs are organized around the hypothesis that both syndromes—bingeing (and, for some, purging) and substance abuse—are the result of addictive behaviors or unsuccessful attempts to diminish anxiety. Other theories are based on the fact that some medications seem to be effective in the treatment of both alcohol abuse and bulimia nervosa. For example, narcotic blockers are now being used to treat narcotic abuse, alcohol abuse, and bulimia (Jonas and Gold 1988).

■ Psychological and Family Hypothesis

Many anecdotal accounts as well as some research studies reveal a huge variety in premorbid psychological functioning of bulimic patients. What seems clear from all of them is the undeniable impingement of the developmental process's characteristics in the genesis of the condition. Personality traits, family dysfunctionality, psychological trauma, physical and sexual abuse, self-starvation side effects, and media influence have all been partially linked to the genesis or the maintenance of bulimia.

Psychoanalytic researchers have long explored the possible symbolic meaning of eating disorder symptoms. They have also investigated a number of theories about the genesis of the disorders. Most theories have centered on anorexia nervosa, yet many of the conjectures are equally applicable to bulimic patients. Disturbances in the early mother–child interactive dyad have been linked to a variety of later psychological problems. Attachment and separation predicaments, inability or incomplete ability to decode external and internal stimuli effectively, and internalization aberrations are more contemporary explanations of the genesis of the old triad of 1) disturbance in body image, 2) cognitive and perceptive misinterpretations of stimuli, and 3) lack of control and impulsivity.

Fassino et al. (2001) designed a study to see how anger, temperament, and character profiles would differ across different eating disorders and in comparison with healthy control subjects. The researchers found greater levels of anger in patients with bulimia nervosa than in those with anorexia nervosa. They also found different personality profiles and differences in the expression of anger, eating attitudes, and personality dimensions for these groups. Borderline personality disorders have been found in patients with bulimia nervosa, but other Cluster B personality disorders (antisocial, histrionic, and narcissistic) are common as

well (Wonderlich et al. 1994). Evidence also suggests that even though heterogeneous personality structures are found in patients with eating disorders, they probably have no special etiological role (Herzog et al. 1992).

The etiological participation of self-representation and self-perception has also been the object of research. Given that many women are concerned about their body weight and contours, some studies have relied heavily on self-valuation, as this appears to be even a greater concern in patients with diagnosable eating disorders (Garner et al. 1992). The American Association of University Women (1991) study, which described girls' loss of self-worth and competence, showed that for most girls, certain aspects of their appearance is what matters most. As Orenstein (1994) reported, many girls still adopt traditional roles that reflect their low self-image and self-doubt, diminishing their creative and intellectual potential and their chances for professional success.

Family environment has traditionally been seen as central in the etiology of eating disorders. Inconsistencies in the study results, however, have hindered the advances regarding this dynamic. Among the factors believed to influence bulimia, eating disorders in family members, mood disorders, obesity, sexual abuse, diabetes mellitus, and drug abuse (Marcus 1995; Peveler 1995) are the most relevant. Offner (1997) explored the discrepancies between theory and research evidence. Her findings summarize the current conclusions of family environment research and are consistent with accounts from family practitioners and clinicians. Eating-disordered families are less cohesive, less emotionally expressive, more conflictual, less independent, and more achievement-oriented than nondisordered families. A word of caution is important here: Given that controlled studies are very difficult to conduct within a family setting, causality should not be assumed. The fact that family dysfunction and eating disorders are linked has been established; however, more research is needed to define the nature of this association.

Barnett (1997) confirmed, in a 5-year follow-up study, the importance of the following risk factors in the etiology of eating disorders (especially bulimia nervosa): 1) overinternalization of the value that a culture places on thinness in women, 2) inordinate dissatisfaction with body form, 3) depression, and 4) irrational beliefs and cognitions about thinness and the benefits of dieting.

A history of sexual abuse has been reported as an etiological factor in bulimia nervosa (Connors and Morse 1993; Kearney-Cooke and Striegel-Moore 1994; Waller 1992). Folsom et al. (1993) and Smolak et al. (1990) investigated the relationship between sexual and physical abuse and psychiatric symptoms; Deep (1999) studied the comorbidity of sexual abuse with substance abuse; and Welch and Fairburn (1994) studied the link between sexual abuse and a higher incidence of smoking and other psychological markers of distress. On the basis of the findings of these studies, one could speculate that sexually abusive experiences may relate to the development of psychological stress, which can, in vulnerable people, induce the development of eating disorders, but the question remains as to how specific this factor is and how direct its influence on the etiology of eating disorders is.

Clinical Description

Bulimia nervosa frequently occurs in people with a history of anorexia nervosa. Both male and female patients express general dissatisfaction and unhappiness, which tends to be displaced and expressed in concerns related to body form, size, shape, and weight. Restrictive dieting is initiated very often in early adolescence, usually—for females—after onset of menarche. Efforts at restricting calories and increasing exercise, which begin as attempts to deal with self-dissatisfaction, produce semistarvation states. Patients eat fewer than 1,000 calories per day and avoid all foods they believe to be fattening. After some time, patients become vulnerable and capitulate to their feeling of hunger and their thoughts of food. As these intensify, they secretly begin to snack and very soon they engage in high-calorie bingeing episodes. Bingeing has been described as the outcome of a conflict when the cultural demand to diet meets the internal biological systems responsible for regulation of body weight (Barber 1997). Purging and vomiting appears to be both a guilty reaction to having gorged and a compensatory technique to prevent further weight gain. There are also some cases reported in which the binge/purge behavior begins de novo. This seems to happen mostly in normal-weight patients who use it as a way to control their weight. Overeating is sporadic and is usually followed by vomiting. This pattern may easily become a frequent occurrence, producing the same physical and metabolic complications that other purging patients have.

The condition may therefore range from very mild, with a nonsignificant weight change and little metabolic compromise, to purging after each bingeing episode, every day or several times a day, with severe consequences affecting basically all biological systems.

■ Physical Examination Findings

Bulimic patients have a characteristic appearance. The face is usually round, with swollen cheeks (chipmunk face) because of enlarged salivary glands (especially the parotids), testifying to a habit of frequent vomiting. Also, fluid retention, a common side effect of electrolytic disturbances, adds to the bloated facial appearance. Commonly, the body is, in contrast, relatively thin, and the patient looks generally unwell. Amenorrhea or irregular menses is seen in both low- and normal-weight patients, and sexual drive is also diminished in patients of both groups who are hypometabolic. During history taking, most patients will describe some or all of the following symptoms: bradycardia, shallow breathing (especially in low-weight patients or in those who vomit repeatedly), fatigability, hypotension, cold intolerance and difficulty regulating temperature, muscle pain, gastrointestinal dysfunction with epigastric fullness, a sensation of bloating, and abdominal pain. Polyuria is common and is usually accompanied by an urgent need to urinate and by amenorrhea or change in frequency, regularity, and quantity of menses. Some psychological symptoms that should be explored are sleep disorders, changes in libido and sexuality, dysphoria or depression, reduced attention and concentration, irritability, social withdrawal and isolation, and obsessive-compulsive symptoms (especially a relentless, unremitting preoccupation with weight, body shape, and food).

On examination, dental problems of various degrees are found, including enamel erosion and loss, gum recession, cavities, and sometimes actual tooth loss. The skin is often dry and cold and has reduced turgor due to dehydration and hypometabolism, and general body temperature is likely to be low. The skin may have cuts, scars, and abrasions, particularly over the knuckles (Russell's sign), an indication of self-gagging.

Hypotension, orthostatic hypotension, and bradycardia can be confirmed on physical examination. Abdominal fullness and bloating is also a common complaint, but it is rarely observed. On neurological examination, one can often find sluggish tendon reflexes, which is usually due to hypometabolism. The patient's weight, degree of starvation, and frequency of purging usually define the severity of physical symptoms.

A bleeding esophagus, a ruptured stomach, and ruptured esophagus are among the most serious complications of bulimia. Sore throats, ulcerated esophagi, and laryngeal tumors can also be found. Some bulimic patients still abuse ipecac to induce vomiting, which may cause cardiomyopathy, cardiac arrhythmias, and heart failure. Other complications include subconjunctival hemorrhages and kidney failure.

Mental status examination results vary from being within normal limits to cognitive problems (attention and concentration) and delirium. Lower-weight patients may be irritable, and all patients may be short-tempered, particularly when questioned about their diets, bingeing or purging, and vomiting. Dysphoria can become chronic, and there may be changes in the level of consciousness.

Many of these findings are probably secondary to dehydration, electrolyte abnormalities, and the general tendency in bulimic patients to be hypometabolic. As patients enter states of starvation and semistarvation, compensatory processes commence for adaptation and life preservation. Body weight does not always reflect the degree of malnutrition, and it is not atypical to see normal-weight bulimic individuals who are significantly hypometabolic. This probably happens as energy conservation becomes essential and is best accomplished by lowering the metabolic rate and exerting changes that protect the brain from the low-calorie state induced by the restricted intake—hence the electrolyte changes, the lowering of triiodothyronine levels, and the autonomic neuropathy (Calloway 1988). As insulin levels decline and glucose uptake is reduced in peripheral tissue so the brain can use it, fatty acids become the dominant energy source for muscles and the liver through increased lipolysis. The central nervous system also responds by altering the turnover and reuptake of neurotransmitters. Research on neurotransmitters is also discussed above, under "Biological Hypothesis."

■ Psychological Symptoms

Most bulimic patients are constantly preoccupied with weight, food, and body size and shape; they are usually dissatisfied and very unhappy. Most patients develop acute anxiety states that may become chronic and severe. It is the combination of the anxiety state and self-induced starvation, with the ensuing hunger, that is responsible for the bingeing episodes. Binge eating has been described as an escape from self-awareness, and its function as a blocking out of cognition and emotions (Heartherton and Baumeister 1991). However, many bulimic patients, especially in long-term treatment, can explore and describe the aggressive and sexual content of the fantasies that accompany their bingeing attacks and vomiting episodes (Szydlo 2000). The typical answer they give when asked about their emotions is "My mind is a blank," and yet many of them jump at the opportunity to address their self-destructive feelings and aggressive impulses directed toward themselves and others.

Bulimic patients frequently report being depressed. They feel disheartened, apparently because their attempts to control their bingeing and purging fail. However, as therapeutic exploration continues and their general dissatisfaction with themselves becomes apparent, they often feel enraged at what they see as their incapacity to have the perfect bodies that they want. Their lack of impulse control adds to their sense of guilt and their frustration intolerance. Therapeutic endeavors usually uncover manifestations of self-reproach and self-criticism for failing to have meaningful relationships and for having lives that the patients perceive as empty and lacking in goals. Therefore, it is typical that patients report low self-esteem and that they need others' opinions to enhance their self-worth. However, as time passes, they will tend to find in the outside world the same level of criticism that they direct at themselves, which is probably partly provoked by their own behaviors and partly the result of overpersonalization and misunderstanding of others' behavior or statements. As a result, patients may become socially withdrawn, isolation that for some becomes both a reinforcer of and a justification for the bulimic cycle.

As described above (see "Etiology"), psychological processes are an etiological component in the development of bulimia nervosa. Regardless of how effective premorbid coping skills are, they become insufficient as bulimic patients are overwhelmed by internal struggles and attempts to deal with anxiety. Patients then make extreme, desperate attempts to regain self-control: Emotional paralysis, somatization, and acting out become alternative ways of managing the internal and external pressure. Perfectionism, obsessive-compulsive symptoms, and erratic behavior are frequently seen, manifested through an inability to make decisions about life goals or by making inconsistent and self-damaging choices about the future. These difficulties, as we have said, serve a dual function in the patients' mind. On the one hand, they are seen as the result of the all-consuming preoccupation with body shape. On the other hand, they are the justifications for not having to make decisions of any kind, closing a vicious circle in which self-blame and defense feed each other.

Families of bulimic patients are often dysfunctional, and their dynamics repeatedly reveal excessive concern about weight and appearance in parents and siblings, mood disorders in first-degree relatives, and commonly, sexual and physical abuse (Schmidt et al. 1997; Welch and Fairburn 1994). Many studies have focused on identifying family factors that potentially contribute to the development of an eating disorder. Some have attempted to organize these characteristics into prototypes for the "anorexic family" or the "bulimic family." Although research has been unable to define a clear picture of family characteristics, certain traits have emerged as typical of the eating-disordered family. Some of those described include overpowering mothers; weak, absent, or ineffective fathers; a family tendency to somatize; and exaggerated expression of emotion, especially overt criticism and open hostility (Szydlo 1999).

Few studies approach the problem of alcohol and drug abuse as a covariable with eating disorders. Kendler (2000) reported in a recent study that women who have experienced childhood sexual abuse have a substantially increased risk for developing a wide range of psychopathology and psychiatric disorders in adulthood. Self-reported childhood sexual abuse was positively associated with all disorders, the highest correlations being with bulimia and with alcohol and other drug dependence. Welch and Fairburn (1998) showed, in another study, that bulimic patients smoked more than either matched healthy control subjects or women with other mental disorders. They also found that bulimics were more likely to resume smoking after a period of abstinence.

■ Laboratory Examination Findings

All the expected effects of malnutrition and hypometabolic states can be found in bulimic patients. However, none of them is specific to bulimia nervosa. Electrolyte and acid–base imbalance, which can lead to heart failure, is a frequent complication in patients who vomit or use laxatives or diuretics.

Anemia, a finding sometimes masked by volume depletion, is also common in this group. Volume decrease becomes the source of a number of observable complications. An increase in serum renin and aldosterone levels promotes renal loss of potassium. Hypokalemic and hypochloremic alkalosis is generated by the reduced chloride availability, which in turn increases bicarbonate and sodium resorption. Sodium retention may be severe enough to produce a rapid uncontrollable weight gain if purging is stopped abruptly. On top of the medical risks involved with this reaction, the psychological response would be enough to start the purging cycle again. Another complication of potassium depletion is cardiac arrhythmia. Premature ventricular contractions or elongations of the QT interval seen on electrocardiogram may identify individuals at risk.

Hypoproteinemia can lead to edema, which increases the sensation of bloating and raises the accumulation of fluid in the serous cavities. Magnesium and zinc levels have been reported to be borderline or low (Casper 1980). Magnesium depletion has been found to be related to cardiac and vascular diseases, diabetes, bone deterioration, renal failure, hypothyroidism, and stress, all of which are complications of bulimia too. One study (Peeters and Meijboom 2000) of 31 female patients in a community mental health center concluded that electrolyte abnormalities, hypomagnesemia, and hypoalbuminemia were not significant enough to justify routine performance of laboratory studies in ambulatory bulimic patients with normal weight. Amylase levels may be elevated in bulimic patients. A low basal metabolic rate is common, with thyroid function characterized by low levels of thyroid-stimulating hormone and triiodothyronine, the most powerful thyroid hormone, which affects almost every process in the body, including body temperature, growth, and heart rate.

Serotonin (5-hydroxytryptamine [5-HT]) studies have captured the interest of researchers for many years. The involvement of brain serotonin systems in the pathophysiology of eating disorders has been repeatedly demonstrated. Abnormal serotonergic regulation has also been linked to depressed mood and impulsivity. Jimerson et al. (1992) reported low levels of serotonin and dopamine precursors in cerebrospinal fluid, suggesting that this phenomenon explains the blunted satiety seen in binge eaters and their abnormal responses to food. Steiger et al. (2001) linked altered serotonin activity in the brain to bulimia nervosa and to increased propensity for parasuicidality and self-injury. They measured serum prolactin and cortisol levels after administration of a 5-HT agonist to assess serotonin functioning. Blunting of prolactin and cortisol responses was remarkable in women with a history of self-destructiveness. Jimerson (2000), also using serotonin-mediated prolactin responses to compare individuals whose bulimia nervosa had remitted and those with current bulimia, showed a state-related abnormality with a diminished serotonergic neuroendocrine response in patients with current bulimia.

Anorexic patients may develop low bone density, detectable by bone-density studies, in as short a time as 2 years. Bulimic patients suspected of having been anorexic or who have previously been given a diagnosis of anorexia nervosa should undergo dual-energy X-ray absorptiometry to determine bone density, particularly if they have been amenorrheic for longer than 6 months. Low-weight bulimic patients should also undergo absorptiometry after 2 symptomatic years. Because osteoporosis has been associated with amenorrhea, and because low bone density has been found to be related to a history of anorexia nervosa, prolonged amenorrhea, and persistent low body mass index (Newton et al. 1993), it used to be common practice to start hormone replacement therapy (HRT) 6 months to 1 year after cessation of menstruation. However, in the light of numerous studies that describe the risks of using HRT (Gambacciana et al. 2003; Gupta et al. 2002; Menon et al. 2003), this practice should be evaluated on an individual-case basis. In any case, hormone replacment–induced menses does not protect against osteoporosis; supplemental calcium, phosphorus, and vitamin D are essential for reducing the onset of osteoporosis in later life.

Determining the resting metabolic rate can be very helpful in understanding symptomatology in bulimic patients. Muscle wasting is common, especially in low-weight patients, in whom chest X rays may show reduced heart size.

Differential Diagnosis

All medical and psychiatric conditions that cause dysregulation of the eating cycles, produce weight loss, or are associated with chronic vomiting must be differentiated from bulimia nervosa. The following groups of disorders must be considered in making a differential diagnosis:

- *Upper gastrointestinal disorders:* Malabsorption syndromes, gastrointestinal ulcers, and enteritis have to be considered. Gastrointestinal disorders are especially important when they lead to repeated vomiting; however, the characteristic bulimic psychopathology is usually absent.
- *Neurological disorders:* Brain tumors' signs and symptoms (especially prolactin-secreting pituitary tumors and hypothalamic tumors) may resemble the physical symptoms of bulimia nervosa. On occasion, it is the tumor itself that may also be responsible for the psychiatric manifestations, which makes the diagnostic process more complex. Kleine-Levin syndrome and Klüver-Bucy syndrome have to be ruled out as well. Rare cases of total starvation and/or unstoppable appetites with weight gain have been seen in patients who have had mild strokes.
- *Hormonal disorders:* Any condition that produces malnutrition and hypometabolic states must be considered, as well as adrenal disease, diabetes mellitus, anterior pituitary dysfunction, and hyperparathyroidism. (For a report of successful surgical treatment of hyperparathyroidism, see Ozawa et al. [1999].) The fact that electrolyte imbalance, anemia, and skin changes are common medical complications of many hormonal conditions further clouds the clinical picture.
- *Major depressive disorder:* Bulimic patients frequently experience depressive symptoms, which may make difficult the distinction between major depressive disorder and bulimia, especially if the patient does not admit to vomiting or if there are no signs of the binge–purge dyad. When present, the bulimic symptoms of vomiting and bingeing and purging and the vegetative symptoms of major depression can help to distinguish the two disorders. The fact that patients with low self-esteem, self-criticism, and low satisfaction with weight, body shape, and body contour often have dysphoric mood but also develop eating disorders seems to indicates a connection between bulimia and major depressive disorder.
- *Personality abnormalities:* Bulimic patients are often found to have borderline personality disorder (and other personality disorders) as well.
- *Other eating disorders:* As stated earlier, anorexia ner-

vosa often progresses to bulimia nervosa; however, a differential diagnosis is necessary, given that restricting and binge-eating/purging subtypes for anorexia nervosa and purging and nonpurging subtypes for bulimia nervosa can be confused. Using the DSM-IV-TR diagnostic criteria and body mass index can make this differentiation easier. Another condition to be considered in the differential diagnosis is binge-eating disorder, purging type.

- *Comorbidity:* Eating disorders may coexist with alcohol and drug dependence, psychiatric illness such as schizophrenia, and sociopathic behaviors that range from minor offenses such as shoplifting to more destructive conduct such as aggressive, perverse, and violent interactions. (See "Etiology" and "Research Issues" for further discussion of comorbidity.)

Treatment

The treatment of bulimia nervosa has been explored in a variety of modalities that include pharmacological approaches; nutritional rehabilitation; psychoeducational interventions; various individual, group, and family psychological methods; and a combination of all of these with multidisciplinary teams.

Outpatient treatment is generally favored except in severe cases in which

- Complications such as hypokalemia, electrolyte imbalance, or dehydration are life-threatening (see discussions of complications under both "Laboratory Examination Findings" and "Differential Diagnosis"), especially if binge-eating and purging is out of control
- Stronger support is needed by the patient, family dysfunction is endangering the therapeutic process, or there is a risk of suicide or of a psychotic breakdown
- When outpatient treatment has failed, motivation is poor, or closer monitoring is required

Clinicians must tailor treatment strategies to each patient on the basis of specific characteristics, individual differences, family configuration, presence of comorbidity, and symptom presentation.

Research on the pharmacological treatment of bulimia nervosa has produced additional theories about and better understanding of the etiology of the disorder and the complexity of its treatment. Failure of satiety has been linked to neuroendocrine processes, placing serotonin—which is believed to be linked to satiety—at the center of complex studies since the 1990s. Accordingly, selective serotonin reuptake inhibitors (SSRIs) have been used in treating bulimia nervosa (Fluoxetine Bulimia Nervosa Collaborative Study Group 1992). A multitude of projects have been aimed at demonstrating the efficacy of using SSRIs to treat bulimia nervosa. Krueger and Kennedy (2000) found SSRIs effective in treating binge urges and binge-eating behavior. Mitchell et al. (2001) found the use of fluoxetine in combination with self-help manuals to be more effective, whereas Walsh et al. (2000) found fluoxetine effective in reducing the frequency of binge-eating and of purging behavior in patients who did not respond to psychotherapy. Barlow et al. (1988), the Fluoxetine Bulimia Nervosa Collaborative Study Group (1992), and Goldstein et al. (1999) reported the usefulness of treatment with fluoxetine regardless of whether there was comorbid depression. On the basis of the findings of SSRI studies, Kaye et al. (1998) challenged the theory that cultural environment causes the disorder, instead proposing the concept of a biological diathesis that places people at risk for developing bulimia nervosa.

Other antidepressants found to be effective in treating bulimia are tricyclics and monoamine oxidase (MAO) inhibitors. Bacaltchuk et al. (2000) reported no difference in efficacy using different classes of antidepressants.

However, not all researchers agree on the effectiveness of these compounds. In her study, Krueger and Kennedy (2000) indicated that more trials are needed to investigate the use of SSRIs for maintenance treatment and for the management of partial remissions. Earlier studies also showed that after an initial response to antidepressants, only a minority of patients were free of binge eating/purging at the end of treatment. As many as 70% showed an initial reduction of symptoms, but only 22% were reported to be symptom free after a medication-only treatment plan (Mitchell et al. 1989; Pyle et al. 1981). Placebo response reports have also varied; some claimed minimal differences in symptom reduction between medication and placebo groups, whereas others found significant differences between both groups (Alger et al. 1991; Bacaltchuk et al. 2000; Mitchell and Groat 1984).

In a review, Freeman (1998) found that there is enough evidence to support consideration of treating bulimic patients with such drugs as anticonvulsants (Knable 2001), amphetamines (methylphenidate), amphetamine-like compounds such as phentermine, fenfluramine and other appetite suppressants (Sokol et al. 1999), and lithium. Given that there has been a link between the reduction of anxiety in people who use opiates and alcohol and in those who binge-eat, opiate antagonists have also been used to treat bulimia nervosa. Opiate blockers (naloxone, naltrexone, nalmefene) have been used successfully for this disorder, although hepatotoxicity is a high risk because the dosage needed in bulimia nervosa is four to five times greater than that used in the treatment of opiate abuse or alcoholism (Alger et al. 1991; Jonas and Gold 1988).

Cognitive-behavioral therapy (CBT) was proven to be a very effective treatment in the early 1980s (Fairburn 1982). Since then, researchers have designed sophisticated trials to compare this psychotherapeutic modality with other approaches or to test their combined effectiveness. A number of component variations have been used to address two basic principles: 1) the self-monitoring of food intake and binge-eating episodes and 2) the identification of triggers for binge episodes. Some early designs of outcome studies were based on the inclusion of three or more meals per day, introduction of feared food into the meal plan, and identification and rectification of distorted cognitions about food, weight, and body contour (Rossiter et al. 1988). After a 19-session program, 40% of patients were symptom free, 44% (Agras et al. 1992) were somewhat improved, and 16% dropped out. Agras et al. (2000a), in a more recent multisite study on outcome predictors, compared dropouts with maintainers and found that dropouts had more severe bulimic cognition and greater impulsivity but could not identify clinically useful predictors. Those for whom treatment failed shared poor social adjustment and lower body mass index. Early progress in treatment was a good outcome predictor. Bulik et al. (1999) found that both frequency of bingeing and self-directedness were useful predictors of a good response to a brief course of CBT. In reporting another study (Bulik et al. 1998), the same researchers suggested that setting goals that address 1) abstinence from bingeing and restricting and 2) decreases in urges to binge in response to high-risk cues predicts a better outcome.

Interpersonal psychotherapy (Klerman et al. 1984), a short-term therapeutic modality that focuses on modifying current interpersonal problems, not only has been shown to be as effective as CBT in nor-mal-weight bulimic patients (Fairburn et al. 1991) but also has become a promising alternative to CBT (Fairburn 1998). Typically, issues about binge eating/purging are not addressed directly; instead, efforts are concentrated on interpersonal problem areas. In a recent study, Agras et al. (2000a) compared CBT with interpersonal psychotherapy and reported a statistical and clinical advantage of CBT over interpersonal psychotherapy.

Sequencing studies have been published in which treatment models are investigated to assess their efficacy. Nevonen et al. (1999) developed a model for group therapy that included CBT and interpersonal psychotherapy. At 1-year follow-up evaluation, clinical and self ratings showed sustained improvement and progress. Davis et al. (1999) investigated the value of psychoeducation and CBT. They found that the group that received psychoeducation and CBT had greater reductions in specific eating symptoms of bingeing and purging and significantly higher remission rates than did the group that received psychoeducation alone.

Dialectical behavioral therapy, an affect-regulation model used to teach emotion regulation skills, has also been claimed to be useful in the treatment of bulimic patients (Safer et al. 2001a, 2001b).

Psychodynamic therapy has not been found to be helpful, on its own, for younger patients with bulimia but has been used successfully with older patients and with patients of all ages in combination with family therapy, medication, and group therapy. Its main value resides in the fact that an enormous amount of published information exists describing individual treatment accounts, as well as addressing etiological, developmental, and gender issues and their concomitant psychodynamic explanations, thus shedding some light on the complexities of these patients, their families, and the progression of their symptoms. This therapeutic modality has been under increasing pressure to justify the time and cost that it involves.

Psychoeducation and psychoeducational therapy (Olmstead et al. 1991) have been suggested as a cost-effective group program for the treatment of patients with less severe bulimia. CBT is also effective for patients with mildly severe bulimia, and sit is equally beneficial over longer periods of time with more disturbed patients. Even though some consider cost-effectiveness the best feature of psychoeducation—because treatment duration is short yet the results approximate those of longer-term therapy—psychoeducational therapy has also found acceptance in multimodal treatment plans: If psychoeducational therapy alone does not prove satisfactory, interpersonal therapy or CBT, with or without medication, can be used. Other designs bring psychoeducation into the picture in conjunction with individual and family therapies (Szydlo 2000).

Family therapy has been part of the treatment armamentarium for all eating disorders for a very long time (K. Mitchell and Carr 2000). A classic study investigating the effects of family therapy versus individual therapy in bulimic patients (Russell et al. 1987) was replicated by Eisler et al. (1997). Family therapy was seen to be more effective with younger girls and in those with earlier disorder onset. Johnson et al. (1998) attempted to create more secure attachments in families with an emotionally focused family intervention using Bowlby's attachment theory principles. Offner (1997) looked into the relationship between family environment and outcome and reported, contrary to others' findings, that perceived family environment did not influence outcome and did not predict degree of recovery as assessed at a two-year follow-up evaluation.

Prognosis

Despite the increasingly immense body of research on bulimia nervosa, defining and predicting successful treatment, or treatment combinations, remains confusing, unclear, and at times, contradictory. Anecdotal accounts based on clinical experience suggest that late onset, a long duration of symptoms (bingeing and purging), a history of unsuccessful treatments, comorbid substance abuse, and the existence of Cluster B personality disorders predict a poor prognosis. Other predictors of a poor prognosis are family configurations with weaker or absent fathers and overpowering mothers; individual psychological symptoms such as feelings of inadequacy, overconcern about being liked, and inability to deal with and express negative feelings; and a previous history of anorexia nervosa. The presence of comorbid affective disorders has been linked to a higher rate of death and suicide. Herzog et al. (2000) reported a crude mortality rate of 5.1% with standardized mortality rates of 9.6 for death and 58.1 for suicide. Fatal outcome was correlated to longer duration of illness, binging and purging, comorbid sub-

stance abuse, and comorbid affective disorders. Predictors of a good outcome have been linked to combination strategies that include an educational component, a grouping or sequence of individual therapeutic modalities, family interventions, and sometimes psychopharmacotherapy.

Research Issues

Three areas characterize the research efforts in relation to bulimia nervosa: biology, psychology, and culture. Biological research attempts to better define three areas: 1) the etiology and physiopathology of the disease, 2) the genetic implications of the disease, and 3) pharmacological interventions. Psychological investigation is aimed at achieving a higher degree of understanding of personality development, psychopathogenesis, and effective treatment modalities. Research on cultural influences examines the effect that society has on today's children and adolescents, their values, and their expectations of themselves and others.

Being a multifaceted problem with complex interactions that derive from a variety of sources, bulimia nervosa poses a challenge to professionals from many disciplines. Researchers must not only address the specific questions pertinent to their area of expertise but also undertake the difficult task of conceptualizing the intricate and elaborate set of interactions that define this condition. Some have already begun this process. Serotonin research, for example, has reached the fascinating area of genetic studies. Nishiguchi et al. (2001) showed that binge-eating and/or purging behavior with comorbid borderline personality disorder is linked with increased frequency of a specific allele of the 5-HT receptor gene, suggesting its association with pathological features of both eating disorders and borderline personality disorders. Biology and psychology are also being linked. Carrasco et al. (2000), for example, compared platelet MAO activity (index of brain serotonin activity) and impulsive personality features in bulimic patients and in healthy control subjects. They found that platelet MAO activity was significantly lower in bulimic patients than in healthy control subjects and that the values for MAO activity were inversely and significantly correlated with scores on impulsivity scales and with the presence of borderline personality disorder characteristics. The authors also suggested that because platelet MAO activity has a genetic component, there is a need for studies to link low platelet MAO activity and higher risk for developing eating disorders.

The etiological, diagnostic, and therapeutic implications of these associations are far-reaching. The classification disagreements and inconsistencies that surround eating disorders will subside as adequate criteria are established for bulimia and its subsyndromes.

References

Abraham SF, Beaumont PJV: How patients describe bulimia or binge eating. Psychol Med 12:625–635, 1982

Agras WS, Rossiter EM, Arnow B, et al: Pharmacologic and cognitive behavioral treatment for bulimia nervosa: a controlled comparison. Am J Psychiatry 149:82–87, 1992

Agras WS, Crow SJ, Halmi KA, et al: Outcome predictors for the cognitive behavior treatment of bulimia nervosa: data from a multisite study. Am J Psychiatry 157:1302–1308, 2000a

Agras WS, Walsh T, Fairburn CG, et al: A multicenter comparison of cognitive-behavioral therapy and interpersonal psychotherapy for bulimia nervosa. Arch Gen Psychiatry 57:459–466, 2000b

Albert U, Venturello S, Maina G, et al: Bulimia nervosa with and without compulsive syndromes. Compr Psychiatry 42:456–460, 2001

Alger SA, Schwalbert MD, Bigaoutte JM, et al: Effects of a tricyclic antidepressant and opiate antagonist in normal weight bulimic and obese binge-eating subjects. Am J Clin Nutr 53:865–871, 1991

American Association of University Women: American Association of University Women Report: Short-Changing Girls, Short-Changing America. Washington, DC, American Association of University Women, 1991

American Psychiatric Association: Diagnostic and Statistical Manual of Mental Disorders, 3rd Edition. Washington, DC, American Psychiatric Association, 1980

American Psychiatric Association: Diagnostic and Statistical Manual of Mental Disorders, 3rd Edition, Revised. Washington, DC, American Psychiatric Association, 1987

American Psychiatric Association: Diagnostic and Statistical Manual of Mental Disorders, 4th Edition, Text Revision. Washington, DC, American Psychiatric Association, 2000

Bacaltchuk J, Hay P, Mari JJ: Antidepressants versus placebo for the treatment of bulimia nervosa: a systematic review. Aust N Z J Psychiatry 34:310–317, 2000

Barber JK: Bulimia nervosa, in Textbook of Child and Adolescent Psychiatry, 2nd Edition. Edited by Wiener JM. Washington, DC, American Psychiatric Press, 1997, pp 563–572

Barlow J, Blouin JH, Blouin AG, et al: Treatment of bulimia with desipramine: a double-blind crossover study. Can J Psychiatry 33:129–133, 1988

Barnett TE: Risk factors and bulimia outcomes in adolescent women: a longitudinal and retrospective analysis. Unpublished doctoral dissertation, Utah State University, 1996 [Dissertation Abstracts International: 57:9-B, 5905, 1997]

Becker AE, Grinspoon SK, Klibanski A, et al: Eating disorders. N Engl J Med 340:1092–1098, 1999

Bulik CM, Sullivan PF, Carter FA, et al: Predictors of one-year treatment outcome in bulimia nervosa. Compr Psychiatry 39:206–214, 1998

Bulik CM, Sullivan PF, Carter FA, et al: Predictors of rapid and sustained response to cognitive-behavioral therapy for bulimia nervosa. Int J Eat Disord 26:137–144, 1999

Bulik CM, Sullivan PF, Wade TD, et al: Twin studies of eating disorders: a review. Int J Eat Disord 27:2–20, 2000

Button EJ, Whitehouse A: Subclinical anorexia nervosa. Psychol Med 11:509–516, 1981

Calloway CW: Biologic adaptations to starvation and semi-starvation, in Obesity and Weight Control. Edited by Frankle RT, Yang M. Rockville, MD, Aspen, 1988

Carrasco JL, Diaz-Marsa M, Hollander E, et al: Decreased platelet monoamine oxidase activity in female bulimia nervosa. Eur Neuropsychopharmacol 10:113–117, 2000

Casper RC: An evaluation of trace minerals, vitamins, and taste function in anorexia nervosa. Am J Clin Nutr 33:1801–1808, 1980

Casper RC, Eckert ED, Halmi KA, et al: Bulimia: its incidence and clinical importance in patients with anorexia nervosa. Arch Gen Psychiatry 37:1030–1035, 1980

Connors ME, Morse W: Sexual abuse and eating disorders: a review. Int J Eat Disord 13:1–12, 1993

Covasa M, Marcuson JK, Ritter RC: Diminished satiation in rats exposed to elevated levels of endogenous or exogenous cholecystokinin. Am J Physiol Regul Integr Comp Physiol 280:331–337, 2001

Davis R, McVey G, Heinmaa M, et al: Sequencing of cognitive behavioral treatment for bulimia nervosa. Int J Eat Disord 25:361–374, 1999

Deep AL, Lilenfeld LR, Plotnicov KH, et al: Sexual abuse in eating disorder subtypes and control women: the role of comorbid substance dependence in bulimia nervosa. Int J Eat Disord 25:1–10, 1999

Drewnowski A, Hopkins SA, Kessler RC: The prevalence of bulimia nervosa in the U.S. college student population. Am J Public Health 78:1322–1325, 1988

Eisler I, Dare C, Russell GFM, et al: Family and individual therapy in anorexia nervosa: a 5-year follow-up. Arch Gen Psychiatry 54:1025–1030, 1997

Fairburn CG: A cognitive-behavioral approach to the management of bulimia. Psychol Med 11:707–711, 1982

Fairburn CG: Interpersonal psychotherapy for bulimia nervosa, in Interpersonal Psychotherapy. Edited by Markowitz JC. (Review of Psychiatry Series; Oldham JM and Riba MB, series eds.). Washington DC, American Psychiatric Press, 1998, pp 99–128

Fairburn CG, Cooper PJ: The clinical features of bulimia nervosa. Br J Psychiatry 144:238–246, 1981

Fairburn CG, Jones R, Peveler RC, et al: Three psychological treatments for bulimia nervosa: a comparative trial. Arch Gen Psychiatry 48:463–469, 1991

Fairburn CG, Cowen PJ, Harrison PJ: Twin studies and the etiology of eating disorders. Int J Eat Disord 26:349–358, 1999

Fassino S, Daga GA, Piero A, et al: Anger and personality in eating disorders. J Psychosom Res 51:757–764, 2001

Fluoxetine Bulimia Nervosa Collaborative Study Group: Fluoxetine in the treatment of bulimia nervosa: a multicenter, placebo-controlled, double-blind trial. Arch Gen Psychiatry 49:139–145, 1992

Folsom V, Krahn D, Nairn K, et al: The impact of sexual and physical abuse on eating disordered and psychiatric symptoms: a comparison of eating disordered and psychiatric inpatients. Int J Eat Disord 13:249–257, 1993

Freeman C: Drug treatment for bulimia nervosa. Neuropsychobiology 37:72–79, 1998

Gambacciani M, Monteleone P, Sacco A, et al: Hormone replacement therapy and endometrial, ovarian and colorectal cancer. Best Pract Res Clin Endocrinol Metab 17:139–147, 2003

Garfinkel PE, Lin E, Goering P, et al: Bulimia nervosa in a Canadian community sample: prevalence and comparison of subgroups. Am J Psychiatry 152:1052–1058, 1995

Garner DM, Garner MV, Van Egeren LF: Body dissatisfaction adjusted for weight: the body illusion index. Int J Eat Disord 12:263–271, 1992

Ghadirian AM, Marini N, Jabalpurwala S, et al: Seasonal mood patterns in eating disorders. Gen Hosp Psychiatry 21:354–359, 1999

Goleman D: Eating disorder rates surprise the experts. New York Times, October 4, 1995, p 31

Goldstein DJ, Wilson MC, Ascroft RC, et al: Effectiveness of fluoxetine therapy in bulimia nervosa regardless of comorbid depression. Int J Eat Disord 25:19–27, 1999

Gupta G, Aronow WS: Hormone replacement therapy: an analysis of efficacy based on evidence. Geriatrics 57(8):18–20, 23–24, 2002

Heartherton TF, Baumeister RF: Binge eating as an escape from self-awareness. Psychol Bull 110:86–108, 1991

Herzog DB, Keller MB, Lavori PW, et al: The prevalence of personality disorders in 210 women with eating disorders. J Clin Psychiatry 53:147–152, 1992

Herzog DB, Dorer DJ, Keel PK, et al: Recovery and relapse in anorexia and bulimia nervosa: a 7.5-year follow-up study. J Am Acad Child Adolesc Psychiatry 38:829–837, 1999

Herzog DB, Greenwood DN, Dorer DJ, et al: Mortality in eating disorders: a descriptive study. Int J Eat Disord 28:20–26, 2000

Hill AJ, Bhatti R: Body shape perception and dieting in preadolescent British Asian girls: links with eating disorders. Int J Eat Disord 17:175–183, 1995

Hill AJ, Oliver S, Rogers PJ: Eating in an adult world: the rise of dieting in childhood and adolescence. Br J Clin Psychol 31:95–105, 1992

Jimerson DC: Serotonin function following remission from bulimia nervosa. Neuropsychopharmacology 22:257–263, 2000

Jimerson DC, Lesem MD, Kaye WH, et al: Low serotonin and dopamine metabolite concentrations in cerebrospinal fluid from bulimic patients with frequent binge episodes. Arch Gen Psychiatry 49:132–138, 1992

Johnson C, Powers P, Dick R: Athletes and eating disorders: the National Collegiate Athletic Association Study. Int J Eat Disord 26:179–188, 1999

Johnson SM, Maddeaux C, Blouin J: Emotionally focused family therapy for bulimia: changing attachment patterns. Psychotherapy 35:238–247, 1998

Jonas JM, Gold MS: The use of opiate antagonists in treating bulimia: a study of low-dose versus high-dose naltrexone. Psychiatry Res 24:195–199, 1988

Kaltiala-Heino R, Rimpelae M, et al: Bulimia and bulimic behavior in middle adolescence: more common than thought? Acta Psychiatr Scand 100:22–29, 1999

Kaye WH, Berrettini W, Gwirtzman H, et al: Altered cerebrospinal neuropeptide Y and peptide YY immunoreactivity in anorexia and bulimia nervosa. Arch Gen Psychiatry 47:548–556, 1990

Kaye WH, Gendall K, Strober M: Serotonin neuronal function and selective serotonin reuptake inhibitor in anorexia and bulimia nervosa. Biol Psychiatry 44:825–838, 1998

Kaye WH, Klump KL, Frank GKW, et al: Anorexia and bulimia nervosa. Annu Rev Med 51:299–313, 2000

Kearney-Cooke A, Striegel-Moore RH: Treatment of childhood sexual abuse in anorexia nervosa and bulimia nervosa: a feminist psychodynamic approach. Int J Eat Disord 15:305–319, 1994

Kendler KS: Childhood sexual abuse and adult psychiatric and substance use disorders in women: an epidemiological and Cotwin control analysis. Arch Gen Psychiatry 57:953–959, 2000

Kendler KS, MacLean C, Neale M, et al: The genetic epidemiology of bulimia nervosa. Am J Psychiatry 148:1627–1637, 1991

Killen JD, Hayward C, Wilson DM, et al: Factors associated with eating disorder symptoms in a community sample of 6th and 7th grade girls. Int J Eat Disord 15:357–376, 1995

Klerman GL, Weissman MM, Rounsaville BJ, et al: Interpersonal Psychotherapy of Depression. New York, Basic Books, 1984

Klump KL., Kaye WH, Strober M: The evolving genetic foundations of eating disorders. Psychiatr Clin North Am 24:215–225, 2001

Knable MB: Topiramate for bulimia nervosa in epilepsy. Am J Psychiatry 158:322–323, 2001

Kortegaard LS, Hoerder K, Joergensen J, et al: A preliminary population-based twin study of self-reported eating disorder. Psychol Med 31:361–365, 2001

Krueger S, Kennedy SH: Psychopharmacotherapy of anorexia nervosa, bulimia nervosa and binge-eating disorder. J Psychiatry Neurosci 25:497–508, 2000

Lester R, Petrie TA: Prevalence of disordered eating behaviors and bulimia nervosa in a sample of Mexican American female college students. Journal of Multicultural Counseling and Development 26:157–165, 1998

Marcus MD: Binge eating in obesity, in Eating Disorders and Obesity: A Comprehensive Handbook. Edited by Brownell KD, Fairburn CG. New York, Guilford, 1995

Menon KV, Angulo P, Boe GM, et al: Safety and efficacy of estrogen therapy in preventing bone loss in primary biliary cirrhosis. Am J Gastroenterol 98:889–892, 2003

Mitchell JE, deZwaan M: Pharmacological treatments of binge eating, in Binge Eating: Nature, Assessment, and Treatment. Edited by Fairburn CG, Wilson CT. New York, Guilford, 1993, pp 250–269

Mitchell JE, Groat R: A placebo-controlled double-blind trial of amitriptyline in bulimia. J Clin Psychopharmacol 4:186–192, 1984

Mitchell JE, Pyle RL, Ekert ED, et al: Response to alternative antidepressants in imipramine non-responders with bulimia nervosa. J Clin Psychopharmacol 9:291–293, 1989

Mitchell JE, Fletcher L, Hanson K, et al: The relative efficacy of fluoxetine and manual-based self-help in the treatment of outpatients with bulimia nervosa. J Clin Psychopharmacol 21:298–304, 2001

Mitchell K, Carr A: Anorexia and bulimia, in What Works With Children and Adolescents? A Critical Review of Psychological Interventions with Children, Adolescents and Their Families. Edited by Carr A. London, Routledge, 2000, pp 233–257

Nevonen L, Broberg AG, Lindstroem M, et al: A sequenced group psychotherapy model for bulimia nervosa patients: a pilot study. European Eating Disorders Review 7:17–27, 1999

Newton JR, Freeman CP, Hannan WJ, et al: Osteoporosis and normal weight bulimia nervosa—which patients are at risk? J Psychosom Res 37:239–247, 1993

Nishiguchi N, Matsushita S, Suzuki K, et al: Association between 5-HT$_{2A}$ receptor gene promoter region polymorphism and eating disorders in Japanese patients. Biol Psychiatry 50:123–128, 2001

Offner D: Eating disorders: family environment and outcome. Unpublished doctoral dissertation, Boston University, 1997 [Dissertation Abstracts International: 57:9-B, 5927, 1997]

Olivardia R, Harrison GP, Mangweth B, et al: Eating disorders in college men. Am J Psychiatry 192:1279–1285, 1995

Olmstead MP, Davis R, Rochert W, et al: Efficacy of a brief psychoeducational intervention for bulimia nervosa. Behav Res Ther 29:71–83, 1991

Orenstein P: School Girls. New York, Doubleday, 1994

Ozawa Y, Koyano H, Akama T: Complete recovery from intractable bulimia nervosa by the surgical cure of primary hyperparathyroidism. Int J Eat Disord 26:107–110, 1999

Peeters F, Meijboom A: Electrolyte and other blood serum abnormalities in normal weight bulimia nervosa: evidence for sampling bias. Int J Eat Disord 27:358–362, 2000

Peveler RC: Eating disorders and diabetes, in Eating Disorders and Obesity: A Comprehensive Handbook. Edited by Brownell KD, Fairburn CG. New York, Guilford, 1995

Powell AD, Kahn AS: Racial differences in women's desire to be thin. Int J Eat Disord 17:191–195, 1995

Pyle RL, Mitchell JE, Eckert ED: Bulimia: report of 31 cases. J Clin Psychiatry 42:60–64, 1981

Ratan D, Gandhi D, Palmer R: Eating disorders in British Asians. Int J Eat Disord 24:101–105, 1998

Rosen JC, Leitenbert H, Fisher C, et al: Binge eating episodes in bulimia nervosa: the amount and type of food consumed. Int J Eat Disord 5:255–257, 1986

Rossiter EM, Agras WS: An empirical test of DSM-III-R definition of a binge. Int J Eat Disord 9:513–518, 1990

Rossiter EM, Agras WS, Losch M: Dietary restraint of bulimic subjects following cognitive-behavioral or pharmacological treatment. Behav Res Ther 26:495–498, 1988

Russell GFM: Bulimia nervosa: an ominous variant of anorexia nervosa. Psychol Med 9:429–448, 1979

Russell GFM, Szmukler GI, Dare C, et al: An evaluation of family therapy in anorexia nervosa and bulimia nervosa. Arch Gen Psychiatry 44:1047–1056, 1987

Safer DL, Telch CF, Agras WS: Dialectical behavioral therapy adapted for bulimia: a case report. Int J Eat Disord 30:101–106, 2001a

Safer DL, Telch CF, Agras WS: Dialectical behavioral therapy for bulimia nervosa. Am J Psychiatry 158:632–634, 2001b

Schmidt U, Humfress H, Treasure J: The role of general family environment and sexual and physical abuse in the origins of eating disorders. Int J Eat Disord 5:184–207, 1997

Shotte DE, Stunkard AJ: Bulimia vs bulimic behaviors on a college campus. JAMA 258:1213–1215, 1987

Smolak L, Levine MP, Sullins E: Are child sexual experiences related to eating disordered attitudes and behavior in a college sample? Int J Eat Disord 10:167–178, 1990

Sokol MS, Gray NS, Goldstein A, et al: Methylphenidate treatment for bulimia nervosa associated with cluster B personality disorder. Int J Eat Disord 25:233–237, 1999

Steiger H, Koerner N, Engelberg MJ, et al: Self-destructiveness and serotonin function in bulimia nervosa. Psychiatry Res 103:15–26, 2001

Strober M, Freeman R, Lampert C, et al: Males with anorexia nervosa: a controlled study of eating disorders in first-degree relatives. Int J Eat Disord 29:264–269, 2001

Sullivan PF, Bulik CM, Kendler KS: Genetic epidemiology of binging and vomiting. Br J Psychiatry 173:75–79, 1998

Szydlo D: Psychological and familial determinants of eating disorders: causes and effects. Keynote lecture, National Conference on Psychiatric Disorders, American British Cowdray Medical Center, Mexico City, October 1999

Szydlo D: Eating disorders, a public health problem in underdeveloped countries. Keynote lecture, National Conference on Eating Disorders, American British Cowdray Hospital, Mexico City, October 2000

Timmerman MG, Wells LA, Chen S: Bulimia nervosa and associated alcohol abuse among secondary school students. J Am Acad Child Adolesc Psychiatry 29:118–122, 1990

Turnbull J, Freeman CP, Barrie F, et al: The clinical characteristics of bulimia nervosa. Int J Eat Disord 8:399–409, 1989

Waller G: Sexual abuse and the severity of bulimic symptoms. Br J Psychiatry 161:90–93, 1992

Walsh BT, Agras WS, Delvin MJ, et al: Fluoxetine for bulimia nervosa following poor response to psychotherapy. Am J Psychiatry 157:1332–1334, 2000

Welch SL, Fairburn CG: Sexual abuse and bulimia nervosa: three integrated case-control comparisons. Am J Psychiatry 151:402–407, 1994

Welch SL, Fairburn CG: Smoking and bulimia nervosa. Int J Eat Disord 23:433–437, 1998

Whitaker A, Johnson J, Sheffer D, et al: Uncommon troubles in young people: prevalence estimates of selected psychiatric disorders in a nonreferred adolescent population. Arch Gen Psychiatry 47:487–496, 1990

Willie JT, Chernelli RM, Sinton CM, et al: To eat or to sleep? Orexin in the regulation of feeding and wakefulness. Annu Rev Neurosci 24:429–459, 2001

Wonderlich SA, Fullerton D, Swift WJ, et al: Five-year outcome from eating disorders: relevance of personality disorders. Int J Eat Disord 15:513–518, 1994

Woodside DB, Field LL, Garfinkel PE, et al: Specificity of eating disorders diagnoses in families of probands with anorexia nervosa and bulimia nervosa. Compr Psychiatry 39:261–264, 1998

World Health Organization: International Statistical Classification of Diseases and Related Health Problems, 10th Revision. Geneva, World Health Organization, 1992

Ziolko HU: Bulimia: a historical outline. Int J Eat Disord 20:345–358, 1996

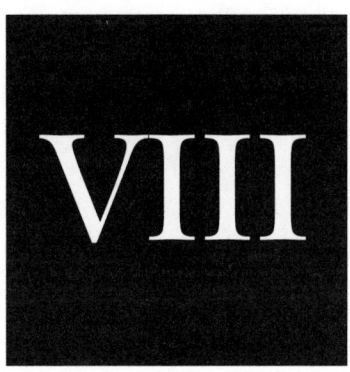

Disorders Affecting Somatic Function

Tic Disorders

Robert A. King, M.D.
James F. Leckman, M.D.

Definition

Tics are abrupt, purposeless, recurrent, stereotyped movements or sounds. They are frequently experienced as being involuntary or as occurring in response to an irresistible impulse (Leckman et al. 1999a). Tics can sometimes, with effort, be suppressed or deferred for brief periods of time. The frequency of tics can vary considerably over the course of a day in response to changing environmental circumstances. Over the course of weeks to months, a pattern of waxing and waning of tic symptoms is common. Tics may exactly mimic voluntary movements or speech, or they may have an exaggerated or more forceful character.

Simple tics are sudden, brief, meaningless tics occurring singly; in contrast, complex tics involve movements or vocalizations orchestrated into longer or more purposeful-appearing constellations. Common simple motor tics include grimaces, rapid head or limb jerks, shrugs, and abdominal tensing. Among the most common simple vocal tics are sniffs, barks, coughs, guttural throat clearing, and other expiratory vocalizations. Examples of complex motor tics are biting, throwing, hitting, skipping, touching objects or self, dystonic postures, and gestures, which may be obscene (copropraxia) or compulsive imitations (echopraxia). Complex vocal tics range from dysfluencies and aberrations in prosody through formed syllables, words, or phrases; such phrases often take the form of stereo-

typed ejaculations (e.g., "shut up!," "you bet!"), obscenities (coprolalia), or echoing others (echolalia) or one's self (palilalia).

Among affected individuals, the intensity, frequency, and diversity of tics combine to create a wide gamut of severity. At one end of the spectrum stand transient simple tics that occur passingly in a large number of school-age children. At the other extreme stand the persistent, variegated multiple vocal and motor tics of Tourette's disorder. In some individuals, tics appear as apparently isolated phenomena. In others, they may be associated with learning difficulties, impulsivity, inattentiveness, emotional lability, or obsessive-compulsive phenomena (King and Scahill 2001).

The current classification of tic disorders in DSM-IV-TR (American Psychiatric Association 2000) distinguishes three specific disorders: transient tic disorder (Table 37–1), chronic motor or vocal tic disorder (Table 37–2), and Tourette's disorder (Table 37–3). The DSM-IV-TR schema distinguishes these disorders by means of precise criteria for frequency, persistence, and variety of tics. However, these criteria are more or less arbitrary; despite their apparent precision, it is unclear to what extent the frequency and duration criteria demarcate distinctive syndromes with differing etiologies, symptomatic concomitants, or clinical courses. It may be that the various tic disorders do not represent discrete entities but rather points on a spectrum of symptomatic severity in the expression of a common underlying genetic vulnerability.

This chapter reflects the work of the late Donald J. Cohen, M.D., and his decades of research, clinical care, and advocacy on behalf of individuals affected by Tourette's syndrome.

Table 37–1. DSM-IV-TR diagnostic criteria for transient tic disorder

A. Single or multiple motor and/or vocal tics (i.e., sudden, rapid, recurrent, nonrhythmic, stereotyped motor movements or vocalizations)

B. The tics occur many times a day, nearly every day for at least 4 weeks, but for no longer than 12 consecutive months.

C. The onset is before age 18 years.

D. The disturbance is not due to the direct physiological effects of a substance (e.g., stimulants) or a general medical condition (e.g., Huntington's disease or postviral encephalitis).

E. Criteria have never been met for Tourette's disorder or chronic motor or vocal tic disorder.

Specify if:

Single Episode or **Recurrent**

Source. Reprinted from American Psychiatric Association: *Diagnostic and Statistical Manual of Mental Disorders*, 4th Edition, Text Revision. Washington, DC, American Psychiatric Association, 2000. Copyright 2000 American Psychiatric Association. Used with permission.

Clinical Findings

■ Transient Tic Disorder

Transient tics are very common in prepubertal children, with boys being more often affected than girls. The most common transient tics involve the face, head, neck, or arms. Transient vocal tics are much more rare. Transient tics run a waxing and waning course, which is often exacerbated by stress, excitement, or fatigue. Children are often unaware of their tics or may try to rationalize them away (e.g., "I just sniffed because I had a cold"). Indeed, forceful, repetitive blinking, sniffing, or throat clearing often results in visits to the optometrist, allergist, or pediatrician. Transient tics in childhood are by definition time-limited and in most cases are nonimpairing. In the absence of a positive family tic history, however, there are no clear clinical guidelines to predict which mild motor tics of recent onset are likely to remit and which are likely to persist or effloresce. Family studies suggest that in some individuals transient tic disorder represents a mild phenotypical expression of the Tourette's syndrome gene and a marker of genetic risk for that individual's offspring (Kurlan et al. 1988). Whether

other forms of transient tics exist that are not genetically determined ("phenocopies") or that have alternate genetic determinants remains to be determined.

Table 37–2. DSM-IV-TR diagnostic criteria for chronic motor or vocal tic disorder

A. Single or multiple motor or vocal tics (i.e., sudden, rapid, recurrent, nonrhythmic, stereotyped motor movements or vocalizations), but not both, have been present at some time during the illness.

B. The tics occur many times a day nearly every day or intermittently throughout a period of more than 1 year, and during this period there was never a tic-free period of more than 3 consecutive months.

C. The onset is before age 18 years.

D. The disturbance is not due to the direct physiological effects of a substance (e.g., stimulants) or a general medical condition (e.g., Huntington's disease or postviral encephalitis).

E. Criteria have never been met for Tourette's disorder.

Source. Reprinted from American Psychiatric Association: *Diagnostic and Statistical Manual of Mental Disorders*, 4th Edition, Text Revision. Washington, DC, American Psychiatric Association, 2000. Copyright 2000 American Psychiatric Association. Used with permission.

Table 37–3. DSM-IV-TR diagnostic criteria for Tourette's disorder

A. Both multiple motor and one or more vocal tics have been present at some time during the illness, although not necessarily concurrently. (A *tic* is a sudden, rapid, recurrent, nonrhythmic, stereotyped motor movement or vocalization.)

B. The tics occur many times a day (usually in bouts) nearly every day or intermittently throughout a period of more than 1 year, and during this period there was never a tic-free period of more than 3 consecutive months.

C. The onset is before age 18 years.

D. The disturbance is not due to the direct physiological effects of a substance (e.g., stimulants) or a general medical condition (e.g., Huntington's disease or postviral encephalitis).

Source. Reprinted from American Psychiatric Association: *Diagnostic and Statistical Manual of Mental Disorders*, 4th Edition, Text Revision. Washington, DC, American Psychiatric Association, 2000. Copyright 2000 American Psychiatric Association. Used with permission.

■ Chronic Motor or Vocal Tic Disorder

By definition chronic motor or vocal tic disorder is more persistent than transient tic disorder. As with other tic disorders, it runs a waxing and waning course; manifests a broad range of severity; and appears to be exacerbated by stress, arousal, or fatigue. The most common chronic tics are motor tics, especially those of the face, head, neck, and arms. In evaluating adults with chronic tics, a careful history often reveals that the tics have been present since childhood; in fact, in retrospect some such individuals may have met the criteria for Tourette's syndrome as children, but after an amelioration of their symptoms in late adolescence, they now manifest only either chronic motor or vocal tics as a residual condition.

■ Tourette's Syndrome (Chronic Motor and Phonic Tic Disorder)

Chronic motor and phonic tic disorder was first described in 1885 by Georges Gilles de la Tourette (Goetz and Klawans 1982), who described what he considered its cardinal features: convulsive muscular jerks, inarticulate shouts, and coprolalia. He also noted that individual symptoms waxed and waned and that, although some patients' tic symptoms worsened over time, there was no general mental deterioration.

The initial symptoms of Tourette's syndrome most frequently appear in prepuberty between ages 5 and 8 years. Initially, they may resemble the transient motor tics of childhood in that they are often mild and transient and involve the face, head, or upper extremities. With time, however, the tics become persistent and increase in diversity and distribution, often progressing from the upper parts of the body to involve the trunk and legs (rostral-caudal progression). Initially most motor tics are simple ones (e.g., blinks, arm or head jerks, grimaces), but with time more complex motor tics such as biting, clapping, touching, or orchestrated simultaneous multiple movements may appear as well.

The onset of motor tics usually precedes that of vocal tics by a year or two. However, in some cases simple vocal tics such as sniffing or compulsive throat clearing may be the first harbingers of the disorder. Initial vocal tics are most often simple and include clicks, chirps, throat clearing, grunts, coughs, or squeaks. Later, vocal tics may increase in complexity, with inappropriate blurting out of formed syllables, words, and phrases or compulsive repetition of either the patient's own utterances (palilalia) or those of others (echolalia). Speech fluency and prosody may be paroxysmally altered. Despite its traditional association with the syndrome, coprolalia does not usually appear until around puberty and occurs in only about one-third of cases.

The variety and temporal patterning of tics is virtually limitless (Leckman et al. 1999a). Individual tics may wax and wane over weeks or months; they may even disappear, only to be replaced in time by others. Tics may occur singly or as part of complex combinations of motor and vocal tics involving many parts of the body. Their frequency may range from isolated occurrences a few times a week to torrential bouts that last for hours and leave the patient and those nearby frightened and exhausted. Analysis of the temporal patterning of tics reveals a fractal character; regardless of the time scale examined, tics occur in bouts (or bouts of bouts, or bouts of bouts of bouts), a distribution that may underlie the characteristic waxing and waning of tics over weeks and months (Peterson and Leckman 1998). The intensity of tics may vary from those so minimal that only the patient is aware of them to explosive outbursts that resound throughout the house or result in physical damage to the self or to surroundings. In rare cases, disfigurement or even blindness may result from violent motor tics (e.g., self-hitting.)

Children, especially young ones, may be unaware of or may deny or minimize their symptoms. Efforts may be made to camouflage the tic-like nature of a gesture (e.g., by disguising a head toss as a brushing back of the hair) or to substitute a less objectionable exclamation for an offensive one (e.g., "Sh-sh!" or "Sugar!"). Patients may be able to suppress tics more or less successfully for a period of time (e.g., in church or while performing), but they may experience a paroxysm of tics once they relax their guard. As a result, teachers and parents may have divergent impressions of tic severity or be misled into thinking that the tics are voluntary and could be eliminated if only the child would exert more willpower. Tics markedly decrease or disappear during sleep and are exacerbated by stress, excitement, fatigue, and illness (Silva et al. 1995; Surwillo et al. 1978).

Although the course of tics in any individual case is unpredictable, early adolescence is usually the period of greatest severity, with most individuals experiencing a diminution or even disappearance of tics by early adulthood (Leckman et al. 1998). (Comorbid difficulties, however—such as obsessions, compulsions, anxiety, and attention-deficit disorder–like symptoms—may persist unabated.) Identifying the factors that predispose individuals to the persistence of tics into adulthood is an important area of clinical research.

On careful inquiry, most patients with Tourette's syndrome of a few years' duration report that their tics are often preceded by a premonitory sensation or urge to perform the tic (Bliss 1980; Leckman et al. 1993). These bodily urges—often described as an intense urge, pressure, or itch—and the effort necessary to suppress them are often more debilitating and distracting than the tic actions themselves. Performing the tic, which is experienced as being at least partially voluntary, produces transient relief. Some patients report the need to repeat a complex tic "one more time" or until they have gotten the action "just right" (e.g., complete or symmetrical) (Leckman et al. 1994b).

When tic symptoms are prominent, they frequently take a serious toll on children's self-esteem and social confidence. Beyond exposing the child to gibes and reproaches, the tics leave the child feeling out of control of his or her own body and mental processes. The very boundaries of the self and the distinction between what is actively willed versus what is involuntarily experienced are called into question (Cohen 1980, 1991).

■ Associated Conditions

Not all of the psychological difficulties of the child with Tourette's syndrome result from stigma or shame. Impulsivity, distractibility, anxiety proneness, mood lability or depression, and learning difficulties are often associated with the syndrome and may even antedate the onset of tics (King and Scahill 2001). Indeed, for many children these associated symptoms, especially symptoms of attention-deficit/hyperactivity disorder (ADHD), are potentially greater sources of social and functional impairment than are the tics themselves (Stokes et al. 1991).

The increased rates of anxiety seen in individuals with Tourette's syndrome may be a reflection of their increased autonomic reactivity (Chappell et al. 1994). Individuals with Tourette's syndrome also frequently have impairments in various neuropsychological domains, such as visuomotor integration and executive functioning. In the school setting, these are often manifested in poor handwriting, disorganized papers, and difficulty copying figures and designs (Schultz et al. 1999).

By adolescence, compulsions and obsessions may make their appearance. Some compulsions—such as tapping, kissing, biting, and sexual touching—may be impossible to distinguish from complex motor tics. Other obsessions and compulsions may range from ordering behaviors (e.g., "evening up") or needing to get an action "just right" through full-blown egodystonic obsessions and compulsions such as repetitive washing and checking. Careful inquiry often reveals recurrent, intrusive, and unwanted thoughts or images (frequently concerning aggression, sex, or other emotionally charged issues), as well as a relentless preoccupation with resisting compulsive urges. By adulthood, as many as 40% of patients with Tourette's syndrome also meet the criteria for an associated diagnosis of obsessive-compulsive disorder (OCD). Tic-related OCD appears to differ from cases of OCD without a history of tics in terms of phenomenology, neurobiological features, and treatment response (King et al. 1999a; Leckman et al. 1995; Miguel et al. 2001). Compared with non-tic-related OCD, tic-related OCD appears to have a greater male preponderance, earlier onset, and a greater predominance of 1) obsessions and compulsions concerning religion, sex, and aggression; and 2) compulsions involving repeating, counting, ordering, arranging, and symmetry; in addition, tic-related compulsions are more likely to feel driven by "just-right" phenomena and urges rather than by anxiety.

Andy first developed eye blinking and facial grimaces at age 9, about 6 months after the tragic accidental death of a beloved older brother. Over the next several months Andy developed additional motor tics that included head jerks, shoulder shrugs, and hand and arm movements; in addition, he began to grunt and make throat-clearing sounds. About 2 years later, after his father had seen a television program on the disorder, the diagnosis of Tourette's syndrome was finally made. Andy was initially given haloperidol, which markedly decreased his symptoms, but he felt sedated and complained of "feeling like a zombie." At school Andy's performance was mediocre because of attentional difficulties, the disruption of his tics, and fights with peers who teased him. During the next 7–8 years Andy and his family maintained regular contact with the Tourette Syndrome Clinic team, who came to be important sustaining figures for him. His vocal tics remained simple ones, but at times his motor tics included pounding and hitting objects. Over the years, Andy's motor tics waxed and waned, but they were only partially controlled by trials of clonidine, clonazepam, and neuroleptics. In the face of an unsettled home situation and economic hardship, Andy finished high school, obtained a job as a maintenance worker, and moved into an apartment of his own. Despite his tics, Andy was popular with girls and maintained a close circle of friends. However, his ability to drive, on which his job depended, was periodically compromised by violent arm jerks.

One day, at age 19, while having lunch with an infirm elderly aunt, Andy was suddenly seized by an intrusive urge and mental image of smashing her in the face with his fist. Although no stranger to fistfights with peers, Andy was dismayed by what he felt to be a horrific, repugnant urge and quickly found a pretext to flee the room. Similar ego-alien thoughts and urges began to trouble Andy at work and at home; these were most often directed toward weak or infirm figures for whom he in fact had fond feelings. For example, Andy had to flee a family gathering when he found himself preoccupied with thoughts of kicking his pregnant cousin in the abdomen. These intrusive thoughts and urges became so upsetting that Andy feared he was going insane, and he even contemplated killing himself or moving across the country to protect his loved ones. Screwing up his courage to confide these thoughts to the clinic's nurse specialist, Andy was greatly relieved to learn that such obsessions and compulsions represented a facet of Tourette's syndrome. However, despite the addition of fluoxetine to his neuroleptic regimen, these thoughts remained both deeply upsetting and distracting and finally culminated in Andy's quitting his job.

Differential Diagnosis

In its fully developed form, with both simple and complex motor and phonic tics present, Tourette's syndrome is easily distinguished from other neurological conditions. However, when motor tics occur in isolation, as in the other tic disorders or prodromal phase of Tourette's syndrome, the differential diagnosis must include a variety of other dyskinesias: myoclonus, choreoathetosis, dystonia, akathisia, paroxysmal and tardive dyskinesias, and excessive startle syndromes (Jankovic 2001). The presentation and natural history of the tic disorders are usually sufficiently distinctive to permit diagnosis on clinical grounds without extensive diagnostic tests. In few other conditions besides the tic disorders does one find the confluence of childhood onset and abrupt but intermittent movements that are temporarily suppressible. The distribution, timing, and kinesthetics of tics usually distinguish them from the unilateral pattern of ballismus; the twisting, frequently sustained movements of dystonia; and the inability to sustain contractions that characterizes chorea.

Clinical context is also a helpful guide. For example, acute and tardive akathisia and dyskinesias are usually associated with starting or stopping neuroleptic medication. Chorea often occurs in the context of a genetic or metabolic disorder (e.g., Wilson's disease or Huntington's chorea) or, in the case of Sydenham's chorea (Marques-Dias et al. 1997), a poststreptococcal autoimmune reaction.

Children with OCD may sometimes have to touch, tap, blink, or look in certain compulsive patterns, but these movements are usually deliberate and associated with specific ideation or situations, with an absence of sporadic, random tics. (In children who have both Tourette's syndrome and OCD, however, it may be difficult or impossible to determine whether a given compulsive repetitive act is best considered a complex tic or a simple compulsion.) Psychogenic tics (conversion disorder) usually lack the characteristic pattern of early simple tics that wax and wane over time. Stereotypies are repetitive behaviors most often found in children with pervasive developmental disorders or other poorly related children (Rapin 2001) (although they may also occur occasionally in children with good social relations); in contrast to the multiplicity of waxing and waning tics seen in Tourette's syndrome, stereotypies typically remain unchanged over years or months and appear to be soothing or pleasurable, rather than intrusive or distressing. The lack of self-reflection, limited intellectual capacity, and impaired social language seen in such children often hamper the task of determining whether the behaviors are volitional, pleasurable, or unwished for. Children with frequent cursing sometimes raise the question of coprolalia; it is rare, however, to see tic-related coprolalia without a plethora of simple motor or vocal tics. Although coprolalia may occur in the context of anger or upset, it is most distinctive in contexts where there is no apparent motivation to curse.

Epidemiology

Tics are common among children, with the highest apparent prevalence between ages 7 and 11 years. Community surveys find that as many as 18% of boys and 11% of girls are reported by their parents to have "tics" (Zohar et al. 1999). Community prevalence estimates vary widely with the survey method and the question wording used. Most existing estimates are probably overly inclusive and do not indicate casesness.

At one time, Tourette's syndrome was considered extremely rare. With greater public and professional awareness, many more cases now come to clinical attention. At the same time it has become clearer that there exist many mild, previously undiagnosed cases. Thus, clinical surveys are likely to underestimate the true prevalence of tic disorders in the general population. Most population-based surveys yield prevalence estimates of Tourette's syndrome in the range of 5–10 per 10,000, with children being more likely to be identified than adults and males more commonly affected than females (Scahill et al. 2001b); a few studies, such as those by Comings et al. (1990) and Mason et al. (1998), have found substantially higher rates when school-based observational techniques are used. Community-based studies (Apter et al. 1993; Peterson et al. 2001a) also point to significant co-occurrence of Tourette's syndrome and OCD, suggesting that the association is not simply an artifact of referral bias.

An interesting longitudinal study (Peterson et al. 2001a) assessed the presence of tics, OCD, ADHD, and other comorbid disorders in an epidemiological sample of children at four time points beginning in childhood and continuing into early adulthood. When the subjects were seen at age 1–10 years, the prevalence of tics was 17.7%; in adolescence the rate of tics in the same children was 2%–3%, suggesting that most childhood tics remit by adolescence. Childhood tics were associated with increased rates in adolescence of OCD and other anxiety symptoms. Adolescents with tics were more likely to have or develop OCD, depressive symptoms, and conduct disorder. In young adolescents with tics, the presence of comorbid ADHD predicted the persistence of tics into later adolescence; the presence of comorbid OCD and phobias predicted persistence of tics into early adulthood. However, tics were not significantly associated with ADHD either cross-sectionally or prospectively.

Etiology

Recent advances in understanding the pathogenesis of Tourette's syndrome provide a working model that may serve as a paradigm for other childhood-onset neuropsychiatric disorders: an apparent genetically determined vulnerability, age-dependent expression of symptoms reflecting maturational factors, sexual di-

morphism, stress-dependent fluctuations in symptom severity, and apparent environmental influences on the phenotypical expression of the underlying genotype (Leckman and Cohen 1999).

■ Genetic Factors

Monozygotic twin pairs show a markedly higher concordance rate for Tourette's syndrome (53%) than do dizygotic twins (only 8%); if concordance is measured by the broader criteria of the presence of *any* tics in the co-twin, the monozygotic concordance rate increases to 77% versus 23% for dizygotic twin pairs (Price et al. 1985). These figures suggest a strong genetic factor in Tourette's syndrome as well as a common genetic determinant for both Tourette's syndrome and milder tic symptoms. The existence of monozygotic pairs discordant for the presence of tics or tic severity, however, also suggests that nongenetic factors play a role in determining the phenotypical expression of the presumed genetic vulnerability to Tourette's syndrome.

Family studies indicate that at least 60% of cases of Tourette's syndrome are familial. However, these same studies suggest that what is transmitted in the families of probands with Tourette's syndrome is not simply vulnerability to Tourette's syndrome per se but rather vulnerability to a broad range of tic or obsessive-compulsive symptoms (Pauls et al. 1990). Thus, the phenotypical expression of the presumed Tourette's syndrome genotype is highly variable, with the inherited diathesis manifesting itself in the form of either tics or obsessive-compulsive symptoms of varying severity. Gender-related, stress-related, and other as yet poorly understood factors appear to modify the form and severity of phenotypical expression.

Although some family data are consistent with a single autosomal locus, other polygenic models may need to be considered. For example, whereas a single locus may confer vulnerability to tic-spectrum disorders, other loci may help determine the severity or phenotypical presentation (Pauls et al. 1999).

The family data also point to common genetic factors at work in both tic disorders and some cases of OCD (Pauls et al. 1995, 1999). As previously noted, OCD is a common associated diagnosis in patients with Tourette's syndrome. Furthermore, first-degree relatives of patients with Tourette's syndrome have an increased prevalence of OCD that may occur unaccompanied by any tic symptoms. This increased risk of OCD among first-degree relatives is unaffected by whether the probands have both Tourette's syndrome and obsessive-compulsive disorder or Tourette's syndrome alone. This suggests that the OCD seen in such families represents an alternative phenotypical expression of the Tourette's syndrome gene.

The Tourette Syndrome International Consortium for Genetics (1999) is using genomewide scans of affected sibling pairs and various well-characterized high-density families to develop high-density maps of genomic regions of interest; among these are two areas on chromosomes 4q and 8p. A complementary approach of examining rare cases of cytogenetic abnormalities co-segregating with Tourette's syndrome and related disorders has pointed to regions on chromosomes 3p, 7q, 8q, 9p, and 18q (State et al., submitted for publication). Other investigators from South Africa (Simonic et al. 2001) and Quebec (Merette et al. 2000) have identified a promising site located at 11q23.

■ Neuroanatomical Correlates

Several converging lines of evidence suggest that the basal ganglia and their cortical, thalamic, and midbrain connections provide the neuroanatomical substrate of Tourette's syndrome (and related obsessive-compulsive phenomena) (Leckman and Riddle 2000; Peterson et al. 1999). With their extensive connections to the sensorimotor and associational cortex, the basal ganglia appear to play a crucial role in integrating sensorimotor information and motor control. Functionally, these structures are organized into multiple parallel cortico-striato-thalamo-cortical circuits that appear to process information associated with the planning and performance of motor routines. It is these neural loops that permit the adaptive formation of habits—acquired semiautomatic routines linking sensory cues and motor actions (Leckman and Riddle 2000). Failure of inhibition in specific subcircuits may produce the premonitory sensations and urges, compulsions, and movements associated with Tourette's syndrome and related forms of OCD (as well as the basis of attention and impulsivity found in patients with comorbid ADHD).

Leckman and Riddle (2000) propose that "tics or stereotypies may be best seen as those prewired bits of behavior that are available to be assembled into habits" (p. 350). The work of Canales and Graybiel (2000) and others suggests that the relative functional balance between the striosomal and matrix compartments of the striatum may determine the vulnerability to tic-like dopamine-mediated stereotypies; these two compartments receive their respective inputs from limbic structures and from motor and sensorimotor areas. Hence, changes in the activity of the neurons at the striosomal-matrix boundary could potentially tune this striatal system to respond more selectively to either internal somatosensory or external perceptual cues (Leckman and Riddle 2000). Dysregulation of this striatal tuning function, due either to intrinsic striatal defects or perturbations in the relative strength of inputs received from other structures, could theoretically result in the too-ready release of (or failure to inhibit) preformed motor routines in response to external or internal stimuli.

The basal ganglia are rich in dopamine and other neurotransmitters implicated in the pathogenesis of Tourette's syndrome by neuropharmacological evidence. For example, a single-photon emission computed tomographic (SPECT) study of monozygotic twins with Tourette's syndrome revealed increased dopamine receptor availability in the caudate nuclei of the more severely affected co-twins (Wolf et al. 1996). (Postmortem studies of a small number of brains of Tourette's syndrome patients have also suggested altered neurotransmitter levels in the basal ganglia [Anderson et al. 1999].)

Early imaging studies showed that some adults with Tourette's syndrome have reduced basal ganglia volumes, with loss of the normal left–right asymmetry found in right-handed control subjects (Peterson 1995). More recent studies find specifically that caudate nucleus volumes are significantly smaller in children and adults with Tourette's syndrome (Peterson et al., submitted for publication). Lenticular nucleus volumes are especially decreased in adults and children with a diagnosis of comorbid OCD, suggesting that this abnormality may be a marker for the presence of comorbid OCD and for the persistence of tic symptoms into adulthood. However, basal ganglia volumes or asymmetries did not correlate significantly with severity of tic, OCD, or ADHD symptoms.

In addition to basal ganglia abnormalities, subjects with Tourette's syndrome also have altered cortical volumes, with larger dorsal prefrontal and parieto-occipital regions and smaller inferior occipital volumes (Peterson et al. 2001b). Smaller orbitofrontal and parieto-occipital volumes are associated with greater worst-ever tic severity, suggesting decreased inhibitory reserves to help suppress tic impulses (Peterson et al.

2001b). Functional magnetic resonance imaging studies of Tourette's syndrome subjects during voluntary tic suppression reveal activation of the ventral prefrontal cortex and caudate nucleus associated with bilateral deactivation of the putamen and globus pallidus, which are likely substrates for the generation of tic activity (Peterson et al. 1998).

Evidence of intracortical deficits in inhibition in Tourette's syndrome is seen in the decreased duration in adults with Tourette's syndrome (relative to control subjects with no tic disorder) of the usual silencing of spontaneous cortical discharge produced by transcranial magnetic stimulation over the motor cortex (Ziemann et al. 1997).

■ Neurochemical Correlates

One of the most promising areas of research into the pathogenesis of tic disorders concerns possible defects in neurotransmitter or neuromodulator regulation. The most intensively studied systems are those mediated by various amino acid and monoamine neurotransmitters and the neuropeptides located in the basal ganglia and related brain structures (Anderson et al. 1999).

Support for the role of altered dopaminergic functioning in Tourette's syndrome comes from the clinical observation that neuroleptics, which preferentially block central dopaminergic receptors, are clinically useful in partially suppressing tics in most patients with Tourette's syndrome. In contrast, dopaminergic agonists such as levodopa, dextroamphetamine, methylphenidate, and cocaine frequently exacerbate tics. The relative roles of the various dopamine receptor subsystems located in different cortical and subcortical structures remain unclear.

Dopaminergic fibers originating in the substantia nigra and the ventral tegmental area connect these nuclei and related portions of the basal ganglia to the associative cortex, the limbic system, and the locus ceruleus (the principal regulator of noradrenergic tone in the central nervous system). A preliminary SPECT study of unmedicated adults with Tourette's syndrome found a significantly increased density of striatal presynaptic dopamine uptake sites in the basal ganglia (Malison et al. 1995). The nature of the altered dopaminergic functioning implicated in Tourette's syndrome remains unclear, as does the question of whether this abnormality is primary or secondary to defects in other neurotransmitter systems.

A possible modulating role for the noradrenergic system in the course of Tourette's syndrome is suggested by the observations that stress exacerbates many tics (Silva et al. 1995; Surwillo et al. 1978) and that α_2-adrenergic receptor blockers, such as clonidine and guanfacine, may ameliorate some tics as well as the impulsivity seen in some patients with ADHD (Tourette's Syndrome Study Group 2002). Individuals with Tourette's syndrome show a heightened reactivity of the adrenergic sympathetic system and of the hypothalamic-pituitary-adrenal axis in response to stress. For example, compared with healthy control subjects, individuals with Tourette's syndrome receiving lumbar puncture showed elevated cerebrospinal fluid levels of norepinephrine; cerebrospinal fluid norepinephrine levels were correlated with motor tic severity (Chappell et al. 1994). This apparent increase in noradrenergic response to stress may help account for the exacerbation of tics in response to stress.

The endogenous opioid system (including dynorphin and met-enkephalin), which is known to interact with central dopaminergic neurons and to have a broad range of motor effects, has also been implicated in the pathophysiology of Tourette's syndrome, as well as those of other movement disorders involving the basal ganglia (Anderson et al. 1999). Other neuropeptides, such as oxytocin and arginine vasopressin, whose brain distribution is sexually dimorphic, have also been studied. Cerebrospinal fluid levels of oxytocin are markedly elevated in non-tic-related OCD but not in tic-related OCD, underlining the pathophysiological distinctiveness of these two forms of OCD (Leckman et al. 1994a).

The ambiguity of the evidence regarding the roles of specific neurotransmitters in the pathogenesis of Tourette's syndrome reflects the complexity of the pathophysiological mechanisms involved and the relative crudeness of the investigational methods currently available. The interactions between the various neurotransmitter systems in the basal ganglia and associated structures are complex. For example, although dopamine-receptor blockers diminish tics in many individuals, their ultimate therapeutic effect may be exerted many synapses removed from the dopaminergic neurons on which they have their immediate impact.

■ Perinatal Factors

The lack of complete concordance for tics among monozygotic twins provides additional evidence that nongenetic factors influence the phenotypical expression of the Tourette's syndrome gene (Peterson et al. 1995). Supporting the notion that prenatal factors exert an important mediating role is the finding that among monozygotic twin pairs discordant for Tourette's syndrome, the twin who subsequently develops tics appears to be usually the twin with the lower birth weight (Leckman et al. 1990). Furthermore, SPECT studies show that monozygotic co-twins with more severe tics have greater numbers of dopamine receptor sites in the caudate nucleus (Wolf et al. 1996). Stressful maternal life circumstances during pregnancy and the severity of first-trimester nausea and vomiting appear to be risk factors for the later development of tic disorder (Leckman et al. 1990). Such perinatal stressors have been shown to produce enduring heightened neurobiological responsivity to stress and are suspected to play a role in the pathophysiology of other neuropsychiatric disorders.

Gender-specific prenatal hormonal factors may also account for some of the sexually dimorphic aspects of the phenotypical expression of the putative Tourette's syndrome gene, such as its apparently greater penetrance in males. Prenatal androgen levels are known to have dramatic and permanent effects on the functional organization of the developing nervous system, and it is therefore possible that androgens or other gender-related factors favoring symptomatic expression of the Tourette's syndrome gene exert their effects prenatally on the developing male nervous system (Peterson et al. 1995).

■ Autoimmune Factors

A theoretically and potentially clinically important biological subtype of tic disorder has been proposed by Swedo and colleagues (1998). These researchers have suggested that aberrant autoimmune mechanisms triggered by group A β-hemolytic streptococcal infection may produce a spectrum of disorders including tics and OCD; they have termed this putative group of disorders *pediatric autoimmune neuropsychiatric disorders associated with streptococcal infection* (PANDAS) (Swedo et al. 1998) (see also Chapter 30, "Obsessive-Compulsive Disorder," in this volume). Sydenham's chorea (St. Vitus' dance), now recognized as a late sequela of rheumatic fever, is often accompanied by the appearance of tics, mood changes, OCD, ADHD, and anxiety (Marques-Dias et al. 1997; Mercadante et al. 2000, 2001; Swedo et al. 1993). Swedo et al. have reported on

a series of children in whom exacerbations of OCD or tics were accompanied by positive streptococcal throat cultures and increased antistreptococcal and antineuronal antibodies without any evidence of rheumatic fever. This clinical syndrome appears to be characterized by sudden onset of symptoms, episodic course, and abrupt symptom exacerbations, which may also be accompanied by adventitious movements.

After the observations of Kiessling et al. (1993) and Swedo et al. (1994), other studies noted the presence of antineuronal or antinuclear antibodies in patients with Tourette's syndrome or OCD (Morshed et al. 2001; Singer et al. 1998). Elevated levels of the B-cell surface protein D8/17 (a proposed genetic marker for rheumatic vulnerability) have also been reported in patients with Tourette's syndrome, OCD, or PANDAS. Questions remain, however, about the diagnostic specificity and causal significance of these findings (Mercadante et al. 2001). Infusion of sera with autoantibodies from patients with Tourette's syndrome into the striatum of rats has been found to produce stereotypies and vocalizations that may be analogous to tics (Hallett et al. 2000; Taylor et al. 2002); efforts to replicate and expand these animal models continue. Given the existence of genetic vulnerability factors for rheumatic fever and other autoimmune disorders, it will be important to determine whether genetic factors also play a role in possible autoimmune or streptococcal-related forms of tics.

The existence of autoimmune or streptococcal-related forms of tic disorder may have important clinical and preventive implications. In their series of PANDAS cases, Swedo et al. (1998) observed that symptoms tended to become more chronic and intractable to pharmacological treatment with repeated streptococcal infections. In a systematic treatment trial in a series of children meeting the criteria for PANDAS, plasmapheresis or intravenous immunoglobulin infusion produced a dramatic improvement, sustained for up to a year, that was significantly superior to placebo infusion (Perlmutter et al. 1999). Because promiscuous use of antibiotics carries its own individual and public health risks, antibiotic prophylaxis should be reserved only for cases with well-documented recurrent streptococcal-linked exacerbations (Garvey et al. 1999). At present, it seems prudent to maintain a readiness to culture children with Tourette's syndrome or OCD who complain of sore throat or who have been exposed to streptococcus.

Because streptococcal infections, tics, and obsessive-compulsive symptoms are all common in the school-age population, further research is needed to refine the identification of cases where there is a causal link and to clarify the pathophysiological mechanisms involved (Mercadante et al. 2001; Singer et al. 2000).

Treatment

Treatment must begin with a careful, comprehensive evaluation of the patient's psychological, social, and educational or vocational adjustment. The diagnosis of an identifiable tic disorder does not obviate the need for a thorough medical, developmental, family, and psychosocial history and assessment. The impact of the symptoms on the patient's self-concept, family and peer relations, and classroom participation must be assessed in the context of the patient's and family's overall strengths and weaknesses (Leckman et al. 1999b).

Structured instruments are helpful adjuncts in collecting and summarizing symptom data and provide useful baseline information for any therapeutic intervention (Goetz and Kompoliti 2001; Scahill et al. 1999). The Yale Global Tic Severity Scale (Leckman et al. 1989) and the Shapiro Tourette Syndrome Severity Scale (Shapiro et al. 1988) are two reliable and valid clinical rating instruments that are used to inventory and quantify current tic symptoms. Although standardized videotaping may be useful in assessing and recording current tic behavior, fluctuations in a patient's tic behavior in response to the clinical setting may make it difficult to obtain a representative sample of tic behavior. The challenges facing patients with tic disorders (and their families) vary with both the changing manifestations of the disorder and the vicissitudes of normal development. Because chronic tic disorder and Tourette's syndrome are chronic conditions, the ongoing availability of a supportive clinician is an invaluable asset for both patient and family in anticipating and dealing with difficulties (King et al. 1999b; Leckman et al. 1999b).

■ Supportive, Educational, and Psychotherapeutic Interventions

By the time consultation is sought, the child's symptoms are often already caught up in a web of anxious apprehensions or blameful attributions. Education about the nature and course of tic disorders can ameliorate this burden, but it is essential to learn what shared and private meanings the symptoms and diagnosis carry for the patient and family. These idiosyncratic meanings may become apparent only in course of extended clinical contact. For example, helping the child, parents, and school understand the child's symptoms as manifestations of a neuropsychiatric disorder can help "decriminalize" symptoms previously regarded as willful, provocative, or crazy. Parents are usually relieved to learn that, in contrast to the extreme picture often presented in the lay press, most cases are not relentlessly progressive and improve by adulthood. When the condition is familial, its heritable aspects may be painful for families to contemplate. Parents often feel guiltily responsible for a condition that appears to come from their side of the family. When one of the parents also has symptoms of the disorder, his or her own experiences may provide either a valuable source of empathy or a burdensome impetus to repudiate or overidentify with the child's difficulties. Ongoing attention to such issues and support for the parents and child in coping with symptoms are essential elements of care.

Collaboration with the school can be very helpful in further destigmatizing the child's behavior, obtaining needed special educational services, and gaining the teachers' support in dealing with peer ostracism or teasing.

It is now generally accepted that chronic tic disorders are not *caused* by psychological factors. However, symptoms are often exacerbated by stress or emotional arousal, and in turn, the tic disorders are themselves the source of considerable psychosocial difficulty. Thus, although psychotherapy cannot be expected to eliminate chronic tics, it may nonetheless play an important role in reducing stress, addressing low self-esteem, and ameliorating family or internal conflicts that relate to the tics.

Cognitive-behavioral interventions such as exposure and response prevention may be useful for obsessive-compulsive symptoms associated with Tourette's syndrome, although tic-related compulsions that are apparently more driven by "just right" phenomena and premonitory urges, rather than by anxiety, may benefit more from a habit-reversal approach (King et al. 1999b; Piacentini and Chang 2001). Habit-reversal techniques have also been successfully employed with tics, but in light of doubts about the generalizability of benefits beyond the specific tic targeted and the considerable energy that must be deployed for self-monitoring and response substitution, the technique appears to be best suited to specific, especially bothersome, tics or compulsions (King et al. 1999b)

The local and national Tourette Syndrome Association can provide educational materials, advocacy resources, and valuable emotional support through contact with other children with Tourette's syndrome and their families.

■ Pharmacological Treatment

As with other disorders, medication is indicated in tic disorder only when potential benefits appear to outweigh potential side effects. For a detailed review of the pharmacotherapy of tic disorders, see King et al. (2003). In children with Tourette's syndrome, the indications and choice of medication will differ depending on whether the target symptoms are the tics themselves or the associated symptoms of inattention, impulsivity, or obsessive-compulsive disorder. There is no evidence that medication affects the prognosis or underlying course of the illness.

Physical discomfort, social stigmatization, and interference with classroom participation are all indications for a trial of medication for tics.

Although the most potent tic-suppressing medications are neuroleptics and related dopamine blocking agents (see below), their frequent side effects warrant limiting their use to more severe cases of Tourette's syndrome or to those who are unresponsive to other medication. A more benign first-choice medication for tics, especially in mild cases, is one of the α-adrenergic agents, such as clonidine or guanfacine; although they are less potent and less consistently effective than the neuroleptics, these agents have fewer serious side effects (Leckman et al. 1991; Scahill et al. 2001a; Tourette's Syndrome Study Group 2002). Unlike the neuroleptics, which are usually given in a single bedtime dose to reduce sedation, clonidine or guanfacine must be given in divided doses (usually 3–4 times a day for clonidine, 2–3 times a day for guanfacine) to maintain tic control. Clonidine is best started with a single 0.05-mg dose (0.025 mg for younger children) each morning. If this is tolerated well, additional doses of 0.025–0.05 mg are added at weekly intervals, first at lunch or early afternoon and then after school. If tics are troublesome in the evening, an additional supper-time dose may be added. If necessary, the strength of each dose may be gradually increased in small increments up to a daily total of about 0.3 mg; beyond this level, side effects usually become problematic. (The corresponding starting dose for guanfacine is 0.5 mg, with increases in 0.25-mg increments up to a total of 3 mg, if necessary, in three divided doses.) The response to clonidine or guanfacine is usually gradual, sometimes requiring several weeks to become apparent. Beyond reducing tics, clonidine and guanfacine also frequently have a beneficial effect on the inattentiveness, distractibility, and emotional lability found in many children with Tourette's syndrome (Leckman et al. 1991; Tourette's Syndrome Study Group 2002); guanfacine may be superior to clonidine in this regard, with less sedation and longer duration of action (Scahill et al. 2001a).

The principal side effect of clonidine is sedation, which occurs in about 10%–20% of patients; this drowsiness is dose related and usually decreases over time. Other side effects of guanfacine and clonidine include irritability, dry mouth, orthostatic hypotension, and, rarely, cardiac arrhythmias.

The most potent medications for tics are the various neuroleptics. Of these, the typical neuroleptics—haloperidol, fluphenazine, and pimozide, which are relatively specific dopamine type 2 receptor (D_2) antagonists—have been most widely studied and used the longest. About 60%–90% of patients with Tourette's syndrome respond to these medications and experience a mean reduction in symptom severity of about 65% (Shapiro et al. 1989).

Despite their potency, the neuroleptic drugs' frequent side effects limit their usefulness. Acute dystonias, akathisia, drowsiness, cognitive blunting, medication-induced dysphoria, or separation anxiety often necessitate reducing or discontinuing these medications or lead to patient noncompliance. The possibility of tardive dyskinesias, especially with the older typical neuroleptics, also makes their long-term use potentially worrisome.

The recent availability of the newer atypical neuroleptics has provided more acceptable alternatives to the typical neuroleptics. Of these, there are systematic data supporting the usefulness of risperidone (Bruggeman et al. 2001; Scahill et al. 2003), olanzapine (Onofrj et al. 2000), and ziprasidone (Sallee et al. 2000) for suppressing tics and the lack of efficacy of clozapine. Although these agents promise to carry a lower long-term risk of tardive dyskinesias than do the typical neuroleptics, acute dyskinesias, sedation, and dysphoria can occur with the atypical agents as well. Excessive weight gain is especially a problem with risperidone and olanzapine. As with pimozide, ziprasidone may cause cardiac conduction abnormalities (such as prolonged QTc interval); hence, electrocardiographic monitoring before and after initiating medication is desirable, as is caution regarding coadministration of medications (such as macrolide antibiotics) that may interfere with cytochrome metabolism.

Neuroleptic medication is best started at a low dose (e.g., 0.25 mg of haloperidol, 0.5 mg of risperidone, or 1 mg of pimozide) with gradual increments of the same amount every 1–2 weeks if the tic symptoms remain bothersome. Increases and decreases in dosage should be made slowly because the therapeutic response to medication is often gradual, and rebounds in tic severity after abrupt withdrawal of medication can obscure the underlying course of the symptoms.

Other dopaminergic agents that have proved useful for treating tics include sulpiride, tiapride, and tetrabenazine; however, these agents are not currently available or approved for use in the United States.

Many patients with Tourette's syndrome continue to suffer troublesome tics even on optimal doses of neuroleptic or α-adrenergic drugs. Because of the side effects associated with polypharmacy, these individuals pose a difficult therapeutic challenge.

Pergolide is a mixed D_2/D_1 agonist that in lower doses is believed to reduce dopaminergic transmission through its effect on presynaptic D_2 autoreceptors. In a 6-week placebo-controlled crossover study in children, Gilbert et al. (2000) found that pergolide (mean dose, 200 μg; range, 150–300 μg) produced a significant decrease in total tic severity scores relative to placebo. Because of limitations in the study design, however, further studies are needed.

Nicotinergic agents, such as nicotine or mecamylamine, may augment the tic-suppressing effectiveness of neuroleptics, perhaps by prolonged inactivation of acetylcholinergic nicotinic receptor subtypes (Young et al. 2001). For example, in several open trials (Silver et al. 1996) and one placebo-controlled trial (Silver et al. 2001a), application of a transdermal nicotine patch (7 mg/day) for one to several days produced a substantial reduction of tics in patients whose tics were inadequately controlled with an optimal maintenance dose of neuroleptic. (Longer periods of application are undesirable because they may produce

nicotine addiction.) Improvement may be maintained for up to a month after a single period of nicotine patch application, but it appears to dissipate over longer periods. Some individuals may experience nausea or vomiting from the nicotine transdermal patch, in some cases severe enough to require its removal.

Because of their designs, studies of mecamylamine for the treatment of tics have been difficult to interpret. However, a recent double-blind, placebo-controlled study of mecamylamine, up to 7.5 mg/day, as a monotherapy for subjects with Tourette's syndrome found no significant differences between the effects of mecamylamine and placebo on tic severity (Silver et al. 2001b).

Baclofen, a muscle relaxant that influences γ-aminobutyric acid neurotransmission, has been studied for the treatment of tics, with equivocal results. In one double-blind, placebo-controlled trial in 10 children with Tourette's syndrome, Singer et al. (2001) found baclofen (20 mg 3 times a day) to be superior to placebo in improving patients' impairment scale scores; however, there was no significant difference between baclofen and placebo in tic severity scores, leaving it unclear what aspect of the subjects' functioning or subjective experience actually improved with baclofen (Kurlan 2001; Scahill et al. 1999).

Injections of dilute botulinum toxin have been studied in several open trials (reviewed by Kwak et al. 2000) and one randomized, double-blind study with Tourette's syndrome patients (Marras et al. 2001). In most cases, benefit was limited to the anatomical areas injected. The most common side effects were soreness, often bothersome muscle weakness, ptosis, and mild transient dysphagia. Injection appeared to be most effective for eyelid and vocal tics. Direct injection of the vocal cords was reported to be effective in several cases of severe vocal tics, but it also produced the adverse effect of hypophonia (Kwak et al. 2000). These studies thus suggest that botulinum toxin injection may be useful for ameliorating specific severe or impairing tics but do not produce overall improvement of tics at untreated sites. Botulinum toxin treatment also has the disadvantage that injections usually have to be repeated every few weeks.

Apart from the tics themselves, the inattention, distractibility, or obsessions and compulsions that accompany Tourette's syndrome may require pharmacological intervention.

Pharmacological Treatment of ADHD in Individuals With Tourette's Syndrome

The ADHD symptoms that accompany Tourette's syndrome are often more impairing for children than the tics themselves (Stokes et al. 1991). Because stimulants may increase tics (or precipitate de novo tics) in a small number of children, the approach to treating comorbid tics and ADHD has been controversial. Some studies (e.g., Gadow et al. 1995) have found no increase in tics in children with ADHD and tics who were treated with methylphenidate; other trials have found little or no increase in *average* tic scores, but clinically significant increases in a handful of subjects (Castellanos et al. 1997; Gadow et al. 1999; Law and Schachar 1999; Varley et al. 2001).

Alternatives to stimulant medication that have proved useful in controlled trials for the treatment of comorbid ADHD and tics include clonidine (Leckman et al. 1991; Tourette's Syndrome Study Group 2002); guanfacine (Scahill et al. 2001a); and deprenyl (Feigin et al. 1996). Tricyclic antidepressants such as desipramine (Singer et al. 1995) and perhaps nortriptyline (Spencer et al. 1993) also appear to be useful, although careful electrocardiographic monitoring appears warranted in light of concerns about possible arrhythmias and cardiac conduction effects (Riddle et al. 1993).

Our own personal preference for the treatment of children with ADHD and moderately severe tics is first to try an α-adrenergic agent, preferably guanfacine, because this may helpful both for tics and ADHD symptoms. If ADHD symptoms remain impairing, however, a low dose of a stimulant might be tried next, after appropriate discussion of the potential risks and benefits. A recent randomized study (Tourette's Syndrome Study Group 2002) compared methylphenidate alone, clonidine alone, methylphenidate and clonidine combined, and placebo alone in children with ADHD and tics. Clonidine alone and methylphenidate alone were more effective than placebo in reducing ADHD symptoms, with combined clonidine and methylphenidate producing the greatest benefit; clonidine appeared to be most helpful for impulsivity and hyperactivity, whereas methylphenidate appeared most useful for inattention. The authors concluded that methylphenidate, alone or in combination, did not increase tics over the short-term period of the trial, and that, aside from some drowsiness in about a quarter of the children taking clonidine, the medications were well tolerated. Although the lack of adverse cardiac effects in this study was reassuring, further studies are warranted in light of the controversy over the safety of such drug combinations (Popper 1995; Swanson et al. 1999; Wilens and Spencer 1999) and the very large number of children to whom they are being prescribed (Jensen et al. 1999).

Treatment of OCD in Individuals With Chronic Tic Disorder

Obsessive-compulsive symptoms plague many patients with Tourette's syndrome, even when their tics have diminished spontaneously or in response to medication. Depending on the type of OCD symptoms experienced, exposure and response-prevention or habit-reversal techniques may be an important component in their treatment (King et al. 1999b; Piacentini and Chang 2001).

The various selective serotonin reuptake inhibitors (SSRIs) have been used successfully in children with combined tic disorder and OCD (Kurlan et al. 1993; Riddle et al. 1990; Scahill et al. 1997; Wehr and Namerow 2001). As with other children, the SSRIs are generally well tolerated in children with combined tics and OCD, with behavioral activation (Riddle et al. 1991) the most common troublesome side effect. Although tic exacerbations or de novo tics have been reported with SSRI administration (Fennig et al. 1994), this is relatively uncommon (Scahill et al. 1997).

As noted above under "Associated Conditions," however, tic-related forms of OCD appear to differ from non-tic-related OCD in terms of phenomenology and treatment response (King et al. 1999a; Leckman et al. 1995; Miguel et al. 2001). For example, compared with non-tic-related OCD, tic-related OCD is less responsive to SSRI monotherapy (McDougle et al. 1993, 1994). Addition of a neuroleptic—such as haloperidol (McDougle et al. 1994), risperidone (McDougle et al. 2000), or olanzapine (Bogetto et al. 2000)—appears to be useful in improving treatment response to an SSRI.

Patients with tic disorders and their families should be cautioned about all drug use, both licit and illicit. Sympathomimetics ranging from decongestants through speed and cocaine markedly exacerbate tics. Older patients may experiment with alcohol, nicotine, or cannabinoids in an attempt to self-medicate their tics.

Research

Research into the pathogenesis and treatment of tics is progressing on many fronts. Advances in imaging techniques such as magnetic resonance imaging and spectroscopy, positron emission tomography, and SPECT of regional cerebral blood flow promise to shed light on the pathophysiology and neuroanatomy of Tourette's syndrome and related disorders. The development of brain banks and new immunohistochemical techniques will facilitate postmortem neuropathological studies of Tourette's syndrome. Basic neurophysiological research into the functioning of the basal ganglia and their neurotransmitter systems will be an important adjunct to understanding the pathophysiology of Tourette's syndrome, as will the development of animal models for these disorders.

Ongoing studies of affected sibling pairs and high-risk families with high prevalences of tic disorder or obsessive-compulsive disorder serve several goals. First, studies of such families utilizing new molecular genetic techniques may permit locating and characterizing the putative Tourette's syndrome gene or genes, as well as clarifying how the pathogenic effects of the gene or genes are exerted; this in turn may facilitate the development of therapeutic agents. Second, identification of individuals who are genetically at risk for Tourette's syndrome and related conditions will facilitate the study of how nongenetic factors influence the pathogenesis of these conditions (Carter et al. 1994). However, the development of markers that can prospectively identify as-yet asymptomatic children who are genetically at risk for Tourette's syndrome will pose the double challenge of how to avoid stigmatization and how to intervene preventively to minimize the development of symptomatic illness.

References

American Psychiatric Association: Diagnostic and Statistical Manual of Mental Disorders, 4th Edition, Text Revision. Washington, DC, American Psychiatric Association, 2000

Anderson GM, Leckman JF, Cohen DJ: Neurochemical and neuropeptide systems, in Tourette's Syndrome—Tics, Obsessions, Compulsions: Developmental Psychopathology and Clinical Care. Edited by Leckman JF, Cohen DJ. New York, Wiley, 1999, pp 261–281

Apter A, Pauls DL, Bleich A, et al; An epidemiological study of Gilles de la Tourette's syndrome in Israel. Arch Gen Psychiatry 50:734–738, 1993

Bliss J: Sensory experiences of Gilles de la Tourette syndrome. Arch Gen Psychiatry 37:1343–1347, 1980

Bogetto F, Bellino S, Vaschetto P, et al: Olanzapine augmentation of fluvoxamine-refractory obsessive-compulsive disorder (OCD): a 12-week open trial. Psychiatry Res 96:91–98, 2000

Bruggeman R, van der Linden C, Buitelaar JK, et al: Risperidone versus pimozide in Tourette's disorder: a comparative double-blind parallel-group study. J Clin Psychiatry 62:50–56, 2001

Canales JJ, Graybiel AM: A measure of striatal function predicts motor stereotypy. Nat Neurosci. 3: 377–383, 2000

Carter AS, Pauls DL, Leckman JF, et al: A prospective longitudinal sudy of Gilles de la Tourette's syndrome. J Am Acad Child Adolesc Psychiatry 33:377–385, 1994

Castellanos FX, Giedd JN, Elia J, et al: Controlled stimulant treatment of ADHD and comorbid Tourette's syndrome: effects of stimulants and dose. J Am Acad Child Adolesc Psychiatry 36:589–596, 1997

Chappell PB, Riddle M, Anderson G, et al: Enhanced stress responsivity of Tourette syndrome patients undergoing lumbar puncture. Biol Psychiatry 36:35–43, 1994

Cohen DJ: The pathology of the self in primary childhood autism and Gilles de la Tourette syndrome. Psychiatr Clin North Am 3:383–402, 1980

Cohen DJ: Tourette's syndrome: a model disorder for integrating psychoanalytic and biological perspectivs. Int Rev Psychoanal 18:195–209, 1991

Comings DE, Himes JA, Comings BG: An epidemiological study of Tourette's syndrome in a single school district. J Clin Psychiatry 51:463–469, 1990

Feigin A, Kurlan R, McDermott MP, et al: A controlled trial of deprenyl in children with Tourette's syndrome and attention deficit hyperactivity disorder. Neurology 46:965–968, 1996

Fennig S, Naisberg Fennig S, Pato M, et al: Emergence of symptoms of Tourette's syndrome during fluvoxamine treatment of obsessive-compulsive disorder. Br J Psychiatry 164:839–841, 1994

Gadow KD, Sverd J, Sprafkin J, et al: Efficacy of methylphenidate for attention-deficit hyperactivity disorder in children with tic disorder. Arch Gen Psychiatry 52:444–455, 1995

Gadow KD, Sverd J, Sprafkin J, et al: Long-term methylphenidate therapy in children with comorbid attention-deficit hyperactivity disorder and chronic multiple tic disorder. Arch Gen Psychiatry 56:330–336, 1999

Garvey MA, Perlmutter SJ, Allen AJ, et al: A pilot study of penicillin prophylaxis for neuropsychiatric exacerbations triggered by streptococcal infection. Biol Psychiatry 45:1564–1571, 1999

Gilbert DL, Sethuraman G, Sine L, et al: Tourette's syndrome improvement with pergolide in a randomized, double-blind, crossover trial. Neurology 54:1310–1315, 2000

Gilles de la Tourette G: Etude sur une affection nerveuse caractérisée par de l'incoordination motrice accompagnée d'echolalie et de coprolalie. Arch Neurol (Paris) 9:19–42, 158–200, 1885

Goetz CG, Klawans HL: Gilles de la Tourette on Tourette syndrome, in Gilles de la Tourette Syndrome (Advances in Neurology Series, Vol 35). Edited by Friedhoff AJ, Chase TN. New York, Raven, 1982, pp 1–16

Goetz CG, Kompoliti K: Rating scales and quantitative assessment of tics, in Tourette Syndrome and Associated Disorders (Advances in Neurology Series, Vol 85). Edited by Cohen DJ, Jankovic J, Goetz C. Philadelphia, PA, Lippincott Williams & Wilkins, 2001, pp 31–42

Hallett JJ, Harling-Berg CJ, Knopf PM, et al: Anti-striatal antibodies in Tourette syndrome cause neuronal dysfunction. J Neuroimmunol 111:195–202, 2000

Jankovic J: Differential diagnosis and etiology of tics, in Tourette Syndrome and Associated Disorders. (Advances in Neurology Series, Vol 85). Edited by Cohen DJ, Jankovic J, Goetz C. Philadelphia, PA, Lippincott Williams & Wilkins, 2001, pp 15–29

Jensen PS, Bhatara VS, Vitiello B, et al: Psychoactive medication prescribing practices for U.S. children: gaps between research and clinical practice. J Am Acad Child Adolesc Psychiatry 38:557–565, 1999

Kiessling LS, Marcotte AC, Culpepper L: Antineuronal antibodies: tics and obsessive compulsive symptoms. J Dev Behav Pediatr 14:281–282, 1993

King RA, Scahill L: Emotional and behavioral difficulties associated with Tourette's syndrome, in Tourette Syndrome and Associated Disorders (Advances in Neurology Series, Vol 85). Edited by Cohen DJ, Jankovic J, Goetz C. Philadelphia, PA, Lippincott Williams & Wilkins, 2001, pp 79–88

King RA, Leckman J, Scahill L: Associated forms of psychopathology: obsessive-compulsive disorder, anxiety, and depression, in Tourette's Syndrome—Tics, Obsessions, Compulsions: Developmental Psychopathology and Clinical Care. Edited by Leckman JF, Cohen DJ. New York, Wiley, 1999a, pp 43–62

King RA, Scahill L, Findley D: Psychosocial and behavioral treatments in Tourette's syndrome, in Tourette's Syndrome—Tics, Obsessions, Compulsions: Developmental Psychopathology and Clinical Care. Edited by Leckman JF, Cohen DJ. New York, Wiley, 1999b, pp 338–359

King RA, Scahill L, Lombroso PJ, et al: Tourette's syndrome and other tic disorders, in Pediatric Psychopharmacology: Principles and Practice. Edited by Martin A, Scahill L, Charney DS, Leckman JF. New York, Oxford University Press, 2003, pp 526–542

Kurlan R: New treatments for tics? Neurology. 56:580–581, 2001

Kurlan R, Behr J, Medved L, et al: Transient tic disorder and the spectrum of Tourette's syndrome. Arch Neurol 45:1200–1201, 1988

Kurlan R, Como PG, Deeley C, et al: A pilot controlled study of fluoxetine for obsessive-compulsive symptoms in children with Tourette's syndrome. Clin Neuropharmacol 16:167–172, 1993

Kwak CH, Hanna PA, Jankovic J: Botulinum toxin in the treatment of tics. Arch Neurol 57:1190–1193

Law SF, Schachar RJ: Do typical clinical doses of methylphenidate cause tics in children treated for attention-deficit hyperactivity disorder? J Am Acad Child Adolesc Psychiatry 38:944–951, 1999

Leckman JF, Cohen DJ: Evolving models of pathogenesis, in Tourette's Syndrome—Tics, Obsessions, Compulsions: Developmental Psychopathology and Clinical Care. Edited by Leckman JF, Cohen DJ. New York, Wiley, 1999, pp 155–176

Leckman JF, Riddle M: Tourette's syndrome: when habit forming systems form habits of their own? Neuron 28:349–354, 2000

Leckman JF, Riddle MA, Hardin MT, et al: The Yale Global Tic Severity Scale (YGTSS): initial testing of a clinician-rated scale of tic severity. J Am Acad Child Adolesc Psychiatry 28:566–573, 1989

Leckman JF, Dolnansky ES, Hardin MT, et al: Perinatal factors in the expression of Tourette's syndrome: an exploratory study. J Am Acad Child Adolesc Psychiatry 29:220–226, 1990

Leckman JF, Hardin MT, Riddle MA, et al: Clonidine treatment of Gilles de la Tourette's syndrome. Arch Gen Psychiatry 48:324–328, 1991

Leckman JF, Walker DE, Cohen DJ: Premonitory urges in Tourette's syndrome. Am J Psychiatry 150:98–102, 1993

Leckman JF, Goodman WK, North WG, et al: Elevated levels of CSF oxytocin in obsessive compulsive disorder: comparison with Tourette's syndrome and healthy controls. Arch Gen Psychiatry 51:782–792, 1994a

Leckman JF, Walker DE, Goodman WK, et al: "Just right" perceptions associated with compulsive behaviors in Tourette's syndrome. Am J Psychiatry 151, 675–680, 1994b

Leckman JF, Grice DE, Barr LC, et al: Tic-related vs. non-tic related obsessive compulsive disorder. Anxiety 1:208–215, 1995

Leckman JF, Zhang H, Vitale A, et al: Course of tic severity in Tourette syndrome: the first two decades. Pediatrics 102:14–19, 1998

Leckman JF, King RA, Cohen DJ: Tics and tic disorders, in Tourette's Syndrome—Tics, Obsessions, Compulsions: Developmental Psychopathology and Clinical Care. Edited by Leckman JF, Cohen DJ. New York, Wiley, 1999a, pp 23–42

Leckman JF, King RA, Scahill L, et al: Yale approach to assessment and treatment, in Tourette's Syndrome—Tics, Obsessions, Compulsions: Developmental Psychopathology and Clinical Care. Edited by Leckman JF, Cohen DJ. New York, Wiley, 1999b, pp 285–308

Malison RT, McDougle CJ, van Dyck CH, et al: [123I]Beta-CIT SPECT imaging demonstrates increased striatal dopamine transporter binding in Tourette's syndrome. Am J Psychiatry 152:1359–1361, 1995

Marques-Dias MJ, Mercandante MT, Tucker D, et al: Sydenham's chorea. Psychiatr Clin North Am 20:809–820, 1997

Marras C, Andrews D, Sime E, et al: Botulinum toxin for simple motor tics: a randomized, double-blind, controlled clinical trial. Neurology 56:605–610, 2001

Mason A, Banerjee S, Eapen V, et al: The prevalence of Tourette syndrome in a mainstream school population. Dev Med Child Neurol 40:292–296, 1998

Miguel EC, do Rosario-Campos MC, Shavitt RG, et al: The tic-related obsessive-compulsive disorder: phenotype and treatment implications, in Tourette Syndrome and Associated Disorders (Advances in Neurology Series, Vol 85). Edited by Cohen DJ, Jankovic J, Goetz C. Philadelphia, PA, Lippincott Williams & Wilkins, 2001, pp 43–56

McDougle CJ, Goodman WK, Leckman JF, et al: The efficacy of fluvoxamine in obsessive compulsive disorder: effects of comorbid chronic tic disorder. J Clin Psychopharmacol 13:354–358, 1993

McDougle CJ, Goodman WK, Leckman JF, et al: Haloperidol addition in fluvoxamine-refractory obsessive compulsive disorder: a double blind placebo-controlled study in patients with and without tics. Arch Gen Psychiatry 51:302–308, 1994

McDougle CJ, Epperson CN, Pelton GH, et al: A double-blind, placebo-controlled study of risperidone addition in serotonin reuptake inhibitor-refractory obsessive-compulsive disorder. Arch Gen Psychiatry 57:794–801, 2000

Mercadante MT, Busatto GF, Lombroso PJ, et al: The psychiatric symptoms of rheumatic fever. Am J Psychiatry 157:2036–2038, 2000

Mercadante MT, Hounie AG, Diniz JB, et al: The basal ganglia and immune-based neuropsychiatric disorders. Psychiatr Ann 31:534–540, 2001

Merette C, Brassard A, Potvin A, et al: Significant linkage for Tourette syndrome in a large French Canadian family. Am J Hum Genet 67:1008–1013, 2000

Morshed SA, Parveen S, Leckman JF, et al: Antibodies against neural, nuclear, cytoskeletal, and streptococcal epitopes in children and adults with Tourette's syndrome, Sydenham's chorea, and autoimmune disorders. Biol Psychiatry 50:566–577, 2001

Onofrj M, Paci C, D'Andreamatteo G, et al: Olanzapine in severe Gilles de la Tourette syndrome: a 52-week double-blind cross-over study vs. low-dose pimozide. J Neurol 247:443–446, 2000

Pauls DL, Pakstis AJ, Kurlan R, et al: Segregation and linkage analyses of Gilles de la Tourette's syndrome and related disorders. J Am Acad Child Adolesc Psychiatry 29:195–203, 1990

Pauls DL, Alsobrook J, Goodman W, et al: A family study of obsessive-compulsive disorder. Am J Psychiatry 152:76–84, 1995

Pauls DL, Alsobrook JP II, Gelernter J, et al: Genetic vulnerability, in Tourette's Syndrome—Tics, Obsessions, Compulsions: Developmental Psychopathology and Clinical Care. Edited by Leckman JF, Cohen DJ. New York, Wiley, 1999, pp 194–212

Perlmutter SJ, Leitman SF, Garvey MA, et al: Therapeutic plasma exchange and intravenous immunoglobulin for obsessive-compulsive disorder and tic disorders in childhood. Lancet 354:1153–1158, 1999

Peterson BS: Neuroimaging in child and adolescent neuropsychiatric disorders. J Am Acad Child Adolesc Psychiatry 34:1560–1576, 1995

Peterson BS, Leckman JF: The temporal dynamics of tics in Gilles de la Tourette syndrome. Biol Psychiatry 44:1337–1348, 1998

Peterson BS, Leckman JF, Cohen DJ: Tourette's syndrome: a genetically predisposed and an environmentally specified developmental psychopathology, in Developmental Psychopathology. Vol 2, Risk, Disorder, and Adaptation. Edited by Cicchetti D, Cohen DJ. New York, Wiley, 1995, pp 213–242

Peterson BS, Skudlarski P, Anderson AW, et al: A functional magnetic resonance imaging study of tic suppression in Tourette syndrome Arch Gen Psychiatry 55:326–333, 1998

Peterson BS, Leckman JF, Arnsten A, et al: Neuroanatomical circuitry, in Tourette's Syndrome—Tics, Obsessions, Compulsions: Developmental Psychopathology and Clinical Care. Edited by Leckman JF, Cohen DJ. New York, Wiley, 1999, pp 230–260

Peterson BS, Pine DS, Cohen P, et al: Prospective, longitudinal study of tic, obsessive-compulsive, and attention-deficit/hyperactivity disorders in an epidemiological sample. J Am Acad Child Adolesc Psychiatry 40:685–695, 2001a

Peterson BS, Staib L, Scahill L, et al: Webster R. Regional brain and ventricular volumes in Tourette syndrome. Arch Gen Psychiatry 58:427–440, 2001b

Peterson BS, Thomas P, Kane M, et al: Basal ganglia volumes in patients with Gilles de la Tourette's syndrome. Arch Gen Psychiatry 60:415–424, 2003

Piacentini J, Chang S: Behavioral treatments for Tourette syndrome and tic disorders: state of the art, in Tourette Syndrome and Associated Disorders (Advances in Neurology Series, Vol 85). Edited by Cohen DJ, Jankovic J, Goetz C. Philadelphia, PA, Lippincott Williams & Wilkins, 2001, pp 319–331

Popper CW: Combining methylphenidate and clonidine: pharmacologic questions and new reports about sudden death. J Child Adolesc Psychopharmacol 5:157–166, 1995

Price RA, Kidd KK, Cohen DJ, et al: A twin study of Tourette syndrome. Arch Gen Psychiatry 42:815–820, 1985

Rapin I: Autism spectrum disorders: relevance to Tourette syndrome, in Tourette Syndrome and Associated Disorders (Advances in Neurology Series, Vol 85). Edited by Cohen DJ, Jankovic J, Goetz C. Philadelphia, PA, Lippincott Williams & Wilkins, 2001, pp 89–101

Riddle MA, Hardin MT, King R, et al: Fluoxetine treatment of children and adolescents with Tourette's and obsessive-compulsive disorders: preliminary clinical experience. J Am Acad Child Adolesc Psychiatry 29:45–48, 1990

Riddle MA, King RA, Hardin MT, et al: Behavioral side effects of fluoxetine in children and adolescents. J Child Adolesc Psychopharmacol 3:193–198, 1991

Riddle MA, Geller B, Ryan N: Another sudden death in a child treated with desipramine. J Am Acad Child Adolesc Psychiatry 32:792–797, 1993

Sallee FR, Kurlan R, Goetz CG, et al: Ziprasidone treatment of children and adolescents with Tourette's syndrome: a pilot study. J Am Acad Child Adolesc Psychiatry 39:292–299, 2000

Scahill L, Riddle MA, King RA, et al: Fluoxetine has no marked effect on tic symptoms in patients with Tourette's syndrome: a double-blind placebo-controlled study. J Child Adolesc Psychopharmacol 7:75–85, 1997

Scahill L, King RA, Schultz RT, et al: Selection and use of diagnostic and clinical rating instruments, in Tourette's Syndrome—Tics, Obsessions, Compulsions: Developmental Psychopathology and Clinical Care. Edited by Leckman JF, Cohen DJ. New York, Wiley, 1999, pp 310–324

Scahill L, Chappell PB, Kim YS, et al: A placebo-controlled study of guanfacine in the treatment of children with tic disorders and attention deficit hyperactivity disorder. Am J Psychiatry 158:1067–1074, 2001a

Scahill L, Tanner C, Dure L: The epidemiology of tics and Tourette syndrome in children and adolescents, in Tourette Syndrome and Associated Disorders (Advances in Neurology Series, Vol 85). Edited by Cohen DJ, Jankovic J, Goetz C. Philadelphia, PA, Lippincott Williams & Wilkins, 2001b, pp 261–271

Scahill L, Leckman JF, Schultz RT, et al: A placebo-controlled trial of risperidone in Tourette syndrome. Neurology 60:1130–1135, 2003

Schultz RT, Carter AS, Scahill L, et al: Neuropsychological findings, in Tourette's Syndrome—Tics, Obsessions, Compulsions: Developmental Psychopathology and Clinical Care. Edited by Leckman JF, Cohen DJ. New York, Wiley, 1999, pp 80–103

Shapiro AK, Shapiro ES, Young JG, et al: Measurement in tic disorders, in Gilles de la Tourette Syndrome, 2nd Edition. Edited by Shapiro AK, Shapiro ES, Young JG, et al. New York, Raven, 1988, pp 451–480

Shapiro E, Shapiro AK, Fulop G, et al: Controlled study of haloperidol, pimozide, and placebo for the treatment of Gilles de la Tourette's syndrome. Arch Gen Psychiatry 46:722–730, 1989

Silva RR, Munoz DM, Barickman J, et al: Environmental factors and related fluctuation of symptoms in children and adolescents with Tourette's disorder. J Child Psychol Psychiatry 36:305–312, 1995

Silver AA, Shytle RD, Philipp MK, et al: Case study: long-term potentiation of neuroleptics with transdermal nicotine in Tourette's syndrome. J Am Acad Child Adolesc Psychiatry 35:1631–1636, 1996

Silver AA, Shytle RD, Philipp MK, et al: Transdermal nicotine and haloperidol in Tourette's disorder: a double-blind placebo-controlled study. J Clin Psychiatry 62:707–714, 2001a

Silver AA, Shytle RD, Sheehan KH, et al: Multicenter, double-blind, placebo-controlled study of mecamylamine monotherapy for Tourette's disorder. J Am Acad Child Adolesc Psychiatry 40:1103–1110, 2001b

Simonic I, Nyholt DR, Gericke GS, et al: Further evidence for linkage of Gilles de la Tourette syndrome (GTS) susceptibility loci on chromosomes 2p11, 8q22 and 11q23–24 in South African Afrikaners. Am J Med Genet 105:163–167, 2001

Singer H, Brown J, Quaskey S, et al: The treatment of attention-deficit hyperactivity disorder in Tourette's syndrome: a double-blind placebo-controlled study with clonidine and desipramine. Pediatrics 95:74–81, 1995

Singer HS, Giuliano JD, Hansen BH, et al: Antibodies against human putamen in children with Tourette syndrome. Neurology 50:1618–1624, 1998

Singer HS, Giuliano JD, Zimmerman AM, et al: Infection: a stimulus for tic disorders. Pediatr Neurol 22:380–383, 2000

Singer HS, Wendlandt J, Krieger M, et al: Baclofen treatment in Tourette syndrome: a double-blind, placebo-controlled, crossover trial. Neurology 56:599–604, 2001

Spencer T, Biederman J, Wilens T, et al: Nortriptyline treatment of children with attention-deficit hyperactivity disorder and tic disorder or Tourette's syndrome. J Am Acad Child Adolesc Psychiatry 32:205–210, 1993

State M, Greally JM, Cuker A, et al: Epigenetic abnormalities associated with a chromosome 18(q21-q22) inversion and a Gilles de la Tourette syndrome phenotype. Proc Natl Acad Sci USA 100:4684–4689, 2003

Stokes A, Bawden HN, Camfield PR, et al: Peer problems in Tourette's disorder. Pediatrics 87:936–942, 1991

Surwillo WW, Shafii M, Barrett CL: Gilles de la Tourette syndrome: a 20-month study of the effects of stressful life events and haloperidol on symptom frequency. J Nerv Ment Dis 166:812–816, 1978

Swanson JM, Connor DF, Cantwell D: Combining methylphenidate and clonidine: ill-advised. J Am Acad Child Adolesc Psychiatry 38:617–619, 1999

Swedo SE, Leonard HL, Schapiro MB, et al: Sydenham's chorea: physical and psychological symptoms of St Vitus Dance. Pediatrics 91:706–713, 1993

Swedo SE, Leonard HL, Kiessling LS: Speculations on antineuronal antibody-mediated neuropsychiatric disorders of childhood. Pediatrics 93:323–326, 1994

Swedo SE, Leonard HL, Garvey M, et al: Pediatric autoimmune neuropsychiatric disorders associated with streptococcal infections: clinical description of the first 50 cases. Am J Psychiatry 155:264–271, 1998

Taylor JR, Morshed SA, Parveen S, et al: An animal model of Tourette's syndrome. Am J Psychiatry 159:657–660, 2002

Tourette Syndrome International Consortium for Genetics: A complete genome screen in sib pairs affected by Gilles de la Tourette syndrome. Am J Hum Genet 65:1428–1436, 1999

Tourette's Syndrome Study Group: Treatment of ADHD in children with Tourette's syndrome: a randomized controlled trial. Neurology 58:527–536, 2002

Varley CK, Vincent J, Varley P, et al: Emergence of tics in children with attention deficit hyperactivity disorder treated with stimulant medications. Compr Psychiatry 42:228–233, 2001

Wehr AM, Namerow LB: Citalopram for OCD and Tourette's syndrome. J Am Acad Child Adolesc Psychiatry 40:740–741, 2001

Wilens TE, Spencer TJ, Swanson JM, et al: Combining methylphenidate and clonidine: a clinically sound medication option. J Am Acad Child Adolesc Psychiatry 38:614–616; discussion 619–622, 1999

Wolf SS, Jones DW, Knable MB, et al: Tourette syndrome: prediction of phenotypic variation in monozygotic twins by caudate nucleus D_2 receptor binding. Science 273:1225–1227, 1996

Young JM, Shytle RD, Sanberg PR, et al: Mecamylamine: new therapeutic uses and toxicity/risk profile. Clin Ther 23:532–565, 2001

Ziemann U, Paulus W, Rothenberger A: Decreased motor inhibition in Tourette's disorder: evidence from transcranial magnetic stimulation. Am J Psychiatry 154:277–284, 1997

Zohar AH, Apter A, King RA, et al: Epidemiological studies, in Tourette's Syndrome—Tics, Obsessions, Compulsions: Developmental Psychopathology and Clinical Care. Edited by Leckman JF, Cohen DJ. New York, Wiley, 1999, pp 177–193

Sleep Disorders in Infancy Through Adolescence

Thomas F. Anders, M.D.

Since the 1950s, polysomnographic recordings of sleeping subjects have been used to acquire knowledge about the organization and regulation of sleep and waking states. The evaluation of sleep disorders in a sleep laboratory has also become a helpful clinical diagnostic tool for some disorders. The American Sleep Disorders Association certifies clinical laboratories and the technicians who conduct polysomnographic recordings; the American Board of Sleep Disorders Medicine and Clinical Polysomnography certifies clinicians. This relatively new sleep disorders specialty comprises an active group of interdisciplinary professionals. Unfortunately, child and adolescent psychiatrists continue to be underrepresented in this group.

A number of psychophysiological systems are routinely recorded by polysomnography in a sleep laboratory. Typically, electrodes record peripheral muscle tone, eye movements, cardiac and respiratory activity, and the electroencephalogram (EEG). Eye movement, muscle tone, and electroencephalographic patterns are the primary parameters used to score rapid eye movement (REM) and non–rapid eye movement (NREM) sleep states. Patterns of obstructed breathing, heart rate irregularity, and episodic behavior during sleep are associated features that are useful in diagnosing specific sleep disorders.

Until recently, polysomnographic recordings were largely confined to nighttime in a laboratory. Sleeping in an unfamiliar sleep laboratory disrupts normal sleep and requires adaptation by recording over several nights. These constraints have made sleep research with young subjects especially difficult. Both children and their parents are reluctant to sleep away from home for multiple nights. Ambulatory polysomnogra-phy, actigraphy, and time-lapse video recording have greatly expanded the scope of sleep evaluations by providing opportunities both for home recording and for 24-hour recording.

Physiology of Sleep States

Aserinsky and Kleitman (1955) are credited with the first modern descriptions of the two states of sleep, now widely known as REM and NREM sleep. REM sleep has been called active or paradoxical sleep because, in contrast to patterns of slowed neurophysiological and neurochemical activity expected in sleep, metabolic processes are paradoxically active (Kales 1969). The electrical activity of the brain recorded by the EEG during REM sleep resembles wakefulness. Neuronal firing, neurotransmitter release and uptake, and metabolic rates also resemble patterns during waking. Mental activity during REM sleep is vigorous and is reported as dreams. Thus, during REM sleep, an individual appears asleep, but for the most part the central nervous system is highly activated.

Studies from sleep laboratories demonstrate why individuals appear so peaceful during REM sleep when their brains are so active (Berger 1969). During REM sleep, the limbs are "paralyzed" by the active inhibition of peripheral muscle tone. Animal studies have shown that when the brain centers responsible for this inhibition of peripheral muscle tone are transected, the lesioned animals show motor disinhibition. They are behaviorally active during REM sleep, seeming to act out the content of their visual imagery. Transected cats will hiss and use defensive posturing, as if attacking a predator or defending themselves (Jouvet and DeLorme 1965). One of the parasomnias, REM behavior disorder, seems to represent a clinical analogy of this experimental transection in humans (Mahowald and Rosen 1990).

In contrast to the psychophysiological activation of the REM state, the NREM state is characterized by the more expected basal organized patterns of physiological inhibition. The active inhibition of muscle tone characteristic of the REM state ceases, as do the REM bursts. Both respiratory rate and heart rate are slowed and are more regular in rhythm. The EEG is synchronized with specific lower-frequency waveforms. Sleep spindles, K complexes, and delta waves define four distinct NREM sleep stages. The EEG of stage 1 NREM sleep resembles the tracing of REM sleep; however, respiratory and heart rate patterns and eye movement patterns are inhibited. The EEG of stage 2 NREM sleep contains K complexes and sleep spindles. Stages 3 and 4 NREM sleep have varying amounts of slow, high-voltage synchronized delta waves. In newborns, only two sleep states—REM sleep and NREM sleep—can be distinguished. During the first 6 months of an infant's life, during NREM sleep the specific electroencephalographic waveforms emerge that are used to subclassify NREM sleep.

Development of Sleep–Wake State Organization

The maturation reflected in the appearance of electroencephalographic waveforms is only one of the developmental changes in sleep–wake organization that occurs during infancy. The proportional relationships between REM sleep and NREM sleep, the lengths of REM and NREM sleep cycles, the initial wake-to-sleep state, and diurnal influences on sleep–wake organization are four other areas that mature during childhood (Anders et al. 2000).

Proportionally, in adults REM sleep occupies about 20% and NREM sleep about 80% of total sleep time. Stages 3 and 4 NREM sleep account for approximately 20% of all NREM sleep. In newborns, REM sleep occupies 50% of total sleep time, and stage 4 NREM sleep does not occur (Roffwarg et al. 1966). Adult proportions are achieved by adolescence. REM and NREM sleep states alternate with each other in sleep cycles that recur periodically. In adults, sleep cycles recur every 90 minutes on average, whereas in infants the cycle

length is approximately 50 minutes.

In adults, sleep typically begins with NREM stage 4 sleep, and the first third of the sleep period contains most of the total night's stage 4 NREM sleep. That is, although REM–NREM cycles recur at 90-minute periods throughout the night, the percentage of stage 4 NREM sleep in a single cycle is greater during the early part of the night than later in the night. The proportion of REM sleep in a single sleep cycle is greater during the latter part of the night. In infants, sleep begins with an initial REM period, and sleep cycles throughout the night include as much REM sleep as NREM sleep. No early and late-night differences in REM–NREM proportions are found. Thus, these shifts in the temporal organization of states during the course of a night's sleep further reflect the maturation of internal central nervous system timing mechanisms. That is, biological clocks mature to regulate both the ultradian and circadian control mechanisms to achieve sleep–wake state consolidation. An understanding of these changes in the organization and regulation of REM and NREM sleep is important for understanding the presentation of specific sleep disorders that affect infants, children, and adolescents.

Sleep Disorders in Infants, Children, and Adolescents

Sleep disorders in infants, children, and adolescents can be viewed from a developmental perspective. Although age distinctions are not ironclad, a developmentally oriented evaluation is useful in differential diagnosis, treatment planning, and prognosis. In general, an age-appropriate, short-lived disturbance is less serious and requires less intervention than a disorder that appears earlier or persists beyond the usual age limits. The former most often reflects environmental disruptions or perturbations; the latter may reflect more significant organic or psychopathological dysfunction.

Studies refute the myth that children "outgrow" their "trivial" developmental sleep problems. Several investigators who have studied infants longitudinally into the childhood years have observed that almost half of infants with sleep problems continue to exhibit those problems later (Kataria et al. 1987; Zuckerman et al. 1987). However, investigators who conducted a recent longitudinal study reported less stability; they

Table 38–1. Classification systems for sleep disorders

	ICSD-DCM	DSM-IV-TR	DC 0–3
Dyssomnias	Intrinsic disorders Extrinsic disorders Circadian disorders	Primary insomnia Primary hypersomnia Narcolepsy Breathing-related sleep disorder Circadian rhythm sleep disorder	Sleep behavior disorder
Parasomnias	Arousal disorders Sleep–wake transition REM parasomnias	Nightmare disorder Sleep terror disorder Sleepwalking disorder	Sleep behavior disorder
Medical/psychiatric disorders	Mental disorders Neurological disorders Other medical disorders	Mental disorders General medical condition Substance-induced	Regulatory disorder with sleep problem

Note. ICSD-DCM=International Classification of Sleep Disorders: Diagnostic and Coding Manual; DC 0–3=Diagnostic Classification, Zero to Three; REM=rapid eye movement.

found that 30% of full-term infants who experienced night waking at 5 months were also experiencing night waking at 20 months. Only 17% of these night-waking infants were reported to be having night waking at 56 months (Wolke et al. 1995).

■ Classification of Sleep Disorders

Several competing nosologic systems for classifying sleep disorders are currently available, although none of these systems adequately meet criteria for younger children. They are the International Classification of Sleep Disorders: Diagnostic and Coding Manual (ICSD-DCM) (American Sleep Disorders Association 1990), DSM-IV-TR (American Psychiatric Association 2000), and Diagnostic Classification, Zero to Three (DC 0–3) (Zero to Three 1994). Table 38–1 summarizes some of the principal similarities and differences between these systems.

In ICSD-DCM (American Sleep Disorders Association 1990), three major categories of disordered sleep are defined: dyssomnias, parasomnias, and sleep disorders associated with medical or psychiatric conditions. Because the most common sleep problems of infants and young children are characterized by night waking, difficulty in falling asleep, or both, these problems are classified in this nosologic system as dyssomnias. Some specific subclasses of dyssomnia—such as limit-setting sleep disorder, sleep-onset association disorder, or food allergy insomnia—point to possible etiologies. However, few studies support these subclasses. Moreover, the distinction between disorder and normal

variation is not clearly specified, especially as it pertains to changing developmental norms.

In DSM-IV-TR (American Psychiatric Association 2000), sleep disorders are classified into four major subtypes, listed in Table 38–2. Primary sleep disorders are subdivided into dyssomnias (insomnias, hypersomnias, and circadian rhythm sleep disorders) and parasomnias (REM and NREM parasomnias). In infants and young children, DSM-IV-TR diagnostic criteria often are not met, especially for primary insomnia and primary hypersomnia (Tables 38–3 and 38–4). In an attempt to improve the classification of early childhood sleep disorders, a new research-based, clinically relevant, diagnostic scheme for classifying sleep problems in young infants and toddlers has been proposed (Gaylor et al. 2001). This nosologic system classifies disorders in terms of initiating or maintaining sleep, and therefore they fall in the general DSM-IV-TR class of primary sleep disorders and in the ICSD-DCM class of dyssomnias. Because they do not meet full adult criteria of DSM-IV-TR for functional impairment, they are referred to as *protodyssomnias.*

DC 0–3 (Zero to Three 1994) is a multiaxial classification system developed specifically for use in infancy and early childhood. DC 0–3 was designed to complement DSM-IV (American Psychiatric Association 1994) by extending diagnostic criteria downward to younger ages and by focusing on problems and behaviors that were not addressed in DSM-IV. Axis I identifies primary diagnoses that reflect the most prominent features of a disorder. DC 0–3 provides several opportunities to classify sleep problems either as a primary entity or as

Table 38–2. DSM-IV-TR sleep disorders

Primary sleep disorders
   Dyssomnias
      Insomnias
      Hypersomnias
      Circadian rhythm sleep disorders
   Parasomnias
      REM parasomnias
      NREM parasomnias
Sleep disorders related to another mental disorder
Sleep disorder due to a general medical condition
Substance-induced sleep disorder

Note. NREM=non–rapid eye movement; REM=rapid eye movement.

Table 38–3. DSM-IV-TR diagnostic criteria for primary insomnia

A. The predominant complaint is difficulty initiating or maintaining sleep, or nonrestorative sleep, for at least 1 month.
B. The sleep disturbance (or associated daytime fatigue) causes clinically significant distress or impairment in social, occupational, or other important areas of functioning.
C. The sleep disturbance does not occur exclusively during the course of narcolepsy, breathing-related sleep disorder, circadian rhythm sleep disorder, or a Parasomnia.
D. The disturbance does not occur exclusively during the course of another mental disorder (e.g., major depressive disorder, generalized anxiety disorder, a delirium).
E. The disturbance is not due to the direct physiological effects of a substance (e.g., a drug of abuse, a medication) or a general medical condition.

Source. Reprinted from American Psychiatric Association: *Diagnostic and Statistical Manual of Mental Disorders,* 4th Edition, Text Revision. Washington, DC, American Psychiatric Association, 2000. Copyright 2000, American Psychiatric Association. Used with permission.

a symptom of another Axis I disorder such as traumatic stress disorder, adjustment disorder, regulatory disorder, anxiety disorder, or mood disorder. The primary sleep disorder is called *sleep behavior disorder.*

■ Taking a Sleep History

It is not only important to obtain a careful sleep history when evaluating children with sleep problems; it is also

Table 38–4. DSM-IV-TR diagnostic criteria for primary hypersomnia

A. The predominant complaint is excessive sleepiness for at least 1 month (or less if recurrent) as evidenced by either prolonged sleep episodes or daytime sleep episodes that occur almost daily.
B. The excessive sleepiness causes clinically significant distress or impairment in social, occupational, or other important areas of functioning.
C. The excessive sleepiness is not better accounted for by insomnia and does not occur exclusively during the course of another sleep disorder (e.g., narcolepsy, breathing-related sleep disorder, circadian rhythm sleep disorder, or a parasomnia) and cannot be accounted for by an inadequate amount of sleep.
D. The disturbance does not occur exclusively during the course of another mental disorder.
E. The disturbance is not due to the direct physiological effects of a substance (e.g., a drug of abuse, a medication) or a general medical condition.

  Specify if:

    Recurrent: if there are periods of excessive sleepiness that last at least 3 days occurring several times a year for at least 2 years

Source. Reprinted from American Psychiatric Association: *Diagnostic and Statistical Manual of Mental Disorders,* 4th Edition, Text Revision. Washington, DC, American Psychiatric Association, 2000. Copyright 2000, American Psychiatric Association. Used with permission.

important to inquire about sleep habits in all children with behavior problems. Some attention-deficit and hyperactivity syndromes may represent disordered sleep; growth retardation may also be associated with sleep disorder (Stores and Wiggs 2001).

A sleep history requires a detailed description of all sleep-related symptoms in the child and a thorough history of sleep problems and patterns in other family members. What is the age at onset of the problem? What is the frequency of the symptom in terms of events per week or per night, and what has been its course (stable, worsening, improving)? What time during the night or day does the symptom occur, in terms of both clock time and time since falling asleep? For example, parasomnias are related to sleep onset and not to clock time. They generally occur 90–120 minutes after falling asleep. Phase delay syndromes are related to clock time. Sleep onset usually occurs at times that are later than usual. Night terrors can be distinguished from nightmares in that the former occur during the first third of the sleep period in stage 4 NREM sleep, and the latter occur later in the night when REM sleep predominates.

It is important to establish the child's customary sleep habits. What is the usual bedtime and rise time? How regular are sleep habits? What are the sleeping arrangements? With whom does the child share a room or bed? Do the child's symptoms disturb others? Are bedtime rituals present? How common are dreams and nightmares? How common are night waking and bed-wetting? All sleep histories need to include data about breathing during sleep. In the absence of colds, is breathing labored? Are pauses in breathing audible? Is snoring prominent, regular? Is mouth breathing common, regular? Finally, it is important to assess the effects of a nighttime sleep problem on daytime functioning. Is the child sleepy during the day, or is the child alert and active? Does the child nap regularly? Do the nighttime symptoms encroach on normal social functions? For example, is the child embarrassed to sleep at a friend's house or away at camp because of the sleep problem?

■ Sleep Disorders in Infants and Toddlers (Birth to Age 2 Years)

"My infant is not sleeping through the night" is one of the most common concerns of parents who bring their child to a health care professional. Parents of newborns expect continuous sleep periods of 3–4 hours punctuated by brief awakenings for feedings for the first 2–3 months of life, with longer periods of sleep at night and shorter periods (naps) during the day by age 4 months.

Some parents expect their infants to sleep through the night shortly after birth. Occasionally, health professionals prescribe hypnotics or antihistamines for 6- to 12-month-old infants who "don't sleep through the night." More often, they counsel parents to let their babies cry.

From a developmental perspective, night-waking problems precede falling-asleep problems, which in turn precede problems with going to bed. At young ages, falling asleep often occurs outside of the bed, and awakenings in the middle of the night are normal. Feeding, rocking, and being held are commonly associated with falling asleep, even though newborns shortly after birth are able to fall asleep on their own and do not need these soothing interventions to help them. This pattern of rocking or holding at bedtime

until sleep onset continues to occur in approximately 15%–20% of children ages 6 months to 3 years (Mindell 1993; Burnham et al. 2002).

Difficulty in returning to sleep following a nighttime awakening often repeats the pattern of sleep onset at bedtime. When assessing night-waking problems in a clinical setting it is important to obtain a detailed history of bedtime interactions that occur at the beginning of the night. Assessment of falling asleep at nap time also may shed light on the middle-of-the-night problem. At older ages, some children when going to bed may exhibit nonspecific anxiety, or they may show specific fears of the dark or of being alone. When transient, such common fears benefit from reassurances from parents and the use of night lights.

Using all-night, time-lapse videotape recording in the infant's home, in contrast to obtaining morning-after maternal reports, Anders and colleagues found that babies stay asleep for less time than their parents report (Anders 1979). Because parents are usually asleep during the night and report only on infants who awaken and cry, infants who awaken and return to sleep on their own are reported as having slept through the night. Videotape studies show that almost all infants after age 6 months awaken once or twice during the night after 5–6 hours of sleep. One-third to one-half of these awakenings result in a return to sleep without crying.

These findings have led to the designation of nighttime awakenings as signaled (those associated with a call for help when they awaken) and self-soothing (those associated with a return to sleep). By age 1 year, infants can themselves be classified as signalers or self-soothers. No discernible differences in REM-NREM sleep state organization distinguished signalers from self-soothers. However, significant differences were seen in the way parents of signalers handled their infants at bedtime. In general, parents of signalers placed their infants into the crib when they were already asleep. Self-soothers were more likely to be placed into the crib while awake and allowed to fall asleep on their own. Self-soothers were more likely to use a sleep aid, such as a pacifier, to help them fall asleep on their own. Signalers, in contrast, did not use a sleep aid because they were already asleep. In the middle of the night, after an awakening, the process was repeated. Self-soothers awakened for 3–5 minutes but fell asleep on their own; they frequently used their sleep aid. Signalers awakened, became fussy, and began to cry. They seemed to use their parents as their sleep aid (Anders et al. 1992). These findings have been replicated and expanded in longitudinal studies of a large sample of 80 infants over the course of their first year of life (Burnham et al. 2002; Goodlin-Jones et al. 2001).

During the second year of life, infants commonly resist going to bed and separating from their parents and develop bedtime routines that make the transition easier. Infants with significant problems have severe and intractable battles at bedtime that are associated with frequent and prolonged bouts of night waking that begin shortly after sleep onset and persist until morning rise time. These more serious disorders become a major source of family tension and are usually associated with significant parental conflict about managing the infant's sleep.

A number of strategies to assist families have been devised. These range from letting the infant cry for 5–7 nights, to withdrawing parental presence gradually by waiting a longer time before intervening (Ferber 1985), to shaping bedtime behaviors such as getting ready for bed and sleep (Moore and Ucko 1957). Because night waking at this age seems to be associated with whether an infant is put into the crib awake or asleep at sleep onset, the night-waking problem sometimes can be better understood as a problem of separation. Parents may benefit by "teaching" their children to separate and fall asleep on their own.

■ Sleep Disorders in Preschool-Age Children (Ages 3–5 Years)

The common problems of the preschool-age child are related to being told to go to bed and to having nightmares. Preschoolers—especially if there are older siblings in the family—enjoy participating in the family's evening activities. When asked, they fervently deny being tired. Although separation anxiety per se does not play a major role at bedtime after children are 3 years old, separation struggles or fears of the dark are frequently associated with insecure attachments (Benoit et al. 1992; Owens et al. 2000). Because daytime experiences for preschoolers are frequently exciting and overstimulating, calming down at bedtime may be difficult. Day-care settings may be associated with overstimulation, leading to troubled sleep. Because many families have irregular schedules, time with a parent may be a precious commodity that the child wishes to prolong. These families commonly have two working parents or a working single parent who usually works

away from the home. The role of television in overstimulation and fear arousal has also been posited.

Whatever the causes, the preschool child may protest vigorously, attempting to delay bedtime. Examples of protestation include requesting bedtime stories to be repeated, returning for more goodnight hugs and kisses, asking for another glass of water or a snack, and pleading for "5 more minutes" until bedtime. A child may also insist on falling asleep in the parents' bed or while lying next to and holding the parents.

Dreams are normally reported by children after age 3 years (Foulkes 1982), and nightmares shortly thereafter. Dream content before children are age 8 years is usually short and concrete. Dream symbolization and elaboration are uncommon. Nightmares are anxiety dreams that awaken the sleeping child. Nightmares occur during REM sleep and result in a fully awake and oriented child who remembers and recounts the content of the dream. Because REM sleep occurs most commonly in the latter third of the night, nightmares are generally noted in the early-morning hours, after 2:00 A.M. Nightmares must be distinguished from night terrors. The DSM-IV-TR criteria for nightmare disorder are listed in Table 38–5.

Table 38–5. DSM-IV-TR diagnostic criteria for nightmare disorder

A. Repeated awakenings from the major sleep period or naps with detailed recall of extended and extremely frightening dreams, usually involving threats to survival, security, or self-esteem. The awakenings generally occur during the second half of the sleep period.

B. On awakening from the frightening dreams, the person rapidly becomes oriented and alert (in contrast to the confusion and disorientation seen in sleep terror disorder and some forms of epilepsy).

C. The dream experience, or the sleep disturbance resulting from the awakening, causes clinically significant distress or impairment in social, occupational, or other important areas of functioning.

D. The nightmares do not occur exclusively during the course of another mental disorder (e.g., a delirium, posttraumatic stress disorder) and are not due to the direct physiological effects of a substance (e.g., a drug of abuse, a medication) or a general medical condition.

Source. Reprinted from American Psychiatric Association: *Diagnostic and Statistical Manual of Mental Disorders,* 4th Edition, Text Revision. Washington, DC, American Psychiatric Association, 2000. Copyright 2000, American Psychiatric Association. Used with permission.

A nightmare is frightening. Its content often involves being injured, lost, or abandoned. If nightmares are frequent, they can be another source of the child's reluctance to go to bed. For preschool-age children, nightmares often include images of monsters and frightening animals; for older school-age children, nightmares typically include more comprehensible human imagery.

Most commonly, nightmares and bedtime protestations are transient, ordinary occurrences that do not seriously disrupt family functioning. In treating frequent, recurrent nightmares and nightly prolonged struggles at bedtime, the clinician must explore sources of anxiety and interventions that can address, as well as possible, the child's needs for comfort, security, regularity of sleep habits, and protection from overstimulation.

A sleep disorder that may make its appearance in the preschooler, albeit rarely, can be classified as a disorder of excessive somnolence. Specifically, sleep apnea syndromes are the most common intrinsic (biologically based) sleep disorders of young children. Two distinct central nervous system mechanisms control breathing in humans. A voluntary cortical mechanism functions during wakefulness and synchronizes breathing with vocalization; an involuntary subcortical mechanism maintains oxygen saturation during sleep. When the involuntary system fails during sleep, blood and brain oxygen saturation fall, triggering a brief arousal, which is sufficient to return control of breathing to the voluntary system. Once the "central" sleep apnea episode has ended with an awakening, the subject returns to sleep. The awakening during sleep is most often a micro-arousal that is unnoticed by the sleeper. However, the sequence of apnea, arousal, and return to sleep may recur many times during the night.

Sleep apnea may result from mechanical or physical anomalies—such as enlarged tonsils and adenoids; excessive obesity; or structural narrowing of the airway, which reduces airflow during sleep (Guilleminault and Stoohs 1990). Again, only an arousal restores breathing. Such "obstructive" sleep apnea is characterized by expiratory snoring and mouth breathing. Obstructive sleep apnea should be suspected in any child who snores. Sleep apnea can also result from neurological conditions or medical conditions of the cardiopulmonary system or from combinations of central and peripheral mechanisms.

Both obstructive and central sleep apnea syndromes can produce chronic sleep loss. The multiple arousals fragment sleep and may lead to sleepiness during daytime. Consequently, such children may not present with complaints of a sleep disorder but rather with symptoms of daytime sleepiness or chronic fatigue. Because young children rarely complain of sleepiness or feeling tired, they may present with inattention or even "hyperactivity" as they fidget to fight off their sleepiness.

If the awakenings significantly interfere with the secretion of growth hormone, which normally occurs during NREM stage 4 sleep, a young, growing child may present with mild growth retardation or, in extreme cases, a full-blown failure-to-thrive syndrome (Stores and Wiggs 2001). To help diagnose apnea, a cassette recorder at the bedside can be used to record snoring. However, sleep apnea should be investigated by polysomnographic technology in a sleep laboratory so that its specific cause and severity can be identified and so that an appropriate intervention can be prescribed. DSM-IV-TR criteria for breathing-related sleep disorder are listed in Table 38–6.

Table 38–6. DSM-IV-TR diagnostic criteria for breathing-related sleep disorder

---

A. Sleep disruption, leading to excessive sleepiness or insomnia, that is judged to be due to a sleep-related breathing condition (e.g., obstructive or central sleep apnea syndrome or central alveolar hypoventilation syndrome).

B. The disturbance is not better accounted for by another mental disorder and is not due to the direct physiological effects of a substance (e.g., a drug of abuse, a medication) or another general medical condition (other than a breathing-related disorder).

Coding note: Also code sleep-related breathing disorder on Axis III.

Source. Reprinted from American Psychiatric Association: *Diagnostic and Statistical Manual of Mental Disorders,* 4th Edition, Text Revision. Washington, DC, American Psychiatric Association, 2000. Copyright 2000, American Psychiatric Association. Used with permission.

Whereas the cause of the obstruction associated with sleep apnea in adults is often unknown, in preschoolers the obstruction is often associated with hypertrophied tonsils and adenoids. Clinicians should always inquire about sleep habits in evaluating failure-to-thrive and hyperactivity syndromes in children.

■ Sleep Disorders in School-Age Children (Ages 6–13 Years)

During latency, infants' and toddlers' sleep problems often subside; however, some children's bedtime rituals continue as habits. For example, the need for a night light might persist, or a stuffed animal may continue to be a nighttime companion. A relatively uncommon but dramatic group of disorders, the parasomnias, may appear during this age period. Parasomnias are sleep disorders in which episodes of non-waking activity interrupt sleep suddenly and intermittently. The three most common parasomnias in childhood are night terrors (pavor nocturnus), sleepwalking (somnambulism), and sleep talking (somniloquy). Night terrors often begin during the toddler and preschool period but may persist into the school years. Night terrors are often misdiagnosed as nightmares.

Until recently, all the parasomnias were considered to share a set of common physiological properties unique to stage 4 NREM sleep (Anders and Keener 1983; Mahowald and Schenck 1998; Stores 2001; Wise 1997). In an expanded classification, however, both REM and NREM parasomnias have been defined (Mahowald and Rosen 1990). The REM parasomnias, also known as REM sleep behavior disorders, are not commonly seen in children. The NREM parasomnias are more common. They generally occur at a particular point in the sleep cycle, at the end of an NREM stage 4 sleep period, just before a transition to REM sleep. Physiologically, NREM stage 4 sleep is the deepest stage of sleep. Sensory thresholds are highest, and it is difficult to arouse the sleeper. Thus, when aroused from an NREM parasomnia, subjects are generally disoriented, their thinking is confused, and there is no verbal recounting of mental activity. This contrasts sharply with awakenings from REM nightmares, which are characterized by alertness, rapid orientation, and articulate recall of dream experiences. Awakening from NREM stage 1 and 2 sleep is similar to awakening from REM sleep.

Broughton (1968) suggested that REM sleep following NREM stage 4 sleep may arouse the subject from deep sleep. He speculated that in children who present with NREM stage 4 parasomnias, the central nervous system mechanisms that trigger the transition from stage 4 NREM sleep to REM sleep are immature or dysfunctional. The failure to enter REM sleep leads to a parasomnia arousal, which substitutes for the standard activating effects of REM sleep. Therefore,

NREM stage 4 parasomnias have also been called disorders of arousal (Broughton 1968).

In addition to the unique timing of NREM stage 4 parasomnias (just before an expected REM period), other common features of NREM parasomnias are 1) a predominance in males versus females (6–8:1), 2) a strongly positive family history (along male lines), and 3) a retrograde amnesia for the event on the following morning. Children who have parasomnias distress their families but often are not aware of the episode. They usually do not awaken; if they do, they are disoriented and confused and fall rapidly back to sleep. In the morning, they have no recollection of the event.

In general, NREM stage 4 parasomnias are easy to diagnose. The time of the episode after sleep onset is a key differential diagnostic feature because NREM stage 4 sleep is often limited to the first 3 hours of sleep. Therefore, a night terror attack or a sleepwalking episode usually occurs approximately 90–120 minutes after sleep onset. Individuals are difficult to awaken; when they awaken, they are disoriented and confused, and there are no reports of dreaming. The following parasomnias are commonly seen in children:

- *Night terrors.* Night terrors are characterized by a toddler's or preschool child's sudden arousal, accompanied by screaming and thrashing uncontrollably in bed. The child may appear glassy-eyed and may stare without seeing; there is no response to visual or verbal cues. In the laboratory, such an episode is characterized by continuous high-voltage delta waves on the EEG, characteristic of NREM stage 4 sleep. During a night terror attack, the child is not awake but may appear to be highly agitated. Autonomic arousal, characterized by tachypnea, tachycardia, and diaphoresis, is obvious. Consolation by parents is not effective. The attack terminates spontaneously after approximately 3–5 minutes, and a transition to REM sleep occurs. Occasionally, an attack may last up to 30 minutes. If parental intervention is sustained and vigorous, the child may awaken but then is confused, disoriented, and unable to relate dream material. The child quickly returns to sleep and does not remember the episode on the following morning. DSM-IV-TR criteria for sleep terror disorder are listed in Table 38–7.

The clinical presentation of night terrors is distinct from that of nightmares. Nightmares are associated with vivid dream imagery; a fully alert, frightened, and

Table 38–7. DSM-IV-TR diagnostic criteria for sleep terror disorder

A. Recurrent episodes of abrupt awakening from sleep, usually occurring during the first third of the major sleep episode and beginning with a panicky scream.

B. Intense fear and signs of autonomic arousal, such as tachycardia, rapid breathing, and sweating, during each episode.

C. Relative unresponsiveness to efforts of others to comfort the person during the episode.

D. No detailed dream is recalled and there is amnesia for the episode.

E. The episodes cause clinically significant distress or impairment in social, occupational, or other important areas of functioning.

F. The disturbance is not due to the direct physiological effects of a substance (e.g., a drug of abuse, a medication) or a general medical condition.

Source. Reprinted from American Psychiatric Association: *Diagnostic and Statistical Manual of Mental Disorders,* 4th Edition, Text Revision. Washington, DC, American Psychiatric Association, 2000. Copyright 2000, American Psychiatric Association. Used with permission.

Table 38–8. DSM-IV-TR diagnostic criteria for sleepwalking disorder

A. Repeated episodes of rising from bed during sleep and walking about, usually occurring during the first third of the major sleep episode.

B. While sleepwalking, the person has a blank, staring face, is relatively unresponsive to the efforts of others to communicate with him or her, and can be awakened only with great difficulty.

C. On awakening (either from the sleepwalking episode or the next morning), the person has amnesia for the episode.

D. Within several minutes after awakening from the sleepwalking episode, there is no impairment of mental activity or behavior (although there may initially be a short period of confusion or disorientation).

E. The sleepwalking causes clinically significant distress or impairment in social, occupational, or other important areas of functioning.

F. The disturbance is not due to the direct physiological effects of a substance (e.g., a drug of abuse, a medication) or a general medical condition.

Source. Reprinted from American Psychiatric Association: *Diagnostic and Statistical Manual of Mental Disorders,* 4th Edition, Text Revision. Washington, DC, American Psychiatric Association, 2000. Copyright 2000, American Psychiatric Association. Used with permission.

oriented youngster; and recollection of the episode in the morning. As described previously, nightmares are also more likely to occur during the latter third of the night when REM sleep predominates.

- *Sleepwalking disorder.* Sleepwalking (Table 38–8), like night terrors, occurs approximately 90–120 minutes after sleep onset. The child sits up in bed and may fidget for a time or may leave the bed and walk to another location. The child generally does not scream, so he or she may be found in a new location in the morning. If sitting up or moving around the bed is the only manifestation of the parasomnia, then no one may be aware of the episode in the morning. The child does not recall the episode.

A popular misconception is that sleepwalking is purposeful. In general, sleepwalkers are poorly coordinated and are unable to carry out complex behaviors. In fact, sleepwalkers are in danger of injuring themselves, and parents should be advised to accident-proof their child's sleeping environment to protect the child from harm. It is highly unlikely that a child or adolescent who leaves the house and takes a drive in the family car or who wanders to the kitchen to consume a midnight snack is sleepwalking. Sleepwalkers are unable to perform such complex behaviors.

- *Sleep talking.* Like sleepwalking and night terror attacks, sleep talking is generally confined to NREM stage 4 sleep. Short cries or garbled utterances can be heard; usually, the sleep utterances are unintelligible. The episode is short and is not remembered in the morning.

NREM stage 4 parasomnias are considered to be familial, developmental immaturities of sleep state transition mechanisms. The most parsimonious treatment is reassuring the child and family that the problem is transient, is not serious, and requires no specific pharmacological or psychotherapeutic intervention. Often the child outgrows the parasomnia by the onset of adolescence. Protecting the sleeping child from accidental injury is critical.

Both excessive sleep loss and fatigue related to overexertion are associated with an increased need for NREM stage 4 sleep. Thus, these two daytime conditions may predispose a susceptible child to an increase in the frequency and intensity of NREM parasomnias. Parents should be advised of the importance of regular sleep habits, particularly sufficient amounts of nighttime sleep. An after-school nap also may reduce any NREM stage 4 sleep deficit.

In extreme cases in which the parasomnia is so frequent that the child becomes too embarrassed to sleep at a friend's house or becomes inhibited in other usual daytime social activities, a benzodiazepine may be tried at bedtime. These drugs are usually effective, but termination of pharmacotherapy often results in a recurrence of the parasomnia. When parasomnias persist into adolescence or present initially in adolescence, neurological consultation and further medical evaluation are warranted to rule out a seizure disorder. Parasomnias frequently resemble seizures, and an EEG with nasopharyngeal electrodes may be warranted for persistent, intractable cases before prescribing benzodiazepines (Zucconi and Ferine-Strambi 2000).

A clinical disorder that has expanded the definition of parasomnias beyond NREM stage 4 sleep is the REM sleep behavior disorder (Mahowald and Rosen 1990). The normal tonic inhibition of peripheral muscle tone characteristic of REM sleep results in sleep paralysis. However, in affected subjects, this atonia is absent during REM sleep, resulting in vigorous and sometimes violent self-directed or other-directed motor attacks. REM sleep behavior disorder is rare; it is most commonly reported in older adult men (Schenck et al. 1997). Two cases in childhood have been reported: one in a child with associated brainstem pathology and the other in a child with undetected neuropathology to date (Schenck et al. 1986). The pathophysiology seems to be related to tumors or vascular malformations in brainstem areas associated with REM muscle tone inhibition (Rye et al. 1999; Sheldon and Jacobsen 1998). Medical and supportive treatment are indicated for this disorder.

■ Sleep Disorders in Adolescents (Puberty to Age 18 Years)

Two classes of sleep disorder commonly affect adolescents: disorders of excessive somnolence and phase delay syndromes. The disorder of excessive somnolence that begins in adolescence is narcolepsy, and the most common initial complaint is feelings of sleepiness while awake.

To quantitatively assess the amount of excessive daytime sleepiness that patients with disorders of excessive somnolence experience, the Multiple Sleep Latency Test should be performed (Carskadon and Dement 1987). The test is done in a sleep laboratory and uses polysomnography to measure the amount of sleep that is obtained during five 20-minute trials, from midmorning to early evening. At each 20-minute period, the subject tries to fall asleep, and the latency to sleep onset for each attempted nap represents how sleepy the individual is. The test, standardized for use in adults and in adolescents at different Tanner stages of puberty (Tanner 1962), has been a sensitive indicator of sleepiness and is significantly correlated with the performance decrement associated with sleepiness.

Narcolepsy is a REM sleep hypersomnia attributed to dysfunction of brainstem mechanisms associated with sleep–wake regulation (Broughton 2000a, 2000b; Guilleminault 1987) (Table 38–9). The definitive diagnosis of narcolepsy requires polysomnographic evaluation in a sleep laboratory. Epidemiological studies have reported the prevalence of narcolepsy to be 0.04%–0.07%, making narcolepsy twice as common as multiple sclerosis and half as common as Parkinson's disease.

Table 38–9. DSM-IV-TR diagnostic criteria for narcolepsy

A. Irresistible attacks of refreshing sleep that occur daily over at least 3 months.

B. The presence of one or both of the following:

(1) cataplexy (i.e., brief episodes of sudden bilateral loss of muscle tone, most often in association with intense emotion)

(2) recurrent intrusions of elements of rapid eye movement (REM) sleep into the transition between sleep and wakefulness, as manifested by either hypnopompic or hypnagogic hallucinations or sleep paralysis at the beginning or end of sleep episodes

C. The disturbance is not due to the direct physiological effects of a substance (e.g., a drug of abuse, a medication) or another general medical condition.

Source. Reprinted from American Psychiatric Association: *Diagnostic and Statistical Manual of Mental Disorders,* 4th Edition, Text Revision. Washington, DC, American Psychiatric Association, 2000. Copyright 2000, American Psychiatric Association. Used with permission.

The peak age at onset is in adolescence and young adulthood, although cases of childhood onset have been reported (Guilleminault and Pelayo 1998; Wise 1998). Genetic factors are important. First-degree probands of narcoleptic patients are at eight times greater risk of having some disorder of excessive sleepiness than are individuals in the general population.

Recently, speculation regarding pathophysiology has focused on genetically mediated dysfunction in cholinergic–dopaminergic interactions (Guilleminault et al. 1998).

Human leukocyte antigen (HLA) testing is essentially 85% positive for the *HLA-DQB1*0602* and *HLA-DR2* alleles for patients with narcolepsy compared with 12%–38% of the general population. Genetic factors other than HLA are also likely to be involved. In narcoleptic dogs, a specific narcolepsy gene has been identified, and it is likely that the discovery of the human gene (or genes) is soon to follow (Honda et al. 1986; Matsuki et al. 1987; Takahashi 1999). Nevertheless, the importance of environmental factors is evidenced by the reported 70%–75% of monozygotic twins who are discordant for narcolepsy (Mignot 1998).

The narcoleptic adolescent naps for 20- to 40-minute periods, awakening refreshed. The cycle is repeated again within 2–3 hours. This refreshed feeling contrasts with the disorientation and persistent fatigue associated with disorders of excessive somnolence secondary to other causes.

Full-blown narcolepsy is characterized by the narcoleptic tetrad: 1) irresistible attacks of REM sleep intruding on wakefulness, 2) cataplexy, 3) hypnagogic hallucinations, and 4) sleep paralysis. Cataplexy—characterized by sudden loss of bilateral peripheral muscle tone, often provoked by strong affect—reflects the peripheral muscle inhibition of REM sleep. Consciousness and memory remain intact. Cataplectic attacks are brief, rarely more than several minutes, with immediate and complete recovery. Attacks may occur only several times a year or as frequently as many times in one day. Both hypnagogic hallucinations (vivid, dreamlike mentation at sleep onset) and sleep paralysis (immobility of limbs as sleep begins) similarly represent REM sleep EMG inhibition and dreaming, occurring during sleep onset, when REM sleep is normally not prominent. Although cataplexy, hypnagogic hallucinations, and sleep paralysis diminish in frequency over time, narcolepsy, once present, is a lifelong chronic condition.

The treatment of narcolepsy is symptomatic and must be individualized depending on the severity of specific symptoms (Thorpy 2001). Stimulant medications are used most commonly for the treatment of excessive daytime sleepiness, and tricyclic antidepressant medications are used for the treatment of cataplexy. Because psychostimulants are often used in the treatment of attention-deficit/hyperactivity disorder, children who combat sleep attacks with fidgetiness and motor restlessness often receive the proper treatment for the wrong reason. In a retrospective study of adult patients with narcolepsy, a significant number had been misdiagnosed as having attention-deficit/hyperactivity disorder in adolescence but had been treated appropriately with amphetamines or methylphenidate, with good symptom improvement (Navelet et al. 1976). Although narcolepsy is a rare disorder, occurring in only 4 in 10,000 (0.04%) individuals, and hyperactivity is a more common disorder, estimated to occur in 7%–10% of school-age children, in all children who present with attention-deficit/hyperactivity disorder or other hyperactivity syndromes, a careful sleep history should be obtained. The therapist should ask specific questions that focus on symptoms of the narcoleptic tetrad and on a family history of sleep disorders.

Clomipramine 10–20 mg/day in divided doses has been used successfully to manage cataplexy. Monoamine oxidase inhibitors may be used to manage both cataplexy and the REM sleep onset symptoms of sleep paralysis and hypnagogic hallucinations. A new wakefulness-promoting drug, modafinil, which activates orexin-containing neurons, is reported to be more effective and to have fewer side effects than the customary stimulants (Chemelli et al. 1999; Fry 1998).

Patients with narcolepsy usually adjust poorly to their disorder. They exhibit problems in school and in social relationships. Associated psychiatric disorders include major depression, generalized anxiety, and substance abuse. Behavioral management with psychosocial support and counseling is an essential component of treatment. Patients must be encouraged to follow regular bedtimes and rise times. Regularly scheduled naps for 20–30 minutes two or three times daily should be encouraged. School and work schedules need to be designed to accommodate the sleep needs of the patient. Patients are advised to attend self-help support groups. The American Narcolepsy Association publishes a newsletter that keeps members informed of recent advances.

Another more common sleep disorder that occurs in adolescents meets the criteria for circadian rhythm sleep disorder (Thorpy et al. 1988) (Table 38–10).

Careful studies of the sleep needs of adolescents have repeatedly reported that adolescents after puberty need more sleep, particularly NREM stage 4 sleep, than do younger children. The increased physiologi-

Table 38–10. DSM-IV-TR diagnostic criteria for circadian rhythm sleep disorder

A. A persistent or recurrent pattern of sleep disruption leading to excessive sleepiness or insomnia that is due to a mismatch between the sleep–wake schedule required by a person's environment and his or her circadian sleep–wake pattern.

B. The sleep disturbance causes clinically significant distress or impairment in social, occupational, or other important areas of functioning.

C. The disturbance does not occur exclusively during the course of another sleep disorder or other mental disorder.

D. The disturbance is not due to the direct physiological effects of a substance (e.g., a drug of abuse, a medication) or a general medical condition.

Specify type:

Delayed Sleep Phase Type: a persistent pattern of late sleep onset and late awakening times, with an inability to fall asleep and awaken at a desired earlier time

Jet Lag Type: sleepiness and alertness that occur at an inappropriate time of day relative to local time, occurring after repeated travel across more than one time zone

Shift Work Type: insomnia during the major sleep period or excessive sleepiness during the major awake period associated with night shift work or frequently changing shift work

Unspecified Type

Source. Reprinted from American Psychiatric Association: *Diagnostic and Statistical Manual of Mental Disorders,* 4th Edition, Text Revision. Washington, DC, American Psychiatric Association, 2000. Copyright 2000, American Psychiatric Association. Used with permission.

cal need for sleep seems to be related to the endocrinological changes of pubertal development (Carskadon et al. 1980). This endocrine-associated sleep need is coupled with heightened social pressures, including staying up late to study or socialize. The combination leads to a significant sleep deficit in many adolescents. Typically, adolescents begin to complain of feeling tired and frequently sleep longer hours on weekends than on school days. Adolescents may often fall asleep at any time. These behaviors contrast sharply with the tireless, high-energy preadolescent child who never wants to go to bed.

The circadian rhythm sleep disorder, however, results because, as adolescents stay up later at night, they then tend to awaken later in the morning. The circadian regulation of sleep, including the many physiological functions that are triggered by sleep onset, becomes progressively delayed. As the body's timing mechanisms shift, it becomes more difficult physiologically to fall asleep and wake up at the usual hours. Adolescents thus find themselves in a perpetual condition of jet lag. That is, their biological clocks become reset at a time different from the demands of their social and academic lives.

Sufficient sleep—at least 8 hours each night at regular, socially acceptable times—is particularly important during adolescence. When sleep debts accumulate by force of circumstances, napping should be encouraged. Once a phase-delay syndrome is chronic and persistent, phase-advance methods of resetting the biological clock may be necessary (Ferber 1987). This condition usually can be diagnosed from the history alone. Occasionally, however, adolescents are poor reporters and misrepresent both the degree of their sleepiness and the phase disturbances of their sleep. Multiple Sleep Latency Test evaluations and spending a night in a sleep laboratory may clarify confusing pictures.

■ Disordered Sleep in Medical and Psychiatric Conditions

Less information is available about sleep–wake state disorganization in children and adolescents who have medical and psychiatric conditions than in adults (Kales and Tan 1969). However, a recent book provides an excellent summary of what is known (Stores and Wiggs 2001). Even the disruptions of sleep presumably associated with common childhood illnesses are, in general, anecdotal reports not supported by systematic research. Because several laboratory conditions, such as ambient temperature and unfamiliar surroundings, have been shown to affect sleep, it is likely that children with fevers or obstructed breathing or who are sleeping in new settings will experience fragmented sleep.

Children who live in institutions are reported to have short sleep periods, repeated nighttime awakenings, and phase-delay disorders. Children with mental retardation and autistic-like syndromes also experience frequent night awakenings and phase shifts (Okawa and Sasaki 1987; Stores and Wiggs 2001). In general, however, disorganization of REM and NREM sleep parameters per se is associated only with profound syndromes of brain damage (Feinberg 1969).

Similarly, sleep disruption in children with psychiatric disorders remains controversial. Although it has been clearly demonstrated that adults with major depressive disorder have characteristic indicators of disturbed sleep, including disruptions of sleep-related endocrine regulation, these indicators are not regularly present in the sleep of children and adolescents with major depressive disorder (Dahl and Puig-Antich 1990). The sleep of depressed adults is characterized by a short initial REM latency and by fragmented ultradian regulation with multiple arousals and early-morning awakening. The circadian peak of early-morning cortisol excretion is blunted. Although a few studies of depressed children and adolescents have suggested changes comparable to those noted in depressed adults, these studies are characterized by small sample sizes, failure to provide for laboratory recording effects, and inadequately diagnosed subjects. More carefully controlled, larger studies have failed to replicate the disrupted patterns of sleep-wake disorganization noted in depressed adults, although the endocrine changes have been noted in children (Dahl and Puig-Antich 1990; Dahl et al. 1994; Waterman et al. 1994).

Similarly, in the few studies of children with attention-deficit disorder (or hyperactivity), despite complaints from parents about disturbed sleep, sleep studies conducted in a sleep laboratory showed the children's sleep-wake state organization to be unaffected (Greenhill et al. 1983; Kaplan et al. 1987; Small et al. 1971). Again, the paucity of studies, characterized by small samples and heterogeneous diagnostic groupings, contributes to inadequate definitive conclusions. The waking behavioral hyperactivity associated with excessive somnolence, both from narcolepsy and from obstructive sleep apnea syndrome, is described above (see "Sleep Disorders in Preschool-Age Children").

Finally, studies examining the effects of alcohol and other chemicals on sleep generally report two patterns of sleep-wake state disorganization (Lumley et al. 1987): 1) decreased REM sleep and fragmented sleep resulting from multiple arousals during agitated states of hallucinosis and withdrawal, and 2) periods of prolonged atypical "drugged" sleep during states of intoxication. However, these results are difficult to interpret. The pharmacological effects of chemicals, both prescription and nonprescription, vary by dosage, chronicity of use, and chemical structure of the compound. Initially, most sedatives lead to increased sleep; habituation and tolerance then develop, leading to chronic sleep deprivation, particularly REM deprivation.

Both hypnotic drugs and alcohol are frequently misused for insomnia that reflects underlying disorders of anxiety and depression. After periods of drug misuse, it is often unclear whether inappropriate drug use has led to disordered sleep or whether disordered sleep-wake organization precipitated the course of self-medication. Careful studies of the effects of substance abuse on sleep-wake state organization in children and adolescents have not been done.

Research Issues

Researchers have learned a great deal about sleep-wake state maturation, regulation, and organization in children and adolescents. This research allows clinicians to be more informed. Many disorders, such as parasomnias and disorders of excessive somnolence, previously were overlooked entirely or misdiagnosed. Often, symptoms of these disorders were labeled as psychogenic and were treated predominantly by psychotherapy. Although the pathogenesis of some syndromes is uncertain, the ability to diagnose them more accurately and, on occasion, to prescribe more specific, palliative treatments provides reassurance to children and their families and prevents the stigma of inappropriate or inaccurate diagnoses.

However, other than physical restitution primarily associated with NREM stage 4 sleep, the functions of sleep in general and of REM sleep in particular are unclear. Why is there more REM sleep in immature individuals, and why is NREM stage 4 sleep seemingly so important in early childhood and adolescence? It is speculated that information processing occurs during REM sleep so that daytime experiences, especially novel experiences, are converted from short-term to long-term memories during REM sleep. Because infants and young children presumably experience more novel bits of information each day than do adults, perhaps they require relatively more time in REM sleep for this information-processing function.

Similarly, it is known that growth hormone is secreted primarily during NREM stage 4 sleep. Because early childhood and adolescence are periods of rapid growth, it is possible that the increased need for this state during these developmental periods provides the substrate for increased growth hormone secretion.

The relationships between sleep-state organization and physical and mental health in children and adolescents are only beginning to be explored. The informed clinician must be concerned about sleep–wake state organization in all children who present with physical and psychological disorders. A careful sleep history examining regularity of sleep habits, amounts of sleep, disruptions of sleep, and behaviors associated with going to bed each night should be obtained in every evaluation. When disruptions of sleep are reported, careful timing of the event as it relates to going to bed and falling asleep is critical in making a diagnosis. Recognizing associated characteristics of specific parasomnias, in terms of alertness and orientation surrounding the event, also helps to substantiate a clinical impression. Occasionally, a bedside cassette tape recorder or camcorder, activated by the child's parents, helps capture sleep disruptions for clinical review.

It is necessary to understand nighttime sleep–wake state organization in the broader context of daytime activity and circadian regulation. The emerging field that investigates these disorders from the 24-hour perspective is known as chronobiology. As polysomnographic and actigraphic recording equipment becomes more miniaturized and automated for long-term recording, it will soon be possible to study larger groups of children over longer periods in their home environments. Only then will it be possible to make more definitive statements about the etiology, natural history, and treatment efficacy of childhood sleep disorders.

References

American Psychiatric Association: Diagnostic and Statistical Manual of Mental Disorders, 4th Edition. Washington, DC, American Psychiatric Association, 1994

American Psychiatric Association: Diagnostic and Statistical Manual of Mental Disorders, 4th Edition, Text Revision. Washington, DC, American Psychiatric Association, 2000

American Sleep Disorders Association: The International Classification of Sleep Disorders: Diagnostic and Coding Manual. Rochester, MN, American Sleep Disorders Association, 1990

Anders T: Night waking in infants during the first year of life. Pediatrics 63:860–864, 1979

Anders T, Keener M: Sleep–wake state development and disorders of sleep in infants, children and adolescents, in Developmental-Behavioral Pediatrics. Edited by Levine M, Carey W, Crocker A, et al. Philadelphia, PA, WB Saunders, 1983, pp 596–606

Anders T, Halpern L, Hua J: Sleeping through the night: a developmental perspective. Pediatrics 90:554–560, 1992

Anders T, Goodlin-Jones B, Sadeh A: Sleep disorders, in Handbook of Infant Mental Health, 2nd Edition. Edited by Zeanah C. New York, Guilford, 2000, pp 326–338

Aserinsky E, Kleitman N: A motility cycle in sleeping infants as manifested by ocular and gross bodily activity. J Appl Physiol 8:11–13, 1955

Benoit D, Zeanah C, Boucher C, et al: Sleep disorders in early childhood: association with insecure maternal attachment. J Am Acad Child Adolesc Psychiatry 31:86–93, 1992

Berger R: Physiological characteristics of sleep, in Sleep: Physiology and Pathology. Edited by Kales A. Philadelphia, PA, JB Lippincott, 1969, pp 66–79

Broughton R: Sleep disorders: disorders of arousal? Science 154:1070–1078, 1968

Broughton R: The Berger Lecture: Chronobiology of sleep/wake and of sleepiness/alertness states in normal and sleep disordered human subjects. Suppl Clin Neurophysiol 53:9–18. 2000a

Broughton RJ: The treatment of narcolepsy. Suppl Clin Neurophysiol 53:371–374, 2000b

Burnham M, Goodlin-Jones B, Gaylor E, et al: Nighttime sleep–wake patterns and self-soothing from birth to one year of age: a longitudinal intervention study. J Child Psychol Psychiatry 43:713–725, 2002

Carskadon M, Dement W: Sleepiness in normal adolescents, in Sleep and Its Disorders in Children. Edited by Guilleminault C. New York, Raven, 1987, pp 53–66

Carskadon M, Harvey K, Duke P, et al: Pubertal changes in daytime sleepiness. Sleep 3:453–460, 1980

Chemelli R, Willie J, Sinton C, et al: Narcolepsy in orexin knockout mice: molecular genetics of sleep regulation. Cell 98:47–51, 1999

Dahl R, Puig-Antich J: Sleep disturbances in child and adolescent psychiatric disorders. Pediatrician 17:32–37, 1990

Dahl RE, Ryan ND, Perel J, et al: Cholinergic REM induction test with arecoline in depressed children. Psychiatry Res 51:269–282, 1994

Feinberg I: Sleep in organic brain conditions, in Sleep: Physiology and Pathology. Edited by Kales A. Philadelphia, PA, JB Lippincott, 1969, pp 131–147

Ferber R: Solve Your Child's Sleep Problem. New York, Simon & Schuster, 1985

Ferber R: Circadian and schedule disturbances, in Sleep and Its Disorders in Children. Edited by Guilleminault C. New York, Raven, 1987, pp 165–180

Foulkes D: Children's Dreams: Longitudinal Studies. New York, Wiley, 1982

Fry J: Treatment modalities in narcolepsy. Neurology 50 (suppl 1):S43–S48, 1998

Gaylor E, Goodlin-Jones B, Anders T: Classification of young children's sleep problems: a pilot study. J Am Acad Child Adolesc Psychiatry 40:61–67, 2001

Goodlin-Jones BL, Burnham MM, Gaylor EE, et al: Night waking, sleep–wake organization, and self-soothing in the first year of life. J Dev Behav Pediatr 22:226–233, 2001

Greenhill L, Puig-Antich J, Goetz R, et al: Sleep architecture and real sleep measures in prepubertal children with attention-deficit disorder with hyperactivity. Sleep 6:91–101, 1983

Guilleminault C: Narcolepsy and its differential diagnosis, in Sleep and Its Disorders in Children. Edited by Guilleminault C. New York, Raven, 1987, pp 181–194

Guilleminault C, Pelayo R: Narcolepsy in prepubertal children. Ann Neurol 43:135–142, 1998

Guilleminault C, Stoohs R: Obstructive sleep apnea syndrome in children. Pediatrician 17:46–51, 1990

Guilleminault C, Heinzer R, Mignot E, et al: Investigations into the neurologic basis of narcolepsy. Neurology 50 (suppl 1):S8–S15, 1998

Honda Y, Juji T, Matsuki K, et al: HLA-DR2 and Dw2 in narcolepsy and in other disorders of excessive somnolence without cataplexy. Sleep 9:133–242, 1986

Jouvet M, DeLorme F: Locus coeruleus et Sommeil paradoxical. C R Soc Biol (Paris) 159:895–899, 1965

Kales A (ed): Sleep: Physiology and Pathology. Philadelphia, PA, JB Lippincott, 1969

Kales A, Tan T: Sleep alterations associated with medical illnesses, in Sleep: Physiology and Pathology. Edited by Kales A. Philadelphia, PA, JB Lippincott, 1969, pp 148–157

Kaplan B, McNicol J, Conte R, et al: Sleep disturbances in preschool-aged hyperactive and nonhyperactive children. Pediatrics 80:839–844, 1987

Kataria S, Swanson MS, Trevathan GE: Persistences of sleep disturbances in preschool children. J Pediatr 110:642–646, 1987

Lumley M, Roehrs T, Askel D, et al: Ethanol and caffeine effects on daytime sleepiness/alertness. Sleep 10:306–312, 1987

Mahowald M, Rosen G: Parasomnias in children. Pediatrician 17:21–31, 1990

Mahowald M, Schenck C: Parasomnias including the restless legs syndrome. Clin Chest Med 19:183–202, 1998

Matsuki K, Honda Y, Juji T: Diagnostic criteria for narcolepsy and HLA-DR2 frequencies. Tissue Antigens 30:155–160, 1987

Mignot E: Genetic and familial aspects of narcolepsy. Neurology 50 (suppl 1):S16–S22, 1998

Mindell JA: Sleep disorders in children. Health Psychol 12:151–162, 1993

Moore T, Ucko L: Night waking in early infancy, I. Arch Dis Child 32:333–342, 1957

Navelet Y, Anders T, Guilleminault C: Narcolepsy in children, in Narcolepsy (Advances in Sleep Research, Vol 3). Edited by Guilleminault C, Dement W, Passouant P. Holliswood, NY, Spectrum, 1976, pp 171–177

Okawa M, Sasaki H: Sleep disorders in mentally retarded and brain impaired children, in Sleep and Its Disorders in Children. Edited by Guilleminault C. New York, Raven, 1987, pp 171–177

Owens JA, Spirito A, McQuinn M: The children's sleep habits questionnaire: psychometric properties of a survey instrument for school-aged children. Sleep 23:1043–1051, 2000

Roffwarg H, Muzio J, Dement W: Ontogenetic development of the human sleep–dream cycle. Science 152:576–582, 1966

Rye D, Johnston L, Watts R, et al: Juvenile Parkinson's disease with REM sleep behavior disorder. Neurology 63:1868–1870, 1999

Schenck C, Bundlie S, Patterson A, et al: Chronic behavior disorders in a 10-year-old girl and episodic REM and NREM sleep movements in an 8-year-old brother (abstract). Sleep Research 15:162, 1986

Schenck C, Boyd J, Mahowald M: A parasomnia overlap disorder involving sleep walking, sleep terrors, and REM sleep behavior disorder in 33 polysomnographically confirmed cases. Sleep 20:972–981, 1997

Sheldon S, Jacobsen J: REM-sleep motor disorder in children. J Child Neurol 13:257–260, 1998

Small A, Hibi S, Feinberg I: Effects of dextroamphetamine sulfate on EEG sleep patterns of hyperactive children. Arch Gen Psychiatry 25:369–380, 1971

Stores G: Dramatic parasomnias. J R Soc Med 94:173–176, 2001

Stores G, Wiggs L (eds): Sleep Disturbance in Children and Adolescents with Disorders of Development: Its Significance and Management (Clinics in Developmental Medicine Series, No 155). London, Mac Keith, 2001

Takahashi J: Narcolepsy genes wake up the sleep field. Science 285:2076–2077, 1999

Tanner J: Growth at Adolescence, 2nd Edition. Oxford, UK, Blackwell Scientific, 1962

Thorpy M, Korman E, Spielman A, et al: Delayed sleep-phase syndrome in adolescents. J Adolesc Health Care 9:22–27, 1988

Waterman G, Dahl R, Birmaher B, et al: The 24-hour pattern of prolactin secretion in depressed and normal adolescents. Biol Psychiatry 35:440–445, 1994

Wise M: Parasomnias in children. Pediatr Ann 26:427–433, 1997

Wise M: Childhood narcolepsy. Neurology 50 (suppl 1):S37–S42, 1998

Wolke D, Meyer R, Ohrt B, et al: The incidence of sleeping problems in preterm and fullterm infants discharged from neonatal special care units: an epidemiological longitudinal study. J Child Psychol Psychiatry 36:203–223, 1995

Zero to Three: Diagnostic Classification, 0–3: Diagnostic Classification of Mental Health and Developmental Disorders of Infancy and Early Childhood. Arlington, VA, Zero To Three, 1994

Zuckerman B, Stevenson J, Bailey V: Sleep problems in early childhood: continuities, predictive factors, and behavioral correlates. Pediatrics 80:664–671, 1987

Zucconi M, Ferine-Strambi L: NREM parasomnias: arousal disorders and differentiation from nocturnal frontal epilepsy. Clin Neurophysiol 111(suppl 2):S129–S135, 2000

Disorders of Elimination

Thomas Walsh, M.D.

Edgardo Menvielle, M.D.

The disorders of elimination—enuresis and encopresis—represent an inability to achieve or maintain control of bodily functions. These disorders are not uncommon and can cause significant distress for both the child and the family. The presenting symptoms of elimination disorders are seen by a variety of health professionals, occasionally as symptoms of other disorders. In this chapter we review the causes, sequelae, and treatment of each of these disorders.

Enuresis

Enuresis is the repeated involuntary or intentional discharge of urine beyond the expected age for controlling urination (in the absence of a definable physical disorder). According to DSM-IV-TR (American Psychiatric Association 2000), the disorder is present when voiding of urine occurs at least twice a week for at least 3 months or causes clinically significant distress or impairment in functioning (Table 39–1). Primary enuresis occurs in children who have never controlled their wetting for an extended period; secondary enuresis is the reemergence of wetting after a continuous period of control of 6 months or longer. Enuresis may be characterized as *nocturnal* (the most common), *diurnal* (more frequent in children younger than 5 years), and *mixed.*

■ Clinical Features

About 80% of patients with enuresis have primary enuresis. Left untreated, the remission rate is 10%–20% per year, which gradually increases with age. Primary enuresis therefore can be viewed as a self-limiting dis-

order, with enuresis continuing into adulthood in 1% of patients (Forsythe and Redmond 1974).

Although most children with enuresis do not have a coexisting psychiatric disorder, the prevalence of emotional-behavioral disorders is greater than in the general population (Friman et al. 1998; Rutter 1989). Associations have been demonstrated with attention deficit/hyperactivity disorder (Biederman et al. 1995) and with anxiety disorders, specifically selective mutism (Kristensen 2000). Coexisting disorders include encopresis and developmental delays. No association has been demonstrated between enuresis and tics, nail biting, temper tantrums, fire setting, or cruelty to animals (Felthous and Bernhard 1978; Oppel et al. 1968).

Psychosocial impairment in children with enuresis can result from the effect of enuresis on the child's self-esteem, the degree to which the disorder causes social isolation and ostracism by peers, and the negative response of caregivers (e.g., anger, punishment, and rejection). Impairment also may be a result of coexisting disorders. Although the number of enuretic children with coexisting emotional-behavioral problems is small, children for whom help is sought may have more behavioral symptoms (Couchells et al. 1981).

■ Differential Diagnosis

A diagnosis of enuresis assumes the absence of identifiable physical causes. Any condition causing increased urine output can cause enuresis; therefore, diabetes mellitus and diabetes insipidus must be considered, as well as increased fluid intake with psychogenic causes. Urinary tract infection, especially in girls, must be ruled out, as must seizure disorders, renal insufficiency,

Table 39–1. DSM-IV-TR diagnostic criteria for enuresis

A. Repeated voiding of urine into bed or clothes (whether involuntary or intentional).

B. The behavior is clinically significant as manifested by either a frequency of twice a week for at least 3 consecutive months or the presence of clinically significant distress or impairment in social, academic (occupational), or other important areas of functioning.

C. Chronological age is at least 5 years (or equivalent developmental level).

D. The behavior is not due exclusively to the direct physiological effect of a substance (e.g., a diuretic) or a general medical condition (e.g., diabetes, spina bifida, a seizure disorder).

Specify type:

Nocturnal Only
Diurnal Only
Nocturnal and Diurnal

Source. Reprinted from American Psychiatric Association: *Diagnostic and Statistical Manual of Mental Disorders,* 4th Edition, Text Revision. Washington, DC, American Psychiatric Association, 2000. Copyright 2000, American Psychiatric Association. Used with permission.

neurological disorders that affect bladder innervation, neuroleptic-induced enuresis, and urinary tract anatomical dysfunctions. All of these can be readily ruled out by careful clinical assessment based on history, physical examination, urinalysis, and urine culture when necessary, with further assessment only as clinically indicated.

■ Epidemiology

Enuresis is as common in girls as in boys between ages 4 and 6 years. Beyond that age range the difference in prevalence increases steadily; by age 11 boys are twice as likely as girls to be symptomatic. Nocturnal enuresis occurs in 15% of 5-year-olds, with a decrease of about 15% per year thereafter. At age 7, 15% of boys have involuntary wetting less often than once a week, and 7% have involuntary wetting at least once a week. Commonly, boys from the latter group are those referred for treatment (Shaffer 1985).

Approximately 75% of enuretic children have a first-degree relative with a history of enuresis. When both parents have a positive history, 77% of the children are enuretic; when one parent is affected, 44% of the children are enuretic (Bakwin 1973). The relationship of enuresis to a range of psychosocial factors—

including family, social, and economic background—once was thought to be significant but has since been questioned (Fergusson et al. 1986).

■ Etiology

No single cause of enuresis has been identified. Primary enuresis has been viewed as representing a maturational delay, with multiple factors contributing to this theory. Genetic studies have demonstrated a high incidence of enuresis in parents and siblings of bed wetters, with the suggestion of subtypes based on a variety of modes of genetic transmission (von Gontard et al. 1999). Investigation of the endogenous production of the antidiuretic hormone arginine vasopressin initially indicated that enuresis might be a result of a failure to achieve the expected diurnal variation of antidiuretic hormone (Medel et al. 1998; Norgaard et al. 1989). Although this has led to better understanding of the physiology of the disorder, the findings have been inconclusive. Physiological research has been extended to the role of urine osmolality and renal tubular function (Mikkelsen 2001).

Investigations of enuresis as a disorder of sleep have determined that no association exists between enuresis and any particular stage of sleep (Mikkelsen et al. 1980). A better understanding of the role of sleep may lead to the identification of subtypes of the disorder (Neveus et al. 1999). Enuresis has been related to abnormalities in bladder size, function, or anatomy, but these anatomical factors appear to account for only a minority of patients.

Secondary enuresis can be a manifestation of stress in children, especially those between ages 4 and 6 years. Environmental stressors, such as a move to a new home, birth of a sibling, hospitalization, or child abuse, may cause a transient regression in bladder control. Although there is no evidence to support the notion that enuresis has a symbolic meaning, a relationship can be found between psychiatric disorders and enuresis, with cause and effect being different in individual cases (Rutter 1989). In some children with daytime wetting, a lack of awareness of internal cues may be an etiological factor.

■ Treatment

Multiple treatment modalities exist for functional enuresis. However, one point is central to applying all modalities: enuresis is mostly a self-limited, benign disorder. It is necessary to provide reassurance and support to prevent secondary emotional effects on self-esteem and family relationships and to prevent shame and guilt from developing from the symptoms. Excessive investigation and overaggressive treatment of all types should be avoided.

Treatment should be preceded by a period of observation during which there is open discussion of the problem, tracking of symptoms by using a chart, and positive reinforcement of dry periods. Simple interventions such as late fluid restrictions and encouragement of nighttime urination may be tried. This pretreatment period sometimes produces significant and lasting remission of symptoms.

The most effective treatment for primary enuresis is the enuresis alarm, a conditioning device with an alarm triggered by the child's voiding. Various designs of this apparatus are available, ranging from the conventional bell and pad to more compact and sensitive systems. Explanations for the success of this treatment are based on behavioral theories—including classical conditioning, avoidance learning, and social learning—but these are not adequate explanations of its efficacy. The success rate for the enuresis alarm is good: 60%–80% of patients initially respond to the alarm, with some relapse. Because of the relapse rate, a second course of treatment is often necessary (Forsythe and Butler 1989). Dry bed training (including positive reinforcement for inhibiting urination, retention-control training, positive-practice nighttime awakening, cleanliness training, and aversive consequences) has been used but does not appear to be effective when used without the enuresis alarm (Butler 1998). For maximum effect, compliance in using the enuresis alarm must be addressed. When a family fails to continue using the alarm, the clinician must be sensitive to the family's difficulties in sustaining treatment and must offer guidance and support.

A number of pharmacologic agents have been used with some success to treat enuresis. Tricyclic antidepressants and desmopressin (deamino-8-D-arginine vasopressin [DDAVP]) have proved beneficial (Monda and Husmann 1995); stimulants, sedatives, and anticholinergic agents have not.

Tricyclic antidepressants, especially imipramine, have been widely studied and used in the treatment of enuresis (Bindelglas and Dee 1978; Fritz et al. 1994). The mechanism of action of imipramine is uncertain. Effective doses are in the 25–75-mg range, with a decrease in frequent wetting in most cases, but total re-mission in only about 30%; significant relapse occurs after discontinuing imipramine. Potential cardiac conduction abnormalities and other unwanted side effects and risk of fatal toxicity on overdose, intentional or otherwise, must be considered when using imipramine.

DDAVP, an analog of the antidiuretic hormone vasopressin, has been found to be effective in the treatment of enuresis and has replaced imipramine as the most-used pharmacologic agent (Thompson and Rey 1995). The postulated mechanism is decreased nighttime urine output to a point that does not exceed bladder capacity, thus eliminating nighttime wetting. DDAVP is administered in doses of 200–400 μg orally (20–40 μg intranasally) and produces a remission of symptoms comparable to that of imipramine with a similarly significant relapse rate (Hjalmas et al. 1998). The relatively rare occurrence of hyponatremia and possible seizures is a consideration in its use.

In general, pharmacologic interventions are useful when rapid, short-term relief from symptoms must be achieved, when symptoms become the source of conflict in relationships within a family, or when symptoms create or exacerbate maladaptive behavior in the child and other methods have failed.

The clinician's decision to treat is an important one for each child; the benefits need to justify a sometimes prolonged and complex treatment process. Because it appears that children have improved self-concept following successful treatment and that treatment failure does not have adverse emotional effects, treatment of this condition should be considered (Moffatt 1989).

■ Prognosis

Because enuresis is mostly self-limiting and effective treatment is available, prognosis is good. In children with coexisting disorders or significant secondary emotional complications, appropriate intervention is necessary for successful outcome.

Encopresis

According to DSM-IV-TR, encopresis is the repeated involuntary or intentional passage of feces into inappropriate places by children older than 4 years or with a mental equivalent to age 4 years. Encopresis is not exclusively due to the effect of a substance, such as a lax-

Table 39–2. DSM-IV-TR diagnostic criteria for encopresis

A. Repeated passage of feces into inappropriate places (e.g., clothing or floor) whether involuntary or intentional.

B. At least one such event a month for at least 3 months.

C. Chronological age is at least 4 years (or equivalent developmental level).

D. The behavior is not due exclusively to the direct physiological effects of a substance (e.g., laxatives) or a general medical condition except through a mechanism involving constipation.

Code as follows:

787.6   With Constipation and Overflow Incontinence
307.7   Without Constipation and Overflow Incontinence

Source. Reprinted from American Psychiatric Association: *Diagnostic and Statistical Manual of Mental Disorders*, 4th Edition, Text Revision. Washington, DC, American Psychiatric Association, 2000. Copyright 2000, American Psychiatric Association. Used with permission.

ative, or to a medical condition, except when medical conditions result in constipation. The frequency required to meet DSM-IV-TR criteria is at least one event per month for at least 3 months (Table 39–2).

■ Clinical Features

In primary encopresis, the disturbance is not preceded by a period of fecal continence; secondary encopresis is preceded by a period of fecal continence lasting at least 1 year. The secondary type may account for as many as 50%–60% of all cases (Walker et al. 1988). Different types of encopresis can be described based on the outcome of bowel training, awareness of defecation, presence of chronic constipation, and psychological precipitants of soiling episodes. In children who achieve adequate bowel control but who deposit feces in inappropriate places in response to family stress or as a purposeful act, the soiling episode may represent episodic behavioral disorganization or regression under stress or an act of defiance or reprisal toward caregivers. Children who have never achieved appropriate bowel control and who may have a history of inadequate, unsuccessful toilet training may be unaware of the soiling or may be aware but unable to control it.

Encopresis with constipation and overflow incontinence is the most common type (85%–95%). Children with this disorder either have never achieved bowel control or have achieved control but proper functioning is not maintained because of constipation leading to fecal impaction and overflow. This group has infrequent bowel movements and frequent accidents (often more than two a day) in the form of small stains of liquid stool (Doleys 1983; Levine 1982).

Cases not involving constipation and feces overflow are characterized by intentional depositing or smearing of feces in a prominent location. This type of encopresis is associated with defiant behaviors, that is, as a covert expression of anger. Smearing may occur accidentally in the child's attempt to clean or hide feces passed involuntarily.

Some children want to avoid embarrassing situations, and they may hide soiled clothes and deny the soiling, appearing mortified when the problem is discussed. Others appear either unconcerned, unaware, or indifferent to the offensive odor. Most children with functional encopresis do not appear to have significant behavioral problems (Gabel et al. 1986). However, the social ostracism that many children with encopresis experience may lead to low self-esteem and poor peer relationships. Because primary care providers may manage many cases of encopresis associated with underlying constipation, children who are referred to psychiatrists may represent either a more severely affected group or those who have comorbid behavior disorders (Friman et al. 1988).

■ Differential Diagnosis

Functional encopresis must be distinguished from structural organic causes of encopresis, such as aganglionic megacolon (Hirschsprung's disease). Although severe cases of aganglionic megacolon are detected soon after birth, mild cases may go undetected until later in life. Functional encopresis also should be distinguished from chronic or intermittent diarrhea due to organic disorders such as Crohn's disease or irritable bowel syndrome or the use of laxatives. A medical condition that causes constipation allows for a concurrent diagnosis of encopresis; however, the diagnosis is not warranted when fecal incontinence is related to nonconstipating conditions such as chronic diarrhea. A plain abdominal roentgenogram can aid diagnosis and management of encopresis (Rockney et al. 1995).

■ Epidemiology

Functional encopresis is estimated to affect between 1.5% and 7.5% of children of elementary school age

(Walker et al. 1988). This range of reported incidence results from the various diagnostic criteria used in these studies. In children, secondary encopresis rarely starts after age 8 years. Primary encopresis apparently is more common in lower socioeconomic classes and is three to four times more common in boys than in girls. It is generally believed that encopresis is underreported (Doleys 1983; Hersov 1985).

■ Etiology

No single pathophysiological or psychodynamic explanation accounts for all cases of encopresis. Combinations of maturational and psychosocial factors may be involved, including precipitating psychosocial stressors such as parental divorce, sibling rivalry, or starting school. In one case series of 63 children, boys with primary encopresis were more likely to have developmental delays and enuresis, whereas boys with secondary encopresis were more likely to have conduct disorders (Foreman and Thambirajah 1996).

Anismus, the lack of relaxation of the external anal sphincter during defecation, is observed in 75% of cases of encopresis (Sentovich et al. 1998). However, it remains unclear whether this neuromuscular dysfunction precedes or follows constipation. Chronic constipation may result from a combination of factors. The retention of feces may result from painful defecation because of an anal fissure, a struggle between the parent and the child over bowel training, or a phobic avoidance of the toilet based on a real or imaginary negative experience. Constipation leads to fecal impaction, and liquid feces tend to leak around the impaction. The child's attempts to prevent involuntary passage of feces by anal contraction may increase the amount of retained feces. With rectal distention, the internal anal sphincter becomes weak and underresponsive, and the sensation of passage of feces through the rectum decreases. The child may lose awareness of the passage of stools, and his or her sense of smell becomes habituated to the foul odor (this may be most relevant for older children who appear to lack an age-appropriate social concern). In primary encopresis, constipation is often established before the child has mastered bowel control skills.

Psychodynamic factors generally focus on the mother-child relationship or on a fixation on anal self-stimulation as a source of pleasure (Clarck et al. 1990). Proposed causes include rigid, perfectionist parents; coercive training; and the mother's ambivalence to-ward the child's need for autonomy (Anthony 1957; Easson 1960; Pinkerton 1958). Family-constellation factors—such as an uninvolved, passive father and a domineering, overinvolved, or depressed mother—have been implicated as well (Bemporad et al. 1971). Posttraumatic encopresis associated with anal sexual assault has been observed (Boon 1991).

■ Treatment

The goal of treatment is the child's regular independent use of the toilet and the resolution of coexisting problems. The therapeutic approach should be based on the type of encopresis, and medical, behavioral, and psychotherapeutic interventions should be used as indicated. Careful evaluation, including both medical and psychosocial assessment, and a period of observation to record soiling, accompanied by open discussion of the symptoms, should precede any intervention. Medical and behavioral interventions vary according to the characteristics of each child's soiling. The treatment principles for children who retain feces include educating the child and parents about the problem, disimpacting the bowel, and training the child in bowel control. Education about the symptom, the mechanism of retention, and the rationale for the intervention is used as the initial strategy to recruit both parent and child as active participants collaborating to solve the problem (Landman and Rappaport 1985).

A necessary medical intervention is to remove the blockage of feces in the bowel, which is usually done with laxatives or enemas. After the bowel is clean, several management measures are used to prevent reimpaction and to gain continence control (Seth and Heyman 1994). Diet modification with an increase in the child's intake of dietary fiber and water helps to facilitate bowel function and to prevent impaction. To increase the chance of bowel movements in the toilet utilizing the gastroileal reflex, 10-minute sittings 20 minutes after meals are prescribed. Appropriate bowel movements and accident-free days are reinforced through praise or tangible rewards. Aversive consequences for soiling accidents, such as showering and washing the soiled clothes, also reinforce the child's self-monitoring (Doleys 1983; Gerber and Meyer 1965; Houts and Peterson 1986; Young 1973). The initial promise of biofeedback therapy was not supported by subsequent studies that failed to demonstrate superiority to the conventional approach of catharsis, diet modification, educational intervention, and behavioral training (Loening-Baucke 1990, 1995; Nolan et al. 1998). Biofeedback may still have a use as an adjunctive treatment. Because of the chronic nature of constipation, ongoing medical management of recurring constipation may be required for months or years.

Pharmacologic agents may have some role in the treatment of nonretentive encopresis. Some studies have reported symptomatic improvement with imipramine and amitriptyline (Dossetor et al. 1998; Mikkelsen 1996). Tricyclic antidepressants exacerbate constipation and therefore are contraindicated in retentive encopresis.

When significant comorbid psychopathology is present in the individual and family, appropriate psychotherapeutic intervention is indicated. Associated psychopathology may be a factor in the etiology of encopresis, especially in children who have shown adequate bowel control. In other cases, psychopathology may result from the encopresis and may impede the effectiveness of bowel control training. Although psychiatric intervention may be needed to treat coexisting primary psychiatric disorders, psychotherapy may also be needed to treat secondary maladaptive patterns, even though self-esteem may improve with simple relief of the symptoms. Family therapy is useful when the child and family must disengage from interactions that perpetuate the problem (Margolies and Gilstein 1983–1984).

■ Prognosis

The prevalence of functional encopresis gradually declines from a peak at age 6 years in boys and 8 years in girls to almost complete disappearance by age 16 years in both boys and girls (Rex et al. 1992). Soiling at night is associated with a poorer prognosis than is soiling during the day. Other indicators of poor prognosis are nonchalant attitude, associated conduct problems, and soiling as an expression of aggression (Landman and Rappaport 1985; Levine 1982).

Research Issues

Compared with enuresis, there is a paucity of research on encopresis, possibly reflecting the relative rarity of encopresis (Mikkelsen 2001). Because maturational factors are so important in diagnosing both enuresis and encopresis, further research is needed to explore the relationship between the two, to define the pathophysiology of each, and to explore common links to other developmental disorders. In addition, the relationship between maturational and emotional factors needs further investigation. Because these disorders are treated by primary-care physicians, urologists, gastroenterologists, and psychiatrists, issues related to developing common definitions and integrated treatment approaches must be explored. More data need to be collected to understand whether the types of disorders treated differ among various practitioners and whether the various treatment approaches are efficacious.

References

American Psychiatric Association: Diagnostic and Statistical Manual of Mental Disorders, 4th Edition, Text Revision. Washington, DC, American Psychiatric Association, 2000

Anthony EJ: An experimental approach to the psychology of childhood: encopresis. Br J Med Psychol 30:146–175, 1957

Bakwin H: The genetics of enuresis, in Bladder Control and Enuresis. Edited by Kolvin L, MacKeith RC, Meadow SR. London, Heinemann Medical, 1973, pp 73–77

Bemporad JR, Pfeifer CM, Gibbs L, et al: Characteristics of encopretic patients and their families. J Am Acad Child Psychiatry 10:272–292, 1971

Biederman J, Santangelo SL, Faraone SV: Clinical correlates of enuresis in ADHD and non-ADHD children. J Child Psychol Psychiatry 36:865–877, 1995

Bindelglas PM, Dee G: Enuresis treatment with imipramine hydrochloride: a 10-year follow-up study. Am J Psychiatry 135:1549–1552, 1978

Boon F: Encopresis and sexual assault (letter). J Am Acad Child Adolesc Psychiatry 30:509–510, 1991

Butler RJ: Annotation: night wetting in children: psychological aspects. J Child Psychol Psychiatry 39:453–463, 1998

Clarck AF, Tayler PJ, Bhate SR: Nocturnal fecal soiling and anal masturbation. Arch Dis Child 65:1367–1368, 1990

Couchells SM, Johnson SB, Carter R, et al: Behavioral and environmental characteristics of treated and untreated enuretic children and matched nonenuretic controls. J Pediatr 99:812–816, 1981

Doleys DM: Enuresis and encopresis, in Handbook of Child Psychopathology. Edited by Ollendick TH, Hersen M. New York, Plenum, pp 201–226, 1983

Dossetor D, Stiefel I, Gomes L: A case of predominantly nocturnal soiling treated with amitriptyline. Eur Child Adolesc Psychiatry 7:114–118, 1998

Easson RL: Encopresis-psychogenic soiling. Can Med Assoc J 82:624–628, 1960

Felthous AR, Bernhard H: Enuresis, firesetting, and cruelty to animals: the significance of two-thirds of this triad. J Forensic Sci 45:240–246, 1978

Fergusson DM, Horwood LJ, Shannon FT: Factors related to the age of attainment of nocturnal bladder control: an 8-year longitudinal study. Pediatrics 78:884–890, 1986

Foreman DM, Thambirajah MS: Conduct disorder, enuresis and specific developmental delays in two types of encopresis: a case-note study of 63 boys. Eur Child Adolesc Psychiatry 5:33–27, 1996

Forsythe WL, Butler RJ: Fifty years of enuretic alarms. Arch Dis Child 64:879–885, 1989

Forsythe WL, Redmond A: Enuresis and spontaneous cure rate of 1,129 enuretics. Arch Dis Child 49:259–265, 1974

Friman PC, Mathews JR, Finney JW, et al: Do encopretic children have clinically significant behavioral problems? Pediatrics 82 (3 pt 2):407–409, 1988

Friman PC, Handwerk ML, Swerer SM, et al: Do children with primary nocturnal enuresis have clinically significant behavior problems? Arch Pediatr Adolesc Med 152:537–539, 1998

Fritz GK, Rockney RM, Yeung AS: Plasma levels and efficacy of imipramine treatment for enuresis. J Am Acad Child Adolesc Psychiatry 33:60–64, 1994

Gabel S, Hegeders AM, Wald A, et al: Prevalence of behavior problems and mental health utilization among encopretic children: implications for behavioral pediatrics. J Dev Behav Pediatr 7:293–297, 1986

Gerber H, Meyer V: Behavior therapy and encopresis: the complexities involved in treatment. Behav Res Ther 2:227–231, 1965

Hersov L: Faecal soiling, in Child and Adolescent Psychiatry: Modern Approaches, 2nd Edition. Edited by Rutter M, Hersov L. St. Louis, MO, CV Mosby, 1985, pp 482–489

Hjalmas K, Hanson E, Hellstrom AL, et al: Long-term treatment with desmopressin in children with primary monosymptomatic nocturnal enuresis: an open multicentre study. Swedish Enuresis Trial (SWEET) Group. Br J Urol 82:704–709, 1998

Houts AC, Peterson JK: Treatment of a retentive encopretic child using contingency management and diet modification with stimulus control. J Pediatr Psychol 11:375–383, 1986

Kristensen H: Selective mutism and comorbidity with developmental disorder/delay, anxiety disorder, and elimination disorder. J Am Acad Child Adolesc Psychiatry 39:249–256, 2000

Landman GB, Rappaport L: Pediatric management of severe treatment-resistant encopresis. J Dev Behav Pediatr 6:349–351, 1985

Levine MD: Encopresis: its potentiation, evaluation and alleviation. Pediatr Clin North Am 29:315–330, 1982

Loening-Baucke V: Modulation of abnormal defecation by biofeedback treatment in chronically constipated children with encopresis. J Pediatr 116:214–222, 1990

Loening-Baucke V: Biofeedback treatment for chronic constipation and encopresis in childhood, I: long-term outcome. Pediatrics 96:105–110, 1995

Margolies R, Gilstein K: A systems approach to the treatment of chronic encopresis. Int J Psychiatry Med 13:141–151, 1983–1984

Medel R, Dieguez S, Brindo M, et al: Monosymptomatic primary enuresis: differences between patients responding or not responding to oral desmopressin Br J Urol 81:46–49, 1998

Mikkelsen EJ: Modern approaches to enuresis and encopresis, sleep stage, and drug response, in Child and Adolescent Psychiatry, 2nd Edition. Edited by Lewis M. Baltimore, MD, Williams & Wilkins, 1996, pp 593–601

Mikkelsen EJ: Enuresis and encopresis: ten years of progress. J Am Acad Child Adolesc Psychiatry 40:1146–1158, 2001

Mikkelsen EJ, Rapoport JL, Nee L, et al: Childhood enuresis, I: sleep patterns and psychopathology. Arch Gen Psychiatry 37:1139–1145, 1980

Moffatt MEK: Nocturnal enuresis: psychologic implications of treatment and nontreatment. J Pediatr 114(4, pt 2): 697–704, 1989

Monda JM, Husmann DA: Primary nocturnal enuresis: a comparison among observation, imipramine, desmopressin acetate and bed-wetting alarm systems. J Urol 154:745–748, 1995

Neveus T, Hetta J, Cnattingius S, et al: Depth of sleep and sleep habits among enuretic and incontinent children. Acta Paediatr 88:748–752, 1999

Nolan T, Castro-Smith T, Coffey C, et al: Randomized control trial of biofeedback training in persistent encopresis with anismus. Arch Dis Child 79:131–135, 1998

Norgaard JP, Rittig S, Djurhuus JC: Nocturnal enuresis: an approach to treatment based on pathogenesis. J Pediatr 114 (4 pt 2):705–710, 1989

Oppel WC, Harper PA, Rider RV: Social, psychological and neurological factors associated with enuresis. Pediatrics 42:627–641, 1968

Pinkerton P: Psychogenic megacolon in children: the implications of bowel negativism. Arch Dis Child 33:371–398, 1958

Rex DK, Fitzgerald JF, Goulet RJ: Chronic constipation with encopresis persisting beyond 15 years of age. Dis Colon Rectum 35:242–244, 1992

Rockney RM, McQuade WH, Days AL: The plain abdominal roentgenogram in the management of encopresis. Arch Pediatr Adolesc Med 149:623–627, 1995

Rutter M: Isle of Wight revisited: twenty-five years of child psychiatric epidemiology. J Am Acad Child Adolesc Psychiatry 28:633–653, 1989

Sentovich SM, Kauffman SS, Cali RL: Pudendal nerve function in normal an encopretic children. J Pediatr Gastroenterol Nutr 26:70–72, 1998

Seth R, Heyman MB: Management of constipation and encopresis in infants and children. Gastroenterol Clin North Am 23:621–636, 1994

Shaffer D: Enuresis, in Child Psychiatry: Modern Approaches, 2nd Edition. Edited by Rutter M, Hersov L. Oxford, UK, Blackwell Scientific, pp 465–481, 1985

Thompson S, Rey JM: Functional enuresis: is desmopressin the answer? J Am Acad Child Adolesc Psychiatry 34:266–271, 1995

von Gontard A, Eiberg H, Hollmann E, et al: Molecular genetics of nocturnal enuresis: linkage to a locus on chromosome 22. Scand J Urol Nephrol Suppl 202:76–80, 1999

Walker CE, Milling L, Bonner B: Incontinence disorders: enuresis and encopresis, in Handbook of Pediatric Psychology. Edited by Routh D. New York, Guilford, pp 263–298, 1988

Young GC: The treatment of childhood encopresis by conditioned gastro-ileal reflex training. Behav Res Ther 11:499–503, 1973

Somatoform Disorders

Larry K. Brown, M.D.
Kristin Bruning, M.D.
Gregory K. Fritz, M.D.
David B. Herzog, M.D.

Since Socrates and Hippocrates, physicians have concerned themselves with the enigmatic interaction between psyche and soma. Lipowski (1977) noted that Hieronymus David Gaub, a professor of chemistry and medicine in Leiden in the mid-1700s, wrote, "The reason why a sound body becomes ill or an ailing body recovers very often lies in the mind. Contrariwise, the body can frequently both beget mental illness and heal its offspring" (p. 234). The term *psychosomatic* has since been used to categorize a number of disorders in which there appears to be a loss or alteration of physical function secondary to psychological factors (Graham 1985).

The psychosomatic movement began in Germany and Austria in the 1920s and 1930s in response to the increasing mechanization of medicine. Franz Alexander brought the psychosomatic movement to the United States from Germany and focused his psychoanalytical research energies on psychosomatic problems. Alexander's group studied patients with seven disorders (asthma, peptic ulcer, rheumatoid arthritis, ulcerative colitis, neurodermatitis, thyrotoxicosis, and essential hypertension) that had been identified in the past as the psychosomatic diseases. Each of the seven was postulated to have a specific psychodynamic conflict as its etiological base. For example, in asthma, strong, unconscious dependency wishes and a concomitant fear of separation were thought to constitute its psychological roots; the wheezing was seen as a suppressed cry for the mother. Alexander's (1950) "specificity theories" have received little empirical validation over the years, but the creativity of his concepts makes

his book *Psychosomatic Medicine: Its Principles and Applications* an enduring contribution to the field. At about the same time, Flanders Dunbar (1954) pursued her own specificity theory, in which she proposed that particular personality types characterized patients with a specific psychosomatic disease. Her description of the "ulcer personality," the "arthritic personality," and so on predated the currently postulated type A personality. In contrast to specificity theories, more recent studies have shown that the presence of a chronic illness in general, rather than characteristics of a specific disorder, accounts for much of the significant psychological variation between chronically ill and healthy children (Hilliard et al. 1985; Lavigne and Faier-Routman 1992).

Currently, psychosomatic theories of disease emphasize the complexity and nonlinearity of the mind–body relationship. Each chronic disease is seen as a heterogeneous entity comprising subforms, each with a different clinical picture. Individuals with the same disorder may vary genetically, physiologically, and psychologically. Their own reactions to the illness, their personal habits and behavior, and the reactions and behaviors of individuals in their social setting contribute to the predisposition, presentation, and course of the disease. The complexity of these relationships—as well as our relative ignorance about them—is highlighted by questions that commonly arise in consultation in pediatric units. Is a child at greater risk for illness if he or she is depressed or living in a home stressed by parental discord? How is the stress mediated? What are the interactive changes in neurotransmitters, neuroendocrine pathways, and immunologically related susceptibility? How do these factors interact with a child's genetic vulnerability to a chronic disease such as asthma (Mrazek et al. 1991) or diabetes mellitus (Brand et al. 1986; Johnson 1988)? Confusing the issue further is the fact that many children with organic disease have secondary emotional consequences that often lead to further physical consequences—for example, diabetic ketoacidosis resulting from poor compliance with treatment, "volitional" or "manipulative" asthma attacks (Matus 1981), or pseudoseizures. In addition, many children with psychiatric disorders also have multiple physical complaints. Livingston et al. (1988) found that between 25% and 39% of children admitted to a psychiatric hospital had physical symptoms, including headache, food intolerance, abdominal pain, nausea, and dizziness.

Biopsychosocial Model

The biopsychosocial model (Engel 1980) focused attention on interactions among all of the contextual levels in an illness, from the organ to the societal level. As vividly described by Engel, even something as apparently physical as a venipuncture interacts with the patient's psychological state (e.g., frustration, self-blame) and caregivers' attitudes and, in a spiral of interactions, ultimately affects further physical states, hospital course, and relations with peers and family. An understanding of these transactional effects requires that every illness be viewed as psychosomatic in nature. The complex interplay between mind and body is further reinforced by research in oncology, immunology, and wellness behavior that challenges conventional views of cause and effect. The vast majority of recent research has been conducted on adults and is summarized in the following paragraphs. These tantalizing findings provide many suggestive clues about the complicated relationship between the mind and body in children and adolescents.

Psychological forces, it is speculated, play important roles in a wide range of diverse major somatic illnesses, from cancer progression to immune functioning. For example, in a well-controlled follow-up study of women with metastatic breast cancer, Spiegel et al. (1989) found that psychotherapy could improve the quality and length of life for patients. At the 10-year follow-up of a random sample of 86 cancer patients,

the psychotherapy group had lived an average of 18 months longer than the control group.

Ader (1974) first presented data showing that immunological reactivity could be classically conditioned. Rats prone to develop autoimmune disease were given cyclophosphamide paired with a saccharin-flavored solution. The saccharin solution subsequently functioned as an immune suppressant. Data indicate that immune conditioning can also occur in humans (Smith and McDaniel 1983). In this research, psychological factors have been implicated in modifying the delayed hypersensitivity or tuberculin reaction. When tuberculin was substituted for saline in the saline bottle and was injected into the arms of adult volunteers who had previously received saline injections, the resulting hypersensitivity response was markedly diminished. It appears likely that the immune system is integrated with psychological processes and that this regulatory balance helps explain the effect of psychological factors in disease progression (Rogers 1989), although the role of psychological forces in the progression of human immunodeficiency virus (HIV) disease appears exceedingly complex (Saks et al. 1994). The converse—the extent to which immune functioning influences behavior—has received little exploration. A small study of adults with cancer found that depression was associated with elevated plasma levels of interleukin-6 (Musselman et al. 2001). Interleukin-6 is a proinflammatory cytokine that is believed to induce a syndrome of "sickness behavior" with many features of depression, such as anhedonia, fatigue, and anorexia. Thus, an altered immune response may influence psychiatric symptoms.

An example of immune–psychological relationships in humans is provided by research on the health implications of psychotherapy. In 45 children with a history of frequent upper respiratory tract infections, psychotherapy using relaxation exercises and guided imagery was associated with increases in secretory immunoglobulin A levels and decreases in symptoms of upper respiratory tract infections during the next year (Hewson-Bower and Drummond 2001). Pennebaker et al. (1988) asked healthy college students to write about either traumatic or trivial events for 4 days. Writing about a traumatic experience was associated with a decrease in health center use and an improvement in blastogenic response of T lymphocytes to two mitogens. These examples, and more detailed studies (Rogers 1989; Weiner 1989), illustrate the complex relationships between mind, brain, and body. Such research suggests not only that these relationships exist but that psychotherapy could be cost-effective in improving health care.

Stages of Psychosomatic Involvement

The biopsychosocial model emphasizes interactions at any level and in any direction among components. Linear cause-and-effect models do not adequately explain the diversity of findings described above. For many aspects of the interaction between psyche and soma, we do not yet know what questions to ask and have no valid and reliable biochemical, behavioral, or psychological measures. Studies tend to be retrospective and focus on numbers too small for multifactorial analysis; therefore, clinical judgment must be used to determine the importance of psychological involvement in each case (Esman et al. 1985). For the purpose of clinical practice, it is useful to delineate phases of the illness as 1) vulnerability to disease, 2) symptom onset, 3) recurrence, 4) chronicity of the disease state, and 5) adaptation or reaction to the illness. The extent to which psychological factors exert a significant influence on a particular illness phase will vary from patient to patient. Together, these influential factors constitute the psychosomatic component for an individual patient.

There is abundant evidence that certain behaviors increase one's vulnerability to future disease. The adverse health consequences of smoking, overeating, and drug abuse are recognized. In fact, the three leading causes of death in teenagers—accident, homicide, and suicide—are due to "behavioral misadventures" (Paulson 1988). The clear relationship between behavioral risks (needle sharing, unprotected sexual intercourse) and HIV infection is a current, poignant, and lethal example illustrating the importance of behavior in determining vulnerability to disease. A change in psychological state, even without altering observable behavior, may also influence health. Individuals who have experienced a major stress are more susceptible to illness. This relationship is clear in adults: changes in immune functioning have been documented following the death of a spouse (Rogers 1989). Similar immune changes in children can be presumed to occur after parental death or divorce or even after less significant but additive life upsets.

Biopsychological factors may precipitate the onset of a disorder or may influence the timing of symptom presentation. Failure to thrive in infancy secondary to mother–child attachment dysfunction is perhaps the clearest example (Benoit et al. 1989; Chatoor and Egan 1983). The types of attachment dysfunctions are varied and are largely nonspecific. During adolescence, the onset of eating disorders is undoubtedly a result of psychological, sociocultural, and biological forces (Herzog 1988; Yates 1989). The interaction between biological and psychological factors is highlighted by the fact that one-third to one-half of young women who develop anorexia cease to menstruate before significant weight loss occurs (Halmi 1974). One study emphasizes the impact that family stress has on those at risk for subsequent illness. In a longitudinal study of 150 children at genetic risk for asthma, the development of asthma by age 2 years was significantly associated with early problems in maternal coping and parenting (Mrazek et al. 1991).

Psychological dysfunction may increase the recurrence of illness. In teenagers with diabetes mellitus, stress has been associated with poor short-term (fasting blood sugar) and long-term (glycosylated hemoglobin) measures of glucose control (Hanson and Pichert 1986; Schwartz et al. 1986). In children with asthma, psychological stress sometimes precipitates asthma attacks, and reports of childhood fatalities reveal the frequent emotional triggers of episodes in those patients (Fritz et al. 1987). Similarly, some skin disorders, particularly atopic dermatitis, are thought to multiply because of genetic factors, increases in immunoglobulin E antibodies, and emotional precipitants. Flare-ups in dermatitis often occur in conjunction with emotionally stressful periods, perhaps mediated by the immune system (Engels 1982). In hemophilia, high emotional arousal can increase the tendency for bleeding, apparently without trauma. Whether this tendency is due to changes in the vascular bed caused by neuroendocrine changes or is due to inadvertent, unrecognized self-injury is unclear (Mattson and Kim 1982).

Psychological factors can sustain chronic illnesses by a diverse set of mechanisms. When there is a common underlying biological dysfunction, psychological factors may act synergistically with the physical factors. In addition, psychological factors may influence patient or family noncompliance with the medical regimen, resulting in increased morbidity. Depression and asthma, for example, have both been associated with relative increases in cholinergic activity (Nadi et al. 1984). In severe depression, the increased activity has been reported in metabolites of central cholinergic neurotransmitters; in asthma, increased peripheral parasympathetic tone results in bronchoconstriction. A similar imbalance in both conditions could account for the worsening of both states concurrently and additively. One study demonstrated that for children with asthma, increased emotional reactivity (assessed after they viewed the movie *E.T.*) was associated with increased airway reactivity and decreased pulmonary functioning, consistent with mediation by cholinergic pathways (Miller and Wood 1994). In patients with cystic fibrosis, the family and health care staff must pay substantial attention to diet (Roy et al. 1984). For a small group of teenage girls with cystic fibrosis, the disease interacts with their developing self-image and eating behavior to produce an atypical eating disorder, further complicating treatment of the original medical disorder (Pumariega et al. 1986).

Somatoform disorders, sometimes labeled functional disorders, have psychological components that affect the recurrence and maintenance of symptoms (Bernstein et al. 1997; Fritz et al. 1997; Herzog and Harper 1981). A study by Campo and Fritsch (1994) reported that although unexplained disabilities are frequent in childhood, children's symptoms seldom met the necessary DSM-III-R (American Psychiatric Association 1987) criteria for somatization disorder. Another study identified somatizers in a cohort of 21,000 children in pediatric care and found that somatizers were at risk for psychiatric disorders, family dysfunction, functional impairment, and frequent use of health services (Campo et al. 1999). Children with recurrent abdominal pain, for example, continue complaining of pain despite the absence of indications of organic etiology after comprehensive pediatric evaluations (Ernst et al. 1984; Hodges et al. 1984; McGrath et al. 1983). For some children, abdominal pain may be present only during the day, preventing school attendance and secondarily impairing peer relationships. These children may have emotional conflicts in the intrapsychic, dyadic, or family arena. If a child's illness serves to resolve an intrapsychic conflict, the child will seem too ready to accept the consequences of the illness. If there is an unconscious dyadic purpose, then the illness will lead to increased, often regressive, enmeshment between a parent (often the mother) and the child. If symptoms of the illness arise among family tensions, then the parents will unite by focusing too narrowly on the child's medical needs. All these solutions to intrapsychic and interpersonal conflicts prevent anger, sadness, and disclosure of secrets, but at the price of normal development and the risk of medical intervention.

Psychological Aspects of Chronic Disease and Their Impact on Development

For the child and family, chronic disease is experienced as a major loss that has a substantial impact on day-to-day life. The impact of the disease varies by the child's age, the nature of the illness, and the secondary effects on family life (Geist 1979; Knapp and Harris 1997, 1998; Taylor 1985). In the following discussion, we summarize the psychological aspects of specific chronic illnesses and the potential psychological consequences of having a chronic illness during different phases of development.

■ Chronic Disease

The toddler with a serious seizure disorder faces daily medication, restricted activities, low self-esteem (e.g., because of the stigma of a helmet), and learning difficulties either because of the seizures or as a side effect of the medication. For a young child, seizures may limit activities and peer interactions. Instead of having school as a place to build self-esteem and social skills, every day may be a struggle to gain self-confidence and not feel inferior or rejected. For an adolescent, the years of being supported and sheltered by the family give way to the desperate need for autonomy and acceptance by peers. Seizures are frightening to the adolescent trying to achieve a sense of autonomy and control and to peers who think their friend may suddenly die before their eyes. Seizure disorders interrupt common but critical activities such as driving a car. The medications may seem a burden—a daily symbol of inferiority and of being different.

The child with diabetes is faced with daily injections, diet restrictions, and blood testing (Feinkelstein 1986). The very young diabetic patient needs to gain the earliest sense of autonomy in the midst of "good control" of his or her blood sugar level. Parents are forced by the illness to be more involved at every developmental stage of childhood than otherwise would be dictated. Parents must cope with their own feelings about control and of guilt for passing on the genetic vulnerability. They are faced with numerous questions: How should they instill the needed discipline? How much is needed? How responsible will they feel when their child becomes ketotic or hypoglycemic? How can they help their adolescent face the limits of diabetes amid the developmental need for power and limitlessness? How can they best prevent or delay and then help their child and themselves adjust to complications and permanent limitations? A recent study that underscores the importance of family factors found better glycemic control among preadolescents in families with a parenting style characterized by warmth and support rather than by restrictiveness (Davis et al. 2001).

Cystic fibrosis presents a different set of challenges (Drotar et al. 1981). For all but the most severely affected children, the diagnosis is made early, followed by a long period of good health. Nevertheless, this long grace period depends on frequent physical therapy, an exercise program, and multiple medications. Sustained parental involvement is required: parents take on the role of physical therapist several times a day, cheerleader during exercise that by adolescence is a burdensome reminder of respiratory limitations, and pharmacist for the dozen or more pills needed every day. Even family functioning during mealtime may be different because of the explicit dietary guidelines for cystic fibrosis than in families without the illness (Spieth et al. 2001). Although antibiotic therapy and nutrition are increasing the life expectancy of children with cystic fibrosis so that many will live into their 20s and 30s, older adolescents face noisy breathing, shortness of breath, repeated hospitalizations, hemoptysis, and deaths of clinic friends.

Children with cancer are faced with the overall life-and-death struggle, the intense sickness with repeated chemotherapy, and the dread of recurrence (Selter 1990).

Those with inflammatory bowel disease have a fear of embarrassment, a need to be near a bathroom, extended bouts of pain, and the likely prospect of major surgery.

For many families, the stresses of illness are sadly compounded by the burdens of repeated hospitalizations and multiple medications. Remarkably, most children who are given information, empathic care, and parental support adapt very well to these burdens of their illness. Although regression, depression, poor

compliance, and anger or frustration may ensue in times of stress, children with chronic disease can continue their emotional development with remarkably little dysfunction. Orr et al. (1984) found that most children with chronic disease did well psychosocially but that those with ongoing impairment were at higher risk for dysfunction. Studies of specific disorders, such as diabetes (Frisch and Bode 1990) and cystic fibrosis (Khaw 1990), show only a mildly increased risk of psychosocial dysfunction. Psychosocial follow-up studies, however, report difficulties in measuring intrapsychic distress, self-esteem, and social functioning. School grades or attendance records are convenient but superficial measures; assessing peer relationships, self-esteem, or the deeper emotional effect of the disease on the child and family is methodologically more difficult.

■ Illness at Developmental Levels

The child's level of psychosocial development influences reactions to a new illness or the progression of a chronic disorder. More detailed reviews show the relationship between developmental stage and chronic illness (McCollum 1981) and acute hospitalization (Mrazek 1986). The nature and extent of reaction are impossible to predict. No single factor causes poor adjustment, and in fact most children and families continue to function well (Pless and Pinkerton 1975; Stabler 1988).

Severe illnesses in infants may produce intense emotional reactions in new parents at the same time they are trying to become a family. Parents with little child-rearing experience have great difficulty separating problems with their baby into illness-related and normal disturbances. In some cases, the predictable guilt, horror, and disbelief associated with illness or handicap in an infant can damage parent–child attachment, leading to chronic dysfunction. Ultimately, adaptation is generally good, and some follow-up studies of cancer survivors have found that the earlier the illness, the better the long-term functioning (Koocher et al. 1980).

Preschoolers are verbal and increasingly motoric. Chronic illnesses and repeated hospitalizations restrict activities and may impair early, needed socialization experiences. Because of preschoolers' egocentrism, illnesses may be psychologically associated with a sense of wrongdoing or punishment. At the same time, parents may become confused about the degree of strictness to use with an ill child. Misbehavior, which normally emerges in this stage, may become extreme, or the wish to be naughty may be overly controlled in the "perfect" child. In both cases, the usual balanced internalization of family rules has been interrupted.

Latency-age children use causal thinking and are more observant of their own bodily reactions. Consequently, they can understand their illness in some logical detail. However, dramatic misconceptions can result if professionals are not careful to use developmentally appropriate words; for example, a frightened boy in the X-ray department thought the computed axial tomography (CAT) scanner contained a ferocious feline. When children reach latency age, their reports of symptoms are increasingly used to make treatment decisions. Research with asthmatic children has shown a high degree of variation among individuals in their ability to perceive accurate changes in peak flow rate (Fritz et al. 1990). The accuracy of these children may be influenced by their cognitive level and by emotional factors. A sense of mastery and achievement, especially in school, is usually acquired by children at this age. Illness that interferes with school peformance or disrupts normal peer activities can damage selfesteem. For latency-age children who are ill, efforts to improve academics (e.g., tutoring, teacher conferences, or neuropsychiatric assessment) or to enhance allowed physical activities (e.g., noncontact sports for hemophilia patients) may prove beneficial.

In teenagers, illnesses can affect their autonomy, physical-sexual development, and peer relationships. Illness can force dependence on parents and physicians to a degree not found in healthy teenagers. The perception by adults of immaturity (because of delayed growth in secondary sexual characteristics) can reinforce this dependence. Compliance problems often result when the illness and its treatment affect a teenager's struggle for independence. Full autonomy actually enhances adoption of reasonable therapeutic goals. For example, one study showed that compliance with salicylate therapy in teenagers with rheumatoid arthritis increases with better-developed autonomy (Litt et al. 1982). Physical and sexual maturation may be delayed by chronic illness. Boys who are late in developing are rated as less mature, popular, or confident than their peers; for girls, being more confident is associated with maturing at the same rate as their peers (Gross and Duke 1980). Many reports document the tendency of healthy people to ignore the emerging sexuality of those with physical disabilities. Being treated as asexual can greatly inhibit sexual exploration. The importance of adequate, timely medical care to sexual development is highlighted in a follow-up report of 80 women with congenital adrenal hyperplasia (Mulaikal et al. 1987). Of patients whose vaginal reconstruction had resulted in an inadequate introitus, 64% had not had any sexual experiences, compared with 23% in those with an adequate repair.

Adolescents with HIV infection proceed with sexual development in the context of a chronic, lethal sexually transmitted illness associated with societal stigma and multiple losses within families (Brown et al. 2000). Adaptation to the illness may be disrupted by unresolved anger (Brown et al. 1995). To cope, some HIV-infected teenagers avoid sex, and others engage in high-risk behaviors.

The family's reactions to an ill child are equally complex and depend on prior family patterns, coping styles, and experiences with illness. Fear, anger, loneliness, and guilt seem to be universal feelings (Featherstone 1980). Marital strain seems inevitable, and some research (Breslau and Davis 1986) has found a greater rate of divorce and depressive symptoms in mothers of children with chronic illness. For many illnesses, such as cancer and acquired immunodeficiency syndrome (AIDS), the ambiguities of diagnosis and treatment coupled with social stigma are unsettling (Comaroff and Maguire 1981; Krener and Miller 1989). When children have an acute illness, their siblings can be relatively neglected by parents and health care workers. Feelings of jealousy, overprotectiveness, and survival guilt are common among siblings of ill children. Often the needs and concerns of siblings are overlooked by health-care providers. Fortunately, some programs have been developed for the families of chronically ill children that focus on the reactions and concerns of siblings (Lobato and Kao, in press). It is to be hoped that more of these programs will be developed and will become a routine part of care for children with chronic illness.

Assessment

A comprehensive medical examination assesses the role of psychological factors in the course of a chronic illness or the occurrence of a physical symptom. The psychological component of the diagnostic process should be as important as physical and laboratory components. The psychological component should be introduced directly as a relatively routine part of the process, and this component should take place concurrently with other diagnostic studies rather than be withheld as a last resort. The nature of psychosomatic interactions dictates that physicians involved in the comprehensive evaluation communicate effectively with one another before, during, and after the diagnostic process. This fact seems too obvious to emphasize, but adequate communication is hardly the rule in most settings.

The child psychiatrist assessing psychosocial factors in a pediatric patient must keep several principles in mind. First, a significant psychosomatic element is possible in every disorder; there are no diagnostic categories that, when discovered, rule out an associated major psychological component. Second, even in diseases in which psychosocial factors have been widely recognized, such as asthma, diabetes, and ulcerative colitis, it is possible for the psychological components to be minimally important for a particular child's illness. Individuals, not disorders, have psychosomatic relationships. Third, a lack of satisfying findings on physical or laboratory examination is not adequate evidence for ascribing a psychological explanation to a specific case. Psychiatric examination should identify a combination of intrapsychic and environmental factors of sufficient magnitude and likelihood to affect the course of the disorder before psychosocial intervention is undertaken. Finally, a lack of typical major psychopathology diagnosable in either the child or the family does not preclude the possibility that psychological factors are influencing the illness to a significant degree.

The child psychiatrist's approach to the family must be gentle, patient, and nonconfrontational. Rather than etiology, the consequences of the disorder and the dysfunction should be the focus. The pediatric follow-up and diagnostic workup should continue at an appropriate level of intensity and invasiveness. Ancillary medical services, such as dietetics or physical therapy, should be used to treat the symptoms. At a minimum, such medical treatment gives the child respect, understanding, and a way to form an alliance with mental health professionals without acknowledging an exclusively psychological explanation. Sometimes, there is tension during the evaluation because the family considers the psychiatric assessment as an indicator that their primary care physician or even subspecialist has missed a causative factor. Parents may press for further medical diagnostic procedures. Every test cannot be done, and the broader pediatric or psychiatric examination may be conducted amid nagging doubts. Children and families may be reluctant to talk about psychological issues if they express emotional conflicts in actions, symptoms, and dysfunctions rather than words. "Doctor shopping" is common and often ignores the needs of the child.

Psychological evaluation of a child with a physical illness entails essentially the same thorough approach described in Part II of this volume, with an additional focus on the assessment of somatic symptoms. Especially important in the history is a chronology of the relationship between physical symptoms and emotional or stressful periods. Having the child or parents keep a journal in which daily entries track important variables can be an asset in understanding a complicated picture. Standard assessment instruments, which are becoming increasingly common in psychiatric practice, may be of limited use with children who are physically ill, because disease-related symptoms (e.g., fatigue, somatic concerns, sleep disturbances, medication side effects) complicate efforts to quantify psychological phenomena such as depression and anxiety. However, several questionnaires have been developed specifically for assessing children and families with medical problems, and they may be useful in the evaluation process. Examples include the following:

- *The Eating Attitudes Test* (Garner and Garfinkel 1979) is a 40-item measure of the symptoms of eating disorders that is readily applicable in a clinical setting.
- *The High Sensitivity Cognitive Screen* (Faust and Fogel 1989) is a 20-minute interview-based test designed to detect subtle or delineated cognitive deficits in an assessment short of formal neuropsychological examination. This test is useful for patients age 13 years and older.
- *The Coping Health Inventory for Parents* (McCubbin et al. 1983) is an 80-item checklist on which parents report their responses to the management of family life with a chronically ill child. Different coping patterns are quantified.
- *The Varni-Thompson Pediatric Pain Questionnaire* (Thompson and Varni 1986) is an instrument developed to quantify pain in children. Easy to administer at the bedside, the questionnaire is an adjunct to clinical assessment.

In addition to these and other standardized questionnaires, physiological measures can be helpful in the psychosomatic assessment of specific children. Examples include pulmonary function testing (especially the peak flowmeter used at home), ambulatory electroencephalogram monitoring (used to distinguish various types of seizure disorders and pseudoseizures), and videotaping at home to record unusual episodes or symptoms.

Treatment

The early specificity theorists were motivated by the hope that if they could identify a psychological etiology for a psychosomatic disease, then psychological therapy could treat or cure it. Psychoanalysis and dynamic psychotherapy proved not to be as effective as expected. It remains true that the multifactorial etiology of chronic illness means that even intensive psychological intervention will not "cure" the disorder. However, a number of approaches are available to the child psychiatrist that, singly or in combination, can be of major benefit to patients with a particular illness. These interventions are described in order of increasing intensity and investment of time and money (Fritz 1983).

■ Education

The most straightforward psychologically based intervention to modify the psychosomatic component of an illness is education. Misunderstanding, nonadherence to the regimen, poor judgment about symptom management, and faulty communication with medical professionals frequently contribute to much of the morbidity associated with chronic pediatric illnesses. Therefore, effective education is increasingly seen as worthwhile and cost-effective for patients and their families. Formal educational programs; educational tapes, books, and coloring books; computer programs; and videotapes have been developed for many chronic illnesses, although their availability is uneven. In more recent years, the Internet has become a rich source for educational and therapeutic resources for children with chronic illness and their families. Internet chat rooms exist whereby patients with an illness can communicate on-line with others who have the same ailment. Starbright is an especially innovative Internet-based program that is available in many children's hospitals.

This program enables a child, while hospitalized, to communicate in real time and to see the other child on the computer monitor. In addition, such programs help decrease the sense of aloneness and isolation that many children with severe chronic medical illness experience.

Child psychiatrists consulting on pediatric units frequently encounter patients whose understanding of their illness and its treatment is inadequate. Arranging for the appropriate education is a critical step toward improving the child's situation. Educational programs for chronically ill children and their parents should strive to make them experts on their illness (consistent with levels of development) to help them become sophisticated partners with the physician in managing the illness, minimizing morbidity, and maximizing normal functioning. Guidance can be provided on stress management, environmental manipulation, communication with physicians, and peer contact.

■ Consultation

Adding to the complexity of the evaluation and treatment plan is the child psychiatrist's relationship with the referring pediatrician. The families of children with functional disorders, for example, may have intimidated one or more pediatricians and may have refused previous child psychiatric referrals. The pediatrician's first call often is marked by frustration and requests for help in convincing the family to accept a referral. The following eight suggestions may be useful for clinicians working with families who resist psychiatric evaluation:

1. Avoid making a final etiological diagnosis. The pediatrician should suggest that both the physical and the psychological components require further exploration.
2. Focus on the psychosocial history, common sources of stress, family psychiatric history, and emotional consequences of the dysfunction. By gathering sufficient detailed information, the pediatrician may be able to identify clear psychological needs that are quite distinct from the symptoms.
3. Suggest focusing on dysfunction rather than diagnosis. Thus, the child psychiatric evaluation is justified clearly by the dysfunction rather than by the etiology.
4. Suggest patience, with the hope that time will foster a sufficient relationship.

5. Suggest an "if…, then…" approach. The pediatrician should note concern and doubt about future diagnostic procedures but willingness to pursue additional noninvasive efforts. The family should agree in advance to accept a referral if this last round of diagnostic test results are negative.

6. Initiate the child psychiatric consultation on day 1 if pediatric hospitalization is necessary. Delaying a child psychiatric evaluation until the other workups have been completed communicates to the family that the child psychiatric evaluation is a last resort, not as important as the other referrals, and, given the short length of stay, not a priority.

7. Some families, despite the best efforts of both the pediatrician and the child psychiatrist, refuse the referral. The pediatrician should recognize that this refusal is part of the family's problem and not a reflection of the pediatrician's competency.

8. In some extreme cases, the pediatrician may need to express concern that the child may be at risk for abuse if the family continues to pursue high-risk, invasive evaluations. Rarely, referral to the state social services department is the only approach that will protect the child from needless surgery.

If the pediatrician makes a successful referral, then prompt action and careful communication are essential. In outpatient settings, the child psychiatrist should call the pediatrician and discuss the key stages of the assessment process. For inpatient consultations, the child psychiatrist should suggest a team meeting involving himself or herself, the primary care nurse, pediatrician, ancillary medical services such as physical therapy, and house staff (Fritz 1990). Bringing the team together and developing a comprehensive, unified, structured treatment plan is helpful to the child and family in following through with treatment efforts. A breakdown in communication or the family's poor compliance with a treatment plan is a serious concern that should be addressed immediately. Ignoring such signals leads to discharges against medical advice, time-consuming arguments among the team, and, ultimately, poor care of the child.

■ Outpatient Psychosomatic Intervention

Outpatient psychiatric intervention is recommended for a substantial group of patients seen in consultation. The mode of treatment is determined on an individual basis; no particular disorder implies or rules out a given intervention.

Individual and family therapy are commonly used in treating psychosomatic problems as well as psychiatric disorders. However, the therapist must remember several caveats when beginning therapy with a child who has a chronic pediatric illness and his or her family. First, the therapist must respect the reality of the medical situation. Although intrapsychic factors are always relevant, the stressors associated with a chronic or potentially fatal illness should not be underestimated or minimized. Second, the therapist must respect the need for somatic language and symptoms. When outpatient therapy does not "take" with psychosomatic cases, the problem often results from language differences between the therapist, who uses psychological language, and the patient and family, who think and speak in terms of physical illness, medical problems, and somatic dysfunction. Confronting this somatic disposition early in therapy and attempting to deal with the "real" or underlying issues can often lead to the patient feeling misunderstood or out of place. Finally, the therapist must respect the patient's creativity in discovering coping solutions. The same standards used for judging mental health, defenses, and developmental progression that have evolved for physically healthy children often do not apply or are only partially relevant to children with chronic illness.

Behavioral techniques are being used more frequently for children with chronic illnesses. Relaxation training is the most common of these, and it has been applied in treating a number of chronic disorders, including asthma, pain syndromes, cystic fibrosis, and cancer. The usefulness of relaxation training is disputed because outcome studies vary in the results they report (Erskine and Schonell 1979; Richter and Dahme 1982). The major concern about relaxation training is the clinical relevance of small but statistically significant changes in a given psychological parameter. When biofeedback is added to the relaxation training—typically, information on frontalis muscle tension is provided—the result may be improved. Cognitive-behavioral therapy, which adds coping skill and behavior shaping to relaxation techniques, is a well-established treatment for procedure-related pain (Powers 1999). Behavior therapy with contingent reinforcement is also used to enhance compliance and to reduce the illness behavior that impairs functioning. The behavioral approaches have been so generally effective that most large pediatric centers use health care psychologists working in conjunction with psychiatrists.

The patient's school life may be compromised by a variety of factors operative in chronic illness: frequent school absence, cognitive impairment, disfigurement, or delay in physical maturation. The psychiatrist's contact with school personnel must be active, ranging from telephone contact to teacher conferences to planning an educational program on chronic illness for classmates of the patient (Henning and Fritz 1983). A current example of community alarm and anxiety associated with pediatric illness is reentry into the classroom by children with HIV infection. Physician involvement can decrease fear regarding the initial case and can include, as a primary prevention, helping schools plan for longer-range issues and consulting with school personnel regarding appropriate curriculum development (Brown and Fritz 1988).

■ Inpatient Psychosomatic Treatment

Hospitalization on a pediatric psychosomatic unit, the most intensive psychological intervention for treating children with chronic illness, has been described in detail by Steiner et al. (1982). The service is designed for patients with symptoms that disrupt development and are refractory to outpatient medical and psychological interventions. The staffs of acute pediatric wards usually have neither the time nor the training to attend to the psychological complexities these cases present. Similarly, the staffs of most psychiatric wards cannot provide the acute medical care needed to manage the medical crises or provide the medical treatment that various chronic illnesses require. The psychosomatic unit provides daily group and individual therapy; a highly structured milieu that incorporates behavior-modification approaches, such as contracting and a token economy; and frequent family sessions. The specific goals and therapeutic strategies are individually tailored, and close communication between pediatricians and psychiatrists is assiduously maintained. Psychosomatic inpatient units are now common in many medical centers, and they have made an important contribution to the care of children with psychosomatic disorders.

Research Issues

Although the future promises a greater understanding of the treatment of psychological aspects of chronic ill-ness, future treatments are also likely to be more complex than those currently in use. In addition to what is already known about psychodynamics and family systems, there will be major contributions from the fields of genetics, endocrinology, and immunology. Studies on depression, alcoholism, and attention-deficit/hyperactivity disorder have found strong genetic factors, suggesting that the transmission of somatic vulnerabilities goes beyond psychological identification and includes a major genetic component. Research on the interaction of endocrinologic and immunological humoral factors means that we are likely to redefine our views on most of the disorders currently thought to be psychosomatic and on some that now are considered purely organic (Olweus et al. 1988). The hint of what is to come may be evident in research on the suppression of immunological function in depressed adults (O'Donnell et al. 1988). Obviously, more research is needed to confirm and expand these findings and to determine whether they apply to children. Other areas in need of further investigation include the impact of cultural and ethnic factors on somatic presentation and disease management. In the book *The Spirit Catches You and You Fall Down* (Fadiman 1997), the clash between traditional Hmong culture and modern Western medicine is poignantly demonstrated through the story of a girl with a seizure disorder. Another resource concerning the influence of different cultural backgrounds on treatment is the landmark book *Ethnicity and Family Therapy* (McGoldrick et al. 1982). Future research integrating contributing environmental factors such as stress, the parents' behavior, and the child's personality and development will continue to challenge the child psychiatrist functioning as researcher, consultant, or clinician.

References

Ader R: Behaviorally conditioned immunosuppression (letter). Psychosom Med 36:183–184, 1974

Alexander F: Psychosomatic Medicine: Its Principles and Applications. New York, WW Norton, 1950

American Psychiatric Association: Diagnostic and Statistical Manual of Mental Disorders, 3rd Edition, Revised. Washington, DC, American Psychiatric Association, 1987

Benoit D, Zeanah C, Barton M: Maternal attachment disturbances in failure to thrive. Infant Ment Health J 10:185–202, 1989

Bernstein G, Massie E, Thras P, et al: Somatic symptoms in depressed school refusers. J Am Acad Child Adolesc Psychiatry 36:661–668, 1997

Brand AH, Johnson JH, Johnson SB: Life stress and diabetic control in children and adolescents with insulin-dependent diabetes. J Pediatr Psychol 11:481–495, 1986

Breslau N, Davis G: Chronic stress and major depression. Arch Gen Psychiatry 43:309–314, 1986

Brown LK, Fritz GK: AIDS education in the schools: literature review as a guide for curriculum planning. Clin Pediatr (Phila) 27:311–316, 1988

Brown LK, Schutz JR, Gragg RA: HIV-infected adolescents with hemophilia: adaptation and coping. Pediatrics 96:459–463, 1995

Brown LK, Lourie KJ, Pao M: Children and adolescents living with HIV and AIDS: a review. J Child Psychol Psychiatry 41:81–96, 2000

Campo JV, Fritsch SL: Somatization in children and adolescents. J Am Acad Child Adolesc Psychiatry 33:1223–1235, 1994

Campo JV, Jansen-McWilliams L, Comer DM, et al: Somatization in pediatric primary care: association with psychopathology, functional impairment, and use of services. J Am Acad Child Adolesc Psychiatry 38:1093–1101, 1999

Chatoor I, Egan J: Nonorganic failure to thrive and dwarfism due to food refusal: a separation disorder. J Am Acad Child Psychiatry 22:294–301, 1983

Comaroff J, Maguire P: Ambiguity and the search for meaning: childhood leukemia in the modern clinical context. Soc Sci Med 15:115–123, 1981

Davis CL, Delamater AM, Shaw KH, et al: Parenting styles, regimen adherence, and glycemic control in 4- to 10-year-old children with diabetes. J Pediatr Psychol 26:123–129, 2001

Drotar D, Doershuk CF, Stern RC, et al: Psychosocial functioning of children with cystic fibrosis. Pediatrics 67:338–343, 1981

Dunbar F: Emotions and Bodily Changes. New York, Columbia University Press, 1954

Engel G: The clinical application of the biopsychosocial model. Am J Psychiatry 137:535–544, 1980

Engels W: Dermatologic disorders. Psychosomatics 23:1209–1219, 1982

Ernst AR, Routh DK, Harper DC: Abdominal pain in children and symptoms of somatization disorder. J Pediatr Psychol 9:77–86, 1984

Erskine J, Schonell M: Relaxation therapy in bronchial asthma. J Psychosom Res 23:131–137, 1979

Esman A, Hertzig ME, Lewis NB, et al: Grand rounds in child psychiatry: a case of psychogenic pain. J Am Acad Child Psychiatry 24:781–787, 1985

Fadiman A: The Spirit Catches You and You Fall Down. New York, Noonday Press, 1997

Faust D, Fogel B: The development and initial validation of a sensitive bedside cognitive screening test. J Nerv Ment Dis 177:25–30, 1989

Featherstone H: A Difference in the Family: Living With a Disabled Child. New York, Basic Books, 1980

Feinkelstein R: Living with insulin-dependent diabetes mellitus, in Clinical Diabetes Mellitus: A Problem-Oriented Approach. Edited by Davidson JK. New York, Thieme-Stratton, 1986, pp 544–550

Frisch L, Bode H: Diabetes mellitus, in Massachusetts General Hospital Handbook of Psychiatric Aspects of General Hospital Pediatrics. Edited by Jellinek MS, Herzog DB. Chicago, IL, Year Book Medical, 1990, pp 124–131

Fritz GK: Childhood asthma: a psychosomatic review. Psychosomatics 24:959–967, 1983

Fritz GK: Consultation-liaison in child psychiatry and evolution of pediatric psychiatry. Psychosomatics 31:85–90, 1990

Fritz GK, Rubinstein S, Lewiston N: Psychological factors in fatal childhood asthma. Am J Orthopsychiatry 57:253–257, 1987

Fritz GK, Klein RB, Overholser JC: Accuracy of symptom perception in childhood asthma. J Dev Behav Pediatr 11:69–73, 1990

Fritz GK, Fritsch S, Hagino O: Somatoform disorders in children and adolescents: a review of the past 10 years. J Am Acad Child Adolesc Psychiatry 36:1329–1338, 1997

Garner D, Garfinkel P: The Eating Attitudes Test: an index of the symptoms of anorexia nervosa. Psychol Med 9:273–279, 1979

Geist RA: Onset of chronic illness in children and adolescents: psychotherapeutic and consultative intervention. Am J Orthopsychiatry 49:4–23, 1979

Graham PF: Psychosomatic relationships, in Child and Adolescent Psychiatry: Modern Approaches, 2nd Edition. Edited by Rutter M, Hersov L. St. Louis, MO, Blackwell Scientific, 1985, pp 599–613

Gross R, Duke P: The effect of early versus late physical maturation on adolescent behavior. Pediatr Clin North Am 27:71–77, 1980

Halmi K: Anorexia nervosa: demographic and clinical features in 94 cases. Psychosom Med 36:18–26, 1974

Hanson S, Pichert J: Perceived stress and diabetes control in adolescents. Health Psychol 5:439–452, 1986

Henning J, Fritz GK: School reentry in childhood cancer. Psychosomatics 24:261–269, 1983

Herzog DB: Eating disorders, in The New Harvard Guide to Psychiatry. Edited by Nicholi A. Cambridge, MA, Harvard University Press, 1988, pp 434–445

Herzog DB, Harper G: Unexplained disability: diagnostic dilemmas and principles of management. Clin Pediatr (Phila) 22:29–33, 1981

Hewson-Bower B, Drummond P: Psychological treatment of recurrent symptoms of colds and flus in children. J Psychosom Res 51:369–377, 2001

Hilliard JP, Fritz GK, Laviston NJ: Levels of aspiration of parents for their asthmatic, diabetic and healthy children. J Clin Psychol 41:587–597, 1985

Hodges K, Kline JJ, Barbero G, et al: Life events occurring in families of children with recurrent abdominal pain. J Psychosom Res 28:185–186, 1984

Johnson SB: Psychological aspects of childhood diabetes. J Child Psychol Psychiatry 29:729–738, 1988

Khaw KT: Cystic fibrosis, in Massachusetts General Hospital Handbook of Psychiatric Aspects of General Hospital Pediatrics. Edited by Jellinek MS, Herzog DB. Chicago, IL, Year Book Medical, 1990, pp 132–137

Knapp P, Harris E: Consultation-liaison in child psychiatry: a review of the past 10 years, I: clinical findings. J Am Acad Child Adolesc Psychiatry 36:1329–1338, 1997

Knapp P, Harris E: Consultation-liaison in child psychiatry: a review of the past 10 years, II: research and treatment approaches and outcomes. J Am Acad Child Adolesc Psychiatry 37:139–146, 1998

Koocher G, O'Malley J, Gogan J, et al: Psychological adjustment among pediatric cancer survivors. J Child Psychol Psychiatry 21:163–173, 1980

Krener P, Miller F: Psychiatric response to HIV spectrum disease in children and adolescents. J Am Acad Child Adolesc Psychiatry 28:596–605, 1989

Lavigne JV, Faier-Routman J: Psychological adjustment to pediatric physical disorders: a meta-analytic review. J Pediatr Psychol 17:133–157, 1992

Lipowski Z: Psychosomatic medicine in the seventies: an overview. Am J Psychiatry 134:233–244, 1977

Litt I, Cuskey W, Rosenberg A: Role of self-esteem and autonomy in determining medication compliance among adolescents with juvenile rheumatoid arthritis. Pediatrics 69:15–17, 1982

Livingston R, Taylor JL, Crawford SL: A study of somatic complaints and psychiatric diagnosis in children. J Am Acad Child Adolesc Psychiatry 27:185–187, 1988

Lobato DJ, Kao BT: Sibling-parent group intervention to improve sibling knowledge and adjustment to chronic illness and disability. J Pediatr Psychol 27:711–716, 2002

Mattson A, Kim S: Blood disorders. Psychiatr Clin North Am 5:345–356, 1982

Matus I: Assessing the nature and clinical significance of psychological contributions to childhood asthma. Am J Orthopsychiatry 51:327–341, 1981

McCollum A: The Chronically Ill Child: A Guide for Parents and Professionals. New Haven, CT, Yale University Press, 1981

McCubbin MA, Patterson JM, Cauble E, et al: CHIP: Coping Health Inventory for Parents: an assessment of parental coping patterns in the care of the chronically ill child. J Marriage Fam 45:359–370, 1983

McGoldrick M, Pearce JK, Giordano J (eds): Ethnicity and Family Therapy. New York, Guilford, 1982

McGrath PJ, Goodman JT, Firestone P, et al: Recurrent abdominal pain: a psychogenic disorder? Arch Dis Child 58:888–890, 1983

Miller BD, Wood BL: Psychophysiologic reactivity in asthmatic children: a cholinergically mediated confluence of pathways. J Am Acad Child Adolesc Psychiatry 33:1236–1245, 1994

Mrazek D: Pediatric hospitalization: understanding the stress from a developmental perspective, in The Psychosomatic Approach: Contemporary Practice of Whole-Person Care. Edited by Christie M, Mellett P. New York, Wiley, 1986, pp 164–196

Mrazek DA, Klinnert MD, Mrazek P, et al: Early asthma onset: consideration of parenting issues. J Am Acad Child Adolesc Psychiatry 30:277–282, 1991

Mulaikal R, Migeon C, Rock J: Fertility rates in female patients with congenital adrenal hyperplasia due to 21-hydroxylase deficiency. N Engl J Med 316:178–182, 1987

Musselman DL, Miller AH, Porter MR, et al: Higher than normal plasma interleukin-6 concentrations in cancer patients with depression: preliminary findings. Am J Psychiatry 158:1252–1257, 2001

Nadi N, Nurnberger J, Gershon E: Muscarinic cholinergic receptors on skin fibroblasts in familial affective disorder. N Engl J Med 311:225–230, 1984

O'Donnell M, Silove D, Wakefield D: Current perspectives on immunology and psychiatry. Aust N Z J Psychiatry 22:366–382, 1988

Olweus D, Mattsson A, Schalling D, et al: Circulating testosterone levels and aggression in adolescent males: a causal analysis. Psychosom Med 50:261–272, 1988

Orr DP, Weller SC, Satterwhite B, et al: Psychosocial implications of chronic illness in adolescence. J Pediatr 104:152–157, 1984

Paulson JA: The epidemiology of injuries in adolescents. Pediatr Ann 17:84–96, 1988

Pennebaker J, Kiecolt-Glaser J, Glaser R: Disclosure of traumas and immune function: health implications for psychotherapy. J Consult Clin Psychol 56:239–245, 1988

Pless I, Pinkerton P: Chronic Childhood Disorder: Promoting Patterns of Adjustment. Chicago, IL, Year Book Medical, 1975

Powers SW: Empirically supported treatments in pediatric psychology: procedure-related pain. J Pediatr Psychol 24:131–145, 1999

Pumariega A, Pursell J, Spock A, et al: Eating disorders in adolescents with cystic fibrosis. J Am Acad Child Psychiatry 25:269–275, 1986

Richter R, Dahme B: Bronchial asthma in adults: there is little evidence for the effectiveness of behavioral therapy and relaxation. J Psychosom Res 26:533–540, 1982

Rogers M: The interaction between brain behavior and immunity, in Psychosomatic Medicine: Theory, Physiology and Practice, Vol 1. Edited by Cheren S. Madison, CT, International Universities Press, 1989, pp 279–330

Roy C, Darling P, Weber A: A rational approach to meeting macro- and micronutrient needs in cystic fibrosis. J Pediatr Gastroenterol Nutr 3(suppl 1):154–162, 1984

Saks JA, Goetz R, Reddy N, et al: Psychological distress and natural killer cells in gay men with and without HIV infection. Am J Psychiatry 151:1479–1491, 1994

Schwartz L, Springer J, Flaherty J, et al: The role of recent life events and social support in the control of diabetes mellitus. Gen Hosp Psychiatry 8:212–216, 1986

Selter L: Oncology, in Massachusetts General Hospital Handbook of Psychiatric Aspects of General Hospital Pediatrics. Edited by Jellinek MS, Herzog DB. Chicago, IL, Year Book Medical, 1990, pp 142–149

Smith G, McDaniel S: Psychologically mediated effect on the delayed hypersensitivity reaction to tuberculin in humans. Psychosom Med 45:65–70, 1983

Spiegel D, Bloom J, Kraemer H, et al: Effect of psychosocial treatment on survival of patients with metastatic breast cancer. Lancet 2:888–891, 1989

Spieth LE, Stark LJ, Mitchell MJ, et al: Observational assessment of family functioning at mealtime in preschool children with cystic fibrosis. J Pediatr Psychol 26:215–224, 2001

Stabler B: Perspectives on chronic health problems, in Child Health Psychology. Edited by Melamed B, Matthews K, Routh D, et al. Hillsdale, NJ, Erlbaum, 1988, pp 251–263

Steiner H, Fritz G, Hilliard D, et al: A psychosomatic approach to childhood asthma. J Asthma 19:111–121, 1982

Taylor DC: Psychological aspects of chronic sickness, in Child and Adolescent Psychiatry: Modern Approaches, 2nd Edition. Edited by Rutter M, Herzov L. St. Louis, MO, Blackwell Scientific, 1985, pp 614–619

Thompson K, Varni J: A developmental cognitive-behavioral approach to pediatric pain assessment. Pain 25:283–296, 1986

Weiner H: Dynamics of the organism: implications of recent biological thought for psychosomatic theory and research. Psychosom Med 51:608–635, 1989

Yates A: Current perspectives on the eating disorders, I: history, psychological and biological aspects. J Am Acad Child Adolesc Psychiatry 28:813–828, 1989

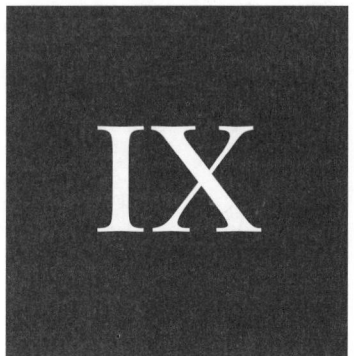

IX

Other Disorders and Special Issues

Adjustment and Reactive Disorders

Gloria Reeves, M.D.
David Pruitt, M.D.

The diagnosis of adjustment disorder does not align easily with other categories of psychiatric illness. Although clinical practice teaches us to link stressors with presenting symptoms, most psychiatric diagnoses do not require a specific stressor to be identified or characterized. Diagnostic criteria tend to emphasize observable behaviors and internalized experiences, independent of environmental factors and external events. In contrast, the diagnostic criteria for adjustment disorder focus on the connection between stressors and psychological distress. This unique perspective offers an important option for clinicians who treat children and adolescents. Pediatric patients are often exposed to stressors beyond their control (e.g., parental divorce, financial stressors, relocation to a new home). The diagnosis of adjustment disorder elevates the importance of involving families and outside systems in treatment because it focuses on the impact of psychosocial stressors. This shift in focus may serve to destigmatize the individual patient and offer support to the child's family and community network.

The usefulness of the adjustment disorder diagnosis is challenged by the low volume of research available to characterize this disorder. The extensive review by Despland et al. (1995) of the adult literature on adjustment disorder between 1974 and November 1992 identified only 16 articles, with only 9 articles described as actual studies. Further research is warranted to help characterize the natural course of adjustment disorder as well as the unique features of this disorder during childhood.

Definition

DSM-IV-TR (American Psychiatric Association 2000) diagnostic criteria (Table 41–1) define adjustment disorder as the development of emotional or behavioral symptoms in response to a recent stressor and further define the disorder as occurring within 3 months of the onset of the stressor. Symptoms must be beyond what would be expected for the given stressor and must result in significant impairment in social or academic functioning. Other Axis I conditions and bereavement must be excluded as a cause of the clinical presentation, and symptoms should resolve within 6 months of the termination of the stressor or its consequences. The course can be specified as either acute or chronic, depending on whether the duration of symptoms is less than or greater than 6 months. The diagnostic subtypes include adjustment disorder with either depressed mood, anxiety, mixed anxiety and depressed mood, disturbance of conduct, or mixed disturbance of emotions and conduct.

Differential Diagnosis

Stress-related diagnostic categories include posttraumatic stress disorder (PTSD) and bereavement. In PTSD, the stressor is specified as a traumatic event in which there is a serious threat to the safety of self or

Table 41–1. DSM-IV-TR diagnostic criteria for adjustment disorders

A. The development of emotional or behavioral symptoms in response to an identifiable stressor(s) occurring within 3 months of the onset of the stressor(s).

B. These symptoms or behaviors are clinically significant as evidenced by either of the following:

   (1) marked distress that is in excess of what would be expected from exposure to the stressor

   (2) significant impairment in social or occupational (academic) functioning

C. The stress-related disturbance does not meet the criteria for another specific Axis I disorder and is not merely an exacerbation of a preexisting Axis I or Axis II disorder.

D. The symptoms do not represent bereavement.

E. Once the stressor (or its consequences) has terminated, the symptoms do not persist for more than an additional 6 months.

Specify if:

Acute: if the disturbance lasts less than 6 months
Chronic: if the disturbance lasts for 6 months or longer

Adjustment disorders are coded based on the subtype, which is selected according to the predominant symptoms. The specific stressor(s) can be specified on Axis IV.

309.0	**With Depressed Mood**
309.24	**With Anxiety**
309.28	**With Mixed Anxiety and Depressed Mood**
309.3	**With Disturbance of Conduct**
309.4	**With Mixed Disturbance of Emotions and Conduct**
309.9	**Unspecified**

Source. Reprinted from American Psychiatric Association: *Diagnostic and Statistical Manual of Mental Disorders,* 4th Edition, Text Revision. Washington, DC, American Psychiatric Association, 2000. Copyright 2000 American Psychiatric Association. Used with permission.

others and there is a well-defined profile of hyperarousal, avoidance, and reexperiencing symptoms. Bereavement is a diagnostic category used when the focus of stress is the loss of a loved one, particularly if "normal" grief reactions occur within the first few months after the death.

Depression and anxiety disorders should also be considered in the differential diagnosis. The distinction from adjustment disorder may not be readily apparent. Both disorders may cause prominent shifts in mood or behavior, and both may be associated with psychosocial stressors. However, the diagnoses of anxiety or depressive disorders require more specific behavior and emotional symptom profiles, and symptoms are not necessarily linked to a specific stressor. With depressive and anxiety disorders, the symptoms do not have to occur within a specific time frame after onset of the stressor.

Cultural Syndromes and Issues

Cultural syndromes may be quite striking in presentation, but they are not considered to be pathological disorders. For example, "brain fag" is a term originating in West Africa to describe concentration, memory, and energy deficiencies associated with students undergoing school pressures. If the symptoms remain within culturally accepted behavior and belief systems, the individual would not be considered to meet criteria for a reactive disorder. This characterization of cultural syndromes as nonpathological conditions raises some interesting questions about how cultural beliefs may mediate psychological distress. If an individual's mood or behavior changes can be attributed to a culturally defined experience, negative sequelae from the event may be minimized and the return to a normal mood state may occur much faster. For example, in the cultural syndrome described above, a student may have marked changes in mood or behavior while experiencing school stressors. Yet if those changes are attributed to an accepted cultural phenomenon, they often evoke less distress because the behavior is considered normal and is known to occur in other healthy individuals.

Bird et al. (1989) conducted a large community study of Puerto Rican children, ages 4–16 years, to gather information about the prevalence of psychiatric disorders and risk factors for maladjustment. A unique finding in the Puerto Rican sample, compared with the United States mainland community subset, was that single parenthood was not associated with any of the psychopathology variables in the Puerto Rican children. The authors suggest that it may be a culturally specific finding, in that the prominent role of the extended family in Puerto Rico may serve as a protective factor in single-parent families, shielding the child and family unit from the development of symptoms.

Etiology

Although the diagnostic criteria clearly state that symptoms are associated with an identifiable stressor, there are important intrinsic factors that modulate the impact of a distressing event. Woolston (1988) discusses how an individual's level of cognitive development influences the interpretation of stressful events. For example, he points out that children are more likely than adults to link unrelated events as a cause-and-effect phenomenon. This may generate greater feelings of guilt or distress if the child feels involved in causing an uncontrollable event. Sanger et al. (1993) surveyed a group of 50 children with idiopathic epilepsy, ages 5–16 years, to ask what was the cause of their seizures. Only 41% of the respondents identified their seizure disorder as a dysfunction of the brain. One child assumed her seizures were related to overeating.

A child's level of psychological development also will modulate the response to stressors. An external stressor may have greater impact in causing distress if it amplifies preexisting issues, such as poor self-esteem (Woolston 1988). The capacity to engage adaptive defense mechanisms will also modulate the impact of a stressor. A child using more primitive defense mechanisms may be less effective in managing distress and thus more vulnerable to developing symptoms.

At a physiological level, individual neurohormonal responses to stressors may alter the subjective sense of distress after an event. If the stressor is adjustment to a chronic illness, the physiological changes related to the illness may mimic psychiatric symptoms (e.g., anemia causing fatigue or hypoglycemia causing anxiety or poor concentration). Side effects of treatment can also be mislabeled as psychiatric symptoms (e.g., increased sleep from a sedating medication).

Prevalence

Initial studies of adjustment disorder in clinical populations have generally shown its prevalence to be high (Newcorn and Strain 1992). A retrospective study of all psychiatric patients admitted in 1989 through a suburban hospital emergency department revealed that 7.1% of adults and 34.4% of adolescents had an adjustment disorder admission diagnosis. The most common subtype in adults and adolescents was adjustment disorder with depressed mood (Greenberg et al. 1995). In a sample of more than 11,000 patients at a university-based clinic, 10% of all patients and 16% of patients under age 18 years were diagnosed with adjustment disorder. There was no significant difference in prevalence between male and female patients (Mezzich et al. 1989). Follow-up prevalence rates of adjustment disorder in clinical samples may be underestimated, however, because insurance companies and managed-care systems often do not authorize inpatient admission or extensive treatment follow-up if adjustment disorder is identified as the primary diagnosis.

Clinical Presentation and Course of Illness

Kovacs et al. (1994) conducted a prospective study of 30 child psychiatric patients, ages 8–13 years, with a research-defined diagnosis of adjustment disorder. To meet criteria, subjects needed to have at least three clinically significant symptoms in the relevant symptom domain. Because the DSM-IV (American Psychiatric Association 1994) criteria do not require a specific number of symptoms to be present, the research team defined a uniform threshold number of symptoms necessary to make the diagnosis. For example, all patients were required to have at least three clinically significant symptoms of depression to be diagnosed with adjustment disorder with depressed mood. These patients were compared with 26 control subjects, who were also matched for comorbidity rates. For patients diagnosed with adjustment disorder with depressed mood, the most common symptoms were sadness, decreased pleasure, self-deprecation, and irritability. More than half (58%) indicated a history of suicidal ideation at some point after onset of the stressor. The identified stressors included new school year (30%), change in family situation (23%), peer rejection (13%), parental illness (10%), death of parent or grandparent (7%), move (7%), or other (10%). Median time to recovery after onset of symptoms was 7 months, and close to 100% of the study population had resolution of symptoms within 2 years. Compared with the control group, there was no evidence of long-term sequelae over an 8-year follow-up assessment.

Andreasen and Hoenk (1982) examined the predictive value of the adjustment disorder diagnosis by conducting a 5-year follow-up of a cohort of adolescents (n=52) and adults (n=48) who were diagnosed with the disorder. The adults fared better than the adolescents; 71% of adults and 44% of the adolescents were assessed to be free from psychiatric illness at follow-up (an additional 13% of adolescents were well but had intervening problems during the 5-year period). With regard to diagnostic subtypes, patients with disturbance of conduct tended to have poorer outcomes than patients with depressed mood. Whether the initial adjustment disorder diagnosis was made in an inpatient or an outpatient setting was not significant in predicting good outcome. The most common follow-up diagnoses in the adolescent group were major depressive disorder (19%), antisocial personality disorder (19%), alcoholism (17%), and substance abuse (12%).

Fabrega et al. (1987) addressed the specificity of the adjustment disorder diagnosis by examining symptomatology in more than 5,000 patients who were assessed in a walk-in psychiatric clinic (15% of the patients were under age 19). Diagnostic evaluations were completed using a semistructured interview format. Patients were divided into three groups: those with no psychiatric diagnosis (1.6%), those with a sole diagnosis of adjustment disorder (2.3%), and those with specific Axis I or Axis II diagnoses (96.1%). The third group included patients with adjustment disorder diagnoses and a comorbid psychiatric diagnosis. Data on these three groups were organized by categories of symptom profiles, including 1) mood and affect symptoms; 2) thought content and perception symptoms; 3) behavior, speech, and cognitive symptoms; and 4) vegetative, substance abuse, and characterologic symptoms. The groups were also assessed for severity of psychosocial stressors and adaptive functioning. The results indicated that patients with a sole diagnosis of adjustment disorder rated higher on measures of psychosocial stressors than did patients with specific diagnoses (i.e., other than adjustment disorder), but the adjustment disorder patients rated lower on all indicators of psychopathology. Patients with diagnoses of adjustment disorder also scored higher on psychopathology measures than did patients with no diagnosable mental illness. The authors concluded that adjustment disorder serves a useful purpose as a transitional illness category because it describes a population with psychopathology intermediate between people with psychosocial stressors but no diagnosable disorder and people with stressors who meet criteria for a disorder other than adjustment disorder.

Specific Stressors and Resilience Factors

Because adjustment disorder is related specifically to stressors, investigation of children's reactions to different types of stressors may help to determine prevention and treatment interventions. Two major stressors experienced by many children are disruption of the family unit (e.g., parental separation or divorce) and adjustment to illness.

Weitzman and Adair (1988) outlined three major phases of divorce: the acute phase, the transitional phase, and the postdivorce phase. The acute phase was described as the period from when the family acknowledges that the divorce will occur to approximately 2 years after the divorce occurs. This may be the time when maladjustment between the child and parent is most likely to occur because it is a period of dramatic change. Children are forced to adapt to new routines, changes in the household, and disruption in time spent with each parent. The transition phase marks the establishment of single-parent households. Children usually experience a stronger sense of control as a result of having more choices and more input about what happens in their single-parent household. For example, children may be involved in setting up their room in a new home or may get to select which days they are to visit with the noncustodial parent. The authors state that children may be prone to maladjustment in this phase if the parents continue to be embroiled in conflict. Prolonged marital conflict interferes with child rearing because parents are less likely to agree on uniform expectations and consequences of the child's behaviors. The inconsistency of the parenting and uncertainties created by ongoing conflict create confusion in the child, which interferes with the ability to develop a sense of mastery and control of the situation. The final phase, postdivorce, can be hoped to mark the achievement of relative stability. The separate households are generally well established, and many parents start to consider the possibility of new relationships and even remarriage. Maladjustment during this final phase can occur if unrealistic expectations are placed on the child's relationships with new sibling or parent figures. The child may be reluctant to accept new relationships, so he or she may not attach to new family members initially.

Newcorn and Strain (1992) point out the challenge of reconciling adjustment disorder criteria with the stressor of divorce. Because divorce produces irreversible and enduring changes in the child's life, it is often difficult to place a stressor into a specific time period. Kelly's (2000) literature review supports the notion that marital conflict is a more important predictor of child maladjustment than divorce itself. Thus, the stressor may be an ongoing experience that is not marked by a specific event or time of onset.

Adjustment to illness is another stressor experienced by many during childhood. Siegel et al. (1992) assessed a population of 62 children, ages 7–16, whose parents had terminal cancer. In these cases, the physician estimated that the parent had less than 6 months to live. Not surprisingly, the children of terminally ill parents scored significantly higher than a control group of community children on internalizing and externalizing symptoms on the Child Behavior Checklist. A less expected finding, however, was that these children scored significantly lower than the control group on measures of social competence. The authors suggest that social competence may be useful to target in interventions of children with very ill parents. Maintaining and providing positive social interactions with peers may be difficult during intense periods of parental illness and death, but it possibly provides stability in the child's long-term adjustment to this loss.

Chronic illness is a risk factor for behavioral and emotional problems in children (Kovacs et al. 1995; Newcorn and Strain 1992; Perrin et al. 1993). Kovacs et al. (1995) investigated childhood adjustment to the onset of juvenile diabetes. The study assessed a cohort of 92 children hospitalized for acute-onset diabetes. Within 6 months of the hospitalization, the most common psychiatric diagnosis was adjustment disorder. The first month after the diagnosis was the period of greatest vulnerability; 73% of the adjustment disorder diagnoses were made during that time frame. This increased vulnerability may be related to physiological factors, because a patient's glucose levels often have not stabilized during this early phase of treatment. This period is also the time when patients and families need the greatest support and when prevention efforts are the most critical. The short-term psychiatric outcomes for the children in this study were good. All children eventually recovered from the adjustment disorder, and the average time to recovery was 3 months. However, the presence of adjustment disorder was a risk factor for other psychiatric illnesses during the next 5 years. The authors discussed the importance of assessing for stressors beyond the obvious medical condition. Although the physical illness of diabetes attracts a lot of attention by families and health professionals, there may be concurrent stressors that have a cumulative or greater impact on the child's emotional health. For example, children experiencing a combination of diabetes and parental marital conflict were at greater risk for developing a reactive disorder than those dealing solely with diabetes.

Perrin et al. (1993) investigated perceptions of adjustment in children with chronic health conditions, including grand mal and petit mal seizure disorders, cerebral palsy, and visible orthopedic conditions (e.g., rheumatoid arthritis, scoliosis). The investigators attempted to recruit subjects who were not in an acute health crisis, so they excluded children who had been diagnosed with a chronic illness less than 6 months before, or had been hospitalized less than 6 months previously, or did not attend school regularly. Measures of psychosocial adjustment were completed by the children, their parents, and their teachers. Children with chronic illness were compared with a community control group.

All three observers (child, parent, and teacher) rated children with chronic orthopedic conditions (including rheumatoid arthritis and scoliosis) as equally or better adjusted than same-age peers. The overall assessment of child adjustment in this group was higher than for other health conditions The authors suggest that a visible condition may elicit more support from others to alleviate stress. All the teachers were aware of health problems in this group, whereas only half the teachers knew about the health condition in the epileptic group. However, children with cerebral palsy received higher ratings of adjustment from self and teacher reports than from parental reports. The authors hypothesized that patients with cerebral palsy have had their conditions most of their lives, so they probably do not think of themselves as being ill, whereas the parents are acutely aware of how many services and how much care the children needed throughout their development.

The investigators also surveyed mothers about their beliefs regarding control of their children's epilepsy. Mothers who felt they had control over the prevention of their children's seizures tended to rate their epileptic children as better adjusted than did mothers who felt they had little impact on the prevention of their children's seizures. Thus, parental perceptions involved a complex interaction between the parents' experience of observing and interacting with their child and their individual beliefs about their capacity to control the child's health condition.

Treatment

There are few research data available on treatment options for adjustment disorder. However, it can be ascertained from the review described in the previous section that treatment should be strongly influenced by the child's situation. Because family members may be involved in the identified stressor and they have considerable influence on a child's perception and experience of stressors, they are an important part of the treatment equation. Family interventions can help eliminate labeling of the child in the "sick role" and may provide relief to others affected by the stress. Unlike with PTSD, in which the stressor may be more extreme and less common, stressors identified in adjustment disorder may occur quite frequently in a given population. This allows for easier identification of patients for group interventions and prevention efforts. Pharmacological treatment of adjustment disorder may be considered to target the child's reactive symptoms and alleviate immediate distress around the onset of a stressor. However, adjustment disorder is usually short-lived, and little is known about any long-term benefit in pharmacological treatment to prevent later onset of other psychiatric illnesses. Longer-term follow-up of children with adjustment disorder may be helpful in understanding the merits of various interventions.

Justin is a 14-year-old male with a history of attention-deficit/hyperactivity disorder (ADHD) and stuttering. He has been seen by a child psychiatrist for medication management for several years and receives speech and language services at school. His mood and behavior have been relatively stable for 2 years. However, at a routine follow-up appointment, Justin's mother expresses concern that his school performance has declined over the past quarter. He has trouble completing classwork, and he recently got in a fight at school. Justin's mood is more irritable and he has some problems with insomnia, but he still enjoys activities with peers and has no change in appetite or energy level. Justin denies any periods of hopelessness, but he admits to feeling more frustrated lately. Review of recent stressors reveals that Justin's parents separated at the beginning of the school quarter, and he now stays with his mother on weekdays and visits his father on the weekends. When Jus-

tin is asked about the divorce, he complains, "I hate it, I don't want to talk about it."

This case is consistent with an episode of adjustment disorder. The child has had a marked change in functioning after a significant stressor, namely divorce. The patient has some mood symptoms, but not enough to warrant an Axis I mood disorder diagnosis. This patient may be at particular risk for a reactive disorder if his difficulties with language interfere with his ability to express his emotional distress. The comorbid ADHD condition and prominent difficulties with school also raise questions about whether the ADHD condition has destabilized or whether a subtle learning disorder has been missed. Psychosocial stressors can contribute to destabilization of psychiatric conditions, because adherence to treatment may be more difficult when these stressors are present. For example, in this case the patient may not have taken his medication consistently during the initial separation because the parents were experiencing more stress and were learning how to manage parenting issues between two households. Because of the possibility that a mood or anxiety disorder may develop, the child needs to be monitored closely. Comorbidity between ADHD and affective disorders is high, and the patient may be presenting early in the natural course of a mood disorder. Because the patient does not meet full criteria for an Axis I mood disorder at this time, his distress may be managed initially with a combination of individual and family therapy sessions to help him adjust to the parents' separation. However, additional stressors or more prominent mood symptoms may come to light as treatment progresses. A final point illustrated by this case is the importance of involving the child's support network in his or her treatment. The child may be the identified patient, but the identified stressor affects the entire family; the child's distress over the stressor is unlikely to resolve without the parents being involved in treatment.

Conclusion

The diagnostic category of adjustment disorder appears to describe a unique reaction to stress, distinct from those experienced by children with other psychiatric illnesses. The adjustment disorder diagnosis offers clinicians the option of conceptualizing a child's difficulties in the framework of a stress reaction, which may be helpful in destigmatizing the child's problems and enlisting the participation of families and other systems in treatment.

However, it is not always clear how to operationally define the diagnosis. Researchers developed more stringent diagnostic criteria (e.g., presence of four or more active symptoms) to help distinguish these patients more clearly from children who experience stress but who function reasonably well. The time frame defined for symptomatology is also problematic. The judgment of when a stressor began and when it has resolved is often subjective and is therefore susceptible to poor interrater reliability. Longitudinal research is needed to clarify the usefulness of this diagnosis in predicting future risk of maladjustment and psychiatric illness. This information could be applied in developing prevention efforts and in planning treatment interventions.

References

American Psychiatric Association: Diagnostic and Statistical Manual of Mental Disorders, 4th Edition. Washington, DC, American Psychiatric Association, 1994

American Psychiatric Association: Diagnostic and Statistical Manual of Mental Disorders, 4th Edition, Text Revision. Washington, DC, American Psychiatric Association, 2000

Andreasen NC, Hoenk PR: The predictive value of adjustment disorders: a follow-up study. Am J Psychiatry 139:584–590, 1982

Bird HR, Gould MS, Yager T, et al: Risk factors for maladjustment in Puerto Rican children. J Am Acad Child Adolesc Psychiatry 28:847–850, 1989

Despland JN, Monod L, Ferrero F: Clinical relevance of adjustment disorder in DSM-III-R and DSM-IV. Compr Psychiatry 36:454–460, 1995

Fabrega H, Mezzich JE, Mezzich AC: Adjustment disorder as a marginal or transitional illness category in DSM-III. Arch Gen Psychiatry 44:567–572, 1987

Greenberg WM, Rosenfeld DN, Ortega EA: Adjustment disorder as an admission diagnosis. Am J Psychiatry 152:459–461, 1995

Kelly JB: Children's adjustment in conflicted marriage and divorce: a decade of research. J Am Acad Child Adolesc Psychiatry 39:963–973, 2000

Kovacs M, Gatsonis C, Pollock M, et al: A controlled prospective study of DSM-III adjustment disorder in childhood. Arch Gen Psychiatry 51:535–541, 1994

Kovacs M, Ho V, Pollock MH: Criterion and predictive validity of the diagnosis of adjustment disorder: a prospective study of youths with new-onset insulin-dependent diabetes mellitus. Am J Psychiatry 152:523–528, 1995

Mezzich JE, Fabrega H Jr, Coffman GA, et al: DSM-III disorders in a large sample of psychiatric patients: frequency and specificity of diagnoses. Am J Psychiatry 146:212–219, 1989

Newcorn JH, Strain J: Adjustment disorder in children and adolescents. J Am Acad Child Adolesc Psychiatry 31:318–326, 1992

Perrin EC, Ayoub CC, Willett JB: In the eyes of the beholder: family and maternal influences on perceptions of adjustment of children with a chronic illness. J Dev Behav Pediatr 14:94–105, 1993

Sanger MS, Perrin EC, Sandler HA: Development in children's causal theories of their seizure disorders. J Dev Behav Pediatr 14:88–93, 1993

Siegel K, Mesagnso FP, Karus D, et al: Psychosocial adjustment of children with a terminally ill parent. J Am Acad Child Adolesc Psychiatry 31:327–333, 1992

Weitzman M, Adair R: Divorce and children. Pediatr Clin North Am 35:1313–1323, 1988

Woolston JL: Theoretical considerations of the adjustment disorders. J Am Acad Child Adolesc Psychiatry 27:280–287, 1988

Personality Disorders

Paulina F. Kernberg, M.D.

Jerry M. Wiener, M.D.

The diagnosis of personality disorders in childhood and adolescence remains controversial. Only a few textbooks on child psychiatry even include personality disorder, regardless of the author's theoretical orientation (Adams and Fras 1988; Finch and Green 1979; Josephson and Porter 1979; P.F. Kernberg 1988; Lewis 1986).

As Lewis (1986) asserted, although the rate of change of personality in childhood and adolescence appears to be faster than in subsequent stages of the life cycle, this does not mean that a personality does not exist. If one finds numerous personality traits in a child or adolescent that are maladaptive, inflexible, or rigid with continuity in time and across situations, the possibility of a specific personality disorder should be considered.

Frequently the thrust of development is not sufficient to counterbalance early or chronic deformations or distortions of the child's personality. Development proceeds, but it does so along pathological lines. All too often, the psychiatrist addresses only a DSM-IV-TR (American Psychiatric Association 2000) Axis I diagnosis in a child's diagnostic evaluation and overlooks an underlying Axis II personality disorder or developmental disorder, which will significantly affect the child's ultimate prognosis (Plakun 1989; Weissman et al. 1978). The current diagnostic nomenclature in DSM-IV-TR contributes to the controversy because it sets severe limits on the use of the personality disorder diagnosis in children, so that children's chronic, maladaptive ways of dealing with themselves and their environment are not specifically addressed in Axis II. Some equivalent categories—social phobia, oppositional defiant disorder, and severe conduct disorders—are placed in Axis I.

Definition of Personality in Children and Adolescents

To consider the existence of personality disorders in children, the concept of personality first needs to be defined. As stated in DSM-IV-TR, personality traits "are enduring patterns of perceiving, relating to, and thinking about the environment and oneself that are exhibited in a wide range of social and personal contexts" (p. 686). Another useful conception comes from Fenichel (1945), who referred to personality as the ego's habitual modes of adjusting to the external world, the id, and the superego, and the characteristic ways of combining these modes with one another. Using the DSM-IV-TR definition, clinicians can identify in children personality traits such as egocentricity, inhibition, cautiousness, self-confidence, sociability, activity, resentfulness, and oppositionalism in various combinations. If such traits become inflexible, maladaptive, and chronic across time and situations, causing significant impairment in the child's functioning, then a personality disorder is suspected, regardless of age. Indeed, DSM-IV-TR indicates that personality disorder categories may be applied to children or adolescents in the relatively unusual instances in which the individual's particular maladaptive personality traits appear to be pervasive and persistent; in an individual younger than age 18 years, the features must have been present for at least 1 year. Moreover, a requirement for the diagnosis of antisocial disorder is a severe, chronic conduct disorder and a pattern of irresponsible and antisocial behavior since age 15 years.

As Rutter (1981) indicated, some concept of personality is needed that goes beyond the notion that child psychopathology is simply a persistence of habits or behaviors. The concept of personality in children serves as the anchoring point for the organization of constitutional factors, experiences, traumas, and symptoms. Thus, Rutter (1984) considered various kinds of continuity in his study of personality. Most relevant for personality development is the continuity of structural process or mechanism, which refers not to the form or quality of the personality but to the underlying psychological process. This continuity may link patterns of behavior related to early experiences with some psychological outcome at a later date, such as a relationship between sexual abuse and borderline personality disorders.

Certainly, personality traits and their expression are affected by situational and interpersonal factors, such as the presence or absence of the father in the attachment phase; the arrival of a new sibling; or observation of the child at home, at school, or with peers. Trait theories, however, recognize situational variability (Epstein 1979). Here it is important to consider the effective environment. Rutter and Garmezy (1983), for example, demonstrated that institutionally reared children experience lasting effects through their late 20s, even though they are by then in entirely different environments. The concept of cumulative trauma, such as repeated separations or long-term sexual abuse, implies a consideration of personality development. Also, the concept of personality is needed before one can understand how a child may actively induce, as it were, negative or positive environments, according to early experiences. For example, Pedersen et al. (1978) discussed the effect that a particular teacher may have on children. The effect of positive attitudes and work habits and the promotion of self-esteem increase the capacity of these children to profit from later education. Negative experiences in childhood, when not counteracted by positive supports later on, expose a lack of resilience and resourcefulness if circumstances again become unfavorable.

Personality Development

There is evidence of significant genetic contributions to personality disorders such as obsessive-compulsive personality disorder (Flament et al. 1988) and antisocial personality disorder (Shields 1975; Shulsinger 1972). Biologically determined disorders, such as attention-deficit/hyperactivity disorder, or cognitive deficits that are due to perinatal factors also contribute to the development of personality disorders (Andrulonis et al. 1981). Attention, memory, affect modulation, and spatial orientation are cognitive functions that contribute to the formation of the child's representational world (Sandler and Rosenblatt 1962) and thus to personality. Attachment seems to have been confirmed as a determinant of personality development (Rutter 1985). Neglect, sexual abuse, physical violence, multiple separations, and psychiatric illness in the parents frequently contribute to the genesis of personality disorders, especially the impulsive character disorders (histrionic, borderline, narcissistic, and antisocial personality disorders). Indeed, one could start from the premise that any factor—genetic, constitutional, or environmental—that interferes with the normal integration and differentiation of the child's representational world (i.e., the self-representations and representations of others in interaction with the self, including affect links) will place the child at risk for a personality disorder. Traumatic experiences, as well as developmental disorders, also affect the formation of the representational world and in turn distort ego functions, superego functions, and the adaptive expression of affects, impulses, and wishes (Fenichel 1945).

Beres (1969) referred to character or personality development as a consistent pattern of adaptation to reality, whether normal or pathological. Consider, for example, the excessive use of projection in the paranoid character, action-proneness in the acting-out character, reaction formations in the obsessive character, and repression in the hysterical character. What is important is the precocious fixity of these defense patterns.

Hartmann (1958) linked individual differences in the early emerging ego functions to later choice of defense and, by implication, to choice of illness. He also introduced the hypothesis of individual differences at birth with regard to the infant's state of adaptiveness. Years later, Brazelton (1973) illustrated the extent of individual differences in processing internal and external stimuli. Although it is difficult to bridge neonatal and adult behavior, research findings show that it is possible to observe continuities in some personality traits (Bronson 1967; Kagan 1984; Korner 1964; Looney et al. 1981; Rutter 1984). In this regard, Korner proposed that the style of development should be studied instead of particular developmental processes—an approach that might contribute to the understanding of personality development in children.

Longitudinal Studies

Moss and Susman (1980) summarized longitudinal studies of personality that, despite methodological differences, all indicated that infants have a personality profile. The New York longitudinal study showed that in the period from age 3 months to at least 2 years, mood, adaptability, approach behavior, and intensity were most stable, and the activity level and distractibility were least stable. The National Institute of Mental Health longitudinal study (Halverson and Waldrop 1976; Yang and Moss 1978) examined the role of environmental and biological factors. For males, biological and temperamental influences were most important, whereas for females, environmental stimuli, such as the mother's interest in social behavior, seemed to account for behaviors such as social responsiveness. Escalona and Heider (1959) predicted personality styles in preschool children from observations conducted between ages 4 and 32 weeks; sex role, interest patterns, activity patterns, and expressive behavior were successfully predicted. The Purdue longitudinal study (Martin 1964), which followed up four preschool cohorts from ages 2 to 5 years, showed a high degree of stability in the relative amount of aggression and control dominance, as well as stability in dependency, autonomous achievement, and friendship-affiliation behavior.

Of children showing aggression at age 3 years, 68% showed this trait 5 years later (Richman et al. 1982). In another longitudinal study of personality development, children were seen yearly between ages 2.5 and 6 years, then seen again and followed up each year from ages 6 to 12 years, during adolescence, and again as young adults (Kagan and Moss 1962). During the first 10 years of life, passivity was highly stable for boys and girls, and independent orientation showed a moderate degree of stability. Independence was stable for females during the 11-year span from age 3 to age 14; it was stable for males only from middle childhood to adolescence. Girls who were dependent on female adults during middle childhood established a dependent and passive relationship with males during adulthood.

In the same study it was found that aggression to peers but not to mother was highly stable during the first 10 years of life. Indirect aggression to peers, such as verbal attacks, was stable from the preschool years through adolescence. During the span from childhood to adulthood, aggression was more stable for males than for females.

Nearly three-quarters of the severe conduct disturbances persisted between ages 10 and 15 years in the Isle of Wight study (Rutter and Graham 1973). Whereas passivity (an acceptable behavior for females but not for males) was stable from childhood to adulthood only for females, achievement (an acceptable behavior for both females and males) was stable for both sexes. There also was a high degree of continuity between preschool sex-role behavior and adolescent behavior. Fixed sex interests were stable from childhood to adulthood for both sexes, but especially for males. Social interaction traits were also predictive. Lack of spontaneity and social withdrawal during middle childhood and adolescence were predictive of adult social anxiety. Last, introspectiveness was predictive of a similar tendency during adulthood.

Diagnosis of Personality Disorder in Childhood

DSM-IV-TR is used as a framework for organizing observations on child personality disorders. Children younger than age 18 years who have the essential features of any of the conditions described for adults as personality disorders can be so diagnosed (taking modifications from developmental considerations into account). Cohen et al. (1983) reported that children may manifest persistent, unstable patterns of developmental deviations by the fourth year of life. From another perspective, Rapoport and Ismond (1990) indicated that equivalent "symptoms" diagnosed in childhood and persisting after age 18 are then classified under the corresponding adult personality disorder. General DSM-IV-TR diagnostic criteria for a personality disorder are listed in Table 42–1.

As further clinical research evidence accumulates and the concept of personality disorders in childhood becomes more familiar, the nomenclature in DSM-IV-TR for certain diagnoses in childhood or adolescence might be replaced with the corresponding personality disorder. For example, if all criteria are met, including those of severity and chronicity, social phobia beginning in childhood or adolescence (subsuming the previous category

Table 42–1. DSM-IV-TR general diagnostic criteria for a personality disorder

A. An enduring pattern of inner experience and behavior that deviates markedly from the expectations of the individual's culture. This pattern is manifested in two (or more) of the following areas:

(1) cognition (i.e., ways of perceiving and interpreting self, other people, and events)
(2) affectivity (i.e., the range, intensity, lability, and appropriateness of emotional response)
(3) interpersonal functioning
(4) impulse control

B. The enduring pattern is inflexible and pervasive across a broad range of personal and social situations.
C. The enduring pattern leads to clinically significant distress or impairment in social, occupational, or other important areas of functioning.
D. The pattern is stable and of long duration, and its onset can be traced back at least to adolescence or early adulthood.
E. The enduring pattern is not better accounted for as a manifestation or consequence of another mental disorder.
F. The enduring pattern is not due to the direct physiological effects of a substance (e.g., a drug of abuse, a medication) or a general medical condition (e.g., head trauma).

Source. Reprinted from American Psychiatric Association: *Diagnostic and Statistical Manual of Mental Disorders,* 4th Edition, Text Revision. Washington, DC, American Psychiatric Association, 2000. Copyright 2000, American Psychiatric Association. Used with permission.

of avoidant disorder) may lead to or correspond with avoidant personality disorder (Rapoport and Ismond 1990); oppositional defiant disorder, to passive-aggressive personality disorder; and pervasive developmental disorder, to schizotypal personality disorder. All of the conduct disorders (solitary aggressive type and undifferentiated) may be subsumed in the Cluster B personality disorders (i.e., borderline, narcissistic, and antisocial personality disorders). At present, antisocial personality disorder requires that the conduct disorder start before age 15, and there is an injunction that the diagnosis of antisocial personality disorder not be given before age 18. However, if a patient fulfills the criteria for antisocial personality disorder for 3 years or more, it would seem to be justified for that diagnosis to be made before age 18. In sum, if the diagnostic criteria for antisocial personality disorder are met and if the disturbance is pervasive and persistent, it is unlikely that the disorder will be limited to a developmental stage. In particular, from a developmental perspective the differences between a 15-year-old, a 16-year-old, and a 17-year-old are not sufficient to warrant withholding a diagnosis of antisocial personality disorder.

Spectrum of Childhood Personality Disorders

In DSM-IV-TR, personality disorders are grouped into three clusters. Cluster A includes paranoid, schizoid, and schizotypal personality disorders, referred to by O.F. Kernberg (1976a) as *psychotic personality disorders.*

Cluster B (considered a developmentally and functionally intermediate level of personality pathology) includes antisocial, borderline, histrionic, and narcissistic categories. Cluster C (considered the most adaptive or least pathological of the personality disorders and also referred to as *neurotic*) includes avoidant, dependent, and obsessive-compulsive categories. O.F. Kernberg (1976a) also includes categories of passive-aggressive, self-defeating, and sadistic personality disorders. To receive any of these diagnoses, children should meet the corresponding DSM-IV-TR criteria for adults in a descriptive sense, but they also should be viewed from a functional and structural perspective. For example, does the child have a sense of age-appropriate identity and cope with internal and external stresses by using more advanced mechanisms of defense such as repression, rationalization, or isolation? Most important, does the child have a sense of and a relationship to reality with intact reality testing?

The more severe disorders include the schizoid, paranoid, borderline, narcissistic, antisocial, and histrionic personality disorders, all of which conceptually have a borderline personality organization (O.F. Kernberg 1976b). There is a lack of integration of identity both of the self and of others.

Sense of Identity

The sense of identity—the child's self-concept and representation or working schema of others—must be considered here as an important anchor or organizer of personality traits. Although identity consolidation is a predominant developmental task of adolescence, the school-age child already has an age-appropriate sense of identity. Between ages 6 and 12 years, children have a sense of "me-ness." They have a sense of who they are and of their own continuity throughout various activities (e.g., school, home, camp), through time (past, present, future), and with different persons. Disturbances in identity development and consolidation occur in all the Cluster A and B disorders. At one phase, lower-level defense mechanisms predominate, such as splitting, denial, projection, primitive idealization, devaluation, and omnipotent control. Moreover, the relationship to reality may be lost, but the capacity to test reality is preserved, and the child can regain reality contact with the clinician's support.

At the most severe end is the psychotic personality organization, which includes the schizotypal personality disorder. Children with this disorder have a fragmented and bizarre sense of identity, with psychotic defense mechanisms, such as severe constriction, deanimation of animate objects (e.g., considering other people to be machines), and animation of inanimate objects (e.g., assuming that stuffed animals have a life of their own). These defenses are an attempt to keep massive anxiety and depression under control. In addition, there is a loss of the capacity to test reality and a loss of a relationship to reality.

In general, treatment recommendations follow this spectrum of personality disorders. For the neurotic personality disorders, clinicians tend to use psychosocial interventions, with the exception of obsessive-compulsive personality disorder; the medication treatment is described by Rapoport and Ismond (1990) and by Leonard et al. elsewhere in this volume (see Chapter 30, "Obsessive-Compulsive Disorder"). For the borderline personality organization, individual supportive-expressive psychotherapy (P.F. Kernberg 1983b), group therapy (Scheidlinger 1982), or family therapy (Shapiro et al. 1975) is indicated, whereas medication may be used for specific target symptoms (Cantwell and Carlson 1978; O.F. Kernberg 1976b; Petti 1981; Rockland 1989; Wiener 1995).

Finally, in the psychotic personality organization, treatment is a combination of neuroleptics with psychosocial interventions of a supportive nature, including environmental changes.

The application of adult criteria for personality disorders to children and adolescents has not yet been explored systematically in all categories. It is possible, for example, that Cluster A diagnoses, which include paranoid personality disorder, can be seen in adolescence as part of a mixed personality disorder with schizoid, schizotypal, or borderline personality disorder. Such is the case of Maria, a 15-year-old girl hospitalized for trying to kill her parents by cooking stews and muffins with rat poison and setting fires outside their bedroom door. Her parents, who came from Latin America, were deprecated by Maria as "minority WASPs." Except for one girlfriend, Maria felt there was nobody she could count on. Her own parents, she explained, deliberately annoyed her by ignoring her sensitivity to their "disgusting" eating habits and the way they talked. Moreover, she felt she could never forgive her parents for not controlling her older brother, who had physically abused her. She did not care what others thought of her; even when praised, she was convinced this was done solely for exploitation.

The diagnostic impression here was of a personality disorder not otherwise specified with paranoid, schizoid, and sadistic features. The recommended treatment in such cases is individual and family psychotherapy. Neuroleptic medications may be useful in modulating the paranoid and more bizarre thinking.

Histrionic Personality Disorder

DSM-IV-TR criteria for histrionic personality disorder (Table 42–2) are a compromise between the older hysterical personality disorder and the histrionic personality disorder of DSM-III (American Psychiatric Association 1980), which overlapped with borderline personality disorder. Children with this disorder appear outgoing, engaging, and charming but are soon perceived as irritating and intrusive, impulsive, and more selfish than is normal for their age (P.F. Kernberg 1981). They crave attention, stimulation, and excitement. Hyperemotional, but in a superficial way, these children have a fickle and capricious quality. They lose friends as quickly as they gain them. Their emotions are labile, erupting in theatrical outbursts or undergoing equally abrupt withdrawal.

The provocative seductiveness is only superficially sexual; it also expresses identifications with seductive parents as a means of retrieving or maintaining love, or as an acting out of hostile manipulations. The hysterical child or adolescent seldom seeks a sexual part-

Table 42–2. DSM-IV-TR diagnostic criteria for histrionic personality disorder

A pervasive pattern of excessive emotionality and attention seeking, beginning by early adulthood and present in a variety of contexts, as indicated by five (or more) of the following:

(1) is uncomfortable in situations in which he or she is not the center of attention

(2) interaction with others is often characterized by inappropriate sexually seductive or provocative behavior

(3) displays rapidly shifting and shallow expression of emotions

(4) consistently uses physical appearance to draw attention to self

(5) has a style of speech that is excessively impressionistic and lacking in detail

(6) shows self-dramatization, theatricality, and exaggerated expression of emotion

(7) is suggestible, i.e., easily influenced by others or circumstances

(8) considers relationships to be more intimate than they actually are

Source. Reprinted from American Psychiatric Association: *Diagnostic and Statistical Manual of Mental Disorders,* 4th Edition, Text Revision. Washington, DC, American Psychiatric Association, 2000. Copyright 2000, American Psychiatric Association. Used with permission.

ner in the adult sense, but instead absorbs an eroticized positive or negative attention from the parents or others. If the mother herself is hysterical or infantilizing or encourages competitiveness in her child, the child will identify with her. A histrionic personality disorder also can result if a girl manages to turn her father into a substitute mother by developing abnormally close ties with him because she is (or feels) deprived of adequate mothering. If this relationship becomes sexualized (because of her father's conflict), the child later may use this technique to obtain dependent gratification from other father figures at the cost of submission and passivity.

Most patients with histrionic personality disorder have some deficit in their cognitive development with inevitable limitations in learning tasks. They are so busy both acting on and repressing their sexual and aggressive impulses that they have little attention left for sublimated interest or learning. In addition, their cognitive style is characterized by lack of discrimination and a global approach to learning.

The main mechanisms of defense in the patient

with histrionic personality disorder are repression of the awareness of sexual elements in their own behavior, reaction formation, and intellectualization to handle the anger and frustration. In more severe forms of histrionic personality disorder, defenses are more primitive, including splitting, projection, and somatization.

Case 1

Jeannie, 14½ years old, was described temperamentally as an expressive, easily excitable baby. Later, she generally seemed able to control her affects but had intense temper tantrums if something did not go her way. As a teenager, she was provocative but prudish, exhibiting herself in a bikini but expressing outrage if boys commented on her looks. Despite her attractive appearance, she behaved as a sexless, frozen person. She complained, as is frequent in personality disorders, of feelings of depression. During treatment, Jeannie demonstrated a global cognitive style. "I never seem to grasp the idea of a conversation," she complained. "I want to make sure that people will like me.... Usually, this results in my feeling forced.... What else can I say? I can never tell what is fair and what is unfair. It is a defense against really knowing."

"Almost everything I do, I drop out of," she continued. "My older brother has kept his interest throughout the years, and by now he is a good piano player. I have it all there, but I can't seem to do anything with it.... I haven't done anything with my talents. It is almost as if [I] didn't have them."

In sum, Jeannie fit several criteria for histrionic personality disorder, including overstatement and hyperbole in her speech, her constant search for praise and approval, inappropriate sexual seductiveness, exaggerated emotional expression (her temper outbursts and changing moods), a feeling of lack of genuineness, and self-centeredness.

Case 2

Tina, a 6-year-old, showed some characteristics of the histrionic personality disorder despite her much younger age. Tina's parents consulted me because of her extremely negative reactions to her brother, 3 years her junior. Since his birth, she had become very demanding and chronically dissatisfied. She also antagonized and alienated her peers. Her desk was a mess, and she was forever losing her possessions and money. During the diagnostic evaluation, Tina drew herself quite large, almost 20 inches tall, while she made her brother a fragment of a stick figure only 2 inches tall. There was a theatrical quality about her. Overall, Tina showed constant need for praise and approval, problems in her relationships with others, exaggerated emotional expression, overconcern with physical appearance, and intense penis envy, as reflected in her intense negative reaction to her brother's genitals. Her seductive relationship to her father was evident in her kissing him on the mouth to say good night; with her mother, she complained of aches and pains to obtain nurturing reactions.

■ Treatment

For histrionic personality disorder, analysis or psychoanalytic psychotherapy two or three times a week is the treatment of choice, aimed at the maladaptive defenses, oral demandingness, envy of children of the opposite sex, and guilt about sexual feelings (P.F. Kernberg 1981). Specifically, the child's oedipal rivalry, as well as the misuse of sexualized interactions to fulfill dependency needs, should be addressed. As the treatment progresses, character traits may be slowly transformed into symptoms of depression, anxiety, or even dissociation, which can be resolved through interpretive work in a therapeutic atmosphere of supportiveness and understanding.

Parental counseling also is advisable. Although cultural and individual differences play a role in hysterical pathology, the main contributing factor seems to be the parent–child relationship (Metcalf 1977). The hysterical patient's insatiable attention seeking may originate in part in partially frustrated attachment behaviors in infancy. In the two cases described above, the mothers were uncomfortable and uncertain about their maternal role and were emotionally unavailable.

Often, for example, the mother shows hysterical traits herself. Moreover, the parents may seem to overtly encourage the child to expect help or guidance from others, yet they may covertly signal that obtaining this help is beyond the child's competence and that it can be supplied only by the parents. They may discourage the expression of anger, assertiveness, or anxiety and may encourage dependency and passivity instead. Further problems arise when parents are physically overstimulating or infantilize the child. As a result, the child may show an early and intense sexuality or eroticization, and in later life he or she may need to maintain a high level of egocentric and sexually oriented interactions to satisfy dependency needs.

There are somewhat different recommendations for treatment of patients at the more severe range of the spectrum, where histrionic personality overlaps with borderline personality disorder. Here the treatment should follow supportive-expressive approaches with psychotherapy twice a week for 1–3 years. Structured limits should be established. Parental counseling should include clarification of primitive defense mechanisms operating within the family.

Borderline Personality Disorder

Borderline personality in childhood has been described by various authors (Aarkrog 1977; Ekstein and Wallerstein 1954; Frijling-Schreuder 1969; Geleerd 1958; P.F. Kernberg 1983a; Kestenbaum 1983; Mahler and Kaplan 1977; Masterson 1980; Pine 1974, 1983; Rosenfeld and Sprince 1963; Weil 1953). The descriptive symptomatology bears a resemblance to the diagnostic category for adult borderline personality disorder (Table 42–3), namely 1) a pattern of unstable and intense interpersonal relationships, alternating between idealization and devaluation; 2) impulsiveness; 3) affective instability, or marked shifts in mood, usually lasting a few hours and only rarely lasting more than a few days; 4) inappropriate intense anger or lack of control of anger, frequent displays of temper, and recurring physical fights; 5) recurring suicidal threats, gestures, or behavior, or self-mutilating behavior; 6) marked and persistent identity disturbance, manifested by uncertainty about self-image, sexual orientation, type of friends, long-term goals, and/or preferred values; 7) chronic feelings of emptiness or boredom; and 8) frantic efforts to avoid real or imagined abandonment.

Petti and Law (1982), Dr. Jerome Liebowitz (personal communication, July 1981), and Bemporad et al. (1982) have demonstrated the applicability of diagnostic criteria for borderline personality disorder to children in inpatient and outpatient settings. Similarly, Rapoport and Ismond (1990) recommended that borderline personality disorder "be diagnosed in children and adolescents, rather than the corresponding childhood category of identity disorder, provided that the personality disorder criteria are met and the nature of the disturbance is pervasive, persistent, and not limited to a developmental stage" (p. 61).

From a developmental perspective, children with borderline personality disorder have not accomplished tasks that nonborderline preschool children have achieved; namely, they cannot tolerate separation from the mother, lack established standards of bad and good, have an inability to express a wide variety of

Table 42–3. DSM-IV-TR diagnostic criteria for borderline personality disorder

A pervasive pattern of instability of interpersonal relationships, self-image, and affects, and marked impulsivity beginning by early adulthood and present in a variety of contexts, as indicated by five (or more) of the following:

(1) frantic efforts to avoid real or imagined abandonment.   **Note:** Do not include suicidal or self-mutilating behavior covered in Criterion 5.

(2) a pattern of unstable and intense interpersonal relationships characterized by alternating between extremes of idealization and devaluation

(3) identity disturbance: markedly and persistently unstable self-image or sense of self

(4) impulsivity in at least two areas that are potentially self-damaging (e.g., spending, sex, substance abuse, reckless driving, binge eating).   **Note:** Do not include suicidal or self-mutilating behavior covered in Criterion 5.

(5) recurrent suicidal behavior, gestures, or threats, or self-mutilating behavior

(6) affective instability due to a marked reactivity of mood (e.g., intense episodic dysphoria, irritability, or anxiety usually lasting a few hours and only rarely more than a few days)

(7) chronic feelings of emptiness

(8) inappropriate, intense anger or difficulty controlling anger (e.g., frequent displays of temper, constant anger, recurrent physical fights)

(9) transient, stress-related paranoid ideation or severe dissociative symptoms

Source.   Reprinted from American Psychiatric Association: *Diagnostic and Statistical Manual of Mental Disorders,* 4th Edition, Text Revision. Washington, DC, American Psychiatric Association, 2000. Copyright 2000, American Psychiatric Association. Used with permission.

modulated feelings, and are uncertain about sexual distinctions (P.F. Kernberg 1979). Compared with their school-age peers, children with borderline personality disorder are not able to maintain a sense of sex and role identity through play, fantasy, and learning tasks. Impulse control is poor, and they do not enjoy peer interactions or increased independence from parents. The oedipal period is prolonged, with delays in sublimation and repression.

The adolescent with borderline personality disorder has not acquired a stable sense of identity or developed age-appropriate abstract thinking. There is little indication of emancipation and autonomy from the family, and the perceptions of the family tend to be unrealistic. Gender identity with the capacity for intimacy and heterosexual adjustment is not established, and masturbatory fantasies are primarily connected with various pregenital themes, such as sadistic or excretory activities. Identity disorder is an important predicting factor in the diagnosis of personality disorders in general and borderline personality disorders in particular. Currently, more systematized studies to evaluate identity in children are in progress with instruments derived from E. Erikson's, M. Mahler's, S. Akhtar's, and O. Kernberg's theories (P. Kernberg and S. Kondrashin, "Assessing Personality Disorders in Adolescence," unpublished manuscript, June 2002).

Children with borderline personality disorder, in contrast to adults with this personality, may report visu-

al and auditory hallucinations, but kinesthetic and tactile hallucinations are rare. Visual and auditory hallucinations may be fostered if children are unable to express their aggression because their parents cannot contain or handle it. If these children have poor models for reality testing (Pine 1974), they may lose contact with reality (Geleerd 1958) while preserving the capacity for reality testing.

Play should be considered as an additional diagnostic descriptor in children with borderline personality disorder. These children do not play in an age-appropriate manner. The play is compulsive (Weil 1953) with little evidence of enjoyment or of the capacity to resolve conflict through elaborations of fantasies. Games may be endlessly repeated, and the child may enter into elementary fantasy play more typical of much younger children (e.g., playing at eating or flying and falling). Aggressive and sexual impulses infiltrate the play, so that intense anxiety follows, and the child is unable to continue playing. In their fantasies, these children see themselves as omnipotent, and oral and anal-sadistic themes predominate.

Relationships with peers are characterized by a sense of coercion and possessiveness with idealization or abrupt devaluations and, occasionally, a phenomenon called "shadowing" (echoing and borrowing from a peer's identity). There is no empathy for others, because these youngsters relate to others as "props" or projections of part of themselves.

The most important diagnostic criteria include an identity disorder; shifting levels of ego organization involving motor, cognitive, and affect modulation; and an inability to assume responsibility for one's own actions. There is a lack of a sense of "me-ness" and of gender identity, as well as an incapacity to be alone or a longing and fear of being left. Shifting levels of ego function account for the abrupt regressions, sudden lack of judgment, and impulsivity, as well as the disturbed relationship to reality (although the capacity to test reality is preserved). The use of primitive defenses—particularly splitting, projection, and denial—explains the difficulties these children have in assuming responsibility for their actions; formation of an integrated conscience or superego is impaired. In addition, children with borderline personality disorder tend to show extreme ambivalence toward their siblings; sibling rivalry can become outright hatred with sibling abuse. The splitting mechanism affects the relationship with the parents, not only in terms of bad and good but also in establishing a relationship to the parents on a one-to-one basis. The child relates to the mother to the exclusion of the father or to the father to the exclusion of the mother. A normal transitional object, in terms of timing and the kind of object, tends to be absent.

An unstable sense of identity is reflected in a sense of dependence on the "other" for survival, illustrating the personality disorder problem underlying severe separation anxiety problems. An alternative is to resort to narcissistic defenses, indicating a lack of need for anybody and denial of danger. These patients try at times to control others totally or to submit entirely to another's control to gain some sense of identity (P.F. Kernberg 1983a). Another attempt to gain identity can frequently be seen during treatment when the patient attributes the role of patient to the therapist while assuming the role of therapist. This can be done so vividly that the therapist literally feels as if he or she is the patient.

Depression frequently accompanies a borderline personality disorder (Gorton and Akhtar 1990). Children with borderline personality disorder perceive themselves as being without continuity, so they fail to anticipate gratification or even show it. They lack an age-appropriate capacity for realistic self-esteem or mastery. Their chronic feeling tone is one of apathy and anhedonia or worthlessness. They do not derive gratification because of lack of reciprocity in maternal/paternal or peer relationships. To the contrary,

they are rejected and disliked for their primitive ways of relating to others. These children are unable to derive pleasure from play or to use play to discharge their frustrations and aggressions, which adds to their helplessness and hopelessness.

Finally, the frequent coexistence of organicity (Andrulonis et al. 1981) makes for difficulties in learning and social interaction that compound the child's depression. This multidetermined depression, coexisting with impulsivity and other characteristics, may account for the fact that suicide attempts are a frequent cause for hospitalization (Pfeffer 1983).

Case 3

Velia, cited by Kestenbaum (1983), had no friends at age 5 and by age 7 was prone to severe and uncontrollable rages, did not get along with other children, and abused younger children if she did not get her way. She had begun lying to her parents, stealing from her mother's purse, and tearing up her own clothes and hiding them. Despite high intelligence, Velia lacked the concentration to complete homework. She seemed constantly nervous but denied that she had any problems. At times, she betrayed her anger and hostility in comments such as "How would you like it if I put a live rattlesnake on your plate?" This 7-year-old often became violently upset with her therapist, exclaiming "You are dead; I killed you!" or "You are a mind reader and a witch; you made me think of awful things!" In this way, she showed her shifting levels of functioning, her tendency for projections, and her paranoid ideation. Abrupt regressions in ego states also existed, such as when she soiled herself during sessions. Yet, in other sessions, Velia displayed positive emotions, telling the therapist that she wished to adopt her because she loved her as much as her grandmother. When followed up in adult life (Kestenbaum 1983), Velia had low achievement not commensurate with her intelligence, drug abuse, promiscuity, manipulative suicidal threats, and disturbances in close relationships. Beneath her seemingly good socialization lay a disturbed identity, shifting identifications with others, and a predominance of rageful affect rather than emotional warmth. There were also brief micropsychotic episodes under stress. In all, she fulfilled the criteria for adult borderline personality disorder as outlined by Gunderson and Kolb (1978).

Case 4

Nick, 7½ years old, had severe separation anxiety marked by an inability to sleep in his own room or to be left alone day or night. Nick had no friends. Indeed, a school transfer was necessary because he was continually scapegoated. He refused to bathe, wore his clothes backward, chewed his shirts, swallowed his nasal mucus, and occasionally soiled his pants. Depressed and moody, he frequently talked about suicide. (At the time, the parents were talking about divorce, although this was kept from the child.) At age 2, Nick had been evaluated by a developmental specialist. He showed accelerated development in certain areas and retardation in others. Although his intellectual ability placed him in the superior range, he differed from most 2-year-olds in the way he used his abilities, illustrating the deficit in adaptive capacity described by Leichtman and Nathan (1983). For example, he conceptualized his environment to such a degree that his response to blocks did not reflect their potential use in building houses. His capacity for imaginative play was already lagging. At age 2, he was considered to be at risk for borderline personality disorder.

Family Assessment

The families of adolescents (Shapiro et al. 1975) and children with borderline personality disorder tend to foster and maintain borderline functioning. There is anxiety about supporting the child's autonomy and a denial of his or her independence. The defense mechanisms of splitting, devaluation, idealization, denial, and primitive forms of projection seen in the individual also operate in the family group.

In a well-designed pilot study, children of mothers with borderline personality disorder were compared with children of mothers with a nonborderline personality disorder (Weiss et al. 1996). All the subjects were patients at a psychiatric outpatient department. The children whose mothers had borderline personality disorder had significantly more diagnoses of attention deficit disorder, disruptive behavior disorder, and borderline personality disorder than did the control subjects. Their scores on the Child Global Assessment Schedule (CGAS) were significantly lower compared with the control subjects and tended to be in the nonfunctional range.

Trauma did not differentiate the two groups. Trauma included all forms of abuse (physical, sexual, and verbal), neglect, witnessing of domestic violence, and placement in an institution. The increased psychopathology in the offspring of mothers with borderline personality could be accounted for by shared temperamental factors such as impulsivity and by family characteristics. Indeed, compared with the families of control subjects, the families of the mothers with borderline personality had lower cohesion, less organization, and less stability. Parental drug abuse and suicide attempts and unprotective fathers were also significantly more prevalent. Thus, both biological and psychological factors appeared to play roles in the increased psychopathology in the children (Weiss et al. 1996).

Protective factors that mitigate the increased risk of psychopathology that results from having a parent with manifest borderline pathology are self-understanding, sublimation, ability to form positive relationships with other caretakers, and constructive use of fantasy (Glickhauf-Hughes and Mehlman 1998).

Psychological Testing

In both structured and projective tests, children with borderline personality disorder show fluidity of associations, peculiar logic, and flights into fantasy, although not formal thought disorder. Even if their perceptual, motor, and intellectual capacities are intact, these children do not use them creatively or effectively. Overall, there is a deficit in adaptation (Leichtman and Nathan 1983). Object representations seem to be unrealistic and unidimensional. Human precepts tend to split into all-bad or all-good figures. Partial merger, in the sense of one person being attached to another, seems rather typical: for example, a patient may describe two-headed people or two elephants joined together at the tail. Themes of loss, separation, and abandonment, with helplessness and primitive aggression, appear. The tenuous sense of identity is illustrated by body-image distortions, anxiety about disappearance, strong identification with extraterrestrial beings, and visions of people about to explode.

Differential Diagnosis

Borderline personality disorder should be considered in Axis I syndromes such as severe conduct disorders, separation anxiety disorder, anorexia nervosa, bulimia nervosa, gender identity disorder, and selective mutism. In adolescents, as with adults, major affective disorder is frequently associated with borderline personality disorder. The specific developmental disorders have all been found in a significant percentage of adolescents and young adults with borderline personality disorder (Andrulonis et al. 1981).

Children with borderline personality disorder may have brief psychotic episodes related to stress with paranoid symptoms, depersonalization, derealization, dissociation, and suicide attempts. However, these are different from psychosis (P.F. Kernberg 1983a). Typical psychotic processes include fragmentation, extreme hypochondriasis, animation of inanimate objects, deanimation of animate objects, formation of bizarre objects, and persistent delusions and hallucinations. The anxieties go beyond the ones of annihilation but are characterized by fears of falling, losing oneself through dissolving, or disappearing. Lack of capacity to test reality, given the supports of clarification and confrontation, further delineates psychosis from borderline conditions. The psychotic patient's regressions to a symbolic state, with no boundaries between self and object, are to be contrasted with the fusion fantasies of the patient with borderline personality (P.F. Kernberg 1983a). Children with borderline personality illustrate failures in the separation-individuation process but not regression to an undifferentiated self. This formulation has practical implications in clarifying and understanding the reactions of the patient to the therapist.

■ Treatment

The treatment of the patient with borderline personality disorder should be multimodal, with the therapist giving attention to both the child and the environment. Day hospitals, inpatient settings, and special school programs are reserved for the more severe forms of this disorder.

Family Therapy

Family work should address the correction of intrafamilial interactions—especially splitting, projection, and denial among different family members—and the child's acceptance of the parents' relationship as a couple. The child also needs help in seeing the parents objectively in both their positive and their negative aspects, as well as support in grieving for what the parents are not. In this way, the child becomes able to see that parents have their own separate limitations, which are not caused by the child.

Psychotherapy

Psychoanalytically oriented psychotherapy should be conducted two or three times a week for a minimum of 1–2 years. Play materials should be simple and should lend themselves to gross motor activities (e.g., sponge

balls, dart games, bowling equipment). Interventions should emphasize the here and now as a way of enhancing the child's reality-testing capacity. The child's perception of the therapist's actions and verbal interventions should also be clarified on an ongoing basis. Fantasy distortions need to be verbalized and shared to allow for secondary verbalization and clarification. The possibility of sharing primitive fantasies with the therapist will lower the child's anxiety and will permit fantasies to be channeled through play, dreams, or even daydreams rather than impulse-ridden, self-destructive behaviors.

Working with the lack of ego and superego integration requires discussion of attempts at splitting, denial, omnipotent control, primitive projection, idealization, and devaluation. Often the child's body language evidences the splitting defense, and this should be clarified. Integration of the split sense of self is another important goal. Facilitating a sense of continuity across time and situations helps correct the unstable sense. The therapist serves as the container of different states and different frames of mind that belong to one person—the child.

A focus on superego functions can help to neutralize aggressive impulses toward self and others as well as omnipotent traits that prompt the child to antisocial behaviors. The child's ability to empathize with others can be improved by providing feedback on the effect of the child's shifting functioning onto the therapist.

The various vicissitudes of differentiation, rapprochement, and pathological symbiosis should be dealt with in the relationship between therapist and child. The so-called preoedipal conflicts around issues of trust or distrust, remaining the same or daring to become different, following or running away, being controlled or being in control, remaining dependent or becoming autonomous, being a boy or a girl or an undifferentiated neuter—all are aspects that can be discussed to enable the child to proceed with development into later stages.

Children with borderline personality disorder also may need help with their sense of body ego, especially given the frequent association with attention-deficit disorders and associated cognitive disorders, which can augment their sense of instability. These children need to be able to talk realistically about such deficits.

Finally, treatment should account for ego weakness and lack of impulse control. The ego defect or arrest is seen as resulting from defenses such as splitting, denial, projection, and regression; these can be interpreted in terms of their meanings and functions during therapeutic work. In contrast, if the ego weakness is seen as irreversible, rather than as a form of defense, the possibility of change will not be considered, thus contributing to a self-fulfilling prophecy.

Through interactions with another child, in a group of two or with a small therapy group, the child learns how to listen, respond, maintain contact, negotiate, and conclude interactions in a step-by-step manner.

Medication

Medication also can be an important adjunct for the child with a borderline personality disorder. The choice depends on the target symptoms. Low-dosage, high-potency neuroleptics may be helpful in reducing the child's disorganization and facilitating the internalization of therapeutic interventions. If the target symptom is depression, appropriate psychopharmacological agents may be indicated. In general, the effects of medication should be reassessed from time to time as the child's psychological reorganization becomes stabilized.

■ Prognosis

The prognosis of children with borderline personality is from guarded to good, depending on environmental factors and the possibility of access to effective treatment. Without treatment, however, the general consensus is that these children are at severe risk for the continuation of their borderline personality disorder, antisocial personality disorder, substance abuse, or other forms of more serious disorders in the schizophrenic and manic-depressive range (Kestenbaum 1983).

The continuity of childhood borderline conditions into adulthood has been addressed, although as yet not in a conclusive manner (Blum 1974; O.F. Kernberg 1978; Mahler and Kaplan 1977; Pine 1974). In an ongoing study of borderline personality disorders in adults, Dr. John Clarkin (personal communication, May 1989) found that patients with borderline personality typically reported that their symptoms started in childhood, a finding supported by Dr. Martha Linehan (personal communication, March 1988).

Narcissistic Personality Disorder

McGlashan and Heinssen (1989) described an overlap between narcissistic, antisocial, and borderline personality disorders; all share certain features of borderline personality and a relative absence of schizophrenic and manic symptoms. They differ, however, in terms of narcissistic and antisocial traits. The three basic criteria for narcissistic personality disorder are a pervasive pattern of grandiosity, lack of empathy, and a hypersensitivity to the evaluation of others.

In more detail, DSM-IV-TR criteria (Table 42–4) are that the patient 1) reacts to criticism with feelings of rage, shame, or humiliation; 2) is interpersonally exploitive, taking advantage of others to achieve his or her own needs; 3) has a grandiose sense of self-importance, expects to be noticed as "special," and exaggerates achievements and talents; 4) believes that his or her problems are unique and can be understood only by other "special" people; 5) is preoccupied with fantasies of unlimited success, power, brilliance, beauty, or ideal love; 6) has a sense of entitlement; 7) requires constant attention and admiration; 8) lacks empathy, being unable to recognize and experience how others feel; and 9) is preoccupied with feelings of envy.

Frequently, many of the features of histrionic, borderline, and antisocial personality disorders are also present in narcissistic personality disorder (McGlashan and Heinssen 1989). Depressed mood is extremely common. Personal defeats or irresponsible behavior may be justified by rationalization or lying. There is no gratification in achievement. The superego is not well integrated and tends to be projected either to the outside (through paranoid anxieties) or to the body (through somatic and hypochondriacal symptoms. Typically, exploitiveness is also projected to the outside, resulting in extreme distrust of others.

Case 5

Cathy was 9 years old when I first saw her. She was described by her parents as overcontrolling, prone to temper outbursts, derogatory toward adults, and insulting to her parents, calling them "dumb" and "stupid." Because of her haughty and controlling manner, she did not have any friends. She was seen for 7 months, and most of these traits appeared to recede, but 3 years later, her parents consulted me again. Although Cathy was now doing very well at school, she did not have close friends. Her mother commented on Cathy's self-centeredness and indicated that she did not know the subtleties of discretion or "loyalty." There was intense rivalry with her sister, 3 years her junior. She was prone to temper tantrums and made her parents feel incompetent. She also devalued her mother's relationship with her father, saying she couldn't understand why her mother had married

Table 42–4. DSM-IV-TR diagnostic criteria for narcissistic personality disorder

A pervasive pattern of grandiosity (in fantasy or behavior), need for admiration, and lack of empathy, beginning by early adulthood and present in a variety of contexts, as indicated by five (or more) of the following:

(1) has a grandiose sense of self-importance (e.g., exaggerates achievements and talents, expects to be recognized as superior without commensurate achievements)

(2) is preoccupied with fantasies of unlimited success, power, brilliance, beauty, or ideal love

(3) believes that he or she is "special" and unique and can only be understood by, or should associate with, other special or high-status people (or institutions)

(4) requires excessive admiration

(5) has a sense of entitlement, i.e., unreasonable expectations of especially favorable treatment or automatic compliance with his or her expectations

(6) is interpersonally exploitative, i.e., takes advantage of others to achieve his or her own ends

(7) lacks empathy: is unwilling to recognize or identify with the feelings and needs of others

(8) is often envious of others or believes that others are envious of him or her

(9) shows arrogant, haughty behaviors or attitudes

Source. Reprinted from American Psychiatric Association: *Diagnostic and Statistical Manual of Mental Disorders*, 4th Edition, Text Revision. Washington, DC, American Psychiatric Association, 2000. Copyright 2000, American Psychiatric Association. Used with permission.

her father. Cathy had a poor body image and liked to cover herself with oversized sweatshirts. She had problems going away from home and felt chronically homesick at camp. Described as arrogant by her teachers, she avoided eye contact with adults. She did only things she could do easily and well. Left to her own devices, she was easily bored. Indeed, there was a constant sense of dissatisfaction and dysphoria, which she verbally denied.

■ Clinical Manifestations

Some clinical and developmental manifestations are characteristic of narcissistic children (P.F. Kernberg 1989). They may have severe learning problems. Despite superior intelligence, these children can fail. Teachers report that these youngsters can be arrogant and haughty, believing that nobody is entitled to tell them what to do. They either get the best grades or the worst, for they find it difficult to apply themselves to any study they feel is beneath their dignity. They do not enjoy their learning experience. All their activities have a "driven" quality, without interest in the activity for its intrinsic value. Activities and achievements are only means to satisfy the ongoing need for attention and admiration.

Problems with peers are codetermined by an inability to empathize with others and by intense feelings of envy. Any acknowledgment of difference is haughtily denied. Friends can be friends only when they are clones. Peers are related to with a feeling of entitlement that justifies exploitiveness. Friends can be over-

idealized or can be devalued if they become a source of envy, so that the whole relationship is disavowed. These youngsters tend to choose either a popular, pretty, or handsome partner to reflect on their grandiosity or someone who is considered extremely ugly or "a freak," in that way enhancing their sense of worth by contrast with the devalued partner, who is under their control.

Narcissistic children may show gaze aversion. For children with narcissistic personality disorder, avoiding eye contact helps to avoid the traumatic experience of not being acknowledged. In addition, it helps to avoid confrontation between their own grandiosity and the reflection from adults, who see them as vulnerable and self-deceiving.

The play of narcissistic children is disturbed. Between ages 3.5 and 11 years, these children quickly become bored with new toys and are inhibited in their play, particularly their fantasy play. Even in structured games, however, these children react to any defeat with rule changes, temper tantrums, and regressive reactions. As treatment proceeds and the narcissistic child engages in fantasy, the play is characterized by raw aggression: toys and dolls are dismembered and bleed to death, or the whole earth is massacred by a gun-wielding murderer without mercy. Initially, the play is pleasureless, but later sadistic enjoyment may occur. There is a proclivity to cheat and to change rules if the game does not go in their direction. The need for constant attention and admiration can disguise an inability to be alone. Separation anxiety may be covered up by haughtiness and devaluation. One 4-year-old patient dragged his mother into the playroom, only to have her sit there while he conducted himself in an aloof manner, as if he did not care about her existence. However, if the mother attempted to leave the room or refused to accompany him into the playroom, he had a temper outburst. In adolescence, these patients may refuse to participate in sleep-overs or to go away to camp, claiming a lack of interest in these activities.

A preoccupation with self-image can be seen at times in a compulsive need to look in the mirror. There is an acute sense of vulnerability in self-regard, both psychological and physical.

■ Additional Developmental Considerations

In the diagnosis of narcissistic personality disorder in childhood, it is important to differentiate between infantile narcissism and pathological narcissism. Young children, for instance, normally have grandiose fantasies and make angry efforts to control their mother and to keep themselves at the center of her attention. Fantasies of great power, wealth, and beauty are common in the preschool years. However, the nonnarcissistic child does not need to be universally admired as the sole owner of everything that is enviable and valuable. The demands are related to realistic needs and incapacities. When these needs are gratified, the child is satisfied. In contrast, in pathological narcissism, the demands are excessive and can never be fulfilled.

Nonnarcissistic children are capable of warm gratitude when their demands are met, but narcissistic children tend to be cold and aloof, "entitled" at best. In the nonnarcissistic child, achievements enhance self-esteem and self-regard, are enjoyed, and enable the child to set new realistic goals. In contrast, in narcissistic children, successes or achievements offer fleeting satisfaction, as long as attention from others is obtained. Nonnarcissistic young children show genuine attachment and interest in others, at least when they are not frustrated, and they have the capacity to trust or depend on significant objects. The narcissistic child is unable to depend on other people and does not show genuine attachment and interest in others; on the contrary, these feelings are pretended to obtain gratification and to exploit others.

At least from school age on, nonnarcissistic children accept their positive and negative aspects and begin striving toward ideals provided by parents or friends. In narcissistic children, the accepted aspects

of the self are coalesced with the ideals, leading to the formation of a grandiose self, with projection of the negative aspects of the self onto the external world.

Rinsley (1989) postulated that although narcissistic personality disorder has overlapping characteristics with borderline personality disorder, it is developmentally different in the relationship to the mother. In the child with borderline personality, there is an arrest of both separation and individuation processes. In contrast, in narcissistic personality disorder there is a dissociation of these two processes, so a significant degree of individuation may be achieved in the face of separation failure. This leads to a pseudomature child and explains the separation anxiety.

Various developmental influences may present a risk for the formation of narcissistic personality disorder, such as having narcissistic parents, being adopted, being abused, being overindulged, losing a parent through death, or having a divorced parent who attempts to erase any traces of the child's identification with the other parent.

■ Treatment

The choice of treatment for narcissistic personality disorder is either psychoanalysis or intensive expressive-supportive psychotherapy two or three times a week. The goals are to uncover the primitive fantasies connected with the grandiose self and replace this pathological self with normal infantile narcissism or, in adolescence, with normal narcissism. This requires the systematic clarification, confrontation, and interpretation of the narcissistic defenses, including omnipotent control, devaluation, idealization, and denial in their expression in the relationship between the patient and the therapist (Egan and Kernberg 1984). Empathy with both the patient's libidinal, dependent wishes and his or her envious destructiveness is necessary. The therapist must be extremely cautious given the vulnerability of these patients; as one of them explained, "I feel like a turtle without a shell."

Concomitant parental counseling or family therapy is strongly recommended. Often the child is seen as an extension of the parents and not as a separate and different person in his or her own right. On the other hand, at times these children may exert such control on family members with such effectiveness that the family submits to them; the child then becomes the "monster who needs to be appeased," fueling the sense of grandiosity. Counseling with the parents includes enabling them to empathize with the child's contradictory, subjective experience of grandiosity and vulnerability, including the child's intense envy of those who can enjoy things.

Antisocial Personality Disorder

The diagnosis of antisocial personality disorder requires evidence of a full-fledged conduct disorder with onset before age 15 and a pattern of irresponsible and antisocial behavior since age 15 (Table 42–5).

Case 6

Adams and Fras (1988) described the case of Sharwell, an 11-year-old boy who met the criteria for borderline personality disorder and, it could be added, for antisocial personality disorder (except for age). This child had been seen by psychiatrists since age 5, which points to the chronicity and severity of his problems. He was assaultive and, by age 11, had beaten and raped a 6-year-old girl. His anger was uncontrollable, and he had bizarre fantasies about violence, death, and destructiveness. He occasionally lapsed into baby talk. On admission to the inpatient unit, Sharwell was ingratiating and overly complimentary to the therapist, whom he considered the only good person; in contrast, he was abusive to the rest of the staff, threatening to kill them. He had no ability to control his cravings: he overate and had the table manners of a 2-year-old. He conned other children; similarly, he begged or borrowed from any gullible adult. Yet, despite his show of bravado, he described himself as "bad, dumb, fat, weird looking, weak, and ugly."

Case 7

Because he was 16 years old at the time of his evaluation, Sam was given a diagnosis of severe conduct disorder, solitary type, rather than antisocial personality disorder. He had been stealing and lying since grammar school. Sam was the biological son of a man who had beaten and raped his mother. His mother was a substance abuser. In kindergarten, Sam was evaluated professionally when he poked a schoolmate with scissors. Although he was never officially charged with a crime, he was arrested by the police because of vandalism. He had day and night dreams of shooting and stabbing people. He also cut himself, stating "I feel relieved....I had a weight on my shoulders and [now] I don't feel it anymore."

In his mental status examination, Sam did not show any formal thought disorder. Cognitive function was intact clinically, as was his reality testing, although he had heard voices inside his head: "They tell me I am bad." Despite his fantasies of suicide and homicide, he denied he would act on these. He was aware of his lack of remorse when he did hurt someone: "I am so cold. Things don't affect me. I have no conscience." He had some insight into the nature of his difficulties, commenting that if he had a lot of feelings, he just could not hold everything in: "It builds up and I explode."

Table 42–5. DSM-IV-TR diagnostic criteria for antisocial personality disorder

A. There is a pervasive pattern of disregard for and violation of the rights of others occurring since age 15 years, as indicated by three (or more) of the following:

    (1) failure to conform to social norms with respect to lawful behaviors as indicated by repeatedly performing acts that are grounds for arrest

    (2) deceitfulness, as indicated by repeated lying, use of aliases, or conning others for personal profit or pleasure

    (3) impulsivity or failure to plan ahead

    (4) irritability and aggressiveness, as indicated by repeated physical fights or assaults

    (5) reckless disregard for safety of self or others

    (6) consistent irresponsibility, as indicated by repeated failure to sustain consistent work behavior or honor financial obligations

    (7) lack of remorse, as indicated by being indifferent to or rationalizing having hurt, mistreated, or stolen from another

B. The individual is at least age 18 years.

C. There is evidence of conduct disorder (see [DSM-IV-TR] p. 98) with onset before age 15 years.

D. The occurrence of antisocial behavior is not exclusively during the course of schizophrenia or a manic episode.

Source. Reprinted from American Psychiatric Association: *Diagnostic and Statistical Manual of Mental Disorders,* 4th Edition, Text Revision. Washington, DC, American Psychiatric Association, 2000. Copyright 2000, American Psychiatric Association. Used with permission.

During the psychiatric assessment, this boy murdered a neighbor. He did not complete the evaluation, because he was sent to a reform school.

■ Treatment

Psychotherapy is not effective for the child with antisocial personality disorder, because psychotherapy depends on the capacities for relationship and honesty, which are impaired in these patients. Behavior modification has had some positive results in attempts to control aggression with token economy and time-out procedures or contingency programs in which cessation of the behavior (e.g., stealing) leads to home visits. Parent training has also been relatively successful based on parent reporting. Pharmacotherapy has been used for target symptoms, but the findings from these trials are inconclusive.

Berlin (unpublished manuscript, October 1988) reported on a noncontingency milieu approach in which all contingencies are unpredictable and inconsistent in terms of punishment and rewards. The youngster is thrown into acute anxiety or depression, or even acute disorganization, which makes the child more dependent on the staff and more treatable. The treatment lasts from a few weeks to 2 months.

Research Issues

The systematic exploration of personality disorders in childhood and adolescence remains to be done. Gutterman et al. (1987) reviewed five structured diagnostic interviews keyed to DSM-III criteria for psychiatric disorders in childhood and adolescence. Only one of the five interview schedules for children included the assessment of borderline, compulsive, histrionic, and schizotypal personality disorders. Yet treatment outcome may depend on the diagnosis of personality disorder.

It is important to clarify the Axis II category and the relationship between Axis II and Axis I diagnoses. To compound the problem, there is overlap within Axis II (Gorton and Akhtar 1990; McGlashan and Heinssen 1989). In the overlap between Axis I and Axis II there is coexistence of affective disorders with a spectrum of disorders, including borderline, antisocial, dependent, narcissistic, and histrionic personality disorders; hypomanic episode; and other self-defeating disorders. Schizophrenic disorders and even paranoid disorders may exist on a spectrum with Cluster A (or psychotic) personality disorders, whereas the anxiety disorders and social phobias coexist on a continuum with Cluster C (or neurotic) personality disorders. Organic brain disorders such as attention-deficit/hyperactivity disorder seem to be frequently associated with the spectrum of borderline personality disorders. What is most interesting is that Axis II diagnoses may indicate a vulnerability to certain psychiatric illnesses, but they also may be the expression of chronic subsyndromal forms of specific psychiatric illnesses. Both conditions could be attributed to a specific or particular developmental experience or genetic predisposition. What is most important is that personality comorbidity often predicts the disease course and treatment outcome in a variety of patients (Weissman et al. 1978).

In sum, the consideration of personality disorders in children and adolescents provides the clinician with a potentially useful tool for treatment planning, as well as for coordinating research efforts within the adult psychiatry field.

Conclusion

A study of personality development is closely linked with the issues of continuities and discontinuities in development, as summarized by Emde and Harmon (1984). Although discontinuities often concern specific times of developmental transformation or change, there are also times of qualitative shifts with the formation of new patterns of behavior. From a genetic point of view, there are processes that switch on and switch off in development, so genetic mechanisms not only form the basis for stabilities but also can account for discontinuities. Discontinuity, however, does not imply a lack of connectedness between early developments and later ones, as described by Rutter (1984). From a different perspective, Korner (1964) described continuities in style that are related to temperament and dyadic relationships and continuities concerning competencies or skill, such as cognition.

Even biological models have to address these new perspectives on continuities. Despite the notion of critical periods, it has been found that adults can undergo structural alterations as a result of experience. The plasticity of the brain is greater than anticipated.

Longitudinal studies may clarify issues of continuity and discontinuity. For example, when the representational self emerges, an internalized set of intentions and role structures also begins to appear, so that it should then be more possible than before to identify continuities and behavioral connectedness. Another approach looks in more detail at heterotypical continuities, which relate to a given behavior that appears different at a later age because of developmental transformations.

Which aspects of personality are chosen for study certainly affects the outcome. Personality traits organize themselves, and it is this organization that shows continuity, not the isolated traits. It is also important to appreciate the mutual influences of the observation of behavioral traits and the environment, taking into account, for example, role expectations for the different sexes at school or at home. To talk about continuities requires that these continuities be related to the context in which they are studied.

■ Assessing Normality and Abnormality

Discussions of personality and personality disorders in the adult psychiatric literature (Frances 1986; Gorton and Akhtar 1990) indicate the controversy between categorical and dimensional taxonomy. Categorical taxonomy draws sharp boundaries between normality (no disorder present) and abnormality (disorder present). In contrast, dimensional taxonomy requires a quantitative assessment across a number of continuous dimensions, such as self-concept, interpersonal relations, and cognitive styles. Indeed, personality disorders viewed from a categorical perspective do not include patients who may have significant pathology, such as those who overlap Axis I and Axis II categories or have mixed atypical disorders. Moreover, more than one personality diagnosis may be present.

The same considerations can be applied to childhood psychopathology, with certain modifications. Any boundary between normality and abnormality needs to be related to the developmental stage. State versus trait confusion can be significantly reduced if clinicians base their assessment on collateral historical information and repeated interviews and observations rather than on a single interview. Any diagnosis of personality disorder should fulfill these criteria: 1) that there are inflexible and maladaptive behaviors causing significant impairment in social or occupational functioning, as well as subjective distress, and 2) that these

behaviors have been characteristic of the child's or adolescent's functioning for a period of 2 years or more and have been exhibited in a wide range of important social and personal contexts. This proviso should reassure clinicians who rightfully are concerned about overdiagnosis in childhood and adolescence.

References

Aarkrog T: Borderline and psychotic adolescents: borderline symptomatology from childhood—actual therapeutic approach. J Youth Adolesc 6:187–197, 1977

Adams PL, Fras I: Beginning Child Psychiatry. New York, Brunner/Mazel, 1988

American Psychiatric Association: Diagnostic and Statistical Manual of Mental Disorders, 3rd Edition. Washington, DC, American Psychiatric Association, 1980

American Psychiatric Association: Diagnostic and Statistical Manual of Mental Disorders, 4th Edition, Text Revision. Washington, DC, American Psychiatric Association, 2000

Andrulonis PA, Glueck BC, Stroebel CF, et al: Organic brain dysfunction and the borderline syndrome. Psychiatr Clin North Am 4:47–66, 1981

Bemporad JR, Smith HE, Hanson G, et al: Borderline syndromes in childhood: criteria for diagnosis. Am J Psychiatry 139:596–602, 1982

Beres D: Character formation in adolescence, in Psychoanalytic Approach to Problems and Therapy. Edited by Lorand S, Schneer H. New York, Delta Books, 1969, pp 1–9

Blum HF: The borderline childhood of the wolfman. J Am Psychoanal Assoc 22:721–742, 1974

Brazelton TB: Neonatal Behavioral Assessment Scale. Philadelphia, PA, JB Lippincott, 1973

Bronson WC: Adult derivatives of emotional expressiveness and reactivity control: developmental continuities from childhood to adulthood. Child Dev 38:801–817, 1967

Cantwell DP, Carlson GA: Stimulants, in Pediatric Psychopharmacology. Edited by Werry JS. New York, Brunner/Mazel, 1978, pp 171–207

Cohen DJ, Slaywitz SE, Young G, et al: Borderline syndromes and attention-deficit disorders of childhood, in The Borderline Child: Approaches to Etiology, Diagnosis and Treatment. Edited by Robson KS. New York, McGraw-Hill, 1983, pp 197–222

Egan J, Kernberg PF: Pathologic narcissism in childhood. J Am Psychoanal Assoc 32:39–62, 1984

Ekstein R, Wallerstein J: Observations on the psychology of borderline and psychotic children. Psychoanal Study Child 11:303–311, 1954

Emde RN, Harmon RJ: Entering a new era in the search for developmental continuities, in Continuities and Discontinuities in Development. Edited by Emde RN, Harmon RJ. New York, Plenum, 1984, pp 1–14

Epstein S: The stability of behavior: on predicting most of the people much of the time. J Pers Soc Psychol 37:1097–1126, 1979

Escalona SK, Heider GM: Prediction and Outcome. New York, Basic Books, 1959

Fenichel O: The Psychoanalytic Theory of the Neuroses. New York, WW Norton, 1945

Finch SM, Green JM: Personality disorders, in Basic Handbook of Child Psychiatry, Vol 2. Edited by Noshpitz J. New York, Basic Books, 1979, pp 235–248

Flament M, Whitaker A, Rapoport JL, et al: Obsessive-compulsive disorder in adolescence: an epidemiological study. J Am Acad Child Adolesc Psychiatry 27:764–771, 1988

Frances AJ: Introduction to personality disorders, in Psychiatry, Vol 1. Edited by Michels R, Cavenar JO Jr, Brodie HKH, et al. New York, Basic Books, 1986, pp 1–6

Frijling-Schreuder E: Borderline states in children. Psychoanal Study Child 24:307–327, 1969

Geleerd E: Borderline states in childhood and adolescence. Psychoanal Study Child 13:279–295, 1958

Glickauf-Hughes C, Mehlman E: Non-borderline patients with mothers who manifest borderline pathology. British Journal of Psychotherapy 14:295–302, 1998

Gorton G, Akhtar S: The literature on personality disorders, 1985–1988: trends, issues and controversies. Hosp Community Psychiatry 41:39–51, 1990

Gunderson J, Kolb J: Discriminating features of borderline patients. Am J Psychiatry 135:792–796, 1978

Gutterman EM, O'Brien JD, Young JG: Structured diagnostic interview for children and adolescents: current status and future directions. J Am Acad Child Adolesc Psychiatry 25:621–630, 1987

Halverson CF, Waldrop MF: Relations between preschool activity and aspects of intellectual and social behavior at age $7\frac{1}{2}$. Dev Psychol 12:107–112, 1976

Hartmann H: Ego Psychology and the Problem of Adaptation. New York, International Universities Press, 1958

Josephson MM, Porter RT (eds): Clinicians Handbook of Childhood Psychopathology. Northvale, NJ, Jason Aronson, 1979

Kagan J: Continuity and change in the opening years of life, in Continuities and Discontinuities in Development. Edited by Emde RN, Harmon RJ. New York, Plenum, 1984, pp 15–39

Kagan J, Moss A: Birth to Maturity. New York, Wiley, 1962

Kernberg OF: Borderline Conditions and Pathological Narcissism. Northvale, NJ, Jason Aronson, 1976a

Kernberg OF: Object Relations Theory and Clinical Psychoanalysis. New York, Jason Aronson, 1976b

Kernberg OF: The diagnosis of borderline conditions in adolescence, in Adolescent Psychiatry, Vol 6. Edited by Feinstein S, Giovacchini P. Chicago, IL, University of Chicago Press, 1978, pp 298–319

Kernberg PF: Psychoanalytic profile of the borderline adolescent, in Adolescent Psychiatry, Vol 7. Edited by Feinstein S, Giovacchini P. Chicago, IL, University of Chicago Press, 1979, pp 234–256

Kernberg PF: Hysterical personality in child and adolescent analysis, in Three Further Clinical Faces of Childhood. Edited by Anthony EJ. Jamaica, NY, Spectrum, 1981, pp 27–28

Kernberg PF: Borderline conditions: child and adolescent aspects, in The Borderline Child: Approaches to Etiology, Diagnosis and Treatment. Edited by Robson KS. New York, McGraw-Hill, 1983a, pp 101–119

Kernberg PF: Issues in the psychotherapy of borderline conditions in children, in The Borderline Child: Approaches to Etiology, Diagnosis and Treatment. Edited by Robson KS. New York, McGraw-Hill, 1983b, pp 224–234

Kernberg PF: Children with borderline personality organization, in Handbook of Clinical Assessment of Children and Adolescents, Vol 2. Edited by Kestenbaum CJ, Williams DT. New York, New York University Press, 1988, pp 604–625

Kernberg PF: Narcissistic personality disorder in childhood. Psychiatr Clin North Am 12:671–694, 1989

Kestenbaum C: The concept of the borderline child as a child at risk for major psychiatric disorder in adult life, in The Borderline Child: Approaches to Etiology, Diagnosis and Treatment. Edited by Robson KS. New York, McGraw-Hill, 1983, pp 49–82

Korner A: Significance of primary ego and drive endowment for later development in the exceptional infant, in The Normal Infant, Vol 1. Edited by Helmuth J. New York, Brunner/Mazel, 1964, pp 192–207

Leichtman M, Nathan S: A clinical approach to the psychological testing of borderline children, in The Borderline Child: Approaches to Etiology, Diagnosis and Treatment. Edited by Robson KS. New York, McGraw-Hill, 1983, pp 121–170

Lewis M: Personality and personality disorder, in Psychiatry, Vol 2. Edited by Michels R, Cavenar JO Jr, Brodie HKH, et al. New York, Basic Books, 1986, p 108

Looney JG, Kramer J, Milich R: The hyperactive child grows up: prediction of symptoms, delinquency, and achievement at follow-up, in Psychosocial Aspects of Drug Treatment for Hyperactivity. Edited by Gadow K, Looney J. Boulder, CO, Westview Press, 1981, pp 212–241

Mahler M, Kaplan L: Developmental aspects in the assessment of narcissistic and so-called borderline personalities, in Borderline Personality Disorders: The Concept, the Syndrome, the Patient. Edited by Hartocollis P. New York, International Universities Press, 1977, pp 71–86

Martin WE: Singularity and stability of profiles of social behavior, in Readings in Child Behavior and Development. Edited by Stendler DB. New York, Harcourt, Brace, and World, 1964, pp 92–117

Masterson J: From Borderline Adolescent to Functioning Adult: The Test of Time. New York, Brunner/Mazel, 1980

McGlashan TH, Heinssen RK: Narcissistic, antisocial and noncomorbid subgroups of borderline disorder. Psychiatr Clin North Am 12:653–670, 1989

Metcalf A: Childhood process to structure, in Hysterical Personality. Edited by Horowitz MJ. Northvale, NJ, Jason Aronson, 1977, pp 223–282

Moss HA, Susman EJ: Longitudinal study of personality development, in Constancy and Change in Human Development. Edited by Brim OG Jr, Kagan J. Cambridge, MA, Harvard University Press, 1980, pp 530–595

Pedersen E, Faucher TA, Eaton WW: A new perspective on the effects of first grade teachers on children's subsequent adult status. Harv Educ Rev 48:1–31, 1978

Petti AT: Imipramine treatment of borderline children: case reports with a controlled study. Am J Psychiatry 138:515–518, 1981

Petti AT, Law W: Borderline psychotic behavior in hospitalized children: approaches to assessment and treatment. J Am Acad Child Psychiatry 21:197–202, 1982

Pfeffer CR: Clinical observations of suicidal behavior in a neurotic, a borderline and a psychotic child: common processes of symptom formation. Child Psychiatry Hum Dev 13:120–133, 1983

Pine F: On the borderline concept in children. Psychoanal Study Child 29:341–368, 1974

Pine F: A working nosology of borderline syndromes in children, in The Borderline Child: Approaches to Etiology, Diagnosis and Treatment. Edited by Robson KS. New York, McGraw-Hill, 1983, pp 83–100

Plakun EM: Narcissistic personality disorder: a validity study and comparison to borderline personality disorder. Psychiatr Clin North Am 12:3, 1989

Rapoport JL, Ismond DR: DSM-III-R Training Guide for Diagnosis of Childhood Disorders. New York, Brunner/Mazel, 1990

Richman N, Stevenson J, Graham P: Preschool to School: A Behavioral Study. London, Academic Press, 1982

Rinsley DB: Notes on the developmental pathogenesis of narcissistic personality disorder. Psychiatr Clin North Am 12:695–707, 1989

Rockland LH: Supportive Therapy: A Psychodynamic Approach. New York, Basic Books, 1989

Rosenfeld K, Sprince M: An attempt to formulate the meaning of the concept "borderline." Psychoanal Study Child 18:603–635, 1963

Rutter M: Stress, coping and development: some issues and some questions. J Child Psychol Psychiatry 22:323–356, 1981

Rutter M: Continuities and discontinuities in socio-emotional development: empirical and conceptual perspectives, in Continuities and Discontinuities in Development. Edited by Emde RN, Harmon RJ. New York, Plenum, 1984, pp 41–68

Rutter M: Psychopathology and development: links between childhood and adult life, in Child and Adolescent Psychiatry: Modern Approaches. Edited by Rutter M, Hersov L. Oxford, UK, Blackwell Scientific, 1985, pp 720–739

Rutter M, Garmezy N: Developmental psychopathology, in Handbook of Child Psychology, Vol 4: Socialization, Personality and Social Development. Edited by Hetherington EM. New York, Wiley, 1983, pp 775–991

Rutter M, Graham P: Psychiatric disorder in the young adolescent: a follow-up study. Proc R Soc Med 66:1226–1229, 1973

Sandler V, Rosenblatt B: The concept of the representational world. Psychoanal Study Child 17:128–145, 1962

Scheidlinger S: Focus on Group Psychotherapy: Clinical Essays. New York, International Universities Press, 1982

Shapiro ER, Zinner J, Shapiro RL: The influence of family experience on borderline personality development. Int Rev Psychoanal 2:399–412, 1975

Shields J: Some recent developments in psychiatric genetics. Arch Gen Psychiatry 22:347–360, 1975

Shulsinger F: Psychopathy: heredity and environment. Journal of Mental Health 1:190–206, 1972

Weil AM: Certain severe disturbances of ego development in childhood. Psychoanal Study Child 8:271–286, 1953

Weiss M, Zelkowitz P, Feldman RB, et al: Psychopathology in offspring of mothers with borderline personality disorder: a pilot study. Can J Psychiatry 41:285–290, 1996

Weissman MM, Prusoff BA, Klerman GL: Personality and the prediction of long-term outcome of depression. Am J Psychiatry 135:797–800, 1978

Wiener JM: Diagnosis and Psychopharmacology of Childhood and Adolescent Disorders. New York, Wiley, 1995

Yang RK, Moss HA: Longitudinal study of personality development, in Constancy and Change in Human Development. Edited by Brim OG Jr, Kagan J. Cambridge, MA, Harvard University Press, 1978, pp 530–595

Substance Abuse Disorders

Steven L. Jaffe, M.D.

Ramon Solhkhah, M.D.

Substance use and abuse continue to constitute an epidemic in the adolescent population. Most teenagers use drugs or alcohol occasionally without negative consequences (71% of high school seniors drank alcohol during 2001), which gives parents and adolescents the impression that alcohol and drug use is normal. The reality is that half of these alcohol-using adolescents (35% of the seniors) have had a binge episode (five or more drinks at one time) in the past month, and 3.6% drink daily (Johnson et al. 2001). These adolescents become the group in which high-risk behaviors (e.g., driving after drinking, unprotected sex, and violence) will occur, with their associated morbidity and mortality. Whereas 13% of high school students drive a car after drinking, another 33% ride in cars in which the driver has been drinking (Levy et al. 2002). Homicides, suicides, and injuries account for 80% of teenage deaths, and more than half of these are associated with alcohol (Rogers and Adger 1993).

Substance abuse disorder and substance dependence disorder are specific DSM-IV-TR diagnoses defined by essential clinical criteria (American Psychiatric Association 2000). (Note: the DSM-IV-TR terminology has been modified for use in this chapter, as explained below under "Diagnostic Criteria.") Substance abuse disorder involves alcohol or drug usage that causes recurrent school, legal, and social failures and other high-risk behavior. A recent survey of 31,000 high school seniors (Harrison et al. 1998) reported that 15% met criteria for substance abuse disorder. Substance dependence disorder involves compulsive seeking and using alcohol or drugs despite negative physical or psychological problems. In the community survey of high school seniors, 7% met criteria for sub-

stance dependence disorder. Thus, more than 20% of seniors in high school are significantly involved with using alcohol and drugs and are in need of an intervention.

Significant substance abuse is a major or complicating factor in adolescents with severe psychiatric problems. Grunebaum and colleagues (1991) found that 40% of adolescents treated in psychiatric day or residential programs were comorbid for substance abuse disorder or substance dependence disorder related to alcohol or marijuana. In a study of adolescents admitted to an acute psychiatric impatient unit, Deas-Nesmith et al. (1998) found that 33% met criteria for substance abuse or dependence disorder that had not been identified during the hospitalization. Even higher rates, up to 80%, are found in adolescents in the juvenile justice system (Neighbors et al. 1992). These studies demonstrate that mental health professionals treating adolescents need to be knowledgeable and proficient in the assessment and treatment of adolescent substance use disorder.

Adolescents with psychiatric disorders also frequently have substance abuse disorders, and because 40%–90% of adolescents with substance use disorders have comorbid psychiatric disorders—specifically attention-deficit/hyperactivity disorder (ADHD), conduct disorders, anxiety disorders, and affective disorders (Jaffe 1996a)—the common practice of separating community psychiatric services from alcohol and drug services is inappropriate for adolescents. Substance abuse assessment and treatment services for adolescents need to be integrated with psychiatric services so that a higher level of therapeutic success can be attained.

Diagnostic Criteria

Adolescent substance abuse is a general nonspecific term that includes any use of alcohol or drugs by teenagers. This includes the entire range from occasional recreational use without negative consequences to the full syndrome of substance dependence disorder. The term *substance use* is rarely employed because all use by minors is illegal and therefore fits under *substance abuse*. In DSM-IV-TR under "Substance Use Disorders," *substance dependence* and *substance abuse* are listed. We recommend that the word *disorder* be appended to these terms (as we have done in this chapter) because it defines specific criteria and differentiates the DSM-IV-TR diagnosis from the general meaning of *substance abuse*. Tables 43–1 and 43–2 list the DSM-IV-TR diagnostic criteria for substance abuse disorder and substance dependence disorder.

Table 43–1. DSM-IV-TR diagnostic criteria for substance abuse

A. A maladaptive pattern of substance use leading to clinically significant impairment or distress, as manifested by one (or more) of the following, occurring within a 12-month period:

(1) recurrent substance use resulting in a failure to fulfill major role obligations at work, school, or home (e.g., repeated absences or poor work performance related to substance use; substance-related absences, suspensions, or expulsions from school; neglect of children or household)

(2) recurrent substance use in situations in which it is physically hazardous (e.g., driving an automobile or operating a machine when impaired by substance use)

(3) recurrent substance-related legal problems (e.g., arrests for substance-related disorderly conduct)

(4) continued substance use despite having persistent or recurrent social or interpersonal problems caused or exacerbated by the effects of the substance (e.g., arguments with spouse about consequences of intoxication, physical fights)

B. The symptoms have never met the criteria for substance dependence for this class of substance.

Source. From American Psychiatric Association: *Diagnostic and Statistical Manual of Mental Disorders,* 4th Edition, Text Revision. Washington, DC, American Psychiatric Association, 2000. Copyright 2000, American Psychiatric Association. Used with permission.

These diagnostic categories were developed from adult studies, and their validity in adolescents has not been demonstrated. Winters (2001) summarizes the problems in applying DSM-IV-TR criteria to adolescents: 1) withdrawal and drug-related medical problems are rare; 2) one abuse symptom yields a diagnosis; 3) abuse symptoms often do not precede dependence symptoms; and 4) two dependence symptoms with no abuse symptoms yields no diagnosis, but these "diagnostic orphans" do need therapeutic intervention. Substance dependence disorder that corresponds to addiction results from induced neurological changes in brain functioning in the reward circuitry (Roberts and Koob 1997). This results in the inability to moderate substance use despite severe harmful consequences even when the person tries to regulate use. This is often problematic to apply to adolescents who are heavily involved with substances but have made no acknowledged effort to control their use. Despite these problems, DSM-IV-TR does define clinically useful categories that require intensive treatment with the goals of abstinence, decreasing risks, and minimizing impairments.

Epidemiology

There are two major population-based surveys of substance abuse in adolescents. The Monitoring the Future Survey (Johnson et al. 2001) is school based and surveys about 50,000 students in grades 8, 10, and 12. The National Household Survey (Office of Applied Studies 2000) involves face-to-face interviewers and may include school dropouts but will still miss adolescents in juvenile justice and psychiatric residential settings. Data from these settings are used to demonstrate past and current general trends. Because overall abuse varies directly with availability and inversely with perceived risk of harm, these factors have recently been surveyed.

Information from the Monitoring the Future Survey reveals the following data and trends. Use of alcohol, the most commonly abused drug, has been fairly consistent over the past 25 years. (An apparent decrease in 1993 resulted from a change in the wording of the question defining a drink to "more than a few sips.") (Harrison 2001). Annual use by seniors has remained at about 73% since 1994. Use of marijuana in the previous year by seniors peaked in 1979 at 50.8%

Table 43–2. DSM-IV-TR diagnostic criteria for substance dependence

A maladaptive pattern of substance use, leading to clinically significant impairment or distress, as manifested by three (or more) of the following, occurring at any time in the same 12-month period:

(1) tolerance, as defined by either of the following:
   (a) a need for markedly increased amounts of the substance to achieve intoxication or desired effect
   (b) markedly diminished effect with continued use of the same amount of the substance
(2) withdrawal, as manifested by either of the following:
   (a) the characteristic withdrawal syndrome for the substance (refer to Criteria A and B of the criteria sets for withdrawal from the specific substances)
   (b) the same (or a closely related) substance is taken to relieve or avoid withdrawal symptoms
(3) the substance is often taken in larger amounts or over a longer period than was intended
(4) there is a persistent desire or unsuccessful efforts to cut down or control substance use
(5) a great deal of time is spent in activities necessary to obtain the substance (e.g., visiting multiple doctors or driving long distances), use the substance (e.g., chain-smoking), or recover from its effects
(6) important social, occupational, or recreational activities are given up or reduced because of substance use
(7) the substance use is continued despite knowledge of having a persistent or recurrent physical or psychological problem that is likely to have been caused or exacerbated by the substance (e.g., current cocaine use despite recognition of cocaine-induced depression, or continued drinking despite recognition that an ulcer was made worse by alcohol consumption)

Specify if:

   With Physiological Dependence: evidence of tolerance or withdrawal (i.e., either Item 1 or 2 is present)
   Without Physiological Dependence: no evidence of tolerance or withdrawal (i.e., neither Item 1 nor 2 is present)

Course specifiers (see text for definitions):

   Early Full Remission
   Early Partial Remission
   Sustained Full Remission
   Sustained Partial Remission
   On Agonist Therapy
   In a Controlled Environment

Source. From American Psychiatric Association: *Diagnostic and Statistical Manual of Mental Disorders,* 4th Edition, Text Revision. Washington, DC, American Psychiatric Association, 2000. Copyright 2000, American Psychiatric Association. Used with permission.

and reached a low of 21.8% in 1992, but it has increased rapidly with a recent high of 38.5% in 1997 and 37% in 2001. The perceived harmfulness of marijuana use significantly decreased in the 1990s.

Cigarette smoking by adolescents peaked in the late 1970s, dropped in the 1980s, and remained just below the 1980s level in the 1990s. After a relative increase in 1997, the rate returned to the low of 1992. Of course the rate of 29.5% of seniors who smoked cigarettes in the past month in 2001 is much too high. Nonprescription amphetamine use peaked in 1981, reached a low in 1992, and has shown a small increase recently. Methamphetamine use has increased in recent years. LSD use peaked in 1975 and reached a low between 1988 and 1990, but returned to almost peak use in 1997, when annual use by seniors was 8.4%. Inhalant use, which peaks in early adolescence, has slowly decreased in the 1990s, with the annual rate for eighth-graders decreasing to 9.1% in 2001. This steady decline appears to be related to increased perception of the high risk of harm. Heroin use has recently declined after some years of growth, and cocaine use moderately increased after a low in 1999.

Of much concern is the recent sharp increase in the use of 3,4-methylenedioxymethamphetamine (MDMA; "ecstasy"). The annual rate for seniors increased from 3.6% in 1998 to 9.2% in 2001. There has also been a sharp increase in availability. A hopeful sign is that the perceived risk increased during 2001. Another area of significant concern is the continued increase in the use of anabolic steroids, with the annual rate of use among seniors of 1.3% in 1994 increasing to 2.4% in 2001. These statistics indicate that although there is some variability in extent and drug of choice, during the past 25 years adolescents have continued to abuse substances at frightening levels.

Assessment

■ Domains and Stages to Be Assessed

All adolescents presenting with mental health problems should be screened for substance abuse. Any change in behavior, mood, or cognitive functioning may indicate that substance abuse is a major or contributing factor. Tarter (1990) presents the importance of exploring problems in all the domains of the adolescent's life. These include physical health status, aggressive-behavior problems, psychiatric disorders, social skills, family relationships, school adjustment, peer relationships, work adjustment, and recreation.

In terms of these domains, the severity of substance use and the consequences for the adolescent (including physical, emotional, and cognitive areas as well as school, peer, and family functioning) need to be defined. Patterns of use—including age at onset, amount, frequency, types of agents, and negative consequences—should be explored. Adolescents tend to move along a specific progression, with fewer individuals using each agent in the sequence (Kandel 1975). Thus many adolescents begin with cigarettes, beer, and wine; some progress to marijuana; some of those progress to problem drinking; and fewer still move on to hallucinogens, stimulants, and opiates. Adolescents tend not to stop using the substances used earlier in the sequence, which results in the characteristic that adolescents are multiple drug users. Assessment involves defining the times, places, peer use, antecedents, consequences, and attempts and failures to control use for each type of substance used. Because the adolescent may not be fully honest in what is revealed, information from the family, school, peers, and legal authorities is essential.

In addition to a progression of specific substances used, there is a progression of stages that describes increased involvement, effects, and consequences of substances on the life of the adolescent (Chatlos 1996; Macdonald 1984; Nowinski 1990). These stages are outlined below. Assessing the stage of substance involvement helps in specific treatment planning.

1. *Experimental or social stage.* This is the beginning stage of use, in which the important factors are curiosity and doing what one's peers may be doing. Teenagers are often told that drugs are fun, and they seek the thrill of doing something they are not supposed to be doing. They often find that drug use helps them gain acceptance by specific peers. As they become somewhat more involved in using alcohol and drugs they may then enter the second stage.

2. *Substance misuse.* In this stage the teenager is actively seeking the pleasurable experiences of using alcohol and drugs. Often he or she has also learned that the misuse helps him or her to escape from feelings of frustration, anger, depression, and inadequacy. At this stage the teenager tends to use substances primarily on weekends, and there will be some deterioration in grades and in conforming with rules. Increased usage and involvement may then lead to the third stage.

3. *Substance abuse disorder.* At this stage the teenager is clearly harmfully involved and preoccupied with using alcohol and drugs. Drugs and alcohol are now being used during the week. The peer group is primarily a drug and alcohol using group. The adolescent knows where and how to obtain alcohol and drugs and is increasingly involved in these activities. Alcohol and drugs are now significantly taking over the teenager's life, and there are significant impairments in functioning at school and at home. The teenager has become secretive, deceptive, and dishonest. DSM-IV-TR criteria of substance abuse disorder will be met. This involves a maladaptive pattern of failure of major role obligations at work, school, or home because of substance use; recurrent use in physically hazardous situations; recurrent substance-related legal problems; or continued use despite recurrent social or interpersonal problems. Further involvement in the progression may lead to the fourth stage of substance dependence disorder.

4. *Substance or chemical dependence disorder (also described as addiction).* This is the stage of harmful dependence. DSM-IV-TR criteria of substance dependence will be met. Usually tolerance has developed. Withdrawal symptoms, which tend to be infrequent in the adolescent population, may be present. Attempts to control usage have been unsuccessful. Use of larger amounts than were intended and failure in attempts to stop or reduce usage have occurred. Obtaining, using, and dealing with the consequences of use of alcohol and drugs have taken over most of the teenager's life, and he or she continues to use despite knowledge of the severe con-

sequences. Addiction involves an inability to use alcohol and drugs in moderation. An adolescent at this stage of drug involvement might be able to have some periods of not using drugs at all, but when or if he or she begins to use, the use rapidly goes out of control, with return of severe negative consequences.

■ Standardized Assessment Instruments

The well-known CAGE screening questions were developed for adults and are not very useful for adolescents. During the past several years, a number of screening and evaluation instruments have been developed that specifically assess adolescent substance abuse. These include the following:

- *The CRAFFT.* This screening instrument, developed in a medical office setting, consists of the following questions:

  C—Have you ever ridden in a **C**ar driven by someone (including yourself) who was high or had been using alcohol or drugs?

  R—Do you ever use alcohol/drugs to **R**elax, feel better about yourself, or fit in?

  A—Do you ever use alcohol/drugs while you are by yourself or **A**lone?

  F—Do you ever **F**orget things you did while using alcohol/drugs?

  F—Do your **F**amily or **F**riends ever tell you that you should cut down on your drinking or drug use?

  T—Have you ever gotten into **T**rouble while you were using alcohol or drugs?

  Two or more "yes" answers suggest serious problems with substances and indicate that further evaluation is needed (Knight et al. 1999).
- *Drug Use Screening Inventory (DUSI).* This self-report instrument, which consists of 149 yes/no questions, identifies specific problem areas in the 10 domains that need further evaluation (Tarter 1990).
- *Problem Oriented Screening Instrument for Teenagers (POSIT).* This self-report questionnaire, consisting of 139 true/false questions, identifies problems in 10 domains. It is available at no charge from the National Institute on Drug Abuse.
- *Personal Experience Screening Questionnaire (PESQ).* An initial screening instrument, the self-report PESQ consists of 38 questions. It measures problem sever-

ity and drug use history and includes a validity scale for lying (Center for Substance Abuse Treatment 1999a; Winters 2001).
- *Personal Experience Inventory (PEI).* A self-report questionnaire with 300 items, the PEI measures problem severity of substance use and personal risk factors; it includes a validity scale (Center for Substance Abuse Treatment 1999a; Winters 2001).
- *Adolescent Diagnostic Interview (ADI).* The ADI is a structured interview to evaluate DSM-III-R (American Psychiatric Association 1987) substance abuse diagnosis, school and interpersonal functioning, and psychosocial stresses (Center for Substance Abuse Treatment 1999a; Winters 2001).
- *Teen-Addiction Severity Index.* This is a semistructured interview that rates severity in seven domains. It is intended for use in follow-up studies (Kaminer 1991).
- *Urine drug screens.* Urine drug tests are commonly used to detect recent use of illegal drugs. Mental health professionals and parents need to be aware of the uses and limitations of the urine drug screen. The urine must be obtained under observed conditions to make sure that it is the test subject's sample, that a foreign substance such as apple juice has not been substituted, and that it has not been adulterated. The accuracy of the urine drug test is limited to the length of time the specific drug stays in the body and will therefore be present in the urine. Stimulants may be detected up to 48 hours after the last use; cocaine and its metabolite benzoylecgonine may be detected up to 3 days; and opiates (morphine, codeine) may be detected up to 2 days after last use. Short-acting barbiturates can be detected for 1 day, diazepam, up to 4 days, and methaqualone, up to 2 weeks. Marijuana, which is stored in fatty tissue, may be detected in the urine up to 4 days in recreational users and up to a month in daily users (Schwartz 1993). A negative urine test result does not prove that the adolescent does not use drugs, although many parents use a negative test to confirm their denial. A positive test result should be confirmed by more specific testing. A positive test result only demonstrates use and not a substance use disorder. Results of the urine drug screen need to be integrated into the entire assessment of the adolescent and the family and should be used as important but not conclusive data.

Table 43–3. Risk factors for development of substance abuse disorders

Genetic factors

- Presence of a substance abuse problem in one or both parents

Constitutional and psychological factors

- Psychiatric comorbidity
- History of physical, sexual, or emotional abuse
- History of attempted suicide

Sociocultural factors

Family

- Parental experiences and positive attitudes toward drug use
- History of parental divorce (or separation)
- Low expectations for the child

Peers

- Friends who use drugs
- Friends' positive attitudes toward drug use
- Antisocial or delinquent behavior

School

- School failure or dropping out

Community

- Positive attitudes toward drug use
- Economic and social deprivation
- Availability of drugs and alcohol (including cigarettes)

Etiology

Certain factors put children and adolescents at risk for the development of a substance use disorder. These factors are summarized in Table 43–3.

No one risk factor leads to substance abuse. In fact, the more risk factors an individual has, the greater the risk of developing the disorder. Different combinations of risk factors can lead to different potentials for negative outcomes, based on the strength and nature of the individual risk factors. Some protective factors, however, may cushion the effect of the risk factor and modify the severity or prevent negative outcome. Some researchers have begun to identify the interaction between risk factors and protective factors (Pandina et al. 1992; Newcomb 1995).

Some studies highlight the complexity of these interacting factors with biopsychosocial development. Certain genetic factors may not come into play until after substances have begun to be used. In adoption studies on 485 monozygotic and 335 dizygotic female twins, Kendler and Prescott (1998a) demonstrated

that cannabis use was influenced by genetic and familial environmental factors, whereas cannabis abuse and dependence were solely related to genetic factors. The same was also true for cocaine use versus abuse and dependence (Kendler and Prescott 1998b). Inherited susceptibility can be explained by the neurobiological research done by Nestler (1994, 1995). Those who have a greater genetic predisposition to develop substance abuse may be more susceptible to the influence of alcohol on gene expression. Consistent exposure of the ventral tegmentum and nucleus accumbens to alcohol and other drugs may form permanent changes in the second messenger system inside the cell. This may influence the turning on of genes, which may in turn influence the drive mechanism to use substances.

The age and developmental level of beginning substance use are important factors. Rapid progression of alcohol and drug disorders occurred often with earlier age at onset and with greater frequency, not longer duration, of use (DeWitt et al. 2000; Kandel 1992). Individuals with earlier onset had a shorter time span from first exposure to dependence than did individuals in adult-onset groups (Clark et al. 1998). Age at onset of heavy drinking also predicted alcohol-related problems (Lee and DiClimente 1985).

Peer issues are some of the strongest factors of risk. Peer attitudes about use of substances predicted initiation of use of alcohol and other substances (Bauman and Ennett 1994; Kandel 1975). In fact, strong peer attachment rather than parent attachment has been shown to be more influential during adolescence in predicting susceptibility to substance abuse (Brook 1980; Kandel 1978). Peer influence also plays a strong role in predicting relapse. Ninety percent of teenagers who relapse do so due to peer pressure (Brown 1993).

Treatment

After careful evaluation, the clinician should make a determination of the stage of substance abuse involvement. In the framework outlined below, each stage of substance abuse involvement is described along with the corresponding treatment approaches. This framework provides an initial strategy for relating treatment to the degree of involvement in substance abuse (Chatlos 1996; Jaffe 1996b) (Figure 43–1).

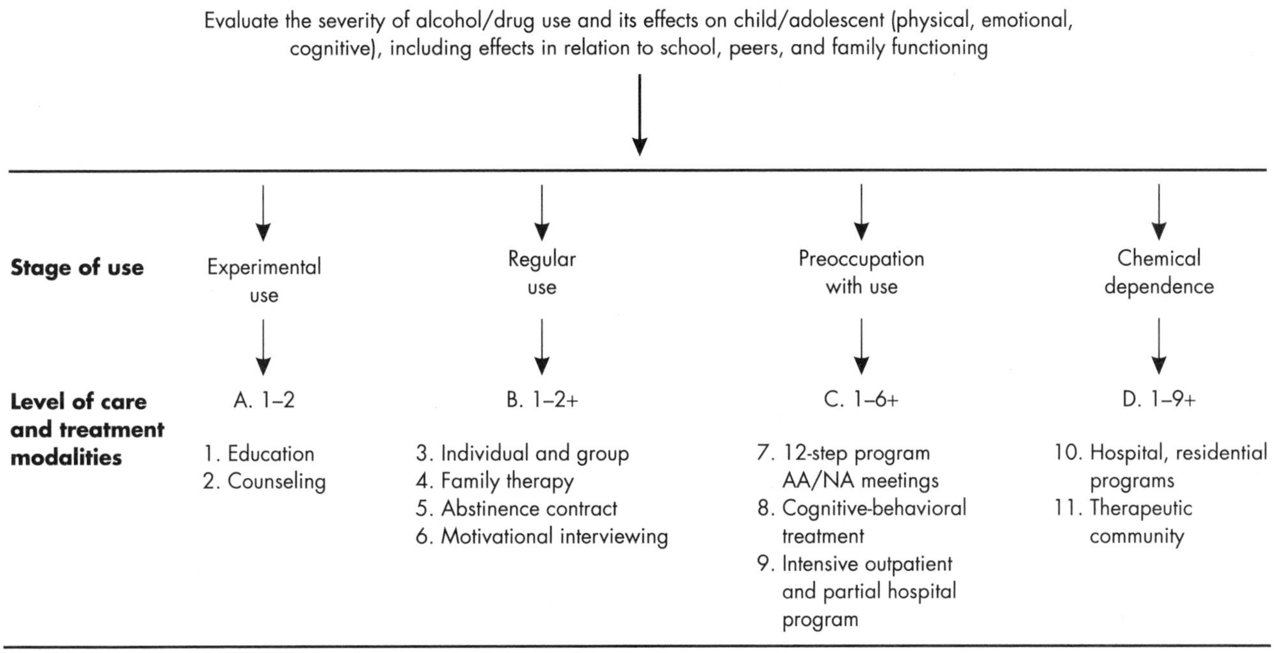

Evaluate the severity of alcohol/drug use and its effects on child/adolescent (physical, emotional, cognitive), including effects in relation to school, peers, and family functioning

Stage of use	Experimental use	Regular use	Preoccupation with use	Chemical dependence
Level of care and treatment modalities	A. 1–2	B. 1–2+	C. 1–6+	D. 1–9+
	1. Education 2. Counseling	3. Individual and group 4. Family therapy 5. Abstinence contract 6. Motivational interviewing	7. 12-step program AA/NA meetings 8. Cognitive-behavioral treatment 9. Intensive outpatient and partial hospital program	10. Hospital, residential programs 11. Therapeutic community

Figure 43–1. Substance abuse decision tree.

Note. AA=Alcoholics Anonymous; NA=Narcotics Anonymous.

■ Treatment Strategies for Experimental or Social Use

For adolescents at the stage of experimental or social use, education and counseling are appropriate. Teenagers use drugs in direct proportion to the availability and perceived safety of the drug. Learning about the realistic dangers of drugs and alcohol is helpful. For example, although adolescents tend to view marijuana as a benign drug, they should be taught that marijuana use poses a serious threat to brain functioning. Marijuana has been clearly demonstrated to cause loss of short-term memory, decreased concentration, and decreased motivation (Schwartz et al. 1989). Marijuana has been demonstrated to be addictive (Budney et al. 1999), but this information is usually not helpful in discussions with teenagers. More meaningful is the fact that as teenagers increase their consumption of marijuana to two or three times a week, their school work declines; their motivation decreases; and they spend more time being preoccupied with obtaining, smoking, and thinking about marijuana and tend to lose goals and productivity. Impairment, such as reduced ability to drive after smoking marijuana, may last up to 24 hours and is often not recognized by the adolescent (Leirer et al. 1991).

In addition to education, counseling is needed for adjustment issues, and parents may need help regarding how to set appropriate limits with rewards and consequences. Much educational material appropriate for teenagers may be obtained from the National Institute on Drug Abuse (http://www.drugabuse.gov; 1-888-644-6432) and the National Clearinghouse for Alcohol and Drug Information (http://www.health.org; 1-888-729-6686) of the Substance Abuse and Mental Health Services Administration.

■ Treatment Strategies for Substance Misuse

At the substance misuse stage, individual and group therapies, family treatments, and an abstinence contract may be needed in addition to education and counseling. At this stage family therapies—such as strategic, structural, systemic, and behavioral therapy—will be important interventions. Behavioral family therapy involves parent management training as well as contingency contracting. Specific, clear rules are established between parents and adolescents so that there are negative consequences for any drug use. Positive reinforcement is given for going to school, doing homework, avoiding peers who use drugs, and developing other recreational activities that are incompatible with drug use.

The abstinence or "honest look" contract is often helpful (Bailey 1996). In this situation, the teenager expresses a willingness to stop using drugs and alcohol and to stop "druggie" types of behavior. Specific rewards and punishments are contracted between the adolescent and the parents. Unannounced urine drug screens are included. If the teenager is unable to abide by the contract, specific consequences are dictated; these can include undergoing treatment at a more intense level of care.

Brief interventions using a combination of motivational interviewing, education, and development of coping skills have been developed as a harm reduction approach for the prevention and treatment of heavy alcohol use at college (Dimeff et al. 1999).

■ Treatment Strategies for Substance Abuse Disorder and Substance Dependence Disorder

In 1990, Catalano and colleagues (1990–1991) extensively reviewed the literature on adolescent drug abuse treatment and found that in residential programs, time in treatment was related to reduced alcohol and drug use. Family participation was associated with better outcome. No treatment modality was significantly better than any other, leading the researchers to conclude that some treatment was better than no treatment.

During the past several years, significant progress has been made. The National Institute on Drug Abuse has specifically increased support and direction for controlled studies on adolescent drug abuse treatment. Standards for clinical assessment and treatment, called *practice parameters,* have been published (Bukstein 1997). Deas and Thomas (2001) reviewed controlled studies on adolescent substance abuse and concluded that no treatment modality was shown to be more effective than any other. They recommended increased use of standardized assessment instruments and improved adolescent-specific outcome measures. A number of different treatment approaches have been used alone or in various combinations for the treatment of adolescent substance abuse and dependence disorders. The three most common are family therapy, 12-step–based programs, and therapeutic communities (Center for Substance Abuse Treatment 1999b). These and other treatment modalities are reviewed in the following sections.

Family Treatments

Treatment studies have demonstrated strong empirical support for the efficacy of family therapy (Stanton and Shadish 1997). Classic family therapy is based on the hypothesis that there is a connection between family relationships and the development and maintenance of drug abuse. Family therapy targets these specific interpersonal family processes. With structural-strategic family therapy, the emphasis is on establishing a coherent family hierarchy with appropriate rules and authority. Lewis et al. (1990) combined a number of different family therapy models to develop a 12-session treatment called the Purdue model. The goals included redefining substance use as a family problem, reestablishing parental influence, interrupting dysfunctional sequences of family behavior, and assessing the interpersonal function of the drug abuse. Families receiving this treatment model significantly decreased adolescent drug abuse compared with families receiving parent skill training.

Azrin and colleagues (1994) combined family therapy with behavior therapy techniques. The most important treatment component was the social–family contract, in which parents reinforced drug-incompatible activities, supervised home urge-control assignments, and employed written specification of desired behavior with contingent reinforcers. The control group received only supportive counseling. Significant results were demonstrated, with abstinence rates after 6 months of treatment being 73% for the treatment group and only 9% for the supportive-counseling group. Treated youths also had improved schoolwork and family relationships.

Multisystemic Therapy

Henggeler's multisystemic therapy integrates family therapy with direct interventions in the multiple interacting systems involving the individual, school, peer group, and community (Henggeler et al. 1993). Responsible behavior among all family members is promoted, and individuals develop the capacity to manage their own problems. Therapists work intensively with each adolescent and family and see them within their home, school, and even neighborhood peer group. Randomized studies in which multisystemic therapy was compared with individual counseling or probation for chronic juvenile offenders demonstrated reduced criminal activity continuing through a 4-year follow-up period. Preliminary data from a current study on multisystemic therapy for substance-abusing delinquents demonstrate excellent retention rates and favorable outcomes (Pickrel and Henggeler 1996).

Twelve-Step-Based Programs

Treatment based on the 12-step program is the treatment model that has been most commonly applied in adolescents. There are many misunderstandings about this treatment modality. The mental health professional who wishes to use and understand it not only needs to read the important literature but also needs to attend Alcoholics Anonymous (AA) or Narcotics Anonymous meetings, participate in adolescent substance abuse groups, and learn from counselors in recovery. Working the 12 steps is a very concrete process that does not require abstract thinking.

In the development of AA, Bill Wilson set up clear guidelines that enable AA to avoid problematic issues of money, politics, and powerful leaders. AA owns no property, does no fund raising, accepts no outside contributions, and is open and free to anyone who wants to stop drinking. The 12 steps, conceived by Wilson and other early members, were first published in *Alcoholics Anonymous* in 1939 (Alcoholics Anonymous 1976). The 12 steps are the guide for the changes in actions, thoughts, feelings, and belief that an individual addict slowly undergoes so that he or she can establish a stage of recovery and abstain from drinking. Because an addict cannot use alcohol and drugs in moderation, abstinence is the necessary goal.

Presented below are the first five steps and descriptions of ways they can be modified to make them meaningful for adolescents. Jaffe (1990) uses a workbook format whereby the adolescent writes answers to specific questions, which are reviewed by counselors and may be presented to a group.

1. *We admitted we were powerless over alcohol—that our lives had become unmanageable.* The workbook instructs the adolescents to examine in detail the negative consequences of their alcohol and drug use. Various issues are explored, such as the ways that drug and alcohol use puts their own and others' lives in danger and the effects it has on family, school, work, mood, and self-esteem. The major issue is whether drugs and alcohol are destroying their lives such that they need to stop using to make their lives better. Because adolescents desire to become more powerful, the workbook emphasizes that by abstaining from alcohol and drugs the individual becomes powerful to have a life. Although many adult programs emphasize the concept of "surrendering" and admitting one is an addict,

these are not useful for adolescents. Rather, enhancing power by doing what one needs to do (i.e., stop using alcohol and drugs) instead of what one wants to do (i.e., use alcohol and drugs) is emphasized.

2. *We came to believe that a power greater than ourselves could restore us to sanity.* This step is approached in the adolescent workbook by recognizing that the first higher power in a child's life is the person that raised him or her. For many drug-abusing or drug-addicted adolescents, their parental figures were neglectful or abusive. Mourning—eliciting the pain and sadness caused by the disappointments of their childhood higher powers—enables them to begin to develop a sense of something positive in the universe that they can turn to for help. The concept of a higher power is not a religious belief but a spiritual feeling that one can trust something positive (i.e., the group, another person, nature, etc.) to take care of those aspects of one's life that one cannot control. One needs to have trust in the stability of the world and realize one controls one's own behavior but not what others say or do. For many adolescents, the concrete positive feelings of their relationships with other members becomes their 12-step higher power.

3. *We made a decision to turn our will and our lives over to the care of God as we understood Him.* The adolescent workbook presents an interpretation of this step that involves having the adolescents make a decision to commit themselves to working the steps and having a positive spiritual power. The teenagers are helped to recognize that they had turned over their lives to alcohol and drugs. Now they are being asked to turn their lives over to a positive program.

4. *We made a searching and fearless moral inventory of ourselves.* The workbook instructs the adolescents to answer numerous detailed questions covering all aspects of their childhood and present life.

5. *We admitted to God, to ourselves, and to another human being the exact nature of our wrongs.* At this point the adolescents verbalize their inventories to a counselor or to their sponsor.

Twelve-step programs provide the opportunity to attend free AA or Narcotics Anonymous meetings, which are conducted several times a day in almost every city and town in the United States and most other countries. It is well recognized that adolescents will return to using alcohol and drugs if they return to contact with their alcohol- and drug-using friends (Jaffe 1992). Twelve-step programs provide the opportunity to meet other recovering peers and to provide "big brother" or "big sister" relationships in the form of sponsors. In this relationship, an older member with at least a year of sobriety provides a relationship and guidance on how to work the program toward sobriety. For many adolescents, it can be helpful for them to view themselves as being "on the way to becoming an addict" if they do not see themselves as already being one.

Although research on 12-step programs for adolescents has been sparse, the Chemical Abuse Treatment Outcome Registry (CATOR) (Harrison and Hoffman 1989) residential treatment follow-up program indicated that teenagers who attend two or more meetings a week were almost six times more likely to report abstinence at 1 year than were those who never attended. A more recent follow-up study by Winters (Center for Substance Abuse Treatment 1999b) used improved methodology with a high follow-up contact rate and meaningful comparison groups. At 12-month follow-up, those completing 12-step-based treatment had an abstinence/minor relapse rate of 53% compared with 27% of those who needed but did not receive treatment.

Therapeutic Communities

The therapeutic community involves long-term treatment (12–18 months) for youths with the most severe problems. Under this model the community itself becomes the treatment process. Residents move through stages of increasing responsibility and privileges. Work, education, group activities, seminars, meals, job functions, and formal and informal interactions with peers and staff become the experiences of self-development. Staff members who are recovering and family members have important functions. Outcome studies indicated that 31% completed the residential phase of treatment and 52% dropped out. Treatment completers at 1 year after treatment had more positive outcomes, with reduction in substance use and decreased criminal activity (Center for Substance Abuse Treatment 1999b).

Cognitive-Behavioral Therapy

Cognitive-behavioral therapy (CBT) uses the learning principles of classical and operant conditioning along with approaches to correct cognitive distortions and underlying negative belief systems. This treatment includes having the adolescent learn specific techniques to deal with drugs and alcohol. Skills to refuse alcohol and drugs are taught and practiced through role-playing exercises. For example, adolescents are taught to immediately say "no" in a firm manner, making direct eye contact with the person offering them alcohol or drugs. They are then to suggest an alternative activity, or if that is not successful, to simply tell the person to stop asking. Cognitive-behavioral coping skills to deal with urges, to manage using thoughts, and to handle emergencies and lapses are taught and practiced. Because deficits in coping skills for negative feelings and life stresses contribute to continued substance abuse, more general coping skills—such as communication skills, problem-solving strategies, anger, and mood management—as well as relaxation training are taught and practiced. CBT is being studied in random clinical trials (e.g., Botvin et al. 1990). Kaminer and Burleson (1999) compared CBT group therapy with interactional group therapy in adolescents with dual disorders. CBT demonstrated a decrease in severity of substance use but was not shown to be superior to interactional therapy at the 15-month follow-up evaluation.

Motivational Treatment

According to Prochaska and DiClemente (1982), in stopping an addictive behavior a person goes through a series of stages of change: 1) pre-contemplation, in which the person is not even thinking about stopping and does not recognize any problem with alcohol or drug use; 2) contemplation, which is the stage of ambivalence wherein the person goes back and forth between reasons to change and reasons not to change; 3) preparation, in which the person increases his or her commitment to change; 4) action, in which the person stops using alcohol and drugs; and 5) maintenance, in which the person develops a lifestyle to avoid relapse. People have different levels of motivation depending on their stage of change.

Therapeutic intervention involves helping the patient in an empathetic, nonconfrontational manner to move along the stages. Brief motivational interventions consist of one to four sessions in which, after an assessment, direct feedback and advice are given in a nonconfrontational manner respecting the person's personal responsibility for making a decision. Monti and colleagues (2001) studied the use of a single 45-

minute emergency room brief motivational interview for adolescents with accidents related to alcohol use. Follow-up revealed fewer alcohol-related problems. Jaffe's (2001) *Adolescent Substance Abuse Intervention Workbook* instructs the adolescent to concretely explore how 12 areas of his or her life have been negatively affected by substances in an effort to move them from pre-contemplation into contemplation.

The Community-Reinforcement Approach

The community-reinforcement approach is an adult alcohol treatment approach with strong empirical research support whereby the person's life is rearranged so that abstinence is more rewarding than drinking. The community-reinforcement approach closely resembles the "enthusiastic sobriety" adolescent program developed by Bob Meehan (2000). This 12-step-based program uses young, energetic, enthusiastic, recovering, well-trained counselors. They are role models demonstrating that one can have fun without drugs or alcohol. The adolescent participates in daily groups, meetings, and social functions with recovering peers who make sobriety more fun and rewarding than using drugs and alcohol.

Level of Care

Adolescents rarely need medical detoxification. Reasons for this seem to be related to the fact that adolescents tend to use multiple drugs in an episodic time course. Also, adolescents are usually in better general physical health than adults. Despite this, physical addiction to alcohol, sedatives, or minor tranquilizers may occur with life-threatening withdrawal symptoms that necessitates detoxification in an inpatient setting. Adolescents are usually not very honest about the types, amounts, and frequency of their alcohol or drug use. The physician needs to clarify the importance of honesty in relation to the use of these physically addictive substances, especially the benzodiazepines (i.e., diazepam, clonazepam, and alprazolam), because this could be a life-and-death issue. Other indications for inpatient hospitalization include danger to self or others, psychotic symptoms, and high-risk behavior that could be life-threatening.

Adolescents with substance abuse disorder or substance dependence disorder often need a short period of inpatient hospitalization so that they can be fully evaluated and stabilized. Then they may be stepped down to a day patient or intensive outpatient program. Within these programs family therapy, 12-step facilitation therapy, CBT, and motivational interviewing may be used. Full biopsychosocial evaluation is needed because comorbid disorders are present in 40%–90% of these patients (Bukstein et al. 1989). These comorbid affective, behavioral, and anxiety disorders should be defined and considered for concurrent treatment. The major issue for adolescents with substance abuse disorder or substance dependence disorder who are to be treated in day or intensive outpatient program is whether they can resist returning to contact with their peers who are using drugs.

The American Society of Addiction Medicine has developed treatment levels of care (Hoffman et al. 1993), which include the dimensions of treatment resistance, relapse potential, and recovery environment. These levels for adolescents are currently being revised.

Comorbid Psychiatric Disorders

In this section, the terms *dual diagnosis* and *comorbidity* are used as general terms to refer to patients who meet the criteria for a psychoactive substance use disorder and for another psychiatric diagnosis on Axis I or II using DSM-IV-TR (American Psychiatric Association 2000).

■ Prevalence

In different patients with the same two comorbid disorders, the course and treatment may vary depending on which disorder is primary (i.e., which one preceded the other) (Miller and Fine 1993) and on their relative severity (Bukstein 1997; Caton et al. 1989; King et al. 1996; Ries et al. 1994; Schuckit 1985; Weiss et al. 1992). It is unhelpful to assume that all patients with dual diagnoses are the same and require the same treatment (Weiss et al. 1992). Although a high prevalence of comorbidity has been reported among adolescent inpatients with drug use disorders (Clark et al. 1995, 1997; Grilo et al. 1995; Hovens et al. 1994; Kaminer et al. 1991), it is unclear how many exhibit psychiatric symptoms secondary to the substance abuse disorder and how many have a primary or coexisting psychiatric diagnosis. Miller and Fine (1993) argue that methodological considerations—including the length of abstinence required before the diagnosis is made, the population sampled, and the perspective of the examiner—affect prevalence rates for psychiatric disorders in persons who abuse substances and that these considerations account for the variability. These authors see the prevalence rates for psychiatric disorders as being artificially elevated by the tendency to make a diagnosis before abatement of some of the psychiatric symptoms that are secondary to substance use.

Until very recently, studies involving adolescents were smaller and involved clinical populations. Stowell and Estroff (1992) studied 226 adolescents receiving inpatient treatment in private psychiatric hospitals for a primary substance abuse disorder. Psychiatric diagnoses were made 4 weeks into treatment by using a semistructured diagnostic interview. Of the total, 82% of the patients met DSM-III-R criteria for an Axis I psychiatric disorder; 61% had mood disorders; 54% had conduct disorders; 43% had anxiety disorders; and 16% had substance-induced organic disorder. Seventy-four percent of the patients had two or more psychiatric disorders. Westermeyer et al. (1994) studied 100 adolescents ages 12–20 years who sought care at two university-based outpatient substance abuse treatment programs; the researchers found similar high rates of comorbidity and multiple diagnoses. Of the 100 adolescents, 22 had eating disorders, 8 had conduct disorders, 7 had major depressive disorder, 6 had minor depressive disorder, 5 had bipolar disorder, 5 had schizophrenia, and 4 had anxiety disorders. Three had another psychotic disorder, 3 had an organic mental disorder, and 2 had ADHD. The distribution of diagnoses as a function of age showed that older adolescents had increased eating disorder diagnoses and depressive symptoms (Westermeyer et al. 1994).

Burke et al. (1990) studied data from the Epidemiologic Catchment Area Study of the National Institute of Mental Health to determine hazard rates for the development of disorders. They concluded that 15–19 years were the peak ages for the onset of depressive disorders in females and for the onset of substance use disorders and bipolar disorders in both sexes. The National Comorbidity Study included a large noninstitutional sample of persons ages 15–24 years, although adolescents were not studied separately from young adults (Kessler et al. 1996). Compared with older adults, 15- to 24-year-olds had the highest prevalence of three or more disorders occurring together and of any disorders, including substance use disorders. The Methods for the Epidemiology of Child and Adolescent Mental Disorders Study obtained data for 401

subjects ages 14–17 years (Kandel et al. 1999). Adolescents with substance use disorders had much higher rates of mood and conduct disorders than those without substance use disorders.

■ Major Diagnostic Categories

Depressive Disorders

Studies of adults who abused substances showed that the substance-induced mood disorder dissipated with abstinence, but the primary depressive disorder did not, and if left untreated it could interfere with treatment and recovery (Burke et al. 1990; Miller 1993; Miller and Fine 1993; Schuckit 1985). Deykin et al. (1992) interviewed 223 adolescents in residential treatment for substance abuse and found that almost 25% met the DSM-III-R (American Psychiatric Association 1987) criteria for depression. Of these, 8% met the criteria for primary depression; the other 16% had a secondary mood disorder. Bukstein et al. (1992) studied adolescent inpatients on a dual-diagnosis unit and reported that almost 31% had comorbid major depression, with secondary depressive disorder much more common than primary depressive disorder. Unlike findings reported for adults, Bukstein et al. (1992) found that the secondary depression did not remit with abstinence. This finding, if replicated, would argue for more vigorous treatment of depressive syndromes in adolescents.

Depression interferes with treatment, owing to the lack of concentration, motivation, and hope and the tendency toward isolation. Kempton et al. (1994) found cognitive distortions, including magnification (all-or-nothing thinking) and personalizing, to be particularly prominent among adolescents with the multiple diagnoses of conduct disorder, depressive disorder, and substance abuse. A depressed adolescent may benefit from a specific cognitive intervention for depression (Beck et al. 1979; Kaminer 1994).

If the adolescent has a depressive disorder that predates the substance abuse, has a family history of depression, and has a mood disorder that interferes with treatment several weeks into abstinence despite cognitive interventions, pharmacotherapy is indicated. Serotonergic agents such as fluoxetine have a relatively safe profile for side effects and may be most appropriate considering reports that young substance abusers have a preexisting serotonin deficit (Crowley and Riggs 1995; Horowitz et al. 1992; Riggs et al. 1997).

Bipolar Disorder

The diagnosis of bipolar disorder may be among the hardest to make in children and adolescents, and it is even more difficult in teenagers with substance abuse. Issues such as change in sleeping patterns and mood swings can be symptoms of bipolar disorder, substance abuse, or even normal adolescence. The diagnosis of bipolar disorder should certainly be considered in substance-abusing youths, particularly those with a binge pattern.

Wilens et al. (1999) found an increased risk for substance use disorders in adolescents with bipolar disorder. Children who were diagnosed and treated appropriately at a younger age had a lower risk for substance abuse. Some patients use substances, particularly alcohol, to calm themselves during a manic phase. Clearly, some of these symptoms are also seen with substance intoxication. If a patient exhibits these symptoms after a period of abstinence, the diagnosis of bipolar disorder should be considered. Bipolar disorders are most often treated with mood stabilizers, the most common of which is lithium carbonate (Geller et al. 1998).

Anxiety Disorders and Posttraumatic Stress Disorder

Anxiety disorders are among the most common psychiatric conditions coexisting in adolescents and adults with substance use disorders. Anxiety disorders are often not detected or treated, especially when they are present with depression or psychoactive substance use disorders (Burke et al. 1990; Clark and Bukstein 1998). Because some of the symptoms of panic attacks might be seen in substance intoxication or withdrawal, it is important to establish abstinence before making a diagnosis. Patients with social phobia may isolate themselves on an inpatient unit or within a group. Behavioral treatment, including relaxation training, is often helpful for anxiety disorders (Kaminer 1994). The issue of pharmacotherapy is controversial. Buspirone hydrochloride and serotonin reuptake inhibitors have been recommended as nonaddictive antianxiety agents (Wilens et al. 1998).

In clinical reports on adolescents, the incidences of severe trauma and symptoms of posttraumatic stress disorder are surprisingly high (Clark et al. 1995, 1997; Deykin and Buka 1997; Kandel et al. 1999). An adolescent who has been acting out and abusing substances may not have dealt with previous trauma, such as physical and sexual abuse or exposure to violence, or with the trauma that may be incurred when abusing substances (Clark et al. 1997). Symptoms and memories of trauma may manifest themselves only during abstinence.

Care should be taken to acknowledge the trauma without arousing anxiety that will interfere with abstinence and substance abuse treatment. Groups that support self-care and a first-things-first attitude may be the best approach; the patient needs to learn to stay safe, and treatment for substance abuse is a most important aspect of safety.

Organic Mental Disorders

The abuse of substances—including alcohol, marijuana, cocaine, ecstasy, hallucinogens, and inhalants—is associated in some patients with acute and residual cognitive damage (American Psychiatric Association 2000; Kempton et al. 1994; Stowell and Estroff 1992). Acute symptoms may include impaired concentration and receptive and expressive language abilities, as well as irritability. Long-term interference with memory and other executive functions occurs. The possibility of substance-induced dementia should be considered in adolescents who have difficulty coping with the cognitive and organizational demands of a structured and supportive program. Some of the adolescents will be able to use the program if instructions are simplified and if they comprehend information accurately. There may be rapid improvement in cognitive functioning, but the cognitive functioning of some patients continues to improve for as long as a year or more after cessation of the chemical assault to the brain. Some may be left with residual impairment.

Schizophrenia

Because the late adolescent years are a time when many schizophrenic disorders begin, and the use of substances may precipitate incipient psychosis, patients with this disorder may seek treatment during early stages of schizophrenia (Kaminer 1991; Miller and Fine 1993; Ries 1993a). Increasingly, younger schizophrenic patients abuse substances (Buckley 1999; Minkoff 1989; Ries 1993b), sometimes in an attempt to manage or deny their psychotic symptoms. Their abuse of substances often interferes with treatment for their psychotic disorder. These patients are best managed in special dual-diagnosis programs for psychotic patients (Buckley 1999; Caton et al. 1989; Mason and Siris 1992; Ries 1993a; Ries et al. 1994).

Attention-Deficit/Hyperactivity Disorder

Many involved in the treatment of adolescents who abuse substances have noted the large numbers of adolescents who also have ADHD (Bukstein 1997; Bukstein et al. 1989; Riggs 1998; Wilens et al. 1996). Treatment should include behavioral and educational intervention. Pharmacotherapy for adolescents has been controversial, particularly because some have argued that the use of psychostimulants might predispose adolescents to abuse other substances (Riggs 1998). Riggs et al. (1998) reported some success with the use of bupropion. Wilens et al. (1996) suggest that the successful treatment of adolescents with ADHD with stimulants may actually lower the probability that they will develop a substance use disorder. Because the successful treatment of substance abuse involves teaching patients to plan and to delay impulses, the effective treatment of ADHD is necessary in an integrated plan.

Conduct Disorder and Antisocial Personality Disorder

Conduct disorder and antisocial personality disorder are the most common comorbid diagnoses with substance abuse, particularly in males (Bukstein 1997; Crowley and Riggs 1995; Kandel et al. 1999; King et al. 1996; Rao et al. 1999; Schuckit 1985; Stowell and Estroff 1992; Westermeyer et al. 1994; Wilens et al. 1996). Cloninger (1987) presented an interesting scheme of hereditary factors on three axes that may account for many psychiatric diagnoses and their interrelationships. The three axes are reward dependence, harm avoidance, and novelty seeking. Based on these axes, Cloninger (1987) distinguished type 1 and type 2 alcoholic patients. Type 2 alcoholic patients score low on reward dependence and harm avoidance and high on novelty seeking. Younger alcoholic patients with antisocial personality disorder fit the type 2 classification. The higher prevalence of antisocial personality disorder and conduct disorder among younger alcoholic patients may explain why many clinicians find adolescent substance abusers more difficult to treat. Adolescents with conduct disorders and antisocial personality disorder need a strong behavioral program with clear limits. If there is a comorbid disorder (such as a mood

or attention disorder) that can be treated successfully, the adolescents are more likely to do well (Crowley and Riggs 1995; Riggs 1998; Wilens et al. 1996).

Eating Disorders

Because the incidences of eating disorders and substance abuse have increased in the adolescent population (Katz 1990; Ross and Ivis 1999; Westermeyer and Specker 1999; Westermeyer et al. 1994), it is not uncommon to find them together. In fact, one-quarter of all patients with an eating disorder have a history of substance abuse or are currently abusing substances (Katz 1990). Anorexia nervosa is not as prevalent as bulimia in the general population and among persons who abuse substances (Westermeyer and Specker 1999).

Psychiatric disorders and substance abuse frequently occur together. This leads to difficulty in both assessment and treatment. An awareness of the prevalence and manifestations of psychiatric diagnoses is essential for the quality treatment of adolescents who abuse substances. Frequently, the use of psychiatric medications such as antidepressants, mood stabilizers, psychostimulants, and others is of benefit. However, care must be taken to avoid potential interactions between the illicit drugs and the prescribed medications (Wilens et al. 1997). In addition, the use of groups such as AA, Narcotics Anonymous, or "double trouble" groups that deal with issues of mental illness and chemical abuse or of dual diagnosis can often be a useful adjunct to treatment with a mental health professional (Brown 1993; Hohman and LeCroy 1996; Simkin 1996).

Prevention

Prevention of substance abuse in adolescents has proved to be a complex problem. Reducing availability—for example, by increasing the drinking age or increasing the cost of cigarettes—has had some positive effect in decreasing substance use in adolescents. The widely used prevention strategy of increasing the knowledge of consequences (as in the DARE program) was shown in a controlled study to result in no short-term or long-term effects (Ennett et al. 1994). In a review of the effectiveness of program components, Hansen (1996) demonstrated that programs with an informational or affective component had little effect.

Programs that enhanced social skills and drug refusal skills were more successful. The life skills training developed by Botvin and colleagues (1995) used an intervention in the seventh grade and booster sessions during the following 2 years. Significant decreases in drug use were found when these students reached the twelfth grade. Prevention programs that target high-risk youth (e.g., those with poor academic achievement) are being developed and studied.

Research Issues

In the future, research should continue to build on the foundations laid in the past decade. Much still needs to be done in the areas of etiology, diagnostic and nosological issues, and, of course, treatment. Although treatments have generally been shown to be effective, there may be certain subpopulations of adolescents who might benefit from one approach over another. Moreover, it is not clear that treatments designed for use in adults are necessarily developmentally appropriate for adolescents.

Perhaps the greatest need for research is in prevention. Stopping substance use before it begins may perhaps be the most effective strategy in the "war on drugs." A better understanding of the progression from experimentation to recreational use to abuse and ultimately to dependence may help tailor interventions specific to each stage. Lastly, a developmentally appropriate understanding of treatment also needs to be refined with future research endeavors. How does a substance abusing 12-year-old differ from a substance abusing 18-year-old? Are different genetic factors at play? Different psychiatric comorbidities? Different sociocultural factors? It can be hoped that future research will begin to find answers for these and other questions.

References

Alcoholics Anonymous: The Story of How Many Thousands of Men and Women Have Recovered From Alcoholism, 3rd Edition. New York, Alcoholics Anonymous World Services, 1976

American Psychiatric Association: Diagnostic and Statistical Manual of Mental Disorders, 3rd Edition, Revised. American Psychiatric Association, Washington, DC, 1987

American Psychiatric Association: Diagnostic and Statistical Manual of Mental Disorders, 4th Edition, Text Revision. Washington, DC, American Psychiatric Association, 2000

Azrin NH, Donohue B, Besale VA, et al: Youth drug abuse treatment: a controlled outcome study. Journal of Child and Adolescent Substance Abuse 3(3):1–16, 1994

Bailey GW: Helping the resistant adolescent enter substance abuse treatment: the office intervention. Child Adolesc Psychiatr Clin N Am 5:149–164, 1996

Bauman KE, Ennett S: Peer influence on adolescent drug use. Am Psychol 49:820–822, 1994

Beck AT, Rush AJ, Shaw BF, et al: Cognitive Therapy of Depression. New York, Guilford, 1979

Botvin GJ, Baker E, Dusenbury L, et al: Preventing adolescent drug abuse through multimodal cognitive behavioral approach: results of a three year study. J Consult Clin Psychol 58:437–446, 1990

Botvin GJ, Baker E, Dusenbury L, et al: Long-term follow-up of randomized drug abuse prevention trial in a white middle-class population. JAMA 273:1106–1112, 1995

Brook JS, Lukoff IF, Whiteman M: Initiation into adolescent marijuana use. J Genet Psychol 137:133–142, 1980

Brown SA: Recovery patterns in adolescent substance abusers, in Addictive Behavior Across the Life Span: Prevention, Treatment and Policy Issues. Edited by Baer JS, Marlatt, GA, McMahon, RJ. Beverly Hills, CA, Sage, 1993, pp 161–163

Buckley PF: Substance abuse in schizophrenia: a review. J Clin Psychiatry 59(suppl 3):26–30, 1999

Budney AJ, Novy PL, Hughes JR: Marijuana withdrawal among adults seeking treatment for marijuana dependence. Addiction 94:1311–1322, 1999

Bukstein O: Practice parameters for the assessment and treatment of children and adolescents with substance use disorders. J Am Acad Child Adolesc Psychiatry 36(10, suppl):140S–156S, 1997

Bukstein OG, Brent DA, Kaminer Y: Comorbidity of substance abuse and other psychiatric disorders in adolescents. Am J Psychiatry 146:1131–1141, 1989

Bukstein OG, Glancy LJ, Kaminer Y: Patterns of affective comorbidity in a clinical population of dually diagnosed adolescent substance abusers. J Am Acad Child Adolesc Psychiatry 31:1041–1045, 1992

Burke KC, Burke JD Jr, Regier DA, et al: Age at onset of selected mental disorders in five community populations. Arch Gen Psychiatry 47:511–518, 1990

Catalano RF, Hankins JD, Wells EA, et al: Evaluation of the effectiveness of adolescent drug abuse treatment, assessment of risk for relapse, and promising approaches for relapse prevention. Int J Addict 25:1085–1140, 1990–1991

Caton CL, Gralnick A, Bender S, et al: Young chronic patients and substance abuse. Hosp Community Psychiatry 40:1037–1040, 1989

Center for Substance Abuse Treatment: Screening and assessing adolescents for substance use disorders (Treatment Improvement Protocol Series, No 31). Rockville, MD, Substance Abuse and Mental Health Services Administration, 1999a

Center for Substance Abuse Treatment: Treatment of adolescents with substance abuse disorder (Treatment Improvement Protocol Series, No 32). Rockville, MD, Substance Abuse and Mental Health Services Administration, 1999b

Chatlos JC: Recent trends and a developmental approach to substance abuse in adolescents. Child Adolesc Psychiatr Clin North Am 5:1–28, 1996

Clark DB, Bukstein OG: Psychopathology in adolescent alcohol abuse and dependence. Alcohol Health Res World 22:117–126, 1998

Clark DB, Bukstein O, Smith MG, et al: Identifying anxiety disorders in adolescents hospitalized for alcohol abuse and dependence. Psychiatr Serv 46:618–620, 1995

Clark DB, Lesnick L, Hegedus AM: Traumas and other adverse life events in adolescents with alcohol use and dependence. J Am Acad Child Adolesc Psychiatry 36:1744–1751, 1997

Clark DB, Kirisci L, Tarter RE: Adolescent versus adult onset and the development of substance use disorders in males. Drug Alcohol Depend 49:115–121, 1998

Cloninger CR: Neurogenetic adaptive mechanisms in alcoholism. Science 236:410–416, 1987

Crowley TJ, Riggs PD: Adolescent substance use disorder with conduct disorder and comorbid conditions. NIDA Res Monogr 156:49–111, 1995

Deas D, Thomas SE: An overview of controlled studies of adolescent substance abuse treatment. Am J Addict 10:178–189, 2001

Deas-Nesmith D, Campbell S, Brady KT: Substance use disorders in adolescent inpatient psychiatric population: J Natl Med Assoc 90:233–238, 1998

DeWitt DJ, Adlaf EM, Offord DR, et al: Age of first alcohol use: a risk factor for the development of alcohol disorders. Am J Psychiatry 157:745–750, 2000

Deykin EY, Buka SL: Prevalence and risk factors for posttraumatic stress disorder among chemically dependent adolescents. Am J Psychiatry 154:752–757, 1997

Deykin EY, Buka SL, Zeena TH: Depressive illness among chemically dependent adolescents. Am J Psychiatry 149:1341–1347, 1992

Dimeff LA, Baer JS, Kivlahan DR, et al: Brief Alcohol Screening and Intervention for College Students. New York, Guilford, 1999

Ennett ST, Rigwatt C, Flewelling RL: How effective is drug abuse resistance education? A meta-analysis of project DARE evaluations. Am J Public Health 84:1394–1401, 1994

Geller B, Cooper TB, Sun K, et al: Double-blind and placebo-controlled study of lithium for adolescent bipolar disorders with secondary substance dependency. J Am Acad Child Adolesc Psychiatry 37:171–178, 1998

Grilo CM, Becker DF, Walker ML, et al: Psychiatric comorbidity in adolescent inpatients with substance use disorders. J Am Acad Child Adolesc Psychiatry 34:1085–1091, 1995

Grunebaum PE, Prange ME, Friedman RM, et al: Substance abuse prevalence and comorbidity with other psychiatric disorders among adolescents with severe emotional disturbances. J Am Acad Child Adolesc Psychiatry 30:575–583, 1991

Hansen WB: Pilot test results comparing the All Stars program with seventh grade DARE: program integrity and mediating variable analysis. Subst Use Misuse 31:1359–1377, 1996

Harrison PA: Epidemiology, in Manual of Substance Abuse Treatment. Edited by Estroff TW. Washington DC, American Psychiatric Publishing, 2001, pp 1–12

Harrison PA, Hoffman NC: CATOR Report: Adolescent Treatment Completion One Year Later. St. Paul, MN, Ramsey Clinic, 1989

Harrison PA, Fullerson JA, Beebe TJ: DSM-IV substance use disorder criteria for adolescents: a critical examination based on a statewide school survey. Am J Psychiatry 155:486–492, 1998

Henggeler SW, Melton GB, Smith LA, et al: Family preservation using multisystemic treatment: long-term follow-up to a clinical trial with serious juvenile offenders. Journal of Child and Family Studies 2:283–293, 1993

Hoffman NG, Mee-Lee D, Arrowood AA: Treatment issues in adolescent substance use and addictions: options, outcome, effectiveness, reimbursement and admission criteria. Adolesc Med 4:371–390, 1993

Hohman M, LeCroy CW: Predictors of adolescent A.A. affiliation. Adolescence 31:339–352, 1996

Horowitz HA, Overton WF, Rosenstein D, et al: Comorbid adolescent substance abuse: a maladaptive pattern of self-regulation. Adolesc Psychiatry 18:465–483, 1992

Hovens JG, Cantwell DP, Kiriakos R: Psychiatric comorbidity in hospitalized adolescent substance abusers. J Am Acad Child Adolesc Psychiatry 33:476–483, 1994

Jaffe SL: Step Workbook for Adolescent Chemical Dependency Recovery: A Guide to the First Five Steps. Washington, DC, American Psychiatric Press, 1990

Jaffe SL: Pathways to relapse in chemically dependent adolescents. Adolescent Counselor 55:42–44, 1992

Jaffe SL (ed): Adolescent Substance Abuse and Dual Disorders. Child Adolesc Psychiatr Clin N Am 5:1–261, 1996a

Jaffe SL: The substance abusing youth, in Child and Adolescent Psychiatry. Edited by Parmelee DX. St. Louis, MO, Mosby, 1996b, pp 237–244

Jaffe SL: Adolescent Substance Abuse Intervention Workbook: Taking a First Step. Washington, DC, American Psychiatric Press, 2001

Johnston LD, O'Malley PM, Bachman JG: National Survey Results on Drug Use From the Monitoring the Future Study, 1975–2000, Vol 1: Secondary School Students (NIH Publ No 01-4924). Rockville, MD, National Institute on Drug Abuse, 2001

Kaminer Y: Adolescent Substance Abuse: A Comprehensive Guide to Theory and Practice. New York, Plenum, 1994

Kaminer Y, Burleson J: Psychotherapies for adolescent substance abusers: 15-month follow-up of a pilot study. Am J Addict 8:114–119, 1999

Kaminer Y, Bukstein OG, Tarter RE: The Teen Addiction Severity Index: rationale and reliability. Int J Addict 26:219–226, 1991

Kandel D: Stages in adolescent involvement in drug use. Science 190:912–914, 1975

Kandel DB, Yamaguchi K, Chen K: Stages of progression in drug involvement from adolescence to adulthood: further evidence for the gateway theory. J Stud Alcohol 53:447–457, 1992

Kandel DB, Johnson JG, Bird HR, et al: Psychiatric comorbidity among adolescents with substance use disorders: findings from the MECA study. J Am Acad Child Adolesc Psychiatry 38:693–699, 1999

Katz JL: Eating disorders: a primer for the substance abuse specialist, I: clinical features. J Subst Abuse Treat 7:143–149, 1990

Kempton T, Van Hasselt VB, Bukstein OG, et al: Cognitive distortions and psychiatric diagnosis in dually diagnosed adolescents. J Am Acad Child Adolesc Psychiatry 33:217–222, 1994

Kendler KS, Prescott CA: Cannabis use, abuse, and dependence in a population-based sample of female twins. Am J Psychiatry 155:1016–1022, 1998a

Kendler KS, Prescott CA: Cocaine use, abuse and dependence in a population-based sample of female twins. Br J Psychiatry 173:345–350, 1998b

Kessler RC, Nelson CB, McGonagle KA, et al: The epidemiology of co-occurring addictive and mental disorders: implications for prevention and service utilization. Am J Orthopsychiatry 66:17–31, 1996

King C, Ghaziuddin N, McGovern L, et al: Predictors of comorbid alcohol and substance abuse in depressed adolescents. J Am Acad Child Adolesc Psychiatry 35:743–751, 1996

Knight JR, Shrier LA, Bravender TD, et al: A new brief screen for adolescent substance abuse. Arch Pediatr Adolesc Med 153:591–596, 1999

Lee GP, DiClimente CC: Age of onset versus duration of problem drinking on the Alcohol Use Inventory. J Stud Alcohol 46:298–402, 1985

Leirer VO, Yesavage JA, Morrow DG: Marijuana carry-over effects on aircraft pilot performance. Aviat Space Environ Med 62:221–227, 1991

Levy S, Vaughan BL, Knight JR: Office-based intervention for adolescent substance abuse. Pediatr Clin North Am 49:329–343, 2002

Lewis RA, Piercy FP, Sprenkle DH, et al: Family based interventions for helping drug abusing adolescents. J Adolesc Res 5:82–95, 1990

Macdonald DI: Drugs, drinking and adolescence. Am J Dis Child 138:117–125, 1984

Mason SE, Siris SG: Dual diagnosis: the case for case management. Am J Addict 1:77–82, 1992

Meehan B: Beyond the Yellow Brick Road: Revised. Kersey, CO, Meek, 2000

Miller NS: Comorbidity of psychiatric and alcohol/drug disorders: interactions and independent status. J Addict Dis 12:5–16, 1993

Miller NS, Fine J: Current epidemiology of comorbidity of psychiatric and addictive disorders. Psychiatr Clin North Am 16:1–10, 1993

Minkoff K: An integrated treatment model for dual diagnosis of psychosis and addiction. Hosp Community Psychiatry 40:1031–1036, 1989

Monti PM, Barnett NP, O'Leary JA, et al: Motivational enhancement for school-involved adolescents, in Adolescents, Alcohol, and Substance Abuse. Edited by Monti PM, Colby SM, O'Leary TA. New York, Guilford, 2001, pp 145–182

Neighbors B, Kempton D, Forehand R: Co-occurrence of substance abuse with conduct, anxiety and depressive disorders in juvenile delinquents. Addict Behav 17:379–386, 1992

Nestler EJ: Molecular neurobiology of drug addiction. Neuroscientist 11:77–87, 1994

Nestler EJ: Molecular basis of addiction states. Neuroscientist 1:212–220, 1995

Newcomb MD: Identifying high-risk youth: prevalence and patterns of adolescent drug abuse. NIDA Res Monogr 156:7–38, 1995

Nowinski J: Substance Abuse in Adolescents and Young Adults: A Guide to Treatment. New York, WW Norton, 1990 pp 38–65

Office of Applied Studies: Summary of Findings From the 1999 National Household Survey on Drug Abuse (DHHS Publ No [SMA] 00-3466). Rockville, MD, Substance Abuse and Mental Health Services Administration, 2000

Pandina RJ, Johnson V, Labouvie EW, et al: Affectivity: a central mechanism in the development of drug dependence, in Vulnerability to Drug Abuse. Edited by Glantz M, Pickens R. Washington, DC, American Psychological Association, 1992

Pickrel SG, Henggeler SW: Multisystemic therapy for adolescent substance abuse and dependence. Child Adolesc Psychiatr Clin N Am 5:201–211, 1996

Prochaska JO, DiClemente CC: Transtheoretical therapy: toward a more integrated model of change. Psychotherapy: Theory, Research and Practice 19:276–288, 1982

Rao U, Ryan N, Dahl DE, et al: Factors associated with the development of substance use disorders in depressed adolescents. J Am Acad Child Adolesc Psychiatry 38:1109–1117, 1999

Ries RK: Clinical treatment matching models for dually diagnosed patients. Psychiatr Clin North Am 16:167–175, 1993a

Ries RK: The dually diagnosed patient with psychotic symptoms. J Addict Dis 12:103–122, 1993b

Ries R, Mullen M, Cox G: Symptom severity and utilization of treatment resources among dually diagnosed inpatients. Hospital Community Psychiatry 45:562–568, 1994

Riggs PD: Clinical approach to treatment of ADHD in adolescents with substance use disorders and conduct disorder. J Am Acad Child Adolesc Psychiatry 37:331–332, 1998

Riggs PD, Mikulich SC, Coffman L, et al: Fluoxetine in drug-dependent delinquents with major depression: an open trial. J Child Adolesc Psychopharmacol 7:87–95, 1997

Riggs PD, Mikulich SC, Pottle LC: An open trial of bupropion for ADHD in adolescents with substance use disorder and conduct disorder. J Am Acad Child Adolesc Psychiatry 37:1271–1278, 1998

Roberts AJ, Koob GF: The neurobiology of addiction. Alcohol Health Res World 21:101–106, 1997

Rogers PD, Adger H Jr: Alcohol and adolescents. Adolesc Med 4:295–304, 1993

Ross HE, Ivis F: Binge eating and substance abuse among male and female adolescents. Int J Eat Disord 26:245–260, 1999

Schuckit MA: The clinical implications of primary diagnostic groups among alcoholics. Arch Gen Psychiatry 42:1043–1049, 1985

Schwartz RH: Testing for drugs of abuse: controversies and techniques. Adolesc Med 4:353–370, 1993

Schwartz RH, Gruenwald PJ, Klitzner M, et al: Short-term memory impairment in cannabis-dependent adolescents. Am J Dis Child 143:1214–1219, 1989

Simkin DR: Twelve-step treatment from a developmental perspective. Child Adolesc Psychiatr Clin N Am 5:165–175, 1996

Stanton MD, Shadish WR: Outcome, attrition and family-couples treatment for drug abuse: a meta-analysis and review of the controlled, comparative studies. Psychol Bull 122:170–191, 1997

Stowell JA, Estroff TW: Psychiatric disorders in substance-abusing adolescent inpatients: a pilot study. J Am Acad Child Adolesc Psychiatry 31:1036–1040, 1992

Tarter RE: Evaluation and treatment of adolescent substance abuse: a decision tree method. Am J Drug Alcohol Abuse 16:1–46, 1990

Weiss RD, Mirin SM, Frances RJ: Alcohol and drug abuse: the myth of the typical dual diagnosis patient. Hospital and Community Psychiatry 43:107–108, 1992

Westermeyer J, Specker S: Social resources and social function in comorbid eating and substance disorder: a matched-pairs study. Am J Addict 8:332–336, 1999

Westermeyer J, Specker S, Neider J, et al: Substance abuse and associated psychiatric disorder among 100 adolescents. J Addict Dis 13:67–89, 1994

Wilens TE, Biederman J, Spencer TJ: Attention deficit hyperactivity disorder and psychoactive substance use disorders. Child Adolesc Psychiatr Clin N Am 5:73–91, 1996

Wilens TE, Biederman J, Spencer TJ: Case study: adverse effects of smoking marijuana while receiving tricyclic antidepressants. J Am Acad Child Adolesc Psychiatry 36:45–48, 1997

Wilens T, Spencer T, Frazier J, et al: Psychopharmacology in children and adolescents, in Handbook of Child Psychopathology. Edited by Ollendick T, Hersen M. New York, Plenum, 1998, pp 603–636

Wilens TE, Biederman J, Millstein RB, et al: Risk for substance use disorders in youths with child- and adolescent-onset bipolar disorder. J Am Acad Child Adolesc Psychiatry 38:680–685, 1999

Winters KC: Assessing adolescent substance use problems and other areas of functioning: state of the art, in Adolescents, Alcohol, and Substance Abuse. Edited by Monti PM, Colby SM, O'Leary TA. New York, Guilford, 2001, pp 80–108

Gender Identity and Psychosexual Disorders

Kenneth J. Zucker, Ph.D.

Susan J. Bradley, M.D.

This chapter provides an overview of gender identity and psychosexual problems in children and adolescents. Three terms—*gender identity, gender role,* and *sexual orientation*—are useful in organizing a conceptual framework in thinking about these issues.

Gender identity refers to a person's basic sense of self as male or female. It includes both the awareness that one *is* male or female and an affective appraisal of such knowledge. In the clinical literature, the term *gender dysphoria* has been used to characterize a person's sense of discomfort or unease about his or her status as male or female. Based on clinical work with children born with physical intersexual conditions, Money et al. (1957) concluded that gender identity typically appears in its nascent form between ages 2 and 3 years. During the past four decades, this original clinical observation has been buttressed by normative empirical studies, which have demonstrated that children in this age range—typically by about 30–36 months—are able to categorize people by sex on the basis of phenotypic social cues, such as clothing and hairstyle (for reviews, see Ruble and Martin 1998; Zucker et al. 1999). According to some researchers, this ability likely precedes the ability to self-categorize oneself as a boy or a girl.

Gender role refers to a person's behavioral adoption of cultural markers of masculinity and femininity. In children, gender role preference can be measured in a variety of ways, including playmate affiliations, toy interests, role and fantasy play, and endorsement of various personality attributes. Conceptually, one can consider a child to be primarily masculine or feminine based on the pattern of gender role behavior. Alterna-

tively, one can view a child as both masculine and feminine (androgynous) or as neither masculine nor feminine (undifferentiated). Over the past 50 years, many studies have been conducted on gender role behavior in children (Ruble and Martin 1998). Almost without exception, these studies have shown that boys and girls differ significantly with regard to several sex-typed attributes, including toy and fantasy play (Fagot 1977), peer affiliation preference (Maccoby 1998; Maccoby and Jacklin 1987), aggression (Maccoby and Jacklin 1974, 1980), activity level (Benenson et al. 1997; Campbell and Eaton 1999; Eaton and Enns 1986), and rough-and-tumble play (DiPietro 1981).

Sexual orientation refers to the pattern of a person's erotic responsiveness. Heterosexual, bisexual, and homosexual are the three sexual orientations most commonly described by contemporary nosologists in sexology, although it is also important to consider the age of the sexual partner (either in fantasy or in behavior), as in heterosexual or homosexual pedophilia. Gender identity and gender role are typically viewed as developing before the emergence of sexual orientation, although this view is not held universally (Isay 1989).

Diagnostic Criteria

In DSM-IV-TR (American Psychiatric Association 2000), four diagnoses are of relevance with regard to gender identity and psychosexual problems during childhood and adolescence:

Table 44–1. DSM-IV-TR diagnostic criteria for gender identity disorder

A. A strong and persistent cross-gender identification (not merely a desire for any perceived cultural advantages of being the other sex).

In children, the disturbance is manifested by four (or more) of the following:

(1) repeatedly stated desire to be, or insistence that he or she is, the other sex

(2) in boys, preference for cross-dressing or simulating female attire; in girls, insistence on wearing only stereotypical masculine clothing

(3) strong and persistent preferences for cross-sex roles in make-believe play or persistent fantasies of being the other sex

(4) intense desire to participate in the stereotypical games and pastimes of the other sex

(5) strong preference for playmates of the other sex

In adolescents and adults, the disturbance is manifested by symptoms such as a stated desire to be the other sex, frequent passing as the other sex, desire to live or be treated as the other sex, or the conviction that he or she has the typical feelings and reactions of the other sex.

B. Persistent discomfort with his or her sex or sense of inappropriateness in the gender role of that sex.

In children, the disturbance is manifested by any of the following: in boys, assertion that his penis or testes are disgusting or will disappear or assertion that it would be better not to have a penis, or aversion toward rough-and-tumble play and rejection of male stereotypical toys, games, and activities; in girls, rejection of urinating in a sitting position, assertion that she has or will grow a penis, or assertion that she does not want to grow breasts or menstruate, or marked aversion toward normative feminine clothing.

In adolescents and adults, the disturbance is manifested by symptoms such as preoccupation with getting rid of primary and secondary sex characteristics (e.g., request for hormones, surgery, or other procedures to physically alter sexual characteristics to simulate the other sex) or belief that he or she was born the wrong sex.

C. The disturbance is not concurrent with a physical intersex condition.

D. The disturbance causes clinically significant distress or impairment in social, occupational, or other important areas of functioning.

Code based on current age:

302.6　　**Gender Identity Disorder in Children**
302.85　　**Gender Identity Disorder in Adolescents or Adults**

Specify if (for sexually mature individuals):

Sexually Attracted to Males
Sexually Attracted to Females
Sexually Attracted to Both
Sexually Attracted to Neither

Source. From American Psychiatric Association: *Diagnostic and Statistical Manual of Mental Disorders,* 4th Edition, Text Revision. Washington, DC, American Psychiatric Association, 2000. Copyright 2000, American Psychiatric Association. Used with permission.

1. Gender identity disorder (GID) (Table 44–1)
2. Gender identity disorder not otherwise specified (GIDNOS) (Table 44–2)
3. Transvestic fetishism (Table 44–3)
4. Sexual disorder not otherwise specified (Table 44–4)

During childhood, only the first two of these four diagnoses are of relevance. In adolescence, however, all of these diagnoses may be utilized as gender identity and psychosexual concerns become more differentiated, in part because of the increased salience of erotic behavior. Therefore, in addition to concerns about gender identity proper (which can be diagnosed with either GID or its residual diagnosis, GIDNOS), the clinician must also be attentive to paraphilic behavior (transvestic fetishism) or distress regarding one's sexual orientation, most typically in homosexuality (sexual disorder not otherwise specified).

Only one study has formally evaluated the reliability of the GID diagnosis in children, which was based on the criteria from DSM-III (American Psychiatric Association 1980). Based on chart data from 36 consecutive referrals to a child and adolescent gender identity clinic, Zucker et al. (1984) found high agreement with DSM-III criteria for GID. Validity evidence was also

Table 44–2. DSM-IV-TR diagnostic criteria for gender identity disorder not otherwise specified

This category is included for coding disorders in gender identity that are not classifiable as a specific gender identity disorder. Examples include

1. Intersex conditions (e.g., partial androgen insensitivity syndrome or congenital adrenal hyperplasia) and accompanying gender dysphoria
2. Transient, stress-related cross-dressing behavior
3. Persistent preoccupation with castration or penectomy without a desire to acquire the sex characteristics of the other sex

Source. From American Psychiatric Association: *Diagnostic and Statistical Manual of Mental Disorders,* 4th Edition, Text Revision. Washington, DC, American Psychiatric Association, 2000. Copyright 2000, American Psychiatric Association. Used with permission.

Table 44–3. DSM-IV-TR diagnostic criteria for transvestic fetishism

A. Over a period of at least 6 months, in a heterosexual male, recurrent, intense sexually arousing fantasies, sexual urges, or behaviors involving cross-dressing.
B. The fantasies, sexual urges, or behaviors cause clinically significant distress or impairment in social, occupational, or other important areas of functioning.

Specify if:

With Gender Dysphoria: if the person has persistent discomfort with gender role or identity

Source. From American Psychiatric Association: *Diagnostic and Statistical Manual of Mental Disorders,* 4th Edition, Text Revision. Washington, DC, American Psychiatric Association, 2000. Copyright 2000, American Psychiatric Association. Used with permission.

found: the children who met the complete diagnostic criteria were, on average, more cross-gendered in their behavior than were the children who did not meet the complete diagnostic criteria. Subsequent analyses with larger numbers of children have verified this distinction (Zucker and Bradley 1995; Zucker et al. 1992, 1993b).

Among demographic variables, age of the child at assessment has been most consistently associated with the GID diagnosis. Based on 488 consecutive referrals from two specialized gender identity clinics (one in Toronto, Ontario, Canada, and the other in Utrecht, the Netherlands), Cohen-Kettenis et al. (2003) found that the children who met the complete criteria for GID

Table 44–4. DSM-IV-TR diagnostic criteria for sexual disorder not otherwise specified

This category is included for coding a sexual disturbance that does not meet the criteria for any specific sexual disorder and is neither a sexual dysfunction nor a paraphilia. Examples include

1. Marked feelings of inadequacy concerning sexual performance or other traits related to self-imposed standards of masculinity or femininity
2. Distress about a pattern of repeated sexual relationships involving a succession of lovers who are experienced by the individual only as things to be used
3. Persistent and marked distress about sexual orientation

Source. From American Psychiatric Association: *Diagnostic and Statistical Manual of Mental Disorders,* 4th Edition, Text Revision. Washington, DC, American Psychiatric Association, 2000. Copyright 2000, American Psychiatric Association. Used with permission.

(mean age, 6.8 years) were significantly younger than the children who were subthreshold (mean age, 8.6 years). Elsewhere it was shown that children who met the complete diagnostic criteria were from a higher social class and were more likely to come from an "intact" two-parent family. Sex of the child and IQ were not associated with the presence or absence of the complete diagnostic criteria for GID (Zucker and Bradley 1995).

To test which variables contributed to the correct classification of the children in the two diagnostic groups, a discriminant-function analysis was performed (Zucker and Bradley 1995). Age, sex, IQ, and parents' marital status contributed to the discriminant function, with age showing the greatest power. In the DSM-III group, 82.6% were correctly classified, and in the non-DSM-III group, 68.8% were correctly classified.

The data regarding age appear to be related to older children's tendency not to verbalize the wish to be of the opposite sex, which was a distinct criterion for GID in both DSM-III and DSM-III-R (American Psychiatric Association 1987). Clinical evidence may suggest continued discomfort with gender identity issues, but the older child may be more aware of social convention and thus may not verbalize concerns, at least during an initial diagnostic assessment.

These findings led to the question of whether it was appropriate to retain the wish to be the opposite sex as a distinct criterion in DSM-IV (Bradley et al. 1991; Zucker et al. 1998). The DSM-IV Subcommittee on

Gender Identity Disorders recommended that the verbalized wish to be the opposite sex should be collapsed with several other behavioral criteria to index the child's cross-gender identification (see Criterion A in Table 44–1) (Bradley et al. 1991). In a reanalysis of an existing data set, Zucker et al. (1998) showed that this change somewhat reduced the influence of age on the likelihood of a child meeting the requirements in Criterion A.

Table 44–1 also shows Criterion B for the diagnosis of GID: the child's sense of discomfort about his or her sex and the sense of inappropriateness in the gender role of that sex. At present, formal studies to fully evaluate the reliability and validity of the modified GID diagnosis for children have not been conducted.

Perhaps the most substantive change in the diagnostic criteria for GID in DSM-IV and DSM-IV-TR pertains to the inclusion of age-related criteria so that the diagnosis can be applied to all phases of the life cycle. This change resulted in the elimination of two diagnoses from DSM-III-R: 1) transsexualism and 2) gender identity disorder of adolescence or adulthood, nontranssexual type.

From a clinical point of view, the establishment of the GID diagnosis in adolescents requires that one pay close attention to the descriptors *strong and persistent* (Criterion A) and *persistent discomfort* (Criterion B). Unfortunately, no gold standard is available to make this kind of clinical judgment and, to date, there has been little in the way of systematic empirical research regarding the reliability and validity of the diagnosis in adolescents (see, however, Smith et al. 2001; Zucker and Bradley 1995).

No formal empirical studies have been conducted to examine the reliability and validity of the diagnosis of transvestic fetishism in adolescents; however, the DSM-IV-TR diagnostic criteria for transvestic fetishism (see Table 44–3) are sufficiently loose to make their use with adolescents not particularly difficult (Zucker and Blanchard 1997; Zucker and Bradley 1995). Clinically, one encounters adolescents who display a range of fetishistic cross-dressing (e.g., from wearing women's underwear while masturbating to complete cross-dressing accompanied by erotic arousal). Conceptually, clinicians should be interested in whether such behavior represents an erotic preference (Zucker and Blanchard 1997). With adolescents, this is not always clear, because many adolescent boys also display considerable heterosexual arousal and interaction without the use of feminine apparel. However, DSM-IV-TR criteria for transvestic fetishism do not address the issue of erotic preference.

In DSM-IV-TR, the term *autogynephilia* was introduced as a new descriptive construct, giving recognition to its increased clinical use in understanding the linkage between transvestic fetishism and GID. The term *autogynephilia* was constructed from Greek roots meaning "love of oneself as a woman" and has been defined as a male's propensity to be sexually aroused by the thought or image of himself as a female (for review, see Zucker and Blanchard 1997). It is most commonly the case that transvestic adolescents who experience autogynephilic feelings and fantasies are the ones who will present with the request for sex-reassignment surgery.

Clinical Findings

■ Phenomenology

Children with GID present with a rather coherent set of behavioral signs. In a boy, these signs include making verbal statements that he is, or would like to be, a girl; cross-dressing in girls' or women's clothing; having a preference for culturally stereotypical feminine toys and activities; emulating females in fantasy play; having a preference for girls as playmates; expressing dislike of his sexual anatomy (e.g., concealing his penis, sitting to urinate in order to embellish the fantasy of having female genitalia); and being averse to rough-and-tumble play and group sports. In a girl, the inverse is observed. Of particular note is the intense aversion to culturally stereotypical girls' clothing and the desire to have her hairstyle look like that of a boy, such that a naive observer would perceive her as male. Taken together, these characteristics point to the child's very strong cross-gender identification, and several research studies have established their discriminant validity or relative uniqueness (Green 1974, 1987; Zucker 1985, 1992; Zucker and Bradley 1995).

Apart from the features of GID described in the formal DSM diagnostic criteria, there are other aspects that have been noted clinically and empirically. For example, many clinicians have observed how intense and rigid cross-gender identification can be in these youngsters (Coates 1990, 1997; Coates and Wolfe 1995, 1997), and sometimes this extends into domains that surprise even the most sophisticated practitioner. One example of this pertains to sex-typed color preferences, which some gender theorists might characterize as an overelaborated gender schema (Ruble and Martin 1998). Clinically, one is often impressed by the rigidity of color choices by children with GID. For example, the boys invariably prefer pink and purple, as exemplified, perhaps, in the critically acclaimed film *Ma Vie en Rose* (My Life in Pink), about a boy with GID (Kline 1998). One can observe this in the type of clothing that they request and in their drawings, which are often of idealized, beautiful, and benevolent females. Girls with GID invariably reject colors like pink and purple and will often prefer dark colors, such as blue and black. About 10% of boys with GID appear preoccupied not with benevolent females but with malevolent ones: they endlessly draw pictures of angry, hostile females, such as the Wicked Witch of the West, Cruella De Vil from *101 Dalmatians*, or Ursula from *The Little Mermaid*.

The study of the child's actual sense of gender identity has been somewhat more complicated. Most children with GID "know" that they are male or female; that is, if they are asked the question "Are you a boy or a girl?" they answer correctly (Zucker et al. 1993b). Some of these youngsters, however, do not seem to know the answer or else appear to be confused about their gender status (i.e., whether they are male or female). In part, this may be a developmental phenomenon, but it also may be a sign of the severity of the overall condition (Stoller 1968a). Indeed, Zucker et al. (1999) reported evidence for a developmental lag in acquisition of gender constancy among children with GID.

The child's internal representation of gender has been more difficult to study, although clinical experience suggests that the stability of the gender sense can be quite labile in some children. Zucker et al. (1993b) reported the results of a gender identity interview schedule that identified two factors, tentatively labeled cognitive gender confusion and affective gender confusion, both of which discriminated children referred for gender identity problems from clinical and nonclinical control subjects. The following responses were given by an 8-year-old boy (IQ, 133) who, by parent report, met DSM-IV criteria for GID:

Interviewer (I): Are you a boy or a girl?
Child (C): Both.
I: Are you a girl?
C: Kind of.
I: When you grow up, will you be a mom or a dad?

C: Don't know.
I: Could you ever grow up to be a mom?
C: Yes.
I: Are there any good things about being a boy?
C: Yes.
I: Tell me some of the good things about being a boy.
C: Boys don't have to have babies and get their spine ripped open…
I: Are there any things that you don't like about being a boy?
C: Yes.
I: Tell me some of the things that you don't like about being a boy.
C: …Everything. Please don't make me tell.
I: Do you think it is better to be a boy or a girl?
C: Girl.
I: Why?
C: There are so many reasons. Girls are more mature…positive…better…
I: In your mind, do you ever think that you would like to be a girl?
C: Yes.
I: Can you tell me why?
C: Because the guys don't accept me for what I am.…Girls have better bands, like the Spice Girls.
I: In your mind, do you ever get mixed up and you're not really sure if you are a boy or a girl?
C: Yes.
I: Tell me more about that.
C: Practically all the time. I think the doctor was totally wrong and deformed me. I am a woman in a man's body. He gave me a girl's mind and switched brains or bodies.
I: Do you ever feel more like a girl than like a boy?
C: Yes.
I: Tell me more about that.
C: Well, I do lots of times, especially when I'm in the bath.…This is going way too deep.…Well, usually girls want me to play their games.…Then I get mixed up being a girl or a boy.
I: You know what dreams are, right? Well, when you dream at night, are you ever in the dream?
C: Yes.
I: In your dreams, are you a boy, a girl, or sometimes a boy and sometimes a girl?
C: Both.…it's just me as a girl, me and my friends…find out the secret of being trapped in a boy's body. We go to the doctor's to find out, look into his files and find nothing about me. Then we destroy him.
I: Do you ever think that you really are a girl?
C: Yes.
I: Tell me more about that.
C: …Practically all the time…because of my feelings.…I want to be a lead singer of a girls' band when I grow up.

■ Age at Onset

Green (1976) reported that the age at onset of cross-gender behaviors in GID is typically during the preschool years. In his sample of boys, for example, 55% were cross-dressing by their third birthday, 80% were cross-dressing by their fourth birthday, and 90% were cross-dressing by their fifth birthday. Many experienced clinicians have observed that repetitive, intense cross-gender behaviors appear even before a child's second birthday. Clinical data on girls reveal a similar age at onset (Zucker and Bradley 1995). It is important to note that among more typical children, a display of various gender role behaviors can also be observed during this period in the life cycle. This similarity suggests that the underlying mechanisms for both patterns may be the same, albeit mirror images.

■ Associated Psychopathology

In DSM-IV-TR, it is noted that children with GID may have co-occurring behavioral difficulties, including social isolation, low self-esteem, separation anxiety, and depression. What are the data regarding the presence of other types of psychopathology in children with GID? If other forms of psychopathology are present, how is the association with GID to be understood?

Unfortunately, omnibus structured interview schedules that cover the gamut of childhood psychopathology have not been utilized in this clinical population. However, several more narrowly focused empirical studies have reported on the presence of general psychopathology in both boys and girls with GID (Coates and Person 1985; Cohen-Kettenis et al. 2003; Zucker and Bradley 1995). These studies have shown that both boys and girls with GID display levels of general psychopathology similar to those of demographically matched psychiatric control subjects and levels greater than those of control subjects without psychiatric disorders. For example, children with GID have been shown to display behavior problems at a level comparable to the clinic-referred standardization sample (Coates and Person 1985; Cohen-Kettenis et al. 2003; Zucker and Bradley 1995), as measured with the Child Behavior Checklist (CBCL) (Achenbach and Edelbrock 1981), a parent-report instrument of behavior problems. In boys with GID, internalizing problems were somewhat more common than externalizing problems, a finding that is consistent with clinical observations that many of these boys experience anxiety, depression, and social withdrawal (see also Zucker et al. 1996a). More generally, it should be noted that the overall functioning of children with GID varies considerably. Some of these youngsters show pervasive behavioral difficulties and often require intensive intervention for these problems in their own right; on the other hand, some youngsters show minimal behavioral psychopathology and function quite well in the different environments of daily life.

How might these associated behavioral difficulties be best understood? Zucker and Bradley (1995) provided data that showed that in boys with GID, behavioral difficulties based on CBCL measures increased with age. This was interpreted as being consistent with the influence of social ostracism, which becomes more pronounced over time. Two subsequent studies, utilizing a more direct measure of poor peer relations, confirmed this inference empirically; indeed, in a multiple regression analysis, it was the measure of poor peer relations, not age, that accounted for the most variance in predicting CBCL behavior problems in both boys and girls with GID (Cohen-Kettenis et al. 2003; Zucker et al. 2002).

A study by S.R. Fridell (unpublished doctoral dissertation, 2001) provided further evidence that the cross-sex-typed behavior of boys with GID may well be related to how well they are liked by other children. Fridell created 15 age-matched experimental play groups consisting of one boy with GID and two nonreferred boys and two nonreferred girls (age range, 3–8 years). After two 60-minute play sessions, conducted a week apart, each child was asked to select their favorite playmate from the group. The nonreferred boys most often chose the other nonreferred boy as their favorite playmate, thus indicating a distinct preference over the boy with GID. The nonreferred girls chose the other girl as their favorite playmate, thus showing a relative disinterest in either the boy with GID or the two nonreferred boys.

In another line of research, Zucker and Bradley (1995) showed that a composite measure of maternal psychopathology also predicted the extent of behavioral difficulties detected with the CBCL, which suggests that generic familial emotional and psychiatric factors also contribute to the degree of general psychopathology (see also Cohen-Kettenis et al. 2003; Zucker et al. 2002).

Another perspective on the nature of the associated psychopathology has been advanced by Coates and Person (1985), who provided data on a high rate of separation anxiety disorder in boys with GID. These researchers argued that the high rate of separation anxiety could be accounted for by a great deal of familial psychopathology, which rendered the mothers of these boys unpredictably available. The authors claimed that the emergence of the separation anxiety actually preceded the first appearance of the feminine behavior, which was understood to serve a representational coping function of recapturing an emotionally unavailable mother.

As noted elsewhere (Zucker and Green 1992), Coates and Person (1985) did not have empirical evidence available to document the putative temporal relation between separation anxiety and GID, because both diagnoses were made concurrently at the time of assessment. Rather, the temporal relation was inferred on the basis of clinical evidence. Subsequently, Zucker et al. (1996a) confirmed the high rate of co-occurring traits of separation anxiety disorder in boys with GID, and A.S. Birkenfeld-Adams (unpublished doctoral dissertation, 1999) has shown a rate of insecure attachment to the mother, but the temporal aspect of the hypothesis of Coates and Person (1985) remains to be tested.

■ Biophysical Markers

By observation, it is apparent that the vast majority of children with GID do not have abnormalities in physical sex differentiation—such as in the various physical intersexual disorders—that might, on theoretical grounds, contribute to the condition (Meyer-Bahlburg 1994; Zucker 1999c). Because sex hormone levels are so low during childhood (Sizonenko 1980), it is unlikely that a standard endocrine assessment would detect abnormalities. Green (1976) and Rekers et al. (1979) reported normal XY karyotypes in boys with GID. Green also found that the feminine boys he studied did not differ in height and weight from nonfeminine boys at the time of assessment (Roberts et al. 1987), although they were hospitalized more often before their participation in the study.

However, if one starts with a sample of children or adolescents with certain physical intersexual conditions, such as genetic females with congenital adrenal hyperplasia (CAH) raised as girls, genetic males with partial androgen insensitivity syndrome raised as girls, and genetic males with cloacal exstrophy raised as girls, gender identity problems or gender dysphoria appears to be present in a subgroup of these young-sters (for reviews, see Zucker 1999c, 2002). However, these conditions are invariably already known to the clinician at the time of diagnostic assessment.

Differential Diagnosis

■ Diagnostic Issues in Children

Several diagnostic issues require consideration in relation to GID. A small number of boys engage in a type of cross-dressing that appears to be quite different from the type of cross-dressing that is part of the clinical picture in GID. In the latter, cross-dressing encompasses a range of behaviors, including the wearing of dresses, women's shoes, and jewelry, all of which enhance the fantasy or desire to be like the opposite sex. In the former, cross-dressing is limited to the use of undergarments, such as panties and nylons. As with boys with GID, the cross-dressing has a compulsive and self-soothing flavor to it. However, it is not accompanied by other signs of cross-gender identification; in fact, apart from the cross-dressing, these boys are conventionally masculine (Zucker and Blanchard 1997). Many male adolescents and adults who have a diagnosis of transvestic fetishism recall such cross-dressing during childhood (Zucker and Bradley 1995); however, no prospective studies of prepubertal boys engaging in this form of cross-dressing have been conducted to determine what proportion, if any, of these boys develop transvestic fetishism.

When all of the clinical signs of GID are present, there is little difficulty in making the diagnosis. If one accepts the idea of a spectrum of cross-gender identification, then there is more room for ambiguity, and one must be prepared to identify what Meyer-Bahlburg (1985) referred to as the "zone of transition between clinically significant cross-gender behavior and mere statistical deviation from the gender norm" (p. 682).

Friedman (1988), for example, suggested that there is a subgroup of boys who are "unmasculine" but not feminine. Based on clinical experience, Friedman argued that these boys have a "persistent, profound feeling of masculine inadequacy which leads to negative valuing of the self" (p. 199). Although it is not described in the formal clinical literature, there is also probably a subgroup of girls who are "unfeminine" but not masculine and may have similar feelings. Such youngsters would not meet DSM-IV-TR criteria for

GID, but the residual diagnosis of GIDNOS could be used in such cases.

For girls, the main differential diagnostic issue concerns the distinction between GID and what is known in popular culture as tomboyism. According to *Webster's Ninth New Collegiate Dictionary,* a tomboy is "a girl of boyish behavior." Green et al. (1982) studied a community sample of tomboys and found that, compared with a control group of nontomboys, tomboys displayed a greater number of masculine traits, such as a preference for boys as playmates, interest in rough-and-tumble play, and play with guns and trucks. In many respects, the cross-gender behavior of such tomboys is similar to the masculine gender role preferences of girls who are referred clinically for gender identity concerns (Bailey et al. 2002; Zucker and Bradley 1995).

Based on critiques of DSM-III criteria for GID in girls (Zucker 1982), DSM-III-R and DSM-IV (American Psychiatric Association 1994) criteria for girls were modified in the hope of better differentiating these two groups. Clinical experience suggests that at least three characteristics are useful in making a differential diagnosis. First, girls with GID express a profound unhappiness with their female gender status; in contrast, Green (1980) noted that his sample of tomboys were "generally content being female" (p. 262). Second, girls with GID display a marked aversion to culturally defined feminine clothing and will do their utmost to avoid having to wear it. Their refusal to wear "girls' clothes" under any circumstance often precipitates clinical referral. Although tomboys prefer functional and casual clothing (Green et al. 1982), they do not display the same type of rigid rejection of feminine clothing. Third, girls with GID, unlike tomboys, often express discomfort with or dislike of their sexual anatomy.

■ Diagnostic Issues in Adolescents

The clinician will encounter at least four types of psychosexual problems among adolescents (Bradley and Zucker 1990; Zucker and Bradley 1995). First, clinical experience suggests that persistent cross-gender identification throughout childhood is a risk factor for the continuation of GID into adolescence and adulthood. As noted earlier, it is important to evaluate the fixedness of the desire to change sex, because therapeutic decisions will be influenced, at least to some extent, by the adolescent's openness to consider alternatives to

sex reassignment (Newman 1970). From a differential diagnostic standpoint, the residual diagnosis of GID-NOS can be used for individuals whose desire to change sex does not quite fit the criteria for GID.

The second psychosexual problem that can be observed in adolescents involves individuals who have a history of GID or a subclinical variant. These adolescents show various signs of cross-gender identification but do not voice a desire to change sex. They are circumspect about their sexual orientation, so it is not possible to classify them as homosexuals. These youngsters often are referred because of continued social ostracism. Many of these adolescents are able to acknowledge distress about not "fitting in" because of their cross-gender behavior. In these cases, the residual diagnosis of GIDNOS could be used to indicate that the adolescent continues to struggle with gender identity concerns.

A third type of psychosexual problem involves adolescents who have been referred because of homosexual behavior or orientation. Many of these adolescents have a history of GID or a variation of it, perhaps akin to the unmasculinity described by Friedman (1988; see also Friedman and Downey 2002; Friedman and Stern 1980). Although the reason for referral varies, it is important to rule out continuing concerns about gender identity. For adolescents distressed about their sexual orientation, the diagnosis of sexual disorder not otherwise specified can be given.

The last type of psychosexual problem is, as far as we know, the exclusive domain of adolescent males: cross-dressing associated with sexual arousal. As noted earlier, the extent of the cross-dressing varies and there is no problem, in principle, in employing the diagnosis of transvestic fetishism. As noted with adults with transvestic fetishism, a heterosexual orientation predominates. A history of GID is not part of the clinical picture, although some of these boys think about sex-reassignment surgery and are at risk for GID. Although the clinical course of GID in males with a history of transvestic fetishism seems to develop more slowly than does GID in males who are sexually attracted to other biological males (Blanchard 1994; Blanchard et al. 1987), there is now considerable clinical evidence to suggest that even among adolescents with transvestic fetishism the presence of autogynephilic feelings can be substantial, thus resulting in rather intense gender dysphoria, leading to the desire for sex-reassignment surgery.

In DSM-III-R, the diagnosis of transsexualism (GID

in DSM-IV) was an exclusionary criterion for transvestic fetishism, but this was shown to be clinically inaccurate (Blanchard and Clemmensen 1988). In DSM-IV-TR, the diagnosis of transvestic fetishism allows the co-occurrence of gender dysphoria to be specified (see Table 44–3).

Epidemiology

■ Prevalence

No studies have been designed to specifically assess the prevalence of GID in children. Nevertheless, the characterization of GID by Meyer-Bahlburg (1985) as a rare phenomenon is not unreasonable. If one accepts the assumption that GID in childhood is associated with its continuation into adulthood, then conservative estimates of prevalence in childhood might be inferred from epidemiological data on GID in adults. Bakker et al. (1993) inferred the prevalence of GID in adults in the Netherlands from the number of persons receiving cross-gender hormonal treatment at the main adult gender identity clinic in that country: 1 in 11,000 men and 1 in 30,400 women.

However, this approach has at least three limitations: first, it relies on the number of persons who attend specialty clinics serving as gateways for surgical and hormonal sex reassignment, which may not include all gender-dysphoric adults. Second, the assumption that GID in children will in fact persist into adulthood is not necessarily true (see "Prognosis" section below). Nevertheless, prevalence estimates of GID in children derived from data on adults support the notion of its rarity. Last, unlike adult women with gender dysphoria, who are predominantly sexually attracted to biological females (but see Chivers and Bailey 2000), adult men with gender dysphoria are about equally likely to be sexually attracted to biological males or females (Blanchard et al. 1987). A childhood history of GID or its subclinical manifestation occurs largely among adults with gender dysphoria and a homosexual sexual orientation. Estimates of the prevalence of childhood GID inferred from the prevalence of GID in men should take this into account.

Current prospective evidence indicates that GID in childhood is associated with subsequent homosexuality (see "Prognosis" below). There also is substantial retrospective evidence that homosexual men and women are more likely than heterosexual men and women to recall engaging in various cross-gender behaviors during childhood (Bailey and Zucker 1995). Accordingly, the literature on the epidemiology of homosexuality might also help to gauge the prevalence of GID.

Unfortunately, the true prevalence of exclusive, or nearly exclusive, homosexuality is a source of contention. Many authorities now acknowledge that the widely quoted 10% prevalence rate of homosexuality in men, which was culled from the work of Kinsey et al. (1948), is erroneous but has continued to be cited for political reasons (Begley 1991). Scholars who have reworked the Kinsey terrain suggest much lower prevalence rates, typically between 2% and 6% for men and about 2% for women (Diamond 1993; Rogers and Turner 1991). Even lower estimates for men and women have emerged from studies pertaining to the acquired immunodeficiency syndrome (AIDS) epidemic (Laumann et al. 1994; Spira et al. 1994; Wellings et al. 1994).

Another problem is that the retrospective literature on childhood cross-gender behavior in homosexual men and women often does not indicate how to classify individuals as either cross-gendered or not cross-gendered. Moreover, patients classified as cross-gendered would not necessarily meet the complete DSM-IV-TR diagnostic criteria for GID (Friedman 1988).

Liberal estimates of prevalence can be derived from studies on children in whom individual cross-gender behaviors have been assessed. For example, in one study of parents' responses on the CBCL (Achenbach and Edelbrock 1981), the percentage of mothers of nonreferred 4- to 13-year-old boys grouped at 2-year intervals who endorsed the item "behaves like opposite sex" ranged from 0.7% in boys ages 12–13 to 6.0% in boys ages 4–5 years. Among nonreferred girls, maternal endorsement of this item was higher, ranging from 9.6% to 12.9%. For the item "wishes to be of opposite sex," the endorsement was lower for both sexes, ranging from 0% to 5.0% in specific sex-by-age groupings. Similar results were obtained from another parent report questionnaire—the Achenbach-Connors-Quay Behavior Checklist (Achenbach et al. 1991)—which contained 3 items pertaining to cross-gender identification out of a total of 215 (2 from the original CBCL and a third, "dresses like or plays at being opposite sex"). If anything, endorsement of these items appeared to be less common on the new questionnaire than on the original CBCL, which supports the general point that extreme cross-gender behavior is relatively uncommon. This kind of information no doubt overestimates caseness, although the method of data collection might be a reasonable screening device for more intensive evaluation (Pleak et al. 1989).

■ Incidence

No adequate epidemiological data are available to address the question of whether the incidence of GID has changed over the years.

■ Referral Rates

Prevalence and incidence issues aside, there has been a consistent observation that boys are more often referred than girls for gender identity concerns. In two specialized gender identity clinics for children—one in Toronto, Canada, and the other in Utrecht, the Netherlands—the sex ratio was 4.7:1 favoring boys over girls (*N*=488) (Cohen-Kettenis et al. 2003). However, the sex ratio was significantly larger in the Toronto clinic than in the Utrecht clinic (5.8:1 versus 2.9:1).

There are at least two explanations for this strong sex difference in referral rates. First, it may well be that boys are more vulnerable to GID than are girls, much as they are to a variety of other child psychiatric conditions (Eme 1979). Second, cultural factors appear to be related to differential tolerance of cross-gender behavior in boys versus girls. In childhood, cross-gender behavior in girls is less subject to negative sanctions than it is in boys by both peers and parents (Fagot 1985; Langlois and Downs 1980; Zucker et al. 1995). In fact, Cohen-Kettenis et al. (2003) showed that boys with GID had significantly poorer peer relations than girls with GID in both the Toronto clinic and in the Utrecht clinic. Moreover, adults are more likely to link cross-gender behavior in boys to atypical outcomes, such as homosexuality, than they are in girls (Antill 1987; Martin 1990). Both Cohen-Kettenis et al. (2003) and Zucker et al. (1997a) provided data to suggest that girls with GID need to display more extreme cross-gender behaviors than do boys to elicit a referral. Therefore, cases of GID in girls may be under-referred because of greater acceptance of girlhood masculinity.

Etiology

■ Biological Mechanisms

The search for biological determinants of human psychosexual development—gender identity, gender role,

and sexual orientation—has been a slow and complex endeavor, despite a great deal of effort on the part of many researchers. These researchers disagree on several issues. Do biological factors exert fixed versus predisposing influences on the components of psychosexual development? Can animal models be useful in understanding human phenomena? Are there unwanted political implications of advancing a biological explanation for human psychosexual development? These questions and others have been subject to intense debate within the field of sexual science over the years.

At present, researchers have been unable to identify a clear biological anomaly or variant associated specifically with GID. There is evidence, however, that certain behavioral traits linked to biological processes may characterize children with GID. The relation to biological variables also relies on data from allied populations from which generalizations might be made.

Prenatal Sex Hormones

Although circulating sex hormones probably have little causal effect on gender identity, gender role, and sexual orientation, considerable attention has been accorded to the influential role of the prenatal hormonal environment and its effect on psychosexual differentiation. Experimental studies—conducted in animal models ranging from mice to monkeys—have shown quite clearly how manipulation of the prenatal hormonal milieu can affect postnatal sex-dimorphic behavior (Meyer-Bahlburg 1984). Is there evidence that prenatal hormonal variations in humans, due to either endogenous anomalies or exogenous manipulation, exert effects that are consistent with those that have been observed in lower animals? Reviews of this complex literature suggest that there is enough consistency to pursue the lead (Collaer and Hines 1995).

One may consider, for example, studies of CAH, the most common physical intersexual condition that affects genetic females. This autosomal recessive disorder is associated with enzyme defects that result in abnormal adrenal steroid biosynthesis. Because of the high level of androgen production during fetal development, masculinization of the external genitalia is common. Based on data from lower animals and from theory, it has been presumed that some masculinization of the organ of behavior, the brain, may also have occurred.

As reviewed elsewhere (Collaer and Hines 1995; Zucker 1999c), there is evidence that the gender role behavior of girls with CAH is more masculine or less feminine than that of unaffected control subjects. The impact of CAH on gender identity is less clear, although the percentage of affected individuals who express some ambivalence about being female or who have been reared as boys (in part because the condition was untreated) is probably higher than among girls in the general population (Meyer-Bahlburg 1994; Meyer-Bahlburg et al. 1996). Adult follow-up studies of girls with CAH suggest that they have higher rates of bisexuality and homosexuality (particularly in fantasy) and lower rates of marriage and sociosexual experiences than would be expected otherwise (Dittmann et al. 1992; Money et al. 1984; Mulaikal et al. 1987; Zucker et al. 1996b).

Despite the rather obvious role of the hormonal anomaly in explaining the overall pattern, it is important to note that individual differences in outcome occur, and the determinants of such variation remain open to debate (Berenbaum 1990; Dittmann et al. 1992; Ehrhardt and Baker 1974). It is not clear, for instance, to what extent differences result from the severity of the disorder, from biomedical sequelae of the condition, or from social factors, such as how parents' understanding of the condition might affect their socialization techniques vis-à-vis gender.

Can this body of data help us understand the genesis of GID? As noted above (see "Biological Mechanisms"), no identifiable hormonal anomaly seems to characterize children with this disorder. Perhaps, however, less pronounced variations in the prenatal hormonal milieu that do not affect genital differentiation but that do account in part for intrasex differences in the expression of sex-dimorphic behavior play a role. For example, an avoidance of rough-and-tumble play and a low activity level both appear to be part of the clinical picture in boys with GID (Green 1987; Zucker and Bradley 1995). Both of these behaviors show a strong sex dimorphism (Eaton and Enns 1986) and are probably partly determined by biological factors. Such behavioral traits, coupled with the anxiety often observed clinically in such boys (Coates 1990; Zucker and Bradley 1995), may set in motion a complex chain of psychosocial sequelae that predispose to cross-gender identification (Green 1987).

Physical Appearance

In a small-scale clinical study of extremely feminine boys, Stoller (1968b, 1975) noted that the mothers commented on their sons' extreme physical beauty as infants, particularly the face. Although Stoller (1975) suggested that this description may have been a bit of an exaggeration, he was impressed by these boys' physical appearance: "We have noticed that they often have pretty faces, with fine hair, lovely complexions, graceful movements, and—especially—big, piercing, liquid eyes" (p. 43). In Stoller's view, the physical beauty of the boy fueled the mother's conscious and unconscious desires to feminize her son.

Green and colleagues (Green 1987; Green et al. 1985; Roberts et al. 1987) systematically studied physical attractiveness in a larger sample of feminine and control boys. Masked ratings of audiotaped interviews showed that the parents of the feminine boys were more likely than the parents of the control boys to describe their sons during infancy as "beautiful" and "feminine." Green (1987) found that the degree of recalled beauty correlated with ratings of maternal encouragement of feminine behavior. Green's data suggest that these boys may well have had objective physical properties that distinguished them from control subjects. On the other hand, it is easy to see how retrospective distortion can be implicated in explaining these data.

Zucker et al. (1993c) reported physical attractiveness data on a group of boys with GID and clinical control boys. Color photographs of both groups of boys were taken at the time of assessment (mean age, 8.1 years). College students then made ratings of their pictures for five traits: attractive, beautiful, cute, handsome, and pretty. The raters were masked to group status, being informed only that they would be viewing pictures of boys. The boys with GID were rated as significantly more attractive than the clinical control boys on all five traits.

In a subsequent study, Fridell et al. (1996) reported physical attractiveness data on a group of girls with GID and clinical and nonclinical control girls (mean age, 6.6 years). College students rated the girls' pictures for five traits: attractive, beautiful, cute, pretty, and ugly. On all traits except "ugly," the girls with GID were rated as significantly less attractive than the clinical and nonclinical control girls. In a third study, boys with GID were judged to be significantly less "all-boy," masculine, and rugged than control boys, whereas girls with GID were judged to be significantly more masculine, rugged, and tomboyish in appearance than control girls (McDermid et al. 1998).

The attractiveness/appearance data on boys complement and extend the previous findings of Stoller (1968b) and Green (1987). Nevertheless, interpretation of the data for both the boys and girls remains complex. On the one hand, these findings may reflect objective, biophysical differences in the appearance of GID and control children. On the other hand, they may reflect the effects of social shaping of physical appearance. In other words, physical appearance may be a predisposing factor in the development of GID or it may serve to perpetuate the disorder as a result of social shaping.

Handedness

Slightly more males than females show a preference for using the left hand in unimanual behavioral tasks such as writing. There is no established consensus for understanding the basis of this sex difference. Genetic factors clearly play a role in determining hand preference. Another line of research implicates adverse prenatal or perinatal events that result in an increase in left-handedness above the approximate gold standard of 10% in the general population.

Zucker et al. (2001) found that boys with GID (n=205) had a significantly elevated rate of left-handedness (19.5%) compared with three separate quasi-epidemiological samples of boys (11.8%, total n= 13,253) and with a diagnostically heterogeneous sample of clinical control boys (8.3%, n=205). This finding parallels studies of adult males with GID, who also appear to have an elevated rate of left-handedness (e.g., Green and Young 2001; Herman-Jeglinska et al. 1997), as well as studies of adult men with a homosexual sexual orientation (Lalumière et al. 2000). At present, the explanation for the elevation remains unclear, but candidate factors have centered on some type of perturbation in prenatal development that in some way affects sex-dimorphic behavioral differentiation.

Sibling Sex Ratio and Birth Order

Boys with GID have an excess of brothers to sisters (sibling sex ratio) and have a later birth order (Blanchard et al. 1995; Zucker et al. 1997b). Some additional evidence shows that boys with GID are born later in relation to brothers but not to sisters. In the study by Blanchard and colleagues, clinical control boys showed no evidence for an altered sibling sex ratio or a late birth order. One biological explanation to account for these

results pertains to maternal immune reactions during pregnancy. The male fetus is experienced by the mother as more "foreign" (i.e., antigenic) than the female fetus. Based on studies with lower animals, it has been suggested that one result of this is that the mother produces antibodies that have the consequence of demasculinizing or feminizing the male fetus but produce no corresponding masculinizing or defeminizing of the female fetus (Blanchard and Klassen 1997). This model predicts that males born later in a line of siblings might be more affected because the mother's antigenicity increases with each successive male pregnancy, which is consistent with the empirical evidence on sibling sex ratio and birth order among GID probands. At present, however, this proposed mechanism has not been formally tested in humans.

Birth Weight

On average, males weigh more than females at the time of birth (Arbuckle et al. 1993). There are, of course, many factors that influence variations in birth weight. One hypothesized factor is the sex difference in prenatal exposure to androgens. In one study, girls with CAH had a higher mean birth weight than unaffected girls (Qazi and Thompson 1971). In another study, genetic males with the complete form of the androgen insensitivity syndrome had comparable birth weights to genetic females (de Zegher et al. 1998).

Blanchard et al. (2002) compared the birth weights of boys with GID (n=250) and clinical control boys (n=739) and girls (n=261). The clinical control subjects showed the expected sex difference in birth weight. The boys with GID had birth weights that were intermediate to those of the clinical control boys and the control girls and did not differ significantly from either group. Further analysis of the birth weight data indicated an effect of sibling sex and birth order. The boys with GID who had two or more older brothers weighed significantly less at birth than did the control boys with two or more older brothers. In contrast, the GID and control boys with fewer than two older brothers did not differ in birth weight. Given the interactive effect of sibling sex and birth order, a simple prenatal hypoandrogenization influence among the GID probands is unlikely. Although it was speculative, Blanchard et al. (2002) suggested that the mechanism may be immunological, that is, that antimale antibodies produced by human mothers in response to immunization by male fetuses could decrease the birth weights of subsequent male children and could increase the odds of those children developing behavioral femininity (i.e., GID).

Biological Mechanisms Summary

Research conducted during the past decade has begun to identify some characteristics of children (particularly boys) with GID that may well have a biological basis. Corresponding studies of girls have been less numerous, largely because of problems in sample size that limit statistical power. In many respects it has been easier to rule out candidate biological explanations, such as the influence of gross anomalies in prenatal hormonal exposure, than it has been to identify the relevant biological mechanisms that are involved in affecting sex-dimorphic behavioral differentiation, but not sex-dimorphic genital differentiation. However, the identification of new potential biological markers may open up avenues for further empirical inquiry.

■ Psychosocial Mechanisms

Several psychosocial factors have been thought to play a role in either the genesis or the perpetuation of GID. Most of these factors have been better studied in boys than in girls, and some of them have been held to be sex-specific. Below we discuss a few of the more prominent hypotheses.

Social Reinforcement

Do parents shape or influence sex-dimorphic behavior in their children? This very simple question has proved exceedingly difficult to answer. If one turns to the normative literature, it becomes apparent how complicated the matter actually is (Fagot 1985; Fagot and Leinbach 1989; Lytton and Romney 1991; Ruble and Martin 1998). Perhaps a general conclusion is that parents do play a role in influencing patterns of sex-dimorphic behavior but not in the simplistic way that social learning theorists so readily expected.

When the parents of children with GID are asked to recall their initial responses to cross-gender behaviors, such as cross-dressing and cross-sex toy play, tolerance and nonresponsiveness appear to be very common, as suggested by reasonable evidence (Green 1987; J.N. Mitchell, unpublished doctoral dissertation, 1991; Zucker and Bradley 1995). Actual encouragement of these behaviors appears to be more common than negative or discouraging reactions.

Initial parental tolerance or encouragement of cross-gender behavior may therefore be of some etiological significance. The reasons for such tolerance appear to be quite variable, including parental values and goals regarding psychosexual development; feedback from professionals that the behavior is within normal limits and is only a phase; parental conflicts about issues of masculinity and femininity; and parental psychopathology and discord, which leave the parents relatively preoccupied and thus unresponsive to their child's behavior.

Parental Preference for Sex of Offspring

Some clinicians have suggested that parents' tolerance of cross-gender behavior in boys is related to their preference for the sex of the child before its birth. Therefore, one line of empirical research has explored whether parents of boys with GID had disproportionately hoped that the child would be a girl. There was no evidence that this had occurred (Green et al. 1985; Zucker et al. 1994). However, Zucker and Bradley (1995) noted that among mothers of boys with GID who had desired daughters, a small subgroup appeared to experience what might be termed pathological gender mourning (Zucker et al. 1993a). The wish for a daughter was acted out (by cross-dressing the boy) or was expressed in other ways (see Zucker and Bradley 2000). These mothers often had severe depression, which was lifted only when the boy began to act in a certain feminine manner. This clinical observation, however, must be examined in much greater detail, including understanding how the wish for a girl, when it occurs, is resolved in most cases.

Mother–Child and Father–Child Relationships

In clinical studies of boys with GID, Stoller (1968b, 1975, 1979) described an overly close relationship between mother and son and a distant, peripheral father–son relationship. Stoller (1985) claimed that such qualities were of etiological relevance: "The more mother and the less father, the more femininity" (p. 25). He argued that GID in boys was a "developmental arrest…in which an excessively close and gratifying mother-infant symbiosis, undisturbed by the father's presence, prevents a boy from adequately separating himself from his mother's female body and feminine behavior" (p. 25).

Green (1987) assessed the amount of shared time between parents of feminine boys and control subjects during the first 5 years of life. The fathers of feminine boys reported spending less time with their sons from the second to the fifth year than did the fathers of control subjects. In contradiction to the overcloseness hypothesis, the mothers of feminine boys also reported spending less time with their sons than did the mothers of control subjects.

The data on father–son shared time are quite consistent with a large body of clinical literature, whereas the mother–son data are not. Negative findings are difficult to interpret, particularly when they have not been consistently replicated. In this instance, they are difficult to reconcile with data showing that feminine boys feel closer to their mothers than to their fathers (Green 1987). Perhaps qualitative features of the mother–son relationship, such as attunement to each other's feelings, would have been a more sensitive index of the nature of the dyad. It is also possible that relative time spent with mother versus father would have yielded differences between Green's feminine boys and the control subjects.

Systematic studies on parent–child relationships have not yet been conducted for girls with GID. Preliminary clinical observations (Green 1974; Stoller 1975; Zucker and Bradley 1995) suggest that the mother–daughter relationship is often conflictual and not close, leading to what might be described as a disidentification from the mother (Greenson 1968). In some instances, femininity is devalued and masculinity is overvalued, which seem to be encouraged by the parents. Many of these girls tend to admire what their fathers do. In other cases, they appear to be quite frightened of their fathers and seem to develop the belief that they need to be quite strong and powerful to be safe. These preliminary clinical studies suggest that marked differences in the qualitative aspects of the parent–child relationship may exist between gender-disturbed boys and girls.

Maternal Psychosexual Development

Based on clinical data, Stoller (1968b) reported that the mothers of very feminine boys had childhood psychosexual conflicts. Although these women were initially feminine, he argued that "a degree of masculinity beyond what usually [would] be called tomboyishness" (p. 298) developed after a breach in the father–daughter relationship. A desire to be male was relinquished

at puberty, yet sociosexual experience was minimal, and, as adults, these women married distant men with whom sexual relations were poor. These women appeared to be uncomfortable with their femininity: "While these women have a feminine quality, inextricably woven in is this other, difficult to describe but easy to observe use of certain boyish or 'neuter' external features" (Stoller 1968b, p. 298).

Green's effort to verify Stoller's observations yielded mixed results. Mothers of feminine boys were more likely than mothers of control boys to describe themselves as tomboys (Green et al. 1985), but the mothers did not differ with regard to their recall of specific sex-typed behaviors (Green 1987). In a subsequent study using a factor-analyzed questionnaire, Zucker and Bradley (1995) did not find any differences in recalled childhood gender dysphoria or cross-gender behavior between mothers of boys with GID and clinical and nonclinical control mothers. In Green's (1987) study, the two groups of mothers also did not differ with regard to the extent of adolescent sociosexual experience. Trait assessment of childhood masculinity and femininity did not provide strong support for the possibility that less severe signs of cross-gender behavior were present (Green 1987). Taken as a whole, these data suggest that mothers of very feminine boys, on average, do not have grossly atypical psychosexual histories. Perhaps other aspects of psychosexuality should be studied, such as the mother's current attitude toward men and her concurrent views regarding masculinity and femininity.

General Psychopathology

Little systematic study has been given to the presence of general dysfunction, such as psychiatric disorder and marital discord, in the parents of children with GID. However, the evidence to date suggests that these parents display more psychiatric and emotional difficulties than parents of control subjects (Marantz and Coates 1991; S.M. Wolfe, unpublished doctoral dissertation, 1990; Zucker and Bradley 1995, 2000). Assuming these preliminary data hold up, there will be two main questions to pursue. First, will there be any specificity to the parental difficulties, or will they simply be typical of what is observed in the parents of other children with psychiatric difficulties? Second, how, if at all, do these difficulties play a direct role in the development of the child's GID? A rather simple hypothesis might be that the degree of parental dysfunction and marital discord is associated with tolerance of cross-gender behavior, perhaps because the parents are not functioning optimally and thus are less sensitive about developments in the child. If large enough samples could be generated, causal-modeling techniques could be used to test different hypothesized pathways leading to the development of GID in the child.

Treatment

■ Ethical Issues

Any contemporary child clinician responsible for the therapeutic care of children and adolescents with GID will quickly be introduced to complex social and ethical issues pertaining to the politics of sex and gender in postmodern Western culture and will have to think them through carefully. Is GID really a disorder or is it just a normal variant of gendered behavior? Is marked cross-gender behavior inherently harmful or is it simply harmful because of social factors? If a teenager requests immediate cross-sex hormonal and surgical intervention as a therapeutic treatment for gender dysphoria, should the clinician comply? If parents request treatment for their child with GID to divert the probability of a later homosexual sexual orientation, what is the appropriate clinical response? All these questions force the clinician to think long and hard about theoretical and treatment issues.

Perhaps the most acute ethical issue concerns the relation between GID and a later homosexual sexual orientation. As noted below, follow-up studies of boys with GID, who were largely untreated, indicate that homosexuality is the most common long-term psychosexual outcome. Some parents of children with GID request treatment, in part, with an eye toward preventing subsequent homosexuality in their child, whether this is because of personal values, concerns about stigmatization, or other reasons.

In the 1990s, this rationale for treatment was subject to intense scrutiny (Minter 1999; Sedgwick 1991). Some critics, for example, have argued that clinicians, consciously or unconsciously, accept the prevention of homosexuality as a legitimate therapeutic goal (Pleak 1999). Minter (1999) has claimed, as have others (Scholinski 1997), that some adolescents in the United States are being hospitalized against their will because of their homosexual sexual orientation but under the guise of the GID diagnosis. To our knowledge, howev-er, these allegations have not been verified in any systematic manner, and we are personally aware of no such case in which this has occurred (see also Meyer-Bahlburg 1999). Others have asserted, albeit without direct empirical documentation, that treatment of GID results in harm to children who are "homosexual" or "pre-homosexual" (Isay 1997). Lastly, some clinicians have raised questions about differential diagnosis, arguing that there is not always an adequate distinction between children who truly have GID and those who are merely pre-homosexual (Corbett 1996; Richardson 1996, 1999; cf. Zucker 1999a).

The various issues regarding the relation between GID and homosexuality are complex—both clinically and ethically. Three points, albeit brief, can be made. First, until it has been shown that any form of treatment for GID during childhood affects later sexual orientation, the issue is moot. From an ethical standpoint, however, the clinician has an obligation to inform parents about the state of the empirical database. Second, we have argued elsewhere that some critics incorrectly conflate gender identity and sexual orientation, regarding them as isomorphic phenomena (Zucker 1999b), as do some parents. Psychoeducational work with parents can review the various explanatory models regarding the statistical linkage between gender identity and sexual orientation (Bailey and Zucker 1995; Bem 1996), but also clarify their distinctness as psychological constructs. Third, many contemporary clinicians emphasize that the primary goal of treatment of children with GID is to resolve the conflicts that are associated with the disorder per se, regardless of the child's eventual sexual orientation. Most clinicians who have worked with children and adolescents with GID believe that these youngsters experience a great deal of suffering—many of them are preoccupied with gender identity issues, they experience increased social ostracism and alienation as they get older, and they show evidence of other behavioral and psychiatric difficulties. Most clinicians, therefore, take the position that therapeutics designed to reduce the gender dysphoria, to decrease the degree of social ostracism, and to reduce the degree of psychiatric comorbidity constitute legitimate goals of intervention. How, then, might one go about reaching these therapeutic goals?

■ Developmental Considerations

One aspect of the clinical literature suggests that there are important developmental considerations to bear in mind. For example, there is some evidence to suggest that GID is less responsive to psychosocial inter-ventions during adolescence, and certainly by young adulthood, than it is during childhood. Therefore, the lessening of malleability and plasticity over time in gender identity differentiation is an important clinical consideration.

■ Treatment of Children

For children with GID, clinical experience suggests that psychosocial treatments can be relatively effective in reducing the gender dysphoria. Therapeutic approaches have included the most commonly used interventions for children in general, including be-havior therapy, psychodynamic therapy, parent coun-seling, and group therapy (for detailed reviews, see Zucker 1985, 1990, 2001). In considering these various therapeutic approaches, there is one important, sober-ing fact to contemplate: apart from a series of intra-subject behavior therapy case reports from the 1970s, one will find not a single randomized, controlled treat-ment trial in the literature (Zucker 2001). Therefore, the treating clinician must rely largely on the clinical wisdom that has accumulated in the case report litera-ture and the conceptual underpinnings that inform the various approaches to intervention.

Treatment for children with GID often proceeds on two fronts: 1) individual therapy with the child, in which efforts are made to understand the factors that seem to fuel the fantasy of wanting to become a mem-ber of the opposite sex and then to resolve them; 2) parent counseling, in which efforts are made to help the child, in the naturalistic environment, to feel more comfortable about being a boy or a girl. Treat-ment can address several issues: for youngsters who are quite confused about their gender identity, one can fo-cus on the mastery of basic cognitive concepts of gen-der, including correct identification of the self as a boy or a girl; encouragement in the development of same-sex friendships, in which areas of mutual interest can be identified; and exploration of factors within the family that might be contributing to the gender iden-tity conflict.

With parents, treatment issues include the following: limit setting of cross-gender behavior and encourage-ment of gender-neutral or sex-typical activities; factors within the family matrix that may be contributing to the child's gender identity conflict; and parent factors, in-cluding psychiatric impairment, that may be compromis-ing functioning in the parental role in general.

Here we focus on some technical aspects of limit setting that are often misunderstood in the clinical lit-erature and that therefore require further explication. A common error committed by some clinicians is to simply recommend to parents that they impose limits on their child's cross-gender behavior without atten-tion to context. This kind of authoritarian approach is likely to fail, just as it will with regard to any behavior, because it does not take into account systemic factors, both in the parents and in the child, that fuel the "symptom." At the very least, a psychoeducational ap-proach is required, but in many cases limit setting needs to occur within the context of a more global treatment plan.

From a psychoeducational point of view, one ratio-nale for limit setting is that if parents allow their child to continue to engage in cross-gender behavior, the GID is in effect being tolerated, if not reinforced. Therefore, such an approach contributes to the per-petuation of the condition. Another rationale for limit setting is that it is in effect an effort to alter the GID from the "outside in," whereas individual therapy for the child can explore the factors that have contributed to the GID from the "inside out." At the same time that they attempt to set limits, parents also need to help their child with alternative activities that might help consolidate a more comfortable same-gender identifi-cation. Encouragement of same-sex peer group rela-tions can be an important part of such alternatives; for example, some boys with GID develop an avoidance of male playmates because they are anxious about rough-and-tumble play and fantasy aggression. Such anxiety may be fueled by parent factors (e.g., where mothers conflate real aggression with fantasy aggression), but it may also be fueled by temperamental characteristics of the child (Zucker 2000a). Efforts on the part of par-ents to be more sensitive to their child's temperamen-tal characteristics may be quite helpful in planning peer group encounters that are not experienced by the child as threatening and overwhelming. It is not unusual to encounter boys with GID who have a genu-ine longing to interact with other boys, but because of their shy and avoidant temperament they do not know how to integrate themselves with other boys, particu-larly if they experience the contextual situation as threatening. Over time, with the appropriate thera-peutic support, such boys are able to develop same-sex peer group relationships and begin to identify more with other boys as a result.

Another important contextual aspect of limit setting is to explore with parents their initial encouragement or tolerance of the cross-gender behavior. Some parents will tolerate the behavior initially because they have been told, or believe themselves, that the behavior is only a phase that their child will grow out of. Such parents become concerned about their child once they begin to recognize that the behavior is not merely a phase (Zucker 2000b). For other parents, the tolerance or encouragement of cross-gender behavior can be linked to some of the systemic and dynamic factors described earlier. In these more complex clinical situations, one must attend to the underlying issues and work them through. Otherwise, it is quite likely that parents will not be comfortable in shifting their position.

Although many contemporary clinicians have emphasized the important role of working with the parents of children with GID, one can ask if there is any empirical evidence demonstrating that this is effective. Again, systematic information on the question is scanty. The most relevant study (Zucker et al. 1985) found some evidence that parental involvement in therapy was significantly correlated with a greater degree of behavioral change in the child at 1-year follow-up, but this study did not make random assignment to different treatment protocols, so one has to interpret the findings with caution.

■ Treatment of Adolescents

If GID in adolescence is not responsive to psychosocial treatment, should the clinician recommend the same kinds of physical interventions that are used with adults (Harry Benjamin International Gender Dysphoria Association 1998)? Before making such a recommendation, many clinicians will usually encourage adolescents with GID to consider alternatives to this invasive and expensive treatment. One area of inquiry can thus explore the meaning behind the adolescent's desire for sex reassignment and whether there are viable alternative lifestyle adaptations. In this regard, the most common area of exploration pertains to the patient's sexual orientation. Almost all adolescents with GID recall that they always felt uncomfortable growing up as boys or as girls, but that the idea of undergoing a sex change did not occur to them until they became aware of homoerotic attractions. For some of these youngsters, the idea that they might be gay or homosexual is abhorrent. For some such adolescents, psychoeducational work can explore their attitudes and feel-

ings about homosexuality. Group therapy, in which such youngsters have the opportunity to meet gay adolescents, can be a useful adjunct in such cases. In some cases, the gender dysphoria will be resolved and a homosexual adaptation will ensue (Zucker and Bradley 1995). For others, however, a homosexual adaptation is not possible and the gender dysphoria does not abate.

For adolescents in whom the gender dysphoria appears to be chronic, the clinician can consider two main options: 1) management until the adolescent turns 18, when he or she then can be referred to an adult gender identity clinic; or 2) early institution of contrasex hormonal treatment. Regarding the latter option, Gooren and Delemarre-van de Waal (1996) recommended that one option with gender-dysphoric adolescents is to prescribe puberty-blocking luteinizing hormone-release agonists (e.g., depot leuprolide or depot triptorelin) that facilitate more successfully passing as the opposite sex. Thus, for example, in male adolescents, such medication can suppress the development of secondary sex characteristics, such as the growth of facial hair and deepening of the voice, which makes it more difficult to pass in the female social role. Cohen-Kettenis and van Goozen (1997, 1998) reported that early cross-sex hormone treatment for adolescents under age 18 years who are judged to be free of gross psychiatric comorbidity facilitates the complex psychosexual and psychosocial transition to living as a member of the opposite sex and results in a lessening of the gender dysphoria (see also Smith et al. 2001, 2002).

Although such early hormonal treatment is controversial (Cohen-Kettenis 1994, 1995; Meyenburg 1994, 1999), it may well be the treatment of choice once the clinician is confident that other options have been exhausted. One issue that is not yet resolved concerns determining who the best candidates for early hormonal treatments are. Cohen-Kettenis and van Goozen (1997) suggested that the least risky subgroup of adolescents with GID are those who show little evidence of psychiatric impairment (Smith et al. 2001). In our own clinic, a substantial majority of adolescents with GID would not qualify on this basis (Zucker et al. 2002). However, by adolescence, the issue is a tricky one because it is not clear to what extent the psychiatric impairment is a consequence of the chronic gender dysphoria (Newman 1970). A randomized controlled trial would be useful in resolving the matter.

Prognosis

Green (1987) has provided the most detailed information regarding long-term follow-up of boys with GID vis-à-vis gender identity and sexual orientation (for other follow-up reports, see Zucker and Bradley 1995). Green originally assessed 66 extremely feminine boys and 56 control boys at a mean age of 7.1 years (range, 4–12). About two-thirds of the boys in each of these groups were reevaluated at a follow-up mean age of 18.9 years (range, 14–24). A semistructured interview schedule was used to assess sexual orientation in fantasy and behavior. Using Kinsey scale criteria, all 35 reevaluated control boys were heterosexual in fantasy at follow-up. Of the 25 control boys who had experienced overt sexual relations, 1 was classified as bisexual, and the remainder were classified as heterosexual. In contrast, 33 of the 44 feminine boys (75%) were classified as either bisexual or homosexual; of the 30 feminine boys who had experienced overt sexual relations, 24 (80%) were classified as either bisexual or homosexual. Only 1 of the feminine boys, who was sexually attracted to males, was seriously entertaining the notion of sex-reassignment surgery. Thus, homosexuality rather than GID persisting into late adolescence or young adulthood appears to be the most common long-term outcome associated with GID.

Other more recent follow-up studies suggest a higher rate of persistent gender dysphoria. For example, Cohen-Kettenis (2001) reported that of 74 children with GID who had been initially assessed before age 12 (mean age, 9 years; range, 6–12) and had now reached adolescence 17 (23.0%) applied for sex-reassignment surgery. At present, then, it is clear that more information is needed regarding the natural history of GID, particularly when one starts with a prospective sample of children. Although homosexuality without co-occurring gender dysphoria is probably the most common outcome, heterosexuality appears to develop in a minority of youngsters, and persistent gender dysphoria occurs in others. A key research issue will be to attempt to identify predictors of these variations in outcome.

Research Issues

The phenomenology of GID has now been well described. Excellent assessment tools are available for diagnostic workups (Green 1987; Zucker 1992; Zucker and Bradley 1995). Perhaps what needs to be better understood is the concept of gender dysphoria as it applies to young children, because it is this feeling state that is the sine qua non of its expression during adulthood.

The psychobiology of gender identity, gender role, and sexual orientation remains an area of intense study. The exact effects of prenatal sex hormones on postnatal sex-dimorphic behavior will continue to be an area of great importance. More recent studies, particularly in relation to sexual orientation, may yield new insights regarding the role of biological phenomena. These domains of research include molecular genetics (Hamer et al. 1993; Hu et al. 1995; see also Rice et al. 1999), behavior genetics (Mustanski et al. 2002), cognitive abilities and neuropsychological function (reviewed in Zucker and Bradley 1995), neuroanatomical structures (Allen and Gorski 1992; Byne et al. 2001; LeVay 1991; Zhou et al. 1995), dermatoglyphics (e.g., Brown et al. 2002; Hall and Kimura 1994; Williams et al. 2000), and the demographic variables of sibling sex ratio and birth order (Blanchard and Bogaert 1996; Blanchard and Sheridan 1992; Blanchard et al. 1996). Much of this research has focused on sexual orientation per se, so its precise relevance for GID in children is unclear. Elsewhere, Zucker and Bradley (1995) examined the evidence for convergence and divergence in the biological studies of sexual orientation and GID.

Psychosocial research has also yielded important leads. It is now clear how complex early social interaction is with regard to gender (Fagot and Leinbach 1989). Microsocial observations of the behavior of children with GID may help to elucidate the complexities in early interactions with significant others. The assessment of general psychopathology, in both the child and the parents, requires greater attention. Elucidating how general psychopathology serves as a risk factor in this disorder will be of great importance. Finally, the connection between GID and later sexual orientation suggests that a better understanding of the development of eroticism is required in its own right (Bailey and Zucker 1995). To date, the processes underlying erotic development have not been well described (Bem 1996; Green 1987). It is hoped that advances on all of these fronts will sharpen our understanding of psychosexual differentiation and its disorders as we begin the third millennium.

References

Achenbach TM, Edelbrock CS: Behavioral problems and competencies reported by parents of normal and disturbed children aged four through sixteen. Monogr Soc Res Child Dev 46(1):1–82, 1981

Achenbach TM, Howell CT, Quay HC, et al: National survey of problems and competencies among four- to sixteen-year-olds: parents' reports for normative and clinical samples. Monogr Soc Res Child Dev 56(3):1–131, 1991

Allen LS, Gorski RA: Sexual orientation and the size of the anterior commissure in the human brain. Proc Natl Acad Sci USA 89:7199–7202, 1992

American Psychiatric Association: Diagnostic and Statistical Manual of Mental Disorders, 3rd Edition. Washington, DC, American Psychiatric Association, 1980

American Psychiatric Association: Diagnostic and Statistical Manual of Mental Disorders, 3rd Edition, Revised. Washington, DC, American Psychiatric Association, 1987

American Psychiatric Association: Diagnostic and Statistical Manual of Mental Disorders, 4th Edition. Washington, DC, American Psychiatric Association, 1994

American Psychiatric Association: Diagnostic and Statistical Manual of Mental Disorders, 4th Edition, Text Revision. Washington, DC, American Psychiatric Association, 2000

Antill JK: Parents' beliefs and values about sex roles, sex differences, and sexuality: their sources and implications, in Sex and Gender. Edited by Shaver P, Hendrick C. Newbury Park, CA, Sage, 1987, pp 294–328

Arbuckle TE, Wilkins R, Sherman GJ: Birth weight percentiles by gestational age in Canada. Obstet Gynecol 81:39–48, 1993

Bailey JM, Zucker KJ: Childhood sex-typed behavior and sexual orientation: a conceptual analysis and quantitative review. Dev Psychol 31:43–55, 1995

Bailey JM, Bechtold KT, Berenbaum SA: Who are tomboys and why should we study them? Arch Sex Behav 31:333–341, 2002

Bakker A, van Kesteren PJM, Gooren LJG, et al: The prevalence of transsexualism in the Netherlands. Acta Psychiatr Scand 87:237–238, 1993

Begley S: What causes people to be homosexual? Newsweek, September 9, 1991, p 52

Bem DJ: Exotic becomes erotic: a developmental theory of sexual orientation. Psychol Rev 103:320–335, 1996

Benenson JF, Liroff ER, Pascal SJ, et al: Propulsion: a behavioural expression of masculinity. British Journal of Developmental Psychology 15:37–50, 1997

Berenbaum SA: Congenital adrenal hyperplasia: intellectual and psychosexual functioning, in Psychoneuroendocrinology: Brain, Behavior, and Hormonal Interactions. Edited by Holmes CS. New York, Springer-Verlag, 1990, pp 227–260

Birkenfeld-Adams AS: Quality of attachment in young boys with gender identity disorder: a comparison to clinic and nonreferred control boys. Unpublished doctoral dissertation, York University, Downsview, Ontario, 1999

Blanchard R: A structural equation model for age at clinical presentation in nonhomosexual male gender dysphorics. Arch Sex Behav 23:311–320, 1994

Blanchard R, Bogaert AF: Homosexuality in men and number of older brothers. Am J Psychiatry 153:27–31, 1996

Blanchard R, Clemmensen LH: A test of the DSM-III-R's implicit assumption that fetishistic arousal and gender dysphoria are mutually exclusive. J Sex Res 25:426–432, 1988

Blanchard R, Klassen P: H-Y antigen and homosexuality in men. J Theor Biol 185:373–378, 1997

Blanchard R, Sheridan PM: Sibship size, sibling sex ratio, birth order, and parental age in homosexual and nonhomosexual gender dysphorics. J Nerv Ment Dis 180:40–47, 1992

Blanchard R, Clemmensen LH, Steiner BW: Heterosexual and homosexual gender dysphoria. Arch Sex Behav 16:139–152, 1987

Blanchard R, Zucker KJ, Bradley SJ, et al: Birth order and sibling sex ratio in homosexual male adolescents and probably prehomosexual feminine boys. Dev Psychol 31:22–30, 1995

Blanchard R, Zucker KJ, Cohen-Kettenis PT, et al: Birth order and sibling sex ratio in two samples of Dutch gender-dysphoric homosexual males. Arch Sex Behav 25:495–514, 1996

Blanchard R, Zucker KJ, Cavacas A, et al: Fraternal birth order and birth weight in probably prehomosexual feminine boys. Horm Behav 41:321–327, 2002

Bradley SJ, Zucker KJ: Gender identity disorder and psychosexual problems in children and adolescents. Can J Psychiatry 35:477–486, 1990

Bradley SJ, Blanchard R, Coates S, et al: Interim report of the DSM-IV subcommittee for gender identity disorders. Arch Sex Behav 20:333–343, 1991

Brown WM, Finn CJ, Cooke BM, et al: Differences in finger length ratios between self-identified "butch" and "femme" lesbians. Arch Sex Behav 31:123–127, 2002

Byne W, Tobet S, Mattiace L, et al: The interstitial nuclei of the human anterior hypothalamus: an investigation of variation with sex, sexual orientation, and HIV status. Horm Behav 40:86–92, 2001

Campbell DW, Eaton WO: Sex differences in the activity level of infants. Infant and Child Development 8:1–17, 1999

Chivers ML, Bailey JM: Sexual orientation of female-to-male transsexuals: a comparison of homosexual and nonhomosexual types. Arch Sex Behav 29:259–278, 2000

Coates S: Ontogenesis of boyhood gender identity disorder. J Am Acad Psychoanal 18:414–438, 1990

Coates S: Gender identity disorder in boys: the search for a constitutional factor, in A Queer World: The Center for Lesbian and Gay Studies Reader. Edited by Duberman M. New York, New York University Press, 1997, pp 108–133

Coates S, Person ES: Extreme boyhood femininity: isolated behavior or pervasive disorder? J Am Acad Child Psychiatry 24:702–709, 1985

Coates S, Wolfe S: Gender identity disorder in boys: the interface of constitution and early experience. Psychoanalytic Inquiry 15:6–38, 1995

Coates S, Wolfe S: Gender identity disorders of childhood, in Infants and Preschoolers: Development and Syndromes. Edited by Greenspan S, Wieder S, Osofsky J (Handbook of Child and Adolescent Psychiatry, Vol 1; Noshpitz JD, series ed). New York, Wiley, 1997, pp 452–473

Cohen-Kettenis PT: Die Behandlung von Kindern und Jugendlichen mit Geschlechtsidentitätsstörungen an der Universität Utrecht [Clinical management of children and adolescents with gender identity disorders at the University of Utrecht]. Z Sexualforschung 7:231–239, 1994

Cohen-Kettenis PT: Replik auf Bernd Meyenburg's "Kritik der hormonellen Behandlung Judendlicher mit Geschlechtsidentitätsstörungen" [Rejoinder to Bernd Meyenburg's "Criticism of hormone treatment for adolescents with gender identity disorders"] Z Sexualforschung 8:165–167, 1995

Cohen-Kettenis PT: Gender identity disorder in DSM? (letter). J Am Acad Child Adolesc Psychiatry 40:391, 2001

Cohen-Kettenis PT, van Goozen SHM: Sex reassignment of adolescent transsexuals: a follow-up study. J Am Acad Child Adolesc Psychiatry 36:263–271, 1997

Cohen-Kettenis PT, van Goozen SHM: Pubertal delay as an aid in diagnosis and treatment of a transsexual adolescent. Eur Child Adolesc Psychiatry 7:246–248, 1998

Cohen-Kettenis PT, Owen A, Kaijser VG, et al: Demographic characteristics, social competence, and behavior problems in children with gender identity disorder: a cross-national, cross-clinic comparative analysis. J Abnorm Child Psychol 31:41–53, 2003

Collaer ML, Hines M: Human behavioral sex differences: a role for gonadal hormones during early development? Psychol Bull 118:55–107, 1995

Corbett K: Homosexual boyhood: notes on girlyboys. Gender and Psychoanalysis 1:429–461, 1996

de Zegher F, Francois I, Boehmer ALM, et al: Androgens and fetal growth. Horm Res 50:243–244, 1998

Diamond M: Homosexuality and bisexuality in different populations. Arch Sex Behav 22:291–310, 1993

DiPietro JA: Rough-and-tumble play: a function of gender. Dev Psychol 17:50–58, 1981

Dittmann RW, Kappes ME, Kappes MH: Sexual behavior in adolescent and adult females with congenital adrenal hyperplasia. Psychoneuroendocrinology 17:153–170, 1992

Eaton WO, Enns LR: Sex differences in human motor activity level. Psychol Bull 100:19–28, 1986

Ehrhardt AA, Baker SW: Fetal androgens, human central nervous system differentiation, and behavior sex differences, in Sex Differences in Human Behavior. Edited by Friedman RC, Richart RM, Vande Wiele RL. New York, Wiley, 1974, pp 33–51

Eme RF: Sex differences in childhood psychopathology. Psychol Bull 86:574–595, 1979

Fagot BI: Consequences of moderate cross-gender behavior in preschool children. Child Dev 48:902–907, 1977

Fagot BI: Beyond the reinforcement principle: another step toward understanding sex-role development. Dev Psychol 21:1097–1104, 1985

Fagot BI, Leinbach MD: The young child's gender schema: environmental input, internal organization. Child Dev 60:663–672, 1989

Fridell SR, Zucker KJ, Bradley SJ, et al: Physical attractiveness of girls with gender identity disorder. Arch Sex Behav 25:17–31, 1996

Fridell SR: Sex-typed play behavior and peer relationships in boys with gender identity disorder. Unpublished doctoral dissertation, Ontario Institute for Studies in Education of the University of Toronto, Toronto, Ontario, 2001

Friedman RC: Male Homosexuality: A Contemporary Psychoanalytic Perspective. New Haven, CT, Yale University Press, 1988

Friedman RC, Downey JI: Sexual Orientation and Psychoanalysis: Sexual Science and Clinical Practice. New York, Columbia University Press, 2002

Friedman RC, Stern LO: Juvenile aggressivity and sissiness in homosexual and heterosexual males. J Am Acad Psychoanal 8:427–440, 1980

Gooren L, Delemarre-van de Waal H: The feasibility of endocrine interventions in juvenile transsexuals. J Psychol Human Sex 8(4):69–84, 1996

Green R: Sexual Identity Conflict in Children and Adults. New York, Basic Books, 1974

Green R: One hundred ten feminine and masculine boys: behavioral contrasts and demographic similarities. Arch Sex Behav 5:425–446, 1976

Green R: Patterns of sexual identity development in childhood: relationship to subsequent sexual partner preference, in Homosexual Behavior: A Modern Reappraisal. Edited by Marmor J. New York, Basic Books, 1980, pp 255–266

Green R: The "Sissy Boy Syndrome" and the Development of Homosexuality. New Haven, CT, Yale University Press, 1987

Green R, Young R: Hand preference, sexual preference, and transsexualism. Arch Sex Behav 30:565–574, 2001

Green R, Williams K, Goodman M: Ninety-nine "tomboys" and "non-tomboys": behavioral contrasts and demographic similarities. Arch Sex Behav 11:247–266, 1982

Green R, Williams K, Goodman M: Masculine or feminine gender identity in boys: developmental differences between two diverse family groups. Sex Roles 12:1155–1162, 1985

Greenson RR: Dis-identifying from mother. Int J Psychoanal 49:370–374, 1968

Hall JA, Kimura D: Dermatoglyphic asymmetry and sexual orientation in men. Behav Neurosci 108:1203–1206, 1994

Hamer DH, Hu S, Magnuson VL, et al: A linkage between DNA markers on the X chromosome and male sexual orientation. Science 261:321–327, 1993

Harry Benjamin International Gender Dysphoria Association: The Standards of Care for Gender Identity Disorders, 5th Version. Düsseldorf, Symposon Publishing, 1998

Herman-Jeglinska A, Dulko S, Grabowska AM: Transsexuality and adextrality: do they share a common origin?, in Sexual Orientation: Toward Biological Understanding. Edited by Ellis L, Ebertz L. Westport, CT, Praeger, 1997, pp 163–180

Hu S, Pattatucci AML, Patterson C, et al: Linkage between sexual orientation and chromosome Xq28 in males but not in females. Nat Genet 11:248–256, 1995

Isay RA: Being Homosexual: Gay Men and Their Development. New York, Farrar Straus Giroux, 1989

Isay RA: Remove gender identity disorder in DSM. Psychiatr News 32(9):13, 1997

Kinsey AC, Pomeroy WB, Martin CE: Sexual Behavior in the Human Male. Philadelphia, PA, WB Saunders, 1948

Kline TJ: Alain Berliner's *Ma Vie en Rose* (1997): crossing dress, crossing boundaries. Gender and Psychoanalysis 3:435–449, 1998

Lalumière ML, Blanchard R, Zucker KJ: Sexual orientation and handedness in men and women: a meta-analysis. Psychol Bull 126:575–592, 2000

Langlois JH, Downs AC: Mothers, fathers, and peers as socialization agents of sex-typed play behaviors in young children. Child Dev 51:1237–1247, 1980

Laumann EO, Gagnon JH, Michael RT, et al: The Social Organization of Sexuality: Sexual Practices in the United States. Chicago, IL, University of Chicago Press, 1994

LeVay S: A difference in hypothalamic structure between heterosexual and homosexual men. Science 253:1034–1037, 1991

Lytton H, Romney DM: Parents' differential socialization of boys and girls: a meta-analysis. Psychol Bull 109:267–296, 1991

Maccoby EE: The Two Sexes: Growing Up Apart, Coming Together. Cambridge, MA, Harvard University Press, 1998

Maccoby EE, Jacklin CN: The Psychology of Sex Differences. Stanford, CA, Stanford University Press, 1974

Maccoby EE, Jacklin CN: Sex differences in aggression: a rejoinder and reprise. Child Dev 51:964–980, 1980

Maccoby EE, Jacklin CN: Gender segregation in childhood. Adv Child Dev Behav 20:239–287, 1987

Marantz S, Coates S: Mothers of boys with gender identity disorder: a comparison with matched controls. J Am Acad Child Adolesc Psychiatry 30:310–315, 1991

Martin CL: Attitudes and expectations about children with nontraditional and traditional gender roles. Sex Roles 22:151–165, 1990

McDermid SA, Zucker KJ, Bradley SJ, et al: Effects of physical appearance on masculine trait ratings of boys and girls with gender identity disorder. Arch Sex Behav 27:253–267, 1998

Meyenburg B: Kritik der hormonellen Behandlung Judendlicher mit Geschlechtsidentitätsstörungen [Criticisms of hormone treatment for adolescents with gender identity disorders]. Z Sexualforschung 7:343–349, 1994

Meyenburg B: Gender identity disorder in adolescence: outcomes of psychotherapy. Adolescence 34:305–313, 1999

Meyer-Bahlburg HFL: Psychoendocrine research on sexual orientation: current status and future options. Prog Brain Res 61:375–398, 1984

Meyer-Bahlburg HFL: Gender identity disorder of childhood: introduction. J Am Acad Child Psychiatry 24:681–683, 1985

Meyer-Bahlburg HFL: Intersexuality and the diagnosis of gender identity disorder. Arch Sex Behav 23:21–40, 1994

Meyer-Bahlburg HFL: Review of *The Last Time I Wore A Dress: A Memoir*. Arch Sex Behav 28:431–434, 1999

Meyer-Bahlburg HFL, Gruen RS, New MI, et al: Gender change from female to male in classical congenital adrenal hyperplasia. Horm Behav 30:319–332, 1996

Minter S: Diagnosis and treatment of gender identity disorder in children, in Sissies and Tomboys: Gender Nonconformity and Homosexual Childhood. Edited by Rottnek M. New York, New York University Press, 1999, pp 9–33

Mitchell JN: Maternal influences on gender identity disorder in boys: searching for specificity. Unpublished doctor dissertation, York University, Downsview, Ontario, 1991

Money J, Hampson JG, Hampson JL: Imprinting and the establishment of gender role. Archives of Neurology and Psychiatry 77:333–336, 1957

Money J, Schwartz M, Lewis VG: Adult erotosexual status and fetal hormonal masculinization and demasculinization: 46,XX congenital virilizing adrenal hyperplasia and 46,XY androgen-insensitivity syndrome compared. Psychoneuroendocrinology 9:405–414, 1984

Mulaikal RM, Migeon CJ, Rock JA: Fertility rates in female patients with congenital adrenal hyperplasia due to 21-hydroxylase deficiency. N Engl J Med 316:178–182, 1987

Mustanski BS, Chivers ML, Bailey JM: A critical review of recent biological research on human sexual orientation. Annu Rev Sex Res 13:89–140, 2002

Newman LE: Transsexualism in adolescence: problems in evaluation and treatment. Arch Gen Psychiatry 23:112–121, 1970

Pleak RR: Ethical issues in diagnosing and treating gender-dysphoric children and adolescents, in Sissies and Tomboys: Gender Nonconformity and Homosexual Childhood. Edited by Rottnek M. New York, New York University Press, 1999, pp 34–51

Pleak RR, Meyer-Bahlburg HFL, O'Brien JD, et al: Cross-gender behavior and psychopathology in boy psychiatric outpatients. J Am Acad Child Adolesc Psychiatry 28:385–393, 1989

Qazi QH, Thompson MW: Birthweight in congenital virilizing adrenal hyperplasia. Arch Dis Child 46:350–352, 1971

Rekers GA, Crandall BF, Rosen AC, et al: Genetic and physical studies of male children with psychological gender disturbances. Psychol Med 9:373–375, 1979

Rice G, Anderson C, Risch N, et al: Male homosexuality: absenceof linkage to microsatellite markers at Xq28. Science 284:665–667, 1999

Richardson J: Setting limits on gender health. Harv Rev Psychiatry 4:49–53, 1996

Richardson J: Response: finding the disorder in gender identity disorder. Harv Rev Psychiatry 7:43–50, 1999

Roberts CW, Green R, Williams K, et al: Boyhood gender identity development: a statistical contrast of two family groups. Dev Psychol 23:544–557, 1987

Rogers SM, Turner CF: Male–male sexual contact in the U.S.A.: findings from five sample surveys, 1970–1990. J Sex Res 28:491–519, 1991

Ruble DN, Martin CL: Gender development, in Social, Emotional, and Personality Development. Edited by Eisenberg N (Handbook of Child Psychology, 5th Edition, Vol 3; Damon W, series ed). New York, Wiley, 1998, pp 933–1016

Scholinski D: The Last Time I Wore A Dress: A Memoir. New York, Riverhead Books, 1997

Sedgwick EK: How to bring your kids up gay. Social Text 9:18–27, 1991

Sizonenko PC: Endocrinology in preadolescents and adolescents, I: hormonal changes during normal puberty. Am J Dis Child 132:704–712, 1980

Smith YLS, van Goozen SHM, Cohen-Kettenis PT: Adolescents with gender identity disorder who were accepted or rejected for sex reassignment surgery: a prospective follow-up study. J Am Acad Child Adolesc Psychiatry 40:472–481, 2001

Smith YLS, Cohen L, Cohen-Kettenis PT: Postoperative psychological functioning of adolescent transsexuals: a Rorschach study. Arch Sex Behav 31:255–261, 2002

Spira A, Bajos N, and the ACSF Group: Sexual Behaviour and AIDS. Aldershot, England, Avebury, 1994

Stoller RJ: Male childhood transsexualism. J Am Acad Child Psychiatry 7:193–209, 1968a

Stoller RJ: Sex and Gender, Vol 1: The Development of Masculinity and Femininity. New York, Science House, 1968b

Stoller RJ: Sex and Gender, Vol 2: The Transsexual Experiment. London, Hogarth Press, 1975

Stoller RJ: Fathers of transsexual children. J Am Psychoanal Assoc 27:837–866, 1979

Stoller RJ: Presentations of Gender. New Haven, CT, Yale University Press, 1985

Wellings K, Field J, Johnson AM, et al: Sexual Behaviour in Britain: The National Survey of Sexual Attitudes and Lifestyles. London, Penguin, 1994

Williams TJ, Pepitone ME, Christensen SE, et al: Finger length patterns indicate an influence of fetal androgens on human sexual orientation. Nature 404:455–456, 2000

Wolfe S: Psychopathology and psychodynamics of parents of boys with a gender identity disorder of childhood. Unpublished doctoral dissertation, City University of New York, 1990

Zhou J, Hofman MA, Gooren LJG, et al: A sex difference in the human brain and its relation to transsexuality. Nature 378:68–70, 1995

Zucker KJ: Childhood gender disturbance: diagnostic issues. J Am Acad Child Psychiatry 21:274–280, 1982

Zucker KJ: Cross-gender-identified children, in Gender Dysphoria: Development, Research, Management. Edited by Steiner BW. New York, Plenum, 1985, pp 75–174

Zucker KJ: Treatment of gender identity disorders in children, in Clinical Management of Gender Identity Disorders in Children and Adults. Edited by Blanchard R, Steiner BW. Washington, DC, American Psychiatric Press, 1990, pp 25–47

Zucker KJ: Gender identity disorder, in Child Psychopathology: Diagnostic Criteria and Clinical Assessment. Edited by Hooper SR, Hynd GW, Mattison RE. Hillsdale, NJ, Lawrence Erlbaum, 1992, pp 305–342

Zucker KJ: Commentary on Richardson's (1996) "Setting Limits on Gender Health." Harv Rev Psychiatry 7:37–42, 1999a

Zucker KJ: Gender identity disorder in the DSM-IV (letter). J Sex Marital Ther 25:5–9, 1999b

Zucker KJ: Intersexuality and gender identity differentiation. Annu Rev Sex Res 10:1–69, 1999c

Zucker KJ: Commentary on Walters and Whitehead's (1997) "Anorexia Nervosa in a Young Boy with Gender Identity Disorder of Childhood: A Case Report." Clinical Child Psychology and Psychiatry 5:232–238, 2000a

Zucker KJ: Gender identity disorder, in Handbook of Developmental Psychopathology, 2nd Edition. Edited by Sameroff AJ, Lewis M, Miller SM. New York, Kluwer Academic/Plenum, 2000b, pp 671–686

Zucker KJ: Gender identity disorder in children and adolescents, in Treatments of Psychiatric Disorders, 3rd Edition, Vol 2. Edited by Gabbard GO. Washington, DC, American Psychiatric Press, 2001, pp 2069–2094

Zucker KJ: Intersexuality and gender identity differentiation. J Pediatr Adolesc Gynecol 15:3–13, 2002

Zucker KJ, Blanchard R: Transvestic fetishism: psychopathology and theory, in Sexual Deviance: Theory, Assessment, and Treatment. Edited by Laws DR, O'Donohue W. New York, Guilford, 1997, pp 253–279

Zucker KJ, Bradley SJ: Gender Identity Disorder and Psychosexual Problems in Children and Adolescents. New York, Guilford, 1995

Zucker KJ, Bradley SJ: Gender identity disorder, in Handbook of Infant Mental Health, 2nd Edition. Edited by Zeanah CH. New York, Guilford, 2000, pp 412–424

Zucker KJ, Green R: Psychosexual disorders in children and adolescents. J Child Psychol Psychiatry 33:107–151, 1992

Zucker KJ, Finegan JK, Doering RW, et al: Two subgroups of gender-problem children. Arch Sex Behav 13:27–39, 1984

Zucker KJ, Bradley SJ, Doering RW, et al: Sex-typed behavior in cross-gender-identified children: stability and change at a one-year follow-up. J Am Acad Child Psychiatry 24:710–719, 1985

Zucker KJ, Lozinski JA, Bradley SJ, et al: Sex-typed responses in the Rorschach protocols of children with gender identity disorder. J Pers Assess 58:295–310, 1992

Zucker KJ, Bradley SJ, Ipp M: Delayed naming of a newborn boy: relationship to the mother's wish for a girl and subsequent cross-gender identity in the child by the age of two. J Psychol Human Sex 6(1):57–68, 1993a

Zucker KJ, Bradley SJ, Sullivan CB, et al: A gender identity interview for children. J Pers Assess 61:443–456, 1993b

Zucker KJ, Wild J, Bradley SJ, et al: Physical attractiveness in boys with gender identity disorder. Arch Sex Behav 22:23–34, 1993c

Zucker KJ, Green R, Garofano C, et al: Prenatal gender preference of mothers of feminine and masculine boys: relation to sibling sex composition and birth order. J Abnorm Child Psychol 22:1–13, 1994

Zucker KJ, Wilson DNS, Kurita JA, et al: Children's appraisals of sex-typed behavior in their peers. Sex Roles 33:703–725, 1995

Zucker KJ, Bradley SJ, Lowry Sullivan CB: Traits of separation anxiety in boys with gender identity disorder. J Am Acad Child Adolesc Psychiatry 35:791–798, 1996a

Zucker KJ, Bradley SJ, Oliver G, et al: Psychosexual development of women with congenital adrenal hyperplasia. Horm Behav 30:300–318, 1996b

Zucker KJ, Bradley SJ, Sanikhani M: Sex differences in referral rates of children with gender identity disorder: some hypotheses. J Abnorm Child Psychol 25:217–227, 1997a

Zucker KJ, Green R, Coates S, et al: Sibling sex ratio of boys with gender identity disorder. J Child Psychol Psychiatry 38:543–551, 1997b

Zucker KJ, Green R, Bradley SJ, et al: Gender identity disorder of childhood: diagnostic issues, in DSM-IV Sourcebook, Vol 4. Edited by Widiger TA, Frances AJ, Pincus HA, et al. Washington, DC, American Psychiatric Association, 1998, pp 503–512

Zucker KJ, Bradley SJ, Kuksis M, et al: Gender constancy judgments in children with gender identity disorder: evidence for a developmental lag. Arch Sex Behav 28:475–502, 1999

Zucker KJ, Beaulieu N, Bradley SJ, et al: Handedness in boys with gender identity disorder. J Child Psychol Psychiatry 42:767–776, 2001

Zucker KJ, Owen A, Bradley SJ, et al: Gender-dysphoric children and adolescents: a comparative analysis of demographic characteristics and behavioral problems. Clinical Child Psychology and Psychiatry 7:398–411, 2002

Physical Abuse of Children

Paramjit T. Joshi, M.D.

Peter T. Daniolos, M.D.

Jay A. Salpekar, M.D.

Definitions

Child abuse continues to be a serious pediatric and social problem all over the world. In the Child Abuse Prevention, Adoption and Family Services Act of 1988, physical abuse was defined as "the physical injury of a child under 18 years of age by a person who is responsible for the child's welfare, under circumstances which indicate that the child's health or welfare is harmed or threatened" (Kaplan 1996, p. 1034). For the National Incidence Study, physical abuse was defined as being present when a child younger than age 18 experiences nonaccidental injury (harm standard) or risk of injury (endangerment standard) as a result of having been hit with a hand or other object or having been kicked, shaken, thrown, burned, stabbed, or choked by a parent or parent substitute (Sedlak and Broadhurst 1996).

Child neglect is differentiated from child abuse and refers to the failure of the responsible caretaking adults to provide adequate physical care and supervision. This chapter focuses on physical abuse.

Epidemiology

The work of Kempe (1962), who first described the battered child syndrome, led to the recognition of child abuse as a major pediatric, psychiatric, and social problem. By 1965 child protective services were established throughout the United States, and all 50 states passed laws requiring mandatory medical reporting of child abuse and neglect.

A report issued by the National Child Abuse and Neglect Data System of the U.S. Department of Health and Human Services in 2001 noted 826,000 victims of maltreatment nationwide, declining from over 900,000 children in 1998. In a trend starting in 1993, the number of victimized children decreased by 19.2% from a record of 1,018,692 in 1993. Parents continue to remain the main perpetrators. The most common maltreatment was a child victimized by a female parent. Almost 60% of all victims experienced neglect, whereas 21.3% experienced physical abuse and 11.3% were sexually abused. The number of child fatalities caused by maltreatment remained unchanged at about 1,100. Fisher and colleagues (1997) studied a community probability sample of 665 youngsters, ages 9–17 years, interviewing the young person and a parent. The authors found that an alarming 25.9% had experienced abuse as defined by behaviors such as severe punishment or infliction of physical injury.

Younger children seem to be at greatest risk for fatal maltreatment. In a 1998 report by the U.S. Department of Health and Human Services (cited by Kaplan et al. 1999) it was documented that more than 75% of maltreatment fatalities in 1996 involved children younger than age 3. Homicides occurring during the first week of life are almost exclusively perpetrated by mothers. Mothers and fathers were equally likely to fatally injure their children ages 1 week to 13 years. However, fathers committed 63% of parent-perpetrated homicides among 13- to 15-year-olds and were responsible for 80% of those occurring in 16- to 19-year-olds (Kunz and Bahr 1996). Powers and colleagues (1990) noted that the gender distributions varied with age, with a greater representation of females as victims of adolescent physical abuse.

Etiology

The prevailing model of the etiology of abuse is an ecological one (Belsky 1980). Most experts believe that child abuse occurs as a result of the combined outcome of various forces that may occur both in the parents and in the child in conjunction with the environment. Parental mental illness and substance abuse and child vulnerabilities such as low birth weight and difficult temperament are all risk factors. Furthermore, toddlers and adolescents appear to be more vulnerable. Other etiological factors include lack of social supports, poverty, single parenthood, minority ethnicity, lack of acculturation, the presence of four or more children in a family, young parental age, stressful events, and exposure to family violence.

Over the years, several investigators have examined a number of etiological risk factors. Risk factors that may predict recurrence of abuse include young age of the victim; number of previous referrals to child protective services; and caretaker characteristics such as emotional impairment, substance abuse, lack of social support, presence of domestic violence, and history of childhood abuse (English et al. 1999). Furthermore, Cicchetti and Toth (1995) believe that the probability of abuse could be increased by risk factors in the child such as prematurity, mental retardation, and physical handicaps. Martin and Elmer (1992) found a history of low birth weight in 19% of an abused cohort compared with a 9.2% general prevalence at the time. These children may be more vulnerable to abuse due to excessive crying or behavior that is difficult to control, with the abuse in turn leading to a greater likelihood of the child becoming aggressive. On the other hand, the probability of maltreatment may be reduced by protective factors such as parental support systems.

Children with cognitive or neuropsychiatric deficits are even more vulnerable to maltreatment resulting in aggressive behaviors in the child, partly because of impaired judgment compounded by a decreased ability to tolerate feelings and to put them into words rather than actions (Lewis 1992). Child maltreatment has been shown to be strongly correlated with poverty, less parental education, underemployment, poor housing, reliance on welfare, and single parenting.

Child abuse tends to occur in multiproblem families—that is, families in which domestic violence, social isolation, parental mental illness, and parental substance abuse occur (Thompson 1994).

Green (1980) examined the role of low socioeconomic status in increasing the risk for physical abuse and found that environmental stress is increased by family disorganization, unemployment, inadequate income, poor housing, and large numbers of children. When traditional use of physical punishment and authoritarian forms of child rearing are common, such practices may be transmitted from one generation to the next. Green believed that environmental stress, compounded by parental personality traits and characteristics of the child, created a climate leading to abuse. Egeland et al. (1993) found that maltreated mothers who were able to break the intergenerational cycle of abuse reported receiving emotional support from a foster parent or relative when they were children, which in turn enhanced their self-worth and ability to be effective parents. These positive experiences challenged their negative caregiving models and helped them work through their own experiences of being abused.

It is widely believed that abuse during childhood can lead to victims abusing their own offspring (Kaufman and Zigler 1987; Oliver 1993; Straus et al. 1980). However, Ertem et al. (2000) comprehensively reviewed empirical studies published in English between 1965 and 2000 and found only 10 controlled studies of this phenomenon over two generations. In only 4 studies were the relative risks of maltreatment in the children of parents who had been abused during childhood found to be significantly increased. Furthermore, only one study that met all eight methodological standards (derived from the randomized controlled trial) provided evidence for the intergenerational continuity of child physical abuse. The authors also noted limitations in the generalizability of these studies, with the latest studies involving populations from the 1980s.

The one study identified by Ertem and colleagues that met the methodological standards (Egeland et al. 1988) can be generalized only to primiparous mothers of low socioeconomic status and their children up to age 24 months. Ertem et al. (2000) note that the researchers found that "primiparous mothers of low socioeconomic status who reported clearly defined severe physical abuse during childhood were 12.6 times more likely to abuse their children than mothers who had emotionally supportive parents." This study viewed abuse within an ecological model, recognizing the significance of the role played by the characteristics of the mother and the child in the genesis of abuse (i.e., their relationship and environment). The researchers used attachment theory as a theoretical frame, examining whether the individual's interpersonal relationships could explain the occurrence of child abuse. Egeland et al. (1988) also examined the important question of how intergenerational continuity of abuse is interrupted. By including women who "broke the cycle of abuse," the research emphasizes that continuity is not the rule. Many abused children grow up to be competent, nonabusive parents, a theory supported by other investigators, including Herman (1992).

Two categories of trauma have been described by Terr (1991). Type I trauma produces typical symptoms of posttraumatic stress disorder (PTSD) after a one-time, sudden traumatic event. Type II trauma is the result of long-term repeated exposure to trauma, similar to what many physically abused youths experience. Type II trauma often results in an array of coping mechanisms such as denial and dissociation rather than symptoms characteristic of PTSD. Terr also noted conduct disorder, attention-deficit/hyperactivity disorder (ADHD), depression, and dissociative disorders to be common conditions in children with histories of type II trauma. Pelcovitz et al. (1994) likewise found higher prevalences of depression, conduct disorders, and oppositional defiant disorder (ODD) in their sample of physically abused youths.

Profiles of Perpetrators

Earlier descriptions of parents who were abusive toward their children were based on clinical observations of a relatively small number of parents. However, the personality traits or psychological disorders that were attributed to these abusive parents were also found in parents who were not abusive toward their children. As was pointed out by Ertem and colleagues (2000), the lack of control groups in these studies contributed to faulty generalizations and conclusions being made about parents who were abusive toward their children.

Green (1997) described characteristics of abusive parents, including a background of deprivation and

abuse and a high prevalence of psychopathology and psychiatric impairment (especially antisocial personality disorder, alcoholism, and major depression). Abusive fathers were often characterized by extreme jealousy of their spouse's attention toward the targeted child, stemming from their own maternal deprivation in childhood and unresolved sibling rivalry.

Furthermore, Smith et al. (1973) reported that half of their sample of abusive mothers were of borderline or subaverage intelligence. Several controlled studies of abusive mothers showed significantly lower self-esteem compared with the control mothers (Anderson and Lauderdale 1982; Evans 1980; Rosen and Stein 1980). Parental social isolation and poverty were also noted to exert a cumulative negative effect on parenting ability, making physical abuse of children more likely. It is postulated that social isolation reduces exposure of the parent to other parents who could provide a normal and corrective parenting model.

Clinical Presentation of Physical Child Abuse

One must consider the possibility of physical abuse in every child who presents with an injury. The clinician should perform a careful history and physical examination in every injured child, including radiological and laboratory studies.

Indicators suggesting possible abuse include lack of a reasonable explanation for the injury; contradictory, changing, or vague history of the injury; observation of an inappropriate history for the injury; an excessive or inadequate level of concern; and delay in seeking medical attention (Cheung 1999).

In addition, a parent blaming an injury on a sibling or claiming that it was self-inflicted, or a parent with unrealistic and premature expectations of the child could also be suggestive of abuse (Green 1997).

Although there is no clinical finding or diagnostic procedure that can confirm child abuse with absolute certainty, the behavioral observations and findings on clinical examination of the child described below should suggest an inflicted injury.

■ Behavioral Observations

The clinician needs to be sensitive to and aware of certain frequently observed behaviors that have been associated with abuse in children. Some of these characteristics were succinctly described by DeAngelis (1992):

- A child who is unusually fearful and docile, distrustful, and/or guarded
- A child with no expectation of being comforted
- A child who is wary of physical contact
- A child who is on the alert for danger
- A child who attempts to meet parents' needs by role reversal
- A child who is afraid to go home

■ Physical Findings in Children and Adolescents

The physician should closely examine an injured child for suspicious physical findings suggesting abuse (Cheung 1999):

- Cutaneous injuries, such as bruises or lacerations in the shape of an object or multiple bruises in areas that are difficult to injure in play (e.g., upper arms, medial thighs)
- Stocking-glove distribution burns suggesting immersion, burns on the perineum, burns in recognizable shapes (e.g., an iron), cigarette burns, and especially multiple burns in various stages of healing
- Head injuries, including complex skull fractures with intracranial hemorrhage, retinal hemorrhage, bilateral ocular injury, dental injury, or traumatic hair loss with scalp hematomas
- Ear injuries, including twisting injuries of the lobe and ruptured tympanic membranes
- Skeletal injuries, including posterior rib fractures (especially when there are multiple fractures), multiple fractures in different stages of healing, metaphyseal fractures in long bones of infants, spiral fractures, and femur fractures in a nonambulatory child; also, radiological signs of subperiosteal hemorrhage, epiphyseal separation, periosteal shearing, and periosteal calcification
- Abdominal injuries, including hepatic hematoma, laceration, or hemorrhage and duodenal hematoma or perforation
- Anogenital injuries such as lacerations, scarring or bruising of genitalia, and anal dilatation or scarring
- Chest injuries, including pulmonary contusion, pneumothorax, pleural effusion, and tracheobronchial injuries

■ Physical Findings in Infants and Toddlers

Special attention needs to be paid when examining an infant or toddler for physical abuse. In 1972, pediatric radiologist John Caffey coined the term *whiplash shaken baby syndrome* to describe a constellation of clinical findings in infants and toddlers, including retinal hemorrhages, subdural or subarachnoid hemorrhages, and little or no evidence of external cranial trauma. It was postulated that whiplash forces caused subdural hematomas by tearing cortical bridging veins. Shaking the infant usually results from the adult's frustration with the baby's crying. Caretakers often have unrealistic expectations for their infant, with a role reversal whereby the adult expects the child to meet the adult's needs.

Serious injuries in infants are rarely accidental unless there is a clear explanation. Head injuries are the leading cause of traumatic childhood death and of child abuse fatalities. Sublethal shaking may result in poor feeding, vomiting, lethargy, and irritability. A caretaker who violently shakes an infant to the point of unconsciousness may put the infant to bed, hoping that he or she will recover, thereby losing any opportunity for early therapeutic intervention. Permanent brain injury may then result. Bruce (1992) noted that of shaken babies presenting with an alteration of consciousness, one-third of victims will have a good outcome, one-third will be physically or mentally disabled, and one-third will die of their injuries.

■ Evaluation Guidelines

A good evaluation starts with obtaining a thorough history and completing a comprehensive physical examination of the child. Documentation of all injuries is crucial, with photographic documentation of cutaneous findings. Radiologic documentation of skeletal injuries may be the best and first source of evidence of alleged abuse. High-definition radiographs read by a pediatric radiologist are optimal. A skeletal survey to identify recent and old fractures is indicated in a child less than age 2 years with suspicious bruising or fractures. Such surveys are not as helpful in children over age 5 years (American Academy of Pediatrics 2001). Bone scans should be performed to identify subtle fractures in children less than age 5 years. A magnetic resonance imaging (MRI) study can better identify epiphyseal separations if they are suspected from the plain films. Ultrasound may also be indicated to identify epiphyseal injury (Toomey and Bernstein 2001). Both MRI and computed tomographic (CT) scans can assist in determining when the injuries occurred and can also substantiate repeated injuries by documenting changes in the chemical states of hemoglobin in affected areas (Sato et al. 1989).

In the event of suspected brain or head injury, a CT scan is the first-line imaging investigation, with its sensitivity to intraparenchymal, subarachnoid, subdural, and epidural hemorrhage and also to mass effect. Due to its relative insensitivity to subarachnoid blood and fractures, an MRI study is considered complementary to a CT scan and should ideally be obtained 2–3 days later if possible. Because MRI may fail to detect acute bleeding, its use should be delayed for 5–7 days in acutely ill children (Cheung 1999). Thoracoabdominal trauma is best evaluated initially by CT scanning (Toomey and Bernstein 2001).

In a study examining the etiology of rib fractures in children under age 1 year, Bulloch et al. (2000) found that of 39 cases of rib fractures in infants, 32 (82%) were caused by child abuse. In a retrospective study, Cadzow and Armstrong (2000) found that 15 of the 18 rib fractures (83%) reviewed in children less than age 2 years were due to child abuse. Scherl et al. (2000) found that a significant proportion of femur fractures due to abuse were transverse, although spiral fractures are slightly more common in abused children compared with accidental causes (36% versus 27%). The authors found, however, that spiral fractures were more typically investigated for abuse.

The American Academy of Pediatrics (2000) states that the use of radiographic imaging "is not only to identify the extent of physical injury when abuse has occurred, but also to elucidate all imaging findings that point to alternative diagnoses" (p. 1345). The report adds that there are published standards for skeletal survey imaging in cases of suspected abuse, with "recent evidence suggesting that a follow-up skeletal survey approximately 2 weeks after the initial study increased the diagnostic yield" (p. 1346). This technique helps to identify new fractures that may not be radiologically apparent until they begin to heal, possibly 7–10 days after the injury. This facilitates more precise determination of the age of the injuries. If there are no changes during this interval, this suggests that the initial finding is a normal anatomical variant or is related to bone dysplasia.

■ Differential Diagnosis

Differential diagnosis includes bone diseases (such as osteogenesis imperfecta), congenital syphilis, osteomyelitits, infantile cortical hyperostosis, and spina bifida. All of these conditions may result in fractures and pathological alterations in bones that may resemble lesions caused by physical abuse. Proper radiological imaging can identify characteristic findings for each of these diseases (Green 1997). Bleeding disorders, such as hemophilia, might simulate inflicted injuries and can be detected by coagulation studies. Because children by nature are quite active, true accidental injuries are common in this age group. However, these accidental injuries can usually be distinguished from those that occur secondary to physical abuse by information obtained in the clinical history and by findings on clinical examination that are described above.

Diagnostic Considerations, Clinical Findings, and Comorbidity of Physical Abuse

There is increasing evidence that children who are victims of abuse are prone to behavioral and emotional difficulties. In reviewing the psychological effects of physical abuse, Cicchetti and Toth (1995) noted a wide range of effects, such as affective dysregulation, disruptive and aggressive behaviors, insecure and atypical attachment patterns, impaired peer relationships with either increased aggression or social withdrawal, and academic underachievement. The same authors also found a high rate of other comorbid psychiatric disorders, including depression, conduct disorder, ADHD, ODD, and PTSD. Others have reported abuse to be significantly associated with global impairment, poor social competence, major depression, conduct disorder, ODD, agoraphobia, overanxious disorder, ADHD, and substance abuse (Famularo et al. 1992; Fisher et al. 1997; Kaplan et al. 1998; Livingston et al. 1993).

■ Neurodevelopmental Impact of Physical Abuse

Neuroanatomical and neurophysiological changes secondary to physical abuse may directly decrease a child's ability to express feelings in words. Abused children seem to lack empathy, which may be linked to trauma-induced expressive deficits coupled with a conditioned higher pain threshold. Others have identified significantly lower pain thresholds in abused subjects, who more frequently blamed themselves for their pain and exhibited more maladaptive pain coping strategies (Scarinci et al. 1994). A study of abused children did, however, find a capacity for moral thought, with the children believing it was wrong to harm another person (Smetana and Kelly 1989).

Cognitive and academic impairment in maltreated youths have been consistently documented in a number of studies (Cahill et al. 1999; Coster et al. 1989; Fox et al. 1988; McFadyen and Kitson 1996). Language delays have been reported in abused youths (Fox et al. 1988). Studies of preschool children report significantly decreased intelligence compared with control subjects (Vondra et al. 1990). Perez and Widom (1994) reported on a cohort of abused children, finding that the formerly abused and neglected individuals had significantly lower IQ scores. Wodarski and colleagues (1990) studied a group of physically abused youths and found that 60% of the neglected youths and 55% of the abused youths had repeated at least one grade, compared with 24% of the comparison group. A 3-year follow-up study of this population found that the language and mathematics scores dropped in the abused group. Those who had been neglected, on the other hand, had shown some academic improvement.

In their comprehensive review of neurodevelopmental responses to trauma, Perry and Pollard (1998) discuss how abuse can result in neuropsychiatric problems, including depressive disorders, ADHD, dissociative disorders, and developmental disorders. PTSD is not the inevitable outcome, although posttraumatic dissociative-like symptoms or hyperarousal commonly coexist with the other resulting disorders in abused children. By definition, a traumatic event overwhelms the child, disrupting homeostasis and creating a compensatory response that leads to a less functional new state of equilibrium (Perry and Pollard 1998). All parts of the brain are affected—cortex, limbic system, midbrain, and brainstem—with different types of traumatic memories created. Altered cortical homeostasis results in cognitive or narrative memory, altered limbic homeostasis results in emotional memory, altered midbrain homeostasis results in motor memory, and altered brainstem homeostasis results in physiological-state memories (Castro-Alamancos and Connors

1996; LeDoux et al. 1989; Perry and Pollard 1998; Phillips and LeDoux 1992). These altered brain equilibria and the resulting memories are the foundation of abuse-related neuropsychiatric signs and symptoms.

Adults with PTSD due to severe sexual or physical abuse exhibit decreased hippocampal size, which may explain the memory impairment in victims of abuse (Bremner et al. 1995, 1997). Sapolsky (1996) reviewed how sustained stress leads to stimulation of the hypothalamic-pituitary-adrenal (HPA) axis and subsequently to elevated cortisol levels, which in turn damage the hippocampus. In children with histories of physical or sexual abuse, frontotemporal and anterior brain electrophysiological abnormalities have also been noted. In a subsequent study, electroencephalographic examination of severely abused children revealed decreased cortical differentiation (Ito et al. 1993, 1998).

Two primary human responses to stress are hyperarousal and dissociative reactions. Hyperarousal, or "fight or flight," involves activation of the sympathetic nervous system via the midbrain norepinephrine-neuron-containing locus ceruleus. Arousal, startle responses, vigilance, irritability, and sleep are all affected by this activation. Physically abused youths exhibit impaired sleep efficiency with prolonged sleep latency and increased activity during sleep (Glod et al. 1997). In addition, interaction between the locus ceruleus and the HPA axis results in increase in the release of adrenocorticotropin and cortisol to prepare the body for defense (Perry and Pollard 1998). As described above, chronic activation of the HPA axis may have negative consequences, including hippocampal damage. Studies of abused children have revealed hippocampal and limbic abnormalities, which in turn predispose to memory deficits and emotional dysregulation. Following the acute fear response, the brain creates a set of memories that can be triggered by reminders of the trauma. Affected children thus remain in a persistent state of fear, with hypersensitivity and reactivity (Perry and Pollard 1998).

Fight or flight is rarely an option for a child, who may be physically unable to defend himself or herself or to escape. The only response to the pain of the abuse may be to activate dissociative mechanisms involving disengagement from the external world by using primitive defenses such as depersonalization, derealization, numbing, and—in extreme cases—catatonia (Perry and Pollard 1998). Dissociation is protective and allows the child to psychologically survive the abuse. Over time, it often becomes maladaptive, emerging at inappropriate times, for example during situations that may trigger verbal or nonverbal (bodily) memories of earlier trauma. During dissociative episodes, the child may stare off briefly and appear as if he or she is daydreaming. Such children may be misdiagnosed as having ADHD, inattentive type. Other children may freeze in response to certain activating stimuli. Caregivers or teachers may misinterpret this reaction as an act of defiance. If confronted, more anxious children can quickly escalate to feeling threatened or "frozen" and may ultimately resort to a classic fight or flight by becoming aggressive or combative over relatively minor events. Other children may react to stressors by dissolving into regressed, dissociative states that may contain micropsychotic episodes and may lead clinicians to misdiagnose a psychotic disorder. According to Perry and Pollard, males tend to use hyperarousal responses, whereas females are much more likely to dissociate.

The specific outcome of physical abuse depends on many variables, such as the nature, duration, and severity of the trauma and the age of the child. Infants and young children have immature central nervous system development—an infant can have a startle response and distress but may be unable to formulate a plan or to use words as an outlet for distressing feelings. Infants' primary mechanism to elicit help is to cry—a behavior that can lead to abuse. Ultimately, learned helplessness sets in, and the child may sink into apathetic silence and withdrawal. Clinicians sometimes misinterpret an abused child's silence and outward calm as resilience, when in fact the child is much more affected by the abuse then is apparent (Perry and Pollard 1998).

■ Attachment Dysregulation

According to attachment theory (Bowlby 1969, 1973, 1980, 1982), infants between ages 6 and 12 months are developmentally predisposed to forming attachments that allow the child to survive. A child's internal representation of his or her attachment figure depends on how available and responsive the caregiver is. Research has shown that the way a child thinks about his or her relationship with the primary caregivers is related to the child's self-esteem, social competence, peer relationships, arousal, distress, and psychopathology (Crowell 1995). Over time, the infant develops a set of expectations about future interactions based on previous

experiences of interactions with the primary caregiver (Bowlby 1980).

Ainsworth and colleagues (1978) proposed that an infant securely attaches to a mother who is sensitive to the infant's needs. Insensitive or unresponsive parenting leads to insecure attachments. These researchers further subcategorized insecure attachments as anxious/avoidant and anxious/ambivalent. They later identified a third insecure pattern, disorganized attachment. Rejecting and intrusive parenting were believed to lead to an avoidant attachment pattern in the infant, with inconsistent, underinvolved parenting leading to an ambivalent pattern.

Abusive parenting is associated with insecure attachments, often of the disorganized type, which in turn often leads to later psychopathology in the infant. Main and Hesse (1990) postulated that the presence of fear in a caregiving relationship promotes the disorganized pattern of attachment. In a review of the impact of child maltreatment on subsequent attachment patterns (Morton and Browne 1998), 11 of 13 studies found that compared with control children, significantly more maltreated infants displayed insecure attachments. The review included a study by Carlson et al. (1989) that found that 82% of maltreated infants were classified as "disorganized" in their attachment pattern, the most impaired of the attachment classifications. Children exposed to abusive parenting are excessively sensitized in their arousal level, emotional regulation, and behavioral reactivity and are at risk for later developing neuropsychiatric problems (Perry and Pollard 1998).

Conversely, Gunnar (1998) suggests that the security of attachment between an infant and caregiver buffers stress by downregulating the HPA axis. Compared with insecurely attached infants, 18-month-old children with secure attachments to their mothers were found to have decreased cortisol levels when frightened by a clown (Nachmias et al. 1996). Numerous studies have identified the key role of a responsive, predictable, and nurturing caregiver in the development of a healthy neurobiological stress response (Perry and Pollard 1998). During the first 2 years of life, there is a genetically programmed overproduction of axons, dendrites, and synapses in the brain, with subsequent pruning of those not used (Singer 1995). The environment thus regulates which synaptic connections survive (Glaser 2000), possibly explaining the power of physical abuse in derailing attachment and developmental outcomes and of nurturance in sustaining secure attachments and healthy outcomes. Other authors, including Kagan (1984, 1998), suggest that these attachment patterns are more due to a child's temperament than to the environment, although he concedes that a negative environment can worsen an inhibited/anxious temperament. Finally, as the work of Lyons-Ruth et al. (1990) and Beardslee et al. (1997) has shown, healthy infant–parent attachment promotes optimal development and protects against adverse outcomes.

■ Peer and Adult Relationships

Lewis (1996) highlighted the negative reactions that abused children tend to evoke in clinicians:

> The capacity of abused children to repress or deny their own painful feelings as well as the pain of others, their inability to articulate emotions, their emotional lability and impulsivity, their distortions of reality, their perceptions of threat where no threat exists, and their resultant tendency to put angry feelings into actions rather than words can become a relatively enduring adaptational style. This constellation of unlovable characteristics accounts in great measure for the tendency of clinicians to dismiss severely abused, aggressive children and adolescents as simply conduct disordered or sociopathic. (p. 340)

Salzinger et al. (1993) found that physically abused children are more disliked and less popular than their nonabused peers. They tend to exhibit less intimacy, more conflict, and more negative affect with peers than do nonabused children (Parker and Herrera 1996).

■ Aggression

The most frequent outcome of abuse is aggression. Abused preschool children engage in aggressive behavior more frequently than their peers (Klimes-Dougan and Kistner 1990), and they more often attribute hostile intent to their peers (Dodge et al. 1990). Abused children have also been reported to be at risk for violent criminal behavior in adolescence (Herrenkohl et al. 1997) and in adulthood (Widom 1989). Adolescents with a history of abuse are also reported to engage in more aggression with their peers and within their dating relationships (Wolfe et al. 1998).

Lewis (1992) summarizes how physical abuse begets violence:

> In short, whatever increases impulsivity and irritability, engenders hypervigilance and paranoia, diminishes judgement and verbal competence, and curtails the ability to recognize one's own pain and the pain of others, also enhances the tendency toward violence. Abusive, neglectful caretaking does all of these things. In a resilient child, maltreatment...may not engender aggression. In an already vulnerable child with tendencies toward impulsivity, hypervigilance, expressive difficulties, and dissociation from painful feelings, maltreatment is often sufficient to create a very violent individual. (pp. 388–389)

The etiology of this aggression is complex, with the environment believed to play the major role. Pathological defense mechanisms may also play a role, including identification with the aggressor. It is known that the repeated infliction of pain can lead to aggression, well illustrated in the training of fighting dogs and bulls (Berkowitz 1984). Lewis (1996) writes that abusive experiences provide a model for violence, teach aggression through reinforcement, inflict pain, and cause central nervous system injuries associated with impulsivity, emotional lability, and impaired judgment. Furthermore, this experience creates a sense of being endangered and thus increases paranoid feelings and diminishes the child's capacity to recognize feelings and put them into words, not actions.

■ Substance Abuse and Self-Injurious Behavior

Children may resort to behaviors that facilitate opioid-mediated dissociation, such as rocking, head banging, and self-mutilation, with these painful stimuli activating the brain's endogenous opiates. Abused children are also more likely to develop substance abuse, likely in a self-medicating fashion. Alcohol serves to reduce anxiety, opiates trigger soothing dissociation, and stimulants such as cocaine activate dopaminergic reward mesolimbic areas in children with few true rewards in their lives (Perry and Pollard 1998).

■ Attention-Deficit/Hyperactivity Disorder

Studies of abused children have documented a higher prevalence of ADHD in abused children and adolescents. It has been postulated that there may be two explanations for this. It is possible that children who have ADHD are more likely to provoke abusive behaviors in adults. Impulsive parents could also genetically transmit ADHD to their children. However, it is also plausible that the trauma of abuse itself plays a causal role in the development of ADHD symptoms. (Famularo et al. 1992; Kaplan et al. 1994).

■ Depression and Suicide

Abused infants are prone to affective withdrawal, diminished capacity for pleasure, and a tendency to exhibit negative affects such as sadness and distress (Green 1997). Major depression or dysthymia was also reported in 27% of children of latency age who had been abused (Green 1997). Approximately 8% of children and adolescents with documented physical abuse have a current diagnosis of major depressive disorder, 40% have lifetime major depressive disorder diagnoses, and at least 30% have lifetime disruptive disorder diagnoses (ODD or conduct disorder). These prevalence rates are several times higher than those found in community samples of children and adolescents (Kaplan et al. 1999). Depression may be a consequence of abuse or may result in a child being more vulnerable to abuse.

Studies are also reporting an association between physical abuse in childhood and subsequent suicidal behavior and risk taking (Kaplan et al. 1999). Furthermore, Green (1997) reported self-mutilation and suicidal ideation and attempts in children subjected to parental beatings or threatened abandonment by their adult caretakers. Sexual risk taking leads to increased teenage parenthood and exposure to human immunodeficiency virus and sexually transmitted diseases (Kaplan et al. 1999).

■ Dissociative Disorders

Dissociative disorders may result from physical abuse. Children who dissociate may experience brief psychotic symptoms, for example hearing command auditory hallucinations. It is relatively common for severely physically abused children to hear voices commanding them to harm themselves or others. Because of this, they can be misdiagnosed as having a primary psychotic disorder such as schizophrenia. At other times a dissociating child is misdiagnosed as being an externalizing child—that is, as having ADHD, ODD, or an impulse control disorder. A study of a group of severely abused youngsters in residential treatment found that 23% of the boys met DSM-IV criteria for dissociative identity disorder (American Psychiatric Association 1994; Yeager and Lewis 2000).

■ Anxiety Disorders and Posttraumatic Stress Disorder

Green (1997) described anxiety states, sleep disturbances, nightmares, and psychosomatic complaints in abused children, with some children meeting criteria for PTSD. The children demonstrated repetitive traumatic play expressing themes of the abuse, flashbacks, constriction of affect, and avoidance of events associated with the abuse in addition to symptoms of increased autonomic arousal. Famularo et al. (1992) reported that 39% of a cohort of maltreated children were given a diagnosis of PTSD.

Talbott (2001) recently reported on the presentation of PTSD in children. Children often display disorganized or agitated behavior rather than the fear, helplessness, and horror described in adults. Repetitive play involving themes of the trauma is common, rather than the classic flashbacks or recurrent and intrusive recollections of the trauma. Children may have vague frightening dreams that are often not of the abusive event itself. Others (e.g., Bursztajn et al. 1999) have found similar presentations in traumatized youth.

In her review of trauma leading to PTSD, Terr (1996) wrote that traumatic events, including physical abuse, cause psychic trauma when the child understands that something terrible is happening and that he or she is in danger, senses his or her own helplessness, and registers and stores an implicit or explicit traumatic memory. Terr cites protective factors, including intelligence, humor, and relatedness. Soon after a traumatic event, Terr notes the possible clinical finding of posttraumatic play, which can be "grim, monotonous, and at times, dangerous." The child often does not make a connection between the play and the trauma. Only later does the clinician typically see more clearly intrusive thoughts, fears, and repeated dreams. A foreshortened sense of the future is common in abused children and can lead to reckless risk taking. Unconscious reenactment of the trauma can lead to retraumatization of the child. In some cases, this reenactment can be dangerous to the child or to others.

Pelcovitz and colleagues (1994) studied the prevalence of PTSD in physically abused adolescents and found that these youths may be more at risk for behavioral, emotional, and social difficulties than for clear PTSD. This is in contrast to the previous work of Green (1997), who found that physically abused adolescents were at risk for developing PTSD. Pelcovitz et al. (1994) suggest that physically abused adolescents may "enact" the results of their victimization rather than express their reactions to the abuse via symptoms of PTSD. All the physically abused adolescents who received a PTSD diagnosis in this study reported these symptoms in response to extrafamilial sexual assaults. The authors point out the differences between physical and sexual assaults, with sexual abuse often accompanied by a higher level of secrecy and shame, which may reinforce the emergence of PTSD symptoms. External signs of physical abuse, such as bruises and fractures, may lead to more support, facilitating integration of the trauma. Pelcovitz et al. add that an alternative possibility is that the physically abused youths in their study did not manifest PTSD symptoms because they remained in an abusive environment. There can be a delay in the onset of PTSD symptoms until after the trauma has ended. In his classic trauma studies, Krystal (1968) reported that holocaust survivors frequently did not manifest PTSD symptoms until years after leaving the concentration camps.

Treatment

■ Prevention

The cornerstone of treatment of children who are victims of abuse is first to make certain that the child is protected from further injury. Even more important is to prevent abuse from occurring at all. Kaplan (1996) reviews three types of child abuse primary prevention strategies: 1) competency enhancement with parent education programs; 2) media campaigns, hotlines, and parent socialization programs; and 3) targeting high-risk groups, such as single parents and teenage parents. Other high-risk groups of parents include those of low socioeconomic status and those with neurocognitively compromised children.

Research has shown that maltreated children with healthier ego resiliency, ego overcontrol, and self-esteem fared better in their overall adjustment compared with abused peers lacking these strengths (Glaser 2000). A focus of treatment should therefore be helping abused youths gain better control over their urges and actions and better self-awareness, ultimately creating a coherent narrative of their life story. This is a complex undertaking, due in part to the likelihood that ego control and ego resilience are at least in part temperamentally determined and that self-esteem is influenced by nurturance (Glaser 2000). Abuse dam-

ages nurturance and therefore self-esteem and can shift a child's neurodevelopment, including possibly temperament, resulting in a child who is less able to develop ego control and resilience and who is less responsive to psychotherapy. Because brain development is related to environmental forces, intense and early intervention offers the greatest hope for healthier outcomes.

Leventhal (2001) described two home-based models for preventing child abuse and neglect: Healthy Families, using a trained paraprofessional supervised by a social worker and health personnel, and the Olds model, in which the home visitor is a nurse supervised by a social worker. The paraprofessionals are less skilled than the nurse or the social worker in making clinical assessments and are less knowledgeable about health and development. However, they often come from the community being served and may be better able to ally with families, thereby forming a stronger link and alliance with the parents. Both models focus on high-risk families. The Healthy Families model uses the Kempe Family Stress Inventory to identify high-risk families, covering areas such as a parental history of abuse, violence, substance abuse, mental illness, or criminal acts. In the Olds model, first-time mothers are eligible if they have two of the following characteristics: 1) have less than 12 years of education, 2) are unmarried, or 3) are of low socioeconomic status.

Research on the effectiveness of these two models has shown that families can be helped and that the effects are sustained over many years. However, home visiting does not cure all difficulties. When high levels of domestic violence are present, it is difficult for parents to improve their parenting by the use of home visits. Leventhal (2001) writes that fathers need specific attention, because as much as two-thirds of serious physical abuse is caused by males in the family. Typically these men have little experience caring for young children, have difficulties with their own impulse control, and tend to be violent toward their partners. One strategy is to empower women to leave their partners and to make better future decisions. Another strategy is to help men be more nurturing and effective as parents.

Prevention strategies based on attachment theory focus on improving the caregiver–child relationship, which in turn buffers the child against life stressors. A number of studies have attempted to change insecure attachment relationships to secure ones (Morton and Browne 1998). Interventions focusing on enhancing parental sensitivity were more successful in changing attachment status than were more in-depth interventions that focused on the intrapsychic representational model.

Lyons-Ruth et al. (1990) examined attachment patterns among infants at social risk, measuring development, mother–infant interaction, and maternal depression and social contacts while also evaluating the efficacy of home visits in improving the security of a child's attachment to the caregiver. The home-visiting service had four goals:

1. Providing an accepting relationship
2. Increasing the family's competence in accessing resources
3. Modeling and reinforcing more interactive, positive, and developmentally appropriate exchanges between mother and infant, emphasizing the mother's dual role as teacher and source of emotional security for her infant
4. Decreasing social isolation with a weekly parenting group or a monthly social hour. Psychodynamic interventions, based on the work of Fraiberg (1980), and behavioral interventions were used.

The authors found that "at 18 months of age, infants of depressed mothers who received home-visiting services outperformed unserved infants of depressed mothers by a mean of 10 points on the Bayley Mental Development Index, and were twice as likely to be classified as securely attached in their relationships with their mothers" (Lyons-Ruth et al. (1990, p. 95). Because a secure attachment has been associated with lower risk of abuse, this could be a powerful intervention to decrease the risk of physical maltreatment.

■ Child and Parent Treatment

The major goals of treatment are first to protect the child and strengthen the family, and then to address the impact of past abuse in treatment of the child and the family. If possible, the child should remain at home unless his or her physical or psychological safety is in jeopardy.

The ecological model calls for a focus on the multidimensional aspects of child abuse, rather than just on the abusive parent (as has been done in traditional child abuse programs). Attachment theory has emphasized the interactive aspects of maltreatment and the importance of intervening in changing the parent–child

relationship, with the hope of facilitating a more secure attachment between child and parent.

Family-based therapy needs to improve the parents' devalued self-image, reverse distortions of their child that can lead to scapegoating, interpret any links between the current abuse and the parent's own abuse history, and provide the parent with a positive model of raising children. Green (1997) suggests using therapeutic nurseries to treat infants and pathological parent–child interactions, with dyadic parent–child therapy serving as the foundation of treatment.

Psychotherapy of the child should include creating a therapeutic environment, either in individual or group settings, which allow the child to master the trauma, in part though controlled repetitions of the event using symbolic reenactments with dolls, puppets, drawings, etc. According to Green (1997), "The retrieval and integration of traumatic memories will gradually enable the child to verbalize memories and feelings associated with the abuse rather than acting them out in a repetitive manner. Impulse control is strengthened by imposing limits on the direct expression of aggression, such as hitting or destroying play materials, and encouraging the verbalization of anger. Self-esteem gradually improves during the child's exposure to the climate of acceptance generated by the therapist, which gradually neutralizes the child's mistrust and hypervigilance" (p. 694). The child must be told that the abuse is not his or her fault and that he or she is not to be blamed. Terr (1996) reminds clinicians of the need to explore issues of betrayal, overexcitement, and personal responsibility, especially in children who have been abused within their own families.

Play therapy is useful in the treatment of a traumatized child (Terr 1996). Pynoos and Eth (1986) reviewed the utility of drawings in unlocking feelings associated with the abuse. Play and drawing allow the abused child to use nonverbal and symbolic expressions of events that are either too painful to be expressed in words or that are carefully buried and masked with defenses such as acting out, projecting, splitting, repression, or dissociation. The play therapy session allows for safe displacement of the complex thoughts and feelings stemming from the abuse so that the child can begin to work through them and can eventually heal. A goal of therapy should be helping the child use healthier coping responses.

Pharmacotherapy can also improve the outcome of abused children, especially if they are manifesting symptoms of PTSD. A full review of psychopharmacological interventions is beyond the scope of this chapter. According to anecdotal reports (Kaplan et al. 1999; Terr 1991), propranolol decreased hyperarousal and hypervigilance in abused children. Clonidine has also helped to reduce symptoms of hyperarousal, aggression, and insomnia in abused preschool children with PTSD (Harmon and Riggs 1996). Guanfacine was found to help alleviate sleep disturbances in boys with PTSD (Leonard 1999).

Individual child and parental vulnerability, family dysfunction, and environmental stress variables all need to be addressed if the treatment is to be successful. In most states, abused and neglected children who are involved in court proceedings receive court-appointed guardians. Kaplan and colleagues (1999) note that children and parents in maltreatment cases are often not routinely screened for psychopathology and substance abuse. These authors recommend that psychiatrists should be routinely involved as members of hospital child protection committees.

■ Resilience

Heller et al. (1999) reviewed the literature on resilience to the effects of child maltreatment. Dispositional or temperamental attributes of the child include above-average intelligence, high self-esteem, internal locus of control, external attribution of blame, presence of spirituality, ego resilience, and high ego control. Familial cohesion (including competent foster care) with the presence of caring adults has also been related to developing resilience in children. Extrafamilial support such as a positive school experience promotes resilience, which in turn likely increases individual self-worth and sense of control over one's destiny.

Rutter (1990) has argued that the field must move beyond focusing on single resilience factors to considering the developmental processes that promote adaptive functioning. Rutter has also suggested that resilience is probably not a fixed state but is rather a malleable and organic trait, which can be enhanced with a nurturing environment. The total number of risk factors affecting the child-caregiver dyad better predicts outcome. Furthermore, rather than being a fixed trait, resilience may be fluid over time and may be dependent on environmental context such as external support systems, which may buffer the impact of physical maltreatment and promote a positive sense of one's worth.

■ Prognosis

Positive outcomes can be enhanced with rapid, early, and effective psychotherapeutic interventions. Therapeutic day-care programs for abused youngsters have been shown to improve their social and cognitive skills and self-esteem (Kaplan et al. 1999). Kaplan and colleagues (1999) found positive outcomes from a psychotherapeutic approach using peers to work with withdrawn physically abused young children, which in turn helped the abused children play in a healthier and more interactive fashion.

Research Issues

Future research will need to expand the current understanding of the etiology of maltreatment. As Ertem et al. (2000) noted, widespread assumptions about abuse—such as the adage "once abused, an abuser you will become"—need to be challenged, and when they are found to be fictitious should be discarded. It is likely that the ecological model represents the current best understanding of the complex interactive web of factors that may lead to abuse, taking into account the child's constitution, the mother's psychological well-being, and environmental factors such as poverty, stigma, and isolation. As each of these factors becomes better understood, more effective interventions can be fashioned.

Resilience, a major protective factor, needs to be better studied and better understood. Future studies could examine how resilience can be fostered and supported to minimize the impact of an adverse environment. A better understanding is needed of the complex interactions between risk and protective factors and the protective role of the caregiving relationship in mediating both extrinsic and intrinsic risk factors (Glaser 2000).

Neurodevelopmental research must continue to explore the impact of abuse and neglect on the developing child's brain and the subsequent emotional and behavioral dysregulation and derailment of social development. This understanding can support the development of more effective psychotherapeutic interventions, for example working with nonverbal or expressive interventions (using techniques such as drawing or drama) to compensate for verbal memory deficits caused by trauma.

The role of dissociation in the symptoms displayed

by the abused child also needs to be better understood. Stress has also been shown to have a suppressive effect on hippocampal neurogenesis, which in turn likely negatively affects the consolidation of memory and may play a role in the development of dissociation.

There is great variability in the various measures of juvenile victimization that have been developed. These measures were developed for a variety of specific research, clinical, and public policy needs. Juvenile victimization would greatly benefit from assessment instruments that are comprehensive, methodologically sound, and relevant to settings such as health and mental health clinics, criminal justice institutions, and child protection agencies (Hamby and Finkelhor 2000). It is critically important that future efforts focus on the development of a well-defined, reliable measurement tool.

Finally, early intervention preventive programs must be developed to work with at-risk parents to promote a secure attachment pattern, which has been associated with later psychological well-being. As Bowlby (1973) wrote in his classic work on loss, "The disruption of attachment is itself a primary form of trauma, which may intensify the effects of other stressors, particularly if disruption occurs at critical stages of development."

References

Ainsworth MDS, Blehar MC, Waters E, et al: Patterns of Attachment: A Psychological Study of the Strange Situation. Hillsdale NJ, Erlbaum, 1978

American Academy of Pediatrics: Diagnostic imaging of child abuse. Pediatrics 105:1345–1348, 2000

American Academy of Pediatrics, Committee on Child Abuse and Neglect: Shaken baby syndrome: rotational cranial injuries—technical report. Pediatrics 108:206–210, 2001

American Psychiatric Association: Diagnostic and Statistical Manual of Mental Disorders, 4th Edition. Washington, DC, American Psychiatric Association, 1994

Anderson S, Lauderdale M: Characteristics of abusive parents: a look at self-esteem. Child Abuse Negl 6:285–293, 1982

Beardslee WR, Salt P, Versage EM, et al: Sustaining change in parents receiving preventive interventions for families with depression. Am J Psychiatry 154:510–515, 1997

Belsky J: Child maltreatment: an ecological integration. Am Psychol 35:320–335, 1980

Berkowitz L: Physical pain and the inclination to aggression, in Biological Perspectives on Aggression. Edited by Flannelly KJ, Blanchard RJ, Blanchard DC. New York, Alan R Liss, 1984, pp 27–47

Bowlby J: Attachment and Loss, Vol 1: Attachment. London, Hogarth Press, 1969

Bowlby J: Attachment and Loss, Vol 2: Separation: Anxiety and Anger. London, Hogarth Press, 1973

Bowlby J: Attachment and Loss, Vol 3: Loss: Sadness and Depression. London, Hogarth Press, 1980

Bowlby J: Attachment and Loss, 2nd Edition, Vol 1: Attachment. London, Hogarth Press, 1982

Bremner JD, Randall P, Scott TM, et al: Deficits in short-term memory in adult survivors of childhood abuse. Psychiatry Res 59:97–107, 1995

Bremner JD, Randall P, Vermetten E, et al: MRI-based measurement of hippocampal volume in PTSD related to childhood physical and sexual abuse: a preliminary report. Biol Psychiatry 41:23–32, 1997

Bruce D: Neurosurgical aspects of child abuse, in Child Abuse: A Medical Reference. Edited by Ludwig S, Kornberg AE. New York, Churchill Livingstone, 1992, pp 117–130

Bulloch B, Schubert CJ, Brophy PD, et al: Cause and clinical characteristics of rib fractures in infants. Pediatrics 105:E48, 2000

Bursztajn HJ, Joshi PT, Sutherland SM, et al: Update: recognizing post-traumatic stress. Patient Care, October 15, 1999, pp 171–186

Cadzow SP, Armstrong KL: Rib fractures in infants: red alert! The clinical features, investigation, and child protection outcomes. J Paediatr Child Health 36:322–326, 2000

Caffey J: On the theory and practice of shaking infants: its potential residual effects of permanent brain damage and mental retardation. Am J Dis Child 124(2):161–169, 1972

Cahill LT, Kaminer RK, Johnson PG: Developmental, cognitive, and behavioral sequelae of child abuse. Child Adolesc Psychiatr Clin N Am 8:827–843, 1999

Carlson V, Cicchetti D, Barnett D, et al: Disorganized/disoriented attachment relationships in maltreated infants. Dev Psychol 25:382–383, 1989

Castro-Alamancos MA, Connors BW: Short-term plasticity of a thalamocortical pathway dynamically modulated by behavioral state. Science 272:274–276, 1996

Cheung KK: Identifying and documenting findings of physical child abuse and neglect. J Pediatr Health Care 13:142–143, 1999

Cicchetti D, Toth SL: A developmental psychopathology perspective on child abuse and neglect. J Am Acad Child Adolesc Psychiatry 34:541–565, 1995

Coster WJ, Gersten MS, Beeghly M, et al: Communicative functioning in maltreated toddlers. Dev Psychol 25:777–793, 1989

Crowell JA: A review of adult attachment measures: implications for theory and research. Social Development 4:294–327, 1995

DeAngelis C: Clinical indicators of child abuse, in Clinical Handbook of Child Psychiatry and the Law. Edited by Schetky DH, Benedek EP. Baltimore, MD, Williams & Wilkins, 1992

Dodge KA, Bates JE, Pettit GS: Mechanisms in the cycle of violence. Science 250:1678–1683, 1990

Egeland B, Jacobvitz D, Sroufe LA: Breaking the cycle of abuse. Child Dev 59:1080–1088, 1988

Egeland B, Carlson E, Sroufe LA: Resilience as process. Dev Psychopathol 5:517–528, 1993

English DJ, Marshall DB, Brummer S, et al: Characteristics of repeated referrals to child protective services in Washington State. Child Maltreatment 4:297–307, 1999

Ertem IO, Leventhal JM, Dobbs S: Intergenerational continuity of child physical abuse: how good is the evidence? Lancet 356:814–819, 2000

Evans A: Personality characteristics and disciplinary attitudes of child-abusing mothers. Child Abuse Negl 4:179–187, 1980

Famularo R, Kinscherff R, Fenton T: Psychiatric diagnoses of maltreated children: preliminary findings. J Am Acad Child Adolesc Psychiatry 31:863–867, 1992

Fisher AJ, Kramer RA, Hoven CW, et al: Psychosocial characteristics of physically abused children and adolescents. J Am Acad Child Adolesc Psychiatry 36:123–131, 1997

Fox L, Long SH, Anglois A: Patterns of language comprehension deficit in abused and neglected children. J Speech Hear Disord 53:239–244, 1988

Fraiberg S (ed): Clinical Studies in Infant Mental Health. New York, Basic Books, 1980

Glaser D: Child abuse and neglect and the brain: a review. J Child Psychol Psychiatry 41(1):97–116, 2000

Glod CA, Teicher MH, Hartman CR, et al: Increased nocturnal activity and impaired sleep maintenance in abused children. J Am Acad Child Adolesc Psychiatry 36:1236–1243, 1997

Green AH: Child Maltreatment: A Handbook for Mental Health and Child Care Professionals. New York, Jason Aronson, 1980

Green AH: Physical abuse of children, in Textbook of Child and Adolescent Psychiatry, 2nd Edition. Edited by Weiner JM. Washington DC, American Psychiatric Press, 1997, pp 687–697

Gunnar M: Quality of early care and buffering of neuroendocrine stress reactions: potential effects on the developing human brain. Prev Med 27:208–211, 1998

Hamby SL, Finkelhor D: The victimization of children: recommendations for assessment and instrument development. J Am Acad Child Adolesc Psychiatry 39:829–840, 2000

Harmon RJ, Riggs PD: Clonidine for posttraumatic stress disorder in preschool children. J Am Acad Child Adolesc Psychiatry 35:1247–1249, 1996

Heller SS, Larrieu JA, D'Imperio R, et al: Research on resilience to child maltreatment: empirical considerations. Child Abuse Negl 23:321–338, 1999

Herman JL: Trauma and Recovery. New York, Basic Books, 1992

Herrenkohl RC, Egolf BP, Herrenkohl EC: Preschool antecedents of adolescent assaultive behavior: a longitudinal study. Am J Orthopsychiatry 67:422–432, 1997

Ito Y, Teicher MH, Glod CA, et al: Increased prevalence of electrophysiological abnormalities in children with psychological, physical and sexual abuse. J Neuropsychiatry Clin Neurosci 5:401–408, 1993

Ito Y, Teicher MH, Glod CA, et al: Preliminary evidence for aberrant cortical development in abused children: a quantitative EEG study. J Neuropsychiatry Clin Neurosci 10:298–307, 1998

Kagan J: The Nature of the Child. New York, Basic Books, 1984

Kagan J: Three Seductive Ideas. Cambridge, MA, Harvard University Press, 1998

Kaplan SJ: Physical abuse and neglect, in Child and Adolescent Psychiatry: A Comprehensive Textbook, 2nd Edition. Edited by Lewis M. Baltimore, MD, Williams & Wilkins 1996, pp 1033–1041

Kaplan SJ, Pelcovitz D, Weiner M: Adolescent physical abuse. Child Adolesc Psychiatr Clin N Am 3:695–711, 1994

Kaplan SJ, Pelcovitz D, Salzinger S, et al: Adolescent physical abuse: risk for adolescent psychiatric disorders. Am J Psychiatry 155:954–959, 1998

Kaplan SJ, Pelcovitz D, Labruna V: Child and adolescent abuse and neglect research: a review of the past 10 years, I: physical and emotional abuse and neglect. J Am Acad Child Adolesc Psychiatry 38:1214–1222, 1999

Kaufman J, Zigler E: Do abused children become abusive parents? Am J Orthopsychiatry 57:186–192, 1987

Kempe CH, Silverman R, Steele B, et al: The battered child syndrome. JAMA 181:17–24, 1962

Klimes-Dougan B, Kistner J: Physically abused preschoolers' responses to peers' distress. Dev Psychol 26:599–602, 1990

Krystal H: Massive Psychic Trauma. New York, International Universities Press, 1968

Kunz J, Bahr SJ: A profile of parental homicide against children. J Fam Violence 11:347–362, 1996

LeDoux JE, Romanski L, Xagoraris A: Indelibility of subcortical emotional memories. J Cogn Neurosci 1:238–243, 1989

Leonard H: Guanfacine alleviates sleep disorders in boys with PTSD. Brown University Child and Adolescent Psychopharmacology Update, October 1999, p 1

Leventhal JM: The prevention of child abuse and neglect: successfully out of the blocks. Child Abuse Negl 25:431–439, 2001

Lewis DO: From abuse to violence: psychophysiological consequences of maltreatment. J Am Acad Child Adolesc Psychiatry 31:383–391, 1992

Lewis DO: Development of the symptom of violence, in Child and Adolescent Psychiatry: A Comprehensive Textbook, 2nd Edition. Edited by Lewis M. Baltimore, MD, Williams & Wilkins, 1996, pp 334–344

Livingston R, Lawson L, Jones JG: Predictors of self-reported psychopathology in children abused repeatedly by a parent. J Am Acad Child Adolesc Psychiatry 32:948–953, 1993

Lyons-Ruth K, Connell DB, Grunebaum H: Infants at social risk: maternal depression and family support services as mediators of infant development and security of attachment. Child Dev 61:85–98, 1990

Main M, Hesse E: Parents' unresolved traumatic experiences are related to infant disorganized attachment status: is frightened and/or frightening parent behavior the linking mechanism? In Attachment in the Preschool Years: Theory, Research, and Intervention. Edited by Greenberg M, Cicchetti D, Cummings E. Chicago, IL, University of Chicago Press, 1990, pp 161–182

Martin JA, Elmer E: Battered children grown up: a follow-up study of individuals severely maltreated as children. Child Abuse Negl 16:75–87, 1992

McFadyen RG, Kitson WJH: Language comprehension and expression among adolescents who have experienced childhood physical abuse. J Child Psychol Psychiatry 37:551–562, 1996

Morton N, Browne KD: Theory and observation of attachment and its relation to child maltreatment: a review. Child Abuse Negl 22:1093–1104, 1998

Nachmias M, Gunnar M, Mangelsdorf S, et al: Behavioral inhibition and stress reactivity; the moderating role of attachment security. Child Dev 67:508–522, 1996

Oliver JE: Intergenerational transmission of child abuse: rattles, research, and clinical implications. Am J Psychiatry 150:1315–1324, 1993

Parker JG, Herrera C: Interpersonal processes in friendship: a comparison of abused and nonabused children's experiences. Dev Psychol 32:1025–1038, 1996

Pelcovitz D, Kaplan S, Goldenberg B, et al: Post-traumatic stress disorder in physically abused adolescents. J Am Acad Child Adolesc Psychiatry 33:305–312, 1994

Perez CM, Widom CS: Childhood victimization and long-term intellectual and academic outcomes. Child Abuse Negl 18:617, 1994

Perry BD, Pollard R: Homeostasis, stress, trauma and adaptation—a neurodevelopmental view of childhood trauma. Child Adolesc Psychiatr Clin N Am 7:33–51, 1998

Phillips RG, LeDoux JE: Differential contribution of amygdala and hippocampus to cued and contextual fear conditioning. Behav Neurosci 106:274–285, 1992

Powers JL, Eckenrode J, Jaklitsch B: Maltreatment among runaway and homeless youth. Child Abuse Negl 14:87–98, 1990

Pynoos R, Eth S: Witness to violence: the child interview. J Am Acad Child Adolesc Psychiatry 25:306–319, 1986

Rosen B, Stein M: Women who abuse their children. Am J Dis Child 134:947–950, 1980

Rutter M: Psychosocial resilience and protective mechanisms, in Risk and Protective Factors in the Development of Psychopathology. Edited by Rolf J, Masten AS, Cicchetti K, et al. New York, Cambridge University Press, 1990, pp 181–214

Salzinger S, Feldman RS, Hammer M, et al: The effects of physical abuse on children's social relationships. Child Dev 64:169–187, 1993

Sapolsky R: Why stress is bad for your brain. Science 273:749–750, 1996

Sato Y, Yuh WT, Smith WL, et al: Head injury in child abuse: evaluation with MR imaging. Radiology 173:653–657, 1989

Scarinci IC, McDonald-Haile J, Bradley LA, et al: Altered pain perception and psychosocial features among women with gastrointestinal disorders and a history of abuse: a preliminary model. Am J Med 97:108–118, 1994

Scherl SA, Miller L, Lively N, et al: Accidental and nonaccidental femur fractures in children. Clin Orthop 376:96–105, 2000

Sedlak AJ, Broadhurst DD: The Third National Incidence Study of Child Abuse and Neglect. Washington, DC, U.S. Department of Health and Human Services, 1996

Singer W: Development and plasticity of cortical processing architectures. Science 270:758–764, 1995

Smetana JG, Kelly M: Social cognition in maltreated children, in Child Maltreatment: Theory and Research on Causes and Consequences of Child Abuse and Neglect. Edited by Cicchetti D, Carlson V. New York, Cambridge University Press, 1989, pp 620–646

Smith SM, Hanson R, Noble S: Parents of battered babies: a controlled study. Br Med J 4:388–391, 1973

Straus M, Gelles R, Steinmets S: Behind Closed Doors: Violence in the American Family. New York, Anchor Press, 1980

Talbott JA: Look beyond classic symptoms to spot PTSD in affected kids. Clinical Psychiatry News, October 2001, p 26

Terr LC: Childhood traumas: an outline and overview. Am J Psychiatry 148:10–20, 1991

Terr LC: Acute responses to external events and posttraumatic stress disorder, in Child and Adolescent Psychiatry: A Comprehensive Textbook, 2nd Edition. Edited by Lewis M. Baltimore, MD, Williams & Wilkins, 1996

Thompson RA: Social support and the prevention of child maltreatment, in Protecting Children From Abuse and Neglect: Foundations for a New National Strategy. Edited by Melton GB, Barry FD. New York, Guilford, 1994, pp 40–130

Toomey S, Bernstein H: Child abuse and neglect: prevention and intervention. Curr Opin Pediatr 13:211–215, 2001

U.S. Department of Health and Human Services: HHS reports new child abuse and neglect statistics. HHS News, April 2, 2001. Available at: http://www.hhs.gov/news/press/2001pres/20010402.html. Accessed July 21, 2003

Vondra JI, Barnett D, Cicchetti D: Self-concept, motivation, and competence among preschoolers from maltreating and comparison families. Child Abuse Negl 14:525–540, 1990

Widom CS: Child abuse, neglect, and adult behavior. Criminology 27:251–271, 1989

Wodarski JS, Kurtz PD, Gaudin JM Jr, et al: Maltreatment and the school age child: major academic, socioemotional, and adaptive outcomes. Soc Work 35:506–513, 1990

Wolfe DA, Wekerle C, Reitzel-Jaffe D, et al: Factors associated with abusive relationships among maltreated and non-maltreated youth. Dev Psychopathol 10:61–85, 1998

Yeager CA, Lewis DO: Mental illness, neuropsychologic deficits, child abuse, and violence. Child Adolesc Psychiatr Clin N Am 9:793–813, 2000

Sexual Abuse of Children

Paramjit T. Joshi, M.D.

Jay A. Salpekar, M.D.

Peter T. Daniolos, M.D.

Definitions

Sexual abuse is a general term that refers to the involvement of children in sexual activity that is developmentally inappropriate and that violates laws or social taboos (American Academy of Pediatrics 1999). Sexual abuse most commonly refers to any activity within a spectrum ranging from inappropriate physical touching to sexual intercourse or rape. For decades child sexual abuse has continued to elude specific definition despite the efforts of researchers, therapists, and child advocates (Haugaard 2000).

Important considerations include the wide range of normative sexual behavior and development among children and adolescents (Ryan 2000). Children may exhibit a wide range of sexual behaviors, even in circumstances where abuse may not be present (Friedrich et al. 1998). Children are very impressionable and model behavior that they see in adults. Eroticized behavior, increased sexual interest, and sexual play may result from numerous influences beyond potential abuse, including inadvertent observation of adults engaged in sexual activity, oedipal fantasies, manic or hypomanic states, or exposure to pornographic materials and television (Yates 1997). *Sexual play* generally involves mutually interested children at similar ages and developmental stages and does not involve coercion (American Academy of Pediatrics 1999). *Incest* refers to the sexual abuse of children within the context of the nuclear family, generally involving sexual activity between a parent and child or among siblings.

Legal definitions of abuse generally involve sexual contact between an adult and a minor child (Green 1993). Sexual abuse is understood to have occurred in any such adult–child contact, and it generally involves the forced participation or exploitation of the child in the context of gross inequality of the power of the participants. If both the perpetrator and the victim are minors, abuse can be understood to have occurred, provided that there is a significant discrepancy in age or there is coercion involved. Some have defined age discrepancies of 4–5 years as being more definitive for an abuse scenario, but there is not a commonly accepted age difference defining abuse of a minor by another minor. Particularly when coercion, multiple simultaneous perpetrators, developmental asymmetry, or intimidation by physical strength is involved, age differences are less relevant.

Abusive acts include physical fondling of the genitalia, anus, or breasts; genital or anal intercourse; oral-genital contact; and penetration using objects. These acts may be performed by or on the abused child; in some circumstances, perpetrators may force victims to perform abusive acts on other victims.

Children may be victims of nontouching abuse as well, especially in the context of coerced exhibitionism or exploitation. Abusers may engage children in exhibitionism for the purposes of producing child pornography. Such photographic or video-recorded rendition of children in eroticized situations is ultimately nonconsensual and falls within the designation of sexual abuse. Children may likewise be considered victims of abuse when they are forced to view pornographic material. Sexual abusers commonly solicit children by such methods. Perpetrators may also solicit children via the Internet by use of email or chat rooms and by seeking personal information from children who visit child-oriented web sites (Hlaing 2001).

Ritual abuse involves sexual abuse of children in a context of ceremonial religious beliefs generally involving satanic worship (Nurcombe and Unutzer 1991). Despite its high media profile during past decades, the extent to which this type of abuse actually occurs remains controversial.

Historical Perspective

Inappropriate sexual activity and possibly abuse have been documented since the days of antiquity. Most cultures through history have prohibited incest or have in some way restricted procreative activity between close blood relatives. Cases of sexual abuse were documented in the literature from the Byzantine Empire between A.D. 324 and 1453 (Lascaratos and Poulakou-Rebelakou 2000). The empire was characterized by strict legal and religious laws; however, sexual assaults were described in all social classes, including the ruling class (Lascaratos and Poulakou-Rebelakou 2000). Ruling classes routinely engaged in consanguineous or incestuous relationships and arranged marriages to preserve ruling power.

Before the seventeenth century, sexual contact with children was not commonly regarded as a criminal act. The age of consent for sexual activity was often as low as 12 years, and the reality of psychosexual development was not well appreciated (Jackson 1993). In the eighteenth and nineteenth centuries, childhood sexual abuse became increasingly viewed as criminal or inappropriate (Jackson 1993).

In 1896, Freud associated a history of sexual abuse with the symptomatology of some of his early cases of "hysteria" (Green 1993), although controversy regarding the validity of his observations persists (Gleaves and Hernandez 1999; Martin 1995).

In the early twentieth century, legal prohibitions of incest were developed (Jackson 1993). Awareness of the physical abuse of children increased tremendously after the publication of the paper "Battered Child Syndrome" by Kempe and colleagues in 1962. During the 1970s, cases of incest and sexual abuse were increasingly reported (Green 1993). Kempe continued his groundbreaking efforts to increase awareness by identifying sexual abuse as a profoundly underrecognized problem (Kempe 1978). Methodologically sophisticated research in child sexual abuse became more common during the 1980s (Green 1993). Child protective services were developed by states throughout the United States to investigate and pursue legal action against perpetrators of both physical and sexual abuse.

The advent of the acquired immunodeficiency syndrome (AIDS) epidemic brought sexual behavior to the focus of national discussion (Lindegren et al. 1998). However, sexual abuse is still significantly underreported, and awareness has not reached the required level, even among physicians, to ensure safety for children. In response to this reality, attempts have recently been made to identify childhood sexual abuse as a key national public health issue.

Epidemiology

Sexual abuse is unfortunately not rare, and the prevalence is routinely shown to be higher than is commonly perceived. Overall, government studies tend to report lower incidences of sexual abuse than do nongovernment studies (Yates 1997). Some retrospective studies have indicated that 10%–25% of girls are sexually victimized in some manner before age 18 (Fergusson et al. 1996b). Other studies report that as many as 34% (Wyatt et al. 1999) of women had been victimized by sexual abuse before age 18. The age of child victims ranges from infancy to adolescence. The most common age range of victims at the first incidence of abuse is between 8 and 11 years (Kempe 1978; Muram 2001).

As reported in Chapter 45 of this volume ("Physical Abuse of Children"), 1999 U.S. Department of Health and Human Services statistics note an overall decline in the incidence of child maltreatment. Still, more than 90,000 children were determined to be victims of sexual abuse as evaluated by child protective services organizations nationwide (U.S. Department of Health and Human Services 2001). This compares with approximately 114,000 cases of sexual abuse in 1994 (Finkelhor and Berliner 1995). Male parents or male parent figures were reported to be the most common perpetrators of sexual abuse among these victims, consistent with findings in previous years (U.S. Department of Health and Human Services 2001). Women are reported as abusers in a distinct minority of cases, and adolescents are reported to be the perpetrators in 20% of cases (American Academy of Pediatrics 1999).

Sexual abuse of boys has been less well studied than sexual abuse of girls and may be more significantly underreported and untreated (Moody 1999). Retrospective surveys have found that as many as 18% of males over age 18 reported having been victims of childhood sexual abuse (Finkelhor et al. 1990; Holmes and Slap 1998). Boys seem less likely to disclose abuse, generally for fear of disbelief, retribution, or social stigma and reluctance to admit vulnerability (Holmes and Slap 1998; Yates 1997). Perpetrators of abuse against boys are most likely to be male and unrelated to the victim (Holmes and Slap 1998). When the perpetrator is male, adolescent boys may worry about being considered homosexual, may be embarrassed by the implication, and hence may be even less likely to report such an occurrence. This can also lead to subsequent aggressive and homophobic behavior (Watkins and Bentovim 1992). Studies have also shown that sexually abused boys are more likely to ultimately express a homosexual identity compared with boys without such a history (Fromuth and Burkhart 1989). However, if the perpetrator is female, boys may be even more disinclined to report abuse and also may be less likely to be supported by caregivers when abuse is reported (Holmes and Slap 1998; Peluso and Putman 1996).

Etiology

The etiology of sexual abuse is considered to be multifactorial. Certain family characteristics have been described that can lead to child sexual abuse, although a specific family psychopathology has eluded reliable description. Despite the range of family characteristics, common themes of social isolation, enmeshment, and role confusion emerge, particularly in incestuous families in which the father sexually abuses a daughter. A rigid patriarchal structure and a poor marital relationship have been frequently described. As with many abusive households, social isolation may be perpetuated to prevent discovery. Fathers have been reported as being more likely to have an unstable job history, to abuse alcohol, and to be sexually and emotionally rejected by the spouse (Yates 1997). The incestuous father then seeks gratification from the daughter as an alternative to pursuing extramarital affairs (Mrazek and Mrazek 1981; Schetky and Green 1988). Some reports suggest that deep religiosity or social inhibition may lead to the selection of intrafamilial sexual abuse

rather than adulterous affairs (Yates 1997).

One recent study reports that households with impaired parenting and parents having adjustment problems are most often associated with sexual abuse. Specific findings include impaired parental bonding, increased frequency of divorce, parents having been raised by stepparents, and parental engagement in illicit or criminal behavior (Fergusson et al. 1996b). Overall patterns of sexual abuse more consistently occur in families that have significant instability and dysfunction associated with character or personality disorders versus major mental illness.

It is commonly believed that abusers were often themselves abused as children. Although the studies often have methodological difficulties, many authors have reported this to be the case, especially when studying adults. One study indicates that 35% of male perpetrators were themselves abused, and the likelihood of male victims becoming perpetrators was increased if the abuser was a female relative (Glasser et al. 2001). Mothers who were abused as children may unconsciously recreate scenarios of abuse by transferring parental roles to a daughter, who ultimately becomes incestuously involved with an abusive father (Yates 1997).

Sexual abuse is similarly prevalent in all socioeconomic classes (Fergusson et al. 1996b), whereas neglect and physical abuse may be more common in lower socioeconomic classes (Wissow 1995). Abusers have a racial, religious, and ethnic profile that is similar to that of the general population (Ryan et al. 1996). Domestic violence and other sorts of physical or emotional abuse are frequently present in families of a sexually victimized child. Child sexual abuse may fit into a global pattern of abuse within such households (Bowen 2000).

■ Profiles of Perpetrators

Perpetrators have a wide variety of character and personality pathology. However, a common theme among abusers is that they regard their victims not as independent but instead as narcissistic extensions of themselves, existing only for the purposes of their own gratification (Glasser et al. 2001). Abusers select children based on age, gender, and physical characteristics—all of which primarily reflect their emotional needs more than sexual attraction. Those who have been abused may select victims with characteristics that match their own appearance or age when they were first abused.

Abusers have been described as passive and inadequate in most aspects of their lives; contact with children gives them feelings of power and control (Hilton and Mezey 1996).

Perpetrators may associate themselves with events or circumstances where they have access to children. Examples include youth group activities, schools, recreational facilities, or locations near playgrounds or other areas that youths may frequently be found. Abusers may seek to "groom" victims, offering them gifts or money in order to gain their trust prior to engaging in any abusive behavior (Hilton and Mezey 1996). Perpetrators may also encourage individual children to recruit other children to participate in abusive activities along with the perpetrator.

Perpetrators of sexual abuse are most often male and most often select female victims (U.S. Department of Health and Human Services 2001). Perpetrators are usually gender specific regarding their victims; those who select both male and female victims may have more severe psychopathology (Hilton and Mezey 1996). Intrafamilial victimization or victimization by known perpetrators is generally more common than sexual abuse from an unknown or extrafamilial source (Faller 1994). Less is known about female perpetrators of abuse. Women are less likely to be reported as sexual abusers (Bell 1999). Up to half of female perpetrators reported were adolescent babysitters (Holmes and Slap 1998). Women were less likely to sexually abuse younger boys, and the boys were far less likely to report the abuse or believe themselves to have been abused (Bell 1999).

Children and adolescents constitute a significant percentage of the perpetrators of sexual abuse. Approximately 30%–50% of the instances of sexual abuse are perpetrated by those under age 18, and most initially engage in abusive acts before age 15 (Shaw 1999). The Federal Bureau of Investigation indicates that 15% of those arrested for forcible rape were under age 18 (Ryan et al. 1996). The Uniform Data Collection System developed by the National Adolescent Perpetrator Network has extensively collected sociodemographic information on perpetrators (Ryan et al. 1996). In the study by Ryan and colleagues, nearly 40% of abusive youths reported having been sexually abused themselves. More than 60% were known to school systems as having truancy or behavior or learning problems at school. The majority of female adolescents who abuse have been abused themselves. These adolescents were generally abused at younger ages and

were three times as likely to have been abused by a female (Shaw 1999; Mathews et al. 1997). Sexually abusive youths most frequently have comorbid conduct disorder, mood disorders, and anxiety disorders (Shaw 1999). The number of psychiatric diagnoses increases as the age of first offense decreases (Shaw et al. 1996).

■ Theoretical Models of Psychopathology

Four factors have been suggested to describe the extent to which a child is traumatized by sexual abuse. These include traumatic sexualization, powerlessness, stigmatization, and betrayal. Premature stimulation leads to the inappropriate traumatization of early sexual behavior in the service of nonsexual as well as sexual needs. In such a situation the youngster is rendered powerless, and the lack of control leads to feelings of fear, anxiety, and helplessness. Stigmatization occurs, especially after the abuse is discovered. Negative reactions from caregivers or other adults can lead the child to believe that he or she is bad or damaged, which exacerbates feelings of shame and guilt. Disillusionment and anger result secondarily from the betrayal that stems from mistreatment by a person who is trusted (Finkelhor and Browne 1986).

Schetky and Green (1988) cite a somewhat different list of factors that influence the sexually abused child's symptomatology and outcome. These are the age and developmental level of the child; the onset, duration, and frequency of the abuse; the degree of coercion and physical trauma; the relationship between the child and the perpetrator; the child's preexisting personality; and the interaction between acute and long-term variables. The manner in which the system handles the case and the family's reaction after disclosure are also very important determinants of outcome.

A transactional model has been proposed by Spaccarelli (1994) in which the stress of sexual abuse emerges from a series of abuse events, abuse-related events, and disclosure-related events that all influence the outcome. The child's cognitive appraisal and response to the events, as well as developmental and environmental factors, mitigate the damage. This model takes into consideration the broad range of immediate reactions and long-term outcomes that can be found after sexual abuse. A similar model is proposed by Briere and Elliott (1994), in which the distress manifested by a given individual is a function of many abuse-specific variables as well as of individual and environmental factors operating before or after the abuse. Such approaches may effectively demythologize sexual abuse, equating it to a number of other stressors that can affect children.

Clinical Presentation

■ Behavioral Findings

Children who are victims of sexual abuse exhibit a variety of emotional and behavioral symptoms. Presentation to mental health professionals is often varied and may mask underlying sexual abuse. The age at onset of the sexual abuse plays an important role in subsequent presenting symptoms. Many authors have reported aggression and disruptive behaviors in children who are victims of abuse. However, younger children seem more likely to have angry reactions and externalizing symptoms. Victims under age 7 tend to have more hypersexual behavior, self-exposing, and victimizing sexual behaviors toward others (McClellan et al. 1996). Older children may be more likely to engage in substance abuse or delinquent behavior (Yates 1997). Cultural background may play a role in differing symptom presentation. Asian victims have been reported to have less externalizing behavior and more suicidality (Rao et al. 1992). Boys have been described as having more externalizing problems than girls have, but that notion is likely an oversimplification. Boys may in fact have more complex problems than do girls (Garnefski and Diekstra 1997).

Eroticized behavior or sexual acting out is commonly seen in victims of abuse. Exhibitionism, excessive masturbation, simulated sexual activity, or sexually provocative behavior may be prominent. (Kolko et al. 1988; Mrazek and Mrazek 1981) Sexual preoccupation may be evident in victims' play or conversations at inappropriate times with both adults and peers. Artwork or play may reflect themes of sexual activity or sexual aggression.

Fire-setting behavior has also been noted in abused children (Lowenstein 1989). Some reports indicate that sexually abused children are overrepresented among fire setters (Puri et al. 1995). Clinical anecdotes have been noted involving sexually abused children who preferentially set fire to beds or mattresses.

Although externalizing behaviors are frequently seen, sexually abused children commonly exhibit internalizing behaviors as well, such as being withdrawn or isolatory. In addition, depression and anxiety are commonly reported. Many children have feelings of guilt and the notion that they are responsible for or deserving of the abusers' behavior. Alternatively, children may feel as if the abusive relationship is idyllic and constitutes evidence of their positive regard on the part of the abuser. This may lead to difficulty in interrupting the abuse and may provide significant resistance to treatment. Behavioral symptoms such as phobias, anxiety reactions, or disruptive behaviors may initially be presented to pediatricians or other primary care providers.

■ Medical Findings

Victims of sexual abuse commonly present to pediatricians. Frequently, the presenting complaints are vague and may take the form of abdominal pain, headaches, enuresis, encopresis, and sleep dysregulation. Children are often highly secretive or vague regarding such complaints for fear of reprisals coming from the perpetrator.

Certain physical findings such as irritation of the vulva, repeated urinary tract infections, hematuria, blood in the stool, or anal fissures can be commonly identified in sexually abused children but are nevertheless nonspecific. Pediatric consultation is of paramount importance to appropriately consider alternative diagnostic possibilities. Sometimes the presenting symptoms, such as rectal or genital bleeding or sexually transmitted diseases, are highly suggestive of sexual abuse. Specific findings such as a dilated hymen or anus, bruising, scarring, or perianal tearing are important findings to discern and to document appropriately (Atabaki and Paradise 1999; Hobbs et al. 1995; Shaw 1999).

The presence of sexually transmitted diseases may or may not confirm the occurrence of sexual activity or abuse. Generally, gonorrhea, genital herpes, or syphilis definitively diagnosed in a child outside of the perinatal period usually confirms the occurrence of sexual activity and possible sexual abuse. The presence of human immunodeficiency virus (HIV), chlamydia, or anogenital condylomata acuminata should raise suspicion for sexual abuse but may not represent diagnostic certainty (Atabaki and Paradise 1999; Shaw 1999). Definitive findings confirming sexual activity include pregnancy or the presence of semen. Pregnancy in an adolescent should always lead to an inquiry as to the possibility of sexual abuse. A sexual abuse history is often present in adolescents who become sexually active early, and some reports indicate that up to two-thirds of pregnant adolescents have experienced sexual abuse (Elders and Albert 1998).

Emergency room physicians are commonly called on to perform acute evaluations that include crisis management and evidence collection. Physical examination should be done promptly. However, if the abuse has occurred in the previous 72 hours, physical examinations should be performed immediately with the goal of obtaining reliable physical evidence. It is recommended that a physician trained in conducting sexual abuse evaluations perform the examination. The examination should be done a minimum number of times by the smallest possible number of clinicians. The assessment should be done as part of a comprehensive physical examination to deemphasize the genital findings. Sexually abused children frequently do not have corroborating physical findings (Bernet 1997). Obtaining evidence from a physical examination is exquisitely important; if physical evidence is present, perpetrators are 2.5 times as likely to receive legal consequences (Palusci et al. 1999).

The American Academy of Pediatrics (Shaw 1999) has outlined comprehensive guidelines for the necessary physical examination after sexual abuse; among them are the following:

- The examination should not cause additional emotional trauma. Appropriate time must be allowed to account for the child's anxiety.
- Careful explanation of every step should precede the examination.
- Particular attention needs to be given to examination of the mouth, genitals, perineal region, anus, buttocks, and thighs.
- A supportive adult known to the child as well as a nursing chaperone should be present.
- The examination should be thorough, including developmental, growth, mental, and emotional factors as well as physical findings.
- History taking should be thorough and ideally should be obtained before the physical examination. Care should be taken not to suggest answers to questions.
- If collection of forensic samples is imperative and the child is unable to cooperate, use of sedation should be considered.
- Appropriate agency reporting and thorough documentation of findings as well as the child's statements and behavior are essential.

- The physician should offer reassurance, such as "your body will heal and recover" [Elders and Albert 1998].

■ Diagnostic Considerations and Comorbidity

Children who are victims of sexual abuse do not have a well-defined postabuse symptom profile. Sexual abuse may also yield limited or mild symptoms that may not require psychiatric attention. Symptoms and sequelae vary widely, stemming from the variability in timing, duration, frequency, and specific characteristics of the abuse as well as an individual child's resilience and vulnerability to particular major mental illness. Many children and adolescents who are hospitalized with other presenting problems have underlying and often undisclosed histories of sexual abuse. An abuse history is an integral component of any psychiatric evaluation, particularly in hospitalized patients.

Several sophisticated assessment tools offer standardized methods to assess normative and nonnormative sexual behavior or occurrence of trauma. Such measures include the Child Sexual Behavior Inventory (Friedrich 1997; Friedrich et al. 2001) and the Childhood Trauma Questionnaire (Bernstein et al. 1997). However, caution must be employed when using any single method of screening to identify abuse. A multidimensional assessment approach is vastly preferable (Babiker and Herbert 1998).

Depression has frequently been observed in sexually abused children, particularly among adolescents (Brand et al. 1996; Wozencraft et al. 1991). Victims often feel hopeless and helpless to prevent further victimization, and such feelings can be the core of their symptom profiles of major depression. Suicidal gestures and self-injurious behavior have been shown to be prominent in the months following the initiation of an incestuous relationship (Wozencraft et al. 1991). Depression and suicidal behavior are overrepresented among adolescent inpatients with a history of sexual abuse (Brand et al. 1996; Rew et al. 2001). Depression may be refractory to treatment, especially if appropriate attention is not given to disclosing the abuse history and ensuring safety.

Bipolar disorder is an important diagnosis to consider in children or adolescents who are hypersexual and even sexually abusive of others. Children and adolescents with manic states of bipolar disorder may be more impulsive and sexually provocative. This can lead them to be reckless in terms of seeking social interaction or sexual activity and to be vulnerable to the actions of abusers. Excessive gregarious behavior and curiosity may be misinterpreted as sexual interest or consent.

Disruptive behavior disorders are common in younger children who have been sexually abused. Symptoms of hyperactivity, aggression, and motor restlessness may be especially prominent, particularly when such behavior represents a change from baseline functioning. This may reflect a history of abuse versus a primary diagnosis of attention-deficit/hyperactivity disorder (ADHD). The symptom profiles may be so similar that it is important to rule out any kind of abuse before definitively diagnosing ADHD (Weinstein et al. 2000).

Anxiety disorders may take many forms, including phobias, social anxiety, generalized anxiety disorder, and posttraumatic stress disorder (PTSD). Symptoms of PTSD include fear reactions, reexperiencing phenomena, flashbacks, sleep disruption, exaggerated startle response, and hyperacuity, as well as general anxiety and deterioration of premorbid functioning. Sexual abuse is one of a number of traumatic situations that can lead to the occurrence of PTSD in children and adolescents. Studies in adolescents have shown that chronicity and severity of abuse increases the likelihood of a PTSD diagnosis (Brand et al. 1996).

Dissociative disorders are difficult to discern in younger children, especially before age 7 when faculties of concrete reasoning are generally less well developed. It is important to discern the subject of the dissociation. Dissociation may be present in victims of sexual abuse more often than in victims of physical abuse (Kisiel and Lyons 2001). Some children may have dissociative experiences as defense mechanisms or as a manner of reexperiencing or gaining understanding and mastery over the abusive experience.

Eating disorders, including bulimia nervosa and anorexia nervosa, have been identified in sexual abuse victims. Some authors report that eating disorders stem from an early history of sexual abuse (Wonderlich et al. 2000, 2001), although others have found no such association (Kinzl et al. 1994; Pope 1992). Family background is likely to be a more significant predictor of the development of an eating disorder than the presence or absence of sexual abuse (Kinzl et al. 1994).

Treatment

Treatment of sexually abused children is complicated and usually must be multidisciplinary. The most important concern must be the current and future safety of the child, and this should be communicated early on to the child and caregivers. The treatment must first begin with the assessment of the nature of the abuse and the identification of whether the abuse occurs inside or outside the child's family (American Academy of Child and Adolescent Psychiatry 1988). The next step is generally to ensure the safety of the child both from becoming victimized by further abuse and from potential sequelae of the abuse. Reporting to child protective services needs to occur as soon as possible, preferably in the context of the initial evaluation or first disclosure.

Therapeutic techniques vary depending on the developmental level of the child. The manner of interaction is critical for a successful intervention. Children must be comfortable to reveal details of abuse. The clinician should take care to avoid asking leading questions, suggesting answers, or reacting with shock or surprise when children discuss abuse experiences. Clinicians should be sensitive to the consequences that may ensue following the results of such disclosure and should not make impossible promises regarding reporting events to the appropriate authorities.

Selection of an appropriate clinician is key to ensuring success in treatment. Gender and age issues cannot be ignored. Given that the sexually abused child may be traumatized catastrophically, every effort should be made to improve the likelihood of a successful therapeutic alliance. This may mean selecting therapists of the same gender or selecting age to the degree that can facilitate rapport and avoid undue physical similarity to perpetrators. Adolescent girls may be more resistant to discussing certain topics of abuse with a male counselor (Moon et al. 2000). Therapists must be conscious of the transference and countertransference issues that may emerge in the course of therapy. Appropriate care of the patient demands that therapists have adequately reconciled any of their own personal issues of trauma or abuse.

Treatment of ensuing psychiatric disorders should be done promptly and should involve consultation with a child and adolescent psychiatrist. Particular attention should be given to diagnosing potential life-threatening psychiatric illness such as depression and to identifying clear target symptoms for any type of pharmacological or nonpharmacological treatments. Treatment for depression and PTSD not only can provide symptom relief but may also allow the child to be more available for psychotherapeutic interventions.

Treatment models are varied and continue to be controversial (Finkelhor and Berliner 1995). Some questions remain regarding whether general supportive psychotherapy is preferable to abuse-specific psychotherapy. However, cognitive-behavioral therapy that is somewhat more abuse specific was superior to supportive counseling in a 12-month follow-up study (Cohen and Mannarino 1998). Cognitive-behavioral treatment may have particular utility in children who have PTSD symptoms (Deblinger et al. 1999).

In any abuse-specific therapy it is important to consider the notion of retraumatization. Therapists must be exceedingly sensitive to issues of resistance and the pace that is necessary for successful treatment. Many victims may not directly confront the realities of their abuse but instead may benefit sufficiently from a problem-oriented approach or supportive approach. Despite this fact, it is prudent for the therapist early on to make clear the reason for the initiation of the therapy and to point out behavior patterns that may be maladaptive as a result.

Perception and attribution of the abuse are key elements to be identified in therapy and have important implications in treatment planning and course (Cohen and Mannarino 2000). Children may not regard the particular acts as malevolent and in fact may not consider that they have been abused. The focus of individual therapy frequently includes efforts to reduce self-blame and to attribute responsibility for the abusive acts to the perpetrator (Celano et al. 2002). The overall goals of treatment have to be clearly focused on behavioral and functional issues that need improvement. A significant number of children may not require protracted courses of treatment immediately after the occurrence of abuse. Individual cases merit specific consideration in terms of the mode, duration, and frequency of therapy; flexibility on the part of the therapist is essential.

Group therapy may benefit older adolescents who have relatively positive self-esteem. Ideal candidates for group therapy have emotional and cognitive capacities both to benefit from the experience and not to impair the treatment of others (Sturkie 1994). Specific activities, including role-playing and games to improve communication skills, can be effective in group settings (Celano 1990). When recommending group treatment, consideration also depends on pending legal proceedings (Faller 1994). It may be inadvisable to involve a victim in group treatment before the individual is to give legal testimony because the information

may be rejected or perceived as having been contaminated by suggestion from others.

Family therapy or individual therapy for a parent is often necessary to assist caregivers in coming to terms with their own responses to the child's victimization (Grosz et al. 2000). Nonoffending parents often have issues of guilt or depression regarding the fact that they were unable to prevent the child's victimization. Treatment that includes individual therapy for nonoffending parents can improve the psychosocial functioning of the abused child (Celano et al. 1996). Furthermore, a parent's own issues of childhood sexual abuse may emerge and may ultimately be disclosed coincidentally with the child's treatment. Family therapy can help to establish appropriate boundaries and roles for family members and can help avoid scapegoating the victim (Hilton and Mezey 1996).

False Accusations

False accusations of sexual abuse and recantation of previous disclosures of abuse are not uncommon (Bernet 1997). Children may make false accusations of sexual abuse for a wide range of conscious or unconscious reasons. In general, children have imperfect memories for events, and memories of abuse become more inaccurate over time, particularly in younger children (Goodman and Saywitz 1994). Children are suggestible and may prefer to recount events in a manner that will please a parent or other adult.

In circumstances of divorce or custody dispute, a parent may initiate allegations of child sexual abuse against a spouse with or without corroborating evidence from the child. Contentious spouses or ex-spouses may coach children to make unfounded disclosures. Such children may have vague or changing narratives and may even look to the parent for assistance in perpetuating the false account. Older children may make accusations regarding sexual abuse to exact revenge or express anger toward a parent or other adult.

Such occurrences emphasize the need for careful evaluation, interviewing, and documentation procedures as well as sophisticated treatment and support for victims and their family members. Children who are genuinely victims of abuse most often are embarrassed, ashamed, and less willing to reveal details of the events. In contrast, children who falsely accuse may embellish events, incorporate unrealistic details, and have relatively little discomfort in revealing the alleged abusive acts (Yates 1997).

Legal Considerations

Legal considerations are important in the initial stages of evaluation. Physicians and mental health clinicians are mandated by all 50 states to report suspected cases of child sexual abuse. The specific requirements in terms of timing, level of suspicion, and other details vary according to state guidelines. Most important is prompt referral to a child protective services organization to ensure appropriate collection and validation of forensic information. The forensic evaluation should be performed by a clinician who is trained in forensic assessment; this individual usually should not be the physician or therapist who is involved in ongoing treatment. This increases the level of objectivity and the quality of evidence and may preserve the child's perceived safety and alliance with the treating clinician.

Confidentiality issues must be clarified before a forensic evaluation. The fact that an evaluation is being done for purposes of court proceedings needs to be made clear to the parents and child from the outset. The usual handling of medical records must be adjusted to provide requisite information to reporting agencies and to make legal procedures effective. Treating clinicians should document direct statements of disclosure in the medical record, preferably as quotations. Depending on specific legal circumstances, such information may obviate the need for direct testimony from the child victim (Kermani 1993).

Guidelines for forensic evaluation of children have been published by the American Academy of Child and Adolescent Psychiatry (1988; Bernet 1997) and by the American Professional Society on the Abuse of Children (1990). Although there is no absolute standard for forensic evaluations, some of the key points include the following:

- The overall goals of the assessment are to maintain objectivity, to avoid biasing or leading questions, and ultimately to discover the truth about what occurred during incidents of suspected abuse.
- A gentle, nonthreatening demeanor that avoids retraumatization is essential.
- Assessment of a child's developmental level, medical or psychiatric conditions, and basic cognitive function should be made.

- A stepwise interview approach that begins with nonabuse topics and general questions then progresses to abuse topics and specific questions is most effective (Bernet 1997).
- Specialized techniques requiring special training, such as use of drawings or anatomical dolls, may be necessary for younger children but are not essential. The information must be considered only as a part of the comprehensive interview, because there is controversy about low sensitivity and specificity of these techniques.
- Psychological testing and screening checklists may be useful for treatment purposes but do not provide definitive evidence of sexual abuse.

Physician Awareness

Sexual abuse is often undetected by physicians. Some physicians miss cases because of discomfort related to discussing sexual topics. Primary care pediatricians attribute lack of recognition of sexual abuse to a lack of focus on such topics during their training (Leder et al. 1999). Commonly, physicians do not appreciate the fact that abusers themselves are frequently minors (Olsen and Kalbfleisch 2001). Clinicians may also find it difficult to isolate the occurrence of sexual abuse in the context of severe family disruption and existing involvement by social services agencies for other reasons. Educational interventions for pediatricians, family practitioners, and gynecologists have yielded positive results (Leder et al. 1999; Olsen and Kalbfleisch 2001). Educational strategies to improve physician documentation of critical examination findings have also proved to be worthwhile efforts (Socolar et al. 1998).

Prognosis

Childhood sexual abuse is well recognized to be associated with long-term psychiatric and emotional difficulties (Green 1993; MacMillan et al. 2001; Paolucci et al. 2001). Some controlled and prospective outcome studies have identified positive outcomes related to successful treatment. Many reports that find more negative outcomes are retrospective surveys of victims who were identified long after the abuse, often as adults.

Positive outcomes are possible despite egregious abuse scenarios. Prognosis after sexual abuse depends on many factors, including familial, demographic, and treatment characteristics. A degree of stability within the family plays an important role. In general, parent support and involvement in treatment along with the affected child yields a significantly better outcome (Cohen and Mannarino 1996, 1998; Tremblay et al. 1999).

A 5-year follow-up treatment study revealed a worse outcome for children who initially present with depression or low self-esteem (Tebbutt et al. 1997). Family variables and abuse characteristics were observed to be less important predictors of dysfunction. Hypersexuality and aggressive behavior may be particularly resistant to change (Finkelhor and Berliner 1995). Adolescent victims may have continuing problems of increased sexual activity and increased behaviors that carry high risk for exposure to HIV (Brown et al. 1997).

Many studies, including the National Comorbidity Survey, report an increased risk in adulthood among victims of childhood sexual abuse for the subsequent development of mood, anxiety, and substance use disorders (Bulik et al. 2001; Dinwiddie et al. 2000; Fergusson et al. 1996a; Kendler et al. 2000; Merry and Andrews 1994; Molnar et al. 2001b; Pribor and Dinwiddie 1992; Stevenson 1999). Abuse factors that increase the likelihood of subsequent psychopathology include a higher degree of violence, completed intercourse, and a negative response when the abuse was disclosed (Bulik et al. 2001). Adults with depression and a history of childhood sexual abuse more commonly report an initial suicide attempt in adolescence (Molnar et al. 2001a) or have prolonged episodes of depression (Zlotnick et al. 2001). Adults who have a personality disorder have an increased likelihood of reporting sexual abuse in childhood (Johnson et al. 1999). Furthermore, coping styles, social interaction styles, and defense mechanisms may be significantly more immature in adults with a history of childhood sexual abuse (Romans et al. 1999; Tong et al. 1987).

The long-term outcome may also vary depending on the attribution of the sexual abuse. In a study of incarcerated men, those who had experienced sexual abuse but did not perceive the activity as abusive had increased levels of alcohol abuse. Those who did perceive the acts as abusive had increased prevalence of PTSD (Fondacaro et al. 1999). Adult women who had been victims of incest were significantly more depressed if they perceived the abuse as attributable to their own qualities versus the result of circumstances external to themselves

or beyond their control (Morrow 1991).

Adults with a history of childhood sexual abuse can also be vulnerable to subsequent victimization as adults (Coid et al. 2001; Messman-Moore et al. 2000). Low self-esteem, self-blame, and reexperiencing phenomena can lead adult victims to engage in high-risk activity and revictimization (Arata 2000). College-age women with a history of sexual abuse have an increased likelihood to be victims of aggression in a dating relationship (Banyard et al. 2000).

Adult victims may have unsatisfactory relationships or difficulties with intimacy or sexual functioning of their own. Mothers who were sexually abused may have problematic parenting styles. One study reports an increased likelihood of overly permissive parenting practices, similar to those found in adult children of alcoholics (Ruscio 2001).

Prevention

The Centers for Disease Control and Prevention recently developed important summary recommendations to raise awareness of and improve efforts for primary prevention (McMahon and Puett 1999). This includes educating children about "bad touch" and empowering them to resist abusers (Durfee 1989). School-based primary prevention programs have been shown to be effective in raising awareness, particularly when used over a long term and with older as well as younger children (Adler and McCain 1994; Davis and Gidycz 2000; Hebert et al. 2001; MacIntyre and Carr 1999). Recent efforts have included providing outreach to adults who are abusers or victims themselves (Chasan-Taber and Tabachnick 1999).

Research Issues

Recent research has increased understanding of the neurophysiological changes associated with trauma in maltreated children. Cortisol is an important regulatory hormone related to chronic and acute stress. Children who have experienced both physical and sexual abuse had substantial elevations in morning cortisol levels (Cicchetti and Rogosch 2001). Adult women with a history of childhood sexual abuse may have persisting irregular cortisol levels or impaired hypothalamic-pituitary-adrenal (HPA) reactivity (Heim et al.

2000; Steiger et al. 2001). The HPA axis has been most recently suspected to play an important role in the pathogenesis of depressive symptoms (Weiss et al. 1999). It has also been shown that growth hormone response patterns are markedly impaired in boys who have been sexually abused (Jensen et al. 1991).

Neuroanatomical changes have been studied in women with histories of childhood sexual abuse, some with resultant PTSD. Two small studies using positron emission tomography have reported increased activity in some key prefrontal and temporal brain regions (Bremner et al. 1999; Shin et al. 1999). The prefrontal cortex and other regions in the temporal lobe and cingulate gyrus have been suspected to be important in the pathophysiology of PTSD.

Unfortunately, funded research on sexual abuse of children has not kept pace with other efforts in medical research (Finkelhor 1998). These studies are difficult to conduct. The determination that sexual abuse has occurred is often elusive even for well-trained mental health clinicians. It is often impractical or even unethical to involve abused children in controlled research protocols, particularly if there are acute treatment needs or necessary legal proceedings that can confound the clinical study. Retrospective studies are frequently insufficient to describe the full impact of the problem. The wide variety of sexual abuse phenomena as well as varying characteristics and circumstances of victims make homogeneous samples for study difficult to obtain. Furthermore, it is difficult to generalize the impact from restrictive samples to larger clinical samples (Finkelhor and Berliner 1995).

It is clear, however, that childhood sexual abuse is widely prevalent and that the impact of abuse is far-reaching. Many adult sexual offenders begin patterns of abusive behavior in childhood, and significant sequelae continue for victims of abuse. Providing grounds for optimism, outcome studies have shown that treatment programs for victims as well as abusers yielded improvement in symptoms and prevented subsequent victimization. Therefore, future research efforts need to expand and focus on early prevention, identification, and intervention strategies.

References

Adler NA, McCain JL: Prevention of child abuse: issues for the mental health practitioner. Child Adolesc Psychiatr Clin N Am 3:679–693, 1994

American Academy of Child and Adolescent Psychiatry: Perspective: guidelines for the clinical evaluation of child and adolescent sexual abuse. J Am Acad Child Adolesc Psychiatry 27:655–657, 1988

American Academy of Pediatrics Committee on Child Abuse and Neglect: Guidelines for the evaluation of sexual abuse of children: subject review. Pediatrics 103:186–191, 1999

American Professional Society on the Abuse of Children: Guidelines for Psychosocial Evaluation of Suspected Sexual Abuse in Young Children. Chicago, IL, American Professional Society on the Abuse of Children, 1990

Arata CM: From child victim to adult victim: a model for predicting sexual revictimization. Child Maltreat 5:28–38, 2000

Atabaki S, Paradise JE: The medical evaluation of the sexually abused child: lessons from a decade of research. Pediatrics 104:178–186, 1999

Babiker G, Herbert M: Critical issues in the assessment of child sexual abuse. Clin Child Fam Psychol Rev 1:231–252, 1998

Banyard VL, Arnold S, Smith J: Childhood sexual abuse and dating experiences of undergraduate women. Child Maltreat 5:39–48, 2000

Bell K: Female offenders of sexual assault. J Emerg Nurs 25:241–243, 1999

Bernet W: Practice parameters for the forensic evaluation of children and adolescents who may have been physically or sexually abused. American Academy of Child and Adolescent Psychiatry. J Am Acad Child Adolesc Psychiatry 36 (10, suppl):37S–56S, 1997

Bernstein DP, Ahluvalia T, Pogge D, et al: Validity of the childhood trauma questionnaire in an adolescent psychiatric population. J Am Acad Child Adolesc Psychiatry 36:340–348, 1997

Bowen K: Child abuse and domestic violence in families of children seen for suspected sexual abuse. Clin Pediatr (Phila) 39:33–40, 2000

Brand EF, King CA, Olson E, et al: Depressed adolescents with a history of sexual abuse: diagnostic comorbidity and suicidality. J Am Acad Child Adolesc Psychiatry 35:34–41, 1996

Bremner JD, Narayan M, Staib LH, et al: Neural correlates of memories of childhood sexual abuse in women with and without posttraumatic stress disorder. Am J Psychiatry 156:1787–1795, 1999

Briere JN, Elliott DM: Immediate and long-term impacts of child sexual abuse. Future Child 4:54–69, 1994

Brown LK, Kessel SM, Lourie KJ, et al: Influence of sexual abuse on HIV-related attitudes and behaviors in adolescent psychiatric inpatients. J Am Acad Child Adolesc Psychiatry 36:316–322, 1997

Bulik CM, Prescott CA, Kendler KS: Features of childhood sexual abuse and the development of psychiatric and substance use disorders. Br J Psychiatry 179:444–449, 2001

Celano MP: Activities and games for group psychotherapy with sexually abused children. Int J Group Psychother 40:419–429, 1990

Celano M, Hazzard A, Webb C, et al: Treatment of traumagenic beliefs among sexually abused girls and their mothers: an evaluation study. J Abnorm Child Psychol 24:1–17, 1996

Celano M, Hazzard A, Campbell SK, et al: Attribution retraining with sexually abused children: review of techniques. Child Maltreat 7:65–76, 2002

Chasan-Taber L, Tabachnick J: Evaluation of a child sexual abuse prevention program. Sex Abuse 11:279–292, 1999

Cicchetti D, Rogosch FA: Diverse patterns of neuroendocrine activity in maltreated children. Dev Psychopathol 13:677–693, 2001

Cohen JA, Mannarino AP: Factors that mediate treatment outcome of sexually abused preschool children. J Am Acad Child Adolesc Psychiatry 34:1402–1410, 1996

Cohen JA, Mannarino AP: Factors that mediate treatment outcome of sexually abused preschool children: six and 12 month follow-up. J Am Acad Child Adolesc Psychiatry 37:44–51, 1998

Cohen JA, Mannarino AP: Predictors of treatment outcome in sexually abused children. Child Abuse Negl 24:983–994, 2000

Coid J, Petruckevitch A, Feder G, et al: Relation between childhood sexual and physical abuse and risk of revictimisation in women: a cross-sectional survey. Lancet 358:450–454, 2001

Davis MK, Gidycz CA: Child sexual abuse prevention programs: a meta-analysis. J Clin Child Psychol 29:257–265, 2000

Deblinger E, Steer RA, Lippman J: Two-year follow-up study of cognitive behavioral therapy for sexually abused children suffering post-traumatic stress symptoms. Child Abuse Negl 23:1371–1378, 1999

Dinwiddie S, Heath AC, Dunne MP, et al: Early sexual abuse and lifetime psychopathology: a co-twin-control study. Psychol Med 30:41–52, 2000

Durfee M: Prevention of child sexual abuse. Psychiatr Clin North Am 12:445–453, 1989

Elders JM, Albert AE: Adolescent pregnancy and sexual abuse. JAMA 280:648–649, 1998

Faller KC: Extrafamilial sexual abuse. Child Adolesc Psychiatr Clin North Am 3:713–727, 1994

Fergusson DM, Horwood LJ, Lynskey MT: Childhood sexual abuse and psychiatric disorder in young adulthood, II: psychiatric outcomes of childhood sexual abuse. J Am Acad Child Adolesc Psychiatry 34:1365–1374, 1996a

Fergusson DM, Lynskey MT, Horwood LJ: Childhood sexual abuse and psychiatric disorder in young adulthood, I: prevalence of sexual abuse and factors associated with sexual abuse. J Am Acad Child Adolesc Psychiatry 34:1355–1364, 1996b

Finkelhor D: Improving research, policy, and practice to understand child sexual abuse. JAMA 280:1864–1865, 1998

Finkelhor D, Berliner L: Research on the treatment of sexually abused children: a review and recommendations. J Am Acad Child Adolesc Psychiatry 34:1408–1423, 1995

Finkelhor D, Browne A: Initial and long-term effects: conceptual framework, in Sourcebook on Child Sexual Abuse. Edited by Finkelhor D. Beverly Hills, CA, Sage, 1986, pp 180–198

Finkelhor D, Hotaling G, Lewis IA, et al: Sexual abuse in a national survey of adult men and women: prevalence, characteristics, and risk factors. Child Abuse Negl 14:19–28, 1990

Fondacaro KM, Holt JC, Powell TA: Psychological impact of childhood sexual abuse on male inmates: the importance of perception. Child Abuse Negl 23:361–369, 1999

Friedrich WN: CSBI: Child Sexual Behavior Inventory. Professional Manual. Odessa, FL, Psychological Assessment Resources, 1997

Friedrich WN, Fisher J, Broughton D, et al: Normative sexual behavior in children: a contemporary sample. Pediatrics 101(4):E9, 1998

Friedrich WN, Fisher JL, Dittner CA, et al: Child Sexual Behavior Inventory: normative, psychiatric, and sexual abuse comparisons. Child Maltreat 6:37–49, 2001

Fromuth ME, Burkhart BR: Long-term psychological correlates of childhood sexual abuse in two samples of college men. Child Abuse Negl 13:533–542, 1989

Garnefski N, Diekstra RFW: Child sexual abuse and emotional and behavioral problems in adolescence: gender differences. J Am Acad Child Adolesc Psychiatry 36:323–329, 1997

Glasser M, Kolvin I, Campbell D, et al: Cycle of child sexual abuse: links between being a victim and becoming a perpetrator. Br J Psychiatry 179:482–494, 2001

Gleaves DH, Hernandez E: Recent reformulations of Freud's development and abandonment of his seduction theory: historical/scientific clarification or a continued assault on truth? Hist Psychol 2:304–354, 1999

Goodman GS, Saywitz KJ: Memories of abuse: interviewing children when sexual victimization is suspected. Child Adolesc Psychiatr Clin N Am 3:645–661, 1994

Green AH: Child sexual abuse: immediate and long-term effects and intervention. J Am Acad Child Adolesc Psychiatry 32:890–902, 1993

Grosz CA, Kempe RS, Kelly M: Extrafamilial sexual abuse: treatment for child victims and their families. Child Abuse Negl 24:9–23, 2000

Haugaard JJ: The challenge of defining child sexual abuse. Am Psychol 55:1036–1039, 2000

Hebert M, Lavoie F, Piche C, et al: Proximate effects of a child sexual abuse prevention program in elementary school children. Child Abuse Negl 25:505–522, 2001

Heim C, Newport DJ, Heit S, et al: Pituitary-adrenal and autonomic responses to stress in women after sexual and physical abuse in childhood. JAMA 284:592–597, 2000

Hilton MR, Mezey GC: Victims and perpetrators of child sexual abuse. Br J Psychiatry 169:408–421, 1996

Hlaing WM: Sexual solicitation of youth on the Internet (letter). JAMA 286:1176–1177, 2001

Hobbs CJ, Wynne JM, Thomas AJ: Colposcopic genital findings in prepubertal girls assessed for sexual abuse. Arch Dis Child 73:465–469, 1995

Holmes WC, Slap GB: Sexual abuse of boys: definition, prevalence, correlates, sequelae, and management. JAMA 280:1855–1862, 1998

Jackson S: Childhood and sexuality in historical perspective. Child Adolesc Psychiatr Clin N Am 2:355–367, 1993

Jensen JB, Pease JJ, Bensel RT, et al: Growth hormone response patterns in sexually or physically abused boys. J Am Acad Child Adolesc Psychiatry 30:784–790, 1991

Johnson JG, Cohen P, Brown J, et al: Childhood maltreatment increases risk for personality disorders during early adulthood. Arch Gen Psychiatry 56:600–606, 1999

Kempe CH: Sexual abuse, another hidden pediatric problem: the 1977 C. Anderson Aldrich Lecture. Pediatrics 62:382–389, 1978

Kempe CH, Silverman FN, Steele BF, et al: The battered child syndrome. JAMA 181:17–24, 1962

Kendler KS, Bulik CM, Silberg J, et al: Childhood sexual abuse and adult psychiatric and substance use disorders in women: an epidemiological and cotwin control analysis. Arch Gen Psychiatry 57:953–959, 2000

Kermani EJ: Child sexual abuse revisited by the U.S. Supreme Court. J Am Acad Child Adolesc Psychiatry 32:971–974, 1993

Kinzl JF, Traweger C, Guenther V, et al: Family background and sexual abuse associated with eating disorders. Am J Psychiatry 151:1127–1131, 1994

Kisiel CL, Lyons JS: Dissociation as a mediator of psychopathology among sexually abused children and adolescents. Am J Psychiatry 158:1034–1039, 2001

Kolko DJ, Moser JT, Weldy SR: Behavioral/emotional indicators of sexual abuse in child psychiatric inpatients: a controlled comparison with physical abuse. Child Abuse Negl 12:529–541, 1988

Lascaratos J, Poulakou-Rebelakou E: Child sexual abuse: historical cases in the Byzantine empire (324–1453 A.D.). Child Abuse Negl 24:1085–1090, 2000

Leder MR, Emans SJ, Hafler JP, et al: Addressing sexual abuse in the primary care setting. Pediatrics 104:270–275, 1999

Lindegren ML, Hanson IC, Hammett TA, et al: Sexual abuse of children: intersection with the HIV epidemic. Pediatrics 102(4):E46, 1998

Lowenstein LF: The etiology, diagnosis and treatment of the fire-setting behaviour of children. Child Psychiatry Hum Dev 19:186–194, 1989

MacIntyre D, Carr A: Evaluation of the effectiveness of the stay safe primary prevention programme for child sexual abuse. Child Abuse Negl 23:1307–1325, 1999

MacMillan HL, Fleming JE, Streiner DL, et al: Childhood abuse and lifetime psychopathology in a community sample. Am J Psychiatry 158:1878–1883, 2001

Martin EJ: Incest/child sexual abuse: historical perspectives. J Holist Nurs 13:7–18, 1995

Mathews R, Hunter JA, Vuz J: Juvenile female sexual offenders: clinical characteristics and treatment issues. Sex Abuse 9:187–199, 1997

McClellan J, McCurry C, Ronnel M, et al: Age of onset of sexual abuse: relationship to sexually inappropriate behaviors. J Am Acad Child Adolesc Psychiatry 35:1375–1383, 1996

McMahon PM, Puett RC: Child sexual abuse as a public health issue: recommendations of an expert panel. Sex Abuse 11:257–266, 1999

Merry SN, Andrews LK: Psychiatric status of sexually abused children 12 months after disclosure of abuse. J Am Acad Child Adolesc Psychiatry 33:939–944, 1994

Messman-Moore TL, Long PJ, Siegfried NJ: The revictimization of child sexual abuse survivors: an examination of the adjustment of college women with child sexual abuse, adult sexual assault, and adult physical abuse. Child Maltreat 5:18–27, 2000

Molnar BE, Berkman LF, Buka SL: Psychopathology, childhood sexual abuse and other childhood adversities: relative links to subsequent suicidal behaviour in the US. Psychol Med 31:965–977, 2001a

Molnar BE, Buka SL, Kessler R: Child sexual abuse and subsequent psychopathology: results from the National Comorbidity Survey. Am J Public Health 91:753–760, 2001b

Moody CW: Male child sexual abuse. J Pediatr Health Care 13:112–119, 1999

Moon LT, Wagner WG, Kazelskis R: Counseling sexually abused girls: the impact of counselor. Child Abuse Negl 24:753–765, 2000

Morrow KB: Attributions of female adolescent incest victims regarding their molestation. Child Abuse Negl 15:477–483, 1991

Mrazek DA, Mrazek PB: Psychosexual development within the family, in Sexually Abused Children and Their Families. Edited by Mrazek PB, Kempe CH. Oxford, UK, Pergamon, 1981, pp 17–32

Muram D: The medical evaluation in cases of child sexual abuse. J Pediatr Adolesc Gynecol 14:55–64, 2001

Nurcombe B, Unutzer J: The ritual abuse of children: clinical features and diagnostic reasoning. J Am Acad Child Adolesc Psychiatry 30:272–276, 1991

Olsen ME, Kalbfleisch JH: Sexual abuse knowledge base among residents in family practice, obstetrics/gynecology, and pediatrics. J Pediatr Adolesc Gynecol 14:89–94, 2001

Palusci VJ, Cox EO, Cyrus TA, et al: Medical assessment and legal outcome in child sexual abuse. Arch Pediatr Adolesc Med 153:388–392, 1999

Paolucci EO, Genuis ML, Violato C: A meta-analysis of the published research on the effects of child sexual abuse. J Psychol 135:17–36, 2001

Peluso E, Putman N: Case study: sexual abuse of boys by females. J Am Acad Child Adolesc Psychiatry 35:51–54, 1996

Pope HG, Hudson JI: Is childhood sexual abuse a risk factor for bulimia nervosa? Am J Psychiatry 149:455–463, 1992

Pribor EF, Dinwiddie SH: Psychiatric correlates of incest in childhood. Am J Psychiatry 149:52–56, 1992

Puri BK, Baxter R, Cordess CC: Characteristics of fire-setters: a study and proposed multiaxial psychiatric classification. Br J Psychiatry 166:393–396, 1995

Rao K, DiClemente RJ, Ponton LE: Child sexual abuse of Asians compared with other populations. J Am Acad Child Adolesc Psychiatry 31:880–886, 1992

Rew L, Taylor-Seehafer M, Fitzgerald ML: Sexual abuse, alcohol and other drug use, and suicidal behaviors in homeless adolescents. Issues Compr Pediatr Nurs 24:225–240, 2001

Romans SE, Martin JL, Morris E, et al: Psychological defense styles in women who report childhood sexual abuse: a controlled community study. Am J Psychiatry 156:1080–1085, 1999

Ruscio AM: Predicting the child-rearing practices of mothers sexually abused in childhood. Child Abuse Negl 25:369–387, 2001

Ryan G: Childhood sexuality: a decade of study, I: research and curriculum development. Child Abuse Negl 24:33–48, 2000

Ryan G, Miyoshi TJ, Metzner JL, et al: Trends in a national sample of sexually abusive youths. J Am Acad Child Adolesc Psychiatry 35:17–25, 1996

Schetky D, Green A: Child Sexual Abuse: A Handbook for Health Care and Legal Professionals. New York, Brunner/Mazel, 1988

Shaw JA: Practice parameters for the assessment and treatment of children and adolescents who are sexually abusive of others. American Academy of Child and Adolescent Psychiatry Working Group on Quality Issues. J Am Acad Child Adolesc Psychiatry 38 (12, suppl):55S–76S, 1999

Shaw JA, Applegate B, Rothe E: Psychopathology and personality disorders in adolescent sex offenders. Am J Forensic Psychiatry 17:19–37, 1996

Shin LM, McNally RJ, Kosslyn SM, et al: Regional cerebral blood flow during script-driven imagery in childhood sexual abuse-related PTSD: a PET investigation. Am J Psychiatry 156:575–584, 1999

Socolar RR, Raines B, Chen-Mok M, et al: Intervention to improve physician documentation and knowledge of child sexual abuse: a randomized, controlled trial. Pediatrics 101:817–824, 1998

Spaccarelli S: Stress, appraisal, and coping in child sexual abuse: a theoretical and empirical review. Psychol Bull 116:340–362, 1994

Steiger H, Gauvin L, Israel M, et al: Association of serotonin and cortisol indices with childhood abuse in bulimia nervosa. Arch Gen Psychiatry 58:837–843, 2001

Stevenson J: The treatment of the long-term sequelae of child abuse. J Child Psychol Psychiatry 40:89–111, 1999

Sturkie K: Group treatment for sexually abused children: clinical wisdom and empirical findings. Child Adolesc Psychiatr Clin N Am 3:813–829, 1994

Tebbutt J, Swanston H, Oates RK, et al: Five years after child sexual abuse: persisting dysfunction and problems of prediction. J Am Acad Child Adolesc Psychiatry 36:330–339, 1997

Tong L, Oates K, McDowell M: Personality development following sexual abuse. Child Abuse Negl 11:371–383, 1987

Tremblay C, Hebert M, Piche C: Coping strategies and social support as mediators of consequences in child sexual abuse victims. Child Abuse Negl 23:929–945, 1999

U.S. Department of Health and Human Services: Abuse and neglect (section HC 210), in Trends in the Well-Being of America's Children and Youth 2001. Washington, DC, Office of the Assistant Secretary for Planning and Evaluation, U.S. Department of Health and Human Services, 2001, pp 142–143

Watkins B, Bentovim A: The sexual abuse of male children and adolescents: a review of current research. J Child Psychol Psychiatry 33:197–248, 1992

Weinstein D, Staffelbach D, Biaggio M: Attention-deficit hyperactivity disorder and posttraumatic stress disorder: differential diagnosis in childhood sexual abuse. Clin Psychol Rev 20:359–378, 2000

Weiss EL, Longhurst JG, Mazure CM: Childhood sexual abuse as a risk factor for depression in women: psychosocial and neurobiological correlates. Am J Psychiatry 156:816–828, 1999

Wissow LS: Child abuse and neglect. N Engl J Med 332:1425–1431, 1995

Wonderlich SA, Crosby RD, Mitchell JE, et al: Relationship of childhood sexual abuse and eating disturbance in children. J Am Acad Child Adolesc Psychiatry 39:1277–1283, 2000

Wonderlich SA, Crosby RD, Mitchell JE, et al: Pathways mediating sexual abuse and eating disturbance in children. Int J Eat Disord 29:270–279, 2001

Wozencraft H, Wagner W, Pellegrin A: Depression and suicidal ideation in sexually abused children. Child Abuse Negl 15:505–511, 1991

Wyatt GE, Loeb TB, Solis B, et al: The prevalence and circumstances of child sexual abuse: changes across a decade. Child Abuse Negl 23:45–60, 1999

Yates A: Sexual abuse of children, in Textbook of Child and Adolescent Psychiatry, 2nd Edition. Edited by Wiener JM. Washington, DC, American Psychiatric Press, 1997, pp 699–709

Zlotnick C, Mattia J, Zimmerman M: Clinical features of survivors of sexual abuse with major depression. Child Abuse Negl 25:357–367, 2001

HIV and AIDS

Global and United States Perspectives

Kerim M. Munir, M.D., M.P.H., D.Sc.

Myron L. Belfer, M.D., M.P.A.

Acquired immunodeficiency syndrome (AIDS) is a complex illness with a strong psychological and developmental impact on children and adolescents. It also has strong effects on families and other caregivers, on institutions, and on society. The impact of the AIDS epidemic is increasingly felt in many countries worldwide. Although the absolute number of children and adolescents infected with the human immunodeficiency virus (HIV) in the United States remains relatively small, the number of uninfected children and adolescents who are affected—that is, youths with one or more parents, siblings, or family members who have been infected with HIV, have developed AIDS, or have died from AIDS—is vastly greater than those themselves infected. It has been estimated that 28% of persons with AIDS in the United States have children under age 18 (Knodel and Van Landingham 2000; Schuster et al. 2000).

Globally the incidence of HIV infection is increasing at an alarming pace, mostly because of new infections in developing countries that have the least resources and least adequate societal structures to cope with its impact (Epstein and Chen 2002). As the global HIV/AIDS epidemic continues to evolve, the consequences are becoming urgently evident in the developing world. This dimension is likely to reverberate for years to come because countries that are heavily affected by the HIV/AIDS epidemic are susceptible to political instability. Many of these countries are already burdened by socioeconomic challenges, and AIDS

threatens their stability and welfare on an unprecedented scale (Joint United Nations Programme on HIV/AIDS 2002). The HIV/AIDS epidemic has had a devastating impact on societal organization and family structure, making recovery even more difficult. The needs for long-term international financing and for leadership by the United States have therefore become increasingly important. These needs have recently been partially addressed by the establishment of the Global Fund to Fight AIDS, Tuberculosis and Malaria (http://www.globalfundatm.org).

As of December 2002, there were 42 million persons (19.2 million women and 3.2 million children under age 15 years) living with HIV/AIDS worldwide (Joint United Nations Programme on HIV/AIDS 2002). People newly infected with HIV in 2002 alone total 4.4 million, of whom 2 million are women and 800,000 are children under age 15 years (2,000 children per day). During 2002 a total of 3.1 million persons died of AIDS, of whom 1.2 million were women and 610,000 were children under age 15 years (1,200 children per day).

AIDS has become the leading cause of death in sub-Saharan Africa (accounting for 85% of deaths) and has become the fourth-largest cause worldwide (Joint United Nations Programme on HIV/AIDS 2001). It has become increasingly clear that in many parts of the developing world, the majority of new infections occur in young women of childbearing age and in young children, who are especially vulnerable.

This work was supported by National Institutes of Health Grants MH59257 and D43 TW05807 (K.M.M.). The authors also gratefully acknowledge the assistance of Kay Lee Park.

Furthermore, it is estimated that by 2010 nearly 15 million children under age 5 will be orphaned by AIDS, and many more will live with sick parents or caregivers in impoverished conditions. The children and adolescents are the most vulnerable to feeling the impact of the disease on their families and communities as well as its direct effects on their nurturance, growth, and future development.

From the outset of the HIV/AIDS epidemic, the influence of parental death and disability on children from this stigmatizing illness has generated a pressing set of social and psychological issues (Stuber 1992). With the entry of the United Nations General Assembly and leaders such as former South African president Nelson Mandela—who has made it his mission to get AIDS policies changed—the stigma has now been challenged head on in the fight against AIDS, especially with promotion of the development of nationwide and regional programs to prevent mother-to-child transmission (Lamont and Innocenti 2002). Life expectancy at birth in southern Africa, which rose from 44 years in the early 1950s to 59 in the early 1990s, is expected to drop to just 45 from 2000 to 2010. Mandela has recently described HIV/AIDS as "the biggest threat facing our future" to prompt immediate action on the issue. South Africa has one of the highest HIV infection rates in the world, with 4.7 million HIV-infected citizens. This has led Mandela to state, "This is a war. It has killed more people than has been the case in all previous wars and in all natural disasters. We must not continue to be debating when people are dying" (Lamont and Innocenti 2002).

The roles of child and adolescent psychiatrists and of training in child mental health are essential in the diagnosis of specific psychopathology, the support of systems of care, and the evolution of effective prevention strategies. HIV/AIDS is both an epidemic and a chronic illness in the mainstream of global concern. HIV/AIDS can no longer be viewed as a condition rarely affecting children and youths, and the adoption of national and international policies and care strategies represents an important paradigm shift. Such strategies involve not only the provision of antiretroviral drugs but also the development of health care infrastructure and ongoing measures to prevent further infection.

Mental health service providers for children and adolescents must continue to be knowledgeable and active in the fight against AIDS. They all need to be aware of the critical care issues in the counseling of individuals and families with HIV/AIDS and to be involved in coordinated and interdisciplinary prevention and care activities. HIV/AIDS represents long-term psychological, cognitive, and social hazards for children and adolescents. In the United States within the relatively short course of two decades, progress has been made in improving quality and duration of life in young children with HIV/AIDS. One of the greatest successes has been the reduction of the rate of mother-to-child transmission in the United States below 2%. This reflects the availability not only of effective treatments but also of an advanced health care infrastructure. Yet the prevention of HIV transmission to women and children worldwide has remained a major challenge.

Mother-to-child transmission of HIV is reducible with the use of antiretroviral agents during early pregnancy (Connor et al. 1994). A promising development in recent years is the availability in developing countries of an inexpensive antiretroviral agent, nevirapine, that significantly reduces mother-to-child transmission. Currently about 95% of newly infected children in sub-Saharan Africa and 10%–15% of all new HIV infections worldwide are acquired through mother-to-child vertical transmission. However, at the present time treatments to prevent mother-to-child transmission reach fewer than 5% of women in sub-Saharan Africa.

Mother-to-child transmission has the potential to take place at three different points in time: before birth, during labor and delivery, and (less commonly) after birth through breastfeeding. The greatest proportion of transmission occurs during labor and delivery. Antiretroviral agents given to HIV-positive mothers at the onset of labor have shown substantial effectiveness in reducing the likelihood of HIV transmission to the newborn. A joint study conducted by Uganda and the United States showed that nevirapine reduces transmission of HIV by 47% and perinatal transmission of HIV by 41% at age 18 months in a breastfeeding population. Nevirapine is administered in a single dose to the mother at the onset of labor and in a single dose to the baby during its first 3 days of life. Although the cost had been estimated to be less than $4 at the time the study was completed, nevirapine can now be made available at a much lower cost.

However, beyond potentially successful therapeutic interventions, the key to interrupting HIV transmission is the understanding and modification of the behaviors that put infants and adolescents at risk (Auerbach et al. 1994). Preventive interventions to halt mother-to-child transmission of HIV, however crucial, represent the final common pathway in the prevention cycle. If HIV/AIDS is to be stopped, the preventive efforts need to target a broad array of behavioral, sexual, and drug use determinants (Allen and Curran 1988; Peckham and Gibb 1995). In this regard, as well as in aspects of long-term care, child and adolescent psychiatrists and mental health personnel have a crucial role to play.

The United Nations General Assembly Special Session on HIV/AIDS established a framework for both national and international accountability in the fight against AIDS. This framework includes a series of requisite benchmarks relating to prevention, care, support, and alleviation of disproportionate impact on vulnerable groups as part of a comprehensive response. Incorporated as major parts of these targets are young adults, women, and children. The goals include the provision of "highest attainable standard of treatment for HIV/AIDS, including antiretroviral therapy in a careful and monitored manner." A further goal involves the development of multisectoral strategies to address the impact of HIV/AIDS at the individual, family, community, and national levels (Joint United Nations Programme on HIV/AIDS 2002).

The social conditions that maintain the epidemic of AIDS in children and adolescents include poor education, inadequate access to health and social services, homelessness, illicit drug use, poor attitudes about sexual responsibility, sexual abuse, and teenage prostitution (American Public Health Association 1989). Social and economic factors remain at the forefront of planning mental health services for affected children, adolescents, and families.

Global HIV/AIDS in Children and Adolescents

The poorest regions of the developing world represent the epicenter of the HIV/AIDS pandemic. The region with the highest impact by far is sub-Saharan Africa, followed by South and Southeast Asia. Most persons in these regions do not know that they carry the virus and even many more know very little or nothing at all to protect themselves from HIV.

■ Sub-Saharan Africa

With an estimated 3.5 million new infections in 2002, about 29.4 million Africans are now living with HIV. If the recent trends continue, many of these individuals will not survive the decade. Several parts of sub-Saharan Africa now have prevalence rates among pregnant women exceeding 30%. There is evidence that the regional HIV incidence among young adults slightly decreased by 5% between 1999 and 2000. However, the incidence among children during the same period continued to increase. A stabilizing trend in new HIV incidence may be partly due to the fact that the long-standing African epidemics have already reached large numbers of people whose behavior exposes them to HIV, leaving a smaller population of people who are still able to acquire infection. However, as the infection continues to strike women at a younger age, and as women continue to have sex and reproduce without any precautionary measures, the incidence of pediatric cases continues to rise. Furthermore, the loss of an infected caregiver profoundly affects children whether or not they are infected with the disease. Of the cumulative number of 13.2 million children (under age 15 years) estimated to have been orphaned by AIDS at the end of 1999, about 12.1 million were from sub-Saharan Africa.

■ South and Southeast Asia

The total number of adults and children living with HIV/AIDS in South and Southeast Asia at the end of 2002 was 6 million. During 2000, an estimated 700,000 adults, 250,000 of them women, became infected in the region, with about 210,000 children living with HIV/AIDS. These estimates reflect the current transmission pattern whereby men serve as vectors and contribute to the transmission—much of it through commercial sex and injection drug use practices. In Thailand and Cambodia political leadership and large-scale prevention programs are beginning to hold the epidemic at bay, lowering the HIV prevalence among pregnant women to 2.7%—reduced by a third from 1997 levels.

■ Latin America and the Caribbean

At the end of 2002, about 1.5 million adults and children were living with HIV/AIDS in Latin America, and 440,000 in the Caribbean. The transmission pattern of

HIV in this region is a complex mosaic of male-to-male sex, sex between men and women, and injection drug use. In the Caribbean, HIV is transmitted primarily through heterosexual sex, placing a far larger proportion of the population at immediate risk. HIV rates in the Caribbean are the second highest in the world outside Africa. During 2002, 210,000 adults and children were newly infected in Latin America and the Caribbean, of whom 5.5% were children.

■ Western European Countries

In the high-income European countries, the annual number of children who have acquired HIV has remained stable. Overall, HIV prevalence has slightly risen as a result of antiretroviral therapy, with individuals living longer. However, among high-risk groups an optimistic view of antiretroviral therapy as a cure has led to growing complacency, with increased risk-taking behavior. A majority of new infections have been among injecting drug users and their families. The estimated number of children living with HIV/AIDS is 15,100 of a total of 570,000 infected people, with about 30,000 acquiring the infection in 2002.

■ Eastern Europe and Central Asia

The estimated number of adults and children living with HIV/AIDS in Eastern Europe and Central Asia has increased dramatically, with the Russian Federation experiencing the fastest-growing epidemic in the world. In fact, in 2000, more new HIV infections were registered in the Russian Federation than in all the previous years combined. In 2002, there were an estimated 250,000 new infections in this region, bringing the total living with HIV/AIDS to 1.2 million. The fight against HIV/AIDS is being waged against a backdrop of socioeconomic instability, fueling HIV transmission through unsafe injection drug use and commercial sex practices. The number of children estimated to be living with HIV/AIDS by the end of 2000 was 15,000.

■ East Asia and the Pacific Region

In 2002 the estimated total number of people living with HIV/AIDS in East Asia and the Pacific region was 1.2 million, with prevalence much lower than in South and Southeast Asia. Although the East Asian AIDS epidemic has remained at a deceptively low level, there is

potential for growth with extensive sex trading and drug use, along with increased migration and mobility within and across borders. In China, 100 million people are now on the move, more people than at any other time in history. A recent steep rise in rates of sexually transmitted diseases could translate into higher HIV spread in the future. There is continuing complacency about the danger of HIV. Another major challenge facing this region is the need for attaining higher rates of condom use than those that now prevail.

■ North Africa and the Middle East

Due to insufficient data, few estimates of HIV infection in the Middle East and North Africa were produced between 1994 and 1999. In more recent years, the number of new reported HIV cases has increased dramatically—between 1999 and 2002, from 220,000 to 550,000. The reported HIV infections in children increased 5.5 fold. The recent evidence suggests that new infections are on the rise in this region. The epidemic is most marked in Djibouti, Somalia, and Sudan. Localized rates in southern Algeria are around 1% in pregnant women attending antenatal clinics, whereas surveillance sites in northern and southern Sudan indicate increasing HIV rates in the general population.

■ Worldwide: AIDS Orphans

One of the most dramatic consequences of HIV/AIDS worldwide is the evidence of neglect of the young, largely invisible population of children under age 15 who have lost one or both parents to AIDS. In sub-Saharan Africa alone, the total number of AIDS orphans of all ages is expected to reach 25 million by 2010 (Children on the Brink 2002). The alternatives for these AIDS orphans are grim. In some societies decisions are made at the earliest age to let them die because there are no available caregivers. Thus, neglect becomes institutionalized. Others find their way to orphanages, where marginal support is provided, but the children remain largely rejected by family and community and therefore have uncertain outcomes at best. This is not solely a problem of sub-Saharan Africa. It is a problem in the Caribbean, in South Asia, in Eastern Europe—in short, it is a growing world problem. In 2015 more than one-third of the children of Zimbabwe under age 15 will be orphaned. In Western Kenya every fifth household is caring for at least one orphan.

The United Nations General Assembly Special Session on HIV/AIDS (Joint United Nations Programme on HIV/AIDS 2002) has targeted benchmarks by 2003 to develop and by 2005 to implement national multisectoral strategies in these countries to provide a supportive environment for orphans and children infected with and affected by HIV/AIDS. The challenge, however, is to build on the much-promised assistance and convert it to sustained future action.

HIV/AIDS in U.S. Children

As of June 2001, a cumulative total of 793,026 adult and pediatric cases of HIV/AIDS were reported in the United States; 40% of these individuals have died. Children (age under 13 years) constitute 1.3% of the overall total, with young children (age under 5 years) representing 75% of all reported pediatric AIDS cases (age under 13 years) (Centers for Disease Control and Prevention 2001). The reduction in pediatric case fatality rate over the years, however, is attributable to the greater efforts at early recognition and treatment of acute AIDS-related infections in young children, who traditionally have had the highest case fatality rates. The case fatality rates remain significantly higher for children under age 13 years (46.1%). As of June 2001, a cumulative total of 8,994 pediatric AIDS cases (age under 13 years) had been reported in the following exposure groups:

- Behavior risk: children born to mothers who are injection drug users or the sexual partners of males infected with HIV (91% of all pediatric cases)
- Transfusion, blood components, or tissue recipients (4% of all pediatric cases)
- Hemophilia and coagulation factor patients (3% of all pediatric cases)
- Undetermined risk (2% of all pediatric cases)

Although both the number of newly diagnosed cases and case fatality rates of HIV/AIDS have been falling, the decreases among the African American and Hispanic populations are disproportionately lower. Of the total pediatric AIDS cases by race or ethnicity, African American children currently represent 56%; Hispanic children, 23%; and Caucasian children, 17%.

The metropolitan areas with populations greater than 500,000 persons continue to comprise 85% of all pediatric AIDS cases, with an annual incidence of 18.3

in 100,000 from July 2000 to June 2001 (versus 20 per 100,000 a year earlier). The cumulative number of pediatric cases has been highest for New York City, accounting for approximately 23% of the total (Centers for Disease Control and Prevention 2001). Among other metropolitan areas with populations greater than 500,000, the largest numbers of pediatric cases (in descending order) occur in Miami, Florida; Newark, New Jersey; Washington, D.C.; Philadelphia, Pennsylvania; Fort Lauderdale, Florida; San Juan, Puerto Rico; Chicago, Illinois; Los Angeles, California; Baltimore, Maryland; and West Palm Beach, Florida. The first nine metropolitan areas (excluding New York City) account for 26% of the pediatric AIDS cases. Metropolitan areas with populations between 50,000 and 500,000 persons account for 9%, with the remaining 6% accounted for by nonmetropolitan areas. The annual incidence for these metropolitan areas between July 2000 and June 2001 was 9.4 in 100,000 (versus 9.6 in 100,000 a year earlier).

■ Transmission

Mother With or at Risk for HIV Infection

Virtually all new cases of HIV infection in children are transmitted vertically from HIV-seropositive mothers by three possible routes: 1) in utero through maternal-fetal circulation (Lapointe et al. 1985; Marion et al. 1986); 2) during labor and delivery by exposure to the mother's blood or secretions (Macchi et al. 1986; Pyun et al. 1987); and 3) postnatally through breast milk, as suggested by case reports (Thiry et al. 1985; Weinbreck et al. 1988; Ziegler et al. 1985). Breastfeeding has been shown to be independently associated with increased risk of HIV transmission (Eichberg et al. 1988; European Collaborative Study 1992; French Collaborative Study Group 1994). The meta-analysis of a number of prospective studies suggests that the risk attributable to breast transmission may be as high as 7%–22% (Dunn et al. 1992).

The rate of vertical transmission ranges between 10% and 40% (Blanche et al. 1989; European Collaborative Study 1988; Newell and Peckham 1993; Pizzo 1995). The average transmission rate is about 25%. The transmission rates of human immunodeficiency virus type 1 (HIV-1) and human immunodeficiency virus type 2 (HIV-2) differ. HIV-1 is more prevalent worldwide, whereas HIV-2 is very rare outside West Africa. Only about 1% of mothers infected with HIV-2 pass the infection on to their children. Up to 42% of mothers infected with HIV-1 pass the infection to their children by all routes. Postnatal transmission of HIV-1 by breast milk is more important than was previously believed and doubles the risk of mother-to-child transmission. (A.D. Grant and DeCock 2001).

A threshold historic study conducted under Pediatric AIDS Clinical Trials Group Protocol 076, funded by the National Institutes of Health (NIH), demonstrated that the rate of vertical transmission can be reduced as low as 8% when mothers take zidovudine during pregnancy and at delivery and when the infant is given zidovudine for the first 6 weeks of life (Connor et al. 1994). Although this important trial left many questions unanswered (Peckham and Gibb 1995), the results raised the question of an expanded role for voluntary prenatal HIV testing in the United States, where zidovudine is available to pregnant mothers. However, because the proportion of infants acquiring HIV in utero compared with those acquiring it during delivery or labor is still relatively unknown, the time of administration has both practical and ethical implications. These issues are particularly relevant in less economically advantaged areas in the United States, where access to primary and prenatal care is limited, and in developing countries, where costs are high and resources are severely restricted.

The Working Group on Antiretroviral Therapy and Medical Management of Infants, Children and Adolescents with HIV Infection (1993) published recommendations for the use of zidovudine in pregnancy and in childhood. Recent advances have led to major changes in the treatment and monitoring of pediatric HIV infection in the United States. The guidelines for the therapy and management of the HIV-infected child by the Working Group on Antiretroviral Therapy were subsequently updated by the National Pediatric HIV Resource Center, the Health Resources and Services Administration, and the NIH-convened Working Group on Antiretroviral Therapy and Medical Management of HIV-Infected Children (1998), consisting of pediatric HIV experts and government agency representatives. Published in *Morbidity and Mortality Weekly Reports* (Centers for Disease Control and Prevention 1998), the new guidelines are regularly updated as new clinical information and experience become available, with the information being made available on the U.S. Department of Health and Human Services AIDSinfo web site (http://www.aidsinfo.nih.gov).

The following guidelines are considered in the formulation of treatment of pediatric HIV infection (Centers for Disease Control and Prevention 1998):

- HIV-infected women should be identified before and during pregnancy so that optimal therapy can be provided for both infected women and their children and so that perinatal transmission can be prevented. Prenatal counseling and consent are therefore the standard of care for all pregnant women in the United States (American Academy of Pediatrics 1995; Centers for Disease Control and Prevention 1995b).

- Enrollment into clinical trials is recommended because it offers the best means of determining safe and effective therapies. Information about clinical trials for HIV-infected adults and children can be obtained from the U.S. Department of Health and Human Services AIDSinfo Web site (http://www.aidsinfo.nih.gov).

- Pharmaceutical companies and the federal government should work in tandem so that pediatric drug formulations suitable for administration to infants and children are made available.

- Concurrent clinical trials for children are needed in addition to extrapolation from clinical trials involving adults for the use of any approved antiretroviral drug in children.

- Management of HIV infection in children, whenever possible, should be directed by a specialist in the treatment of pediatric and adolescent HIV infection.

- A multidisciplinary team approach is also needed that includes physicians, nurses, social workers, psychologists, psychiatrists, nutritionists, outreach workers, and pharmacists.

- Assays to measure HIV RNA and CD4+ T-cell levels are essential for monitoring and modifying treatment.

- The following factors should be considered in adherence to antiretroviral regimens: 1) availability and palatability of pediatric formulations; 2) impact of medication schedule on quality of life, including number and coadministration of medications and frequency of administration; 3) ability of the caregiver to administer complex medication regimens and availability of resources that might be effective in facilitating adherence; and 4) potential for drug interactions.

- HIV resistance assays should be made available for perinatally infected children; however, the usefulness of such assays in pediatric populations should be interpreted cautiously.

- Monitoring of growth and development and nutritional support therapy are essential for the care of HIV-infected children.

Blood Transfusion and Hemophilia/ Coagulation Disorders

Screening of donated blood and plasma, heat treatment of clotting factor concentrates, and donor screening were begun in April 1985. These methods reduced the risk of HIV infection associated with transfused blood products from 1 in 100,000 to 1 in 1,000,000 per transfused unit of blood (Centers for Disease Control 1985b). The seroprevalence of HIV infection is high in patients with severe hemophilia as well as in their childbearing-age spouses or partners. Four percent of cumulative pediatric AIDS cases occur in children with hemophilia or coagulation disorder. Of these children, 67% are Caucasian, 16.5% are Hispanic, and 14.5% are African American (Centers for Disease Control and Prevention 1995a).

Sexual Transmission

The problem of child prostitution needs to be considered. It exists virtually worldwide. Poverty, the disintegration of family life, urban migration, drug use, and parental unemployment are common contributors to the rise in child prostitution and the increasing spread of HIV through this route (Kandela 2000).

■ Detection and Classification

Early identification of maternal HIV infection is crucial both for the health of the mother and for the care of HIV-exposed and HIV-infected children. Such knowledge can enable 1) provision of HIV-infected women with antiretroviral therapy and prophylaxis against opportunistic infections; 2) provision of antiretroviral prophylaxis with zidovudine to HIV-infected women during pregnancy and labor and to newborns to reduce the risk for mother-to-child transmission (Centers for Disease Control and Prevention 1994, 1998; Connor et al. 1994); 3) counseling of HIV-infected women about the risk of HIV transmission through breast milk; 4) initiation of prophylaxis against *Pneumocystis carinii* pneumonia in all HIV-exposed infants beginning at ages 4–6 weeks (Centers for Disease Con-

trol and Prevention 1998); and 5) early diagnostic evaluation of HIV-infected infants to permit initiation of more aggressive antiretroviral therapy.

HIV infection can be diagnosed in most infants by age 1 month and in virtually all infected infants by age 6 months by means of viral diagnostic assays; that is, HIV is detected by culture or by DNA or RNA polymerase chain reaction (PCR) assay and is then confirmed by an additional virological test on a second specimen. It is recommended that testing be performed before the infant is 48 hours old, at age 1–2 months, and at age 3–6 months with the consent of the mother unless state law allows testing without consent. The DNA PCR assay is the preferred method for diagnosing HIV in infancy. The HIV RNA assay in plasma may be more sensitive than DNA PCR testing for early diagnosis, and data are more limited regarding their sensitivity and specificity. HIV culture has a similar sensitivity but is more complex and expensive to perform than the DNA PCR assay.

One issue that had confounded HIV detection in children younger than 15 months involved the presence of maternal antibodies passively acquired from an HIV-infected mother (Rogers et al. 1989; Rubinstein 1986). These HIV antibodies could then be detected by enzyme-linked immunosorbent assay (ELISA) or Western blot screening tests. If the child is uninfected, seroconversion to negative HIV status occurs by age 15–18 months; children who seroconvert are almost invariably not infected with HIV.

The Centers for Disease Control and Prevention (CDC) considers children older than 15 months to be infected if they have had at least one positive assay. However, because children younger than 15 months are particularly vulnerable to potentially fatal infections during the first month of life, it has become important to establish the diagnosis as swiftly as possible. Virus-specific assays (e.g., measurement of virus load by DNA PCR assay, quantitative HIV culture techniques, analysis of the plasma RNA by the PCR assay, and p24 detection assays) have therefore been variably used in early diagnosis of HIV infection in young children (Pezzela et al. 1989; Pizzo 1995; Pizzo et al. 1988; Rogers et al. 1989). However, the use of p24 antigen testing alone to exclude infection in infants less than a month old is not recommended because of a high frequency of false-positive tests during this period (Nesheim et al. 1997). As costs have become more manageable, the PCR tests have become the diagnostic standard in the United States. In the past a much less sensitive test, particularly during the first few months of life, involved assaying virus-specific immunoglobulin A antibodies in an infant's saliva. Although they are much less expensive and need not be done on blood, these tests have now been superseded by PCR methodology (Quinn et al. 1991).

Despite the availability of the more sensitive and specific assays, only 25%–30% of infants truly infected with HIV test positive in the first 48 hours after birth. Those who do so most likely have acquired HIV in utero. The remainder will test positive by viral culture or PCR by the first month of life and at the latest by the first 6 months. The majority of this infected group are thought to have acquired the infection at the time of labor or delivery, most likely by means of contamination through the mother's blood or secretions.

The definition of HIV/AIDS in children younger than 13 years is based on three essential factors: 1) history of a risk factor associated with HIV/AIDS, 2) laboratory evidence of immunodeficiency, and 3) evidence of HIV infection (Centers for Disease Control and Prevention 1987, 1994). Multiple or recurrent bacterial infections, lymphoid interstitial pneumonia, and pulmonary lymphoid hyperplasia are accepted as indicative of AIDS in children.

The incubation period, or the time from transmission to first detectable clinical disease, appears to be relatively shorter in children with intrauterine transmission. Data taken from the New York City and New York State case registries suggest that there may be a short incubation period (median, 4.1 months) and a long incubation period (median, 6.1 years) (Auger et al. 1988).

■ Differential Diagnosis

The common presentations of AIDS in young children are failure to thrive, loss of developmental milestones, fever, recurrent bacterial infections (pneumonia, septicemia, meningitis, or cellulitis), *Pneumocystis carinii* pneumonia or other opportunistic infections, chronic unexplained diarrhea, persistent oral candidiasis, and wasting (McLoughlin et al. 1987). Other symptoms include lymphadenopathy (larger than 1 cm) at two or more noncontiguous sites, hepatomegaly, splenomegaly, recurrent otitis media, parotitis, or evidence of neuroencephalopathy (Pawha et al. 1986).

HIV can directly infect cells in the central nervous system (CNS) (Barnes 1986; Ho et al. 1985; Shaw et al. 1985). CNS manifestations of AIDS in children include motor dysfunction, encephalopathy, meningitis, seizures, and neoplastic involvement (Rogers et al. 1987). Neoplastic involvement includes primary CNS lymphomas; systemic lymphomas invading the meninges; and cerebral metastases secondary to Kaposi's sarcoma, otherwise very rare in children. An embryopathy attributed to in utero HIV infection has been described (Iosub et al. 1987; Marion et al. 1986), but other researchers have not confirmed the presence of craniofacial dysmorphism in children exposed to intrauterine HIV (Qazi et al. 1987), and the possibility of HIV-related dysmorphism is now abandoned by many clinicians. Neurological symptoms or evidence of encephalopathy related to HIV infection have consistently been noted in about 65% of children with HIV (Pizzo et al. 1988). A devastating complication is neuropsychological deterioration characterized by progressive loss of developmental milestones and cognitive functioning (Belman et al. 1988). Apathy and psychomotor retardation may also be presentations of HIV infection in young children.

■ Antiretroviral and Supportive Therapy

Unfortunately, the lack of adherence to prescribed regimens of antiretroviral agents enhances the development of drug resistance. The adherence to these complex drug regimens is problematic for children, who are dependent on others for administration of medications. The assessment of caregivers, their environments, and supports is therefore an essential component of treatment planning. These evaluations may include nursing, social services, and behavioral and psychological assessments. An intensive follow-up is required, especially during the initial phase of treatment. Coordinated, comprehensive, family-based, culturally sensitive care is crucial. Case management, mental health counselors, peer educators, outreach workers, and other members of the multidisciplinary team need to work in a flexible manner to address the barriers to adherence and sustenance of therapeutic interventions in the long term (Centers for Disease Control and Prevention 1998).

The level of HIV RNA considered to be indicative of increased risk for disease progression is not well defined for children. Factors to consider in deciding to initiate therapy include 1) high or increasing HIV RNA levels, 2) rapidly declining CD4+ T-cell count or percentage to values approaching those indicative of moderate immune suppression, or 3) developmental or clinical symptoms (Centers for Disease Control and Prevention 1998).

Based on clinical, immunological, and virological data from clinical trials, antiretroviral drug regimens are listed by the CDC as "strongly recommended," "recommended as an alternative," "offered in special circumstances," or "not considered." Combination therapy is recommended for all infants, children, and adolescents who are treated with antiretroviral agents (Centers for Disease Control and Prevention 1998 [updated regularly; see http://www.aidsinfo.nih.gov]). Monotherapy with any of the available antiretroviral drugs is no longer recommended. Use of zidovudine as a single agent is appropriate only in infants of indeterminate HIV status during the first 6 weeks of life to prevent perinatal transmission.

The initial antiretroviral regimen chosen is influenced by the maternal regimen during pregnancy, especially because maternal therapy with multiple antiretroviral agents is becoming more common and the prevalence of resistant strains may increase over time. Aggressive therapy with at least three drugs is recommended for initial treatment of infected children because it provides the best opportunity to preserve immune function and delay disease progression. (Centers for Disease Control and Prevention 1998). The strongly recommended regimen includes initial triple therapy with dual nucleoside reverse transcriptase inhibitors (NRTIs) with one of the recommended protease inhibitors. These combinations have reduced HIV RNA to undetectable levels in a substantial proportion of children. The combination of two NRTIs with a protease inhibitor has proved to be more effective than only one NRTI with a protease inhibitor. Antiretroviral regimens that are recommended as an alternative for initial therapy include the combination of nevirapine with two NRTIs and the triple nucleoside analog regimen of abacavir, zidovudine, and lamivudine.

Because antiretroviral therapy is expected to continue for many years, the choices need to consider barriers to adherence in the context of complex schedules, nutritional requirements, and palatability issues.

However, when HIV infection is suspected or determined—especially in children under age 12 months—there is urgency to prevent serious and potentially life-threatening infections, particularly *Pneumocystis carinii* pneumonia. For HIV-infected children older than 1 year, the prophylactic antibiotic treatment is guided by age-corrected CD4+ cell counts (Pizzo 1995). As part of the protocol, all infected children should receive nutritional supplements and a full battery of immunizations. The most significant results have been obtained in children whose HIV-induced encephalopathy improved with combination therapy. In summary, the medical management of HIV infection in children emphasizes supportive care (e.g., nutrition, passive immunization, and antibiotic therapy). As in adults with AIDS, there is evidence that treatment with antiretroviral agents reduces morbidity in children, especially in those with AIDS encephalopathy (Pizzo et al. 1988). Infants who were infected with HIV-1 in utero, especially those with AIDS at less than 6 months, have a worse prognosis (Novick and Rubinstein 1987).

HIV/AIDS in U.S. Adolescents

In 1990, there were 500 adolescent cases of AIDS in the United States. By June 1995, this figure surpassed 2,000—a fourfold increase. By June 2001 the numbers of adolescents had increased threefold compared with June 1995 levels; adolescents and young adults (ages 13–24 years) now jointly constitute 3.2% of cumulative United States AIDS cases. The incidence of AIDS increases with age through adolescence and young adulthood. Given the long incubation period (more than 8 years), it seems likely that many of those with AIDS in the 20- to 24-year age group and some in the 25- to 29-year age group may have been infected during adolescence.

Statewide and CDC surveillance data invariably underreport adolescent AIDS cases, particularly from regions with low HIV seroprevalence. The incidence rate is also underestimated in view of the competing risks for mortality among adolescents from accidents, homicide, and suicide, which may be proportionally higher among adolescents at highest risk for HIV infection.

As of June 2001, a cumulative total of 5,893 AIDS cases in adolescents (ages 13–19 years) and 19,269 cases in young adults (ages 20–24 years) were reported to the CDC. AIDS in adolescents (ages 13–19 years) can be categorized into three groups that emphasize the presence or absence of risk behaviors:

1. Known behavior risk group—infected through high-risk sexual contact or injection drug use (69% of male patients and 57% of female patients)
2. Blood transfusion or coagulation disorder risk group—infected by receipt of HIV-contaminated

blood transfusion, blood components, tissue, or clotting factors (4% of male patients and 1% of female adolescent patients)

3. Undetermined risk group or "risk not reported or identified" (27% of male patients and 42% of female adolescent patients)

It is noteworthy that there are currently more females than males with AIDS in the 13–19 year age group (3,360 females, 2,532 males) compared with the 2:1 ratio of males to females among young adults ages 20–24 years. Fifty percent of female adolescents have predominantly acquired AIDS through heterosexual contact. The proximity of the ratio among adolescent populations has always signaled a greater role of heterosexual transmission and has been particularly evident in large metropolitan areas from the outset of the HIV/AIDS epidemic (Vermund et al. 1989).

Of particular concern is the apparent recent rise in new cases of HIV/AIDS among adolescents after a period of stable or declining numbers. This likely represents an increased denial of vulnerability with a sense that the epidemic is under better control in the United States.

■ Transmission

Transmission data on adolescent AIDS cases reported to the CDC by state health departments have customarily been presented in seven categories: 1) sexual contact with men; 2) injection drug use; 3) sexual contact with men and injection drug use; 4) hemophilia or coagulation disorder; 5) heterosexual contact (includes sex with injection drug user, sex with bisexual male, sex with person with hemophilia, sex with transfusion recipient, sex with HIV-infected person risk unspecified); 6) recipient of blood transfusion, blood components, or tissue; and 7) other risk not reported or identified.

As of June 2001, among male adolescents (ages 13–19 years), category 1 (sexual contact with men) constituted 35% of the cumulative total number of AIDS cases, and category 3 (sexual contact with men and injection drug use) constituted 5% of the cumulative total. Among young men (ages 20–24 years), category 1 constituted 74% of the total and category 3 constituted 8% (Centers for Disease Control and Prevention 2001). Given the long incubation period for AIDS, these figures highlight sexual contact with men with or without injection drug use as a promi-

nent risk factor during the adolescent period.

Category 2 (injection drug use alone) accounted for 6% of AIDS cases among male adolescents compared with 9% of cases among male young adults and adolescents. However, among adolescents residing in large metropolitan areas, injection drug use has consistently been much more prevalent (e.g., in New York City, 23%; outside New York City, 14%) (Vermund et al. 1989) and has been associated with unsafe sex practices, such as teen prostitution or exchanging sex for drugs (Fullilove et al. 1990).

As of June 2001, category 4 (hemophilia or coagulation disorder) represented the largest cumulative total among male adolescents (31%) (Centers for Disease Control and Prevention 2001; Goedert et al. 1989), but the incidence of new cases was reaching saturation. Category 5 (heterosexual contact) was the largest group among female adolescents (51%) and young women ages 20–24 years (55%). Heterosexual transmission cumulatively constituted 2% of male adolescent cases in 1990, increasing to 5% in 1994; this proportion remained stable through 2001.

Category 6 (receipt of blood transfusion, components, or tissue) cumulatively constitutes 4% of male and 5% of female adolescent cases. HIV screening begun in the spring of 1985 across all blood banks in the United States has largely eliminated this problem (Centers for Disease Control [and Prevention] 1985b, 2000). Since the implementation of these precautions, a handful of adults, adolescents, and children have developed AIDS after receiving blood that was tested negative for HIV antibody. A major issue of concern has been the high proportion of adolescents in category 7 (risk not identified), which in 1997 included 6% of males and 20% of females. As of June 2001, this proportion was 15% for male and 29% for female adolescents. There does appear to be a major gender difference in June 2001 between adolescents in category 2 (injecting drug use): 13% of females versus 6% of males (compared with 10% of females and 7% of males in 1997).

The gender difference in the distribution of adolescent AIDS cases is no longer predominantly due to hemophilia and coagulation disorder being overrepresented among males (31% males versus 1% females in 2001 compared with 43% of males versus 1% of females in 1995) and the risk of male-to-male transmission (category 1) among male adolescents (35% in 2001 versus 33% in 1995). There is now a clearly greater prevalence of AIDS being acquired through heterosexual contact, with an overrepresentation among female adolescents and also in particular among those in injecting drug use or unidentified risk groups. Females remain at high risk of HIV transmission by heterosexual contact, and the present distribution of AIDS cases therefore reflects this change.

From a behavioral and psychosocial risk perspective, adolescents who are at highest risk for HIV infection (with the possible exceptions of the transfusion and the coagulation disorder groups) are disenfranchised inner-city youths who engage in unprotected sex practices or injection drug use (Deisher et al. 1989; Eisenberg 1989; Hein 1989; Vermund et al. 1989). The numbers of cases in adolescents who are black but not Hispanic, particularly females, have continued to climb unabated, and the cumulative total number of cases in females has now surpassed the cumulative total number of cases in males (Centers for Disease Control and Prevention 2001).

■ Comorbidity

Preexisting or co-occurring high rates of mental disorders, high incidence of HIV-related neurological and psychiatric syndromes, psychosocial stress, and negative societal reactions are common accompaniments of AIDS in adolescent populations. The neuropsychological effects of HIV infection in adolescents have not been studied separately from those in adults. AIDS dementia complex associated with primary HIV infection of the brain is likely to be a leading cause of cognitive, motor, and behavioral impairment (I. Grant et al. 1987; Navia et al. 1986). Initial complaints may include poor concentration and impairment of short-term memory and coordination. The psychological and behavioral symptoms may precede the sensory and motor neurological deficits. As in adults, organic brain syndromes caused by HIV infection (Beckett et al. 1987; Ostrow et al. 1988) may mimic functional psychiatric disorders such as major depression (Faulstich 1987), paranoid or schizophreniform psychosis (Thomas and Szabaldi 1987), mania (Gabel et al. 1986), or obsessive-compulsive disorder (Fenton 1987; Nurnberg et al. 1984; Perry and Jacobsen 1986; Rundell et al. 1986).

The increased relative risk of suicide, either as an acute reaction to the distress of being informed about the infection or as a consequence of an HIV-related psychiatric disorder (e.g., depression), has been documented in young men (ages 20–39 years) in New York City and California (Kizer 1988; Marzuk et al. 1988). Adolescents at risk for HIV infection are also likely to be at high risk for suicide, which underscores the need for vigilant psychiatric follow-up. This is particularly relevant among male adolescents ages 15–19 years because suicide represents the second most frequent cause of death in this age group (Brent et al. 1988; Shaffer 1988). High rates of affective disorder, antisocial behavior, and substance abuse also co-occur.

Psychological and Developmental Aspects

The precise nature of the impact of HIV infection on development is not well understood. Neplaz et al. (1991) showed that HIV infection did not appear to affect psychomotor function in early life. However, the developmental milestones of infants from drug-addicted mothers lagged behind those of infants from mothers who contracted HIV through heterosexual contact. Interaction with psychosocial problems in drug-injecting mothers is likely to be important because these factors independently affect the early psychological and cognitive development of infants irrespective of HIV infection. However, seropositivity of the infants seems to play an overriding role in the prediction of cognitive and motor development. For example, among infants born to women at risk for HIV infection, Aylward and colleagues (1992) found that compared with HIV-seronegative infants, the HIV-seropositive children scored significantly lower on the Mental Development Index and the Psychomotor Development Index of the Bayley Scales, but the seropositive and seronegative groups did not differ in race/ethnicity, infant age at initial testing, maternal age, maternal educational level, maternal history of intravenous drug use, or percentage of children in foster care.

Neurodevelopmental delays in infants and persistent neuropsychological deficits in youths have been reported to occur in more than 75% of cases of HIV infection. Most of these deficits are considered to be the direct result of a primary HIV infection in the brain, although prenatal exposure to drugs and nutritional deficiency may contribute to the observed deficits (Belman et al. 1988). Comprehensive neuropsychological assessments appropriate to the child's age or stage of development are essential. These should include measures of general ability, adaptive behavior, language, attention, memory, and learning, as well as visual and perceptual abilities and problem solving. HIV-related neuropsychological syndromes are difficult to recognize in the early stages of infection (Nurnberg et al. 1984; Perry and Jacobsen 1986). Infants and children born to mothers who use injected drugs are likely to have developmental delays irrespective of HIV infection; therefore, documentation of progressive loss of milestones (or a decline in psychometric scores) is important.

The psychological reactions of young children with AIDS are comparable to those seen in children with catastrophic medical illness or cancer. Although features such as anxiety, sadness, nightmares, irritability, and "battle fatigue" (depending on the duration and severity of the disease and its treatment) are common, young children with AIDS face a unique set of adverse conditions. These conditions include the presence of physical illness in one or more major attachment figures (i.e., the presence of AIDS in a parent); a family history of psychiatric illness in one or both parents (e.g., substance abuse, depression, HIV-related organic brain disorders); major life events (e.g., death of a parent, foster care placement); and poverty and social alienation.

Children who are old enough to attend school may experience estrangement, avoidance, and rejection by peers; disfiguring effects of wasting; ensuing lesions; and the complications of treatment. These burdens extend to their most intimate relationships at home, at school, and among peers and are exaggerated by the extreme uncertainty that characterizes the entire process. All these factors affect the psychological life of the child and adolescent.

In cases of perinatal AIDS, the emotions in the transmitting parent also have a significant effect on the child. These emotions range from the parent's own fear of the disease to guilt about passing the virus to the child to the anger and shame of being a victim. These feelings are compounded by the uncertainty (until the child reaches age 15 months) that an antibody-positive child may be truly infected. This period of uncertainty may seriously affect the character of the relationship between the child and parents or other caregivers (Adnopoz et al. 1994). Anticipatory grief needs to be worked through openly and needs to be sanctioned by the caregiving system, because it can temper the severity of the grief reaction. Parents of infected children may benefit from talking to others in the same situation. In this respect, support groups for parents provide a safe environment for open discussion.

Because early treatment, supportive care, and nutritional supplementation are considered essential in prolonging the quality and length of survival in perinatal AIDS, extraordinary efforts are necessary to provide and maintain treatment for these children (Centers for Disease Control 1985a). It is important to encourage a therapeutic alliance with a key caregiver; to establish support teams, including counselors and social workers who will follow the family throughout the vicissitudes of illness; and to provide institutional care sensitive to the needs of these patients. Older siblings without HIV infection face the prospect of multiple losses of family members to AIDS and therefore need counseling as well as placement with other family members, friends, or foster parents. In some instances, the older siblings become the primary caregivers, with all the attendant problems faced by young parents and compounded by their own experience of loss.

AIDS as a Chronic Illness

With the recognition that children with AIDS will be living longer comes the need to consider long-term support for families and children. Central to this support is the recognition that even in remission AIDS remains a disease with high lethality. An irony is that successful treatment for AIDS, as evidenced by adult outcomes in terms of long-term risk for the development of malignancy, is perhaps secondary to the vulnerability conveyed by the treatments themselves (Biggar et al. 2000). There is an increased risk of non-Hodgkin's lymphoma of varying types. Therefore, the therapist who works with families and children must decide how to balance recognized ongoing risk with the desire to promote a positive future outlook.

In recognition of AIDS now being seen as a chronic illness, Sherman et al. (2000) studied self-disclosure among children with HIV/AIDS. In this study (which has certain methodological weaknesses but nevertheless addresses an important issue), it was demonstrated that self-disclosure to friends did not affect the child's behavior or self-concept. Interestingly, self-disclosure was associated with increased CD4 cell counts among recent disclosers.

Psychiatric Treatment Guidelines

According to guidelines of the American Academy of Child and Adolescent Psychiatry (1995), the presence or risk of HIV infection should not be a reason to deny admission to inpatient psychiatric or substance abuse treatment settings. The child and adolescent psychiatrist can serve as an advocate for children and adolescents with respect to the most appropriate interventions irrespective of HIV status. The American Academy of Child and Adolescent Psychiatry recommends that all inpatients be treated with universal precautionary measures. This assumes that the patients who are HIV positive or at risk for HIV should not be segregated from other patients (e.g., assigned to individual rooms or separate toilets). Indeed, these patients should participate in all aspects of the inpatient program. In addition, adolescent substance abuse programs must provide concurrent psychosocial support and medical care for HIV-positive patients (American Academy of Child and Adolescent Psychiatry 1995).

Children and adolescents should not be routinely tested, and such requirements for testing cannot be a condition for inpatient admission. There are specific state and federal laws regarding authorization for HIV testing and informed consent in minors, as well as for the protection of confidentiality and disclosure of HIV-antibody test results. Involvement of the minor in the consent process is strongly recommended (American Academy of Child and Adolescent Psychiatry 1995). Ultimately, HIV testing (with pretest and posttest counseling) should be reserved for patients with risk factors for HIV infection and should be done with written informed consent of the parent(s) or guardian(s). Because substance abuse is strongly correlated with adolescent HIV risk behaviors, HIV risk assessment and psychoeducational programs should be part of all substance abuse and inpatient units (DiClemente and Ponton 1993; Ponton et al. 1991).

Psychological Issues in Uninfected Children

In a program for uninfected children in AIDS-affected families (i.e., families with affected children), Adnopoz and Nagler (1992) reported that 36% of children with HIV-infected mothers interviewed had problems severe enough to require some form of intervention. To date, no controlled studies have been done to determine the extent of the psychological impact on affected siblings and children (Adnopoz et al. 1994). The range of symptoms in affected children is likely to be similar to that seen in children with family members who have developed terminal illness (e.g., cancer) or other chronic or life-threatening illness.

Another psychological phenomenon is the heightened fear about AIDS in children in affected and unaffected families. Fisman and Walsh (1994) reported on the fear of AIDS in children with obsessive-compulsive disorder. In the children with obsessive-compulsive disorder who were studied, a trigger for their fears was exposure to potentially AIDS-contaminated materials in a classroom setting. The relationship between AIDS information (as well as AIDS misinformation) and the incidence rate of obsessive-compulsive disorder and other psychiatric disorders in childhood and adolescence has yet to be clearly elucidated (Fassler et al. 1990; Fisman and Walsh 1994).

AIDS Orphans

As noted above under "Global HIV/AIDS," the number of AIDS orphans in the United States and worldwide is presenting a significant challenge for caregivers and systems of care. The issues in the United States and those in other countries are not substantively different, but they differ in magnitude and in the available financial resources (Schuster et al. 2000).

HIV/AIDS in more than one family member is a frequent occurrence in affected families. Therefore, a large proportion of AIDS orphans may already have lost multiple attachment figures. A child's developmental level and cognitive capacities to understand death, as well as the availability of substitute parenting and psychosocial supports, shape adaptation (Siegel and Gorey 1994).

Because of the perceived risks associated with the disclosure of HIV infection, secrecy is an important concern for all infected and affected children and adolescents. Immediate family members may frequently choose to keep the diagnosis secret from other extended family members and friends because of the powerful cultural stigma attached to homosexuality or intravenous drug abuse. A consequence is that AIDS orphans may not be able to talk openly about the loss of a parent within or outside the family. This may lead to isolation associated with feelings that something shameful has occurred (Michaels and Levine 1992).

Multidisciplinary and Family-Centered Care

There is a need to provide comprehensive and interdisciplinary care using case management to address medical and social needs and to ensure adequate health care financing, access to services, and flexible responsiveness to needs of all children and families (Association for the Care of Children's Health 1989; Stuber 1992). Outside the hospital setting, where multidisciplinary neonatal and infant nurseries are being established, a variety of foster-care, day-care, and home-support programs for children with AIDS are being developed. Child and adolescent psychiatrists, along with other mental health professionals, have an important role to play. Support needs to be extended to all surrogate caregivers of children affected by HIV/ AIDS and their siblings.

Where there has been effective preparation in the community and school by educators and mental health professionals, integration of children into schools has been possible. Where children have been excluded and have become homebound, limited tutoring and restricted activities have invariably isolated them. Although special care centers are designed to meet the specific needs of HIV-infected children, their purpose is not infection control, and they should not become a means to segregate infected children.

Trad et al. (1994) provided examples of the assessment and psychotherapeutic intervention needed with youngsters who are HIV positive or who have AIDS. These researchers emphasize the potential for the psychotherapist to be the coordinator of services for the child and surviving family members. To facilitate treatment, a protocol for interventions must be established. This will yield a more orderly approach to the clinical care of the child and the family. The protocol helps the therapist who takes on the integrating role to deal with the overwhelming needs of the patient, the family, and other caregivers.

It is particularly challenging to provide programming for adolescents because of limited information on HIV-infected gay youths, street youths, and youths in institutions (DiClemente et al. 1988; Goodman and Cohall 1989; Hein 1989). HIV identification and treatment efforts for adolescents will need to be closely linked to drug treatment programs; family planning, sexually transmitted disease, and perinatal clinics; programs for runaway and homeless youths; child protective services; and the juvenile courts.

Provider Support

So far, the lack of AIDS care training among psychiatrists has been of little consequence in some regions because of the low incidence of HIV infection in children and adolescents. This will change as child psychiatrists are increasingly called on to be consultants for hospitals, schools, and day-care centers. As AIDS in children and adolescents becomes a chronic illness because of earlier and more effective but palliative interventions, child and adolescent psychiatrists as therapists are more likely to work directly with young AIDS patients. The hospital staff members caring for critically ill or bereaved children with AIDS are likely to feel unusually vulnerable to their own anxieties about death and failure. In the tradition of consultation services of general hospitals (Cassem 1987), psychiatrists can foster close working relationships with other hospital staff members, becoming significant members of support teams in the comprehensive care of AIDS patients (Krener 1987; Krener and Miller 1989). Widespread educational and preventive programs remain the only hope of containing the epidemic. Child psychiatrists and other mental health professionals will need to be increasingly involved in this new frontier.

Prevention

■ Risk Behaviors

Efforts to control HIV infection in children and adolescents involve focusing on at-risk sexual behavior and on needle sharing among injection drug users as well as addressing a number of complex issues, including use of alcohol and other substances by adolescents, pregnancy, homelessness, prostitution, urban poverty, inadequate social services, poor education, and deficient health care services (Conway et al. 1993). As of this writing, no consistently effective means are available for altering the behaviors that relate to the most common modes of HIV transmission: unprotected sexual intercourse (heterosexual and homosexual) and injection drug use.

There are parallels between the risk factors for teenage pregnancy and adolescent risk factors for transmission of HIV-1 infection: minority status, low socioeconomic status, low educational attainment, and history of poor family relationships (Maciak et al. 1987; Zuckerman et al. 1984). Continued efforts aimed at both delaying early sexual experiences and encouraging the use of contraception are necessary to reduce the pregnancy rate and the risk of HIV seroconversion in teenagers.

Short-term behavior change has been achieved among adolescents as a result of AIDS education, but this varies with sexual experience. For example, studies that have assessed the long-term effects on risk-behavior reduction of interventions focusing on high school students have demonstrated that intensive sex education delays the onset of intercourse among those who have never had sex but not among sexually experienced teenagers (Eisen et al. 1990; Howard and Mc-Cabe 1990; Kirby et al. 1991).

Some adolescents, such as runaway youths, are particularly difficult to reach with AIDS behavioral interventions. Runaway or "throwaway" youths are characterized by multiple and often overlapping problems, including substance abuse, drug dealing, prostitution, and a history of legal and mental health interventions. One group of researchers engaged runaway youths in AIDS education and coping skills training combined with individual risk-reduction counseling. Following up both 3 and 6 months later, researchers found a higher increase in condom use and safer sex among those who attended the intervention site than among those at the control site (Rotheram-Borus et al. 1991). The long-term efficacy of this shelter-based intervention has yet to be assessed; however, the results of this study suggest that, at least on a short-term basis, adolescents with multiple risks in their lives, including vulnerability for HIV infection, can modify their sexual risk taking. School- and community-based HIV prevention programs need to go beyond the transfer of factual information to interactive teaching of adolescents on issues such as safe sex practice strategies and perceptions of invulnerability (DiClemente et al. 1992).

Children and adolescents who have been sexually abused or raped by individuals infected with HIV may themselves become infected (Gellert and Mascola 1989). Sexual abuse of children and adolescents is a se-

rious and increasing public health problem (see Chapter 46, "Sexual Abuse of Children," in this volume). At least 250,000 cases of child sexual abuse are reported annually (Krugman 1986). Furthermore, a single molester or rapist may commit an astonishingly high number of abusive acts (American Academy of Pediatrics 1988; Gellert and Mascola 1989).

■ Education and Prevention Programs

Efforts to intercept the AIDS epidemic rest on the development of effective health education to change behavior that leads to disease transmission (Eisenberg 1989; Sandberg et al. 1988). Yet educational efforts to date have been more successful in heightening awareness about AIDS than in producing sufficient changes in transmission behavior (Becker and Joseph 1988; Hingson et al. 1990).

Any educational intervention aimed at imparting knowledge or promoting prevention must be repeated in a meaningful fashion at each evolving developmental stage. A one-time imparting of knowledge is virtually useless; sequential, reinforced teaching is needed. HIV transmission is a complex issue to communicate to young children, and very few age-appropriate materials currently exist (Fassler and McQueen 1990; Hausherr 1989; Quackenbush and Villarreal 1988, 1989). AIDS should be identified as an illness and should be placed in the context of other known illnesses. Over time, issues of transmission are introduced, as are issues related to the transmission of other familiar illnesses. By age 10, for a child with average intelligence, educators can move beyond imparting knowledge about transmission to address changing behavior. Ten-year-olds represent an important target group because in many high-risk locales, sexual activity and substance abuse may be beginning or, more rarely, may have begun. Thus by this age, there is a small window of opportunity for preventive education and behavior change. Soon thereafter, with the onset of adolescent risk-taking activity, emphasis must be placed on remediation rather than education or prevention.

In terms of psychological development, there needs to be a sense of self-esteem and a healthy sense of vulnerability. Unfortunately, development may already be compromised in at-risk children and adolescents because of other realities of daily life. The conditions that place the adolescent at risk begin early and are affected by traumatic experiences. For adolescents with histories of sexual abuse or rape, information about AIDS is emotionally compounded (Gellert and Mascola 1989). Professionals who counsel sexual abuse victims are concerned that the paucity of data on HIV-1 infection acquired through sexual abuse will delay preventive action. A survey of Maryland hospitals suggested that topical anti-HIV spermicidal agents such as nonoxynol-9 should be used as soon as possible after an assault on a female, perhaps by the victim herself, or soon after arrival at the hospital (Foster and Bartlett 1989). The issue of HIV testing should also be approached with caution in this risk group.

The knowledge of HIV infection is likely to cause panic, acting-out, or suicidal behavior in some adolescents. In one study, 21% of the adolescents spontaneously reported that they would commit suicide if they had positive test results, highlighting the level of anxiety associated with the issue of testing in this age group (Goodman and Cohall 1989). Because teenagers usually have difficulty in perceiving probable future risks and think of the present in concrete terms, it may be difficult to help them understand concepts such as an incubation time that may take years before the development of AIDS (Haffner 1987).

An essential part of every preventive or educational program is to meet with a person with AIDS (Klitzner 1989). Adolescents at the greatest risk for HIV infection are those who are likely to see themselves as invulnerable to death or disease and who tend to resist traditional preventive strategies. Correlates of non-maintenance of safer sex techniques include youth, depression, and heavy drug or alcohol use (Kelly et al. 1990; Stall et al. 1990).

Behavioral change in the potentially vulnerable heterosexual adolescent and young adult populations is uncommon, as is risk reduction in urban minorities (Becker and Joseph 1988). Only a few studies investigate the relationship of knowledge and attitudes to risk reduction (Fullilove et al. 1990; Hingson et al. 1990). As AIDS spreads beyond the initial risk groups, the ability to assess risk by sexual history becomes less meaningful. For adolescents and young adults, this has led some investigators to recommend the use of condoms and spermicide containing nonoxynol-9 for all sexual encounters except long-standing monogamous relationships. Reduction in number and careful selection of partners are also recommended (Francis and Chin 1987; Hearst and Hulley 1988).

One encouraging finding that has emerged in some prevention programs is the increased level of worry about contracting AIDS reported by adolescents who engage in one or more high-risk behaviors. Programs should help build the skills necessary for safer sex practices and should be targeted to specific, identifiable high-risk groups (Goodman and Cohall 1989; Kegeles et al. 1989; Sandberg et al. 1988). Newer programs are emphasizing peer education, peer-staffed hot lines, and other peer-related support activities accompanied by close supervision, reinforcement, and emotional support by responsible adults (Klitzner 1989).

Conclusion

During the last two decades, which correspond with the course of the HIV/AIDS epidemic, the United States and much of the developed world experienced unprecedented economic progress. Yet in many communities in the developed world and much of the developing countries and emerging democracies, the HIV/AIDS epidemic in children and adolescents—and especially in women and youth—has made dramatic inroads. In recent years, the fact that the international community may be awakening to the global surge of HIV/AIDS is evidenced by the establishment of a global fund to fight AIDS. The leadership in the developed world is cautious regarding how such a fund, even if it were imminently adequate, could be well spent. Other diseases—such as measles, smallpox, typhoid, and malaria—have claimed many lives worldwide (Epstein and Chen 2002). However, as in the case of these other global infections, addressing HIV/AIDS in the developing countries will involve more than antiretroviral drugs alone, even if they were to be made available cheaply. A systematic approach by the global fund will need to empower developing communities, alleviate poverty and despair, and help build and motivate the human infrastructure for sustainable care that is necessary to fight the illness. In fact, in the United States and much of the developed world, HIV/ AIDS is as much a chronic debilitating illness as an acute illness ending in death, and in those regions it is raising a distinct set of complex psychological and developmental issues. Both nationally and worldwide, however, HIV/AIDS affects individuals, families, and communities. It creates despair and loneliness and impoverishes the livelihoods of affected persons. Such conditions, in turn, fuel more risky and self-destructive behaviors. Child and adolescent psychiatrists and their colleagues can greatly ease the burden of illness associated with the infected individual and his or her affected relatives and friends and need to be more actively involved in international and nongovernmental relief work worldwide, especially with the new impetus to fight HIV/AIDS globally.

In the United States, progress in detection, diagnosis, treatment, and supportive services over the past decade has been remarkable. Although hope for cure and prevention is the key to keeping HIV infection from further affecting children and adolescents, there is evidence that the disease has become more resistant among youths and women in particular than in other risk groups. Child and adolescent psychiatrists and their colleagues must persist in their efforts to understand the psychological, physical, and social determinants and consequences of the illness and must be more actively available to provide the needed support both nationally and internationally. In particular, the involvement of trainees in the fight against HIV/AIDS should be encouraged. This presents unique opportunities not only for the understanding of the new paradigm of care for diseases of globalization but also for important public service. These ailments of infectious, environmental, and behavioral origin undoubtedly will require extensive global cooperation for their ultimate control and will be increasingly important in the future (Epstein and Chen 2002).

References

Adnopoz JA, Nagler S: Supporting HIV infected children in their own families through family centered practice, in Advancing Family Preservation Practice. Edited by Grigsby KR, Morton ES. Newbury Park, CA, Sage, 1993, pp 119–128

Adnopoz JA, Forsyth BWC, Nagler SF: Psychiatric aspects of HIV infection and AIDS on the family. Child Adolesc Psychiatr Clin N Am 3:543–555, 1994

Allen JR, Curran JW: Prevention of AIDS and HIV infection: needs and priorities for epidemiologic research. Am J Public Health 78:381–386, 1988

American Academy of Child and Adolescent Psychiatry: Policy statement: HIV and treatment issues in children and adolescents. Washington, DC, HIV Issues Committee, American Academy of Child and Adolescent Psychiatry, 1995

American Academy of Pediatrics: Rape and the adolescent. Pediatrics 81:595–597, 1988

American Academy of Pediatrics, Provisional Committee on Pediatric AIDS: Perinatal human immunodeficiency virus testing. Pediatrics 95:303–307, 1995

American Public Health Association: Pediatric HIV infection: report of the special initiative on AIDS (APHA/SIA Report 6). Washington, DC, American Public Health Association, 1989

Association for the Care of Children's Health: Building Systems of Care for Children with HIV Infection and Their Families. Washington, DC, Health Resources and Services Administration, Office of Maternal and Child Health, 1989

Auerbach JD, Wypijewska C, Brodie HKH: AIDS and Behavior: An Integrated Approach. Washington, DC, National Academy Press, 1994

Auger I, Thomas P, De Grutolla V, et al: Incubation periods for paediatric AIDS patients. Nature 336:575–577, 1988

Aylward EH, Butz AM, Hutton N, et al: Cognitive and motor development in infants at risk for human immunodeficiency virus. Am J Dis Child 146:218–222, 1992

Barnes DM: Brain function decline in children with AIDS (abstract). Science 232:1196, 1986

Becker MH, Joseph JG: AIDS and behavioral change to reduce risk: a review. Am J Public Health 78:394–410, 1988

Beckett A, Summergrad P, Manscreck T, et al: Symptomatic HIV infection of the CNS in a parent without clinical evidence of immunodeficiency. Am J Psychiatry 144:1342–1344, 1987

Belman AL, Diamond G, Dickson D, et al: Pediatric acquired immunodeficiency syndrome: neurologic syndromes. Am J Dis Child 149:29–35, 1988

Biggar RJ, Frisch M, Goedert JJ: Risk of cancer in children with AIDS. AIDS–Cancer Match Registry Study Group. JAMA 284:205–209, 2000

Blanche S, Rouzioux C, Moscato MG, et al: A prospective study of infants born to women seropositive for human immunodeficiency virus type 1. N Engl J Med 320:1643–1648, 1989

Brent DA, Perper IA, Goldstein CE, et al: Risk factors for adolescent suicide: a comparison of adolescent suicide victims with suicidal inpatients. Arch Gen Psychiatry 45:581–588, 1988

Cassem NH: The consultation service, in Psychiatry in a General Hospital: The First Fifty Years. Edited by Hackett TP, Weisman AD, Kucharski A. Littleton, MA, PSG Publishing, 1987, pp 33–39

Centers for Disease Control: Education and foster care of children infected with human T-lymphotropic virus type-III/lymphadenopathy-associated virus. MMWR Morb Mortal Wkly Rep 34:517–521, 1985a

Centers for Disease Control: Provisional Public Health Service inter-agency recommendations for screening donated blood and plasma for antibody to the virus causing acquired immunodeficiency syndrome. MMWR Morb Mortal Wkly Rep 34:1–5, 1985b

Centers for Disease Control: Classification system for human immunodeficiency virus (HIV) infection in children under 13 years of age. MMWR Morb Mortal Wkly Rep 36:225–230, 235–236, 1987

Centers for Disease Control and Prevention: 1994 revised classification system for human immunodeficiency virus infection in children less than 13 years of age. MMWR Recomm Rep 43 (RR-12):1–10, 1994

Centers for Disease Control and Prevention: HIV/AIDS Surveillance Report: U.S. HIV and AIDS Cases Reported Through June 1995, Vol 7, No 1. Atlanta, GA, Centers for Disease Control and Prevention, 1995a

Centers for Disease Control and Prevention: U.S. Public Health Service recommendations for human deficiency virus counseling and voluntary testing for pregnant women. MMWR Recomm Rep 44 (RR-7), 1995b

Centers for Disease Control and Prevention: Guidelines for the use of antiretroviral agents in pediatric HIV infection. MMWR Recomm Rep 47 (RR-4):1–43, 1998. June 2003 update available at: http://www.aidsinfo.nih.gov/guidelines. Accessed July 21, 2003

Centers for Disease Control and Prevention: HIV/AIDS Surveillance Report: U.S. HIV and AIDS Cases Reported Through June 2001, Vol 13, No 1. Atlanta, GA, Centers for Disease Control and Prevention, 2001

Connor EM, Sperling RS, Gelber R, et al: Reduction of maternal-infant transmission of human immunodeficiency virus type 1 with zidovudine treatment. Pediatric AIDS Clinical Trials Group Protocol 076 Study Group. N Engl J Med 331:1173–1180, 1994

Conway G, Epstein M, Hayman C: Trends in HIV prevalence among disadvantaged youth: survey results from a national job training program, 1988 through 1992. JAMA 269:2887–2889, 1993

Deisher RW, Farrow JA, Hope K, et al: The pregnant adolescent prostitute. Am J Dis Child 143:1162–1165, 1989

Dennis M, Ross J, Smith S (eds): Children on the Brink: A Joint Report on Orphan Estimates and Program Strategies. Geneva, Switzerland, UNAIDS, July 2002. Available at: http://www.unaids.org/barcelona/presskit/childrenonthebrink

DiClemente RJ, Ponton L: HIV-related risk behaviors among hospitalized adolescents and school-based adolescents. Am J Psychiatry 150:324–325, 1993

DiClemente RJ, Boyer CB, Morales ES: Minorities and AIDS: knowledge, attitudes, and misconceptions among black and Latino adolescents. Am J Public Health 78:55–57, 1988

DiClemente RJ, Durbin M, Siegel D, et al: Determinants of condom use among junior high school students in a minority, inner-city school district. Pediatrics 89:197–202, 1992

Dunn DT, Newell ML, Ades AE, et al: Risk of human immunodeficiency virus type 1 transmission through breast-feeding. Lancet 340:585–588, 1992

Eichberg JW, Allan JS, Cobb KE, et al: In utero transmission of an infant chimpanzee with HIV. N Engl J Med 319:722–723, 1988

Eisen M, Zellman G, McAlister A: Evaluating the impact of a theory-based sexuality and contraceptive education program. Fam Plann Perspect 22:261–271, 1990

Eisenberg L: Health education and the AIDS epidemic. Br J Psychiatry 154:754–767, 1989

Epstein H, Chen L: Can AIDS be stopped? New York Review of Books, March 14, 2002, pp 29–31

European Collaborative Study: Mother-to-child transmission of HIV infection. Lancet 2:1039–1043, 1988

European Collaborative Study: Risk factors for mother-to-child transmission of HIV-1. Lancet 339:1007–1009, 1992

Fassler D, McQueen K: What's a Virus, Anyway? The Kids Book About AIDS. Burlington, VT, Waterfront Publications, 1990

Fassler D, McQueen K, Duncan P, et al: Children's perceptions of AIDS. J Am Acad Child Adolesc Psychiatry 29:459–462, 1990

Faulstich ME: Psychiatric aspects of AIDS. Am J Psychiatry 144:551–556, 1987

Fenton TW: AIDS-related psychiatric disorder. Br J Psychiatry 151:579–588, 1987

Fisman SN, Walsh L: Obsessive-compulsive disorder and fear of AIDS contamination in childhood. J Am Acad Child Adolesc Psychiatry 33:349–353, 1994

Foster IM, Bartlett J: Anti-HIV substances to rape victims (letter). JAMA 261:3407, 1989

Francis DP, Chin J: The prevention of AIDS in the United States. JAMA 257:1357–1366, 1987

French Collaborative Study Group of HIV Infection in Newborns: Comparison of vertical human immunodeficiency virus type 2 and human immunodeficiency virus type 1 transmission in the French prospective cohort. Pediatr Infect Dis J 13:502–506, 1994

Fullilove RE, Fullilove MT, Bowser BP, et al: Risk of sexually transmitted disease among black adolescent crack users in Oakland and San Francisco, Calif. JAMA 263:851–855, 1990

Gabel RH, Barnard N, Norko M, et al: AIDS presenting as mania. Compr Psychiatry 27:251–254, 1986

Gellert GA, Mascola L: Rape and AIDS (letter). Pediatrics 83 (suppl):644, 1989

Goedert JJ, Kessler CM, Aledort LM, et al: A prospective study of human immunodeficiency virus type-1 infection and the development of AIDS in subjects with hemophilia. N Engl J Med 321:1141–1148, 1989

Goodman E, Cohall AT: Acquired immunodeficiency syndrome and adolescents: knowledge, attitudes, beliefs, and behaviors in a New York City adolescent minority population. Pediatrics 84:36–42, 1989

Grant AD, DeCock KM: ABC of AIDS: HIV infection and AIDS in the developing world. BMJ 322:1475–1478, 2001

Grant I, Atkinson JH, Hesselink JR, et al: Evidence for early central nervous system involvement in the acquired immunodeficiency syndrome (AIDS) and other human immunodeficiency virus (HIV) infections: studies with neuropsychologic testing and magnetic resonance imaging. Ann Intern Med 107:828–836, 1987

Haffner DW: AIDS and Adolescents: The Time for Prevention Is Now. Washington, DC, The Center for Population Options, 1987

Hausherr R: Children and the AIDS Virus: A Book for Children, Parents and Teachers. New York, Clarion Books, 1989

Hearst N, Hulley SB: Preventing the heterosexual spread of AIDS: are we giving our patients the best advice? JAMA 259:2428–2432, 1988

Hein K: Commentary on adolescent acquired immunodeficiency syndrome: the next wave of the human immunodeficiency virus epidemic? J Pediatr 114:144–149, 1989

Hingson RW, Strunin L, Berlin B, et al: Beliefs about AIDS, use of alcohol and drugs, and unprotected sex among Massachusetts adolescents. Am J Public Health 80:295–299, 1990

Ho DD, Rota TR, Schooley RT, et al: Isolation of HTLV-III from cerebrospinal fluid and neural tissues of patients with neurological syndromes related to acquired immunodeficiency syndrome. N Engl J Med 313:1493–1497, 1985

Howard M, McCabe J: Helping teenagers postpone sexual involvement. Fam Plann Perspect 22:21–26, 1990

Iosub S, Bamji M, Stone RK, et al: More on the immunodeficiency virus embryopathy. Pediatrics 80:512–516, 1987

Joint United Nations Programme on HIV/AIDS: AIDS Epidemic Update: December 2001. Geneva, Joint United Nations Programme on HIV/AIDS and World Health Organization, 2002

Kandela P: Child prostitution and the spread of AIDS (news item). Lancet 356:1991, 2000

Kegeles SM, Adler NE, Irwin CE: Adolescents and condoms. Am J Dis Child 143:911–915, 1989

Kelly JA, St. Lawrence JS, Betts R, et al: A skills-training group intervention model to assist persons in reducing risk behaviors for HIV infection. AIDS Educ Prev 2:24–35, 1990

Kirby D, Barth R, Leland N: Reducing the risk: impact of a new curriculum on sexual risk-taking. Fam Plann Perspect 23:253–263, 1991

Kizer KW: AIDS and suicide in California (letter). JAMA 260:1881, 1988

Klitzner M: AIDS prevention and education: recommendations of the work group. J Adolesc Health Care 10:458–478, 1989

Knodel J, Van Landingham M: Children and older persons: AIDS' unseen victims. Am J Public Health 90:1024–1025, 2000

Krener PK: Impact of the diagnosis of AIDS on hospital care of an infant. Clin Pediatr (Phila) 26:30–34, 1987

Krener PK, Miller FB: Psychiatric response to HIV spectrum disease in children and adolescents. J Am Acad Child Adolesc Psychiatry 28:596–605, 1989

Krugman RD: Recognition of sexual abuse in children. Pediatr Rev 8:25–30, 1986

Lamont J, Innocenti ND: Mandela makes it his mission to get AIDS policy changed. Financial Times, February 19, 2002, p 16

Lapointe N, Michaud J, Pekovic D, et al: Transplacental transmission of HTLV-III virus. N Engl J Med 312:1325–1326, 1985

Macchi B, Verani P, Lazzarin A, et al: Evidence of HTLV-III/LAV intrauterine infection. Paper presented at the 2nd International Conference on AIDS, Paris, June 23–25, 1986

Maciak BJ, Spitz AM, Strauss LT, et al: Pregnancy and birth rates among sexually experienced U.S. teenagers: 1974, 1980, 1983. JAMA 258:2069–2071, 1987

Marion RW, Wiznia AA, Hutcheon RG, et al: Human T-cell lymphotrophic virus type-III (HTLV-III) embryopathy: a new dysmorphic syndrome associated with intrauterine HTLV-III infection. Am J Dis Child 140:638–640, 1986

Marzuk PM, Tierney H, Tardiff K, et al: Increased risk of suicide in persons with AIDS. JAMA 259:1333–1337, 1988

McLoughlin LC, Nord KS, Joshi VV, et al: Severe gastrointestinal involvement in children with the acquired immunodeficiency syndrome. J Pediatr Gastroenterol Nutr 6:517–524, 1987

Michaels D, Levine C: Estimates of the number of motherless youth orphaned by AIDS in the United States. JAMA 268:3456–3461, 1992

Navia BA, Jordan B, Price RW: The AIDS dementia complex, 1: clinical features of the AIDS dementia complex. Ann Neurol 19:525–535, 1986

Neplaz MC, Blay O, Caron A, et al: Study of psychological development of infants born from HIV infected mothers (abstract WC 3178). Paper presented at the Paris International AIDS Conference, June 16–21, 1991

Nesheim S, Lee F, Kalish ML, et al. Diagnosis of perinatal human immunodeficiency virus infection by polymerase chain reaction and p24 antigen detection after immune complex dissociation in an urban community hospital. J Infect Dis 175:1333–1336, 1997

Newell ML, Peckham C: Risk factors for vertical transmission of HIV-1 and early markers of HIV-1 infection in children. AIDS 7 (suppl 1):S91–S97, 1993

Novick BE, Rubinstein A: AIDS: the paediatric perspective. AIDS 1:3–7, 1987

Nurnberg HG, Prudic J, Fiori M, et al: Psychopathology complicating acquired immunodeficiency syndrome (AIDS). Am J Psychiatry 141:95–96, 1984

Ostrow D, Grant I, Atkinson H: Assessment and management of the AIDS patient with neuropsychiatric disturbances. J Clin Psychiatry 49 (suppl):14–22, 1988

Pawha S, Kaplan M, Fikrig S, et al: Spectrum of human T-cell lymphotropic virus type-III infection in children. JAMA 255:2299–2305, 1986

Peckham C, Gibb D: Mother-to-child transmission of the human immunodeficiency virus (current concepts). N Engl J Med 333:298–302, 1995

Perry S, Jacobsen P: Neuropsychiatric manifestations of AIDS spectrum disorders. Hosp Community Psychiatry 37:135–142, 1986

Pezzela M, Rossi P, Lombardi V, et al: HIV viral sequences in seronegative people at risk detected by in situ hybridization and polymerase chain reaction. BMJ 298:713–716, 1989

Pizzo PA: HIV infection and AIDS in children, in Clinical Research. Washington, DC, National Cancer Institute, Summer/Fall 1995, pp 1–3

Pizzo PA, Eddy J, Falloon J, et al: Effect of continuous intravenous infusion of zidovudine (AZT) in children with symptomatic HIV infection. N Engl J Med 319:889–896, 1988

Ponton LE, DiClemente RJ, McKenna S: An AIDS education and prevention program for hospitalized adolescents. J Am Acad Child Adolesc Psychiatry 30:729–734, 1991

Pyun KH, Ochs HD, Dufford MTW, et al: Perinatal infection with human immunodeficiency virus: specific antibody responses by the neonate. N Engl J Med 317:611–614, 1987

Qazi QH, Sheikh TM, Fikrig S, et al: Lack of evidence for craniofacial dysmorphism in prenatal human immunodeficiency virus infection. J Pediatr 112:7–11, 1987

Quackenbush M, Villarreal S: Does AIDS Hurt? Educating Young Children About AIDS. Santa Cruz, CA, Network Publications, 1988

Quackenbush M, Villarreal S: Talking About AIDS With Young Children: Focus, AIDS Health Project. San Francisco, University of California, 1989

Quinn TC, Kline RL, Halsey N, et al: Early diagnosis of perinatal HIV infection by detection of viral-specific IgA antibodies. JAMA 266:3439–3442, 1991

Rogers MF, Thomas PA, Stracher ET, et al: Acquired immunodeficiency syndrome in children: report of the Centers for Disease Control national surveillance, 1982 to 1985. Pediatrics 79:1008–1014, 1987

Rogers MF, Ou CY, Rayfield M, et al: Use of polymerase chain reaction for early detection of the proviral sequences of human immunodeficiency virus in infants born to seropositive mothers. N Engl J Med 320:1649–1654, 1989

Rotheram-Borus M, Koopman C, Haignere C, et al: Reducing HIV sexual risk behaviors among runaway adolescents. JAMA 266:1237–1241, 1991

Rubinstein A: Pediatric AIDS. Curr Probl Pediatr 16:361–409, 1986

Rundell JR, Wise MG, Ursano RJ: Three cases of AIDS-related psychiatric disorders. Am J Psychiatry 143:777–778, 1986

Sandberg DE, Rotheram-Borus MJ, Bradley J, et al: Methodological problems in assessing AIDS prevention programs. J Adolesc Res 3:413–418, 1988

Schuster MA, Kanouse DE, Morton SC et al: HIV-infected parents and their children in the United States. Am J Public Health 90:1074–1081, 2000

Shaffer D: The epidemiology of teen suicide: an examination of risk factors. J Clin Psychiatry 49 (suppl):36–41, 1988

Shaw GM, Harper ME, Hahn BE, et al: HTLV-III infection in brains of children and adults with AIDS encephalopathy. Science 227:177–181, 1985

Sherman BF, Bonanno GA, Wiener LS, et al: When children tell their friends they have AIDS: possible consequences for psychological well-being and disease progression. Psychosom Med 62:238–247, 2000

Siegel K, Gorey EG: Childhood bereavement due to parental death from acquired immunodeficiency syndrome. J Dev Behav Pediatr 15:866–870, 1994

Stall R, Ekstrand M, Pollack L, et al: Relapse from safer sex: the next challenge for AIDS prevention efforts. J Acquir Immune Defic Syndr Hum Retrovirol 3:1181–1187, 1990

Stuber ML: Children and AIDS. Washington, DC, American Psychiatric Press, 1992

Thiry L, Sprecher-Goldberger S, Jonckheer T, et al: Isolation of AIDS virus from cell-free breast milk of three healthy virus carriers. Lancet 2:891–892, 1985

Thomas CT, Szabaldi E: Paranoid psychosis as the first presentation of a fulminating lethal case of AIDS. Br J Psychiatry 151:693–695, 1987

Trad PV, Kentros M, Solomon GE, et al: Assessment and psychotherapeutic intervention for an HIV-infected preschool child. J Am Acad Child Adolesc Psychiatry 33:1338–1345, 1994

Vermund SH, Hein K, Gayle HD, et al: Acquired immunodeficiency syndrome among adolescents: case surveillance profiles in New York City and the rest of the United States. Am J Dis Child 143:1220–1225, 1989

Weinbreck P, Loustaud V, Denis F, et al: Post-natal transmission of HIV-1 infection (letter). Lancet 1:482, 1988

Working Group on Antiretroviral Therapy, National Pediatric HIV Resource Center: Antiretroviral therapy and medical management of the human immunodeficiency virus-infected child. Pediatr Infect Dis J 12:513–522, 1993

Working Group on Antiretroviral Therapy and Medical Management of Infants, Children and Adolescents with HIV Infection: Antiretroviral therapy and medical management of Pediatric HIV infection. Pediatrics 102 (4, suppl):1005–1062, 1998

Ziegler JB, Cooper DA, Johnson RO, et al: Postnatal transmission of AIDS-associated retrovirus from mother to infant. Lancet 1:896–898, 1985

Zuckerman BS, Walker DK, Frank DA, et al: Adolescent pregnancy: behavioral determinants of outcome. J Pediatr 105:857–863, 1984

Suicide and Suicidality

Cynthia R. Pfeffer, M.D.

Since the late 1970s and early 1980s, when suicidal behavior was initially recognized to be a national mental health problem of youth, many advances have been made in the understanding of this behavior in children and adolescents. Identification of the multifaceted features of risk, concepts of prevention, and goals of treatment have been described in the increasing number of scientific papers published about this significant morbid condition. The application of scientific techniques has provided information about the longitudinal course of suicidal children and adolescents and those at risk for suicidal behavior. The Surgeon General of the United States published a "call to action" in which he outlined important principles for identification, assessment, treatment, and prevention of suicidal behavior among youths (U.S. Public Health Service 1999). Also notable is the publication of the "Practice Parameter for the Assessment and Treatment of Children and Adolescents With Suicidal Behavior" (American Academy of Child and Adolescent Psychiatry 2001). This important document provides clinicians with up-to-date information about suicidal behavior among youths to enable the clinicians to effectively provide psychiatric care to children and adolescents who are at risk for suicidal behavior. Much is still to be learned, especially about the developmental specificity of neurobiological characteristics of childhood and adolescent suicidal behavior and about effective treatments for those at risk.

This chapter provides a review of current empirical information about the characteristics of childhood and adolescent suicidal behavior, including risk and protective factors, assessment and identification of those at risk, and strategies for intervention and prevention. There is now a consistent conclusion that suicidal behavior among children and adolescents is a distinct, prevalent, and valid phenomenon and that

medical professionals should be skilled at recognizing it and at intervening to prevent the morbidity and death of children who are at risk.

Diagnostic Criteria, Course, and Prognosis

Suicidal behavior is not a psychiatric diagnosis but is considered a psychiatric symptom. Suicidal behavior has the same definition for children and adolescents as it does for adults: it is a preoccupation or act that intentionally aims to inflict injury or death on oneself. Suicidal behavior is episodic. An episode of suicidal ideation or action may be acute and brief or may last several hours or days. Repeated suicidal acts occur. Suicidal ideation or acts may occur in the preschool or preadolescent periods or in adolescence. Although an intent to cause self-injury or to die is an essential element of the definition, it is not necessary that a child have a mature concept of the finality of death. The aim of the suicidal preoccupation or act is to die, regardless of what the concept of death means to the child (Pfeffer 1997).

Another important developmental concern is appraisal of the lethality of suicidal intent, an issue that is complicated in children because of their cognitive immaturity. Objective lethality involves the actual potential for death or serious injury if a self-destructive method is enacted. However, children often do not understand the extent or severity of a suicide method and as a result may not appreciate the outcome of their self-destructive intentions. In assessing the level of risk, clinicians should evaluate the objective and perceived lethality of an intended suicidal act. A child who considers a suicide plan to be lethal may be considered to be at high risk even if the objective lethality is low. A variety of factors are relevant in determining the degree of lethality of a suicidal act; these may include demographic characteristics and psychosocial factors. In one study, charts of 131 adolescents consecutively hospitalized in a psychiatric unit for suicide attempts were reviewed to identify factors associated with lethality (Brent 1987). The results suggested that high medical lethality was most strongly associated with being male and having a diagnosis of an affective or substance abuse disorder and definite suicidal intent. Furthermore, these factors were similar to those in adolescents who committed suicide. The study also revealed that the lethality of an impulsive suicide attempt was most strongly associated with the availability of lethal suicide methods (e.g., firearms). However, suicide intent and the severity of psychopathology were most greatly associated with the lethality of nonimpulsive suicide attempts.

The diagnosis of suicidal behavior is made by direct information from the child and by information from other sources. Direct inquiry about the presence of suicidal phenomena involves inquiry about thoughts of wishing to kill oneself and a plan of carrying out suicidal intent. This assessment may be complicated by the child's immature understanding of the cause and effect of implementing a plan or by the child's inability to clearly discuss suicidal thinking because of the presence of psychiatric symptoms such as anhedonia, psychomotor retardation, psychosis, impulsivity, or poor concentration (Jacobsen et al. 1994). Among the reasons why others may not report reliably about children's suicidal intent or acts are that parents may feel responsible for their child's morbid condition and may minimize its extent; parents' openness in reporting the behavior may be impaired by the stigma of having a suicidal child; and the parents' lack of knowledge about their child's inner motives and overt suicidal acts may decrease identification of the level of risk based on parental reports (Jacobsen et al. 1994). Prediction of suicidal behavior is not reliable, although prospective research suggests that previous suicidal ideation or suicide attempts can predict suicidal acts. Specifically, a study of 133 prepubertal psychiatric inpatients and nonsuicidal children living in the community suggested that prepubertal children who had reported suicidal ideation were three times more likely to attempt suicide in adolescence than the nonsuicidal children, and those who had attempted suicide as children were six times more likely to attempt suicide in

adolescence than the nonsuicidal children (Pfeffer et al. 1993).

Research suggests that children who had initial suicidal ideation or attempts within the previous 2 years are more likely to attempt suicide than are previously nonsuicidal children (Pfeffer et al. 1994a). Furthermore, empirical research suggests that repeated episodes of suicidal ideation or acts are prevalent (Pfeffer et al. 1994a). Psychological "autopsy" studies, in which individuals who knew suicide victims report on the psychological condition of the deceased before the suicide, strongly suggest that approximately 26%–33% of children and adolescents who commit suicide had a history of a suicide attempt (Brent et al. 1993; Shaffer et al. 1996). Specifically, among 67 adolescent suicide victims, 25.8% had a previous suicide attempt (relative risk [RR], 17.0; 95% confidence interval [CI], 2.3–127.7) compared with 1.5% of 67 nonsuicidal adolescents selected from the community (Brent et al. 1993).

In summary, developmental considerations in the assessment of child and adolescent suicidal behavior are essential to diagnosis. The course of early-onset suicidal behavior involves recurrent episodes and potential for death.

Differential Diagnosis and Comorbidity

The differential diagnosis for suicidal behavior involves primarily other forms of self-injury (such as self-mutilation involving superficially cutting oneself or pulling out hair or eyelashes), sexual asphyxiation, high-risk behaviors (including eating disorders; substance abuse involving alcohol, drugs, or cigarettes; unprotected sexual activities; and motor vehicle accidents), and homicide. Superficial cutting is often associated with suicidal intent, and in this regard it is considered a suicidal act. However, when overwhelmed with feelings of anger and anxiety, children and adolescents may exhibit self-mutilation. Such behavior—involving superficial cutting of the arms, legs, and other body areas—is often associated with stress, dissociative phenomena, and anger and is not associated with the distinct intent to kill oneself. In such cases, these behaviors are not distinctly suicidal. Children and adolescents with intense anxiety may exhibit trichotillomania involving pulling out hair or eyelashes and eyebrows. Such behaviors usually do not involve suicidal intent and are not considered suicidal behaviors. Sexual asphyxiation involves behavior in which the airway is obstructed while involved in sexual self-stimulation. Adolescents, especially males, have hung themselves during acts of sexual self-stimulation. Often sexually stimulating pictures or other objects are found at the scene of death, and this enables differentiating suicide from sexual asphyxiation behavior. Excessive high-risk behaviors, such as motor vehicle speeding or promiscuous sexual behavior, should be differentiated from suicidal behavior. It is essential to acquire comprehensive details about the context of such behaviors and to determine if they involved suicidal intent.

The suicidal symptoms of ideation and acts are listed in DSM-IV and DSM-IV-TR (American Psychiatric Association 1994, 2000) as criterion items only for the diagnoses of major depressive disorder and borderline personality disorder. Regarding major depressive disorder, DSM-IV-TR includes recurrent thoughts of death, recurrent suicidal ideation without a plan, or a suicide attempt or a specific plan for committing suicide as the criterion for suicidal state. It includes recurrent suicidal behavior, gestures, or threats, or self-mutilating behavior as the criterion for self-destructive behavior associated with borderline personality disorder. Although suicidal ideation and acts are integral diagnostic criteria for these disorders, not all individuals with these disorders exhibit suicidal ideation or acts.

Suicidal behavior is frequently comorbid with a variety of other psychiatric disorders, including anxiety, conduct, substance abuse, developmental, and personality disorders. In fact, the presence of these disorders increases the risk for suicidal behavior. Psychological autopsy studies of adolescent suicide victims suggest the relative risks for suicide imparted by specific psychiatric disorders. In a study of 67 adolescent suicide victims compared with 67 demographically matched adolescents selected from the community, the relative risks for suicide imparted by psychiatric disorders were as follows: for major depression, 27.0 (95% CI, 3.6–199.8); for alcohol abuse, 7.5 (95% CI, 1.7–32.8); for drug abuse, 9.0 (95% CI, 1.1–71.0); and for conduct disorder, 6.0 (95% CI, 1.8–20.4) (Brent et al. 1993). The presence of any psychiatric disorder increased risk 35-fold (95% CI, 4.8–255.4). Similar results of another psychological autopsy study supported the significance of psychiatric disorders, especially mood disorders, as important risk factors for adolescent suicide

(Shaffer et al. 1996). This study of 120 adolescent suicide victims and 147 demographically matched nonsuicidal adolescents indicated that among the psychiatric disorders, mood disorders (RR, 12.10; 95% CI, 5.12–28.57) were risk factors for suicide in males and females. In addition, among males, any substance abuse (RR, 5.76; 95% CI, 1.61–20.6) and prior suicide attempt (RR, 19.39; 95% CI, 2.32–162.13) increased the risk for suicide.

In addition to the effects of psychopathology on suicide risk, a study comparing 120 adolescent suicide victims with 147 adolescents from the community who were matched for age, gender, and ethnicity or race suggested that environmental factors increased risk for youth suicide (Gould et al. 1996). Specifically, risk for suicide was increased by lack of an intact family (odds ratio [OR], 1.9; 95% CI, 1.1–3.3), poor communication with mother (OR, 4.3; 95% CI, 1.6–11.6) or father (OR, 4.0; 95% CI, 1.8–9.0), mother with a history of mood disorder (OR, 2.0; 95% CI, 1.1–3.7), father having problems with police (OR, 4.0; 95% CI, 1.5–10.9), family history of suicidal behavior (OR, 4.6; 95% CI, 1.8–11.7), disciplinary crises (OR, 5.1; 95% CI, 2.7–9.5), loss (OR, 1.9; 95% CI, 1.1–3.3), failing a grade (OR, 3.3; 95% CI, 1.4–7.7), suspension from school (OR, 6.1; 95% CI, 1.6–23.4), dropping out of school (OR, 5.1; 95% CI, 1.2–20.7), neither working nor in school (OR, 44.1; 95% CI, 4.5–432.0), and lack of a college education (OR, 7.8; 95% CI, 2.2–27.3). These stressful life events should be considered in evaluating risk for suicidal behavior among youths.

Studies of nonfatal child and adolescent suicidal behavior indicate increased risk for suicidal acts when specific psychiatric disorders are present. For example, when characteristics of 27 adolescent suicide victims were compared with those of 56 adolescent psychiatric inpatients who reported suicidal ideation or a suicide attempt, both groups showed similar rates of mood disorders, family history of mood disorders, suicidal behavior, and antisocial disorder (Brent et al. 1988). However, the suicide victims had higher prevalences of bipolar disorder, mood disorder with comorbid psychiatric disorders, lack of prior psychiatric treatment, and availability of firearms in the home.

Strong associations between suicidal behavior and specific psychiatric disorders in children and adolescents have been found in other studies as well. For example, a prospective follow-up study of prepubertal children included psychiatric inpatients—of whom 25 reported a recent suicide attempt, 28 reported recent suicidal ideation, and 16 had no history of suicidal ideation or suicide attempt—and 64 prepubertal children selected from the community who had no history of suicidal ideation or suicide attempt (Pfeffer et al. 1993). These children were evaluated at an initial time when they were 6–12 years old and again 6–8 years later when they were adolescents. Relative risk factors for a suicide attempt or suicidal ideation in adolescence were identified as follows: for mood disorder, 3.54 (95% CI, 1.35–9.28) initially, 5.28 (95% CI, 1.76–15.82) at follow-up; for substance abuse disorder measured at follow-up, 2.84 (95% CI, 1.18–6.83); for life event stress, 1.69 (95% CI, 1.10–2.59) initially, 1.71 (95% CI, 1.11–2.64) at follow-up; and for poor social adjustment, 4.14 (95% CI, 2.18–7.84) initially, 4.32 (95% CI, 2.15–8.66) at follow-up. These results add information to the data available for adolescent suicide victims by suggesting the importance of early-onset mood disorders and their chronicity as risk factors for suicidal behavior in youths. In addition, the risk imparted by substance abuse disorders, especially when comorbid with mood disorders, increases the risk for suicidal behavior in adolescence.

Personality traits and cognitive styles have also been identified as correlates of nonfatal suicidal behavior in individuals younger than age 25 years who participated in the Canterbury Suicide Project from September 1, 1991, to May 31, 1994, in Christchurch, New Zealand (Beautrais et al. 1999). Among 129 youths who attempted suicide, compared with 153 youths who reported no suicidal behavior, hopelessness (OR, 18.5; 95% CI, 4.9–10.0), neuroticism (OR, 5.4; 95% CI, 3.9–7.6), and external locus of control (OR, 2.9; 95% CI, 2.1–4.0) were significant risk factors for suicide attempts. These results suggest that features of long-standing traits and styles influence risk for suicidal behavior and that prevention of suicidal behavior may be effective when such factors are identified and treated. Furthermore, other studies suggested that among adolescent suicide attempters, poor self-esteem is correlated with hopelessness, a factor that is highly associated with suicidal behavior in youths (Donaldson et al. 2000). Risk for repetition of suicide attempts is predicted most strongly by severity of depressive symptoms, although symptoms of hopelessness, poor self-esteem, anger, or difficulties in problem solving are contributing risk factors for suicidal behavior (Hawton et al. 1999).

Epidemiology

With the recognition of high suicide rates among 15- to 24-year-olds, which peaked at 13.6 per 100,000 in 1977 (Pfeffer 1986), other epidemiological trends in suicide rates became apparent. Age or cohort effects suggest that as individuals age, suicide rates increase, especially among white males (Klerman 1989). However, this relationship is not strictly linear but is bimodal, with a peak in suicide rates in the 35- to 44-year-old group, a slight decrease thereafter, and a subsequent increase among those older than 65.

Table 48–1 presents the suicide rates for different age groups per 100,000 population in 1979, 1992 (Kochanek and Hudson 1994), 1998, and 1999 (Hoyert et al. 2001). Among children and adolescents ages 5–14 years and 15–24 years, the suicide rates increased between 1979 and 1992 but decreased in 1998 and 1999. Suicide is the third leading cause of death in youths ages 15–24, after accidents and homicide. In 2000, 3,877 youths ages 15–24 committed suicide, which accounted for a suicide rate of 10.1 per 100,000 population (Minino and Smith 2001). In 1999, 3,901 adolescents and young adults ages 15–24 died by suicide (age-adjusted suicide rate, 10.3 per 100,000 population), and among them, 59.3% died by the use of firearms (Hoyert et al. 2001). Suicide is the fifth leading cause of death for children and young adolescents ages 5–14, after accidents, malignancies, congenital anomalies, and homicide. In 2000, 297 children and young adolescents ages 5–14 committed suicide, which accounted for a suicide rate of 0.7 per 100,000 population (Minino and Smith 2001). In 1999, 244 children and young adolescents ages 5–14 died by suicide (age-adjusted suicide rate, 0.6 per 100,000 population), and among them 42.2% died by the use of firearms (Hoyert et al. 2001). There was a consistent decrease in suicide between 1979 and 1999 for individuals ages 25–34. In general, for other age groups, there was a decrease in suicide rates between 1979 and 1999. People age 65 and older have had the highest suicide rates. Also, between 1986 and 1991, suicide among black youths increased more rapidly than it did among white youths (Shaffer et al. 1994).

The increase in rates of youth suicide is associated with greater availability and use of firearms (Boyd and Moscicki 1986). Use of firearms is the most lethal method of suicide attempt. In 1999, 28,874 individuals died from self-inflicted firearm injuries; of these

Table 48–1. Suicide rates in 1979, 1992, 1998, and 1999 by age groups

Age group (years)	Suicide rate (per 100,000 population)			
	1979[a]	1992[a]	1998[b]	1999[b]
1–4	—	—	—	—
5–14	0.6	0.9	0.8	0.6
15–24	12.8	13.0	11.1	10.3
25–34	15.5	14.5	13.8	13.5
35–44	14.3	15.1	15.4	14.4
45–54	14.8	14.7	14.8	14.2
55–64	15.7	14.8	13.1	12.4
65–74	16.8	16.5	14.1	13.6
75–84	28.9	22.8	19.7	18.3
85 and older	19.7	21.9	21.0	19.2

[a]Data from Kochanek and Hudson 1994.
[b]Data from Hoyert et al. 2001.

deaths, 416 were 5- to 14-year-olds and 2,896 were 15- to 19-year-olds (Hoyert et al. 2001). In 1999, the rates per 100,000 individuals of suicide by use of firearms for both sexes were 0.5 for 10- to 14-year-olds, 4.9 for 15- to 19-year-olds, 7.4 for 20- to 24-year-olds, and 6.1 for all ages. In 10- to 14-year-olds, the rate per 100,000 individuals of suicide by use of firearms was greater for males (0.8) than for females (0.2). In 1999, rates per 100,000 population of suicide by use of firearms were greater for males (8.5 for 15- to 19-year-olds and 13.2 for 20- to 24-year-olds) than for females (1.1 for 15- to 19-year-olds and 1.4 for 20- to 24-year-olds) (Hoyert et al. 2001). It has also been reported that adolescent suicide victims who use firearms as a suicide method were 4.9 times more likely to have been drinking than were adolescents who used other suicide methods (Brent et al. 1987). The greater availability of firearms and increased use of alcohol among teenagers were significant factors in the increased rates for youth suicide. Furthermore, compliance of relatives with removing firearms from the home is problematic and therefore is a challenge to strategies for suicide prevention (Brent et al. 2000).

Another trend in suicide rates is period effects, which indicate changes in suicide rates during particular historical periods (Holinger 1989). Period effects cannot be identified for 10- to 14-year-olds because the suicide rates for this age group have been consistently low. For the 15- to 24-year age group, period effects are indicated by high rates in the 1930s, decreases in the 1940s to mid-1950s, and increases during the mid-

1950s to 1980s. Mechanisms underlying age or period effects for suicide rates have been proposed. One is that the recent increase in youth suicide rates is correlated with increases in rates of depression, substance abuse, and divorce (Klerman 1989). Changes in the number of youths in the population are directly associated with changes in suicide rates among youths: a higher number of youths in the population is associated with higher suicide rates (Holinger and Offer 1982). A proposed mechanism for this relationship is the greater intensity of competition (e.g., for jobs or school openings) when there is a larger youth population. Such competition produces stress and feelings of anxiety, despair, hopelessness, and worthlessness among those who are less successful.

In 1988, Oregon became the first state to require hospital-based reporting of suicide attempts in adolescents younger than age 18 (Andrus et al. 1991). When the 644 suicide attempters in 1988 were compared with 137 adolescents who committed suicide between 1979 and 1988, the most significant predictor of suicide was the method used in the suicide attempt. Use of firearms was the most lethal method. The prevalence of suicide attempts has been estimated to be 9% for adolescents in the general population (Harkavy-Friedman et al. 1987; Smith and Crawford 1986). Approximately 1% of preadolescents report a recent suicide attempt (Pfeffer et al. 1984). In a study of 3,294 youngsters in the Ontario Child Health Study, among 14- to 16-year-olds suicide attempts and suicidal ideation were more prevalent among girls than among boys (Joffe et al. 1988). In girls the prevalence of suicide attempts was 7.1% and that of suicidal ideation was 14.5%; in boys the prevalences were 2.4% for suicide attempts and 3.3% for suicidal ideation. The Youth Risk Behavior Surveillance System is a survey that monitors health-risk behaviors among a nationally representative sample of 1,270 youths and young adults in the ninth through the twelfth grades in the United States (Kann et al. 2000). Based on this survey, in 1999, 19.3% of students seriously considered attempting suicide, with females (24.9%) being significantly more likely than males (13.7%) to have considered attempting suicide. In addition, 8.3% of the students attempted suicide at least once in the year before the survey (Kann et al. 2000). Female students (10.9%) were more likely to have attempted suicide than were males (5.7%). Approximately 2.6% of students attempted suicide that resulted in injury or need for medical attention.

In the Methods for the Epidemiology of Child and Adolescent Mental Disorders Study sponsored the National Institute of Mental Health, a representative sample of 1,285 randomly selected children and adolescents ages 9–17 years was studied to evaluate psychopathology in children and adolescents. Forty-two (3.3%) had attempted suicide, and 67 (5.2%) reported only suicidal ideation (King et al. 2001). When children and adolescents who reported suicidal ideation were compared with those who had attempted suicide at some time in their lifetime, those who had attempted suicide were more likely to have experienced stressful life events, to have become sexually active, to have smoked more than one cigarette daily, and to have smoked marijuana. In addition, suicidal ideation or suicide attempt was significantly associated with the presence of current mood disorder (OR, 12.6; 95% CI, 7.7–20.5), anxiety disorder (OR, 6.1; 95% CI, 4.0–9.3), or disruptive disorder (OR, 5.0; 95% CI, 3.2–7.9). After adjustments were made for demographic features and the presence of psychiatric disorders (such as mood, anxiety, or disruptive disorder), there was a significantly higher prevalence among those reporting suicidal ideation or suicidal attempts—compared with those without suicidal behavior—of poor family environment (OR, 3.6; 95% CI, 2.2–5.8); low parental monitoring (OR, 5.0; 95% CI, 2.4–10.4); low youth competence (OR, 5.4; 95% CI, 2.8–10.7); and high-risk behaviors such as sexual activity (OR, 3.4; 95% CI, 2.3–5.2), recent drunkenness (OR, 4.3; 95% CI, 2.6–7.0), current smoking (OR, 6.6; 95% CI, 3.5–12.5), and physical fighting (OR, 2.8; 95% CI, 1.9–4.2). The significance of this study is that independent of psychiatric disorders, family environment and high-risk behaviors are significant risk factors for suicidal behavior among children and adolescents and should be focused on in developing strategies for suicide prevention.

The risk of suicide attempts in late adolescence and young adulthood among individuals who were ages 19–23 years was examined in a study of a representative sample of 1,709 adolescents ages 14–18 years who lived in western Oregon between 1987 and 1989 (Lewinsohn et al. 1995, 2001). The risk for suicide attempts was found to be higher for females, but by age 19 years the risk for suicide attempts for females dropped to that for males. However, females continued to have a higher risk for depression than males. Furthermore, adolescent suicide attempts predicted suicide attempts in young adulthood for females but not for males. Other factors that predicted suicide attempts in young adulthood for males and females were major depression (OR for males, 3.61; 95% CI, 1.02–12.78; OR for females, 3.04; 95% CI, 1.15–8.04), negative cognitions (OR for males, 2.51; 95% CI, 1.07–5.86; OR for females, 2.12; 95% CI, 1.18–3.81), and coping skills (OR for males, 1.12; 95% CI, 1.02–1.23; OR for females, 1.07; 95% CI, 1.01–1.13). Furthermore, the lifetime prevalence of bipolar disorder was 1%. These adolescents reported high rates of psychopathology, including suicide attempts and anxiety and disruptive disorders. This study highlighted the fact that the transition to young adulthood imparts different risks for suicidal behavior than the period of adolescence.

Rates of suicide and suicide attempts are higher among psychiatric patients than in the general population. In a 4- to 15-year follow-up of 1,331 formerly hospitalized child psychiatric patients, suicide was nine times more frequent than was expected in the general population (Kuperman et al. 1988). It has been reported that 34% of adolescent psychiatric inpatients were hospitalized because of a recent suicide attempt (Pfeffer et al. 1988).

The effect of sexual orientation on risk for suicidal behavior has received recent attention. In one study 56 lesbian, gay, or bisexual youths ages 16–21 years were compared with an age- and gender-matched sample of heterosexual youths. The results indicated that sexual orientation was not associated with higher risk for suicidal behavior when psychosocial factors—such as the severity of depression, hopelessness, substance abuse, and social support—were considered as potential risk factors in analyses of the data (Safren and Heimberg 1999). However, 30% of the youths with minority sexual orientation (compared with 13% of the heterosexual youths) reported a previous suicide attempt. Despite the controlled nature of the study, this sample was relatively small. In a study of 1,265 children who were followed up for 21 years, 28 participants (2.2%) reported being gay, lesbian, or bisexual (Fergusson et al. 1999). The sexual-minority adolescents were at increased risk for suicidal ideation (OR, 5.4; 95% CI, 2.4–12.2) and suicide attempts (OR, 6.2; 95% CI, 2.7–14.3). That higher rates of suicidal ideation (OR, 3.61; 95% CI, 1.40–9.36) and suicide attempts (OR, 7.10; 95% CI, 3.05–16.53) were associated with sexual-minority adolescents was also suggested by a study in which 394 sexual-minority adolescents were compared with 336 gender- and age-matched heterosexual adolescents (Remafedi et al. 1998). Additional research is needed to understand risk indicators in youths who are gay, lesbian, or bisexual.

Etiology

The basic etiological elements of suicidal behavior are thought to be genetic. However, there is relatively little definitive information about the specific aspects of the genetics of suicidal behavior. Efforts to understand the genetics of suicidal behavior have focused on abnormalities in the serotonergic neurotransmitter system, which is believed to be partly under genetic control (Mann et al. 2001). Genetic factors that are independent of the genetics of psychiatric disorders may be associated with risk for suicidal behavior. These genetic factors have not been identified. It is also hypothesized that intermediate phenotypes—involving impulsivity, pathological aggression, psychomotor change, and biological abnormalities including gene products—may be related to genetic variants, which thereby increase risk for suicidal behavior (Mann et al. 2001). Candidate genes involving the serotonergic neurotransmitter system are being studied with regard to risk for suicidal behavior. These include the 5-hydroxytryptamine (serotonin) type 1B (5-HT$_{1B}$) receptor and gene, the tryptophan hydroxylase gene, the serotonin transporter gene, the serotonin type 2A (5-HT$_{2A}$) receptor and gene, the serotonin type 1A (5-HT$_{1A}$) receptor and gene, and the monoamine oxidase A gene (Mann et al. 2001).

Reports have focused on neurobiological indices that are associated with childhood and adolescent suicidal behavior, and these provide some validation for the focus on the genetics of the serotonergic neurobiological system. For example, in the first study of children for levels of whole blood tryptophan, platelet serotonin content, and serotonin-amplified platelet aggregation, 75 prepubertal psychiatric inpatients—of whom 30% had no history of suicidal ideation or suicide attempts, 43% had recent suicidal ideation, and 27% had a recent history of at least one suicide attempt—were compared with 35 nonsuicidal prepubertal children living in the community (Pfeffer et al. 1998). The mean whole blood tryptophan content was significantly lower among children with a history of a recent suicide attempt than among the nonsuicidal community children or inpatients with recent suicidal ideation. The inpatients with a mood disorder had significantly higher platelet serotonin content than inpatients without a mood disorder. These results suggested that serotonergic indices may be predictive of risk for suicidal behavior among children and that such factors should be studied further.

Other etiological factors involve risk factors that increase the likelihood of the incidence and prevalence of suicidal behavior. Because major depressive disorder is considered to be among the most important risk factors, it is important to identify factors that may increase the likelihood of occurrence of depression. A study of a representative sample of 3,617 noninstitutionalized adults living in the United States who were age 25 years and older was utilized to understand the role of specific childhood adverse events on the incidence and prevalence of symptoms of depression (Kessler and Magee 1993). Among these individuals, 281 (7.8%) had the onset of depression before age 20 years. The effects of specific childhood adversities on the incidence and prevalence of depression were evaluated. In the entire population, adverse events that occurred before age 16 years included early death of mother (3.8%), early death of father (6.3%), serious parental marital problems (17.5%), parental divorce (7.5%), family violence (11.2%), serious family drinking problems (18.4%), family mental illness (7.0%), and absence of a close and confiding relationship with any adult (17.7%). All factors except parental divorce (OR, 1.17; 95% CI, 0.93–1.48) predicted first onset of depression before age 20 years. The strongest risk factor was mother's death (OR, 2.90; 95% CI, 1.56–5.37) followed by family violence (OR, 2.61; 95% CI, 1.88–3.63), death of father (OR, 1.65; 95% CI, 1.01–2.70), absence of a close and confiding relationship with any adult (OR, 1.59; 95% CI, 1.16–2.17), family mental illness (OR, 1.56; 95% CI, 1.01–2.40), serious family drinking problems (OR, 1.48; 95% CI, 1.27–1.72), and serious parental marital problems (OR, 1.47; 95% CI, 1.26–1.71). If identified among children and adolescents, these factors should be a focus of intervention to decrease risk for depression and should thereby potentially be an important intervention to decrease risk for youth suicidal behavior.

The National Comorbidity Survey, a nationally representative survey of the prevalence and correlates of DSM-III-R psychiatric disorders in people ages 15–54 years in the United States, provided information about the prevalence of depressive disorders among 1,769 youths ages 15–24 years (Kessler and Walters 1998). The lifetime prevalence of major depression was

15.3%, and the lifetime prevalence of minor depression was 9.9%. Recurrent depression was reported in 73.9% of those with major depression and in 69.2% of those with minor depression. Among those with major depression, 21.9% reported a suicide attempt. Among those with lifetime major depression (76.7%) and those with lifetime minor depression (69.3%), comorbid psychiatric disorders antedated the depressive disorders. Generalized anxiety disorder (OR, 2.0; 95% CI, 1.1–3.8) was the strongest predictor of major depressive disorder, whereas the effects of other disorders in predicting subsequent major depression or minor depression were nonspecific. Another study of 1,580 high school students suggested independent associations between adolescent suicidal ideation or suicide attempts and major depressive disorder (OR for suicidal ideation, 6.21; 95% CI, 2.58–14.90; OR for suicide attempts, 4.85; 95% CI, 1.86–12.60) and panic attacks (OR for suicidal ideation, 3.34; 95% CI, 2.38–4.68; OR for suicide attempts, 1.93; 95% CI, 1.23–3.03) (Pilowsky et al. 1999). The high prevalence of depressive symptoms and comorbid disorders suggested that enhanced understanding of methods of identifying such disorders early in life may enable interventions to reduce risk for other problems, such as suicidal behavior.

A 3-year longitudinal study of 138 children and adolescents ages 7–17 years highlighted the notion that children and adolescents with major depressive disorder and who attempted suicide may be a subgroup of youngsters with major depression who have higher levels of impulsivity that were associated with conduct problems (Myers et al. 1991). This study illustrated the importance of identifying risk factors for suicidal behavior in such youths because they have major depressive disorder. The effects of major depressive disorder were highlighted in another longitudinal study of 73 adolescents with major depression and 37 adolescents without psychopathology who were followed up 10–15 years later (Weissman et al. 1999). Among the adolescents with major depressive disorder, approximately 7.7% committed suicide, and no adolescent without psychopathology committed suicide. The adolescents with major depressive disorder, compared with those without psychopathology, were significantly more likely to attempt suicide at least once in their lifetimes (OR, 14.3; 95% CI, 3.1–65.4) and at least once during the follow-up period (OR, 5.6; 95% CI, 1.2–25.2). An earlier study of adolescents who committed suicide and who had mood disorder identified predictors of suicide among these youths (Brent et al. 1994). Among 63 adolescent suicide victims with mood disorder and 23 adolescents with a lifetime history of a mood disorder, risk for suicide was evaluated for major depressive disorder, comorbid substance abuse, history of a suicide attempt, family history of major depressive disorder, treatment with a tricyclic antidepressant, history of legal problems, and availability of a handgun in the home. The significant predictors of suicide were current major depressive disorder (OR, 6.3; 95% CI, 1.8–22.4) and family history of major depressive disorder (OR, 10.0; 95% CI, 2.0–50.7).

Family history of suicidal behavior has been identified as being associated with suicide in children and adolescents (Brent et al. 1996a; Pfeffer et al. 1994b). A study of 58 adolescent suicide victims and 55 demographically matched nonsuicidal adolescents indicated that the rates of suicide attempts and completed suicides were significantly higher among first-degree relatives, such as parents and siblings (OR, 5.3; 95% CI, 2.0–14.3), and second-degree relatives (OR, 3.7; 95% CI, 1.6–8.7) of suicide victims than among nonsuicidal adolescents (Brent et al. 1996a). These increased rates of suicidal behaviors among relatives of suicide victims were independent of the rates of psychiatric disorders among these relatives. A family study of 488 first-degree and 1,062 second-degree relatives of 69 prepubertal psychiatric inpatients (of whom 25 had reported recent suicide attempts, 28 had reported recent suicidal ideation, and 16 had no history of suicidal ideation or suicide attempts) and of 54 prepubertal children with no history of suicidal ideation or suicide attempts who were selected from the community focused on identifying the rates of suicidal and violent behaviors and psychiatric disorders among the relatives of these children (Pfeffer et al. 1994b). The results suggested that children's suicidal ideation and suicide attempts were significantly associated with suicidal acts of the first-degree relatives, including parents and siblings. In addition, compared with the first-degree relatives of the nonsuicidal community children, the first-degree relatives of the suicidal children had higher rates of antisocial personality disorder, assaultive behavior, and substance abuse (Pfeffer et al. 1994b). These family studies imply that family history of suicidal behavior should be evaluated in all assessments of suicidal risk in children and adolescents.

Treatment

There have been relatively few empirical studies of treatment of suicidal children or adolescents. The importance of effective treatment of risk factors for suicidal behavior is one of the key features of suicide prevention.

A barrier to suicide prevention is the lack of consistent use of treatment services. Depression is a key risk factor for youth suicide and suicide attempts (Flisher 1999). However, utilization of treatment among depressed youths is not common, as illustrated by a study of a representative sample of 206 children and adolescents ages 9–17 years who had diagnoses of major depression or dysthymia and who were in a community with five treatment service delivery systems (Wu et al. 2001). Notably, 36% never received professional care, and of those who were treated, only 31% were treated with antidepressants. Parents' perceptions of their children's mental health treatment needs were associated with whether the children received treatment. The mother's level of education, whether the children had health insurance, and whether the children had suicidal or other severe symptoms were associated with whether the children received antidepressant treatment. Important implications of this study were that treatment utilization was affected by parental perceptions of need, socioeconomic factors, and clinicians' and parents' identification and appreciation of the severity of children's symptoms. Suicide prevention strategies should incorporate education about youth depression and improvement of insurance coverage for children's psychiatric problems.

Children and adolescents who attempt suicide are frequently first evaluated in emergency services. Therefore, attention to the quality of emergency room procedures to assist suicidal children and adolescents may enhance their outcomes. An 18-month follow-up of 140 adolescent female suicide attempters—who received either emergency service treatment as usual or a special emergency service intervention intended to enhance adherence to outpatient treatment by providing psychoeducation about suicidal behavior, a family session, and staff training—suggested that the specialized emergency service approach lowered parental emotional distress, enhanced family cohesion, and improved the outcomes of the adolescent suicide attempters (Rotheram-Borus et al. 2000). Further research is needed to evaluate the types of effective emergency service treatment for suicidal youths.

Suicidal behavior has been identified as being associated with family dysfunction. Intervention focused on family issues may be important in decreasing suicidal ideation or suicide attempts in children and adolescents. However, few empirical studies have evaluated the effects of family intervention on suicidal behavior among children and adolescents. The results of one randomized study, in which an experimental home-based family intervention was compared with routine treatment, suggested that reduction of suicidal ideation occurred in adolescents who received the experimental family treatment and who did not have mood disorders (Harrington et al. 2000). However, among those with mood disorders, there was no difference in outcome between those who received the experimental family intervention and those who received routine treatment. This study pointed out that treatment planning should consider the characteristics of suicidal children and adolescents and that treatments may need to be different for various subgroups of suicidal youths.

Cognitive-behavioral treatments that focus on dysfunctional cognitions and impulsive behaviors in adults and suicidal adolescents have received empirical attention (Brent 1997). It has been recommended that treatments for suicidal youths should focus on coexisting psychopathology, such as mood disorders, remediation of social and problem-solving deficits, and family psychoeducation and intervention (Brent 1997). Furthermore, specific psychopharmacological treatment studies for suicidal youths have not been undertaken. However, medications that have been shown to be effective in reducing major depression (such as the selective serotonin reuptake inhibitors), bipolar disorders (such as mood stabilizers), and psychoses (such as typical and atypical antipsychotics) should be utilized to decrease the symptoms of psychiatric disorders that are risk factors for suicidal behavior.

Research Issues

Psychological autopsy studies (Brent et al. 1996a) and studies of prepubertal children who reported nonfatal suicidal behavior (Pfeffer et al. 1994b) have suggested that rates of suicidal behavior were higher among parents and siblings of these children than in the general population. However, other reports (Mercy et al.

2001) suggest no significant associations between adolescent suicide attempts and exposure to the suicidal behavior of relatives or friends. Furthermore, prospective studies of children and adolescents who were bereaved by the suicide of a parent or acquaintance suggested that bereaved children and adolescents did not exhibit an increased rate of suicidal behavior within 1 year (Pfeffer et al. 1997, 2000b) or within 3 years of the relatives' deaths (Brent et al. 1996b). Further research is necessary to understand the developmental course of children and adolescents whose relatives commit or attempt suicide.

Identification of risk for suicidal behavior is one of the hallmarks of suicide prevention. Methods of early identification require further development and study. Recent research has been focused on developing screening methods that utilize reliable and valid self-report measures (Pfeffer et al. 2000a). For example, the Child–Adolescent Suicidal Potential Index (CASPI) was developed to identify features of suicide risk, including anxious-impulsive depression, suicidal ideation or suicide attempts, and family distress (Pfeffer et al. 2000a). This 30-item measure is reliable and valid in discriminating between children and adolescents who reported recent suicidal ideation or suicide attempts and those without a history of suicidal behavior. As with all self-report measures of a low-prevalence behavior, such as suicidal behavior, there is often a high rate of false-positive findings. As a result, it is recommended that screening with the CASPI and other self-report screening measures be performed in conjunction with a direct interview that is given to children and adolescents who score high on the self-report measure. This approach will validate the results of the self-report screen and will identify those who appear to provide false-positive results. Other methods to identify children and adolescents at risk for suicidal behavior should include methods of educating parents, school professionals, medical professionals, and others who work with children about the risk factors for suicidal behavior, how to identify them, and when to make a referral for additional evaluation by a child and adolescent psychiatrist or other trained and skilled mental health professionals.

Extensive research is necessary to develop and evaluate the efficacy of treatments involving psychosocial and psychopharmacological methods to reduce suicidal behavior in children and adolescents (American Academy of Child and Adolescent Psychiatry 2001).

Studies should focus on the utilization of treatment services such as psychiatric hospitalization and outpatient methods, including individual and family treatments involving cognitive-behavioral, interpersonal, and psychodynamic orientations. Utilization of follow-up methods should be studied as a means of identifying and treating risk for recurrent suicidal states. There should be an intervention focus on treating risk factors, such as psychiatric disorders (especially mood, disruptive, and substance abuse disorders) and other psychosocial factors (such as family distress, poor coping behaviors, and dysfunctional cognitive styles). Studies should aim to acquire understanding of indices that involve developmental and aberrant neurobiological variations that may be associated with suicidal behavior. In this way, the results may lead to the development of innovative methods to treat and prevent suicidal behavior in children and adolescents.

References

American Academy of Child and Adolescent Psychiatry: Practice parameter for the assessment and treatment of children and adolescents with suicidal behavior. J Am Acad Child Adolesc Psychiatry 40 (7, suppl):24S–51S, 2001

American Psychiatric Association: Diagnostic and Statistical Manual of Mental Disorders, 4th Edition. Washington, DC, American Psychiatric Association, 1994

American Psychiatric Association: Diagnostic and Statistical Manual of Mental Disorders, 4th Edition, Text Revision. Washington, DC, American Psychiatric Association, 2000

Andrus JK, Fleming DW, Heumann MA, et al: Surveillance of attempted suicide among adolescents in Oregon, 1988. Am J Public Health 81:1067–1069, 1991

Beautrais AL, Joyce PR, Mulder RT: Personality traits and cognitive styles as risk factors for serious suicide attempts among young people. Suicide Life Threat Behav 29:37–47, 1999

Boyd JH, Moscicki EK: Firearms and youth suicide. Am J Public Health 76:1240–1242, 1986

Brent DA: Correlates of the medical lethality of suicide attempts in children and adolescents. J Am Acad Child Adolesc Psychiatry 26:87–89, 1987

Brent DA: Practitioner review: the aftercare of adolescents with deliberate self-harm. J Child Psychol Psychiatry 38:277–286, 1997

Brent DA, Perper JA, Allman CJ: Alcohol, firearms, and suicide among youth: temporal trends in Allegheny County, Pennsylvania, 1960 to 1983. JAMA 257:3369–3372, 1987

Brent DA, Perper JA, Goldstein CE, et al: Risk factors for adolescent suicide: a comparison of adolescent suicide victims with suicidal inpatients. Arch Gen Psychiatry 45:581–588, 1988

Brent DA, Perper JA, Moritz G, et al: Psychiatric risk factors for adolescent suicide: a case-control study. J Am Acad Child Adolesc Psychiatry 32:521–529, 1993

Brent DA, Perper JA, Moritz G, et al: Suicide in affectively ill adolescents: a case-control study. J Affect Disord 31:193–202, 1994

Brent DA, Bridge J, Johnson BA, et al: Suicidal behavior runs in families: a controlled family study of adolescent suicide victims. Arch Gen Psychiatry 53:1145–1152, 1996a

Brent DA, Moritz G, Bridge J, et al: Long-term impact of exposure to suicide: a three-year controlled follow-up. J Am Acad Child Adolesc Psychiatry 35:646–653, 1996b

Brent DA, Baugher M, Birmaher B, et al: Compliance with recommendations to remove firearms in families participating in a clinical trial for adolescent depression. J Am Acad Child Adolesc Psychiatry 39:1220–1226, 2000

Donaldson D, Spirito A, Farnett E: The role of perfectionism and depressive cognitions in understanding the hopelessness experienced by adolescent suicide attempters. Child Psychiatry Hum Dev 31:99–111, 2000

Fergusson DM, Horwood LJ, Beautrais AL: Is sexual orientation related to mental health problems and suicidality in young people? Arch Gen Psychiatry 56:876–880, 1999

Flisher AJ: Annotation: mood disorder in suicidal children and adolescents: recent developments. J Child Psychol Psychiatry 40:315–324, 1999

Gould MS, Fisher P, Parides M, et al: Psychosocial risk factors of child and adolescent completed suicide. Arch Gen Psychiatry 53:1155–1162, 1996

Harkavy-Friedman JM, Asnis GM, Boeck M, et al: Prevalence of specific suicidal behaviors in a high school sample. Am J Psychiatry 144:1203–1206, 1987

Harrington R, Kerfoot M, Dyer E, et al: Deliberate self-poisoning in adolescence: why does a brief family intervention work in some cases and not others? J Adolescence 23:13–20, 2000

Hawton K, Kingsbury S, Steinhardt K, et al: Repetition of deliberate self-harm by adolescents: the role of psychological factors. J Adolesc 22:369–378, 1999

Holinger PC: Epidemiologic issues in youth suicide, in Suicide Among Youth: Perspectives on Risk and Prevention. Edited by Pfeffer CR. Washington, DC, American Psychiatric Press, 1989, pp 41–62

Holinger PC, Offer D: Prediction of adolescent suicide: a population model. Am J Psychiatry 139:302–307, 1982

Hoyert DL, Arias E, Smith BL, et al: Deaths: final data for 1999. Natl Vital Stat Rep 49(8):1–113, 2001

Jacobsen LK, Rabinowitz I, Popper MS, et al: Interviewing prepubertal children about suicidal ideation and behavior. J Am Acad Child Adolesc Psychiatry 33:439–452, 1994

Joffe RT, Offord DR, Boyle MH: Ontario Child Health Study: suicidal behavior in youth 12–16 years. Am J Psychiatry 145:1420–1423, 1988

Kann L, Kinchen SA, Williams BI, et al: Youth Risk Behavior Surveillance—United States, 1999. J Sch Health 70:271–285, 2000

Kessler RC, Magee WJ: Childhood adversities and adult depression: basic patterns of association in a US national survey. Psychol Med 23:679–690, 1993

Kessler RC, Walters EE: Epidemiology of DSM-III-R major depression and minor depression among adolescents and young adults in the National Comorbidity Survey. Depress Anxiety 7:3–14, 1998

King RA, Schwab-Stone M, Flisher AJ, et al: Psychosocial and risk behavior correlates of youth suicide attempts and suicidal ideation. J Am Acad Child Adolesc Psychiatry 40:837–846, 2001

Klerman GL: Suicide, depression, and related problems among the baby boom cohort, in Suicide Among Youth: Perspectives on Risk and Prevention. Edited by Pfeffer CR. Washington, DC, American Psychiatric Press, 1989, pp 63–81

Kochanek KD, Hudson BL: Advance report of final mortality statistics, 1992. Mon Vital Stat Rep 43(6, suppl):1–76, 1994

Kuperman S, Black DW, Burns TL: Excess suicide among formerly hospitalized child psychiatry patients. J Clin Psychiatry 49:88–93, 1988

Lewinsohn PM, Klein DM, Seeley JR: Bipolar disorders in a community sample of older adolescents: prevalence, phenomenology, comorbidity, and course. J Am Acad Child Adolesc Psychiatry 34:454–463, 1995

Lewinsohn PM, Rohde P, Seeley JR, et al: Gender differences in suicide attempts from adolescence to young adulthood. J Am Acad Child Adolesc Psychiatry 40:427–434, 2001

Mann JJ, Brent DA, Arango V: The neurobiology and genetics of suicide and attempted suicide: a focus on the serotonergic system. Neuropsychopharmacology 24:467–477, 2001

Mercy JA, Kresnow MJ, O'Carroll PW, et al: Is suicide contagious? A study of the relation between exposure to the suicidal behavior of others and nearly lethal suicide attempts. Am J Epidemiol 154:120–127, 2001

Minino AM, Smith BL: Deaths: preliminary data for 2000. Natl Vital Stat Rep 49(12):1–40, 2001

Myers K, McCauley E, Calderon R, et al: The 3-year longitudinal course of suicidality and predictive factors for subsequent suicidality in youths with major depressive disorder. J Am Acad Child Adolesc Psychiatry 30:804–810, 1991

Pfeffer CR: The Suicidal Child. New York, Guilford, 1986

Pfeffer CR: Childhood suicidal behavior: a developmental perspective. Psychiatr Clin North Am 20:551–562, 1997

Pfeffer CR, Zuckerman S, Plutchik R, et al: Suicidal behavior in normal school children: a comparison with child psychiatric inpatients. J Am Acad Child Psychiatry 23:416–423, 1984

Pfeffer CR, Newcorn J, Kaplan G, et al: Suicidal behavior in adolescent psychiatric inpatients. J Am Acad Child Adolesc Psychiatry 27:357–361, 1988

Pfeffer CR, Klerman GL, Hurt SW, et al: Suicidal children grow up: rates and psychosocial risk factors for suicide attempts during follow-up. J Am Acad Child Adolesc Psychiatry 32:106–113, 1993

Pfeffer CR, Hurt SW, Kakuma T, et al: Suicidal children grow up: suicidal episodes and effects of treatment during follow-up. J Am Acad Child Adolesc Psychiatry 33:225–230, 1994a

Pfeffer CR, Normandin L, Kakuma T: Suicidal children grow up: suicidal behavior and psychiatric disorders among relatives. J Am Acad Child Adolesc Psychiatry 33:1087–1097, 1994b

Pfeffer CR, Martins P, Mann J, et al: Child survivors of suicide: psychosocial characteristics. J Am Acad Child Adolesc Psychiatry 36:65–74, 1997

Pfeffer CR, McBride A, Anderson GM, et al: Peripheral serotonin measures in prepubertal psychiatric inpatients and normal children: associations with suicidal behavior and its risk factors. Biol Psychiatry 44:568–577, 1998

Pfeffer CR, Jiang H, Kakuma T: Child-Adolescent Suicidal Potential Index (CASPI): a screen for risk for early onset suicidal behavior. Psychol Assess 12:304–318, 2000a

Pfeffer CR, Karus D, Siegel K, et al: Child survivors of parental death from cancer or suicide: depressive and behavioral outcomes. Psychooncology 9:1–10, 2000b

Pilowsky DJ, Wu LT, Anthony JC: Panic attacks and suicide attempts in mid-adolescence. Am J Psychiatry 156:1545–1549, 1999

Remafedi G, French S, Story M, et al: The relationship between suicide risk and sexual orientation: results of a population-based study. Am J Public Health 88:57–60, 1998

Rotheram-Borus MJ, Piacentini J, Cantwell C, et al: The 18-month impact of an emergency room intervention for adolescent female suicide attempters. J Consult Clin Psychol 68:1081–1093, 2000

Safren SA, Heimberg RG: Depression, hopelessness, suicidality, and related factors in sexual minority and heterosexual adolescents. J Consult Clin Psychol 67:859–866, 1999

Shaffer D, Gould M, Hicks RC: Worsening suicide rate in black teenagers. Am J Psychiatry 151:1810–1812, 1994

Shaffer D, Gould MS, Fisher P, et al: Psychiatric diagnosis in child and adolescent suicide. Arch Gen Psychiatry 53:339–348, 1996

Smith K, Crawford S: Suicidal behavior among "normal" high school students. Suicide Life Threat Behav 16:313–325, 1986

U.S. Public Health Service: The Surgeon General's Call to Action to Prevent Suicide. Washington, DC, U.S. Public Health Service, 1999

Weissman MM, Wolk S, Goldstein RB, et al: Depressed adolescents grown up. JAMA 281:1707–1713, 1999

Wu P, Hoven CW, Cohen P, et al: Factors associated with use of mental health services for depression by children and adolescents. Psychiatr Serv 52:189–195, 2001

Forensic Psychiatry

John B. Sikorski, M.D.

Anlee D. Kuo, J.D., M.D.

Forensic psychiatry is a field within psychiatry in which scientific and clinical expertise is applied to legal issues in legal contexts (Rosner 1989, p. 323). Within forensic psychiatry, child and adolescent forensic psychiatry emerged in the last two decades of the twentieth century as a subspecialized area of increased activity, complexity, and utilization (Nurcombe and Partlett 1994; Schetky and Benedek 1985, 1992, 2002). This development paralleled the maturation of the field of child and adolescent psychiatry as a medical specialty with its own research-oriented database (Institute of Medicine 1989), fund of knowledge of human neurobiological development and psychopathology (Cicchetti and Cohen 1995), and more specific clinical application, such as those reflected in the practice parameters published by the American Academy of Child and Adolescent Psychiatry (1995, 1997b, 1997c). This rapidly expanding area of forensics is complex and multifaceted and involves a diverse range of topics paralleling the changes and concerns in American society such as the legal rights of children and adolescents, custody and visitation disputes, child abuse and neglect evaluations, delinquent behavior and the juvenile justice system, mental disability, civil commitment of youths, and special education issues.

In response to the growing demands for recognized competence in this area, the American Board of Medical Specialties officially established forensic psychiatry as a subspecialty in 1992 and directed the American Board of Psychiatry and Neurology to offer certification in this field. The examination requires completion of a 1-year fellowship from a program certified by the Accreditation Council for Graduate Medical Education (ACGME). Currently, there are 37 ACGME-accredited certified fellowships in the United States. The Accreditation Council for Graduate Medical Education (1988) also revised its requirements for child psychiatry training programs to include forensic psychiatry as part of training in consultation. However, teaching and content in forensic psychiatry vary widely among residency programs (Marrocco et al. 1995).

The intent of this chapter is

- To increase awareness and understanding of children's rights
- To provide an overview of relevant legal processes and forensic psychiatry concepts
- To provide an understanding of the essential elements of a forensic evaluation
- To provide an overview of relevant ethical and legal issues in the treatment of minors and to highlight important professional liability concerns
- To highlight some areas of particular activity and concern to child and adolescent forensic psychiatry practice, including issues involving child custody and divorce, child abuse and neglect, the role of children as witnesses, youth violence, the juvenile justice system, civil commitment of minors, and special education
- To provide some guidance for further study and encouragement for seeking consultation with colleagues and counsel

The Changing Status of Children's Rights

Many changes have occurred within American society and the legal system with regard to the recognition and protection of children's needs, well-being, and rights. One can more fully appreciate these changes by examining the status of children before the twentieth century. For example, children have historically been viewed as property of the family, particularly the father, or wards of the state with no political power and few legal rights (Rodham 1973). They were valued for their economic contributions and were often fully exploited in the workforce before the existence of child labor laws (Nurcombe and Partlett 1994, p. 42). Until 1875, no organization existed for the protection of abused or mistreated children. The first prosecuted case of child abuse had to be taken to the Society for the Prevention of Cruelty to Animals (American Academy of Child and Adolescent Psychiatry 1997c, p. 425). Further evidence of disregard for the special needs of children is apparent in the treatment of juvenile delinquents before the twentieth century, when children over age 7 who were charged with misconduct were subject to the same criminal proceedings and sanctions as adults (Schetky 2002b, p. 4).

Beginning in the later part of the nineteenth century and during much of the twentieth century, private, professional, and political leadership in the United States increasingly expressed its concern for the care and well-being of children. In 1909, the establishment of the first White House Conference on Children and Youth reflected a growing concern for the care of dependent children following the sociocultural changes in American society at the turn of the century. Subsequent White House conferences in each decade focused on child welfare standards; child health and protection; and the rights, needs, and well-being of children (Beck 1974). The White House Conference on Children, convened in 1970 (U.S. Government Printing Office 1971), asserted the following specific rights as central to a child's well-being:

1. The right to grow in a society that respects the dignity of life and is free of poverty, discrimination, and other forms of degradation
2. The right to be born and to be healthy and wanted through childhood
3. The right to grow up nurtured by affectionate parents
4. The right to be a child during childhood, to have meaningful choices in the process of maturation and development, and to have a meaningful voice in the community
5. The right to be educated to the limits of one's capa-

bility and through processes designed to elicit one's full potential
6. The right to have societal mechanisms to enforce the foregoing rights

The recent publication of *Mental Health: A Report of the Surgeon General* (U.S. Department of Health and Human Services 1999) and the subsequent *Report of the Surgeon General's Conference on Children's Mental Health* (U.S. Public Health Service 2000) highlighted a national agenda to promote awareness of children's mental health issues and needs. This included the reduction of stigma associated with mental illness, continuing to utilize scientifically proven prevention and treatment services in the field of children's mental health; improving the recognition of the mental health needs of children; eliminating racial, ethnic, and socioeconomic disparities in access to mental health care; improving the infrastructure for children's mental health services across professions; and increasing the quality of mental health care services and training providers to recognize and manage mental health issues.

The changes in society's perception and treatment of children during the twentieth century is similarly reflected in the legal system, in which two legal doctrines—*parens patriae* and *the best interests of the child*—were increasingly used by the courts to intervene in private family life for the protection of the child. Parens patriae empowers the state to protect citizens who are unable to protect themselves and has been used to justify state interference with parental prerogatives. The concept of the child's best interest was originally acknowledged in *Chapsky v. Wood* (1881) and has guided lawmakers and courts to prioritize the child's best interests over those of other involved persons, including the parents. Although these concepts have infused the vision of much federal legislation and many appellate court decisions regarding some aspects of child care, education, health, welfare, and juvenile justice, much remains to be accomplished in implementing these principles at a practical and universal level.

Overview of the Legal System

On a pragmatic and somewhat oversimplified level, law can be viewed as anything that a court having jurisdiction will enforce. This process protects an individual's claim to the possession of property or authority or to the enjoyment of privilege or immunity (Rodham 1973). Law in the United States is derived from the U.S. and state constitutions and from federal and state legislation and case law.

Structurally, the court system can be divided into two main categories: state courts and federal courts. The state court system consists of lower courts (or trial courts), higher courts (or appellate courts), and the state's supreme court, which serves a supervisory function over trial court decisions. Most of these courts have general jurisdiction, which means they hear both civil and criminal cases arising under state law. However, some state courts are considered to be specialized and exercise jurisdiction over specific types of cases. Some of the specialized courts especially pertinent to the child forensic psychiatrist include the juvenile and family courts and surrogate courts. Juvenile courts have statutory authority over matters relating to juvenile delinquency, abuse, and neglect. Family courts have statutory authority over divorce and child custody issues. Surrogate courts have authority over matters relating to civil commitment, guardianship, adoption, administration of trusts and estates, and contested wills.

The federal court system consists of federal trial courts, 13 U.S. Courts of Appeal and the U.S. Supreme Court. These courts decide civil and criminal cases arising under the United States Constitution and federal statutes, as well as civil actions in which the parties are of diverse state citizenship. As in the state court system, appellate courts serve a supervisory function over trial court decisions. Unique to the federal court system is the existence of the U.S. Supreme Court, which serves a supervisory function over federal appellate court decisions and has appellate jurisdiction to review any final state judicial decision.

Legal proceedings are essentially of two types: civil and criminal cases. Civil cases consist of breach of contract; property and financial disputes; and torts, including injury, negligence, professional liability, libel, and slander. These cases involve disputes between the plaintiff and defendant, third parties, cross plaintiffs, and cross defendants. The plaintiff must prove the elements of the cause of action. In criminal cases, the state lodges the complaint against the defendant, who is the alleged criminal. As a result of the presumption of innocence, the state has the burden of proving the elements of the charged crime. Both civil and criminal

proceedings operate under standard rules of civil procedure and evidence, which provide the mechanism for fact finding, decision making, and enforcement.

One important aspect of the legal process is the standard of proof or the level of certainty required for a judicial decision. The standard of *preponderance of evidence* (or *more likely than not*) is used in most civil litigation. The intermediate standard, *clear and convincing evidence,* is required in cases of deprivation of rights or liberty, such as involuntary civil commitment (*Addington v. Texas* 1979), and in cases of termination of parental rights (*Santosky v. Kramer* 1982). The highest standard of proof, *beyond a reasonable doubt,* is required by law in criminal cases, including juvenile court and delinquency proceedings (*In re Winship* 1970). Physicians who testify in court may also be asked if their opinions are given with a *reasonable degree of medical certainty.* The concept of reasonable medical certainty is not necessarily synonymous with any of the legal standards of proof but rather reflects "that level of certainty equivalent to what a physician uses when making a diagnosis and starting treatment" (Rappeport 1985, p. 9). Clinicians must understand the particular standard of proof that is required by the legal matter at hand and must be able to articulate and demonstrate their medical opinions relative to that standard.

Evidence is of two types: 1) legal fact (i.e., what the court accepts as fact) and 2) expert opinion. Both are presented in the form of witness testimony and exhibits. In this regard, the forensic psychiatrist may be called to testify as a fact witness or as an expert witness. As a fact witness, the psychiatrist testifies to a matter perceived or witnessed. As an expert witness, he or she testifies to matters of special learning and knowledge. Mental health professionals frequently participate as expert witnesses in the legal arena. However, their appropriate role in the courtroom continues to be highly controversial, as demonstrated by the case law on the admissibility of expert testimony.

The traditional standard for acceptance of scientific evidence by expert witnesses has become known as the Frye rule, an opinion that stated in part that "while courts will go a long way in admitting expert testimony deduced from a well recognized scientific principle or discovery, the thing from which the deduction is made must be sufficiently established to have gained general acceptance in the particular field in which it belongs" (*Frye v. United States* 1923). In 1975, a new set of federal rules of evidence was adopted. Rule 702 states, in part, "[I]f scientific, technical or other specialized knowledge will assist the trier of fact to understand the evidence or to determine a fact in issue, a witness qualified as an expert by knowledge, skill, expertise, training or education may testify thereto in the form of an opinion or otherwise" (Zonana 1994, p. 311). The U.S. Supreme Court concluded that the expanded federal rule of evidence superseded the Frye rule and that trial judges have the obligation to ensure that "any and all scientific testimony or evidence admitted is not only relevant, but reliable" (*Daubert v. Merrell Dow* 1993, p. 8). This in effect expands the trial judge's gatekeeping and decision-making functions over the admissibility of scientific knowledge and increases the risk that "junk science" or personal opinions will be admitted into the judicial process through expert witnesses.

In subsequent cases, the Supreme Court upheld the *Daubert* ruling and further elaborated on its proper application. In *General Electric Co. et al. v. Joiner* (1997), the Supreme Court decided that "abuse of discretion" is the proper standard of review of a district court's decision to admit or exclude scientific evidence under the Daubert principles. In *Kumho Tire Co.* (1999), the U.S. Supreme Court held that the Daubert principles apply to all types of expert testimony, gave the trial judge broad latitude in determining the reliability of expert testimony, and emphasized that the Daubert rules should be applied in a flexible manner to the extent relevant in each case. During the past two decades, there has been a burgeoning of civil litigation involving expert opinion, including psychiatric expert opinion, in cases ranging from product liability to abuse and harassment. The full impact of these changes is yet to be felt. Suffice it to say that these changes, while allowing for a larger inclusion of scientific knowledge and expert opinion, also allow for a much closer scrutiny of methodology, validity, relevance, and demonstration of the reasoning supporting the expert conclusions (Zonana 1994).

The Supreme Court discussed psychiatric testimony in *Ake v. Oklahoma* (1985):

> Psychiatry is not, however, an exact science, and psychiatrists disagree widely and frequently on what constitutes mental illness, on the appropriate diagnosis to be attached to given behavior and symptoms, on cure and treatment, and on likelihood of future dangerousness. Perhaps because there often is no single, accurate psychiatric conclusion on legal insanity in a given case, juries remain the primary fact finders on this issue, and they must resolve differences in opinion within the psychiatric profession on the basis of the evidence offered by each party.... It is for this reason that States rely on psychiatrists as examiners, consultants, and witnesses, and that private individuals do so as well, when they can afford to do so. (p. 7)

The Forensic Evaluation

A child and adolescent psychiatrist may become involved in a legal matter as 1) an evaluating or treating psychiatrist of a patient who is coincidentally involved in a lawsuit; 2) as a court-appointed expert for a specific case; or 3) as a forensic expert contracted by one party or attorney for the purpose of providing consultation, evaluation, or testimony for one side in a lawsuit.

In the first instance, the requirement for confidentiality may be waived by the patient, parent, or legal guardian; in other circumstances, the therapist or evaluator may be legally required to report or testify, such as when a case falls under mandatory reporting requirements for neglect, abuse, or threat of specific violence, or when a patient places his or her mental condition at issue in a civil suit.

If a subpoena, which is a valid court order, is served, the psychiatrist may be required to release the patient's records to a designated person, and the psychiatrist may also be required to give a deposition or court testimony as to his or her evaluation, course of treatment, or role in the legal matter. It should be noted that this process does not automatically make the treating psychiatrist's opinion expert evidence. To be an expert witness, the court must qualify the psychiatrist as an expert witness in the specific case before the court.

In the second instance, courts may choose from a panel of qualified professionals and appoint an expert to serve as a consultant; to evaluate records or an individual; or to provide consultation, reports, or testimony to the court in regard to a specific matter before the court. Child psychiatrists working in family and juvenile court matters are frequently appointed in this way. Psychiatrists are also chosen by agreement of the opposing attorneys, and a stipulated agreement is made to the court. The psychiatrist should request that this stipulation or court order include

- A statement of the appointment of the expert professional to proceed with the work
- The purpose of the evaluation, including persons to be evaluated and the scope of the evaluator's authority regarding collateral information

- The specification of the person to whom the report is to be made
- The method of payment of fees for the professional services rendered

As in any highly skilled and hazardous professional work, psychiatrists working in the forensic arena are entitled to reasonable and customary professional fees prevailing in their communities for those specific professional services. Fee schedules and methods of payment, including retainer fees, should be arranged in advance of the work provided. If a fee is dependent on the successful outcome of a case, the goal of objectivity and honesty is defeated. According to the Opinions of the Council on Ethical and Judicial Affairs of the American Medical Association (1994), contingency fees are unethical.

In the third instance, litigants or their attorneys frequently contact forensic experts to become partisan experts for their particular side in a case. The work of the psychiatrist may fall under the duties and obligations of the attorney-client privilege, which is different from the doctor-patient privilege. This may present the psychiatrist with professional and ethical dilemmas that must be clarified with the contracting attorney, sometimes assisted by consultation with professional colleagues or with one's own attorney.

When a psychiatrist is engaged or appointed as a consultant or evaluator in a legal matter, it is essential that the persons being evaluated or interviewed be told and clearly understand the nature and purpose of the interview—it is not a confidential or doctor–patient privileged interview, and the information obtained may be used in a report, deposition, or testimony that the psychiatrist may be required to produce in the legal matter. The expert opinion developed by the forensic expert is rendered in the form of a written report, deposition, or court testimony.

A forensic report should include the following five elements:

1. How one was referred or became involved in the case
2. What the purpose was of the evaluation or the legal issues to be addressed (not an attorney's theory of the case)
3. What procedures were performed, including the dates and locations of interviews, documents reviewed, and collateral information obtained
4. What observations and findings were made

5. What conclusions—in the form of diagnosis, prognosis, opinions, and recommendations—were made based on what specific data and relative to the law and legal guidelines obtaining to the legal matter under consideration

The psychiatrist should clarify any questions or ambiguities regarding the relevant laws, procedures, or legal guidelines with the attorney involved in the case if that communication is appropriate, with the court if the expert is court appointed, or with the expert's own counsel if in doubt.

If a formal diagnosis is used in the report, it should follow DSM-IV-TR format and should be referenced as such (American Psychiatric Association 2000). In developing the expert opinion, the report should reflect the particular case data, relevant scientific knowledge, and applicable law or legal guidelines. The clinical data should show the mental, emotional, and psychological relevance to the legal issues at hand. The opinion should be articulated in a way that clearly reveals to the trier of fact the reasoning and formulation in the matter rather than a simple summary and conclusive opinion. The report should be comprehensive enough to cover the relevant topics, document what occurred, support the conclusions, and reflect the clinical judgment and reasoning, but it should not be so long as to become argumentative, jargonistic, boring, or unintelligible to the court.

A deposition provides court-ordered or subpoenaed testimony under oath to discover or preserve information to be used at trial or to ascertain information that might be used to impugn the credibility of a witness at trial. When an expert is sworn in to a trial, his or her qualifications are presented to be accepted by the court. Only after such acceptance is the direct examination and opinion rendered, followed by cross-examination by the opposing attorney. Redirect questions, recross questions, and sometimes the judge's own questions may follow.

An expert who is to testify in court should 1) be prepared; 2) be professional; 3) be precise; 4 anticipate adverse, hypothetical, and adversarial cross-examination; 5) speak to the finders of fact; and 6) be aware of personal, professional, clinical, and legal pitfalls and vulnerabilities, such as arrogance, ideological argumentation, countertransference issues, or ignorance of the legal and ethical directives and boundaries of the case.

Ethical Issues in the Clinician's Practice

The province of ethics is generally considered the study of moral principles and values that govern behavior rather than statutes or legal regulations. Unfortunately, ethical guidelines for conducting child and adolescent forensic consultations and evaluations have not been firmly established. Therefore, the child forensic psychiatrist must look to a patchwork of resources to find guidance on ethical dilemmas arising in his or her work. The American Psychiatric Association and the American Academy of Child and Adolescent Psychiatry have established ethical standards; however, these standards are limited by the fact that they are based on the guidelines of the American Medical Association with its traditional physician–patient relationship and the hippocratic principles of beneficence and nonmaleficence, which do not exist in the forensic setting (Simon and Wettstein 1997). As described by Applebaum (1990, 1997), in forensic psychiatry no physician–patient relationship is established and the forensic psychiatrist acts not as a healer but as a provider of testimony in court to further the interests of truth and justice. More recently, the American Psychiatric Association has demonstrated an awareness of the critical need for ethical guidelines specific to the rapidly expanding field of forensic psychiatry. Although they are limited in scope, some forensic ethical issues are now addressed by the American Psychiatric Association in its *Principles of Medical Ethics With Annotations Especially Applicable to Psychiatry* (American Psychiatric Association 2001b) and in its periodic publishing of the *Opinions of the Ethics Committee on the Principles of Medical Ethics With Annotations Especially Applicable to Psychiatry* (American Psychiatric Association 2001a).

Despite the limitations in the code of ethics of the American Academy of Child and Adolescent Psychiatry, it is relevant and useful because it recognizes the special ethical tension present in a clinician's work with children and adolescents. The preamble to the code of ethics states, in part, "The [ethical] issues... must be viewed within the context of the overlapping and potentially conflicting rights of the child or adolescent, of the parents, and of society" (American Academy of Child Psychiatry 1980, p. 2) This tension between legal obligations and ethical responsibilities in the treatment of adolescents has also been highlighted by Berland et al. (1990) and Shields and Johnson (1992), who provide some guidelines for difficult clinical judgment. A landmark special section of the *Journal of the American Academy of Child and Adolescent Psychiatry* (1992) was devoted to ethical issues. Articles contained in this section highlighted the integrity and vigilance needed in clinical practice (O'Rourke et al. 1992) and the ethical and legal conflicts wrought by developing managed care systems and other constraints on the parameters of care imposed by third parties (Geraty et al. 1992); they further explored a variety of other general ethical issues in forensic psychiatry (Schetky 1992). Ethical principles governing research (Munir and Earls 1992) include, among numerous other specific considerations, guidelines for protection of children, appropriate risk–benefit analysis, informed consent and confidentiality issues, and issues regarding scientific integrity. Approaches to teaching ethics in child and adolescent psychiatry (Sondheimer and Martucci 1992) tend to focus on three distinguishing dimensions involved in the care and treatment of children:

1. The child is a minor and parental involvement is necessary to some degree.
2. The child's developmental maturation expands the capacity for understanding and judgment and responsibility for behavior.
3. The child is involved with school and perhaps other social agencies and institutions that require exchange of information and collaboration in the care and treatment efforts.

Perhaps the most significant and comprehensive contribution in this field was the publication of *Ethics and Child Mental Health* (Hattab 1994). This book assembles the work of 35 international child and adolescent mental health authorities and provides a cross-cultural perspective on the vexing ethical issues confronting professionals in their vast array of clinical work, research, and advocacy for children and families.

After the official recognition of forensic psychiatry as a subspecialty in 1992, the American Academy of Psychiatry and the Law (AAPL) established ethical guidelines applicable to general forensic evaluations and developed the AAPL Ethics Committee to assist district branch ethics committees in cases involving forensic psychiatry issues. Although they are lacking in guidance on many ethical issues unique to child forensics, the AAPL guidelines (American Academy of Psychiatry and the Law 1995b) and the published opinions of the AAPL Ethics Committee (American Academy of Psychiatry and the Law 1995a) highlight useful general principles such as the importance of striving for honesty and objectivity in the consultation, avoiding role confusion and conflict of interest, obtaining fully informed consent, and protecting the examinee's privacy and confidentiality to the maximum extent legally possible. Other useful resources further elaborate on these topics (American Psychological Association 1994; Simon and Wettstein 1997) or provide more comprehensive overviews on the variety of ethical issues confronting the forensic psychiatrist (Rosner and Weinstock 1990). With regard to child and adolescent forensics, Schetky (2002a, p. 15) reviewed some important ethical principles and set the stage for further exploration.

Legal Issues in the Clinician's Practice

Although ethics codes govern the moral behavior in a clinician's practice, statutes define and regulate the business and legal aspect of his or her work. Clinical practice is a licensed professional business governed by statutes that define and regulate the nature of the practice as well as the duties and responsibilities of the practitioner (California Medical Association 2003; Caudill and Pope 1995). Professional business practices are subject to a variety of state, city, and county ordinances, as well as federal government regulating bodies such as the Drug Enforcement Administration, Medicare, and the Internal Revenue Service. States vary with regard to laws and rulings governing issues such as confidentiality; informed consent to various types of procedures and treatments; and duties to report, warn, or protect various individuals (Erikson 1995; Neinstein 1987). Clinicians should become familiar with the specific laws governing these issues in their state and locality.

■ Confidentiality, Privilege, and Duty

Although confidentiality and privileged communication in the healing arts have a long ethical tradition, they also are in fact duties and responsibilities created by state statutes to facilitate the communication, trust, and confidence that are necessary for a patient or cli-

ent to attain health or improvement through seeking professional treatment. The term *confidentiality* refers to the clinician's obligation to hold in confidence information obtained from the patient in the course of the professional relationship. Confidentiality rules govern disclosure of a patient's information to any person other than the patient (Bernet 1998, p. 463). The legal right of confidentiality belongs to the patient and can be waived only by the patient except as provided for by statutory exceptions or court order (e.g., when there is a duty to report or a duty to warn or protect a specific third party or when the patient puts his or her own mental condition at issue in a lawsuit). This basic legal right of the adult person becomes complicated with the legal status of the minor and raises an issue as to who holds the right. In general, a parent legally entitled to authorize treatment for a minor child holds the legal right to full information disclosed by the minor (Macbeth 2002, p. 314). In addition, for most purposes, minors cannot consent to or refuse treatment (Ash and Derdeyn 1997). However, a general trend in the law has increasingly afforded adolescents the rights and responsibilities of adults (Ash and Derdeyn 1997), so psychiatrists must be alert to exceptions and must carefully review the statutes specific to each state. Some jurisdictions now allow minors to hold confidentiality rights based on their age or their ability to consent to certain treatments on their own. In 1990, a California appellate court upheld the principle that even if the patient is a minor, that patient is still the holder of the psychotherapist–patient privilege (*Silva v. Haney* 1990). The increasingly common situations of separation and divorce further complicate this issue. Traditionally, the parent with legal custody held the right, but laws have shown an increasing trend toward protecting the rights of the noncustodial parent to such information (Macbeth 2002, p. 315).

Regardless of whether the parent or the minor holds the right, a clinician may have a legal duty to breach confidentiality, to report the condition to the designated persons or authorities, and to take appropriate actions to restrain the patient and protect others from danger of violence if a patient presents an imminent physical danger to self or others or makes a specific threat of violence against a particular person. Clinicians should familiarize themselves with the specific procedures for notifying authorities and providing involuntary evaluation and treatment in their particular jurisdiction (Caudill and Pope 1995).

During the past two decades, public policy in the

form of legislative enactments and appellate court decisions has tended to shift the scope of duty that requires licensed clinicians to supersede the obligations of confidentiality in favor of duties to report abuse, neglect, or threat of violence. In the landmark case on the duty to protect (*Tarasoff v. Regents of the University of California* 1976), the California Supreme Court ruled

> When a therapist determines, or pursuant to the standards of his profession should determine, that his patient presents a serious danger of violence to another, he incurs an obligation to use reasonable care to protect the intended victim against such danger. The discharge of this duty may require the therapist to take one or more of various steps, depending on the nature of the case. Thus, it may call for him to warn the intended victim or others likely to apprise the victim of the danger, to notify the police, or to take whatever steps are reasonably necessary under the circumstances. (p. 425)

Subsequent appellate court and various state statutes have attempted to define the nature of the dangerousness, its predictability, and procedures for warning or attempting to protect individuals from the threats of dangerous behavior. It appears that the trend is not to require therapists to predict dangerousness or violence in general but rather to impose the duty to protect specifically identifiable individuals who are intended victims by warning them and local police authorities of specific threats of violence. In reference to the behavior of minors in this regard, a California appellate court (*Thompson v. Alameda County* 1980) ruled that a history of delinquent or violent behavior reflecting nonspecific threats of violence not against specific identifiable victims does not give rise to a duty to warn or a duty to protect the community at large.

Makers of public policy continue efforts to balance the rights of patients' privileged communication against the need for disclosure to protect the public, to protect disturbed individuals from themselves, or to protect vulnerable individuals from abuse or neglect by persons responsible for their care. The Child Abuse Prevention and Treatment Act of 1978 provided incentives for states to develop statutes addressing child abuse and neglect. By the early 1980s, each state had in place detailed statutes setting forth specific definitions of reportable conditions, including sexual abuse, sexual assault, sexual exploitation, neglect, maltreatment, willful cruelty, unlawful or unjustifiable corporal punishment, and abuse in out-of-home care (ten Bensel et al. 1985). These statutes (e.g., California Pe-

nal Code No. 11165 et seq.) are very specific with regard to the duty of licensed professionals to report what they "know or reasonably suspect" to the locally designated child protective agency, immediately or within a specified time frame. The statutes are equally specific regarding the mode of reporting the suspected abuse or neglect and the duties, procedures, protections, and immunities of the various parties and agencies (California Medical Association 2003; Caudill and Pope 1995). These statutes provide for the conditions of immunity to the licensed professional regarding mandatory reporting, as well as misdemeanor penalties for failure to report. Civil suits against professionals for failure in their duty to report and protect minors have been successful.

Finally, a court may mandate disclosure of confidential information and require the clinician to disclose privileged communication in certain legal proceedings. There is much overlap between the rules of confidentiality and those of privilege, but privilege rules apply more specifically to the disclosure of confidential information in judicial, quasi-judicial, and administrative proceedings. Rules and exceptions to confidential rights and privileges vary between different states, so clinicians should familiarize themselves with the relevant statutes in their jurisdiction. In cases arising under federal law, the federal courts uniformly recognize a psychotherapist–patient privilege (*Jaffe v. Redmond* 1996); however, the scope and limits of this privilege and its exceptions are still evolving in appellate court decisions (Nelken 2000). Frequent exceptions to privileged communication between a psychiatrist and his or her patient include commitment proceedings, will contests, criminal matters, child custody cases, and implicit or explicit waiver of the privilege by the patient or the person authorized to act on his or her behalf (Macbeth 2002).

■ Informed Consent and Competence

In law, a competent person's prior consent is required before any medical procedure or treatment is undertaken, based on the principle of the patient's right of self-determination. In general, when the patient is a minor, the consent of the parent(s) or legal guardian is required for consultation, evaluation, treatment, or release of information for the minor child unless there are statutory or appellate court exceptions, which are increasingly numerous and varied. Furthermore, the leading appellate court case in the area of consent

(*Cobbs v. Grant* 1972) requires that patients be given sufficient information about complicated procedures to make an informed choice. In clinical practice, informed consent requires several elements, including the following:

- The clinician must inform the patient of the nature of the condition and the recommended treatment, including potential benefits, risks, and potential serious harm explained in layperson's terms. Alternatives to the recommended treatment along with their risks and benefits should also be given.
- The patient's choice is voluntary and is not coerced by the providers of the service.
- The patient has competence and capacity to consent.

In addition to statutory definitions and case law interpretation, the professional practice standard prevailing at the time and in the community is the standard of proof for matters involving informed consent (*Arato v. Avedon* 1993).

Informed consent from the parent(s) or legal guardian for minors should be reflected in the medical records and should include indications for the use of the medication relative to the patient's condition, potential short- and long-term effects, possible side effects, and specific consent for the administration of the medication. As part of obtaining consent for the treatment plan, there should be an explanation of the nature of and necessity for the privileged communication between patient and therapist and, where appropriate, an articulation of the legal requirements that set forth when confidentiality must be broken and when information about abuse or threat or danger to self or others must be reported by the therapist to specific persons or agencies.

In considering a minor's competence to consent to treatment, states provide various statutory exceptions to the general requirement of parental consent. In most jurisdictions, emancipated minors can consent to their own treatment. These include minors who are older than age 15, living away from parents, and economically self-sufficient; married (or divorced) minors; minors on active duty in the United States armed services; and minors who have been emancipated for cause with a specific court order. A "mature" minor or one whom the courts determine is sufficiently mature to appreciate the nature, extent, and consequences of the medical treatment may also consent to his or her

own treatment (*Cardwell v. Bechtol* 1987). Following a general trend in the direction of treating minors more as adults, state legislatures are also allowing minors to consent to specific types of medical and psychiatric treatment such as treatment related to sexual behavior (abortion, birth control, sexually transmitted diseases) and time-limited outpatient mental health treatment (Ash and Derdeyn 1997).

The issue of informed consent with minors is problematic because minors may not have sufficient maturity, understanding, or worldly exposure to make an informed judgment about the nature of the condition, complicated procedures, or potential consequences. Explanations should be adapted to their level of comprehension and ability to consent. As a practical matter, psychiatric consultation, evaluation, and treatment with most children and adolescents usually takes place in the interactive context of involvement and consent of the child and parents (or legal guardian), who have usually arranged for the initial consultation and evaluation and who participate in the treatment planning and pay for the services.

■ Civil Commitment

The occasional clinical necessity for hospital treatment of seriously disturbed children and adolescents may bring their rights to liberty and self-determination into conflict with the rights, responsibilities, and duties of parents, legal guardians, and state agencies. Clinical guidelines (American Academy of Child and Adolescent Psychiatry 1989) for such hospitalization includes 1) a qualified psychiatrist's evaluation; 2) diagnosis by DSM criteria; 3) severity of impairment in two or more areas of daily functioning; 4) likelihood of benefit from the proposed treatment; 5) prior consideration of less-restrictive treatment procedures and the judgment that they are inappropriate or inadequate to meet the patient's needs; 6) the child's encouragement to voluntarily participate in the admission, treatment planning, and discharge process; and 7) parents' full information about and participation in the hospitalization and treatment planning decisions.

In the governing U.S. Supreme Court case regarding hospitalization of minors (*Parham v. J.R.* 1979), the right of parents to seek and secure hospital treatment for their minor children was affirmed, provided that independent medical reviews—and not necessarily an adversarial due process legal review—confirm the nature of the illness and the likelihood of benefit from the proposed treatment. Moreover, this independent medical review must have the power to deny admission if medical standards and legal requirements are not met. In addition, the youth has the right to periodic reviews of treatment procedures and of the hospital confinement. The findings in *Parham* were subsequently extended to a Pennsylvania case, *Secretary of Public Welfare of Pennsylvania v. Institutionalized Juveniles* (1979), in which the Supreme Court decided that the *Parham* procedural safeguards offered sufficient protection of the minors' "liberty interests." However, the Court also concluded that parents cannot waive the rights of minors to due process civil commitment procedures and that minors have the right to challenge the psychiatric diagnosis within 72 hours and a right to a formal adversary hearing within 14 days of hospitalization.

States can afford more extensive due protections than those required in *Parham v. J.R.* (1979). In a California Supreme Court case, *In re Roger S.* (1977), the court gave minors age 14 and over the following procedural safeguards: entitlement to administrative hearing by a neutral fact finder before commitment, notice of the reasons for the proposed action, right to counsel, the opportunity to present evidence and cross-examine witnesses, and proof by a preponderance of the evidence that the minor has a mental illness and will be benefited by the treatment.

■ Professional Liability

During the past two decades, the increase in claims and awards for professional malpractice has not bypassed psychiatrists and other mental health providers. Because of recently expanding case law and legislation in matters such as psychic trauma and legal liability, mental health professionals are increasingly vulnerable to claims and suits based on matters such as abandonment of patients, battery, breach of confidentiality or duty, failure to follow established or community standards of care, failure of duty to report or protect against harassment or abuse of patients, negligence, improper treatment, wrongful injury, or other alleged violations of federal or state laws regarding professional responsibilities and practice.

In accordance with the principles and precedents of tort law or civil wrongful behavior rather than of criminal behavior, a professional practitioner may be liable for behavior that unintentionally resulted in harm or injury to a patient or to a third party that could have or should have been reasonably prevented.

The essential elements of professional negligence or malpractice are sometimes referred to as the four *D*'s of negligence:

- **D**uty—a duty of care was owed to the patient by the physician.
- **D**ereliction—the duty of care was breached.
- **D**amages—the patient experienced actual damage due to the breach of duty.
- **D**irect causation—the dereliction was the direct cause of the damages.

The plaintiff's case must demonstrate these elements to the trier of fact, whereas the defense attempts to demonstrate that one or more of these elements did not or could not have occurred according to the standard of care prevalent in the community at the time. The standard of proof in malpractice cases is preponderance of evidence (i.e., more likely than not). As concepts regarding civil liability have been expanding (Guyer 1990), mental health professionals involved in civil litigation are increasingly involved in the evaluation, treatment, and damage assessments regarding other plaintiffs and defendants (Schetky and Guyer 1990). By the same processes, mental health professionals are having their own professional procedures and behaviors scrutinized for negligence or breach of duty and may find themselves vulnerable to claims for inadequate evaluations, failure to obtain informed consent, or a myriad of other improper actions or omissions. Residency training programs in child and adolescent psychiatry have also been successfully sued for patient mismanagement and other claims involving faculty and trainees (Wagner et al. 1993).

The increasing involvement of mental health professionals in child sexual abuse cases and a growing body of literature on repressed memories and the suggestibility of child witnesses has fueled the emergence of new areas of litigation. One evolving area of litigation involves third-party claims brought by parents against their child's therapists. In 1994, a California superior court allowed a father to successfully sue his daughter's therapist for negligence and intentional infliction of emotional distress after the therapist had suggested memories of sexual abuse to the daughter and encouraged her to confront the father (*Ramona v. Isabella* 1994) The court found that the therapist owed a duty of care to the parent because he was involved in the therapy of the child and had become a client along with the daughter. However, in *Althaus v. Cohen* (1998), the court found no such duty of care to the parents of an alleged victim of abuse because it would create a breach of the therapist's fundamental duty to her patient and would destroy the therapeutic process. Other new areas of litigation involve claims for implanting false memories of abuse and attempts to overturn previous convictions based on the suggestibility of child witnesses (*Commonwealth of Massachusetts v. Amirault LeFave* 1999). This is a new and evolving area of case law, and the full impact of these decisions is yet to be known.

Another rapidly emerging area of ethical and legal vulnerability for mental health professionals involves the cost-containment purposes of managed care overriding the independent clinical judgment of attending physicians with regard to patient-care decisions. When a managed care company denies coverage for a service for "lack of medical necessity," the physician has four duties: First, the physician should appeal the decision (*Wickline v. California* 1986). Second, the physician should discuss the issues raised by the managed care company with the patient. The patient should be informed that the insurer has refused to pay and that the patient has the option of paying out-of-pocket or appealing the decision. Third, there is always the duty to treat the patient in an emergency, even without payment. Fourth, the physician should develop alternative treatment plans in the face of the denial of a preferred treatment plan by the managed care company.

■ Child Custody and Divorce

In the past generation, there has been an increase in divorce, remarriage, single-parent families, stepparenting families, and alternative families (Shiono and Quinn 1994). As a result, there is perhaps no issue at the interface of psychiatry and the law that has grown more in volume, permutations of detail, and hostile conflict than the law in regard to child custody, child access, and perhaps parental responsibility and financial obligations (Hyde 1984). This has occurred in the context of the recently burgeoning social science research data on children and families undergoing the process and effects of divorce, especially high-conflict custody divorce cases, which pose a significant workload for the courts (Behrman 1994; Hetherington 1989; Kelly 1988, 2000; Roseby and Johnston 1998; Wallerstein 1991).

The legal doctrine of the best interests of the child is the current guiding principle in deciding child cus-

tody disputes (Nurcombe and Partlett 1994, p. 91). The model legislation of the Uniform Marriage and Divorce Act approved by the American Bar Association in 1974 (Group for the Advancement of Psychiatry 1980) contains a section regarding the best interests criteria. According to the relevant section (Section 402), the court shall determine custody in accordance with the best interests of the child and shall consider all relevant factors, including the wishes of the parents and the child; the interactions of the child with those who may significantly affect his or her best interests; the child's adjustment to his or her home, school, and community; and the mental and physical health of all individuals involved (Group for the Advancement of Psychiatry 1980; Nurcombe and Partlett 1994, p. 92).

The majority of states have adapted their statutes (either wholly or in modified form) from the concept and language of the Uniform Marriage and Divorce Act. For example, California Family Code, Section 3011 et seq., concerning the custody of children, provides, in part, "it is the public policy of this state to assure minor children frequent and continuing contact with both parents...and to encourage parents to share the rights and responsibilities of child rearing." In awarding child custody, the court makes a determination in the best interests of the child, considering—among other factors it finds relevant—the health, safety, and welfare of the child; allegations of abuse and neglect; and the habitual or continued illegal use of controlled substances or the continual abuse of alcohol (California Family Code 3011). "The court shall also consider, among other factors, which parent is more likely to allow the child frequent and continued contact with the noncustodial parent...and shall not prefer a parent custodian because of that parent's sex" (California Family Code 3040). Family Code 3042 also states, in part, "if a child is of sufficient age and capacity to reason so as to form an intelligent preference as to custody, the court shall consider and give weight to the wishes of the child in making an order granting or modifying custody."

Despite the general acceptance of the "best interests" principle (Goldstein et al. 1996), the concept remains ambiguous and indeterminate, leaving judges with wide discretion to interpret it in a variety of ways. As a result of this vagueness, the courts have increasingly relied on the expertise of child mental health professionals to assist in the determination of best interests (American Academy of Child and Adolescent Psychiatry 1997b). To promote and maintain standards of care and assist those engaged in this specialized work, guidelines for evaluating child custody disputes have been published by the American Psychological Association (1994), the American Association of Family and Conciliation Courts (1994), the American Psychiatric Association (1988), and the Judicial Council of California (2002). A number of mental health professionals have also published important guiding principles (Bernet 1998; Herman 1999).

While clinicians and court personnel struggle to ascertain and articulate the "best interests of the child" in any particular case, they may be guided by the commentary of the California Supreme Court's perception (*In re Marriage of Carney* 1979) that

> The essence of parenting...lies in the ethical, emotional, and intellectual guidance the parent gives to the child throughout his formative years, and often beyond. The source of this guidance is the adult's own experience of life; its motive power is parental love and concern for the child's well-being; and its teachings deal with such fundamental matters as the child's feelings about himself, his relationships with others, his system of values, his standards of conduct, and his goals and priorities in life (p. 739).

The application of such wisdom requires careful clinical observation and judgment in the exceedingly complex labyrinth of child custody evaluations and procedures (Ames and Huntington 1991; Ash and Guyer 1986; Herman 1990; Kelly 1991).

Current social forces have engendered special issues in child custody disputes that complicate the evaluation and present additional challenges to the forensic expert. The special issues involve a diverse range of topics such as infant placement and custody (Horner and Guyer 1993), homosexual parenting, rights of stepparents and grandparents, parental kidnapping, the mentally ill parent, sexual abuse allegations, parental relocation (Shear 1996), and controversies arising from advances in reproductive technologies (Bernet 1998; Herman 1990; Nurcombe and Partlett 1994). The highly controversial issue of alienation in children of divorce is currently being reformulated (Kelly and Johnston 2001).

The emotionally charged topic of homosexual parenting is particularly complex and challenging. The mental health literature on homosexual parenting appears to suggest no appreciable differences in parenting abilities or in the psychological health and sexual orientation of the child (Binder 1998). Despite these findings in the literature, legal jurisdictions have taken varied approaches to the issue. Some jurisdictions equate homosexuality with parental unfitness, whereas other jurisdictions have opposed the use of sexual orientation in determining the outcome of visitation or custody disputes (*In re Birdsall* 1988).

Grandparents, stepparents, and other third parties are increasingly seeking visitation rights or custody of children. States vary in their approach to these issues. With regard to stepparents obtaining custody of a child, the general trend in the courts appears to favor the natural parent over the nonbiological parent unless "clear and convincing evidence" (Herman 1990) or "exceptional circumstances" (Herman 1990) support placement with the nonbiological parent. All 50 states have enacted some form of grandparent visitation legislation, but the visitation statutes vary in their degree of permissiveness (Scott 2000). In a recent ruling on this controversy, the U.S. Supreme Court (*Troxel v. Granville* 2000) concluded that the broad language of a Washington State visitation statute allowing "any person" to petition for visitation rights "at any time" unconstitutionally infringed on the parents' "fundamental right" under the Fourteenth Amendment to raise their family free from governmental interference (*Troxel v. Granville* 2000). Future cases will likely continue to attempt to define the boundary between parental autonomy and the state's authority to impose visitation or custody rights of stepparents, grandparents, and other third parties in furthering the best interests of the child.

A tragic outcome of child custody disputes is the serious problem of parental kidnapping. An underground network has even developed to assist parents who are fleeing with their children from what is perceived as an unjust legal system (Herman 1990). Schetky and Haller (1983) reviewed the agonizing conflicts created in the child, the legal aspects of the problem, and attempts to deal with the issue. The forensic examiner confronted with this type of case should be familiar with the relevant state laws, federal laws (Uniform Child Custody Jurisdiction and Enforcement Act and the Parental Kidnapping Prevention Act) and international agreements (1988 International Child Abduction Remedies Act and the 1980 Hague Convention on the Civil Aspects of International Child Abduction) that provide some procedures and sanctions to address this issue (Weiner 2000).

Regardless of whether the evaluation involves general issues or more complex situations as described previously, the examiner should be prepared to deal with a potentially high-conflict, emotionally intense process. Divorcing parents are often dissatisfied with the adversarial nature, high costs, and inefficiencies of the court system involved with divorce litigation (Pruett and Jackson 2001). Studies have also shown significant negative outcomes on child and parent from the adversarial process (Kelly 2000).

Mediation provides an important alternative to the adversarial process and has increased in availability and utilization in the past decade (Kelly 2000). In several states—including California, Maine, New Mexico, Connecticut, and Maryland—mediation is mandated by the court before custody litigation begins (Herman 2002). The process of mediation differs in the legal jurisdictions throughout the country, but the current literature suggests increased overall satisfaction among the involved parties and more frequent joint custody and cooperation between parents (Ash and Derdeyn 1997).

The child custody evaluator should be knowledgeable about the two usual outcomes of a custody dispute—that is, joint custody or sole custody—and the potential effects of these outcomes on the child. In joint legal custody, both parents have legal decision-making powers regarding the child. In joint physical custody, the parents have responsibility for co-parenting. In sole custody, one parent has this power. Current literature reflects a lack of consensus on the best custody arrangement for children (Binder 1998), but relevant research studies support certain generalizations on this topic. Interparental conflict, the psychological health of the parents, and the quality of parent–child relationships appear to be among the most important predictors of a child's adjustment to divorce (Ash and Derdeyn 1997; Kelly 2000). High levels of interparental conflict—whether in the conflict of the marriage or in high-conflict divorce situations—appear to have an especially negative influence on the psychological adjustment of children (Roseby and Johnston 1998). The effect of the parent's and child's gender on postdivorce adjustment is another increasingly important area of study. The literature appears to suggest that girls are less well adjusted in families with father and stepfather custody, and boys are less well adjusted in mother-custody families (Binder 1998). Furthermore, in mother-custody families, boys may have improved adjustment with regular paternal contact, provided the father is reasonably healthy (Binder 1998).

Child custody evaluations involve a dynamic, exceedingly complicated area of family law. In May 2000, the American Law Institute approved a project called the Principles of the Law of Family Dissolution to examine the present state of legal development in this area of the law; to clarify underlying principles; and to suggest future direction for public policy in the issues of dissolution, child and spousal support, property division, and custody of children (Kay 2000). Twenty-first-century lawmakers should consider the proposed legal framework and standards as they continue to address the constant challenges and complexities of this rapidly evolving area of the law.

■ Child Abuse and Neglect

The apparent incidence of child abuse and neglect has dramatically risen since the passage of the Child Abuse Prevention and Treatment Act in 1978 (Larner et al. 1998). After implementation of the federally mandated guidelines, all states passed laws requiring designated persons to report child abuse and neglect (Nurcombe and Partlett 1994, p. 137). Reporting of allegations continues to rise as a result of this federal legislation and increased media attention (Quinn 2002). Failure to report can result in civil liability for negligence and malpractice (*Landeros v. Flood* 1976) or even in criminal penalties as specified by statutes (Nurcombe and Partlett 1994, p. 138). The mandated reporting is an exception to confidentiality, and the reporter is granted immunity from suits for negligence or defamation if the suspected case of abuse is reported in good faith (Quinn 2002). State laws vary in their legal definition of terms related to the maltreatment of children, so clinicians should familiarize themselves with the statutes in their specific jurisdiction. Variability is especially wide in sexual abuse definitions, in which the age of both the child and the perpetrator as well as their relationship determines the nature of the offense and the penalties involved (Quinn 2002).

In child maltreatment cases, the forensic evaluator can perform a variety of functions, including assessment of the nature and extent of harm to the child; evaluation of parental fitness; and recommendations regarding placement, treatment, or termination of parental rights (American Academy of Child and Adolescent Psychiatry 1997c). The forensic evaluation may be used in a variety of legal proceedings, including criminal prosecution, dependency and guardianship actions, custodial dispute, termination of parental rights, and tort litigation (Barnum 1997).

To address questions related to the nature and extent of harm, the forensic examiner should familiarize himself or herself with the clinical patterns associated with child maltreatment. Several authors have provided reviews of the most recent literature regarding the clinical patterns, differential diagnosis, and long-term consequences associated with child abuse and neglect (American Academy of Child and Adolescent Psychiatry 1997c; Bernet 1993; Kaplan et al. 1999; Nurcombe and Partlett 1994). In addition to the clinical patterns of physical abuse, sexual abuse victims manifest a wider and greater frequency of inappropriate sexual behaviors than nonabused children (Bernet 1998). Although physical and sexual abuse have been the focus of most studies, emotional maltreatment is likely the most frequent form of abuse and neglect, with the strongest relationship to long-term psychological functioning (Kaplan et al. 1999). However, relevant studies are lacking because of the perception that it is less damaging than physical and sexual abuse (Kaplan et al. 1999).

Assessment of parental capacity and prognosis is a challenging task, because a clinical consensus on this standard remains to be developed. Barnum (2002), providing the most recent guidance on this issue, offers a theoretical framework for understanding parenting, discusses the impact of developmental issues and parental strengths and weaknesses on parenting capacity, and describes specific techniques for assessment. Clinical opinions regarding this issue will be central to the adjudication and disposition of a child maltreatment case. Based on the findings, the juvenile court may decide to return the child home with further diagnostic or therapeutic interventions or commit the child to custody of the state with a requirement of home-based services and periodic reports to the court (Nurcombe and Partlett 1994, p. 143). However, if parents are deemed incapable of providing a safe environment for the child, the child may be removed from the home and placed in foster care or institutional care with plans for eventual reunification (Wasserman et al. 2002).

Foster care is an increasingly utilized temporary placement option for the child who is removed from the home. Social policy and increasing prevalence of substance abuse, human immunodeficiency virus infection, and homelessness in the late 1980s led to a dramatic increase in the foster care population (Wasserman et al. 2002) and growing concern for the future welfare of these children. Appropriate consulta-tion in these cases requires awareness of the complexities in the system and an understanding of its potential impact on the child. For example, numerous studies have described the difficulties in this population of children, including physical problems, psychological and emotional issues, and academic difficulties (Rosenfeld et al. 1997). The emotional impact of the parent–child separation on the child, contradictory demands on the biological and foster parents, and a system that lacks the resources to address the special needs of this population create an especially difficult situation for a child who already has problems (Rosenfeld et al. 1997). Yet despite this negative perspective, evidence also indicates that foster care can have positive outcomes, including improved health, social functioning, and academic performance (Rosenfeld et al. 1997). The literature also suggests that certain risk factors (e.g., poverty, alcoholism, parent mental illness, low education) and protective factors (e.g., intelligence, positive emotional ties, external support system) likely influence the outcomes of a child's foster care experience (Rosenfeld et al. 1997). Numerous confounding variables make definitive conclusions on this issue difficult. However, the government and social agencies have made some efforts to improve the plight of these children. To address concern about the lack of stable, healthy, consistent attachments in this population, the federal government enacted the Adoption Assistance and Child Welfare Act of 1980 (P.L. 96-272) "to end the drift of children in foster care and encourage plans for permanency." The law mandates social agencies to make "reasonable efforts" to help the biological family remedy the issues leading to removal of the child and, in case family reunification efforts fail, to begin permanency plans within 18–20 months of foster care placement (Rosenfeld et al. 1997, p. 449). Other promising developments include the increasingly popular use of kinship care and therapeutic foster care programs (Rosenfeld et al. 1997; U.S. Public Health Service 2000, p. 176; Wasserman et al. 2002). Unfortunately, positive changes in the foster care system are undermined by a managed care system that seeks to decrease child welfare expenses. Ultimately, public policy makers will have the difficult if not impossible task of allocating diminished resources to provide high levels of special care for a growing population in an already overburdened system.

Although the law mandates that reasonable efforts be made to encourage reunification with the family, the state is entitled to petition for termination of parental rights if family reunification has failed and the child has been in foster care for 18 months (Adoption Assistance and Child Welfare Act of 1980, P.L. 96-272). Certain crimes (e.g., murder, rape, sexual abuse) even warrant the automatic pursuit of termination of parental rights (Schetky 2002d). The legal standard for termination of parental rights is *clear and convincing evidence* (*Santosky v. Kramer* 1982). Nurcombe and Partlett (1994, p. 147) and Schetky (2002d) described specific criteria to be considered in termination proceedings such as the child's need for permanency, continuity of relationships with siblings and extended family members, special needs of the child, quality of the parent–child relationship, and capacity for attachment and adoptability. The forensic examiner should also be familiar with the various possible outcomes of termination proceedings, including long-term foster care; legal guardianship; emancipation; and closed, open, or kinship adoptions (Schetky 2002d).

The Child as Witness

Because of a frequent lack of physical corroboration, allegations of sexual abuse often require a child's testimony. This is less likely to be the case in allegations of physical abuse because the physician can testify to the abuse based on his or her observations or a medical diagnosis of the battered child syndrome. In sexual abuse cases, the child's testimony can be critical to determining the likelihood of sexual abuse.

A number of widely publicized cases of allegations of sexual abuse in the 1980s and 1990s led to much research on the accuracy of children's memory and the reliability and suggestibility of their statements. From a developmental perspective, the literature suggests that memory—especially short-term memory—and retention begin to exist functionally at age 3, undergo a major developmental shift at age 6, and continue to improve with age (Clark 2002, p. 130). Although research has shown that children are capable of accurately recalling information, studies also indicate that they are highly susceptible to suggestion (American Academy of Child and Adolescent Psychiatry 1997c; Ceci and Bruck 1993). There appear to be significant age differences in suggestibility, with preschool children being disproportionately more vulnerable to suggestion than either school-age children or adults, but the age differences are a matter of degree (American

Academy of Child and Adolescent Psychiatry 1997c; Ceci and Bruck 1993). Even adults are susceptible to suggestion, as evidenced by research on the phenomena of "recovered memories" and "repressed memories"(Corelli et al. 1997). The negative consequence of suggestive interviewing techniques includes errors about the source of the information as well as major details of the peripheral and central events, such as falsely reporting that a person had touched their private parts (Bruck and Ceci 2002, p. 139). Several significant contributors to this literature include Loftus (1997), Loftus and Pickrell (1995), and Poole and Lindsay (1995, 2001).

These controversies have led to a large body of literature on the appropriate assessment of allegedly abused children, including appropriate interview techniques to minimize bias and distortion (American Academy of Child and Adolescent Psychiatry 1997c; Bernet 1998). In general, the current literature suggests that interviewers should start with an open-ended question; progress to more focused questions if necessary; and avoid leading questions, repetitive questioning, questions promoting speculation or fantasy, and manipulation of the emotional tone to direct the interviewee (Ceci and Bruck 1993; Schetky and Benedek 2002, p. 154). These studies suggest that memory appears to be most accurate when elicited through free recall without the use of cueing, leading questions, suggestive interviewing, or multiple interviews. Trained child clinicians will find their knowledge of child development most valuable in these interviews, because children have age-related differences in memory, cognitive abilities, language skills, range of experience, and emotional maturity.

The child's credibility is ultimately determined by the judge or jury and not the forensic expert. However, the forensic expert may give expert testimony on this topic. Several authors have described factors that can assess the credibility of a child (American Academy of Child and Adolescent Psychiatry 1997c; Benedek and Schetky 1987a, 1987b; Green 1986; Nurcombe and Partlett 1994, p. 172; Raskin and Esplin 1991). Some of these factors include spontaneity of statements, age-appropriate terminology, general consistency in statements, appropriate affect, and consideration of motivational factors (such as in divorce-related circumstances) (American Academy of Child and Adolescent Psychiatry 1997b; Derdeyn et al. 1994). However, studies have shown that even well-trained professionals cannot reliably differentiate between true and false reports when these reports have been influenced by suggestive interviewing techniques (Ceci and Bruck 1993). This may be explained by the current scientific literature, which suggests that memory is constructive rather than reconstructive in nature and that retrieval is influenced by current attitudes, feelings, and beliefs (Corelli et al. 1997). Therefore, the factors for assessing credibility cannot be used definitively to determine whether abuse has occurred.

A child's testimony is only valuable if he or she is competent. *Competence* refers to the child's ability to testify in court in a reliable and meaningful manner. Several authors have contributed to the literature on this topic (American Academy of Child and Adolescent Psychiatry 1997c; Nurcombe and Partlett 1994, p. 168). In general, a child's competence is determined by four criteria: the capacity to register the event, the ability to accurately recall and recount the event, the ability to distinguish truth from falsehood, and the capacity to communicate based on personal knowledge of the facts (Nurcombe and Partlett 1994, p. 169).

The evaluation and prosecution of maltreatment cases may subject the child victim to multiple assessments and evaluations in home, school, clinical, or police settings (Arthur 1986) and may require the child to participate in depositions and pretrial hearings and to testify in court as a witness (Office of Juvenile Justice and Delinquency Prevention 1994). In addition to child protective services and juvenile court dependency proceedings, these evaluations and sometimes the child's own testimony as a witness may be required in criminal proceedings against the perpetrator, as well as in civil litigation for claims of psychic damages. There has been concern about the effect of this process on the child witness because of the child's particular level of cognitive and emotional development. A number of suggestions and attempts have been made to reduce the number of evaluations and to modify prosecutorial procedures (Arthur 1986; Office of Juvenile Justice and Delinquency Prevention 1994). The precedent-setting U.S. Supreme Court decision in this area (*Wheeler v. United States* 1895) indicated that a 5-year-old boy "was not by reason of his youth, as a matter of law, absolutely disqualified as a witness" and further ruled that the question of competence "depends on the capacity and intelligence of the child, his appreciation of the difference between truth and falsehood, as well as his duty to tell the former" (p. 254).

During the past decade, the U.S. Supreme Court has decided eight cases that balanced the best interests and cognitive and emotional capabilities of a child witness against the constitutional rights of defendants to protections against self-incrimination (Fifth Amendment), the right to confront and cross-examine witnesses (Sixth Amendment), and due process (Fourteenth Amendment) (Kermani 1991, 1993). In the most recent decision in this series (*White v. Illinois* 1992), the court recognized what amounts to a specific hearsay exception: The testimony of a physician was admitted and did not violate the defendant's Sixth Amendment rights because the child's statement to the physician was "a spontaneous declaration" made to the physician for the purpose of medical diagnosis and treatment. Clinicians working in this area should be aware of additional state and local jurisdiction rulings and of current standards of assessment related to the particular case and status of the child witness.

Youth Violence

The current surge in youth violence in the United States has permeated the national consciousness and media and has prompted school administrators, law enforcement officials, policy makers, and mental health professionals to more closely examine this complex issue. The forensic psychiatrist may serve as a consultants in risk assessment, risk management, and prevention of violence.

A growing body of literature has recently developed, beginning with the neurodevelopmental impact of violence in childhood. Results of the studies suggest that exposure to violence and trauma and the neurophysiological adaptations to this exposure can alter normal development of the child's brain and can lead to changes in physiological, emotional, behavioral, cognitive, and social functioning (Perry 2002, p. 192). Children raised in violent communities or in homes with chronic parental violence appear to be at higher risk for psychiatric disturbances, delinquent behavior, and an increased likelihood of becoming perpetrators of aggressive and violent behavior themselves (Perry 2002, p. 208). A large number of studies on the impact of media violence on children reveal that it increases risk for aggressive behavior (Singer et al. 1998), desensitizes youths to violence in the real world (American Medical Association 1996), creates a perception of the world as a dangerous and unfriendly place (Singer et al. 1998), and potentially leads to greater risks of psychological and social problems (Singer et al. 1998). However, not all children are similarly affected by violence, and protective factors such as the parent–child relationship and age have also been described (Al-Mateen 2002, p. 220).

The wave of school shootings in the mid and late 1990s fueled a growing concern about school violence and led to much inquiry about risk assessment and prevention of violence in children and adolescents. A growing body of literature has attempted to identify factors associated with aggressive, violent, antisocial, or delinquent behavior. Disruptions in early development, abnormal neurotransmitter levels, mental illness, learning disabilities, exposure to violence, certain parenting styles, substance use, neurological impairment, and socioeconomic class are among some of the causal factors implicated in an increased risk of delinquent or aggressive behavior (Schetky 2002c, p. 234). The wide diversity of the associative factors speaks to the complexity of this issue and may explain why clinicians face a daunting task when trying to identify youths at high risk for violence. Several authors have discussed the limits of the ability to make long-term predictions of violence and have offered more realistic approaches to the problem, such as more ongoing involvement with high-risk students; more frequent assessments targeting risk of imminent danger (rather than long-term predictions); and the creation of a supportive, positive school environment with good communication between school administration and students (Mulvey and Cauffman 2001).

The heightened awareness of school violence has prompted school administrators, policy makers, and mental health professionals to implement a variety of prevention and intervention programs. Schetky and Benedek (2002, p. 239) and Pittel (1998) delineated guidelines for taking a violence and weapons history. Some of the preventive programs that have resulted in positive outcomes include conflict resolution, interpersonal problem-solving techniques, bullying reduction programs, supervised recreation after school hours, mentoring programs, parent management training, and family therapy (U.S. Department of Health and Human Services 2001). Because all of these described programs have practical and methodological limitations that curtail their effectiveness, further research is warranted.

Dependency, Delinquency, and the Juvenile Court

The juvenile court system in the United States originated as a result of the progressive and reform movements at the end of the nineteenth century. The system was seen as a way to move minors out of the adult criminal justice system and into specialized procedures and programs to meet their best interests and rehabilitative needs. This specialized system was developed in every state through enabling legislation that established a local county court with original jurisdiction over the care, rehabilitation, treatment, supervision, and disposition of minors who came to the attention of the juvenile court for the following reasons: 1) dependency, neglect, or abuse; 2) incorrigibility or truancy, now called status offenses; or 3) delinquency offenses, that is, violation of laws that if committed by an adult would be subject to the jurisdiction of the criminal court.

The prevailing concepts of parens patriae in common law provided the justification for the development of this juvenile court and probation system, which exercised responsibility for minors who violated the law, were not properly cared for, or could not otherwise exercise proper control over themselves. Juvenile courts in each county (Edwards 1992; Guyer 1985) had wide discretion, latitude, and encouragement to act in an informal, highly individualized fashion, utilizing a wide variety of procedures and interventions in the care, rehabilitation, "reform," or treatment of the abused, abandoned, neglected, incorrigible, or delinquent minors within their jurisdictions.

If a youth was deemed to be beyond the rehabilitative capabilities of the local juvenile court detention, probation, or state training school facilities, the youth was transferred—or waived—to the jurisdiction of the adult criminal court in that county. In the first juvenile court intervention ruling (*Kent v. United States* 1966), the Supreme Court held that the decision to transfer or waive a juvenile to adult criminal court is "critically important." It therefore must provide fairness and due process involving a fair (though informal) hearing, assistance of counsel with access to social service records, a written record of the proceedings indicating the findings of the court, and a reason for the transfer or certification to the adult criminal court so that the proceedings may be reviewed on appeal.

Substantial reform was brought to the operation of

the juvenile court system in the Supreme Court's second decision on proceedings (*In re Gault* 1967). The court articulated five basic constitutional rights in the adjudicatory phase of the juvenile court procedures:

1. Adequate notice of trial at all stages
2. Right to counsel
3. Right to confront witnesses in cross-examination
4. Privilege against self-incrimination, both before and during trial
5. Proper appellate review, including the right to transcripts of the proceedings

Concerning other procedural matters, the Supreme Court held that a higher standard of proof (i.e., beyond a reasonable doubt) was required in juvenile delinquency adjudications (*In re Winship* 1970). However, there is no constitutional right to a trial by jury in juvenile delinquency adjudication (*McKeiver v. Pennsylvania* 1971). Moreover, state statutes may provide for juvenile pretrial detention when it is determined that a particular juvenile presents a "serious risk" or that the juvenile "may before the return date commit an act which, if committed by an adult, would constitute a crime" (*Schall v. Martin* 1984, p. 2405). Many unresolved and ongoing procedural due process concerns continue to challenge the juvenile justice system, particularly as more juveniles are tried in adult courts. The issue of search and seizure has become increasingly pertinent as schools seek to deal with the presence of weapons and drugs in schools. In *New Jersey v. T.L.O.* (1985), the Supreme Court found no violation of Fourth Amendment rights when a principal searched a student's purse for drugs without a search warrant. Other important controversial areas include confessions and the limits of interrogation.

An alarming increase in youth violence in the past decade had led to a movement away from the rehabilitative ideal of the original juvenile court system toward the direction of holding more violent youths responsible as adults. Many states have passed "get tough" laws allowing more juveniles to be tried in adult court (Snyder and Sickmund 1995). Some of these laws—such as the 1996 Michigan Juvenile Justice Reform Legislation (Clark 1996)—automatically place a juvenile in adult court for certain violent offenses, and others increase the number of offenses for which a juvenile could be waived at the discretion of the district attorney (direct file waiver) or after a judicial hearing. Most recently, the California Supreme Court affirmed

that specific charges against minors age 14 years and older may be filed directly in a court of criminal jurisdiction without a judicial determination of unfitness under the juvenile court law (*Manduley v. Superior Court of San Diego* 2002).

The increased readiness to waive juveniles to adult court has resulted in a heightened concern about the issue of competence in the juvenile. The current standard for competence to stand trial is "whether a defendant has sufficient present ability to consult with his lawyer with a reasonable degree of rational understanding and whether he has a rational as well as factual understanding of the proceedings against him" (*Dusky v. United States* 1960). A number of screening instruments can assist the examiner in determining a juvenile's competence: the Georgia Court Competency Test, the MacArthur Competence Assessment Tool, and McGarry's Competency Assessment Interview. Other authors have also made important contributions to the literature on this topic (Grisso 1998a; Ratner 1992).

Although competence to stand trial is the most common competence referral, competence to waive Miranda rights and to be executed are becoming significantly more important as more juveniles are transferred to adult court. In *Fare v. Michael* (1979), the U.S. Supreme Court determined that the juvenile's waiver of his Miranda rights must be determined in light of the totality of the circumstances, including factors such as the individual's comprehension of the warning and the context surrounding the confessions. Grisso (1998b) elaborated on this issue and developed four standardized tools to assist the examiner in this question. The constitutionality of executing a juvenile is variable based on the juvenile's age and the jurisdiction. In two separate cases, the U.S. Supreme Court held that execution of an offender age 15 or younger is unconstitutional (*Thompson v. Oklahoma* 1988) and that a juvenile may be subject to the death penalty for crimes committed at age 16 or 17 (*Stanford v. Kentucky* 1989). States with the death penalty statute vary in their minimum age requirement, but the range is between ages 16 and 18 years.

In many of these waiver cases, child and adolescent psychiatrists are often called on to evaluate and provide testimony to the court regarding the juvenile's degree of dangerousness to the community, risk assessment, and the juvenile's amenability to treatment or rehabilitation (Barnum 1987). Although realistic limitations prevent mental health professionals from making actual predictions about an individual's future violent behavior, several studies have identified both risk factors and protective factors that are generally associated with chronic delinquency and increased rates of violence (Deprato and Hammer 2002, p. 268; Hoge et al. 1996; Kirkish et al. 2000; Steiner 1997). Many studies have focused on the high prevalence of mental disorders in this population (Deprato and Hammer 2002, p. 269; Foley et al. 1996; O'Shaughnessy 1992). Although no assessment instrument exists to accurately predict future violence, several instruments assess mental and personality disorders, including the Minnesota Multiphasic Personality Inventory—Adolescent, the Millon Adolescent Clinical Inventory, the Child Behavior Checklist, the Hare Psychopathy Checklist—Youth Version, and the Massachusetts Youth Screening Instrument (Grisso et al. 2001; Scott 2002, p. 293). Practice guidelines have also been developed for assessing these youths and can assist the forensic examiner in his or her work in these cases (Ash and Derdeyn 1997, p. 1498).

Consultation on the disposition of the youth from the juvenile court system involves a comprehensive knowledge of both current disposition options and effective treatment models. Dispositions to be considered include waiver to adult court as described above, diversion before adjudication, probation, community placement, and commitment to a correctional facility (Sacks and Reader 1992). Diversion programs defer the youth's adjudication and offer an opportunity for dismissal of the charges if the juvenile can successfully complete a treatment program such as an individual and family counseling, educational, vocational, or recreational intervention or rehabilitation for substance abuse in cooperation with the juvenile drug court (Nurcombe and Partlett 1994). Probation is multifaceted and can include drug counseling, weekend confinement in a local detention center, and community and victim restitution (Snyder and Sickmund 1995). Twenty years ago, the literature on delinquency presented a pessimistic view on the outcomes of treatment and interventions. Treatment programs such as residential treatment centers failed to consider the multifaceted nature of delinquency and tended to approach the problem in a fragmented and unidimensional manner (Deprato and Hammer 2002, p. 274). The youth often reverted to antisocial, delinquent behavior once he or she returned to his community. As described in the report of the Surgeon General's Conference on Children's Mental Health (U.S. Public Health Service 2000), the development of newer interventions such as multisystemic therapy and therapeutic foster care has improved outcomes and has led to a more optimistic outlook on the future of this growing population.

Clinicians providing consultation, forensic assessment (O'Shaughnessy 1992), evaluation, or treatment services in the juvenile court system (Kalogerakis 1992) should be familiar not only with the general philosophy of laws and procedures but also with the local complexities and cross-currents that animate or confound cities and communities and that are reflected and acted out—sometimes with a vengeance—by the participants in the juvenile court setting. The Task Force on Juvenile Justice Reform (American Academy of Child and Adolescent Psychiatry 2001) provided the most recent initiative, with specific recommendations regarding areas such as determinations of competence and standards for treatment within the juvenile justice system.

School-Related Legal Issues

In the American tradition, education of children and adolescents has been the province and responsibility of families and local government through parochial or nonsectarian private schools or through the local public school districts, which operate through enabling state legislation. It was not until the latter half of the twentieth century that the federal government provided more than statistical information about the condition of education (U.S. Department of Education 1993).

In the landmark Supreme Court decision ending segregation as a legal policy in public school (*Brown v. Board of Education* 1954), the court affirmed the principle that education is a "right which must be made available to all on equal terms." The rights of the handicapped were established by Congress with the passage of the Civil Rights Act of 1973, Section 504, which states, in part, "No otherwise qualified handicapped individual in the United States...shall solely by reason of her or his handicap be excluded from participation in, be denied the benefits of, or be subject to discrimination under any program or activity receiving federal financial assistance." These principles were articulated relative to schools and handicapped children by Congress in the Education for All Handicapped Children

Act of 1975 (P.L. 94-142, Section 611, 88 stat 579 et seq), which stated that the purpose of the act was to ensure that "all handicapped children have available to them a free appropriate public education which emphasizes special education and related services designed to meet their unique needs." Public Law 94-142 provided for the definition of various handicapping conditions, including but not limited to learning disabilities, serious emotional disturbance, mental retardation, and speech and language impairment. It also provided numerous procedural processes, including that "free and appropriate public education" and "related services" be assessed and provided through an "individualized educational plan" in the "least restrictive environment" with procedural rights and protections, including written notice, parental consent, due process administrative review, and judicial review after all administrative remedies are eliminated. In 1991, Congress amended this law, changing the name of the statute to the Individuals With Disabilities Education Act (IDEA) (P.L. 102-119), and declared its purposes:

1. To provide assistance to states to develop early intervention services for infants and toddlers with disabilities and their families and to assure free appropriate public education to all children and youth with disabilities.
2. To ensure that the rights of children and adolescents with disabilities from birth to age 21 and their families are protected.
3. To assist states and localities to provide for early intervention services and the education of all children with disabilities.
4. To assess and assure the effectiveness of efforts to provide early intervention services and educate children with disabilities.

IDEA also requires yearly reports to Congress on the progress of these special education programs (U.S. Department of Education 1998). The specific meaning and applicability of these concepts have been the subject of numerous appellate court decisions (*Board of Education v. Rowley* 1982; *Polk v. Central Susquehanna Intermediate Unit 16* 1988). Further federal legislation (Americans With Disabilities Act of 1990, P.L. 101-336) may be utilized to provide accommodations within school and institutional settings.

Clinicians evaluating or treating children and adolescents with disabilities under Social Security (U.S. Department of Health and Human Services 2003) must follow guidelines and procedures published periodically by the Social Security Administration (Ameri-can Academy of Child and Adolescent Psychiatry 1997a). Clinicians consulting with school programs (Behrman 1996; Berkovitz 2001a, 2001b; Berkovitz and Sinclair 2001; Jellinek 1990; Sikorski 1996) should be aware that DSM-IV-TR diagnostic criteria are not synonymous or interchangeable with the educational code definitions used by the local and state educational authority (California Department of Education 2002). Each state must develop implementing legislation and codes of regulations that follow federal law to be eligible to receive federal supplemental education funding. In 2002 the 108th Congress was scheduled to reauthorize these and other discretionary programs and the federal funding stream to these programs that define, support, and advance the educational and related services to children with defined disabilities.

Conclusion

Clinicians working at the interface of law and psychiatry should proceed with caution, maintain a current knowledge base in their areas of clinical work, develop systems of maintaining awareness of the relevant laws in their local jurisdiction, and exercise sound clinical judgment. If in doubt, they should seek the consultation of experienced colleagues or the advice of their own counsel.

References

Accreditation Council for Graduate Medical Education: Special Requirements for Residency Training in Child Psychiatry. Chicago, IL, Accreditation Council for Graduate Medical Education, 1988

Addington v Texas, 441 US 418, 99 S Ct 1804 (1979)

Adoption Assistance and Child Welfare Act of 1980, Pub. L. No. 96-272, 94 stat 501–535

Ake v Oklahoma, 105 S Ct (1985)

Al-Mateen C: Effects of witnessing violence on children and adolescents, in Principles and Practice of Child and Adolescent Forensic Psychiatry. Edited by Schetky D, Benedek E. Washington, DC, American Psychiatric Publishing, 2002, pp 213–233

Althaus v Cohen, 710 A2d 1147 (Pa Sup Ct 1998)

American Academy of Child and Adolescent Psychiatry: Policy Statement: Inpatient Hospital Treatment of Children and Adolescents. Washington, DC, American Academy of Child and Adolescent Psychiatry, 1989

American Academy of Child and Adolescent Psychiatry: Policy Statement: Practice Parameters for the Forensic Evaluation of Children and Adolescents Who May Have Been Physically or Sexually Abused. Washington, DC, American Academy of Child and Adolescent Psychiatry, 1995

American Academy of Child and Adolescent Psychiatry: Guidelines for Reviewing SSI Disability Benefits for Children and Adolescents With Mental Disorders. Washington, DC, American Academy of Child and Adolescent Psychiatry, Department of Government Affairs, 1997a

American Academy of Child and Adolescent Psychiatry: Practice parameters for child custody evaluation. J Am Acad Child Adolesc Psychiatry 36:57S–67S, 1997b

American Academy of Child and Adolescent Psychiatry: Practice parameters for the forensic evaluation of children and adolescents who may have been physically or sexually abused. J Am Acad Child Adolesc Psychiatry 36:423–442, 1997c

American Academy of Child and Adolescent Psychiatry: Recommendation for Juvenile Justice Reform. Washington, DC, American Academy of Child and Adolescent Psychiatry, Task Force on Juvenile Justice Reform, 2001

American Academy of Child Psychiatry: Code of Ethics. Washington, DC, American Academy of Child Psychiatry, 1980

American Academy of Psychiatry and the Law: Additional opinions. Committee on Ethics. Bull Am Acad Psychiatry Law 20:49–51, 1995a

American Academy of Psychiatry and the Law: Ethics Guidelines for the Practice of Forensic Psychiatry (adopted May 1987; revised October 1989, 1991, and 1995). Bloomfield, CT, American Academy of Psychiatry and the Law, 1995b

American Association of Family and Conciliation Courts: Model Standards of Practice for Child Custody Evaluations. Madison, WI, American Association of Family and Conciliation Courts, 1994

American Medical Association: Physician Guide to Media Violence. Chicago, IL, American Medical Association, 1996

American Psychiatric Association: Task Force on Clinical Assessment in Child Custody Disputes, Child Custody Consultation. Washington, DC, American Psychiatric Association, 1988

American Psychiatric Association: Diagnostic and Statistical Manual of Mental Disorders, 4th Edition, Text Revision. Washington, DC, American Psychiatric Association, 2000

American Psychiatric Association: Opinions of the Ethics Committee on the Principles of Medical Ethics With Annotations Especially Applicable to Psychiatry, 2001 Edition. Washington, DC, American Psychiatric Association, 2001a

American Psychiatric Association: The Principles of Medical Ethics With Annotations Especially Applicable to Psychiatry, 2001 Edition. Washington, DC, American Psychiatric Association, 2001b

American Psychological Association: Guidelines for Child Custody Evaluations in Divorce Proceedings. Am Psychol 49:677–680, 1994

Americans With Disabilities Act of 1990, Pub. L. No. 101-336, 42 USC 12101 et seq

Ames JT, Huntington DS: Child Custody Evaluation. San Francisco, Judicial Council of California, 1991

Applebaum PS: The parable of the forensic psychiatrist: ethics and the problem of doing harm. Int J Law Psychiatry 13:249–259, 1990

Applebaum PS: A theory of ethics for forensic psychiatry. J Am Acad Psychiatry 25:233–246, 1997

Arato v Avedon, 5 Cal 4th 1172 (1993)

Arthur LG: Child sexual abuse: improving the system's response. Juv Fam Court J 37:1–75, 1986

Ash P, Derdeyn A: Forensic child and adolescent psychiatry: a review of the past 10 years. J Am Acad Child Adolesc Psychiatry 36:1493–1501, 1997

Ash P, Guyer M: The functions of psychiatric evaluation in contested child custody and visitation cases. J Am Acad Child Adolesc Psychiatry 25:554–561, 1986

Barnum R: Child psychiatry and the law. J Am Acad Child Adolesc Psychiatry 26:922–925, 1987

Barnum R: A suggested framework for forensic consultation in cases of child abuse and neglect. J Am Acad Psychiatry Law 25:581–593, 1997

Barnum R: Parenting assessment in cases of neglect and abuse, in Principles and Practice of Child and Adolescent Forensic Psychiatry. Edited by Schetky D, Benedek E. Washington, DC, American Psychiatric Publishing, 2002, pp 81–96

Beck R: The White House conferences on children: an historical perspective, in The Rights of Children. Cambridge, MA, Harvard Educational Review, 1974, pp 88–103

Behrman RE: Children and divorce. Future Child 4:1–255, 1994

Behrman RE: Special education for students with disabilities: analysis and recommendations. Future Child 6:4–24, 1996

Benedek EP, Schetky DH: Problems in validating allegations of sexual abuse, 1: factors affecting perception and recall of events. J Am Acad Child Adolesc Psychiatry 26:912–915, 1987a

Benedek EP, Schetky DH: Problems in validating allegations of sexual abuse, 2: clinical evaluation. J Am Acad Child Adolesc Psychiatry 26:916–921, 1987b

Berkovitz IH: The benefits of a clinician consulting in schools of education. Child Adolesc Psychiatr Clin N Am 10:199–204, 2001a

Berkovitz IH: Evaluations of outcome in mental health consultation in schools. Child Adolesc Psychiatr Clin N Am 10:93–103, 2001b

Berkovitz IH, Sinclair E: Training programs in school consultation. Child Adolesc Psychiatr Clin N Am 10:83–92, 2001

Berland DI, Pinazzola VL, Brayer E, et al: Ethical, legal and psychodynamic considerations in intervention of a possible cult member. J Am Acad Child Adolesc Psychiatry 29:975–981, 1990

Bernet W: False statements and the differential diagnosis of abuse allegations. J Am Acad Child Adolesc Psychiatry 32:903–910, 1993

Bernet W: The child and adolescent psychiatrist and the law, in Handbook of Child and Adolescent Psychiatry. Edited by Adams P, Bleiberg E. New York, Wiley, 1998, pp 438–468

Binder R: American Psychiatric Association resource document on controversies in child custody: gay and lesbian parenting, transracial adoptions, joint versus sole custody and custody gender issues. J Am Acad Psychiatry Law 26:267–276, 1998

Board of Education v Rowley, 458 US 176, 102 S Ct 3034, 73 L Ed 2d 690 (1982)

Brown v Board of Education, 347 US 483 (1954)

Bruck M, Ceci S: Reliability and suggestibility of children's statements, in Principles and Practice of Child and Adolescent Forensic Psychiatry. Edited by Schetky D, Benedek E. Washington, DC, American Psychiatric Publishing, 2002, pp 137–145

California Department of Education: California Special Education Programs: A Composite of Laws. Sacramento, California Department of Education, 2002

California Family Code, 3011 et seq

California Medical Association: California Physician's Legal Handbook, Vol 1–6. San Francisco, CA, California Medical Association, 2003

California Penal Code, 11165 et seq

Cardwell v Bechtol, 724 SW 2d 739 (Tenn 1987)

Caudill OB, Pope KS: Law and Mental Health Professionals: California. Washington, DC, American Psychological Association, 1995

Ceci S, Bruck M: Suggestibility of the child witness: a historical review and synthesis. Psychol Bull 113:403–439, 1993

Chapsky v Wood, 26 Kan 650 (1881)

Child Abuse Prevention and Treatment Act of 1978, 42 USC 5706(g)(4)

Cicchetti D, Cohen DJ: Developmental Psychopathology, Vols 1 and 2. New York, Wiley, 1995

Civil Rights Act of 1973, 29 USC 794 et seq

Clark B: Developmental aspects of memory in children, in Principles and Practice of Child and Adolescent Forensic Psychiatry. Edited by Schetky D, Benedek E. Washington, DC, American Psychiatric Publishing, 2002, pp 129–145

Clark P: 1996 Juvenile Justice Reform Legislation. Criminal Defense Newsletter (Detroit [MI] State Appellate Defender Office) 19(9–10), June–July, 1996

Cobbs v Grant, 8 Cal 3d, 229 (1972)

Committee for Economic Development: Children in Need: Investment Strategies for the Educationally Disadvantaged. New York, Committee for Economic Development, 1987

Commonwealth of Massachusetts v Amirault LeFave, 403 Mass 169, 714 NE 2nd 805 (1999)

Corelli T, Hoag M, Howell R: Memory, repression and child sexual abuse: forensic implications for the mental health professional. J Am Acad Psychiatry Law 25:31–45, 1997

Daubert v Merrell Dow, 61 NSLW 4805, 113 S Ct 2786 (1993)

Deprato D, Hammer JH: Assessment and treatment of juvenile offenders, in Principles and Practice of Child and Adolescent Forensic Psychiatry. Edited by Schetky D, Benedek E. Washington, DC, American Psychiatric Publishing, 2002, pp 267–278

Derdeyn AP, Poehailos A, Seigle E: Adequate evaluation of divorce-related child sexual abuse allegations. Bull Am Acad Psychiatry Law 22:280–287, 1994

Dusky v United States, 362 US 402 (1960)

Education for All Handicapped Children Act of 1975, Pub. L. No. 94-142, 20 USC 1401 et seq, Section 611, 88 stat 579 et seq

Edwards LP: The juvenile court and the role of the juvenile court judge. Juv Fam Court J 43:1–45, 1992

Erikson JT: California Laws Relating to Minors. Los Angeles, CA, Legal Books Distributing, 1995

Fare v Michael C, 442 US 707 (1979)

Foley H, Carlton C, Howell R: The relationship of attention deficit hyperactivity disorder and conduct disorder to juvenile delinquency: legal implications. Bull Am Acad Psychiatry Law 24:333–345, 1996

Frye v United States, 293 F 1013, DC Cir (1923)

General Electric Co et al v Joiner, 118 S Ct 512 (1997)

Geraty RD, Hendrin RL, Flaa CJ: Ethical perspectives on managed care as it relates to child and adolescent psychiatry. J Am Acad Child Adolesc Psychiatry 31:398–402, 1992

Goldstein J, Freud A, Solnit AJ, et al: In the Best Interests of the Child. New York, Free Press, 1996

Green AH: True and false allegations of sexual abuse in child custody disputes. J Am Acad Child Psychiatry 25:449–456, 1986

Grisso T: Juvenile's competency to stand trial, in Forensic Evaluation of Juveniles. Sarasota, FL, Professional Resources Press, 1998a, pp 83–126

Grisso T: Juveniles' waiver of Miranda rights, in Forensic Evaluation of Juveniles. Sarasota, FL, Professional Resources Press, 1998b, pp 37–82

Grisso T, Barnum R, Fletcher K, et al: Massachusetts Youth Screening Instrument for mental health needs of juvenile justice youths. J Am Acad Child Adolesc Psychiatry 40:541–548, 2001

Group for the Advancement of Psychiatry: Divorce, Child Custody and the Family. New York, Mental Health Materials Center, 1980

Guyer MJ: Commentary: the juvenile justice system, in Emerging Issues in Child Psychiatry and the Law. Edited by Schetky DH, Benedek EP. New York, Brunner/Mazel, 1985, pp 159–179

Guyer MJ: Child psychiatry and legal liability: implications of recent case law. J Am Acad Child Adolesc Psychiatry 29:958–962, 1990

Hattab JY (ed): Ethics and Child Mental Health. Hewlett, NY, Gefen Books, 1994

Herman S: Special issues in child custody evaluations. J Am Acad Child Adolesc Psychiatry 29:969–974, 1990

Herman S: Child custody evaluations and the need for standards of care and peer review. Journal of the Center for Children and the Courts 1:139–150, 1999

Herman SP: Child custody evaluations, in Principles and Practice of Child and Adolescent Forensic Psychiatry. Edited by Schetky D, Benedek E. Washington, DC, American Psychiatric Publishing, 2002, pp 69–79

Hetherington EM: Coping with family transitions: winners, losers and survivors. Child Dev 60:1–14, 1989

Hoge RD, Andrews DA, Leschied AW: An investigation of risk and protective factors in a sample of youthful offenders. J Child Psychol Psychiatry 37:419–424, 1996

Horner TM, Guyer MJ: Infant placement and custody, in Handbook of Infant Mental Health. Edited by Zeanah C. New York, Guilford, 1993, pp 462–479

Hyde LM: Child custody in divorce. Juv Fam Court J 35:1–71, 1984

Individuals With Disabilities Education Act of 1991, Pub. L. No. 102-119, 20 USC 1401 et seq

In re Birdsall, No G004537, CA Ct App 4th District (1988)

In re Gault, 371 US 187, 83 S Ct 1428 (1967)

In re Marriage of Carney, 24 Cal 3d, 725 (1979)

In re Roger S, 19 Cal 3d, 921 (1977)

In re Winship, 397 US 358, 90 S Ct 1068 (1970)

Institute of Medicine: Research on Children and Adolescents With Mental, Behavioral and Developmental Disorders. Washington, DC, National Academy Press, 1989

Jaffe v Redmond, 518 US 1 (1996)

Jellinek MS: School consultation: evolving issues. J Am Acad Child Adolesc Psychiatry 29:311–314, 1990

Judicial Council of California: Uniform Standards of Practice for Court Ordered Child Custody Evaluations, Rule 5.220, 2003

Kalogerakis MG: Handbook of Psychiatric Practice in the Juvenile Court. Washington, DC, American Psychiatric Association, 1992

Kaplan S, Pelcovitz D, Labruna V: Child and adolescent abuse and neglect research: a review of the past 10 years, I: physical and emotional abuse and neglect. J Am Acad Child Adolesc Psychiatry 38:1214–1222, 1999

Kay H: From the second sex to the joint venture: an overview of women's rights and family law in the United States during the twentieth century. California Law Review 88:2017–2093, 2000

Kelly JB: Longer-term adjustment in children of divorce: converging findings and implications for practice. J Fam Psychol 2:119–140, 1988

Kelly JB: Parent interaction after divorce: comparison of mediated and adversarial divorce processes. Behav Sci Law 9:387–398, 1991

Kelly JB: Children's adjustment in conflicted marriage and divorce: a decade review of research. J Am Acad Child Adolesc Psychiatry 39:963–973, 2000

Kelly JB, Johnston J: The alienated child. Family Court Review 39:249–266, 2001

Kent v United States, 383 US 541, 86 S Ct 1045 (1966)

Kermani EJ: The U.S. Supreme Court on victimized children: the constitutional rights of the defendant versus the best interests of the child. J Am Acad Child Adolesc Psychiatry 30:839–844, 1991

Kermani EJ: Child sexual abuse revisited by the U.S. Supreme Court. J Am Acad Child Adolesc Psychiatry 32:971–974, 1993

Kirkish P, Sreenivasan S, Welsh R, et al: The future of criminal violence: juveniles tried as adults. J Am Acad Psychiatry Law 28:38–46, 2000

Kumho Tire Company, 119 S Ct 1167 (1999)

Landeros v Flood, 551 P2d 389 (Cal 1976), 138, 236, 516 nn.27, 34:529n.102

Larner MB, Stevenson CS, Behrman RE: Protecting children from abuse and neglect: analysis and recommendations. Future Child 8:4–22, 1998

Loftus E: Creating false memories. Sci Am 277(3):70–75, 1997

Loftus E, Pickrell J: The formation of false memories. Psychiatr Ann 25:720–725, 1995

Macbeth J: Legal issues in the treatment of minors, in Principles and Practice of Child and Adolescent Forensic Psychiatry. Edited by Schetky D, Benedek E. Washington, DC, American Psychiatric Publishing, 2002, pp 309–323

Manduley v Superior Court of San Diego, 27 Cal 4th 537, 41 P3d 3; 2002 Cal LEXIS 622; 117 Cal Rptr 2d 168 (2002)

Marrocco MK, Uecker JC, Ciccone JR: Teaching forensic psychiatry to psychiatric residents. Bull Am Acad Psychiatry Law 23:83–91, 1995

McKeiver v Pennsylvania, 403 US 528, 91 S Ct 1976 (1971)

Mulvey E, Cauffman E: The inherent limits of predicting school violence. Am Psychol 56:797–802, 2001

Munir K, Earls F: Ethical principles governing research in child and adolescent psychiatry. J Am Acad Child Adolesc Psychiatry 31:408–414, 1992

Neinstein LS: Consent and confidentiality laws for minors in the western United States. West J Med 147:217–224, 1987

Nelken M: The limits of privilege: the developing scope of federal psychotherapist-patient privilege law. Review of Litigation 20:1–42, Austin, Texas, 2000

New Jersey v TLO, 469 US 325 (1985)

Nurcombe B, Partlett DF: Child Mental Health and the Law. New York, Free Press, 1994

Office of Juvenile Justice and Delinquency Prevention: The Child Victim as a Witness. Washington, DC, U.S. Department of Justice, 1994

O'Rourke K, Snider BW, Thomas JM, et al: Knowing and practicing ethics. J Am Acad Child Adolesc Psychiatry 31:393–396, 1992

O'Shaughnessy RJ: Clinical aspects of forensic assessment of juvenile offenders. Psychiatr Clin North Am 15:721–735, 1992

Parham v JR, 442 US 584, 99 S Ct 2493, 61 L Ed 2d 101 (1979)

Perry B: Neurodevelopmental impact of violence in childhood, in Principles and Practice of Child and Adolescent Forensic Psychiatry. Edited by Schetky D, Benedek E. Washington, DC, American Psychiatric Publishing, 2002, pp 191–204

Pittel E: How to take a weapons history: interviewing children at risk for violence at school. J Am Acad Child Adolesc Psychiatry 37:1100–1102, 1998

Polk v Central Susquehanna Intermediate Unit 16, 853 F2d 171 (1988)

Poole DA, Lindsay DS: Interviewing preschoolers: effects of nonsuggestive techniques, parental coaching and leading questions on reports of nonexperienced events. J Exp Child Psychol 60:129–154, 1995

Poole DA, Lindsay DS: Children's eyewitness reports after exposure to misinformation from parents. J Exp Psychol Appl 7:27–50, 2001

Pruett MK, Jackson TD: Perspectives on the divorce process: parental perceptions of the legal system and its impact on family relations. J Am Acad Psychiatry Law 29:18–28, 2001

Quinn K: Interviewing children for suspected sexual abuse, in Principles and Practice of Child and Adolescent Forensic Psychiatry. Edited by Schetky D, Benedek E. Washington, DC, American Psychiatric Publishing, 2002, pp 149–159

Ramona v Isabella, 61898 Napa Cty Cal Sup Ct (1994)

Rappeport JR: Reasonable medical certainty. Bull Am Acad Psychiatry Law 13:5–15, 1985

Raskin D, Esplin P: Statement validity assessment: interview procedures and content analysis of children's statements of sexual abuse. Behavioral Assessment 13:265–291, 1991

Ratner R: Role of the psychiatrist, in Handbook of Psychiatric Practice in the Juvenile Court. Edited by Kalogerakis MG, Workgroup on Psychiatric Practice in the Juvenile Court of the American Psychiatric Association. Washington, DC, American Psychiatric Association, 1992, pp 25–35

Rodham H: The rights of children. Harv Educ Rev 43:487–514, 1973

Roseby V, Johnston J: Children of Armageddon: common developmental threats in high-conflict divorcing families. Child Adolesc Psychiatr Clin N Am 7:295–309, 1998

Rosenfeld A, Pilowsky D, Fine P, et al: Foster care: an update. J Am Acad Child Adolesc Psychiatry 36:448–456, 1997

Rosner R: Forensic psychiatry: a subspecialty (the presidential address at the nineteenth annual meeting of the American Academy of Psychiatry and the Law). Bull Am Acad Psychiatry Law 17:323–333, 1989

Rosner R, Weinstock R (eds): Ethical Practice in Psychiatry and the Law. New York, Plenum, 1990

Sacks H, Reader WD: Procedures in the juvenile court, in Handbook of Psychiatric Practice in the Juvenile Court. Edited by Kalogerakis MG, Workgroup on Psychiatric Practice in the Juvenile Court of the American Psychiatric Association. Washington, DC, American Psychiatric Association, 1992, pp 13–19

Santosky v Kramer, 455 US 745, 102 S Ct 1388 (1982)

Schall v Martin, 467 US 253, 104 S Ct 2403 (1984)

Schetky DH: Ethical issues in forensic child and adolescent psychiatry. J Am Acad Child Adolesc Psychiatry 31:403–407, 1992

Schetky DH: Forensic ethics, in Principles and Practice of Child and Adolescent Forensic Psychiatry. Edited by Schetky D, Benedek E. Washington, DC, American Psychiatric Publishing, 2002a, pp 15–20

Schetky DH: History of child and adolescent psychiatry, in Principles and Practice of Child and Adolescent Forensic Psychiatry. Edited by Schetky D, Benedek E. Washington, DC, American Psychiatric Publishing, 2002b, pp 3–6

Schetky DH: Risk assessment of violence in youths, in Principles and Practice of Child and Adolescent Forensic Psychiatry. Edited by Schetky D, Benedek E. Washington, DC, American Psychiatric Publishing, 2002c, pp 231–244

Schetky DH: Termination of parental rights, in Principles and Practice of Child and Adolescent Forensic Psychiatry. Edited by Schetky D, Benedek E. Washington, DC, American Psychiatric Publishing, 2002d, pp 109–116

Schetky DH, Benedek EP (eds): Emerging Issues in Child Psychiatry and the Law. New York, Brunner/Mazel, 1985

Schetky DH, Benedek EP (eds): Clinical Handbook of Child Psychiatry and the Law. Baltimore, MD, Williams & Wilkins, 1992

Schetky DH, Benedek EP: Principles and Practice of Child and Adolescent Forensic Psychiatry. Washington, DC, American Psychiatric Publishing, 2002

Schetky DH, Guyer MJ: Civil litigation and the child psychiatrist. J Am Acad Child Adolesc Psychiatry 29:963–968, 1990

Schetky DH, Haller LH: Parental kidnapping. J Am Acad Child Psychiatry 22:279–285, 1983

Scott C: Troxel, et vir, Petitioners v. Granville: grandparents' rights or parental autonomy? J Am Acad Psychiatry Law 28:465–468, 2000

Scott C: Juvenile waivers to adult court, in Principles and Practice of Child and Adolescent Forensic Psychiatry. Edited by Schetky D, Benedek E. Washington, DC, American Psychiatric Publishing, 2002, pp 289–295

Secretary of Public Welfare of Pennsylvania v Institutionalized Juveniles, 99 S Ct 2523 (1979)

Shear L: Life stories, doctrines and decision making. Fam Concil Courts Rev 34:439–459, 1996

Shields JM, Johnson A: Collision between law and ethics: consent for treatment with adolescents. Bull Am Acad Psychiatry Law 20:309–323, 1992

Shiono PH, Quinn LS: Epidemiology of divorce. Future Child 4(1):15–28, 1994

Sikorski JB: Academic underachievement and school refusal, in Handbook of Adolescent Health Risk Behavior. Edited by DiClemente RJ, Hansen W, Ponton LE. New York, Plenum, 1996, pp 393–411

Silva v Haney, Cal App 3d 90 CDOS 3595 (1990)

Simon R, Wettstein R: Toward the development of guidelines for the conduct of forensic psychiatric examinations. J Am Acad Psychiatry Law 24:17–30, 1997

Singer M, Slovak K, Frierson T, et al: Viewing preferences, symptoms of psychological trauma, and violent behaviors among children who watch television. J Am Acad Child Adolesc Psychiatry 37:1041–1048, 1998

Snyder H, Sickmund M: Juvenile Offenders and Victims: A National Report. Washington, DC, Office of Juvenile Justice and Delinquency Prevention, 1995

Sondheimer A, Martucci LC: An approach to teaching ethics in child and adolescent psychiatry. J Am Acad Child Adolesc Psychiatry 31:415–422, 1992

Stanford v Kentucky, 109 S Ct 2969 (1989)

Steiner H, the Work Group on Quality Issues: Practice parameters for the assessment and treatment of children and adolescents with conduct disorder. J Am Acad Child Adolesc Psychiatry 36(10, suppl):122S–139S, 1997

Tarasoff v Regents of the University of California, 17 Cal 3d 425, 551 P2d 334, 131 Cal Rptr 14 (1976)

ten Bensel RW, Arthur LG, Brown L, et al: Child abuse and neglect. Juv Fam Court J 35:1–51, 1985

Thompson v Alameda County, 614 P2d 728 (1980)

Thompson v Oklahoma, 56 USLW 4892 (1988)

Troxel v Granville, 530 US 57, 120 S Ct 2054, US Wash (2000)

U.S. Department of Education, Office of Educational Research and Improvement: Educational Reforms and Students at Risk: A Review of the Current State of the Art. Washington, DC, U.S. Government Printing Office, 1993

U.S. Department of Education: 20th Annual Report to Congress on the Implementation of the Individuals With Disabilities Education Act. Washington, DC, U.S. Department of Education, 1998

U.S. Department of Health and Human Services: Mental Health: A Report of the Surgeon General. Rockville, MD, Substance Abuse and Mental Health Administration, Center for Mental Health Services, National Institute of Mental Health, 1999

U.S. Department of Health and Human Services: Youth Violence: A Report of the Surgeon General. Rockville, MD, U.S. Department of Health and Human Services, 2001. Available at: http://www.surgeongeneral.gov/library/youthviolence/youvioreport.htm

U.S. Department of Health and Human Services, Social Security Administration: Disability Evaluation Under Social Security (SSA Publ No 64-039). Rockville, MD, U.S. Department of Health and Human Services, 2003

U.S. Government Printing Office: Report to the President: White House Conference on Children. Washington, DC, U.S. Government Printing Office, 1971

U.S. Public Health Service: Report of the Surgeon General's Conference on Children's Mental Health: A National Action Agenda. Washington, DC, U.S. Department of Health and Human Services, 2000. Available at: http://www.surgeongeneral.gov/cmh/childreport.htm

Wagner KD, Pollard R, Wagner RF: Malpractice litigation against child and adolescent psychiatry residency programs, 1981–1991. J Am Acad Child Adolesc Psychiatry 32:462–465, 1993

Wallerstein JS: The long-term effects of divorce on children: a review. J Am Acad Child Adolesc Psychiatry 30:349–360, 1991

Wasserman S, Rosenfeld A, Nickman S: Foster care and adoption, in Principles and Practice of Child and Adolescent Forensic Psychiatry. Edited by Schetky D, Benedek E. Washington, DC, American Psychiatric Publishing, 2002, pp 97–108

Weiner MH: International child abduction and the escape from domestic violence. Fordham Law Review 69(2):593–706, 2000

Wheeler v United States, 159 NS 523 S Ct (1895)

White v Illinois, 112 S Ct 736 (1992)

Wickline v California, 192 Cal App 3d 1630, 239 Cal Rptr 810 (1986)

Zonana H: Daubert v Merrell Dow Pharmaceuticals: a new standard for scientific evidence in the courts? Bull Am Acad Psychiatry Law 22:309–325, 1994

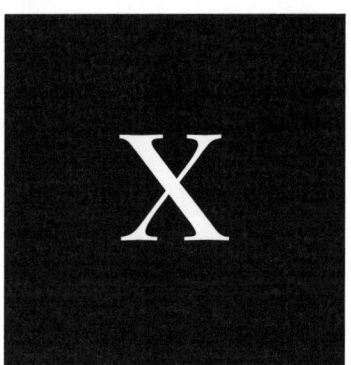

Treatment

Psychopharmacology

Joseph Biederman, M.D.
Thomas Spencer, M.D.
Timothy Wilens, M.D.

In modern pediatric psychopharmacology, diagnostic hypotheses guide intervention. Diagnostic information should be gathered from the child, the parents or caretakers, and, whenever possible, the teachers, and a diagnosis based on DSM-IV-TR criteria (American Psychiatric Association 2000) should be made. Careful attention should be paid to comorbidity and differential diagnosis, including both medical/neurological and psychosocial factors contributing to the clinical presentation. Because psychiatric disorders of children and adolescents can be associated with additional cognitive deficits (e.g., learning disabilities), which may not respond to psychotropics, it is important to pinpoint these deficits to help define appropriate remedial interventions. Pharmacotherapy should be part of a treatment plan in which consideration is given to all aspects of the child's or adolescent's life. It should not be used instead of other interventions or after other interventions have failed. Realistic expectations of pharmacotherapy based on knowledge of what it can and cannot do, as well as careful definition of target symptoms, are major ingredients for a successful intervention.

Therapeutic intervention should be started early—before the occurrence of complications, chronicity, and social incapacitation, which can make treatment and restabilization of functional life habits more difficult. In addition to pharmacotherapy, treatment of behavioral and emotional disorders of youths may need to involve a variety of psychosocial methods, such as individual psychotherapy, family and group therapy, behavioral and cognitive-behavioral therapy, and parental counseling. These interventions should also be based on diagnostic hypotheses and careful selection of target symptoms. The closer the match between the treatment and the spectrum of difficulties the child and his or her family face, the more successful the intervention will be. In severe cases, hospitalization may be required.

Before treatment with a psychotropic is initiated, the family and the child need to be made familiar with the risks and benefits of the intervention, the availability of alternative treatments, and the likely adverse effects, including short-term, long-term, and withdrawal adverse effects. Certain adverse effects can be anticipated on the basis of known pharmacological properties of the drug (e.g., the anticholinergic effects of tricyclic antidepressants [TCAs]); other adverse effects, generally rare, are unexpected (idiosyncratic) and are difficult to anticipate. Short-term adverse effects can be minimized by introducing the medication at low doses and titrating slowly. Patients receiving drugs with known adverse effects should be monitored for long-term adverse effects (e.g., patients taking lithium carbonate should be monitored for changes in kidney and thyroid functions). Idiosyncratic adverse effects require drug discontinuation and selection of alternative treatment modalities.

Treatment should be started at the lowest possible dose, usually the lowest manufactured dose. Frequent (e.g., weekly) contact with the patient and family is necessary during the initial phase of treatment, to monitor response to the intervention and adverse effects. Evaluation of adverse effects should include subjective reports by the patient and family (e.g., reports of stomachaches or appetite changes) as well as objective measurements (e.g., measurement of heart rate and blood pressure). After a sufficient period of clinical stabilization (e.g., 6–12 months), it is prudent to evaluate the need for continued psychopharmacological intervention. Withdrawal symptoms should be distinguished from exacerbation of symptoms of the disorder for which the psychotropic was prescribed. To minimize withdrawal reactions, it is important to discontinue medications gradually. Because most psychiatric disorders are chronic or recurrent, timely follow-up after drug discontinuation is necessary. Despite recent progress, insufficient information exists regarding the efficacy, safety, and pharmacology of most psychotropics in children and adolescents, a situation that necessitates continued reliance on adult data to guide pediatric psychopharmacology.

Major Classes of Drugs Used in Pediatric Psychiatry

■ Stimulants (Tables 50–1 and 50–2)

Stimulant drugs were the first class of compounds reported to be effective in the treatment of behavioral disturbances in children with attention-deficit/hyperactivity disorder (ADHD). Stimulants are sympathomimetic drugs that are structurally similar to endogenous catecholamines. The most commonly used compounds in this class include methylphenidate, dextroamphetamine, the mixed amphetamine salts product Adderall, and magnesium pemoline. These drugs are thought to act both in the central nervous system (CNS) and peripherally by enhancing dopaminergic and noradrenergic neurotransmission. Because the various stimulants have somewhat different mechanisms of action, some patients may respond preferentially to one or another (Greenhill et al. 1999).

Because of their short half-lives, the short-acting stimulants (methylphenidate and dextroamphetamine) are given in divided doses throughout the day, typically 4 hours apart. The total daily dose ranges from 0.3 to 2 mg/kg (0.3–1.0 mg/kg for dextroamphetamine). The starting dosage is generally 2.5–5 mg/day, given once daily in the morning. If necessary, the dose is increased every few days by 2.5–5 mg in a divided-dose schedule. Given the anorexigenic effects of the stimulants, it may be beneficial to administer the medicine after meals. The therapeutic effects of magnesium pemoline, which has a longer half-life, generally last through the school period. For full-day coverage, pemoline is typically given twice daily (e.g., at 8:00 A.M. and 2:00 P.M.), with total daily doses ranging from 1 to 3 mg/kg. Because magnesium pemoline is a longer-acting compound with greater potential for hepatotoxicity, this drug is a second- or third-line agent. The therapeutic effects of Adderall (a mixed amphetamine salts formulation), like those of pemoline, last through most or all of the school day. For full-day coverage, Adderall is usually administered twice a day (e.g., at 8:00 A.M. and 2:00 P.M.), with total daily doses ranging from 0.5 to 1.5 mg/kg. Typically, stimulants have a rapid onset of action; therefore, a clinical response will be evident when a therapeutic dose has been achieved.

A new generation of highly sophisticated, well-developed, safe, effective, and long-acting stimulants has reached the market and revolutionized the treatment of ADHD. These compounds use novel delivery systems to overcome acute tolerance (tachyphylaxis). The methylphenidate preparation Concerta uses an osmotic pump mechanism that creates an ascending profile of methylphenidate in the blood, providing effective treatment for 10–12 hours. Concerta is available in 18-, 36-, and 54-mg tablets, approximating the 5-, 10-, and 15-mg thrice-daily doses of immediate-release (IR) methylphenidate. The methylphenidate preparations Metadate CD and Ritalin LA both take the form of capsules containing a mixture of immediate- and delayed-release beads, providing effective treatment for 8–9 hours. In Metadate CD capsules, 30% of the beads are immediate release and 70% are delayed release. Metadate CD is available in 20-mg capsules, approximating the 10-mg twice-daily doses of IR methylphenidate. In Ritalin LA capsules, there is a 1:1 ratio of IR beads to delayed-release beads. Ritalin LA is available in 20-, 30-, and 40-mg capsules, approximating 10-, 15-, and 20-mg twice-daily doses of IR methylphenidate. Adderall XR is manufactured as capsules with a 1:1 ratio of IR beads to delayed-release beads, providing effective amphetamine (Adderall) treatment for 10–12 hours. Adderall XR is available in 10-, 20-, and 30-mg capsules, approximating 5-, 10-, and 15-mg twice-daily doses (at 0 and 4 hours) of Adderall. Formulations consisting of beads in capsules (i.e., all the aforementioned drugs but Concerta) may be used as sprinkle preparations for children unable to swallow pills.

Methylphenidate as a secondary amine gives rise to four optical isomers: D-*threo*, L-*threo*, D-*erythro*, and L-*erythro*. There is stereoselectivity in receptor site binding and its relationship to response. The standard preparation is composed of the D,L-*threo* racemate, the

Table 50–1. Stimulants

Drug	Daily dose (mg/kg)	Dosage schedule	Main indications	Adverse effects and comments
Dextroamphetamine				*Stimulants:*
Dexedrine	0.3–1.0	bid–tid	• ADHD • Mental retardation + ADHD	• Insomnia, decreased appetite, weight loss • Depression, psychosis (rare, with very high doses) • Mild increase in heart rate and blood pressure
Mixed amphetamine salts formulation				• Possible reduction in growth velocity with long-term use • Withdrawal effects and rebound phenomena
Adderall	0.5–1.5	Once daily or bid	• ADHD • Adjunct therapy in refractory depression	*Adderall:* 6 hours of action *Pemoline:* Rare serious hepatotoxicity; monitoring of
Methylphenidate				liver function required
Focalin	0.5–1.0	bid–tid	• ADHD	
Methylin	1.0–2.0	bid–tid		
Ritalin	1.0–2.0	bid–tid		
Magnesium pemoline				
Cylert	1.0–3.0	Once daily or bid	• ADHD	

Note. Doses are general guidelines. All doses must be individualized, and appropriate monitoring should be performed. Weight-corrected doses are less appropriate for obese children. ADHD = attention-deficit/hyperactivity disorder.

Table 50–2. New long-acting stimulants

Drug	Daily dose (mg/kg)	Dosage schedule	Duration of behavioral effect (hours)	Comments
Methylphenidate				
Concerta	1.0–2.0	Once daily or bid	10–12	Ascending profile, OROS technology
Metadate CD	1.0–2.0	Once daily or bid	8–9	Capsule with 3:7 ratio of IR beads to DR beads
Ritalin LA	1.0–2.0	Once daily or bid	8–9	Capsule with 1:1 ratio of IR beads to DR beads
Mixed amphetamine salts formulation				
Adderall XR	0.5–1.5	Once daily or bid	10–12	Capsule with 1:1 ratio of IR beads to DR beads

Note. Doses are general guidelines. All doses must be individualized, and appropriate monitoring should be performed. Weight-corrected doses are less appropriate for obese children. DR=delayed-release; IR=immediate-release; OROS=osmotic release oral system.

form apparently active in the CNS. Moreover, recent data suggest that the D-methylphenidate isomer is the active form (Ding et al. 1995). This has led to the development of a purified D-*threo*-methylphenidate compound, Focalin. Studies have shown Focalin to be at least as effective as the racemate, at half the dose (Conners et al. 2001; Novartis, data on file). Focalin is available in 2.5-, 5-, and 10-mg doses, approximating the 5-, 10-, and 20-mg doses of D,L-methylphenidate.

The early concern that optimal clinical efficacy is attained at the cost of impaired learning ability has not been confirmed (Gittelman-Klein 1987). In fact, studies indicate that both behavior and cognitive performance improve with stimulant treatment, in a dose-dependent fashion (Douglas et al. 1988; Klein 1987; Kupietz et al. 1988; Pelham et al. 1985; Rapport et al. 1987, 1989a, 1989b; Tannock et al. 1989). Findings on the association between clinical benefits in ADHD and plasma levels of stimulants have been equivocal and complicated by wide inter- and intraindividual variability in plasma levels at constant oral doses (Gittelman-Klein 1987).

The most commonly reported side effects of stimulant medications are appetite suppression and sleep disturbances. The sleep disturbance commonly reported is delay of sleep onset; this side effect is usually associated with late-afternoon or early-evening administration of stimulant medications. Although less often reported, mood disturbances ranging from increased tearfulness to a full-blown major depression–like syndrome can be associated with stimulant treatment (Wilens and Biederman 1992). Other infrequent side effects include headaches, abdominal discomfort, increased lethargy, and fatigue.

Although the adverse cardiovascular effects of stimulants—beyond effects on heart rate and blood pressure—have not been examined, mild increases (of unclear clinical significance) in pulse and blood pressure have been observed (Brown et al. 1984). Increases in blood pressure that can occur with stimulant therapy may be of greater clinical significance in adults with ADHD than in children with the disorder. A stimulant-associated toxic psychosis has also been (very rarely) observed, usually in the context of either a rapid increase in dose or very high doses. The reported psychosis in children in response to stimulant medications resembles a toxic phenomenon (e.g., visual hallucinosis) and is dissimilar to the exacerbation of psychotic symptoms in schizophrenia. Development of psychotic symptoms in a child exposed to stimulants necessitates careful evaluation to rule out a preexisting psychotic disorder. Administration of magnesium pemoline over several months has been associated with rare hypersensitivity reactions involving the liver, accompanied by increases in aspartate transaminase (AST) and alanine transaminase (ALT) levels. Thus, baseline and repeat liver function studies are recommended with administration of this compound. Because of increasing concerns about hepatotoxicity, the U.S. Food and Drug Administration (FDA) is now requiring biweekly liver function monitoring when pemoline is used.

Early reports indicated that children with a personal or family history of tic disorders were at greater risk of developing a tic disorder when exposed to stimulants (Lowe et al. 1982). However, more recent work has challenged this view (Comings and Comings 1988; Gadow et al. 1992, 1995). For example, in a controlled study involving 34 children with ADHD and tics, methylphenidate effectively suppressed ADHD symptoms and had only a weak effect on the frequency of tics (Gadow et al. 1995). In a study involving 128 boys with ADHD, there was no evidence of earlier onset, higher rates, or worsening of tics in the subgroup exposed to stimulants (Spencer et al. 1999a). Although this work is reassuring, more information is needed, obtained in a larger number of subjects over a longer time period. Until more is known, it seems prudent to weigh risks and benefits on a case-by-case basis. The physician should discuss with the child and family the benefits and pitfalls of the use of stimulants in children with ADHD and tics.

Similar uncertainties remain about the abuse potential of stimulants in ADHD children. Despite the concern that ADHD may increase the risk of abuse by adolescents and young adults (or their associates), there is no clear evidence to date of abuse of prescribed stimulant medication by children with appropriately diagnosed ADHD who are carefully monitored. The most commonly abused substance among adolescents and adults with ADHD is marijuana, not stimulant medication (Biederman et al. 1995c). Furthermore, the use of stimulants and other pharmacological treatments for ADHD was recently found to significantly decrease the risk of subsequent substance use disorders among ADHD youth (Biederman et al. 1999c).

Although concerns continue regarding the effect of long-term administration of stimulants on growth, investigators have begun to question this issue. Stimulants are known to routinely produce anorexia and weight loss, but their effect on growth in height is much less certain. Although initial reports suggested that a persistent stimulant-associated decrease in growth in height occurred in children (Mattes and Gittelman 1983; Safer et al. 1972), other reports have failed to substantiate this claim (Gross 1976; Satterfield et al. 1979). Moreover, several studies showed that ultimate height appears to be unaffected if treatment is discontinued in adolescence (Klein and Mannuzza 1988). A more recent study suggested that deficits in growth in height are transient maturational delays associated with ADHD, rather than stunting of growth (Spencer et al. 1998b). If this hypothesis is confirmed, the common practice of drug holidays for ADHD children would appear unnecessary. However, it seems prudent to institute drug holidays or alternative treatment in the case of children suspected of stimulant-associated growth deficits. This recommendation should be carefully weighed against the risk of

exacerbation of symptoms due to drug discontinuation. A transient behavioral deterioration occurs in some children after abrupt discontinuation of stimulant medications. The prevalence of this phenomenon and the etiology are unclear. Rebound phenomena also occur between doses in some children, creating an uneven, often disturbing clinical course. In those cases, consideration should be given to alternative treatments.

■ Antidepressants (Table 50–3)

There are several main families of antidepressant medications: tricyclic antidepressants (TCAs) (mixed neurotransmitter profile); selective serotonin reuptake inhibitors (SSRIs); monoamine oxidase inhibitors (MAOIs) (mixed neurotransmitter profile); and atypical antidepressants such as bupropion (dopaminergic/noradrenergic profile), venlafaxine (serotonergic/noradrenergic profile), nefazodone (serotonergic/noradrenergic profile), mirtazapine (serotonergic/noradrenergic profile), noradrenergic-specific reuptake inhibitors, and reboxetine.

In open and controlled studies involving children and adolescents, noradrenergic antidepressant medications and TCAs were beneficial in treating ADHD (Biederman et al. 1989a, 1989b), SSRIs were beneficial in treating obsessive-compulsive disorder (OCD) (De-Veaugh-Geiss et al. 1992; D. A. Geller et al. 1995) and depression (Emslie et al. 1997; Wagner et al. 1998), and TCAs were beneficial in treating enuresis (Gittelman 1980). Other childhood conditions that may benefit from antidepressant treatment include anxiety (serotonergic drugs) and tic disorders (TCAs, possibly other noradrenergic compounds) (Singer et al. 1994; Spencer 1997).

Antidepressant drugs appear to act by exerting various effects on pre- and postsynaptic receptors, affecting the release and reuptake of brain neurotransmitters, including norepinephrine, serotonin, and dopamine. The effect and adverse-effect profiles of the various classes of antidepressant drugs differ greatly. Because a substantial interindividual variability in metabolism and elimination has been demonstrated in children, doses should always be individualized. Studies have begun to document striking similarities between children and adults in terms of pharmacokinetic profiles of sertraline (Alderman et al. 1998), venlafaxine (Derivan 1995), and paroxetine (Findling et al. 1999).

Table 50–3. Antidepressants

Drug	Daily dose (mg/kg)	Dosage schedule	Main indications	Adverse effects and comments
Tricyclics (TCAs)				• Mixed mechanism of action (noradrenergic and serotonergic); secondary amines more noradrenergic; clomipramine primarily serotonergic
Tertiary amines			• ADHD	• Narrow therapeutic index
Amitriptyline	2.0–5.0[a]	Once daily or bid	• Enuresis	• Overdoses can be fatal
Clomipramine	2.0–5.0[a]	Once daily or bid	• Tic disorder	• Anticholinergic symptoms (dry mouth, constipation, blurred vision)
Imipramine	2.0–5.0[a]	Once daily or bid	• ? Anxiety disorders	• Weight loss
Secondary amines			• OCD (clomipramine)	• Serum level and electrocardiographic monitoring needed
Desipramine	2.0–5.0[a]	Once daily or bid		• At daily doses >3.5 mg/kg, electrocardiographic and blood pressure monitoring needed
Nortriptyline	1.0–3.0[b]	Once daily or bid		• No known long-term side effects
				• Possible withdrawal effects (severe gastrointestinal symptoms, malaise)
				• Risk of seizures
Monoamine oxidase inhibitors (MAOIs)			• Atypical depression	• Difficult to use in juvenile patients
Phenelzine	0.5–1.0	bid–tid	• Refractory depression	• Reserved for refractory cases
Seleginine	0.2–0.4	bid–tid		• Severe dietary restrictions (high-tyramine foods)
Tranylcypromine	0.5–1.0	bid–tid		• Drug–drug interactions
				• Hypertensive crisis with dietetic transgression or with certain drugs
				• Weight gain
				• Drowsiness
				• Changes in blood pressure
				• Insomnia
				• Rare hepatotoxicity
Selective serotonin reuptake inhibitors (SSRIs)			• MD	• Serotonergic
Citalopram	0.3–0.9	Once daily (in A.M.)	• Dysthymia	• Large margin of safety
Fluoxetine	0.3–0.9	Once daily (in A.M.)	• OCD	• No cardiovascular effects
Fluvoxamine	1.0–4.5	Once daily (in A.M.)	• Anxiety disorders	• Irritability
Paroxetine	0.3–0.9	Once daily (in A.M.)	• Eating disorders	• Insomnia
Sertraline	1.5–3.0	Once daily (in A.M.)	• ? PTSD	• Gastrointestinal symptoms
				• Headaches
				• Sexual dysfunction
				• Withdrawal symptoms more common with short-acting SSRIs
				• Potential drug–drug interactions (P450 enzymes)

Table 50–3. Antidepressants (continued)

Drug	Daily dose (mg/kg)	Dosage schedule	Main indications	Adverse effects and comments
Bupropion (SR)	3–6	bid	• ADHD • MD • Smoking cessation • ?Bipolar depression	• Mixed mechanism of action (dopaminergic and noradrenergic) • Irritability • Insomnia • Drug-induced seizures at doses >6 mg/kg • Contraindicated in bulimic patients
Mirtazapine	0.2–0.9	Once daily (in P.M.)	• MD • Anxiety disorders • ?Stimulant-induced insomnia • ?Bipolar depression	• Mixed mechanism of action (serotonergic and noradrenergic) • Sedation • Weight gain • Dizziness • ?Less likely to induce mania
Nefazodone	4.0–8.0	bid	• MD • Anxiety disorders • ?OCD • ?Bipolar depression	• Mixed mechanism of action (serotonergic and noradrenergic) • Dizziness • Nausea • Potential interactions with nonsedating antihistamines, cisapride (P450 enzymes) • Rare serious hepatotoxicity • ?Less likely to induce mania
Venlafaxine (XR)	1–3	Once daily	• MD • Anxiety disorders • ?ADHD • ?OCD	• Mixed mechanism of action (serotonergic and noradrenergic) • Adverse effects similar to SSRIs • Irritability • Insomnia • Gastrointestinal symptoms • Headaches • Potential withdrawal symptoms • Blood pressure changes

Note. Doses are general guidelines. All doses must be individualized, and appropriate monitoring should be performed. Weight-corrected doses are less appropriate for obese children. When high doses are used, serum levels may be obtained to avoid toxicity. ADHD = attention-deficit/hyperactivity disorder; MD = major depression; OCD = obsessive-compulsive disorder; PTSD = posttraumatic stress disorder; SR = sustained-release; XR = extended-release.
[a]Dose adjusted according to serum levels.
[b]Dose adjusted according to serum levels; therapeutic window.

TCAs include tertiary (imipramine and amitriptyline) and secondary (desipramine and nortriptyline) amine compounds. Treatment with a TCA should be initiated with a 10-mg or 25-mg dose, and the dose should be increased by 20%–30% every 4–5 days. When a daily dose of 3.0 mg/kg (or a lower effective daily dose, or, in the case of nortriptyline, a daily dose of 1.5 mg/kg) is reached, steady-state serum levels and an electrocardiogram (ECG) should be obtained. Typical dose ranges for TCAs are 2.0–5.0 mg/kg (for nortriptyline, 1.0–3.0 mg/kg). Common short-term adverse effects of TCAs include anticholinergic effects, such as dry mouth, blurred vision, and constipation. However, chronic administration of these drugs has no known deleterious effects. Gastrointestinal symptoms and vomiting may occur when TCAs are discontinued abruptly; thus, slow tapering of these medications is recommended. Because the anticholinergic effects of TCAs limit salivary flow, the drugs may promote tooth decay.

Evaluations of short- and long-term effects of therapeutic doses of TCAs on the cardiovascular system in children have shown TCAs to be generally well tolerated, with only minor electrocardiographic changes associated with daily oral doses as high as 5.0 mg/kg. TCA-induced electrocardiographic abnormalities (conduction defects) have been consistently reported in children receiving doses higher than 3.5 mg/kg (Biederman et al. 1989a) (nortriptyline dose, 1.0 mg/kg). Although of unclear hemodynamic significance, the development of conduction defects in children receiving TCAs merits closer electrocardiographic and clinical monitoring, especially when relatively high doses of these medicines are used. In the context of cardiac disease, conduction defects may have more serious clinical implications. When there is doubt about the cardiovascular state of a patient, a more comprehensive cardiac evaluation is suggested—including cardiac consultation and 24-hour electrocardiographic monitoring—before initiation of treatment with a TCA, to help determine the risk-to-benefit ratio of such an intervention. In a recent controlled study of heart rate variability, investigators examined the cardiac risk associated with use of desipramine in children (Prince et al., unpublished data, May 2003). Although changes in individual markers of heart rate variability were noted in ADHD youths treated with desipramine, the agent did not appear to adversely affect the overall balance of sympathetic or parasympathetic input into the myocardium.

In the 1980s, several case reports of sudden death in children being treated with desipramine raised concern about the potential cardiotoxic risk associated with TCA therapy in the pediatric population (Riddle et al. 1991). Despite uncertainty and imprecise data, an epidemiological evaluation suggested that the risk of desipramine-associated sudden death is slightly increased but is not much greater than the baseline risk of sudden death among children not taking medication (Biederman et al. 1995b). Nevertheless, treatment with a TCA should be preceded by a baseline ECG, with serial ECGs at regular intervals throughout treatment. Because of the potential lethality of TCA overdose, parents should be advised to store the medication in a place that is inaccessible to children.

SSRIs include fluoxetine, paroxetine, sertraline, fluvoxamine, and citalopram. The SSRIs are structurally dissimilar to each other and vary in their pharmacokinetics and side-effect profiles. Because of their pharmacological profiles, these medications have fewer anticholinergic, sedative, cardiovascular (in terms of blood pressure and electrocardiographic changes) (Leonard et al. 1998; Wilens et al. 1996b), and weight-related adverse side effects than do TCAs.

Fluoxetine comes in capsules of 10 and 20 mg and in a scored 10-mg tablet. Fluoxetine and its active metabolite have long half-lives (approximately 7–9 days). In contrast, paroxetine, sertraline, and citalopram have medium half-lives (approximately 24 hours), as does fluvoxamine (approximately 15 hours). Paroxetine comes in 10-, 20-, 30-, and 40-mg tablets, and citalopram comes in 20- and 40-mg tablets. Fluoxetine, paroxetine, and citalopram are all available in liquid form. Fluoxetine, paroxetine, and citalopram have similar potencies, and suggested daily doses range from 0.3 to 0.9 mg/kg. Sertraline comes in 25-, 50-, and 100-mg scored tablets, and the usual daily dose range is 1.5–3.0 mg/kg (≤200 mg/day). Fluvoxamine comes in 25-, 50-, and 100-mg scored tablets, and the usual daily dose range is 1.0–4.5 mg/kg (≤300 mg/day). Among the common adverse effects of SSRIs are agitation, gastrointestinal symptoms, irritability, insomnia, and sexual dysfunction, including decreased libido and anorgasmia.

The atypical antidepressants include venlafaxine, nefazodone, bupropion, and mirtazapine. Venlafaxine is chemically unrelated to other antidepressants and has both SSRI and TCA properties (i.e., is serotonergic and noradrenergic). IR venlafaxine has a short half-life (approximately 5 hours; the half-life of O-desmethylvenlafaxine is approximately 11 hours), but venlafaxine was recently reformulated into a long-acting compound that allows once-daily administration. The long-acting preparation of venlafaxine comes in 37.5, 75, 150, and 225 mg. Venlafaxine lacks significant activity at muscarinic, cholinergic, α-adrenergic, and histaminergic sites and therefore has fewer side effects (sedation, anticholinergic effects) than other antidepressants. Because venlafaxine therapy has been associated with changes in blood pressure in adults, it is advisable to monitor blood pressure when using this antidepressant.

Mirtazapine is an atypical mixed antidepressant with complex and unique pre- and postsynaptic effects affecting both serotonergic and noradrenergic neurotransmission. Because of its strong effects on histaminergic neurotransmission, it has potent hypnotic effects. Use of the agent has been also associated with weight gain. Mirtazapine is available in 15-, 30-, and 45-mg tablets.

Nefazodone is a novel-structured, mostly serotonergic antidepressant with complex pre- and postsynaptic effects on serotonergic neurotransmission. Because it has little effect on cholinergic or α$_2$- or β-adrenergic systems, it has a relatively mild side-effect profile. Recently, use of nefazodone has been associated with liver failure. Patients should be advised to be alert to signs and symptoms of liver dysfunction. In addition, nefazodone therapy appears to be associated with a lower incidence of sexual dysfunction compared with SSRI therapy. Nefazodone comes in 50-, 100-, and 200-mg capsules, and the usual dose range is 4–8 mg/kg/day, given in two divided doses.

Bupropion is a novel-structured antidepressant of the aminoketone class and is related to the phenylisopropylamines but pharmacologically distinct from known antidepressants. Although its specific site or mechanism of action remains unknown, bupropion seems to have an indirect mixed agonist effect on dopamine and norepinephrine neurotransmission. Bupropion is indicated for depression and smoking cessation in adults (Hurt et al. 1997). It is rapidly absorbed, with peak plasma levels usually achieved after 2 hours, and its average elimination half-life is 14 hours (range, 8–24 hours). The usual dose range is 3.0–6.0 mg/kg/day, given in divided doses. Side effects include irritability, anorexia, insomnia, and, rarely, edema, rashes, and nocturia. Exacerbation of tic disorders has also been reported with bupropion therapy. Compared with use of other antidepressants, use of bupropion appears to be associated with a somewhat higher rate (0.4%) of drug-induced seizures, particularly at daily doses greater than 6.0 mg/kg, as well as in patients with preexisting seizure disorder and patients with bulimia. Bupropion was recently formulated as a long-acting (sustained-release) preparation that can be administered twice daily, and this form of the drug appears to be associated with a lesser risk of seizures than the IR compound. A once-daily formulation of bupropion is being developed.

MAOIs include hydrazines (phenelzine) and non-hydrazines (tranylcypromine), and selegiline. In adults, MAOIs have been found to be helpful in the treatment of atypical depressive disorders with reverse endogenous features and depressive disorders with prominent anxiety features (Quitkin et al. 1991). Daily doses of phenelzine and tranylcypromine, which range from 0.5 to 1.0 mg/kg/day (and of selegiline, 0.2–0.4 mg/kg/day) should be carefully titrated according to response and adverse effects. Short-term adverse effects include orthostatic hypotension, weight gain, drowsiness, and dizziness. Major limitations for the use of MAOIs in children and adolescents are the severe dietetic restrictions (patients must not eat tyramine-containing foods, including most cheeses) and severe drug interactions (e.g., with pressor amines, most cold medicines, and amphetamines); incorrect use of MAOIs can induce a hypertensive crisis and a serotonergic syndrome. A new family of reversible inhibitors of monoamine oxidase A, used in Europe and Canada but not currently available in the United States, may be free of these difficulties. Currently being developed is a new generation of MAOIs, administered transdermally to avoid dietetic and drug–drug interactions.

Antidepressants and many other psychotropics are metabolized in the liver by the cytochrome P450 system (see the section "Combined Therapy" below) (DeVane 1998; Greenblatt et al. 1998; Nemeroff et al. 1996). Because of genetic polymorphism, patients may be slow or extensive (rapid) metabolizers. In addition, exogenous compounds can dramatically affect the efficacy of these enzymes and lead to drug–drug interactions. Coadministration of a TCA and an SSRI (paroxetine, fluoxetine, or sertraline; fluvoxamine; and, to a lesser extent, nefazodone) may result in increased levels of the TCA. Some compounds metabolized by the P450 enzyme 3A4 have been associated with QT prolongations when combined with drugs that inhibit 3A4, and such coadministration could lead to potentially lethal ventricular arrhythmias (torsade de pointes). Thus, great caution should be exercised when using the drugs that affect 3A4 activity (i.e., fluvoxamine, nefazodone, and, to a lesser degree, fluoxetine and sertraline). Citalopram, venlafaxine, and mirtazapine minimally inhibit P450 enzymes. Caution should be exercised when using combination treatments, because an increase to dangerous levels is possible with any drug that is metabolized by a P450 enzyme whose activity is inhibited by another drug (DeVane 1998; Greenblatt et al. 1998; Nemeroff et al. 1996).

■ Antipsychotics (Table 50–4)

On the basis of their mechanisms of action, antipsychotics can be divided into typical (blocking dopamine D_2 receptors) and atypical (having mixed dopaminergic and serotonergic [5-HT$_2$]) activity). Typical antipsychotic drugs include low-potency phenothiazines (which must be given at high daily doses), high-potency phenothiazines (given at low daily doses), butyrophenones (haloperidol and pimozide), thioxanthenes (thiothixene), and indole derivatives (molindone). Low-potency phenothiazines (e.g., chlorpromazine, thioridazine) are particularly likely to have unwanted autonomic side effects, such as hypotension and sedation, whereas high-potency compounds are associated with a higher risk of extrapyramidal adverse effects. Their in vitro receptor binding properties and their in vivo effects confirm that the typical antipsychotic drugs in current use block the binding of dopamine at the dopamine D_2 receptor. The best evidence that the observed dopamine D_2 receptor antagonism is relevant to the therapeutic effects of antipsychotic drugs (in psychotic disorders) is the finding that their rank order of clinical potency (e.g., haloperidol>perphenazine>chlorpromazine) is the same as their rank order of in vitro binding affinity for the dopamine D_2 receptor but not for other receptors. Even if the dopamine D_2 receptor is the primary site of action of typical antipsychotic drugs, much remains to be learned. In particular, the afferents and efferents of the mesolimbic dopamine projections and the role of dopaminergic transmission in healthy as well as psychotic individuals must be better understood before an understanding of what dopamine D_2 receptor blockade actually accomplishes can be gained. Because most psychotic patients improve over a period of days to weeks, it is likely that blockade of the dopamine D_2 receptor initiates a slow-onset change in some other component of the synaptic machinery or in the postsynaptic neuron (Hyman and Nestler 1993).

The atypical antipsychotics include dibenzazepines (loxapine, clozapine), risperidone, olanzapine, quetiapine, and ziprasidone. These chemically varied drugs differ in clinical activity and adverse effects. Atypical antipsychotic agents have relatively strong antagonistic interactions with serotonergic (5-HT$_2$) receptors and perhaps more variable activity at central α_1-adrenergic, cholinergic, and histaminic (H$_1$) sites, which may account for the varying adverse-effect profiles of these compounds. Although clozapine exerts only weak antagonism of dopaminergic (D$_2$) transmission, it has a high affinity for dopamine D_4 receptors, with a greater specificity for mesolimbic and mesocortical tracts. Thus, these compounds are associated with a low risk of acute extrapyramidal adverse effects and can be effective in treatment-resistant cases or in children who develop tardive dyskinesia. Risperidone, olanzapine, and quetiapine are novel atypical antipsychotic medications that combine dopaminergic (D$_2$) and serotonergic (5-HT$_2$) antagonist properties and are also associated with a lower incidence of acute extrapyramidal adverse effects and perhaps a lower risk of tardive dyskinesia.

Target symptoms that most commonly respond to typical antipsychotics are so-called positive symptoms (see "Psychotic Disorders"). In contrast, atypical antipsychotics are more effective agents for "negative symptoms." In addition to use in childhood psychotic disorders, antipsychotics have been used to control symptoms of agitation, aggression, and self-injurious behaviors that occur in children with mental retardation and pervasive developmental disorders (autistic and autistic-like disorders). Because of their serotonergic (5-HT$_2$) antagonist activity, atypical antipsychotics possess thymoleptic properties that are helpful in mood regulation. In recent years, atypical antipsychotics have been found to be efficacious in the treatment of adult and pediatric mania, having beneficial effects on both manic and depressive symptoms (Frazier et al. 1999). However, because of this thymoleptic activity, these agents may also precipitate or worsen mania.

The typical antipsychotic drugs haloperidol and pimozide have been widely used in the treatment of Tourette's disorder, with equivocal results (Shapiro et al. 1988). QTc prolongations of unclear clinical significance have been reported with pimozide treatment.

Table 50–4. Antipsychotics

Drug	Daily dose (mg/kg)	Dosage schedule	Main indications	Adverse effects and comments
Typical antipsychotics				• Primarily dopaminergic (D$_2$) antagonism
Butyrophenones			• Psychosis	• Anticholinergic effects (dry mouth, constipation, blurred vision); more common with low-potency agents
Haloperidol, others	0.1–0.3	Once daily or bid	• Mania	
Indole derivatives			• Tourette's disorder	• Weight gain (lower risk associated with molindone)
Molindone, others	0.1–0.5	Once daily or bid	• Hyperaggressive behavior, severe agitation, severe insomnia, severe self-injurious behavior	• Extrapyramidal reactions (dystonia, rigidity, tremor, akathisia); higher risk associated with high-potency agents
Phenothiazines				• Drowsiness
Low-potency				• Risk of TD with chronic administration
Chlorpromazine, thioridazine, others	3.0–6.0	Once daily or bid		• Withdrawal dyskinesia
High-potency				
Fluphenazine, perphenazine, others	0.1–0.5	Once daily or bid		
Thioxanthenes				
Thiothixene, others	0.1–0.5	Once daily or bid		
Atypical antipsychotics				• Dopaminergic- and serotonergic-like typical antipsychotics
Loxapine[a]	0.5–2.0	Once daily or bid	• Psychosis	• Lower incidence of extrapyramidal adverse effects than associated with typical antipsychotics
Olanzapine	0.1–0.2	Once daily or bid	• Positive and negative symptoms	• With ziprasidone, QTc monitoring needed
Quetiapine	0.7–4.0	Once daily or bid	• Mania	• Serotonergic, adrenergic, histaminergic
Risperidone	0.01–0.1	Once daily or bid		• Low incidence of extrapyramidal adverse effects; does not induce dystonia
Ziprasidone	0.5–1.5	Once daily or bid		• Low risk of TD
Clozapine	3.0–7.0	bid–tid	• Refractory psychosis	• Granulocytopenia or agranulocytosis (treatment involves constant monitoring of blood count)
			• Refractory mania	• Seizure risk is dose related

Note. Doses are general guidelines. All doses must be individualized, and appropriate monitoring should be performed. Weight-corrected doses are less appropriate for obese children. When high doses are used, serum levels may be obtained to avoid toxicity. TD = tardive dyskinesia.
[a]Loxapine has features similar to atypicals.

Pimozide at doses up to 0.3 mg/kg is recommended for use in patients with Tourette's disorder who fail to respond to more conventional treatments. In addition to typical antipsychotics, clonidine and guanfacine have been found to be useful in the treatment of some children with this disorder (Leckman et al. 1991).

The usual oral dose of antipsychotic drugs ranges between 3.0 and 6.0 mg/kg/day for low-potency phenothiazines and between 0.1 and 0.3 (up to 1.0) mg/kg/day for high-potency phenothiazines, butyrophenones, thioxanthenes, and indole derivatives. The daily dose range of clozapine is 3.0–7.0 mg/kg; that of risperidone is up to 85 µg/kg. Antipsychotic medications have relatively long half-lives and therefore should be administered not more than twice daily. Most antipsychotic preparations are available in either tablet or capsule form. In addition, at least one compound from each class of antipsychotics is available in a liquid concentrate form, including risperidone (1 mg/mL). Several compounds, including chlorpromazine, haloperidol, and fluphenazine, are available in injectable form for intramuscular administration.

Common short-term adverse effects of antipsychotic drugs are drowsiness, increased appetite, and weight gain. It is not entirely clear why weight gain, a particularly thorny adverse effect, is associated with use of atypical antipsychotics. Anticholinergic effects such as dry mouth, nasal congestion, and blurred vision are more commonly seen with use of low-potency phenothiazines. Extrapyramidal effects such as acute dystonia, akathisia (motor restlessness), and parkinsonism (bradykinesia, tremor, facial inexpressiveness) are more commonly seen with administration of high-potency compounds (phenothiazines, butyrophenones, and thioxanthenes). Treatment with thioridazine and with ziprasidone has been associated with increases in QTc and may necessitate electrocardiographic monitoring.

Although children appear generally less vulnerable to tardive dyskinesia (and tardive dystonia) than adults, long-term administration of typical antipsychotic drugs in children and adolescents may be associated with tardive dyskinesia. Tardive dyskinesia should be distinguished from the more common, generally benign, withdrawal dyskinesia that is associated with abrupt cessation of antipsychotic drugs and tends to subside several months after drug discontinuation. In children with mental retardation and pervasive developmental disorders, tardive dyskinesia should be differentiated from the commonly occurring stereotypies. One approach to minimize withdrawal reactions is to taper antipsychotic drugs very slowly over several months. Early detection with regular monitoring is the only available approach for tardive dyskinesia. It appears that treatment with atypical antipsychotics is less likely to be associated with tardive dyskinesia.

Increases in prolactin levels have occurred with the use of typical antipsychotics because of dopamine D_2 receptor–blocking effects on prolactin release, but the risk of hyperprolactinemia appears to be particularly high with the use of the atypical antipsychotic risperidone. The clinical implications of hyperprolactinemia remain unknown, but given the potential for disruption of the pituitary-gonadal axis, more efforts are needed to evaluate this problem in children and adolescents. In a recent case series, antipsychotic-induced hyperprolactinemia was successfully treated with cabergoline (Cohen and Biederman 2001). The serum prolactin levels normalized in all four subjects at a mean cabergoline dose of 2 mg/week. The cabergoline dose was reduced to 1 mg/week in three of four subjects. Cabergoline was well tolerated and had no adverse effects.

The atypical antipsychotic clozapine is associated with an increased risk of leukopenia and agranulocytosis, necessitating weekly monitoring of blood counts for the first 6 months and biweekly thereafter.

Another serious idiosyncratic reaction to antipsychotics is neuroleptic malignant syndrome, which is potentially lethal and consists of muscle rigidity, delirium, and autonomic instability (instability of blood pressure and pulse, diaphoresis, and hyperpyrexia), often accompanied by high creatine phosphokinase levels and less commonly accompanied by rhabdomyolysis. Preliminary evidence indicates that its presentation in juvenile patients is similar to that in adult patients. This syndrome may be difficult to distinguish from primary CNS pathology, concurrent infection, or other, more benign side effects of antipsychotic treatment, including extrapyramidal involvement or anticholinergic toxicity. Treatment of neuroleptic malignant syndrome involves intensive medical surveillance, immediate discontinuation of the antipsychotic, symptomatic treatment, and aggressive treatment of concomitant medical conditions, such as rhabdomyolysis. Although there is no general agreement about specific pharmacological treatment for neuroleptic malignant syndrome, dantrolene and bromocriptine have been used.

Short-term adverse effects of antipsychotics are

more easily managed. Excessive sedation can be avoided by using less sedating antipsychotics and managed by prescribing most of the daily dose at night. Drowsiness should not be confused with impaired cognition and can usually be eliminated by adjusting the dose and the timing of administration. In fact, there is no evidence that antipsychotics adversely affect cognition when given at low doses. Anticholinergic adverse effects can be minimized by choosing a medium- or high-potency compound or atypical antipsychotics. Extrapyramidal reactions can be avoided in most cases by slowly titrating the antipsychotic dose. Antiparkinsonian agents (i.e., anticholinergic drugs, antihistamines, amantadine) should be avoided unless strictly necessary, because of the added adverse effects that these drugs may produce. Extrapyramidal reactions can be prevented in many cases by avoiding rapid increase in neuroleptic dose or the use of high-potency typical antipsychotics such as haloperidol. When a child or adolescent taking antipsychotics develops an acutely agitated clinical picture with associated inability to sit still and aggressive outbursts, akathisia should be rapidly considered in the differential diagnosis. If akathisia is suspected, the dose of the antipsychotic may need to be decreased. β-Blockers (e.g., propranolol) and high-potency benzodiazepines have been found helpful in relieving symptoms of antipsychotic-induced akathisia in adults and may help relieve similar symptoms in juvenile patients (Ananth and Lin 1986).

■ Mood Stabilizers (Table 50–5)

Lithium Carbonate

Lithium is a simple solid element, and it bears chemical similarities to sodium, potassium, calcium, and magnesium. As with other psychotropic agents, the precise cellular mechanism of action by which lithium produces its beneficial effect is unknown. Lithium has diverse cellular actions that alter hormonal, metabolic, and neuronal systems. Proposed theories for lithium's mechanism of action relate to neurotransmission (i.e., interaction with catecholamine, indolamine, cholinergic, and endorphin systems; inhibition of β-adrenoreceptors), endocrine effects (i.e., blocking of testosterone synthesis and the release of thyroid hormone), circadian rhythm (i.e., normalization of altered sleep-wake cycles), and cellular processes (i.e., ionic substitution, inhibition of adenylate cyclase).

In children, the elimination half-life of lithium is approximately 18 hours, and it takes 5–7 days to reach steady state (Alessi et al. 1994). Aside from a shorter elimination half-life and a higher total clearance, the pharmacokinetics of lithium in children seem to be the same as in adults. Because work done to determine therapeutic ranges of lithium has been based on a 12-hour sampling interval, blood samples for determination of serum lithium levels should be obtained 12 hours after the last dose. Micromethods permit use of the finger-stick technique to obtain samples. Recent data suggest that lithium levels in saliva correlate with serum lithium levels (Weller et al. 1987). If this proves to be the case, monitoring of lithium therapy in young children, in whom venipuncture may be problematic, could become easier.

The usual lithium starting dose ranges from 10 to 30 mg/kg, given once a day or in divided doses twice a day. There is no known therapeutic serum lithium level in pediatric psychiatry. Suggested guidelines, based on the adult literature, include serum levels of 0.8–1.5 mEq/L for acute episodes and 0.6–0.8 mEq/L for maintenance or prophylactic therapy. Nevertheless, as with any other intervention, the lowest effective dose or serum level should always be chosen. Slow- and controlled-release lithium carbonate preparations are available. Lithium is also available in a liquid form, lithium citrate, which contains 8 mEq of lithium per 5 mL, equivalent to the amount in 300 mg of lithium carbonate.

Common short-term adverse effects include gastrointestinal symptoms such as nausea and vomiting, renal symptoms such as polyuria and polydipsia, and CNS symptoms such as tremor, sleepiness, and memory impairment. Chronic administration of lithium may be associated with metabolic (weight gain, decreased calcium metabolism), endocrine (decreased thyroid functioning), and possible renal damage. Data collected over the last 10 years, however, suggest that maintenance lithium therapy does not lead to serious nephrotoxicity, at least in adults. Nevertheless, renal function (blood urea nitrogen and creatinine levels) and thyroid function should be measured in children before lithium treatment is started, and these tests should be repeated at least every 6 months. Particular caution should be exercised when lithium is used in patients with neurological, renal, or cardiovascular disorders. In addition, nonsteroidal anti-inflammatory agents, certain diuretics, and angiotensin-converting enzyme inhibitors may increase plasma lithium levels.

Table 50–5.　Mood stabilizers

Drug	Daily dose (mg/kg)	Dosage schedule	Main indications	Adverse effects and comments
Lithium carbonate	10–30[a]	Once daily or bid	• Bipolar disorder	• *Lithium:* Polyuria, polydipsia; tremor, nausea, diarrhea; weight gain, drowsiness, skin abnormalities; possible effects on thyroid and renal functioning with chronic administration; monitoring of lithium levels and thyroid and renal function needed; lithium toxicity (level>2 mEq/L) can be life-threatening
Typical antiepileptic drugs			• Bipolar disorder prophylaxis	• *Antiepileptic drugs:* Sedation, nausea, dizziness, rashes
Carbamazepine	10–20[a]	bid	• Hyperaggressive behavior	• *Carbamazepine:* Bone marrow suppression (monitoring of blood counts and levels needed, initially and during treatment); may increase metabolism of low-dose oral contraceptives; rare liver toxicity
Oxcarbazepine	15–35	bid	• Adjunct therapy in refractory MD	• *Oxcarbazepine:* Little effect on P450 system, few drug–drug interactions
Valproic acid	15–60[a]	bid–tid	• ?Dysphoric conduct disorder	• *Valproic acid:* Rare liver toxicity; monitoring of blood counts and liver and renal function needed, initially and during treatment
Atypical antiepileptic drugs			• Bipolar disorder	• *Gabapentin, tiagabine, and topiramate:* Renally excreted; little effect on P450 system, few drug–drug interactions, large margin of safety; laboratory monitoring usually not necessary
Gabapentin	10–30	bid–tid	• Bipolar disorder prophylaxis	• *Lamotrigine:* Hepatically metabolized; interactions with typical antiepileptic drugs; associated with potentially life-threatening toxic epidermal necrolysis (Stevens-Johnson syndrome) in 2% of children
Lamotrigine	3–7	bid	• Hyperaggressive behavior	• *Tiagabine:* Risk of kidney stones (weak carbonic anhydrase inhibitor)
Tiagabine	0.8–0.8	bid–qid	• Adjunct therapy in refractory MD	
Topiramate	3–6	bid	• ?Dysphoric conduct disorder	

Note.　Doses are general guidelines. All doses must be individualized, and appropriate monitoring should be performed. Weight-corrected doses are less appropriate for obese children. When high doses are used, serum levels may be obtained to avoid toxicity. MD = major depression.
[a]Dose adjusted according to serum levels.

Concomitant use of these drugs necessitates closer monitoring of plasma lithium levels.

Anticonvulsants

Alternative mood-stabilizing antimanic agents include the typical antiepileptic drugs carbamazepine, oxcarbazepine, and valproic acid, as well as atypical antiepileptic drugs.

Carbamazepine. Carbamazepine is structurally related to TCAs. The plasma half-life after chronic administration is between 13 and 17 hours. The therapeutic plasma concentration is variably reported at 4–12 µg/mL, and recommended daily doses in children range from 10 to 20 mg/kg, administered twice a day. Because the relationship between dose and plasma level is variable and uncertain, with marked interindividual variability, close plasma level monitoring is recommended. Common short-term side effects include dizziness, drowsiness, nausea, vomiting, and blurred vision. Idiosyncratic reactions such as bone marrow suppression, liver toxicity, and skin disorders (including Stevens-Johnson syndrome) have been reported but appear to be rare. However, given the seriousness of these reactions, careful monitoring of blood counts and liver and renal function is warranted, initially and during treatment. Carbamazepine should be used with care in females because it is teratogenic and may increase the metabolism of low-dose oral contraceptives, resulting in an increased risk of unwanted pregnancy. Carbatrol is a carbamazepine formulation that consists of immediate-release, extended-release, and enteric-release beads, allowing twice-daily dosing. It is available in 200- and 300-mg capsules that can be opened and used as a sprinkle preparation.

Oxcarbazepine. Oxcarbazepine is chemically similar to carbamazepine, with some important differences. Because there is little interaction between oxcarbazepine and the P450 system, few drug–drug interactions are associated with administration, and the drug does not induce its own metabolism. It also does not share the hepatic and hematological liability of carbamazepine, and thus laboratory monitoring is not required. The drug is given twice daily. In adults, the maximum suggested dose is 2,400 mg/day. Controlled trials of oxcarbazepine in pediatric epilepsy led to development of weight-based dosing guidelines. Oxcarbazepine is available in 150-, 300-, and 600-mg scored tablets.

Valproic acid. Valproic acid is another anticonvulsant with well-documented efficacy in adult mania, particularly the mixed or dysphoric subtype of mania (Pope et al. 1991). Valproic acid is primarily metabolized by the liver and has a plasma half-life of 8–16 hours. The therapeutic plasma concentration range is 50–100 µg/mL. The recommended initial daily dose is 15 mg/kg, gradually increased to a maximum of 60 mg/kg, administered three times a day. Common short-term side effects include sedation, thinning of hair, anorexia, nausea, and vomiting. Idiosyncratic reactions such as bone marrow suppression and liver toxicity have been reported but appear to be rare. Asymptomatic increases in AST levels usually resolve spontaneously. Although hepatic fatalities have been reported in children less than 10 years old who were receiving monotherapy, most of these children were less than 2 years old. The risk of serious hepatic involvement is increased by concomitant use of other antiseizure medications and may be dose related. Careful monitoring of blood counts and liver and renal function is warranted, initially and during treatment. Valproate should be used with care in females because it is teratogenic.

Atypical antiepileptic drugs. A generation of atypical antiepileptic drugs with potential mood-stabilizing effects has emerged. These drugs include gabapentin (available in 100, 300, and 400 mg), tiagabine (4, 12, 16, and 20 mg), topiramate (25, 100, and 200 mg), and lamotrigine (25, 100, 150, and 200 mg). Their roles in the treatment of mania are being actively investigated, and initial case reports and published case series are encouraging. Gabapentin, tiagabine, and topiramate are postulated to act on γ-aminobutyric acid (GABA) levels, with little effect on the P450 system. Considering their wide margin of safety, the lack of a need for laboratory monitoring, and their renal excretion, they may represent major additions to the therapeutic armamentarium if they are found to be effective in the treatment of pediatric mania. Topiramate may be anorectic and therefore may be helpful as an adjunct to atypical antipsychotics, with their associated weight gain side effects. Unlike other atypical antiepileptic drugs, lamotrigine acts by inhibiting use-dependent sodium channels and is hepatically metabolized; therefore, serum levels are affected by coadministration of lamotrigine and typical antiepileptic drugs. Lamotrigine has been associated with a high risk of potentially life-threatening toxic epidermal necrolysis (Stevens-Johnson syndrome) and should be used with extreme

Table 50–6. Antianxiety drugs

Drug	Daily dose (mg/kg)	Dosage schedule	Main indications	Adverse effects and comments
High-potency benzodiazepines *Long-acting* Clonazepam *Short- to intermediate-acting* Alprazolam Lorazepam	0.01–0.04 0.02–0.06 0.04–0.09	Once daily or bid tid tid	• Anxiety disorders • Adjunct in refractory psychosis • Adjunct in mania • Severe agitation • Tourette's disorder • Severe insomnia • MD+anxiety	• Drowsiness, disinhibition, agitation • Confusion • Depression • Potential risk of abuse and dependence • Risk of rebound and withdrawal reactions greater with short-acting benzodiazepines
Nonbenzodiazepines Buspirone	0.20–0.65	bid	• Anxiety disorders • ?Agitated states	• Large margin of safety, laboratory monitoring usually not necessary

Note. Doses are general guidelines. All doses must be individualized, and appropriate monitoring should be performed. Weight-corrected doses are less appropriate for obese children. MD = major depression.

caution in children and be titrated extremely slowly over several weeks.

■ Antianxiety Drugs (Table 50–6)

The major agents in the antianxiety drug class are the benzodiazepines. Related compounds include barbiturates, several compounds structurally related to alcohol (i.e., chloral hydrate, paraldehyde, meprobamate), and sedative antihistamines (i.e., diphenhydramine, hydroxyzine, promethazine). The first nonbenzodiazepine antianxiety medicine to come on the market was buspirone. Buspirone is a novel nonbenzodiazepine anxiolytic without anticonvulsant, sedative, or muscle relaxant properties. The anxiolytic effects of buspirone may relate to reduction in serotonergic neurotransmission (Eison 1989). Clinical experience suggests that this drug has limited antianxiety efficacy. The daily dose is estimated to range from 0.2 to 0.65 mg/kg. Buspirone may be effective in the treatment of aggressive behaviors in children with pervasive developmental disorders (Realmuto et al. 1989).

Benzodiazepines (along with other sedatives, hypnotics, and antihistamines) are widely used in children, mostly to treat poorly diagnosed symptoms of agitation and insomnia, because of their pharmacological properties (clinical effects), toxicological properties (comfortable margin of safety), and minimal pharmacokinetic interactions with other drugs (D. M. Quinn 1986). Most benzodiazepines are lipophilic and are highly bound to plasma membranes; most have ac-

tive metabolites that dominate their course of activity. Most benzodiazepines are absorbed at an intermediate rate, with peak plasma levels appearing 1–3 hours after ingestion. Benzodiazepines and related sedative drugs can produce tolerance (and cross-tolerance with other benzodiazepines), physiological dependence (addiction), and psychological dependence (habituation).

GABA A receptors are the primary sites of action of benzodiazepines and barbiturates in the CNS. Some of the intoxicating effects of ethanol also occur at GABA A receptors. Benzodiazepines and barbiturates act at separate binding sites on the receptor, to potentiate the inhibitory action of GABA. Barbiturates and ethanol, but not benzodiazepines, can also independently open the chloride ion channel within the receptor. The fact that benzodiazepines, barbiturates, and ethanol all have related actions on a common receptor type explains their pharmacological synergy and cross-tolerance. It is not yet clear how benzodiazepines function as anxiolytics. The general belief, based on animal models, is that the anxiolytic properties of benzodiazepines reflect their actions on the limbic system, including the hippocampus and amygdala. The drugs' anticonvulsant actions may be primarily cortical, and their sedative actions may be primarily mediated in the brainstem. Neurons inhibited by benzodiazepines to produce anxiolysis may include serotonin (5-HT) and noradrenergic neurons. The pharmacological effects of buspirone include inhibition of serotonin neurons and the decrease of striatal levels of serotonin binding sites.

Because the pharmacological profiles of antianxiety drugs include behavioral disinhibition, and because many childhood psychiatric disorders are characterized by behavioral disinhibition, use of these agents in the absence of a specific indication may worsen the clinical picture (Wilens et al. 1998). Possible indications for use of antianxiety agents in pediatric psychiatry include childhood anxiety symptoms and disorders (Leonard and Rapoport 1989). The high-potency benzodiazepines alprazolam and clonazepam have received increasing attention as effective and safe agents for the treatment of adult panic disorder with or without agoraphobia (Biederman 1990; Herman et al. 1987). Reports suggest that children also may manifest adult-type anxiety disorders such as panic disorder and agoraphobia, which may respond to treatment with high-potency benzodiazepines (Biederman 1987). Possible additional uses of benzodiazepines include adjunct treatment of acute psychotic episodes, treatment of refractory schizophrenia, and treatment of antipsychotic-induced akathisia (Kutcher et al. 1989). The chlorinated benzodiazepines clonazepam and clorazepate may be particularly helpful in the treatment of complex partial seizures. Lorazepam and oxazepam do not have active metabolites and do not tend to accumulate in tissue; this makes them preferable for short-term symptomatic use. When long-term use is anticipated, longer-acting benzodiazepines (such as clonazepam) are preferable. It has been suggested that buspirone is beneficial in agitated states such as those occurring in patients with developmental disorders (Realmuto et al. 1989).

In general, the clinical toxicity of benzodiazepines is low. The most commonly encountered short-term adverse effects are sedation, drowsiness, and decreased mental acuity. When these drugs are given at high doses, patients can become confused. In adults, benzodiazepines have been reported to be associated with depressogenic adverse effects. With the exception of the potential risk of tolerance and dependence (this risk is suspected but not well studied in adults and is unknown in children), benzodiazepines have no known long-term adverse effects. Adverse withdrawal effects can occur, and benzodiazepines should always be tapered slowly.

In recent years, however, serotonergic antidepressants (including paroxetine, sertraline, and venlafaxine) have been increasingly found to have strong antianxiety effects in juvenile patients with OCD or other anxiety disorders. Clomipramine, sertraline, and fluvoxamine underwent large-scale, multisite clinical trials, and positive results were achieved in children and adolescents. Considering the safety profiles of serotonergic drugs, their long half-lives, the absence of addictive potential, and their antidepressant properties, serotonergic antidepressants should be considered first-line agents in the treatment of juvenile anxiety disorders.

The P450 enzyme 2C19 is involved in the biotransformation of diazepam and is inhibited by fluoxetine, sertraline, and fluvoxamine. In addition, 3A4 is involved in the biotransformation of triazolobenzodiazepines (triazolam, alprazolam, and midazolam) and is affected by fluoxetine, sertraline, fluvoxamine, and nefazodone. Thus, administration of benzodiazepines with these other drugs could affect serum levels of the benzodiazepines.

■ Other Drugs (Table 50–7)

Alpha-Adrenergic Agents

Clonidine. Clonidine, a presynaptic α_2-adrenergic agonist, has been widely used in pediatric psychiatry, despite extremely limited safety and efficacy data supporting its use. Clonidine is an imidazoline derivative with α-adrenergic agonist properties that has been primarily used in the treatment of hypertension. At low doses, the drug appears to stimulate inhibitory, presynaptic autoreceptors in the CNS. In pediatric psychiatry, clonidine is most commonly used in the treatment of Tourette's disorder and other tic disorders (Leckman et al. 1991), ADHD, and ADHD-associated sleep disturbances (Hunt et al. 1990; Prince et al. 1996). In addition, the agent has been reported to be useful in controlling aggression toward self and others in patients with developmental disorders.

Clonidine is a relatively short-acting compound with a plasma half-life ranging from approximately 5.5 hours (in children) to 8.5 hours (in adults). Daily doses should be titrated and individualized. Usual daily doses range from 3 to 10 µg/kg, given generally in two, three, or sometimes four divided doses. Therapy is usually initiated with a full or half 0.1-mg tablet (the lowest manufactured dose), depending on the size of the child (for a dose of approximately 1–2 µg/kg), and the dose is increased depending on clinical response and adverse effects. Because of clonidine's sedative effect, initial doses are best given in the evening hours or before bed.

Sedation is the most common short-term adverse

Table 50–7. Other drugs

Drug	Daily dose	Dosage schedule	Main indications	Adverse effects and comments
α₂-Adrenergic agonists				
Clonidine	3–10 μg/kg	bid–qid	• Tourette's disorder	• Sedation (very frequent)
Guanfacine	15–90 μg/kg	Once daily or bid	• ADHD • Aggression, self-abuse • Severe agitation • Withdrawal syndromes	• Hypotension (rare) • Dry mouth • Confusion (with high dose) • Depression • Rebound hypertension • Localized irritation with transdermal preparation • *Guanfacine:* Same effects as above, but less sedation and less hypotension
β-Blockers				
Propranolol	1–7 mg/kg	bid	• Aggression, self-abuse • Severe agitation • Akathisia	• Sedation • Depression • Risk of bradycardia and hypotension (dose dependent) and rebound hypertension • Bronchospasm (propranolol contraindicated in asthmatic patients) • Rebound hypertension with abrupt withdrawal
Naltrexone	1–2 mg/kg	Once daily or bid	• Self-injurious behavior • Addiction	• Long-acting opioid antagonist • Minimal adverse effects • Hepatotoxicity (rare)
DDAVP (Desmopressin)	20–40 μg intranasally 0.2–0.4 mg orally	Once daily hs Once daily hs	• Enuresis	• Headache • Nausea
Noradrenergic-specific reuptake inhibitors				
Atomoxetine	0.5–1.8 mg/kg	Once daily or bid	• ADHD with or without comorbidity	• Mild increase in pulse and diastolic blood pressure • Mild decrease in appetite • No insomnia • No cardiac conduction or repolarization delays • Not abusable

Note. Doses are general guidelines. All doses must be individualized, and appropriate monitoring should be performed. Weight-corrected doses are less appropriate for obese children. ADHD=attention-deficit/hyperactivity disorder; DDAVP=1-desamino-8-D-arginine-vasopressin.

effect. Hypotension, dry mouth, depression, and confusion may also occur. Clonidine is not known to have long-term adverse effects. In hypertensive adults, abrupt withdrawal of clonidine has been associated with rebound hypertension. Thus, slow tapering must precede discontinuation of the drug. Clonidine should not be administered concomitantly with β-blockers because adverse interactions have been reported with this combination. Recent reports of death in several children taking the combination of methylphenidate and clonidine have generated new concerns about clonidine's safety. Although more work is needed to determine whether an increased risk exists with this combination, a cautious approach is advised, including increased surveillance and cardiovascular monitoring.

Guanfacine. There has been anecdotal evidence that the more selective α-adrenergic agonist guanfacine (an α_{2a}-adrenergic agonist) has benefits similar to those of clonidine, with less sedation and longer duration of action (Chappell et al. 1995; Horrigan and Barnhill 1995; Hunt et al. 1995). Usual daily doses range from 15 to 90 µg/kg, given generally in two or three divided doses.

Propranolol

Propranolol is a nonselective (affecting both β_1 and β_2 receptors) β-adrenergic antagonist. It has received considerable attention for its potential use in psychiatric disorders, including drug-induced akathisia, anxiety disorders, and schizophrenia, as well as in aggressive and self-abusive behavior disorders (Ananth and Lin 1986; Sorgi et al. 1986). Propranolol effects are mediated through the drug's blocking of β-adrenergic receptors at multiple sites in the body. Propranolol also crosses the blood–brain barrier, which probably accounts for some of its efficacy in psychiatric disorders but also contributes to concerns regarding potential CNS toxicity. It is unclear whether the benefits of propranolol therapy are primarily due to peripheral or to central effects of the drug. In pediatric psychiatry, propranolol has been used in the management of severe aggressive and self-injurious behaviors (the drug is administered in daily doses of 2–5 mg/kg).

Short-term adverse effects of propranolol include nausea, vomiting, constipation, and mild diarrhea. Propranolol can cause bradycardia and hypotension as well as increase airway resistance and is contraindicated in asthmatic and certain cardiac patients. Chronic administration of propranolol has no known long-term effects. Because abrupt cessation of this drug can be associated with rebound hypertension, gradual tapering is recommended. Coadministration of β-blockers such as propranolol and SSRIs could affect serum levels of β-blockers.

Naltrexone

Naltrexone is a potent, long-acting opioid antagonist with a rapid onset of action. It has been administered in daily doses of 1–2 mg/kg to children with pervasive developmental disorders and to children with self-abuse (Lienemann and Walker 1989). Although naltrexone is relatively free of serious adverse effects, there have been some rare reports of hepatotoxicity. Naltrexone has been used in the treatment of alcohol craving (O'Malley et al. 1996).

Desmopressin

Desmopressin (1-desamino-8-D-arginine-vasopressin; DDAVP), a synthetic antidiuretic hormone peptide analogue, was recently approved by the FDA for the treatment of enuresis. Daily doses are 0.1–0.2 mL by intranasal spray, given at bedtime. Although desmopressin suppresses urine production for 7–10 hours, it lacks the pressor effects of antidiuretic hormone. Adverse effects are minimal. The drug's safety has been established in patients requiring long-term therapy (Rew and Rundle 1989).

Atomoxetine

Atomoxetine is a potent noradrenergic-specific reuptake inhibitor that has been studied in more than 1,800 children and more than 250 adults and has been submitted for FDA approval (Michelson et al. 2001; Spencer 2002). Atomoxetine has been shown to be effective for ADHD at all ages and has a favorable adverse-effect profile, consisting of mild appetite suppression and no insomnia. As with tricyclics, there are mild increases in diastolic blood pressure and heart rate. Unlike tricyclics, atomoxetine does not affect electrocardiographic intervals. In a study involving children and adolescents, response was best at 1.2 or 1.8 mg/kg/day and superior to 0.5 mg/kg/day; all three doses were superior to placebo (Kratochvil et al. 2001). Safety and efficacy data at 1 year revealed that atomoxetine continued to be effective and well tolerated. The acute mild increases in diastolic blood pressure and heart rate persisted but did not worsen. Growth in height and weight was normal, and there were no significant differences between atomoxetine and placebo in terms of laboratory parameters and electrocardiographic intervals.

Main Diagnostic Categories and Clinical Considerations

■ Attention-Deficit/Hyperactivity Disorder (Table 50–8)

ADHD is defined in DSM-IV-TR as a behavioral disorder of childhood onset (by age 7 years) characterized by symptoms of inattentiveness and impulsivity-hyperactivity. DSM-IV-TR includes three types: 1) a combined type, in which both inattention and hyperactivity-impulsivity symptoms are present; 2) a predominantly inattentive type; and 3) a predominantly hyperactive-impulsive type. In addition, DSM-IV-TR also includes the category ADHD not otherwise specified, used for individuals presenting with atypical features.

ADHD is one of the major clinical and public health problems in the United States in terms of morbidity and disability in children and adolescents. ADHD is estimated to affect at least 5% of school-age children. Its effect on society is enormous in terms of financial cost, stress on families, effect on schools, and damaging effects on self-esteem. Although the etiology of ADHD remains unknown, data from family, genetic, twin, adoption, and segregation analyses strongly suggest a genetic etiology. Indeed, the genetic contribution appears to be substantial, as suggested by the very high heritability coefficients (mean, 0.8) associated with this disorder. Preliminary molecular genetic studies have implicated several candidate genes, including the dopamine D_2 receptor gene (*DRD2*) and the dopamine D_4 receptor gene (*DRD4*), as well as the dopamine transporter gene (*DAT1*) (Faraone and Biederman 1999). Both dopamine and norepinephrine, neurotransmitters thought to mediate the response to anti-ADHD medications, are potent agonists of the dopamine D_4 receptor.

Data from follow-up studies indicate that children with ADHD are at risk of maintaining and developing new psychiatric disorders in adolescence and adulthood, including antisocial and substance use (tobacco, alcohol, drugs) disorders. Follow-up data also indicate that the disorder persists into adulthood in a substantial number of individuals and may be a common adult diagnosis (Spencer et al. 1998a). In recent years, ADHD has been increasingly recognized as highly heterogeneous, occurring at high levels in conjunction with psychiatric disorders (conduct and oppositional defiant disorders, unipolar and bipolar mood disorders, and anxiety disorders), cognitive problems (learning disability), and social problems (social disability, nonverbal learning disability). Neuroimaging studies have identified subtle anomalies in the frontal cortex and in projecting subcortical structures (Faraone and Biederman 1999), and it has been posited that dysregulation of catecholamine neurotransmission underlies ADHD's pathophysiology (Zametkin and Rapoport 1987).

There is extensive, clear documentation of the short-term efficacy of methylphenidate treatment, mostly in latency-age Caucasian boys (Spencer et al. 1997). The literature on stimulants administered at other ages or to females or ethnic minorities is more limited. The few studies of stimulants in adolescents found rates of response highly consistent with response rates among latency-age children. In contrast, the few studies involving preschoolers appear to indicate that young children respond less well to stimulant therapy, which suggests that ADHD in preschoolers may be more refractory. It has been clearly documented that treatment with stimulants improves not only abnormal behaviors of ADHD but also self-esteem and cognitive, social, and family function, findings that support the importance of treating ADHD patients beyond school or work hours. Three controlled clinical trials indicated the efficacy of methylphenidate, Adderall, and pemoline in adults with ADHD (Spencer et al. 1995, 1999b; Wilens et al. 1999a). In these trials, there was a highly clinically and statistically significant difference between study drug and placebo, and the magnitude of effects was consistent with that in pediatric trials.

New long-acting stimulant preparations have revolutionized ADHD treatment. An analogue classroom paradigm was used to test the fine-grained pharmacodynamic and pharmacokinetic profiles of some of these medications. Developed by Swanson and colleagues (2000), these settings simulate real-life demands and distractions of a typical classroom. Trained observers hourly record frequencies of behaviors as well as academic production and accuracy. Sequential

Table 50–8. Pharmacotherapy for disruptive behavior disorders

Disorder	Main characteristics	Pharmacotherapy
Attention-deficit/ hyperactivity disorder (ADHD)	• Inattentiveness, impulsivity, hyperactivity • Persists into adulthood in 50% of individuals	*First-line* • Stimulants (70% response; for uncomplicated ADHD; caution advised in patients with tic disorders) • Atomoxetine *Second-line* • TCAs (70% response; first-line therapy for patients with comorbid MD or anxiety disorders and for patients with ADHD+tics) • Serum level and cardiovascular monitoring needed • Bupropion *Third-line* • Clonidine, guanfacine (both first-line therapy for patients with ADHD+tics) *Fourth-line* • MAOIs • Combined pharmacotherapy for treatment-resistant cases
Conduct disorder (CD)	• Persistent and pervasive patterns of aggressive and antisocial behaviors • Often associated with ADHD, MD, and bipolar disorder	• No specific pharmacotherapy available for core disorder • Behavior therapy • Conduct disorder in conjunction with other Axis I disorders (e.g., ADHD, MD, mania, psychosis, anxiety): treat underlying disorder (anti-ADHD agents for ADHD, SSRIs for MD, antimanic agents for mania, antianxiety agents for anxiety, α-adrenergic agents and β-blockers for agitation, aggression, and self-abuse)

Note. MAOI = monoamine oxidase inhibitor; MD = major depression; SSRI = selective serotonin reuptake inhibitor; TCA = tricyclic antidepressant.

serum sampling from catheters allows correlation of blood levels to behavioral activity.

The first medication developed was the methylphenidate preparation Concerta. Concerta uses an osmotic pump mechanism that creates an ascending profile of methylphenidate in the blood, providing effective treatment for 10–12 hours. Concerta is available in 18-, 36-, and 54-mg tablets, approximating the 5-, 10-, and 15-mg thrice-daily doses of IR methylphenidate. A laboratory classroom study involving 68 children found that a single morning dose of Concerta was effective for 12 hours with regard to social and task behaviors and academic performance (Pelham et al. 2001). A large multicenter, randomized clinical trial was used to determine the safety and efficacy of Concerta in an outpatient setting (Wolraich et al. 2001). Two hundred eighty-two children with ADHD (ages 6–12 years) were randomized to placebo administration (*n*=90), IR methylphenidate three times a day (*n*=97), or Concerta once a day (*n*=95) in a double-blind, 28-day trial. Throughout the study, children in the Con-

certa and IR methylphenidate treatment groups showed significantly greater reductions in core ADHD symptoms than did children receiving placebo. Concerta was well tolerated; there was mild appetite suppression, but study subjects experienced no sleep abnormalities. A 1-year follow-up study involving 407 children treated with Concerta found no marked effects on weight, height, blood pressure, or pulse and no tic exacerbation (Wilens and Group 2000).

A new extended-release form of the methylphenidate preparation Ritalin (Ritalin LA) provides effective methylphenidate treatment for 8–9 hours. Ritalin LA's bimodal release system produces, in single-dose administration, pharmacokinetic characteristics that resemble those of two doses of Ritalin administered 4–5 hours apart. Ritalin LA consists of a mixture of immediate- and delayed-release beads in a 1:1 ratio. The delayed-release beads are coated with an absorption-delaying polymer. Ritalin LA is available in 20-, 30-, and 40-mg capsules, approximating 10-, 15-, and 20-mg twice-daily doses of IR methylphenidate. Ritalin LA may be used as a sprinkle preparation for children unable to swallow pills. The initial analogue classroom study evaluated the pharmacodynamic (efficacy) profile, safety, and tolerability of Ritalin LA (Spencer et al. 2000). Compared with placebo, single doses of all variants of Ritalin LA improved classroom behavior and academic productivity over the 9-hour period after dosing. Ritalin LA had a rapid onset of effect, and the improvement relative to placebo was statistically significant during both the morning (0–4 hours after dosing) and the afternoon (4–9 hours after dosing).

Ritalin LA was further tested in a multicenter, double-blind trial involving 160 children (Biederman et al. 2001). There was a 2- to 4-week titration to optimal dose, followed by a 1-week placebo washout period. A total of 137 subjects with persistent ADHD symptoms during the washout were randomized to treatment with Ritalin LA or placebo. Compared with children taking placebo, children taking Ritalin LA were rated (by teachers and parents) on the Conners' ADHD/ DSM-IV Scale as greatly improved. Scores on the subscales of inattention and hyperactivity indicated equally robust improvements. Significant drug-specific improvement was also noted by clinicians in scores on the Clinical Global Impression Scale. Ritalin LA was well tolerated, having minimal side effects. Rates of mild appetite suppression and mild insomnia were both low (3.1%).

Metadate CD comes in capsules with a mixture of immediate- and delayed-release beads containing methylphenidate. In Metadate CD capsules, 30% of the beads are immediate release and 70% are delayed release, to provide effective methylphenidate treatment for 8–9 hours. The efficacy and safety of Metadate CD were tested in a multicenter, randomized, double-blind, placebo-controlled trial conducted at 32 sites and involving 316 children with ADHD (Greenhill et al. 2002). The trial consisted of a 1-week single-blind, placebo run-in, followed by a 3-week double-blind titration and treatment period. Improvement compared with placebo was equally good morning and afternoon as measured by teachers on the Conners' Global Index. The medication was well tolerated, with relatively low rates of decreased appetite (9.7% in the treated group vs. 2.5% in the placebo group) and insomnia (7.1% vs. 2.5%). Metadate CD is available in 20-mg capsules, approximating the 10-mg twice-daily doses of IR methylphenidate. Recently, a study found that the bioavailability and tolerability of Metadate CD are not altered when the capsule is opened and the beads are sprinkled on food (Pentikis et al. 2002).

Adderall XR (a mixed amphetamine salts formulation) comes in capsules with a 1:1 ratio of IR beads to delayed-release beads, to release drug content in a time course similar to that of Adderall given twice daily (at 0 and 4 hours). Adderall XR is available in 10-, 20-, and 30-mg capsules. An analogue classroom study compared various doses of Adderall XR with Adderall given twice daily and placebo (McCracken et al. 2000). Behavioral and academic improvement were documented to 12 hours after dosing. The efficacy and safety of Adderall XR were further tested in a multicenter, randomized, double-blind, placebo-controlled trial conducted at 47 sites (Biederman et al. 2002). A total of 584 children with ADHD were randomized to administration of once-daily morning doses of placebo or Adderall XR 10 mg, 20 mg, or 30 mg for 3 weeks. Continuous, significant improvement was determined in morning and afternoon assessments by teachers (using the Conners' Global Index Scale for Teachers) and in morning, afternoon, and late-afternoon assessments by parents (using the Conners' Global Index Scale for Parents). All active-treatment groups showed significant dose-related improvement in behavior from baseline. The medication was well tolerated, with rates of adverse events similar for active treatments and placebo. A 1-year follow-up study involving 411 children taking Adderall XR examined long-term safety and efficacy (Chandler et al. 2001). Efficacy was maintained for 12 months, as measured by the Conners' Global Index. The medication was safe and well tolerated, with a low frequency of mild adverse events and no evidence of untoward cardiovascular effects.

Methylphenidate as a secondary amine gives rise to four optical isomers: D-*threo*, L-*threo*, D-*erythro*, and L-*erythro*. There is stereoselectivity in receptor site binding and its relationship to response. The standard preparation is composed of the D,L-*threo* racemate, the form apparently active in the CNS. Moreover, recent data suggest that the D-methylphenidate isomer is the active form. In a positron emission tomography study, D-*threo*-methylphenidate was found to bind specifically to the basal ganglia, rich in dopamine transporter receptors, whereas L-*threo*-methylphenidate widely distributed with only nonspecific binding (Ding et al. 1995). These findings led to the development of a purified D-*threo*-methylphenidate compound, Focalin. When given in equimolar doses, D-*threo*-methylphenidate and D,L-*threo*-methylphenidate were found to have similar pharmacokinetic profiles. That is, the maximum concentration, the time to maximum concentration, and the half-life of D-methylphenidate were the same for the two racemates.

The efficacy of Focalin was established in two controlled studies. In the first trial, 132 children and adolescents were randomized to administration of D-*threo*-methylphenidate, D,L-*threo*-methylphenidate, or placebo at 8 A.M. and noon for 4 weeks (Conners et al. 2001). At week 4, teacher ratings on the Swanson, Nolan, and Pelham, version IV (SNAP-IV), scale revealed robust improvement with active treatment. The average improvement from baseline was equivalent to one standard deviation on the SNAP-IV scale—a clinically important change. Parent ratings on the SNAP-IV scale revealed superiority of both treatments over placebo 3 hours after dosing, but only superiority of D-methylphenidate (not D,L-methylphenidate) 6 hours after dosing. In a second controlled study, investigators tested the specificity of response to D-*threo*-methylphenidate (data on file, Novartis). A total of 116 patients were treated openly with D-*threo*-methylphenidate to determine the optimal dose. At the end of 6 weeks, 75 responders were randomized to blinded treatment with D-*threo*-methylphenidate or placebo over 2 weeks. Subjects randomized to placebo administration had a high rate of relapse (62%) compared with those who continued taking D-*threo*-methylphenidate (17%). In addition, the parent SNAP-IV scale ratings indicated persistent effect 6 hours after D-*threo*-methylphenidate dosing. In both studies, adverse effects of D-*threo*-methylphenidate were consistent with those of D,L-*threo*-methylphenidate. These studies showed Focalin to be as effective as the racemate at half the dose. Focalin is available in 2.5-, 5-, and 10-mg doses, approximating the 5-, 10-, and 20-mg doses of D,L-methylphenidate.

Treatment with stimulants improves a wide variety of cognitive abilities (Barkley 1977; Klein 1987; Rapport et al. 1988), increases school-based productivity (Famularo and Fenton 1987), and improves performance on academic tests (H. Abikoff, personal communication, June 1965). Patients with ADHD may also manifest learning disabilities that are not responsive to pharmacotherapy (Bergman et al. 1991; Faraone et al. 1993) but respond to educational remediation.

It is estimated that at least 30% of individuals with ADHD do not respond adequately to or cannot tolerate stimulant treatment (Barkley 1977; Gittelman 1980; Spencer et al. 1996). In addition, stimulants are short-acting drugs that must be administered multiple times during the day, necessitating treatment during school or work hours and affecting compliance. Although this problem may be offset by the development of an effective long-acting stimulant, that class of drugs often affects sleep, making use in evening hours difficult when children and adults need to be able to concentrate in order to deal with daily demands and interact with family members and friends. In addition to these problems, the fact that stimulants are controlled substances continues to create worries in children, families, and the treating community, further inhibiting their use. These feelings are based on lingering concerns about the potential for abuse of stimulant drugs by the child or his or her family members or associates; concerns about the possibility of diversion; and safety concerns regarding the use of a controlled substance by patients who are impulsive and frequently have antisocial tendencies (Goldman et al. 1998). Similarly, the controlled nature of stimulant drugs creates important medicolegal concerns for the treating community that further increase the barriers to treatment.

In addition to these unresolved problems, it is increasingly evident that ADHD frequently occurs with mood or anxiety disorders, conditions that may affect response to stimulant drugs. For example, six of eight pediatric studies (75%) that examined ADHD children with depression or anxiety found a lesser response to stimulants in terms of improvement of ADHD symptoms (DuPaul et al. 1994; Pliszka 1989; Swanson et al. 1978; Tannock et al. 1995; Taylor et al. 1987; Voelker et al. 1983). Moreover, a recent report indicated that stimulants are poorly effective in the treatment of ADHD in the context of coexisting manic symptomatology and that their use in such patients may result in increased mood instability (Biederman et al. 1999b).

Noradrenergic and dopaminergic active antidepressants such as MAOIs (Zametkin et al. 1985), secondary amine TCAs (Biederman et al. 1989a; Donnelly et al. 1986; Wilens et al. 1993), and bupropion (Barrickman et al. 1995; Casat et al. 1989; Conners et al. 1996) have been found to be superior to placebo in controlled clinical trials. (See "Antidepressants" for details on specific drugs and Table 50–3 for doses and side effects.) Possible advantages of these compounds over stimulants include a longer duration of action without symptom rebound or insomnia, greater flexibility in dosage, the option (with TCAs) of monitoring plasma drug levels, minimal risk of abuse or dependence, and potential treatment of comorbid internalizing symptoms. Although beneficial effects of the SSRI fluoxetine in the treatment of ADHD were noted in one open case series (Barrickman et al. 1991), little other clinical or scientific evidence implicates serotonergic systems in the pathophysiology of ADHD.

Perhaps the best established of the second-line agents for ADHD are the TCAs. Of 33 studies (21 controlled, 12 open) evaluating TCA therapy in children, adolescents (N=1,139), and adults (N=78), 91% found that TCAs had positive effects on ADHD symptoms (Spencer et al. 1997). Of the studies of TCA therapy in ADHD, the studies of imipramine treatment and of desipramine treatment are the most numerous; a handful of studies focusing on other TCAs have been conducted. Although most TCA studies (73%) were relatively brief, lasting a few weeks to several months, 9 studies (27%) found enduring effects of up to 2 years. Outcomes in both short- and long-term studies were equally positive. Although one study found that the drop-out rate after 1 year was 50%, it is noteworthy that subjects who continued taking imipramine experienced sustained improvement (P.O. Quinn and Rapoport 1975). More recent studies using aggressive doses of TCAs found sustained improvement for up to 1 year with desipramine therapy (>4 mg/kg) (Biederman et al. 1986; Gastfriend et al. 1985) and nortriptyline therapy (2.0 mg/kg) (Wilens et al. 1993). Although response was equally positive at all the dose ranges, it was more sustained in studies in which higher doses were administered. A high interindividual variability in serum TCA levels has been consistently reported for imipramine and desipramine, with little relationship between serum level and daily dose, response, or side effects. In contrast, dose and serum level appear to be positively associated in nortriptyline therapy (Wilens et al. 1993).

In the largest controlled study of TCA therapy in children, our group reported favorable results with desipramine in 62 clinically referred children with ADHD, most of whom had previously failed to respond to psychostimulant treatment (Biederman et al. 1989a). The study was a randomized, placebo-controlled, parallel-design, 6-week clinical trial. Clinically and statistically significant differences in behavioral improvement were found for desipramine over placebo, at an average daily desipramine dose of 5 mg/kg. Although the presence of comorbidity increased the likelihood of a placebo response, neither comorbidity with conduct disorder (CD), depression, or anxiety

nor a family history of ADHD yielded differential responses to desipramine treatment. In addition, desipramine-treated patients with ADHD showed a substantial reduction in depressive symptoms compared with placebo-treated patients.

Similar results were obtained in a similarly designed controlled clinical trial of desipramine therapy in 41 adults with ADHD (Wilens et al. 1996c). Desipramine, at an average daily dose of 150 mg (average serum level, 113 ng/mL), was statistically and clinically more effective than placebo. Sixty-eight percent of desipramine-treated patients responded, compared with none of the placebo-treated patients (P<0.0001). Moreover, at the end of the study, the average severity of ADHD symptoms in patients receiving desipramine was reduced to below the level required to meet diagnostic criteria. Importantly, although the full desipramine dose was achieved at week 2, clinical response improved further over the following 4 weeks, indicating a latency of response. Response was independent of dose, serum desipramine level, sex, or lifetime comorbidity with anxiety or depressive disorders.

In a recent prospective, placebo-controlled discontinuation trial, we demonstrated the efficacy of nortriptyline at doses of up to 2 mg/kg/day in 35 school-age youths with ADHD (Prince et al. 1999). In that study, 80% responded by week 6 in the open phase. During the discontinuation phase, subjects randomized to placebo administration lost the anti-ADHD effect, whereas those receiving nortriptyline maintained a robust anti-ADHD effect. Youths receiving nortriptyline also were found to have more modest but statistically significant reductions in oppositionality and anxiety. Nortriptyline was well tolerated, with some weight gain. (Weight gain is frequently considered a desirable side effect in this population.) Less favorable results were obtained in a systematic study involving 14 youths with refractory ADHD who received protriptyline (mean dose, 30 mg). Because of adverse effects, only 45% of subjects responded to or could tolerate protriptyline (Wilens et al. 1996a).

Thirteen (40%) of the 33 TCA studies compared TCAs and stimulants. Five studies found stimulants to be superior to TCAs (Garfinkel et al. 1983 [studied two TCAs]; Gittelman-Klein 1974; Greenberg et al. 1975; Rapoport et al. 1974), five studies found stimulants to be equal to TCAs (Gross 1973; Huessy and Wright 1970; Kupietz and Balka 1976; Rapport et al. 1993; Yepes et al. 1977), and three studies found TCAs to be superior to stimulants (Watter and Dreyfuss 1973; Werry 1980; Winsberg et al. 1972). Analyses of response profiles indicate that TCAs more consistently improve behavioral symptoms—as rated by clinicians, teachers, and parents—than they affect cognitive function as measured through neuropsychological testing (Gualtieri and Evans 1988; P. O. Quinn and Rapoport 1975; Rapport et al. 1993; Werry 1980). Studies of TCAs have uniformly found a robust rate of response of ADHD symptoms in ADHD subjects with comorbid depression or anxiety (Biederman et al. 1993; Cox 1982; Wilens et al. 1993, 1995a). In addition, studies of TCAs have consistently found a robust rate of response in ADHD subjects with comorbid tic disorders (Dillon et al. 1985; Hoge and Biederman 1986; Riddle et al. 1988; Singer et al. 1994; Spencer et al. 1993a, 1993b). For example, in a controlled study, Spencer and colleagues (Spencer 1997) replicated data from a retrospective chart review indicating that desipramine has a robust beneficial effect on ADHD and tic symptoms. The potential benefits of TCAs in the treatment of ADHD have been clouded by safety concerns stemming from reports of sudden unexplained death in four ADHD children treated with desipramine ("Sudden Death in Children Treated With a Tricyclic Antidepressant" 1990), although the causal link between desipramine and these deaths remains uncertain.

The mixed dopaminergic/noradrenergic antidepressant bupropion was shown to be effective in treating ADHD in children in a controlled multisite study (N=72) (Casat et al. 1987, 1989; Conners et al. 1996) and in a comparison with methylphenidate (N=15) (Barrickman et al. 1995). In an open study involving adults with ADHD, sustained improvement was documented at 1 year at an average dose of 360 mg administered for 6–8 weeks (Wender and Reimherr 1990). In a recent double-blind, controlled clinical trial of bupropion in adults with ADHD, bupropion was found to be superior to placebo (Wilens et al. 1999c), with an effect size highly consistent with the effect sizes in the pediatric trials. Although bupropion has been associated with a slightly increased risk (0.4%) of drug-induced seizures relative to other antidepressants, this risk has been linked to high doses, a history of seizures, and eating disorders.

Although a small number of studies suggested that MAOIs may be effective in juvenile and adult ADHD, the potential for hypertensive crisis associated with use of irreversible MAOIs (e.g., phenelzine, tranylcypromine), with dietetic transgressions (con-

sumption of tyramine-containing foods [e.g., most cheeses]), and with drug interactions (interactions with pressor amines, most cold medicines, and amphetamines) seriously limits their use. The "cheese effect" might be obviated with reversible MAOIs such as moclobemide (not available in the United States), which has shown promise in one open trial (Trott et al. 1991, 1992). Although a single small, open study suggested that fluoxetine may be beneficial in the treatment of ADHD in children (Barrickman et al. 1991), the usefulness of SSRIs in the treatment of core ADHD symptoms is not supported by clinical experience ("Alternative Pharmacology of ADHD" 1996). Similarly uncertain is the usefulness of the mixed serotonergic/noradrenergic atypical antidepressant venlafaxine in the treatment of ADHD. Although a response rate of 77% was reported for subjects who completed treatment in four open studies involving 61 adults with ADHD, 21% of subjects dropped out because of side effects (Adler et al. 1995; Findling et al. 1996; Hornig-Rohan and Amsterdam 1995; Reimherr et al. 1995). Additionally, in a single open study of venlafaxine therapy in 16 children with ADHD, the response rate for subjects who completed therapy was 50%, and the rate of dropping out because of side effects (most prominently, increased hyperactivity) was 25% (Olvera et al. 1996).

Atomoxetine, a potent noradrenergic-specific reuptake inhibitor, has been studied in more than 1,800 children and more than 250 adults and has been submitted for FDA approval. Three acute, randomized, double-blind, placebo-controlled studies have been conducted: two involving children, and two involving children and adolescents (Michelson et al. 2001; Spencer et al. 2002). A total of 291 ADHD children, ages 7 through 13, were randomized in two trials (combined: atomoxetine therapy, n=129; placebo treatment, n=124; and methylphenidate therapy, n=38) (Spencer et al. 2002). The acute treatment period was 9 weeks. The stimulant-naive patients were randomized to double-blind treatment with atomoxetine (n=56), placebo (n=53), or methylphenidate (n=38). Patients with previous exposure to stimulants were randomized to double-blind treatment with atomoxetine (n=73) or placebo (n=71). Atomoxetine significantly reduced total scores on an investigator-rated DSM-IV ADHD rating scale. Response was defined as a ≥25% decrease in scores on the ADHD rating scale. Response rates were greater in the atomoxetine treatment group than in the placebo treatment group (61.4% vs. 32.3%,

$P<0.05$). In the stimulant-naive stratum, 69.1% of atomoxetine-treated patients, 73% of methylphenidate-treated patients, and 31.4% of placebo-treated patients were considered responders. Atomoxetine was well tolerated. Mild appetite suppression was reported in 22% of patients receiving atomoxetine, compared with 32% of methylphenidate-treated patients and 7% of placebo-treated patients. Less insomnia was associated with atomoxetine treatment than with methylphenidate treatment (7.0% vs. 27.0%, $P<0.05$). Mild increases in diastolic blood pressure and heart rate were noted in the atomoxetine treatment group, with no significant differences in electrocardiographic intervals or laboratory parameters between the atomoxetine and placebo treatment groups.

In an additional controlled study, 297 children and adolescents were randomized to different doses of atomoxetine or placebo for 8 weeks (Michelson et al. 2001). Atomoxetine was associated with a graded dose response: response was best at 1.2 or 1.8 mg/kg/day, poorer at 0.5 mg/kg/day, and poorer still with placebo. There was also a dose-dependent enhancement of social and family function. The Child Health Questionnaire was used to assess the well-being of the child and the family. Parents of children taking atomoxetine reported fewer emotional difficulties and behavioral problems, as well as greater self-esteem, in their children and less emotional worry and fewer limitations on their personal time in themselves.

Safety and efficacy data were evaluated in a yearlong, open follow-up study involving atomoxetine-treated children and adolescents ($N=325$) (Kratochvil et al. 2001). Atomoxetine treatment continued to be effective and well tolerated. The acute mild increases in diastolic blood pressure and heart rate persisted without a change in severity. Growth in height and weight were normal, and there were no significant differences between atomoxetine and placebo treatment groups in laboratory parameters and electrocardiographic intervals.

Despite its wide use in children with ADHD, only four studies ($N=122$ children; two studies were controlled) have supported the efficacy of clonidine (Gunning 1992; Hunt 1987; Hunt et al. 1985; Steingard et al. 1993). Clonidine appears to have mostly behavioral effects on disinhibited and agitated youth; the drug has limited effect on cognition. Several cases of sudden death have been reported in children treated with clonidine plus methylphenidate, raising concerns

about the safety of this combination (see "Clonidine") (Wilens et al. 1999d).

Only three small open studies of guanfacine in children and adolescents with ADHD have been conducted (Chappell et al. 1995; Horrigan and Barnhill 1995; Hunt et al. 1995). In these studies, beneficial effects on hyperactive behaviors and attentional abilities were noted.

Use of β-adrenergic blockers in ADHD has also been studied. An open study of propranolol in ADHD adults with temper outbursts found improvement at daily doses of up to 640 mg (Mattes 1986). Another report indicated that β-blockers may be helpful in combination with stimulants (Ratey et al. 1991). In a controlled study of pindolol in 52 children with ADHD, symptoms of behavioral dyscontrol and hyperactivity were improved, with less apparent cognitive benefit (Buitelaar et al. 1996). However, prominent adverse effects such as nightmares and paresthesias led to discontinuation of the drug in all test subjects. An open study of nadolol in aggressive, developmentally delayed children with ADHD symptoms found effective diminution of aggression, with little apparent effect on ADHD symptoms (Connor et al. 1997).

In an open study involving 12 ADHD children, the nonbenzodiazepine anxiolytic buspirone, administered at 0.5 mg/kg/day, improved both ADHD symptoms and psychosocial function in ADHD youths (Malhotra and Santosh 1998). Buspirone has a high affinity for 5-HT$_{1A}$ receptors, both pre- and postsynaptic, as well as a modest effect on the dopaminergic system and α-adrenergic activity. However, in a recent multisite, controlled clinical trial involving a large number of children with ADHD, the response to transdermal buspirone was not different from the response to placebo (Bristol-Myers Squibb, unpublished data, June 1996). Although old literature suggested that typical antipsychotics are effective in the treatment of children with ADHD, the drugs' short-term (extrapyramidal reactions) and long-term (tardive dyskinesia) adverse effects greatly limit their usefulness. More recently, a meta-analysis of data from 10 studies provided preliminary evidence that carbamazepine may have activity in ADHD (Silva et al. 1996).

Evidence has emerged that nicotinic dysregulation may contribute to the pathophysiology of ADHD. This is not surprising, given that nicotinic activation enhances dopaminergic neurotransmission (Mereu et al. 1987; Westfall et al. 1983). Independent lines of investigation have demonstrated that ADHD is associated with an increased risk and earlier age at onset for cigarette smoking (Milberger et al. 1997; Pomerleau et al. 1996); that maternal smoking during pregnancy increases the risk of ADHD in the offspring (Milberger et al. 1996); and that in animals, in utero exposure to nicotine confers a heightened risk of an ADHD-like syndrome in the newborn (Fung 1988; Fung and Lau 1989; Johns et al. 1982). In subjects without ADHD, central nicotinic activation has been shown to improve temporal memory (Meck and Church 1987), attention (Jones et al. 1992; Peeke and Peeke 1984; Wesnes and Warburton 1984), cognitive vigilance (Jones et al. 1992; Parrott and Winder 1989; Wesnes and Warburton 1984), and executive function (Wesnes and Warburton 1984).

Support for a "nicotinic hypothesis" for ADHD is derived from a study of the therapeutic effects of nicotine in adults with ADHD (Levin et al. 1996). Although this controlled clinical trial found that use of a commercially available transdermal nicotine patch significantly improved ADHD symptoms, working memory, and neuropsychological functioning (Levin et al. 1996), the trial was short (2 days long) and included only a handful of patients. The usefulness of nicotinic drugs in ADHD was more substantially demonstrated in a recent controlled clinical trial of ABT-418 in adults with ADHD (Wilens et al. 1999b). ABT-418 is a CNS cholinergic nicotinic activating agent that is structurally similar to nicotine. Phase 1 studies of this compound in humans indicated its low abuse liability, as well as adequate safety and tolerability in elderly adults (Abbott Laboratories, unpublished data, June 1998). In a double-blind, placebo-controlled, randomized, crossover trial comparing a transdermal patch of ABT-418 (75 mg daily) and placebo in adults with a DSM-IV diagnosis of ADHD, a significantly higher proportion of ADHD adults were much improved while receiving ABT-418 than while receiving placebo (40% vs. 13%; $\chi^2=5.3$, $P=0.021$) (Wilens 1999b). Although preliminary, these results suggest that nicotinic analogues may have activity in ADHD.

Several other compounds have been evaluated and found to be ineffective in the treatment of ADHD; they include dopamine agonists (amantadine and L-dopa) (Gittelman-Klein 1987) and amino acid precursors (DL-phenylalanine and L-tyrosine) (Reimherr et al. 1987). In addition, a controlled study of the antiserotonergic, anorectic drug fenfluramine failed to find therapeutic benefits in patients with ADHD (Donnelly et al. 1989).

■ Other Disruptive Behavior Disorders: Conduct Disorder (Table 50–8) and Oppositional Defiant Disorder

In DSM-IV-TR, conduct disorder is conceptualized as a childhood-onset disorder characterized by antisocial and aggressive behaviors. Children with CD are at high risk of developing adult antisocial personality disorder and substance use disorders. Oppositional defiant disorder (ODD) is characterized by oppositional and obstinate behaviors. Although very taxing to families, ODD does not share CD's serious adult outcome. There is no specific pharmacotherapy for CD or ODD, but several controlled investigations have found mood stabilizers and antipsychotics to be effective in reducing aggression and explosiveness (but not sociopathy) in children with CD (Campbell et al. 1992; Platt et al. 1984). These findings are consistent with mounting evidence linking some forms of CD and ODD with bipolar and nonbipolar mood disorders (hence "dysphoric") (Biederman et al. 1999a; Frazier et al. 1999). Studies have also shown a significant decrease in aggressive behaviors with the use of behavioral management techniques, whether focused on the child's coping skills or the parents' management skills (Greene 1998; Quay 1986). When CD or ODD occurs with ADHD, mood disorders, or anxiety disorders, treatment of the comorbid disorder can result in substantial clinical stabilization and facilitate psychosocial treatment of CD or ODD.

■ Tic Disorders (Table 50–9)

Tic disorders are common and may occur in 5%–10% of children. The best known of these disorders is Tourette's disorder, a rare but more severe neuropsychiatric syndrome of childhood onset and lifelong duration that consists of multiform motor and phonic tics and associated behavioral and psychological symptoms. Affected patients commonly have spontaneous waxing, waning, and symptomatic fluctuation. Tourette's disorder is commonly associated with ADHD (in about 50% of cases) and OCD (in about 30% of cases) (Pauls et al. 1986). In many cases, the comorbid disorder, rather than the tic disorder, is the major source of distress and disability. The association with ADHD is particularly problematic because ADHD appears earlier in life than the tics and because the use of stimulants may be detrimental in some cases.

The noradrenergic modulators clonidine (Leck-

Table 50–9. Pharmacotherapy for tic disorders

Disorder	Main characteristics	Pharmacotherapy
Tourette's disorder	• Multiple motor tics and one or more vocal tics • Frequently associated with ADHD or obsessive-compulsive disorder	*First-line* • Treatment unclear • Atypical (blocking dopamine D_2 receptors) and typical antipsychotics • α-Adrenergic agents • TCAs *Second-line* • High-potency benzodiazepines • β-Blockers • Cholinergic agents • Combined pharmacotherapy for treatment-resistant cases

Note. ADHD = attention-deficit/hyperactivity disorder; TCA = tricyclic antidepressant.

man et al. 1991) and guanfacine (Chappell et al. 1995) have proven effective in some children with Tourette's disorder. For severe or treatment-resistant conditions, antipsychotic drugs—particularly haloperidol, pimozide, and, more recently, risperidone (Lombroso et al. 1995)—appear to be the most effective medications. However, antipsychotics have limited effects on the frequently associated comorbid disorders, and the drugs carry a risk of development of tardive dyskinesia when they are administered chronically (Riddle et al. 1987). In addition, clonazepam, β-blockers, nortriptyline, and desipramine (Singer et al. 1994; Spencer 1997) have been reported to be helpful in some children with Tourette's disorder. Clonidine, guanfacine, and TCAs may be particularly helpful in patients with Tourette's disorder and ADHD. Patients with comorbid OCD may need additional pharmacotherapy, in the form of serotonergically active drugs such as clomipramine or SSRIs.

■ Childhood Anxiety Disorders (Table 50–10)

The category of childhood anxiety disorders includes a subclass of disorders in which anxiety that is not due to psychosocial stressors is the predominant feature. In addition to separation anxiety disorder and selective mutism, the family of anxiety disorders affecting the young also includes panic disorder, agoraphobia (Biederman 1990; Leonard and Rapoport 1989), social and specific phobias, generalized anxiety disorder, OCD, posttraumatic stress disorder, and the atypical anxiety disorders termed *anxiety disorders not otherwise specified*. This continuity of adult- and childhood-onset

anxiety disorders is recognized in DSM-IV-TR; disorders formerly coded as childhood disorders (overanxious disorder and avoidant disorder) are now subsumed under the corresponding adult diagnoses (generalized anxiety and social phobia, respectively).

Although childhood anxiety disorders are common disorders that bear striking similarities to the adult anxiety disorders and in many cases persist into adult life, not much is known about their treatment, with the notable exception of treatment of OCD. TCAs and MAOIs can be effective in the treatment of anxiety disorders, but their adverse-effect profiles, multiple drug–drug interaction problems, and narrow margins of safety, as well as the dietetic restrictions of MAOIs, make these compounds less desirable for use in management of anxiety disorders in youths. Similarly, although the high-potency benzodiazepines clonazepam, lorazepam, and alprazolam are important therapeutic agents in the management of anxiety disorders (Bernstein et al. 1987; Biederman 1987), their sedative properties, their potential for addiction and misuse, and their potential for negative cognitive adverse effects make them less desirable agents in the management of pediatric anxiety disorders. Of the high-potency benzodiazepines, clonazepam may be particularly useful in the treatment of children and adolescent patients, because of the drug's high potency and long duration of action. Although it has not been tested in youth, the nonbenzodiazepine anxiolytic buspirone may also have a role to play in the management of some forms of juvenile anxiety disorders.

Several controlled clinical trials have clearly demonstrated that the serotonergic-specific antidepressants

Table 50–10. Pharmacotherapy for anxiety disorders

Disorder	Main characteristics	Pharmacotherapy
Separation anxiety disorder	• Excessive anxiety on separation from caretakers or familial surroundings • Inability to separate from the parent or from major attachment figures	*First-line* • SSRIs (particularly when MD is present) • Atypical antidepressants (serotonergic)
Selective mutism	• Similar to agoraphobia • Persistent failure to speak in specific social situations • Similar to social phobia	*Second-line* • Benzodiazepines
Panic disorder (with or without agoraphobia)	• Recurrent discrete periods of intense fear (panic attacks) • Frequent comorbidity with MD (50%) and ADHD (30%)	*Third-line* • Buspirone for mild anxiety • Combined pharmacotherapy for refractory illness or patients with comorbid diagnoses (e.g., ADHD)
Agoraphobia	• Fear of being in places or situations with limited escape possibilities (e.g., school); because of this fear, adolescent restricts travel or needs a companion or caretaker when away from home	
Social phobia	• Fear of social situations in which individual may be exposed to scrutiny or endure humiliation	
Generalized anxiety disorder	• Excessive or unrealistic worry about future events	
Adjustment disorder with anxiety (severe)	• Maladaptive short-term reaction to a severe stressor	
Obsessive-compulsive disorder	• Recurrent, severe, and distressing obsession and/or compulsion	• SSRIs, clomipramine • Combined pharmacotherapy for refractory illness or patients with comorbid diagnoses (e.g., MD, ADHD, psychosis)

Note. ADHD = attention-deficit/hyperactivity disorder; MD = major depression; SSRI = selective serotonin reuptake inhibitor.

clomipramine, sertraline, and fluvoxamine are superior to placebo in the treatment of juvenile OCD, and the responses achieved in those studies were strikingly similar to documented responses in adults with this disorder. Because of the findings of these investigations, use of clomipramine, sertraline, and fluvoxamine in pediatric OCD has FDA approval. Although not yet tested in children and adolescents, the serotonergic antidepressants have been found to be superior to placebo in the treatment of panic disorder and agoraphobia in adults, and paroxetine and venlafaxine have been found to be superior to placebo in the treatment of social phobia and generalized anxiety disorder in adults. Thus, serotonergic antidepressants may play a similarly beneficial therapeutic role in the treatment of pediatric forms of generalized anxiety disorder, social phobia, panic disorder, agoraphobia, and perhaps posttraumatic stress disorder. Because of their favorable adverse-effect profiles and large margins of safety, serotonergic antidepressants should be considered first-line agents in the treatment of anxiety disorders.

■ Mood Disorders (Table 50–11)

Depressive Disorders

Pediatric depression is recognized in DSM-IV-TR as a family of conditions with core symptoms similar to those found in adult depression. In DSM-IV-TR, major (major depression), minor (dysthymic disorder), and atypical (depression not otherwise specified) forms of depression are recognized as affecting the young. Core features of depression in youths include a sad or irritable mood, a persistent loss of interest or pleasure in favorite activities, physiological disturbances such as changes in appetite and weight, abnormal sleep patterns, psychomotor abnormalities, fatigue, diminished ability to think and concentrate, feelings of worthlessness or guilt, and suicidal preoccupation. Also recognized in DSM-IV-TR are developmentally specific associated features in depression affecting youth, including academic difficulties, school refusal, negativism, aggression, and antisocial behavior. In addition, emerging evidence indicates that depression in youths may have unique features, compared with adult depression, that can complicate its identification. These include dysphoria and irritability as predominant mood disturbances, rather than sadness and melancholia (Biederman et al. 1995a); "mood reactivity" as

seen in atypical forms of adult depression (Nierenberg et al. 1998); insidious onset and a chronic course rather than acuteness and an episodic course (Biederman et al. 1995a; Kovacs et al. 1984); male preponderance or equal gender representation (Angold and Costello 1993), rather than female preponderance; and an increased personal and familial risk of bipolar disorder (B. Geller et al. 1994). In addition, pediatric depression is characterized by a much larger spectrum of comorbidity than is seen in adult depression (Angold and Costello 1993; Biederman et al. 1995a); comorbid conditions in juvenile patients with depression include not only anxiety disorders but also ADHD, CD, and ODD (Angold and Costello 1993; Biederman et al. 1995a, 1996).

Controlled clinical trials failed to document efficacy for TCAs in pediatric depression (Bostic et al. 1999). In contrast, a number of studies have obtained more promising results with SSRIs. In a controlled study, Emslie and colleagues (1997) found that improvement with fluoxetine (in 57% of subjects) was significantly superior to placebo (33%) in a sample of nearly 100 depressed youths. Important features of this study were that 1) children with comorbid ADHD were not excluded as in previous investigations and 2) both children and adolescents were included. A very large multisite trial of paroxetine in 275 adolescents with depression also found that although paroxetine (improvement in 66%) was superior to placebo (43%), imipramine (57%) was not (Wagner et al. 1998). Furthermore, 32% of subjects receiving imipramine dropped out of the study because of adverse events, compared with 10% of the paroxetine treatment group and 7% of the placebo treatment group (P<0.05). Finally, in a recent open but prospective trial of sertraline in a sample of depressed adolescents, there was a positive response to sertraline therapy (Ambrosini et al. 1999). These studies, plus the more advantageous adverse-effect profiles and large margins of safety of these compounds, suggest that SSRIs should be considered first-line agents in the treatment of depression in the young.

Pediatric Mania

There is emerging evidence that children not only have unipolar depressions but also develop mania. Recent studies have begun to challenge the long-held notion that mania is nonexistent or rare in children. In fact, a recent report documented that mania was

Table 50–11. Pharmacotherapy for mood disorders

Disorder	Main characteristics	Pharmacotherapy
Major depression	• Sad or irritable mood and associated cognitive, psychological, and vegetative symptoms occurring together for a time	*First-line* • SSRIs *Second-line* • Atypical antidepressants (serotonergic) *Third-line* • TCAs • Combined pharmacotherapy for refractory illness or patients with comorbid diagnoses (e.g., ADHD) • ECT for refractory illness
Bipolar disorder		
Manic	• Elevated or severely irritable or angry mood with or without associated psychotic symptoms • Often violent • Frequent comorbidity with conduct disorder • Very dysfunctional	• Atypical antipsychotics (risk of weight gain and hyperprolactinemia necessitate monitoring) • Mood stabilizers (lithium, oxcarbazepine, carbamazepine, valproic acid, atypical AEDs) • Combined therapy for refractory illness (i.e., atypical antipsychotics+mood stabilizers) • ECT for refractory illness
Depressed	• Potential for worsening of mania or induction of rapid cycling	• Antidepressants that may be less likely to induce mania: bupropion, paroxetine, nefazodone, mirtazapine
Mixed	• Mixed depressive and manic symptoms • Most common presentation of bipolar disorder in juvenile patients • Very severe clinical picture	• Atypical antipsychotics and/or mood stabilizers+antidepressants

Note. ADHD = attention-deficit/hyperactivity disorder; AED = antiepileptic drug; ECT = electroconvulsive therapy; SSRI = selective serotonin reuptake inhibitor; TCA = tricyclic antidepressant.

diagnosed in 15% of preadolescents referred to a pediatric psychopharmacology clinic (Wozniak et al. 1995), indicating that mania may be far more common than previously thought. When diagnosed, mania was characterized by extreme and persistent irritability and explosiveness, a mixed presentation (symptoms of mania and depression, dysphoric mania), and a chronic course (Wozniak et al. 1995). In addition, a high degree of comorbidity (ADHD, CD, anxiety disorders, and psychosis) characterized these manic children.

Because of the misguided assumption that juvenile mania does not exist, there is a paucity of information on pharmacological treatment of the condition. Although mood stabilizers (lithium, carbamazepine, valproic acid) are generally considered the mainstays of treatment for adult bipolar disorders, their therapeutic role is less certain in pediatric mania. A recent systematic review of records of youths with mania con-

firmed that mood stabilizers are selectively associated with improvement of manic symptoms, but their beneficial effects were exceedingly slow to unfold, and children who improved rapidly deteriorated (Biederman et al. 1998a). In contrast, a systematic exploration of the effectiveness of the atypical antipsychotic risperidone revealed that this compound had a more effective, rapid, and sustained response in pediatric mania than previously observed with mood stabilizers (Frazier et al. 1999). A particularly thorny issue in the treatment of youths with bipolar disorders is the management of comorbid ADHD, which is very prevalent in children with juvenile mania (Biederman et al. 1998b). In a recent report, we documented that in the treatment of patients who have bipolar disorder and ADHD, mood stabilization must precede attempts to treat ADHD (Biederman et al. 1999b). Children with active manic symptoms failed to respond to anti-

ADHD treatments until mood was stable. Because bipolar disorder with or without comorbid disorders (depression, ADHD) must commonly be treated aggressively, with several therapeutic agents targeting the various comorbid disorders, special attention should be given to potential drug–drug interactions.

■ Psychotic Disorders (Table 50–12)

The term *psychosis* is used in DSM-IV to describe abnormal behaviors of individuals with grossly impaired reality testing. The term is also used when the individual's behavior is grossly disorganized and it can be inferred that reality testing is impaired. A diagnosis of psychosis involves the presence of either delusions, false implausible beliefs, or hallucinations (false perceptions that may be visual, auditory, or tactile). Psychotic disorders in children, as in adults, can be functional or organic. Functional psychotic syndromes include schizophrenia and related disorders and the psychotic forms of mood disorders. Organic psychosis can develop as a result of lesions in the CNS as a consequence of medical illnesses, trauma, or drug use, both licit and illicit.

The early literature on childhood schizophrenia overlapped with that on autism, and hallucinations or delusions were not requirements (McClellan and Werry 1994). Beginning with DSM-III (American Psychiatric Association 1980), the criteria for childhood- and adult-onset schizophrenia were identical, and psychotic symptoms became the hallmark of the disorder. In DSM-IV-TR, a diagnosis of schizophrenia now involves a 1-month period of two symptoms (or a single symptom, if very bizarre) such as delusions, hallucinations, disorganized speech or behavior, or negative symptoms. It continues to be a problem to distinguish, in children, true psychotic phenomena from nonpsychotic idiosyncratic thinking and perceptions caused by developmental delays or language disorders. However, psychotic features such as hallucinations and delusions are required for a diagnosis of schizophrenia to be made, and these features are usually associated with a marked change in mental status and lowered level of function (McClellan and Werry 1994).

Antipsychotics are indicated in the treatment of childhood psychotic disorders. Positive symptoms are the target symptoms most likely to respond to antipsychotics. These symptoms include hallucinations,

delusions, formal thought disorder (incoherence), catatonic symptoms (stupor, negativism, rigidity, excitement, and posturing), and bizarre affect. In contrast, negative symptoms include affective blunting, poverty of speech and thought, apathy, anhedonia, and poor social functioning. Negative symptoms are associated with 1) insidious onset, positive premorbid history, and chronic deterioration and 2) atrophy as shown by computed tomography, abnormalities indicated by neuropsychological testing, and poor response to or worsening during treatment with typical antipsychotics. The atypical antipsychotics clozapine and risperidone appear to be more effective agents for negative symptoms.

When the psychotic process occurs in the context of a mood disorder, concomitant use of specific treatments for mood disorders is crucial for clinical stabilization. When psychosis is associated with severe agitation, adjunctive use of high-potency benzodiazepines, such as lorazepam or clonazepam, can facilitate management of the patient and may lead to use of lower doses of antipsychotics. The extent to which antiparkinsonian agents should be used prophylactically when antipsychotics are introduced is controversial. Whenever possible, use of antiparkinsonian agents should be reserved until extrapyramidal symptoms emerge. Extrapyramidal reactions can be prevented in many cases by avoiding rapid increase in neuroleptic dose or the use of high-potency typical antipsychotics such as haloperidol. When a child or adolescent taking antipsychotics develops an acutely agitated clinical picture with associated inability to sit still and aggressive outbursts, akathisia should be rapidly considered in the differential diagnosis. If akathisia is suspected, the dose of the antipsychotic may need to be decreased. β-Blockers (e.g., propranolol) and high-potency benzodiazepines have been found helpful in relieving symptoms of antipsychotic-induced akathisia in adults and may help relieve similar symptoms in juvenile patients (Ananth and Lin 1986).

In recent years, postpsychotic depression has received increasing attention. Initial trials of antidepressant drugs added to the antipsychotic treatment appear to be promising in terms of elimination of associated depression, thus fostering rehabilitation efforts. Postpsychotic depression should be distinguished from akinesia, an adverse extrapyramidal effect that may respond to treatment with antiparkinsonian agents.

Table 50–12. Pharmacotherapy for psychotic disorders

Disorder	Main characteristics	Pharmacotherapy
Psychotic disorders	• Delusions and hallucinations • Negative symptoms	• Atypical antipsychotics (risk of weight gain and hyperprolactinemia necessitate monitoring) • Typical antipsychotics (risk of tardive dyskinesia) • Combined therapy for treatment-resistant cases • Clozapine for treatment-resistant cases

Developmental Disorders (Table 50–13)

In DSM-IV-TR, the developmental disorders are mental retardation (Axis II), pervasive developmental disorders (autistic and autistic-like disorders), and learning disorders. Autism is discussed in detail in Chapter 20 in this volume ("Autistic Disorder"). No specific treatment alters the natural history of this disorder. The learning disorders represent a mixed group of cognitive dysfunctions in the context of no overall intelligence deficit and adequate educational opportunities.

Children with mental retardation or pervasive developmental disorders often have other psychiatric disorders and behavioral problems, including hyperactive, aggressive, distractible, and self-abusive behaviors. They also often manifest multiple neurological abnormalities. Psychotropics are primarily used in this population for the treatment of agitation, aggression, and self-injurious behaviors. Antipsychotics have been commonly used to control these symptoms. In recent years, the atypical antipsychotics have been used in the management of affective dysregulation, manic-like symptoms, and aggressive symptoms in this population. β-Blockers and clonidine have also been used in the management of aggression and dyscontrol in patients with developmental disorders.

Antidepressant drugs and antimanic agents can also be effective in controlling mood dysregulation of the bipolar and nonbipolar types, and stimulants may improve symptoms of ADHD in children and adolescents with mental retardation or pervasive developmental disorders. With the increasing popularity of serotonergic-specific drugs in recent years, there has been rising interest in their use in patients with pervasive developmental disorders. This interest stems in part from the hypothesis linking repetitive stereotypical behaviors in these patients to OCD shown to be responsive to serotonergic-specific drugs. Gordon et al. (1993) reported results of a controlled clinical trial evaluating the efficacy and tolerability of the serotonergic TCA clomipramine, the noradrenergic tricyclic desipramine, and placebo in patients with pervasive developmental disorders. They found that clomipramine was superior to placebo and desipramine in terms of ratings of autistic symptoms including stereotypies, anger, and compulsive ritualized behaviors. However, clomipramine and desipramine were equally effective in controlling symptoms of hyperactivity in this group.

Antianxiety agents should be used with caution in children with developmental disorders because these drugs tend to produce disinhibition, which may result in increased restlessness and more disturbed behavior. The anorectic drug fenfluramine has been reported to have beneficial effects in some children with autism; however, more recent studies obtained equivocal results (Aman and Kern 1989; Campbell et al. 1988a). An open study found that use of the nonbenzodiazepine antianxiety drug buspirone was associated with reduced aggression and hyperactivity in four autistic children (Realmuto et al. 1989). In an open study, Campbell et al. (1988b) evaluated the efficacy and safety of naltrexone, a potent and long-acting opioid antagonist, in the treatment of autistic children; daily doses of 1–2 mg/kg were administered. In this open trial, naltrexone was associated with improvement in social and language behaviors and was well tolerated.

The treatment of learning disorders is largely remedial and supportive. Psychotropics have not been effective in altering the basic course of the disorder. Children with learning disabilities and ADHD or major depression can benefit from treatments directed at the associated psychiatric disorder.

Children with functional enuresis usually respond to nonpharmacological therapies (e.g., behavior modification, psychotherapy), and these treatments should

Table 50–13. Pharmacotherapy for developmental disorders

Disorder	Main characteristics	Pharmacotherapy
Mental retardation (MR)	• Significant subaverage global intellectual functioning and deficits in adaptive functioning	• No specific pharmacotherapy for core disorder • Nonspecific treatment for aggression and self-abuse: β-blockers (e.g., propranolol), α-adrenergic agents, antimanic agents, opioid antagonist (naltrexone), typical and atypical antipsychotics • SSRIs for OCD-like repetitive behaviors • MR in conjunction with Axis I disorders (e.g., ADHD, mania, psychosis, anxiety): treat underlying disorder
Pervasive developmental disorders (PDDs)	• Qualitative impairment of social interactions and acquisition of cognitive, language, and motor skills • Can be global or exist in specific or multiple areas	• Same as for MR
Specific developmental disorders (learning disabilities)	• Inadequate development of specific academic, language, and motor skills that is not due to physical or neurological disorders, PDDs, or deficient educational opportunities	• No specific pharmacotherapy for core disorder • Remedial help and special education remain main treatments • Specific developmental disorders in conjunction with other Axis I disorders (e.g., ADHD, major depression, anxiety): treat underlying disorders
Enuresis	• Bed-wetting	• Behavior therapy • DDAVP (Desmopressin) • TCAs (low doses)

Note. ADHD=attention-deficit/hyperactivity disorder; DDAVP=1-desamino-8-D-arginine-vasopressin; OCD=obsessive-compulsive disorder; SSRI=selective serotonin reuptake inhibitor; TCA=tricyclic antidepressant.

be considered first. When an immediate therapeutic effect is necessary, an antidepressant drug, commonly imipramine, may be used. In most cases, symptoms reappear after the drug is withdrawn. Antidepressant therapy should not be continued for more than 6 months, because enuresis may remit spontaneously. In addition, the FDA has approved the use of the synthetic antidiuretic hormone desmopressin for the treatment of enuresis.

Combined Therapy

Although in clinical practice, many juvenile patients receive multiple treatments, the literature on combined pharmacotherapy is sparse and thus does not permit development of clear therapeutic guidelines. In contrast to polypharmacy, rational combined pharmacological approaches can be used for the treatment of psychiatric comorbidity, as augmentation strategies for patients with insufficient response to a single agent, and for the management of treatment-emergent adverse effects. Examples of the rational use of combined treatment include the use of an antidepressant plus a stimulant for ADHD and comorbid depression, the use of clonidine to ameliorate stimulant-induced insomnia, and the use of lithium plus an anti-ADHD agent to treat ADHD occurring with bipolar disorder (Wilens et al. 1995b). All psychotropics except lithium are metabolized by the P450 system. When multiple medications are used, there must be monitoring for drug–drug interactions, with careful evaluation of adverse effects and serum levels.

The hepatic P450 system consists of more than 40 enzymes that metabolize psychotropics and similar compounds. Because of genetic polymorphism, 5%–10% of Caucasians have innate deficiencies in this metabolic capacity and thus are slow metabolizers. Likewise, 5%–10% of Caucasians have duplicate copies and are extensive (rapid) metabolizers (DeVane 1998; Greenblatt et al. 1998; Nemeroff et al. 1996). Efficiency of these enzymes can be affected by competing substrates or by inhibition or enhancement (induction) by exogenous compounds, which often leads to drug–drug interactions in which serum levels of psychotropics are dramatically increased (or decreased).

The P450 enzyme 1A2 is involved in the demethylation of tertiary TCAs to secondary TCAs and is inhibited by fluvoxamine. 2C19 is involved in the demethylation of tertiary TCAs and biotransformation of diazepam and is inhibited by fluoxetine, sertraline, and fluvoxamine. 2D6 is involved in the hydroxylation of secondary TCAs (desipramine and nortriptyline) (Preskorn et al. 1994) and is affected by paroxetine, fluoxetine, and sertraline, with a lesser effect of nefazodone; thus, coadministration of these SSRIs and TCAs results in increased levels of the TCAs. In addition, 2D6 is involved in the metabolism of antipsychotics (haloperidol, thioridazine, perphenazine, clozapine, risperidone) and hydroxylation of β-blockers; thus, serum levels could be affected if any of the following are coadministered: an antipsychotic, β-blocker, TCA, or SSRI (paroxetine, fluoxetine, sertraline). 3A4 is involved in the demethylation of tertiary TCAs and biotransformation of benzodiazepines (triazolam, alprazolam, midazolam, carbamazepine), and the nonsedating antihistamine loratadine (Claritin) is affected by fluvoxamine, nefazodone, and, to a lesser degree, fluoxetine and sertraline (DeVane 1998; Greenblatt et al. 1998; Nemeroff et al. 1996). Citalopram, venlafaxine, and mirtazapine minimally inhibit P450 enzymes. Similarly, there is little drug–drug interaction between lithium and TCAs or SSRIs, or between stimulants and antidepressants (Cohen et al. 1999).

Conclusion

Although the origins of pediatric psychopharmacology date from more than 50 years ago, the long-term outlook for pediatric psychopharmacology is dependent on careful clinical applications and future re-search. It is essential to apply a careful differential diagnostic assessment that considers psychiatric, social, cognitive, educational, and medical or neurological factors, all of which may contribute to the child's clinical presentation. It is therefore also essential to consider the use of pharmacotherapy as part of a broader treatment plan that encompasses all aspects of a child's life. Major ingredients of a successful pharmacological intervention include realistic expectations regarding the intervention, careful definition of target symptoms, and careful assessment of the potential risks and benefits of this type of intervention for psychiatrically disturbed children. The lack of FDA approval for pediatric use of many of the medications, although it imposes a restriction on general use, does permit the careful introduction of innovative therapy. It is to be hoped that an increasing number of referral centers will explore the appropriate use of psychopharmacological agents in pediatric psychiatry through high-quality research protocols.

References

Adler LA, Resnick S, Kunz M, et al: Open-label trial of venlafaxine in adults with attention deficit disorder. Psychopharmacol Bull 31:785–788, 1995

Alderman J, Wolkow R, Chung M, et al: Sertraline treatment of children and adolescents with obsessive-compulsive disorder or depression: pharmacokinetics, tolerability, and efficacy. J Am Acad Child Adolesc Psychiatry 37:386–394, 1998

Alessi N, Naylor M, Ghaziuddin M, et al: Update on lithium carbonate therapy in children and adolescents. J Am Acad Child Adolesc Psychiatry 33:291–304, 1994

Alternative Pharmacology of ADHD (NIMH Report). Rockville, MD, National Institute of Mental Health, 1996

Aman MG, Kern RA: Review of fenfluramine in the treatment of the developmental disabilities. J Am Acad Child Adolesc Psychiatry 28:549–565, 1989

Ambrosini PJ, Wagner KD, Biederman J, et al: Multicenter open-label sertraline study in adolescent outpatients with major depression. J Am Acad Child Adolesc Psychiatry 38:566–572, 1999

American Psychiatric Association: Diagnostic and Statistical Manual of Mental Disorders, 3rd Edition. Washington, DC, American Psychiatric Association, 1980

American Psychiatric Association: Diagnostic and Statistical Manual of Mental Disorders, 4th Edition, Text Revision. Washington, DC, American Psychiatric Association, 2000

Ananth H, Lin K: Propranolol in psychiatry. Neuropsychobiology 15:20–27, 1986

Angold A, Costello EJ: Depressive comorbidity in children and adolescents: empirical, theoretical and methodological issues. Am J Psychiatry 150:1779–1791, 1993

Barkley RA: A review of stimulant drug research with hyperactive children. J Child Psychol Psychiatry 18:137–165, 1977

Barrickman L, Noyes R, Kuperman S, et al: Treatment of ADHD with fluoxetine: a preliminary trial. J Am Acad Child Adolesc Psychiatry 30:762–767, 1991

Barrickman L, Perry P, Allen A, et al: Bupropion versus methylphenidate in the treatment of attention-deficit hyperactivity disorder. J Am Acad Child Adolesc Psychiatry 34:649–657, 1995

Bergman A, Winters L, Cornblatt B: Methylphenidate: effects on sustained attention, in Ritalin: Theory and Patient Management. Edited by Greenhill L, Osman B. New York, Mary Ann Liebert, 1991, pp 223–231

Bernstein GA, Garfinkel B, Borchart C: Imipramine versus alprazolam for school phobia. Paper presented at the annual meeting of the American Academy of Child and Adolescent Psychiatry, Washington, DC, October 1987

Biederman J: Clonazepam in the treatment of prepubertal children with panic-like symptoms. J Clin Psychiatry 48:38–41, 1987

Biederman J: The diagnosis and treatment of adolescent anxiety disorders. J Clin Psychiatry 51:20–26, 1990

Biederman J, Gastfriend DR, Jellinek MS: Desipramine in the treatment of children with attention deficit disorder. J Clin Psychopharmacol 6:359–363, 1986

Biederman J, Baldessarini RJ, Wright V, et al: A double-blind placebo-controlled study of desipramine in the treatment of attention deficit disorder, I: efficacy. J Am Acad Child Adolesc Psychiatry 28:777–784, 1989a

Biederman J, Baldessarini RJ, Wright V, et al: A double-blind placebo-controlled study of desipramine in the treatment of attention deficit disorder, II: serum drug levels and cardiovascular findings. J Am Acad Child Adolesc Psychiatry 28:903–911, 1989b

Biederman J, Baldessarini RJ, Wright V, et al: A double-blind placebo controlled study of desipramine in the treatment of ADD, III: lack of impact of comorbidity and family history factors on clinical response. J Am Acad Child Adolesc Psychiatry 32:199–204, 1993

Biederman J, Faraone S, Mick E, et al: Psychiatric comorbidity among referred juveniles with major depression: fact or artifact? J Am Acad Child Adolesc Psychiatry 34:579–590, 1995a

Biederman J, Thisted R, Greenhill L, et al: Estimation of the association between desipramine and the risk for sudden death in 5- to 14-year-old children. J Clin Psychiatry 56:87–93, 1995b

Biederman J, Wilens T, Mick E, et al: Psychoactive substance use disorder in adults with attention deficit hyperactivity disorder: effects of ADHD and psychiatric comorbidity. Am J Psychiatry 152:1652–1658, 1995c

Biederman J, Faraone SV, Mick E, et al: Child behavior checklist (CBCL) findings further support comorbidity between ADHD and major depression in a referred sample. J Am Acad Child Adolesc Psychiatry 35:734–742, 1996

Biederman J, Mick E, Bostic J, et al: The naturalistic course of pharmacologic treatment of children with manic-like symptoms: a systematic chart review. J Clin Psychiatry 59:628–637, 1998a

Biederman J, Russell R, Soriano J, et al: Clinical features of children with both ADHD and mania: does ascertainment source make a difference? J Affect Disord 51:101–112, 1998b

Biederman J, Faraone S, Chu M, et al: Further evidence of a bidirectional overlap between juvenile mania and conduct disorder in children. J Am Acad Child Adolesc Psychiatry 38:468–476, 1999a

Biederman J, Mick E, Prince J, et al: Systematic chart review of the pharmacologic treatment of comorbid attention deficit hyperactivity disorder in youth with bipolar disorder. J Child Adolesc Psychopharmacol 9:247–256, 1999b

Biederman J, Wilens T, Mick E, et al: Pharmacotherapy of attention-deficit/hyperactivity disorder reduces risk for substance use disorder. Pediatrics (serial online) 104:20, 1999c. Available at: http://www.pediatrics.org/cgi/content/full/104/2/e20. Accessed May 12, 2003

Biederman J, Quinn D, Weiss M, et al: Methylphenidate HCL extended-release capsules (Ritalin LA): a new once-daily therapy for ADHD, in Scientific Proceedings of the 48th Annual Meeting of the American Academy of Child and Adolescent Psychiatry. Edited by Villani S. Honolulu, HI, American Academy of Child and Adolescent Psychiatry, October 2001, p A41

Biederman J, Lopez FA, Boellner SW, et al: A randomized, double-blind, placebo-controlled, parallel-group study of SLI381 (Adderall XR) in children with attention-deficit/hyperactivity disorder. Pediatrics 110:258–266, 2002

Bostic J, Wilens T, Spencer T, et al: Pharmacologic treatment of juvenile depression. Psychiatr Clin North Am 6:175–191, 1999

Brown RT, Wynne ME, Slimmer LW: Attention deficit disorder and the effect of methylphenidate on attention, behavioral, and cardiovascular functioning. J Clin Psychiatry 45:473–476, 1984

Buitelaar JK, van der Gaag RJ, Swaab-Barneveld H, et al: Pindolol and methylphenidate in children with attention-deficit hyperactivity disorder: clinical efficacy and side-effects. J Child Psychol Psychiatry 37:587–595, 1996

Campbell M, Adams P, Small AM, et al: Efficacy and safety of fenfluramine in autistic children. J Am Acad Child Adolesc Psychiatry 27:434–439, 1988a

Campbell M, Adams P, Small AM, et al: Naltrexone in infantile autism. Psychopharmacol Bull 24:135–139, 1988b

Campbell M, Gonzalez NM, Silva RR: The pharmacologic treatment of conduct disorders and rage outbursts. Psychiatr Clin North Am 15:69–85, 1992

Casat CD, Pleasants DZ, Van Wyck Fleet J: A double-blind trial of bupropion in children with attention deficit disorder. Psychopharmacol Bull 23:120–122, 1987

Casat CD, Pleasants DZ, Schroeder DH, et al: Bupropion in children with attention deficit disorder. Psychopharmacol Bull 25:198–201, 1989

Chandler M, Lopez F, Boeliner S: Long-term safety of SLI381 in children with ADHD, in Scientific Proceedings of the 48th Annual Meeting of the American Academy of Child and Adolescent Psychiatry. Edited by Villani S. Honolulu, HI, American Academy of Child and Adolescent Psychiatry, October 2001, p B12

Chappell P, Riddle M, Scahill L, et al: Guanfacine treatment of comorbid attention-deficit hyperactivity disorder and Tourette's syndrome. J Am Acad Child Adolesc Psychiatry 34:1140–1146, 1995

Cohen LG, Biederman J: Treatment of risperidone-induced hyperprolactinemia with a dopamine agonist in children. J Child Adolesc Psychopharmacol 11:435–440, 2001

Cohen LG, Prince J, Biederman J, et al: Absence of effect of stimulants on the pharmacokinetics of desipramine in children. Pharmacotherapy 19:746–752, 1999

Comings DE, Comings BG: Tourette's syndrome and attention deficit disorder, in Tourette's Syndrome and Tic Disorders: Clinical Understanding and Treatment. Edited by Cohen DJ, Bruun RD, Leckman JF. New York, Wiley, 1988, pp 119–136

Conners CK, Casat CD, Gualtieri CT, et al: Bupropion hydrochloride in attention deficit disorder with hyperactivity. J Am Acad Child Adolesc Psychiatry 35:1314–1321, 1996

Conners CK, Casat C[D], Coury D, et al: Randomized trial of dex-methylphenidate (D-MPH) and D,L-MPH in children with ADHD, in Scientific Proceedings of the 48th Annual Meeting of the American Academy of Child and Adolescent Psychiatry. Edited by Villani S. Honolulu, HI, American Academy of Child and Adolescent Psychiatry, October 2001, p C49

Connor D, Ozbayrak K, Benjamin S, et al: A pilot study of nadolol for overt aggression in developmentally delayed individuals. J Am Acad Child Adolesc Psychiatry 36:826–834, 1997

Cox W: An indication for the use of imipramine in attention deficit disorder. Am J Psychiatry 139:1059–1060, 1982

Derivan A: Venlafaxine metabolism in children and adolescents, in Scientific Proceedings, American Academy of Child and Adolescent Psychiatry, XI, New Orleans, LA, 1995, NR162 p 128

DeVane CL: Differential pharmacology of newer antidepressants. J Clin Psychiatry 59(suppl 20):85–93, 1998

DeVeaugh-Geiss J, Moroz G, Biederman J, et al: Clomipramine hydrochloride in childhood and adolescent obsessive-compulsive disorder: a multicenter trial. J Am Acad Child Adolesc Psychiatry 31:45–49, 1992

Dillon DC, Salzman IJ, Schulsinger DA: The use of imipramine in Tourette's syndrome and attention deficit disorder: case report. J Clin Psychiatry 46:348–349, 1985

Ding YS, Fowler JS, Volkow ND, et al: Carbon-11-D-*threo*-methylphenidate binding to dopamine transporter in baboon brain. J Nucl Med 36:2298–2305, 1995

Donnelly M, Zametkin AJ, Rapoport JL, et al: Treatment of childhood hyperactivity with desipramine: plasma drug concentration, cardiovascular effects, plasma and urinary catecholamine levels, and clinical response. Clin Pharmacol Ther 39:72–81, 1986

Donnelly M, Rapoport JL, Potter WZ, et al: Fenfluramine and dextroamphetamine treatment of childhood hyperactivity. Clinical and biochemical findings. Arch Gen Psychiatry 46:205–212, 1989

Douglas V, Barr R, Amin K, et al: Dosage effects and individual responsivity to methylphenidate in attention deficit disorder. J Child Psychol Psychiatry 29:453–475, 1988

DuPaul GJ, Barkley RA, McMurray MB: Response of children with ADHD to methylphenidate: interaction with internalizing symptoms. J Am Acad Child Adolesc Psychiatry 33:894–903, 1994

Eison MS: The new generation of serotonergic anxiolytics: possible clinical roles. Psychopathology 22:13–20, 1989

Emslie GJ, Rush AJ, Weinberg WA, et al: A double-blind, randomized, placebo-controlled trial of fluoxetine in children and adolescents with depression. Arch Gen Psychiatry 54:1031–1037, 1997

Famularo R, Fenton T: The effect of methylphenidate on school grades in children with attention deficit disorder without hyperactivity: a preliminary report. J Clin Psychiatry 48:112–114, 1987

Faraone SV, Biederman J: The neurobiology of attention deficit hyperactivity disorder, in Neurobiology of Mental Illness. Edited by Charney DS, Nestler EJ, Bunney BS. New York, Oxford University Press, 1999, pp 788–801

Faraone SV, Biederman J, Lehman BK, et al: Intellectual performance and school failure in children with attention deficit hyperactivity disorder and in their siblings. J Abnorm Psychol 102:616–623, 1993

Findling RL, Schwartz MA, Flannery DJ, et al: Venlafaxine in adults with attention-deficit/hyperactivity disorder: an open trial. J Clin Psychiatry 57:184–189, 1996

Findling RL, Reed MD, Myers C, et al: Paroxetine pharmacokinetics in depressed children and adolescents. J Am Acad Child Adolesc Psychiatry 38:952–959, 1999

Frazier JA, Meyer MC, Biederman J, et al: Risperidone treatment for juvenile bipolar disorder: a retrospective chart review. J Am Acad Child Adolesc Psychiatry 38:960–965, 1999

Fung YK: Postnatal behavioural effects of maternal nicotine exposure in rats. J Pharm Pharmacol 40:870–872, 1988

Fung YK, Lau YS: Effects of prenatal nicotine exposure on rat striatal dopaminergic and nicotinic systems. Pharmacol Biochem Behav 33:1–6, 1989

Gadow KD, Nolan EE, Sverd J: Methylphenidate in hyperactive boys with comorbid tic disorder, II: short-term behavioral effects in school settings. J Am Acad Child Adolesc Psychiatry 31:462–471, 1992

Gadow KD, Sverd J, Sprafkin J, et al: Efficacy of methylphenidate for attention-deficit hyperactivity disorder in children with tic disorder. Arch Gen Psychiatry 52:444–455, 1995

Garfinkel BD, Wender PH, Sloman L, et al: Tricyclic antidepressant and methylphenidate treatment of attention deficit disorder in children. J Am Acad Child Adolesc Psychiatry 22:343–348, 1983

Gastfriend DR, Biederman J, Jellinek MS: Desipramine in the treatment of attention deficit disorder in adolescents. Psychopharmacol Bull 21:144–145, 1985

Geller B, Fox L, Clark K: Rate and predictors of prepubertal bipolarity during follow-up of 6- to 12-year-old depressed children. J Am Acad Child Adolesc Psychiatry 33:461–468, 1994

Geller DA, Biederman J, Reed ED, et al: Similarities in response to fluoxetine in the treatment of children and adolescents with obsessive-compulsive disorder. J Am Acad Child Adolesc Psychiatry 34:36–44, 1995

Gittelman R: Childhood disorders, in Drug Treatment of Adult and Child Psychiatric Disorders. Edited by Klein D, Quitkin F, Rifkin A, et al. Baltimore, MD, Williams & Wilkins, 1980, pp 576–756

Gittelman-Klein R: Pilot clinical trial of imipramine in hyperkinetic children, in Clinical Use of Stimulant Drugs in Children. Edited by Conners C. The Hague, The Netherlands, Excerpta Medica, 1974, pp 192–201

Gittelman-Klein R: Pharmacotherapy of childhood hyperactivity: an update, in Psychopharmacology: The Third Generation of Progress. Edited by Meltzer HY. New York, Raven, 1987, pp 1215–1224

Goldman L, Genel M, Bezman R, et al: Diagnosis and treatment of attention-deficit/hyperactivity disorder in children and adolescents. JAMA 279:1100–1107, 1998

Gordon C, State R, Nelson J, et al: A double-blind comparison of clomipramine, desipramine, and placebo in the treatment of autistic disorder. Arch Gen Psychiatry 50:441–447, 1993

Greenberg L, Yellin A, Spring C, et al: Clinical effects of imipramine and methylphenidate in hyperactive children. International Journal of Mental Health 4:144–156, 1975

Greenblatt D, Moltke L, Harmatz J, et al: Drug interactions with newer antidepressants: role of human cytochromes P450. J Clin Psychiatry 59:19–27, 1998

Greene R: The Explosive Child: A New Approach for Understanding and Parenting Easily Frustrated, "Chronically Inflexible" Children, 1st Edition. New York, HarperCollins, 1998

Greenhill LL, Halperin JM, Abikoff H: Stimulant medications. J Am Acad Child Adolesc Psychiatry 38:503–512, 1999

Greenhill LL, Findling RL, Swanson JM: A double-blind, placebo-controlled study of modified-release methylphenidate in children with attention-deficit/hyperactivity disorder. Pediatrics (serial online) 109:39, 2002. Available at: http://www.pediatrics.org/cgi/content/full/109/3/e39. Accessed May 12, 2003

Gross M: Imipramine in the treatment of minimal brain dysfunction in children. Psychosomatics 14:283–285, 1973

Gross M: Growth of hyperkinetic children taking methylphenidate, dextroamphetamine, or imipramine/desipramine. J Pediatr 58:423–431, 1976

Gualtieri CT, Evans RW: Motor performance in hyperactive children treated with imipramine. Percept Mot Skills 66:763–769, 1988

Gunning B: A controlled trial of clonidine in hyperkinetic children. Unpublished thesis, Department of Child and Adolescent Psychiatry, Academic Hospital Rotterdam–Sophia Children's Hospital Rotterdam, Rotterdam, The Netherlands, 1992

Herman JB, Rosenbaum JF, Brotman AW: The alprazolam to clonazepam switch for the treatment of panic disorder. J Clin Psychopharmacol 7:175–178, 1987

Hoge SK, Biederman J: A case of Tourette's syndrome with symptoms of attention deficit disorder treated with desipramine. J Clin Psychiatry 47:478–479, 1986

Hornig-Rohan M, Amsterdam J: Venlafaxine vs. stimulant therapy in patients with dual diagnoses of ADHD and depression. Poster 92, presented at the New Clinical Drug Evaluation Unit Program, Orlando, FL, June 1995

Horrigan JP, Barnhill LJ: Guanfacine for treatment of attention-deficit hyperactivity disorder in boys. J Child Adolesc Psychopharmacol 5:215–223, 1995

Huessy HR, Wright AL: The use of imipramine in children's behavior disorders. Acta Paedopsychiatr 37:194–199, 1970

Hunt RD: Treatment effects of oral and transdermal clonidine in relation to methylphenidate: an open pilot study in ADD-H. Psychopharmacol Bull 23:111–114, 1987

Hunt RD, Minderaa RB, Cohen DJ: Clonidine benefits children with attention deficit disorder and hyperactivity: report of a double-blind placebo-crossover therapeutic trial. J Am Acad Child Psychiatry 24:617–629, 1985

Hunt RD, Capper L, O'Connell P: Clonidine in child and adolescent psychiatry. J Child Adolesc Psychopharmacol 1:87–102, 1990

Hunt RD, Arnsten AF, Asbell MD: An open trial of guanfacine in the treatment of attention-deficit hyperactivity disorder. J Am Acad Child Adolesc Psychiatry 34:50–54, 1995

Hurt RD, Sachs DP, Glover ED, et al: A comparison of sustained-release bupropion and placebo for smoking cessation. N Engl J Med 337:1195–1202, 1997

Hyman SE, Nestler EJ: The Molecular Foundations of Psychiatry, 1st Edition. Washington, DC, American Psychiatric Press, 1993

Johns JM, Louis TM, Becker RF, et al: Behavioral effects of prenatal exposure to nicotine in guinea pigs. Neurobehav Toxicol Teratol 4:365–369, 1982

Jones GM, Sahakian BJ, Levy R, et al: Effects of acute subcutaneous nicotine on attention, information processing and short-term memory in Alzheimer's disease. Psychopharmacology (Berl) 108:485–494, 1992

Klein RG: Pharmacotherapy of childhood hyperactivity: an update, in Psychopharmacology: The Third Generation of Progress. Edited by Meltzer HY. New York, Raven, 1987, pp 1215–1225

Klein RG, Mannuzza S: Hyperactive boys almost grown up, III: methylphenidate effects on ultimate height. Arch Gen Psychiatry 45:1131–1134, 1988

Kovacs M, Feinberg TL, Crouse-Novak M, et al: Depressive disorders in childhood, I: a longitudinal prospective study of characteristics and recovery. Arch Gen Psychiatry 41:229–237, 1984

Kratochvil C, Wernicke J, Michelson D, et al: Long-term study of atomoxetine in the treatment of ADHD, in Scientific Proceedings of the 48th Annual Meeting of the American Academy of Child and Adolescent Psychiatry. Edited by Villani S. Honolulu, HI, American Academy of Child and Adolescent Psychiatry, October 2001, p 119

Kupietz SS, Balka EB: Alterations in the vigilance performance of children receiving amitriptyline and methylphenidate pharmacotherapy. Psychopharmacology (Berl) 50:29–33, 1976

Kupietz SS, Winsberg BG, Richardson E, et al: Effects of methylphenidate dosage in hyperactive reading-disabled children, I: behavior and cognitive performance effects. J Am Acad Child Adolesc Psychiatry 27:70–77, 1988

Kutcher S, Williamson P, MacKenzie S, et al: Successful clonazepam treatment of neuroleptic-induced akathisia in older adolescents and young adults: a double-blind, placebo-controlled study. J Clin Psychopharmacol 9:403–406, 1989

Leckman JF, Hardin MT, Riddle MA, et al: Clonidine treatment of Gilles de la Tourette's syndrome. Arch Gen Psychiatry 48:324–328, 1991

Leonard H, Rapoport J: Anxiety disorders in childhood and adolescence, in American Psychiatric Press Review of Psychiatry, Vol 9. Edited by Tasman A, Hales R, Frances A. Washington, DC, American Psychiatric Press, 1989, pp 162–179

Leonard H, March J, Rickler K, et al: Pharmacology of the selective serotonin reuptake inhibitors in children and adolescents. J Am Acad Child Adolesc Psychiatry 36:725–736, 1998

Levin E, Conners C, Sparrow E, et al: Nicotine effects on adults with attention-deficit/hyperactivity disorder. Psychopharmacology (Berl) 123:55–63, 1996

Lienemann J, Walker F: Naltrexone for treatment of self-injury (letter). Am J Psychiatry 146:1639–1640, 1989

Lombroso P, Scahill L, King R, et al: Risperidone treatment of children and adolescents with chronic tic disorders: a preliminary report. J Am Acad Child Adolesc Psychiatry 34:1147–1152, 1995

Lowe TL, Cohen DJ, Detlor J: Stimulant medications precipitate Tourette's syndrome. JAMA 247:1168–1169, 1982

Malhotra S, Santosh PJ: An open clinical trial of buspirone in children with attention deficit/hyperactivity disorder. J Am Acad Child Adolesc Psychiatry 37:364–371, 1998

Mattes JA: Propranolol for adults with temper outbursts and residual attention deficit disorder. J Clin Psychopharmacol 6:299–302, 1986

Mattes JA, Gittelman R: Growth of hyperactive children on maintenance regimen of methylphenidate. Arch Gen Psychiatry 40:317–321, 1983

McClellan J, Werry J: Practice parameters for the assessment and treatment of children and adolescents with schizophrenia. J Am Acad Child Adolesc Psychiatry 33:616–635, 1994

McCracken JT, Biederman J, Greenhill LL, et al: Analog classroom assessment of SLI381 for treatment of ADHD, in Scientific Proceedings of the 47th Annual Meeting of the American Academy of Child and Adolescent Psychiatry. Edited by Villani S. New York, American Academy of Child and Adolescent Psychiatry, October 2000, Poster 114

Meck W, Church R: Cholinergic modulation of the content of temporal memory. Behav Neurosci 101:457–464, 1987

Mereu G, Yoon K, Gessa G, et al: Preferential stimulation of ventral tegmental area dopaminergic neurons by nicotine. Eur J Pharmacol 141:395–399, 1987

Michelson D, Faries D, Wernicke J, et al: Atomoxetine in the treatment of children and adolescents with attention-deficit/hyperactivity disorder: a randomized, placebo-controlled, dose-response study. Pediatrics (serial online) 108:83, 2001. Available at: http://www.pediatrics.org/cgi/content/full/108/5/e83. Accessed May 12, 2003

Milberger S, Biederman J, Faraone SV, et al: Is maternal smoking during pregnancy a risk factor for attention deficit hyperactivity disorder in children? Am J Psychiatry 153:1138–1142, 1996

Milberger S, Biederman J, Faraone SV, et al: ADHD is associated with early initiation of cigarette smoking in children and adolescents. J Am Acad Child Adolesc Psychiatry 36:37–43, 1997

Nemeroff CB, DeVane CL, Pollock BG: Newer antidepressants and the cytochrome P450 system. Am J Psychiatry 153:311–320, 1996

Nierenberg A, Alpert J, Pava J, et al: Course and treatment of atypical depression. J Clin Psychiatry 59:5–9, 1998

Olvera RL, Pliszka SR, Luh J, et al: An open trial of venlafaxine in the treatment of attention-deficit/hyperactivity disorder in children and adolescents. J Child Adolesc Psychopharmacol 6:241–250, 1996

O'Malley SS, Jaffe AJ, Chang G, et al: Six-month follow-up of naltrexone and psychotherapy for alcohol dependence. Arch Gen Psychiatry 53:217–224, 1996

Parrott AC, Winder G: Nicotine chewing gum (2 mg, 4 mg) and cigarette smoking: comparative effects upon vigilance and heart rate. Psychopharmacology (Berl) 97:257–261, 1989

Pauls DL, Towbin KE, Leckman JF, et al: Gilles de la Tourette's syndrome and obsessive-compulsive disorder: evidence supporting a genetic relationship. Arch Gen Psychiatry 43:1180–1182, 1986

Peeke S, Peeke H: Attention, memory, and cigarette smoking. Psychopharmacology (Berl) 84:205–216, 1984

Pelham WE, Bender ME, Caddell J, et al: Methylphenidate and children with attention deficit disorder. Arch Gen Psychiatry 42:948–952, 1985

Pelham WE, Gnagy EM, Burrows-Maclean L, et al: Once-a-day Concerta methylphenidate versus three-times-daily methylphenidate in laboratory and natural settings. Pediatrics (serial online) 107:105, 2001. Available at: http://www.pediatrics.org/cgi/content/full/107/6/e105. Accessed May 12, 2003

Pentikis HS, Simmons RD, Benedict MF, et al: Methylphenidate bioavailability in adults when an extended-release multiparticulate formulation is administered sprinkled on food or as an intact capsule. J Am Acad Child Adolesc Psychiatry 41:443–449, 2002

Platt JE, Campbell M, Green WH, et al: Cognitive effects of lithium carbonate and haloperidol in treatment-resistant aggressive children. Arch Gen Psychiatry 41:657–662, 1984

Pliszka SR: Effect of anxiety on cognition, behavior, and stimulant response in ADHD. J Am Acad Child Adolesc Psychiatry 28:882–887, 1989

Pomerleau O, Downey K, Stelson F, et al: Cigarette smoking in adult patients diagnosed with ADHD. J Subst Abuse 7:373–378, 1996

Pope HG, McElroy SL, Keck PE Jr, et al: Valproate in the treatment of acute mania. Arch Gen Psychiatry 48:62–68, 1991

Preskorn S, Alderman J, Chung M, et al: Pharmacokinetics of desipramine coadministered with sertraline or fluoxetine. J Clin Psychopharmacol 14:90–98, 1994

Prince J, Wilens T, Biederman J, et al: Clonidine for ADHD related sleep disturbances: a systematic chart review of 62 cases. J Am Acad Child Adolesc Psychiatry 35:599–605, 1996

Prince J, Wilens T, Biederman J, et al: A controlled study of nortriptyline in children and adolescents with attention deficit hyperactivity disorder, in Scientific Proceedings, American Academy of Child and Adolescent Psychiatry, XV. Chicago, IL, May 1999

Quay HC: Conduct disorder, in Psychopathologic Disorders of Childhood. Edited by Quay HC, Werry JS. New York, Wiley, 1986, pp 35–73

Quinn DM: Prevalence of psychoactive medication in children and adolescents. Can J Psychiatry 31:575–580, 1986

Quinn PO, Rapoport JL: One-year follow-up of hyperactive boys treated with imipramine or methylphenidate. Am J Psychiatry 132:241–245, 1975

Quitkin FM, Harrison W, Stewart JW, et al: Response to phenelzine and imipramine in placebo nonresponders with atypical depression. Arch Gen Psychiatry 48:319–323, 1991

Rapoport JL, Quinn P, Bradbard G, et al: Imipramine and methylphenidate treatment of hyperactive boys: a double-blind comparison. Arch Gen Psychiatry 30:789–793, 1974

Rapport MD, Jones JT, DuPaul GJ, et al: Attention deficit disorder and methylphenidate: group and single-subject analyses of dose effects on attention in clinic and classroom settings. J Clin Child Psychol 16:329–338, 1987

Rapport MD, Stoner G, DuPaul GJ, et al: Attention deficit disorder and methylphenidate: a multilevel analysis of dose-response effects on children's impulsivity across settings. J Am Acad Child Adolesc Psychiatry 27:60–69, 1988

Rapport MD, DuPaul GJ, Kelly KL: Attention deficit hyperactivity disorder and methylphenidate: the relationship between gross body weight and drug response in children. Psychopharmacol Bull 25:285–290, 1989a

Rapport MD, Quinn SO, DuPaul GJ, et al: Attention deficit disorder with hyperactivity and methylphenidate: the effects of dose and mastery level on children's learning performance. J Abnorm Child Psychol 17:669–689, 1989b

Rapport MD, Carlson GA, Kelly KL, et al: Methylphenidate and desipramine in hospitalized children, I: separate and combined effects on cognitive function. J Am Acad Child Adolesc Psychiatry 32:333–342, 1993

Ratey JJ, Greenberg MS, Lindem KJ: Combination of treatments for attention deficit hyperactivity disorder in adults. J Nerv Ment Dis 179:699–701, 1991

Realmuto GM, August GJ, Garfinkel BD: Clinical effect of buspirone in autistic children. J Clin Psychopharmacol 9:122–125, 1989

Reimherr FW, Wender PH, Wood DR, et al: An open trial of L-tyrosine in the treatment of attention deficit disorder, residual type. Am J Psychiatry 144:1071–1073, 1987

Reimherr F[W], Hedges D, Strong R, et al: An open-trial of venlafaxine in adult patients with attention deficit hyperactivity disorder. Paper presented at the New Clinical Drug Evaluation Unit Program, Orlando, FL, May 1995

Rew DA, Rundle JS: Assessment of the safety of regular DDAVP therapy in primary nocturnal enuresis. Br J Urol 63:352–353, 1989

Riddle MA, Hardin MT, Towbin KE, et al: Tardive dyskinesia following haloperidol treatment in Tourette's syndrome (letter). Arch Gen Psychiatry 44:98–99, 1987

Riddle MA, Hardin MT, Cho SC, et al: Desipramine treatment of boys with attention-deficit hyperactivity disorder and tics: preliminary clinical experience. J Am Acad Child Adolesc Psychiatry 27:811–814, 1988

Riddle MA, Nelson JC, Kleinman CS, et al: Sudden death in children receiving Norpramin: a review of three reported cases and commentary. J Am Acad Child Adolesc Psychiatry 30:104–108, 1991

Safer DJ, Allen RP, Barr E: Depression of growth in hyperactive children on stimulant drugs. N Engl J Med 287:217–220, 1972

Satterfield JH, Cantwell DP, Schell A, et al: Growth of hyperactive children treated with methylphenidate. Arch Gen Psychiatry 36:212–217, 1979

Shapiro AK, Shapiro ES, Young JG, et al: Gilles de la Tourette Syndrome. New York, Raven, 1988

Silva R, Munoz D, Alpert M: Carbamazepine use in children and adolescents with features of attention-deficit hyperactivity disorder: a meta-analysis. J Am Acad Child Adolesc Psychiatry 35:352–358, 1996

Singer S, Brown J, Quaskey S, et al: The treatment of attention-deficit hyperactivity disorder in Tourette's syndrome: a double-blind placebo-controlled study with clonidine and desipramine. Pediatrics 95:74–81, 1994

Sorgi PJ, Ratey JJ, Polakoff S: Beta-adrenergic blockers for the control of aggressive behavior in patients with schizophrenia. Am J Psychiatry 143:775–776, 1986

Spencer T: A double-blind, controlled study of desipramine in children with ADHD and tic disorders, in Scientific Proceedings, 44th annual meeting of the American Academy of Child and Adolescent Psychiatry, Toronto, Ontario, Canada, October 1997

Spencer T, Biederman J, Kerman K, et al: Desipramine treatment of children with attention-deficit hyperactivity disorder and tic disorder or Tourette's syndrome. J Am Acad Child Adolesc Psychiatry 32:354–360, 1993a

Spencer T, Biederman J, Wilens T, et al: Nortriptyline treatment of children with attention-deficit hyperactivity disorder and tic disorder or Tourette's syndrome. J Am Acad Child Adolesc Psychiatry 32:205–210, 1993b

Spencer T, Wilens T, Biederman J, et al: A double-blind, crossover comparison of methylphenidate and placebo in adults with childhood-onset attention-deficit hyperactivity disorder. Arch Gen Psychiatry 52:434–443, 1995

Spencer T, Biederman J, Wilens T, et al: Pharmacotherapy of attention-deficit hyperactivity disorder across the life cycle. J Am Acad Child Adolesc Psychiatry 35:409–432, 1996

Spencer T, Biederman J, Wilens T: Pharmacotherapy of ADHD: a life span perspective, in American Psychiatric Press Review of Psychiatry, Vol 16. Edited by Oldham J, Riba M. Washington, DC, American Psychiatric Press, 1997, pp 87–128

Spencer T, Biederman J, Wilens TE, et al: Adults with attention-deficit/hyperactivity disorder: a controversial diagnosis. J Clin Psychiatry 59(suppl 7):59–68, 1998a

Spencer T, Biederman J, Wilens T[E]: Growth deficits in children with attention deficit hyperactivity disorder. Pediatrics 102:501–506, 1998b

Spencer T, Biederman J, Coffey B, et al: The 4-year course of tic disorders in boys with attention-deficit/hyperactivity disorder. Arch Gen Psychiatry 56:842–847, 1999a

Spencer T, Wilens T, Biederman J, et al: Efficacy and tolerability of a mixed amphetamine salts compound in adults with attention deficit hyperactivity disorder, in Scientific Proceedings of the American Academy of Child and Adolescent Psychiatry, XV. Chicago, IL, May 1999b

Spencer T, Swanson J, Weidenman M, et al: Pharmacodynamic profile of Ritalin LA, a new extended-release dosage form of Ritalin, in children with ADHD, in Scientific Proceedings of the 47th Annual Meeting of the American Academy of Child and Adolescent Psychiatry. Edited by Villani S. New York, American Academy of Child and Adolescent Psychiatry, October 2000

Spencer T, Heiligenstein J, Biederman J, et al: Results from two proof-of-concept, placebo-controlled studies of atomoxetine in children with ADHD. J Clin Psychiatry 63:1140–1147, 2002

Steingard R, Biederman J, Spencer T, et al: Comparison of clonidine response in the treatment of attention deficit hyperactivity disorder with and without comorbid tic disorders. J Am Acad Child Adolesc Psychiatry 32:350–353, 1993

Sudden death in children treated with a tricyclic antidepressant. Med Lett Drugs Ther 32:53, 1990

Swanson J, Kinsbourne M, Roberts W, et al: Time-response analysis of the effect of stimulant medication on the learning ability of children referred for hyperactivity. Pediatrics 61:21–24, 1978

Swanson J, Agler D, Fineberg E, et al: University of California, Irvine, laboratory school protocol for pharmacokinetic and pharmacodynamic studies, in Ritalin: Theory and Practice, 2nd Edition. Edited by Greenhill L, Osman B. Larchmont, NY, Mary Ann Liebert, 2000, pp 405–430

Tannock R, Schachar RJ, Carr RP, et al: Dose-response effects of methylphenidate on academic performance and overt behavior in hyperactive children. Pediatrics 84:648–657, 1989

Tannock R, Ickowicz A, Schachar R: Differential effects of methylphenidate on working memory in ADHD children with and without comorbid anxiety. J Am Acad Child Adolesc Psychiatry 34:886–896, 1995

Taylor E, Schachar R, Thorley G, et al: Which boys respond to stimulant medication? a controlled trial of methylphenidate in boys with disruptive behaviour. Psychol Med 17:121–143, 1987

Trott GE, Menzel M, Friese HJ, et al: Effectiveness and tolerance of the selective MAO-A inhibitor in children with hyperkinetic syndrome (in German). Z Kinder Jugendpsychiatr 19:248–253, 1991

Trott GE, Friese HJ, Menzel M, et al: Use of moclobemide in children with attention deficit hyperactivity disorder. Psychopharmacology (Berl) 106(suppl):S134–S136, 1992

Voelker S, Lachar D, Gdowski CL: The Personality Inventory for Children and response to methylphenidate: preliminary evidence for predictive validity. J Pediatr Psychol 8:161–169, 1983

Wagner K, Birmaher B, Carlson G, et al: Safety of paroxetine and imipramine in the treatment of adolescent depression. Paper presented at the New Clinical Drug Evaluation Unit Program, Boca Raton, FL, June 1998

Watter N, Dreyfuss FE: Modifications of hyperkinetic behavior by nortriptyline. Virginia Medical Monthly 100:123–126, 1973

Weller EB, Weller RA, Fristad MA, et al: Saliva lithium monitoring in prepubertal children. J Am Acad Child Adolesc Psychiatry 26:173–175, 1987

Wender PH, Reimherr FW: Bupropion treatment of attention-deficit hyperactivity disorder in adults. Am J Psychiatry 147:1018–1020, 1990

Werry J: Imipramine and methylphenidate in hyperactive children. J Child Psychol Psychiatry 21:27–35, 1980

Wesnes K, Warburton DM: The effects of cigarettes of varying yield on rapid information processing performance. Psychopharmacology (Berl) 82:338–342, 1984

Westfall TC, Grant H, Perry H: Release of dopamine and 5-hydroxytryptamine from rat striatal slices following activation of nicotinic cholinergic receptors. Gen Pharmacol 14:321–325, 1983

Wilens TE, on behalf of the Concerta study group: Prospective one-year study of OROS MPH, dosed qd in children with ADHD. Paper presented at the annual meeting of the American Academy of Neurology, San Diego, CA, June 2000

Wilens T[E], Biederman J: The stimulants. Psychiatr Clin North Am 15:191–222, 1992

Wilens TE, Biederman J, Geist DE, et al: Nortriptyline in the treatment of ADHD: a chart review of 58 cases. J Am Acad Child Adolesc Psychiatry 32:343–349, 1993

Wilens TE, Biederman J, Mick E, et al: A systematic assessment of tricyclic antidepressants in the treatment of adult attention-deficit hyperactivity disorder. J Nerv Ment Dis 183:48–50, 1995a

Wilens TE, Spencer T, Biederman J, et al: Combined pharmacotherapy: an emerging trend in pediatric psychopharmacology. J Am Acad Child Adolesc Psychiatry 34:110–112, 1995b

Wilens TE, Biederman J, Abrantes AM, et al: A naturalistic assessment of protriptyline for attention-deficit hyperactivity disorder. J Am Acad Child Adolesc Psychiatry 35:1485–1490, 1996a

Wilens TE, Biederman J, Baldessarini RJ, et al: Cardiovascular effects of therapeutic doses of tricyclic antidepressants in children and adolescents. J Am Acad Child Adolesc Psychiatry 35:1491–1501, 1996b

Wilens TE, Biederman J, Prince J, et al: Six-week, double-blind, placebo-controlled study of desipramine for adult attention deficit hyperactivity disorder. Am J Psychiatry 153:1147–1153, 1996c

Wilens TE, Wyatt D, Spencer TJ: Disentangling disinhibition. J Am Acad Child Adolesc Psychiatry 37:1225–1227, 1998

Wilens TE, Biederman J, Spencer TJ, et al: Controlled trial of high doses of pemoline for adults with attention-deficit/hyperactivity disorder. J Clin Psychopharmacol 19:257–264, 1999a

Wilens TE, Biederman J, Spencer TJ, et al: A pilot controlled clinical trial of ABT-418, a cholinergic agonist, in the treatment of adults with attention deficit hyperactivity disorder. Am J Psychiatry 156:1931–1937, 1999b

Wilens T[E], Spencer T[J], Biederman J, et al: A controlled trial of bupropion SR for attention deficit hyperactivity disorder in adults. Poster presented at the New Clinical Drug Evaluation Unit Program, Boca Raton, FL, 1999c

Wilens TE, Spencer TJ, Swanson JM, et al: Combining methylphenidate and clonidine: a clinically sound medication option. J Am Acad Child Adolesc Psychiatry 38:614–619, 1999d

Winsberg BG, Bialer I, Kupietz S, et al: Effects of imipramine and dextroamphetamine on behavior of neuropsychiatrically impaired children. Am J Psychiatry 128:1425–1431, 1972

Wolraich ML, Greenhill LL, Pelham W, et al: Randomized, controlled trial of OROS methylphenidate once a day in children with attention-deficit/hyperactivity disorder. Pediatrics 108:883–892, 2001

Wozniak J, Biederman J, Kiely K, et al: Mania-like symptoms suggestive of childhood onset bipolar disorder in clinically referred children. J Am Acad Child Adolesc Psychiatry 34:867–876, 1995

Yepes LE, Balka EB, Winsberg BG, et al: Amitriptyline and methylphenidate treatment of behaviorally disordered children. J Child Psychol Psychiatry 18:39–52, 1977

Zametkin AJ, Rapoport JL: Noradrenergic hypothesis of attention deficit disorder with hyperactivity: a critical review, in Psychopharmacology: The Third Generation of Progress. Edited by Meltzer HY. New York, Raven, 1987, pp 837–842

Zametkin A[J], Rapoport JL, Murphy DL, et al: Treatment of hyperactive children with monoamine oxidase inhibitors, I: clinical efficacy. Arch Gen Psychiatry 42:962–966, 1985

51

Psychoanalysis and Psychodynamic Therapy

Jules Bemporad, M.D.

Maurizio Zambenedetti, M.D.

The psychoanalytic treatment of children evolved as an application of psychoanalytic therapy with adults. Although modifications in technique have been recommended to fit the child's stage of psychological development, the primary therapeutic agent in the treatment of both children and adults is the analyst's interpretation of unconscious content, which is performed to bring such material (and its behavioral and emotional derivatives) under greater control of the ego.

Forays into child treatment were made early in the evolution of psychoanalysis and include Sigmund Freud's (1909/1955) own treatment of little Hans via the child's father; Ferenczi's (1913/1950) single consultation with Arpad, a 5-year-old boy who was obsessed with and phobic of chickens; and Hug-Helmuth's (1920) more systematic treatment of children, using drawings and games. However, it was not until the late 1920s that child analysis became established under the guidance of Melanie Klein and Anna Freud, whose influence continues to dominate the field.

Klein and Freud developed greatly disparate systems of treatment derived from the treatment of adults and based on different theoretical modifications of psychoanalytic formulations. This disparity resulted in an unfortunate animosity between the two theorists and between their disciples. A detailed description of the metapsychological directions in which Klein took psychoanalytic theory, as opposed to the more traditional Freudian approach (and the latter's modification as an ego psychology), is beyond the scope of this chapter. Freud's system is more prevalent in the United States. However, Kleinian child analysis is currently a vital and popular form of treatment (particularly in Europe and South America), and a brief presentation of its principles is warranted.

Kleinian Child Psychoanalysis

Klein's technique is based on three fundamental principles: 1) play as the child's mode of free association, 2) the existence of transference in children, and 3) the restriction of the analyst's role solely to interpreting unconscious sources of anxiety (Segal 1972). Klein maintained that play is the natural mode of expression for children and that the patients symbolize their inner wishes, fears, and internalized relationships through this medium. Play is therefore a suitable substitute for the free association of adults. Continuing this analogy, Klein maintained that inhibitions in the ability to play (and subsequently in the ability to learn) demonstrate a fear of letting one's imagination run freely and thus perhaps uncovering disagreeable or terrifying fantasies. Comfort with free, unrestricted play is a sign of psychological health, just as the ability of the adult to truly free-associate indicates a lack of repression or pathological defenses (Klein 1932).

Klein also maintained that children are capable of transference neurosis, despite their still largely dependent and interactive relationships with their parents. Transference is possible even in very young children, according to Klein, because they project onto the therapist aspects of their past internalized parents, with all their inherent distortions, rather than their actual current parents.

Finally, Klein insisted on strict neutrality on the part of the analyst, who is to refrain from reassurance, guidance, or any deviation from supplying only interpretations. The analyst may participate in a game at the child's request but must keep the participation to the barest minimum. The analyst may help a child perform tasks beyond the child's age capacity (e.g., sharpening a pencil) but may not help in actual play or the actual production of drawings. Support or reassurance, for Klein, is sufficiently derived by the child through relief from anxiety as the therapy progresses. It is in this manner that the child realizes that the analyst is helpful, not by the latter's nurturance or encouragement. In a brief retrospective account of her career, Klein (1955) described how she was timid at first about interpreting to the child what she perceived to be the basis for the child's anxiety. When she did so, the child first experienced a momentary increase in anxiety while becoming aware of true, if repressed, motives, but then grew calmer and felt reassured as he or she was able to integrate these wishes into conscious life and no longer live in fear of them.

The purpose of Kleinian analysis is for children to differentiate what is internal and what is external to their psyches so that they no longer confuse significant others in their environment with projections of past internalized objects. By clarifying unconscious fantasies, which are symbolized in play, and bringing these to consciousness, children can realize their own feelings of envy, hatred, greed, lust, or jealousy and no longer need to project them onto others. Similarly, they can discover the sense of guilt over these feelings that causes them to fail or to be victimized in everyday life.

The actual technique of therapy is to explain that the child has come to sessions to play. Children are presented with an assortment of materials that are entirely their own and are kept separate from those of other patients. Klein suggested dolls (child, adult, and animal), toy houses, cars, trains, fences, various containers, scissors, string, balls, paper, pencils, clay, and glue. These items are to be as nondescript as possible so as to allow the freest use of the child's imagination. The therapy is conducted in a safe, plain room without breakable items so that the child can freely vent aggression. A chair and table (used for drawings, for example) and a couch for occasional oral free association are also included. A thorough history is obtained from the parents or others so that the analyst has some idea of problem areas and can use this information as the basis for interpretation. So that the child understands that the relationship with the analyst is different from the child's interchange with other adults, the analyst begins to interpret at the initial visit as indicated by the played-out transference behavior of the child. Sessions last about an hour and are scheduled five times per week.

Klein (1932) wrote detailed accounts of her analysis of children, providing an almost verbatim narrative of the process. She first interpreted to the child that the play figures represented significant people in the child's psychic reality. Then, depending on what the child did with the figures in play, interpretations were directed at the latent meaning beneath the manifest behavior:

Klein described the analysis of Peter, a boy 3 years and 9 months old, who was referred for inability to play, poor frustration tolerance, and other difficulties. His behavior had deteriorated after a summer holiday, when he shared his parents' bedroom and, ostensibly, had witnessed his parents having intercourse. In the first session, Peter had two horse dolls bump into each other, after which Peter proclaimed that they were dead. He then lined up toy cars and smashed them (Klein 1932).

Klein eventually interpreted the play with horses as the child's representation of parental coitus and the play with cars as his damaging his father's genitalia, an act that he feared would subsequently cause damage to himself. She related that these interpretations produced more play material, which in turn was interpreted, thus expanding the child's awareness of his repressed thoughts and wishes. In this process, according to Klein, the child came to understand those emotions and anxieties that he had previously had to keep repressed but that restricted his psychic existence and distorted his appreciation of the external world.

Freudian Child Psychoanalysis

Anna Freud's system of treatment varies markedly from that of Klein, although Freud also considered interpretations of unconscious content the major therapeutic agent. Although she based her system on the traditional psychoanalysis of adults, Freud took great care in detailing the ways in which a child in analysis is quite different from an adult analysand (A. Freud 1965). Among the differences are that children 1) do not seek out therapy on their own and may have little motivation for cure, 2) tend to deny problems and try to externalize their causes rather than accept responsibility for them, 3) will run away from discomfort and so will not easily relinquish fantasy for reality, and 4) prefer the mode of acting to that of talking.

Perhaps the more pertinent characteristics of child analysis that highlight the disparity between Freud's system and Klein's are Freud's questioning whether a child can really free-associate and her rejection of play as a substitute for free association. Freud also differed from Klein in that Freud regarded a mastery of speech as a prerequisite for child analysis; therefore, Freud did not recommend this form of treatment for very young children (A. Freud 1945/1968). Freud also doubted that a child could form a true transference neurosis, with a true reliving of a past relationship toward the analyst, although transference reactions are indeed manifest. In fact, Freud considered these transference reactions to be immediately evident in the overt behavior toward the analyst and contended that they should be interpreted as representing modes of relating to past significant others. These manifestations are of prime importance for Freud's theory and may crowd out most other analytic material, so that, in children, they replace dreams as the "royal road to the unconscious" (A. Freud 1965, p. 37). While expressing transferential repetitions of older relationships, the child also uses the analyst as a new "object" in a thirst for novelty and new experience. The analyst must know how to differentiate these healthier modes of relating from the aggressive and libidinal transferential behaviors, because cure results largely from encouraging the former and interpreting the latter as each occurs in the analytic session. The key to the Freudian system of child analysis is therefore to create a new relationship and to bring to consciousness the automatic repetition of prior relationships that impedes the child's normal urge to complete development. This inherent maturational drive is seen as the most important ally of the analyst in the curative process and separates the analysis of children from that of adults.

Finally, Freud listed other modifications of analytic technique that are often necessary with children, including the analyst's use of the following:

- Verbalization and clarification of the preconscious material, to prepare the child for an interpretation and to lessen the anxiety that may accompany the uncovering process
- Suggestions and educational efforts
- Reassuring of the child as part of a trusting relationship with an adult

In addition, given the role of the analyst as an important new figure in the child's life, the child patient will frequently misuse the therapy as a "corrective emotional experience" rather than benefit only from interpretations.

In summary, Freud developed a system of child analysis that varies greatly in technique from that of adult analysis but that is still based on the interpretation of transference and resistance and the widening of consciousness at the expense of the unconscious, with the consequent increase in ego dominance (A. Freud 1965).

Psychodynamic Psychotherapy

Psychodynamic psychotherapy is a derivative of child analysis and is often difficult to differentiate from analytic therapy, particularly when one considers the modifications in technique suggested by Anna Freud. However, children in psychotherapy are *not* usually seen five times per week; the parents are often greatly involved in treatment; and, in addition, the indications for psychotherapy are more general, encompassing a variety of conditions beyond neurosis.[1] Furthermore, children in psychotherapy are given more active support and practical guidance than are children in analysis, where an almost exclusive reliance on the curative role of interpretations prevails. Corrective emotional experiences are encouraged rather than viewed as obstacles to self-awareness.

It would be a grave error, however, to consider psychodynamic psychotherapy a watered-down or lesser form of treatment compared with child analysis, to be recommended only when financial or time constraints or the limited availability of a more highly trained ther-

---

[1] This last criterion may not be completely valid, for although the ideal patient for Freudian child analysis is one who possesses a strong ego that can easily integrate knowledge of unconscious forces, all too often, as Nagera (1980) commented, this form of intensive treatment is sought as a last resort for very sick children who have not responded to other interventions. Kleinians, also, would consider most nonorganic childhood disorders responsive to analysis to some degree.

apist forces one to opt for a "second-rate" form of treatment. Actually, most psychodynamic therapy has its own inherent logical consistency, techniques, and goals, although extensively utilizing psychoanalytic concepts. The similarities and distinctions between these forms of treatment may be made clearer by an examination of how psychodynamic psychotherapy conceptualizes play, the role of the therapist, and specific curative factors.

In psychodynamic psychotherapy, the play of a young child and the drawings of an older child are viewed as the patient's manner of revealing his or her total life situation. Children do project their inner lives into the play activity, but they also reveal their reality situations. In essence, play is taken as the child's description of his or her perception of the universe, combining actual events and the particular distortions of developmental limitations or of a specific psychopathological attitude. Play is not used predominantly as a substitute for free association, nor is it used for its possible symbolism of unconscious drives or superego sanctions; rather, it is used as a child's mode for communicating the totality of his or her current life. Play is selected as the medium for gathering information because it is the natural activity of the child, who often lacks the ability to describe events in spoken words. Play affords an additional advantage, for it allows the child to present his or her predicament "in displacement," as if it did not particularly pertain to the child. In the 1930s, Jacob Conn (cited in Kanner 1940) described a method of "play interview" in a series of articles, in which he indicated how the child's feelings and wishes were projected (displaced) onto doll figures and thus could be expressed without fear or guilt:

> It is not the child but the doll who is afraid of the dark. It is not he who is envious or hates but the doll character. Therefore, he can give an account of the motives and imaginations which explain the doll's behavior and consequently his own. (cited in Kanner 1940, p. 14)

The play activity can be used to gather information just through observation of the situations and characters created by the child, or the therapist may join in the play, by assuming the role of one or more of the child's characters, to obtain more data. The therapist may also offer suggestions for solving problems or supply interpretations in the guise of a play character to the play figure that represents the child patient. This last technique represents the use of play as treatment, with the therapist confronting the child's usual manner of doing things or the therapist interpreting the child's motives or feelings without breaking down the defensive displacement.

Axline (1947) emphasized the curative aspects of play in itself in a manner similar to Klein's approach but without the use of interpretations. Axline believed that play by a child is a natural and spontaneous activity through which a variety of internal or external obstacles to psychological growth are revealed. These impediments are worked out in the context of a warm relationship with the therapist that allows the child to be his or her true self. The play activity of the child is geared to the developmental level: younger children may prefer the use of dolls to represent their life situations, older children reveal their personal styles of interacting through drawings or through games and other shared activities, and preadolescents may dispense with therapeutic props and insist on describing their circumstances verbally. The mode of communication varies with the age and the cognitive capacities of the child. However, there are no fixed rules regarding the medium of therapy; an older child may on occasion wish to draw or play a game to help in the revelation of his or her life, and, pari passu, a very young child may interrupt play for a significant verbal interchange. Overall, the activity of therapy should be geared to the capacities and limitations of the child's developmental state.

Another view of play is as a means of obtaining information, both from the content of the play and the form it takes in the child's interactions with the therapist. Play is seen as a familiar activity that fosters a relationship with the therapist; the way play is used in the relationship helps to define the task of therapy. This type of treatment, usually termed *relationship therapy*, was extensively described by Allen (1942) in the 1930s and 1940s and constitutes the framework for much of the child psychotherapy that is currently practiced. Allen (1942) believed that the patient "must find new values in himself, not in isolation, but in the relation to another human being" (p. 57). Therapy becomes an active interchange in which patients first use the therapist according to their experiences with prior relationships and then gradually are allowed the freedom to relate in a more autonomous and creative fashion. According to Allen, if the therapist is sufficiently empathic and does not impose his or her values in the therapeutic situation, the patients will sense the potentially liberating atmosphere and will express themselves with increasing authenticity and a willingness to share themselves. Allen commented that the therapeutic value of talking lies less in the particular content expressed and more in the freedom to talk.

The curative factor in Allen's form of psychotherapy would appear to be a type of corrective emotional experience in which a new adult reacts to the child in a manner different from past significant others, to supply the child with a new sense of self in the context of a trusting and liberating relationship. Although all psychotherapists would endorse Allen's emphasis on establishing a therapeutic relationship as the basis for therapy, most would consider it a necessary but not sufficient condition for the entire process. The creation of a close, trusting relationship has value in and of itself, but it also serves to facilitate the child's receptivity to interpretations regarding maladaptive behaviors and distortions of others, as well as the child's acceptance of guidance in finding more productive ways to solve problems.

In summary, psychodynamic psychotherapy does not restrict itself to interpreting derivatives of the unconscious as these appear in play, transference repetitions, or other manifest activities. It tends to deal with the patient's total situation and uses a variety of means to create a therapeutic alliance. The therapist uses a position of influence to allow the child to experience himself or herself in a freer, more realistic fashion and also to work actively with the child to solve reality-based problems (whether these stem from internalized conflicts, deviations of personality, environmental obstacles to psychological growth, or limiting organic or genetic deficits). The therapeutic experience is more similar to the child's activities outside the office as the therapist tries to create a real but influential relationship. As a result, techniques are more varied and less codified. Some therapists use play, others drawings, and others joint activities, from playing catch to building model airplanes.

Gardner (1986), in particular, developed a series of games and techniques that appeal to the child's natural attraction to play and fun while allowing for the investigation and correction of psychological problems. A frequently used therapeutic technique is the Squiggle Game, created by Winnicott (1971) to facilitate the child's expression of feelings or thoughts. In this technique, the therapist and the child exchange drawings, with each drawing initiated by the other person's initial "squiggle." The therapist starts the game by drawing a straight, curved, serpentine, or zigzag line, and

the child has to turn the squiggle into a drawing. He or she is then invited to comment on it. Then the roles are reversed: the child makes the squiggle, and the therapist completes it. Each drawing can be used to tell a story or may stimulate questions. The game can continue as long as it is productive and enjoyable. Often, after many drawings, the child starts to feel more comfortable and spontaneously describes his or her internal psychic life.

This drawing technique is very different from the simple House-Tree-Person Test, in which the child draws a house, a tree, or a person, and the therapist interprets underlying themes. Winnicott (1971) emphasized the use of the Squiggle Game in the development of trust in the therapeutic relationship. The patient "begins to feel that understanding may perhaps be available" (Winnicott 1971, p. 7) and participates more actively in the game. At this point, the therapist can make more active interpretations, which result in the production of more material. Winnicott believed that the Squiggle Game could facilitate the formation of a trusting relationship and shorten the initial period of therapy when a child plays in the presence of the therapist but does not interact or exchange meaningful material.

Unlike in analysis, in which the child is largely left responsible for the unfolding of psychological material, the psychotherapist may bring up specific problems when it is believed that the child is ready to deal with them. Therefore, themes believed to be relevant for an individual child may be introduced gradually at appropriate stages in the therapy. These themes should be expressed in a manner that the child can comprehend according to the child's ontogenetic status. The material can be presented in the play itself, if the patient is a young child, or as part of the style of mutual game playing, in the case of a latency-age child. With a preadolescent, problem areas can be discussed verbally while taking into account the child's still immature appreciation of reality. The frequency of sessions is not specified and may depend on the child's ability to generalize from the therapy sessions to everyday life. Some children can apply to the rest of their waking hours what they gain from only one session per week, whereas others require more frequent meetings to reinforce a problem-solving attitude.

Psychodynamic psychotherapy may be tailored to the individual's particular problem. For example, therapy with a child who has attention-deficit/hyperactivity disorder may focus on learning to live with an organic disorder; therapy with a child who has posttraumatic stress disorder could center on mastering a massive insult to prior adjustment; and therapy with a child who believes he or she must succeed in every undertaking can involve a whole restructuring of evaluations about the self and others.

Siblings, parents, and other adults who affect the psychological life of the child (e.g., teachers, coaches) may be involved at various points during the therapeutic process. Termination usually occurs after the child is relatively free of presenting symptoms; has developed age-appropriate interests, behaviors, and modes of coping; and is progressing along normal developmental paths in a nonpathogenic environment.

Comment

In the preceding descriptions of psychoanalytic and psychodynamic treatments, we accentuated differences and minimized similarities for expository purposes. In practice, however, these systems have a great deal in common.

Analysts recognize the curative value of a close, trusting relationship, and psychotherapists of any persuasion appreciate the essential role of the patient's past, and of motivating forces that are outside awareness, in causing current problems. It is the predominance given to the relationship as a therapeutic instrument and the perceiving of the child in his or her historical context that most differentiates both psychoanalytic and psychodynamic therapies from cognitive or behavioral treatments. The goal of the former therapies is to use the relationship and knowledge about the individual child's situation to remove internal or external obstacles to normal psychological growth and to restore the child to his or her own optimal developmental path.

Effectiveness of Psychotherapy

Evaluating the effectiveness of psychotherapy with children or adolescents is difficult. Unlike adults, who have consolidated a fairly permanent mode of psychological functions, this younger group of individuals is in the process of rapid change. Certain "symptoms" may represent a healthy response to developmental challenges and may subside without treatment when the challenges have been met. This course is most common with minor disturbances, as Anna Freud (1965) observed:

> In fact, where pathology is not too severe, the child analyst will often query after the successful conclusion of a treatment how much of the improvement he can claim as outcome of these therapeutic measures and how much he must ascribe to maturation and to spontaneous developmental moves. (p. 28)

Another complicating characteristic of this population is the significant reliance on parents or other adults to decide if and when a child needs treatment. Children may be brought for therapy when their symptoms are bothersome to others rather than to themselves, and the initiation of therapy may depend on the concern or indifference of parents or other adults (such as school personnel) who interact daily with the children in question. On a similar note, parents or guardians are the ones who decide whether therapy will continue and who ensure that appointments are kept.

A further difficulty encountered in the assessment of therapy in the pediatric population is the relatively strong reactivity to changes within the home environment. When the symptoms of the patient are a reflection of pathogenic family interactions, therapy is doomed to failure unless the appropriate family members are also involved and are motivated to change. This dependence on the child's responsiveness to the environment is especially relevant in efficacy studies carried out in community clinics serving families with social and economic difficulties that directly affect the functioning of the child being seen in therapy. Results of these studies may be poorer than results of studies involving children who come from less troubled families and who are seen in private practice or university settings.

Another factor influencing reported results is the precise treatment effect being measured. In some studies, only one symptom is the therapeutic target; in other studies, improvement of the child's overall psychological functioning is the aim. Other factors that affect results are the person performing the therapy and the setting of the therapy. The skill and experience of the therapist are crucial factors in determining the success or failure of treatment. In addition, the motivation of families participating in the study and the method of recruitment of subjects each play a role. Families that seek out treatment for their children are more apt to cooperate with treatment efforts than, for example, families referred by the courts or other institutions. Similarly, results obtained in studies focusing on treatment of one symptom, with relatively healthy subjects recruited through advertisements in newspapers and elsewhere, are more likely to be positive than results obtained in studies conducted in clinics and involving a variety of referred patients with differing degrees of impairment.

In summary, a number of factors besides the clinical needs of the patient can have a great effect on the results of psychotherapy with children and adolescents. The relative dysfunction of the child's family or everyday environment, the developmental level of the child, the compliance of the parents with therapy recommendations, the extent of treatment goals, and the setting and skill of the practitioner should be considered in evaluating study reports of therapeutic effectiveness.

With these limitations noted, there are sufficient reported studies of the effectiveness of psychotherapy to allow meta-analyses. Meta-analysis involves comparing a specific variable before and after treatment in a treated group and a matched control group, using published studies with clearly defined outcome measures, treatment protocols, and research populations. The degree of difference between groups for the indicated variable is divided by some measure of sample variability, such as the standard deviation of scores, to produce an effect size that indicates whether this difference is attributable to the therapy being studied. Reports considered to lack scientific rigor are not included in the final analysis.

Four relevant meta-analyses have been performed to date, and all demonstrated an appreciable effect size and therefore a significant beneficial result of therapy. These studies will be summarized only briefly here; the interested reader is referred to Weisz and Weiss (1993) for a more detailed exposition.

Casey and Berman (1985) surveyed psychotherapy outcome studies that involved children less than 13 years old and that were published between 1952 and 1983. Sixty-four studies met criteria for inclusion in a meta-analytic calculation, covering a variety of presenting problems, treatment methods, and sources of referral. These authors found an effect size of 0.71, meaning that children assigned to psychotherapy functioned better than 76% of untreated children.

Weisz et al. (1987) surveyed 104 studies published between 1958 and 1984 (32 of these were included in

Casey and Berman's [1985] review). The studies involved children ages 4–18 years. Weisz et al. (1987) found an effect size of 0.79, indicating that 79% of the treated children scored higher on the specific research variable than did the untreated children. However, 5% of the therapy groups yielded negative effect sizes, which means that treated children were worse off than control groups.

Kazdin et al. (1990) conducted a meta-analysis of 105 published reports of therapy outcome in children between ages 4 and 18 years. The studies, published between 1970 and 1988, included some of those examined in the two reviews just mentioned. This review also found an appreciable effect size (0.88)—indicating, again, a beneficial effect of psychotherapy.

Finally, Weisz et al. (1993) surveyed 110 studies, published between 1967 and 1991 and involving children ages 1.5–17.6 years. The obtained effect size was 0.71, indicating that treated children were doing better than 76% of untreated children.

The fact that all four of these large-scale meta-analyses, encompassing more than 200 reported studies, arrived at similar results speaks strongly for the effectiveness of psychotherapy. Using data from different populations, in which various psychotherapeutic interventions and outcome measures were studied, these reviews all showed that approximately three-fourths of children who received psychotherapy functioned better than matched control children who did not receive treatment.

Although meta-analyses may show the overall effectiveness of a specific treatment, they do not indicate where and in which populations response appears to be best. Weisz and Weiss (1993) reviewed these studies in more detail and found that certain factors seem to predict better outcomes than others. The studies with the best results were performed in academic centers with specially trained staff. The subjects were recruited, through advertisements in newspapers and other media, for treatment of only one specific symptom (such as shyness, obesity, or selective phobia). In contrast, studies reporting poor outcomes tended to involve community or publicly funded clinics, which traditionally serve families at lower socioeconomic levels who may have difficulty keeping appointments or be overwhelmed by problems other than those presented by the identified patient. The children treated in these facilities presented with possible organic problems, had extensive histories of prior difficulties, and were often sent for treatment by the courts. In a review of 91 intervention studies involving delinquent youths, Davidson et al. (1986/1993) did not find that traditional psychotherapy had a positive effect, which suggests that this treatment modality may not be appropriate for this population. In a more general review of selected studies, Kazdin (1990) concluded that although psychotherapy may be determined in large meta-analyses to be effective, the relevant priority for research is what *sort* of psychotherapy is most effective, and for what kind of individual.

These reviews indicate that psychotherapy, like most other treatment modalities, has its uses and its limitations and is not universally applicable to all youngsters with psychiatric difficulties. Results obtained in relatively healthy children from motivated, problem-free families who volunteer for a particular project may lead to excessive confidence in the efficacy of psychotherapy. Just as readily, when therapy is attempted with unmotivated patients who have comorbid neurological impairment (such as attention-deficit/hyperactivity disorder), who are burdened with economic disadvantage, and who present with long histories of multiple problems, results may lead to excessive pessimism about the efficacy of this treatment.

The studies summarized in this section are of importance but may not be representative, given that the bulk of psychotherapy is carried out by private practitioners, who generally treat children with problems greater than those seen in special treatment projects but smaller than those reported by community clinics. A more realistic appraisal of psychotherapy as practiced in the community may be found in a series of articles from the Anna Freud Centre in London (Fonagy and Target 1994; Target and Fonagy 1994a, 1994b). The records of 763 children treated with psychodynamic therapy by experienced clinicians were reviewed and assessed to determine symptom reduction and overall psychological functioning. The majority of children were found to benefit from therapy. Specifics of therapeutic response were also delineated. Children with more severe impairment, including both externalizing and internalizing symptoms, responded best to intensive therapy (three to five sessions per week), whereas children with milder impairment responded equally well to less-intensive therapy (one or two sessions per week). Younger children (less than 12 years old) did better with intensive therapy, whereas older children did just as well with less-intensive therapy but required a longer duration of treatment for optimal results. These results suggest that younger children may need more frequent sessions to maintain a new relationship, but because their disturbance may not be as consolidated as that of older children, a shorter period of treatment might suffice. In contrast, older children appear capable of forming a significant therapeutic relationship with less-intensive contact (possibly because they are able to work on therapy issues on their own between appointments) but have so internalized their problems into their everyday functioning that longer treatment is required.

The significant point to be gained from these studies is that psychotherapy, like most forms of treatment, is most applicable in certain cases and is not indicated in others. For some children, psychotherapy alone may suffice. For other children, interventions such as drug therapy, work with the child's family, or treatment in a residential environment should be the major focus (see Chapter 50, "Psychopharmacology"; Chapter 53, "Family Therapy"; and Chapter 56, "Milieu Treatment," in this volume).

References

Allen FH: Psychotherapy With Children. New York, WW Norton, 1942

Axline V: Play Therapy. Boston, MA, Houghton Mifflin, 1947

Casey RJ, Berman JS: The outcome of psychotherapy with children. Psychol Bull 98:388–400, 1985

Davidson WS, Gottschalk R, Gensheimer L, et al: Interventions with juvenile delinquents, unpublished manuscript, 1986. Cited in: Weisz JR, Weiss B: Effects of Psychotherapy With Children and Adolescents. New York, Sage, 1993

Ferenczi S: A little chanticleer (1913), in Sex in Psychoanalysis. New York, Robert Brunner, 1950, pp 240–252

Fonagy P, Target M: The efficacy of psychoanalysis for children with disruptive disorders. J Am Acad Child Adolesc Psychiatry 33:45–55, 1994

Freud A: Indications for child analysis (1945), in The Writings of Anna Freud, Vol 4. New York, International Universities Press, 1968, pp 3–38

Freud A: Normality and Pathology in Childhood: Assessments of Development. New York, International Universities Press, 1965

Freud S: Analysis of a phobia in a five-year-old boy (1909), in The Standard Edition of the Complete Psychological Works of Sigmund Freud, Vol 10. Translated and edited by Strachey J. London, Hogarth Press, 1955, pp 1–149

Gardner RA: The Psychotherapeutic Techniques of Richard A. Gardner. Cresskill, NJ, Creative Therapeutics, 1986

Hug-Helmuth H: On the technique of the analysis of children. Int J Psychoanal 1:361–362, 1920

Kanner L: Play investigation and play treatment of children's behavior disorders. J Pediatr 17:3–16, 1940

Kazdin AE: Psychotherapy for children and adolescents. Annu Rev Psychol 41:21–54, 1990

Kazdin AE, Bass D, Ayers WA, et al: Empirical and clinical focus of child and adolescent psychotherapy research. J Consult Clin Psychol 58:729–740, 1990

Klein M: Psychoanalysis of Children. London, Hogarth Press, 1932

Klein M: The psychoanalytic play technique. Am J Orthopsychiatry 25:223–237, 1955

Nagera H: Child psychoanalysis, in Emotional Disorders in Children and Adolescents. Edited by Sholevar GP, Benson RM, Blinder BJ. New York, Spectrum, 1980, pp 17–23

Segal H: Melanie Klein's technique of child analysis, in Handbook of Child Psychoanalysis. Edited by Wolman BB. New York, Van Nostrand Reinhold, 1972, pp 401–414

Target M, Fonagy P: Efficacy of psychoanalysis for children: prediction of outcome in a developmental context. J Am Acad Child Adolesc Psychiatry 33:1134–1144, 1994a

Target M, Fonagy P: Efficacy of psychoanalysis for children with emotional disorders. J Am Acad Child Adolesc Psychiatry 33:361–371, 1994b

Weisz JR, Weiss B: Effects of Psychotherapy With Children and Adolescents. New York, Sage, 1993

Weisz JR, Weiss B, Alicke MD, et al: Effectiveness of psychotherapy with children and adolescents: a meta-analysis for clinicians. J Consult Clin Psychol 55:542–549, 1987

Weisz JR, Weiss B, Morton G, et al: Unpublished data. Cited in: Weisz JR, Weiss B: Effects of Psychotherapy With Children and Adolescents. New York, Sage, 1993

Winnicott DW: Therapeutic Consultations in Child Psychiatry. New York, Basic Books, 1971

Cognitive-Behavior Modification

52

Alan E. Kazdin, Ph.D.

Behavior modification or behavior therapy (the terms are used synonymously in this chapter) is a treatment approach that emphasizes the empirical evaluation of clinical problems. When behavior modification first emerged as a formal movement in the 1950s, several key characteristics were delineated, including the focus of treatment on overt behavior, the absence of concern with presumed etiology, and the rejection of intrapsychic determinants (Kazdin 1978). Many of these characteristics were proposed as a reaction to prevailing psychoanalytic and psychodynamic views regarding psychopathology and treatment. Behavior modification was an alternative approach, more specifically one that was grounded in basic laboratory research and was committed heavily to empirical evaluation. Embedded in this broader movement were manifold theories, approaches, and treatment techniques. In the ensuing decades, behavior therapy has become even more diverse in terms of available treatments and the scope of applications to clinical problems. Even so, the basic tenets of the approach continue to be evident.

In this chapter, I discuss the scope of behavior modification, including its conceptual views, treatments, and applications. A large number of behavioral treatments for children and adolescents are in use. For illustration, selected treatments for anxiety, major depression, oppositional behavior, and conduct disorder are highlighted. Outcome evidence for these and other treatments is discussed. In addition, I present critical issues and limitations warranting further attention in relation to child treatment.

Scope of Behavior Modification

Many years ago, the standard way to present treatments in textbooks and training programs was to focus on approaches such as psychoanalytic therapy, family therapy, behavior therapy, and others. However, conceptual views and treatments within any approach often embrace conflicting views about what is important in the development of psychopathology and treatment. Consequently, the meaningfulness and alleged uniformity of an approach, even at the broad conceptual level, are easily challenged. The diversity of treatments within behavior modification illustrates this point. Consider the range of conceptual views and interventions and the clinical problems to which they are applied.

■ Conceptual Views

Behavior modification draws heavily on diverse theories to achieve an understanding of affect, cognition, and behavior and the factors that account for their emergence, maintenance, and alteration. Two general conceptual positions are referred to as mediational and nonmediational views. The *mediational view* emphasizes constructs such as affect and cognition that mediate or serve as underpinnings of behavior. A critical role is accorded cognitive processes such as plans, goals, beliefs, attributions, and self-statements. How individuals process the world (i.e., their cognitive

Completion of this chapter was facilitated by support from the Leon Lowenstein Foundation, the William T. Grant Foundation (98-1872-98), and the National Institute of Mental Health (MH59029). Support for this work is gratefully acknowledged.

processes) greatly influences behavior. Cognitive-behavioral theories, and treatments derived from them, fall within a mediational view (Craighead et al. 1994; Kendall 2000).

The *nonmediational view* focuses on direct (i.e., nonmediated) connections between environmental or situational events and behavior. Operant conditioning, which views behaviors as a function of antecedents (e.g., prompts, cues) and consequences (e.g., reactions of others), represents a nonmediational view. Child problems are seen as deficits or excesses in performance and can be altered directly by applying antecedent and consequent events (Kazdin 2001; Sulzer-Azaroff and Mayer 1991). Nonmediational views do not deny cognitive processes. However, intervening processes within the individual are not relied on for achieving therapeutic change.

The mediational and nonmediational views have long traditions in the psychology of learning, including years of theory and programmatic animal laboratory research. Behavioral treatments vary in the extent to which they rely on and integrate mediational views. A number of interventions concentrate almost exclusively on environmental influences and ignore or underplay cognitive processes as a focus of treatment. Techniques derived from operant conditioning (discussed under "Operant Conditioning Techniques" below) illustrate this approach. Other treatments focus primarily on cognitive processes, including various attributions and beliefs. In addition, several interventions rely on both mediational and nonmediational views. For example, many forms of cognitively based treatments emphasize cognitive processes as key to clinical dysfunction and points of intervention to effect change. Cognitively based treatments for anxiety and depression are of this ilk. Yet in the process of changing cognitions, the interventions also rely heavily on practice, overt behavior, and use of environmental sources of influence. For the purpose of changing cognitions, patients are given tasks, are assigned homework, and/or engage in role-play during treatment.

Much of the field is captured by the term *cognitive-behavior modification,* a phrase that reflects the fact that many treatments draw on mediational and nonmediational influences, either in the conceptualization of behavior change or the specific techniques used. How does a therapist change a patient's cognitions (e.g., negative beliefs about the patient or the future)? Merely reasoning with the individual and pointing out misguided thinking and distorted assumptions are

likely to be insufficient. One way to change thought processes is to change behavior—that is, to have the individual practice and engage in activities that promote more adaptive behavior. Practicing self-statements that are positive is one such activity and is designed to alter cognitive processes. The therapist is likely to challenge cognitions as well. Calling the treatment cognitive or behavioral creates an unnecessary and inaccurate dichotomy. In any case, the term *cognitive-behavior modification* better describes many treatments. I use the phrase *behavior modification* throughout the chapter, to encompass the full range of cognitive-behavioral techniques.

■ Intervention Techniques

Hundreds of psychotherapies for children and adolescents are in use. A conservative estimate is more than 550 documented treatments (Kazdin 2001). The number of techniques relating to cognitive-behavior modification is closer to 100–150. A definitive count is difficult because some nonbehavioral treatments have cognitive-behavioral components and a few behavioral treatments use strategies from nonbehavioral approaches. The important point is that there are many behavioral treatments.

A given technique is often identified in ways that mask a large number of variations. For example, *contingency management* is occasionally referred to as a specific intervention in which various rewarding and punishing consequences are used to alter behavior. The intervention refers generally to the alteration of antecedents (e.g., prompts, cues, instructions, discriminative stimuli) and consequences (e.g., reinforcers and schedules for their delivery) in relation to child behavior. Treatments based on contingency management vary in terms of parameters and types of reinforcers (praise, tokens), the persons who administer treatment (parents, teachers, peers, siblings, the children themselves), and the settings in which they are conducted (clinic, home, school, institutions). The variation has allowed application of this one class of treatment to children with a broad range of psychiatric disorders and social and emotional problems. Indeed, variations of contingency management have been applied to scores of clinical populations seen in child, adolescent, and adult psychiatry, as well as community samples (Kazdin 2001).

The full scope of available treatments cannot be presented in a single chapter. Several treatments are highlighted to illustrate the different emphases, foci, and procedures. Extensive evidence exists in support of the treatments covered.

■ Treatment Focus

Behavior modification has been applied to diverse child and adolescent samples and clinical problems (Ammerman and Hersen 1995; Ammerman et al. 1993; Christophersen and Mortweet 2001; Kazdin and Weisz 2003; Mash and Barkley 1998). Applications routinely involve clinical dysfunctions described in DSM-IV-TR (American Psychiatric Association 2000) and meriting treatment referrals. Thus, behavior modification has been applied to children with autism, mental retardation, anxiety or mood disorders, attention-deficit/hyperactivity disorder, conduct disorder, feeding or eating disorders, elimination disorders, learning disorders, tic disorders, substance abuse disorders, and other disorders. For a given clinical dysfunction, the scope of applications may be broad. For example, behavioral techniques have been useful for children with pervasive developmental disorders in the development of language, self-care, interpersonal, educational, and vocational skills (Newsom 1998). Within the area of anxiety disorders in children and adolescents, behavioral techniques have focused on separation anxiety, phobia, obsessive-compulsive disorder, and posttraumatic stress disorder.

Behavioral techniques have addressed several domains of child, adolescent, and indeed adult functioning that would not necessarily be regarded as evidence of clinical dysfunction (Kazdin 2001). The broad scope of applications makes behavior modification somewhat different from other therapies. Table 52–1 includes some of the applications. For each of the areas listed, there have been controlled outcome studies of the intervention. The breadth of applications can be traced to the fact that some of the treatments rely on principles and procedures (e.g., reinforcement, extinction) that can be readily applied across populations. For example, variants of operant conditioning have been used with infants (e.g., to eliminate rumination disorder) and geriatric patients (e.g., to increase engagement in activities or adherence to medication regimens). Although the focus of Table 52–1 is on behavior modification in the context of therapy, it is important to note that behavioral techniques are often used outside that context.

Characteristics of Behavior Modification

Behavior modification is an approach to the assessment, evaluation, and alteration of behavior rather than a specific form of psychotherapy or treatment. It has five broad characteristics, outlined below.

■ Focus on Behavior

In behavior modification, there is an emphasis on actions and performance—that is, what people do in everyday life. Whenever possible, the focus or problem is defined in terms of *overt behavior* that one can see, identify, detect, or observe in some way. Overt behavior is emphasized for three reasons. First, one can often intervene effectively in the case of overt behavior and influence thoughts and feelings. Second, in everyday situations, overt behavior is often the primary concern prompting the need to intervene. Third, the ability to translate problems into behaviors that reflect key aspects of the problem is helpful in evaluating the effectiveness of the intervention. Human functioning entails more than just what people do. Feelings and thoughts are no less important and often are not reducible to observable behaviors. Any given problem may encompass behaviors, feelings, and thoughts. For example, a child who gets into many fights (overt behavior) may be angry with others (affect) and think that others are trying to pick on him or hurt him (cognitions). Behavioral interventions can address all of these components of the problem, but even so, overt behavior is the general focus and is given priority.

Key characteristics of many clinical problems include thoughts (e.g., obsessive thoughts about something) and feelings (e.g., feelings of sadness or worthlessness, as in depression). An emphasis on behavior does not mean an exclusive focus on what people do. Indeed, many people in everyday life are actually "doing" quite well but are miserable and feel stagnant. Often behavior change is an end in itself—for example, in situations in which one wants to reduce criminal behavior and increase adaptive functioning. In other situations, behavior change is a means to an end—that is, changing behavior can help change how people feel and how they perceive the environment. A prevailing assumption has been that changing how people feel and what they think and know will change behavior.

Table 52–1. Some applications of behavior modification

Context or setting	Interventions have been effective in...
Therapy and treatment settings	Treating a broad range of psychological problems and psychiatric disorders, including anxiety (e.g., fears, obsessive-compulsive disorders, panic attacks), depression, substance use and abuse (e.g., use of drugs, alcohol, or cigarettes), conduct problems, hyperactivity, autism, and eating disorders
Education	Improving (in elementary, middle, and high school students) academic performance, studying, achievement, grades, classroom deportment, creative writing, and participation in activities; and improving (in all students, including college students) mastery of subject matter. Many programs in school settings have focused on behaviors beyond the usual domain of education because schools provide a place to deliver interventions. Thus, behavioral programs have been used to reduce or prevent cigarette smoking, alcohol and drug use, and unprotected sex among adolescents.
Medicine and health	Teaching individuals to detect early signs of disease (e.g., self-examination for signs of cancer), protect against sexually transmitted diseases, reduce pain associated with invasive medical procedures (e.g., lumbar taps) or postoperative recovery, and adhere to medical regimens (e.g., for cancer or diabetes)
Business and industry	Teaching workers to engage in practices that reduce accidents (e.g., when using equipment) and to improve health or overcome problems that compete with health and work (e.g., alcohol use, cigarette smoking); and helping individuals to obtain jobs (e.g., teaching how to seek jobs, teaching interview skills), improve job performance, reduce absenteeism and tardiness, improve employee–customer interactions, and reduce shoplifting by customers
Sports and athletics	Improving coaching practices, performance of athletes (e.g., in football, gymnastics, tennis, swimming, and track), and stress management among athletes
Everyday life	Training parents to interact with their children, when parents are in special situations (e.g., have a handicapped child) or have no special difficulties or obstacles or when children are in special situations (e.g., are abused or neglected); training children to engage in safe behaviors (e.g., use seat belts, cross streets safely) or ward off dangerous situations (e.g., respond appropriately to would-be abductors); training the elderly in nursing homes to increase physical activity and have more social interactions with others; and training individuals to drive safely, conserve energy at home, and recycle waste

No doubt this is true in some circumstances, but the opposite also is true—that is, changing what people do can lead to changes in how they feel and what they think. For example, increases in activity and interpersonal interaction have been found to alter depressive symptoms, including feelings and thoughts. As part of treatment, a depressed person may be encouraged to engage in specific activities involving interactions with others and in setting goals for accomplishing specific tasks at home or at work.

In some cases in which the focus or problem is emotions rather than overt behavior, overt behavior will be considered in the evaluation of treatment outcome. For example, an adult or child who is very angry might be treated with techniques that focus on ways to control these feelings. In such instances, the focus of treatment may be on the individual's feelings and in-

ternal cues (e.g., initial feelings of anger, physiological arousal) rather than on overt behavior. However, in the evaluation of treatment effect, overt behavior is likely to be included among the outcome measures.

■ Focus on Current Determinants of Behavior

Behavior modification research focuses on understanding the causes of behavior and the factors that relate to how individuals function and perform in everyday life. Causes of behavior can involve many different facets of functioning. It is useful to distinguish past from present causes or sources of influence. For example, a 20-year-old female college student may seek therapy because she is having problems with relationships. The problem may be due in part to how she was treated as a child. Perhaps as a young child she suffered physical abuse or neglect or just lived with unusual parents. These problems in childhood may play a role in the current problem. Yet the guiding question for any form of intervention is "What can be done now to develop the behaviors of interest and to improve adaptive functioning?" In behavior modification, emphasis is placed on current influences on behavior and how they can be mobilized to make changes.

The focus on current influences and changes does not in any way undermine the importance of understanding how behaviors originally develop. An awareness of how a problem begins can often be used for prevention. Whether the goal is prevention or treatment, there is an urgent need to understand how to change current behavior. Remarkable progress has been made in understanding influences, and this understanding can be brought to bear to develop new behaviors and change maladaptive patterns.

■ Focus on Learning Experiences to Promote Change

Behavioral treatments provide special learning experiences to decrease deviant or maladaptive behavior and to increase adaptive behavior. This learning must be carefully arranged and be much more systematic than in everyday life. It is not accurate in this case to say that practice makes perfect. One can practice endlessly (e.g., practice a musical instrument, practice taking off in a small plane) but make little progress. Practice must be accompanied by other systematic experiences (e.g., instruction, feedback, gradual development of increasingly complex skills), depending on the skill. Much has been learned from research about how to develop, change, increase, reduce, and eliminate behaviors. Theory and research on different types of learning and the conditions under which learning takes place represent active areas of scientific study (for example, see Catania 1997).

Although many problem behaviors can be changed through learning experiences, not all behaviors are learned and can be changed through learning. Biological, behavioral, social, cultural, and other factors influence the development of behavior and also may be relevant to behavior change. The key feature of the behavioral approach is recognition of the amenability of behavior to change when systematic learning experiences are provided. Whether new learning experiences will alter behavior can be determined only by testing what changes occur. The assumption that learning experiences can alter behavior has proven to be extremely helpful in developing effective treatments.

■ Assessment and Evaluation

A central characteristic of behavior modification is a commitment to assessment and evaluation of alternative treatments. In behavior modification research, major emphasis is placed on measuring outcome in controlled studies. Proponents of behavior modification have often viewed the emphasis on outcomes research as the hallmark of the approach. Psychotherapy has increasingly emphasized evidence-based treatments (Christophersen and Mortweet 2001; Lonigan and Elbert 1998).

In clinical work with individuals, evaluation is also important for monitoring progress during treatment. Such evaluation begins with assessment of presenting symptoms or behaviors. The assessment of the child may consist of direct observation of performance at home and at school, evaluations by significant others (parents, peers), and self-evaluations (Mash and Terdal 1997). The focus of the evaluation tends to be on details of the symptoms or behaviors, the conditions associated with their performance (e.g., setting, antecedents, consequences), and resources in the child's repertoire and environment that might be mobilized in specific treatment strategies. Specific measures and evaluation strategies are often used in individual cases to assess effects of treatment and the extent of clinically important changes (Clement 1999; Kazdin 1993). Evaluation of progress in treatment is also facilitated by the existence of clearly specified goals and procedures.

■ Applications in Everyday Life

Many applications of treatment involve meeting a child in individual therapy sessions, as in traditional models of treatment. More commonly, therapy involves working directly with and training those persons responsible for the care, management, and education of the child. Parents and teachers, in particular, frequently serve as agents of change within child behavior therapy.

Several factors point to the need to train those who are in contact with children. First, parents, teachers, institutional staff, and peers unwittingly support many of the problem behaviors identified as worthy of intervention (e.g., obstinacy, tantrums, antisocial behavior). Hence, changing the behaviors of those in contact with the child is often critical to effective treatment. Second, treatment often produces effects more readily in the naturalistic setting than in the therapist's office. Parents and teachers have immediate access to the problems as they occur, and they can bring to bear potent events (e.g., their own attention and affection) to promote appropriate, prosocial behaviors. Third, behavioral problems are often situation specific. For example, a child who is aggressive and oppositional at school may not be so at home. Consequently, treatments are designed for and implemented in situations in which behavior is problematic. When treatment is conducted in a special setting (e.g., in a hospital), the attempt is made to extend the treatment to the settings in which the behaviors ultimately need to be performed.

■ Comment

The previously described characteristics are general, because using more specific characteristics immediately excludes major segments of behavior modification. For example, one might claim that behavioral approaches focus on consequences of behavior (e.g., rewards) to achieve therapeutic change. Although several interventions focus on consequences, many techniques do not. One might also pose that behaviors (e.g., presenting symptoms) are the appropriate treatment focus of behavioral techniques. However, many techniques, particularly those based on cognitive-behavioral procedures, do not have this focus.

Treatment: Illustrations of Selected Interventions

The scope of treatment techniques, clinical problems, and populations to which treatment techniques have been applied precludes even a cursory overview of outcomes research on behavior modification. Five treatments are highlighted here to convey the diversity of interventions and the range of applications in clinical work. These treatments are cognitive-behavioral thera-

py for child anxiety, the Adolescent Coping With Depression Course (CWD-A), cognitive problem-solving skills training, parent management training (PMT), and applications of operant conditioning. The evidence for each of these is extensive and will not be detailed here.[1]

■ Cognitive-Behavioral Therapy for Child Anxiety

Background and Rationale

Cognitive-behavioral therapy for anxiety in children focuses on dysfunctional cognitions and their implications for the child's subsequent thinking and behavior (see reviews by Kendall and Treadwell [1996] and Kendall et al. [2000]). Key components of cognition are distinguished, including cognitive structures (memory and ways in which information is experienced), cognitive content (ongoing self-statements), cognitive processes (how experiences are processed and interpreted), and cognitive products (attributions that result from cognitive structures, content, and processes). Cognitive distortions are considered to play a central role in children with anxiety (Kendall et al. 1997b). The term *cognitive distortions* refers to information processes that lead to misperceptions of oneself or the environment. Treatment helps the child develop new skills, provides new experiences for the child to test dysfunctional as well as adaptive beliefs, and assists the child in processing new experiences. The direct focus of strategies used in treatment is on learning new behaviors through modeling and direct reinforcement. In addition, cognitive strategies, such as the use of self-statements, address processes (information processing style, attributions, and self-talk) that are considered to mediate anxiety.

Characteristics of Treatment

The cognitive-behavioral therapy program consists of 16–20 private sessions with the child. Among the techniques used are modeling, role-playing, in vivo exposure, relaxation training, and reinforcement. In addition, practice efforts are made to extend the treatment

---

[1]Outcomes research on behavior modification is dispersed across many journals in clinical psychology, psychiatry, education, rehabilitation, and health. Journals devoted almost exclusively to behavioral interventions include *Behavior Modification, Behavior Therapy, Behaviour Research and Therapy, Child and Family Behavior Therapy, Cognitive Therapy and Research, Journal of Applied Behavior Analysis*, and *Journal of Behavior Therapy and Experimental Psychiatry*.

to anxiety-provoking situations at home and at school.

Approximately the first half of treatment is devoted to learning steps for coping with anxiety and managing distress. These include recognizing the physiological symptoms of anxiety (e.g., tension), challenging and altering anxiety-provoking cognitions and one's internal dialogue (e.g., expecting bad things to happen and generating ideas about what else might happen); problem solving (e.g., devising a plan to cope with the anxiety, generating other courses of action and selecting one of them); and evaluating the coping plan and engaging in follow-up actions (e.g., self-evaluation and self-reinforcement).

The second half of treatment focuses on applying the newly learned skills in imaginary and low-anxiety-provoking situations and then later in moderate- and high-anxiety-provoking situations. Exposure is also part of homework assignments, with the child applying the steps at home and at school. Rewards are earned for completion of these assignments. In the final session of treatment, the child makes a videotaped "commercial" describing the steps and their use in mastering anxiety-provoking situations.

Evidence and Overall Evaluation

Treatment of children ages 9–13 years has been evaluated in both group and single-case experimental studies (Flannery-Schroeder and Kendall 2000; Kendall et al. 1997b, 2003). In randomized controlled trials, treatment was superior to waiting-list control conditions. Improvements were evident on multiple child, parent, and teacher report measures of anxiety and other symptom domains, including aggression, social problems, hyperactivity, and depression, and in behavioral observations of child distress (Flannery-Schroeder and Kendall 2000; Kendall 1994; Kendall et al. 1997a). Treatment gains were reflected in the return of many youths (64% in one study) to the normative range for anxiety. Follow-up data 1 year and more than 3 years later indicated that treatment effects were maintained (Kendall and Southam-Gerow 1996; Kendall et al. 1997a). Another team of investigators (Barrett 1998; Barrett et al. 1996, 2001; Dadds et al. 1999) replicated the effects of treatment in randomized controlled trials and showed that treatment effects were maintained up to 6 years.

The treatment research is exemplary in a number of ways. First, the studies included children who met DSM criteria for anxiety disorder—primarily generalized anxiety, separation anxiety, and social phobia. Second, the effect of treatment was strong and consistent across studies; in fact, a separate investigative team replicated the main findings. Third, the clinical significance of treatment was demonstrated repeatedly. Clearly, cognitive-behavioral therapy for anxiety disorders is an evidence-based treatment. The availability of a treatment manual (Kendall et al. 1990) allows extension into clinical settings and, of course, further research for developing the treatment.

■ Adolescent Coping With Depression Course

Background and Rationale

The CWD-A Adolescent Coping With Depression Course draws on cognitive and behavioral conceptualizations of major depression (Clarke et al. 2003; Lewinsohn et al. 1996). Depression is associated with multiple cognitions (e.g., hopelessness, helplessness) and restricted behavioral repertoires (e.g., limited participation in pleasant activities, few experiences of reinforcement in the environment). Disruptions of behavioral patterns in everyday life are accorded special importance in terms of initiating depressive cognitions and the symptom patterns of the disorder (Lewinsohn et al. 1985). The CWD-A is a cognitive-behavioral treatment that combines these different views and treatment components. To address cognitive features of depression, the therapist makes the individual aware of his or her often pessimistic, negative thoughts, beliefs, and self-blaming causal attributions. More constructive cognitions are substituted and are practiced outside treatment. To address the behavioral features of depression, activities associated with positive reinforcement from the environment are increased. This is accomplished by the teaching of specific social skills.

Characteristics of Treatment

CWD-A is a group treatment and is conceptualized as a course, with psychoeducational components, so that the stigma of treatment is lessened. The primary focus is on development of skills and the means to cope with problematic situations. Group activities and role-playing are central in the treatment sessions; between sessions, homework assignments extend the treatment beyond the classroom. Treatment includes 16 two-hour sessions over 8 weeks (Lewinsohn et al. 1996).

Up to 10 adolescents are included in the group. The course includes a workbook with brief readings, quizzes, structured learning tasks, and forms for practice (homework) assignments. The sessions focus on specific skills and themes, such as developing social skills, engaging in pleasant activities, and reducing negative cognitions. Throughout the sessions, skills are taught and practiced; skills are also practiced at home.

Other aspects of treatment have been included but are not necessarily central to the main treatment. A parent component has been added in which parents are trained to support and assist skills developed in the adolescent. During these separate sessions for parents, the parents are also taught communication and problem-solving skills. In addition, booster (additional) sessions have been provided to the adolescents at the end of the 16-week course. These sessions, offered for 2 years, address emergent issues specific to each case. There is a brief assessment of how the adolescent is doing in everyday life, of current target complaints, and of the adolescent's use of skills learned in the training course.

Evidence and Overall Evaluation

Randomized controlled clinical trials of the CWD-A in adolescents have demonstrated that the course is significantly more effective than a wait-list control treatment condition in reducing major depression (Lewinsohn and Clarke 1999; Lewinsohn et al. 1990). Treatment effects have been maintained for 2 years of follow-up. The studies have been consistent in demonstrating the effects of the basic treatment. Indeed, many (more than 20) outcome studies—involving adolescents, adults, elderly individuals, minority groups, and caregivers of the elderly, and in the contexts of treatment and prevention—have demonstrated the effectiveness of various forms of this intervention (Cuijpers 1998).

This treatment has several notable features. First, the focus has been on adolescents with diagnosable depression. Second, the effect of treatment has been impressive across a range of outcome domains (e.g., symptoms, functioning in everyday life, coping skills). Third, the clinical effect or significance of treatment has been determined through evaluation of the extent to which youths continue to meet diagnostic criteria for depression. At the end of treatment, the proportion of youths who still meet diagnostic criteria is significantly lower for treated than for wait-list cases (e.g., 33% vs. 52% in Lewinsohn et al. 1996). Fourth, the format of the treatment raises prospects for dissemina-

tion. The intervention is presented as a course and an academic or educational experience, rather than as psychotherapy or treatment. Many depressed individuals who would not otherwise seek treatment—because of the stigma associated with, or perceived to be associated with, seeking therapy or outpatient care—might choose this intervention. The availability of course materials, including a treatment manual, videotapes, and workbooks (Clarke et al. 1990; Lewinsohn et al. 1996), may also make the treatment easily disseminated among practitioners.

■ Cognitive Problem-Solving Skills Training

Background and Rationale

The term *cognitive processes* refers to a broad class of constructs that pertain to how an individual perceives, codes, and experiences the world. Individuals with conduct problem behaviors, particularly aggression, often have distortions of and deficiencies in various cognitive processes. Although selected processes (recall, information processing) are related to intellectual functioning, cognitive problem-solving skills play a separate role in the prediction of behavioral adjustment and social behavior. A variety of cognitive processes have been studied in the context of interpersonal functioning (Crick and Dodge 1994; Shirk 1988). In Table 52–2, several processes are presented that illustrate the focus of cognitively based treatment. The ability to engage in these processes is related to behavioral adjustment, as measured by teacher ratings of disruptive behavior (Spivack and Shure 1982; Spivack et al. 1976). Teacher ratings of disruptive behavior, peer evaluations, and direct assessment of overt behavior point out deficits in and distortion of these processes.

Characteristics of Treatment

Problem-solving skills training (PSST) develops interpersonal cognitive problem-solving skills. Although many variations of PSST have been applied to children with conduct problems, these variations usually share several characteristics.

- The emphasis is on how children approach situations. Although it is important that children ultimately select appropriate means of behaving in everyday life, the primary focus is on the thought processes rather than the outcome or the specific behavioral acts that result.

Table 52–2. Examples of cognitive problem-solving skills

Alternative-solution thinking—the ability to generate different options (solutions) that can solve problems in interpersonal situations

Means–end thinking—awareness of the intermediate steps required to achieve a particular goal

Consequential thinking—the ability to identify what might happen as a direct result of acting in a particular way or choosing a particular solution

Causal thinking—the ability to relate one event to another over time and to understand why one event led to a particular action by another person

Sensitivity to interpersonal problems—the ability to perceive a problem when it exists and to identify the interpersonal aspects of the confrontation that may emerge

- Children are taught to engage in a step-by-step approach to solve interpersonal problems. They make statements to themselves that direct attention to certain aspects of the problem or tasks that lead to effective solutions.
- Treatment includes structured tasks involving games, academic activities, and stories. Over the course of treatment, the cognitive problem–solving skills are increasingly applied to real-life situations.
- Therapists usually play an active role in treatment. They model the cognitive processes by making verbal self-statements, apply the sequence of statements to particular problems, provide cues for prompt use of the skills, and deliver feedback and praise to develop correct use of the skills.
- Treatment usually involves several procedures, including modeling and practice, role-playing, and reinforcement and mild punishment (loss of points or tokens).

Case Example

Cory, a 10-year-old boy, was hospitalized on a short-term children's inpatient unit to begin a treatment regimen designed to control his aggressive, antisocial, oppositional, and disruptive behavior at home and at school. On three occasions, he had been caught playing with matches and setting fires in his room. He had been suspended from school for assaulting and choking a classmate until the child almost passed out. PSST was begun and completed while Cory was in the hospital, because his parents said they could not return for treatment on an outpatient basis once hospitalization ended. Cory underwent 20 individual sessions of PSST; 2–3 sessions were conducted each week. The

sessions began with teaching Cory the problem-solving steps. These consist of specific self-statements, with each statement representing a step for solving a problem and addressing some of the cognitive deficiencies noted in Table 52–2. The self-statements include the following:

1. What am I supposed to do?
2. I have to look at all my possibilities.
3. I have to concentrate and focus.
4. I need to make a choice and select a solution.
5. I need to find out how I did.

In the first session, Cory was taught the steps so that they could be recalled without special reminders or cues from the therapist. In the next several sessions, the steps were applied to simple problems involving various academic tasks (e.g., arithmetic problems) and board games (e.g., checkers). In each of these sessions, Cory's task was to identify the goal, the alternative choices or options and their consequences, the best choice in light of these consequences, and so on. After the steps were applied with facility, the games were withdrawn, and the steps were applied to problems related to interactions with parents, teachers, siblings, peers, and others.

Cory was also given assignments to complete outside treatment. Initially, the assignments were to identify "real" problems (e.g., with another child on the inpatient service) where he could use the steps. When he brought one of these situations to the session, he described how the steps could have been used. He earned points for bringing in such a situation, and these points could be exchanged for small prizes. As the sessions progressed, he received points for using the steps in the actual situations. His use of the steps was checked by the therapist's asking him exactly what he did, by role-playing the situation within the session, and by the therapist's asking other staff on the ward if the events had occurred as Cory described.

The majority of treatment consisted of applying the steps in the session to situations in which Cory's aggressive and antisocial behaviors emerged. A segment of one of these sessions follows:

Therapist: Well, Cory, today we are going to act out some more problem situations using the steps. You have been doing so well with this that I think we can use the steps today in a way that will make it even easier to use them in everyday life. When you use the steps today, I want you to think in your mind what the first steps are. We are going to do the steps in our heads today like this so that it will be easier to use them in everyday life without drawing attention to what we are doing. The same rules apply as in our other sessions. We still want to go slowly in using the steps, and we want to select good solutions.

OK, today I brought in a lot of difficult situations. I think it is going to be hard to use the steps. Let's see how each of us does. I have six stacks of cards here. You can see the stacks are numbered from 1 to 6. We will take turns rolling the die and take a card from the stack with the same number. As we did in the last session, we are going to solve the problem as we sit here, then we will get up and act it out as if it is really happening. OK, why don't you go first and roll the die?

Cory: [Rolls the die] I got a 4.

Therapist: OK, read the top card in that stack. [Points to the fourth stack]

Cory: [Reads the card] "The principal of your school is walking past you in the hall between classes when he notices some candy wrappers that someone has dropped on the floor. The principal turns to you and says in a pretty tough voice, 'Cory, we don't litter in the halls at this school! Now pick up the trash!'"

Therapist: This is a tough one. How are you going to handle this?

Cory: Well, here goes with the steps. [Holds his index finger up and appears to be saying the steps to himself] I would say to him that I did not throw the wrappers down and I would keep walking.

Therapist: Well, it was great that you did not get mad and talk back to him. He was sort of accusing you and you hadn't really thrown the papers down. But if you just say "I didn't do it" and walk away, what might happen?

Cory: Nothing. Because I didn't do it.

Therapist: Yeah, but he may not believe you—maybe especially because you got into trouble before with him. Also, he asked you for a favor and you could help a lot by doing what he asked. Try going through the steps again and see if you can turn your pretty good solution into a great one.

Cory: [Goes through steps 1, 2, 3, and 4] I would say to him that I did not throw the wrappers down but that I would gladly pick them up and toss them in the trash.

Therapist: [With great enthusiasm] That's great—that's a wonderful solution! OK. Go to step 5: How do you think you did?

Cory: I did good because I used the steps.

Therapist: That's right, but you did more than that. You nicely told the principal that you did not do it, and you did the favor he asked. What do you think he will think of you in the future? Very nicely done. OK. Now let's both get up and act this out.

The treatment session continued as this situation was enacted through role-play and several other situations were presented. When Cory did especially well, the situation was made a little more difficult or provocative to help him apply the steps to more challenging circumstances.

Evidence and Overall Evaluation

Several outcome studies have been completed involving children and adolescents with impulsive, aggressive, and conduct problems (see reviews by Baer and Nietzel [1991] and Durlak et al. [1991]). In many of these studies, cognitively based treatment led to significant reductions in aggressive and antisocial behavior at home, at school, and in the community, and these gains were evident up to 1 year later. Some evidence suggests that older children profit more from treatment than younger children, perhaps because of their cognitive development (Durlak et al. 1991). However, the basis for differential responsiveness to treatment as a function of age or severity of symptoms has not been well tested. Moreover, other factors than age appear to play stronger roles in predicting outcome effects. Reading achievement and academic functioning are among these stronger predictors of responsiveness to treatment (Kazdin and Crowley 1997). Children with conduct problems who come from families with high levels of impairment (parent psychopathology, stress, and family dysfunction) respond less well to treatment than do youths from families with less impairment. Whether these factors are specific to PSST or influence the effectiveness of all treatments for youths with conduct problems has yet to be studied.

In the context of treatment for referred cases, evidence supports PSST as a treatment for conduct disorder (Kazdin 2003a). Evidence from outside the context of treatment is quite pertinent to the evaluation of this intervention. PSST has been studied for 20 years in a well-developed program of research (Shure 1997, 1999). In one study, PSST was provided in the classrooms of economically disadvantaged elementary school children. Those who received the training, compared with those who did not, showed decreases in disruptive student behavior and increases in positive, prosocial behavior. Although the effects were evident when training was conducted for 1 year (kindergarten), the impact was greater when training was continued for 2 years (kindergarten and first grade). In either case, the benefits of the intervention were still evident 2 years or more after the program ended. The program is noteworthy because it can be implemented on a large scale in schools and can be used to improve outcomes of children at high risk for academic, social, emotional, and behavioral problems.

Features of PSST make it an extremely promising approach. First, and perhaps most important, several controlled outcome studies with clinical samples have shown that cognitively based treatment leads to therapeutic change. Second, basic research in developmental psychology continues to clarify the relationship between conduct problems and maladaptive cognitive processes among children and adolescents. Third, many variations of treatment are outlined in manuals (e.g., Finch et al. 1993; Shure 1992, 1996). Consequently, the treatment can be evaluated in research and explored further in clinical practice.

Fundamental questions about treatment remain. The role of cognitive processes in clinical dysfunction and treatment warrants further evaluation. It is not entirely evident that a specific pattern of cognitive processes, rather than general disruptive behavioral or adjustment problems, characterizes youth with conduct problems. Also, although it has been shown that cognitive processes change with treatment, it has not been established that change in these processes is responsible for improvements in treatment. Furthermore, developmental constructs, characteristics of children and their families, and parameters of treatment generally have not been explored in relation to treatment outcome. Finally, although reliable changes have been achieved with treatment, the magnitude of change raises questions. Many youths improve but remain outside the range of normative functioning relative to same-age and same-sex peers (Kazdin et al. 1989, 1992). Clearly, central questions about treatment and its effects remain to be resolved. Even so, PSST is highly promising, given that treatment effects have been replicated in several controlled studies involving youth with conduct disorders (Kazdin 2003a; Kazdin, in press).

■ Parent Management Training

Background and Rationale

In PMT, parents are trained to alter their child's behavior in the home. Training is based on the general view that oppositional and aggressive behavior are inadvertently developed and sustained in the home by maladaptive parent–child interactions. Of the many interaction patterns, those involving coercion have received the greatest attention (Patterson 1982; Patterson et al. 1993). The word *coercion* refers to deviant behavior by one person (e.g., the child) that is rewarded by another person (e.g., the parent). Aggressive children are inadvertently rewarded for their aggressive interactions and their escalation of coercive behaviors through discipline practices that sustain aggressive behavior.

The primary goal of PMT is to alter the pattern of interchanges between parent and child so that prosocial, rather than coercive, behavior is directly reinforced and supported within the family. This requires the development of several different parenting behaviors, such as establishing rules for the child to follow, providing positive reinforcement for appropriate behavior, delivering mild forms of punishment to suppress behavior, and negotiating compromises. These parenting behaviors are systematically and progressively developed within the sessions, in which the therapist shapes (develops through successive approximations) parenting skills. The procedures that parents eventually implement in the home are reviewed, modified, and refined in subsequent sessions.

Characteristics of Treatment

Although many variations of PMT exist, several common characteristics can be identified. The parents meet with a therapist who teaches them to use specific procedures to alter interactions with their child, to promote prosocial behavior, and to decrease deviant behavior. Parents are trained to identify, define, and observe problem behaviors in new ways. Careful specification of the problem is essential for delivery of reinforcing or punishing consequences and for determining whether the program is achieving the desired goals. The treatment sessions are opportunities for the parents to see how the techniques are implemented, to practice and refine the techniques (e.g., through extensive role-playing), and to review the behavior-change programs implemented at home.

Parent-managed reinforcement programs for child deportment and performance at school, completion of homework, and activities on the playground are included, with the assistance of teachers, as available.

Case Example

Shawn, a 7-year-old boy, was referred for treatment because of his aggressive outbursts toward his two younger sisters at home and his peers at school. He argued and had severe tantrums at home, stayed out late at night, and occasionally stole from his mother's live-in boyfriend. At school, he fought with peers, argued with the teacher, and disrupted the class. PMT was provided to Shawn's mother. The boyfriend was unable to attend the sessions regularly because of his work as a trucker. The overall goal of treatment was to train the mother to behave differently toward Shawn and her other children. Specifically, she was trained to identify concrete problematic and prosocial behaviors, to observe these behaviors systematically, to implement positive reinforcement programs, to provide mild punishment as needed, and to negotiate such programs directly with the child.

The content of the 16 sessions provided to Shawn's mother (and sometimes her boyfriend) is highlighted in Table 52–3. Each session lasted 1–2 hours. In each session, the therapist reviewed the previous week's observations and implementation of the program. Queries were made to review what the mother and the boyfriend did (e.g., praise, administer points or tokens, send the child to time-out) in response to the child's behavior. The therapist and the mother role-played situations at home in which the mother might have responded more effectively. The mother practiced delivering the consequences and received feedback and reinforcement from the therapist. Problems in the programs, ambiguity about observation procedures, and other facets of treatment were discussed. After the program was reviewed, new material was taught, as outlined in Table 52–3.

Shawn's mother and the therapist developed a program to increase Shawn's compliance with requests. Shawn was asked to do simple chores (e.g., clean his room, set the table) in the first few weeks of the program, to help the mother and the boyfriend apply what they had learned. Time-out from reinforcement (removal of positive reinforcers for a brief period) served as mild punishment for fighting. Over time, several behaviors were incorporated into a program in which Shawn earned points that could purchase special privileges (e.g., staying up 15 minutes beyond bedtime, having a friend sleep over, small prizes, time to play his video game). About halfway through treatment, a home-based reinforcement program was developed to alter behaviors at school. Two teachers at the school were asked to identify behaviors to be developed in class. They were asked to

initial cards that Shawn carried, to indicate how well he behaved in class and whether he completed his homework. On the basis of daily teacher evaluations, Shawn earned additional points at home.

After approximately 5 months, Shawn had improved greatly in his behavior at home. He argued very little with his mother and sisters. His mother and her boyfriend thought they were much better able to manage him. Shawn's teachers reported that he could remain in class like other children. Occasionally, he would not listen to the teacher or would precipitated heated arguments with his peers. However, he was less physically aggressive than he had been before treatment.

Evidence and Overall Evaluation

PMT is one of the best-researched therapy techniques for children and adolescents. Treatment has been evaluated in scores of randomized controlled outcome trials involving children and adolescents varying in age (e.g., 2–17 years old) and severity of oppositional and conduct problems (Kazdin 1997, 2001). Indeed, in a review of treatments for conduct disorder, PMT was identified as the only well-established intervention (i.e., the only intervention shown to be effective in independently replicated controlled clinical trials) (Brestan and Eyberg 1998). PMT has led to marked improvements in child behavior, as reflected in parent and teacher reports of deviant behavior, direct observational measures of behavior at home and at school, and institutional records (e.g., regarding school truancy, police contacts, arrests, and institutionalization). Children and adolescents with conduct problem behaviors who have been treated with PMT have achieved normative levels of functioning at home and at school (levels in keeping with normative data from nonreferred peers [e.g., same age, same sex]). In several studies, treatment gains were maintained 1–3 years after treatment (e.g., Eyberg et al. 2001); one group of investigators reported maintenance of gains 10–14 years after treatment (Long et al. 1994).

In much of the outcomes research, PMT has been administered to individual families in clinic settings. Group administration has been greatly facilitated by the development of videotaped materials that present themes, principles, and procedures to the parents. Use of these tapes has been rigorously evaluated and has been shown to be effective with parents of children with conduct problems (Webster-Stratton 1996; Webster-Stratton and Reid 2003). PMT has been extended

Table 52–3. Parent management training sessions used with Shawn

Session	Topic	Description
1	Introduction and overview	Parents are given an overview of the program, and the demands to be placed on them and the focus of the intervention are outlined.
2	Defining and observing	Parents are trained to pinpoint, define, and observe behavior. Parents and trainer define specific problems that can be observed and develop a specific plan to begin observations.
3	Positive reinforcement	Parents learn about positive reinforcement and factors that contribute to its effective application. Parents rehearse positive reinforcement techniques. Specific programs are outlined in which praise and points are to be provided for the behaviors observed during the week.
4	Review of program and data	Observations of the previous week and application of the reinforcement program are reviewed. Details about administration of praise, points, and backup reinforcers are discussed and enacted as needed so that the trainer can determine how to improve parent performance. The program is changed as needed.
5	Time-out from reinforcement	Parents learn about time-out and factors related to its effective application. Use of time-out is planned for the next week for specific behaviors.
6	Shaping	Parents are trained to develop behaviors in the child by reinforcement of successive approximations, and to use prompts and fading of prompts to develop terminal behaviors.
7	Review and problem solving	Concepts discussed in all prior sessions are thoroughly reviewed. Parents are asked to apply these concepts to hypothetical situations presented in the session. Areas of weakness in understanding or executing the concepts serve as the focus.
8	Attending and ignoring	Parents learn about attending and ignoring and choose undesirable behaviors that they will ignore and a positive opposite behavior to which they will attend. These procedures are practiced.
9	School intervention	Plans are made to implement a home-based reinforcement program to develop school-related behaviors. Before this session, teachers and parents identified specific behaviors to focus on in class (e.g., deportment) and at home (e.g., homework completion). These behaviors are incorporated into the reinforcement system.
10	Reprimands	Parents are trained in effective use of reprimands.
11	Family meeting	Both child and parents attend this session. Programs and problems are discussed. Revisions are made as needed to correct misunderstandings or to alter facets implemented in a way not likely to be effective.
12	Review of skills	Programs and concepts are reviewed. Parents are asked to develop programs for a variety of hypothetical everyday problems at home and at school. Feedback is provided regarding program options and applications.
13	Negotiating and contracting	Child and parents attend this session to negotiate new behavioral programs and to put them in contractual form.
14	Low-rate behaviors	Parents are trained to deal with low-rate behaviors such as fire setting, stealing, and truancy. Specific punishment programs are planned as needed for behaviors characteristic of the case.
15, 16, 17	Review, problem-solving, and practice	Material and procedures from other sessions are reviewed and practiced. Application of individual principles is enacted with the trainer. Parents practice designing new programs, revising ailing programs, and responding to a complex array of situations in which principles and practices discussed in prior sessions are reviewed.

to community settings to bring treatment to those persons least likely to come to or remain in treatment. PMT is effective and highly cost-effective when provided in small parent groups in neighborhoods where the families reside (Cunningham et al. 1995; Thompson et al. 1996). Also, when implemented on a large scale as part of early school intervention (Head Start) programs, PMT has reduced conduct problems and increased positive parenting behaviors (Webster-Stratton 1998).

Perhaps the most important point to underscore is that no other technique for children with oppositional or conduct problems has been studied as often or as well in controlled trials as PMT (Brestan and Eyberg 1998). Moreover, the procedures and practices used in PMT (e.g., various reinforcement and punishment practices) have been widely and effectively applied outside the context of child conduct problems (e.g., in patients with autism, language delays, developmental disabilities, or medical disorders) (Kazdin 2001). Several resources facilitate use of PMT clinically and in research. Treatment manuals are available for clinicians (e.g., Cavell 2000; Forehand and McMahon 1981; Forgatch and Patterson 1989; Patterson and Forgatch 1987; Sanders and Dadds 1993) and convey the structure, content, and flow of treatment sessions. Books and pamphlets for parents (e.g., Forehand and Long 1996; Patterson 1976) convey basic concepts and show how to apply various techniques. Videotapes (mentioned in the previous paragraph) can also be used by professionals to guide group PMT.

PMT has several limitations. First, several demands are made on the parents in PMT, such as mastering educational materials that convey major principles of the program, systematically observing deviant child behavior and implementing specific procedures at home, attending weekly sessions, and responding to frequent telephone contacts made by the therapist. For some families, the demands are too great to allow continued treatment. Second, PMT has been used primarily with parents of children and preadolescents and less often with parents of adolescents. Although treatment has been effective with adolescents (Bank et al. 1991), evidence suggests that treatment is more effective with younger children (Dishion and Patterson 1992). However, the paucity of studies with children of different ages precludes conclusions on the relative effectiveness of PMT for younger and older children.

■ Operant Conditioning Techniques

Background and Rationale

The four treatments highlighted thus far (cognitive-behavioral therapy for child anxiety, the Adolescent Coping With Depression Course, cognitive PSST, and PMT) are specific interventions. Operant conditioning techniques are a large family of interventions that draw heavily on concepts developed and elaborated by Skinner (1938, 1953). A number of concepts underlie operant conditioning; the use of rewards and punishments is one small part of the approach. The full set of change techniques can be conceptualized from the framework of antecedents, behaviors, and consequences. The presentation and alteration of antecedent and setting events (e.g., prompts, cues, aids), the many ways to develop behavior (e.g., shaping, chaining, focusing on response characteristics such as magnitude, intensity, and duration), and the presentation of consequences (e.g., types and schedules of reinforcing events) have resulted in a plethora of treatment variations. Indeed, applications of operant conditioning techniques for purposes of treatment, rehabilitation, and education have been studied in controlled trials across the full developmental span (e.g., in infants, in geriatric patients) (Kazdin 2001).

The emphasis of treatment is on developing positive, prosocial, and adaptive behavior, even in cases in which the primary goal might be viewed as decreasing or eliminating maladaptive or deviant behavior (e.g., self-injury, delinquency, use of drugs). Consequently, positive reinforcement techniques are heavily relied on to promote specific adaptive behaviors. Merely providing incentives for positive, prosocial behavior is not likely to be effective. Laboratory and applied research have established the importance of several parameters of administration (e.g., frequency, immediacy, contingent delivery, schedule of delivery). Punishment procedures are also used in behavioral programs to suppress or eliminate conduct problem behaviors. Such procedures tend to assume a secondary role because of the strong evidence in support of developing positive, prosocial behavior (even when the primary goal may seem to be the elimination of some behavior). The punishment procedures differ from the usual consequences applied to behavior in everyday life; they are also implemented somewhat differently. Punishment in treatment typically involves withdrawal of reinforcers. Three commonly used punishment methods are time-out from reinforcement (removal of positive reinforcers for a short time), applying response cost (removal of a positive reinforcer such as a token or privilege), and overcorrection (correcting the environmental effects of the inappropriate behavior and practicing appropriate performance). Many variations of reinforcement and punishment techniques have been used to reduce conduct problems in children and adolescents at home and at school (Kazdin 2001).

Characteristics of Treatment

Although procedures vary greatly, there is some commonality. First, an effort is made to define goals and carefully assess child functioning. Multiple goals are likely to be of interest, but these are not apt to be worked on simultaneously. Second, a program is developed to change behaviors through reinforcement and perhaps punishment and extinction procedures. Implementation largely determines the success or failure of a program. To determine whether procedures are being implemented, it may be necessary to monitor not only the child's behavior (that is, the behavior to be changed) but also the behaviors of others in relation to the child (e.g., behaviors of staff, parents, and teachers). Multiple techniques may be required, including prompting, fading (gradual removal of prompts), and shaping; administering reinforcers on special schedules; analyzing factors maintaining behavior; and analyzing the requisite behaviors to develop the complex repertoire of interest. Although operant conditioning techniques are conceptually relatively simple, implementation is demanding. It is easy to show that programs delivered in ways that omit important parameters of administration (e.g., immediate, contingent, continuous reinforcement) have little or no effect on child functioning and that programs retaining those parameters do affect performance (Kazdin 2001).

Programs usually combine several reinforcement and punishment contingencies to change behavior. As an example, an intensive behavioral program was provided to young autistic children (age less than 4 years) (Lovaas 1987). The intervention involved multiple operant conditioning procedures and was conducted in the child's home, school, and community for an average of 40 hours per week for 2 or more years. Several college student therapists administered the treatment over this period. In addition, parents were trained ex-

tensively so that treatment could take place at home for almost all the child's waking hours, 365 days a year. The focus of treatment was on eliminating maladaptive behavior (e.g., self-stimulation, aggression) and developing a variety of prosocial (e.g., play) and cognitive/academic (e.g., language, reading, writing) skills. A major goal of treatment was to place children into a regular classroom where they would function largely like other children. For children who entered a regular first-grade class, treatment was reduced from 40 to 10 hours or less per week and was eventually terminated (after which there was minimal contact). For treated children who did not enter regular first grade, the intervention continued up to 6 years (more than 14,000 hours of one-on-one treatment per child).

The results indicated that 47% of the treated group achieved normal intellectual and educational functioning, as reflected by scores in the normal range on standardized intelligence tests and successful completion of first grade in public school. Control children who did not receive the intensive treatment did not show these gains. The effect of treatment was dramatic; compared with control subjects who did not participate in the treatment, treated children scored an average of 30 points higher on standardized intelligence tests (Wechsler Intelligence Scale for Children—Revised, Stanford-Binet Intelligence Scale, or other measure). Follow-up data indicated that after several years (mean, 5 years), more treated youth than control subjects remained in a regular classroom. Treated children's IQ scores and adaptive behaviors were also higher (McEachin et al. 1993). Thus, not only did the program effect marked changes, but these changes were also maintained.

This program has been a source of controversy because of the sample, the ages of the subjects, and the incomplete random assignment of children to conditions. The effects of the program have been replicated in controlled studies and clinical applications (e.g., Sheinkopf and Siegel 1998; Smith et al. 2000). An attempted large-scale replication of the program is under way to provide more definitive information about the scope of the effects (see Lovaas and Smith 2003).

Case Example

John, a 5-year-old boy, lived alone with his mother. He was referred for oppositional defiant disorder and conduct disorder, but part of the clinical picture and the mother's concern was that each night, John insisted on sleeping in his mother's bed. If the mother insisted that he sleep in his own room, a tantrum and an extended argument occurred. John often became so upset that he could not get to sleep for a long time. The problem had begun about a year earlier, when John had a nightmare and came into his mother's bed in the middle of the night and slept through the night. The next night, John insisted on sleeping in his mother's bed again. As this went on, the mother began arguing with him about where to sleep. John had been sleeping in bed with his mother ever since that initial night. The mother wanted this to stop. The therapist elected to begin the treatment with changing the sleeping in the mother's bed, because compared with many behaviors associated with conduct disorder (e.g., stealing, fire setting, fighting), this behavior is fairly easy to change as parenting skills are developed with treatment. Although all the presenting issues were addressed in treatment, only the sleep program is noted here.

As part of the treatment, the mother was trained to interact quite differently with John. Specifically, she was trained to provide clear instructions about what she wanted John to do, to ignore tantrums and not argue, and to provide positive consequences for the behaviors. A behavior-change program was developed for John and included the following: John was told that he could earn stickers ("smiley faces") on a new chart that had been placed on the refrigerator. The stickers would be given for going to bed in his own room. John's mother said that he would earn 2 stickers if they said good night without arguing, 2 if he went into his bed (the lower bunk of a set of bunk beds), and 2 if he remained in his bed through the night. The plan was to provide stickers for the behaviors. John did not have to do all three behaviors to get the stickers. If, for example, he completed the first and second behaviors but got into his mother's bed in the middle of the night, he would still receive 4 stickers. The stickers would be placed on John's chart on the refrigerator in the morning and could be exchanged for rewards right then or later, depending on the reward. The prizes included little toys (4 stickers each), basketball cards (6 stickers each), bedtime 15 minutes later than usual (8 stickers), and a trip to a fast-food restaurant for dinner (12 stickers). His stickers could be saved when he did not spend them all.

John's mother said that for the first few days, she would sleep in the top bunk. When John when to bed the first night, he went into his lower bunk quietly. His mother praised and hugged him enthusiastically for doing this. She reminded him that he would be getting stickers in the morning. The mother had practiced with the therapist to ensure that her comments specified the desired behaviors clearly, were enthusiastic, followed the behavior immediately, and were associated with positive physical contact (hugs, pats, kisses). When John went into his lower bunk, the mother also went to sleep, but in the top bunk.

Having the mother present was considered likely to facilitate the initial transition to John's sleeping in his own room. The plan for the first few nights was to have the mother go to bed in the top bunk but then leave after John fell asleep. (Actually, she slept through the night in the top bunk for the first 2 nights.)

In the morning, the mother mentioned again how well John had done and what a "big boy" he was to sleep in his own bed all night. They went hand in hand to the refrigerator, where she placed the stickers on the chart. She reexplained how the stickers could be used and asked if he wanted one of the rewards he had earned (he had earned 6 stickers). He took one of the toys (a small truck) and saved 2 stickers to be spent at another time.

The program continued like this for 4 nights. Each night, John went to bed without a tantrum and slept through the night. On one of the nights, John could not sleep and kept trying to engage his mother in conversation while they were in their respective bunks. She said she could not talk because it was "sleep time," and she ended the conversation with more praise about how wonderful he was doing by staying in his own bed. On night 5, the mother asked if he could "do the real big boy bedtime" and go into his bunk without her. She asked him to just try it and told him she would check on him after a few minutes. He went into his bed and was tucked in and praised for being such a big boy, for going to his room so nicely, and for getting into bed without her doing the same. About 10 minutes later, John's mother went in to check him and praise him for staying in bed, but he had already fallen asleep. This program addition (sleeping in the room alone) continued for another week. No change was made in the sticker program; the addition was just handled with effusive praise by the mother.

After 15 days, the sticker program was stopped. The mother said John could stay up 15 minutes any night he wanted if he had completed all the bedtime behaviors by himself the previous night. The praise continued, but the sticker program was essentially discontinued. Within less than 3 weeks, the bedtime behaviors had changed and were no longer of concern. Six months later, sleeping was no longer an issue.

Evidence and Overall Evaluation

Analysis of the use of operant conditioning techniques in applied settings, referred to as *applied behavior analysis,* has its own vast literature. The clinical focus is on many disorders in children, including oppositional, conduct, and attention-deficit/hyperactivity disorders; developmental disabilities; autism; and mental retardation (Kazdin 2001; Sulzer-Azaroff and Mayer 1991). Operant conditioning techniques have been applied in many settings, including day care facilities; elementary, middle, and high schools; colleges; correctional institutions; summer camps; and the community. Earlier in the chapter (see "Scope of Behavior Modification"), the scope of applications of behavior modification was mentioned. The wide scope is largely due to the extension of operant conditioning techniques. The basic principles and techniques are easily adapted to different populations in clinical and nonclinical contexts. Thus, the principles and procedures used in PMT can be and have been applied in business and industry (e.g., to teach skills, reduce accidents, or improve performance) and the military (e.g., to improve performance during basic training).

■ Comment

This discussion has highlighted selected treatments for diverse problems. The heterogeneity of the procedures may lead one to wonder why they are unified under the single term *behavior modification*. The characteristics mentioned earlier (see "Characteristics of Behavior Modification") apply to each of the treatments. Also, other features are noteworthy. The different interventions are directive and active, meaning that explicit training experiences are prescribed in treatment. Treatment sessions are frequently used to plan actions for change. Often the actions or activities are assigned as homework, with specific activities being carried out to help achieve desired changes. For example, parents, teachers, and peers often assist the child at home and at school through activities designed to promote therapeutic change. Treatment is conceptualized as learning new behaviors to be performed in everyday life. Activities in which learning needs to take place, and the assistance of others in these settings, serve as the basis for developing new behaviors.

Salient Issues in Current Treatment Research

In developing behavioral treatments and child treatments in general, certain fundamental issues are important to note. The issues relate to the type of treatments developed, their foci, and evaluation of their effect.

■ Magnitude of Therapeutic Change

The criteria for evaluating treatment have expanded in recent years and have placed treatment outcome in a different light. In outcomes research, change (i.e., statistically significant change) and group differences (i.e., between treatment and control conditions) are primary criteria for evaluating interventions. The empirical literature on behavioral techniques for children is extensive. As outcome evidence has accumulated, concern has increased about whether changes achieved in treatment make a difference in everyday life. The term *clinical significance* refers to the practical value or importance of the effect of an intervention—that is, whether the intervention makes any real difference to the clients or to others. Clinical significance can be measured in many ways (see Kazdin 2003b; Kendall 1999). One way is to consider the extent to which referred youths function at normative levels after completion of treatment. The term *normative level* refers to the level of peers of the same age and sex who are functioning adequately or well in everyday life. For example, one would want treated individuals to return to school and not to get into fights or arguments, not to be placed on detention or be suspended, and to be at levels in these behaviors similar to those of their peers functioning well in everyday life. On the positive side, one would want treated youth also to be at normative levels in their prosocial functioning, as reflected in their engagement in social activities with others. Research has shown that treatments can return individuals to normative levels. The broader problem is that in child and adolescent treatment research in general, the importance of the change is rarely evaluated.

Even seemingly marked changes may not be sufficient. For example, in one case familiar to me, treatment reduced the number of times a 12-year-old boy sexually assaulted girls within the hospital. (The boy was under full-time supervision but was able to escape supervision for brief periods.) Treatment seemed to reduce the frequency from about 30 to 2 times per month. Yet his most recent episode was the fondling and attempted rape of a female patient in a closet. Assuming that treatment was responsible for the reduction and that assessments are reliable, one would want greater change than this for treatment to be considered effective.

In a less dramatic case, treatment eliminated the extent to which a 10-year-old boy hit school personnel. He was still extremely verbally aggressive, which had its own consequences (e.g., he was suspended for angrily calling the school principal a "big fat pig"). The issue here is the goals of treatment. What can be achieved with current treatments, and what are the appropriate goals? One might argue for more modest goals. For example, presumably some youths become worse; for these individuals, treatment effects would be important if they kept them from worsening further.

In some cases, the clinical significance of a change is fairly obvious. For example, in the behavioral treatment of the young autistic children mentioned above in "Operant Conditioning Techniques," those who received intensive behavioral treatment, compared with those who did not, showed large gains in IQ and substantially higher rates of entering and remaining in regular first grade (Lovaas 1987). Moreover, the gains in IQ and grade placement were still evident many years later (McEachin et al. 1993). The available outcome evidence from controlled trials involving autistic children is sparse. Changes in school placement and IQ can be regarded as clinically important, particularly if they are maintained. In most studies of treatment, results are not as stark or clear.

In general, magnitude of change is highly important in evaluating treatment. Therapists not only want to achieve change but also have an interest in achieving gains that make a difference in the lives of the individuals being treated, those with whom they are in contact, and society at large. Although cognitive-behavioral treatment outcome studies often use criteria for evaluating clinical significance, such criteria have not been uniformly adopted within the field. In other conceptual approaches to treatment, these criteria receive even less attention. Consequently, basic information about the effect of interventions on the functioning of children in everyday life is sparse.

■ Maintenance of Change

Much more information is needed about the long-term effects of treatment. In most studies of child and adolescent therapy, including studies focusing beyond behavioral treatments, follow-up data are not obtained. Among studies that do include follow-up, the mean duration of assessment is 5–7 months after treatment ends (Durlak et al. 1995; Kazdin et al. 1990). Follow-up assessment is critically important because changes that are present immediately after treatment may not be maintained. Also, when treatments are compared, the one that is considered more (or most)

effective immediately after treatment is not always the most effective in the long run (Kazdin 2000). Consequently, conclusions about treatment may vary depending on the timing of outcome assessment. Apart from conclusions about treatment, follow-up may provide important information that permits differentiation among youngsters. Those who maintain the benefits of treatment may differ in important ways from those who do not. Understanding who responds—and who responds more or less well—to a particular treatment can be helpful in understanding, treating, and preventing conduct disorder.

The study of long-term effects of treatment is difficult. Observing families for an extended period is costly and labor-intensive. Moreover, loss of cases through attrition increases as the duration of follow-up increases. As the sample size decreases over time, conclusions about the effect of treatment become increasingly difficult to draw. Nevertheless, evaluation of the long-term effects of treatment remains a high priority for research.

■ Other Issues

Several other issues remain to be discussed. The criteria chosen to evaluate treatment raise many questions. The usual focus on child symptoms is obviously important. However, most studies fail to assess or treat other domains such as prosocial behavior and academic functioning, which relate to concurrent and long-term adjustment (Kazdin et al. 1990). A broader range of child functioning than symptoms is important to include in treatment evaluation. Also, parent and family functioning (e.g., psychiatric impairment, marital conflict) may be relevant outcomes as well, because they can contribute to and be affected by child dysfunction. The focus of many techniques on parents (e.g., parent training, family approaches) also means that evaluating parent and family functioning may be important in assessing the effect of the intervention (Kazdin and Wassell 2000).

Many outcomes are of interest in evaluating treatment. Existing research indicates that the conclusions reached about a given treatment can vary depending on the outcome criteria. Within a given study, one set of measures (e.g., child functioning) may reveal no differences between two treatments, but another measure (e.g., family functioning) may show that one treatment is clearly better than the other (Kazdin et al. 1992; Szapocznik et al. 1989).

Some critical professional issues warrant mention in passing because they relate to the research evidence, clinical practice, and their interface. There is strong empirical evidence in favor of the treatments highlighted in this chapter, but the majority of treatments in clinical practice are not yet supported in controlled studies. Indeed, most treatments in use have not undergone even open or uncontrolled studies (Kazdin 2001). Among the challenges this presents is the difficulty in influencing the training of mental health professionals, including psychiatrists, psychologists, social workers, and psychiatric nurses. For example, probably no other psychosocial treatment for children has been as well investigated and supported as PMT. Unfortunately, however, mental health professionals working with children are not likely to be exposed to this treatment as part of their training. Presumably, evidence-based practice will filter into clinical settings and training programs in the coming years.

Conclusion

Behavior modification encompasses diverse conceptual views, techniques, and applications. The treatments share a commitment to operationalization, assessment, and evaluation. To illustrate the diversity of techniques, I have highlighted treatments for anxiety, depression, and oppositional and conduct disorders.

Proponents of behavior modification view the commitment to treatment research as the hallmark of the approach. This commitment has led to a large literature on controlled outcome trials. The emphasis of the current movement within psychotherapy research is on evidence-based treatments. Because clinical trials have been emphasized in behavior modification, lists of evidence-based treatments are currently dominated by behavioral treatments (Lonigan and Elbert 1998). It might well be that cognitive-behavioral treatments are among the most effective interventions. The difficulty is that few of the traditional treatments used in clinical practice and the eclectic combinations that clinicians are wont to use have been subjected to randomized controlled trials.

Enormous progress has been made in treatment research concerning children and adolescents (Christophersen and Mortweet 2001; Kazdin and Weisz 2003).

However, dissemination of research findings has been difficult because most professionals in clinical practice have not had access to training. For both research and clinical practice, a large number of treatment manuals have become available that describe how treatment is implemented, key assumptions, and methods for evaluating effectiveness (Kazdin 2000; LeCroy 1994). These treatment manuals facilitate replication and extension of treatment. Of course, manuals do not substitute for supervised training.

There are multiple issues to be addressed in child and adolescent treatment. The goal is to identify interventions that are effective in clinically referred youths and their families. Little research has focused on the factors that influence responsiveness to treatment, whether they relate to characteristics of children, families, or treatment administration. Also, within behavioral and nonbehavioral treatments, little attention has been accorded to therapeutic processes (e.g., alliance, therapeutic bond), particularly in child therapy (Kazdin 2000). Proponents of behavioral treatments have advanced the field by developing concrete interventions and by showing empirically that these interventions can effect change that can be maintained in many areas.

References

American Psychiatric Association: Diagnostic and Statistical Manual of Mental Disorders, 4th Edition. Washington, DC, American Psychiatric Association, 1994

American Psychiatric Association: Diagnostic and Statistical Manual of Mental Disorders, 4th Edition, Text Revision. Washington, DC, American Psychiatric Association, 2000

Ammerman RT, Hersen M (eds): Handbook of Child Behavior Therapy in the Psychiatric Setting. New York, Wiley-Interscience, 1995

Ammerman RT, Last CG, Hersen M (eds): Handbook of Prescriptive Treatments for Children and Adolescents. Needham Heights, MA, Allyn & Bacon, 1993

Baer RA, Nietzel MT: Cognitive and behavioral treatment of impulsivity in children: a meta-analytic review of the outcome literature. J Clin Child Psychol 20:400–412, 1991

Bank L, Marlowe JH, Reid JB, et al: A comparative evaluation of parent-training interventions for families of chronic delinquents. J Abnorm Child Psychol 19:15–33, 1991

Barrett PM: Evaluation of cognitive-behavioral group treatments for childhood anxiety disorders. J Clin Child Psychol 27:459–468, 1998

Barrett PM, Dadds MR, Rapee RM: Family treatment of childhood anxiety: a controlled trial. J Consult Clin Psychol 64:333–342, 1996

Barrett PM, Duffy AL, Dadds MR, et al: Cognitive-behavioral treatment of anxiety disorders in children: long-term (6-year) follow-up. J Consult Clin Psychol 69:135–141, 2001

Brestan EV, Eyberg SM: Effective psychosocial treatment of conduct-disordered children and adolescents: 29 years, 82 studies, and 5275 kids. J Clin Child Psychol 27:180–189, 1998

Catania AC: Learning, 4th Edition. Englewood Cliffs, NJ, Prentice Hall, 1997

Cavell TA: Working With Parents of Aggressive Children: A Practitioner's Guide. Washington, DC, American Psychological Association, 2000

Christophersen ER, Mortweet SL: Treatments That Work With Children: Empirically Supported Strategies for Managing Childhood Problems. Washington, DC, American Psychological Association, 2001

Clarke GN, Lewinsohn PM, Hops H: Adolescent Coping With Depression Course: Leader's Manual for Adolescent Groups. Eugene, OR, Castalia, 1990

Clarke GN, DeBar LL, Lewinsohn PM: Cognitive behavioral group treatment for adolescent depression, in Evidence-Based Psychotherapies for Children and Adolescents. Edited by Kazdin AE, Weisz JR. New York, Guilford, 2003, pp 120–134

Clement PW: Outcomes and Incomes: How to Evaluate, Improve, and Market Your Practice by Measuring Outcomes in Psychotherapy. New York, Guilford, 1999

Craighead L, Craighead WE, Kazdin AE, et al: Cognitive and Behavioral Interventions: An Empirical Approach to Mental Health Problems. Needham Heights, MA, Allyn & Bacon, 1994

Crick NR, Dodge KA: A review and reformulation of social information processing mechanisms in children's social adjustment. Psychol Bull 115:74–101, 1994

Cuijpers P: A psychoeducational approach to the treatment of depression: a meta-analysis of Lewinsohn's "Coping With Depression" course. Behav Ther 29:521–533, 1998

Cunningham CE, Bremner R, Boyle M: Large group community-based parenting programs for families of preschoolers at risk for disruptive behaviour disorders: utilization, cost effectiveness, and outcome. J Child Psychol Psychiatry 36:1141–1159, 1995

Dadds MR, Holland DE, Laurens KR, et al: Early intervention and prevention of anxiety disorders in children: results at 2-year follow-up. J Consult Clin Psychol 67:145–150, 1999

Dishion TJ, Patterson GR: Age effects in parent training outcomes. Behav Ther 23:719–729, 1992

Durlak JA, Fuhrman T, Lampman C: Effectiveness of cognitive-behavioral therapy for maladapting children: a meta-analysis. Psychol Bull 110:204–214, 1991

Durlak JA, Wells AM, Cotten JK, et al: Analysis of selected methodological issues in child psychotherapy research. J Clin Child Psychol 24:141–148, 1995

Eyberg SM, Funderburk BW, Hembree-Kigin TL, et al: Parent-child interaction therapy with behavior problem children: one year maintenance of treatment effects in the family. Child and Family Behavior Therapy 23:1–20, 2001

Finch AJ Jr, Nelson WM, Ott ES: Cognitive-Behavioral Procedures With Children and Adolescents: A Practical Guide. Needham Heights, MA, Allyn & Bacon, 1993

Flannery-Schroeder EC, Kendall PC: Group and individual cognitive-behavioral treatments for youth with anxiety disorders: a randomized clinical trial. Cognit Ther Res 24:251–278, 2000

Forehand R, Long N: Parenting the Strong-Willed Child: The Clinically Proven Five-Week Program for Parents of Two- to Six-Year-Olds. Chicago, IL, Contemporary Books, 1996

Forehand R, McMahon RJ: Helping the Noncompliant Child: A Clinician's Guide to Parent Training. New York, Guilford, 1981

Forgatch M, Patterson GR: Parents and Adolescents Living Together, Part 2: Family Problem Solving. Eugene, OR, Castalia, 1989

Kazdin AE: History of Behavior Modification: Experimental Foundations of Contemporary Research. Baltimore, MD, University Park Press, 1978

Kazdin AE: Evaluation in clinical practice: clinically sensitive and systematic methods of treatment delivery. Behav Ther 24:11–45, 1993

Kazdin AE: Parent management training: evidence, outcomes, and issues. J Am Acad Child Adolesc Psychiatry 36:1349–1356, 1997

Kazdin AE: Psychotherapy for Children and Adolescents. New York, Oxford University Press, 2000

Kazdin AE: Behavior Modification in Applied Settings, 6th Edition. Belmont, CA, Wadsworth, 2001

Kazdin AE: Problem-solving skills training and parent management training for conduct disorder, in Evidence-Based Psychotherapies for Children and Adolescents. Edited by Kazdin AE, Weisz JR. New York, Guilford, 2003a, pp 241–262

Kazdin AE: Research Design in Clinical Psychology, 4th Edition. Needham Heights, MA, Allyn & Bacon, 2003b

Kazdin AE: Child, parent, and family based treatment of aggressive and antisocial child behavior, in Psychosocial Treatments for Child and Adolescent Disorders, 2nd Edition. Edited by Hibbs ED, Jensen PS. Washington, DC, American Psychological Association (in press)

Kazdin AE, Crowley M: Moderators of treatment outcome in cognitively based treatment of antisocial behavior. Cognit Ther Res 21:185–207, 1997

Kazdin AE, Wassell G: Therapeutic changes in children, parents, and families resulting from treatment of children with conduct problems. J Am Acad Child Adolesc Psychiatry 39:414–420, 2000

Kazdin AE, Weisz JR (eds): Evidence-Based Psychotherapies for Children and Adolescents. New York, Guilford, 2003

Kazdin AE, Bass D, Siegel T, et al: Cognitive-behavioral treatment and relationship therapy in the treatment of children referred for antisocial behavior. J Consult Clin Psychol 57:522–535, 1989

Kazdin AE, Bass D, Ayers WA, et al: The empirical and clinical focus of child and adolescent psychotherapy research. J Consult Clin Psychol 58:729–740, 1990

Kazdin AE, Siegel TC, Bass D: Cognitive problem-solving skills training and parent management training in the treatment of antisocial behavior in children. J Consult Clin Psychol 60:733–747, 1992

Kendall PC: Treating anxiety disorders in children: results of a randomized clinical trial. J Consult Clin Psychol 62:100–110, 1994

Kendall PC (ed): Clinical significance. J Consult Clin Psychol 67(special issue):283–339, 1999

Kendall PC (ed): Child and Adolescent Therapy: Cognitive-Behavioral Procedures, 2nd Edition. New York, Guilford, 2000

Kendall PC, Southam-Gerow MA: Long-term follow-up of a cognitive-behavioral therapy for anxiety-disordered youth. J Consult Clin Psychol 64:724–730, 1996

Kendall PC, Treadwell KRH: Cognitive-behavioral group treatment for socially anxious youth, in Psychosocial Treatment Research of Child and Adolescent Disorders: Empirically Based Strategies for Clinical Practice. Edited by Hibbs ED, Jensen PS. Washington, DC, American Psychological Association, 1996, pp 23–41

Kendall PC, Kane M, Howard B, et al: Cognitive-Behavioral Therapy for Anxious Children: Treatment Manual. Philadelphia, PA, Department of Psychology, Temple University, 1990

Kendall PC, Flannery-Schroeder E, Panichelli-Mindel SM, et al: Therapy for anxiety-disordered youth: a second randomized clinical trial. J Consult Clin Psychol 65:366–380, 1997a

Kendall PC, Panichelli-Mindel SM, Sugarman A, et al: Exposure to child anxiety: theory, research, and practice. Clinical Psychology: Science and Practice 4:29–39, 1997b

Kendall PC, Chu BC, Pimentel SS, et al: Treating anxiety disorders in youth, in Child and Adolescent Therapy: Cognitive-Behavioral Procedures, 2nd Edition. Edited by Kendall PC. New York, Guilford, 2000, pp 235–287

Kendall PC, Aschenbrand SG, Hudson JL: Child-focused treatement of anxiety, in Evidence-Based Psychotherapies for Children and Adolescents. Edited by Kazdin AE, Weisz JR. New York, Guilford, 2003, pp 81–100

LeCroy CW (ed): Handbook of Child and Adolescent Treatment Manuals. New York, Lexington Books, 1994

Lewinsohn PM, Clarke GN: Psychosocial treatments for adolescent depression. Clin Psychol Rev 19:329–342, 1999

Lewinsohn PM, Hops H, Teri L, et al: An integrative theory of depression, in Theoretical Issues in Behavior Therapy. Edited by Reiss S, Bootzin RR. San Diego, CA, Academic Press, 1985, pp 331–359

Lewinsohn PM, Clarke GN, Hops H, et al: Cognitive-behavioral treatment for depressed adolescents. Behav Ther 21:385–401, 1990

Lewinsohn PM, Clarke GN, Rohde P, et al: A course in coping: a cognitive-behavioral approach to the treatment of adolescent depression, in Psychosocial Treatment Research of Child and Adolescent Disorders: Empirically Based Strategies for Clinical Practice. Edited by Hibbs ED, Jensen PS. Washington, DC, American Psychological Association, 1996, pp 109–135

Long P, Forehand R, Wierson M, et al: Does parent training with young noncompliant children have long-term effects? Behav Res Ther 32:101–107, 1994

Lonigan CJ, Elbert JC (eds): Empirically supported psychosocial interventions for children. J Clin Child Psychol 27(special issue):138–226, 1998

Lovaas OI: Behavioral treatment and normal educational and intellectual functioning in young autistic children. J Consult Clin Psychol 5:3–9, 1987

Lovaas OI, Smith T: Early and intensive behavioral intervention in autism, in Evidence-Based Psychotherapies for Children and Adolescents. Edited by Kazdin AE, Weisz JR. New York, Guilford, 2003, pp 325–340

Mash EJ, Barkley RA (eds): Treatment of Childhood Disorders, 2nd Edition. New York, Guilford, 1998

Mash EJ, Terdal LG (eds): Assessment of Childhood Disorders, 3rd Edition. New York, Guilford, 1997

McEachin JJ, Smith T, Lovaas OI: Long-term outcome for children with autism who received early intensive behavioral treatment. Am J Ment Retard 97:359–372, 1993

Newsom C: Autistic disorder, in Treatment of Childhood Disorders, 2nd Edition. Edited by Mash EJ, Barkley RA. New York, Guilford, 1998, pp 416–467

Patterson GR: Living With Children: New Methods for Parents and Teachers, Revised. Champaign, IL, Research Press, 1976

Patterson GR: Coercive Family Process. Eugene, OR, Castalia, 1982

Patterson GR, Forgatch M: Parents and Adolescents Living Together, Part 1: The Basics. Eugene, OR, Castalia, 1987

Patterson GR, Reid JB, Dishion TJ: A Social Learning Approach to Family Intervention, Vol 4: Antisocial Boys. Eugene, OR, Castalia, 1992

Sanders MR, Dadds MR: Behavioral Family Intervention. Needham Heights, MA, Allyn & Bacon, 1993

Sheinkopf SJ, Siegel B: Home-based behavioral treatment of young children with autism. J Autism Dev Disord 28:15–23, 1998

Shirk SR (ed): Cognitive Development and Child Psychotherapy. New York, Plenum, 1988

Shure MB: I Can Problem Solve (ICPS): An Interpersonal Cognitive Problem Solving Program. Champaign, IL, Research Press, 1992

Shure MB: Raising a Thinking Child: Help Your Young Child to Resolve Everyday Conflicts and Get Along With Others. New York, Pocket Books, 1996

Shure MB: Interpersonal cognitive problem solving: primary prevention of early high-risk behaviors in the preschool and primary years, in Primary Prevention Works. Edited by Albee GW, Gulotta TP. Thousand Oaks, CA, Sage, 1997, pp 167–188

Shure MB: Preventing Violence the Problem-Solving Way (Juvenile Justice Bulletin). Washington, DC, U.S. Department of Justice, Office of Justice Programs, Office of Juvenile Justice and Delinquency Prevention, 1999

Skinner BF: The Behavior of Organisms. New York, Appleton-Century-Crofts, 1938

Skinner BF: Science and Human Behavior. New York, Free Press, 1953

Smith T, Groen AD, Wynn JW: Randomized trial of intensive early intervention for children with pervasive developmental disorder. Am J Ment Retard 105:269–285, 2000

Spivack G, Shure MB: The cognition of social adjustment: interpersonal cognitive problem solving thinking, in Advances in Clinical Child Psychology, Vol 5. Edited by Lahey BB, Kazdin AE. New York, Plenum, 1982, pp 323–372

Spivack G, Platt JJ, Shure MB: The Problem-Solving Approach to Adjustment. San Francisco, CA, Jossey-Bass, 1976

Sulzer-Azaroff B, Mayer GR: Behavior Analysis for Lasting Change, 2nd Edition. Fort Worth, TX, Holt, Rinehart, Winston, 1991

Szapocznik J, Rio A, Murray E, et al: Structural family versus psychodynamic child therapy for problematic Hispanic boys. J Consult Clin Psychol 57:571–578, 1989

Thompson RW, Ruma PR, Schuchmann LF, et al: A cost-effectiveness evaluation of parent training. Journal of Child and Family Studies 5:415–429, 1996

Webster-Stratton C: Early intervention with videotape modeling: programs for families of children with oppositional defiant disorder or conduct disorder, in Psychosocial Treatment Research of Child and Adolescent Disorders: Empirically Based Strategies for Clinical Practice. Edited by Hibbs ED, Jensen PS. Washington, DC, American Psychological Association, 1996, pp 435–474

Webster-Stratton C: Preventing conduct problems in Head Start children: strengthening parenting competencies. J Consult Clin Psychol 66:715–730, 1998

Webster-Stratton C, Reid MJ: The Incredible Years parents, teachers, and children training series: a multifaceted treatment approach for young children with conduct problems, in Evidence-Based Psychotherapies for Children and Adolescents. Edited by Kazdin AE, Weisz JR. New York, Guilford, 2003, pp 224–240

Family Therapy

G. Pirooz Sholevar, M.D.

Definition

Family theory focuses on human behavior and psychiatric disturbances in the context of interpersonal relationships (Lansky 1989). This theory forms the basis of family therapy, an umbrella term for a number of clinical practices that treat psychopathology within the family system rather than in individuals. Interventions are designed to effect change in family relationships rather than in the individual (Bell 1975; Minuchin 1974; Olson 1970; Shapiro 1986). This approach is based on observations that symptomatic behavior appears in individuals involved in certain dysfunctional processes within their families or with other significant persons.

In family theory, the family is considered an interpersonal system with cybernetic qualities. The relationships among the components of the system are nonlinear (or circular); the interactions are cyclical rather than causative. Complex interlocking feedback mechanisms and patterns of interaction among the members of the system repeat themselves sequentially. Any symptom can be viewed simply as a behavior functioning as a homeostatic mechanism that regulates family interactions (Jackson 1965; Minuchin et al. 1978).

The family system is nonsummative and includes the assets and dysfunctions of the individuals as well as their interactions (Olson 1970). A person's problems cannot be evaluated or treated apart from their context and the functions that they serve. It is assumed, therefore, that an individual cannot be expected to change unless the family system changes (Haley 1963). Treatment addresses the behavioral dysfunctions as manifestations of disturbances within the entire family system; the role of the total family in aiding or in sabotaging treatment is the focus, even when a distinct, diagnosable psychiatric illness is present in one of the family members.

The goals of family therapy as a psychotherapeutic modality are as follows:

- Explore the interactional dynamics of the family and their relation to psychopathology.
- Mobilize the family's internal strength and functional resources.
- Restructure the maladaptive interactional family styles.
- Strengthen the family's problem-solving behavior.

History

Family therapy's roots date back to the child guidance movement in 1909 and to marriage counseling in the late 1920s. Psychoanalytic treatment was applied in confidential parallel sessions with spouses and provided a strong theoretical foundation for early family and marital investigations.

The formal development of family therapy in the United States began in the late 1940s and early 1950s. The major origins of family therapy can be traced to the activities of pioneers such as Ackerman and Bowen; Wynne and Bell; Bateson, Jackson, Haley, and Satir; and Lidz and Flick, and to the semi-independent branch of family therapy that emerged in Milan, Italy, with the work of Selvini Palazzoli. In addition to this initial group of pioneers, a number of charismatic figures have enhanced the development of family therapy, including Whitaker, Minuchin, Boszormenyi-Nagy, and Zuk.

A variety of developments in the field of mental health—developments in psychodynamic, group, and behavior therapies—facilitated family therapy. During the 1920s, sociologists began studying the family and described many family interactional processes and typologies (Burgess 1926). However, the impact of sociology on the field of psychiatry was enhanced by the emergence of social psychiatry, which emphasized the significance of cultural differences and social settings in the development and amelioration of psychiatric disorders (Leighton 1960).

Proponents of psychoanalytic theory and ego psychology believed that symptoms were embedded in the personality and that developing symptomatic behaviors could be an individual's way of adapting to the human and familial environment. Sullivan's (1953) "interpersonal" psychoanalytic school emphasized human relationships and interactions. In the ego-psychological stage of psychoanalytic theory, the significance of social and cultural determinants of behavior was emphasized by Horney (1939), Fromm (1941), and Sullivan (1953). Erikson's (1950) epigenetic theory of human development mapped the interrelationship between individual maturational processes and the social and cultural environment. Interest in the mother–child relationship was expanded through the work of Levy (1943) on "maternal overprotection" and of Fromm-Reichmann (1948) on the "schizophrenogenic mother." The work of Bowlby (1949) on bonding established the theoretical basis for the object relations school of family therapy.

Group therapy expanded throughout the United States after 1924 and enhanced therapists' knowledge of small-group processes, symptomatic behavior within a group, and ways to correct individual behavior within the group setting. Learning theory and behavior therapy emerged and underscored the interconnection between symptomatic behavior and a dysfunctional family environment.

Dissatisfaction with the traditional practices of child psychotherapy inspired a number of early contributors, particularly Bell (1975) and Ackerman (1954). Ackerman, a psychoanalyst, child psychiatrist, and group therapist, was disenchanted with the prevailing practices of child psychotherapists, who generally treated parents and their children in tandem therapy in child guidance clinics. Ackerman's contributions included the concepts of shared unconscious conflicts and defenses; symbiotic relationships; and interpretation, confrontation, and manipulation of metaphors in psychotherapy to delineate characterological defenses of family members (Simon 1985).

The work of Bowen (1961, 1966, 1978), a psychoanalyst and a major independent thinker in the field of family therapy, continues to influence family therapists. Bowen pioneered the investigation and observation of family members hospitalized with schizophrenic patients who were related to them. His observations led to a number of conclusions, some of which strongly influenced the course of family therapy. Although his work was couched in an intergenerational family systems model and psychodynamic concepts, his influence on all schools of family therapy is apparent. His investigations led to the recognition of the *undifferentiation phenomenon* and its relation to the transmission of anxiety within the family system. His early term *undifferentiated ego mass families* has gone through many changes. Differentiation, his foundational concept, is closely related to his other theoretical concepts, such as anxiety, interpersonal triangulation, marital and family fusion, and family projective system.

Wynne and colleagues (Ryckoff et al. 1959; Wynne et al. 1958) investigated psychodynamic aspects of schizophrenia and attempted to identify the characteristic structure of and roles in families of schizophrenic patients. Wynne's work was based on the premise that all humans have a fundamental need to relate to others, as well as a lifelong striving to develop a personal identity. He developed two concepts: *pseudomutuality* and *pseudohostility*. Pseudomutuality is based on a family's intense need to be unified, to the extent that differentiation of identities of persons in the relationship is not permitted and divergence is denied. Pseudohostility is a defensive interactional pattern used to ward off intimacy.

Wynne and Singer studied communication deviance in families of young schizophrenic patients by comparing these families with a group of borderline and neurotic adults. The original work of Wynne and Singer (Singer and Wynne 1965a, 1965b; Wynne 1968; Wynne and Singer 1963) described *communication deviance*, which has been applied in a number of longitudinal studies continuing to the present. The term refers to a lack of clarity in communication.

Lidz et al. (1956) extensively investigated the families of young adult schizophrenic patients and the relationship between parental-marital dysfunctions and the emergence of psychopathology in offspring. They described two family types, schismatic and eschewed, based on the family's display of either constant strife or false harmony resulting from the family's attempts to conceal its dysfunctions. The schismatic family type (characterized by overt marital hostility) can lead to acute schizophrenic breakdown, and the eschewed family type (characterized by covert accommodation to a dysfunctional spouse) can lead to chronic and "process" schizophrenia.

The investigations of the Palo Alto group started in the 1950s through the efforts of Bateson et al. (1956) and, subsequently, Satir (1967). They described communication patterns, cybernetics, systems theory, and the double-bind phenomenon in the early and current life situations of schizophrenic patients. Haley and Weakland both studied the work of Milton Erickson, and Haley (1963) described his observations in *Strategies of Psychotherapy* and other publications.

Jackson established the Mental Research Institute in 1959, which evolved into a major family therapy center and was enriched when Satir and Haley joined the staff in 1962. After Jackson's death in 1968, a number of other directors, including John Bell, Jules Riskin, John Weakland, and Paul Watzlawick, continued the early work of the Mental Research Institute and established the school of brief strategic therapy based on "paradoxical interventions" (Stanton and Todd 1982).

At Emory University in 1946, Whitaker became interested in studying families through his work with families and married couples. His creativity in using unconscious fantasies and countertransference and including all family members resulted in the development of the experiential school of family therapy. His charismatic use of feeling-expression had the goal of self-actualization, and he shied away from distinct theoretical formulations. He became known as one of the most innovative family therapists because he included children in family sessions.

In Europe, family therapy has been investigated particularly in the Milan school of family therapy and in the English school, the Kleinian group within the British Psychoanalytical Society. The English school was based on Melanie Klein's views and is separate from other object relations schools. The Milan school of family therapy was established by Selvini Palazzoli in Italy in the 1960s through her investigation of schizophrenia and anorexia nervosa in collaboration with a number of other investigators (Selvini Palazzoli et al. 1978). The Selvini Palazzoli group was influenced by the studies of Lidz and Wynne and subsequently by the work of the Mental Research Institute group on paradoxical interventions.

The group analytic approach was initiated by a variety of object relations theorists, including Middle-fort, Faulkes, Bion, and Skinner. Recently, the group analytic and object relations approach to families has gained more recognition in the United States.

In 1965, Minuchin moved to the Philadelphia Child Guidance Clinic and, with Haley, established the structural school of family therapy. The structural approach reached its height in theoretical development by defining the term *psychosomatic families*—families of patients with anorexia nervosa and many psychosomatic disorders (Minuchin et al. 1978). The structural approach also has been applied extensively to families of children with behavior disorders and, subsequently, to substance-abusing adults.

An underappreciated approach to family therapy with adolescents and children was attempted by the multiple impact therapy group in Galveston, Texas (MacGregor 1962). The novel intervention by this group included 2 days of family therapy by a number of professionals who alternated their work with different family members during the therapeutic encounter. On the basis of their clinical work with the families, researchers classified the families according to the disorders of the adolescents and children; oppositional defiant disorder, conduct disorder, prepsychotic, and intimidated groups were identified. This classification system predated the current classification initiatives and bridged a significant gap between individual and family psychology.

Major contributors to the study of family therapy with children include Patterson et al. (1982), Forehand and McMahon (1981), Alexander and Parsons (1973), Zilbach (1986), and Scharff and Scharff (1987). Patterson et al. (1982, 1993) and Forehand and McMahon (1981) immeasurably increased knowledge of delinquent behavior, Zilbach (1986) developed a systematic way to include children in family therapy, and Scharff and Scharff's (1987) formulations and recommendations are particularly applicable to families with adolescents.

Twin and adoption studies beginning in the 1960s demonstrated the likely genetic, anatomical, and biochemical contributors to the development of schizophrenia. Paradoxically, some of the studies, such as the Finnish Adoptive Family Study of Schizophrenia (Tienari et al. 1987), also revealed an important family and environmental factor in genetic transmission. These findings facilitated the application of family interventions to major psychiatric disorders.

When initial investigations of family therapy in the context of schizophrenia in psychiatric hospitals yielded disappointing results, the use of such therapy shifted to outpatient settings and to a broader range of psychiatric disorders. More recently, family interventions have been reintroduced in inpatient settings as a cost-effective measure, to reduce length of stay and help prevent relapse (Glick et al. 1987a).

Indications and Contraindications

An apparent and clear indication for family therapy is open and stressful conflicts among family members, with or without symptomatic behaviors in one or more members. Family therapy also can be applicable when there are covert problems within the family, which can give rise to dysfunctional behavior in one or more family members, or when other family members covertly support and perpetuate the disorder. Recognizing covert family problems in the presence of overt dysfunctions in one or more family members is the specific contribution of the field of family therapy.

Recently, family interventions have been used in the treatment of major psychiatric disorders such as schizophrenia, depression, alcoholism, conduct disorders, and somatoform disorders. Family-based interventions used to treat these psychiatric disorders in hospitalized patients are mostly psychoeducational and have beneficial effects when combined with other treatment modalities such as pharmacotherapy.

Therapists should choose family therapy or other treatment modalities on the basis of the nature and adequacy of family communication, structure, boundaries, conflicts, stresses, and resources. Psychodynamic family therapy is frequently used as an intervention for patients with narcissistic or borderline personality disorder.

Contraindications for family therapy are relative rather than absolute. They include discussing long-dormant, charged, or explosive family issues before the family commits to treatment. Another relative contraindication is discussing stressful situations with the family when one or more members are severely destabilized and require hospitalization.

Models of Family Therapy

The diversity of models of family therapy raises questions about the common ground among family therapies. The pioneers in family therapy focused on different dimensions in the family system, and to some degree, these different focuses reflected unrecognized differences among patients treated by these early family therapists. Although family therapists adopted divergent paths, they ignored the likely conclusion that different approaches to family therapy are closely linked to family characteristics commonly observed in different disorders.

Different models of family therapy are applicable to various patient populations. The intergenerational family therapy models of Bowen (1961, 1966, 1978) and Boszormenyi-Nagy (Boszormenyi-Nagy 1987; Boszormenyi-Nagy and Spark 1984) are particularly applicable to families whose members have long-standing disorders and have not negotiated adequate separation and differentiation between the generations. Structural and strategic family therapies are particularly applicable to families confronted with a crisis situation in which there has been adequate separation from previous generations and a reasonably satisfactory precrisis adjustment in the nuclear family. Behavioral family therapy is particularly applicable to marital problems and children with chronic conduct disorders. Psychodynamic and experiential family therapies are exceptionally helpful to family members with narcissistic vulnerability and a broad range of personality and neurotic disorders who have maintained a relatively adequate level of functioning but find little enjoyment in their lives. Social network therapy is particularly applicable to seriously and chronically disabled families with concomitant disintegration in the family and its social network.

Each model of family therapy includes different theoretical concepts and techniques. Some models of family therapy can be grouped on the basis of similarities. The intergenerational models include Bowen's family systems theory and Boszormenyi-Nagy's contextual therapy. The communicational/systems models include structural, strategic (several variations), and triadic-based family therapies and are closely related to behavioral family therapy. The psychodynamic and experiential family therapies are closely aligned.

■ Intergenerational Models

Family Systems Theory

Bowen's family systems theory is one of the most influential theories in family therapy. Many of Bowen's concepts have been adopted in different forms by other schools of family therapy. The foundational concepts are differentiation from the family of origin and establishment of a true self despite familial triangulation. Differentiation and maturation are accomplished when a person defines himself or herself within the context of the relationship. When this process fails, symptomatic phenomena such as undifferentiation and relational cutoff follow. Undifferentiated parents who are emotionally divorced "triangulate" their child between themselves to reduce the anxiety in their relationship. Other major concepts in Bowen's theory include anxiety within the family system, triangulation, transmission of illness across generations, emotional versus cognitive processes, the family projective system, and the overadequate-inadequate couple. The genogram of the family is an especially useful tool in this model, because it allows recognition of similar phenomena across generations.

Bowen's (1978) intervention, called "funneling through the therapist," addresses the family's undifferentiation and counters its attempts to triangulate the therapist. The family members are taught and encouraged to make therapeutic "family voyages" to their families of origin and to resist the senior generation's attempt to triangulate other family members in their conflicts. The strategy for family voyages is planned and discussed in the family session.

Contextual Therapy

Contextual therapy is an intergenerational model developed by Boszormenyi-Nagy (1987). Important in this therapy are the concepts of pathological loyalty, indebtedness, entitlement, and the ethical basis of family relationships. Symptomatic behavior among family members is seen as the by-product of pathology in the aforementioned spheres. Interventions in contextual therapy are based on making family members aware of the pathological loyalties and indebtedness between the generations.

■ Communicational/Systems Models

The communicational/systems models of family therapy combine the principles of general systems theory and cybernetics, which emphasize the circular causality and feedback mechanisms that maintain family homeostasis. The family strives to maintain its homeostasis in the face of environmental forces requiring change. Rigid families attempt to maintain homeo-

stasis at all cost, resulting in the lack of adaptability to environmental demands. Under such circumstances, the heightened tension results in emerging symptomatic interactions and maladaptive behavior in one or more family members. Rigid family boundaries and homeostatic mechanisms also reduce the flexibility needed to adapt to the internal requirements for passage through the life cycle.

Structural, strategic, and triadic-based family therapies are the three major communicational/systems models of family therapy. They are closely aligned with behavioral family therapy.

Structural Family Therapy

Structural family therapy was initially developed by Minuchin (1974), who was working with poor urban families of delinquent children at the Wiltwyck School in New York City. The therapy was later applied to children and adolescents in Philadelphia who had acute behavioral problems and eating disorders. Montalvo and Haley (1973) further enriched Minuchin's approach. The foundational theoretical concept in structural family therapy is the boundary. Clear and flexible boundaries are characteristic of functional families. *Enmeshed* describes families with members who are excessively intrusive, and *disengaged* describes families with members who are unavailable to one another.

Structural family intervention emphasizes establishing boundaries within the family through decisive and sensitive actions of the therapist. Family tasks and homework assignments further enforce this process. These methods of "joining" the family are particularly emphasized to enhance the effect of the therapist in the sessions (see Chapter 11, "Initial and Diagnostic Family Interviews," in this volume). The therapist attempts to "join" the family and shift family members' positions, in order to disrupt dysfunctional patterns and strengthen parental hierarchies. Clear and flexible boundaries are established in the sessions, and the family is encouraged to search for alternative interactional patterns.

Structural family therapy has been used to treat eating disorders, particularly anorexia nervosa, and asthma in children and adolescents. Its effectiveness in treating psychosomatic disorders and behavioral problems has been noted in numerous case reports and observations, as well as in reports of family outcome studies (Minuchin et al. 1978).

Strategic Family Therapy

Strategic family therapy emphasizes the need for a strategy developed by the family therapist to intervene in a family's efforts to maintain homeostasis by adhering rigidly to dysfunctional family patterns and symptoms. Strategic family therapy, like psychodynamic family therapy, has a well-articulated approach to address the resistance within family systems. Dealing with resistance, particularly in the family's response to the therapist's interventions, requires innovative methods. One technique, paradoxical intervention, attempts to reduce resistance and bring about change in the family structure and interactions by discouraging change. Paradoxical interventions facilitate the therapist's "joining" the family, with minimal resistance to restructuring the family's interactional system.

Strategic interventions are based on identifying a family's "rules"—the metacommunicational patterns that underlie symptomatic behaviors. These interventions are applied through directives and homework assignments. The homework can involve a logical, straightforward approach to the behavior or a seemingly illogical, paradoxical approach such as "prescribing the symptom"—a technique requiring family members to do what they have been doing all along in order to reduce family resistance and undermine interactional patterns by supporting the family's communicational pathways. Family life-cycle passages are considered important because they reveal inflexibility in the family's structure that makes the familial response to internal and developmental demands difficult.

The strategic approach of Haley (1973) and Madanes (1981) emphasizes the importance of strengthening the parental alliance to deal effectively with the symptomatic and often challenging behavior of the children. Power struggles between family members and subsequently between the therapist and the family are the focus of the evaluation and treatment.

The Mental Research Institute (Stanton 1986) in Palo Alto, California, emphasizes brief treatment and creative use of paradoxical interventions.

The systems approach of the Milan school of family therapy includes history taking to uncover the function of the symptoms and alter family interactions through positive connotation, reframing, directives, and paradoxical interventions.

The strategic model of family therapy gave rise to a number of new therapeutic approaches at the turn of this century. In stark contrast to traditional strategic approaches, the new models emphasize collaboration between the therapist and the family. Solution-focused therapy concentrates on the "exceptional solution" repertoire already practiced by the patients, to de-emphasize their problem-saturated outlook and enlarge the application of such solutions. Therapeutic effectiveness is enhanced by shifting the focus from "problems" to the "solution" (G.P. Sholevar 2003a, 2003b).

Narrative therapy focuses on the family members' restrictive internal narratives and helps them to reconstruct and coauthor new and empowering ones. The restrictive narratives are formed when the family attempts across the sequence of time to construct a coherent story around its life experience. Such stories are frequently "problem saturated" and restrictive and exclude significant family experiences that are contradictory to the powerful and dominant family narrative. The therapist assists the family to "restory" its experience by constructing alternative accounts that include significant family experiences formerly excluded from the family's dominant narrative. The disempowering influence of stereotypical cultural beliefs on the family is recognized and resolved through exploratory efforts (Browning and Green 2003; Malone 2001; G.P. Sholevar 2003a, 2003b; White and Epston 1990).

Triadic-Based Family Therapy

Zuk (1971) defined the communicational dysfunctions of the family in terms of a "pathological go-between" phenomenon, which develops when a principal in a conflict denies his or her role and promotes conflict between other family members to achieve his or her goal indirectly. Triadic-based family therapy proposes a series of strategies to force the conflict between the original principals into the open to enhance resolution. A major technical maneuver is to resist family members' attempts to engage the therapist in their fight, thereby forcing the family to confront its conflicts.

■ Psychodynamic Family Therapy

Psychodynamic family therapy emphasizes individual maturation, personality development, early childhood experiences, and resolution of symptoms and conflicts in the context of the family system. Special attention is paid to the "unconscious" life of the family members and to the inadequate resolution of prior developmental passages by the family members. Reported traumatic events in the lives of current or previous family members are considered a significant source of feedback about familial dysfunctions leading to symptoms, inhibitions, lack of pleasure, or immaturities. Common theoretical concepts of psychodynamic family therapy include shared unconscious conflicts and defenses, intrafamilial transference reactions, dyadic and triadic family transferences in treatment, projective identification, and a host of object relations psychoanalytic concepts. Holding environment is a particularly relevant concept among object relations theorists, specifically with regard to establishing a highly empathic relationship between the therapist and the family members to allow dormant conflicts to emerge (Scharff and Scharff 1987).

Psychodynamic family therapy is most applicable to families with multiple long-standing but subtle symptomatic behaviors that are intricately interwoven with personality traits. These symptoms include an inability to enjoy life, narcissistic vulnerability, and personality restrictions. Narcissistic relationships are characterized by mutual blaming and preoccupation with, and sensitivity to, shame and guilt, which lend themselves well to psychodynamic family therapy (Lansky 1983). Psychodynamic family interventions also are appropriate for the borderline disorders occurring in families with excessive projective identification, trading of dissociations, and fear of abandonment.

Psychodynamic family therapy can be combined readily and beneficially with individual therapy, simultaneously or sequentially.

Major contributors to psychodynamic family therapy include Ackerman (1958), Stierlin (1974), Shapiro (1986), Zinner (1976), and Framo (1982). A comprehensive application of object relations theory to family therapy has taken place as a result of the work of Zinner and Shapiro (1974) and Scharff and Scharff (1987).

A recent application of the psychodynamic model is the exciting and empirically validated approach of emotionally focused therapy (S.M. Johnson 2002, 2003; S.M. Johnson et al. 2001). In this therapy, attachment theory is applied to differentiate between "defensive" and "attachment affects" to enhance the therapeutic process.

■ Experiential Family Therapy

Experiential family therapy focuses on the expression of feelings, conscious or preconscious fantasies, and intrafamilial transference reactions, as well as the expression of the therapist's emotional experiences within the family, to expand the feeling range of the family. Clear communications, role flexibility, exploration, and spontaneity are encouraged. Carl Whitaker and Virginia Satir are the major pioneers of this approach (Gurman and Kniskern 1981).

■ Behavioral Family Therapy

Behavioral family therapy applies the principles of positive and negative reinforcement to the family unit, with the goal of enhancing reciprocity and minimizing coercive family processes. Coercive family processes generally are in the form of punishment, avoidance, and power play. Enhancing communication and problem-solving skills in the family is emphasized, and family members are discouraged from punishing one another. Contracting and behavioral exchange are enhanced in the family.

Contemporary behavioral family therapy is based on social learning theory and has been applied in the form of parent management training. The parents and children are taught environmental contingencies such as positive and negative reinforcement, or reward and punishment, which shapes behavior. Although alteration of maladaptive and problematic behavior is the focus of intervention, equal attention is paid to enhancing prosocial behavior in the children.

Behavioral family therapy can be combined with communication and problem-solving training. Adaptive and prosocial behavior is rewarded, and coercive family processes such as punishment and avoidance are exchanged for more productive methods of behavioral exchange and control.

■ Psychoeducational Family Intervention

Psychoeducational family intervention includes stress-diathesis theory as its foundational concept and attempts to enhance family adaptation, primarily through informing the family and the patient about the nature of symptomatology and psychopathology in psychiatric disorders. The family and the patient also receive detailed information about the treatment process and outcome. Psychoeducational intervention has been applied extensively in treating major mental illnesses such as schizophrenia, depression, alcoholism, and anxiety disorders. It consists of a series of in-depth instructional sessions by experts on the phenomenology, etiology, and diagnosis of the disorders. Clinical research findings are explained and made user-friendly for the family. Information is also provided about social institutions and systems involved in the care of the patient. Details about housing, crisis management, financial assistance, and other resources are essential for an effective treatment program.

Psychoeducational family therapy can be easily combined with other treatment modalities, particularly pharmacotherapy, crisis intervention, complete or partial hospitalization, residential treatment, and behavior and cognitive psychotherapies. The psychodynamic and exploratory psychotherapies are postponed to the later phases of treatment, when the patient and the family are stabilized.

Psychoeducational approaches make extensive use of empirical findings on expressed emotion, communication deviance, affective styles, and problem solving. These approaches address reducing the stressful family processes to lower the level of stress experienced by the patient. There is also a reduction in illness recurrence and rehospitalization, attributed to improved communication.

The application of psychoeducational models in the treatment of childhood depression and suicidality has been particularly productive (Brent 1997; Brent et al. 1996; Goodman et al. 1993). The model has been applied preventively in a range of stressful and potentially pathogenic situations for children, such as pediatric cancer and death and dying (Koocher 1997; McCreary 1998; Pettle 1998). A model for prevention of depression in children of depressed parents was empirically tested in the past decade and its positive outcome confirmed (Beardslee 1998; Beardslee et al. 1997).

■ Social Network Therapy

Social network therapy, developed by Speck and colleagues (Speck and Attneave 1971; Speck and Rueveni 1969), is applicable to families whose dysfunction and disintegration are closely related to the dysfunction and disintegration of their social network. This therapy focuses on the health and effectiveness of the social network, particularly the more recent constrictions of the family network before the immediate crisis. The size, homogeneity, and heterogeneity of the social network are assessed. The intervention techniques facilitate the emergence of activists within the family social network to enhance leadership, communication, relatedness, functioning, and expansion of the network. These changes can result in the uncovering and resolving of problems involving members of the family or the network.

The Family Life Cycle

The term *family life cycle* was introduced to family theory by Duvall (1977), who proposed that the family moves through a series of developmental stages. Haley (1973) applied the concept of the family life cycle to understanding the clinical problems of families by relating their dysfunctions to their difficulties in moving from one developmental stage to another. Carter and McGoldrick (1980) defined critical emotional issues for the family at different stages of the life cycle.

In Zilbach's (1989) model of the family life cycle, marriage is considered the first stage. The expectable seven stages of the family life cycle are 1) the beginning family, 2) the childbearing family, 3) the family with school-age children, 4) the family with teenagers, 5) the family as a launching center, 6) the family in its middle years, and 7) the aging family.

Combrinck-Graham (1985) proposed the family life spiral, with overlapping developmental issues for different generations. This spiral model emphasizes that the issues of involvement or separation are experienced on parallel levels by each generation. The family has a centripetal shape from the birth of the children through their childhoods and a centrifugal shape when the children move away from the family.

Clinicians use the concept of the family life cycle in different ways. In communicational models of family therapy, the life cycle is important to the explanation of dysfunctional family patterns. Psychodynamic family therapists focus on subtle, complex, reciprocal, and interlocking developmental forces within the individual and the family. Intergenerational family therapists are concerned with deviant family role assignment, which results in the stagnation and role immaturity of the younger generation.

Family Therapy With Children and Adolescents: Overview

■ Theoretical Concepts

All schools of family therapy are founded on theoretical concepts that are specifically applicable to family therapy with children and adolescents. In enmeshed families, there is not sufficient distance and objectivity among family members to allow differentiation of the children through the separation and individuation processes. The children have significant difficulties in school and social relationships, which further curtails their maturation. Overinvolvement between a child and a parent, projective family mechanisms, and triangulation (as described by Bowen) lead to "undifferentiation" that transmits across generations.

Projective identification describes the projection of unresolved parental conflicts onto a child, who assumes an identity based on a historically assigned role. Assumption of this role interferes with the child's appropriate identity formation. Traumatic events such as child neglect and physical or sexual abuse in the early history of the family can result in the repetition of such traumatic situations in subsequent generations. "Parentification," another impediment to the child's development, involves assigning a parental role to a child and depriving him or her of age-appropriate experiences.

Although many schools of family therapy recognize the significance of the separation-individuation process for adolescent family members, few of them describe the intricate network of developmental failures within the family and the adolescent that undermine the separation-individuation process. Stierlin (1974) proposed that binding, delegating, and expulsion are three ways that families negotiate a pathological separation to overcome the fear of prolonged fusion. In the binding mode, the excessive binding of the family to the adolescent can force the adolescent to engage in psychotic or suicidal behavior to free himself or herself from the family unit. In the intricate delegating mode, the family allows the adolescent to depart from the family unit "on a long leash" to return periodically to share the tales of his or her exploits in order to compensate for the restricted life of the parents. In the expulsion mode, the adolescent is rejected by and extruded from the family, to free him or her from the family unit.

■ Techniques

The literature on family therapy with children describes the clinical process and office arrangements that are most welcoming toward children. The office should be equipped with toys that are conducive to imaginative play; paper and crayons provide unlimited possibilities for drawing and expression of fantasies. A special attempt should be made to include the children in the treatment process by using age-appropriate methods of communication. Long and complex discussions discourage children from participating and should be avoided. The observational data on families with young children are especially significant. Techniques for family therapy with children have been described by Zilbach (1986) and Chasin and White (2003).

Family therapy with children frequently consists of two phases. In the first phase, approximately 10–20 sessions, the symptomatic behavior of the child is the focus of treatment, and the child resists the treatment situation on behalf of the parents. This first phase results in an improvement in the child's behavior, leading to enhanced school performance, peer-group relationships, proficiency in sports, and interest in children of the same and opposite sex. Encouraged by therapeutic results with the child, the parents frequently enter the second phase and develop additional goals to enhance their marriage and to resolve their marital dysfunction or parental psychopathology. At times, a third phase of treatment can become necessary when one of the parents decides to pursue a more ambitious therapeutic goal and reach a higher level of productivity, maturity, and creativity.

A common therapeutic mismanagement occurs when the parents succeed in diverting the therapeutic focus away from the child to a premature exploration of marital complaints. This diversion can be a resistance against the child-centered phase of the treatment and can result in an ineffective treatment outcome for both the child and the parents. Montalvo and Haley (1973) recommended recognizing the resistance component of such maneuvers and refraining from entering into marital therapy until the problem with the child is satisfactorily resolved or until there is a clear recontracting for marital rather than child-centered family therapy.

Often family therapy with children discloses child neglect. When family support is potentially available, family intervention can mobilize and rehabilitate family resources to provide the nurturance necessary for resumption of the child's developmental progress. When such resources are not present, it may be necessary to enable the family to search for an alternative living situation with the help of social agencies (Sholevar 1995).

■ Family Therapy and Child and Adolescent Psychiatry

The tensions between the fields of child psychiatry and family therapy were summarized in articles examining the state of "the undeclared war" between child psychiatry and family therapy (Malone 1974; McDermott and Char 1974). Child psychiatrists accused systemic family therapists of lacking appreciation for the individual child, his or her unique developmental characteristics and intrapsychic life, and the effect of early developmental failures, and for not taking a long-term view of child development. In addition, according to child psychiatrists, family therapists were oblivious to biological vulnerabilities and pharmacotherapy. Conversely, family therapists accused child psychiatrists of lacking understanding of the interpersonal dimensions of the child's life and the multiple sources of stress in contemporary family life. Child psychiatrists, according to family therapists, were preoccupied with minute developmental deviations and past events at the expense of present life realities, making treatment costly, lengthy, and frequently ineffective.

In the 1980s, the two camps approached reconciliation. Increasing recognition of family therapy's limitations in the treatment of certain populations, such as substance abusers (Friedman 1990), forced many family therapists to reach beyond family therapy and address peer-group, psychological (intrapsychic and cognitive), educational, and social dimensions of behavior disorders. Pharmacologic agents, such as stimulants, antidepressants, and major tranquilizers, are increasingly being used by many family psychiatrists, with encouraging results. Teaching family therapy has been a requirement in child and adolescent, as well as general, psychiatry residency programs for the past 20 years. The integrative approach in treating major mental illnesses has resulted in the consolidation of a true biopsychosocial approach—namely, family psychiatry (Malone 1979, 1983; G.P. Sholevar 2003a). Psychodynamic and object relations family therapies have demonstrated the many advantages of recognizing the interrelationships between interpersonal and intrapsychic processes (Lansky 1983; Ravenscroft 1991; G.P. Sholevar 2003a), which can be addressed through combined family and individual therapy.

■ Family Intervention and Attention-Deficit/ Hyperactivity Disorder

Family interventions have been used to enhance treatment effectiveness in patients with attention-deficit/ hyperactivity disorder (ADHD). Multiple studies have demonstrated the effectiveness of medications in reducing the core symptoms of ADHD. However, the reduction in negative interaction between parents and children has been greater when parent therapy and family interventions have been provided as primary or adjunctive treatments (Barkley et al. 1992; Diamond and Siqueland 2001; Pelham et al. 1998). Parent training allows the parents to intervene effectively to enhance the capacity of the ADHD child to focus, remain on task, solve problems, act prosocially with peers, and reduce impulsivity and aggression through cognitive processing. Parent therapy and parent management training are effective tools for strengthening the positive parent–child bonds and the ADHD child's fragile self-esteem through reducing negative and counterproductive parental behavior and enhancing skillful and goal-directed intervention by parents in potentially conflictual situations. Treatment manuals by Patterson (1982) and Barkley (1981) serve as useful and flexible guides for training parents to interact productively with their children.

A significant recent study, the Multimodal Treatment Study of Children With Attention Deficit Hyperactivity Disorder, was conducted at multiple sites and involved a large number of children ages 7–9 years (Hinshaw et al. 2000; Diamond and Siqueland 2001). The study featured a comprehensive psychosocial treatment package of school visits, teacher training, and 30 parent-training sessions, with or without the use of medication. The most effective intervention was the combined treatment, which included medication and psychosocial intervention, although pharmacotherapy alone produced impressive results. The combined treatment exhibited the best results in terms of control of ADHD core symptoms, reduction of negative parent–child interaction, enhancement of positive parent–child interaction, and promotion of prosocial behavior in the child.

■ Family Therapy and Conduct Disorders

The high prevalence of conduct disorders in the general population and their occurrence in families with histories of antisocial personality disorder, depression, or criminal behavior have been the focus of family-based investigations and interventions. The role of parents in the genesis of antisocial behavior in their offspring was initially described by A. Johnson and Szurek (1952). Minuchin et al. (1967) described the structural and functional deficiencies in families with aggressive children from deprived socioeconomic backgrounds. The conduct problems could be observed in both enmeshed and disengaged families, although a substantial part of the investigation by structural family therapists focused on enmeshed families.

Patterson et al. (1982) described coercive family processes by which the parents, who generally lack management skills, initiate overly punitive and aggressive actions toward their children but withdraw in the face of strong opposition by the children. The coercive processes result in a high level of aggressive and uncontrollable behavior in the children. In subsequent research, Patterson and colleagues (1982) focused on the relationship between aggressive behavior in children and depression in parents, particularly single mothers.

Patterson et al. (1982) described in detail coercive family processes in families with a high likelihood of producing children with conduct disorders. These families generally have histories of antisocial or criminal behavior, alcoholism, substance abuse, separation or divorce, disruption of education or employment, or related economic hardships. There is a high rate of aggression, resulting in impulsively punitive parental reactions in excess of what can be justified by the children's behavior. The children's equally aggressive response to the parental intervention results in retreat of the parents from the disciplinary course. The repetition of this process, termed *coercive trap*, teaches children that aggressive behavior can result in the withdrawal of punishment and therefore reinforces the disruptive behavior. Depression in the parents of children with conduct disorders commonly occurs as a result of a failure in parenting and further interrupts the parental management practices.

Other researchers have also studied families of children with conduct disorders. Alexander and Barton (1976) examined the function of aggressive behavior in the family and attempted to change the family's interactions from defensive to supportive interactions in order to undermine conduct problems. Reiss (1971, 1982) examined cooperation and cohesiveness in the families, or coordination, which is related to conduct disorders in the children. These researchers' laboratory-based investigations demonstrated the weakness of coordination and cooperation in families of children with conduct disorders, a finding that is consistent with the work of Minuchin, Patterson, Forehand, and Alexander.

Functional family therapy, parent management training, and multisystemic therapy (MST) have produced encouraging therapeutic results in children with conduct disorders.

Functional Family Therapy

Functional family therapy was developed by Alexander and Barton (1976) through an integration of behavioral family therapy and general systems theory. It was initially applied to delinquent children with status offenses, primarily children who run away, and was later applied to children with more severe conduct disorders and delinquent behavior. The approach has proved highly successful in delinquent boys and has been shown to have a preventive effect on conduct problems in younger siblings of the patients and depression in parents.

Parent Management Training

Forehand and McMahon (1981) and Patterson et al. (1982) produced some of the most extensive and experimentally based literature in the area of family therapy, particularly parent management training (see Chapter 52 in this volume, "Cognitive-Behavior Modification," for a complete discussion). The approach developed by Patterson et al. (1993) has been applied in multiple settings by independent teams of investigators and has proved beneficial in altering conduct disorders and enhancing prosocial behavior in children at home and in school. The preventive effect on younger siblings of children with conduct disorders has also been noted (Forehand and Kotchick 1996; Forehand and McMahon 1981; Patterson et al. 1982).

Parent management training has demonstrated significant empirical effectiveness in the treatment of oppositional/defiance and conduct disorders in the past 30 years. It addresses the deficient parental management skills that are intimately correlated with antisocial behavior and arrested socialization in children. It teaches the parents to interact more productively with their children by reinforcing prosocial behavior rather than inadvertently rewarding deviant behavior (Kazdin 1997; Mabe et al. 2001; Patterson 1976; E. Sholevar 2003; G. P. Sholevar 1995).

The basic principles of parent management training are accurate labeling of the child's behavior, emphasis on prosocial behavior, deemphasis of disruptive behavior, administration of tangible reinforcers, use of nonviolent methods of "punishment," and anticipation or resolution of problems. The targeted keystone behavior of the child is noncompliance.

The interventions are based on systematic observation of the child's behavior and include positive reinforcement of prosocial behavior, use of time-out, guidelines for attending or ignoring, shaping the desirable behavior (successive approximation of terminal behaviors), and enhancement of problem solving. Negotiations, compromise formations, and contracting between the parents and the children are encouraged. Coercive family processes (Patterson 1982) are identified and resolved through effective reinforcement.

Extensive research by numerous independent investigators in different settings has demonstrated the effectiveness of parent management training in terms of short- and long-term outcome. There have been decreases in parental (maternal) depression and in subsequent referrals of younger siblings for antisocial behavior. The treatment has been less effective with "insular" mothers, who are socially isolated and depressed and have economic problems (Wahler et al. 1993). A range of behavioral and cognitive interventions, enlargement of the social network, and medication in the case of parental depression can help to enhance maternal functioning.

Multisystemic Therapy

In the past two decades, many attempts have been made to broaden the scope of family interventions to include multiple other systems. The multisystemic therapy (MST) of Henggeler and colleagues is the most widely recognized intervention system of its kind, and a fair amount of empirical evidence supports its effectiveness. It is an intensive family- and community-based treatment that addresses multiple determinants of serious antisocial behavior and substance abuse in juvenile offenders. The intervention is based on the premise that the individual with a conduct disorder is nested within a complex network of interconnected systems that encompass individual, familial, and extrafamilial (peer, school, neighborhood) factors. The target of the family-based intervention has been chronic, violent, or substance-abusing juvenile offenders at high risk for out-of-home placement. The goal of MST is to empower parents through development of the skills and resources needed to raise their teenage children and to empower the youth to cope with family, peer, school, and neighborhood problems. The home-based model of service delivery enhances service access and retention of the family in treatment. The therapists have low caseloads and strong systems

of supervision, supplemented by consultation, to allow the intensive intervention. Treatment generally lasts about 4 months.

In addition to maintaining a clear focus on the risk factors for the youth and their family, peers, and neighborhood, MST emphasizes building youth and family strength (protective factors) on an individualized and comprehensive basis to attenuate risk factors.

- MST emphasizes concrete measures such as removing offenders from deviant peer groups, enhancing school performance, and developing support for the family.
- The program removes barriers to service access by using the home-based model.
- The services are intensive and may include several hours of treatment per week.
- Vigorous efforts are made to measure long-term outcome.
- The program has been applied to male and female adolescents, black and white, between ages 12 and 17 years.

There is a fair amount of evidence of MST's effectiveness. Multiple controlled and randomized clinical trials involving violent or chronic juvenile offenders have been conducted. More than 300 serious, violent, or substance-abusing juvenile offenders and their families participated in these trials.

Evaluation of the MST program yielded the following findings:

- A reduction in the long-term rate of criminal offenses among serious juvenile offenders
- Reduced rates of out-of-home placement
- Reduced rates of drug use and drug-related offenses
- Improvement in family functioning
- A decrease in other mental health problems

Treatment with MST resulted in a lower level of rearrest and reincarceration and a reduction in the number of days of out-of-home placement. The long-term rearrest rate was reduced by 25%–70% in the MST-treated groups in comparison to control groups. In a recent study, MST was used as an alternative to psychiatric hospitalization at the time of crisis. An 85% reduction in the number of days of hospitalization was reported.

Family Therapy and Hospitalization of Children With Conduct Disorders

Hospitalization of children with conduct disorders frequently occurs at the height of the negative escalation between the parents and the children. The child is hospitalized after repetitive fights with the parents, often because of disruptive behavior in school or nonattendance. Through hospitalization, the parents may hope to enlist the assistance of the hospital to make the child compliant. After a few days of compliance with hospital procedures (or absolute refusal to comply), the child may be discharged home without any change in his or her behavioral pattern. In cases in which the pattern of oppositional and rebellious behavior against parental expectation is severe and extreme, it seems unlikely that hospitalization will bring about compliance. The only possible exception to this pattern would be a case in which a dramatic shift in family dynamics occurs whereby the family becomes able to effectively confront issues avoided for many years. If the noncompliance problem is chronic and no resolution of significant emotional issues occurs in treatment, the likelihood of rapid change is low. The task may be better viewed as a search for ways to manage and rehabilitate a chronic and disabling symptom. The parents and the child can be assisted in recognizing that neither side possesses sufficient leverage to win in the situation, and the parents and the child can be encouraged to forge a compromise.

Family Intervention in Residential Treatment Centers

Researchers have determined that the lack of a meaningful conceptual framework to guide intervention with families is the major factor limiting the effectiveness of residential treatment (G.P. Sholevar 2001). Family intervention in a residential treatment center should be guided by two variables: 1) the state of disintegration of the family unit and 2) the level of availability of the family in terms of care provision or participation in psychiatric treatment. Families of patients in residential treatment centers can be divided into four groups: 1) available families, 2) potentially available families, 3) partially available families, and 4) totally unavailable families (G.P. Sholevar 1995, 2001).

Available families. The available family is forced to institutionalize the child after family confrontations occur at the height of negatively escalated interactions. The family and the child are strongly bonded and depend on each other to the point that they cannot live with or without each other. Such families are available for home visits, participation in family sessions, and eventual family reunification.

Potentially available families. The potentially available family has lost its immediate ability to care for the child because of a loss of functional capacity in the nuclear or extended family. A history of divorce, remarriage, physical or psychiatric illness, or death should alert the treatment team to the loss of family resources and capacity. The therapeutic task is to recognize the limitations in the functional and caretaking capacities of these families and protect the families from any unrealistic and premature demands. The functional capacity of the family should be increased by resolving intergenerational conflicts, improving the functional and economic capacities of the parents, and activating the parents' social networks.

Partially available families. The partially available family interacts with the child through erratic telephone calls, occasional visits, or irregular attendance at treatment sessions. Parents in these families have an extreme incapacity to manage life tasks. A realistic treatment strategy is to maintain the family's connection with the child psychologically while making realistic living plans for the child for after discharge from the residential treatment center. The family can serve as a resource to the group home or foster family after the child's discharge from the residential treatment center.

Totally unavailable families. The totally unavailable family is characterized by loss of contact with the child many years before his or her admission to a residential treatment center. There is usually a distorted and unrealistic expectation of a reunion between the family and the child. Such distorted fantasies should be discussed immediately and continually during residential treatment. It is helpful if the family is located early in the course of residential treatment to verify (either in person or by telephone) the family's inability to take care of the child. This strategy helps resolve some of the child's dormant fantasies and conflicts and facilitates his or her adaptation to other living possibilities.

Family Therapy and Psychosomatic Disorders

Minuchin et al. (1978) described several common characteristics of families with children and adolescents who have psychosomatic disorders such as anorexia nervosa, other eating disorders, or asthma. The families with psychosomatic disorders present were enmeshed, overprotective, and rigid; avoided conflict; and used the child's problems to detract attention from parental conflict. The treatment corrects defensive interactional patterns to enhance separation and individuation in the child.

G.P. Sholevar (1986b), Bahnson (1986), and other researchers addressed the characteristics of families with chronic psychosomatic disorders present, including lack of recognition of affect, avoidance of conflict resolution, and superficial and limited object relations. Collectively, these defenses maintain the patient and the family in a chronically stressful and unsatisfying environment that interferes with the quality of life and normative development.

Studies have demonstrated the impressive effect of structural family therapy on families with younger adolescents who have eating disorders or other psychosomatic reactions. However, the utility of the model among older patients who have bulimia has not been supported (Russell et al. 1987).

Family Therapy and Adolescent Substance Abuse

Clinical investigations involving addicted adult populations have examined the dysfunctional family boundaries and structures that lead to a coalition between the addicted family member (usually a young adult or adolescent) and at least one of the parents, usually the mother, who acts as the enabler and supplier for the addicted person. The support of the enabling parent is covert and usually unacknowledged. Stanton (1986) recommended that parents' contributions to the drug addiction be brought into the open to reduce their pathogenic impact on the addicted person.

Family therapy with substance-abusing adolescents was described by Friedman (1989) and Liddle (1991). Friedman (1989) used functional family therapy to increase supportiveness and decrease defensiveness within the family unit. The results achieved with their model have been encouraging. The multidimensional family therapy model of Liddle (1991) addresses a wide range of problematic behaviors in the adolescent in addition to the underlying family interactional patterns that support the addictive behavior.

Engagement of the drug-abusing adolescent can be enhanced by intensive pretreatment family intervention on the telephone or through a home visit (Szapocznik et al. 1989). Liddle and Dakof (Liddle 2000; Liddle and Dakof 1995; Liddle et al. 2001) applied multidimensional, multicomponent, and multisystemic comprehensive family intervention to substance-abusing adolescents. They investigated the links between reductions in adolescent drug abuse and changes in parenting, improvement of the therapist-adolescent alliance, and addressing cultural and gender issues in treatment. Their preliminary findings indicated the effectiveness of family interventions compared with other treatment modalities.

Multisystemic therapy (MST) has been applied in the treatment of substance abuse among adolescents with encouraging results (Henggeler and Santos 1997; Henggeler and Schoenwald 1998; Henggeler et al. 1998, 1999; Multisystemic Treatment Services 2003). It has been effective in reducing drug use and the number of rearrests and days of out-of-home placement.

Recent Developments in Family Theory and Therapy

Family therapy has followed the overall movement of the mental health field in the direction of a more precise and multidimensional definition of psychopathology and disability. The emphasis of DSM-III-R (American Psychiatric Association 1987), DSM-IV (American Psychiatric Association 1994), and DSM-IV-TR (American Psychiatric Association 2000) on classifying psychiatric disorders has heightened the importance of diagnosis. Although DSM-III-R, DSM-IV, and DSM-IV-TR do not address etiology or process, the family therapy movement has already made significant findings in examining the interface between family functioning and individual diagnosis, particularly the diagnoses of schizophrenia, depression, and alcoholism (Clarkin and Miklowitz 2003).

The field of family therapy has moved toward more empirically derived measures, such as expressed emotion, and away from theoretically driven constructs. There has been a close adherence to the stress-diathesis model (Rosenthal 1970; Zubin and Spring 1977), particularly in reference to major mental illnesses. This model recognizes the presence of reasonably convincing evidence for a strong genetic predisposition to a number of major psychiatric disorders, such as schizophrenia, bipolar disorders, and alcoholism, which, in interaction with various life events within and outside the family, can affect the risk of emerging or recurring disorder in a family member. Contemporary family therapy also clearly recognizes the efficacy of psychopharmacology in schizophrenia and depression.

Family interventions based on new clinical research findings have resulted in reduced recurrences of chronic schizophrenia and depression, improved therapeutic results with regard to alcoholism and conduct disorders, and prevention of transmission of alcoholism and conduct disorders to the next generation (Clarkin and Carpenter 2003).

■ The Birth of Family Psychiatry

Progress in genetics, biological psychiatry, and pharmacotherapy has broadened knowledge about the etiological factors associated with the inception, maintenance, and recurrence of major mental illnesses and emotional disorders. Progress in these fields also has substantiated the combined role of various biological, interpersonal, and psychological factors. A true field of family psychiatry has emerged.

Stress-diathesis theory (Rosenthal 1970) and the Finnish Adoptive Family Study of Schizophrenia (Tienari et al. 1987), among others, have provided significant data on the combined role of biological and interpersonal variables in psychiatric disorders. Family psychiatry, with its new integrative orientation, provides a comprehensive framework for understanding the contributions of the family unit to disorders such as schizophrenia and depression. Special attention is paid to the genetic vulnerability of the family members. Therapeutic interventions with such families include multiple treatment modalities such as pharmacotherapy; individual, behavior, group, and milieu therapy; and family therapy. Preventive efforts are particularly geared toward reducing vulnerability in younger children.

Stress-Diathesis Theory

Stress-diathesis or stress-vulnerability theory was first proposed by Rosenthal (1970) and was further refined by Zubin and Spring (1977). In stress-diathesis theory, the disorder is regarded as a product of two sets of variables: vulnerability and stressors. The vulnerability can be the result of genetic and psychobiological factors, although psychological and interpersonal vulnerability can function in a similar fashion. Genetic factors have been studied in schizophrenia, depression, and alcoholism. Stress can be caused by external factors or be the result of stressful psychological mechanisms or interpersonal patterns. The perspective of stress-diathesis theory is that illness is the result of heightened vulnerability and stress and can be best prevented, managed, and treated by altering both sets of factors. Psychotropic medications function by reducing vulnerability, and family interventions focus on lowering interpersonal sources of stress and enhancing coping and problem-solving capacities.

Finnish Adoptive Family Study of Schizophrenia

The Finnish Adoptive Family Study of Schizophrenia (Tienari et al. 1987) produced data supporting the combined and interconnected role of genetic and familial variables in schizophrenia and other psychiatric disorders. Researchers studied the level of family functioning, adaptability, and organization of adoptive families and divided them into five groups, ranging from "optimally functioning" to "inadequately functioning." Although all families adopted children with comparable genetic vulnerability to schizophrenia, the outcome of the children was significantly correlated with the level of family functioning. There were no psychotic or borderline children in the two groups of families with optimal or close to optimal functioning. In contrast, there was a preponderance of schizophrenic and borderline patients in the two groups with the lowest levels of functioning. The Finnish study findings strongly support the notion that genetic risk can be enhanced or decreased according to the level of functioning and adequacy of the family.

■ Family Variables in Schizophrenia

A significant change has occurred in conceptualizing the family dimension of schizophrenia. The family is viewed as a major resource whose availability to the patient can make a crucial difference in positive outcome. Negative interaction between the patient and the family now is seen as largely reactive to the patient's symptoms rather than causative. Blaming family interactions (double bind) or the parents (schizophrenogenic mother) has become obsolete.

In family studies based on the stress-vulnerability model, researchers have investigated variables that can differentiate families of schizophrenic patients from families of nonschizophrenic patients. Studies of indicators of risk have focused particularly on three variables: 1) expressed emotion, 2) communication deviance, and 3) affective style (Goldstein 1987).

Expressed Emotion

Brown et al. (1962) reported that male patients with chronic schizophrenia who returned to live with their families after psychiatric hospitalization were more prone to rehospitalization than were patients who went to other living arrangements. Brown and his colleagues then designed a prospective study to examine the affective atmosphere of the family, including the presence of critical, hostile, or emotionally overinvolved attitudes. He proposed the term *expressed emotion*, a composite variable with the values of high and low, as an index of the family's criticism of and overinvolvement with the patient. *Expressed emotion* refers to negative emotional attitude. A number of subsequent British and American studies indicated that the rate of relapse among schizophrenic and depressed patients in families with high expressed emotion is four times higher than that in families with low expressed emotion (Hahlweg et al. 1987; Hooley et al. 1986; Vaughn and Leff 1976). The interventions with families having high expressed emotion, with specific goals for reducing familial hostility and overinvolvement, have provided experimental evidence that expressed emotion is indeed causally related to the course of illness and that a decrease in the level of expressed emotion results in a decrease in the occurrence of relapse (Hahlweg et al. 1987).

Hooley et al. (1986) proposed that a high level of expressed emotion in family members can be interpreted on the basis of their attitudes toward illness attribution and symptom controllability. Vaughn and Leff (1976) suggested that families who blame the illness rather than the patient for the behaviors typically accompanying psychiatric impairment are likely to be supportive or have low expressed emotion. Families with low expressed emotion do not doubt the legitimacy and nonvolitional nature of the patient's condition. Families with high expressed emotion, in contrast, seem more inclined to attribute the causes of deviant behavior to the patient. These family members often express frustration and anger that the patient does not do more to help himself or herself, and they hold the patient at least partially responsible for the symptoms.

Poor premorbid family relationships and "negative symptoms" increase the likelihood of symptomatic behavior being attributed to internal factors or characterological features of the patient. A satisfactory preillness relationship between the patient and his or her relatives is commonly associated with low expressed emotion.

Communication Deviance

Wynne and Singer (1963) studied communication deviance (i.e., a lack of clarity in parental communication) by comparing parents of schizophrenic patients with parents of nonschizophrenic patients. They found a lack of clarity in communication and disturbances in maintaining attention in the parents of schizophrenic patients. Subsequent studies have indicated that communication deviance is related to the severity of psychopathology in the offspring, although some of the disturbances are nonschizophrenic in nature. Further studies also have indicated that high communication deviance together with high expressed emotion or negative affective style can be a risk factor for schizophrenia spectrum disorders (Wynne 1987).

The nature of the communication deviance is not well recognized, and it may represent a cross-generational shared vulnerability in the parents and children that affects attention, perception, and information processing. The end result is disturbances in attention in the offspring. It also possible that communication deviance in parents is related to the distress of interacting with schizophrenic offspring. Longitudinal studies of communication deviance have shown a high risk of psychopathology among children of parents with high communication deviance, particularly when there is concomitant high expressed emotion and negative affective style.

No studies have focused on how reducing communication deviance in families affects offspring.

Affective Style

Affective style refers to the emotional-verbal behavior of family members during family discussions with patients. It can be classified as either benign or negative.

Affective style is measured by counting the number of criticisms, guilt inductions, intrusions, and supportive statements made by the relatives.

Studies have indicated that expressed emotion and affective style are related to each other and measure different aspects of the same phenomena, such as parental criticism. Data on the predictive value of affective style are sparse but may be of prognostic value. A number of studies have examined the combination of expressed emotion, communication deviance, and affective style in families (Goldstein 1987).

■ Family Intervention and Depression

Deficits in social functioning in depressed patients are common and can persist in the absence of clinical symptoms. Depressed patients tend to be aversive to others and also tend to feel victimized by them. They frequently engage in escalating negative exchanges with their mates. Depressed patients and their spouses tend to verbalize their negative, subjective feelings more frequently than nondepressed couples, whose communications are more task oriented (Haas and Glick 1988; Hinchcliffe et al. 1978). The marriages of depressed women (or men) are characterized by friction, poor communication, dependence, lack of affection, overt hostility, silence, withdrawal, and a tendency for the nondepressed spouse to view his or her spouse's unspoken misery as an accusation (Coyne 1987; Haas and Glick 1988).

The spouses of depressed persons seem vulnerable to disorders: in one study, 40% of spouses had a diagnosable emotional disorder requiring referral during the patient's depression, and 17% had a disorder after the patient's recovery (Coyne et al. 1987). Depressed patients' assortative mating is toward spouses with personal and family histories of psychiatric disturbance (Coyne 1987; Merikangas et al. 1979). However, spouses' psychiatric disturbances did not emerge until after the marriage. The wives of depressed men are particularly vulnerable to depression. Depressed women tend to marry men who have character disturbances or substance abuse problems (Coyne 1987).

An intimate relationship with a spouse may be a protective factor against depression. Specifically, women lacking good marital relationships are significantly more likely to become depressed (Brown and Harris 1978; Coyne 1987). A good marital relationship seems to neutralize the effects of stress, such as the stress of caring for many young children or of unemployment (Brown and Harris 1978).

Children of depressed parents are at risk for many psychological problems. The rate of diagnosable psychiatric disturbance among children of depressed parents can be as high as 40%–50% (Coyne 1987). The risk to children is increased if 1) the depressed person's spouse becomes depressed or is unavailable to the child, 2) there are marital problems or divorce (Coyne 1987), or 3) there is no supportive relationship with another adult. A comprehensive preventive program for the children of depressed parents was described by Beardslee and Schwoeri (1994).

A range of family-based interventions has emerged for treatment and prevention of depression in children and for prevention of transmission of this disorder in the family. Such interventions are based on an integration of family systems theory, psychodynamic theory, and attachment theory within a developmental model (Schwoeri and Sholevar 1994; G.P. Sholevar and Schwoeri 1994). They draw on the psychoeducational model to inform the family and the children of the disruptive effect of this disorder on the family and ways of protecting the family unit. A variety of parent-child and play therapy techniques to be used within the context of the family have been proposed. The nondepressed parent plays a crucial role in enhancing the coping capacity of the family (G.P. Sholevar and Schwoeri 1994). Beardslee's (Beardslee and Schwoeri 1994) comprehensive preventive model to reduce the likelihood of transmission of depression from the parents to the children remains dominant in the field.

Treatment

Pharmacotherapy and a range of interpersonal and cognitive psychotherapies have proved effective in treating depression. Symptoms responding well to medication include early-morning awakening, reduced libido, decreased concentration, and depressed mood. Negative attitude and aversive communication frequently necessitate modification of interpersonal behavior patterns. There usually is no increase in family resistance with the combination of interpersonal therapy and medication, especially if the latter is systematically administered (Haas et al. 1985). Friedman (1975) found the combination of drug and marital therapy more beneficial than exclusive use of one treatment modality. Drug therapy usually was associated with significant early improvement in clinical symptoms, and marital therapy was associated with significant long-term positive changes in family and marital relationships.

■ Psychoeducational Family Intervention

Psychoeducational intervention with families, discussed earlier in this chapter, enhances the family's capacity to cope with the illness (e.g., schizophrenia and depression) in offspring by informing family members about the etiology, phenomenology, and treatment process.

■ Family Intervention and Alcoholism

Alcoholism is a major medical and social disorder, and its high prevalence in families has stimulated significant investigations of genetics and the family (Cadoret et al. 1980, 1986; Goodwin et al. 1973). It is estimated that up to 30% of all families have at least one member who abuses alcohol or drugs (National Institute on Drug Abuse 1991). Numerous studies have found that genetic factors play a definite role in alcoholism (Cadoret et al. 1980, 1986; Goodwin et al. 1973).

Family dynamics, family structure, and alcoholism have been investigated over the past two decades by Steinglass (1979, 1980, 1981) and Wolin et al. (1979, 1988) at the George Washington University. Through their studies, they have defined the "alcoholic family" and the "alcoholic family identity." The alcoholic family identity is formed when alcohol plays a critical role in the day-to-day behavior of the family. The presence of alcohol as an inseparable component in the family's daily life affects the family's growth and development and becomes part of the core family identity. In these families, alcohol becomes the central organizing principle, limits the family's ability to adjust to changes and crises, and affects regulatory family mechanisms, such as rituals, routines, and celebrations.

The alcoholic family identity affects the life cycle of the family. In the early phase, the need for intense activity, the rapid change, and the optimism commonly observed in a nonalcoholic family is affected by the family heritage of alcoholism, which prevents some of the traditional values of the family of origin from being passed on to future family members. In the middle phase, repetitive recycling occurs between states of intoxication and sobriety. The behavior of the family is more predictable in the alcohol-on state, or "wet" state, than when the drinking does not occur. During the intoxicated periods, the family stays away from neighbors and friends and fortifies the boundary between the family and outsiders. In the late phase, the family's orientation toward the future and adjustment to losses and gains can be undermined by the alcoholism. The family has four options: 1) drinking, 2) controlled drinking, 3) alcoholic abstinence, or 4) nonalcoholic abstinence. The stable, dry, or nondrinking pathway can be classified as either alcoholic or nonalcoholic. In the stable, dry alcoholic family, the family continues to use alcohol as an organizing principle, despite the absence of active drinking. In the stable, dry nonalcoholic family, the family has ceased drinking and is no longer preoccupied with alcohol.

The transmission of alcoholism to the next generation is facilitated by an interruption in the family's regulatory mechanisms. These include family rituals and the ritual process, which is a systematized form of communication that establishes and preserves the family's identity and sense of itself (Wolin and Bennett 1984). Family rituals include family celebrations, traditions, and patterned family routines. Preserving family rituals is an effective way to counter the transmission of alcoholism across generations. The undermining of family identity and the related "family myth," the way the family views itself, correlates with the formation of the alcoholic family identity and the transmission of alcoholism to the next generation.

Treatment

Effective treatment of alcoholism involves a multimodal intervention. Removing the alcohol from the family is an essential first step. In addition to family therapy, other interventions such as participation in Alcoholics Anonymous, Al-Anon, or Alateen; hospitalization; community-based programs; and behavior therapies are useful.

Family Classification and Diagnosis

The field of family therapy has been both strongly for and strongly against classifying families on the basis of different theoretical assumptions. Family therapists have described different types of families, such as undifferentiated families, enmeshed families, disengaged families, and psychosomatic families. Some researchers have attempted to classify marital relationships as schismatic or eschewed (Lidz et al. 1956), as well as unstable-unsatisfactory or stable-unsatisfactory (Jackson 1965). A more widely accepted system of classification was proposed by Cuber and Harroff (1992), who described the conflict-habituated marriage, devitalized marriage, and vital and total marriage.

DSM-III-R, DSM-IV, and DSM-IV-TR have rekindled interest in an empirically based family classification and diagnostic system. The family committee of the Group for the Advancement of Psychiatry (1985) proposed a document consistent with DSM-IV to specify diagnostic criteria for family and couple relational disorders. The committee's criteria focus on specific family problems such as sexual or physical abuse, divorce, sexual disorders, failure to thrive, and separation anxiety.

The Global Assessment of Relational Functioning scale (Endicott and Spitzer 1979) has been used by the Group for the Advancement of Psychiatry committee to evaluate the level of a family's dysfunction, analogous to the Axis V rating of global functioning of the individual used in DSM-IV-TR. A second classification system of family relational disorders was proposed by Clarkin and Miklowitz (2003).

Family Intervention in Psychiatric Hospitals

The goals of the family-oriented model of inpatient intervention are to prevent rehospitalization, strengthen fragile ties between the family and the patient, and help the family and the patient reach the highest functional level. This approach is psychoeducationally oriented, emphasizes the rehabilitation of the family for a successful reunion when the patient returns home, and counters the tendency of the hospital to "adopt" the patient by attempting to replace the family psychologically.

Inpatient family intervention focuses on treating the patient's illness, with recognition of the importance of family variables. Based on a stress-diathesis model and guided by recent research on expressed emotion, this type of intervention places the relatively causative biological factors in perspective with the familial and environmental influences (i.e., the primary factors are biological and the secondary factors are familial and environmental). Medication is considered a natural ally of family intervention (Glick et al. 1985).

The multiple functions of the psychiatric hospital in regard to the family include addressing problems that are disturbing the family's homeostasis, assisting other disturbed but resistant family members, and helping the family to regain a "lost," severely dysfunctional family member. Inpatient family intervention also can help change long-standing maladaptive or deteriorating family interactional patterns (Glick et al. 1987b).

In agreement with the tenets of the National Alliance for the Mentally Ill, inpatient family intervention must encourage collaboration and teamwork rather than stigmatize or shut out families of the mentally ill. The family should be considered the most important resource and as such deserves support and respect rather than criticism and blame (Hatfield 1986). The relationship between the family and the psychiatrist should be collaborative on behalf of the patient.

A variety of family therapy approaches have been used in treating hospitalized patients. The psychoeducational model of family intervention is most effective for families with a member who has been hospitalized for schizophrenia or an affective disorder, and this intervention increases the family's knowledge of the illness and enhances the family's ability to deal with the illness. In treating these families, the family therapist refrains from emphasizing changes in the total family unit during the acute phase of the illness, which can increase the level of tension, and avoids exaggerated theoretical notions and claims such as "the family is the patient," which overemphasizes the role of family variables. Treatment planning addresses a range of biological, psychological, and environmental factors that may play a part in the recurrence and genesis of emotional disorders.

In his psychodynamic model of inpatient family intervention, G.P. Sholevar (1983, 1986a) described an "institutionalization process" by which a dysfunctional family in a crisis situation attempts to extrude a vulnerable adolescent to reestablish homeostasis. A variation of the institutionalization process is multiple hospitalization syndrome, whereby the family insists on returning the child home prematurely, to reinvolve him or her in the family's conflicts. Awareness of this institutionalization process can be fostered only through conjoint family therapy evaluation and treatment of the whole family by the hospital staff, including the family therapist.

The family should be involved in the treatment process before the patient's admission to the hospital.

Establishing a mutually supportive relationship with the family is essential to achieve clear goals. The family evaluation should emphasize recognizing the effect of immediate events on the family's interactional pattern that has led to the patient's hospitalization. Including the patient in family therapy from the outset may enhance the therapeutic alliance with the family and the patient.

Research in Family Therapy

Research in the field of family therapy has always been active. Initially, there were uncontrolled studies of interventions with poorly described family types. These uncontrolled studies were followed by controlled investigations of interventions with families having different disorders or family structures. The more recent studies have focused on family interventions in the treatment of individually diagnosed illnesses and on how helpful family therapy is and what place family therapy has in the treatment of childhood and adolescent disorders in comparison with other treatment modalities (Clarkin and Carpenter 2003).

Progress in family therapy research has been apparent in the past two decades. Clarkin and Carpenter (2003) summarized recent advances in family therapy research. In addition to family outcome studies, there has been an interest in family system concepts as they relate to treatment methodology and outcome. The question of whether family therapy is effective has been further refined by examining the effect of specific treatment formats and strategies on specific family problems, individual diagnoses, and mediating therapeutic goals. Studies comparing family therapy with other treatment modalities or combining family therapy with other treatment approaches have focused on the level of responsiveness of different problems to different treatment modalities rather than on family therapy as the superior treatment approach.

Studies on child and adolescent disorders, particularly the treatment of conduct disorders and delinquency, have produced encouraging results. Parent management training (Forehand and McMahon 1981; Patterson et al. 1982, 1993) and functional family therapy (Alexander and Barton 1976) have proved effective. In addition to having a favorable effect on targeted behaviors of adolescent patients, they have produced beneficial results with siblings and parents. These and other cognitive-behavioral studies have shown that family intervention benefits the child patient and reduces anxiety and depression in the parents.

There has been surprisingly less interest in the efficacy of family therapy in treating patients with eating disorders. The findings of Russell et al. (1987) suggest that nonchronic eating disorders in young patients who live at home with their parents are amenable to family interventions.

Research on substance abuse treatment has led to some promising findings. Family intervention may be effective with subgroups of substance abusers, possibly with younger abusers still living at home. Kang et al. (1991) suggested that family therapy may not be effective in treating older cocaine abusers; the patient population in their study was seriously impaired and unamenable to verbal treatment.

Studies involving families of schizophrenic patients have been most impressive in the past decade. The treatment of these families has been documented, and the usefulness and effectiveness of family therapy as part of the overall treatment for these seriously disturbed patients have been demonstrated. The interventions have focused on lowering expressed emotion and increasing the family's coping capacity by using psychoeducational and cognitive-behavioral strategies.

Clarkin and Carpenter (2003) described a number of studies that clearly defined symptomatic behavioral problems in children. The most impressive result was reduced aggressive behavior, in a study by Sayger et al. (1988). Their clinically and statistically meaningful results were continued at 1-year follow-up (Kazdin et al. 1992). Sayger et al. (1988) concluded that family therapy is promising in reducing specific problematic child behaviors, as well as in reducing anxiety and depression in the parents, and that learning parenting skills enhanced parents' effectiveness.

Conclusion

Advances in clinical practice and research on family and marital therapy during the past two decades indicate that the field of family therapy is progressing. The effectiveness of other therapeutic modalities and the roles of psychobiological and genetic factors are acknowledged and used by researchers studying families. Advances in the treatment of schizophrenia, depression, and conduct disorders represent some of the most exciting clinical findings in the field of family and marital therapy.

The need for a better definition of disorders, a classification and diagnostic system that is agreeable to different practitioners and compatible with DSM-IV-TR, and a demonstrated positive treatment outcome has been recognized and accepted by family therapists. Family therapists have joined the broader field of psychiatry by viewing family, marital, and interpersonal therapies as significant treatment modalities rather than as the panacea for all problems.

In the future, family therapy, in collaboration with the broader field of psychiatry, should better define the family variables of different disorders and the responses of those disorders to single or combined treatment modalities or a particular family therapy approach. Given the advances made in biological psychiatry and mapping human genomes, the interactional and psychological correlates of biological vulnerability and dysfunction will present family therapists with an exciting challenge.

Integrating family theory and interventions with other theoretical systems and treatment modalities will address the biological, psychological, and family variables that increase an individual's vulnerability to an emotional dysfunction and disorder. Family therapy has been combined with other treatment modalities, including psychopharmacotherapy, cognitive therapy, and social learning theory.

A major recent development has been the emergence of a true field of family psychiatry based on the investigation of disorders with relatively clear genetic components—namely, schizophrenia, depression, and alcoholism. Recent elaboration of stress-diathesis theory has led to new developments in family psychiatry, especially the focus on genetic vulnerability of different family members to stress and on methods for reducing the likelihood of emotional decompensation or a psychiatric breakdown by reducing the sources of internal and external stress in the family and by using psychotropic or antidepressant medication. Psychoeducational family intervention has been used extensively to enhance family adaptation, without the risk of increasing stresses in the family by stimulating charged conflictual issues.

References

Ackerman NW: Interpersonal disturbances in the family: some unresolved problems in psychotherapy. Psychiatry 17:359–368, 1954

Ackerman NW: The Psychodynamics of Family Life. New York, Basic Books, 1958

Alexander J[F], Barton C: Behavioral systems therapy for families, in Treating Relationships. Edited by Olson D. Lake Mills, IA, Iowa Graphics, 1976

Alexander JF, Parsons BV: Short-term behavioral intervention with delinquent families: impact on family process and recidivism. J Abnorm Psychol 81:219–225, 1973

Alexander JF, Parsons BV: Functional Family Therapy. Monterey, CA, Brooks/Cole, 1982

American Psychiatric Association: Diagnostic and Statistical Manual of Mental Disorders, 3rd Edition, Revised. Washington, DC, American Psychiatric Association, 1987

American Psychiatric Association: Diagnostic and Statistical Manual of Mental Disorders, 4th Edition. Washington, DC, American Psychiatric Association, 1994

American Psychiatric Association: Diagnostic and Statistical Manual of Mental Disorders, 4th Edition, Text Revision. Washington, DC, American Psychiatric Association, 2000

Bahnson C: A historical family systems approach to heart disease and cancer, in A New Image of Man in Medicine. Edited by Shaefer KE. Mount Kisko, NY, Futura, 1986, pp 101–123

Barkley RA: Hyperactive Children: A Handbook for Diagnosis and Treatment. New York, Guilford, 1981

Barkley RA, Anastopoulos AD, Guevremont DC, et al: Adolescents with attention deficit hyperactivity disorder: mother-adolescent interactions, family beliefs and conflicts, and maternal psychopathology. J Abnorm Child Psychol 20:263–288, 1992

Bateson G, Jackson D, Haley J, et al: Toward a theory of schizophrenia. Behav Sci 1:251–264, 1956

Beardslee W, Schwoeri L: Preventive intervention with children of depressed parents, in The Transmission of Depression in Families and Children: Assessment and Intervention. Edited by Sholevar GP, Schwoeri L. Northvale, NJ, Jason Aronson, 1994, pp 285–318

Beardslee WR, Salt P, Versage EM, et al: Sustained change in parents receiving preventive interventions for families with depression. Am J Psychiatry 154:510–515, 1997

Beardslee WR, Versage EM, Gladstone TRG: Children of affectively ill parents: a review of the past 10 years. J Am Acad Child Adolesc Psychiatry 37:1134–1141, 1998

Bell JE: Family Therapy. New York, Jason Aronson, 1975

Boszormenyi-Nagy I: Foundations of Contextual Therapy: The Collected Papers of Ivan Boszormenyi-Nagy. New York, Brunner/Mazel, 1987

Boszormenyi-Nagy I, Spark GM: Invisible Loyalties. New York, Harper & Row, 1984

Bowen M: Family psychotherapy. Am J Orthopsychiatry 31:40–60, 1961

Bowen M: The use of family theory in clinical practice. Compr Psychiatry 7:345–374, 1966

Bowen M: Family Theory in Clinical Practice. New York, Jason Aronson, 1978

Bowlby J: The study and reduction of group tensions in the family. Human Relations 2:123–128, 1949

Brent D: The aftercare of adolescents with deliberate self-harm. J Child Psychol Psychiatry 38:277–286, 1997

Brent D, Holder D, Kolko D, et al: A clinical psychotherapy trial for adolescent depression comparing cognitive, family, and supportive psychotherapy. Arch Gen Psychiatry 54:877–885, 1997

Brown GW, Harris T: Social Origins of Depression. New York, Free Press, 1978

Brown GW, Monck EM, Carstairs GM, et al: Influence of family life on the course of schizophrenic illness. Br J Prev Soc Med 16:55–68, 1962

Browning SW, Green RJ: Constructing therapy: from strategic, to systemic, to narrative models, in Textbook of Family and Couples Therapy: Clinical Applications. Edited by Sholevar GP, Schwoeri LD. Washington, DC, American Psychiatric Publishing, 2003, pp 55–76

Burgess EW: The family as a unit of interacting personalities. Family 7:3–9, 1926

Cadoret RJ, Cain CA, Grove WM: Development of alcoholism of adoptees raised apart from alcoholic biologic relatives. Arch Gen Psychiatry 37:561–563, 1980

Cadoret RJ, Troughton E, O'Gorman TW, et al: An adoption study of genetic and environmental factors in drug abuse. Arch Gen Psychiatry 43:1131–1136, 1986

Carter E, McGoldrick M (eds): The Family Life Cycle. New York, Gardner, 1980

Chasin R, White T: Family therapy with children: a model for engaging the whole family, in Textbook of Family and Couples Therapy: Clinical Applications. Edited by Sholevar GP, Schwoeri LD. Washington, DC, American Psychiatric Publishing, 2003, pp 381–402

Clarkin JF, Carpenter D, Fertuck E: The state of family therapy outcome research: a positive prognosis, in Textbook of Family and Couples Therapy: Clinical Applications. Edited by Sholevar GP, Schwoeri LD. Washington, DC, American Psychiatric Publishing, 2003, pp 771–795

Clarkin J, Miklowitz D: Diagnosis of family relational disorders, in Textbook of Family and Couples Therapy: Clinical Applications. Edited by Sholevar GP, Schwoeri LD. Washington, DC, American Psychiatric Publishing, 2003, pp 341–365

Combrinck-Graham L: A developmental model for family systems. Fam Process 24:131–151, 1985

Coyne JC: Depression, biology, marriage, and marital therapy. J Marital Fam Ther 13:393–407, 1987

Coyne JC, Kessler RC, Tal M, et al: Living with a depressed person. J Consult Clin Psychol 55:347–352, 1987

Cuber J, Harroff P: Five types of marriage, in Family in Transition: Rethinking Marriage, Sexuality, Child Rearing, and Family Organization, 7th Edition. Edited by Skolnick AS, Skolnick JH. New York, HarperCollins, 1992, pp 300–312

Diamond G, Siqueland L: Current status of family intervention science. Child Adolesc Psychiatr Clin North Am 10:641–661, 2001

Duvall E: Marriage and Family Development, 5th Edition. Philadelphia, PA, JB Lippincott, 1977

Endicott J, Spitzer R: Use of research diagnostic criteria for affective disorders and schizophrenia to study affective disorders. Am J Psychiatry 136:52–56, 1979

Erikson EH: Childhood and Society. New York, WW Norton, 1950

Forehand R, Kotchick BA: Cultural diversity: a wake-up call for parent training. Behav Ther 27:187–206, 1996

Forehand R, McMahon R: Helping the Noncompliant Child: A Clinician's Guide to Parent Training. New York, Guilford, 1981

Framo JL: Explorations in Marital and Family Therapy. New York, Springer, 1982

Friedman AS: Interaction of drug therapy with marital therapy in depressive patients. Arch Gen Psychiatry 32:619–637, 1975

Friedman AS: Family therapy vs. parent groups: effects on adolescent drug abusers. Am J Fam Ther 17:335–347, 1989

Friedman AS: The adolescent drug abuser and the family, in Family Therapy for Adolescent Drug Abuse. Edited by Friedman AS. New York, Lexington Books, 1990, pp 3–29

Fromm E: Escape From Freedom. New York, Rinehart, 1941

Fromm-Reichmann F: Notes on the development of treatment for schizophrenia by psychoanalytic therapy. Psychiatry 11:263–273, 1948

Glick I, Clarkin J, Spencer J: Recent developments in family therapy: a review. Hosp Community Psychiatry 33:550–556, 1985

Glick I, Clarkin J, Kessler D: Family intervention and the psychiatric hospital, in Marital and Family Therapy, 2nd Edition. Edited by Glick I, Clarkin J, Kessler D. New York, Grune & Stratton, 1987a, pp 370–391

Glick I, Clarkin J, Spencer J: A controlled evaluation of inpatient family intervention, I: preliminary results of the six month follow-up. Arch Gen Psychiatry 42:882–886, 1987b

Goldstein MJ: Family interaction patterns that antedate the onset of schizophrenia and related disorders: a further analysis of data from a longitudinal prospective study, in Understanding Major Mental Disorder: The Contribution of Family Interaction Research. Edited by Hahlweg K, Goldstein MJ. New York, Family Process Press, 1987, pp 11–32

Goodman S, Brogan D, Lynch M, et al: Social and emotional competence in children of depressed mothers. Child Dev 64:516–531, 1993

Goodwin D, Schulsinger F, Hermansenk L, et al: Alcohol problems in adoptees raised apart from alcoholic biological parents. Arch Gen Psychiatry 28:238–242, 1973

Group for the Advancement of Psychiatry: The Family, the Patient, and the Psychiatric Hospital: Toward a New Model. New York, Brunner/Mazel, 1985, p 24

Gurman A, Kniskern D: Handbook of Family Therapy. New York, Brunner/Mazel, 1981

Haas G, Glick I: Inpatient family intervention: a randomized clinical trial, II: results at hospital discharge. Arch Gen Psychiatry 35:1169–1177, 1988

Haas G, Clarkin J, Glick I: Marital and family treatment of depression, in Handbook of Depression: Treatment, Assessment and Research. Edited by Beckham EE, Leber WR. Homewood, IL, Dorsey, 1985, pp 151–183

Hahlweg K, Neuchterlein K, Goldstein MJ, et al: Parental expressed emotion attitudes and intrafamilial communication behavior, in Understanding Major Mental Disorder: The Contribution of Family Interaction Research. Edited by Hahlweg K, Goldstein MJ. New York, Family Process Press, 1987, pp 156–175

Haley J: Strategies of Psychotherapy. New York, Grune & Stratton, 1963

Haley J: Uncommon Therapy. Toronto, WW Norton, 1973

Hatfield A: The family as partner in the treatment of mental illness. Hosp Community Psychiatry 30:338–340, 1986

Henggeler SW, Santos AB: Innovative Approaches for Difficult-to-Treat Populations. Washington, DC, American Psychiatric Press, 1997

Henggeler SW, Schoenwald SK: The MST Supervisory Manual: Promoting Quality Assurance at the Clinical Level. Charleston, SC, MST Institute, 1998

Henggeler SW, Schoenwald SK, Borduin CM, et al: Multisystemic Treatment of Antisocial Behavior in Children and Adolescents. New York, Guilford, 1998

Henggeler SW, Rowland MD, Randall J, et al: Home-based multisystemic therapy as an alternative to the hospitalization of youths in psychiatric crisis: clinical outcomes. J Am Acad Child Adolesc Psychiatry 38: 1331–1339, 1999

Hinchcliffe M, Hooper D, Roberts F: The Melancholy Marriage. New York, Wiley, 1978

Hinshaw SP, Owens EB, Wells KC, et al: Family processes and treatment outcome in the MTA: negative/ineffective parenting practices in relation to multimodal treatment. J Abnorm Psychol 28:555–568, 2000

Hooley J, Orley J, Teasdale J: Levels of expressed emotion and relapse in depressed patients. Br J Psychiatry 148: 642–647, 1986

Horney K: New Ways in Psychoanalysis. New York, WW Norton, 1939

Jackson DD: The question of family homeostasis. Psychiatr Q 31 (suppl):79–90, 1965

Johnson A, Szurek S: The genesis of anti-social acting out in children and adolescents. Psychoanal Q 21:313–343, 1952

Johnson SM: Emotionally Focused Couple Therapy for Trauma Survivors: Strengthening Attachment Bonds. New York, Guilford, 2002

Johnson SM: Couples therapy research: status and directions, in Textbook of Family and Couples Therapy: Clinical Applications. Edited by Sholevar GP, Schwoeri LD. Washington, DC, American Psychiatric Publishing, 2003, pp 797–814

Johnson SM, Makinen JA, Millikin JW: Attachment injuries in couple relationships: a new perspective on impasses in couples therapy. J Marital Fam Ther 27:145–155, 2001

Kang SY, Kleinman PH, Woody GE, et al: Outcomes for cocaine abusers after once-a-week psychosocial therapy. Am J Psychiatry 148:642–647, 1991

Kazdin AE: Parent management training: evidence, outcomes, and issues. J Am Acad Child Adolesc Psychiatry 36:1349–1356, 1997

Kazdin AE, Siegel TC, Bass D: Cognitive problem-solving skills training and parent management training in the treatment of antisocial behavior in children. J Consult Clin Psychol 60:733–747, 1992

Koocher GP: Pediatric oncology: medical crisis intervention, in Health Psychology Through the Life Span: Practice and Research Opportunities. Edited by Resnick RJ, Rozensky H. Washington, DC, American Psychological Association, 1997, pp 213–225

Lansky MR: Marital therapy for narcissistic disorders, in Handbook of Marital Therapy. Edited by Jacobson N, Gurman A. New York, Basic Books, 1983

Lansky MR: Family therapy, in Comprehensive Textbook of Psychiatry, 5th Edition, Vol 2. Edited by Kaplan HI, Sadock BJ. Baltimore, MD, Williams & Wilkins, 1989, pp 1535–1541

Leighton AH: An Introduction to Social Psychiatry. Springfield, IL, Charles C Thomas, 1960

Levy DM: Maternal Overprotection. New York, Columbia University Press, 1943

Liddle HA: The Adolescents and Families Project: multidimensional family therapy in action, in The First National Conference on the Treatment of Adolescent Drug, Alcohol and Mental Health Problems. Washington, DC, U.S. Government Printing Office, 1991, pp 319–400

Liddle HA: Multidimensional Family Therapy Treatment Manual for the Cannabis Youth Treatment Multisite Collaborative Project. Rockville, MD, Center for Substance Abuse Treatment, 2000

Liddle HA, Dakof G: Family-based treatment for adolescent drug use: state of the science, in Adolescent Drug Abuse: Assessment and Treatment. Edited by Rahdert E. Rockville, MD, National Institute on Drug Abuse, 1995, pp 218–254

Liddle HA, Dakof GA, Parker K, et al: Multidimensional family therapy for adolescent drug abuse: results of a randomized clinical trial. Am J Drug Alcohol Abuse 27:651–688, 2001

Lidz T, Parker B, Cornelison AR: The role of the father in the family environment of the schizophrenic patient. Am J Psychiatry 113:126–132, 1956

Mabe PA, Turner MK, Josephson AM: Parent management training. Child Adolesc Psychiatr Clin North Am 10:451–464, 2001

MacGregor R: Multiple impact psychotherapy with families. Fam Process 1:15–29, 1962

Madanes C: Strategic Family Therapy. San Francisco, CA, Jossey-Bass, 1981

Malone CA: Observations on the role of family therapy in child psychiatry training. J Am Acad Child Psychiatry 13:437–458, 1974

Malone CA: Child psychiatry and family therapy: an overview. J Am Acad Child Psychiatry 18:4–21, 1979

Malone CA: Family therapy and childhood disorders, in Psychiatry Update: The American Psychiatric Association Annual Review, Vol 2. Edited by Grinspoon L. Washington, DC, American Psychiatric Press, 1983, pp 228–241

Malone CA: Child and adolescent psychiatry and family therapy. An overview. Child Adolesc Psychiatr Clin North Am 10:395–414, 2001

McCreary ML, Maffuid J, Stepter TA: Bridges to effective treatment: family therapy and family psychoeducational interventions with maltreating and substance-abusing families, in Substance Abuse, Family Violence and Child Welfare: Bridging Perspecives. Edited by Hampton RI, Senatore V. Thousand Oaks, CA, Sage, 1998, pp 220–248

McDermott JF, Char WF: The undeclared war between child and family therapy. J Am Acad Child Psychiatry 13:422–436, 1974

Merikangas K, Ranelli C, Kupfer D: Marital interaction in hospitalized depressed patients. J Nerv Ment Dis 167:689–695, 1979

Minuchin S: Families and Family Therapy. Cambridge, MA, Harvard University Press, 1974

Minuchin S, Montalvo B, Guerney B, et al: Families of the Slums. New York, Basic Books, 1967

Minuchin S, Rosman B, Baker L: Psychosomatic Families: Anorexia Nervosa in Context. Cambridge, MA, Harvard University Press, 1978

Montalvo B, Haley H: In defense of child therapy. Fam Process 12:227–244, 1973

Multisystemic Treatment Services Multisystemic therapy treatment model. Available at: http://www.mstservices.com/text/treatment.html. Accessed May 21, 2003

National Institute on Drug Abuse: National Household Survey on Drug Abuse: NIDA 1990 findings (DHHS Publ No ADM-91-1732). Washington, DC, U.S. Government Printing Office, 1991

Olson DH: Marital and family therapy: integrative review and critique. J Marriage Fam 32:501–538, 1970

Patterson GR: The aggressive child: victim and architect of a coercive system, in Behavior Modification and Families. Edited by Mash EJ, Hamerlynch LA, Handy LC. New York, Brunner/Mazel, 1976, pp 267–316

Patterson GR: A Social Learning Approach to Family Intervention, Vol 3: Coercive Family Process. Eugene, OR, Castalia, 1982

Patterson G[R], Chamberlain D, Reid J: A comparative evaluation of a parent training program. Behav Ther 13:638–650, 1982

Patterson GR, Reid JB, Dishion TJ: A Social Learning Approach to Family Intervention, Vol 4: Antisocial Boys. Eugene, OR, Castalia, 1993

Pelham WE, Wheeler T, Chronus A: Empirically supported psychological treatments for attention deficit hyperactivity disorder. J Clin Child Psychol 27:190–205, 1998

Pettle S: Thinking about the future when death is inevitable: consultations in terminal care. Clinical Child Psychology and Psychiatry 3:131–139, 1998

Ravenscroft K: Family therapy, in Child and Adolescent Psychiatry. Edited by Lewis M. Baltimore, MD, Williams & Wilkins, 1991, pp 850–869

Reiss D: The nature of consensual experience, III: contrasts between families of normals, delinquents, and schizophrenics. J Nerv Ment Dis 152:73–90, 1971

Reiss D: The working family. Am J Psychiatry 139:1412–1420, 1982

Rosenthal D: Genetic Theory and Abnormal Behavior. New York, Brunner/Mazel, 1970

Russell GFM, Szmukler GI, Dare C, et al: An evaluation of family therapy in anorexia nervosa and bulimia nervosa. Arch Gen Psychiatry 44:1047–1056, 1987

Ryckoff I, Day J, Wynne LC: Maintenance of stereotyped roles in the families of schizophrenics. Arch Gen Psychiatry 1:93–98, 1959

Satir V: Conjoint Family Therapy. Palo Alto, CA, Science and Behavior Books, 1967

Sayger T, Horne A, Walker J, et al: Social learning family therapy with aggressive children: treatment outcome and maintenance. J Fam Psychol 1:261–285, 1988

Scharff D, Scharff J: Object Relations Family Therapy. Northvale, NJ, Jason Aronson, 1987

Schwoeri L, Sholevar GP: A social learning family model of depression and aggression: focus on the single mother, in The Transmission of Depression in Families and Children: Assessment and Intervention. Edited by Sholevar GP, Schwoeri L. Northvale, NJ, Jason Aronson, 1994, pp 145–166

Selvini Palazzoli M, Boscolo L, Cecchin G, et al: Paradox and Counterparadox: A New Model in the Therapy of the Family in Schizophrenic Transaction. Translated by Burt EV. New York, Jason Aronson, 1978

Shapiro R: Psychodynamic family therapy with children and adolescents, in Treatment of Emotional Disorders in Children and Adolescents. Edited by Sholevar GP. Jamaica, NY, SP Medical and Scientific Books, 1986, pp 135–159

Sholevar EH: Parent management training, in Textbook of Family and Couples Therapy: Clinical Applications. Edited by Sholevar GP, Schwoeri LD. Washington, DC, American Psychiatric Publishing, 2003, pp 403–414

Sholevar GP: Family therapy with hospitalized and disabled patients, in Helping Families With Special Problems. Edited by Trexler M. Northvale, NJ, Jason Aronson, 1983, pp 15–35

Sholevar GP: Families of institutionalized children, in Treatment of Emotional Disorders in Children and Adolescents. Edited by Sholevar GP. Jamaica, NY, SP Medical and Scientific Books, 1986a, pp 181–191

Sholevar GP: Psychosomatic disorders and family therapy, in Treatment of Emotional Disorders in Children and Adolescents. Edited by Sholevar GP. Jamaica, NY, SP Medical and Scientific Books, 1986b, pp 343–353

Sholevar GP: Family interventions, in Conduct Disorders in Children and Adolescents. Edited by Sholevar GP. Washington, DC, American Psychiatric Press, 1995, pp 193–209

Sholevar GP: Family intervention with conduct disorders, in Child and Adolescent Psychiatric Clinics of North America, Vol 10, No 3: Current Perspectives on Family Therapy. Edited by Josephson AM. Philadelphia, PA, WB Saunders, 2001, pp 501–518

Sholevar GP: Family theory and therapy: an overview, in Textbook of Family and Couples Therapy: Clinical Applications. Edited by Sholevar GP, Schwoeri LD. Washington, DC, American Psychiatric Publishing, 2003a, pp 3–25

Sholevar GP: Introduction to family theories, in Textbook of Family and Couples Therapy: Clinical Applications. Edited by Sholevar GP, Schwoeri LD. Washington, DC, American Psychiatric Publishing, 2003b, pp 29–33

Sholevar GP, Schwoeri L: The family transmission of depression, in The Transmission of Depression in Families and Children: Assessment and Intervention. Edited by Sholevar GP, Schwoeri LD. Northvale, NJ, Jason Aronson, 1994, pp 123–144

Simon R: Family therapy, in Comprehensive Textbook of Psychiatr, 4th Edition, Vol 2. Edited by Kaplan HI, Sadock BJ. Baltimore, MD, Williams & Wilkins, 1985, pp 1427–1432

Singer MT, Wynne LC: Thought disorder and family relations of schizophrenics, III: methodology using projective techniques. Arch Gen Psychiatry 12:187–200, 1965a

Singer MT, Wynne LC: Thought disorder and family relations of schizophrenics, IV: results and implications. Arch Gen Psychiatry 12:201–212, 1965b

Speck RV, Attneave CL: Social network intervention, in Changing Families. Edited by Haley J. New York, Grune & Stratton, 1971, pp 312–332

Speck RV, Rueveni U: Network therapy: a developing concept. Fam Process 8:182–191, 1969

Stanton MD: Systems approaches to family therapy, in Treatment of Emotional Disorders in Children and Adolescents. Edited by Sholevar GP. Jamaica, NY, SP Medical and Scientific Books, 1986, pp 159–180

Stanton MD, Todd TC: The Family Therapy of Drug Abuse and Addiction. New York, Guilford, 1982

Steinglass P: The Home Observation Assessment Method (HOAM): real-time naturalistic observation of families in their homes. Fam Process 18:337–354, 1979

Steinglass P: A life history model of the alcoholic family. Fam Process 19:211–225, 1980

Steinglass P: The alcoholic family at home: patterns of interaction in dry, wet, and transitional stages of alcoholism. Arch Gen Psychiatry 38:578–584, 1981

Stierlin H: Separating Parents and Adolescents. New York, Quadrangle/New York Times Book Company, 1974

Sullivan HS: The Interpersonal Theory of Psychiatry. New York, WW Norton, 1953

Szapocznik J, Santisteban D, Rio A, et al: Family effectiveness training: an intervention to prevent drug abuse and problem behaviors in Hispanic adolescents. Hispanic Journal of Behavioral Sciences 11:4–27, 1989

Tienari P, Lahti I, Sorri A, et al: The Finnish Adoptive Family Study of Schizophrenia: possible joint effects of genetic vulnerability and family interaction, in Understanding Major Mental Disorder: The Contribution of Family Interaction Research. Edited by Hahlweg K, Goldstein MJ. New York, Family Process Press, 1987, pp 33–54

Vaughn C, Leff J: The influence of family and social factors on the course of psychiatric illness: a comparison of schizophrenic and depressed neurotic patients. Br J Psychiatry 129:125–137, 1976

Wahler RG, Cartor PG, Fleischman J, et al: The impact of synthesis teaching and parent training with mothers of conduct-disordered children. J Abnorm Child Psychol 21:425–440, 1993

White M, Epston D: Narrative means to therapeutic ends. New York, WW Norton, 1990

Wolin SJ, Bennett LA: Family rituals. Fam Process 23:401–420, 1984

Wolin SJ, Bennett LA, Noonan DL: Family rituals and the recurrence of alcoholism over generations. Am J Psychiatry 136:589–593, 1979

Wolin S[J], Bennett L, Jacobs J: Assessing family rituals in alcoholic families, in Rituals in Families and Family Therapy. Edited by Imber-Black E. New York, WW Norton, 1988, pp 199–214

Wynne LC: Methodological and conceptual issues in the study of schizophrenics and their families. J Psychiatr Res 6:185–199, 1968

Wynne LC: Family variables in the longitudinal study of the University of Rochester, in Understanding Major Mental Disorder: The Contribution of Family Interaction Research. Edited by Hahlweg K, Goldstein MJ. New York, Family Process Press, 1987, pp 55–73

Wynne LC, Singer MT: Thought disorder and family relations of schizophrenics, I: a research strategy. Arch Gen Psychiatry 9:191–198, 1963

Wynne LC, Ryckoff IM, Day J, et al: Pseudomutuality in the family relations of schizophrenics. Psychiatry 21:205–220, 1958

Zilbach J: Young Children in Family Therapy. New York, Brunner/Mazel, 1986

Zilbach J: The family life cycle: framework for understanding children in family therapy, in Children in Family Context: Perspectives on Treatment. Edited by Combrinck-Graham L. New York, Guilford, 1989, pp 46–68

Zinner J: The implications of projective identification for marital interaction, in Contemporary Marriage: Structure, Dynamics and Therapy. Edited by Grunebaum H, Christ J. Boston, MA, Little, Brown, 1976, pp 293–308

Zinner J, Shapiro RL: The family as a single psychic entity: implications for acting out in adolescence. Int Rev Psychoanal 1:179–186, 1974

Zubin J, Spring B: Vulnerability: a new view of schizophrenia. J Abnorm Psychol 86:103–126, 1977

Zuk GH: Family Therapy: A Triadic-Based Approach. New York, Behavioral Publications, 1971

Group Psychotherapy

Adelaide S. Robb, M.D.
Lisa A. Efron, Ph.D.

In this chapter we review a variety of theoretical perspectives that offer different types of groups for treatment of children and adolescents. The theories progress from the traditional to the more novel to the self-help movement as ways to approach group therapy in children and adolescents. Each section covers the theory, application, and diagnoses best suited for the type of group treatment. A section on research into group therapy for children and adolescents is included at the end. Table 54–1 provides an overview of different group therapies and their applications.

Children from their earliest ages are members of various groups, such as a preschool playgroup, the fourth-grade class, a swim team, the 4-H club, a family, or the cast of a school play. Individual therapy is an unusual situation in which children are separated and isolated from their peer group and seen as individuals who report on their difficulties in the groups they inhabit outside of the therapeutic hour. Children (and sometimes their parents) are asked to report back to the individual therapist what the problems are outside the office. Group therapy allows the clinician to contrast the individual's report of group interactions with actual group dynamics observed during the therapy sessions. This direct observation allows the therapist to identify peer interactions that may be causing the child difficulties in the real world and allows the child to practice new ways of interacting with peers. Some children call it having a referee watch the behavior, because they feel that the therapist helps them and their peers avoid out-of-bounds or hurtful behaviors. Children can take social risks in the group with the therapist present that they would never try in the real world. With increasing practice in the group comes increasing confidence and new patterns of peer interaction

that can translate to improved functioning in the outside world.

Thus, group therapy is a type of therapy that can be used extensively in child psychiatry for a variety of ages and diagnostic groups. In addition, with the advent of managed care, clinicians face the pressure to see more patients in a shorter period of time. Group therapies allow one clinician to see several patients simultaneously. Group therapy also allows the children to benefit from peer interactions and to learn through their peers. Especially in the adolescent age group, advice given by a peer will often be considered to have much greater validity than the same advice delivered by an adult therapist or parent.

As described in the following sections, groups come from a variety of theoretical perspectives. Each theoretical framework approaches the child in a different manner with specific goals in mind. Most group therapists believe that groups should be composed by age as follows: early school-age, 4–6 years; latency, 6–10 years; preadolescence and early adolescence, 10–14 years; and mid- to late adolescence, 14–19 years. Some child psychiatrists also conduct young adult groups for college students ages 18–21.

Current theory supports mixed-sex groups in all age ranges except early adolescence, when pubertal issues make single-sex groups more effective. Group leaders may be of either sex or work in two-leader groups, one of each sex. Groups may be for a specific diagnosis, such as eating disorders, or for multiple diagnoses. Groups may be open-ended (new members may join at any session) or closed-ended (all members join at the same time). Some groups are time-limited and others are ongoing. A variety of clinical and nonclinical settings may provide group therapies. These

Table 54–1. Comparison of categories of adolescent therapy groups

	Para-analytic group psychotherapy	Therapeutic groups	Educational and sensitivity groups	Self-help groups	Multifamily groups
Leader	Trained mental health professional	Trained mental health professional or counselor	Variable	Recovering group member	Trained mental health professional
Participants	Diagnostic evaluation and patient matched to group	Diagnostic evaluation or screening but less specificity of patient to group	No evaluation	Only criterion: desire to stop addictive behavior	Family who has adolescent in a treatment program
Therapeutic contract	Yes	Yes	No	Yes	Yes
Goals	Define specific individual goals	More defined by nature of group	Personal growth or developmental problems focus	All have same goal: to achieve abstinence	Mutual support; improve adolescent–family relationships
Group frequency	Weekly	Variable	Once or a few times	Daily	Usually weekly
Duration (hours)	1½	1–2	Varies	1–2	1–2
Course	Long-term (6 months to more than 2 years)	Short-term (i.e., inpatient; weeks to a few months) or long-term (i.e., supportive)	One time to a few weeks	For life	May be short-term to long-term
Process	Individual dynamics interface with group dynamics	Varies with group purpose but more ego supportive; cognitive-behavioral and social skills development emphasized	Directive leadership	Working of the 12 steps	Emphasis on family and interpersonal dynamics

Source. Reprinted from Jaffe SL, Dell ML: "Group Therapy," in *Textbook of Child and Adolescent Psychiatry*, 2nd Edition. Edited by Wiener JM. Washington, DC, American Psychiatric Press, 1997, p. 885. Used with permission.

settings include schools, inpatient units, residential treatment facilities, and outpatient departments.

For the longer-term and acute-care settings—such as inpatient and partial-hospitalization settings, schools for behaviorally disturbed children, and residential treatment facilities—group therapy frequently forms the bulk of therapeutic interventions aimed at children. Although individual therapy may take place three times a week and family therapy twice a week in an inpatient unit, as many as nine group therapy sessions may occur during the day. Standing groups in our milieu-based adolescent unit include a patient-run community meeting, a staff-run skills group, psychodynamic group therapy, art therapy or psychodrama, a relaxation exercise group, a review and presentation group (level advancement group), an evening community meeting, an evening group activity, and a relaxation group. This adolescent inpatient unit has additional groups to educate parents about illness, diagnosis, and treatment and special health educational groups on the weekend about sexuality and substance abuse. Our behaviorally oriented child unit runs multiple daily groups led by staff members. These groups include a community meeting, a psychoeducational group (anger management, hygiene, nutrition, fire safety), expressive or art therapy, a relaxation group, school, recreational therapy, an evening activity, and contract review (in which the progress of each child on his or her individual behavior contract for the day is examined). Our partial-hospitalization program also runs a variety of groups to address the difficulties in making the transition from an inpatient setting back into school and the community. These groups are led by staff members and include social skills groups, expressive or art therapy, and a psychoanalytic group.

Psychoanalytic Group Treatment

An understanding of the basic tenets of psychoanalysis is crucial for a review of the psychoanalytic approach to group treatment. First and foremost is the belief that a dynamic unconscious exists that affects an individual's thoughts and behaviors. Along these lines, it is believed that anxiety occurs when the individual experiences the threat of unconscious material coming into conscious awareness. Ego-defense mechanisms (i.e., repression, denial, regression, projection, displacement, reaction formation, and rationalization)

operate outside one's conscious awareness to provide protection from threatening thoughts and feelings; these mechanisms are important for adaptation. In addition, psychoanalytic theory emphasizes the influence of previous experiences on current personality functioning. Specifically, it is believed that there are common developmental events that occur during the first 6 years of life. When the natural resolution of these events is disrupted, dysfunctional thoughts and behaviors result. Finally, a core tenet of psychoanalytic theory is the concept of transference, which reflects the individual's tendency to unconsciously shift to others (e.g., the therapist) feelings and attitudes that stem from his or her interactions with significant others from the past. Interpretation of transference allows the individual to gain insight into the ways in which the past affects present functioning.

The ultimate goal of a psychoanalytic group is to restructure the patient's character and personality system. This task is accomplished by bringing unconscious conflicts to conscious awareness and examining them. This can be achieved through a variety of techniques, several of which are described below. Free association—communicating whatever comes to mind regardless of how irrelevant it may seem—is considered to be the basic tool for uncovering repressed or unconscious material. Foulkes (1965) described this strategy as "free-floating discussion" or "free group association." An extension of this process is the "go-around" technique, in which each member goes around to each of the other members and states the first thing that comes to mind about that person. Another technique, dream analysis, is considered essential for uncovering unconscious material, because dreams are believed to express unconscious needs, conflicts, wishes, fears, and repressed experiences. Therefore, group members are encouraged to share dreams in the context of the group in the hope that by working through dreams, individuals will gain insight into the motivations and unresolved conflicts behind them. Furthermore, interpretation is a therapeutic technique used in the analysis of free associations, dreams, transference feelings, and play (in the case of play therapy). In making interpretations, the group leader points out potential meanings underlying verbalizations and behavior. In doing so, unconscious material is uncovered and new insights occur. As patients develop greater insight into themselves, they become more aware of the ways in which core conflicts are manifested in daily life, and they therefore become better able to change and to develop control over their present behavior.

Although psychoanalytic group therapists hold widely varying opinions regarding the role of the leader, the most traditional approach is to remain relatively anonymous. The rationale is that group members are more likely to project on an anonymous leader their own unconscious images and expectations, which would be a reflection of their past experiences and unconscious needs. Due to the nature of the therapeutic process, traditional psychoanalytical group therapy is generally a long-term, intensive process. It is common for group sessions of 90 minutes to take place once or twice a week over a period of several years. It is generally believed that the optimum size of such a group is between six and eight members.

The psychoanalytic group process described above is most appropriate for adults and older adolescents who are bright, articulate, and motivated. Psychoanalytic group therapy has been adapted to be appropriate for children and younger adolescents. First, traditional psychoanalytic therapy generally uses no medium other than verbal and nonverbal interaction. Although this may be effective with adults, young children may not yet have the vocabulary to articulate their experience. Moreover, children and adolescents may be resistant to opening up in a therapy group. Accordingly, developmentally appropriate activities are considered acceptable in the context of a psychoanalytic group if they facilitate the group process. Thus, many child and adolescent groups incorporate play materials, art activities, and music. Furthermore, it should be noted that children may achieve insight or awareness in very different ways than adults (Ferro 1997). Whereas insight for adults is generally cognitively mediated, in children it tends to be more primitive and experientially grounded. Often, evidence that insight has been achieved by a child is provided by what the child does rather than what the child says. Therefore, by providing children with an alternative to verbalizations, the therapist is likely to obtain more information from the child.

Slavson (1952) pioneered the notion of treating small groups of school-age children in a group format using a psychoanalytic framework. The method he developed became known as activity group therapy. It involved observation of children's behavior, focusing on how they relate and cope with other children in the group and with objects available to them. In this model, the therapist provides little structure and intervenes minimally. Refreshments are provided at the end of the session. Schiffer (1977) then modified this approach, creating activity-interview group psychotherapy. In activity-interview group psychotherapy, children engage in activities selected by the therapist for their potential to promote the expression of internal conflicts. The activity portion of the session is then followed by a group interview conducted by the therapist. During the interview portion of the session, the therapist explores and interprets any fantasy that might have occurred during the activity portion and additionally interprets transference when appropriate. These two models of group therapy represent two specific ways in which psychoanalytic group therapy has been adapted for children.

Cognitive-Behavioral Group Treatment

Cognitive-behavioral therapy (CBT) has become a major approach in the treatment of children and adolescents. The core of this approach is the cognitive model, which focuses on the interactions among thoughts, feelings, and behaviors (Beck et al. 1979). According to this theory, most problematic behaviors, cognitions, and emotions have been learned and therefore can be modified by new learning. The modification process, called therapy, is largely educational, in that individuals learn to develop and internalize self-control skills and problem-solving techniques. The goal of treatment is the development of adaptive modes of responding to problematic situations and the elimination of maladaptive behaviors, thoughts, and feelings.

CBT groups can be adapted for all age groups and can be used in a variety of settings (e.g., schools, outpatient clinics, and hospitals). They are used to treat a variety of presenting problems (e.g., depression, anxiety, social skill deficits, and disruptive behavior problems). Groups tend to meet weekly and are generally short-term and often skills-specific (e.g., anger management training, relaxation training, social skills training). In CBT groups the child is expected to be an active participant in the treatment process.

In planning intervention strategies to be taught in the context of a CBT group, it is crucial to consider the skill levels of the children participating. Specifically, children who are at the preoperational level of cognitive development (preschoolers) are generally capable of thinking only in the here and now; therefore, interventions that focus on planning for a future problem-solving situation would not be appropriate for this age group (Cohen and Schleser 1984). Children who are at the level of concrete operational thought (elementary-school children) can generally appreciate a problem-solving approach but may have difficulty focusing their attention to the task (Petti 1991). Finally, teenagers who reach formal operational thought have the capacity to employ deductive reasoning and problem-solving approaches and can learn to apply various strategies in a flexible manner (Petti 1991). Although cognitive treatments in adults focus on distorted cognitions, in most children and many teenagers the issue of distorted cognitions is de-emphasized relative to the concern about the lack of effective strategies for controlling behavior (Braswell and Kendall 1988). Clearly, as children mature they tend to become more reflective (Leahy 1988; Roberts and Nelson 1984). Therefore, CBT with younger children tends to focus on the acquisition of specific behavioral skills; with older children and adolescents, the focus of CBT generally expands to include more cognitive interventions.

Although many types of CBT models exist, the basic techniques tend to be similar. First it should be noted that—although this is not specifically an intervention—the group offers a variety of models for the individual to imitate, the modeling being performed by the group leader as well as by other members. Throughout the course of the group therapy, the leaders model specific behaviors, and these behaviors often become the focus of role-play exercises. In the context of a cognitive-behavioral group, leaders often coach group members on general principles for performing a particular behavior or series of behaviors (e.g., introducing oneself to a group of unfamiliar others, or anger management procedures). Behavioral rehearsal—practicing a new behavior in the context of the group situation—prepares individuals for engaging in particular behaviors in the real world.

In the group format, reinforcement is provided by the leader as well as by other members of the group through praise, approval, support, and attention. In fact, in the case of children and adolescents, group reinforcement is often more effective than reinforcement provided in a dyadic situation (Rose and Edleson 1987). With younger children, tangible objects (e.g., stickers, small toys) or privileges (e.g., assisting the group leader, choosing the next activity) are often used as reinforcers as well.

Contingency contracts (which specify the specific behaviors to be performed, changed, or discontinued and the rewards associated with those changes) are often implemented with group members. Cognitive restructuring is used where developmentally appropriate. Accordingly, children are taught to be "thought detectives" who identify maladaptive thoughts, evaluate the evidence for those thoughts, consider alternative interpretations, and speculate as to what would really happen if the negative event were to occur. Problem-solving training is another frequently used technique whereby the individual is taught a systematic approach to dealing with problem situations such that the individual will become more capable of solving future problems independently. Self-instructional training is also used; individuals are taught a variety of coping self-statements to guide thinking and behavior during difficult situations. In CBT groups, homework is generally assigned to group members on a regular basis.

Over the years, a number of treatment manuals have been developed. Manualized treatments not only are useful to group leaders as they conduct groups, but they serve to standardize the treatment provided across groups, which then facilitates the evaluation of treatment efficacy. Cognitive-behavioral group therapy for children and adolescents has been found to be effective for a variety of patient populations, including those with depression (Clarke et al. 1999; Rohde et al. 2001), anxiety disorders (Mendlowitz et al. 1999; Thienemann et al. 2001; Toren et al. 2000), disruptive behavior (Kastner 1998; Snyder et al. 1999), and social skills deficits (Blonk et al. 1996).

Group Play Therapy

According to Virginia Axline (1947), play is "the child's natural medium of self-expression." Play therapy, therefore, provides the child with the opportunity to play out his or her feelings and problems just as, in adult-oriented therapy, adults talk out their issues. Schaefer (1985) outlines three main approaches to play therapy. The psychoanalytic approach focuses on the use of the therapist's interpretation of a child's play, as well as on the transference relationship, to assist the child in developing insight into his or her unconscious conflicts. In this approach, children play freely with a variety of toys. In contrast, in the structured approach to play therapy, the therapist controls play by selecting several toys which he or she feels would be useful to assist the child in working out a particular problem. In using such an approach, the therapist poses questions to the child during play, reflects feelings that the child expresses verbally and nonverbally, and plays with or for the child to help the child release certain emotions. It is believed that structuring a child's play so he or she reexperiences a stressful situation not only facilitates a release of pent-up feelings but also assists the child in mastering a particular event. Finally, the relationship approach to play therapy, which is an outgrowth of the work of Carl Rogers and is often associated with the work of Virginia Axline, emphasizes the importance of the therapeutic relationship. In this approach, the therapist creates an atmosphere in which the child feels fully accepted and understood. The setting of such treatment is a well-stocked playroom where the child can play as he or she wishes, without criticism, advice, interpretations, and direction. The therapist observes and reflects the child's thoughts and feelings and attempts to understand the world from the child's perspective. The basic premise of this approach is that when a child's feelings are expressed, identified, and accepted, the child can accept them and is better able to deal with them. Common to all of these approaches to play therapy is the notion that play has tremendous therapeutic value for a child with psychological difficulties.

The techniques of individual play therapy can easily be used in a group format. Axline (1947) suggests that the group format provides the additional element of peer evaluation of behavior as well as the opportunity for peers to interact with each other. She suggests that the group context adds to treatment a realistic element, given that children live in a social world and must learn to interact appropriately with other children. Similarly, in discussing the therapeutic value of group play therapy, O'Connor (1991) states that "For a child to try a new behavior and be reinforced by peers is a more powerful and curative experience than any amount of discussion in which he might engage with…an individual therapist or…group leader" (p. 330).

Group play therapy is usually conducted in a large playroom setting. It is generally recommended that play materials should be simple, generic, and of course safe. Landreth (1991) suggested choosing toys and materials that encourage creative and emotional expression, engage children, facilitate expressive and exploratory play, allow for expression without verbalization, and permit undirected play. In terms of the age range of group participants, it has been recommended that the age difference of group members not exceed 12 months unless developmental delays are an issue (Sweeney and Homeyer 1999). The optimal size of the group will vary as a function of the number of group leaders involved, presenting concerns of participants, and participants' ages, with younger children requiring smaller groups than older children. Sessions generally meet weekly. The ideal length of sessions depends on the developmental level of the child, with younger children requiring shorter sessions; for teenagers, group sessions may last over an hour, whereas for preschoolers, sessions may be most effective if they are limited to 30–40 minutes.

It is generally acknowledged that some children will not respond well to group play therapy. According to Axline (1947), in cases where the child's issues are social, group play therapy may be more helpful than individual play therapy; however, if the child's issues are centered around a "deep-seated emotional difficulty," individual play therapy may be more appropriate. Ginott (1961) suggested that group play therapy would not be appropriate for siblings with severe sibling rivalry, children with very low self-esteem, extremely aggressive children or children who may be inclined to harm others, children who act out sexually, and children with attachment issues.

Expressive and Art Therapies

Art therapy originated with the work of Slavson in 1934 and later in 1944 by adapting play therapy for troubled preadolescents (Bratton and Ferebee 1999). Slavson thought the use of structured and unstructured art activities would allow these children to express their feelings or issues in a developmentally appropriate fashion, rather than in the standard play therapy used with younger children.

Art therapy involves the use of different media to portray a child's feelings through his or her creations. Media can vary from easily controlled materials such as pencils and crayons to less easily controlled media such as watercolors and finger paints. Art therapy can be used to do group projects such as murals or for multiple group members to do individual projects on a specific theme or assignment from the group leader.

Each session has several different phases: for younger children, there is a structured, therapist-directed group activity, followed by unstructured free time, and ending with sharing. For older children and adolescents an art therapy group begins with start-up tasks such as discussing confidentiality and not worrying about the quality of one's product. After this start-up, the group session consists of four phases: motivation (warm-up), the art activity itself, discussion of the process and product (sharing), and closure (Chapman and Appleton 1999).

A variety of different media or tasks have been used as art therapy activities. Drawing and painting activities may include the following exercises: "fighting back," in which children imagine themselves as boats in a storm and describe how they feel; "the rosebush fantasy," wherein they imagine themselves to be a rosebush and draw and describe themselves; and "your world in colors, shapes, and lines," in which they create their world using only colors, shapes, and lines. Collages and photographs may be used to represent a child's feelings, family, or illness. These collections of images allow an adolescent to represent things in his or her inner life without relying so much on manual dexterity and artistic talent. Clay is another medium that can present a three-dimensional representation of a child's life. In one activity, adolescents use clay to sculpt an animal, real or imagined, that represents themselves; they explain why during the sharing part of the group session. Sand play involves the placement of small figurines on a tray filled with sand. The leader usually determines the theme of the play, such as "your best memory." The children usually start with only five or six figures, then go back and add more members to the tableau. This exercise can reveal a great deal about a child's world at home and at school.

Art therapy can be used in a variety of patient populations, using only simple crayons and paints for young children or collages and pen and ink for older adolescents. When people have communication difficulties due to language disorders or inability to speak the native language, art therapy taps a different part of the brain and can allow a window onto the child's inner world. For adolescents with anorexia nervosa who experience alexithymia, art therapy allows the feelings to come out in a nonverbal fashion (Diamond-Raab and Orrell-Valente 2002).

After the September 11th, 2001, attack on the Pentagon, art therapy was used to help children across the Washington, D.C., area work through their worries and concerns. Children at an international school made cards for the police officers and firefighters who had been at the Pentagon and the World Trade Center towers. The cards, from children as young as 5, showed airplanes hitting buildings with flames and smoke pouring from the buildings. On the inside of the cards were messages of "thanks," "get well," and "we love you" surrounded by hearts. Art therapists, psychiatrists, and psychologists from our hospital went to schools that had lost children and teachers on the planes and did group art projects to say goodbye to the lost classmates. Even on the inpatient units, where children and teenagers were shielded from television and the evening news, the artwork reflected the national tragedy. Younger children drew pictures of explosions, bombs, planes, and fires. Teenagers made elaborate drawings of the Pentagon, the Twin Towers, and soldiers fighting. Although these examples of preoccupation with a national tragedy are dramatic, artwork from children frequently reveals worries and concerns that do not come up in verbal therapies. For children who are reluctant to talk about things, art therapy allows progress to occur on issues in a nonverbal fashion.

Psychodrama

J.L. Moreno created psychodrama in Vienna in 1921 as the Theater of Spontaneity. His actors noted release of psychological issues, and he later developed specific techniques as a way to bring about changes in a group setting. Key concepts include reliving and reexperiencing events in the past with the action played out in the present. The group leader functions as the director of the psychodrama (Corey 2000).

This group therapy has three sections to each session: a warm-up, the action stage, and the sharing/wrap-up. In a typical psychodrama one of the group members is the protagonist, who deals with a specific event from his or her past as if it were occurring in the group. Other group members serve as auxiliary egos, important members in the protagonist's life. These auxiliaries help with the warm-up and intensify the feelings of the protagonist. The director may ask one or two members to become doubles or alter egos for the protagonist. These individuals can voice feelings the protagonist may have but is unable to identify or express. The director is free to ask one of the doubles to step in if the protagonist becomes stuck or overwhelmed.

Psychodrama has been a very effective group therapy technique for children and adolescents. It allows individuals who are unable to discuss conflicts in an individual setting to act them out in a group. Shy children may function as auxiliaries (Bratton and Ferebee 1999; Corey 2000); after their confidence builds, they can become protagonists. Because many issues such as identity, conflicts with peers, school difficulties, and problems in the family are common to all children, these themes are common choices for the psychodrama. During the psychodrama children can even be the parents or the popular kid and experience the perspective of others in their lives. Some groups may borrow from strict psychodrama to be used in wider settings, such as role-playing in a high school peer support group. These techniques have been very helpful and are applicable to both children and adolescents with a variety of Axis I disorders. Patients who do not do well in psychodrama include psychotic patients, who might have difficulty with separating roles from reality, and patients with dissociative disorders and posttraumatic stress disorder, whose symptoms might be triggered in such a group setting. Patients with cognitive impairment might benefit from psychodrama when they are in a group of children at a similar cognitive level.

Self-Help and 12-Step Groups

Self-help and mutual support groups grew originally from early trade unions and religious groups (Gazda et al. 2001). The concept of the 12-step group originated with the prototype, Alcoholics Anonymous, which was founded by two recovering alcoholics as a way for those with alcohol abuse to overcome their addiction. The goal is to surrender the addictive behavior and work through a series of 12 steps toward recovery. The 12-step movement has gone beyond alcoholism to drug abuse (Narcotics Anonymous), eating disorders (Overeaters Anonymous), family members of alcoholics (Al-Anon), and adolescent substance abusers (Alateen). The self-help movement is one of the fastest growing in the United States, with the number of members in 12-step groups doubling every 10 years (Gazda et al. 2001).

The self-help groups that are useful for patients look at the individual (rather than the diagnosis) and can be classified into three categories: crisis, permanent, and addiction groups. Crisis groups deal with major life changes (e.g., death of a family member); permanent groups deal with lifelong illnesses that may involve stigma (e.g., schizophrenia); and addiction groups deal with substance and alcohol abuse. Self-help groups have several common characteristics, including peer orientation, problem focus, estrangement from societal norms, and an ideological base. These groups also provide mutual support and mutual aid among the group members. Members of self-help groups have noted a sense of empowerment, use of persuasion to bring about change, giving and getting of help from others in the same situation, fewer interpretations of character, and more empathic responses. Leaders are frequently more senior members with the same problem who have progressed further in the steps, rather than mental health professionals. Mental health professionals may serve as advisors to self-help groups.

Self-help and 12-step groups are useful for children and adolescents. For children, the 12-step groups have been used primarily for alcohol and substance abuse (Alateen). These groups are used as part of larger inpatient and residential treatment programs, as well as in outpatient settings. With many children and adolescents having substance abuse as a comorbid Axis I diagnosis, the 12-step groups have become one way to address substance abuse in pediatric patients. Most mental health professionals do not recommend self-help groups as the only treatment for children and adolescents with substance abuse and comorbid Axis I disorders. They see it as an adjunct to other treatment interventions for their patients, including individual therapy, family therapy, and pharmacotherapy (see Chapter 43 in this volume, "Substance Abuse Disorders," for further details on pharmacotherapy).

Special Populations

Group therapies of many theoretical perspectives have been used to facilitate coping and adjustment in children and teenagers facing specific problems. These include chronic medical illnesses, physical and sexual abuse, and divorce.

Children With Chronic Medical Illness

Children who suffer from a chronic or life-threatening medical illness have a double burden. They have the burden of being medically ill and the burden of coping with pain, social isolation, and possible death. Groups designed especially for medically ill children may focus on one diagnosis such as human immunodeficiency virus infection or on several different diagnoses such as cancer, cystic fibrosis, and epilepsy. These groups are usually ongoing and are offered to any patient with any one of the diagnoses. Medical illness groups also may be more time-limited (e.g., as part of a special summer camp experience for patients with one of the chronic medical illnesses). All these groups allow children with a chronic medical illness to realize that they are not the only child with their illness (e.g., cancer or seizures). Such groups help the children learn how to cope with being different, having to take a lot of medications, and having to miss a lot of school. These groups normalize the experience of being ill and create a community of peers where sharing can take place.

Abused Children

Child protective service departments and community mental health centers frequently provide groups for children and teenagers who are victims of physical and sexual abuse. These groups borrow in format and orientation from groups for adult victims of rape and domestic violence. The pediatric groups are designed to be age-appropriate and to help pediatric abuse victims work through the trauma, learn about inappropriate touching and inappropriate forms of punishment, and avoid becoming violent themselves. Many of these groups have simultaneous groups for parents who are not the abusive adult in the household. Current research shows that parents of children who have been abused have better outcomes if both parents and children have therapy for the abuse (Deblinger et al. 2001).

Children of Divorced Parents

With divorce on the rise in all socioeconomic groups, schools have started to offer divorce groups for children whose parents are separated or divorced (Jaffe and Kahan 1991). School administrators believe that such groups help normalize this as another life transition and help decrease behavioral problems associated with divorce. Groups are led by outside therapists or guidance counselors and aid children in talking about their feelings during this difficult time. When children realize they are not the only ones with divorcing parents, it becomes easier to talk about sad, scared, and angry feelings. Children can then put things in perspective and move forward. Other children who have survived the breakup of a family can help peers in the group move past the self-blame and magical wishing for reunification of the family (Jaffe and Kahan 1991).

Research and Future Directions

Hoag and Burlingame (1997) reviewed 556 outcome studies published between 1974 and 1997 on the effects of group treatment in children and teenagers. Their meta-analysis showed that children and teenagers treated with group therapy were 73% better off than those in control groups. Deblinger et al. (2001) studied the difference in outcome between supportive and cognitive-behavioral group therapy for children who had been sexually abused and their nonoffending parents. The study determined that mothers receiving cognitive-behavioral therapy had greater posttest reductions in intrusive thoughts and negative parental emotions. Children receiving cognitive-behavioral therapy had greater improvement in their knowledge regarding body safety skills.

Groups have become a major form of therapy in a variety of settings for children and adolescents. Each therapeutic approach has its advocates and uses. What the field now needs is more research on outcomes of group psychotherapy for specific pediatric disorders and research comparing group interventions to individual, family, or psychopharmacologic interventions for pediatric disorders. Such outcome research would allow clinicians and families to make informed decisions about what would produce the greatest benefit for a specific child with a specific disorder.

References

Axline V: Play Therapy. New York, Ballantine Books, 1947

Beck A, Rush AJ, Shaw BF, et al: Cognitive Therapy of Depression. New York, Guilford, 1979

Blonk RWB, Prins PJM, Sergeant JA, et al: Cognitive-behavioral group therapy for socially incompetent children: short-term and maintenance effects with a clinical sample. J Clin Child Psychol 25:215–224, 1996

Braswell L, Kendall PC: Cognitive behavioral methods with children, in Handbook of Cognitive Behavioral Therapies. Edited by Dobson KS. New York, Guilford, 1988, pp 167–213

Bratton SC, Ferebee KW: The use of structured expressive art activities in group activity therapy with preadolescents, in Group Play Therapy: How to Do It, How It Works, and Whom It Is Best For. Edited by Sweeney DS, Homeyer LE. San Francisco, CA, Jossey-Bass, 1999, pp 215–233

Chapman L, Appleton V: Art in group play therapy, in Group Play Therapy: How to Do It, How It Works, and Whom It Is Best For. Edited by Sweeney DS, Homeyer LE. San Francisco, CA, Jossey-Bass, 1999, pp 179–191

Clarke GN, Rohde P, Lewinsohn PM, et al: Cognitive-behavioral treatment for adolescent depression: efficacy of acute group treatment and booster sessions. J Am Acad Child Adolesc Psychiatry 38:272–279, 1999

Cohen R, Schleser RS: Cognitive development and clinical interventions, in Cognitive Behavior Therapy With Children. Edited by Meyer AW, Craighead WE. New York, Plenum, 1984, pp 45–68

Corey G: Theory and Practice of Group Counseling, 5th Edition. Belmont, CA, Brooks/Cole, 2000

Deblinger E, Stauffer LB, Steer RA: Comparative efficacies of supportive and cognitive behavioral group therapies for young children who have been sexually abused and their nonoffending mothers. Child Maltreat 6:332–343, 2001

Diamond-Raab L, Orrell-Valente JK: Art therapy, psychodrama, and verbal therapy. An integrative model of group therapy in the treatment of adolescents with anorexia nervosa and bulimia nervosa. Child Adolesc Psychiatr Clin N Am 11:343–364, 2002

Ferro A: The Child and the Psychoanalyst: The Question of Techniques in Child Psychoanalysis. Translated by Faugeras P, Faugeras D. Ramonville Saint-Agne, France, Editions Eres, 1997

Foulkes SH: Therapeutic Group Analysis. New York, International Universities Press, 1965

Gazda GM, Ginter EJ, Horne AM: Group Counseling and Group Psychotherapy: Theory and Application. Boston, MA, Allyn & Bacon, 2001

Ginott H: Group Psychotherapy With Children: The Theory and Practice of Play Therapy. New York, McGraw-Hill, 1961

Hoag MJ, Burlingame GM: Evaluating the effectiveness of child and adolescent group treatment: a meta-analytic review. J Clin Child Psychol 26:234–246, 1997

Jaffe SL, Kahan B: Group therapy, in Textbook of Child and Adolescent Psychiatry. Edited by Wiener JM. Washington, DC, American Psychiatric Press, 1991, pp 617–626

Kastner JW: Clinical change in adolescent aggressive behavior: a group therapy approach. Journal of Child and Adolescent Group Therapy 8:23–33, 1998

Landreth G: Play Therapy: The Art of the Relationship. Muncie, IN, Accelerated Development, 1991, p 116

Leahy RL: Cognitive therapy of childhood depression: developmental considerations, in Cognitive Development and Child Psychotherapy. Edited by Shirk SR. New York, Plenum, 1988, pp 187–204

Mendlowitz SL, Manassis K, Bradley S, et al: Cognitive-behavioral group treatments in childhood anxiety disorders: the role of parental involvement. J Am Acad Child Adolesc Psychiatry 38:1223–1229, 1999

O'Connor KJ: The Play Therapy Primer: An Integration of Theories and Techniques. New York, Wiley, 1991, p 330

Petti TA: Cognitive therapies, in Child and Adolescent Psychiatry: A Comprehensive Textbook. Edited by Lewis M. Baltimore, MD, Williams & Wilkins, 1991, pp 831–841

Roberts RN, Nelson RO: Assessment issues and strategies in cognitive behavioral therapy with children, in Cognitive Behavior Therapy With Children. Edited by Meyers AW, Craighead WE. New York, Plenum, 1984, pp 99–128

Rohde P, Clarke GN, Lewinsohn PM, et al: Impact of comorbidity on a cognitive-behavioral group treatment for adolescent depression. J Am Acad Child Adolesc Psychiatry 40:795–802, 2001

Rose SD, Edleson J: Working With Children and Adolescents: A Multimodal Approach. San Francisco, CA, Jossey-Bass, 1987

Schaefer CE: Play therapy. Early Child Dev Care 19:95–108, 1985

Schiffer M: Activity-interview group psychotherapy: theory, principles and practice. Int J Group Psychother 3:377–388, 1977

Slavson SR: Child Psychotherapy. New York, Columbia University Press, 1952

Snyder KV, Kymissis P, Kessler K: Anger management for adolescents: efficacy of brief group therapy. J Am Acad Child Adolesc Psychiatry 38:1409–1416, 1999

Sweeney DS, Homeyer LE: Group play therapy, in Group Play Therapy: How to Do It, How It Works, and Whom It Is Best For. Edited by Sweeney DS, Homeyer LE. San Francisco, CA, Jossey-Bass, 1999, pp 3–14

Thienemann M, Martin J, Cregger B, et al: Manual-driven group cognitive-behavioral therapy for adolescents with obsessive compulsive disorder: a pilot study. J Am Acad Child Adolesc Psychiatry 40:1254–1260, 2001

Toren P, Wolmer L, Rosental B, et al: Case series: brief parent-child group therapy for childhood anxiety disorders using a manual-based cognitive behavior technique. J Am Acad Child Adolesc Psychiatry 39:1309–1312, 2000

Hypnosis

Daniel T. Williams, M.D.

Human history before the use of hypnosis in psychotherapy abounds with dramatic reports of the healing of disabling symptoms through ceremonies that generated an altered state of consciousness in the patient. In centuries past this healing was believed to result from divine intervention invoked by a spiritual leader (James 1902/1994). Efforts to conceptualize these phenomena in more secular, scientific terms led to a variety of formulations during the eighteenth and nineteenth centuries and to the emergence of the term *hypnosis* to describe them (Ellenberger 1970). An interesting oscillating pattern has subsequently emerged whereby certain clinicians and certain segments of the population have been alternately fascinated with the sometimes dramatic observed benefits of hypnosis and disillusioned with the transience, ineffectiveness, or apparently untoward effects in other cases. This pattern reflects the shift in public perceptions of many therapeutic modalities, from antibiotics to psychotropic medications. For each of these modalities, the public image metamorphoses from panacea to placebo and eventually to poison before people acquire a realistic appreciation of its range of effectiveness, limitations, and contraindications.

As the clinical use of hypnosis in psychotherapy has matured, a sophisticated understanding of its benefits has moved beyond the long-standing tradition of glowing uncontrolled clinical case reports. More recent efforts to conceptualize the therapeutic use of *trance experience,* in contemporary psychological terms, have focused on the intrinsic human trance capacity, which can be seen retrospectively as having been tapped in different ways in different cultures and in different eras. Hypnosis in this context has been understood as a potentially powerful means of actively facilitating therapeutic change by drawing on the patient's trance capacity. This is done in a manner distinctly different

from the nonspecific effects of placebo and suggestion, although hypnosis may also draw on those nonspecific influences, as do all psychotherapeutic modalities.

Hypnosis as a specific means of augmenting psychotherapeutic intervention is a resource that has broad applicability because the vast majority of children and adolescents are hypnotizable. Once its rationale, range of clinical usefulness, techniques of application, and limitations are understood, hypnosis can become a valuable addition to the armamentarium of the child and adolescent psychiatrist.

Definition

Hypnosis can be defined as attentive, receptive focal concentration with diminished peripheral awareness (H. Spiegel et al. 2000). A sophisticated contemporary understanding of hypnosis emphasizes the essential features of absorption, dissociation, and suggestibility. *Absorption* connotes the characteristic state of attentive, receptive focal concentration that is essential to hypnosis. *Dissociation* connotes the relative suspension of peripheral awareness that is a by-product of absorption. An inherent feature of the process of dissociation is that less relevant perceptions that ordinarily would be part of consciousness become split off from consciousness during the trance experience. *Suggestibility* connotes the tendency to accept instructions uncritically in trance, a reflection of the receptive, trusting rapport that is another key feature of hypnosis.

Implicit in the above definition is the observation that overt behavior (as in a hypnotic induction procedure) may be one useful indicator of the trance state, but this indicator requires associated inquiry into the subjective experience of the patient to document that a trance state exists. Also implicit in this formulation—when hypnosis is applied in a clinical setting—is the relevance of *transference*. This term refers to the patient's tendency to elaborate subjectively on the therapy transaction, on the basis of life experiences as well as hopes and expectations regarding the therapy relationship. In contrast to the psychoanalytic approach, in which the transference is gradually fostered nondirectively and then analyzed gradually, hypnosis actively and directively makes use of the transference with a view to expediting therapeutic change (Williams 1997a). By using hypnosis, the therapist provides cues geared to shifting the patient's attention toward relevant goals and strategies. Associated shifts in the emotional and cognitive perspective of the patient take place that will also, it is hoped, engender behavioral change.

The areas of consensus regarding the contemporary definition of hypnosis dispel the common misconception of hypnosis as a form of sleep. There is a superficial similarity between hypnosis and sleep in that peripheral awareness contracts in both. However, in sleep, contraction of peripheral awareness is part of a general withdrawal of attention from the environment. In hypnosis, contracted peripheral awareness enhances heightened focal concentration.

Historically, Freud's (1925/1959) early experiences with hypnosis played an important role in his conceptualization of repression and associated unconscious processes. Interestingly, Freud explained that among the reasons for his early abandonment of hypnosis was the emergence of rather intense (erotic) transference reactions before he had fully formulated his psychodynamic theory and an operational method for handling such transference reactions. In subsequent years, however, he saw that public health needs would reactivate a role for hypnosis to allow more widespread and expeditious therapeutic applications of psychoanalytic insights than could be permitted through psychoanalysis, with its protracted and expensive methods (Freud 1919/1955).

It should be emphasized that psychotherapy administered more actively and directively to facilitate more rapid change should be predicated on a thorough diagnostic assessment, including the psychodynamic, biological, and social considerations that inform any systematic treatment plan. Hypnosis coupled with a poorly conceived treatment plan can expedite untoward results.

Assessing Hypnotizability

Freud and other psychotherapists cited another reason for abandoning hypnosis after initially being enthusiastic about its use: the discovery that not all patients can be hypnotized. In the mesmeric tradition, success in hypnotizing the subject would constitute a tribute to the therapist's charismatic personality and skillful therapeutic prowess; failure to do so would signify a failure by the therapist, with ensuing narcissistic injury. More effective clinical use of hypnosis required both a clearer conceptual basis of understanding its mechanism and a diminished probability of either untoward transference reactions or experiences of "therapeutic failure."

A major contribution to the more recent understanding of hypnosis was the emergence of objective, reproducible measures of hypnotizability (Frankel 1987; D. Spiegel and Maldonado 1999). Although a number of different scales have been developed and standardized, independent researchers who have surveyed large samples of volunteer subjects and patients agree that there are numerous measurable parameters of hypnotizability. It is clear that hypnotizability reflects a psychological capacity of an individual, similar to intellectual capacity; it is not a "spell" projected onto the subject by the mesmeric hypnotist. The common finding of large-sample studies using different standard measures of hypnotizability is that a broad range of hypnotizability exists within the population, with a normal distribution approximating a typical bell-shaped curve. Thus, a minority of subjects will not be hypnotizable, another minority at the other end of the distribution scale will be highly hypnotizable, and the remainder of the population will usually be normally distributed in the midrange. This replicated finding has had important implications. From a research standpoint, it has spawned productive studies elucidating specific effects of hypnosis by allowing comparison of highly hypnotizable with nonhypnotizable subjects. From a clinical standpoint, it allows for appropriate selection of patients for the therapeutic application of hypnosis.

A detailed discussion of hypnotic induction procedures is not included in this chapter, but two scales are noted that are applicable to children and adolescents. The particular induction technique used is relatively unimportant clinically, as long as it is aesthetically and emotionally acceptable to the patient. Of primary importance, by contrast, is the tacit expectation by both the patient and the therapist that the ceremonious transaction between them will lead to a change in the patient's subjective experience. The prerequisite for establishing this shared expectation is creating a trusting rapport during the course of initial diagnostic assessment. If this has been achieved, the induction procedure constitutes a formal signaling to the patient to shift into a state of heightened concentration and receptivity to the therapist's further comments and suggestions.

Morgan and Hilgard (1979) developed the Stanford Hypnotic Clinical Scale for Children, which can be administered in 20 minutes. The form for older children (ages 6–16 years) is based on an eye closure–relaxation induction followed by seven test items. The form for younger children (ages 4–8 years) contains six text items and is based on an active imagination induction because younger children are often resistant to suggestions for eye closure.

The Hypnotic Induction Profile (HIP) can be administered in 5–10 minutes, making it particularly convenient in clinical settings (H. Spiegel and Spiegel 1978; H. Spiegel et al. 2000). The HIP measures and correlates the subject's pattern of responses to instructions for eye roll, dissociation, posthypnotic arm levitation, and posthypnotic subjective experiences. The wording of its instructions can be readily modified according to the age and cognitive level of the child or adolescent.

Aside from ascertaining the patient's hypnotizability, measuring it formally in a clinical setting has the additional advantage of providing the patient with a "practice exposure" to hypnosis without concern about its concomitant therapeutic application. Once hypnotizability has been established, there is a demonstrated new resource with which to tackle the presenting problem. This approach is supported by findings that hypnotizability is a correlate of relative psychological intactness. In contrast to the normal distribution encountered in nonclinical population samples mentioned above, D. Spiegel et al. (1982) found that in groups of severely impaired patients—including those with severe anxiety disorders, affective disorders, and particularly schizophreniform disorders—there is a significant skewing of scores in the direction of nonhypnotizability. One can benefit from this knowledge about nonhypnotizable patients and shift promptly to another therapeutic modality, thus sparing the patient the unnecessary protracted disappointment of an inappropriate treatment.

Special Considerations With Children and Adolescents

Many surveys using the standard measures of hypnotizability in adults have established that about 70% of the adult population is hypnotizable to a clinically significant degree (D. Spiegel and Maldonado 1999). Furthermore, there is impressive stability of hypnotizability within individual adults over time, comparable to that of various measures of adult intellectual capacity.

Surveys of hypnotizability among children and adolescents, using adaptations of adult scales, indicate that children and adolescents are generally more hypnotizable than adults. Assessing 1,232 subjects at various ages, Morgan and Hilgard (1973) found increases in hypnotic responsivity between ages 5 and 10 years, a peak in the preadolescent years (ages 11–12 years), a gradual decline during adolescence, relative stability through early adulthood, then a tailing off again in the older population. As reviewed by Olness and Kohen in 1996 (based on studies done up to that date), one of the reasons for the presumed lesser hypnotic responsivity of younger children (younger than 6 years) may be the inappropriateness of existing scales for assessing this capacity at these younger ages. The consensus of many studies is that there are no overall differences between the sexes in hypnotizability at any age.

Developmental aspects of hypnotizability were explored by Morgan (1973), who studied genetic and environmental influences in 140 twin pairs, ages 5–22 years. In a well-controlled study involving independent testing of each twin, she found significant positive correlations of hypnotizability for monozygotic twins, but not for dizygotic twins. This finding strongly suggests a genetic contribution to hypnotizability. Morgan (1973) further found, however, that personality resemblance as rated by parents on a standardized questionnaire was positively related to similarity in hypnotizability scores for a child and parent of the same sex. No such correlation was found with the opposite-sex parent. Morgan interpreted these latter findings as suggesting an environmental contribution to hypnotizability, based on the child's identification with the same-sex parent and emulation of the latter's emotional-cognitive affinity for trance experience. Thus, evidence indicates that hypnotizability as an indicator of trance capacity derives from both genetic predisposition and subsequent environmental influence, and from their interaction.

Reasoning from clinical experience and theoretical considerations, Gardner (1974) postulated that the greater hypnotizability of children compared with adults was partly due to children's propensity for a narrower cognitive focus. She noted Piaget's observations of the child's tendency toward concrete, literal thinking, helping to explain the child's greater ease in affiliating with the ceremony of hypnosis. Indeed, as is evident cross-culturally in the practice of transmitting religious traditions and concepts through ceremony, children give less consideration than adults to theoretical questions and logical complexities if the experience of the authoritatively sanctioned ceremony is emotionally palatable. As adolescents develop more sophisticated cognitive perspectives, some demonstrate more critical and skeptical styles that may be a source of resistance to hypnosis. However, a therapist's preparedness to respond effectively to questions raised in search of clarification may well defuse potential resistance.

Emotional factors postulated by Gardner (1974) as contributing to the greater hypnotizability of children include their general openness to new experiences, emotional malleability, intrinsic orientation to learning new skills, and greater ease in accepting regressive phenomena. Indeed, psychoanalytic reformulations of hypnosis have viewed it as a circumscribed, guided "regression in the service of the ego" in the psychotherapy setting (Brown and Fromm 1987). In this spirit, the child's greater propensity for trusting responsiveness to suggestions from a respected adult authority is part of a natural developmental progression toward achieving mastery and autonomy.

Enlisting parental understanding and support is essential for the success of any child-centered treatment technique, and this certainly applies to the use of hypnosis. Ensuring parental support frequently requires dispelling misconceptions about hypnosis and explaining how it can play a safe and useful part in the overall treatment strategy. The same principle of enlisting the support of trusted adult authorities applies to other important consensual validators in the hospital setting, including physicians and nurses.

Indications and Applications

Hypnosis, in the hands of enthusiastic proponents, has been used to treat a wide array of psychiatric and medical disorders in children and adolescents, as documented comprehensively by Olness and Kohen (1996). The history of medicine is replete with illustrations of how effective treatments, when first introduced, generate enthusiasm and widespread use, often for inappropriate indications. Indeed, even ineffective and potentially toxic agents and techniques have been known to generate similar waves of initial enthusiasm, followed by disillusionment.

No reasonable contemporary psychiatrist would discard a particular psychopharmacological agent because it was not successful with all patients. However, one does wish for designated indications for specific therapeutic agents. Recent studies on hypnosis, including standardized assessment of hypnotizability, have helped to elucidate these indications for hypnosis (D. Spiegel and Maldonado 1999).

The contemporary standard of demonstrated efficacy of pharmacological agents requires double-blind, placebo-controlled studies to rule out the omnipresent and potentially confusing influence of placebo effect and nonspecific suggestion. Such controlled studies regarding psychotherapeutic interventions have been more difficult to mount for a variety of methodological reasons (Milling and Costantino 2000). Yet the measurability of trance capacity with standardized scales has afforded a unique model for assessing the specificity of psychotherapeutic intervention with hypnosis in treating a variety of psychiatric and medical disorders. This section constitutes a brief outline of the indications for hypnosis in children and adolescents, about which there is some consensus among contemporary clinicians who use hypnosis as a therapeutic adjunct.

■ Pain

Pain is one of the best-established and most systematically studied indications for hypnosis. It is clear that an individual's perception of pain represents both the cortical registering of pain deriving from tissue injury and the ensuing psychological reaction to it. Furthermore, the individual's psychological reaction is influenced by many variables, including preexisting and ongoing affective state, personality, cognitive level, and changing patterns of social reinforcement that are contingent on pain-related behavior. Considering these facts, hypnosis can facilitate altering the subjective experience of pain.

McGlashan et al. (1969) compared highly hypnotizable and essentially nonhypnotizable patients and found that hypnotic analgesia is clearly different from placebo in highly hypnotizable patients and is significantly more effective for them. In contrast, in nonhypnotizable patients, the ceremony of hypnosis functions as the equivalent of placebo. Further distinctions between hypnotic analgesia and the placebo effect have been made possible by the finding that placebo-induced analgesia is mediated by endogenous opioids and can be blocked by the opiate antagonist naloxone. Studies involving both adult volunteers (Goldstein and Hilgard 1975) and adult patients with chronic pain (D. Spiegel and Albert 1983) have shown that hypnotic analgesia is not blocked or reversed by a substantial dose of naloxone given in a double-blind, crossover fashion. In this context, Zelter and LeBaron (1982) demonstrated that hypnosis is superior to an attentional control condition for children with cancer who are undergoing painful procedures.

In a randomized controlled trial, Liossi and Hatira (1999) compared the efficacy of hypnosis with that of cognitive-behavioral coping skills training (CBCST) in alleviating the pain and distress of 30 pediatric cancer patients (ages 5–15 years) who were undergoing bone marrow aspirations. Patients who received either hypnosis or CBCST reported less pain and pain-related anxiety than did control subjects, compared with the subjects' own baseline levels. Although hypnosis and CBCST were similarly effective in the relief of pain, children reported less anxiety and exhibited less behavioral distress in the hypnosis group than in the CBCST group. Similar positive results have been reported from controlled studies of hypnosis for postoperative pain in children (Lambert 1996) and hypnosis for the management of pain associated with sickle cell disease in children, adolescents, and adults (Dinges et al. 1997).

The techniques most often used with children undergoing painful procedures involve focusing the patient's attention on engrossing imagery that provides a distraction from, and hence a diminution of, the painful sensation. Appropriate imagery—geared toward the child's favorite activities, television programs, or current cultural heroes—is combined with supportive communication of the patient's capacity to combat, evade, or otherwise overcome the pain. For example, a boy may be guided in trance to the image of huddling with his favorite football team during a championship game and receiving encouragement from the quarterback to disregard temporary pain as the child focuses on helping

his team to score the game-winning touchdown. Various other strategies and examples are cited by Olness and Kohen (1996) and by Chen et al. (2000).

Operationally, the rationale for hypnosis is initially presented to both the parents and the patient to establish a supportive conceptual framework for its application. In lay terminology, hypnosis may be explained as a relaxation exercise that can harness the power of imagination to help the patient develop a new strategy to diminish and overcome pain and the associated anxiety that can worsen pain. The initial assessment of hypnotizability and development of an individualized hypnosis exercise are generally best done with the patient alone, free from the distracting presence of the parents. Once these have been established, however, particularly with younger children, it is often helpful to review the exercise conjointly with the parents so that they can supportively reinforce it.

Inherent in the format described above is the implication that the patient is being taught a new technique (i.e., self-hypnosis), which can be used even in the absence of the therapist. The therapist has been the teacher, but the newly developed skill resides within the patient, implicitly imparting a newfound sense of mastery with which to confront the challenge of pain. Providing the patient with either an audiotape or written instructions for the self-hypnosis exercise is often helpful in encouraging the patient's sense of autonomy regarding its use.

In clinical situations involving chronic pain, it is extremely important to consider the social reinforcement interacting with pain-related behavior and to deal with this in one's overall treatment strategy. If a state of invalidism (somatization) has been fostered inadvertently, providing a refuge from other life problems, one must address the constellation of pathogenic influences contributing to this state before launching a treatment strategy centered on the pain (Williams 1997b).

■ Psychological Factors Affecting Medical Condition

As elucidated in DSM-IV-TR (American Psychiatric Association 2000), the category "psychological factors affecting medical condition" has broad potential application because current understanding has clarified the probable capacity of one's psychological state to influence the course, and certainly the subjective experience, of virtually any medical disorder. In this regard, it is not surprising that hypnosis has been anecdotally reported as beneficial in a vast array of medical disorders, in both adults and children. In many respects, principles of application are similar to those outlined above for pain. Aside from the mechanisms demonstrated to be operative with diminished pain perception, the presumed associated mechanism of action of hypnosis in this group of disorders involves relaxation. Relaxation is postulated to attenuate or reverse the emotionally based hyperaroused state in response to stress that is thought to mediate a wide variety of psychophysiological disorders. Only a few representative examples are cited here. An important precaution, as in the treatment of pain, is to avoid having one's enthusiasm about addressing psychogenic influences obscure the need to identify and treat possible underlying, undiagnosed organic influences on the patient's condition.

Seizure Disorders

The clinical literature on epilepsy contains many references to the role of psychogenic stress as an excitant of paroxysmal electroencephalographic activity and as a precipitant of seizures (Williams and Bergtraum 2000). This finding has also been demonstrated under controlled conditions in experimental animals (Hoeppner and Smith 2001). A number of clinical reports have pointed to the value of hypnosis as a psychotherapeutic adjunct in improving the control of psychogenically precipitated epileptic seizures, generally based on strategies involving relaxation, distraction, and helping the patient to structure more effective coping strategies to deal with ongoing life stresses. An important diagnostic caveat is the need to distinguish such epileptic seizures from the more common psychogenic nonepileptic seizures (*pseudoseizures*), which may coexist with or exist independent of psychogenically precipitated epileptic seizures (Lancman et al. 2001; Walczak et al. 1994). This distinction is particularly important as a prerequisite to treatment, because uncontrolled seizures tend to elicit aggressive pharmacological treatment with anticonvulsants having substantial potential side effects; if such interventions fail to produce results, seizure surgery is recommended in selected cases (Kanner et al. 2001; Williams et al. 2002).

Gastrointestinal Disorders

Gastrointestinal disorders often present complexities in diagnosis and treatment at the medical–psychiatric interface. Although there are numerous clinical re-

ports of the usefulness of hypnosis in treating children and adolescents with a variety of gastrointestinal problems (Olness and Kohen 1996), two controlled studies involving adults deserve mention. Colgan et al. (1988) reported on a controlled trial of hypnotherapy for preventing relapse of duodenal ulceration. After 30 patients had rapidly relapsing ulcers healed with medication, they were divided into two randomly selected groups that either did or did not receive hypnotherapy. After 1 year, only 8 (53%) of the 15 hypnotherapy patients relapsed compared with 15 (100%) of the control subjects. Further evidence pointing to the capacity of hypnosis to modulate gastric secretion is presented by Klein and Spiegel (1989). These investigators demonstrated, in highly hypnotizable healthy volunteers, the ability of specific hypnotic suggestions either to increase acid secretion (by 89%) or to reduce it (by 39%) compared with basal acid secretion. It is clear that the capacity of hypnosis to modulate pain perception would also be clinically pertinent in this area.

Cancer Chemotherapy Distress

Zelter et al. (1991) conducted a randomized, controlled study of behavioral intervention for chemotherapy distress in 54 children with cancer. After baseline assessment, pediatric cancer patients were randomly assigned to receive either hypnosis, nonhypnotic distraction/relaxation, or attention placebo (control subjects) during a subsequent identical chemotherapy course. Children in the hypnosis group reported the greatest reduction in both anticipatory and postchemotherapy symptoms, including nausea, vomiting, distress, and functional disruption.

Jacknow et al. (1994) similarly studied the effectiveness of hypnosis in treating chemotherapy-related nausea and vomiting in children with cancer. In this controlled, single-blind trial with 20 children receiving cancer chemotherapy, patients were randomly assigned to either a hypnosis or a standard treatment group. Patients in the hypnosis group used less supplemental antiemetic medication than did control subjects during treatment and experienced less anticipatory nausea 1–2 months after diagnosis.

Headache

Much clinical literature supports the potential efficacy of hypnosis in treating various types of headaches in children and adolescents (Olness and Kohen 1996), as well as in adults (Brown and Fromm 1987; Davidson 1987). One study compared self-hypnosis, placebo, and propranolol in the treatment of juvenile classic migraine (Olness et al. 1987). Among 28 children completing the study, a significantly greater reduction in headache frequency occurred with self-hypnosis training than with either propranolol or placebo. Because the pathophysiology of migraine is obscure, the impact of hypnosis in treating migraine, as in other types of headaches, remains speculative.

Asthma

The pathophysiology of asthma is also complex and multidetermined, including genetic vulnerability, allergic sensitivity, infections, and emotional stress (Avery 1994). Here again, the clinical literature suggests the efficacy of hypnosis in controlling apparent psychogenic contributors (Brown and Fromm 1987; Olness and Kohen 1996). Kohen (1986) reported on a prospective study of 28 children with asthma who were randomly placed into groups who either learned self-hypnosis techniques or served as control subjects. Although there were no differences between experimental and control groups with regard to pulmonary function tests from the initial to the postintervention period, the hypnosis-treated group had dramatic improvements at 1- and 2-year follow-up. Further support for this benefit is offered by a systematic, although uncontrolled, study by Morrison (1988). After 1 year of hypnotherapy, 16 patients with chronic asthma whose condition had been inadequately controlled by medications experienced a dramatic, significant decline in frequency and duration of hospital admissions, as well as a significant reduction in use of prednisolone. Hackman et al. (2000) offer a detailed, critical review of hypnosis with both child and adult asthma patients.

■ Somatoform Disorders

Somatoform disorders are characterized by physical symptoms suggesting physical disorder for which there are no demonstrable organic findings or known physiological mechanisms, and for which there is positive evidence, or a strong presumption, that symptoms are linked to psychological factors or conflicts (American Psychiatric Association 2000). The production of symptoms in somatoform disorders is not under voluntary control, implying that an unconscious mechanism

of dissociation influences symptom formation.

Pathological dissociation is thus a key phenomenological feature of somatoform disorders. It can be quite helpful to a patient and family to understand that dissociation is a psychological attribute that can be channeled, through the therapeutic auspices of hypnosis, to alleviate symptoms. Dissociation as a mechanism of maladaptive self-victimization is thereby transformed, with the therapist's help, into a vehicle for self-reparation and mastery.

Effective clinical treatment of somatoform disorders in children and adolescents is often multimodal, corresponding to the multifactorial etiologies that have been discerned as pertinent to this group of disorders (Williams 1997b). Freud saw the limitations of hypnosis when his contemporaries applied hypnosis in treating the somatoform disorders, which were then subsumed under hysteria. At that time, hypnosis was limited to authoritative suggestion of symptom removal, without the dynamic understanding of symptom formation that Freud subsequently developed.

When used in the more enlightened manner that Freud and others later came to advocate, hypnosis can be the vehicle for actively imparting to the patient a summary formulation of the psychodynamics of symptom formation. This summary then becomes the basis of an emotional-cognitive reorientation, in which the therapist supportively suggests to the patient guidelines for a more adaptive mode of coping with ongoing life stresses.

■ Dissociative Disorders

As with somatoform disorders, the central role of dissociation in symptom formation makes hypnosis a logical choice as an adjunct in treating youngsters with dissociative disorders. Currently, the most commonly described dissociative disorder is dissociative identity disorder, formerly called multiple personality disorder. Dissociative identity disorder is now recognized as having frequently documentable antecedents in childhood physical and sexual abuse (Kluft 2001). One way of understanding a central feature of this disorder is that children use this pathological dissociation as a defense, distancing themselves from the terrifying experience of abuse but paying a heavy psychological price for this escape (Butler et al. 1996; D. Spiegel 1986). Dissociative identity disorder is thus conceptualized as a posttraumatic stress disorder that arises in response to repeated trauma imposed by sadistic and double-binding parenting figures.

A host of psychotherapeutic considerations pertain to treating children and adolescents with dissociative disorders (Kluft 2001; Putnam 1989). For many patients with dissociative identity disorder, memories of repressed traumas may be accessible only in the context of certain dissociated states. Hypnosis can be a useful facilitator in this regard, helping patients to recognize the phenomenon of dissociation in a more balanced, supportive frame of reference. Hypnosis may then become a vehicle to help penetrate amnestic barriers, an aid in abreaction, and a resource in the psychotherapeutic endeavor of reintegration (Williams and Velasquez 1996).

■ Anxiety Disorders

In a controlled study, D. Spiegel et al. (1982) demonstrated that adult patients with generalized anxiety disorder are markedly less hypnotizable than adults who do not have the disorder. When such patients are treated with benzodiazepines, they test as more hypnotizable than those who are untreated (D. Spiegel 1980). No comparable controlled studies have been done to date with children or adolescents. However, Olness and Kohen (1996) reviewed a substantial clinical literature that suggests that hypnosis may be a useful adjunct to both behavioral and psychodynamic therapy in children and adolescents. Such applications include the use of hypnosis to facilitate systematic desensitization and the restructuring of the cognitive and emotional response to feared stimuli or situations. When antianxiety medication is needed and is effective, the ceremony of hypnosis can then concretize for the child and family the behavioral and psychological strategies of reorientation that are geared toward gradually obviating the need for medication.

■ Habit Disorders

Childhood habit disorders is a generic term encompassing enuresis, encopresis, thumb sucking, nail biting, and a host of other habits. Clearly, enuresis and encopresis have possible organic etiologies that must be evaluated before embarking on any psychotherapeutic or behavioral intervention (Shaffer 2001). Olness and Kohen (1996) reviewed numerous clinical reports suggesting the potential value of hypnosis for many habit disorders in children and adolescents and developed several guidelines for integrating hypnosis with traditionally advocated behavioral measures for habit disorders.

Banerjee et al. (1993) studied imipramine treatment compared with direct hypnotic suggestions using imagery for the management of functional enuresis. Fifty enuretic children (ages 5–16 years) underwent 3 months of therapy with either imipramine or hypnosis. Positive response to treatment (all dry beds) was obtained in 76% of those treated with imipramine and in 72% of those treated with hypnosis. After termination of active treatment, the hypnosis group continued practicing self-hypnosis daily during a 6-month follow-up period. At the 9-month follow-up, 68% of those in the hypnosis group maintained a positive response, whereas only 24% of the imipramine group did. However, in younger children (ages 5–7 years), hypnosis and self-hypnosis strategies were found to be less effective compared with imipramine treatment.

Trichotillomania may be variously considered a habit disorder or an impulse-control disorder with obsessive-compulsive features. Similar to enuresis, there are numerous controlled studies demonstrating partial response to psychotropic medication (preferentially serotonergic or mixed serotonergic-noradrenergic medications), whereas other studies suggest a partial benefit from cognitive-behavioral interventions or hypnosis (Kohen 1996; McElroy and Arnold 2001). As with anxiety disorders, it may well be reasonable to consider the adjunctive use of hypnosis to enhance symptom response in a partial responder to other therapeutic modalities or to facilitate medication-tapering trials.

Neurophysiological Considerations

The role of the reticular formation in the central nervous system appears to be that of a selective information modulator that filters out stimuli of less interest to the organism, thus accentuating attention to those that are of more interest (Cohen et al. 2002). This capacity provides a plausible conceptual model for understanding the neurophysiological basis of focal attention (absorption) and dissociation, two key phenomenological features of hypnosis.

Empirical support for this formulation is evident in studies demonstrating the capacity of hypnosis to modify cortical evoked responses in highly hypnotizable individuals, with less hypnotizable individuals as control subjects (D. Spiegel et al. 1985, 1989). These findings demonstrate that hypnotically induced subjective changes, such as anesthesia or visual hallucinations, involve alterations in neurophysiological processing. Such findings provide a model for conceptualizing the mechanism of intervention of hypnosis in pain disorders and dissociative disorders. Similar studies of selective attention to somatosensory event-related potentials provide a plausible model for the mechanism of somatoform disorders and the role of hypnosis in their treatment (H. Spiegel et al. 2000).

The effects of hypnosis in altering pain perception have been similarly studied in hypnotizable subjects by using positron emission tomographic measures of regional cerebral blood flow and associated electroencephalographic measures of brain electrical activity (Rainville et al. 1999). These results provide a further enhanced description of the neurobiological basis of hypnosis, demonstrating specific patterns of cerebral activation associated with the hypnotic state and with the processing of hypnotic suggestions. In this domain of research, hypnosis can help to elucidate neurocognitive processes (Raz and Shapiro 2002). In turn, clinicians may thereby be able to use a potentially powerful therapeutic facilitator with greater sophistication and effectiveness.

Precautions and Limitations

As mentioned above, the differential diagnosis of pain, psychological factors affecting a medical condition, and presumptive somatoform disorders should be approached with caution. It is crucial to consider the possible presence of undiagnosed organic pathology before zealously embarking on a presumably relevant psychotherapeutic endeavor with or without hypnosis. This is especially true when evident psychopathology and plausible psychodynamic formulations tempt premature diagnostic closure (Williams 1997b).

Conversely, the presence of documented organic disorder in no way precludes the coexistence of secondarily superimposed somatoform disorder, factitious disorder, malingering, or psychological factors affecting a primary organic disorder. When the diagnosis is initially unclear, it is often useful to pursue a clinical trial of psychotherapeutic intervention, including hypnosis, in close liaison with the physicians responsible for evaluating and treating the apparent organic disorder. A combined assessment, if thorough on both organic and psychological fronts, generally clarifies whether the presenting problem is primarily organic, primarily psychogenic, or a substantial combination of the two (Williams et al. 1995).

Hypnosis is generally not appropriate for psychotic disorders. As noted above (see "Assessing Hypnotizability"), patients with schizophreniform disorders are predominantly nonhypnotizable (D. Spiegel et al. 1982). Because hypnosis involves a relatively intense, trusting rapport with an implicit temporary transfer of executive control of the patient's subjective experience to the therapist, such an experience may be quite threatening to a paranoid patient and is best avoided. Severely depressed or manic patients are also predominantly nonhypnotizable. An apparent exception in this domain is "hysterical psychosis" (D. Spiegel and Fink 1979), which on closer inspection turns out phenomenologically to be a dissociative disorder and not a true psychosis.

One must note the contraindication to using hypnosis coercively rather than collaboratively with the patient. Overzealous attempts at removing a psychodynamically based symptom that has served a defensive function, for example, without helping the patient and family restructure their perspectives for more adaptive coping strategies, will fail. Misguided, heavy-handed interventions, even if transiently effective, undermine the patient's confidence in the therapist and lead to symptom recurrence or symptom substitution. These quagmires can be avoided by a thorough diagnostic assessment that allows a treatment plan to be designed that is sensitive to the individual, to family dynamics, and to the pace at which the patient and family can achieve designated goals. Symptoms may reappear, even after having been relinquished through the appropriate application of hypnosis, if excessive adverse life stresses recur or if psychotherapeutic support needed to consolidate gains is terminated prematurely. However, these observations apply to any psychotherapeutic intervention regardless of whether hypnosis is involved.

Treatment strategies geared to effective and sustained relief of symptoms must address secondary gain features of the symptoms. Thus, in the case of a youngster whose conversion symptom is generating positive attention and solicitude from parents and others and is permitting the child to avoid onerous responsibilities such as school, these untoward consequences must be rectified. This may be accomplished by parental counseling, environmental restructuring, and a behavior modification program. Considering secondary gain features is crucial to the success of any intervention using hypnosis. If one sees no symptomatic improvement in a hypnotizable patient after two or three sessions of treatment with hypnosis, there has probably been some error or omission in either the diagnostic assessment or the treatment formulation, often including inadequate appreciation of the role of secondary gain factors. Reassessment and reformulation in these areas are then in order. On the other hand, partial, gradual improvement (which is often the case) indicates that the patient is communicating both a positive response to treatment and a call for continued support to work through the therapeutic reorientation. In this context, self-hypnosis serves as both a cognitive restructuring homework exercise between sessions and an opportunity to emotionally incorporate the healthier and more mature mode of adaptation suggested by the therapist. Clearly, the therapist should judge the need for frequency and duration of further treatment based on the needs of the individual patient and family.

Forensic Considerations

Although clinicians attempt to be objective in the assessment of psychopathology, including considerations of trauma (Carrion et al. 2002), when legal consequences to the clinical assessment pertain, reporting by the patient and family members will frequently and perhaps inevitably be influenced, either consciously or unconsciously. Although hypnosis has been used by both police and psychotherapists to refresh the recollection of witnesses and victims of crimes, it should be emphasized that hypnosis itself neither validates nor necessarily contaminates the content of what is recalled. Inappropriate use of either hypnosis or any other method of inquiry, such as by suggestive questioning, will of course increase the likelihood of false data retrieval. Nevertheless, because of the capacity of hypnosis to heighten the receptivity of the subject to the hypnotist's suggestions, some courts have excluded testimony of a person who has been previously hypnotized with reference to the event in question (H. Spiegel et al. 2000). Therapists treating trauma or crime victims should therefore be aware that the use of hypnosis may compromise a witness's ability to testify in court. Consultation with counsel is warranted in such situations, preferably before using hypnosis.

Conclusion

Systematic studies have established that the vast majority of children and adolescents are hypnotizable. Hypnosis constitutes a specific and potentially powerful facilitator of therapeutic change, provided that a thorough diagnostic assessment and comprehensive treatment formulation have delineated the appropriate role that hypnosis will play. The effectiveness of hypnosis then depends on the capacities of the patient and family to respond to therapeutic suggestions; on the severity of pathogenic environmental stressors; and on the skill of the therapist in integrating hypnosis with other elements of a well-formulated treatment plan to foster a more healthy mode of adaptation.

References

American Psychiatric Association: Diagnostic and Statistical Manual of Mental Disorders, 4th Edition, Text Revision. Washington, DC, American Psychiatric Association, 2000

Avery ME: Pulmonology, in Pediatric Medicine, 2nd Edition. Edited by Avery ME, First LR. Baltimore, MD, Williams & Wilkins, 1994, pp 217–300

Banerjee S, Srivatav A, Palan BM: Hypnosis and self-hypnosis in the management of nocturnal enuresis: a comparative study with imipramine therapy. Am J Clin Hypn 36:113–119, 1993

Brown DP, Fromm E: Hypnosis and Behavioral Medicine. Hillsdale, NJ, Erlbaum, 1987

Butler LD, Duran RE, Jasuikatis P, et al: Hypnotizability and traumatic experience: a diathesis-stress model of dissociative symptomatology. Am J Psychiatry 153:42–63, 1996

Carrion VG, Weems CF, Ray R, et al: Toward an empirical definition of pediatric PTSD: the phenomenology of PTSD symptoms in youth. J Am Acad Child Adolesc Psychiatry 41:166–173, 2002

Chen E, Joseph MH, Zelter LK: Behavioral and cognitive interventions in the treatment of pain in children. Pediatr Clin North Am 47:523–525, 2000

Cohen RA, Salloway S, Zawacki T: Neuropsychiatric aspects of disorders of attention, in The American Psychiatric Textbook of Neuropsychiatry and Clinical Neurosciences, 4th Edition. Edited by Yudofsky SC, Hales RE. Washington, DC, American Psychiatric Publishing, 2002, pp 489–524

Colgan SM, Faragher EB, Whorwell PJ: Controlled trial of hypnotherapy in relapse prevention of duodenal ulceration. Lancet 1:299–300, 1988

Davidson P: Hypnosis and migraine headache: reporting a clinical series. Australian Journal of Clinical and Experimental Hypnosis 15:111–118, 1987

Dinges DF, Whitehouse WG, Orne EC, et al: Self-hypnosis training as an adjunctive treatment in the management of pain associated with sickle cell disease. Int J Clin Exp Hypn 45:417–432, 1997

Ellenberger HI: The Discovery of the Unconscious. New York, Basic Books, 1970

Frankel FH: Significant developments in medical hypnosis during the past 25 years. Int J Clin Exp Hypn 35:231–247, 1987

Freud S: Lines of advance in psycho-analytic therapy (1919), in The Standard Edition of the Complete Psychological Works of Sigmund Freud, Vol 17. Translated and edited by Strachey J. London, Hogarth Press, 1955, pp 157–168

Freud S: An autobiographical study (1925), in The Standard Edition of the Complete Psychological Works of Sigmund Freud, Vol 20. Translated and edited by Strachey J. London, Hogarth Press, 1959, pp 7–70

Gardner G: Hypnosis with children. Int J Clin Exp Hypn 22:20–38, 1974

Goldstein E, Hilgard E: Failure of opiate antagonist naloxone to modify hypnotic analgesia. Proc Natl Acad Sci USA 72:2041–2043, 1975

Hackman RM, Stern JS, Gershwin ME: Hypnosis and asthma: a critical review. J Asthma 37:1–15, 2000

Hoeppner TJ, Smith MC: Models of psychopathology in epilepsy: lessons learned from animal studies, in Psychiatric Issues in Epilepsy: A Practical Guide to Diagnosis and Treatment. Edited by Ettinger AB, Kanner AM. Philadelphia, PA, Lippincott Williams & Wilkins, 2001, pp 273–288

Jacknow DS, Tschann JM, Link MP, et al: Hypnosis in the prevention of chemotherapy-related nausea and vomiting in children: a prospective study. J Dev Behav Pediatr 15:258–264, 1994

James W: The Varieties of Religious Experience: A Study in Human Nature (1902). New York, Modern Library, 1994

Kanner AM, Palac SM, Lancman ME, et al: Treatment of psychogenic pseudoseizures: what to do after we have reached a diagnosis? In Psychiatric Issues in Epilepsy: A Practical Guide to Diagnosis and Treatment. Edited by Ettinger AB, Kanner MA. Philadelphia, PA, Lippincott Williams & Wilkins, 2001, pp 379–390

Klein KB, Spiegel D: Modulation of gastric acid secretion by hypnosis. Gastroenterology 96:1383–1387, 1989

Kluft RP: Dissociative identity disorder, in Treatment of Psychiatric Disorders, 3rd Edition, Vol 2. Edited by Gabbard GO. Washington, DC, American Psychiatric Publishing, 2001, pp 1653–1694

Kohen DP: Applications of relaxation/mental imagery to the management of asthma: report of behavioral outcomes of a two-year, prospective controlled study (abstract). Am J Clin Hypn 28:196, 1986

Kohen DP: Hypnotherapeutic management of pediatric and adolescent trichotillomania. J Dev Behav Pediatr 17:328–334, 1996

Lambert SA: The effects of hypnosis/guided imagery on the postoperative course of children. J Dev Behav Pediatr 17:307–310, 1996

Lancman ME, Lambrakis CC, Steinhardt MI: Psychogenic pseudoseizures: a general overview, in Psychiatric Issues in Epilepsy: A Practical Guide to Diagnosis and Treatment. Edited by Ettinger AB, Kanner AM. Philadelphia, PA, Lippincott Williams & Wilkins, 2001, pp 341–354

Liossi C, Hatira P: Clinical hypnosis versus cognitive behavioral training for pain management with pediatric cancer patients undergoing bone marrow aspirations. Int J Clin Exp Hypn 47:104–116, 1999

McElroy SL, Arnold LM: Impulse-control disorders, in Treatment of Psychiatric Disorders, 3rd Edition, Vol 2. Edited by Gabbard GO. Washington DC, American Psychiatric Publishing, 2001, pp 2435–2471

McGlashan T, Evans F, Orne M: The nature of hypnotic analgesia and placebo responses to experimental pain. Psychosom Med 31:227–246, 1969

Milling L, Costantino C: Clinical hypnosis with children: first steps toward empirical support. Int J Clin Exp Hypn 48:113–137, 2000

Morgan A: The heritability of hypnotic susceptibility in twins. J Abnorm Psychol 82:55–61, 1973

Morgan A, Hilgard E: Age differences in susceptibility to hypnosis. Int J Clin Exp Hypn 21:78–85, 1973

Morgan A, Hilgard ER: The Stanford Hypnotic Clinical Scale for Children. Am J Clin Hypn 21:148–155, 1979

Morrison JB: Chronic asthma and improvement with relaxation induced by hypnotherapy. J R Soc Med 81:701–704, 1988

Olness K, Kohen D: Hypnosis and Hypnotherapy With Children, 3rd Edition. New York, Guilford, 1996

Olness K, MacDonald JT, Uden DL: Comparison of self-hypnosis and propranolol in the treatment of juvenile classic migraine. Pediatrics 79:593–597, 1987

Putnam FW: Diagnosis and Treatment of Multiple Personality Disorder. New York, Guilford, 1989

Rainville P, Hofbauer RK, Paus T, et al: Cerebral mechanisms of hypnotic induction and suggestion. J Cogn Neurosci 11:110–125, 1999

Raz A, Shapiro T: Hypnosis and neuroscience: a cross talk between clinical and cognitive research. Arch Gen Psychiatry 59:85–90, 2002

Shaffer D: Elimination disorders, in Treatment of Psychiatric Disorders, 3rd Edition, Vol 1. Edited by Gabbard GO. Washington, DC, American Psychiatric Publishing, 2001, pp 211–224

Spiegel D: Hypnotizability and psychoactive medication. Am J Clin Hypn 22:217–222, 1980

Spiegel D: Dissociation, double binds, and posttraumatic stress in multiple personality disorder, in Treatment of Multiple Personality Disorder. Edited by Braun BG. Washington, DC, American Psychiatric Press, 1986, pp 61–77

Spiegel D, Albert L: Naloxone fails to reverse hypnotic alleviation of chronic pain. Psychopharmacology (Berl) 81:140–143, 1983

Spiegel D, Fink R: Hysterical psychosis and hypnotizability. Am J Psychiatry 136:777–781, 1979

Spiegel D, Maldonado J: Hypnosis, in The American Psychiatric Press Textbook of Psychiatry, 3rd Edition. Edited by Hales R, Yudofsky S, Talbott J. Washington, DC, American Psychiatric Press, 1999, pp 1243–1274

Spiegel D, Detrick D, Frischholz E: Hypnotizability and psychopathology. Am J Psychiatry 139:431–437, 1982

Spiegel D, Cutcomb S, Ren C, et al: Hypnotic hallucination alters evoked potentials. J Abnorm Psychol 94:249–255, 1985

Spiegel D, Bierre P, Rootenberg J: Hypnotic alteration of somatosensory perception. Am J Psychiatry 146:749–754, 1989

Spiegel H, Spiegel D: Trance and Treatment: Clinical Uses of Hypnosis. New York, Basic Books, 1978

Spiegel H, Greenleaf M, Spiegel D: Hypnosis, in Kaplan and Sadock's Comprehensive Textbook of Psychiatry, 7th Edition, Vol 2. Edited by Sadock BJ, Sadock VA. Philadelphia, PA, Lippincott Williams & Wilkins, 2000, pp 2128–2146

Walczak TS, Williams DT, Berten W: Utility and reliability of placebo infusion in the evaluation of patients with seizures. Neurology 44:394–399, 1994

Williams DT: Hypnosis, in Textbook of Child and Adolescent Psychiatry, 2nd Edition. Edited by Wiener JM. Washington, DC, American Psychiatric Press, 1997a, pp 893–904

Williams DT: Somatoform disorders, factitious disorders and malingering, in Handbook of Child and Adolescent Psychiatry. Edited by Noshpitz J. New York, Basic Books, 1997b, pp 563–578

Williams DT, Bergtraum M: Epilepsy and nonepileptic seizures, in The Management of Stress and Anxiety in Medical Disorders. Edited by Mostofsky D, Barlow D. Boston, MA, Allyn & Bacon, 2000, pp 240–252

Williams DT, Velasquez L: The use of hypnosis in children with dissociative disorders. Child Adolesc Psychiatr Clin N Am 5:495–508, 1996

Williams DT, Ford B, Fahn S: Psychogenic movement disorders, in Behavioral Neurology of Movement Disorders (Advances in Neurology Series, Vol 65). Edited by Weiner W, Lang A. New York, Raven, 1995, pp 231–248

Williams DT, Pleak RR, Hanesian H: Neurological disorders, in Child and Adolescent Psychiatry: A Comprehensive Textbook, 3rd Edition. Edited by Lewis M. Baltimore, MD, Lippincott Williams & Wilkins, 2002, pp 755–766

Zelter L, LeBaron S: Hypnosis and nonhypnotic techniques for reduction of pain and anxiety during painful procedures in children and adolescents with cancer. J Pediatr 101:1032–1035, 1982

Zelter L, Dolgin M, LeBaron S, et al: A randomized, controlled study of behavioral intervention for chemotherapy distress in children with cancer. Pediatrics 88:34–42, 1991

Milieu Treatment

Inpatient, Partial, Residential

Theodore A. Petti, M.D., M.P.H.

Children and adolescents with severe and persistent psychiatric illness require an extensive and intensive system of services to provide for their health and mental health needs. In this overall continuum of care, inpatient hospital units, partial hospital or day treatment programs, and residential treatment centers (RTCs) play critical roles. Frequently referred to as "restrictive services" or "intensive services," these milieu-focused treatments are among the most costly for families and society. In government reports, statistics on residential and inpatient treatment are frequently considered together, whereas day treatment is detailed separately. This fact highlights the role of day treatment between the highly restrictive interventions of hospital and residential care and the less restrictive outpatient treatments in what has been labeled a continuum or system of care. Each of the three interventions has its own interesting history in the evolution and development of the field. These therapeutic interventions have been both praised and denounced, and providers have come under increasing pressure to demonstrate the relevance of these services in light of the current emphasis on evidence-supported, community-based treatment.

Residential and hospital facilities cover a broad spectrum, from group homes for severely developmentally delayed youths to highly sophisticated university acute hospital units and every conceivable variation in between (Petti 1980). Day treatment programs similarly vary considerably from each other. All three services have a set of guidelines and principles that distinguish them from each other, as well as a common set of values and expectations that allow them to be considered together. The central role played by the milieu is common to each.

When comparing current milieu treatments with those described years ago (Petti 1980) or taking a longitudinal view over decades (Rafferty 1999), one can see that considerable changes have taken place in the past decade. Partial hospital or day treatment is the newest of the three treatments; inpatient hospital care is entering middle age; residential treatment, the oldest of the three, has quietly metamorphosed from orphanages developed to care for parentless children into sophisticated treatment delivery systems operating within a continuum of community services. The latest figures indicate that more children and adolescents are served in residential treatment centers than in psychiatric inpatient hospital units, but the greatest number of youngsters in milieu treatments is found in day treatment or partial hospital programs (Milazzo-Sayre et al. 2000). Inpatient care is considered the most restrictive of all psychiatric treatments for pediatric populations. The decline of fee-for-service covered insurance and the development of managed care have profoundly altered the service delivery landscape (Rafferty 1999). Intermediate-term inpatient lengths of stay have been reduced to weeks or a few months, and acute care is generally measured in days (Masters 1997). The change in decisions by juvenile court judges, appearing to favor punishment over treatment referrals, may also have diminished the use of mental health services (Breda 2001).

This chapter describes common features across the three milieu treatments and considers each modality by defining the intervention and considering its history, organizational structure, unique role, and related issues. Residential services are considered first, followed by inpatient hospital care. Partial hospital or day treatment is the final area reviewed. There is no typical inpatient unit, residential treatment, partial hospital, or day treatment program. However, common features are present across this class of treatments.

Common Issues

The structure and function of a program depend on the system in which it operates. An ideal mental health system has reasonable access to at least one source of each milieu treatment. In the current political, fiscal, and clinical environment, change is a constant with regard to structure and function. This fluidity necessitates the creation of an organizational structure that is sufficiently flexible to allow for accommodation of and adaptation to a rapidly changing environment and that is adequately stable to provide predictability both for referral sources in the external environment and for the staff and patients serving and being served in the program. The type of pressure exerted on an agency or center providing services within a system is highly dependent on several factors. These factors include the parent organization and its philosophy or purpose, the population of patients or clients for which it means to provide care, the mechanisms for financing, and internal and external threats to its functioning and survival. Common to all intensive, restrictive programs providing milieu treatment is the presence of a governing entity or its equivalent, administrative and clinical issues, and the operation of a milieu.

■ Parent or Sponsoring Body

Programs offering milieu treatment have a variety of sponsors or governing bodies and range from state- or government-operated facilities to church-sponsored programs, not-for-profit organizations, operations under university control, and for-profit entities. The church-sponsored programs usually contrast markedly in structure to programs based in universities, which in turn vary depending on whether the program has a public-sector focus; for-profit programs have their own structure that differs from the others. Yet all must have an administration and a link to the governing body and must serve as an organizational component that defines functions within the program and includes supervisory responsibility. Each structure must also be set to deal with regulatory and certifying-body author-

ities as well as with demands of the payers of care. The way a program is structured has a critical influence on the functioning of the program. University-operated and state-operated facilities may have multiple hierarchical layers between the governing body and the facility administration. This may be true with certain for-profit organizations but is unlikely to be the case for programs managed by community mental health centers or those managed by religious and other nonprofit organizations. Structure follows function, which in turn is shaped by program philosophy. The changes in program philosophy have been markedly affected by the current environment in which care is being delivered. Programs of the 1980s and 1990s whose approach to service delivery were inflexible in meeting the changing health care environment have ceased to exist (Woolston 2002).

■ Administrative Issues

Program governance is critical. Each organization can be characterized by specific features outlined by Weisbord (1978). The goals of the organization—the purposes and the degrees to which they are stated, are understood, and shape program practice—are a primary feature. Other features include the formal (e.g., organizational hierarchy) and informal mechanisms (e.g., cafeteria groupings) that operate interdependently and facilitate the program's functioning. Still others are the means by which conflicts are resolved and changes in function are enabled through the management of relationships. Perceptions of reward mechanisms by those leading and working within the system have a decided impact on an agency's ability to grow and thrive. The components that assist in moving the agency forward in a common purpose are called *helping mechanisms* in this schema. Newsletters, forums, and celebrations are typical helping mechanisms. Finally, the style of leadership that is employed to manage conflict and that integrates and coordinates a program's functioning is the critical dimension in the overall structure.

Common structures employed in hospital-based services to achieve a functioning structure depend on the exercise of leadership in the organization. Areas that Woolston (2002) considers critical to the functioning of an inpatient service apply as well to all three milieu treatments. Planning and program development—especially the initial planning—set the stage for future development. This phase includes a needs assessment that should involve hospital administration, senior leadership of the unit, financial consultants, architects, and personnel managers. Their function is to address the content of what is needed and the process of getting the ultimate mission accomplished. This may be accomplished by enlisting community groups directly in the planning or by indirect participation through a needs assessment survey.

It is also important to address factors related to state, federal, and accrediting-body recommendations or criteria. Articulating a program philosophy and mission statement are requisite early activities; scheduled evaluation of adherence to such guidelines is advisable. The critical roles played by financial, legal, regulatory, and staffing considerations cannot be overstated. Nor can the importance of leadership. There has been a decided movement away from physician control of psychiatric programs in favor of administrators with clinical experience. The lack of leadership by physicians may have disastrous consequences for medically oriented programs, such as inpatient units or partial hospital programs, when the psychiatrist is not significantly involved in overseeing the structure and processes related to the delivery of care.

The survival of any program is highly dependent on the relationship and balance between leadership and each of the factors described above. The need to balance program goals with the needs of the population to be served, the constraints of the physical environment, and the requirements of the payer source and associated criteria for eligibility and reimbursement rate seems self-evident. Yet in the managed-care environment of the early twenty-first century, the pendulum has swung to put the payers in a position of disproportionate influence, possibly to the detriment of rational clinical care. A program within a system that is highly penetrated by managed care or is highly dependent on third-party payers will be structured differently and will function differently depending on the demographics and clinical profiles of the population it serves. On the other hand, the increased expectation of accountability for positive outcomes may facilitate the more widespread acceptance of evidence-based treatments and approaches.

Full enrollment or census for many programs may determine their ability to remain solvent and viable. Unpredictable fluctuations in admissions represent a threat to maintaining consistent staffing levels and sustaining morale. The fiscal and managed-care issues affect which patients or residents are admitted to milieu treatment programs, as well as when, why, how, and for how long they are admitted. The programs in turn—in the face of an impending shortage of registered nurses—have needed to develop flexible alternative staffing patterns. At the same time, professional staff members have increased their time spent in completing paperwork to justify initial admission, continued stay, and level of treatment. This decreases time spent in direct work with the patient and hence revenue. These factors, which lead to dilemmas for both administrators and clinicians, should be a focus of attention by policymakers.

Much of the paperwork is related to accountability issues. The requirement by the regulatory and certifying bodies to evaluate outcome is particularly difficult for most milieu treatment programs (Petti et al. 2000). In large measure, the problem emanates from the heterogeneous nature of the populations served, the diversity of programs, and the difficulties in developing operational definitions and measurements of services actually delivered (Kolko 2002). Most available studies are comparisons of patient or family condition on admission, at discharge, and sometimes at a short-term follow-up after 6 months or sometimes longer. The studies frequently employ standardized measures with acceptable psychometric properties. Rarely has there been random assignment to a control or comparison group. Basic methods suggested for studying service outcomes are change analysis, decision analysis, and outcome prediction (Lyons et al. 2001). Most studies to date have employed change analysis, the differences between measures taken before and after service delivery. More basic is the need to better delineate the content of what is delivered by programs being studied, to define parameters of success, to describe the population served, to employ rigorous statistical designs, and to expand the predictors for assessment (Kolko 1992, 2002).

Outcome reviews for each type of program are available, but few generalizations can be made at this time from that body of literature beyond the conclusion that some children and adolescents can benefit from such intensive treatments (Kutash and Rivera 1995). Most reviews suggest approaches for future research that include improved delineation of who can benefit most from milieu treatment and of adequate aftercare service planning. The assumption that the effect of services for youngsters requiring milieu treatment should be evaluated by using an acute illness model (e.g., pneumonia or fever) in contrast to a chronic disease model (e.g., asthma or diabetes) may be mistaken and could be a major barrier to valid and reliable evaluation. Returning to a dysfunctional or abusive family with high expressed emotion or failing to comply with agreed-on aftercare recommendations may easily eradicate any benefits from a highly efficacious milieu treatment. In addition, when aftercare services (i.e., services required after discharge from a program) are limited, unavailable or not easily accessible, and not culturally sensitive to family needs, then even the best, most highly efficacious milieu treatment intervention cannot be expected to have a high probability of producing a long-term positive benefit.

Behavioral health care in the guise of managed care programs significantly affects service delivery. In one study it was found that limitations on almost half of 128 evaluated commercial employment-based behavioral health plans could disrupt the health care of children with mental illness, whose needed services often fell in the realm of aftercare services (Peele et al. 2002). Strategies are needed to induce managed care organizations to accept responsibility for structuring aftercare into their benefit packages.

Lack of evidence demonstrating the effectiveness of milieu treatment may reflect an inability or lack of motivation to conduct the research or evaluations necessary to answer critical questions about these interventions. Such questions include the kinds of milieu treatments that are effective over years and how to combine residential and community-based care to best serve high-risk youths (Whittaker 2000). Aftercare and the role of milieu treatments in the continuum of care and the need for transitional services in step-down processes within the service delivery system are essential to the process, as described below. The role of the therapeutic alliance and family functioning before admission may also be critical (Green et al. 2001). Comparing types of services may prove useful in evaluating milieu treatment programs. The paradigm used to conceptualize the delivery of mental health services to emotionally disturbed children and teenagers needs to be revised so that the effectiveness of those services can be adequately assessed. Likewise, multiple domains in the life of a mentally ill child should be considered (Hoagwood et al. 1996; Jensen et al. 1996).

Milieu treatment programs are the most expensive psychiatric interventions available for children and teenagers. The top 2%–5% of severely and persistently mentally ill juveniles are estimated to use 80%–90% of the available resources for their care. Inpatient and specialized residential treatment account for the bulk of that cost. Effectiveness should be compared in economic as well as clinical terms.

Concerns have been raised about the system of rationally providing services for the most seriously ill juveniles (Jemerin and Philips 1988). Julian and associates (1992) addressed these concerns by enumerating the range and cost of services to 25 randomly selected youths from a regional mental health agency's case register of youths "who required or were candidates for inpatient psychiatric hospitalization." For each child, an average of 16.4 different human services providers or agencies were documented, including 68 hospitalizations (average per participant, 2.7), 48 RTC stays (average, 1.9), and only 7 contacts for day treatment (average, 0.3) over periods ranging from 13 or more years (8 children) to 5–12 years ($n=11$) to 4 years or less ($n=6$). Each subject spent an average of 613.6 days in residential services, and the average stay per residential contact was 43.7 days. The cost of caring for these 25 youths in 1989 dollars was $3,041,000 (including $1,476,000 for inpatient hospitalizations and $684,000 for RTCs). Few support, prevention, or family-oriented treatment services were available to the families or youths studied, and little aftercare was available. However, the needs of youths requiring intermediate-term or long-term hospitalization or RTC interventions are well illustrated by the study. The study also demonstrates that day treatment is sparsely used and that the system fails to adequately address the needs of these youths.

■ Clinical Issues

Quality assurance efforts for program improvement and continuing quality improvement represent the bridge between administrative and clinical issues. Common to all milieu programs are problems with maintaining well-trained and motivated staff, meeting fiscal goals, and maintaining constructive relationships with referral sources. Quality assurance efforts depend on a multitude of factors that range from the program type, philosophy and mission, staffing, leadership, and other aspects of program administration described above. The clinical population served is a rarely considered variable that may significantly affect quality improvement.

Heterogeneous populations receive care in milieu treatment programs. Criteria for admission are surprisingly similar from program to program; they appear to be differentiated arbitrarily between residential, inpatient, and day treatment and are often based on severity of illness, consideration of dangerousness and safety, and need for separation from the family. Criteria for inpatient and residential admission have been widely described (American Academy of Child and Adolescent Psychiatry and American Psychiatric Association 1997; Lewis et al. 2003; Petti 1980; Woolston 2003). The criteria for day treatment or partial hospital care are similar, with the difference being that the child can be safely maintained daily in the community (Evangelakis 1980; Heston et al. 1996).

Some form of formal education takes place in most programs. Partial hospital programs provided after school or on weekends and focusing mainly on social skills and relationship building are one exception. The education component may range from a structured, certified school program offering academic credit to a certified teacher working with schoolbooks and assignments from the child's own school that the family brings in for the few hours each day that the child spends in the school setting. Many children and teenagers admitted for milieu treatment require special education services, and some have received special designation as seriously emotionally disturbed, learning disabled, developmentally delayed (i.e., mentally retarded), or combined handicapped. The legal requirement for an individualized education plan (IEP) must be heeded when the youngster is expected to be in a program for an extended duration and requires special education services. School, home, and the community are the major areas of stress for most juveniles in milieu treatment. Youths in milieu treatment have language disorders, other developmental disabilities, or psychiatric disorders that make learning and academic achievement difficult. These youths represent significant assessment and treatment challenges that are particularly difficult to address during acute psychiatric admissions but are more likely to be recognized and addressed in intermediate- to long-term inpatient and RTC stays. Funding sources for such services are variable and depend on the facility and its particular configuration. Programs are increasingly dependent upon local public school systems to fund or provide school personnel to meet the education requirements of these youths.

Coordination of the school with other components of the milieu is a significant challenge. The importance of the education component is described elsewhere (Heston et al. 1996; Lewis et al. 2003; Petti 1980;

Woolston 2003). Most programs are habilitative rather than rehabilitative. Education for the youngster and family about the illness, its ramifications, and its treatment is understood to be a basic component of care. Social skills training, including anger management, is present in virtually all programs, although the names may differ between programs.

Consideration of nonpsychiatric health care varies between programs. Pediatricians consult on a regular or as-needed basis and are valued members of the treatment teams. Physical illness must be considered with regard to its biopsychosocial impact on individual children. To a varying extent, nursing staff members play a critical role in health and mental health care for juveniles receiving milieu treatment because they bring a medically oriented perspective.

A role for all staff members engaged in milieu treatment is to manage highly aggressive, violent, and destructive youths. This commonly experienced task is directly related to concerns about staff morale, regulations, and fiscal and regulatory issues. Aggressive youths influence everyone's perception of providing, working, or residing in a safe environment (Woolston 2002). There has been an increase in referrals of such youngsters to the more restrictive programs. Aggression by children and teenagers enrolled in programs for those with serious emotional disorders is almost universal and is of grave concern. The American Academy of Child and Adolescent Psychiatry (2002) developed its "Practice Parameter for the Prevention and Management of Aggressive Behavior in Child and Adolescent Psychiatric Institutions, With Special Reference to Seclusion and Restraint" to address this issue. Seclusion and restraint (S&R) had been adopted across most programs as an acceptable means to address the escalating incidence and prevalence of violent and agitated behavior (Gair 1991). Regulatory agencies and advocacy groups have recently become highly involved in this critical area as a result of highly publicized adverse effects associated with mechanical and other forms of restraint (Kennedy and Mohr 2001; Mohr et al. 1998; Ross 1999). Many programs have worked to reduce the utilization of restrictive interventions. The chronicle of one intermediate-term state hospital program may illustrate the advances made in this area (Petti et al. 2002c).

Multiple approaches can reduce the incidence of aggression and agitation that often precede S&R, lower the incidence of seclusion, and eliminate the incidence of restraint (Goren et al. 1996; Petti et al. 2001,

2002, 2003a, 2003b; Singh et al. 1999). Germane to this discussion are the perceptions by the children and adolescents about the use of different types of interventions that are widely accepted and employed throughout milieu treatment programs—for example, S&R, time-out, and as-needed (prn) medications. Contrary to earlier studies extolling the virtues of time out (i.e., time out from reinforcement) (Monkman 1972), the current literature suggests that hospitalized children prefer medication to time outs or seclusion, that time out and other forms of isolation may be counterproductive in children with deviant behavior (Kazdin 1984; Measham 1995; Natta et al. 1990; Petti et al. 2001, 2002, 2003a, 2003b), and that prn medication may not be more effective than placebo (Vitiello et al. 1991). Regrettably, few guidelines exist for the acute treatment of agitation or aggression in pediatric populations (American Academy of Child and Adolescent Psychiatry 2002). The term *chemical restraint* has been introduced to describe the use of psychotropic medications at such times. This term should be given thoughtful consideration before it is accepted as standard usage (Petti et al. 2003b). Aggression and violence will continue to demand considerable attention until more effective interventions are found to decrease or eliminate the agitation and violence of impulsive youngsters with severe mental illness.

It has been suggested that the administration of psychotropic medications on a scheduled basis can decrease agitation and aggression. However, currently available medications are inconsistent in their efficacy for aggression and violence, with notable exceptions (e.g., atypical neuroleptics for psychosis, mood stabilizers for mania, combined neuroleptic and antidepressant treatment for psychotic depression). (See Chapter 50 in this volume, "Psychopharmacology," for more details.) Limiting the utilization of seclusion and mechanical restraint returns responsibility for initiating the use of restrictive interventions back to the health professionals as part of their role in selecting the most appropriate intervention (Petti et al. 2002).

Sexual perpetrators are a subset of aggressive youngsters who are being identified and referred with increasing frequency for intensive, restrictive care. Of equal or greater concern are referrals of children or teenagers who have been sexually or physically abused, because they represent potential victims by peers or, rarely, by deviant staff members. The literature on the care of sexual predators and victims in residential care and group settings has been reviewed. Criteria indicat-

ing the need for more restrictive interventions have been suggested (American Academy of Child and Adolescent Psychiatry 1999).

Safety is an issue for youths who pose a risk for elopement, but this is less true at present than in the past, when inpatient and residential treatment units were long-term facilities and were customarily unlocked. The risk has decreased as programs for the more severely ill have by necessity increased their security. The dynamics related to elopement from treatment programs (McNaught and McKamy 1978) are similar to those found in youths who exhibit self-injurious behavior such as self-cutting, head banging, and ingesting foreign objects. The dynamics leading to elopement or self-injurious behavior are often found in milieu treatment programs: 1) fear of improvement that leads to discomfort and a need to act; 2) lack of insight leading to noncompliance with treatment and discouragement; 3) ambivalence about attachment to or dependence on others; 4) fear that external control is lacking when opportunities for more independent functioning are offered; 5) projection of internal conflicts on the treatment milieu; and 6) perception that the milieu does not allow individual emotional growth. The most frequent cause may be when youths believe that they bear the guilt of a dysfunctional family or peer group outside the milieu. Other reasons include escaping from a peer or several peers' hostility and aggression or being encouraged to elope by another peer (McNaught and McKamy 1978). Elopement and self-injurious behavior represent maladaptive communication and should be addressed as such.

The suicidal youth represents an additional high risk for elopement and overall safety. Slaby and McGuire (1989) discuss the risk factors and associated assessment and management of suicidal adolescents that begins with a preadmission assessment. A high index of suspicion is advised if the youth presents with features related to completed suicide, including associated stresses and "indicants of suicidal intent" such as accidents, risk-taking behavior, and unusual neglect of appearance. Recommended treatment includes a family assessment and a care plan involving team members from the program and caretakers outside the program in coordinated efforts. Addressing comorbid disorders, particularly substance abuse and chemical dependence, is critical in ensuring safety. See Chapter 43, "Substance Abuse Disorders," and Chapter 48, "Suicide and Suicidality," in this volume for more complete discussions.

Dialectical behavior therapy (DBT) and DBT principles are being employed with increasing frequency in milieu treatment programs (Katz et al. 2002). An amalgam of cognitive, behavioral, and numerous other therapeutic approaches, DBT has been found especially useful for parasuicidal youths and those with borderline personality disorder. Employing a multimodal approach, DBT targets impulsive aggression, noncompliance, and engagement in therapy. Hospitalization is generally discouraged when DBT is to be employed, because avoidance of the stressful environment is viewed as counterproductive. However, when hospitalization is used based on severe suicidal or parasuicidal behavior, it is expected to be a brief period (about 2 weeks) during which the assessment and DBT program are instituted. The program may differ from the more traditional DBT outpatient approach by not including parents in the daily skills training group. A DBT focus is expected to work best on a unit with staff members trained in DBT principles who are capable of assisting the youth in using the skills and in developing the ability to generalize the skills to other settings.

Nurcombe (1996) succinctly outlined the critical factors when admitting or discharging youngsters who represent potential danger to themselves and others. This risk resource analysis considers demographic, threat-related, and historical factors that suggest the need for particular caution. These include age; sex; culture; verbalized threats; the presence of or potential for provocation in the environment; access to a weapon; and psychological, social, and other factors. Psychological factors include defense mechanisms that are employed to manage affect; the presence of paranoia, suspicious vigilance, persecutory delusions, or command hallucinations; the strength of inner control; and the extent of impaired executive functioning that would take into account the presence of alcohol or substance abuse. The social environment includes the family's ability to control the patient and the presence of family psychopathology such as abuse, neglect, rejection, violence, or other features of high expressed emotion. The presence or absence of (or the potential to develop) a therapeutic alliance is considered crucial in risk assessment for dangerousness, as are protective factors such as being middle-class, younger, religious, white, female, and from a secure family and having no access to a weapon, no plan or identified victim, and a higher level of intelligence.

Recurrence of S&R, sexualized behavior, and issues concerning safety are all threats to a program's integrity. Programs for mentally ill or developmentally delayed children and teenagers are under the observation of multiple entities. These range from the Centers for Medicare & Medicaid Services (formerly the Health Care Financing Administration) to the Joint Commission on Accreditation of Healthcare Organizations (JCAHO) and related oversight bodies. Safety-related and outcome evaluation issues are high on their list of priorities. These regulatory and certifying bodies are increasingly demanding a structure and process for ensuring the safety and efficacy of the treatment environment. The JCAHO, for example, regularly circulates guidelines for managing what they have categorized as sentinel events. Such events include instances of abuse or neglect and severe adverse reactions to treatment that have death or disability associated with them. Programs requesting JCAHO certification are required to report such events through documented procedures detailed in policy and procedures manuals. Most milieu treatment programs come under the purview of these agencies. In addition, programs must document the manner in which a sentinel event, if it occurs, was managed and the plans to modify policy and procedures to avoid a repetition of the sentinel or a related adverse event.

The master treatment plan (MTP) is required for most milieu treatment programs that are more complex than a group home. The MTP is expected to reflect the multidisciplinary and interdisciplinary nature of its staff and programming. The MTP varies depending on the type of program and the population served. Critical elements include psychiatric symptoms, medical issues, education and psychoeducation, and discharge or disposition. Accrediting, certifying, and other bodies have differing expectations and criteria for an acceptable plan, and most programs struggle to develop plans that balance such competing interests. Various MTP approaches have been advocated (Harper 1989; Nurcombe 1989; Petti 1980). Milieu treatment programs provide some form of therapy; the type depends on the factors described above. The use of psychotropic medications in conjunction with other therapeutic interventions, detailed in most MTPs, is expected to make the child more amenable to utilizing services provided within the treatment milieu.

The Milieu

Milieus are characterized by their predominant environment, social organization, or culture. Rimsley (1980) defines a therapeutic milieu as one having a multidisciplinary staff of professionals and paraprofessionals devoted to the diagnosis and treatment of children with major mental illness within a hospital, residential center, or facility. Facilities have their own unique milieu based on the program's philosophy of care, leadership, history, culture, and staff. Staff includes both professional and front-line workers who provide services for the children and adolescents under their care. The average length of stay or duration of care for a patient also determines the type of milieu and how it operates. The physical environment may play a decisive role in the manner in which the milieu is able to function. Careful attention to safety and aesthetic issues can provide long-term benefits, improve morale, and lead to better outcomes. Staff participation in the planning of any modifications is encouraged; a less-than-ideal physical environment is the rule because seldom-considered variables of building codes, cost, and patient characteristics shape the ultimate design (Davis et al. 1979).

Lyman and Campbell (1996) describe an integrative approach for the therapeutic milieu in residential and psychiatric inpatient settings—a traditional approach that is now more characteristic of day treatment, residential programs, and intermediate-term units. Descriptions of therapeutic milieus and their role in currently functioning acute care units are scarce and are sorely needed. The barriers to developing and maintaining a milieu on such a unit under existing circumstances are enormous.

The Child or Adolescent Requiring Milieu Treatment

Studies and clinical experience indicate that youngsters admitted to milieu treatment programs mainly differ from children in the general population and from other children with emotional illness by the degree of stress they place on the home, school, and community. A distinction must be made between children with psychiatric illness who require milieu treatment and those who have chronic problems with delinquent behavior or whose families are unable to offer a stable, nurturing environment and for whom predominantly custodial care is needed. Undiagnosed or untreated medical conditions are common in referrals to milieu treatment.

The Family

The family is sometimes a forgotten or unavailable resource in intensive, restrictive care. Efforts to clarify parents' perceptions of their ill children's mental health needs (Delaney and Engels-Scianna 1996; Solomon and Evans 1992; Tarico et al. 1989) have been initiated, as have efforts to clarify the responses of facility staff members toward parents' involvement in the treatment process (Baker et al. 1995). The opportunities for youngsters in hospitals or in residential care to have contact with their families or others are inconsistent across programs. There is no common standard for visits by parents. More than half the respondents in one study reported that contact with parents was restricted during the initial adjustment period (Robinson et al. 2003). The JCAHO, the Child Welfare League, and other interested bodies have clearly defined expectations about the rights of residents to have visits or contact with their parents or family members. Restrictions need to be reasonable, and they should be detailed in the treatment plan, explained to the child and family, and reviewed monthly. There are no studies available to guide programs about optimal policies and procedures regarding contacts and visits. Parents are expected to be integral to treatment planning and ongoing care in partial hospital or day treatment programs, just as they are in theory for all milieu treatment.

Residential Treatment Centers

RTCs provide 24-hour mental health and related care for populations of juveniles who often are indistinguishable from those served in hospitals or day treatment programs. The federal government defines RTCs as "psychiatric organizations (exclusive of psychiatric hospitals) that provide residential services primarily to persons under age 18 who have been diagnosed as exhibiting moderate or severe emotional illness or psychiatric disorders" (Stroup et al. 1988, p. 2). They vary in scope and structure from small group homes to highly complex entities offering a full array of services that are equal to and sometimes greater than those found in hospital units.

■ History

Residential treatment programs began as orphanages and boarding schools for youngsters with mental handicaps and psychiatric illness. In the United States they evolved as caregiving facilities beginning with the founding of the first orphanage in 1729 and the establishment of a program for the mentally retarded in 1848. The 1850s were characterized by the proliferation of child care institutions and group foster homes. These facilities were established for the delivery of intensive education to assist emotionally and socially deviant children in an attempt to transform these societal misfits—whose deviant behavior was deemed to be secondary to early abuse and neglect—for at least minimally acceptable functioning in the community (Petti 1980). The 1850s also saw the development of the therapeutic milieu, the evolution of the mental hygiene movement into the mental health movement, and later the specialized care of pediatric psychiatric disorders in the 1900s. From this period, psychoanalytic theories dominated the conceptual arena for diagnosis, assessment, and ascendancy of the therapeutic milieu. In a brief chronology, Jemerin and Philips (1988) compare RTC treatment with inpatient care and with the movement to provide a total therapeutic environment. Zimmerman (1990) considers other conceptual models of care and highlights the current emphasis in residential care on the development of community support networks to ensure postplacement adjustment. He considers the behavioral approach and its limited impact on the therapeutic milieu, the movement toward a positive peer pressure model, and finally a psychoeducational approach based on Hobbs's (1966) Re-Ed model. Zimmerman (1990) also chronicles the evolution of the group home and the shifting of residential care toward a more community-based approach. Whittaker (2000) elaborates on the development of group care and its need to be better integrated into a total continuum of care for the child and family.

To adapt to the changing environment, RTCs have managed to reinvent themselves on a regular basis and to become integral components within systems of care. The RTCs that are most likely to survive are those that have begun partnering with managed care organizations to develop innovative strategies linking all the positive features of a system of care with family involvement and sophisticated technology. These RTCs have modified their programs to provide increasingly shorter lengths of stay and greater flexibility in keeping parents actively involved in the care of their children residing in RTCs. In 1997 there were 32,968 children in RTCs, with 26,322 in RTC programs for emotionally disturbed children—three times the number of children who were in inpatient care but fewer than those

who were receiving care on less than a 24-hour basis (Milazzo-Sayre et al. 2000).

■ Residential Care

RTCs vary considerably in their degree of structure, size, complexity, and services offered. Some offer more comprehensive services than hospital units, and others resemble group homes or halfway houses. These 24-hour facilities are not considered hospitals because nursing and medical care are not available around the clock. Some operate for 5 days a week (Grizenko and Papineau 1992) or have prolonged closures during which services are not provided. Some operate with two or three shifts of staff, whereas others have live-in houseparents or counselors who provide the bulk of supervision and care.

Weintrob (1975) differentiates an RTC from a psychiatric inpatient unit for severely disturbed adolescents requiring long-term treatment. The RTC, he asserts, has group living and individual treatment as its focus. Major differences in perceptions by the youngsters residing in them include the self-perception of being a "resident" of the facility, as contrasted to a sick person in a hospital. Less regression is expected in residential treatment compared with hospital admissions, where total care and meeting of dependence needs are paramount. RTCs expect healthy behavior, rather than the sick behavior that is allowed during a hospital stay. These differences may have been diminished by the brief stays that juveniles are now allowed in acute care units. However, they certainly hold for intermediate- and longer-term hospital care.

The perceptions of parents, the juvenile court, advocates, community workers, academicians, and, importantly, hospital staff seem to perpetuate the expectation that hospitals are a place for sick people. Most youths with a psychiatric illness are able to play the sick role with no difficulty and hence foster the self-fulfilling prophecy of poor functioning. Weintrob (1975) also notes that hospitals emphasize treatment, whereas RTCs offer services that allow the resident to become more self-sufficient.

Except for the most specialized units, per diem costs of RTC treatment are significantly lower than comparable inpatient unit costs but are considerably higher than the costs of comprehensive community care programs (Lyons et al. 1998). Located in communities, RTCs are better able to facilitate the residents' transition back to their home communities and local schools because the RTCs are frequently integrated into a community public school and their residents spend time in the community. This is in contrast to the sheltering experienced in the hospital setting, where patients are exposed to much less stress than are RTC residents.

Youngsters in residential treatment differ significantly from children in the general population, having higher levels of poverty, family dysfunction, and stress and having fewer personal and family resources from which to draw support (Wells et al. 1991). Lyons and associates (1998) commented on the multiple non–mental health–related reasons for RTC placement and reported that more than one-third of residents in randomly selected Illinois RTCs had risk profiles suggesting that they might be better served in community placements because they represented no danger to themselves or others and had limited overall dysfunction and psychopathology. These researchers reported that older teenagers were the most likely to be inappropriately placed in residential care.

Prolonged stays in RTCs after optimal gains have been made are also a major problem for youths in intermediate- and long-term psychiatric hospitals. However, Leichtman and Leichtman (1996) cogently argued that some youngsters need to remain in long-term placement for a variety of reasons, including the need and opportunity for stability in their lives. This view is supported by a follow-up study of youths who had been in an urban RTC for 6 months or more. Ages on admission were 10–17 years (mean age, 14.8 years). The subjects were 14–20 years old (mean, 18.3 years) at follow-up and were doing well in regard to several areas of functioning. Poor adaptation after discharge despite stability in the residence was associated with the absence of adequate family support and with exposure to high levels of perceived stress (Wells et al. 1991).

It has been asserted that mentally ill juveniles who are Caucasian disproportionately receive mental health services, whereas those of minority races are relegated to corrections and juvenile justice facilities. Nevertheless, admission rates for African Americans (overall, and for both males and females to RTCs for emotionally disturbed children) exceeded those for Caucasians in 1997 (Milazzo-Sayre et al. 2000). African American females were admitted at a higher rate than were Hispanic females.

Several theoretical orientations used to classify RTCs are noted above. The RTCs have been variably classified based on their theoretical or functional orientation (e.g., therapeutic communities or token economies, chemical dependency programs, psychoeducational programs, and community-based residential group care). Some are behaviorally oriented, others are psychodynamic/psychoanalytic, and many are cognitive-behaviorally based. A limited number serve juveniles who are dually diagnosed with mental illness and chemical dependence, whereas others serve those who are dually diagnosed with mental illness and mental retardation or related developmental issues. Some are built around the education programs of the facility, with schools on their premises; some have their residents attend school in the community; and others use both these approaches. Many offer outpatient and partial hospital treatment (Milazzo-Sayre et al. 2000; Stroup 1988). Practical aspects of working in or consulting with residential programs are detailed elsewhere (Cohen, in press; Fujita and Arnold, in press).

■ Role in a System of Care

A role for the RTC in the array of services should be unquestioned. Outcome studies have demonstrated RTC care to be a component of a continuum of care. Aftercare has repeatedly been demonstrated as being critical to successful outcome of residential care (Curry 1991). Often the need for long-term involvement, including that provided outside the RTC, can differentiate between successful and unsuccessful response to treatment (Curry 1991; Whittaker 2000). Considerations of the role of long-term residential treatment to complement the short-term care that is now being widely espoused must include the reality that only a limited number of suitable aftercare programs are available for those needing RTC services (Leichtman and Leichtman 1996). The dynamics of unsuccessful return to home or other placements have been poorly studied, and the process of returning to the community deserves attention.

Family involvement in RTC care is problematic, particularly for lower-income families and those receiving welfare, families from rural areas, those living a distance from the facility, and those without adequate support for transportation and child care for other children. In a study of family involvement in three contrasting RTCs (one for those with a psychiatric disorder, one for those diagnosed with mental retardation, and the third for those with a dual diagnosis of psychiatric illness and mental retardation) serving children ages 5–19 years, Baker and associates (1993) reported that almost one-third of the residents had no family contact over a 1-year period. About 50% had three or fewer contacts over the year. The dually diagnosed children experienced lower levels of family involvement than the other two groups. Low socioeconomic status and long driving time between the RTC and the family home were associated with lower levels of involvement by the families of the dually diagnosed.

Even in a program with significant resources allotted to discharge planning, one-third of adolescents consecutively discharged from a comprehensive RTC were homeless within 5 years, more than one-sixth of them within the first year. Risk factors for homelessness included being in state custody at the time of RTC admission, history of physical abuse, and history of drug or alcohol use (Embry et al. 2000). Similar factors were identified in an earlier Ohio study of young adults (Belcher 1991). The relative risk for homelessness was 2.1 for those with a learning disability, 2.81 for those with a history of running away, and 4.79 for those who did not have a thought disorder (Embry et al. 2000). The final risk figure is surprising, because psychosis has generally been considered an indicator of poor clinical outcome (Kutash and Rivera 1995).

■ Outcome and Quality Assessment

Outcome studies of RTC care suggest relative effectiveness within the limitations described above. Factors associated with positive outcomes have been identified in several studies (Kutash and Rivera 1995) and include the absence of the following: psychosis, organic etiology for the psychiatric disorder, below-average level of intelligence, antisocial and bizarre behavior, a dysfunctional family, insufficient duration of residence to allow for consolidation of gains, and inadequate aftercare services. A standardized treatment program delivered in the hospital is a predictor of positive outcome. A stay of less than 1 month is more often associated with a positive outcome (Hoagwood and Cunningham 1992). Defining an adequate length of stay in residential care is difficult, and this may be related to the overall difficulty in evaluating the costs and benefits of RTC care.

Conducting controlled and randomized studies for the evaluation of RTCs has been problematic. Curry (1991) suggested employing research designs that make comparisons between treatments, within programs, and across program designs. He noted that res-

idential treatment cannot be viewed as an isolated event in the life and treatment of an individual child or teenager. He also provided results of comparative outcome studies and emphasized the need to control for the postdischarge environment (Curry 1991). In a quasi-experimental study evaluating prevalent negative beliefs of troubled adolescents about residential placement, Friman and associates (1996) reported that the residential treatment group had significantly more positive views than the comparison group on most measures.

Comparison studies evaluating different types of RTCs have been reported. The course of change was assessed for groups of teenagers with conduct disorder who were treated in publicly funded RTCs that had either a therapeutic community or a token economy orientation. Multiple measures were employed at three points over the time of treatment (Mann-Feder 1996). A trend of overall improvement was noted in the residents of both programs, and few significant differences in progress were found between the programs.

A study by Leon and associates (2000) illustrates a novel prospective approach for assessing the quality of RTCs. A reliable severity measure was used with children (average age, 14 years) referred from an area's 10 largest licensed RTC Medicaid providers for admission for psychiatric hospitalization. Referred youths were categorized as either low risk or high risk, with psychotic symptoms, dangerousness to others, and moderate suicidality constituting the criteria for the high-risk group. The researchers found elevated rates of referrals of low-risk children from five RTCs, with a range of 35%–50%. Further comparisons showed that the same five RTCs had statistically significantly poorer ability to provide adequate supervision to the children under their care and therefore were unable to adequately monitor escalating behavior.

In a related study, the use of antipsychotic medication was evaluated in RTCs located in four states across the United States. Regional differences were noted regarding use and nonuse factors (Rawal et al. 2002). The results were similar to those of an earlier study assessing differences between types of hospitals (Kaplan and Busner 1997). Such studies provide an understanding of actual treatments employed when definable symptom complexes are present and represent a marked advance in providing objective data for use in improving the quality of care.

Similarly, Lyons and associates (2001) examined the clinical status and extent of symptom improvement of 285 adolescents ages 12–17 years from eight RTCs for 2 years. By retrospectively employing a growth-modeling technique with a standardized instrument, these researchers found overall improvement in symptoms but limited improvement in functioning. Variations both in symptom improvement and across sites were noted. Of great interest is the finding that with one exception all sites were comparable in levels of change; the one atypical site showed "reliable worsening." It was also the site that admitted children at healthier levels of functioning.

Inpatient Hospitalization

Psychiatric hospital inpatient programs are defined along several dimensions, including length of stay, type of patient, age range served, and governance (i.e., public, private, or for-profit). Inpatient care has been defined as the most restrictive and expensive of the milieu treatments. Traditionally reserved for the most severely ill who require round-the-clock medical and nursing supervision, inpatient units may exist within psychiatric, pediatric, or general hospitals or in freestanding child and adolescent psychiatric hospitals. They may be obligated to serve within a system of care, be selective in caring for special populations, or be available to all within a certain age range. Similar to RTCs, there is no typical inpatient unit. The American Academy of Child and Adolescent Psychiatry and the American Psychiatric Association (1997) published criteria for the psychiatric hospitalization of children and adolescents. In 1997, 12,402 youngsters under age 18 were admitted for inpatient care. Of these, almost 6,000 were cared for in private psychiatric hospitals and almost 2,700 in state or county hospitals. The remainder were treated in general hospitals or components of mental health organizations (Milazzo-Sayre et al. 2000).

■ History

Inpatient hospital psychiatric treatment of disturbed children and adolescents began in the early 1920s and was undertaken predominantly for behavior problems. The first unit for adolescents was developed in the 1930s for males, who were mainly referred by the courts (Petti 1980; Zimmerman 1990). The history of inpatient and residential care of adolescents is extensively described elsewhere (Zimmerman 1990). Acute inpatient hospital care has changed markedly over the past two decades (Jemerin and Philips 1988; Petti 1980; Woolston 2003).

Judicial decisions may have precipitated the flurry of construction and controversy relating to the phenomenal increases in admissions to private and public facilities for juveniles (predominantly disturbed adolescents) and the increased resources directed to finance such care (Woolston 2003). These increases were accompanied by the ascendancy of a managed care model of mental health care for juveniles, a series of scandals related to the practices of private hospitals, and finally the Child and Adolescent Service System Program movement in conjunction with the initiative by the Robert Wood Johnson Foundation toward family-centered, individualized community care. The result of these current forces has been the closing of a number of the mostly for-profit programs and publicly funded state and county units. "Downsizing" or "rightsizing" resulted in marked decreases in the numbers of psychiatric beds for children and adolescents and led to scarce availability in some areas. This may account for the rising occupancy rates for child and adolescent beds in the year 2000 as part of an overall increase in occupancy for all psychiatric beds of 24.4% over 1996 rates (American Psychiatric Association 2002). The continued relative shortage of public-sector psychiatric beds for children and adolescents has persisted in 2002 and has become problematic for the entire health care system. Low reimbursement rates and failure to provide the resources for alternatives to inpatient care are seen as reasons for the decreasing number of beds (Kanapaux 2002). Managed care has not lessened the problems of access to and appropriate use of inpatient care across geographical areas and has mainly resulted in shortened lengths of stay (Gutterman 1998).

■ Inpatient Care

The focus of inpatient care has become assessment, stabilization, disposition planning, and transition to less restrictive settings. The degree to which each component is emphasized depends on the dimensions described under "Common Issues" above for all the milieu treatments. Acute inpatient units are the most common form of hospital-based care. Intermediate-term units—mainly public sector in governance—and long-term units similarly governed are becoming rare.

Although variations abound, acute hospitalization is reserved for those in need of immediate separation from their family, school, or community. The acute inpatient unit, once limited mainly to university settings, was described as "a specialized setting for comprehensive diagnostic evaluation and brief intervention" (Jemerin and Philips 1988). Recent changes have affected acute inpatient care by folding treatment into the assessment process, blurring boundaries between hospital care and social service and protection, decreasing the ability to understand the patient, and fragmenting care (Jemerin and Philips 1988).

Acute care may be solely for crisis stabilization or for more comprehensive assessment utilizing the resources of larger pediatric, psychiatric, or general hospitals. Intermediate-term facilities offer patients and their families the opportunity for more extensive assessment and for consolidation of gains necessary for successful transition to less restrictive interventions.

Dangerousness was the major reason for hospitalization initiated from emergency units (Gutterman 1998). There are several other factors that determine the need for psychiatric hospitalization; these include the family's or the community's ability to provide for and manage the child's safety (Petti 1998). Therapy beyond resolving the precipitating crisis is frequently not feasible in acute care. Emphasis on therapeutic intervention is expected from intermediate-term and long-term facilities. Altering negative cognitions through various modalities and training in social skills through cognitive, behavioral, and psychodynamic approaches within the milieu are standard in most treatment plans. Efforts devoted to family work are dependent on the availability of the family. Aftercare as a fundamental activity is difficult to implement for most inpatient programs for reasons described above. The concern for "institutionalizing" patients in intermediate-term or longer-term care is real, particularly when the patient feels comfortable in the role of a sick person. Aggression and violence are more likely to occur on inpatient units than in other forms of milieu treatment and are a common focus of attention. Models of inpatient care described elsewhere provide interesting perspectives (Harper 1989; Nurcombe 1989; Woolston 1996).

■ Outcome and Quality Assessment

Defining outcomes and factors specific to inpatient care has been difficult (Blanz and Schmidt 2000).

Moreover, even efforts to standardize definitions of fidelity to types of services provided within inpatient care have not been successful to date. As with RTCs, the conclusions of studies attempting to measure the effectiveness of inpatient care have suggested that these forms of treatment are useful for large numbers of children and adolescents and partially explains their being widely utilized. Kolko (1992) noted a decrease in symptoms among formerly hospitalized children and adolescents on follow-up. His short-term evaluation of 65 children of elementary-school and middle-school ages 2, 4, and 6 months after discharge revealed no differences in outcome as a function of length of stay or time from discharge. He reported that factors including older age, neurological dysfunction, attention-deficit disorder with hyperactivity, a history of physical abuse, and depressive symptoms predicted poorer outcomes compared with those with statistically better outcomes. He suggested attending to factors that parents indicated were improved in the higher-functioning youngsters: decreases in both internalizing and externalizing symptoms, disciplinary effectiveness, adaptive involvement in recreation and leisure activities, positive peer interaction, and improved satisfaction with relationships. Kolko (1992) suggested that the treatments that are most likely to provide the child and family with the skills to achieve such progress should be the focus of therapeutic interventions, for example, parent management training, exposure to group activities fostering prosocial behavior, and cognitive-behavioral skills training. He also emphasized the importance of aftercare planning and the need to sort out parent versus child variables, diagnoses, and other factors that contribute to outcome.

A recent study contributed to the developing methodology for studying outcome from the perspective of health gains. Preadmission status was compared with status after admission, at time of discharge, and at 6-month follow-up. The results showed significant sustained gains on symptoms and adjustment but not on family functioning (Green et al. 2001). There was no change in status between the time of referral (a median of 3 months prior to admission) and the time of hospitalization on the multiple measures of functioning. The amount of time spent in day treatment as part of the care seemed to make little difference in outcome. Mayes and associates (2001) offered a similar ABA design (evaluation during baseline compared with that during intervention and then, after the intervention ends, compared with a return to the baseline condition) to argue for the effectiveness of brief hospitalization.

Studies of multisystemic therapy (MST), a manual-driven system-of-care program, suggest that intermediate-term or long-term inpatient hospital care can be dramatically decreased. In a randomized, controlled study, Henggeler and associates (1999) compared 56 adolescents (average age, 13 years; 64% African American; 65% male) assigned to standard inpatient acute care with 57 youths assigned to MST. Results indicated favorable outcomes from both treatments, but MST including the use of therapeutic foster care and judicious use of hospitalization was at least as effective on several short-term clinical and functional measures of outcome. However, acute hospitalization was required in 44% of patients assigned to MST, thus supporting a putative role for inpatient hospitalization in a total system of care (Henggeler et al. 1999).

Partial Hospitalization and Day Treatment

Multiple variations of partial hospital or day treatment have been described. These treatments are defined as less than 24-hour hospital-level daily care targeted to the diagnosis and treatment of psychiatric disorders for which the prevention of relapse or hospitalization and the chance for improvement in the condition could be expected (Daily and Reddick 1993). The American Association for Partial Hospitalization has defined partial hospitalization as clinical services in an active treatment program offering active ambulatory treatment within a stable therapeutic milieu that is time-limited, therapeutically intensive, coordinated, and structured. It is represented by multiple intensive services between inpatient and outpatient care and has been described as the prototype of a hospital diversion program (Heston et al. 1996). Over time, these programs have been called day care centers, day hospitals, threshold centers, day care clinics, youth day treatment centers, and children's day treatment services (Evangelakis 1980). The differences between partial hospital and day treatment are reviewed elsewhere (Kutash and Rivera 1995). Broadly defined, *partial hospital treatment* refers to less than 24-hour care provided in a hospital setting, whereas *day treatment* refers to school-based care provided for at least 5 hours a day that involves integrated education, counseling, and

family services. In 1997, 517,210 youngsters under age 18 years were admitted to "less than 24-hour care programs" (Milazzo-Sayre et al. 2000). Of these patients, more than 200,000 were cared for in multiservice mental health organizations; 180,000 were cared for in partial care organizations and freestanding outpatient clinics, 75,000 in general hospitals 37,000 in RTCs, 16,000 in private psychiatric hospitals, and almost 5,000 in public mental hospitals.

■ History

Day treatment began in several countries in the 1930s. Organized day hospital treatment began in the United States in 1943 (Zimet and Farley 1985). Few partial hospital programs existed before the 1963 passage of the Community Mental Health Center Act, which mandated it as one of the essential services of community mental health centers. The movement against the perceived antitherapeutic effects of institutional care, the need for cost-effective treatments that could be offered 5 days a week with only a single shift of staff, and a greater role for the family and community gave impetus to partial hospital programs (Evangelakis 1980; Heston et al. 1996). They were meant to provide alternatives to 24-hour care and intensive treatment, to decrease dependence on inpatient and outpatient treatment (Evangelakis 1980), and to minimize the extended sick role that institutional care and long-term outpatient treatment might engender. The therapeutic milieu was meant to alter symptomatic behavior, and the associated special education was to assist in intellectual, social, and emotional development. The day treatment schedule was intended to avoid the problems associated with inconsistent approaches by staff across shifts and the high cost of other restrictive treatments. Parents and their disturbed offspring were expected to work together to foster better communication and parenting skills and to make the transition to less intensive community services.

Since their inception, these programs have been underutilized for children and teenagers with severe psychiatric disorders—often because they are not included in insurance policy coverage. In rural areas, transportation issues can make it difficult to gain access to programs that are not located within the schools. The limitations of having a less structured environment than that provided by inpatient facilities and RTCs were initial concerns of referral sources. Additional problems included the absence of criteria for admission, the absence of clear definitions of outcome, and the reluctance to maintain seriously ill youngsters in the community and home. Many parents expressed their reluctance to engage in regular family therapy. With the emergence of managed care, partial hospital and day treatment programs are expected to grow and to become a more prominent component of the mental health service system (Heston et al. 1996).

■ Partial Hospital and Day Treatment Care

Partial hospital and day treatment programs offer the intensive treatment and therapeutic milieu provided in a hospital or RTC setting while maintaining the youngster in the home and community. A psychoeducational day-school program is the most common type. Evening and after-school programs are also common. The programs may be free-standing or may be part of a hospital clinic, inpatient unit, school, or RTC. Most programs are highly structured, attend to the educational needs of their patients, and provide multimodal treatments. They attempt to avoid the regression frequently found when psychiatrically ill children and adolescents enter inpatient facilities and even some RTCs. The patients are provided the opportunity to work on their issues without needing to assume the sick role, as they would with hospitalization. In keeping with the assumption that the patient is able to exert adequate self-control to avert the risk of dangerous behavior, the expectation for structure to provide for the ultimate safety of the ill patient (as found in inpatient and RTC programs) is minimal.

Care that exceeds multiple weekly outpatient visits is provided on a variable but short-term basis with a crisis focus as an alternative to hospitalization and often serves as a step down from an inpatient or RTC setting. Partial programs are meant for patients who can be managed safely in an intensive setting without the need for 24-hour institutional care. Specialized treatment programs employing the partial hospital model of care are available for those with substance abuse, chemical dependence, and eating disorders; for victims of abuse; and for those who have medical disorders with comorbid psychiatric difficulties (Pruitt 1999).

Inclusion criteria differ from those of the other milieu treatments mainly in that the youngster must have adequate impulse control to remain in the community and does not need the safety and security of an inpatient unit. Disruptive disorders, particularly conduct and attention-deficit/hyperactivity disorders, are gen-

erally the most common diagnoses found in referred children (Doan and Petti 1989; Grizenko 1997). Parents or caretakers must be able to regularly participate in family counseling, training, and therapy and to adequately provide support and exert control over their children during evenings and weekends. Reliable transportation must be available, payment resources must be adequate to complete a course of treatment, and 24-hour care is not required (Heston et al. 1996). Although seclusion and restraint have been standard practice in RTC and inpatient units, partial hospital programs generally do not offer seclusion, and they limit restraint and restrictive practice to those acceptable and available in most home environments. Physical holding and quiet rooms are not customarily used but are available in some programs, but chemical and manual restraints are not (Heston et al. 1996). Exclusion criteria for this type of care include fitting better in a less restrictive outpatient setting (Zimet and Farley 1985).

An approach emphasizing a systems orientation to understanding the development and maintenance of psychopathology with the interplay between the family, the environment, and the child is central for the successful operation of such a program. Thus, day treatment attempts to provide the structure of inpatient and residential care while maintaining an active, functional link to the family and community. In many of these programs, even though they are in educational settings, the academic domain is less dominant than the social and emotional domains, with the school experience serving as the focus around which the therapeutic interactions occur (Zimet and Farley 1985).

Physician involvement varies depending on the type of program and the functions required of the psychiatrist. Programs that function as an alternative to or as a step down from inpatient care require more medical input and greater psychiatrist involvement. Programs that function as intensive outpatient services mainly employ the psychiatrist as a consultant to provide diagnostic assessment and medication monitoring. The practical aspects of work in and consulting to partial hospital and day treatment programs are detailed by Kiser and associates (in press) and by Heston and Paavola (unpublished).

■ Outcome and Quality Assessment

Effectiveness studies of partial or day treatment programs have encountered problems similar to those faced by studies of the other milieu treatments (Doan and Petti 1989; Kutash and Rivera 1995). Measuring successful reintegration into regular school settings, studies showed that day treatment was effective in 65%–70% of cases. Kiser and associates (1996) noted that the primary function of partial hospital programs is to improve the daily level of functioning through ameliorating positive psychiatric symptoms. Identifying and reinforcing family and community strengths so that the family and child become less dependent on more restrictive interventions are secondary goals. Positive perceptions of treatment and outcomes are also important measures of outcome. In comparing two types of partial programs, one academic and urban and the other a suburban general hospital, these researchers found that 1 year after discharge from the programs the children and adolescents were experiencing fewer overall symptoms, including conduct problems; were usually making better grades; and were being better friends. The children were using more (but less intensive) community mental health services, and the parents attributed improvement to participation in the partial hospital programs. Family functioning was improved, particularly in regard to affective involvement and behavior control (Kiser et al. 1996).

Multiple outcome studies of day treatment suggest that a portion of children can benefit from this service or be reintegrated into school settings, that individual and family functioning are improved, that treatment gains are not generalized to the school setting, and that the family plays a critical role in posttreatment outcomes (Grizenko 1997; Kutash and Rivera 1995). In a 5-year follow-up study of 33 children with severe behavior problems, Grizenko (1997) found that the children scored better on global functional assessment measures at discharge and at follow-up 5 years later compared with their admissions scores. Employing repeated-measures analyses of variance, Grizenko found that posttreatment gains were maintained over the duration of the study. These gains included the ability to function in regular classes; scores on total, internalizing, and externalizing scales on the Child Behavior Checklist; improvement in self-esteem; and decrease in depression. Long-term day treatment and inpatient care were required by 3 of the children (9%); social services, including temporary placement, were required by 6 (18%). It was found that the presence of cooperative parents who worked with the program significantly differentiated between those who did not need further social or psychiatric care and those who

did. The study did not have a control group (Grizenko 1997).

Comparing milieu treatments with each other or with other interventions can provide a basis for evaluation. Grizenko and Papineau (1992) performed a comparison of 23 children receiving day treatment with a like number of children who had received inpatient psychiatric treatment at an earlier time. Similarities in characteristics such as baseline diagnoses, symptom severity, family support and functioning, age, and gender between groups were noted. The researchers found that the numbers of children who dropped out of treatment were similar between groups. Also similar between groups were the outcomes of children ages 6–12 years, with the Children's Global Assessment Scale used as the measure of efficacy. The dramatic difference in the average length of stay, 19.6 months for inpatient care (more accurately described as residential care) versus 6.1 months for day treatment, is of import. This dramatic disparity in treatment time was accompanied by a more than sixfold difference in mean cost, CAN\$62,412 for a residential type of inpatient care versus CAN\$9,213 for day treatment. The savings were attributed to shorter episodes in treatment and were probably also related to the close links forged with community schools and the fact that the children resided within the community and family.

In a 10-year follow-up study (Erker et al. 1993) of adolescents and adults who as children had received either residential or day treatment, no differences were reported between the groups in ratings of social and personal adjustment. Improvement at follow-up was present in about 64% of the subjects and was similar to that reported in other studies. Poorer outcomes for both groups were found in those who were more severely impaired at admission to the program. The children who had received day treatment had more sessions involving their parents. The possibility that the parents of the subjects who received residential treatment were less able or willing to engage in treatment is a major variable that could explain the need for more restrictive intervention.

Conclusion

We must rethink the paradigm that views severe child psychiatric illness as an acute illness that can be treated on an episode-by-episode basis. Moreover, as an aid to designing programs and systems of care, we must begin to examine the multiple factors that affect the domains of outcome. We implicitly recognize that in most cases serious psychiatric illness can be categorized as a chronic illness and should be considered in that light (see Looney 1988). The youngsters requiring milieu treatment are most likely to be best served by employing a chronic disease model in their assessment and treatment and in the evaluation of services. Lip service has been given to the need to customize treatment to the individual child; doing this would certainly call for family involvement, especially for youngsters in hospital and residential care. The disconnection between what we know and what we practice is problematic (Lyons et al. 1998; Whittaker 2000).

The milieu treatments have a significant role to play in future service delivery systems. Therefore we must improve our approaches to these treatments, utilize them in the most cost-effective manner, and develop an evidence base to support their use.

References

American Academy of Child and Adolescent Psychiatry: Practice parameters for the assessment and treatment of children and adolescents who are sexually abusive of others. J Am Acad Child Adolesc Psychiatry 38(suppl):55S–76S, 1999

American Academy of Child and Adolescent Psychiatry: Practice parameter for the prevention and management of aggressive behavior in child and adolescent psychiatric institutions, with special reference to seclusion and restraint. J Am Acad Child Adolesc Psychiatry 41(suppl):4S–25S, 2002

American Academy of Child and Adolescent Psychiatry and American Psychiatric Association: Criteria for Short-Term Treatment of Acute Psychiatric Illness. Washington, DC, American Academy of Child and Adolescent Psychiatry and American Psychiatric Association, 1997

American Psychiatric Association: Psychiatric beds filling up fast. Psychiatric Practice and Managed Care 8:1–2, 2002

Baker BL, Blacher J, Pfeiffer S: Family involvement in residential treatment of children with psychiatric disorder and mental retardation. Hosp Community Psychiatry 44:561–566, 1993

Baker BL, Heller TL, Blacher J, et al: Staff attitudes toward family involvement in residential treatment centers for children. Psychiatr Serv 46:60–65, 1995

Belcher J: Moving into homelessness after psychiatric hospitalization. J Soc Serv Res 14(3–4):63–77, 1991

Blanz B, Schmidt MH: Practitioner review: preconditions and outcome of inpatient treatment in child and adolescent psychiatry. J Child Psychol Psychiatry 41:703–712, 2000

Breda CS: The mental health orientation of juvenile courts. J Behav Health Serv Res 28:89–95, 2001

Cohen P: Chemical dependency program, in Community Child and Adolescent Psychiatry: A Manual of Clinical Practice and Consultation. Edited by Petti TA, Salguero C. Washington, DC, American Psychiatric Publishing (in press)

Curry JF: Outcome research on residential treatment: implications and suggested directions. Am J Orthopsychiatry 61:348–357, 1991

Daily S, Reddick C: Adolescent day treatment: an alternative for the future. Adolesc Psychiatry 19:523–540, 1993

Davis C, Glick ID, Rosow I: The architectural design of a psychotherapeutic milieu. Hosp Community Psychiatry 30:453–460, 1979

Delaney KR, Engels-Scianna B: Parent's perceptions of their child's emotional illness and psychiatric treatment needs. J Child Adolesc Psychiatr Nurs 9(4):15–26, 1996

Doan RJ, Petti TA: Clinical and demographic characteristics of child and adolescent partial hospital patients. J Am Acad Child Adolesc Psychiatry 28:66–69, 1989

Embry LE, Evens C, Stoep AV, et al: Risk factors for homelessness in adolescents released from psychiatric residential treatment. J Am Acad Child Adolesc Psychiatry 39:1293–1299, 2000

Erker GJ, Searight HR, Amanat E, et al: Residential versus day treatment for children: a long-term follow-up study. Child Psychiatry Hum Dev 24:31–39, 1993

Evangelakis M: Day treatment, in Emotional Disorders in Children and Adolescents. Edited by Sholevar GP, Benson RM, Blinder BJ. New York, SP Medical & Scientific Books, 1980, pp 235–258

Friman PC, Osgood DW, Smith G, et al: A longitudinal evaluation of prevalent negative beliefs about residential placement for troubled adolescents. J Abnorm Child Psychol 24:299–324, 1996

Fujita M, Arnold V: Community residential programs, in Community Child and Adolescent Psychiatry: A Manual of Clinical Practice and Consultation. Edited by Petti TA, Salguero C. Washington, DC, American Psychiatric Publishing (in press)

Gair DS: Guidelines for children and adolescents, in The Psychiatric Uses of Seclusion and Restraint. Edited by Tardiff K. Washington, DC, American Psychiatric Press, 1991, pp 69–85

Goren S, Abraham I, Doyle N: Reducing violence in a child psychiatric hospital through planned organizational change. J Child Adolesc Psychiatr Nurs 9:(2):27–36, 1996

Green J, Kroll L, Imrie D, et al: Health gain and outcome predictors during inpatient and related day treatment in child and adolescent psychiatry. J Am Acad Child Adolesc Psychiatry 40:325–332, 2001

Grizenko N: Outcome of multimodal day treatment for children with severe behavior problems: a five-year follow-up. J Am Acad Child Adolesc Psychiatry 36:989–997, 1997

Grizenko N, Papineau D: A comparison of the cost-effectiveness of day treatment and residential treatment for children with severe behavior problems. Can J Psychiatry 37:393–400, 1992

Gutterman EM: Is diagnosis relevant in the hospitalization of potentially dangerous children and adolescents? J Am Acad Child Adolesc Psychiatry 37:1030–1037, 1998

Harper G: Focal inpatient treatment planning. J Am Acad Child Adolesc Psychiatry 28:31–37, 1989

Henggeler SW, Rowlan MD, Randall J, et al: Home-based multisystemic therapy as an alternative to the hospitalization of youths in psychiatric crisis: clinical outcomes. J Am Acad Child Adolesc Psychiatry 38:1331–1339, 1999

Heston JD, Kiser LJ, Pruitt DB: Child and adolescent partial hospitalization, in Child and Adolescent Psychiatry: A Comprehensive Textbook, 2nd Edition. Edited by Lewis M. Baltimore, MD, Williams & Wilkins, 1996, pp 883–890

Hoagwood K, Cunningham M: Outcomes of children with emotional disturbance in residential treatment for educational purposes. Journal of Child and Family Studies 1:129–140, 1992

Hoagwood K, Jensen PS, Petti TA, et al: Outcomes of mental health care for children and adolescents, I: a comprehensive conceptual model. J Am Acad Child Adolesc Psychiatry 35:1055–1063, 1996

Hobbs N: Helping disturbed children: psychological and ecological strategies. Am Psychol 21:1105–1115, 1966

Jemerin JM, Philips I: Changes in inpatient child psychiatry: consequences and recommendations. J Am Acad Child Adolesc Psychiatry 27:397–403, 1988

Jensen PS, Hoagwood K, Petti T: Outcomes of mental health care for children and adolescents, II: literature review and application of a comprehensive model. J Am Acad Child Adolesc Psychiatry 35:1064–1077, 1996

Julian DA, Julian TW, Mastrine BJ, et al: Residential and community treatment services utilized by a sample of youth with severe emotional disturbances. Am J Community Psychol 20:799–809, 1992

Kanapaux W: Psychiatric bed shortage puts squeeze on health care systems. Psychiatric Times 19(5):1, 10–11, 2002

Kaplan SL, Busner J: Prescribing practices of inpatient child psychiatrists under three auspices of care. J Child Adolesc Psychopharmacol 7:275–286, 1997

Katz LY, Gunasekara S, Miller AI: Dialectical behavior therapy for inpatient and outpatient parasuicidal adolescents. Adolesc Psychiatry 26:161–178, 2002

Kazdin A: Acceptability of aversive procedures and medication as treatment alternatives for deviant child behavior. J Abnorm Child Psychol 12:289–302, 1984

Kennedy SS, Mohr WK: A prolegomenon on restraint of children: implicating constitutional rights. Am J Orthopsychiatry 71:26–37, 2001

Kiser LJ, Millsap PA, Hickerson S, et al: Results of treatment one year later: child and adolescent partial hospitalization. J Am Acad Child Adolesc Psychiatry 35:81–90, 1996

Kiser L, Heston JD, Paavola M: Day treatment center/partial hospital setting, in Community Child and Adolescent Psychiatry: A Manual of Clinical Practice and Consultation. Edited by Petti TA, Salguero C. Washington, DC, American Psychiatric Publishing (in press)

Kolko DJ: Short-term follow-up psychiatric hospitalization: clinical description, predictors, and correlates. J Am Acad Child Adolesc Psychiatry 31:719–727, 1992

Kolko DJ: Studying the treatment-as-usual setting, in The 14th Annual Research Conference Proceedings, A System of Care for Children's Mental Health: Expanding the Research Base (February 25–28, 2001). Edited by Newman C, Liberton CJ, Kutash K, et al. Tampa, FL, University of South Florida, 2002, pp 385–387

Kutash K, Rivera VR: Effectiveness of children's mental health services: a review of the literature. Education and Treatment of Children 18:443–477, 1995

Leichtman ML, Leichtman ML: Short-term residential treatment and its limits. Treatment Today Spring:12–14, 1996

Leon SC, Lyons JS, Uziel-Miller ND, et al: Evaluating the use of psychiatric hospitalization by residential treatment centers. J Am Acad Child Adolesc Psychiatry 39:1496–1501, 2000

Lewis M, Summerville JW, Graffagnino PN: Residential treatment, in Child and Adolescent Psychiatry: A Comprehensive Textbook, 3rd Edition. Edited by Lewis M. Baltimore, MD, Williams & Wilkins, 2003, pp 1095–1103

Looney JG: Chronic Mental Illness in Children and Adolescents. Washington DC, American Psychiatric Press, 1988

Lyman RD, Campbell NR: Treating Children and Adolescents in Residential and Inpatient Settings. Thousand Oaks, CA, Sage Publications, 1996

Lyons JS, Libman-Mintzer LN, Kisiel CL, et al: Understanding the mental health needs of children and adolescents in residential treatment. Prof Psychol Res Pr 29:582–587, 1998

Lyons JS, Terry P, Martinovich Z, et al: Outcome trajectories for adolescents in residential treatment: a statewide evaluation. Journal of Child and Family Studies 10:333–345, 2001

Mann-Feder VR: Adolescents in therapeutic communities. Adolescence 31(121):17–28, 1996

Masters KJ: Using a coordinated treatment system to minimize child psychiatric hospitalization. J Am Acad Child Adolesc Psychiatry 36:566–568, 1997

Mayes SD, Calhoun SL, Krecko VF, et al: Outcome following child psychiatric hospitalization. J Behav Health Serv Res 28:96–102, 2001

McNaught TR, McKamy LR: Elopement of adolescents: dynamics in the treatment process. Hosp Community Psychiatry 29:303–305, 1978

Measham TJ: The acute management of aggressive behaviour in hospitalized children and adolescents. Can J Psychiatry 40:330–336, 1995

Milazzo-Sayre LJ, Henderson MJ, Manderscheid RW, et al: Persons treated in specialty mental health programs, United States, 1997, in Mental Health, United States, 2000. Edited by Manderscheid RW, Henderson MJ. Rockville, MD, Center for Mental Health Services, 2000, pp 172–217

Mohr WK, Mahon MM, Noone MJ: A restraint on restraints: the need to reconsider restrictive interventions. Arch Psychiatr Nurs 12:95–106, 1998

Monkman MM: A Milieu Therapy Program for Behaviorally Disturbed Children. Springfield, IL, Charles C Thomas, 1972

Natta MB, Holmbeck GN, Kupst MJ, et al: Sequences of staff-child interactions on a psychiatric inpatient unit. J Abnorm Child Psychol 18:1–14, 1990

Nurcombe B: Goal-directed treatment planning and principles of brief hospitalization. J Am Acad Child Adolesc Psychiatry 28:26–30, 1989

Nurcombe B: Malpractice, in Child and Adolescent Psychiatry: A Comprehensive Textbook, 2nd Edition. Edited by Lewis M. Baltimore, MD, Williams & Wilkins, 1996, pp 1134–1145

Peele PB, Lave JR, Kelleher KJ: Exclusions and limitations in children's behavioral health care coverage. Psychiatr Serv 53:591–594, 2002

Petti TA: Residential and inpatient treatment of children and adolescents, in Emotional Disorders in Children and Adolescents. Edited by Sholevar GP, Benson RM, Blinder BJ. New York, SP Medical & Scientific Books, 1980, pp 209–228

Petti TA: Commentary: diagnosis is relevant to psychiatric hospitalization. J Am Acad Child Adolesc Psychiatry 37:1038–1040, 1998

Petti TA, Patrick V, Whitehouse R, et al: Outcome evaluation of state hospital care without funding: lessons learned, in The 12th Annual Research Conference Proceedings, A System of Care for Children's Mental Health: Expanding the Research Base (February 21–24, 1999). Edited by Liberton CJ, Newman C, Kutash K, et al. Tampa, FL, University of South Florida, 2000, pp 83–86

Petti TA, Mohr WK, Somers J, et al: Perceptions of seclusion and restraint by patients and staff in an intermediate-term care facility. J Child Adolesc Psychiatr Nurs 14:115–117, 2001

Petti TA, Sims L, Somers J, et al: Reduction of seclusion and restraint: implications from the Indianapolis experience, in The 14th Annual Research Conference Proceedings, A System of Care for Children's Mental Health: Expanding the Research Base (February 25–28, 2001). Edited by Newman C, Liberton CJ, Kutash K, et al. Tampa, FL, University of South Florida, 2002, pp 441–443

Petti TA, Somers J, Sims LA: Chronicle of seclusion and restraint in an intermediate-term care facility. Adolesc Psychiatry 27:83–116, 2003a

Petti TA, Stigler K, Gardner-Haycox J, et al: Perceptions of PRN psychotropic medications by hospitalized child and adolescent recipients. J Am Acad Child Adolesc Psychiatry 42:434–441, 2003b

Pruitt DB (ed): Your Adolescent: Emotional, Behavioral, and Cognitive Development From Early Adolescence Through the Teen Years. New York, HarperCollins, 1999

Rafferty FT: Changes in the practice of child and adolescent psychiatry (letter). J Am Acad Child Adolesc Psychiatry 38:1211–1212, 1999

Rawal PH, Lyons JS, MacIntyre JC, et al: Regional variation in off-label use of antipsychotic drugs utilized in residential treatment of children and adolescents: a four-state comparison. J Behav Health Serv Res (in press)

Rimsley DB: Principles of therapeutic milieu with children, in Emotional Disorders in Children and Adolescents. Edited by Sholevar GP, Benson RM, Blinder BJ. New York, SP Medical & Scientific Books, 1980, pp 191–208

Robinson A, Jivanjee P, Pullman M: Out of sight, out of mind? Perspectives on parent-child contact during residential treatment, in The 15th Annual Research Conference Proceedings, A System of Care for Children's Mental Health: Expanding the Research Base (March 3–6, 2002). Edited by Newman C, Liberton CJ, Kutash K, et al. Tampa, FL, 2003, pp 165–170

Ross EC: Death by restraint: horror stories continue, but best practices are also being identified. Behav Healthc Tomorrow 8:21–23, 1999

Singh NN, Singh SD, Davis CM, et al: Reconsidering the use of seclusion and restraints in inpatient child and adult Psychiatry. J Child Family Studies 8:243–253, 1999

Slaby AE, McGuire PL: Residential management of suicidal adolescents. Residential Treatment for Children and Youth 7:23–43, 1989

Solomon P, Evans D: Service needs of youths released from a state psychiatric facility as perceived by service providers and families. Community Ment Health J 28:305–315, 1992

Stroup A, Witkin M, Atay J, et al: Residential treatment centers for emotionally disturbed children 1983 (Mental Health Statistical Note No 188). Rockville, MD, National Institute of Mental Health, 1988

Tarico V, Low BP, Trupin E, et al: Children's mental health services: a parent perspective. Community Ment Health J 25:313–326, 1989

Vitiello B, Hill JL, Elia J, et al: P.R.N. medications in child psychiatric inpatients: a pilot placebo-controlled study. J Clin Psychiatry 52:499–501, 1991

Weintrob A: Long-term treatment of the severely disturbed adolescent: residential treatment versus hospitalization. J Am Acad Child Psychiatry 14:436–450, 1975

Weisbord M: Organizational Diagnosis. Reading, MA, Addison-Wesley, 1978

Wells K, Wyatt E, Hobfoll S: Factors associated with adaptation of youths discharged from residential treatment. Child Youth Serv Rev 13:199–216, 1991

Whittaker JK: The future of residential group care. Child Welfare 74:59–74, 2000

Woolston JL: The administration of hospital-based services. Child Adolesc Psychiatr Clin N Am 11:43–65, 2002

Woolston JL: Psychiatric inpatient services, in Child and Adolescent Psychiatry: A Comprehensive Textbook, 3rd Edition. Edited by Lewis M. Baltimore, MD, Williams & Wilkins, 2003, pp 1091–1095

Zimet SG, Farley GK: Day treatment for children in the United States. J Am Acad Child Psychiatry 24:732–738, 1985

Zimmerman DP: Notes on the history of adolescent inpatient and residential treatment. Adolescence 25(97):9–38, 1990

Index

*Page numbers printed in **boldface** type refer to tables or figures.*